CDC
PREVENTION
GUIDELINES

A Guide for Action

Cover Photo: Hygeia, Greek goddess of prevention and health, stands outside the Centers for Disease Control and Prevention headquarters in Atlanta, Georgia (photograph courtesy of Patrick W. O'Carroll, M.D., M.P.H.).

Edited by

Andrew Friede, M.D., M.P.H.

Chief
Public Health Information Systems Branch
Information Resources Management Office
Centers for Disease Control and Prevention
Atlanta, Georgia

Patrick W. O'Carroll, M.D., M.P.H.

Special Assistant to the Director
Public Health Practice Program Office
Centers for Disease Control and Prevention
Atlanta, Georgia
Clinical Associate Professor
Department of Epidemiology and Health Services
University of Washington School of Public Health and Community Medicine
Seattle, Washington

Ray M. Nicola, M.D., M.H.S.A.

Director
Division of Public Health Systems
Public Health Practice Program Office
Centers for Disease Control and Prevention
Associate Clinical Professor
Emory University of Public Health
Atlanta, Georgia
Associate Clinical Professor
University of Washington School of Public Health and Community Medicine
Seattle, Washington

Mark W. Oberle, M.D., M.P.H.

Medical Officer
Public Health Practice Program Office
Centers for Disease Control and Prevention
Atlanta, Georgia

Steven M. Teutsch, M.D., M.P.H.

Chief
Prevention Effectiveness Activity
Epidemiology Program Office
Centers for Disease Control and Prevention
Adjunct Professor
Department of International Health
Emory University School of Public Health
Atlanta, Georgia

CDC
PREVENTION GUIDELINES

A Guide for Action

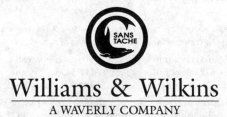

Williams & Wilkins
A WAVERLY COMPANY

BALTIMORE • PHILADELPHIA • LONDON • PARIS • BANGKOK
BUENOS AIRES • HONG KONG • MUNICH • SYDNEY • TOKYO • WROCLAW

Editor: Kathleen Courtney Millet
Production Coordinator: Marette Magargle-Smith
Copy Editor: Richard H. Adin
Designer: Dan Pfisterer
Cover Designer: Tom Scheuerman
Typesetter: Peirce Graphic Services, Inc.
Printer: Vicks Lithograph & Printing Corp.

Accurate indications, adverse reactions and dosage schedules for drugs are provided in this book, but it is possible that they may change. The reader is urged to review the package information data of the manufacturers of the medications mentioned.

Printed in the United States of America

Library of Congress Cataloging-in-Publication Data

CDC prevention guidelines : a guide for action / edited by Andrew
   Friede ... [et al.].
      p.   cm.
   "A compilation of 161 key CDC documents, carefully excerpted from
   larger reports"—Foreword.
   Includes bibliographical references and index.
   ISBN 0-683-30005-9
   1. Medicine, Preventative—Government policy—United States.
   2. Centers for Disease Control and Prevention (U.S.)   I. Friede,
   Andrew.   II. Centers for Disease Control and Prevention (U.S.)
      [DNLM: 1. Preventative Medicine.   2. Public Health.   WA 108 C386
   1997]
   RA445.C34   1997
   614.4'4'0973—dc20
   DNLM/DLC
   for Library of Congress   96-20767
                                                                       CIP

The publishers have made every effort to trace the copyright holders for borrowed material. If they have inadvertently overlooked any, they will be pleased to make the necessary arrangements at the first opportunity.

To purchase additional copies of this book, call our customer service department at **(800) 638-0672** or fax orders to **(800) 447-8438.** For other book services, including chapter reprints and large quantity sales, ask for the Special Sales department.

Canadian customers should call **(800) 268-4178,** or fax **(905) 470-6780.** For all other calls originating outside of the United States, please call **(410) 528-4223** or fax us at **(410) 528-8550.**

Visit Williams & Wilkins on the Internet: http://www.wwilkins.com or contact our customer service department at **custserv@wwilkins.com.** Williams & Wilkins customer service representatives are available from 8:30 am to 6:00 pm, EST, Monday through Friday, for telephone access.

                                                                98 99 00
                                                      2 3 4 5 6 7 8 9 10

Even though it is becoming common knowledge that we can no longer afford the rehabilitative and reparative medicine and surgery that has been our practice for the last three decades, it is still difficult for Americans to come to grips with the prevention of disease and the promotion of good health as an alternative.

In our day, we have become accustomed to the dramatic, life-saving miracles of high-tech medicine, but our greatest strides in prolonging life came not from medical miracles in the late 20th century, but from public health accomplishments of the late 19th and early 20th centuries: vaccination and safer food, water, and housing.

Throughout history, most premature deaths came from things people did not choose: war, work, and infectious disease. Now, in addition to the old, familiar epidemics of infectious disease, we must deal with newer epidemics of self-induced degenerative disease. Now, most premature deaths come from choices that people make. High on the list of these are smoking—the single most preventable cause of death in America—and sexually transmitted diseases.

The great killers of humanity for most of our history, infectious diseases, while under somewhat better control, continue to be with us and at times take new and yet more dangerous forms. The epidemic of acquired immunodeficiency syndrome (AIDS), which began in 1981, was perhaps the first time that Americans have seen a new disease that science and medicine could not readily conquer. In that sense, it has been good for public health because the public is beginning to understand the differences between public health and personal medical care. It is unfortunate that, just at a time when that awakening is beginning to bear fruit among the American people, public health has been put in jeopardy by the combined action of Congress and the Executive Branch in downsizing government.

So, we deal with two types of diseases: those which were developed inadvertently and those which we bring upon ourselves through failure to practice preventive measures. It is a national tragedy that preventable illness makes up approximately 70% of the burden of illness and associated cost. This has major implications in our debate on health care reform and the use of our health care resources. The plain fact is that we Americans do a better job of preventive maintenance on our cars than on ourselves. I might add, parenthetically, that, while I am making that comparison, we do not expect our car insurance to cover preventive maintenance on our cars.

This major new text, *CDC Prevention Guidelines,* comes at a very appropriate time. The book is a compilation of 161 key CDC documents, carefully excerpted from larger reports to retain the recommendations *per se,* but written to enable easy understanding by the reader. Because many of these recommendations were developed on my watch as Surgeon General, I am very pleased to be able to write the foreword to this book.

CDC Prevention Guidelines covers a variety of health topics not usually found in medical or public health texts, such as the preventive program for AIDS and other sexually transmitted diseases, birth defects, environmental and workplace hazards, homicides and suicides, as well as the better-known risks associated with alcohol and tobacco.

Many of these guidelines focus on population-based as well as on individual solutions. And how appropriate that is! Most of us know that Abraham Flexner, in his report of 1910, recommended that medical schools be centered in scientifically-oriented universities, but some of us have forgotten that he declared the purpose of medical education was to benefit the patient, the family, and the *community*.

The authors have nicely included selections from "The Yellow Book," the general guide for travelers, published by the CDC over the years. These are authoritative recommendations from the Centers for Disease Control and Prevention and are designed for clinicians, health departments, hospitals, managed care organizations, program planners, information systems designers, and health science students.

In these days of increasing privatization, many wonder what the role of government might be in health and medicine. There is no doubt in my mind that, because of the enormity of the task, the government must and should have a major role in calling to the public's attention those public health threats that have replaced unsafe water and food, such as addiction to tobacco and the spread of sexually transmitted diseases.

I hope that this volume is widely read, especially by students and beginners in the health and medical professions. because it contains a wealth of information, abbreviated, understandable but, nevertheless, vital.

C. EVERETT KOOP, M.D., Sc.D.
UNITED STATES SURGEON GENERAL, 1981–1989

CDC Prevention Guidelines: A Guide for Action is a selection of CDC guidelines on a variety of public health topics, many of which are not typically covered in medical or public health texts. These authoritative recommendations from CDC are designed for clinicians, health departments, hospitals, managed care organizations, program planners, information systems designers, and health sciences students.

CDC is still often thought of as primarily an infectious diseases agency (as it once was). However, this is no longer true, and so herein you will find recommendations on such noninfectious disease topics as birth defects, diabetes, environmental hazards, homicide and suicide, and the risks associated with tobacco addiction. Of course, CDC still maintains its programs in infectious diseases, most notably AIDS and other sexually transmitted diseases, and other "emerging" infectious diseases; this book covers these, too, as well as guidelines for travelers, immunizations, and workplace hazards.

This book is a very generous selection from the *CDC Prevention Guidelines Database,* an electronic database that contains the full text of over 400 key recommendations. To create the database, the Editors work—on an ongoing basis—with senior scientists and liaisons in each CDC Center to identify candidate articles, selected from many thousands of CDC publications from the past few years. About two-thirds were originally published in CDC's *Morbidity and Mortality Weekly Report (MMWR) Series;* the others were published as CDC monographs, as books or book chapters, as brochures, or as articles in peer-reviewed journals. The database is updated every week with new publications.

CDC Prevention Guidelines: A Guide for Action contains many of the guidelines for the day-to-day practice of preventive medicine. The only ones that were excluded cover general information on public health and laboratory subjects (as these are well covered in other texts) and highly specialized material (e.g., guidelines for the disposal of munitions). To save space, generally only the recommendations *per se* are kept; the background, review of the literature, and many references were deleted (for some more arcane topics, some introductory material was retained). Because of these exclusions, some of the nuances in these recommendations may not be fully appreciated from reading this printed version. Readers are therefore encouraged to review the complete, unedited documents.

In the retained material, essentially no words have been changed, and there has been no in-line editing (except to maintain clarity). We worked closely with the CDC departments that prepared the original to make sure no key information was left out.

HOW DOES CDC DEVELOP RECOMMENDATIONS?

CDC has two mechanisms for developing recommendations. A program (say, the National Immunization Program) can either publish a document, which becomes a *de facto* "official" recommendation, or convene an *advisory committee* to formulate recommendations.

Publication

The principal mechanism by which CDC issues recommendations is via its hundreds of annual scientific publications, which typically conclude with recommendations for action. To assure that authors speak for the Agency, every CDC manuscript is reviewed for scientific and policy content before it may be published. This applies to books and book chapters, pamphlets, symposia proceedings, and government publications, such as the *Morbidity and Mortality Weekly Report (MMWR) Series,* i.e., a host of publication outlets that are often not peer-reviewed, as well as peer-reviewed journals. By tradition, CDC authors of *MMWR* articles are not named. Typically, publications are reviewed by at least two senior scientists who are not co-authors, and who may work in other departments, thereby helping to assure that the opinions expressed represent an agency consensus.

Advisory Committees

Another mechanism for the development of recommendations are advisory committees, which currently include the Advisory Committee on Immunizations Practices (ACIP) (formerly known as Immunizations Practices Advisory Committee); the Advisory Committee of the Elimination of Tuberculosis (ACET); and the new Hospital Infections Control Practices Advisory Committee (HICPAC). The committee members are medical experts who typically work in universities or public health agencies other than CDC; federal scientists serve as *ex officio* (usually non-voting) members of the committees. In addition, major medical and public health organizations are often represented by non-voting liaison members, who, however, participate fully in all discussions. The advisory committees determine the contents of reports, usually after extensive public meetings. CDC scientists staff the committees, and very often write the final reports; hence, they may be cited as authors. (For this book, we included the results of selected advisory committee reports *in toto,* as to avoid excerpting work that originated in an external Advisory Committee; because of this, a smaller type size was used for materials that would have otherwise been deleted.)

However a recommendation is developed, it must be emphasized that CDC is not a regulatory agency (unlike, for example, the Food and Drug Administration), and so its recommendations are just that, recommendations; they do not have the force of administrative regulation or law. Of course, a regulatory agency may use a CDC recommendation as the foundation of a regulation; similarly, Congress or a state legislature may use a CDC recommendation as a source document for a law (say, requiring children to be immunized to attend school). Knowing that this can happen (and often does) makes the authors of CDC recommendations cautious.

ELECTRONIC VERSIONS

The entire database is in searchable form on the *CDC Prevention Guidelines on CD-ROM* (available for Windows), which is available in a version of this book. Additional information is also accessible via CDC WONDER on the Worldwide Web; contact CDC WONDER customer support at 404–332-4569.

ANDREW FRIEDE, M.D., M.P.H.
PATRICK W. O'CARROLL, M.D., M.P.H.
RAY M. NICOLA, M.D., MHSA
MARK W. OBERLE, M.D., M.P.H.
STEVEN M. TEUTSCH, M.D., M.P.H.

ACKNOWLEDGMENTS

We are grateful to the CDC scientists who wrote all this material, and who helped verify that we had excerpted it appropriately. We thank those from each of the CDC offices that helped identify and furnish materials for the database: Gloria Kovach (ACIP); Patti Poindexter (ATSDR); Michael Deming (IHPO); Suzanne Hewitt (EPO); Jennifer Brooks (NCHSTC); Gwen Ingram (NCIPC); Rick Hull (NCCDPHP); Dick Campolucci (NCPS, now NCHSTP); Marilyn Disirio (NCEH); Barbara McCollum (NIP); Polly Potter (NCID); John Whalen and Thomas Ziegler (NIOSH); Jonathan Richmond (OD); and Tom Skinner (OD).

Dixie Snider, M.D., Associate Director for Science, CDC, graciously supported this project. The Associate Directors for Science and other senior scientists in contributing centers devoted many hours to reviewing the selection of articles and the editing: John Andrews, M.D., M.P.H. and Charles Xintaras, Ph.D. (ATSDR); Michael Deming, M.D. (IHPO); Adele Franks, M.D. (NCCD-PHP); Sam Dooley, M.D., Peter Drotman, M.D., and Bess Miller, M.D. (formerly NCPS, now NCHSTP); Thomas Sinks, Ph.D. (NCEH); Stephen Ostroff, M.D. (NCID); and Richard Waxweiler, Ph.D. (NCIPC).

Contributors to constructing and administering the database include: Kathy Grooms and Lisa Elison (database management); Michelle Shaheen and Heitzso (computer programming); Nancy Hughes, Earnestine Dooley, Ron Peterson, and Lesley Peters (editorial assistance); and Sigrid Economou (project coordination).

Many of the items in this book first appeared in the MMWR series of publications, coordinated by the Epidemiology Program Office, directed by Stephen B. Thacker, M.D., M.Sc.; Richard A. Goodman, M.D., M.P.H. is the Editor, MMWR Series. Janis F. Videtto is the Acting Director, Scientific Information and Communications Program, and Karen L. Foster, M.A. is the chief of the MMWR (weekly) Branch, whose writers-editors include David C. Johnson, Patricia A. McGee, Darlene D. Rumph-Person, and Caran R. Wilbanks. Suzanne M. Hewitt, M.P.A. is Chief of the Public Health Publications, whose writers-editors include Nadine W. Martin, Rachel J. Wilson, and Lanette B. Wolcott. Elizabeth E. Rubery is the chief of the Information Resources Management Branch. Visual Information Specialists include Philip C. Bourque, Sandra L. Ford, Morie M. Higgins, and Peter M. Jenkins.

Funding for the database was provided by the Robert W. Woodruff, Jr. Foundation via the CDC INPHO (Information Network for Public Health Officials), under the leadership of David Ross, Sc.D. and Edward Baker, Jr., M.D., M.P.H.; and by the CDC Office of Program Planning and Evaluation via 1% evaluation monies administered by Wilma Johnson and Martha Katz.

It is our pleasure to acknowledge our colleagues at Williams & Wilkins: David Retford, formerly Senior Editor, who immediately saw the potential value of this book and encouraged us to pursue it; and Kathleen Millet, Senior Managing Editor, who managed a very complex and time-consuming project with tremendous skill, judgment, grace, and good humor.

Organizational Abbreviations

Advisory Committee for the Elimination of Tuberculosis (ACET)
Agency for Toxic Substances and Disease Registry (ATSDR)
Epidemiology Program Office (EPO)
Hospital Infection Control Practices Advisory Committee (HICPAC)
Immunizations Practices Advisory Committee (ACIP)
Information Network for Public Health Officials (INPHO)
International Health Program Office (IHPO)
National Center for Chronic Disease Prevention and Health Promotion (NCCDPHP)
National Center for Environmental Health (NCEH)
National Center for Health Statistics (NCHS)
National Center for HIV, Sexually Transmitted Disease, and Tuberculosis Prevention (NCHSTP)
National Center for Infectious Diseases (NCID)
National Center for Injury Prevention and Control (NCIPC)
National Center for Prevention Services (NCPS)
National Immunization Program (NIP)
National Institute for Occupational Safety and Health (NIOSH)
Office of the Director (OD)
Public Health Practice Program Office (PHPPO)

Disclaimer

Use of tradenames is for identification only and does not imply endorsement by the Centers for Disease Control and Prevention or the United States Department of Health and Human Services.

Andrew Friede, M.D., M.P.H. is the Chief of the Public Health Information Systems Branch, Information Resources Management Office, CDC. He leads the development of CDC WONDER, an integrated information and communications system that provides access to some 30 databases for 13,000 users, and provides specialized features used by many CDC surveillance programs. CDC WONDER uses a novel systems architecture that was specifically developed for public health information systems by the CDC WONDER team, and includes specialized end-user communications and graphing software. Dr. Friede is also a principal participant in the CDC INPHO project, which aims to develop a national information network for public health. The first stage of INPHO is the development of a statewide network in Georgia, funded by a $5.2 million grant from the Woodruff Foundation. Twelve states have received additional CDC funding. He has also served as a consultant to the World Bank and the UN for public health and clinical information systems in China and Madagascar.

His epidemiological research interests have focused on maternal and child health conditions, including immunizations, injuries, infant and maternal mortality, teenage pregnancy, and obstetrical complications. His current areas of interest and research include architecting and implementing institution-wide information strategies for medicine and public health.

Patrick W. O'Carroll, M.D., M.P.H. is Special Assistant to the Director of the Public Health Practice Program Office, CDC. He is currently assigned to the State of Washington as part of the CDC Information Network for Public Health Officials (INPHO) project. His responsibilities there include coordinating the development of new information systems applications for the Washington INPHO network, and developing training in public health informatics for mid-career public health managers. He holds Clinical Associate Professor appointments in the Departments of Epidemiology and Health Services at the University of Washington School of Public Health and Community Medicine.

For the past three years, Dr. O'Carroll co-led the development of CDC WONDER with Dr. Friede, and was lead scientist for the CDC Prevention Guidelines Database project. Prior to that, he conducted epidemiologic research at CDC in the areas of suicide and violence prevention. Dr. O'Carroll was chief of the violence research unit at CDC for several years, and is lead author of many of CDC's suicide and violence prevention guidelines. He has received numerous awards for his work in suicide prevention.

Ray M. (Bud) Nicola, M.D., M.H.S.A. is the Director of the Division of Public Health Systems in the Public Health Practice Program Office, CDC. He focuses on supporting the practice of public health at the local level, including the development of leadership within the public health system; the measurement, standards, and guidelines of public health practice; the mobilization of communities to action on health issues; and the role of public health in a changing health system. He currently chairs a CDC Steering Committee on the Los Angeles Fiscal Crisis; he also chairs the CDC Pacific Island Coordinating Committee.

Dr. Nicola has received a PHS Special Recognition Award in 1993 for his effort as part of the Combatting MDR-TB Team, and a 1995 Commissioned Corps and Civil Service Joint Activity Award for the CDC Advisory Committee on the Pacific Islands. He is a member of the Board of Regents of the American College of Preventive Medicine, a clinical faculty member at Emory University School of Public Health and at the University of Washington School of Public Health and Preventive Medicine, an Associate Editor of the Notes from the Field section of the *American Journal of Public Health,* and a Contributing Editor to *Public Health Reports.*

He was formerly at the University of Washington School of Public Health where he directed the Preventive Medicine Residency Program and was Associate Clinical Professor in the Health Services Department. From 1985 through January of 1991 Dr. Nicola was the Director of the Seattle-King County Health Department and previously served as Director of the Tacoma-Pierce County Health Department in Tacoma, Washington, and Associate Director of the Tri-County District Health Department in Englewood, Colorado.

Mark W. Oberle, M.D., M.P.H. is a Medical Epidemiologist with the Public Health Practice Program Office, CDC, working on CDC's Information Network for Public Health Officials (INPHO), a public-private partnership to develop computer networking applications for electronic linkage, data exchange, and information access for public health.

He has directed epidemiological studies and program evaluations in infectious diseases and reproductive health in 14 countries and directed epidemiology programs in the state health departments of Puerto Rico (1975–1977) and Washington State (1992). From 1987 to 1992, he served as Associate Professor and Assistant Dean for Public Health Practice at the University of Washington (UW) School of Public Health and Community Medicine. He founded the Northwest Center for Public Health Practice and was the Director of the UW Preventive Medicine Residency.

Steven M. Teutsch, M.D., M.P.H. is Chief of the Prevention Effectiveness Activity (PEA), Epidemiology Program Office (EPO), CDC. He is responsible for assuring that CDC assesses the effectiveness, safety, and the cost-effectiveness of disease and injury prevention strategies. The PEA develops comparable methodology for studies of the effectiveness and economic impact of prevention programs, provides training in these methods, develops the capacity for conducting necessary studies, and provides technical assistance for conducting economic and decision analysis.

Dr. Teutsch came to CDC in 1977, where he was assigned to the Parasitic Diseases Division and worked extensively on toxoplasmosis. He was then assigned to the Kidney Donor and subsequently the Kidney Disease Program.

He developed the framework for CDC's diabetes control program. He joined EPO and became the Director of the Division of Surveillance and Epidemiology where he was responsible for CDC's disease monitoring activities. Dr. Teutsch is an Adjunct Professor at the Emory University School of Public Health, Department of International Health. His epidemiological research has focused on parasitic diseases, diabetes, technology assessment, health services research, and surveillance.

CONTENTS

SECTION SIX / INJURIES

SECTION EIGHT / MISCELLANEOUS

section one

INFECTIOUS DISEASES

Issues Related to Bovine Spongiform Encephalopathy and the Emergence of a New Variant of Creutzfeldt-Jakob Disease

Original Citation. WHO. World Health Organization Consultation on Public Health Issues Related to Bovine Spongiform Encephalopathy and the Emergence of a New Variant of Creutzfeldt-Jakob Disease. MMWR 1996;45(14):296–302.

Editor's Note: In the United States, the U.S. Department of Agriculture (USDA) has conducted active surveillance for Bovine spongiform encephalopathy (BSE) in cattle since 1990 and has not detected any cases. Nonetheless, because of the concern that variant-Creutzfeldt-Jakob Disease (V-CJD) in the United Kingdom might possibly be linked to BSE, additional safety measures are being instituted, including discontinuation of the use of ruminant tissue in ruminant feeds. A WHO panel of experts concluded that there is no definite link between BSE and V-CJD but that circumstantial evidence suggests exposure to BSE may be the most likely explanation.

BOVINE SPONGIFORM ENCEPHALOPATHY

Bovine spongiform encephalopathy (BSE) is a transmissible spongiform encephalopathy (TSE) in cattle, which was first identified in the United Kingdom in 1986. It is one of a group of similar degenerative diseases that occur in several animal species. Transmission of BSE to cattle appears to have occurred by contaminated meat and bone meal in concentrate feed, sheep or cattle being the original source. The United Kingdom is the only country with a high incidence of the disease and the epidemic there appears to have been due mainly to recycling of affected bovine material back to cattle before the ruminant (cattle, sheep, and goats) feed ban in July 1988 took effect. There is no evidence of either maternal or horizontal transmission of BSE.

VARIANT OF CREUTZFELDT-JAKOB DISEASE

The disease has occurred at younger ages than is usual for classical CJD and shows several clinical and pathologic differences.

RECOMMENDATIONS

Bovine Spongiform Encephalopathy

1. No part or product of any animal that has shown signs of TSE should enter any food chain, human or animal. All countries must ensure the slaughter and safe disposal of TSE-affected animals so that TSE infectivity cannot enter any food chain. All countries should review their rendering procedures to ensure that they effectively inactivate TSE agents.

2. All countries should establish continuous surveillance and compulsory notification for BSE according to recommendations established by the Office
International des Epizooties in Paris. In the absence of surveillance data,
the BSE status of a country must be considered as unknown.
3. Countries should not permit tissues that are likely to contain the BSE
agent to enter any food chain, human or animal.
4. All countries should ban the use of ruminant tissues in ruminant feed.
5. With respect to specific products:
    Tests on milk from BSE infected animals have not shown any BSE infec-
    tivity, and there is evidence from other animal and human spongiform
    encephalopathies to suggest that milk will not transmit these diseases.
    Milk and milk products, even in countries with high incidences of BSE,
    are therefore considered safe.
    Gelatin in the food chain is considered to be safe. The usually applied man-
    ufacturing process has been demonstrated to significantly inactivate any
    residual infective activity that may have been present in source tissues.
6. With respect to medicinal products:
    Removal and inactivation procedures contribute to the reduction of the
    risk of infection, but it must be recognized that the BSE agent is re-
    markably resistant to physico-chemical procedures that destroy the in-
    fectivity of common microorganisms.
    The importance of obtaining bovine materials destined for the pharma-
    ceutical industry only from countries that have a surveillance system in
    place and that report either no or only sporadic cases of BSE is reiter-
    ated.
    Measures recommended to national health authorities to minimize the
    risk of transmitting the agent causing BSE through medicinal products,
    in particular parenteral products, which were developed at a WHO Con-
    sultation in 1991 (1), continue to be generally applicable.
    It is recommended that these measures be reviewed and, if necessary,
    strengthened as more information becomes available.
7. Research on TSE should be promoted, especially on rapid diagnosis, agent
characterization, and epidemiology of TSEs in humans and animals.

Variant of Creutzfeldt-Jakob Disease

1. The full geographic distribution of V-CJD, although reported at present
only in the United Kingdom, needs to be further investigated.
2. While the most likely hypothesis at present for this newly recognized variant is exposure to the BSE agent, further data from scientific studies on
these variant cases are urgently required. More monitoring and surveillance studies on all forms of CJD are required throughout the world, mod-
eled on current European collaborative studies.
3. Exposure to BSE from beef and beef products has already been substantially
reduced by the measures taken in the United Kingdom. Exposure to BSE is
considered lower in other countries. The group considered that implementation of their recommendations will ensure that any continuing risk of exposure to BSE in beef and beef products will be reduced to a minimum.

REFERENCE
1. Bulletin of the World Health Organization 1992;70:183–190.

Encephalitis Associated with Cat Scratch Disease

Original Citation: Centers for Disease Control and Prevention. Epidemiologic Notes and Reports Encephalitis Associated with Cat Scratch Disease—Broward and Palm Beach Counties, Florida, 1994. MMWR 1994;43(49):909, 915–916.

EDITORIAL NOTE

Cat scratch disease (CSD) is caused by infection with Bartonella (formerly Rochalimaea) henselae, an organism that has been associated with bacillary angiomatosis in immunocompromised persons. CSD is associated with exposure to cats infected with B. henselae. An estimated 22,000 cases of CSD occur annually in the United States (1). CSD affects persons of all age groups and both sexes and generally is characterized by a self-limiting, regional lymphadenopathy. Uncommon manifestations of B. henselae infection include Parinaud oculoglandular syndrome, relapsing bacteremia, and endocarditis and bacillary peliosis (2). Affected lymph nodes usually are proximal to the site of a cat scratch or bite, frequently are tender, and may suppurate. Although antimicrobial agents such as trimethoprim-sulfamethoxazole, rifampin, amoxycillin, and tetracycline exhibit in vitro antimicrobial activity against B. henselae, antimicrobial therapy has not been consistently beneficial in reducing the duration or severity of CSD (3). Treatment of CSD is generally supportive, although excision of the affected lymph node(s) and the use of antimicrobials may be indicated for treatment of severe swelling, pain, or suppuration. B. henselae infection in cats is asymptomatic. Cats can be asymptomatically bacteremic for several months and develop detectable antibodies concurrently with bacteremia (4). The seroprevalence of antibodies to B. henselae in cats is 14%–44% (5). Although B. henselae has been detected in fleas, the role of these and other ectoparasites in the transmission of B. henselae is unclear (2). Treatment with tetracycline has reduced bacteremia in cats; however, the effectiveness of treatment on preventing reinfection or recrudescence is unknown.

Recommendations for the prevention of CSD are directed toward the need to minimize contact between infected cats and humans. Cat owners should be encouraged to ensure that their pets receive routine veterinary health care that includes periodic physical examinations to prevent or detect ectoparasite infestations and to maintain current vaccinations against other zoonotic diseases (i.e., rabies). The potential for the transmission of B. henselae also may be reduced by keeping kittens and other pets indoors and by not playing roughly with them. Finally, the public should be educated to avoid contact with stray animals, to wash and disinfect bite and scratch wounds, and to seek appropriate medical care for severe injuries.

REFERENCES: AS NUMBERED IN ORIGINAL PUBLICATION

1. Zangwill KM, Hamilton DH, Perkins BA, et al. Cat scratch disease in Connecticut: epidemiology, risk factors, and evaluation of a new diagnostic test. N Engl J Med 1993;329:8–13.
2. Koehler JE, Glaser CA, Tappero JW. Rochalimaea henselae infection—a new zoonosis with the domestic cat as reservoir. JAMA 1994;271:531–535.
3. Carithers HA, Margileth AM. Cat-scratch disease. Am J Dis Child 1991;145:98–101.
4. Regnery R, Martin M, Olson J. Naturally occurring Rochalimaea henselae infections in domestic cats. Lancet 1992;340:557–558.
5. Childs JE, Rooney JA, Cooper JL, Olson JG, Regnery RL. Epidemiologic observations on infection with Rochalimaea species among cats living in Baltimore, Md. J Am Vet Med Assoc 1994;204:1775–1778.

TOPIC 3 / **CHOLERA**

Defeating Cholera: Clinical Presentation and Management

Original Citation: Defeating Cholera: Clinical Presentation and Management—U.S. Department of Health and Human Services, Public Health Services Centers for Disease Control, National Center for Infectious Diseases Division of Bacterial and Mycotic Diseases, 1992.

DEFEATING CHOLERA: CLINICAL PRESENTATION AND MANAGEMENT

Most persons infected with the cholera bacterium have mild diarrhea or no symptoms at all. Only about 7% of persons infected with the El Tor biotype of Vibrio cholerae O1 have illness requiring treatment at a health center. However, when cholera strikes in areas where practitioners are not acquainted with modern treatment methods, many people die.

Cholera patients should be evaluated and treated quickly. With proper treatment, even severely ill patients can be saved. Prompt restoration of lost fluids and salts is the primary goal of treatment.

SYMPTOMS OF MODERATE OR SEVERE CHOLERA

- Profuse, watery diarrhea
- Vomiting
- Leg cramps

Signs and Symptoms of Dehydration

Some dehydration

- Restlessness and irritability
- Sunken eyes
- Dry mouth and tongue
- Increased thirst
- Skin goes back slowly when pinched

Severe dehydration

- Lethargy or unconsciousness
- Very dry mouth and tongue
- Skin goes back slowly when pinched
- Weak or absent pulse
- Low blood pressure

ORAL REHYDRATION

Dehydrated patients who can sit up and drink should be given oral rehydration salts (ORS) solution immediately and be encouraged to drink. It is important to offer ORS solution frequently, measure the amount drunk, and measure the fluid lost as diarrhea and vomitus. Patients who vomit should be given small, frequent sips of ORS solution, or ORS solution by nasogastric tube.

Guidelines for Treating Patients with Some Dehydration

Approximate amount of ORS solution to give in the first 4 hours to patients with some dehydration.

Age*	< 4 mo.	4–11 mo.	12–23 mo.	2–4 yr.	5–14 yr.	> or = 15 yr.
Weight (kg)	< 5	5–7.9	8–10.9	11–15.9	16–29.9	> or = 30
ml		200–400	400–600	600–800	800–1200	1200–2200	2200–4000

*Use the patient's age only when you do not know the weight. The approximate amount of ORS required (in milliliters) can also be calculated by multiplying the patient's weight in kg by 75.

If the patient requests more than the prescribed ORS solution, give more. Older children and adults should be offered plain water in addition to ORS solution.

For Infants:

- Encourage the mother to continue breast-feeding.
- Give infants under 6 months of age who are not breast-fed an additional 100–200 ml of clean water during this period.

NOTES:

1. The volumes and time shown are guidelines based on usual needs. If necessary, amount and frequency can be increased, or the ORS solution can be given at the same rate for a longer period to achieve rehydration. Similarly, the amount of fluid can be decreased if hydration is achieved earlier than expected.
2. During the initial stages of therapy, while still dehydrated, adults can consume as much as 1000 ml of ORS solution per hour, if necessary, and children as much as 20 ml/kg body weight per hour.
3. Reassess the patient after 1 hour of therapy and then every 1 to 2 hours until rehydration is complete.
4. Resume feeding with a normal diet when vomiting has stopped.

Signs of adequate rehydration

- Skin turgor is normal
- Thirst has subsided
- Urine has been passed
- Pulse is strong

INTRAVENOUS REHYDRATION

Patients with severe dehydration, stupor, coma, uncontrollable vomiting, or extreme fatigue that prevents drinking should be rehydrated intravenously.

Intravenous solutions

- Best: Ringer's Lactate Solution
- Acceptable:* Normal saline
  Half normal saline with 5% glucose
- Unacceptable: Plain glucose (dextrose) solution

*These are acceptable in emergency, but do not correct acidosis and may worsen electrolyte imbalance.

Guidelines for Treating Patients with Severe Dehydration

Start intravenous fluids immediately. If the patient can drink, give ORS solution by mouth while the drip is set up. Give 100 ml/kg Ringer's Lactate Solution divided as follows:

Age	First give 30 ml/kg IV in:	Then give 70 ml/kg IV in:
Infants < 12 mos.	1 hour*	5 hours
Older > 1 yr.	30 minutes*	2½ hours

*Repeat once if radial pulse is still very weak or not detectable.

- Reassess the patient every 1–2 hours. If hydration is not improving, give the IV drip more rapidly.
- Also give ORS solution (about 5 ml/kg per hour) as soon as the patient can drink.
- After 6 hours (infants) or 3 hours (older patients), perform a full reassessment. Switch to ORS solution if hydration is improved and the patient can drink.

ANTIBIOTICS

An antibiotic given orally will reduce the volume and duration of diarrhea. No other drugs for treatment of diarrhea or vomiting should be given.

Appropriate oral antibiotics (give one of these)

- Doxycycline Adult: 300 mg in one dose
- Tetracycline Adult: 500 mg, 4 times a day for 3 days; Child: 12.5 mg/kg, 4 times a day for 3 days

- Trimethoprim-sulfamethoxazole (TMP-SMX) Adult: 160 mg TMP and 800 mg SMX, 2 times a day for 3 days; Child: 5 mg/kg TMP and 25 mg/kg SMX, 2 times a day for 3 days
- Furazolidone Adult: 100 mg, 4 times a day for 3 days; Child: 1.25 mg/kg, 4 times a day for 3 days

Doxycycline is the antibiotic of choice for adults (except pregnant women) because only one dose is required. TMP-SMX is the antibiotic of choice for children. Furazolidone is the antibiotic of choice for pregnant women. Erythromycin may be used when other antibiotics are not available, or the organism is resistant to them.

Cholera Prevention

Original Citation: Cholera Prevention—U.S. Department of Health and Human Services, Public Health Service, Centers for Disease Control and Prevention, National Center for Infectious Diseases Division for Bacterial and Mycotic Diseases, 1991.

CHOLERA PREVENTION

Cholera is an acute, diarrheal illness caused by infection of the intestine with the bacterium Vibrio cholerae. The infection is often mild or without symptoms, but sometimes it can be severe. Approximately 1 in 20 infected persons has severe disease characterized by profuse watery diarrhea, vomiting, and leg cramps. In these persons, rapid loss of body fluids leads to dehydration and shock. Without treatment, death can occur within hours.

What should travelers do to avoid getting cholera?

The risk for cholera is very low for U.S. travelers visiting areas with epidemic cholera. When simple precautions are observed, contracting the disease is unlikely. All travelers to areas where cholera has occurred should observe the following recommendations:

- Drink only water that you have boiled or treated with chlorine or iodine. Other safe beverages include tea and coffee made with boiled water and carbonated, bottled beverages with no ice.
- Eat only foods that have been thoroughly cooked and are still hot, or fruit that you have peeled yourself.
- Avoid undercooked or raw fish or shellfish, including ceviche.
- Make sure all vegetables are cooked—avoid salads.
- Avoid foods and beverages from street vendors.
- Do not bring perishable seafood back to the United States.

A simple rule of thumb is "Boil it, cook it, peel it, or forget it."

Is a vaccine available to prevent cholera?

A vaccine for cholera is available; however, it confers only brief and incomplete immunity and is not recommended for travelers. There are no cholera vacci-

nation requirements for entry or exit in any Latin American country or the
United States.

Can cholera be treated?

Cholera can be simply and successfully treated by immediate replacement of
the fluid and salts lost through diarrhea. Patients can be treated with oral rehydration solution, a prepackaged mixture of sugar and salts to be mixed with
water and drunk in large amounts. This solution is used throughout the world
to treat diarrhea. Severe cases also require intravenous fluid replacement.
With prompt rehydration, fewer than 1% of cholera patients die.

Antibiotics shorten the course and diminish the severity of the illness, but
they are not as important as rehydration. Persons who develop severe diarrhea
and vomiting in countries where cholera occurs should seek medical attention
promptly.

Where can a traveler get information about cholera?

The global picture of cholera changes periodically, so travelers should seek updated information on countries of interest. The Centers for Disease Control
maintains a travelers' information telephone line on which callers can receive
recent information on cholera and other diseases of concern to travelers. Data
for this service are obtained from the World Health Organization. This number is 404–332–4559.

Cholera—Western Hemisphere, and Recommendations for Treatment of Cholera

Original Citation: Centers for Disease Control and Prevention. Current Trends Update:
Cholera—Western Hemisphere, and Recommendations for Treatment of Cholera.
MMWR 1991;40(32):562–565.

EDITORIAL NOTE

Proper treatment of sewage and drinking water in the United States should prevent transmission of cholera by these routes within the United States. With clinical awareness of signs and symptoms of cholera, and knowledge of appropriate
treatment, cholera should not pose a major risk to health in the United States.

Microbiology

Cholera is caused by V. cholerae serogroup O1 strains that produce cholera
toxin. The Latin American epidemic strain is biotype El Tor, serotype Inaba.
This strain can be distinguished from the strain of V. cholerae O1 that is endemic to the U.S. Gulf Coast by hemolysin production and by molecular subtyping techniques (7).

Clinical Suspicion

Cholera should be suspected in a patient with severe watery diarrhea, vomiting, and dehydration. The illness is often accompanied by marked leg cramps, caused by electrolyte disturbances. However, the spectrum of V. cholerae O1 infection ranges from asymptomatic infection (75% of infections) through mild diarrhea to the most severe and clinically recognizable form (5%). Clinical suspicion should be increased for persons returning from areas known to have epidemic cholera or for persons with a recent history of ingestion of raw or undercooked shellfish.

Diagnosis

Cholera is diagnosed by isolation of toxigenic V. cholerae serotype O1 from feces. Other serogroups of V. cholerae, and nontoxigenic V. cholerae O1, may be isolated from stools of patients with diarrhea, but these bacteria are not associated with epidemic cholera. Culture of rectal swabs or fecal specimens on thiosulfate citrate bile salts sucrose (TCBS) medium should be requested for any patient suspected to have cholera. Suspected isolates of V. cholerae should be submitted to public health laboratories for confirmation. Serologic diagnosis may also be made by the presence of a changing titer of vibriocidal antibodies.

Treatment

Patients suspected of having cholera should be treated aggressively while awaiting culture results. In both adults and children, fluid and electrolyte losses should be replaced by rehydration therapy. All but severely dehydrated adults and children can be managed largely or completely with oral rehydration solution (ORS) (8). Patients with mild to moderate vomiting will absorb ORS taken in small sips. At present, World Health Organization ORS packets (WHO-ORS*, Jianas Brothers, St. Louis), Ricelyte® (Mead Johnson), and Rehydralyte® (Ross Laboratories) are the only oral solutions available in the United States that contain the proper balance of electrolytes for treating cholera. WHO-ORS is available from the manufacturer; the other two products are available over the counter. If ORS is not available, rehydration therapy should begin with intravenous fluids.

Intravenous therapy is necessary for patients who are severely dehydrated or in hypovolemic shock. The severely dehydrated cholera patient may have lost more than 10% of body weight and will need rapid volume replacement with Ringer's Lactate solution, the only solution readily available in the United States with the electrolyte composition needed for treating cholera (9, 10). Normal saline is less effective for treatment but can be used if Ringer's Lactate is unavailable (10). Severely dehydrated adults may require several liters of fluid immediately to restore an adequate circulating volume. As soon as the pa-

---

*Use of trade names is for identification only and does not imply endorsement by the Public Health Service or the U.S. Department of Health and Human Services.

tient is hemodynamically stable, oral therapy may be substituted. Patients with cholera have substantial ongoing fluid losses that also need to be replaced.

Antimicrobial drugs are a useful adjunctive therapy, decreasing the duration of both diarrhea and bacterial shedding and diminishing the volume of fluid replacement needed for treatment. Antibiotics with demonstrated effectiveness include doxycycline, tetracycline, trimethoprim-sulfamethoxazole (TMP-SMX), erythromycin, and furazolidone (9, 10). Adults may be treated with a single 300-mg dose of doxycycline. Children may be given TMP-SMX twice a day for 3 days at a dose of 5 mg/kg of TMP and 25 mg/kg of SMX.

Management of Family Contacts

Family members of persons suspected to have cholera should be questioned concerning their health status and advised to seek medical attention immediately if they develop watery diarrhea during the week following illness onset in the index patient. Because secondary transmission in the United States is rare, chemoprophylaxis of family contacts is not necessary. Cholera vaccine is not recommended (4). The family should receive instructions about proper hand washing and about cleaning contaminated clothes and linen with soap and chlorine bleach. The sanitary facilities in a cholera patient's home should be inspected to ensure that the patient's feces are disposed of through adequate sewage treatment or a functioning septic tank or are otherwise decontaminated.

Case Reporting

All suspected or confirmed cases of cholera should be reported immediately to the local and state health department.

REFERENCES: AS NUMBERED IN ORIGINAL PUBLICATION

4. CDC. Cholera—New Jersey and Florida. MMWR 1991;40:287–289.
7. Wachsmuth IK, Bopp CA, Fields PA. Difference between toxigenic Vibrio cholerae O1 from South America and US Gulf Coast [Letter]. Lancet 1991;337:1097–1098.
8. Snyder JS. Use and misuse of oral therapy for diarrhea: comparison of US practices with American Academy of Pediatrics recommendations. Pediatrics 1991;87:28–33.
9. Benenson AS. Cholera. In: Benenson AS, ed. Control of communicable diseases in man. Washington, DC: American Public Health Association, 1990:89–94.
10. World Health Organization. Guidelines for cholera control. Geneva, Switzerland: World Health Organization, Programme for Control of Diarrhoeal Disease, 1991 (WHO/CDD/SER/80.4 rev. 2 (1991)).

Cholera Vaccine

Original Citation: Centers for Disease Control and Prevention. Recommendations of the Immunization Practices Advisory Committee—Cholera Vaccine. MMWR 1988;37(40):617–618, 623–624.

INTRODUCTION

Historically, endemic and epidemic cholera commonly has occurred in parts of southern and southeastern Asia. Since 1961, cholera caused by the El Tor biotype has been epidemic throughout much of Asia, the Middle East, and Africa and in certain parts of Europe. Infection is acquired primarily by consuming contaminated water or food; person-to-person transmission is rare. Travelers who follow the usual tourist itinerary and who use standard accommodations in countries affected by cholera are at virtually no risk of infection.

CHOLERA VACCINE

Cholera vaccines*, whether prepared from Classic or El Tor strains, are of limited usefulness. In field trials conducted in areas with endemic cholera, vaccines have been only about 50% effective in reducing the incidence of clinical illness for 3–6 months. They do not prevent transmission of infection. Therefore, the Public Health Service no longer requires cholera vaccination for travelers coming to the United States from cholera-infected areas, and the World Health Organization (WHO) no longer recommends cholera vaccination for travel to or from cholera-infected areas. Surveillance and treatment are sufficient to prevent spread of the disease if it were introduced into the United States.

Vaccine available in the United States is prepared from a combination of phenol-inactivated suspensions of classic Inaba and Ogawa strains of Vibrio cholerae grown on agar or in broth.

VACCINE USAGE

General Recommendations

Vaccine should not be used to manage contacts of persons with imported cases or to control the spread of infection. Repeated vaccination is required or advised sometimes for laboratory workers and airline and ship crews. However, such groups are unlikely to acquire or transmit cholera. Because information on the long-term safety of repeated vaccination is limited, such practices should be discontinued for airline and ship crews except when resolutely demanded by some countries for international travel. Vaccine is not recommended for infants less than 6 months of age and is not required for travel by most countries.

Vaccination for International Travel

The risk of cholera to U.S. travelers is so low that the vaccine is not likely to benefit most U.S. travelers. Persons using standard tourist accommodations in countries affected by cholera are at virtually no risk of infection. The traveler's best protection against cholera, as well as against many other enteric diseases, is to avoid food and water that might be contaminated.

However, many countries affected or threatened by cholera require evidence of cholera vaccination for entry. One dose of vaccine will usually satisfy entry requirements for persons who anticipate travel to such countries and who will be vaccinated in the United States. With the threat or occurrence of epidemic cholera, health authorities of some countries may require evidence of a complete primary series of two doses or a booster dose within 6 months before arrival. The complete primary series is otherwise suggested only for special high-risk groups that work and live in highly endemic areas under less than sanitary conditions (Table 1). Vaccination requirements published by WHO are regularly updated and summarized for travelers by the Public Health Service and distributed to state and local health departments, airlines, travel agents, many physicians, and others. Physicians and travelers should seek information on requirements from these sources.

---

*Official name: Cholera Vaccine.

Physicians administering vaccine to travelers should emphasize that an International Certificate of Vaccination against cholera must be validated for it to be acceptable to quarantine authorities. Validation can be obtained at most city, county, and state health departments as well as many private clinics and physicians' offices. Failure to secure validation may cause travelers to be revaccinated or quarantined. A properly documented certificate is valid for 6 months, beginning 6 days after vaccination or beginning on the date of revaccination if this revaccination is within 6 months of a previous injection.

Table 1. Recommended doses, by volume, for immunization against cholera

		Route and age		
	Intradermal*	Subcutaneous or intramuscular		
Dose no.	≥ 5 yrs	6 mos–4 yrs	5–10 yrs	> 10 yrs
1 and 2	0.2 mL	0.2 mL	0.3 mL	0.5 mL
Boosters	0.2 mL	0.2 mL	0.3 mL	0.5 mL

*Higher levels of protection (antibody) may be achieved in children < 5 years old by the subcutaneous or intramuscular routes.

Data have indicated that persons given yellow fever and cholera vaccines simultaneously or 1–3 weeks apart had initially lower-titered antibody responses to both vaccines. However, seroconversion rates were unaffected, and the clinical importance of these data are unknown. In view of these data, yellow fever and cholera vaccines ideally should be given at least 3 weeks apart. If that is not possible, and both vaccines must be given, then they can be given simultaneously or at any time within the 3-week interval, although a delay in expected yellow fever protection may occur.

Primary Immunization

Complete primary immunization consists of two doses of vaccine given at least 1 week apart. The intradermal route is satisfactory for persons greater than or equal to 5 years of age (Table 1).

Booster Doses

Booster doses may be given every 6 months if necessary for travel or for residence in highly endemic, unsanitary areas. In areas where cholera occurs in a 2–3 month season, protection is best if the booster dose is given at the beginning of the season. The primary series does not need to be repeated for booster doses to be effective.

PRECAUTIONS AND CONTRAINDICATIONS

Reactions

Vaccination often results in 1–2 days of pain, erythema, and induration at the site of injection. The local reaction may be accompanied by fever, malaise, and headache.

Serious reactions following cholera vaccination are extremely rare. If a person has had a serious reaction to the vaccine, revaccination is not advised. Most governments will permit an unvaccinated traveler to proceed if he/she carries a physician's statement of medical contraindication. However, some countries may quarantine such unvaccinated persons or place them under surveillance if they come from areas with cholera.

Pregnancy

No specific information exists on the safety of cholera vaccine during pregnancy. Its use should be individualized to reflect actual need.

SELECTED BIBLIOGRAPHY

Bart KJ, Gangarosa EJ. Cholera. In: Kelley VC, ed. Brennemann's practice of pediatrics. Vol II, chap. 18c. New York: Harper and Row, 1977:1–12.
Barua D, Burrows W, eds. Cholera. Philadelphia: WB Saunders, 1974.
CDC. Health information for international travel, 1988. Atlanta: US Department of Health and Human Services, Public Health Service, 1988; HHS publication no. (CDC)88–8280.
Felsenfeld O, Wolf RH, Dutta NK. Serological responses of Patas monkeys (Erythrocebus patas) to vaccination against cholera and yellow fever. Proc Soc Exp Biol Med 1973;143:548–550.
Gangarosa EJ, Barker WH. Cholera: implications for the United States. JAMA 1974;227:170–171.
Gateff C, Dodin A, Wiart J. Comparaison des reactions serologiques induites par un vaccin anticholerique classique et une fraction vaccinante purifiee associes ou non au vaccin antiamaril. Ann Microbiol (Paris) 1975;126:231–246.
McCormack WM, Chowdhury AM, Jahangir N, et al. Tetracycline prophylaxis in families of cholera patients. Bull WHO 1968;38:787–792.
Philippines Cholera Committee. A controlled field trial on the effectiveness of the intradermal and subcutaneous administration of cholera vaccine in the Philippines. Bull WHO 1973;49:389–394.
Snyder JD, Blake PA. Is cholera a problem for US travelers? JAMA 1982;247:2268–2269.
Sommer A, Khan M, Mosley WH. Efficacy of vaccination of family contacts of cholera cases. Lancet 1973;1:1230–1232.

Imported Cholera Associated with a Newly Described Toxigenic Vibrio cholerae O139 Strain

Original Citation: Centers for Disease Control and Prevention. Imported Cholera Associated with a Newly Described Toxigenic Vibrio cholerae O139 Strain—California, 1993. MMWR 1993;42(26):501–503.

Original Authors: M Tormey, MPH, L Mascola, MD, L Kilman, P Nagami, MD, E DeBess, DVM, S Abbott, GW Rutherford, III, MD

SUMMARY

Epidemics of cholera-like illness caused by a previously unrecognized organism occurred recently in southern Asia (1). This report documents the first case of cholera imported into the United States that was caused by this organism, the newly described toxigenic Vibrio cholerae O139 strain.

On February 5, 1993, a 48-year-old female resident of Los Angeles County sought care at a local outpatient health-care facility for acute onset of watery diarrhea and back pain. A few hours before seeking medical care, she had returned to the United States from a 6-week visit with relatives in Hyderabad, India.

Her diarrheal illness began in India on February 4 and increased in severity while she traveled to the United States. She reported a maximum of 10 watery stools per day but no vomiting, visible blood or mucous in her stools, or documented fever. The patient was prescribed trimethoprim sulfamethoxazole without rehydration treatment and recovered uneventfully. Duration of illness was approximately 4 days. No secondary illness occurred among family members.

When the patient sought medical care, the physician suspected cholera, and a culture of a stool specimen obtained from the patient at that time yielded colonies suspected of being V. cholerae. This was confirmed by the Los Angeles County Public Health Laboratory. The isolate was identified as V. cholerae non-O1. The isolate produced cholera toxin by Y-1 adrenal cell assay and latex agglutination in the California State Public Health Laboratory. Testing at CDC identified the isolate as toxigenic V. cholerae serogroup O139, resistant to trimethoprim-sulfamethoxazole.

Before this illness, the patient had been in good health. In Hyderabad, she stayed with relatives and did not travel outside the city. Although the source of her infection was not confirmed, on January 30, the patient had eaten fried shrimp and prawns purchased from a local market and prepared by relatives. She also recalled drinking a half glass of unbottled water in Hyderabad on February 3.

Editorial Note

In October 1992, an epidemic of cholera-like illness began in Madras, India, associated with an atypical strain of V. cholerae (2). In early 1993, similar epidemics began in Calcutta (with more than 13,000 cases) and in Bangladesh (with more than 10,000 cases and 500 deaths) caused by similarly atypical strains of V. cholerae (3, 4). These strains could not be identified as any of the 138 known types of V. cholerae and have been designated as a new serogroup, O139 (5). Although the extent of the ongoing epidemic in southern Asia is unclear, this strain is now associated with epidemic cholera-like illness along a 1000-mile coastline of the Bay of Bengal (from Madras, India, to Bangladesh) and appears to have largely replaced V. cholerae O1 strains in affected areas.

The emergence of this new cause of epidemic cholera represents an important shift in the epidemiology of this infectious disease (6). Until 1993, the only recognized causes of epidemic cholera were V. cholerae strains that were part of serogroup O1. V. cholerae isolates from other serogroups (i.e., non-O1) were recognized as causes of sporadic diarrheal and invasive infections but were not considered to have epidemic potential. The relation of the new non-O1 serogroup to typical O1 strains is unclear; except for the presence of O1 antigen, the strains are nearly identical in most characteristics.

Descriptions of the symptoms associated with V. cholerae O139 infection suggest it is indistinguishable from cholera caused by V. cholerae O1 and should be treated with the same rapid fluid replacement (7). Although the illness may be severe, it is treatable with oral and intravenous rehydration therapy. The new organism has been susceptible to tetracycline, which is the recommended antibiotic for treatment of cholera. However, the organism is reportedly resistant to trimethoprim-sulfamethoxazole and furazolidone, other antibiotics used to treat cholera.

Health-care providers should consider the new strain as a possible cause of cholera-like illness in persons returning from the Indian subcontinent. Although previous cases were reported from Madras and Calcutta in India and from Bangladesh, this report suggests that Hyderabad, India—which is inland—is also affected. Because of effective sewerage and water treatment, further spread of this strain is unlikely in the United States. However, the potential for epidemic cholera caused by V. cholerae O139 exists for much of the developing world, and further spread to other parts of Asia is probable.

The emergence of this new strain has at least three other major public health implications. First, it expands the definition of cholera beyond the illness caused exclusively by toxigenic V. cholerae of serogroup O1. Because it appears to cause the same illness and to have similar epidemic potential, the World Health Organization has asked all nations to report illnesses caused by this strain as cholera (1). In the United States, clinicians, laboratorians, and public health authorities should report infections with toxigenic V. cholerae O139 as cholera, in addition to cases of toxigenic V. cholerae O1 infection.

Second, the rapid spread of the V. cholerae O139 epidemic in southern Asia, even among adults previously exposed to cholera caused by V. cholerae O1, suggests that preexisting immunity to toxigenic V. cholerae O1, whether the result of natural infection or cholera vaccine, offers little or no protective benefit. Travelers to areas affected by this epidemic should exercise particular care in selecting food and drink and should not assume that cholera vaccination is protective against the V. cholerae O139 strain.

Third, laboratory identification methods for V. cholerae O1 depend on detection of the O1 antigen on the surface of the bacterium, and therefore do not identify this new strain. A specific diagnostic antiserum for V. cholerae O139 is being prepared for use in U.S. public health laboratories and will be distributed soon. Without such antiserum, this strain might be confused with other non-O1 V. cholerae isolates unrelated to the newly described O139 strain that occasionally cause infections in the United States.

In 1989, a pilot surveillance effort in four states determined that the reported infection rate for non-O1 V. cholerae was 1 per 1 million population (8). Although non-O1 strains can cause illness, non-O1 strains other than the newly described O139 have not been implicated as a cause of epidemics and are not considered a major public health problem. Accordingly, CDC recommends that:

1. Sporadic clinical isolates of non-O1 V. cholerae should be referred to a state public health laboratory for further characterization if there is an epidemiologic link to areas of the world known to be affected by O139 (currently In-

dia and Bangladesh); if the disease is typical of severe cholera (i.e., watery diarrhea with life-threatening dehydration); or if the isolate has been linked to an outbreak (i.e., more than one linked case) of diarrheal illness.

2. Physicians should ask that specimens from persons with suspected cholera be cultured on thiosulfate-citrate-bile salts-sucrose (TCBS) medium for isolation of V. cholerae. All cases of suspected cholera should be reported immediately to local and state health departments.

REFERENCES: AS NUMBERED IN ORIGINAL PUBLICATION

1. World Health Organization. Epidemic diarrhea due to Vibrio cholerae non-O1. Wkly Epidemiol Rec 1993;68:141–142.
2. Ramamurthy T, Garg S, Sharma R, et al. Emergence of novel strain of Vibrio cholerae with epidemic potential in southern and eastern India [Letter]. Lancet 1993;341:703–704.
3. Albert MJ, Siddique AK, Islam MS, et al. Large outbreak of clinical cholera due to Vibrio cholerae non-O1 in Bangladesh [Letter]. Lancet 1993;341:704.
4. Bhattacharya MK, Bhattacharya SK, Garg S, et al. Outbreak of Vibrio cholerae non-O1 in India and Bangladesh [Letter]. Lancet 1993;341:1346–1347.
5. Shimada T, Balakrish Nair G, Deb BC, et al. Outbreak of Vibrio cholerae non-O1 in India and Bangladesh [Letter]. Lancet 1993;341:1347.
6. CDC. Emerging infectious diseases—introduction. MMWR 1993;42:257.
7. Swerdlow DL, Ries AA. Cholera in the Americas: guidelines for the clinician. JAMA 1992;267:1495–1499.
8. Levine WC, Griffin PM, Gulf Coast Vibrio Working Group. Vibrio infections on the Gulf Coast: results of first year of regional surveillance. J Infect Dis 1993;167:479–483.

TOPIC 4 / **DENGUE**

A Program for Prevention and Control of Epidemic Dengue and Dengue Hemorrhagic Fever in Puerto Rico and the U.S. Virgin Islands

Original Citation: Gubler DJ, Casta-Valez A. A Program for Prevention and Control of Epidemic Dengue and Dengue Hemorrhagic Fever in Puerto Rico and the U.S. Virgin Islands. Bulletin of PAHO 1991;25(3):237. Reprinted by U.S. Department of Health and Human Services, Public Health Service, Centers for Disease Control and Prevention.

EPIDEMIC DENGUE AND DENGUE HEMORRHAGIC FEVER

The ongoing resurgence of Aedes aegypti in the Americas—abetted by poor mosquito control, urbanization, and increased air travel—has led to dengue hyperendemicity, more frequent dengue epidemics, and the emergence of dengue hemorrhagic fever (DHF).

Proactive Surveillance

Surveillance for dengue and DHF/DSS can be of two basic types, reactive or proactive (15). Most endemic countries conduct reactive surveillance, with health authorities waiting until the medical community recognizes transmission before reacting to implement control measures. Unfortunately, this type of surveillance is very insensitive—because in the absence of epidemic transmission there is a low index of suspicion among physicians, and dengue is rarely diagnosed. Indeed, in most cases epidemics are near peak transmission before they are recognized and confirmed as dengue. By then it is generally too late to implement effective preventive measures that impact on transmission and thus on the course of the epidemic.

Our program seeks to employ a proactive surveillance system that will permit prediction of epidemic dengue (15). The most important component of this proactive system is virologic surveillance that is designed to monitor dengue virus transmission on the island, especially during interepidemic periods, and to continually provide information on where transmission is occurring, what virus serotype or serotypes are involved, and what type of illness is associated with the dengue infection. If this type of information is available, then without too much delay we should be able to detect the introduction of new dengue virus serotypes.

During periods of low dengue activity, cases of dengue-like illness are frequently not recognized as suspected dengue; many dengue infections present clinically as nonspecific viral illness, and physicians tend not to be on the lookout for dengue during interepidemic periods. For all these reasons, the surveillance program cannot rely on the medical community to monitor dengue virus introductions and transmission. Instead, the program depends upon regular monitoring of patients with viral syndrome to provide increased sensitivity and detect changes in the dengue virus picture.

Each week throughout the year, regardless of dengue activity, Puerto Rico Health Department clinics are asked to take blood samples from selected patients with viral syndrome whose illnesses had their onset three to 14 days earlier. These samples are picked up by Puerto Rico Health Department employees and taken to the laboratory, where they are processed on a weekly basis to isolate dengue virus and detect the presence of dengue-specific IgM antibody (15, 16).

In addition to this clinic work, a collaborative program with a small group of selected private physicians who are interested and who provide high-quality specimens and information has been initiated. All collaborators, both private physicians and clinics, are also asked to take samples from any patient with classical dengue or hemorrhagic manifestations in addition to viral syndrome.

This is a very hard type of surveillance to maintain, because many physicians refuse to take blood samples from patients they are "sure do not have dengue infection." It requires constant communication and encouragement, and even then many physicians do not take the blood samples requested. It is, however, the most critical part of a proactive surveillance system designed to detect new virus introductions.

Because dengue frequently presents as nonspecific febrile illness, especially in children, another component of the proactive system is surveillance designed to detect increased febrile illness in the community (15). Through a network of nurse epidemiologists, physicians, and environmental health workers on the island, any observed increase in febrile illness is reported and investigated immediately. Blood samples are obtained from representative cases, taken to the laboratory, and processed to isolate dengue virus and detect dengue-specific IgM antibody.

The proactive surveillance system also monitors all cases of hemorrhagic disease and all cases of viral illness that have a fatal outcome (17). This is done working in close collaboration with infectious disease physicians who would normally see such cases of severe and fatal disease. All cases reported are investigated, and blood specimens—as well as tissue specimens in fatal cases—are obtained for virologic and serologic study. Fresh-frozen tissue and formalin-fixed tissue may be examined by immunofluorescence, immunoperoxidase, or specific hybridization probes for specific dengue viral antigen.

Each of the above surveillance components has limitations and may not be very sensitive by itself. Collectively, however, they provide a relatively good early warning capability that has been sensitive enough to predict epidemic dengue activity in Puerto Rico. It should be noted that entomologic surveillance is not routinely carried out as part of this program because Ae. aegypti densities are usually well in excess of the level needed for epidemic transmission.

Rapid-Response Emergency Vector Control

The rationale for rapid-response emergency vector control depends on two points. These are as follows: (a) routine mosquito control will not reduce vector populations below the threshold levels required for epidemic transmission; and (b) there is a "lag time" of one to six months between introduction of a new dengue virus and peak epidemic transmission (17). Hence, to follow up on the surveillance program's early warning—if that program is sensitive enough to detect new viruses shortly after their introduction, or to detect increased dengue activity well in advance of epidemic transmission we must have an effective emergency vector control capacity that can be activated quickly. The aim of this activity is to contain an incipient epidemic in a limited area before it spreads to other parts of the island.

Baseline data required for this work include delineation of the most important and productive Ae. aegypti larval habitats in every major town and city, species associations with other potential mosquito vectors, and identification of major problem areas. This island survey was completed in 1985, and the results of the survey were computerized to improve rapid access to information on mosquito breeding sites in all major towns and cities in Puerto Rico and the U.S. Virgin Islands (San Juan Laboratories, unpublished data).

At the time of this writing (1991), details of the rapid-response program had not been fully elaborated. Unfortunately the principal emergency control method, ULV application of insecticide for adult mosquito control, does not work very well (10–13). So, while research to improve the efficacy of adulticiding is under way, we must rely on other approaches as well.

The basic method employed is as follows: When surveillance data suggest increased dengue transmission or introduction of a new dengue virus serotype or strain, the situation is investigated immediately. Epidemiologic data are collected in an attempt to determine where the infection or infections occurred and where it or they may have been transported. At the same time, a fully integrated mosquito control effort is launched on the basis of information taken from the computerized survey results.

This latter control activity, conducted by the environmental health program of the Puerto Rico Department of Health, is directed at the whole community. It uses radio, television, and newspaper public service announcements to inform the people of the problem and what to do about it. A targeted source reduction program is undertaken that emphasizes removing those larval habitats that are the most productive and treating those that cannot be removed with ABATE or other insecticide. In addition, ULV malathion spraying of the entire city where the case was detected may be carried out using truck-mounted equipment. Perifocal ULV spraying in the vicinity of the case, as is done in many countries, is not recommended because it is felt likely that by the time a case is detected and a response mounted the infection will have spread to a wider area.

Other government and civic organizations such as Civil Defense, the Civil Air Patrol, the Boy Scouts, primary and secondary schools, and Rotary Clubs are used in those communities where they are active and agree to participate. Specifically, these organizations help by distributing educational material and providing the public with information about where mosquitoes can be found and how to control them so as to prevent transmission.

In general, it is felt that the response to news of a threatening epidemic should involve community participation. Ultimate success of the program will depend on community participation and cooperation by citizens (most transmission occurs in the home) (10). Therefore, considerable effort is being placed on community education.

One major problem with this approach is the need for government approval in order to use the above community mobilization methods to help control the mosquitoes. Most governments are regrettably reluctant to give such approval, because they like to be 100% sure there is an epidemic before declaring an emergency. This type of thinking must change before an effective emergency response can be mounted.

Contingency Planning, Education of the Medical Community

Because the above long-term program for prevention and control of epidemic dengue will take several years to implement and refine, it has been necessary to develop contingency plans in case a DHF/DSS epidemic should occur before the program is effectively established. One important aspect of these plans is education of the medical community—to make physicians in Puerto Rico and the U.S. Virgin Islands more aware of dengue and to train them in DHF/DSS diagnosis and treatment.

An international seminar on DHF in the Americas was organized in 1985 and was followed by a series of local seminars in all major Puerto Rican cities that gave emphasis to the need for clinical diagnosis and treatment of DHF/DSS. A program continuing these seminars, which has been under way ever since, now relies primarily on a "peer education" system that recruits and trains highly respected physicians in a community to become the local DHF/DSS experts. These physicians give lectures and seminars employing visual materials provided to them by CDC/PRHD, including a video on clinical diagnosis and treatment of DF/DSS written by us and produced by the San Juan Rotary Club for use by physicians and medical associations.

Current plans call for maintaining this program indefinitely. Fortunately, evidence including the improved quality of clinical data received by the surveillance program indicates that progress has been made. In contrast to the situation prevailing in 1985, many physicians now routinely do the official laboratory tests critical for early diagnosis of DHF/DSS. The program has also turned out to have a worthwhile added benefit in that informed physicians are themselves helping to educate the lay community.

Emergency Hospitalization Plan

A second contingency plan dealing with emergency hospitalization has sought to pave the way for making the most effective use of hospital and treatment facilities in case a DHF/DSS epidemic should occur before the medical community is fully aware of the disease and ready for it. This program is being implemented as follows: First, an overall emergency hospitalization plan (see Annex) that outlines basic principles and requirements based on the WHO Technical Guide (4) was drafted and sent to each of the island's eight medical regions. Second, hospitals and potential treatment centers in each region have been identified according to the type of facility and number of beds available. Plans call for entering the names of physicians and paramedics in the area into a computer data base and keeping the list current at the regional level.

Each region will use this information to develop a contingency plan for a "worst case" situation where there is one DHF/DSS case for every 100 cases of dengue infection. If adequate numbers of beds are not available in hospitals and public clinics, plans will be made to convert other public buildings into temporary treatment centers. Each region is responsible for determining needed equipment and supplies and ensuring that these are available in an emergency. Finally, a central committee advises and consults with regional committees appointed to oversee the program.

Long-term, Integrated, Community-Based Mosquito Control

Ultimately, prevention of epidemic dengue and DHF/DSS will depend upon effective, long-term mosquito control. To be cost-effective and sustainable, such control must be achieved through integrated community-based action.

Community participation in Puerto Rico depends upon effective communication with a public that is diverse in terms of its socioeconomic and ethnocultural backgrounds (10). To develop effective community participation, the program seeks to inform the people of Puerto Rico and the U.S. Virgin Islands about DHF/DSS, the potential dangers and consequences of epidemic DHF/DSS, the fact that major epidemics can be prevented, and the fact that it is their responsibility to see that preventive measures are effective. Specifically, the message that must be communicated to all citizens is that (a) DHF/DSS is now endemic in Puerto Rico and the U.S. Virgin Islands; (b) the islands are at high risk of epidemic DHF/DSS because of the high Ae. aegypti densities in all major cities; (c) most dengue transmission occurs in and around the home; (d) this happens because people accumulate excessive trash around their homes, thereby creating mosquito breeding places; (e) dengue can be prevented by controlling these domestic larval habitats, but only the people involved can effectively clean up the areas around their own homes to prevent mosquito breeding; (f) control must be a community effort, because mosquitoes can fly from house to house; (g) insecticide spraying is expensive, is ineffective for routine mosquito control, and at most should only be used in emergency situations; and (h) it is the responsibility of the people, not the government, to prevent epidemic DHF/DSS in Puerto Rico and the U.S. Virgin Islands.

A major effort has been made to develop new and innovative educational materials that can effectively communicate this message to specific population groups. This effort has been based upon ongoing knowledge, attitude, and practices studies conducted by medical anthropologists, social scientists, and health educators who have been attached to the project since 1986 (10). The rationale here is to identify all the major ethnic, social, and cultural elements of the society, study their behavior and attitudes toward dengue and its prevention, and then develop educational materials directed at these groups. (Because one key population group is school-age children, major educational work has been directed toward the schools.) Details of the community-based component of this program will be reported elsewhere (San Juan Laboratories, unpublished data).

Disease control has historically been a responsibility of government. With a disease like dengue, however, most governments do not have the resources to maintain effective control. Because of certain resources available in the private sector, the influence civic organizations can have upon the public, and the marketing skills of those organizations, a plan was developed to involve the business community in dengue prevention and control (10). Briefly, civic organizations such as Rotary International have been encouraged to develop programs that will help government agencies educate the public about its responsibility for environmental sanitation and how to effectively control mosquitoes in the community.

SUMMARY

Our approach has been to identify and involve all segments of the community in Ae. aegypti control. Our rationale is that only a program planned and directed by the community will be truly community-based and sustainable. This does not absolve the government of responsibility, because most of the world's dengue-endemic areas have many larval habitats that require government intervention. Therefore, the programs developed must be integrated to provide government support for the community-based efforts (10). Ultimately, the aim is to develop enforceable legislative control, such as has been successfully implemented in Singapore and Cuba (18, 19)—recognizing that in a democratic society the sort of control program envisaged can only be successful after the public has been educated to a point where it accepts its responsibility for playing the principal role in prevention and control of epidemic dengue and DHF/DSS.

REFERENCES: AS NUMBERED IN ORIGINAL PUBLICATION

4. World Health Organization. Dengue hemorrhagic fever: diagnosis, treatment, and control. Geneva: 1986 (58 pp.).
10. Gubler DJ. Aedes aegypti and Aedes aegypti-borne disease control in the 1990s: top down or bottom up? Am J Trop Med Hyg 1989;40(6):571–578.
11. San Juan Laboratories. Dengue surveillance summary. July 1987; number 44.
12. San Juan Laboratories. Dengue surveillance summary. October 1987; number 47.
13. Chadee DD. An evaluation of malathion ULV spraying against caged and natural populations of Aedes aegypti in Trinidad, West Indies. Cah ORSTOM, Ser Ent Med et Parisitol 1985;23(2):71–74.
15. Gubler DJ. Surveillance for dengue and dengue hemorrhagic fever. Bull Pan Am Health Organ. 1989;23(4):397–404.
16. Gubler DJ, Kuno G, Sather GE, Velez M, Oliver A. Use of mosquito cell cultures and specific monoclonal antibodies for routine surveillance of dengue viruses. Am J Trop Med Hyg 1984;33: 158–165.
17. Gubler DJ, Suharyono W, Sumarmo SPS, et al. Virological surveillance for dengue haemorrhagic fever in Indonesia using the mosquito inoculation technique. Bull WHO 1979;57:931.
18. Chan KL. Singapore's dengue haemorrhagic fever control programme: a case study on the successful control of Aedes aegypti and Aedes albopictus using mainly environmental measures as a part of integrated vector control. Tokyo: SEAMIC, 1985.
19. Armada Gessa JA, Figueredo Gonzalez R. Application of environmental management principles in the program for eradication of Aedes (stegomyia) aegypti (Linneus, 1762) in the Republic of Cuba, 1984. Bull Pan Am Health Organ 1986;20(2):186–193.

ANNEX: HOSPITALIZATION CONTINGENCY PLAN FOR EPIDEMIC DENGUE HEMORRHAGIC FEVER IN PUERTO RICO

Background and Rationale

This section sets forth reasons for the contingency plan that are stated in the foregoing text.

Use of Outpatient Facilities and Indications for Hospitalization

In mild or moderate cases of dehydration or threatened dehydration, oral or parenteral fluid therapy can be given in an outpatient rehydration unit. Establishment of such units in diagnostic treatment centers (DTCs) would reduce the number of hospital beds required for management of the more severe cases. Patients cared for in an outpatient setting must, however, be carefully followed for deterioration and onset of shock, which usually appears toward the end of the febrile period. Indications for hospitalization and immediate treatment are the following signs of shock:

- restlessness/lethargy
- cold extremities, circumoral cyanosis
- rapid and feeble pulse
- narrow pulse pressure (20 mm Hg or less) or hypotension
- elevated or rising hematocrit

Requirements for Inpatient Hospital Facilities

In the worst situations previously encountered, the incidence of seriously ill patients requiring hospitalization has approached one case per 100 dengue infections. This is the situation for which we should be prepared. An overall population of approximately 3.5 million people translates into 35,000 persons hospitalized over a three-month period, or approximately 10,000 per month. Each region should evaluate the number of beds available in existing hospitals and diagnostic treatment centers (DTCs). Based on regional population estimates, contingency plans should be developed to convert schools or public buildings to handle the excess if necessary.

Supplies and Equipment

For Outpatient Departments/Treatment Centers

Diagnostic materials:

- Blood pressure cuffs (adult and pediatric)
- Thermometers
- Hematocrit supplies (lancets, capillary tubes, reader)
- Hematocrit centrifuge
- Compound microscope and materials for white blood cell platelet counts
- Vacutainers or syringes/needles for obtaining dengue and diagnostic test samples

Therapeutic materials:

- Acetaminophen
- WHO oral rehydration solution: 3.5 g sodium chloride (table salt), 2.5 g sodium bicarbonate (baking soda), 1.5 g potassium chloride, and 20.0 g glucose dissolved in 1 liter of potable water
- Lactated Ringer's; 0.85% saline; 5% glucose in water
- Tubing and needles for intravenous therapy

For Hospitals

Diagnostic materials and patient monitoring: Same as Supplies and Equipment, Diagnostic materials, plus:

- Laboratory test equipment and supplies for blood typing and crossmatching, for measuring arterial blood gases and pH, and for measuring serum electrolytes
- Portable X-ray equipment
- Central venous pressure monitoring kits
- Arterial pressure and Swan-Ganz catheters and monitoring equipment when feasible
- Intake-output monitoring charts

Therapeutic materials: Same as Supplies and Equipment, Therapeutic materials, plus:

- Plasma volume expanders (Dextran 40, plasmanate, fresh/frozen plasma, whole blood where available)
- 7.5% sodium bicarbonate for injection
- Chloral hydrate
- Paraldehyde
- Oxygen

Hospitalized patients will require some amount of intravenous fluid therapy with lactated Ringer's or glucose/normal saline. Approximately 20% of all hospitalized patients will require intravascular volume expanders such as dextran 40, plasmanate, or plasma, and about 10% will require the administration of whole blood. The volume of intravenous fluid needed in an individual case will depend on the weight of the patient and the seriousness of the shock state. However, assuming that one-half of the patients are children, an estimate of the supplies required per 10,000 population (100 cases of DHF) in each region can be made:

- 280 liters of normal saline or lactated Ringer's
- 280 liters of 5% glucose in water
- 25 liters of volume expander
- 10 units of whole blood

Organization

A health department coordinating committee should be appointed to organize and advise the community during the emergency. One subcommittee should deal with clinical care. This committee should design and distribute appropriate protocols for the diagnosis and treatment of DHF/DSS, compile and distribute appropriate information and literature on DHF, help develop educational materials for multimedia programs, plan for and implement training programs for health care workers, and oversee usage of supplies and outcome of the clinical care program.

Triage

In the setting of an epidemic, triage of patients with appropriate treatment will be required:

1. Patients with classical dengue fever and without signs of dehydration, hemorrhage, or circulatory failure should be examined by blood pressure measurement, tourniquet test, and hematocrit. In the absence of clinical signs of dehydration, circulatory failure (see below), or hemorrhagic diathesis (positive tourniquet test), patients may be treated with acetaminophen and released with clear instructions to return immediately should signs of decompensation (lethargy, restlessness, cold extremities, skin congestion, hemorrhage, or severe abdominal pain) occur, usually on the third or fourth day after onset.

2. Patients with classical dengue fever and dehydration. Patients with signs described above who are also manifesting severe vomiting, diarrhea, and clinical signs of dehydration, may be given oral or parenteral fluid therapy in the outpatient setting. Such patients should be followed carefully and admitted if clinical criteria are met (see below).

3. Patients with signs of DHF/DSS. Patients with clinical signs of circulatory failures, lethargy, skin congestion, cool and clammy extremities, hypotension, narrowed pulse pressure (< 20 mm Hg, rapid and weak pulse) and with hemorrhagic manifestations (positive tourniquet tests, thrombocytopenia) or elevated hematocrit should be immediately admitted to the hospital.

4. Monitoring and treatment of all these patients should follow guidelines outlined in Dengue Hemorrhagic Fever: Diagnosis, Treatment, and Con-

trol (WHO, 1986). If properly instructed, nurses, medical students, and paramedical workers can carry out triage, but competent laboratory assistance is essential. Patients with similar degrees of severity of illness should be grouped together. Those with shock require intensive 24-hour nursing and physician care. Paramedical workers or parents can assist in oral fluid therapy or in monitoring the rate of intravenous fluid.

ADDITIONAL INFORMATION

1. This article will also be published in Spanish in the Bulletin de la Officina Sanitaria Panamericana, 1992.
2. San Juan Laboratories, Dengue Branch, Division of Vector-Borne Infectious Diseases, Center for Infectious Diseases, Centers for Disease Control, Public Health Service, United States Department of Health and Human Services, San Juan, Puerto Rico. Current address, where reprint requests should be sent: Director, Division of Vector-Borne Infectious Diseases, Center for Infectious Diseases, Centers for Disease Control, P.O. Box 2087, Fort Collins, Colorado 80522, USA.
3. Community Hygiene Division, Environmental Health, Puerto Rico Health Department, Building A, Call Box 70184, San Juan, Puerto Rico.
4. Reprinted by: U.S. Department of Health and Human Services Public Health Service, Centers For Disease Control and Prevention, Atlanta, Georgia 30333.

Dengue Type 3 Infection

Original Citation: Centers for Disease Control and Prevention. International Notes Dengue Type 3 Infection—Nicaragua and Panama, October-November 1994. MMWR 1995;44(02):21–24.

EDITORIAL NOTE

Dengue fever is an acute, mosquito-transmitted viral disease characterized by fever, headache, arthralgia, myalgia, rash, nausea, and vomiting. Infections are caused by any of the four virus serotypes. Although most dengue infections result in relatively mild illness, some can produce DHF. Based on the World Health Organization case definition (1), a case of DHF must meet the following criteria: (a) fever, (b) minor or major hemorrhagic manifestations, (c) thrombocytopenia (less than or equal to 100,000/mm3), and (d) objective evidence of increased capillary permeability (e.g., hemoconcentration [hematocrit increased by greater than or equal to 20%], pleural effusions [evidenced by chest radiography or other imaging method], or hypoproteinemia). A case of dengue shock syndrome (DSS) must meet all the criteria for DHF plus hypotension or narrow pulse pressure (less than or equal to 20 mm Hg); the fatality rate for patients with DSS can be as high as 44% (2).

Health-care providers should consider dengue in the differential diagnosis of all patients who have symptoms compatible with dengue and who reside in or have visited any tropical areas. When dengue is suspected, the patient's blood pressure, hematocrit, and platelet count should be monitored for evidence of hypotension, hemoconcentration, and thrombocytopenia. Acetaminophen products are recommended for management of fever because of the anticoagulant properties of acetylsalicylic acid (i.e., aspirin). Acute- and convalescent-phase serum samples should be obtained for viral isolation and serodiagnosis.

Suspected dengue cases should be reported to the state or territorial health department; the report should include a clinical summary, dates of onset of illness and blood collection, and other epidemiologic information (e.g., a detailed travel history with dates and location of travel). Serum samples should be sent for confirmation through state health department laboratories to CDC's Dengue Branch, Division of Vector-Borne Infectious Diseases, National Center for Infectious Diseases, 2 Calle Casia, San Juan, PR 00921–3200; telephone (809) 766–5181; fax (809) 766–6596.

REFERENCES: AS NUMBERED IN ORIGINAL PUBLICATION

1. World Health Organization. Dengue hemorrhagic fever: diagnosis, treatment, and control. Geneva: World Health Organization, 1986.
2. Tassniyom S, Vasanawathana S, Chirawatkul A, Rojanasuphot S. Failure of high-dose methylprednisolone in established dengue shock syndrome: a placebo-controlled, double-blind study. Pediatrics 1993;92:111–115.

Dengue and Dengue Hemorrhagic Fever

Original Citation: Hayes EB, Gubler DJ. Dengue and Dengue Hemorrhagic Fever. Pediatr Infect Dis J 1992;11:311–317.

Original Authors: Duane J. Gubler, Sc. D, and Edward B. Hayes, MD

DIAGNOSIS

Classical dengue fever may be confused with a variety of febrile illnesses, including influenza, measles, typhoid fever and malaria. DHF may also be confused with sepsis, toxic shock and any of the viral hemorrhagic fevers including yellow fever. Diseases with specific treatments, such as bacterial meningitis, sepsis, malaria and Lassa fever, should be ruled out.

Specific diagnosis of dengue infection is made by isolating the virus from the patient's blood. Acute serum samples are inoculated into tissue cultures of mosquito cells or directly into live *Toxorhynchites* or *Aedes* mosquitoes (66, 67). Isolates can be identified from 2 to 7 days after inoculation depending on the actual technique used (35). Viruses are most likely to be isolated from acute serum samples obtained within 5 days after the onset of illness (34, 35). Specific dengue serotypes can be identified by the indirect fluorescent antibody test, with the use of type-specific monoclonal antibodies on the isolated virus (67).

Immunodiagnostic methods for determining dengue infection include detection of anti-dengue IgM and IgG by enzyme-linked immunosorbent assay

(ELISA) and detection of hemagglutination inhibition antibody. Dengue-induced hemagglutination inhibition antibody cross-reacts broadly with other flaviviruses such as yellow fever and St. Louis encephalitis viruses (35). Complement fixation and neutralization antibody tests are more specific then hemagglutination inhibition (35). Most serologic screening for dengue infection is now done with an IgM ELISA (35, 68). With appropriately timed samples, the sensitivity and specificity of this test in diagnosing dengue infection appear to be high. In a review of 131 patients from whom dengue virus was isolated at the Centers for Disease Control, Dengue branch, 96% of the 76 samples drawn between 7 and 20 days after the onset of illness were positive by IgM capture ELISA (DJ Gubler, G Kuno, I Gomez, et al., unpublished data). A study of the performance of IgM ELISA in Thailand showed the sensitivity of this test in convalescent samples to be 97%, and none of the samples from the 2 groups of noninfected controls (98 soldiers and 39 schoolchildren) were positive (69).

The pattern of HI response has been used to classify dengue infections as primary or secondary, based on the concept that initial, or primary dengue infections tend to elicit lower HI titers than do secondary infections (subsequent infections with a different dengue serotype or antigenically related flavivirus) (28). IgM:IgG ratios as determined by ELISA may be an alternative method of distinguishing primary from secondary infections (69, 70). The rise in neutralizing antibody in primary infection is believed to be relatively type-specific and can be used to determine the infecting serotype (35). In secondary infections, because the immunologic cross-reactivity to different flaviviruses and anamnestic responses may result in heterologous titer elevations, the only reliable method for determining the infecting serotype is virus isolation (35).

In summary, diagnosis of dengue infection is best accomplished by obtaining an acute serum sample within 5 days after the onset of illness for virus isolation and antibody testing and a convalescent serum sample 14 to 21 days after illness onset for detecting IgG antibody titer rise and/or the presence of anti-dengue IgM (35).

TREATMENT

Treatment for classic dengue fever is supportive. Patients should be encouraged to drink plenty of fluids. Acetaminophen may be taken to control fever and aching if necessary. Aspirin is contraindicated both because of its anticoagulant effects and the increased risk of developing Reye syndrome (56, 71, 72). Patients or parents should be carefully instructed of the need to seek medical attention immediately if major or ongoing hemorrhage, signs of impending shock or any change in mental status should occur. The onset of cardiovascular collapse in patients who develop DHF may be sudden (28).

Patients with significant hemorrhage or signs of increased capillary permeability such as hemoconcentration, effusions, edema or low serum albumin, as well as patients with mental status changes or with abnormal fluid and electrolyte balance, should be hospitalized and may require admission to an intensive care unit. Isolation is not necessary in mosquito-free environments. Usual precautions handling blood specimens should be observed.

Intravenous fluid therapy is the mainstay of treatment for patients with DHF (28, 59). Patients with dehydration and hemoconcentration may require intravenous fluids similar in volume and composition to regimens used to treat dehydration due to diarrheal illness (25). Patients in shock should be given fluids and other therapy according to accepted regimens for shock (28, 73). The administration of heparin may need to be considered in patients who develop DIC (28, 59).

There is some controversy over the role of steroids in treatment of severe dengue (74). Studies by Sumarmo, et al. (74, 75), showed no benefit, over fluid therapy alone, of hydrocortisone injection given wither 30 mg/kg/day or 50 mg/kg in a single dose. The potential effect of high dose methylprednisolone in certain severe cases may need further evaluation (74, 76).

PREVENTION AND CONTROL

A. aegypti is an anthropophilic, domestic mosquito which lives intimately with its human hosts (35, 51). These mosquitoes breed primarily in man-made containers such as water storage containers, old tires and flower vases in and around human dwellings. Elimination of these breeding sites is an effective and definitive method of controlling the vector and therefore of preventing transmission of dengue (9, 35, 51). During the 1950s and 1960s widespread control campaigns directed by the Pan American Organization were successful in eradicating *A. aegypti* from many countries of Latin America, with the use of a combination of DDT, which has a long residual activity, and the systematic elimination of larval habitats (9, 51). Unfortunately vigilance and control lapsed during the 1970s, and most of the countries of tropical America have become widely reinfested with *A. aegypti* (9). Nonresidual insecticides such as malathion, which kills mosquitoes on contact, have been used in attempts to control dengue epidemics. However, nonresidual insecticides applied from the truck-mounted and aerial equipment were shown to be ineffective in studies conducted in Puerto Rico, where mosquitoes were found to hide within houses (IP Reiter, DJ Gubler, GC Clark, unpublished data). This approach will likely have similar limitations elsewhere. New efforts are focusing on community education and behavior modification in an attempt to encourage neighborhoods to control the vector through breeding site reduction (9).

There is no dengue vaccine currently available for widespread public health use. Research continues on developing an effective and safe tetravalent vaccine that would circumvent the potential hazards predicted by the immune enhancement theory. Currently the only effective way to avoid dengue infection in areas where the disease is endemic or epidemic is to avoid being bitten by infected mosquitoes through the use of personal insect repellent and other insect barriers.

REFERENCES: AS NUMBERED IN ORIGINAL PUBLICATION

9. Gubler DJ. *Aedes aegypti* and *Aedes aegypti*-borne disease control in the 1990s: top down or bottom up. Am J Trop Med Hyg 1989;40:571–578.
25. Halstead SB. Arboviruses of the Pacific and Southwest Asia. In: Feigin RD, Cherry JD, eds. Textbook of pediatric infectious diseases. Philadelphia: Saunders, 1981:1142.

28. World Health Organization. Dengue hemorrhagic fever: diagnosis, treatment and control. Geneva: WHO, 1986.
34. Gubler DJ, Suharyano W, Tan R, et al. Viraemia in patients with naturally acquired dengue infection. Bull WHO 1981;59:623–630.
35. Gubler DJ. Dengue. In: Monath TP, ed. The arboviruses: epidemiology and ecology. Ch. 23. Boca Raton, FL: CRC Press, 1988:223–260.
51. Halstead SB. Selected primary health care: strategies for control of disease in the developing world. XI. Dengue. Rev Infect Dis 1984;16:251–264.
56. Nimmamitya S. Dengue hemorrhagic fever with unusual clinical manifestations. SE Asian J Trop Med Public Health 1987;18:398–406.
59. Nimmanitya S. Clinical spectrum and management of dengue hemorrhagic fever. In: Proceedings of the International Conference on Dengue and Dengue Hemorrhagic Fever, Kuala Lumpur, 1983:16–33.
66. Rosen L, Gubler DJ. The use of mosquitoes to detect and propagate dengue viruses. Am J Trop Med Hyg 1974;11:1154–1160.
67. Gubler DJ, Kuno G, Sather GE, et al. Mosquito cell cultures and specific monoclonal antibodies in surveillance for dengue viruses. Am J Trop Med Hyg 1984;33:158–165.
68. Gubler DJ. Surveillance for dengue and dengue hemorrhagic fever. PAHO Bull 1989;23:397–404.
69. Innis BL, Nisalak A, Nimmanitya S, et al. An enzyme-linked immunosorbent assay to characterize dengue infections where dengue and Japanese encephalitis co-circulate. Am J Trop Med Hyg 1989;40:418–427.
70. Kuno G, Gomez I, Gubler DJ. An ELISA procedure for the classification of dengue infection. J Clin Microbiol (in press).
71. Hurwitz ES, Barrett MJ, Bregman D, et al. Public health Service study on Reye's syndrome and medications: report of the main study. JAMA 1987;257:1905–1911.
72. Terry S, Golden MHN, Hanchard B, et al. Adult Reye's syndrome after dengue. Gut 1980;21:436–438.
73. Perkin RM, Levin DL. Shock in the pediatric patient: Part II. Therapy. J Pediatr 1982;101:319–332.
74. Sumarmo. The role of steroids in dengue shock syndrome. Southeast Asian J Trop Med Public Health 1987;18:383–389.
75. Sumarmo, Talogo W, Asrin A, et al. Failure of hydrocortisone to affect outcome in dengue shock syndrome. Pediatrics 1982;59:45–49.
76. Futrakul P, Poshyachinda M, Mitrakul C, et al. Hemodynamic response to high-dose methyl prednisolone and mannitol in severe dengue-shock patients unresponsive to fluid replacement. SE Asian J Trop Med Public Health 1987;18:373–379.

Preventing Dengue Fever in Travelers

Original Citation: Centers for Disease Control and Prevention and Agency for Toxic Substances and Disease Registry—Preventing Dengue Fever in Travelers. Brochure, November 1995.

Travelers may acquire dengue fever, a potentially life-threatening viral illness, during visits to tropical and subtropical countries. Dengue is transmitted by the bite of infective *Aedes* mosquitos which are found primarily in urban areas. This disease occurs in most of tropical Asia, the Pacific Islands, the Caribbean Islands, Central and South America, and Africa. There is generally greater risk in urban areas and less risk of dengue in rural areas and at altitudes above 1500 meters (4500 feet).

RISK TO THE TRAVELER

The risk of dengue infection for the international traveler appears to be small, unless an epidemic is currently in progress.

Current data suggest that the strain of dengue virus, and the age, immune status, and genetic background of the human host are important risk factors for developing DHF. In Asia, children under the age of 15 years who are experiencing a second dengue infection appear to have the highest risk of developing DHF. This suggests that most international travelers from nonendemic areas, such as the United States, have a low risk of developing DHF.

PROTECTION AGAINST DENGUE

No vaccine is available for dengue, but travelers can protect themselves by using anti-mosquito measures to avoid being bitten.

General Recommendations to Avoid Mosquito Bites While Traveling

- Apply insect repellent sparingly to exposed skin. An effective repellent will contain 20% to 30% DEET (N,N-diethyl-m-toluamide). DEET in high concentrations (> 30%) may cause side effects, particularly in children. Avoid formulations containing > 30% DEET. Use aerosols in an open space to avoid inhalation. Avoid applying repellent to the hands of young children.
- Wear long-sleeved clothing and long pants if you are outdoors during the day and evening. Spray permethrin or DEET repellents on clothing, as mosquitos may bite through thin clothing.
- Use mosquito netting over the bed if your bedroom is not air conditioned or screened. For additional protection, treat the mosquito netting with the insecticide permethrin.
- Spray permethrin or a similar insecticide in your bedroom before going to bed.

Note: Vitamin B and ultrasound devices are NOT effective in preventing mosquito bites.

REDUCE YOUR RISK FOR INFECTION

Your risk for becoming infected with dengue is lower if you:

- Spend most of your time in air conditioned buildings, hotels, or other closed circulation environments;
- Avoid highly populated residential areas;
- Spend time on beaches or in forested areas.

TOPIC 5 / **DIPHTHERIA, TETANUS, AND PERTUSSIS**

Pertussis Vaccination: Acellular Pertussis Vaccine for the Fourth and Fifth Doses of the DTP Series

Original Citation: Center for Diseases Control and Prevention. Pertussis Vaccination: Acellular Pertussis Vaccine for the Fourth and Fifth Doses of the DTP Series. Update to Supplementary ACIP Statement. MMWR 1992;41(44–15):1–5.

SUMMARY

General recommendations on pertussis prevention were issued August 8, 1991, in the ACIP statement on diphtheria, tetanus, and pertussis (1). A supplementary statement on the use of diphtheria and tetanus toxoids and acellular pertussis vaccine (DTaP) was issued February 7, 1992 (2) after the licensure of ACEL-IMUNE®, prepared by Lederle Laboratories. With the recent licensure of a second DTaP product*, Tripedia™, this statement updates the supplement. Tripedia™ has a formulation that differs from that of ACEL-IMUNE®. Both DTaP vaccines are licensed for use only as the fourth and/or fifth doses of diphtheria, tetanus, and pertussis vaccination; they are not licensed for the initial three-dose series for infants and children, regardless of age. Whole-cell DTP should continue to be used for the initial three-dose series and remains an acceptable alternative for the fourth and fifth doses. For details on the background, indications, use, and precautions and contraindications of DTaP, refer to the earlier supplementary statement (2).

INTRODUCTION

Simultaneous vaccination against diphtheria, tetanus, and pertussis during infancy and childhood has been a recommended routine practice in the United States since the late 1940s. Whole-cell pertussis vaccines in the United States have been and continue to be prepared from suspensions of killed Bordetella pertussis whole bacterial cells. Routine vaccination with whole-cell vaccines has been highly effective in reducing the burden of disease and deaths due to pertussis (3). Whole-cell pertussis vaccines, although safe, are associated with a variety of expected adverse events; these concerns have led to attempts to develop safer pertussis vaccines that have high efficacy.

Several antigenic components of Bordetella pertussis have been identified. Candidate acellular pertussis vaccines, produced by multinational manufacturers, are now available due to advances in the methods of purifying and preparing these components. In general, these vaccines are immunogenic and are less likely to cause common adverse reactions than the current whole-cell preparations. Several clinical trials, which compare relative protective efficacy of primary vaccination utilizing diphtheria and tetanus toxoids and acellular pertussis (DTaP) vaccines with that of whole-cell vaccines administered to infants, are in progress or development. A lack of adequate evidence, until recently, to demonstrate the effectiveness of any single preparation has delayed U.S. licensure for any indication of a candidate acellular pertussis vaccine. On December 17, 1991, the Food and Drug Administration (FDA) licensed the DTaP vaccine ACEL-IMUNE® for use as the fourth and/or fifth doses of the recommended DTP series. The FDA has now licensed a second DTaP vaccine, Tripedia™.

Tripedia™ Information

On August 21, 1992, the FDA licensed Tripedia™ for use as the fourth and/or fifth doses of the recommended DTP series. The acellular pertussis vaccine components are purified from Bordetella pertussis by salt precipitation, ultracentrifugation, and ultrafiltration. After purification, filamentous hemagglutinin (FHA) and pertussis toxin (PT) are combined to obtain a 1:1 ratio and are then treated with formaldehyde to inactivate PT. Each dose of Tripedia™ contains 23.4 mcg protein of FHA and 23.4 mcg protein of inactivated PT (toxoid), as well as 6.7 Lf of diphtheria toxoid and 5.0 Lf of tetanus toxoid. The combined components are adsorbed to aluminum potassium sulfate and preserved with 1:10,000 thimerosal.

Household exposure and ecologic studies among Japanese children vaccinated at greater than or equal to 2 years of age, have suggested efficacy of the BIKEN and other acellular pertussis vaccines when combined with diphtheria and tetanus toxoids as DTaP (4–7). In addition, a randomized, placebo-controlled clinical efficacy trial in Sweden during the period 1985–1987 demonstrated efficacy when two doses of a BIKEN pertussis vaccine—similar to the formulation in Tripedia™—were given to children starting at ages 5–11 months old, an age older than that recommended for initiating whole-cell DTP vaccination in the United States (1, 8). However, the experiences in Sweden and Japan do not satisfactorily define whether acellular pertussis vaccines confer clinical protection when administered early in infancy (i.e., 2, 4, and 6 months of age) and whether protection induced at any age is equivalent to that of whole-cell pertussis vaccine preparations.

The following evidence supports the use of Tripedia™ after the initial three-dose series of whole-cell DTP vaccine in infants:

Immunogenicity

Antibody responses to PT and FHA following administration of Tripedia™ as the fourth and fifth doses of the vaccination series are similar to or higher than those following whole-cell DTP vaccine (Table 1). Data are available to demonstrate the immunogenicity of Tripedia™ among children ages 15–16 months. The standard, single-dose volume of Tripedia™ is 0.5 mL and should be administered intramuscularly (IM).

Table 1. Comparison of immunologic responses to pertussis antigens in children vaccinated with Tripedia™ and in children vaccinated with whole-cell DTP given as the fourth DTP dose at 15–20 months of age and as the fifth DTP dose at 4–6 years of age*

Assay	Percentage with ≥ 4-fold increase 30 days after vaccination at 15–20 months of age		Percentage with ≥ 4-fold increase 30 days after vaccination at 4–6 years of age	
	Tridpedia™ (N = 354)	Whole-cell DTP (N = 175)	Tripedia™ (N = 211)	Whole-cell DTP (N = 65)
Pertussis toxin				
Enzyme immunoassay	92[†]	50	89[†]	55
Filamentous hemagglutinin				
Enzyme immunoassay	73[†]	35	87[†]	55
Agglutination[§]	72	91	NA[¶]	NA[¶]

*BIKEN Acellular DTP Vaccine—Bernstein H, et al. and unpublished data provided by the manufacturer. All children had been previously vaccinated with 3–4 doses of whole-cell DTP. Whole-cell DTP, manufactured by Connaught, was used in the whole-cell comparison group.

[†]P < 0.05.

[§]Sample sizes for each group were 39 and 23, respectively.

[¶]NA—not available.

Clinical Efficacy

The efficacy of two acellular pertussis vaccines developed by the Japan National Institute of Health (JNIH) and prepared by BIKEN was studied in 1985–1987 in a randomized, placebo-controlled clinical trial in Sweden (2,8). One of the vaccines (JNIH-6) contained 23.4 mcg protein/dose each of formaldehyde-treated PT and FHA. The first dose of vaccine or placebo was administered at 5–11 months of age; the second dose was administered 8–12 weeks later. For culture-confirmed disease with cough of any duration, the observed efficacy for JNIH-6 was 69% (95% confidence interval (CI), 47%–82%); for culture-confirmed pertussis with cough lasting greater than 30 days, the observed efficacy was 79% (95% CI, 57%–90%) (8). Non-blinded follow-up studies conducted over a 42-month interval after the trial had ended support the efficacy estimates obtained from the clinical trial (9).

Safety

Local reactions, fever, and other common systemic symptoms occur less frequently after receipt of Tripedia™ vaccine than after whole-cell DTP vaccine. In general, the frequency of local and common systemic events is approximately one-fifth to one-half the frequency of these events after whole-cell DTP vaccination (Table 2).

Table 2. Comparison of frequency (%) of adverse events occurring within 72 hours following vaccination with Tripedia™ or whole-cell DTP in children given the fourth DTP dose at 15–20 months of age and the fifth DTP dose at 4–6 years of age*

Events	Vaccination at 15–20 months of age		Vaccination at 4–6 years of age	
	Tripedia™ (N = 372)	Whole-cell DTP (N = 189)	Tripedia™ (N = 240)	Whole-cell DTP (N = 76)
Local				
Any erythema	18[†]	29	31[§]	61
Erythema > 2.5 cm	3[§]	13	18[§]	47
Any induration	11[§]	40	28[§]	59
Induration > 2.5 cm	2[§]	14	NA[¶]	NA[¶]
Pain/tenderness	14[§]	77	46[§]	93

Table 2.—*continued*

Events	Vaccination at 15–20 months of age		Vaccination at 4–6 years of age	
	Tripedia™ (N = 372)	Whole-cell DTP (N = 189)	Tripedia™ (N = 240)	Whole-cell DTP (N = 76)
Systemic				
Fever ≥ 38 C (100.4 F)**	20§	44	7§	22
Fever ≥ 39 C (102.2 F)**	1‡	6	1	1
Drowsiness	12§	33	15†	33
Fretfulness	21§	68	16§	45
Vomiting	2	3	1.7	1.3

*BIKEN Acellular DTP Vaccine—Bernstein H, et al. and unpublished data provided by the manufacturer. All children had been previously vaccinated with 3–4 doses of whole-cell DTP. Whole-cell DTP, manufactured by Connaught, was used in the whole-cell comparison group.

†$P < 0.05$.

§$P < 0.001$.

¶NA—not available.

**Sample sizes for fever were 361, 186, 209, and 67, respectively.

‡$P < 0.01$.

VACCINE USAGE

See the general ACIP statement on diphtheria, tetanus, and pertussis (1) and the supplementary statement on DTaP for more details (2). DTaP preparations are currently licensed only for use as the fourth and/or fifth doses of the DTP series among children ages 15 months through 6 years (before the seventh birthday). Any of the licensed whole-cell DTP or DTaP preparations can be used interchangeably for the fourth and fifth doses of the routine series of vaccination against diphtheria, tetanus, and pertussis among children greater than or equal to 15 months of age. The ACIP Committee recommends the use of DTaP, if readily available, because it substantially reduces local reactions, fever, and other common systemic events that often follow receipt of whole-cell DTP. There are no specific data to support the use of one particular DTaP vaccine product over the other. No data exist regarding the intermixed use of the two DTaP products at the fourth and fifth doses of the series with respect to safety, immunogenicity, or efficacy.

Tripedia™ can be administered to children as part of the recommended schedule of routine simultaneous vaccination with DTP; oral poliovirus vaccine (OPV); measles, mumps, and rubella vaccine (MMR); and, when appropriate, Haemophilus b conjugate vaccine (HbCV) at 15–18 months of age (9).

SIDE EFFECTS AND ADVERSE REACTIONS

For a complete discussion, see the general ACIP statement on diphtheria, tetanus, and pertussis and the supplementary statement on DTaP (1, 2). Refer to the earlier supplementary statement for details on the precautions and contraindications to DTaP use (2).

Although mild systemic reactions such as fever, drowsiness, fretfulness, and anorexia occur frequently after both whole-cell DTP vaccination and Tripedia™ vaccination, they are less common after Tripedia™ (Table 2). These reactions are self-limited and can be safely managed with symptomatic treatment.

Moderate-to-severe systemic events, including fever greater than or equal to 40.5°C (105°F); persistent, inconsolable crying lasting greater than or equal to 3 hours; and collapse (hypotonic-hyporesponsive episode) have rarely been reported after vaccination with DTaP (8, 10–12). Each of these events appears to occur less often than with whole-cell DTP. When these events occur after the administration of whole-cell DTP, they appear to be without sequelae; the limited experience with DTaP suggests a similar outcome.

Other more severe neurologic events, such as prolonged convulsions or encephalopathy, have not been reported in temporal association after administration of approximately 11,000 doses of Tripedia™ in U.S. studies. This limited experience does not allow conclusions to be drawn as to whether any rare serious adverse events will occur after administration of DTaP. Because DTaP causes fever less frequently than whole-cell DTP, it is anticipated that events such as febrile convulsions will be less common after receipt of DTaP.

REFERENCES: AS NUMBERED IN ORIGINAL PUBLICATION

1. CDC. Diphtheria, tetanus, and pertussis: recommendations for vaccine use and other preventive measures—recommendations of the Immunization Practices Advisory Committee (ACIP). MMWR 1991;40(No. RR-10).
2. CDC. Pertussis vaccination: acellular pertussis vaccine for reinforcing and booster use—supplementary Immunization Practices Advisory Committee (ACIP) statement. MMWR 1992;41(No. RR-1).
3. Aoyama T, Murase Y, Kato M, Iwai H, Iwata T. Efficacy and immunogenicity of acellular pertussis vaccine by manufacturer and patient age. Am J Dis Child 1989;143:655–659.
4. Noble GR, Bernier RH, Esber EC, et al. Acellular and whole-cell pertussis vaccines in Japan; report of a visit by US scientists. JAMA 1987;257:1351–1356.
5. Kimura M, Kuno-Sakai H. Developments in pertussis immunisation in Japan. Lancet 1990;336:30–32.
6. Mortimer EA, Kimura M, Cherry JD, et al. Protective efficacy of the Takeda acellular pertussis vaccine combined with diphtheria and tetanus toxoids following household exposure of Japanese children. Am J Dis Child 1990;144:899–904.
7. Ad hoc group for the study of pertussis vaccines. Placebo-controlled trial of two acellular pertussis vaccines in Sweden—Protective efficacy and adverse events. Lancet 1988;i:955–960.
8. Ad hoc group for the study of pertussis vaccines. Placebo-controlled trial of two acellular pertussis vaccines in Sweden—Protective efficacy and adverse events. Lancet 1988;i:955–960.
9. Olin P. New conclusions and lessons learned from the vaccine trial in Sweden. In: Manclark CR, ed. Proceedings of the Sixth International Symposium on Pertussis. Bethesda, MD: Department of Health and Human Services, 1990; DHHS publication no. (FDA)90–1164:299–301.
10. CDC. Immunization Practices Advisory Committee. General recommendations on immunization. MMWR 1989;38:205–214, 219–227.
11. Blennow M, Granstrom M. Adverse reactions and serologic responses to a booster dose of acellular pertussis vaccine in children immunized with acellular or whole-cell vaccine as infants. Pediatrics 1989;84:62–67.
12. Blumberg DA, Mink CM, Cherry JD, et al. Comparison of acellular and whole-cell pertussis-component diphtheria-tetanus-pertussis vaccines in infants. J Pediatr 1991;119:194–204.

Pertussis Vaccination: Acellular Pertussis Vaccine for Reinforcing and Booster Use

Original Citation: Centers for Disease Control and Prevention. Pertussis vaccination: acellular pertussis vaccine for reinforcing and booster use—supplementary ACIP statement. Recommendations of the Immunization Practices Advisory Committee. MMWR 1992;41(RR-1):1.

This supplementary statement provides information on and recommendations for the use of diphtheria and tetanus toxoids and acellular pertussis vaccine (DTaP). One such vaccine was recently licensed, ACEL-IMUNE. *This vaccine is licensed for use only as the fourth and fifth doses of diphtheria, tetanus,

*Diphtheria and Tetanus Toxoids and Acellular Pertussis Vaccine Adsorbed, prepared and distributed as Tripedia™ by Connaught Laboratories, Inc. (Swiftwater, Pennsylvania), was licensed August 21, 1992. The purified acellular pertussis vaccine component is produced by BIKEN/Tanabe Corporation (Osaka, Japan), and is combined with diphtheria and tetanus toxoids manufactured by Connaught Laboratories.

and pertussis vaccination; it is not licensed for the initial three-dose series in infants and children, regardless of age. At least one other DTaP product is anticipated to be licensed in the future for use as the fourth and fifth doses. The current Immunization Practices Advisory Committee (ACIP) statement on diphtheria, tetanus, and pertussis issued August 8, 1991, gives general recommendations on pertussis prevention, including the use of whole-cell pertussis vaccines for primary and booster vaccination (1).

INTRODUCTION

Current Whole-Cell Pertussis Vaccines

Simultaneous vaccination against diphtheria, tetanus, and pertussis during infancy and childhood has been a routine practice in the United States since the late 1940s. Whole-cell pertussis vaccines in the United States have been and continue to be prepared from suspensions of inactivated or disrupted Bordetella pertussis whole bacterial cells. Routine vaccination with whole-cell pertussis vaccines has been highly effective in reducing the burden of disease and deaths due to pertussis (3). Although the efficacy of each whole-cell vaccine in use in the United States has not been precisely estimated, clear evidence of overall high efficacy is available (4, 5). Whole-cell pertussis vaccines, although safe, are associated with a variety of adverse events, particularly local erythema, swelling and tenderness, fever, and other mild systemic events such as drowsiness, fretfulness, and anorexia (6, 7). Infrequently, febrile convulsions and hypotonic-hyporesponsive episodes can occur after whole-cell DTP vaccination (6). The general concerns about safety have led investigators to attempt to develop safer pertussis vaccines that have high efficacy.

Acellular Pertussis Vaccines

General Information

Efforts have been under way for greater than or equal to 20 years to identify and purify the antigens of B. pertussis that can be incorporated into acellular pertussis vaccines that are protective, yet are less likely to induce reactions. In Japan, the initial impetus for the accelerated development of acellular pertussis vaccines was the occurrence in 1975 of two deaths in infants within 24 hours of DTP vaccination (8, 9). These events led health authorities to temporarily suspend the routine use of whole-cell DTP vaccine in infants (then initiated at 3 months of age). Routine whole-cell DTP vaccination was rapidly reintroduced in most areas but recommended for administration at age greater than or equal to 2 years. However, vaccination coverage of children decreased, and the incidence of reported pertussis increased markedly, reaching a peak in 1979. Meanwhile, efforts to purify antigens of B. pertussis were accelerated. After limited clinical studies of immunogenicity and safety, several DTaP vaccines were licensed in Japan in 1981.

Since 1981, methods of purifying the antigenic components of B. pertussis have continued to improve, additional information on the protection of various antigens in animal models has accumulated, and candidate vaccines have been developed by many multinational manufacturers. Current candidate vaccines contain one or more of the bacterial components thought to provide protection. These components include filamentous hemagglutinin (FHA), pertussis toxin (PT—also known as lymphocytosis promoting-factor, which is inactivated to a toxoid when included in a vaccine), a recently identified 69-kilodalton outer-membrane protein (pertactin; Pn), and agglutinogens of at least two types (fimbriae (Fim) types 2 and 3). Several studies, relating to the immunogenicity and the safety of various candidate acellular pertussis vaccines, are currently being conducted or have been completed among children in the United States and other countries. In general, these vaccines, which are immunogenic, are less likely to cause common adverse reactions than the current whole-cell preparations (10–19).

The efficacy of two acellular pertussis vaccines developed by the Japanese National Institute of Health (JNIH) was studied during the period 1985 through 1987 in a randomized, placebo-controlled clinical trial in Sweden, a country in which pertussis vaccine had not been used routinely since 1979 (20). One vaccine (known in the trial as JNIH-6) contained 23.4 μg/dose each of pertussis toxoid and FHA. Another vaccine (JNIH-7), not similar to any vaccine used in Japan, contained only 37.7 μg/dose of pertussis toxoid. The 3,801 children who participated in this trial were randomly selected to receive two doses of an acellular pertussis vaccine (approximately 1,420 children in each vaccine group) or a placebo (954 children). Neither of the vaccines nor the placebo contained diphtheria and tetanus toxoids. The first dose of vaccine or placebo was administered to children 5–11 months of age; the second dose was administered 8–12 weeks later. Each vaccine demonstrated some degree of efficacy. For culture-confirmed disease with cough of any duration, the observed efficacy was 69% for JNIH-6 (95% confidence interval (CI), 47%–82%) and 54% for JNIH-7 (95% CI, 26%–72%) (20). Levels of estimated efficacy were higher against culture-confirmed pertussis that was more severe and classic. The efficacy of JNIH-6 was 79% (95% CI, 57%–90%) and that of JNIH-7 was 80% (95% CI, 59%–91%) against culture-confirmed pertussis with cough lasting more than 30 days. However, direct comparisons with whole-cell pertussis vaccine were not available to determine whether one or both of these acellular vaccines conferred protection at least equivalent to that of whole-cell vaccine. This trial also demonstrated that the complexities of evaluating pertussis vaccine efficacy had changed substantially depending upon the case definition used (21–23). Specific serologic correlates of immunity were not identified in this study. It remains undetermined which vaccine components are most effective in inducing protection and which types of immune responses are most responsible for protection. During the trial, four participants died of invasive bacterial disease that occurred up to 5 months after vaccination. Three had received the JNIH-6 vaccine and one had received JNIH-7 vaccine; the significance of these findings is uncertain (24). Primarily because of concerns regarding the level of efficacy of the vaccine following vaccination, neither vaccine is licensed for use in Sweden (25).

Until now, acellular pertussis vaccines have been licensed for use only in Japan, where, since 1981, such vaccines have been administered routinely to children greater than or equal to 2 years of age (9). Studies of persons exposed to pertussis in household settings have demonstrated the effectiveness of several acellular pertussis vaccines manufactured in Japan in preventing clinical pertussis among children greater than or equal to 2 years of age (8, 26–28). In Japan, with the continued use of acellular pertussis vaccines, the incidence of disease and death caused by pertussis has declined steadily. However, the reported incidence among children age less than 2 years has remained higher than the incidence among children of that age when whole-cell vaccines were routinely used in infants (9). Since 1989, vaccination of infants with DTaP beginning at 3 months of age has been initiated in many areas of Japan at the recommendation of the Ministry of Health. However, the extent of use among children less than 2 years of age remains low (S. Isomura, personal communication, 1991). Therefore, it is too soon to make conclusions about the effect of this policy on the age-specific incidence of pertussis among children less than 2 years of age.

Based on the experiences in Sweden and Japan, questions remain whether acellular pertussis vaccines confer clinical protection when administered early in infancy, or whether protection induced at any age is equivalent to that of whole-cell pertussis vaccine preparations. Consistent with the licensure of DTaP, the Committee recommends that whole-cell pertussis vaccine be continued for the initial three-dose vaccination series until an alternative vaccine is available that has demonstrated essentially equivalent or higher efficacy. To evaluate the relative protective efficacy of primary vaccination among infants, several clinical trials, which will compare DTaP vaccine with whole-cell DTP vaccine, are in progress or development.

ACEL-IMUNE® Information

On December 17, 1991, the FDA licensed one DTaP vaccine for use as the fourth and fifth doses of the recommended DTP series. ACEL-IMUNE® contains 40 mcg of protein; approximately 86% of this protein is FHA; 8%, PT; 4%, Pn; and 2%, Fim type 2. The acellular pertussis vaccine component is purified by ammonium sulfate fractionation and sucrose density gradient centrifugation; PT is detoxified by treatment with formaldehyde. Each dose of ACEL-IMUNE® contains 7.5 limit of flocculation (Lf) of diphtheria toxoid, 5.0 Lf of tetanus toxoid, and 300 hemagglutinating (HA) units of acellular pertussis vaccine. The FHA and PT components both exhibit HA activity. The combined components are adsorbed to aluminum hydroxide and aluminum phosphate and preserved with 1:10,000 thimerosal.

Household exposure studies have demonstrated efficacy of acellular pertussis vaccines among children in Japan vaccinated at age greater than or equal to 2 years with the Takeda acellular pertussis vaccine component, combined with Takeda-produced diphtheria and tetanus toxoids (27–29). Clinical studies are in progress to examine the relative efficacy of ACEL-IMUNE® in preventing disease when administered to infants at ages 2, 4, and 6 months compared with whole-cell DTP vaccine. The following evidence supports the use of ACEL-IMUNE® after the initial infant three-dose series of whole-cell DTP vaccine.

Immunogenicity

When ACEL-IMUNE® is used for the fourth and fifth doses of the vaccination series, antibody responses after administration are generally similar to those following whole-cell DTP vaccine for the PT, Pn, and Fim components; antibody responses are higher for FHA (Table 1) (17, 18).

Table 1. Comparison of immunologic responses to pertussis antigens among children vaccinated with ACEL-IMUNE® and among children vaccinated with whole-cell DTP given as the fourth DTP dose at 17–24 months of age and as the fifth DTP dose at 4–6 years of age*

Assay	% with ≥ 4-fold increase 30 days after vaccination at 17–24 months of age		% with ≥ 4-fold increase 30 days after vaccination at 4–6 years of age	
	ACEL-IMUNE®	Whole-Cell DTP	ACEL-IMUNE®	Whole-Cell DTP
Pertussis toxin[†]	94 (N = 36)[§]	74 (N = 35)	84 (N = 38)	88 (N = 40)
Filamentous hemagglutinin[†]	92 (N = 36)[§]	60 (N = 35)	97 (N = 38)	85 (N = 40)
Pertactin[†]	81 (N = 16)	89 (N = 18)	86 (N = 36)	68 (N = 34)
Agglutination	82 (N = 34)	86 (N = 35)	47 (N = 32)[§]	72 (N = 36)

*Among children previously vaccinated with whole-cell DTP. The number of specimens tested differ by assay. From Morgan CM, Blumberg DA, Cherry JD, et al. (17), and Blumberg DA, Mink CM, Cherry JD, et al. (18).

[†]By enzyme immunoassay.

[§]$P < 0.05$.

Clinical Efficacy

In Japan, Takeda-manufactured DTaP vaccine has been shown to prevent pertussis disease among children age greater than or equal to 2 years, however, in this retrospective study clinicians and investigators were not blinded to the vaccination status of the participants (28). The occurrence of pertussis was compared in 62 children vaccinated with two to four doses of Takeda DTaP on or after the second birthday and 62 unvaccinated children for the period 7–30 days after household exposure to pertussis. Typical clinical pertussis occurred in one vaccinated child and 43 unvaccinated children; estimated clinical vaccine efficacy: 98% (95% CI, 84%–99%). Minor respiratory illness-possibly representing mild, atypical pertussis-occurred among an additional eight vaccinated and four unvaccinated children. When these children were included, the estimated vaccine efficacy was 81% (95% CI, 64%–90%). None of the vaccinated household contacts in this study were age less than 2 years; by restricting the analysis of results to household contacts who were age greater than or equal to 2 years, the corresponding estimates of efficacy were 97% (95% CI, 82%–99%) and 79% (95% CI, 60%–89%) respectively. In a smaller study of similar design, results were similar (29).

Safety

Local reactions, fever, and other common systemic events occur less frequently after receipt of ACEL-IMUNE® vaccinations than after whole-cell DTP vaccination. In general, local and common systemic events occur approximately one-fourth to two-thirds the frequency after whole-cell DTP vaccination (Table 2) (17, 18). Available data indicate comparable safety for ACEL-IMUNE® and Takeda DTaP packaged in Japan.

Table 2. Comparison of frequency (%) of adverse events occuring within 72 hours after vaccination with ACEL-IMUNE® or whole-cell DTP among children given the fourth DTP dose at 17–24 months of age and the fifth DTP dose at 4–6 years of age*

Events	ACEL-IMUNE® N = 911[†]	Whole-Cell DTP N = 178[†]
Local		
Any erythema	29[§]	50
Erythema > 2 cm	10[§]	21
Any induration	25[§]	40
Induration > 2 cm	7[§]	12
Pain/tenderness	26[§]	73

Table 2.—*continued*

Events	ACEL-IMUNE® N = 911[†]	Whole-Cell DTP N = 178[†]
Systemic		
Fever $\geq$ 38°C (100.4°F)	19[§]	26
Fever $\geq$ 39°C (102.2°F)	1.5	1.7
Antipyretic use	6[§]	17
Drowsiness	6[§]	22
Fretfulness	17[§]	33
Vomiting	2[§]	8

Among children previously vaccinated with whole-cell DTP; from Morgan CM, Blumberg DA, Cherry JD, et al. (17), and Blumberg DA, Mink CM, Cherry JD, et al. (18), and manufacturer's unpublished data.

[†]Of the 911 doses of ACEL-IMUNE®, 778 were given as the fourth dose and 133 were given as the fifth dose; of the 178 doses of whole-cell DTP, the numbers were 89 and 89, respectively.

[§]$P < 0.05$

VACCINE USAGE

See the general ACIP statement on diphtheria, tetanus, and pertussis for more details (1). This vaccine is licensed only for use as the fourth and fifth doses of the DTP series among children ages 15 months through 6 years of age (before the seventh birthday). Use of DTaP is not recommended for children who have received less than three doses of whole-cell DTP, regardless of age. The Committee considers the first four DTP doses as primary immunization against diphtheria, tetanus, and pertussis. The fourth (reinforcing) dose of DTP, generally given at age 15–18 months, is administered to maintain adequate pertussis immunity during the preschool years. The fifth (booster) dose of DTP is administered at ages 4–6 years of age to confer continued protection against exposure during the early years of school.

Either whole-cell DTP or DTaP can be used interchangeably for the fourth and fifth doses of the routine series of vaccination against diphtheria, tetanus, and pertussis among children greater than or equal to 15 months of age. The Committee recommends the use of DTaP, if readily available, because it substantially reduces local reactions, fever, and other common systemic events that often follow receipt of whole-cell DTP.

The standard, single-dose volume of ACEL-IMUNE® is 0.5 mL and should be administered intramuscularly (IM).

Indications for the Fourth (Reinforcing) Dose

Six to 12 months after the third dose of DTP

One dose of DTaP (instead of whole-cell DTP) can be administered IM to children age 15–18 months (or later when necessary); this dose should be administered at least 6 months after the third dose of whole-cell DTP (Table 3). The fourth dose of either DTaP or DTP is an integral part of the primary immunizing course of pertussis vaccination. DTaP is not licensed for use among children age less than 15 months. Although immunogenicity data among children age 15–16 months are not yet available for ACEL-IMUNE®, the Committee suggests that ACEL-IMUNE® be used for children as part of the recommended schedule of routine simultaneous vaccination with DTP, oral poliovirus (OPV), and measles-mumps-rubella (MMR) at age 15–18 months (30).

Table 3. Routine diphtheria, tetanus, and pertussis vaccination schedule summary for children < 7 years of age—United States, 1992

Dose	Age	Customary age/interval	Product
Primary 1	2 months	≥ 6 weeks of age	DTP*
Primary 2	4 months	4–8 weeks after first dose[†]	DTP*
Primary 3	6 months	4–8 weeks after second dose[†]	DTP*
Primary 4	15 months	6–12 months after third dose[†]	DTaP or DTP*[§]
Booster	Age 4–6 years, before entering kindergarten or elementary school (not necessary if fourth primary vaccinating dose administered after fourth birthday)		DTaP or DTP*[§]
Additional boosters	Every 10 years after last dose		Td[¶]

*Use DT if pertussis vaccine is contraindicated. If the child is age ≥ 1 year at the time that primary dose three is due, a third dose 6–12 months after the second dose is administered completes primary vaccination with DT.

[†]Prolonging the interval does not require restarting series.

[§]Either DTaP or whole-cell DTP can be used for the fourth and fifth doses; DTaP is generally preferred, if available.

[¶]Tetanus-diphtheria toxoids absorbed (Td) (for adult use).

Booster Vaccination

Children 4–6 years of age (up to the seventh birthday)

A dose of DTaP can be administered as the fifth dose in the series for children ages 4–6 years who either have received all four prior doses as whole-cell vaccine or for those children who have received three doses of whole-cell DTP and one dose of DTaP. A fifth dose of either DTaP or DTP should be administered before the child enters kindergarten or elementary school. The Committee recommends the use of DTaP, if readily available. This fifth dose is not necessary if the fourth dose in the series is given on or after the fourth birthday.

Special Considerations

Vaccination of infants and young children who have a personal or family history of seizures

Recent data suggest that infants and young children who have had previous seizures (whether febrile or nonfebrile) or who have immediate family members with such histories are at increased risk of seizures following DTP vaccination than those without such histories (1). Because these reactions may be due to the fever induced by whole-cell DTP vaccine and because DTaP is infrequently associated with moderate to high fever, use of DTaP is strongly recommended for the fourth and fifth doses if pertussis vaccination is considered for these children (see Precautions and Contraindications). A family history of seizures or other central nervous disorders does not justify withholding pertussis vaccination. Acetaminophen should be given at the time of DTP or DTaP vaccination and every 4 hours for 24 hours to reduce the possibility of postvaccination fever in these children.

Children with a contraindication to pertussis vaccination (see Precautions and Contraindications)

For children younger than age 7 years who have a contraindication to whole-cell pertussis vaccine, DT should be used instead of DTP; DTaP should not be substituted. If additional doses of pertussis vaccine become contraindicated after a DTP series is begun in the first year of life, DT should be substituted for each remaining scheduled DTP dose.

Pertussis vaccination for persons age greater than or equal to 7 years

Adolescents and adults who have waning immunity are a major reservoir for transmission of pertussis (31). It is possible that booster doses of other preparations of acellular pertussis vaccines will be recommended in the future for persons age greater than or equal to 7 years, although it is not currently recommended.

SIDE EFFECTS AND ADVERSE REACTIONS

For a complete discussion, see the general ACIP statement on diphtheria, tetanus, and pertussis (1).

Although mild systemic reactions such as fever, drowsiness, fretfulness, and anorexia occur frequently after both whole-cell DTP vaccination and ACEL-IMUNE® vaccination, they are less common after ACEL-IMUNE® vaccination (Table 2). These reactions are self-limited and can be safely managed with symptomatic treatment.

Moderate-to-severe systemic events, including fever greater than or equal to 40.5°C (105°F); persistent, inconsolable crying lasting 3 hours or more; and collapse (hypotonic-hyporesponsive episode) have been rarely reported after vaccination with DTaP (16, 20, 32). Each of these events appears to occur less often than with whole-cell DTP. When these events occur after the administration of whole-cell DTP, they appear to be without sequelae; the limited experience with DTaP suggests a similar outcome.

In U.S. studies, more severe neurologic events, such as prolonged convulsions or encephalopathy, have not been reported in temporal association after administration of approximately 6,500 doses of ACEL-IMUNE®. This somewhat limited experience does not allow conclusions to be drawn whether any rare serious adverse events will occur after administration of DTaP. Because DTaP causes fever less frequently than whole-cell DTP, it is anticipated that events such as febrile convulsions will be less common after receiving DTaP.

SIMULTANEOUS ADMINISTRATION OF VACCINES

The simultaneous administration of DTaP, OPV, and MMR has not been evaluated. However, on the basis of studies using whole-cell DTP, the Committee does not anticipate any differences in seroconversion rates and rates of side effects from those observed when the vaccines are administered separately. Although combinations have not been thoroughly studied, simultaneous vaccination with DTaP, MMR, OPV, or inactivated poliovirus vaccine (IPV), and Haemophilus b conjugate vaccine (HbCV) is acceptable; similarly, simultaneous vaccination with DTaP, hepatitis B vaccine (HBV), OPV, IPV, and HbCV is also acceptable. The Committee recommends the simultaneous administration of all vaccines appropriate to the age and the previous vaccination status of the child (30), including the special circumstance of simultaneous administration of DTP or DTaP, OPV, HbCV, and MMR at age greater than or equal to 15 months.

PRECAUTIONS AND CONTRAINDICATIONS

General Considerations

DtaP is licensed only for reinforcing and booster immunization—the fourth and fifth doses in the DTP series. DTaP is not licensed for use among children age less than 15 months, on or after the seventh birthday, or for the initial three-dose series among infants and children regardless of their age.

Contraindications

Because no data currently exist to suggest otherwise, contraindications to further doses of DTaP are the same as those for the whole-cell DTP. If any of the following events occurs in temporal relation with the administration of DTP or DTaP, subsequent vaccination with DTP or DTaP is contraindicated:

1. An immediate anaphylactic reaction.
2. Encephalopathy (not due to another identifiable cause), defined as an acute, severe central nervous system disorder occurring within 7 days after vaccination and generally consisting of major alterations in consciousness, unresponsiveness, or generalized or focal seizures that persist more than a few hours, without recovery within 24 hours.

Precautions (Warnings)

If any of the following events occurs in temporal relation with the receipt of either whole-cell DTP or DTaP, the decision to administer subsequent doses of vaccine containing the pertussis component should be carefully considered. Although these events were once considered absolute contraindications to whole-cell DTP, there may be circumstances, such as a high incidence of pertussis, in which the potential benefits outweigh the possible risks, particularly since the following events have not been proven to cause permanent sequelae:

1. Temperature of greater than or equal to 40.5°C (105°F) within 48 hours, not due to another identifiable cause.
2. Collapse or shock-like state (hypotonic-hyporesponsive episode) within 48 hours.
3. Persistent, inconsolable crying lasting greater than or equal to 3 hours, occurring within 48 hours.
4. Convulsions with or without fever, occurring within 3 days.

If these events occur after receipt of any of the first four doses of whole-cell DTP vaccine and if additional doses of pertussis vaccine are indicated because the potential benefits outweigh the potential risks, consideration should be given to the use of DTaP for the fourth and fifth doses.

REPORTING OF ADVERSE EVENTS AFTER VACCINATION

As with any newly licensed vaccine, surveillance for information regarding the safety of DTaP in large-scale use is important. Surveillance information aids in the assessment of vaccine safety, although its usefulness is limited, by identifying potential events that may warrant further study. Additionally, specific evaluations of DTaP use in larger populations than those studied for license application are being initiated.

The Vaccine Adverse Event Reporting System (VAERS) of the Department of Health and Human Services became operational in November, 1990. VAERS is designed to accept reports of all serious adverse events that occur after receipt of DTaP, as well as any other vaccine, including but not limited to those mandated by the National Childhood Vaccine Injury Act of 1986 (33). Any questions about reporting requirements, completion of the report form, or requests for reporting forms can be directed to 1–800–822–7967.

REFERENCES

1. CDC. Diphtheria, tetanus, and pertussis: recommendations of the immunization practices advisory committee (ACIP) for vaccine use and other preventive measures. MMWR 1991;40: No.RR-10.
2. Food and Drug Administration approval of use of diphtheria and tetanus toxoids and acellular pertussis vaccine. MMWR 1991;40:881–882.
3. Mortimer EA, Jones PK. An evaluation of pertussis vaccine. Rev Infect Dis 1979;1:927–932.
4. Hutchins SS, Cochi SL, Brink EW, et al. Current epidemiology of pertussis in the United States. Tokai J Exp Clin Med 1988;13(Suppl):103–109.
5. Onorato IM, Zell ER, Wassilak SG, Brink EW, Bernier RH. Efficacy of whole-cell pertussis vaccine: estimates from the pertussis multicenter surveillance project. In: Manclark CR, ed. The Sixth International Symposium on Pertussis, Abstracts. Bethesda, MD: Department of Health and Human Services, 1990; DHHS publication no. (FDA)90–1162:213–214.
6. Cody CL, Baraff LJ, Cherry JD, Marcy SM, Manclark CR. The nature and rate of adverse reactions associated with DTP and DT immunization in infants and children. Pediatrics 1981;68:650–660.
7. Long SS, DeForest A, Pennridge Pediatric Associates, Smith DG, Lazaro C, Wassilak SGF. Longitudinal study of adverse reactions following diphtheria-tetanus-pertussis vaccine in infancy. Pediatrics 1990;85:294–302.

---

*Diphtheria and Tetanus Toxoids and Acellular Pertussis Vaccine Adsorbed is prepared and distributed as ACEL-IMUNE® by Lederle Laboratories (Pearl River, New York) and was licensed December 17, 1991 (2). The acellular pertussis vaccine component is produced by Takeda Chemical Industries, Ltd. (Osaka, Japan), and is combined with diphtheria and tetanus toxoids manufactured by Lederle Laboratories.

8. Noble GR, Bernier RH, Esber EC, et al. Acellular and whole-cell pertussis vaccines in Japan; report of a visit by US scientists. JAMA 1987;257:1351–1356.

9. Kimura M, Kuno-Sakai H. Developments in pertussis immunisation in Japan. Lancet 1990;336:30–32.

10. Lewis K, Cherry JD, Holroyd HJ, et al. A double-blind study comparing an acellular pertussis-component DTP vaccine with a whole-cell pertussis-component DTP vaccine in 18-month-old children. Am J Dis Child 1986;140:872–876.

11. Edwards KM, Lawrence E, Wright PF. Diphtheria, tetanus, and pertussis vaccine: a comparison of the immune response and adverse reactions to conventional and acellular pertussis components. Am J Dis Child 1986;140:867–871.

12. Anderson EL, Belshe RB, Bartram J, et al. Clinical and serologic responses to acellular pertussis vaccine in infants and young children. Am J Dis Child 1987;141:949–953.

13. Pichichero ME, Badgett JT, Rodgers GC, et al. Acellular pertussis vaccine: immunogenicity and safety of an acellular pertussis vs. a whole-cell pertussis vaccine combined with diphtheria and tetanus toxoids as a booster in 18- to 24-month-old children. Pediatr Infect Dis J 1987;6: 352–363.

14. Blennow M, Granstrom M, Jaatmaa E, et al. Primary immunization of infants with an acellular pertussis vaccine in a double-blind randomized clinical trial. Pediatrics 1988;82:293–299.

15. Anderson EL, Belshe RB, Bartram J. Differences in reactogenicity and antigenicity of acellular and standard pertussis vaccines combined with diphtheria and tetanus in infants. J Infect Dis 1988;157:731–737.

16. Blennow M, Granstrom M. Adverse reactions and serologic responses to a booster dose of acellular pertussis vaccine in children immunized with acellular or whole-cell vaccine as infants. Pediatrics 1989;84:62–67.

17. Morgan CM, Blumberg DA, Cherry JD, et al. Comparison of acellular and whole-cell pertussis-component DTP vaccines: a multicenter double-blind study in 4- to 6-year-old children. Am J Dis Child 1990;144:41–45.

18. Blumberg DA, Mink CM, Cherry JD, et al. Comparison of an acellular pertussis-component diphtheria-tetanus-pertussis (DTP) vaccine with a whole-cell pertussis-component DTP vaccine in 17- to 24-month-old children, with measurement of 69-kilodalton outer membrane protein antibody. J Pediatr 1990;117:46–51.

19. Kimura J, Kuno-Sakai H, Sato Y, et al. A comparative trial of the reactogenicity and immunogenicity of Takeda acellular pertussis vaccine combined with tetanus and diphtheria toxoids. Am J Dis Child 1991;145:734–741.

20. Ad hoc group for the study of pertussis vaccines. Placebo-controlled trial of two acellular pertussis vaccines in Sweden—Protective efficacy and adverse events. Lancet 1988;i:955–960.

21. Storsaeter J, Hallander H, Farrington CP, et al. Secondary analyses of the efficacy of two acellular pertussis vaccines in a Swedish phase III trial. Vaccine 1990;8:457–461.

22. Blackwelder WC, Storsaeter J, Olin P, Hallander HO. Acellular pertussis vaccine: efficacy and evaluation of clinical case definitions. Am J Dis Child 1991;145:1285–1289.

23. Olin P. New conclusions and lessons learned from the vaccine trial in Sweden. In: Manclark CR, ed. Proceedings of the Sixth International Symposium on Pertussis. Bethesda, MD: Department of Health and Human Services, 1990; DHHS publication no. (FDA)90–1164:299–301.

24. Storsaeter J, Olin P, Renemar B, et al. Mortality and morbidity from invasive bacterial infections during a clinical trial of acellular pertussis vaccines in Sweden. Pediatr Infect Dis J 1988;7:637–645.

25. License application for pertussis vaccine withdrawn in Sweden. Lancet 1989;i:114.

26. Isomura S. Efficacy and safety of acellular pertussis vaccine in Aichi prefecture, Japan. Pediatr Infect Dis J 1988;7:258–262.

27. Aoyama T, Murase Y, Kato M, Iwai H, Iwata T. Efficacy and immunogenicity of acellular pertussis vaccine by manufacturer and patient age. Am J Dis Child 1989;143:655–659.

28. Mortimer EA, Kimura M, Cherry JD, et al. Protective efficacy of the Takeda acellular pertussis vaccine combined with diphtheria and tetanus toxoids following household exposure of Japanese children. Am J Dis Child 1990;144:899–904.

29. Kato T, Goshima T, Nakajima N, Kaku H, Arimoto Y, Hayashi F. Protection against pertussis by acellular pertussis vaccines (Takeda, Japan): Household contact studies in Kawasaki City, Japan. Acta Paediatr Jpn 1989;31:698–701.

30. CDC. Immunization Practices Advisory Committee. General recommendations on immunization. MMWR 1989;38:205–214, 219–227.

31. Mortimer EA Jr. Perspective. Pertussis and its prevention: a family affair. J Infect Dis 1990;161: 473–479.
32. Blumberg DA, Mink CM, Cherry JD, et al. Comparison of acellular and whole-cell pertussis-component diphtheria-tetanus-pertussis vaccines in infants. J Pediatr 1991;119:194–204.
33. CDC. Vaccine Adverse Event Reporting System-United States. MMWR 1990;39(No. 41): 730–733.

Diphtheria, Tetanus, and Pertussis: Recommendations for Vaccine Use and Other Preventive Measures

Original Citation: Centers for Disease Control. Diphtheria, Tetanus, and Pertussis: Recommendations for Vaccine Use and Other Preventive Measures. Recommendations of the Immunization Practices and Advisory Committee (ACIP). MMWR 1991;40(RR-10);1–28.

DEFINITION OF ABBREVIATIONS

ACIP	Immunization Practices Advisory Committee
CDC	Centers for Disease Control
DT	Diphtheria and Tetanus Toxoids Adsorbed (for pediatric use)
DTP	Diphtheria and Tetanus Toxoids and Pertussis Vaccine Adsorbed
HbCV	Haemophilus b Conjugate Vaccine
IM	Intramuscular(ly)
IPV	Inactivated Poliovirus Vaccine
Lf	Limit of flocculation
MMR	Measles-Mumps-Rubella Vaccine
NCES	National Childhood Encephalopathy Study
OPV	Oral Poliovirus Vaccine
SIDS	Sudden Infant Death Syndrome
Td	Tetanus and Diphtheria Toxoids Adsorbed (for adult use)
TIG	Tetanus Immune Globulin
VAERS	Vaccine Adverse Event Reporting System

This revision of the Immunization Practices Advisory Committee (ACIP) statement on diphtheria, tetanus, and pertussis updates the statement issued in 1985, and incorporates the 1987 supplementary statement, which addressed two issues: (a) the risks and benefits of pertussis vaccine for infants and children with family histories of convulsions; and (b) antipyretic use in conjunction with diphtheria and tetanus toxoids and pertussis vaccine absorbed (DTP) vaccination among children with personal or family histories of convulsions (1, 2). This document presents new recommendations for epidemiologic investigation and management of contacts of diphtheria patients.

The updated recommendations include a review of the epidemiology of the three diseases and descriptions of the available immunobiologic preparations with appropriate vaccination schedules. Also included are (a) new information on and reassessment of the possible relation between receipt of DTP and the occurrence of serious acute neurologic illness and permanent brain damage, (b) revisions in the recommendations on precautions for and contraindications to pertussis vaccine use, and (c) revisions on recommendations for chemoprophylaxis for household and other close contacts of pertussis patients.

The Committee has reviewed and taken into consideration the recent report by the Institute of Medicine entitled, "Adverse Effects of Pertussis and Rubella Vaccines" in making these recommendations.

INTRODUCTION

Simultaneous vaccination against diphtheria, tetanus, and pertussis during infancy and childhood has been a routine practice in the United States since the late 1940s. This practice has played a major role in markedly reducing the incidence of cases and deaths from each of these diseases.

DIPHTHERIA

At one time, diphtheria was common in the United States. More than 200,000 cases, primarily among children, were reported in 1921. Approximately 5%–10% of cases were fatal; the highest case-fatality ratios were recorded for the very young and the elderly. Reported cases of diphtheria of all types declined from 306 in 1975 to 59 in 1979; most were cutaneous diphtheria reported from a single state (3). After 1979, cutaneous diphtheria was no longer notifiable. From 1980 to 1989, only 24 cases of respiratory diphtheria were reported; two cases were fatal, and 18 (75%) occurred among persons greater than or equal to 20 years of age.

Diphtheria is currently a rare disease in the United States primarily because of the high level of appropriate vaccination among children (97% of children entering school have received greater than or equal to three doses of diphtheria and tetanus toxoids and pertussis vaccine (DTP)) and because of an apparent reduction in the circulation of toxigenic strains of Corynebacterium diphtheriae. Most cases occur among unvaccinated or inadequately vaccinated persons. The age distribution of recent cases and the results of serosurveys indicate that many adults in the United States are not protected against diphtheria. Limited serosurveys conducted since 1977 indicate that 22%–62% of adults 18–39 years of age and 41%–84% of those greater than or equal to 60 years of age may lack protective levels of circulating antitoxin against diphtheria (4–7). Thus, it appears that further reductions in the incidence of diphtheria would require more emphasis on adult immunization programs. Both toxigenic and nontoxigenic strains of C. diphtheriae can cause disease, but only strains that produce toxin cause myocarditis and neuritis. Furthermore, toxigenic strains are more often associated with severe or fatal illness in noncutaneous (respiratory or other mucosal surface) infections and are more commonly recovered in association with respiratory than from cutaneous infections.

C. diphtheriae can contaminate the skin, usually at the site of a wound. Although a sharply demarcated lesion with a pseudomembranous base often results, the appearance may not be distinctive, and infection can be confirmed only by culture. Usually other bacterial species can also be isolated. Cutaneous diphtheria has most commonly affected indigent adults and certain groups of American Indians.

A complete vaccination series substantially reduces the risk of developing diphtheria, and vaccinated persons who develop disease have milder illnesses. Protection lasts at least 10 years. Vaccination does not, however, eliminate carriage of C. diphtheriae in the pharynx or nose or on the skin.

TETANUS

The occurrence of tetanus in the United States has decreased dramatically from 560 reported cases in 1947, when national reporting began, to a record low of 48 reported cases in 1987 (8). The decline has resulted from widespread use of tetanus toxoid and improved wound management, including use of tetanus prophylaxis in emergency rooms.

Tetanus in the United States is primarily a disease of older adults. Of 99 tetanus patients with complete information reported to CDC during 1987 and 1988, 68% were greater than or equal to 50 years of age, while only six were less than 20 years of age. No cases of neonatal tetanus were reported. Overall, the case-fatality rate was 21% (8). The age distribution of recent cases and the results of serosurveys indicate that many U.S. adults are not protected against tetanus. Serosurveys undertaken since 1977 indicate that 6%–11% of adults 18–39 years of age and 49%–66% of those greater than or equal to 60 years of age may lack protective levels of circulating tetanus antitoxin (4–7). The disease continues to occur almost exclusively among persons who are unvaccinated or inadequately vaccinated or whose vaccination histories are unknown or uncertain (8).

Surveys of emergency rooms suggest that 1%–6% of all persons who receive medical care for injuries that can lead to tetanus receive less than the recommended prophylaxis (9, 10). In 1987–1988, 58% of tetanus patients with acute injuries did not seek medical care for their injuries; of those who did, 81% did not receive prophylaxis as recommended by ACIP guidelines (8).

In 4% of tetanus cases reported during 1987 and 1988, no wound or other condition was implicated. Nonacute skin lesions such as ulcers, or medical conditions such as abscesses were reported in association with 14% of cases.

Neonatal tetanus occurs among infants born under unhygienic conditions to inadequately vaccinated mothers. Vaccinated mothers confer protection to their infants through transplacental transfer of maternal antibody. From 1972 through 1984, 29 cases of neonatal tetanus were reported in the United States (11). No cases of neonatal tetanus were reported in the period 1985–1989. Spores of Clostridium tetani are ubiquitous. Serologic tests indicate that naturally acquired immunity to tetanus toxin does not occur in the United States. Thus, universal primary vaccination, with subsequent maintenance of adequate antitoxin levels by means of appropriately timed boosters, is necessary to protect persons among all age-groups. Tetanus toxoid is a highly effective antigen; a completed primary series generally induces protective levels of serum antitoxin that persist for greater than or equal to 10 years.

PERTUSSIS

Disease caused by Bordetella pertussis was once a major cause of infant and childhood morbidity and mortality in the United States (12, 13). Pertussis became a nationally notifiable disease in 1922, and reports reached a peak of 265,269 cases and 7,518 deaths in 1934. The highest number of reported pertussis deaths (9,269) occurred in 1923. The introduction and widespread use of standardized whole-cell pertussis vaccines combined with diphtheria and tetanus toxoids (DTP) in the late 1940s resulted in a substantial decline in pertussis disease, a decline which continued without interruption for nearly 30 years.

By 1970, the annual reported incidence of pertussis had been reduced by 99%. During the 1970s, the annual numbers of reported cases stabilized at an average of approximately 2,300 cases each year. During the 1980s, however, the annual numbers of reported cases gradually increased from 1,730 cases in 1980 to 4,157 cases in 1989. An average of eight pertussis-associated fatalities was reported each year throughout the 1980s. It is not clear whether the increase in reported pertussis reflects a true increase in the incidence of the disease or improvement in the reporting of pertussis. However, these data underestimate the true number of cases, because many are unrecognized or unreported, and diagnostic tests for B. pertussis-culture and direct-immunofluorescence assay may be unavailable, difficult to perform, or incorrectly interpreted. Because direct-fluorescent-antibody testing of nasopharyngeal secretions has been shown in some studies to have low sensitivity and variable specificity, it should not be relied on as a criterion for laboratory confirmation (14, 15). In addition, reporting criteria have varied widely among the different states. Laboratory diagnosis based on serologic testing is not widely available and is still considered experimental (16). In 1990, to improve the accuracy of reporting, the U.S. Council of State and Territorial Epidemiologists adopted uniform case definitions for pertussis (17).

Before widespread use of DTP, less than 20% of cases and 50%–70% of pertussis deaths occurred among children less than 1 year of age (13, 18). For the period 1980–1989, 47% of reported illnesses from B. pertussis occurred among children less than 1 year of age, and 72% occurred among children less than 5 years of age; 61 (77%) of 79 deaths reported to CDC occurred among children less than 1 year of age (19). Infants less than 2 months of age were at highest risk of complications, with a case-fatality rate of 1.3%. Although incidence based on reported cases increased among all age-groups during the 1980s, the most striking increases occurred among adolescents and adults (19). Whether this represented a true increase or more complete recognition and reporting is not clear.

Pertussis is highly communicable (attack rates of greater than 90% have been reported among unvaccinated household contacts) and can cause severe disease, particularly among very young children. Of 10,749 patients less than 1 year of age reported nationally as having pertussis during the period 1980–1989, 69% were hospitalized, 22% had pneumonia, 3.0% had greater than or equal to one seizure, 0.9% had encephalopathy, and 0.6% died (19). The high rate of hospitalization for infants with pertussis has been observed in several population-based studies (20–22). Because of the substantial risks of complications of the disease, completion of a primary series of DTP vaccine early in life is essential.

Among older children and adults, including those previously vaccinated, B. pertussis infection may result in symptoms of bronchitis or upper-respiratory-tract infection. Pertussis may not be diagnosed because classic signs, especially the inspiratory whoop, may be absent. Older preschool children and school-age siblings who are not fully vaccinated and who develop pertussis can be important sources of infection for infants less than 1 year of age. Adults also play an important role in the transmission of pertussis to unvaccinated or incompletely vaccinated infants and young children (23).

Controversy regarding the safety of pertussis vaccine during the 1970s led to several studies of the benefits and risks of this vaccination during the 1980s. These epidemiologic analyses clearly indicate that the benefits of pertussis vaccination outweigh any risks (24–28).

PREPARATIONS USED FOR VACCINATION

Diphtheria and tetanus toxoids are prepared by formaldehyde treatment of the respective toxins and are standardized for potency according to the regulations of the U.S. Food and Drug Administration. The limit of flocculation (Lf) content of each toxoid (quantity of toxoid as assessed by flocculation) may vary among different products. The concentration of diphtheria toxoid in preparations intended for adult use is reduced because adverse reactions to diphtheria toxoid are apparently directly related to the quantity of antigen and to the age or previous vaccination history of the recipient, and because a smaller dosage of diphtheria toxoid produces an adequate immune response among adults.

Pertussis vaccine is a suspension of inactivated B. pertussis cells. Potency is assayed by comparison with the U.S. standard pertussis vaccine in the intracerebral mouse protection test. The protective efficacy of pertussis vaccines for humans has been shown to correlate with this measure of vaccine potency.

Diphtheria and tetanus toxoids and pertussis vaccine, as single antigens or various combinations, are available as aluminum-salt-adsorbed preparations. Only tetanus toxoid is available in nonabsorbed (fluid) form. Although the rates of seroconversion are essentially equivalent with either type of tetanus toxoid, the adsorbed toxoid induces a more persistent level of antitoxin antibody. The following preparations are currently available in the United States:

1. Diphtheria and Tetanus Toxoids and Pertussis Vaccine Adsorbed (DTP) and Diphtheria and Tetanus Toxoids Adsorbed (DT) (for pediatric use) are for use among infants and children less than 7 years of age. Each 0.5-mL dose is formulated to contain 6.7–12.5 Lf units of diphtheria toxoid, 5 Lf units of tetanus toxoid, and less than or equal to 16 opacity units of pertussis vaccine. A single human immunizing dose of DTP contains an estimated 4–12 protective units of pertussis vaccine.
2. Tetanus and Diphtheria Toxoids Adsorbed for Adult Use (Td) is for use among persons greater than or equal to 7 years of age. Each 0.5-mL dose is formulated to contain 2–10 Lf units of tetanus toxoid and less than or equal to 2 Lf units of diphtheria toxoid.
3. Pertussis Vaccine Adsorbed (P)*, Tetanus Toxoid (fluid), Tetanus Toxoid Adsorbed (T), and Diphtheria Toxoid Adsorbed (D)** (for pediatric use), are single-antigen products for use in special instances when combined antigen preparations are not indicated.

Work is in progress to study the effectiveness of improved acellular pertussis vaccines that have reduced adverse reaction rates. Currently, several candidate vaccines containing at least one of the bacterial components thought to provide protection are undergoing clinical trials. Candidate antigens include filamentous hemagglutinin, lymphocytosis promoting factor (pertussis toxin), a recently identified 69-kiloDalton outer-membrane protein (pertactin), and agglutinogens (23). In published studies, some of these vaccines are less prone to cause common adverse reactions than the current whole-cell preparations, and they are immunogenic (29–36). Whether their clinical efficacy among infants is equivalent to that of the whole-cell preparations remains to be established.

VACCINE USAGE

The standard, single-dose volume of each of DTP, DT, Td, single-antigen adsorbed preparations of pertussis vaccine, tetanus toxoid, and diphtheria toxoid, and of the fluid tetanus toxoid is 0.5 mL. Adsorbed preparations should be administered intramuscularly (IM). Vaccine administration by jet injection may be associated with more frequent local reactions (37).

Primary Vaccination

Children 6 weeks through 6 years old (up to the seventh birthday)

Table 1 details a routine vaccination schedule for children less than 7 years of age. One dose of DTP should be given IM on four occasions-the first three doses at 4- to 8-week intervals, beginning when the infant is approximately 6

---

*Distributed by the Division of Biologic Products, Michigan Department of Public Health Contact Dr. Robert Myers, Chief, Division of Biologic Products, Bureau of Laboratories and Epidemiological Services, Michigan Department of Public Health, Lansing, Michigan 48909 (telephone: 517-335-8120).

**Distributed in the United States by Sclavo, Inc.

Table 1. Routine diphtheria, tetanus, and pertussis vaccination schedule summary for children <7 years of age—United States, 1991

Dose	Customary age	Age/interval	Product
Primary 1	2 months	6 weeks or older	DTP[†]
Primary 2	4 months	4–8 weeks after first dose*	DTP[†]
Primary 3	6 months	4–8 weeks after second dose*	DTP[†]
Primary 4	15 months	6–12 months after third dose*	DTP[†]
Booster	4–6 years old, before entering kindergarten or elementary school (not necessary if fourth primary vaccinating dose administered after fourth birthday)		DTP[†]
Additional boosters		Every 10 years after last dose	Td

*Prolonging the interval does not require restarting series.
[†]Use DT if pertussis vaccine is contraindicated. If the child is ≥1 year of age at the time that primary dose three is due, a third dose 6–12 months after the second completes primary vaccination with DT.

weeks–2 months old; customarily, doses of vaccine are given at 2, 4, and 6 months of age. Individual circumstances may warrant giving the first three doses at 6, 10, and 14 weeks of age to provide protection as early as possible, especially during pertussis outbreaks (38). The fourth dose is given approximately 6–12 months after the third dose to maintain adequate immunity during the preschool years. This dose is an integral part of the primary vaccinating course. If a contraindication to pertussis vaccination exists (see Precautions and Contraindications), DT should be substituted for DTP as outlined (see Special Considerations).

Children greater than or equal to 7 years of age and adults

Table 2 details a routine vaccination schedule for persons greater than or equal to 7 years of age. Because the severity of pertussis decreases with age, and because the vaccine may cause side effects and adverse reactions, pertussis vaccination has not been recommended for children after their seventh birthday or for adults. For primary vaccination, a series of three doses of Td should be given IM; the second dose is given 4–8 weeks after the first, and the third dose 6–12 months after the second. Td rather than DT is the preparation of choice for vaccination of all persons greater than or equal to 7 years of age because side effects from higher doses of diphtheria toxoid are more common than they are among younger children.

Interruption of primary vaccination schedule

Interrupting the recommended schedule or delaying subsequent doses does not lead to a reduction in the level of immunity reached on completion of the primary series. Therefore, there is no need to restart a series if more than the recommended time between doses has elapsed.

Table 2. Routine diphtheria, tetanus, and pertussis vaccination schedule summary for persons ≥7 years of age—United States, 1991

Dose	Age/interval	Product
Primary 1	First dose	Td
Primary 2	4–8 weeks after first dose*	Td
Primary 3	6–12 weeks after second dose*	Td
Booster	Every 10 years after last dose	Td

*Prolonging the interval does not require restarting series.

Booster Vaccination

Children 4–6 years old (up to the seventh birthday)

Those who received all four primary vaccination doses before their fourth birthday should receive a fifth dose of DTP before entering kindergarten or elementary school. This booster dose is not necessary if the fourth dose in the primary series was given on or after the fourth birthday.

Children greater than or equal to 7 years of age and adults

Tetanus toxoid should be given with diphtheria toxoid as Td every 10 years. If a dose is given sooner as part of wound management, the next booster is not needed until 10 years thereafter (See Tetanus Prophylaxis in Wound Management). More frequent boosters are not indicated and can result in an increased occurrence and severity of adverse reactions. One means of ensuring that persons receive boosters every 10 years is to vaccinate them routinely at mid-decade ages, i.e., 15 years old, 25 years old, 35 years old, etc.

Special Considerations

Children with contraindications to pertussis vaccination

For children less than 7 years of age with a contraindication to pertussis vaccine (see Precautions and Contraindications), DT should be used instead of DTP. To ensure that there will be no interference with the response to DT antigens from maternal antibodies, previously unvaccinated children who receive their first DT dose when less than 1 year of age should receive a total of four doses of DT as the primary series, the first three doses at 4- to 8-week intervals and the fourth dose 6–12 months later (similar to the recommended DTP schedule) (Table 1). If additional doses of pertussis vaccine become contraindicated after a DTP series is begun in the first year of life, DT should be substituted for each of the remaining scheduled DTP doses.

Unvaccinated children greater than or equal to 1 year of age for whom pertussis vaccine is contraindicated should receive two doses of DT 4–8 weeks apart, followed by a third dose 6–12 months later to complete the primary series. Children who have already received one or two doses of DT or DTP after their first birthday and for whom further pertussis vaccine is contraindicated should receive a total of three doses of a preparation containing diphtheria and tetanus toxoids appropriate for age, with the third dose administered 6–12 months after the second dose.

Children who complete a primary series of DT before their fourth birthday should receive a fifth dose of DT before entering kindergarten or elementary school. This dose is not necessary if the fourth dose of the primary series was given after the fourth birthday.

Pertussis vaccination for persons greater than or equal to 7 years of age

Routine vaccination against pertussis is not currently recommended for persons greater than or equal to 7 years of age. It should be noted, however, that adolescents and adults with waning immunity, whether derived from disease or vaccination, are a major reservoir for transmission of pertussis (23). For this reason it is possible that booster doses of acellular pertussis vaccine will be recommended in the future for persons ages greater than or equal to 7 years of age.

Persons who have recovered from tetanus or diphtheria

Tetanus or diphtheria infection may not confer immunity; therefore, active vaccination should be initiated at the time of recovery from the illness, and arrangements made to ensure that all doses of a primary series are administered on schedule.

Children who have recovered from pertussis

Children who have recovered from satisfactorily documented pertussis do not need pertussis vaccine. Satisfactory documentation includes recovery of B. pertussis on culture or typical symptoms and clinical course when epidemiologically linked to a culture-proven case, as may occur during outbreaks. When such confirmation of the diagnosis is lacking, DTP vaccination should be completed, because a presumed pertussis syndrome may have been caused by other Bordetella species, Chlamydia, or certain viruses.

Prevention of neonatal tetanus

A previously unvaccinated pregnant woman whose child might be born under unhygienic circumstances (without sterile technique) should receive two doses of Td 4–8 weeks apart before delivery, preferably during the last two trimesters. Pregnant women in similar circumstances who have not had a complete vaccination series should complete the three-dose series. Those vaccinated more than 10 years previously should have a booster dose. No evidence exists to indicate that tetanus and diphtheria toxoids administered during pregnancy are teratogenic.

Adult vaccination with Td

The proportions of persons lacking protective levels of circulating antitoxins against diphtheria and tetanus increase with age; at least 40% of those greater than or equal to 60 years of age may lack protection. Every visit of an adult to a health-care provider should be regarded as an opportunity to assess the person's vaccination status and, if indicated, to provide protection against tetanus and diphtheria. Adults with uncertain histories of a complete primary vaccination series should receive a primary series using the combined Td toxoid. To ensure continued protection, booster doses of Td should be given every 10 years.

Use of Single-Antigen Preparations

A single-antigen adsorbed pertussis vaccine preparation can be used to complete vaccination against pertussis for children less than 7 years of age who have received fewer than the recommended number of doses of pertussis vaccine but have received the recommended number of doses of diphtheria and tetanus toxoids for their age. Alternately, DTP can be used, although the total number of doses of diphtheria and tetanus toxoids should not exceed six each before the seventh birthday.

Available data do not indicate substantially more adverse reactions following receipt of Td than following receipt of single-antigen, adsorbed tetanus toxoid. Furthermore, adults may be even less likely to have adequate levels of diphtheria antitoxin than of tetanus antitoxin. The routine use of Td in all medical settings, including office practices, clinics, and emergency rooms, for all persons greater than or equal to 7 years of age who need primary vaccination or booster doses will improve levels of protection against both tetanus and diphtheria, especially among adults.

SIDE EFFECTS AND ADVERSE REACTIONS FOLLOWING DTP VACCINATION

Local reactions (generally erythema and induration with or without tenderness) are common after the administration of vaccines containing diphtheria, tetanus, or pertussis antigens. Occasionally, a nodule may be palpable at the injection site of adsorbed products for several weeks. Sterile abscesses at the injection site have been reported rarely (6–10/million doses of DTP). Mild systemic reactions such as fever, drowsiness, fretfulness, and anorexia occur frequently. These reactions are substantially more common following the administration of DTP than of DT, but they are self-limited and can be safely managed with symptomatic treatment.

Acetaminophen is frequently given by physicians to lessen fever and irritability associated with DTP vaccination, and it may be useful in preventing seizures among febrile-convulsion-prone children. However, fever that does not begin until greater than or equal to 24 hours after vaccination or persists for more than 24 hours after vaccination should not be assumed to be due to DTP vaccination. These new or persistent fevers should be evaluated for other causes so that treatment is not delayed for serious conditions such as otitis media or meningitis. Moderate-to-severe systemic events, include high fever (i.e., temperature of greater than or equal to 40.5°C (105°F)); persistent, inconsolable crying lasting greater than or equal to 3 hours; collapse (hypotonic-hyporesponsive episode); or short-lived convulsions (usually febrile). These events occur infrequently. These events appear to be without sequelae (39–41). Other more severe neurologic events, such as a prolonged convulsion or encephalopathy, although rare, have been reported in temporal association with DTP administration.

Approximate rates for the occurrence of adverse events following receipt of DTP vaccine (regardless of dose number in the series or age of the child) are shown in Table 3 (42, 43). The frequencies of local reactions and fever are substantially higher with increasing numbers of doses of DTP vaccine, while other mild-to-moderate systemic reactions (e.g., fretfulness, vomiting) are substantially less frequent (41–43).

Concern about the possible role of pertussis vaccine in causing neurologic reactions has been present since the earliest days of vaccine use. Rare but serious acute neurologic illnesses, including encephalitis/encephalopathy and prolonged convulsions, have been anecdotally reported following receipt of whole-cell pertussis vaccine given as DTP vaccine (28, 44). Whether pertussis vaccine causes or is only coincidentally related to such illnesses or reveals an inevitable event has been difficult to determine

Table 3. Adverse events* occurring within 48 hours of DTP vaccinations

Events	Frequency[†]
Local	
redness	1/3 doses
swelling	2/5 doses
pain	1/2 doses
Systemic	
fever ≥ 38°C (100.4°F)	1/2 doses
drowsiness	1/3 doses
fretfulness	1/2 doses
vomiting	1/15 doses
anorexia	1/5 doses
persistent, inconsolable crying	1/100 doses
(duration ≥ 3 hours)	
fever ≥ 40.5°C (≥ 105°F)	1/330 doses
collapse (hypotonic-hyporesponsive episode)	1/1,750 doses
convulsions (with or without fever)	1/1,750 doses

*From Cody CL, Baraff LJ, Cherry JD, et al., 1981 (42).
[†]Rate per total number of doses regardless of dose number in DTP series.

conclusively for the following reasons: (a) serious acute neurologic illnesses often occur or become manifest among children during the first year of life irrespective of vaccination; (b) there is no specific clinical sign, pathological finding, or laboratory test which can determine whether the illness is caused by the DTP vaccine; (c) it may be difficult to determine with certainty whether infants less than 6 months of age are neurologically normal, which complicates assessment of whether vaccinees were already neurologically impaired before receiving DTP vaccine; and (d) because these events are exceedingly rare, appropriately designed large studies are needed to address the question.

To determine whether DTP vaccine causes serious neurologic illness and brain damage, the National Childhood Encephalopathy Study (NCES) was undertaken during 1976–1979 in Great Britain (27, 45–47). This large case-control study attempted to identify every patient with serious, acute, childhood, neurologic illness admitted to a hospital in England, Scotland, and Wales. A total of 1,182 young children 2–36 months of age was identified. Excluding those with infantile spasms, an illness shown in a separate analysis not to be attributable to DTP vaccine, 30 of these children (18 with prolonged convulsions and 12 with encephalitis/encephalopathy) had received DTP vaccine within 7 days of the reported onset of their neurologic illness (48). Analysis of the data from these patients and from age-matched control children showed a significant association (odds ratio = 3.3; 95% confidence interval 1.7–6.5) between the development of serious acute neurologic illness and receipt of DTP vaccine. Most of these events were prolonged seizures with fever. The attributable risk for all neurologic events was estimated to be 1:140,000 doses of DTP vaccine administered. These 30 children were followed up for at least 12 months to determine whether they had neurologic sequelae. Seven of these children presumed to have been previously normal neurologically had died or had subsequent neurologic impairment. A causal relation between receipt of DTP vaccine and permanent neurologic injury was suggested. The estimated attributable risk for DTP vaccine was 1:330,000 doses with a wide confidence interval.

The methods and results of the NCES have been thoroughly scrutinized since publication of the study. This reassessment by multiple groups has determined that the number of patients was too small and their classification subject to enough uncertainty to preclude drawing valid conclusions about whether a causal relation exists between pertussis vaccine and permanent neurologic damage (49–54). Preliminary data from a 10-year follow-up study of some of the children studied in the original NCES study also suggested a relation between symptoms following DTP vaccination and permanent neurologic disability (55). However, details are not available to evaluate this study adequately, and the same concerns remain about DTP vaccine precipitating initial manifestations of pre-existing neurologic disorders.

Subsequent studies have failed to provide evidence to support a causal relation between DTP vaccination and either serious acute neurologic illness or permanent neurologic injury. These include: (a) the 1979 Hospital Activity Analysis of the North West Thames Study in England, in which the hospital records of approximately 17,000 children who each received three doses of DTP vaccine were compared with records of 18,000 children who each received three doses of DT vaccine; (b) a 1974–1983 case-cohort study of children in the Group Health Cooperative of Puget Sound who received a total of 106,000 doses of DTP vaccine; and (c) a 1974–1984 cohort study of 38,171 Medicaid children in Tennessee who received 107,154 doses of DTP vaccine (56–58). An additional study in Denmark of approximately 150,000 children (554 of which had epilepsy) demonstrated no relation between the age at onset of epilepsy and the scheduled age of administration of DTP vaccine (59). Although each of these studies individually contained too few subjects to provide definitive conclusions, taken together they stand in contrast to the original NCES findings. A recent study performed in 1987–1988 in Washington and Oregon of neurologic illness among children did not provide evidence of a significantly increased risk of all serious acute neurologic illnesses within 7, 14, or 28 days of DTP vaccination (60). However, as a pilot effort, this study had limited power to detect significantly increased risks for individual conditions.

The NCES was the basis of prior ACIP statements suggesting that on rare occasions DTP vaccine could cause brain damage. However, on the basis of a more detailed review of the NCES data as well as data from other studies, the ACIP has revised its earlier view and now concludes:

1. Although DTP may rarely produce symptoms that some have classified as acute encephalopathy, a causal relation between DTP vaccine and permanent brain damage has not been demonstrated. If the vaccine ever causes brain damage, the occurrence of such an event must be exceedingly rare. A similar conclusion has been reached by the Committee on Infectious Diseases of the American Academy of Pediatrics, the Child Neurology Society, the Canadian National Advisory Committee on Immunization, the British Joint Committee on Vaccination and Immunization, the British Pediatric Association, and the Institute of Medicine (49–54).
2. The risk estimate from the NCES study of 1:330,000 for brain damage should no longer be considered valid on the basis of continuing analyses of the NCES and other studies.

In addition to these considerations, acute neurologic manifestations related to DTP vaccine are mainly febrile seizures. In an individual case, the role of pertussis vaccine as a cause of serious acute neurologic illness or permanent brain damage is impossible to determine on the basis of clinical or laboratory findings. Anecdotal reports of DTP-induced acute neurologic disorders with or without permanent brain damage can have one of several alternate explanations. Some instances may represent simple coincidence because DTP is administered at a time in infancy when previously unrecognized underlying neurological and developmental disorders first become manifest. Some patients may have short-lived seizures with prompt recovery, and these events represent the first seizure of a child with underlying epilepsy. When epilepsy has its onset in infancy, it is frequently associated with severe mental retardation and developmental delay. These conditions become apparent over a period of several months. The known febrile and other systemic effects of DTP vaccination may stimulate or precipitate inevitable symptoms of underlying central-nervous-system disorders, particularly since DTP may be the first pyrogenic stimulus an infant receives. When children who experience acute, severe central-nervous-system disorders in association with DTP vaccination are studied promptly and carefully, an alternate cause is often found.

Among a subset of NCES children with infantile spasms, both DTP and DT vaccination appeared either to precipitate early manifestations of the condition or to cause its recognition by parents (48). This and other studies suggest that neither vaccine causes this illness (59, 61).

Approximately 5,200 infants succumb to sudden infant death syndrome (SIDS) in the United States each year. Because the peak incidence of SIDS for infants is between 2 and 3 months of age, many instances of a close temporal relation between SIDS and receipt of DTP are to be expected by simple chance. Only one methodologically rigorous study has suggested that DTP vaccine might cause SIDS (62). A total of four deaths were reported within 3 days of DTP vaccination, compared with 1.36 expected deaths. However, these deaths were unusual in that three of the four occurred within a 13-month interval during the 12-year study. These four children also tended to be vaccinated at older ages than their controls, suggesting that they might have other unrecognized risk factors for SIDS independent of vaccination. In contrast, DTP vaccination was not associated with SIDS in several larger studies performed in the past decade (28, 63–65). In addition, none of three studies that examined unexpected deaths among infants not classified as SIDS found an association with DTP vaccination (62, 64, 65).

Claims that DTP may be responsible for transverse myelitis, other more subtle neurologic disorders (such as hyperactivity, learning disorders and infantile autism), and progressive degenerative central-nervous-system conditions have no scientific basis. Furthermore, one study indicated that children who received pertussis vaccine exhibited fewer school problems than those who did not, even after adjustment for socioeconomic status (66).

Recent data suggest that infants and young children who have ever had convulsions (febrile or afebrile) or who have immediate family members with such histories are more likely to have seizures following DTP vaccination than those without such histories (67, 68). For those with a family history of seizures, the increased risks of seizures occurring within 3 days of receipt of DTP or 4–28 days following receipt of DTP are identical, suggesting that these histories are non-specific risk factors and are unrelated to DTP vaccination (68).

Rarely, immediate anaphylactic reactions (i.e., swelling of the mouth, breathing difficulty, hypotension, or shock) have been reported after receipt of preparations containing diphtheria, tetanus, and/or pertussis antigens. However, no deaths caused by anaphylaxis following DTP vaccination have been reported to CDC since the inception of vaccine-adverse-events reporting in 1978, a period during which more than 80 million doses of publically purchased DTP vaccine were administered. While substantial underreporting exists in this passive surveillance system, the severity of anaphylaxis and its immediacy following vaccination suggest that such events are likely to be reported. Although no causal relation to any specific component of DTP has been established, the occurrence of true anaphylaxis usually contraindicates further doses of any one of these components. Rashes that are macular, papular, petechial, or urticarial and appear hours or days after a dose of DTP are frequently antigen-antibody reactions of little consequence or are due to other causes such as viral illnesses, and are unlikely to recur following subsequent injections (69, 70). In addition, there is no evidence for a causal relation between DTP vaccination and hemolytic anemia or thrombocytopenic purpura.

REPORTING OF ADVERSE EVENTS

The U.S. Department of Health and Human Services has established a new Vaccine Adverse Event Reporting System (VAERS) to accept all reports of suspected adverse events after the administration of any vaccine, including but not limited to the reporting of events required by the National Childhood Vaccine Injury Act of 1986 (71).The telephone number to call for answers to questions and to obtain VAERS forms is 1-800-822-7967.

The National Vaccine Injury Compensation Program, established by the National Childhood Vaccine Injury Act of 1986, requires physicians and other health-care providers who administer vaccines to maintain permanent vaccination records and to report occurrences of certain adverse events to the U.S. Department of Health and Human Services. These requirements took effect March 21, 1988. Reportable events include those listed in the Act for each vaccine and events specified in the manufacturer's vaccine package insert as contraindications to further doses of that vaccine (72, 73).

REDUCED DOSAGE SCHEDULES OR MULTIPLE SMALL DOSES OF DTP

The ACIP recommends giving only full doses (0.5 mL) of DTP vaccine; if a specific contraindication to DTP exists, the vaccine should not be given.

Concern about adverse events following pertussis vaccine has led some practitioners to reduce the volume of DTP vaccine administered to less than 0.5 mL/dose in an attempt to reduce side effects. No evidence exists to show that this decreases the frequency of uncommon severe adverse events, such as seizures and hypotonic-hyporesponsive episodes. Two studies have reported substantially lower rates of local reactions with the use of one half the recommended dose (0.25 mL) compared with a full dose (43, 74). However, a study among preterm infants showed that the incidence of side effects was unaltered when a reduced dosage of DTP vaccine was used (75). Two studies also showed substantially lower pertussis agglutinin responses after the second and third half-doses, although in one of the studies the differences were small (74, 75). These investigations used pertussis agglutinins as a measure of clinical protection; however, agglutinins are not satisfactory measures of protection against pertussis disease. Further, no evidence exists to show that the low screening dilution used (1:16) indicates protection. Currently, no reliable measures of efficacy other than clinical protection exist. Other evidence against the use of reduced doses comes from earlier studies of DTP vaccine preparations with potencies equivalent to that of half-doses of current vaccine (76, 77). The risk of pertussis for exposed household members who received these lower potency vaccines was approximately twice as high as the risk of pertussis for those who received vaccines as potent as full doses of current vaccine (29% compared with less than or equal to 14%).

The use of an increased number of reduced-volume doses of DTP in order to equal the total volume of the five recommended doses of DTP vaccine is not recommended. Whether this practice reduces the likelihood of vaccine-related adverse events is unknown. In addition, the likelihood of a temporally associated but etiologically unrelated event may be enhanced by increasing the number of vaccinations.

SIMULTANEOUS ADMINISTRATION OF VACCINES

The simultaneous administration of DTP, oral poliovirus vaccine (OPV), and measles-mumps-rubella vaccine (MMR) has resulted in seroconversion rates and rates of side effects similar to those observed when the vaccines are administered separately (78). Simultaneous vaccination with DTP, MMR, OPV, or inactivated poliovirus vaccine (IPV), and Haemophilus b conjugate vaccine (HbCV) is also acceptable (79). The

ACIP recommends the simultaneous administration of all vaccines appropriate to the age and previous vaccination status of the recipient, including the special circumstance of simultaneous administration of DTP, OPV, HbCV, and MMR at greater than or equal to 15 months of age.

PRECAUTIONS AND CONTRAINDICATIONS

General Considerations

The decision to administer or delay DTP vaccination because of a current or recent febrile illness depends largely on the severity of the symptoms and their etiology. Although a moderate or severe febrile illness is sufficient reason to postpone vaccination, minor illnesses such as mild upper-respiratory infections with or without low-grade fever are not contraindications. If ongoing medical care cannot be assured, taking every opportunity to provide appropriate vaccinations is particularly important.

Children with moderate or severe illnesses with or without fever can receive DTP as soon as they have recovered. Waiting a short period before administering DTP vaccine avoids superimposing the adverse effects of the vaccination on the underlying illness or mistakenly attributing a manifestation of the underlying illness to vaccination.

Routine physical examinations or temperature measurements are not prerequisites for vaccinating infants and children who appear to be in good health. Appropriate immunization practice includes asking the parent or guardian if the child is ill, postponing DTP vaccination for those with moderate or severe acute illnesses, and vaccinating those without contraindications or precautionary circumstances.

When an infant or child returns for the next dose of DTP, the parent should always be questioned about any adverse events that might have occurred following the previous dose.

A history of prematurity generally is not a reason to defer vaccination (75, 80, 81). Preterm infants should be vaccinated according to their chronological age from birth.

Immunosuppressive therapies—including irradiation, antimetabolites, alkylating agents, cytotoxic drugs, and corticosteroids (used in greater than physiologic doses)—may reduce the immune response to vaccines. Short-term (less than 2-weeks) corticosteroid therapy or intra-articular, bursal, or tendon injections with corticosteroids should not be immunosuppressive. Although no specific studies with pertussis vaccine are available, if immunosuppressive therapy will be discontinued shortly, it is reasonable to defer vaccination until the patient has been off therapy for 1 month; otherwise, the patient should be vaccinated while still on therapy (82).

Special Considerations for Preparations Containing Pertussis Vaccine

Precautions and contraindications guidelines that were previously published regarding the use of pertussis vaccine were based on three assumptions about the risks of pertussis vaccination that are not supported by available data: (a) that the vaccine on rare occasions caused acute encephalopathy resulting in permanent brain damage; (b) that pertussis vaccine aggravated preexisting central-nervous-system disease; and (c) that certain nonencephalitic reactions are predictive of more severe reactions with subsequent doses (1). In addition, children from whom pertussis vaccine was withheld were thought to be well protected by herd immunity, a belief that is no longer valid. The current revised ACIP recommendations reflect better understanding of the risks associated not only with pertussis vaccine but also with pertussis disease.

Contraindications

If any of the following events occur in temporal relationship to the administration of DTP, further vaccination with DTP is contraindicated (see Table 4):

1. An immediate anaphylactic reaction. The rarity of such reactions to DTP is such that they have not been adequately studied. Because of uncertainty as to which component of the vaccine might be responsible,

---

Table 4. Contraindications and precautions to further DTP vaccination

Contraindications
    An immediate anaphylactic reaction.
    Encephalopathy occurring within 7 days following DTP vaccination.
Precautions
    Temperature of ≥40.5°C (105°F) within 48 hours not due to another identifiable cause.
    Collapse or shock-like state (hypotonic-hyporesponsive episode) within 48 hours.
    Persistent, inconsolable crying lasting ≥ 3 hours, occurring within 48 hours.
    Convulsions with or without fever occurring within 3 days.

no further vaccination with any of the three antigens in DTP should be carried out. Alternatively, because of the importance of tetanus vaccination, such individuals may be referred for evaluation by an allergist and desensitized to tetanus toxoid if specific allergy can be demonstrated (83, 84).

2. Encephalopathy (not due to another identifiable cause). This is defined as an acute, severe central-nervous-system disorder occurring within 7 days following vaccination, and generally consisting of major alterations in consciousness, unresponsiveness, generalized or focal seizures that persist more than a few hours, with failure to recover within 24 hours. Even though causation by DTP cannot be established, no subsequent doses of pertussis vaccine should be given. It may be desirable to delay for months before administering the balance of the doses of DT necessary to complete the primary schedule. Such a delay allows time for the child's neurologic status to clarify.

Precautions (Warnings)

If any of the following events occur in temporal relation to receipt of DTP, the decision to give subsequent doses of vaccine containing the pertussis component should be carefully considered (Table 4). Although these events were considered absolute contraindications in previous ACIP recommendations, there may be circumstances, such as a high incidence of pertussis, in which the potential benefits outweigh possible risks, particularly because these events are not associated with permanent sequelae (1). The following events were previously considered contraindications and are now considered precautions:

1. Temperature of greater than or equal to 40.5°C (105°F) within 48 hours not due to another identifiable cause. Such a temperature is considered a precaution because of the likelihood that fever following a subsequent dose of DTP vaccine also will be high. Because such febrile reactions are usually attributed to the pertussis component, vaccination with DT should not be discontinued.

2. Collapse or shock-like state (hypotonic-hyporesponsive episode) within 48 hours. Although these uncommon events have not been recognized to cause death nor to induce permanent neurological sequelae, it is prudent to continue vaccination with DT, omitting the pertussis component (40, 85).

3. Persistent, inconsolable crying lasting greater than or equal to 3 hours, occurring within 48 hours. Follow-up of infants who have cried inconsolably following DTP vaccination has indicated that this reaction, though unpleasant, is without long-term sequelae and not associated with other reactions of greater significance (41). Inconsolable crying occurs most frequently following the first dose and is less frequently reported following subsequent doses of DTP vaccine (42). However, crying for greater than 30 minutes following DTP vaccination can be a predictor of increased likelihood of recurrence of persistent crying following subsequent doses (41). Children with persistent crying have a higher rate of substantial local reactions than children who had other DTP-associated reactions (including high fever, seizures, and hypotonic-hyporesponsive episodes), suggesting that prolonged crying was really a pain reaction (85).

4. Convulsions with or without fever occurring within 3 days. Short-lived convulsions, with or without fever, have not been shown to cause permanent sequelae (39, 86). Furthermore, the occurrence of prolonged febrile seizures (i.e., status epilepticus***), irrespective of their cause, involving an otherwise normal child does not substantially increase the risk for subsequent febrile (brief or prolonged) or afebrile seizures. The risk is significantly increased (p = 0.018) only among those children who are neurologically abnormal before their episode of status epilepticus (87). Accordingly, although a convulsion following DTP vaccination has previously been considered a contraindication to further doses, under certain circumstances subsequent doses may be indicated, particularly if the risk of pertussis in the community is high. If a child has a seizure following the first or second dose of DTP, it is desirable to delay subsequent doses until the child's neurologic status is better defined. By the end of the first year of life, the presence of an underlying neurologic disorder has usually been determined, and appropriate treatment instituted. DT vaccine should not be administered before a decision has been made about whether to restart the DTP series. Regardless of which vaccine is given, it is prudent also to administer acetaminophen, 15 mg/kg of body weight, at the time of vaccination and every 4 hours subsequently for 24 hours (88, 89).

Vaccination of infants and young children who have underlying neurologic disorders

Infants and children with recognized, possible, or potential underlying neurologic conditions present a unique problem. They seem to be at increased risk for the appearance of manifestations of the underlying neurologic disorder within 2-3 days after vaccination. However, more prolonged manifestations or increased progression of the disorder, or exacerbation of the disorder have not been recognized (90). In

---

***Any seizure lasting greater than 30 minutes or recurrent seizures lasting a total of 30 minutes without the child fully regaining consciousness.

addition, most neurologic conditions in infancy and young childhood are associated with evolving, changing neurological findings. Functional abnormalities are often unmasked by progressive neurologic development. Thus, confusion over the interpretation of progressive neurologic signs may arise when DTP vaccination or any other therapeutic or preventive measure is carried out.

Protection against diphtheria, tetanus, and pertussis is as important for children with neurologic disabilities as for other children. Such protection may be even more important for neurologically disabled children. They often receive custodial care or attend special schools where the risk of pertussis is greater because DTP vaccination is avoided for fear of adverse reactions. Also, if pertussis affects a neurologically disabled child who has difficulty in handling secretions and in cooperating with symptomatic care, it may aggravate preexisting neurologic problems because of anoxia, intracerebral hemorrhages, and other manifestations of the disease. Whether and when to administer DTP to children with proven or suspected underlying neurologic disorders must be decided on an individual basis. Important considerations include the current local incidence of pertussis, the near absence of diphtheria in the United States, and the low risk of infection with Clostridium tetani. On the basis of these considerations and the nature of the child's disorder, the following approaches are recommended:

1. Infants and children with previous convulsions. Infants and young children who have had prior seizures, whether febrile or afebrile, appear to be at increased risk for seizures following DTP vaccination than children and infants without these histories (68). A convulsion within 3 days of DTP vaccination in a child with a history of convulsions may be initiated by fever caused by the vaccine in a child prone to febrile seizures, may be induced by the pertussis component, or may be unrelated to the vaccination. As noted earlier, current evidence indicates that seizures following DTP vaccination do not cause permanent brain damage. Among infants and children with a history of previous seizures, it is prudent to delay DTP vaccination until the child's status has been fully assessed, a treatment regimen established, and the condition stabilized. It should be noted, however, that delaying DTP vaccination until the second 6 months of life will increase the risk of febrile seizures among persons who are predisposed. When DTP or DT is given, acetaminophen, 15 mg/kg, should also be given at the time of the vaccination and every 4 hours for the ensuing 24 hours (88, 89).

2. Infants as yet unvaccinated who are suspected of having underlying neurologic disease. It is prudent to delay initiation of vaccination with DTP or DT (but not other vaccines) until further observation and study have clarified the child's neurologic status and the effect of treatment. The decision as to whether to begin vaccination with DTP or DT should be made no later than the child's first birthday.

3. Children who have not received a complete series of vaccine and who have a neurologic event occurring between doses. Infants and children who have received greater than or equal to one dose of DTP and who experience a neurologic disorder (e.g., a seizure, for example) not temporally associated with vaccination, but before the next scheduled dose, present a special management challenge. If the seizure or other disorder occurs before the first birthday and before completion of the first three doses of the primary series of DTP, further doses of DTP or DT (but not other vaccines) should be deferred until the infant's status has been clarified. The decision whether to use DTP or DT to complete the series should be made no later than the child's first birthday, and should take into consideration the nature of the child's problem and the benefits and possible risks of the vaccine. If the seizure or other disorder occurs after the first birthday, the child's neurologic status should be evaluated to ensure that the disorder is stable before a subsequent dose of DTP is given. (See the following #4.)

4. Infants and children with stable neurologic conditions. Infants and children with stable neurologic conditions, including well-controlled seizures, may be vaccinated. The occurrence of single seizures (temporally unassociated with DTP) do not contraindicate DTP vaccination, particularly if the seizures can be satisfactorily explained. Parents of infants and children with histories of convulsions should be informed of the increased risk of postvaccination seizures. Acetaminophen, 15 mg/kg, every 4 hours for 24 hours, should be given to children with such histories to reduce the possibility of postvaccination fever (88, 89).

5. Children with resolved or corrected neurologic disorders. DTP vaccination is recommended for infants with certain neurologic problems, such as neonatal hypocalcemic tetany or hydrocephalus (following placement of a shunt and without seizures), that have been corrected or have clearly subsided without residua.

Vaccination of infants and young children who have a family history of convulsion or other central nervous system disorders

A family history of convulsions or other central nervous disorders is not a contraindication to pertussis vaccination (2). Acetaminophen should be given at the time of DTP vaccination and every 4 hours for 24 hours to reduce the possibility of postvaccination fever (88, 89).

Preparations Containing Diphtheria Toxoid and Tetanus Toxoid

The only contraindication to tetanus and diphtheria toxoids is a history of a neurologic or severe hypersensitivity reaction following a previous dose. Vaccination with tetanus and diphtheria toxoids is not known to be associated with an increased risk of convulsions. Local side effects alone do not preclude continued use. If an anaphylactic reaction to a previous dose of tetanus toxoid is suspected, intradermal skin testing with appropriately diluted tetanus toxoid may be useful before a decision is made to discontinue tetanus toxoid vaccination (83). In one study, 94 of 95 persons with histories of anaphylactic symptoms following a previous dose of tetanus toxoid were nonreactive following intradermal testing and tolerated further tetanus toxoid challenge without incident (83). One person had erythema and induration immediately following skin testing, but tolerated a full IM dose without adverse effects. Mild, nonspecific skin-test reactivity to tetanus toxoid, particularly if used undiluted, appears to be fairly common. Most vaccinees develop inconsequential cutaneous delayed hypersensitivity to the toxoid.

Persons who experienced Arthus-type hypersensitivity reactions or a temperature of greater than 103°F (39.4°C) following a prior dose of tetanus toxoid usually have high serum tetanus antitoxin levels and should not be given even emergency doses of Td more frequently than every 10 years, even if they have a wound that is neither clean nor minor.

If a contraindication to using tetanus toxoid-containing preparations exists for a person who has not completed a primary series of tetanus toxoid immunization and that person has a wound that is neither clean nor minor, only passive immunization should be given using tetanus immune globulin (TIG). (See Tetanus Prophylaxis in Wound Management).

Although no evidence exists that tetanus and diphtheria toxoids are teratogenic, waiting until the second trimester of pregnancy to administer Td is a reasonable precaution for minimizing any concern about the theoretical possibility of such reactions.

Misconceptions Concerning Contraindications to DTP

Some health-care providers inappropriately consider certain conditions or circumstances as contraindications to DTP vaccination. These include the following:

1. Soreness, redness, or swelling at the DTP vaccination site or temperature of less than 40.5°C (105°F).
2. Mild, acute illness with low-grade fever or mild diarrheal illness affecting an otherwise healthy child.
3. Current antimicrobial therapy or the convalescent phase of an acute illness.
4. Recent exposure to an infectious disease.
5. Prematurity. The appropriate age for initiating vaccination among the prematurely born infant is the usual chronological age from birth (75, 80, 81). Full doses (0.5 mL) of vaccine should be used.
6. History of allergies or relatives with allergies.
7. Family history of convulsions.
8. Family history of SIDS.
9. Family history of an adverse event following DTP vaccination.

PREVENTION OF DIPHTHERIA AMONG CONTACTS OF A DIPHTHERIA PATIENT

Identification of Close Contacts

The primary purpose of contact investigation is to prevent secondary transmission of C. diphtheriae and the occurrence of additional diphtheria cases. Only close contacts of a patient with culture-confirmed or suspected**** diphtheria should be considered at increased risk for acquiring secondary disease. Such contacts include all household members and other persons with a history of habitual, close contact with the patient, as well as those directly exposed to oral secretions of the patient. Identification of close contacts of a diphtheria patient should be promptly initiated.

Cultures and Antimicrobial Prophylaxis

All close contacts (regardless of their vaccination status) should have samples taken for culture, receive prompt antimicrobial chemoprophylaxis, and be examined daily for 7 days for evidence of disease. Awaiting culture results before administering antimicrobial prophylaxis to close contacts is not warranted. The iden-

---

****For example, a patient for whom the decision has been made to treat with diphtheria antitoxin. Antitoxin can be obtained either from a manufacturer (Connaught Labs, Inc., or Sclavo, Inc.) or the Division of Immunization, CDC (telephone: 404-639-2888).

tification of carriers among close contacts may support the diagnosis of diphtheria for a patient whose cultures are negative either because of prior antimicrobial therapy or because of other reasons. Antimicrobial prophylaxis should consist of either an IM injection of benzathine penicillin (600,000 units for persons less than 6 years old and 1,200,000 units for those greater than or equal to 6 years old) or a 7- to 10-day course of oral erythromycin (children: 40 mg/kg/day; adults: 1 g/day). Erythromycin may be slightly more effective, but IM benzathine penicillin may be preferred, because it avoids possible noncompliance with a multiday oral drug regimen. The efficacy of antimicrobial prophylaxis in preventing secondary disease is presumed but not proven. Identified carriers of C. diphtheriae should have follow-up cultures done after they complete antimicrobial therapy. Those who continue to harbor the organism after either penicillin or erythromycin should receive an additional 10-day course of oral erythromycin and follow-up cultures.

Immunization

Active

All household and other close contacts who have received less than three doses of diphtheria toxoid or whose vaccination status is unknown should receive an immediate dose of a diphtheria toxoid-containing preparation and should complete the primary series according to schedule (Tables 1 and 2). Close contacts who have completed a primary series of greater than or equal to three doses and who have not been vaccinated with diphtheria toxoid within the previous 5 years should receive a booster dose of a diphtheria toxoid-containing preparation appropriate for their age.

Passive

The only preparation available for passive immunization against diphtheria is equine diphtheria antitoxin. Even when close surveillance of unvaccinated close contacts is impossible, use of this preparation is not generally recommended because of the risks of allergic reaction to horse serum. Immediate hypersensitivity reactions occur among approximately 7%, and serum sickness among 5% of adults receiving the recommended prophylactic dose of equine antitoxin. The risk of an adverse reaction to equine antitoxin must be weighed against the small risk that an unvaccinated household contact who receives chemoprophylaxis will contract diphtheria. No evidence exists to support any additional benefit of diphtheria antitoxin use for contacts who have received antimicrobial prophylaxis. If antitoxin is to be used, 5,000–10,000 units IM— after appropriate testing for sensitivity—at a site different from that of the toxoid injection is the dosage usually recommended. Diphtheria antitoxin is unlikely to impair the immune response to simultaneous administration of diphtheria toxoid, but this has not been adequately studied.

A serum specimen collected from a patient with suspected diphtheria (before antitoxin therapy is initiated) may be helpful in supporting the diagnosis of diphtheria if a level of diphtheria antitoxin below that considered to be protective (i.e., less than 0.01 IU/mL) can be demonstrated. Such testing may be particularly helpful with a patient for whom antimicrobial therapy had been initiated prior to obtaining diphtheria cultures.

Cutaneous Diphtheria

Cases of cutaneous diphtheria generally are caused by infections with nontoxigenic strains of C. diphtheriae. If a toxigenic C. diphtheriae strain is isolated from a cutaneous lesion, investigation and prophylaxis of close contacts should be undertaken, as with respiratory diphtheria. If a cutaneous case is known to be due to a nontoxigenic strain, routine investigation or prophylaxis of contacts is not necessary.

TETANUS PROPHYLAXIS IN WOUND MANAGEMENT

Chemoprophylaxis against tetanus is neither practical nor useful in managing wounds. Wound cleaning, debridement when indicated, and proper immunization are important. The need for tetanus toxoid (active immunization), with or without TIG (passive immunization), depends on both the condition of the wound and the patient's vaccination history (Table 5; see also Precautions and Contraindications). Rarely has tetanus occurred among persons with documentation of having received a primary series of toxoid injections.

A thorough attempt must be made to determine whether a patient has completed primary vaccination. Patients with unknown or uncertain previous vaccination histories should be considered to have had no previous tetanus toxoid doses. Persons who had military service since 1941 can be considered to have received at least one dose. Although most people in the military since 1941 may have completed a primary series of tetanus toxoid, this cannot be assumed for each individual. Patients who have not completed a primary series may require tetanus toxoid and passive immunization at the time of wound cleaning and debridement (Table 5).

Available evidence indicates that complete primary vaccination with tetanus toxoid provides long-lasting protection greater than or equal to 10 years for most recipients. Consequently, after complete primary tetanus vaccination, boosters—even for wound management—need be given only every 10 years when wounds are minor and uncontaminated. For other wounds, a booster is appropriate if the patient has not received tetanus toxoid within the preceding 5 years. Persons who have received at least two doses of tetanus toxoid rapidly develop antitoxin antibodies.

Td is the preferred preparation for active tetanus immunization in wound management of patients greater than or equal to 7 years of age. Because a

Table 5. Summary guide to tetanus prophylaxis in routine wound management, 1991

History of adsorbed tetanus toxoid (doses)	Clean, minor wounds		All other wounds*	
	Td([†])	TIG	Td([†])	TIG
Unknown or < three	Yes	No	Yes	Yes
≥Three ([§])	No ([¶])	No	No ([**])	No

*Such as, but not limited to, wounds contaminated with dirt, feces, soil, and saliva; puncture wounds; avulsions; and wounds resulting from missiles, crushing, burns and frostbite.
[†]For children <7 years old; DTP (DT, if pertussis vaccine is contraindicated) is preferred to tetanus toxoid alone. For persons ≥7 years of age, Td is preferred to tetanus toxoid alone.
[§]If only three doses of *fluid* toxoid have been received, then a fourth dose of toxoid, preferably an adsorbed toxoid, should be given.
[¶]Yes, if >10 years since last dose.
**Yes, if >5 years since last dose. (More frequent boosters are not needed and can accentuate side effects.)

large proportion of adults are susceptible, this plan enhances diphtheria protection. Thus, by taking advantage of acute health-care visits, such as for wound management, some patients can be protected who otherwise would remain susceptible. For routine wound management among children less than 7 years of age who are not adequately vaccinated, DTP should be used instead of single-antigen tetanus toxoid. DT may be used if pertussis vaccine is contraindicated or individual circumstances are such that potential febrile reactions following DTP might confound the management of the patient. For inadequately vaccinated patients of all ages, completion of primary vaccination at the time of discharge or at follow-up visits should be ensured (Tables 1 and 2).

If passive immunization is needed, human TIG is the product of choice. It provides protection longer than antitoxin of animal origin and causes few adverse reactions. The TIG prophylactic dose that is currently recommended for wounds of average severity is 250 units IM. When tetanus toxoid and TIG are given concurrently, separate syringes and separate sites should be used. The ACIP recommends the use of only adsorbed toxoid in this situation.

PROPHYLAXIS FOR CONTACTS OF PERTUSSIS PATIENTS

Spread of pertussis can be limited by decreasing the infectivity of the patient and by protecting close contacts. To reduce infectivity as quickly as possible, a course of oral erythromycin (children: 40 mg/kg/day; adults: 1 g/day) or trimethoprim-sulfamethoxazole (children: trimethoprim 8 mg/kg/day, sulfamethoxazole 40 mg/kg/day; adults: trimethoprim 320 mg/day, sulfamethoxazole 1,600 mg/day) is recommended for patients with clinical pertussis. Antimicrobial therapy should be continued for 14 days to minimize any chance of treatment failure. It is generally accepted that symptoms may be ameliorated when effective therapy is initiated during the catarrhal stage of disease (91). Some evidence suggests erythromycin therapy can alter the clinical course of pertussis when initiated early in the paroxysmal stage (19, 92, 93).

Erythromycin or trimethoprim-sulfamethoxazole prophylaxis should be administered for 14 days to all household and other close contacts of persons with pertussis, regardless of age and vaccination status. Although data from controlled clinical trials are lacking, prophylaxis of all household members and other close contacts may prevent or minimize transmission (92, 94–96). All close contacts less than 7 years of age who have not completed the four-dose primary series should complete the series with the minimal intervals (Table 1). Those who have completed a primary series but have not received a dose of DTP vaccine within 3 years of exposure should be given a booster dose.

Prophylactic postexposure passive immunization is not recommended. The use of human pertussis immune globulin neither prevents illness nor reduces its severity. This product is no longer available in the United States.

SELECTED BIBLIOGRAPHY

Combined Diphtheria and Tetanus Toxoids and Pertussis Vaccine

Barkin RM, Pichichero ME. Diphtheria-pertussis-tetanus vaccine: reactogenicity of commercial products. Pediatrics 1979;63:256–260.

Bernier RH, Frank JA Jr, Dondero TJ Jr, Turner P. Diphtheria-tetanus toxoids-pertussis vaccination and sudden infant death syndrome in Tennessee. J Pediatr 1982;101:419–421.

Orenstein WA, Weisfeld JS, Halsey NA. Diphtheria and tetanus toxoids and pertussis vaccine, combined. In: Recent advances in immunization: a bibliographic review. Scientific pub no. 451, Washington: PAHO, 1983:30–51.

Strom J. Further experience of reactions especially of a cerebral nature in conjunction with triple vaccination: a study based on vaccinations in Sweden, 1959–1965. Br Med J 1967;4:320–323.

Taylor EM, Emery JL. Immunization and cot deaths [Letter]. Lancet 1982;2:721.

Diphtheria and Diphtheria Toxoid

Brown GC, Volk VK, Gottshall RY, Kendrick PL, Anderson HD. Responses of infants to DTP-P vaccine used in nine injection schedules. Public Health Rep 1964;79:585–602.

Doull JA. Factors influencing selective distribution in diphtheria. J Prev Med 1930;4:371–404.

Edsall G, Altman JS, Gaspar AJ. Combined tetanus-diphtheria immunization of adults: use of small doses of diphtheria toxoid. Am J Public Health 1954;44:1537–1545.

Ipsen J. Circulating antitoxin at onset of diphtheria in 425 patients. J Immunol 1946;54:325–347.

Gottlieb S, Martin M, McLaughlin FX, Panaro RJ, Levine L, Edsall G. Long-term immunity to diphtheria and tetanus: a mathematical model. Am J Epidemiol 1967;85:207–219.

Koopman JS, Campbell J. The role of cutaneous diphtheria infections in a diphtheria epidemic. J Infect Dis 1975;131:239–244.

Myers MG, Beckman CW, Vosdingh RA, Hankins WA. Primary immunization with tetanus and diphtheria toxoids: reaction rates and immunogenicity in older children and adults. JAMA 1982;248: 2478–2480.

Naiditch MJ, Bower AG. Diphtheria; a study of 1,433 cases observed during a 10-year period at the Los Angeles County Hospital. Am J Med 1954;17:229–245.

Scheibel I, Bentzon MW, Christensen PE, Biering A. Duration of immunity to diphtheria and tetanus after active immunization. Acta Pathol Microbiol Immunol Scand 1966;67:380–392.

Tasman A, Lansberg HP. Problems concerning the prophylaxis, pathogenesis, and therapy of diphtheria. Bull WHO 1957;16:939–973.

Volk VK, Gottshall RY, Anderson HD, Top FH, Bunney WE, Serfling RE. Antigenic response to booster dose of diphtheria and tetanus toxoids. Seven to thirteen years after primary inoculation of noninstitutionalized children. Public Health Rep 1962;77:185–194.

Tetanus and Tetanus Toxoid

Blumstein GI, Kreithen H. Peripheral neuropathy following tetanus toxoid administration. JAMA 1966;198:1030–1031.

Brown GC, Volk VK, Gottshall RY, Kendrick PL, Anderson HD. Responses of infants to DTP-P vaccine used in nine injection schedules. Public Health Rep 1964;79:585–602.

Chen ST, Edsall G, Peel MM, Sinnathuray TA. Timing of antenatal tetanus immunization for effective protection of the neonate. Bull WHO 1983;61:159–165.

Eckmann L, ed. Principles on tetanus: proceedings of the International Conference on Tetanus, 2nd. Bern, 1966. Bern: Huber, 1967.

Edsall G. Specific prophylaxis of tetanus. JAMA 1959;171:417–427.

Edsall G, Elliott MW, Peebles TC, Levine L, Eldred MC. Excessive use of tetanus toxoid boosters. JAMA 1967;202:17–19.

Gottlieb S, Martin M, McLaughlin FX, Panaro RJ, Levine L, Edsall G. Long-term immunity to diphtheria and tetanus:a mathematical model. Am J Epidemiol 1967;85:207–219.

LaForce FM, Young LS, Bennett JV. Tetanus in the United States (1965–1966): epidemiologic and clinical features. N Engl J Med 1969;280:569–574.

MacLennan R, Schofield FD, Pittman M, Hardegree MC, Barile MF. Immunization against neonatal tetanus in New Guinea. Antitoxin response of pregnant women to adjuvant and plain toxoids. Bull WHO 1965;32:683–697.

Myers MG, Beckman CW, Vosdingh RA, Hankins WA. Primary immunization with tetanus and diphtheria toxoids: reaction rates and immunogenicity in older children and adults. JAMA 1982;248: 2478–2480.

Peebles TC, Levine L, Eldred MC, Edsall G. Tetanus-toxoid emergency boosters: a reappraisal. N Engl J Med 1969;280:575–581.

Scheibel I, Bentzon MW, Christensen PE, Biering A. Duration of immunity to diphtheria and tetanus after active immunization. Acta Pathol Microbiol Scand 1966;67:380–392.

Volk VK, Gottshall RY, Anderson HD, Top FH, Bunney WE, Serfling RE. Antigenic response to booster dose of diphtheria and tetanus toxoids. Seven to thirteen years after primary inoculation of noninstitutionalized children. Public Health Rep 1962;77:185–194.

White WG, Barnes GM, Griffith AH, Gall D, Barker E, Smith JWG. Duration of immunity after active immunisation against tetanus. Lancet 1969;2:95–96.

Pertussis and Pertussis Vaccine

Baraff LJ, Wilkins J, Wehrle PF. The role of antibiotics, immunizations, and adenoviruses in pertussis. Pediatrics 1978;61:224–230.

Berg JM. Neurologic complications of pertussis immunization. Br Med J 1958;2:24–27.

British Medical Research Council. The prevention of whooping-cough by vaccination. A Medical Research Council investigation. Br Med J 1951;1:1463–1471.

British Medical Research Council. Vaccination against whooping-cough. A final report. Br Med J 1959;1:994–1000.

Henry RL, Dorman DC, Skinner JA, Mellis CM. Antimicrobial therapy in whooping cough. Med J Aust 1981;2:27–28.

Hinman AR. The pertussis vaccine controversy. Public Health Rep 1984;99:255–259.

Joint Committee on Vaccination and Immunization of the Central Health Services Council and the Scottish Health Service Planning Council. Whooping cough vaccination: review of the evidence on whooping cough vaccination by the joint committee on vaccination and immunization. London: Her Majesty's Stationery Office, 1977:1–33.

Committee on Safety of Medicines and the Joint Committee on Vaccination and Immunisation. Whooping cough. London: Her Majesty's Stationery Office, 1981:79–169.

Lambert HJ. Epidemiology of a small pertussis outbreak in Kent County, Michigan. Public Health Rep 1965;80:365–369.

Manclark CR, Hill JC, eds. International Symposium on Pertussis, 3rd. Bethesda, MD: National Institutes of Health, 1979 (DHEW Publication no. (NIH) 79–1830).

Miller DL, Alderslade R, Ross EM. Whooping cough and whooping cough vaccine: the risks and benefits debate. Epidemiol Rev 1982;4:1–24.

Nelson JD. The changing epidemiology of pertussis in young infants. The role of adults as reservoirs of infection. Am J Dis Child 1978;132:371–373.

Pollard R. Relation between vaccination and notification rates for whooping cough in England and Wales. Lancet 1980;1:1180–1182.

Pollock TM, Miller E, Lobb J. Severity of whooping cough in England before and after the decline in pertussis immunisation. Arch Dis Child 1984;59:162–165.

Royal College of General Practitioners, Swansea Research Unit. Effect of a low pertussis vaccination uptake on a large community. Br Med J 1981;282:23–26.

Sato Y, Izumiya K, Sato H, Cowell JL, Manclark CR. Role of antibody to leukocytosis-promoting factor hemagglutinin and to filamentous hemagglutinin in immunity to pertussis. Infect Immun 1981;31:1223–1231.

Sato Y, Kimura M, Fukumi H. Development of a pertussis component vaccine in Japan. Lancet 1984;1:122–126.

Wilkins J, Williams FF, Wehrle PF, Portnoy B. Agglutinin response to pertussis vaccine. I. Effect of dosage and interval. J Pediatr 1971;79:197–202.

REFERENCES

1. CDC. Diphtheria, tetanus, and pertussis: guidelines for vaccine prophylaxis and other preventive measures: recommendations of the Immunization Practices Advisory Committee (ACIP). MMWR 1985;34:405–414, 419–426.
2. CDC. Pertussis immunization: family history of convulsions and use of antipyretics—supplementary ACIP statement: recommendations of the Immunization Practices Advisory Committee (ACIP). MMWR 1987;36:281–282.
3. Chen RT, Broome CV, Weinstein RA, et al. Diphtheria in the United States, 1971–81. Am J Public Health 1985;75:1393–1397.
4. Weiss BP, Strassburg MA, Feeley JC. Tetanus and diphtheria immunity in an elderly population in Los Angeles County. Am J Public Health 1983;73:802–804.
5. Crossley K, Irvine P, Warren JB, Lee BK, Mead K. Tetanus and diphtheria immunity in urban Minnesota adults. JAMA 1979;242:2298–3000.
6. Ruben FL, Nagel J, Fireman P. Antitoxin responses in the elderly to tetanus-diphtheria (Td) immunization. Am J Epidemiol 1978;108:145–149.

7. Koblin BA, Townsend TR. Immunity to diphtheria and tetanus in inner-city women of childbearing age. Am J Public Health 1989;79:1297–1298.
8. CDC. Tetanus—United States, 1987 and 1988. MMWR 1990;39:37–41.
9. Giangrosso J, Smith RK. Misuse of tetanus immunoprophylaxis in wound care. Ann Emerg Med 1985;14:573–579.
10. Brand DA, Acampora D, Gotlieb LD, et al. Adequacy of antitetanus prophylaxis in six hospital emergency rooms. N Engl J Med 1983;309:636–640.
11. Hinman AR, Foster SO, Wassilak SGF. Neonatal tetanus: potential for elimination in the world. Pediatr Infect Dis J 1987;6:813–816.
12. Gordon JE, Hood RI. Whooping cough and its epidemiological anomalies. Am J Med Sci 1951; 222:333–361.
13. Cherry JD. The epidemiology of pertussis and pertussis immunization in the United Kingdom and the United States: a comparative study. Curr Probl Pediatr 1984;14:1–78.
14. Broome CV, Fraser DW, English WJ. Pertussis-diagnostic methods and surveillance. In: Manclark CR, Hill JC, eds. International Symposium on Pertussis. Bethesda, MD: National Institutes of Health, 1978:19–22.
15. Halperin SA, Bortolussi R, Wort AJ. Evaluation of culture, immunofluorescence and serology for the diagnosis of pertussis. J Clin Microbiol 1989;27:752–757.
16. Onorato IM, Wassilak SGF. Laboratory diagnosis of pertussis: the state of the art. Pediatr Infect Dis J 1987;6:145–151.
17. CDC. Case definitions for public health surveillance. MMWR 1990;39(No. RR-13):26–27.
18. Dauer CC. Reported whooping cough morbidity and mortality in the United States. Public Health Rep 1943;58:661–676.
19. Farizo KM, Cochi SL, Zell ER, Brink EW, Wassilak SG, Patriarca PA. Epidemiologic features of pertussis in the United States, 1980–1989. Rev Infect Dis (in press).
20. Halperin SA, Bortolussi R, MacLean D, Chisholm N. Persistence of pertussis in an immunized population: results of the Nova Scotia Enhanced Pertussis Surveillance Program. J Pediatr 1989;115: 686–693.
21. Miller CL, Fletcher WB. Severity of notified whooping cough. Br Med J 1976;1:117–119.
22. Pollock TM, Miller E, Lobb J. Severity of whooping cough in England before and after the decline in pertussis immunisation. Arch Dis Child 1984;59:162–165.
23. Mortimer EA Jr. Perspective. Pertussis and its prevention: a family affair. J Infect Dis 1990;161:473–479.
24. Hinman AR, Koplan JP. Pertussis and pertussis vaccine: reanalysis of benefits, risks and costs. JAMA 1984;251:3109–3113.
25. Hinman AR, Koplan JP. Pertussis and pertussis vaccine: further analysis of benefits, risks and costs. Dev Biol Stand 1985;61:429–437.
26. Miller DL, Alderslade R, Ross EM. Whooping cough and whooping cough vaccine: the risks and benefits debate. Epidemiol Rev 1982;4:1–24.
27. Miller D, Wadsworth J, Diamond J, Ross E. Pertussis vaccine and whooping cough as risk factors for acute neurological illness and death in young children. Dev Biol Stand 1985;61:389–394.
28. Cherry JD, Brunell PA, Golden GS, Karzon DT. Report of the Task Force on Pertussis and Pertussis Immunization—1988. Pediatrics 1988;81(Suppl):939–984.
29. Lewis K, Cherry JD, Holroyd HJ, et al. A double-blind study comparing an acellular pertussis-component DTP vaccine with a whole-cell pertussis-component DTP vaccine in 18-month-old children. Am J Dis Child 1986;140:872–876.
30. Edwards KM, Lawrence E, Wright PF. Diphtheria, tetanus, and pertussis vaccine: a comparison of the immune response and adverse reactions to conventional and acellular pertussis components. Am J Dis Child 1986;140:867–871.
31. Anderson EL, Belshe RB, Bartram J, et al. Clinical and serologic responses to acellular pertussis vaccine in infants and young children. Am J Dis Child 1987;141:949–953.
32. Pichichero ME, Badgett JT, Rodgers GC, et al. Acellular pertussis vaccine: immunogenicity and safety of an acellular pertussis vs. a whole-cell pertussis vaccine combined with diphtheria and tetanus toxoids as a booster in 18- to 24-month-old children. Pediatr Infect Dis J 1987;6:352–363.
33. Blennow M, Granstrom M, Jaatmaa E, et al. Primary immunization of infants with an acellular pertussis vaccine in a double-blind randomized clinical trial. Pediatrics 1988;82:293–299.
34. Anderson EL, Belshe RB, Bartram J. Differences in reactogenicity and antigenicity of acellular and standard pertussis vaccines combined with diphtheria and tetanus in infants. J Infect Dis 1988;157:731–737.
35. Morgan CM, Blumberg DA, Cherry JD, et al. Comparison of acellular and whole-cell pertussis-component DTP vaccines: a multicenter double-blind study in 4- to 6-year-old children. Am J Dis Child 1990;144:41–45.
36. Blumberg DA, Mink CM, Cherry JD, et al. Comparison of an acellular pertussis-component diphtheria-tetanus-pertussis (DTP) vaccine with a whole-cell pertussis-component DTP vaccine in 17- to 24-month-old children, with measurement of 69-kilodalton outer membrane protein antibody. J Pediatr 1990;117:46–51.

37. CDC. General recommendations on immunization. Immunization Practices Advisory Committee (ACIP). MMWR 1989;205–214, 219–227.
38. Halsey N, Galazka A. The efficacy of DPT and oral poliomyelitis immunization schedules initiated from birth to 12 weeks of age. Bull WHO 1985;63:1151–1169.
39. Hirtz DG, Nelson KB, Ellenberg JH. Seizures following childhood immunizations. J Pediatr 1983;102:14–18.
40. Baraff LJ, Shields WD, Beckwith L, et al. Infants and children with convulsions and hypotonic-hyporesponsive episodes following diphtheria-tetanus-pertusssis immunization: follow-up evaluation. Pediatrics 1988;81:789–794.
41. Long SS, DeForest A, Pennridge Pediatric Associates, Smith DG, Lazaro C, Wassilak SGF. Longitudinal study of adverse reactions following diphtheria-tetanus-pertussis vaccine in infancy. Pediatrics 1990;85:294–302.
42. Cody CL, Baraff LJ, Cherry JD, Marcy SM, Manclark CR. The nature and rate of adverse reactions associated with DTP and DT immunization in infants and children. Pediatrics 1981;68:650–660.
43. Baraff LJ, Cody CL, Cherry JD. DTP-associated reactions: an analysis by injection site, manufacturer, prior reactions and dose. Pediatrics 1984;73:31–36.
44. Kulenkampff M, Schwartzman JS, Wilson J. Neurological complications of pertussis inoculation. Arch Dis Child 1974;49:46–49.
45. Miller DL, Ross EM, Alderslade R, Bellman MH, Rawson NSB. Pertussis immunization and serious acute neurological illness in children. Br Med J 1981;282:1595–1599.
46. Ross E, Miller D. Risk and pertussis vaccine [Letter]. Arch Dis Child 1986;61:98–99.
47. Miller D, Wadsworth J, Ross E. Severe neurological illness: further analyses of the British National Childhood Encephalopathy Study. Tokai J Exp Clin Med 1988;13(Suppl):145–155.
48. Bellman MH, Ross EM, Miller DL. Infantile spasms and pertussis immunisation. Lancet 1983;1:1031–1034.
49. American Academy of Pediatrics, Committee on Infectious Diseases. The relationship between pertussis vaccine and brain damage: reassessment. Pediatrics 1991;(in press).
50. Child Neurology Society. Ad hoc committee for the Child Neurology Society consensus statement on pertussis immunization and the central nervous system. Ann Neurol 1991;29:458–460.
51. Minister of National Health and Welfare, National Advisory Committee on Immunization. Canadian immunization guide. 3rd ed. Canada: Minister of National Health and Welfare, Health Protection Branch;1989:78–83.
52. The British Joint Committee on Vaccination and Immunisation. Immunisation against infectious disease, 1990. London: Her Majesty's Stationery Office, 1990:20–27.
53. British Paediatric Association. Pertussis immunisation. In: Nicoll A, Rudd P, eds. Manual on infections and immunizations in children. Oxford: Oxford University Press, 1989:207–210.
54. Institute of Medicine. In: Howson CP, Howe CJ, Fineberg HV, eds. Adverse effects of pertussis and rubella vaccines. Washington, DC: National Academy Press, August 27, 1991 (in press).
55. Madge N, Miller D, Ross E, Wadsworth J. The National Childhood Encephalopathy Study: a 10-year followup [Abstract]. In: Manclark CR ed. The Sixth International Symposium on Pertussis, Abstracts. Bethesda, MD: Department of Health and Human Services, 1990: DHHS publication no. (FDA)90–1162; 226–227.
56. Pollock TM, Morris J. A 7-year survey of disorders attributed to vaccination in North West Thames region. Lancet 1983;1:753–757.
57. Walker AM, Jick H, Perera DR, Knauss TA, Thompson RS. Neurologic events following diphtheria-tetanus-pertussis immunization. Pediatrics 1988;81:345–349.
58. Griffin MR, Ray WA, Mortimer EA Jr, Fenichel GM, Schaffner W. Risk of seizures and encephalopathy after immunization with the diphtheria-tetanus-pertussis vaccine. JAMA 1990;263:1641–1645.
59. Shields WD, Nielsen C, Buch D, et al. Relationship of pertussis immunization to the onset of neurologic disorders: a retrospective epidemiologic study. J Pediatr 1988;113:801–805.
60. Gale JL, Thapa PB, Bobo JK, Wassilak SGF, Mendelman PM, Foy JM. Acute neurological illness and DTP: report of a case-control study in Washington and Oregon [Abstract]. In: Manclark CR, ed. The Sixth International Symposium on Pertussis, Abstracts. Bethesda, MD: Department of Health and Human Services, 1990; DHHS publication no. (FDA)90–1162; 228–229.
61. Melchior JC. Infantile spasms and early immunization against whooping cough: Danish survey from 1970 to 1975. Arch Dis Child 1977;52:134–137.
62. Walker AM, Jick H, Perera DR, Thompson RS, Knause TA. Diphtheria-tetanus-pertussis immunization and sudden infant death syndrome. Am J Public Health 1987;77:945–951.
63. Hoffman HS, Hunter JC, Damus K, et al. Diphtheria-tetanus-pertussis immunization and sudden infant death: results of the National Institute of Child Health and Human Development Cooperative Epidemiological Study of Sudden Infant Death Syndrome Risk Factors. Pediatrics 1987;79:598–611.
64. Griffin MR, Ray WA, Livengood JR, Schaffner W. Risk of sudden infant death syndrome (SIDS) after immunization with the diphtheria-tetanus-pertussis vaccine. N Engl J Med 1988;319:618–623.
65. Bouvier-Colle MH, Flahaut A, Messiah A, Jougla E, Hatton F. Sudden infant death and immunization: an extensive epidemiological approach to the problem in France-winter 1986. Int J Epidemiol 1989;18:121–126.

66. Butler NR, Haslum M, Golding J, Stewart-Brown S. Recent findings from the 1970 child health and education study: preliminary communication. J R Soc Med 1982;75:781–784.
67. Stetler HC, Orenstein WA, Bart KJ, Brink EW, Brennan J-P, Hinman AT. History of convulsions and use of pertussis vaccine. J Pediatr 1985;107:175–179.
68. Livengood JR, Mullen JR, White JW, Brink EW, Orenstein WA. Family history of convulsions and use of pertussis vaccine. J Pediatr 1989;115:527–531.
69. Mortimer EA Jr, Sorensen RU. Urticaria following administration of diphtheria-tetanus toxoids-pertussis vaccine. Pediatr Infect Dis 1987;6:876–877.
70. Lewis K, Jordan SC, Cherry JD, Sakai RS, Le CT. Petechiae and urticaria after DTP vaccination: detection of circulating immune complexes containing vaccine-specific antigens. J Pediatr 1986;109:1009–1012.
71. CDC. Vaccine adverse event reporting system—United States. MMWR 1990;39:730–733.
72. CDC. National Childhood Vaccine Injury Act: requirements for permanent vaccination records and for reporting of selected events after vaccination. MMWR 1988;37:197–200.
73. Food and Drug Administration. New reporting requirements for vaccine adverse events. FDA Drug Bull 1988;18(2):16–18.
74. Barkin RM, Samuelson JS, Gotlin LP. DTP reactions and serologic response with a reduced dose schedule. J Pediatr 1984;105:189–194.
75. Bernbaum J, Daft A, Samuelson J, Polin RA. Half-dose immunization for diphtheria, tetanus, pertussis: response of preterm infants. Pediatrics 1989;83:471–476.
76. British Medical Research Council. Vaccination against whooping-cough. Relation between protection in children and results of laboratory tests. Br Med J 1956;2:454–462.
77. Cameron J. The potency of whooping cough (pertussis) vaccines in Canada. J Biol Stand 1980; 8:297–302.
78. Deforest A, Long SS, Lischner HW, et al. Simultaneous administration of measles-mumps-rubella vaccine with booster doses of diphtheria-tetanus-pertussis and poliovirus vaccines. Pediatrics 1988;81:237–246.
79. CDC. Haemophilus b conjugate vaccines for prevention of Haemophilus influenzae type b disease among infants and children two months of age and older: recommendations of the Immunization Practices Advisory Committee (ACIP). MMWR 1991;40(no. RR-1):6.
80. Bernbaum J, Anolik R, Polin RA, Douglas SD. Development of the premature infants host defense and its relationship to routine immunizations. Clin Perinatol 1984;11:73–84.
81. Koblin BA, Townsend TR, Munoz A, Onorato I, Wilson M, Polk BF. Response of preterm infants to diphtheria-tetanus-pertussis vaccine. Pediatr Infect Dis J 1988;7:704–711.
82. Gross PA, Lee H, Wolff JA, Hall CB, Minnefore AB, Lazicki ME. Influenza immunization in immunosuppressed children. J Pediatr 1978;92:30–35.
83. Jacobs RL, Lowe RS, Lanier BQ. Adverse reactions to tetanus toxoid. JAMA 1982;247:40–42.
84. Mansfield LE, Ting S, Rawls DO, Frederick R. Systemic reactions during cutaneous testing for tetanus toxoid hypersensitivity. Ann Allergy 1986;57:135–137.
85. Blumberg DA, Mink CM, Lewis K, et al. Severe DTP-associated reactions [Abstract]. In: Manclark CR, ed. The Sixth International Symposium on Pertussis, Abstracts. Bethesda, MD: Department of Health and Human Services, 1990: DHHS publication no. (FDA)90–1162; 223–224.
86. Ellenberg JH, Hirtz DG, Nelson KB. Do seizures in children cause intellectual deterioration? N Engl J Med 1986;314:1085–1088.
87. Maytal J, Shinnar S. Febrile status epilepticus. Pediatrics 1990;86:611–616.
88. Ipp MM, Gold R, Greenberg S, et al. Acetaminophen prophylaxis of adverse reactions following vaccination of infants with diphtheria-pertussis-tetanus toxoids-polio vaccine. Pediatr Infect Dis J 1987;6:721–725.
89. Lewis K, Cherry JD, Sachs MH, et al. The effect of prophylactic acetaminophen administration on reactions to DTP vaccination. Am J Dis Child 1988;142:62–65.
90. Livingston S. Comprehensive management of epilepsy in infancy. Springfield, IL: Charles C Thomas 1972;159–166.
91. Bass JW. Pertussis: current status of prevention and treatment. Pediatr Infect Dis J 1985;4:614–619.
92. Steketee RW, Wassilak SGF, Adkins WN, et al. Evidence for a high attack rate and efficacy of erythromycin prophylaxis in a pertussis outbreak in a facility for the developmentally disabled. J Infect Dis 1988;157:434–440.
93. Bergquist S, Bernander S, Dahnsjo H, Sundelof B. Erythromycin in the treatment of pertussis: a study of bacteriologic and clinical effects. Pediatr Infect Dis J 1987;6:458–461.
94. Biellik RJ, Patriarca PA, Mullen JR, et al. Risk factors for community- and household-acquired pertussis during a large-scale outbreak in central Wisconsin. J Infect Dis 1988;157:1134–1141.
95. Biellik RJ, Patriarca PA, Paul W, Sanden G, Brink EW, Silverman P. Pertussis in an Amish community in Delaware [Abstract]. Presented at the 29th Interscience Conference on Antimicrobial Agents and Chemotherapy, Houston, TX, September 17–20, 1989.
96. Sprauer MA, Cochi SL, Patriarca PA, et al. Use of erythromycin in preventing secondary transmission of pertussis [Abstract]. Presented at the 29th Interscience Conference on Antimicrobial Agents and Chemotherapy, Houston, TX, September 17–20, 1989.

TOPIC 6 / **DRACUNCULIASIS**

Dracunculiasis

Original Citation: Hopkins DR, Ruiz-Tiben E. Strategies for dracunculiasis eradication. Bull WHO 1991;69(5):533–540.

Original Authors: D. R. Hopkins, E. Ruiz-Tiben

In 1991 the Forty-fourth World Health Assembly declared the goal of eradicating dracunculiasis (guinea worm disease) by the end of 1995. This article summarizes the recommended strategies for surveillance and interventions in national dracunculiasis eradication programmes.

The fundamental difference between an eradication programme and a control programme is critical to understanding the need for some of the strategies recommended in this paper. While a control programme may aim to reduce the incidence of a disease until the disease is no longer a public health problem, an eradication programme has a more demanding and specific objective: to reduce the incidence of the disease to zero within a given time period. Control efforts may be limited to areas of moderate or intense transmission, whereas eradication programmes must encompass all areas where transmission occurs, including areas of low incidence. An eradication programme has a fixed endpoint and a limited duration of expenditures, but control programmes and their costs continue indefinitely. Finally, the need for extremely sensitive surveillance to detect all cases, including imported cases, wherever they may occur in the at-risk area, is much more critical in an eradication programme, whereas a control programme may be adequately served by sampling or sentinel surveillance measures.

STRATEGIES

The key necessary activities of dracunculiasis eradication programmes may be grouped into three operational phases.

Phase I: Establishing a National Programme Office and Conducting Baseline Surveys

Each endemic country must designate a national programme coordinator, and establish a small staff/secretariat to support the leadership and coordination roles of the national office of the eradication programme. The two most critical first tasks of this office, if they have not been done already, are to conduct a nationwide, village-by-village survey, and prepare a national plan of action for eradicating dracunculiasis from the country. The main priority of the national survey should be to identify all endemic villages in the country, and secondly to count the number of annual cases of the disease, so as to establish the true extent of the problem (3).

The national survey provides an important basis for preparing or revising a plan of action that reflects the true scope of the national problem. The plan of action provides the basis for mobilizing the necessary national and external support. Countries where the disease occurs nationwide may find it necessary to develop plans of action for each endemic state or region. In most instances, it will be advisable for the programme to also establish, or make use of an existing intersectoral committee or national task force in order to facilitate mobilization and coordination of the diverse governmental and other agencies whose contributions are needed, such as the government ministries concerned with health, water supplies, and information.

Phase II: Implementing Interventions

Active surveillance is also the key to implementing interventions, monitoring progress, and evaluating the impact of the programme, just as it is to planning the attack and mobilizing the necessary resources (3). A vertically organized, quickly conducted national search is the best means of ascertaining the extent of the disease at the outset. In the next phases of the programme it is very desirable to rely on village-based workers, one or more in each known endemic village, to maintain village-based case registers and provide monthly reports of cases as they occur. The advantages of the latter system are that it provides more accurate surveillance, allows monthly tracking of incidence, is compatible with the primary health care (PHC) system to which most countries are already committed, eliminates the need for annual mobilization of active case searches, and provides the documentation of programme impact needed for verifying the absence of transmission, i.e., the attainment of eradication.

Identification and training of village-based workers in each of the known endemic villages is perhaps the most urgent early task of the intervention phase. Where they exist already, primary health care (PHC) workers in endemic villages should be used; where they do not yet exist, an appropriate villager should be designated (who may later be incorporated into the country's PHC programme). In addition to their roles in reporting cases of dracunculiasis monthly, the village-based workers can also be trained to provide health education about the disease to their neighbours, and provide simple topical treatment of wounds caused by the emerging worms. Apart from training, a system for providing regular supervision and supplies for the village-based workers must be established if one does not already exist. The issue of whether such workers are to be volunteers, or paid by the village, or compensated by the programme must be decided by each national authority.

Each endemic country must also decide on the most appropriate mix of the available interventions (health education, provision of rural water supply, use of cloth filters, and vector control) that it can afford or should seek external help for this. No single intervention will work everywhere. "Problem" villages can be dealt with as they become apparent. After most or all of the endemic villages have been identified through the national survey, the goal should be to get interventions started in all these villages as fast as possible. Establishing and training the village-based workers to implement active surveillance and control are probably the first steps in such interventions, which should include the following.

•Health education and community mobilization should be emphasized as a priority because they are the least costly of the interventions available, and are a necessary base for the other interventions. Each country needs to devise an overall plan and comprehensive strategy for health education and community mobilization, taking into account the relevant characteristics and resources of the country and its population. The goal here should be to get the same basic messages to endemic populations repeatedly, using all appropriate channels. The three essential messages are:

- guinea worms come from drinking contaminated water;
- persons with emerging worms or blisters should not contaminate sources of drinking water;
- people can also protect themselves by always filtering or boiling their drinking water, or by only drinking water from safe sources.

The village-based worker, a key source (but not the only one) for the health education messages, should be reinforced by religious and traditional/political leaders in the village, schoolteachers, agricultural and other extension workers, community organizations, and by the mass media (radio, posters, etc.) in the local languages. These activities will create a demand for cloth filters (which can be distributed and their proper use demonstrated by the village-based workers), as well as mobilize support for local participation in the other interventions (water supply, control of copepods). The logistical system should be prepared to meet the increased demand for cloth filters by providing timely supplies to the village-based workers.

•Provision of a safe source of drinking water, such as a bore-hole well with handpump, or a properly constructed hand-dug well, is the other priority intervention. This is the most desirable intervention, since it yields many other important benefits besides eliminating dracunculiasis. But this is also the most expensive of the interventions, especially in smaller communities, and the geological features may not permit this to be used in some affected areas. The overall goal of the eradication programme should be to try to get safe wells provided or rehabilitated in as many of the identified endemic villages as possible and as quickly as possible, especially in the most highly-endemic, densely-populated areas. Among priority areas with the latter characteristics, the highest priority might be given to localities with the greatest agricultural potential.

The programme should seek to get a decision by the government to provide safe water to the endemic villages as a national priority, since such villages are usually the worst off of all the unserved villages. These populations are suffering from dracunculiasis, with its adverse effects on health, agriculture, and school attendance, in addition to the other negative effects of unsafe water that all unserved villages have in common. The villages with dracunculiasis are also only a small fraction of all such unserved villages. Other appropriate technologies such as rainwater harvesting, conversion of step wells into draw wells, or construction of small sand filters, for example, should also be considered, and used where appropriate and necessary.

•The control of copepod populations using Abate* (temephos) is intermediate in cost, relative to the promotion of health education or use of cloth filters and rural water supplies. It should be used only in selected endemic villages, as backup to health education and/or water supply interventions. It should be considered for use in "epidemic control" in very highly affected villages with limited drinking-water sources, to reduce the incidence (while villages wait for a safe water source to be installed) in situations where compliance with health education is poor or where providing a safe water source is not feasible, or to provide a second or third barrier to transmission for additional security in areas where dracunculiasis elimination is imminent or was recently achieved. This intervention is not cost-effective when the volume of the drinking-water source exceeds 500 cubic metres.

The programme in Pakistan has from its inception relied exclusively on health education, use of cloth filters, and temephos to eradicate dracunculiasis, mainly because many residents strongly prefer water from ponds or cisterns, compared to underground water which in many of the endemic areas is brackish. Village implementers are the main providers of health education on dracunculiasis prevention, and they also distribute the cloth filters and monitor their use. Field workers from local health departments were trained by the GWEP to apply temephos.

Ghana and Nigeria began conducting extensive systematic interventions in endemic villages in 1990, although in Nigeria the UNICEF-assisted rural water supply programmes had been giving priority to endemic villages since 1984, and Anambra State had begun health education and community mobilization activities in 1986. Apart from India, so far only Nigeria has established a national policy of priority to endemic villages for sources of safe drinking water (in 1989). In Ghana, the head of state visited 21 villages in 1988 to demonstrate personally the use of cloth filters. Ghana also began distributing tens of thousands of copies of a manual to secondary schools in 1989 for teaching about dracunculiasis. Both Ghana and Nigeria are emphasizing health education, community mobilization, and rural water supply in their interventions so far; more extensive use of temephos in selected villages will be carried out in 1991.

A schematic illustration of the extension of recommended intervention measures is given in Figure 1 [See original document], where the unit of consideration is the endemic village. Whatever the number of endemic villages at the beginning of a programme, towards the end all the residual endemic villages should be included in the case-containment strategy. An appropriately organized and imple-

---

*Use of trade name is for identification only and does not imply endorsement by the Public Health Service or the U.S. Department of Health and Human Services.

mented dracunculiasis eradication programme should be able to mobilize sufficient resources to eliminate all indigenous transmission within five years after the
first national case search is conducted. In some countries, it may be appropriate
to begin using temephos sooner than indicated in Figure 1 [see original docu-
ment], provided the two priority interventions of health education/cloth filters
and water supply are already being implemented. The key activities needed in
national dracunculiasis eradication programmes are summarized in (Table 1).

Phase III: Case Containment

As programmes get closer to achieving eradication, i.e., when the expected case
load of the village-based health worker is one (or less than one) case per worker per day, increasingly stringent surveillance and control measures will be indicated, particularly if transmission is unlikely to be re-established as a result of
introduction of infections from other endemic areas. Of the three programmes
assisted by Global 2000, only Pakistan has reached this stage, although some less
endemic areas of Ghana and Nigeria will begin implementing this strategy in
1991. As applied in the GWEP in Pakistan, this strategy is additive, providing for
rapid attention to each case of the disease, not just to the endemic villages. The
village-based workers, being the best means for immediate detection of new
cases, are essential to this stage of the programme, and for preventing any further transmission from them. In addition to educating the afflicted individual
not to contaminate drinking-water sources and making sure that other inhabi-
tants of the village are aware of the case and have cloth filters to protect themselves (if necessary), the trained village worker can try to determine whether
the patient may have already contaminated a source of drinking water, and also
where the patient acquired the infection the year before.

Table 1. Key activities of dracunculiasis eradication programmes

Phase I:
- Establish a national programme coordinator, office/secretariat
- Conduct complete national village-by-village surveys
- Prepared or revise the national plan of action

Phase II:
- Identify and train village-based workers for each endemic village
- Implement village-based surveillance using case registries
- Implement a comprehensive health education/mobilization strategy
- Provide cloth filters and teach villagers to use them
- Secure priority for endemic villages in provision of rural water supply
- Train and provide for use of temephos in selected endemic villages
- Monitor the coverage, quality of surveillance, and interventions

Phase III:
- Implement the case-containment strategy

Post-eradication:
- Maintain adequate surveillance for 3 years after the last case
- Request WHO to certify eradication

Providing simple medical treatment to patients becomes much more important and feasible at this final stage of the programme. If the resources are available, simple topical treatment should be provided from the outset of the eradication programme, but not if it detracts from providing the other more effective interventions to prevent new infections. Provision of treatment free of charge is a useful incentive for patients to contact the health service, where they can be educated about the disease and where their case can be recorded.

REFERENCES: AS NUMBERED IN ORIGINAL PUBLICATION

3. Muller R. Guinea worm disease: epidemiology, control and treatment. Bull WHO 1979;57:683–689.

TOPIC 7 / **EBOLA**

Update: Ebola-Related Filovirus Infection in Nonhuman Primates and Interim Guidelines for Handling Nonhuman Primates during Transit and Quarantine

Original Citation: Epidemiologic Notes and Reports. Update: Ebola-Related Filovirus Infection in Nonhuman Primates and Interim Guidelines for Handling Nonhuman Primates during Transit and Quarantine. MMWR 1990;39(2):22–24, 29–30.

INTERIM GUIDELINES FOR HANDLING NONHUMAN PRIMATES DURING TRANSIT AND QUARANTINE

All imported nonhuman primates are quarantined for the first 31 days after arrival, including transit time. Nonhuman primates, particularly those recently captured in the wild, may harbor viruses infectious for humans. Although such viruses are usually present in the animal's blood, they may be detected in urine, feces, or saliva. Those at risk for infection include persons working in temporary or long-term holding facilities and persons who transport animals to these facilities (e.g., cargo handlers and inspectors). Although the risk for human infection from these activities is low, guidelines are useful to minimize such risk in persons exposed to nonhuman primates during transport and quarantine.

General Guidelines for Handling Nonhuman Primates during Transit and Quarantine

1. Management of transportation and quarantine facilities should ensure that personnel are instructed as to the hazards of handling nonhuman primates, that protective apparel is available, and that the need for its use

is understood. Management should provide periodic retraining as well as reinforcement of these procedures.

2. Persons working with nonhuman primates should not drink, eat, or smoke while handling animals, cages, crates, or materials from such animals.

3. Access to animal holding areas should be restricted to essential personnel. The number of persons involved in the care, transport, and inspection of nonhuman primates should be the minimum necessary to expedite efficient and humane handling.

4. All staff in direct contact with animals should wear protective clothing (i.e., gloves and surgical masks and gowns) when opening crates, removing foreign materials from crates, feeding the animals, removing dead animals, or handling bedding materials. These persons should remove disposable protective clothing before leaving the animal holding facilities; this clothing should be autoclaved or incinerated. Nondisposable contaminated clothing should be disinfected on site before laundering.

5. Separate nonglass water bottles should be provided for each nonhuman primate during transit and quarantine. Reusable items should be adequately decontaminated between uses.

6. All animal waste, bedding, uneaten food, and other possibly contaminated items should be treated with appropriate disinfectant before removal from the animal holding facilities. All cages, feeding bottles, and other possibly contaminated items should be disinfected between each use or before disposal. Glass items should not be used.

7. A separate disposable needle and syringe (and, if required, infusion equipment) should be used for each animal, then autoclaved or incinerated. A clean needle should be used for any access to multidose vials (e.g., of ketamine) to avoid contamination. After each use on a group of quarantined animals, multidose vials must be autoclaved and discarded. Disposable supplies should be used whenever possible and must not be reused. Nondisposable equipment should be thoroughly disinfected.

8. Caution must be used to prevent infection from potentially contaminated needles, scalpels, or other sharp instruments, particularly during disposal of needles. Used needles should not be recapped by hand; removed from disposable syringes by hand; or bent, broken, or otherwise manipulated. Only one set of disposable syringes, needles, and scalpels should be used per animal. Used disposable syringes and needles, scalpel blades, and other sharp items should be placed in puncture-resistant containers kept · as close to the work site as practical.

9. Nonquarantined animals should never be placed in, or permitted access to, areas with quarantined animals. This includes unrestrained pets, feral animals, and animals temporarily boarded for overseas travelers or destined for export.

10. Management should keep records of all serious febrile illnesses (fever greater than 101.3°F (greater than 38.5°C) for greater than 2 days) in persons having direct contact with nonhuman primates in transit or in quarantine and should promptly notify CDC if such an illness occurs. Management should ensure that the physician providing care is informed that the patient works with and/or has been exposed to nonhuman primates.

Additional Guidelines for Handling Nonhuman Primates during Transit

1. Persons who handle crates or pallets containing nonhuman primates should be protected with elbow-length reinforced leather gloves, long-sleeved shirts and trousers of sufficient thickness to resist minor tears, and sturdy waterproof shoes or boots. The gloves should be of a thickness that prevents penetration of splinters or other crating debris. During warm weather, garments may be of lightweight materials to minimize discomfort. Disposable coverall suits can be used for added protection.

2. Crates should be free of sharp projections that can cause scratches or wounds to workers. Handles should be present on the sides of crates, and mechanical lifting and transporting devices should be used whenever possible.

3. Crates containing nonhuman primates should be separated by a physical or spatial barrier from all other animals and cargo at all times.

4. Wherever possible, nonhuman primates should not be handled directly. Live animals should be removed from cages only when staff can be supervised by a qualified veterinarian. Procedures that may result in bites or scratches should be avoided.

5. Management of holding facilities should maintain records to document the removal of dead animals; documentation should include the date, shipment number, country of origin, species, importer, and disposition of the removed animal. The carcass must be placed in waterproof double bags and incinerated. The Division of Quarantine, Center for Prevention Services (CPS), CDC, should be notified.

6. Temporary holding facilities should document all injections or parenteral infusions administered to nonhuman primates.

7. If animals are removed from a shipment while in transit, facilities retaining these animals should ensure full compliance with these guidelines and should maintain records on the care and disposition of animals. Temporary facilities holding animals in this way must be registered as importers of nonhuman primates.

Additional Guidelines for Care of Nonhuman Primates during Quarantine

1. Quarantine facilities should be secure, with access limited to authorized, trained, and informed personnel.

2. Quarantine facilities should be designed to be adequately disinfected. Management and staff should refer to the Guide for the Care and Use of Laboratory Animals (3) and the CDC/National Institutes of Health Biosafety in Microbiological and Biomedical Laboratories, second edition (Animal biosafety level 2, p. 52) (4), for information on design and operation of animal holding facilities.

3. Staff should use protective clothing, gloves, and masks at all times when in the animal holding facilities; these items should be disinfected or disposed of properly. Staff should use fresh clothing when going from room to room.

4. Adequate equipment and space should be available for discarding and disinfecting all equipment, clothing, and caging.

5. Care should be taken to avoid scratches and bites of animals. All handling of individual animals should be done while the animals are anesthetized or tranquilized, and animals should be maintained in squeeze-back cages wherever possible.
6. Different lots of primates should not be mixed while in quarantine (minimum 31 days).
7. Management should notify the Division of Quarantine, CPS, CDC, of severe illnesses and deaths in recently imported primates. CDC will advise management on collection of specimens for investigation of cause of death.

REFERENCES: AS NUMBERED IN ORIGINAL PUBLICATION

3. National Institutes of Health. Guide for the care and use of laboratory animals. Bethesda, MD: National Institutes of Health, 1985:43–48 (document no. 85–23).
4. CDC/National Institutes of Health. Biosafety in microbiological and biomedical laboratories. 2nd ed. Bethesda, MD: US Department of Health and Human Services, Public Health Service, 1988; DHHS publication no. (CDC)88–8395.

TOPIC 8 / **ENTERICS**

Escherichia coli O157:H7: Procedure for the Isolation and Identification from Stool Specimens

Original Citation: Procedure for the Isolation and Identification of Escherichia coli O157:H7 from Stool Specimens. CDC/NCID brochure, 1994.

DIAGNOSTIC CONSIDERATIONS AND SPECIMEN COLLECTION PROCEDURES

The diagnosis of E. coli O157:H7 infection needs to be considered for all patients who present with diarrhea, especially bloody diarrhea or hemolytic uremic syndrome (HUS) (1). Stool specimens (whole stools, swabs prepared from whole stools or rectal swabs with visible fecal staining) should be collected. Ideally, specimens should be collected as close to the time of onset of diarrhea as possible; however, specimens taken even weeks after the onset of symptoms are sometimes positive (2, 3). Antibiotic treatment decreases the chance of recovery of E. coli O157:H7; therefore, when follow-up specimens are being obtained, the patient should have received no antibiotic for a minimum of 48 hours before culture.

SPECIMEN HANDLING PROCEDURES

Ideally, stool specimens should be examined as soon as they are received in the laboratory. If whole stool specimens will not be processed immediately, they should be either refrigerated or frozen at $-70°C$ as soon as possible after collection. Refrigerated specimens should be examined within 1–2 hours. If stools cannot be examined within this time, they should be placed in transport medium. All rectal swabs should be placed **immediately** into transport medium. If specimens in transport medium will be examined within 2–3 days, they should be refrigerated. If specimens will not be examined within 3 days, they should be frozen immediately, preferably at $-70°C$. Specimens should not be refrigerated for days and then frozen, or placed in transport medium and left at room temperature.

If a transport medium will be used, any of the commercially available transport media (e.g., Cary-Blair, Stuart's, Amie's, buffered glycerol saline) are satisfactory. A swab should be **completely covered** by the transport medium. If the medium does not cover the swab, the swab will not be kept sufficiently moist and recovery of E. coli O157:H7 and other organisms may be compromised.

REFERENCES: AS NUMBERED IN ORIGINAL PUBLICATION

1. Griffin PM, Tauxe RV. The epidemiology of infections caused by Escherichia coli O157:H7, other enterohemorrhagic E. coli, and the associated hemolytic uremic syndrome. Epidemiol Rev 1991; 13:60–98.
2. Belongia EA, Osterholm MT, Soler JT, Ammend DA, Braun JE, MacDonald KL. Transmission of Escherichia coli O157:H7 infection in Minnesota child day-care facilities. JAMA 1993;269:883–888.
3. Pai CH, Ahmed N, Lior H, Johnson WM, Sims HV, Woods DE. Epidemiology of sporadic diarrhea due to verocytotoxin-producing Escherichia coli: a two-year prospective study. J Infect Dis 1988;157: 1054–1057.

Preventing Foodborne Illness: Escherichia coli O157:H7

Original Citation: Preventing Foodborne Illness: Escherichia coli O157:H7. CDC/NCID brochure, April 1993.

ESCHERICHIA COLI O157:H7

Escherichia coli O157:H7 is an emerging cause of foodborne illness. An estimated 10,000 to 20,000 cases of infection occur in the United States each year. Infection often leads to bloody diarrhea, and occasionally to kidney failure. Most illness has been associated with eating undercooked, contaminated ground beef. Person-to-person contact in families and child care centers is also an important mode of transmission. Infection can also occur after drinking raw milk and after swimming in or drinking sewage-contaminated water.

Consumers can prevent E. coli O157:H7 infection by thoroughly cooking ground beef, avoiding unpasteurized milk, and washing hands carefully. Because the organism lives in the intestines of healthy cattle, preventive measures on cattle farms and during meal processing are being investigated.

HOW IS E. COLI O157:H7 SPREAD?

The organism can be found on a small number of cattle farms and can live in the intestines of healthy cattle. Meat can become contaminated during slaughter, and organisms can be thoroughly mixed into beef when it is ground. Bacteria present on the cow's udders or on equipment may get into raw milk.

Eating meat, especially ground beef, that has not been cooked sufficiently to kill E. coli O157:H7 can cause infection. Contaminated meat looks and smells normal. Although the number of organisms required to cause disease is not known, it is suspected to be very small.

Drinking unpasteurized milk and swimming in or drinking sewage-contaminated water can also cause infection.

Bacteria in diarrheal stools of infected persons can be passed from one person to another if hygiene or handwashing habits are inadequate. This is particularly likely among toddlers who are not toilet trained. Family members and playmates of these children are at high risk of becoming infected.

Young children typically shed the organism in their feces for a week or two after their illness resolves. Older children rarely carry the organism without symptoms.

WHAT ILLNESS DOES E. COLI O157:H7 CAUSE?

E. coli O157:H7 infection often causes severe bloody diarrhea and abdominal cramps; sometimes the infection causes nonbloody diarrhea or no symptoms. Usually little or no fever is present, and the illness resolves in 5 to 10 days. In some persons, particularly children under 5 years of age and the elderly, the infection can also cause a complication called hemolytic uremic syndrome, in which the red blood cells are destroyed and the kidneys fail. About 2%–7% of infections lead to this complication. In the United States, hemolytic uremic syndrome is the principal cause of acute kidney failure in children, and most cases of hemolytic uremic syndrome are caused by E. coli O157:H7.

HOW IS E. COLI O157:H7 INFECTION DIAGNOSED?

Infection with E. coli O157:H7 is diagnosed by detecting the bacterium in the stool. Most laboratories that culture stool do not test for E. coli O157:H7, so it is important to request that the stool specimen be tested on sorbitol MacConkey (SMAC) agar for this organism. All persons who suddenly have diarrhea with blood should get their stool tested for E. coli O157:H7.

HOW IS THE ILLNESS TREATED?

Most persons recover without antibiotics or other specific treatment in 5–10 days. There is no evidence that antibiotics improve the course of disease, and it is thought that treatment with some antibiotics may precipitate kidney complications. Antidiarrheal agents, such as loperamide (Imodium), should also be avoided.

Hemolytic uremic syndrome is a life-threatening condition usually treated in an intensive care unit. Blood transfusions and kidney dialysis are often required. With intensive care, the death rate for hemolytic uremic syndrome is 3%–5%.

WHAT ARE THE LONG-TERM CONSEQUENCES OF INFECTION?

Persons who only have diarrhea usually recover completely.

About one-third of persons with hemolytic uremic syndrome have abnormal kidney function many years later, and a few require long-term dialysis.

Another 8% of persons with hemolytic uremic syndrome have other lifelong complications, such as high blood pressure, seizures, blindness, paralysis, and the effects of having part of their bowel removed.

WHAT CAN BE DONE TO PREVENT THE INFECTION?

E. coli O157:H7 will continue to be an important public health concern as long as it contaminates meat. Preventive measures may reduce the number of cattle that carry it and the contamination of meat during slaughter and grinding. Research into such prevention measures is just beginning.

WHAT CAN YOU DO TO PREVENT E. COLI O157:H7 INFECTION?

- Cook all ground beef or hamburger thoroughly. Make sure that the cooked meat is gray or brown throughout (not pink), any juices run clear, and the inside is hot.
- If you are served an undercooked hamburger in a restaurant, send it back for further cooking.
- Consume only pasteurized milk and milk products. Avoid raw milk.
- Make sure that infected persons, especially children, wash their hands carefully and frequently with soap to reduce the risk of spreading the infection.
- Drink municipal water that has been treated with adequate levels of chlorine or other effective disinfectants.

Enhanced Detection of Sporadic Escherichia coli O157:H7 Infections

Original Citation: Enhanced Detection of Sporadic Escherichia coli O157:H7 Infections—New Jersey, July 1994. MMWR 1995;44(22):417–418.

Infection with Escherichia coli O157:H7 causes an estimated 20,000 cases of diarrhea in the United States each year. In 1993, the Council of State and Territorial Epidemiologists recommended that clinical laboratories begin culturing all bloody stools—and optimally all diarrheal stools—for E. coli O157:H7 (1).

A primary strategy for preventing infection with E. coli O157:H7 is reducing risk behaviors through consumer education. The press coverage provided public health officials with an opportunity to inform the public about the risks of eating undercooked ground beef, the need for safe food-handling practices, and the potential for person-to-person transmission.

Although traceback investigations can be important in preventing E. coli O157:H7 infections, they should be undertaken selectively. Traceback investigations are most useful when the implicated vehicle is novel (e.g., salami) (3) or has a long shelf life (e.g., frozen hamburger patties) (4). Because fresh ground beef has a short shelf life and usually is derived from many sources, traceback investigations involving this food item are often unproductive.

An effective public health response to E. coli O157:H7 requires a timely and sensitive national surveillance system.

REFERENCES: AS NUMBERED IN ORIGINAL PUBLICATION

1. Council of State and Territorial Epidemiologists. CSTE position statement #4: national surveillance of Escherichia coli O157:H7. Atlanta: Council of State and Territorial Epidemiologists, June 1993.
3. CDC. Escherichia coli O157:H7 outbreak linked to commercially distributed dry-cured salami—Washington and California, 1994. MMWR 1995;44:157–160.
4. Bell BP, Goldoft M, Griffin PM, et al. A multistate outbreak of Escherichia coli O157:H7-associated bloody diarrhea and hemolytic uremic syndrome from hamburgers: the Washington experience. JAMA 1994;272:1349–1353.

The Management of Acute Diarrhea in Children: Oral Rehydration, Maintenance, and Nutritional Therapy

Original Citation: The Management of Acute Diarrhea in Children: Oral Rehydration, Maintenance, and Nutritional Therapy. MMWR 1992;41(RR-16):1.

PREFACE

Twenty-four years ago, oral rehydration therapy was first proven to be effective in the outpatient management of patients with severe dehydrating diarrhea caused by cholera.

Although diarrhea kills about four million people in developing countries each year, it remains a problem in developed countries as well. Because diarrhea is so common and can be severe, CDC believes the proper management of acute diarrhea in children by parents of small children and by physicians could markedly decrease national rates of hospitalization and death.

This document addresses the treatment of acute diarrhea rather than persistent diarrhea lasting 2 weeks or longer and is aimed primarily at watery diarrhea rather than bloody diarrhea (dysentery). Oral rehydration therapy (ORT) encompasses two phases of treatment: (a) the rehydration phase, in which water and electrolytes are given as oral rehydration solution (ORS) to replace existing losses, and (b) the maintenance phase, which includes both replacement of ongoing fluid and electrolyte losses and adequate dietary intake (7). It is important to emphasize that although ORT implies rehydration alone, in view of present advances, knowledge, and practice, our definition has been broadened to include maintenance fluid therapy and nutrition.

A key factor in the excellent therapeutic and safety record of ORT has been the development of simple rules that can be successfully taught by hospital and community clinic medical staff. These simple rules effectively teach the proper procedure for mixing and administering the solution, when to change to other dietary fluids and foods, and how to avoid therapeutic starvation. Several approaches are effective, but all of them include communicating to the parent or guardian simple guidelines enabling him or her to mix the solution appropriately. These guidelines also permit the amount of oral solution administered to be related to the condition of the child and the frequency of stools. Additionally, all rules encourage the parent or guardian to begin appropriate dietary liquids and foods early in the maintenance phase.

AVAILABILITY OF ORS IN THE UNITED STATES

ORS can be distributed premixed with water or as dry ingredients in packets. Packets are more common in developing countries, where low cost, long shelf life, and ease of transport make them particularly suitable. The disadvantage of packets is the potential for mixing with inappropriate volumes of water, resulting in ORS that is either too diluted or too concentrated. When caretakers are asked to mix ORS from packets at home, detailed written and oral instructions should be given (41). With premixed solutions, the concentration can be ensured, but cost can limit access (42).

Recently, the bicarbonate component of the WHO-ORS has been replaced with the bicarbonate precursor, citrate, because it has a longer shelf life. Citrate-containing solutions are as efficacious as those containing bicarbonate (43), and both components aid in the intestinal absorption of sodium and water (44).

In the United States, several different formulations of premixed ORS are available commercially. In the past 5 years, U.S. manufacturers of ORS have altered their formulations to contain lower, more appropriate concentrations of carbohydrate. The sodium concentrations of the fluids have also increased compared with previously available ORS.

The American Academy of Pediatrics (AAP) (45) recommends that oral solutions used for rehydration should contain 75–90 mEq/L of sodium. However, AAP recommends use of fluids containing 40–60 mEq/L of sodium for the prevention of dehydration or maintenance of hydration status (45). These lower sodium solutions more closely approximate the stool-sodium losses encountered in patients with viral diarrhea, which occurs commonly in the United States. Thus, there is a wide range of sodium content in commercially available products.

When fluids with greater than 60 mEq/L of sodium are used for maintenance, other low-sodium fluids, such as breast milk, diluted or undiluted infant formula, or water, need to be administered as well to prevent sodium overload.

The most widely used solutions in the United States, Pedialyte and Ricelyte, contain 45 and 50 mEq/L of sodium, respectively. These fluids are intended for maintenance of hydration and prevention of dehydration in clinical practice. Ricelyte has been used successfully for rehydration and maintenance therapy in one study; however, the effectiveness of Pedialyte for rehydration has not been studied. Although solutions with higher sodium concentrations (75–90 mEq/L) are preferable, Pedialyte, Ricelyte, and other similar low-sodium solutions can be used for rehydration when the alternative is physiologically inappropriate liquids or IV fluids. When the rate of purging is very high (e.g., greater than 10 ML/kg/hour), solutions with 75–90 mEq/L are recommended for rehydration.

OTHER FORMS OF ORS

Glucose-based ORS does not reduce the duration of illness or the volume of stool output. Early feeding, however, can reduce the severity, duration, and nutritional consequences of diarrhea. A perceived weakness of the glucose-based ORS is its inability to reduce the duration of illness or volume of stool output. Caretakers and practitioners frequently resort to multiple, costly, and often ill-advised therapies to reduce diarrhea. In the past decade, several attempts have been made to improve the standard WHO-ORS by adding other substrates or by replacing glucose with other ingredients. It is anticipated that such formulations will cause an improved clinical response. Many different substrates have been evaluated: sucrose (46–48), glycine (49–51), alanine (52), and, more recently, glutamine (53). Initial studies using glycine-based ORS found the formula superior to glucose-based ORS in efficiency of absorption and in reducing both stool volume and duration of diarrhea. This finding was replicated chiefly for diarrhea associated with cholera. However, in one study (50), the use of a glycine-based ORS predisposed patients to the development of hypernatremia.

With the use of glucose or amino acid substrates for sodium cotransport, there is a limit to the concentration of substrate that can be added. When the concentration of substrate in the solution is too high, then osmolar forces carry water into the gut lumen and exacerbate diarrhea. In contrast, cereal-based ORS contains large polymers that may not create an excessive osmotic load (54–58). Rice-based ORS, for instance, contains cooked rice powder instead of the glucose found in the WHO and other commercially available solutions. Complex carbohydrate molecules are slowly digested by intestinal enzymes and then absorbed as glucose; larger proteins in the cereals are digested and absorbed as smaller peptides and amino acids.

Ricelyte, a commercial preparation containing 30 g/L of rice-syrup solids, differs from a cereal-based solution in that the preparation contains only small glucose polymers derived from rice. In one study, the use of this solution, which differs from rice-based ORS in that it lacks whole rice, reduced stool output during the first 6 hours of therapy when compared with a standard, glucose-based solution (59). No differences in the duration of diarrhea or in total stool output were found, although stool output after 48 hours was not reported. Therefore, it is difficult to draw firm conclusions about the relative efficacy of Ricelyte in comparison with glucose-based ORS.

One advantage of cereal-based ORS, at least in developing countries, is that these solutions can be easily prepared in the home. However, the solutions require time and effort to prepare, and they can become contaminated if left unrefrigerated. Standardization of cereal-based solutions may prove difficult; in India, for example, several food-based solutions made by mothers revealed a wide range of sodium content and generally inadequate amounts of cereal base and glucose (60).

Clinical trials in developing countries have reported that cereal-based ORS reduces stool output and duration of diarrhea (54–58). Critical analysis of these studies, however, reveals that the quantity and quality of the maintenance diet often were not standardized, measured, or described adequately. Therefore, the possibility exists that variations in diet accounted for the differences in results. As discussed below, the practice of early feeding reduces the severity, duration, and nutritional consequences of diarrhea (61–63). In Egypt and Pakistan, large-scale, ongoing studies comparing cereal-based ORS with glucose-based ORS—in which all case-patients receive standardized, early feedings—will address the issue of the comparative efficacies of these two types of solutions.

Home Use of Oral Rehydration and Maintenance Solutions

Management of acute diarrhea should begin at home. Families with infants and small children should be encouraged to keep a supply of ORS at home at all times and use the solution when diarrhea first occurs in the child.

Ideally, management of acute diarrhea should begin at home, since effective early interventions can reduce complications, such as dehydration and poor nutrition. Thus, early home management will result in fewer office or emergency room visits, hospitalizations, and deaths. This type of management is best realized through support and education of mothers by health-care personnel at centers that use oral therapy. All families, particularly those in rural areas or poor urban neighborhoods where access to health care may be delayed, should be encouraged to have a supply of ORS in the home at all times, much in the same way that acetaminophen and syrup of ipecac are viewed as staples of the medicine chest. A recent conference on the household management of acute diarrhea (64) outlined several important points concerning the choice of an appropriate rehydration or maintenance fluid for home use. When diarrhea begins, a commercially available product can be administered at home. Alternatively, food-based fluids (e.g., cereals or gruels) or other plain fluids can be used to prevent dehydration. Regardless of the type of fluid used, an appropriate diet should be administered as well.

The most crucial aspect underlying home management of diarrhea is the need to administer increased volumes of appropriate fluids as well as to maintain adequate caloric intake. Medications, other treatments, or inappropriate home remedies should be avoided. Infants should be offered more frequent feedings at the breast or bottle, and children should also be given more fluids. Further research is needed to identify cultural, dietary, and educational factors that affect the home management of the child with diarrhea (65).

LIMITATIONS AND ADVANTAGES OF ORT

Although ORT is recommended for all age groups and for acute diarrhea caused by any etiologic agent, several limitations to its use exist.

Bloody Diarrhea

ORT is not sufficient therapy for some cases of bloody diarrhea (dysentery) since patients with bloody diarrhea may have a bacterial or parasitic infection requiring treatment with an antimicrobial agent. These patients need to seek medical care immediately.

Severe Dehydration

Patients in shock or near shock should be treated initially with IV solutions. Also, patients with intestinal ileus should not be given oral fluids until bowel sounds are audible.

Intractable Vomiting

Many patients with clinically significant acute diarrhea have concomitant vomiting. Nevertheless, greater than 90% can be successfully rehydrated or maintained with oral fluids when small volumes of ORS (5–10 mL) are administered every 1–2 minutes, with a gradual increase in the amount consumed. A frequent mistake is to allow a thirsty child to drink large volumes of ORS fluids (ad libitum) from a cup or a bottle; the caretaker should be instructed to administer ORS in small amounts via a spoon, syringe, cup, or feeding bottle. Continuous, slow nasogastric infusion of ORS via a feeding tube can be helpful for the child who is vomiting.

High Stool Output

Stool output greater than 10 mL/kg/hour is associated with a lower rate of success of oral rehydration (48), although these data are derived from a study performed among patients who had cholera. In general, no patient should be denied ORT simply because of a high purging rate, since most patients will respond well when administered adequate replacement fluid. In severely purging patients, subtle differences in substrate and electrolyte composition of oral solutions play a critical role in the success of therapy.

Monosaccharide Malabsorption

The presence of glucose or reducing substances in the stools, accompanied by a dramatic increase in stool output with the administration of ORS, is an indication of glucose malabsorption. The presence of stool-reducing substances alone is not sufficient to make the diagnosis, since this is a common finding among patients with diarrhea and does not indicate failure of oral therapy. Patients with true glucose malabsorption will show an immediate reduction in stool output when IV therapy is begun instead of oral therapy. The incidence of clinically evident glucose malabsorption during acute diarrhea is approximately 1%, although rates as high as 8% have been reported among selected populations (43). Malabsorption of lactose, maltose, and sucrose can also occur because of deficiencies of their respective enzymes or starvation associated with the lack of enzyme induction. Nonetheless, ORT is often the optimal method for the treatment of acute diarrhea. Its ability to be administered at home promotes earlier treatment and prevention of dehydration, as well as active involvement of parents in the medical care of their children. Oral fluid administration is safer and more physiologic than IV fluids, and the risks of phlebitis and IV infiltrates are avoided. Finally, the use of ORS with early feeding (discussed below) is not only safer, but more efficacious than IV therapy for the treatment of acute diarrhea.

DIETARY THERAPY OF ACUTE DIARRHEA

Although dehydration is the most serious direct effect of diarrhea, adverse nutritional consequences also can occur when nutritional management is not appropriate.

Acute diarrhea can endanger the nutritional status of affected children for the following reasons: (a) anorexia and food withdrawal interfere with adequate intake; (b) carbohydrates, fats, proteins, and micronutrients are often malabsorbed; (c) excess urinary and stool nitrogen losses are likely, even with subclinical infections; and (d) metabolic demands are generally higher with fever and systemic illness (66). The long-term effects of repeated gastrointestinal tract infections include growth failure and malnutrition (67–69) and possibly impaired cognitive development (70). The nutritional consequences of diarrheal illnesses among well-nourished children or adults in developed countries are less dramatic but have not been extensively investigated.

Reduced Oral Intake Versus Continued Feeding

Two opposing approaches to the nutritional management of acute diarrhea have been recommended (71). One approach favors reducing oral intake during illness to avoid diarrhea that occurs because of intestinal malabsorption, while the other approach favors continued feeding to avoid the nutritional consequences of fasting. The first approach, the tradition of "gut rest," still in wide practice, probably evolved from the observation that stool output was reduced in patients who fasted. However, fasting can reduce enterocyte renewal (72). Enteral nutrition stimulates intestinal cell renewal in several ways. In the short bowel syndrome, for example, villous hypertrophy and increased absorptive capability are stimulated by the direct effects of nutrients on the mucosa and by the nutrient-induced secretion of trophic hormones in the gastrointestinal tract (73). Further, intestinal permeability is increased in fasting (as opposed to fed) children with acute diarrhea (74). Thus, there are several theoretical reasons to avoid fasting.

Until recently, few controlled clinical trials had evaluated the dietary management of acute diarrhea. In one study in Arizona (61), well-nourished Apache infants were administered either a full-strength, lactose-free, soy-based formula immediately upon rehydration, or the infants were first fed ORS for 48 hours, then half-strength, lactose-free, soy-based formula for 24 hours, and finally administered a full-strength formula. Both the stool output and the duration of diarrhea were reduced by approximately 50% for infants who were administered full-strength, lactose-free, soy-based formula immediately after rehydration compared with the stool output and duration of illness for infants whose formula was gradually reintroduced. Similarly, in Peru (62), four different feeding regimens were compared in a group of 128 children ages 3–36 months with acute diarrhea. Two groups were administered a formula containing casein, sucrose, corn-syrup solids, and vegetable oil, either full- or half-strength; two other groups were administered either glucose-based ORS or IV fluids and then advanced to formula feeding. Stool output in the last two groups was noticeably lower than in the other groups for the first 48 hours. However, this difference disappeared when these groups were given food. Moreover, the duration of diarrhea and failure rates among all four groups were similar. More importantly, nitrogen balance, energy absorption, weight gain, and change in arm circumference and skinfold thickness were positively related to the level of dietary energy intake. These studies provide strong evidence for the recommendation that full-strength, lactose-free formulas can be safely introduced immediately after rehydration therapy and that such therapy can improve nutritional outcome as well as reduce stool output.

Lactose Malabsorption

Although recent data support the introduction of a full diet soon after rehydration, the content of this diet, especially for infants receiving most of their calories from milk-based formulas, is controversial. Acquired lactase deficiency, which is a reduction in the intestinal brush border enzyme responsible for lactose digestion, is frequently associated with diarrhea (75). One study reported that 88% of patients hospitalized with rotavirus diarrhea had evidence of lactose malabsorption (76). However, lactase deficiency must be distinguished from lactose malabsorption (a clinical diagnosis based on signs and symptoms of carbohydrate malabsorption), since many infants with lactase deficiency will not have clinical malabsorption.

Despite concerns about lactose malabsorption in breast-fed and bottle-fed children with diarrhea, continued breast-feeding or bottle-feeding during illness is clinically well-tolerated and advantageous. A study of breast-fed children selected at random to receive either ORS or ORS plus, who continued breast-feeding during the first 24 hours of hospital treatment, found that the breast-fed group had reduced stool output (63). The AAP recommends the gradual reintroduction of milk-based formulas in the management of acute diarrhea, beginning with diluted mixtures (45). This recommendation, however, is being reevaluated. Breast-feeding should continue immediately after rehydration.

Continuation of Regular Diet

Older children accustomed to eating a variety of table foods should continue receiving a regular diet; cereal-milk and cereal-legume diets have been used successfully for the dietary management of these children (77–79). Other recommended foods include starches (e.g., rice, potatoes, noodles, crackers, and bananas), cereals (e.g., rice, wheat, and oat cereals), soup, yogurt, vegetables, and fresh fruits. Foods to be avoided are those that are high in simple sugars, which can exacerbate diarrhea by osmotic effects. These foods include soft drinks, undiluted apple juice, Jell-O, and presweetened cereals. In addition, foods high in fat may not be tolerated because of their tendency to delay gastric emptying.

Although there have been no controlled trials concerning its efficacy, the "BRAT" diet (bananas, rice, applesauce, and toast) has long been used as a dietary-management tool among pediatric practices in the United States. To the extent that it includes starches and fruits, it is a reasonable dietary recommendation. However, prolonged use of the BRAT diet, or a protracted course of diluted formulas, can result in inadequate energy and protein content in the recovering child's diet.

PHARMACOLOGIC THERAPY OF ACUTE DIARRHEA

Antimicrobial agents and other drugs have limited usefulness in the management of acute diarrhea. Antimicrobial therapy of acute diarrhea varies depending on the etiologic agent. Since viral agents are the predominant cause of acute diarrhea, antimicrobial agents play only a limited role in case management. Certain diarrheal diseases, however, require appropriate drugs in addition to fluid and nutritional therapy. Identification of patients requiring antimicrobial therapy relies on clinical, epidemiologic, and laboratory evidence. For instance, bloody diarrhea or the presence of white blood cells on methylene blue stain of the stool specimen suggests a bacterial agent causing invasive mucosal damage and indicates that stool cultures should be performed to identify the organism. Other clinical clues suggesting a cause of infectious diarrhea amenable to antimicrobial therapy include a history of recent antibiotic use (in which case Clostridium difficile should be suspected), exposure to children in day care centers where Giardia or Shigella is prevalent, recent foreign travel, and immunodeficiency, in which infectious causes of diarrhea should be diligently evaluated. Conversely, watery diarrhea and vomiting in a child less than 2 years of age most likely represent viral gastroenteritis and therefore do not require antimicrobial therapy. A full discussion of antimicrobial therapy for gastrointestinal tract infections is found in other published reports (80–82). The use of nonspecific antidiarrheal agents such as adsorbents (e.g., kaolin-pectin), antimotility agents (e.g., loperamide), antisecretory drugs, or toxin binders (e.g., cholestyramine) is a common practice in many developed and developing countries (1). Despite the theoretical benefits from their use, available data do not demonstrate their effectiveness in reducing diarrhea volume or duration (80). For example, although stool consistency can be improved by binding agents, stool water losses are unchanged and electrolyte losses may increase (83, 84). Indeed, side effects of these drugs are well-known, including opiate-induced ileus, drowsiness and nausea due to atropine effects, and binding of nutrients and other drugs. One report from Pakistan detailed 18 cases of severe abdominal distention in association with use of loperamide, including at least six deaths (85). Another study reported that even in a controlled clinical setting, six of 28 patients administered loperamide experienced side effects (i.e., ileus, drowsiness) requiring discontinuation of therapy (86). In addition, reliance on antidiarrheal agents shifts the therapeutic focus away from appropriate fluid, electrolyte, and nutritional therapy; can interfere with oral therapy; and can unnecessarily add to the economic cost of the illness. Little evidence exists to support the use of nonspecific drug therapy in children, and much information exists to the contrary.

PRINCIPLES OF CASE MANAGEMENT

Clinical Assessment

Fever, vomiting, and loose stools are the common symptoms of acute gastroenteritis. Among infants and children, however, these can be the symptoms of many nongastrointestinal illnesses as well, including meningitis, bacterial sepsis, pneumonia, otitis media, and urinary tract infection. Vomiting alone can be the first symptom of metabolic disorders, congestive heart failure, toxic ingestions, or trauma. As such, a detailed history and physical examination are important in identifying acute gastroenteritis as a likely diagnosis when symptoms and signs are nonspecific and for ruling out other serious illnesses.

Besides a complete physical examination, an accurate body weight must be obtained. Auscultation for adequate bowel sounds is important before oral therapy is initiated. Visual examination of the stool can confirm abnormal consistency and determine the presence of blood or mucus.

Signs and symptoms of dehydration are crucial in guiding therapy. Infants with acute diarrhea are more apt to dehydrate than are older children because they have a higher body surface-to-weight ratio (i.e., somewhat high insensible loss/kg of body weight), have a higher metabolic rate, and are dependent on others for fluid (87). Although the most accurate assessment of fluid status is acute weight change, the patient's premorbid weight often is not known. The clinical signs and symptoms of mild dehydration (3%–5% fluid deficit) include increased thirst and slightly dry mucous membranes, whereas moderate dehydration (6%–9% fluid deficit) is associated with loss of skin turgor, tenting of skin when pinched, and dry mucous membranes (88). Signs and symptoms of severe dehydration (greater than or equal to 10% fluid deficit) are severe lethargy or altered state of consciousness, prolonged skin tenting and skin retraction time (greater than 2 seconds), cool and poorly perfused extremities, and decreased capillary refill. Rapid, deep breathing (a sign of acidosis), prolonged skin retraction time, and decreased perfusion are more reliably predictive of dehydration than sunken fontanelle or absence of tears (89). A good correlation has been reported between time of capillary refill and fluid deficit (90). However, fever, ambient temperature, and age can affect capillary refill time as well (91).

Supplementary laboratory studies in the assessment of the patient with acute diarrhea are rarely needed. However, serum electrolytes can be measured when the physician recognizes clinical signs or symptoms suggesting abnormal sodium or potassium concentrations. Stool cultures are indicated for dysentery (bloody diarrhea) but are not needed to initiate treatment in the usual case of acute watery diarrhea in the immunocompetent patient.

RECOMMENDATIONS FOR CASE MANAGEMENT

Successful case management of children with diarrhea depends on the principles of appropriate fluid, electrolyte, and nutritional therapy (92). Treatment of symptomatic and dehydrated children who seek medical evaluation should include two phases: rehydration and maintenance. In the rehydration phase, the fluid deficit should be replaced and clinical hydration attained. In the maintenance phase, adequate dietary and fluid intake should be maintained. In both phases, excess fluid losses must be replaced continuously.

Patient Assessment

The patient should be clinically evaluated to assess the degree of dehydration, as well as to rule out other medical conditions, and the patient's body weight should be measured.

Rehydration Therapy Based on Degree of Dehydration

For the mildly dehydrated patient (3%–5% fluid deficit), oral rehydration should commence with a fluid containing 50–90 mEq/L of sodium. The amount of fluid administered should be 50 mL/kg over a period of 2–4 hours. Using a teaspoon, syringe, or medicine dropper, the caregiver should initially provide small volumes of fluid (e.g., one teaspoon) and then gradually increase the amount, as tolerated. After 2–4 hours, hydration status should be reassessed. If the patient is rehydrated, treatment should progress to the maintenance phase of therapy (see below). If the patient is still dehydrated, the fluid deficit should be reestimated and rehydration therapy should begin again.

For the moderately dehydrated patient (6%–9% fluid deficit), ORS should be administered by the same procedures as used for the mildly dehydrated patient. The initial amount of fluid administered for rehydration should be increased to 100 mL/kg, administered over 2–4 hours.

Severe dehydration (greater than or equal to 10% fluid deficit, shock or near shock) constitutes a medical emergency. IV rehydration should begin immediately. Boluses (20 mL/kg) of Ringer's lactate solution, normal saline, or a similar solution should be administered until pulse, perfusion, and mental status return to normal. This treatment may require two IV lines or even alternate access sites (e.g., venous cutdown, femoral vein, intraosseous infusion). When the patient's level of consciousness returns to normal, he or she can take the remaining estimated deficit by mouth. As with less severely ill patients, hydration status should be assessed frequently to monitor the adequacy of replacement therapy.

For patients with acute diarrhea, but without signs of dehydration, the rehydration phase of therapy should be omitted and maintenance therapy started immediately.

Replacement of Ongoing Fluid Losses

During both rehydration and maintenance therapy, ongoing stool and vomit fluid losses must be replaced. If the patient is at a facility where such losses can be measured accurately, 1 mL of ORS should be administered for each gram of diarrheal stool. Alternatively, stool losses can be approximated by administering 10 mL/kg for each watery or loose stool passed, and 2 mL/kg of fluid should be administered for each episode of emesis. Excess fluid losses during maintenance therapy can be replaced with either low-sodium ORS (containing 40–60 mEq/L of sodium) or with ORS containing 75–90 mEq/L of sodium. When the latter type of fluid is used, an additional source of low-sodium fluid is recommended (e.g., breast milk, formula, or water).

Dietary Therapy

Recommendations for maintenance of dietary therapy depend on the age and dietary history of the patient.

Breast-fed infants should continue nursing on demand. For bottle-fed infants, full-strength, lactose-free, or lactose-reduced formulas should be administered immediately upon rehydration in amounts sufficient to satisfy energy and nutrient requirements. When such formulas are unavailable, full-strength, lactose-containing formulas should be used under supervision to assure that carbohydrate malabsorption does not complicate the clinical course. Alternatively, diluted, lactose-containing formulas can be used for the initial infant feedings; however, the concentration of formula should be increased rapidly. Patients with true lactose intolerance will have exacerbation of diarrhea when a lactose-containing formula is introduced. The presence of low pH (less than 6.0) or reducing substances (greater than 0.5%) in the stool in the absence of clinical symptoms is not diagnostic of lactose intolerance; this diagnosis is indicated by more severe diarrhea upon introduction of lactose-containing foods. If lactose intolerance occurs, appropriate therapy includes temporary reduction or removal of lactose from the diet.

Older children receiving semisolid or solid foods should continue to receive their usual diet during diarrhea. Recommended foods include starches, cereals, yogurt, fruits, and vegetables. Foods high in simple sugars and fats should be avoided. Despite the type of dietary regimen chosen, excess fluid losses via vomiting or diarrhea must be replaced with ORS as outlined above.

Drug Therapy

Neither antibiotics nor nonspecific antidiarrheal agents are usually indicated for acute diarrhea. Antibiotics should be considered when dysentery or a high fever is present, when watery diarrhea lasts for greater than 5 days, or when stool cultures, microscopy, or epidemic setting indicate an agent for which specific treatment is required.

Vomiting

In the child with vomiting, oral rehydration should proceed with small, frequent volumes at first (e.g., 5 mL every minute). Administration via a spoon or syringe—with close supervision—helps guarantee a gradual progression in the amount taken. Often, simultaneous correction of dehydration lessens the frequency of vomiting.

Home Management of Acute Diarrhea and Instructions to Parents

Early administration of ORS at home should proceed as described above, with stool and vomit fluid losses replaced with appropriate volumes of ORS and adequate dietary therapy administered. Education of parents and other caretakers should include the fluid and dietary principles noted above. Since morbidity and mortality from diarrhea in the United States usually occur in the first year of life, parents should be taught how to manage diarrhea and dehydration at the first newborn clinic visit or early during the first year of the child's life. Subsequent well-baby examinations should provide an opportunity to emphasize appropriate therapy as part of routine anticipatory guidance and nutritional counseling. During an acute illness, parents should be instructed to telephone or return to the clinic if the patient becomes irritable or lethargic, has decreased urine output, develops intractable vomiting, or has persistent diarrhea.

The management of diarrhea at home can be encouraged by physicians who care for children by supporting efforts to reduce the price and increase the insurance coverage of commercially available ORS. ORS should be available in every household, and a 24-hour supply of ORS should be provided to the parents of children with diarrhea upon clinic visits. Additional efforts regarding proper handwashing techniques, diaper changing practices, and hygiene can help prevent the spread of disease.

CONCLUSION

For many years, the treatment of acute diarrhea has proven that oral therapy, with a fluid-electrolyte solution for rehydration and maintenance, is simple and effective. More recently, the important coprinciple in case management of early refeeding of children immediately upon rehydration has also gained wider acceptance. The combination of oral rehydration and early nutritional support guides a patient through an episode of diarrhea safely and effectively. When the principles of therapy that are outlined are accepted by all levels of the U.S. medical community, and when education of parents includes instructions about how to begin ORT at home, then unnecessary hospitalizations and deaths can be prevented. Meanwhile, improvements in rehydration and maintenance solutions, vaccines, diapering practices, and food safety are anticipated that may help combat one of the most common public health problems of children.

REFERENCES: AS NUMBERED IN ORIGINAL PUBLICATION

 1. Claeson M, Merson MH. Global progress in the control of diarrheal diseases. Pediatr Infect Dis J 1990;9:345–345.
 7. Nalin DR. Nutritional benefits related to oral therapy: an overview. In: Bellanti JA, ed. Acute diarrhea: its nutritional consequences in children. Nestle Nutrition Workshop Series, Vol. 2. New York: Raven Press, 1983:185–190.
41. Santosham M, Foster S, Rousey DB, et al. Outpatient use of oral rehydration solutions in an Apache population: effect of instructions on preparation and contamination. J Pediatr Gastroenterol Nutr 1984;3:687–691.
42. Meyers A, Siegel B, Vinci B. Economic barriers to the use of oral rehydration therapy. JAMA 1991; 265:1724–1725.
43. Salazar-Lindo E, Sack RB, Chea-Woo E, et al. Bicarbonate versus citrate in oral rehydration therapy in infants with watery diarrhea: a controlled clinical trial. J Pediatr 1986;108:55–60.
44. Turnberg LA, Fordtran JS, Carter NW, et al. Mechanisms of bicarbonate absorption and its relationship to sodium transport in the human jejunum. J Clin Invest 1970;49:548–556.
45. American Academy of Pediatrics Committee on Nutrition. Use of oral fluid therapy and post-treatment feeding following enteritis in children in a developed country. Pediatrics 1985;75:358–361.
46. Nalin DR. Sucrose in oral therapy for cholera and related diarrheas. Lancet 1975;1:1400–1403.
47. Nalin DR, Levine MM, Mata L, et al. Comparison of sucrose with glucose in oral therapy of infant diarrhea. Lancet 1978;2:277–279.
48. Sack DA, Islam S, Brown KH, et al. Oral therapy in children with cholera: a comparison of sucrose and glucose electrolyte solutions. J Pediatr 1980;96:20–25.
49. Patra FC, Mahalanabis D, Jalan KN, et al. In search of a super solution: controlled trial of glycine-glucose oral rehydration solution in infantile diarrhea. Acta Paediatr Scand 1984;73:18–21.
50. Santosham M, Burns B, Reid R, et al. Glycine-based oral rehydration solution: reassessment of safety and efficacy. J Pediatr 1986;109:795–801.

51. Nalin DR, Cash RA, Rahman M, Yunus M. Effect of glycine and glucose on sodium and water absorption in patients with cholera. Gut 1970;11:768–771.
52. Patra FC, Sack DA, Islam A, et al. Oral rehydration formula containing alanine and glucose for treatment of diarrhea: a controlled trial. Br Med J 1989;298:1353–1356.
53. Rhoads JM, Keku EO, Quinn J, et al. L-glutamine stimulates jejunal sodium and chloride absorption in pig rotavirus enteritis. Gastroenterology 1991;100:683–691.
54. Molla AM, Sarker SA, Hussain M, et al. Rice-powder electrolyte solution as oral therapy in diarrhea due to Vibrio cholerae and Escherichia coli. Lancet 1982;1:1317–1319.
55. Patra FC, Mahalanabis D, Jalan KN, et al. Is oral rice electrolyte solution superior to glucose electrolyte solution in infantile diarrhea? Arch Dis Child 1982;57:910–912.
56. Santosham M, Fayad IM, Hashem M, et al. A comparison of rice-based oral rehydration solution and "early feeding" for the treatment of acute diarrhea in infants. J Pediatr 1990;116:868–875.
57. Molla AM, Ahmad SM, Greenough WB III. Rice-based oral rehydration solution decreases stool volume in acute diarrhea. Bull WHO 1985;63:751–756.
58. Elliott K, Attawell K, Wilson R, et al. Cereal-based oral rehydration therapy for diarrhea. Aga Khan Foundation and International Child Health Foundation, 1990.
59. Pizarro D, Posada G, Sandi L, Moran JB. Rice-based oral electrolyte solutions for the management of infantile diarrhea. N Engl J Med 1991;324:517–521.
60. Rolston DDK, Mathew P, Mathan VI. Food-based solutions are a viable alternative to glucose-electrolyte solutions for oral hydration in acute diarrhea—studies in a rat model of secretory diarrhea. Trans R Soc Trop Med Hyg 1990;84:156–159.
61. Santosham M, Foster S, Reid R, et al. Role of soy-based, lactose-free formula during treatment of acute diarrhea. Pediatrics 1985;76:292–298.
62. Brown KH, Gastanaduy AS, Saavedra JM, et al. Effect of continued oral feeding on clinical and nutritional outcomes of acute diarrhea in children. J Pediatr 1988;112:191–200.
63. Khin-Maung U, Wai N, Myo-Khin, Mu-Mu-Khin, Tin U, Thane-Toe. Effect on clinical outcome of breast feeding during acute diarrhea. Br Med J 1985;290:587–589.
64. Household Management of Diarrhea and Acute Respiratory Infections. Report of a scientific meeting at the Johns Hopkins School of Hygiene and Public Health in collaboration with the United Nations Children's Fund and the Diarrheal Diseases and Acute Respiratory Infections Control Programmes of the World Health Organization. Occasional Paper No. 12. November 1990.
65. Snyder JD, Molla AM, Cash RA. Home-based therapy for diarrhea. J Pediatr Gastroenterol Nutr 1990;11:438–447.
66. Lifshitz F. Interrelationship of diarrhea and infant nutrition. In: Lebenthal E, ed. Textbook of gastroenterology and nutrition in infancy. 2nd ed. New York: Raven Press Ltd., 1989:659.
67. Black RE, Brown KH, Becker S. Effects of diarrhea associated with specific enteropathogens on the growth of children in rural Bangladesh. Pediatrics 1984;173:799–805.
68. Martorell R, Habicht J-P, Yarbrough C, et al. Acute morbidity and physical growth in rural Guatemalan children. Am J Dis Child 1975;129:1296–1301.
69. Rowland MGM, Cole TJ, Whitehead RG. A quantitative study into the role of infection in determining nutritional status in Gambian village children. Br J Nutr 1977;37:441–450.
70. Galler J, Ramsey F, Soliman G, et al. The influence of early malnutrition on subsequent behavioral development: 1. Degree of impairment in intellectual performance. J Am Acad Child Adolesc Psychiatry 1983;22:8.
71. Brown KH, MacLean WC Jr. Nutritional management of acute diarrhea: an appraisal of the alternatives. Pediatrics 1984;73:119–125.
72. Brown HO, Levine ML, Lipkin M. Inhibition of intestinal cell renewal and migration induced by starvation. Am J Physiol 1963;205:868–872.
73. Vanderhoof JA. Short bowel syndrome. In: Lebenthal E, ed. Textbook of gastroenterology and nutrition in infancy. 2nd ed. New York: Raven Press Ltd., 1989:794.
74. Isolauri E, Juntunen M, Wiren S, et al. Intestinal permeability changes in acute gastroenteritis: effects of clinical factors and nutritional management. J Pediatr Gastroenterol Nutr 1989;8:466–473.
75. Sunshine P, Kretchmer N. Studies of small intestine during development. III. Infantile diarrhea associated with intolerance to disaccharides. Pediatrics 1964;34:38–50.
76. Davidson GP, Goodwin D, Robb TA. Incidence and duration of lactose malabsorption in children hospitalized with acute enteritis: study in a well-nourished urban population. J Pediatr 1984;105:587–590.
77. Brown KH. Dietary management of acute childhood diarrhea: optimal timing of feeding and appropriate use of milks and mixed diets. J Pediatr 1991;118:S92–S98.
78. Brown KH, Perez F, Gastanaduy AS. Clinical trial of modified whole milk, lactose-hydrolyzed whole milk, or cereal-milk mixtures for the dietary management of acute childhood diarrhea. J Pediatr Gastroenterol Nutr 1991;12:340–350.
79. Alarcon P, Montoya R, Perez F, et al. Clinical trial of home available, mixed diets versus a lactose-free, soy-protein formula for the dietary management of acute childhood diarrhea. J Pediatr Gastroenterol Nutr 1991;12:224–232.
80. Pickering LK. Therapy for acute infectious diarrhea in children. J Pediatr 1991;118:S118–S128.
81. American Academy of Pediatrics. Report of the Committee on Infectious Diseases (Red Book). 22nd ed. 1991.

82. World Health Organization. The rational use of drugs in the management of acute diarrhea in children. Geneva: WHO, 1990.
83. Portnoy BL, DuPont HL, Pruitt D, et al. Antidiarrheal agents in the treatment of acute diarrhea in children. JAMA 1976;236:844–846.
84. McClung HJ, Beck RD, Powers P. The effect of a kaolin-pectin adsorbent on stool losses of sodium, potassium, and fat during a lactose-intolerant diarrhea in rats. J Pediatr 1980;96:769–771.
85. Bhutta TI, Tahir KI. Loperamide poisoning in children. Lancet 1990;335:363.
86. Motala C, Hill ID, Mann MD, Bowie MD. Effect of loperamide on stool output and duration of acute infectious diarrhea in infants. J Pediatr 1990;117:467–471.
87. Kooh EW, Metcoff J. Physiologic considerations in fluid and electrolyte therapy with particular reference to diarrheal dehydration in children. J Pediatr 1963;62:107–131.
88. Santosham M, Brown KH, Sack RB. Oral rehydration therapy and dietary therapy for acute childhood diarrhea. Pediatr Rev 1987;8:273–278.
89. Mackenzie A, Barnes G, Shann F. Clinical signs of dehydration in children. Lancet 1989;2:605–607.
90. Saavedra JM, Harris GD, Li S, Finberg L. Capillary refilling (skin turgor) in the assessment of dehydration. Am J Dis Child 1991;145:296–298.
91. Schriger DL, Baraff L. Defining normal capillary refill: variation with age, sex, and temperature. Ann Emerg Med 1988;17:932–935.
92. Santosham M, Greenough WB III. Oral rehydration therapy: a global perspective. J Pediatr 1991;118:S44–S51.

Salmonella enteritis Infection

Original Citation: Salmonella enteritis Infection—National Center for Infectious Diseases, Division of Bacterial and Mycotic Diseases, 1992.

SALMONELLA ENTERITIDIS INFECTION

Egg-associated salmonellosis is an important public health problem in the United States and several European countries. A bacterium, Salmonella enteritidis, can be inside perfectly normal-appearing eggs, and if the eggs are eaten raw or undercooked, the bacterium can cause illness. During the 1980s, illness related to contaminated eggs occurred most frequently in the northeastern United States, but now illness caused by S. enteritidis is increasing in other parts of the country as well. Consumers should be aware of the disease and learn how to minimize the chances of becoming ill.

A person infected with the Salmonella enteritidis bacterium usually has fever, abdominal cramps, and diarrhea beginning 12 to 72 hours after consuming a contaminated food or beverage. The illness usually lasts 4 to 7 days, and most persons recover without antibiotic treatment. However, the diarrhea can be severe, and the person may be ill enough to require hospitalization.

The elderly, infants, and those with impaired immune systems may have a more severe illness. In these patients, the infection may spread from the intestines to the blood stream, and then to other body sites and can cause death unless the person is treated promptly with antibiotics.

How Eggs Become Contaminated

Most types of Salmonella live in the intestinal tracts of animals and birds and are transmitted to humans by contaminated foods of animal origin. Stringent procedures for cleaning and inspecting eggs were implemented in the 1970s and have made salmonellosis caused by external fecal contamination of egg shells extremely rare. However, unlike eggborne salmonellosis of past decades, the current epidemic is due to intact and disinfected grade A eggs. The reason for this is that Salmonella enteritidis silently infects the ovaries of healthy appearing hens and contaminates the eggs before the shells are formed.

Although most infected hens have been found in the northeastern United States, the infection also occurs in hens in other areas of the country. In the Northeast, approximately one in 10,000 eggs may be internally contaminated. In other parts of the United States, contaminated eggs appear less common. Only a small number of hens seem to be infected at any given time, and an infected hen can lay many normal eggs while only occasionally laying an egg contaminated with the Salmonella bacterium.

Who Can Be Infected

Healthy adults and children are at risk for egg-associated salmonellosis, but the elderly, infants, and persons with impaired immune systems are at increased risk for serious illness. In these persons, a relatively small number of Salmonella bacteria can cause severe illness. Most of the deaths caused by Salmonella enteritidis have occurred among the elderly in nursing homes. Egg-containing dishes prepared for any of these high-risk persons in hospitals, in nursing homes, in restaurants, or at home should be thoroughly cooked and served promptly.

What is the Risk

In affected parts of the United States, we estimate that one in 50 average consumers could be exposed to a contaminated egg each year. If that egg is thoroughly cooked, the Salmonella organisms will be destroyed and will not make the person sick. Many dishes made in restaurants or commercial or institutional kitchens, however, are made from pooled eggs. If 500 eggs are pooled, one batch in 20 will be contaminated and everyone who eats eggs from that batch is at risk. A healthy person's risk for infection by Salmonella enteritidis is low, even in the northeastern United States, if individually prepared eggs are properly cooked, or foods are made from pasteurized eggs.

What You Can Do to Reduce Risk

Eggs, like meat, poultry, milk, and other foods, are safe when handled properly. Shell eggs are safest when stored in the refrigerator, individually and thoroughly cooked, and promptly consumed. The larger the number of Salmonella present in the egg, the more likely it is to cause illness. Keeping eggs adequately refrigerated prevents any Salmonella present in the eggs from growing to higher numbers, so eggs should be held refrigerated until they are needed. Cooking reduces the number of bacteria present in an egg; however, an egg with a runny yolk still poses a greater risk than a completely cooked egg. Undercooked egg whites and yolks have been associated with outbreaks of Salmonella enteritidis infections. Both should be consumed promptly and not be held in the temperature range of 40 degrees to 140 degrees for more than 2 hours.

Reducing the Risk of Salmonella Enteritidis Infection

- Keep eggs refrigerated.
- Discard cracked or dirty eggs.
- Wash hands and cooking utensils with soap and water after contact with raw eggs.
- Eat eggs promptly after cooking.
- Do not keep eggs warm for more than 2 hours.
- Refrigerate unused or leftover egg-containing foods.
- Avoid eating raw eggs (as in homemade ice cream or eggnog). Commercially manufactured ice cream and eggnog are made with pasteurized eggs and have not been linked with Salmonella enteritidis infections.
- Avoid restaurant dishes made with raw or undercooked, unpasteurized eggs. Restaurants should use pasteurized eggs in any recipe (such as Hollandaise sauce or Caesar salad dressing) that calls for pooling of raw eggs.

What Else is Being Done

Government agencies and the egg industry have taken steps to reduce Salmonella enteritidis outbreaks. These steps include the difficult task of identifying and removing infected flocks from the egg supply and increasing quality assurance and sanitation measures.

The Centers for Disease Control has advised state health departments, hospitals, and nursing homes of specific measures to reduce Salmonella enteritidis infection. Some states now require refrigeration of eggs from the producer to the consumer. The U.S. Department of Agriculture is testing the breeder flocks that produce egg-laying chickens to ensure that they are free of Salmonella enteritidis. Eggs from known infected commercial flocks will be pasteurized instead of being sold as grade A shell eggs. The U.S. Food and Drug Administration has issued guidelines for handling eggs in retail food establishments and will be monitoring infection in laying hens.

Research by these agencies and the egg industry is addressing the many unanswered questions about Salmonella enteritidis, the infections in hens, and contaminated eggs. Informed consumers, food-service establishments, and public and private organizations are working together to reduce, and eventually eliminate, disease caused by this infectious organism.

Viral Agents of Gastroenteritis: Public Health Importance and Outbreak Management

Original Citation: Viral Agents of Gastroenteritis: Public Health Importance and Outbreak Management. MMWR 1990;39(RR-5):1–24.

SUMMARY

Each year, infectious gastroenteritis causes greater than 210,000 children in the United States to be hospitalized and 4–10 million children to die worldwide. Since the mid-1970s, knowledge has increased dramatically concerning the viral agents that are responsible for much of this public health burden. Rotavirus, the most common cause of diarrhea among children, infects virtually every child in the United States by the age of 4 years and causes potentially lethal dehydration in 0.75% of children less than 2 years of age. Other recently identified pathogens include the enteric adenoviruses, calicivirus, astrovirus, and the Norwalk family of agents. Conclusive diagnosis of these viruses requires electron microscopic examination of stool specimens, a laboratory technique that is available only at a few large centers, including CDC. Stool samples from an outbreak that are submitted to CDC for detection of viral pathology should be collected in bulk from 10 ill persons during their first 48 hours of illness, while feces are still liquid, and should be stored at 4°C (not frozen). Acute- and convalescent-phase serum samples should be collected from the same persons, plus from an equal number of controls, during the first week of illness and 3 weeks thereafter. Control measures for outbreaks of viral gastroenteritis should focus on the removal of an ongoing common source of infection (e.g., an ill food handler or the contamination of a water supply) and on the interruption of person-to-person transmission that can perpetuate an outbreak in a population after the common source has been removed. Because improvements in environmental hygiene may not be accompanied by reductions of endemic diarrhea caused by viruses, immunization may play an important role in future control; vaccine trials for rotavirus are in progress. In anticipation of vaccine development and use, CDC recently began national surveillance for the viral agents of gastroenteritis. Health-care facilities involved in the detection of rotavirus or the other viral agents of diarrhea can participate.

METHODS OF VIRAL DETECTION

Antigen Detection

Commercial antigen-detection kits for rotavirus are widely available, inexpensive, and permit rapid viral diagnosis. Only small amounts of stool are required for the tests, and samples may be frozen before testing. Kits vary widely in range of sensitivities (70%–100%) and specificities (50%–100%) (64, 65). Newborns and breast-feeding children have particularly high false-positive rates. Such kits are most useful for childhood diarrhea during the normal rotavirus season; they have less diagnostic value in situations in which rotavirus is probably rare, as in community outbreaks involving adults or in outbreaks of pediatric diarrhea outside the rotavirus season. Confirmatory testing should be performed in any case in which rotavirus disease would be unusual (e.g., among children in the summer or among adults at any time) as well as periodically to validate the reliability of the assay employed.

A commercial kit for enteric adenoviruses is also available, but because adenoviral diarrhea affects mainly children less than 2 years of age and because outbreaks involving adults have never been reported, the diagnostic value outside the preschool-age group is also limited.

Antigen-detection systems have been used for research on calicivirus, Norwalk, Snow Mountain agent, and astrovirus. Rapid assays for these and other agents are under development at the Viral Gastroenteritis Section, REB, DVRD, CID, CDC. Such techniques would allow the testing of large numbers of samples in a short period of time, an essential condition for determining the contribution of specific viruses to the incidence of diarrhea among populations and for identifying an etiologic agent during an outbreak.

Antibody Detection

Persons infected with a viral agent of gastroenteritis will usually have a rise in antibodies to that virus.

For the Norwalk agent (the most commonly identified agent of outbreaks involving persons greater than 4 years of age), approximately half of adult Americans have preexisting IgG antibodies to the virus, so that a single specimen is insufficient to document recent infection. But if at least half of affected persons in an outbreak have a fourfold rise in specific antibody titers, the Norwalk agent can be designated as etiologic. Titers may begin to rise by the fifth day after onset of symptoms, peak at approximately the third week, and often begin to fall by the sixth week. Hence, the acute-phase serum should be drawn within the first week and the convalescent-phase serum during the third to sixth weeks. Diagnostic assays for IgM and IgA antibodies to Norwalk virus have been used on an experimental basis (66, 67).

One disadvantage of serologic diagnosis is that patients are often reluctant to have serum drawn a month after a brief, self-limited illness. Furthermore, because this class of viruses cannot be cultivated, the supply of antigen for antibody testing is limited to a few research laboratories and cannot be offered for routine screening. In addition, antibodies can be detected to the Norwalk virus only, not the full spectrum of Norwalk-like agents that may cause disease. In a survey of 100 gastroenteritis outbreaks thought to be of viral origin submitted to CDC from 1985 to 1988, the Norwalk agent was identified by antibody rise (i.e., half or more of the persons showed a fourfold rise) in approximately 20% of outbreaks. Approximately 40% showed partial rises (less than half of the persons with a fourfold rise), suggesting that an antigenically related agent may have been involved. The remaining 40% showed no titer rises at all, indicating that an agent completely distinct from Norwalk virus caused the outbreak (68).

Adequate supplies of antigen are essential to any virus-testing system. Although rotavirus and astrovirus have been cultivated, the Norwalk family of viruses has proved resistant, and it may be several years before a panel of molecular diagnostic assays for known enteric viruses is available.

Electron Microscopy

Under an electron microscope, a virus can be identified by its characteristic morphology in a stool specimen. The technique is highly specific but requires substantial resources. Since an electron microscope scans a field of approximately 1 millionth of a milliliter, there must be at least 1 million viruses/milliliter of stool for a detection to be made. Such levels of excretion are normally present only during the first 48 hours of viral diarrhea.

With a specialized technique called immune electron microscopy (IEM), the sensitivity of normal transmission electron microscopy can be improved 10–100 times. In one technique, the grid to be examined is coated with convalescent-phase serum before the stool specimen is applied; a high titer of virus-specific antibody tends to hold aggregates of homologous virus in the field, thereby enhancing diagnostic yield. Because reagents are scarce, this technique for diagnosing viral gastroenteritis is limited to a few centers in the United States.

Other Techniques

Culture

Rotavirus, enteric adenoviruses, and astrovirus can be cultured in research centers, but the techniques are not well suited for routine diagnosis. The other known major viral enteric pathogens cannot yet be cultivated. Enteroviruses can be cultivated but are not thought to be important causes of diarrhea.

Electropherotyping

Rotavirus multiplies in the gut with such efficacy that, during infection, its genome dominates the ribonucleic acid (RNA) content of stool. When this RNA is extracted from stool and run on a gel, an electric field will cause the separate rotavirus genes to migrate in characteristic patterns. The presence of these patterns is diagnostic of rotaviral infection, and pattern variations provide insight into strain differences. Sensitivity is comparable with antigen detection (greater than 90% in the first few days of illness), and specificity is 100%; in addition, atypical rotaviruses (Groups B and C) can be detected, which is not possible with antigen-detection systems for rotavirus A. Electropherotyping has long been used as the principal diagnostic technique for rotavirus in many nations, but in the United States it is used mainly as a research tool.

Hybridization Probes

Dot-hybridization assays have been developed for rotavirus that are considerably more sensitive than conventional antigen-detection techniques and at least equally specific (69, 70), but they are currently available in only a few research centers. Hybridization assays have also been developed for adenoviruses, but they are less sensitive than antigen-detection techniques (26).

Polymerase Chain Reaction (PCR)

Enzymatic amplification of a viral gene to raise its concentration in a specimen to the level of detectability would represent an ideal diagnostic technique for viral gastroenteritis, because at present agents can be identified only when they are excreted at maximal levels (millions of viruses/milliliter of stool). The development of PCR reagents, however, requires cloning and sequencing of viral genes. Cloning and sequencing have been accomplished only with rotavirus, but PCR techniques are being actively developed for the other agents.

ENDEMIC CONTROL

Although essential in outbreak management, improved environmental hygiene (i.e., food, water, and sanitation) may be ineffective in endemic control of some of the known viral agents of gastroenteritis (e.g., rotavirus), perhaps because person-to-person transmission is the principal mechanism for the spread of infection. As a result, the population-based attack rate for these agents is thought to be the same (100%) in developed and developing countries, although disease caused by known agents tends to be acquired earlier in developing countries. The risk of death is highest in areas where medical care is least available and malnutrition is most prevalent.

Vaccines may prove to be the most effective method of endemic control. Because rotavirus is the leading cause of diarrheal mortality in the world and because natural infection appears to induce lifetime immunity, rotavirus has been the main focus of efforts at vaccine development: within 10 years of its discovery in 1973, trials were already under way. Although four major serotypes affect humans, three prototype vaccines have each been of a single serotype, and the results have been inconsistent (71–75). These inconsistencies have been ascribed by some investigators to differences between the vaccine serotype and the strain of rotavirus in the community. A large, multicenter, 2-year, efficacy trial of a vaccine that incorporates all four major serotypes that affect humans is now under way in the United States.

The endemic disease incidence and the nature of immunity for the other viruses is less well defined, and vaccine development for them must await advances in knowledge of their epidemiology and molecular virology.

ENVIRONMENTAL PROTECTION

Although person-to-person transmission is an important aspect of endemic disease, the initiating event for most outbreaks of viral gastroenteritis is contamination of a common source. In contrast to bacterial pathogens, enteric viruses cannot multiply outside their host; hence, the original inoculum into the common source determines infectivity.

Food

Shellfish

Shellfish that grow in fecally contaminated water concentrate enteric viruses in their tissues, and even harvests meeting bacteriologic standards of hygiene may contain viral agents. In addition, depuration (a technique in which shellfish are flushed with clean water treated with ultraviolet light) is less effective in viral than in bacterial decontamination (76). Finally, steaming for as long as 10 minutes may fail to inactivate all viral agents (77). Although boiling shellfish will inactivate viruses, such preparation is not popular with consumers.

The difficulties of assuring virus-free shellfish and the common preference for eating them raw have contributed to their prominent role in gastroenteritis outbreaks. Approximately 50% of Norwalk-confirmed foodborne outbreaks reported to CDC from 1976 to 1980 involved shellfish (52). A continent-wide epidemic of gastroenteritis in Australia in 1978 was attributed to oysters (78). Shellfish were implicated in 103 outbreaks of viral gastroenteritis in New York State in 1982, and similar outbreaks have occurred in the Northeast since then (79). Of 13 outbreaks of Norwalk virus documented in Britain during the period 1984–1985, seven were related to shellfish (57).

Ill Food Handlers

When foods other than shellfish are implicated in viral gastroenteritis outbreaks, the contamination has usually taken place near the point of consumption. An ill food handler was identified in nine of the 15 documented Norwalk outbreaks reported to CDC from 1985 to 1988 for which adequate epidemiologic data were available (CDC, unpublished data). Foods that require handling and no subsequent cooking (e.g., salads) constitute the greatest risk. Among Norwalk-confirmed foodborne outbreaks from 1976 to 1980 that were not attributable to shellfish, salad was the most commonly implicated food (52).

Other Aspects of Foodborne Transmission

The long list of foods implicated in outbreaks of viral gastroenteritis reflects the variety of foods that are handled by food-service personnel and the low infectious dose (10–100 particles) of most viral agents of gastroenteritis, rather than peculiar viral tropisms. In contrast to the factors important in amplifying bacterial contamination, practices such as leaving foods unrefrigerated or warming them for prolonged periods are not direct risk factors for increased viral transmission because the viruses do not multiply outside the human host. Such practices, however, may be indicators of poor food hygiene in general.

The Norwalk agent can remain infective even if frozen for years or heated to 60°C for 30 minutes (80); however, cooking temperatures at boiling or above are probably adequate to inactivate Norwalk and most other enteric viral pathogens.

Water

Outbreaks of viral gastroenteritis have been associated with various sources of contaminated water, including municipal water, well water, stream water, commercial ice, lake water, and pool water.

The most recent U. S. Environmental Protection Agency guidelines (June 29, 1989) for municipal water systems recommend residual chlorine concentrations of greater than or equal to 0.2 milligrams/liter (mg/L) (81), and in many localities peak levels of 5 mg/L are administered. Studies have documented that the Norwalk agent can remain highly infective despite 30-minute exposure to concentrations of chlorine as high as 6.25 mg/L, and levels of 10 mg/L appear necessary to inactivate it (82). This resistance may explain why the Norwalk agents are prominent in outbreaks of waterborne disease. Of 96 waterborne outbreaks with sufficient data reported to CDC from 1976 to 1979, 23% met epidemiologic criteria of a Norwalk virus outbreak (83), and subsequent surveillance data on waterborne outbreaks have been consistent with this finding. Of 38 serologically confirmed Norwalk virus outbreaks between 1976 and 1980, 13 were waterborne (52). Rotavirus, for which only one waterborne outbreak has been documented in the United States, is more sensitive to chlorine than the Norwalk agent and is inactivated by a 30-minute exposure to 3.75 mg/L (82). All viral agents of gastroenteritis are thought to be inactivated by boiling for 10 minutes.

Surfaces

Because rotavirus can survive for several days on nonporous materials in conditions of low temperature and humidity, fomites may contribute to its nosocomial transmission (84). A recent study of a Norwalk viral outbreak on a cruise ship implicated toilets shared between staterooms as a risk factor for infection, suggesting that surfaces contaminated by Norwalk particles from spattered or aerosolized material may play a role in transmission of Norwalk-like viruses (85). Data are lacking on the efficacy of disinfectants against Norwalk-like agents, but a number of germicidal chemicals have been shown in laboratory tests to be ineffective in reducing rotavirus activity (86–88). However, detergents do inactivate rotavirus (89) and should be used for laundering fecally contaminated linens and clothing. Thorough cleaning of environmental surfaces is required, as a minimum, to control spread of the viral agents of gastroenteritis.

Hands

Hands that have been contaminated directly or from surfaces may be the most important means by which enteric viruses are transmitted. Because the active ingredients in some commercial handwashing preparations are ineffective against rotavirus (90), the use of special handwashing products is not indicated. Vigorous handwashing with soap, performed consistently at appropriate intervals, is necessary to control the spread of all enteric pathogens.

Aerosols

Aerosolized or splattered Norwalk-like particles have been implicated in the transmission of gastroenteritis (91). Aerosolized rotavirus has caused diarrheal illness in mice (92), and airborne transmission of this agent among humans has been suspected. Studies are needed to address the efficacy of barrier precautions (e.g., face shields, respirators) in interrupting transmission of these agents.

Zoonoses

Nearly all the agents of viral gastroenteritis in humans have related strains that can cause diarrhea in animal species. But these strains appear to be highly host-specific, and zoonotic transmission has not been documented as having an important role in human disease, either endemically or in outbreaks (93).

TREATMENT

For most humans, viral gastroenteritis is a self-limited illness of a few days' duration, with virus replication restricted to the mucosa of the gut. The main risk is of dehydration and electrolyte imbalance.

Children, in whom the risk of fluid loss is greatest, respond well to oral rehydration therapy (ORT). Hospitalization and treatment with intravenous fluids are required only for cases in which dehydration is severe, or in which the parent or caretaker cannot provide adequate oral rehydration. Analysis of geographic and demographic patterns of diarrheal mortality in the United States suggests that lack of access to medical care, rather than disease virulence, is a principal risk factor for death from gastroenteritis (2). Although infants with diarrhea may manifest subsequent mild lactose intolerance (often 10–14 days for rotavirus infection) (94), most infants completely recover. Breast milk may have a protective effect against bacterial or viral enteric infection, and most infants can be "fed through" an episode (95).

For adults, maintenance of good hydration is also important, particularly among the elderly and those receiving diuretic medication. In one study, bismuth subsalicylate reduced duration of Norwalk infection from 27 to 20 hours (96).

OUTBREAK CONTROL MEASURES

Most outbreaks of viral gastroenteritis are self-limited; however, certain factors create risks of intense or prolonged transmission that may require aggressive intervention. These risk factors include a closed environment (e.g., nursing home), a constantly renewing population of susceptible persons (e.g., children at camp), or persons at special risk (e.g., the elderly). Whatever the initial source of the outbreak, subsequent viral transmission is often person-to-person, with both direct fecal-oral and airborne transport probably involved. Although interruption of this transmission may be difficult, the following measures may be helpful in controlling the spread of infection.

Identify and Eliminate a Common Source

For Norwalk virus outbreaks, an ill food handler is a likely source, although water, ice, and shellfish are other common sources. When a water supply is thought to be contaminated with Norwalk virus, shock chlorine concentrations (greater than or equal to 10 mg/L for 30 minutes or longer) may be helpful.

Prevent Employee Transmission of Illness

In many settings, employees (e.g., health-care providers, staff of day-care centers) are at highest risk for transmitting disease because of their many contacts with ill persons. Any staff member with symptoms that suggest infection should be excluded from contact with potentially susceptible persons for at least 2 days after resolution of illness. This exclusion is particularly important for food handlers, who also should not be involved in preparing food for the same period.

Prevent Employee Acquisition of Illness

Personnel coming into direct contact with ill persons should wear disposable plastic gloves. When contamination of clothing with fecal material is possible, personnel should also wear gowns. Hands, which are the most likely means by which viral spread occurs, should be washed after each contact. The recommended procedure is to rub all surfaces of lathered hands together vigorously for at least 10 seconds, with plain soap or an antimicrobial-containing product, and then thoroughly rinse the hands under a stream of water. Since spattering or aerosols of infectious material may be involved in disease transmission, wearing of masks should be considered, particularly by persons who clean areas grossly contaminated by feces or vomitus.

Use Safeguards with Laundry

Soiled linens and clothes should be handled as little as possible and with minimum agitation to prevent microbial contamination of the air and of persons handling the linen. Laundry should be transported in an enclosed and sanitary manner (e.g., in a plastic bag if the laundry is wet or moist), promptly machine washed with a detergent in water at the maximum cycle length, and then machine dried (109).

Clean Soiled Surfaces

Because environmental surfaces in certain settings have been implicated in the transmission of enteric viruses, bathrooms and rooms occupied by ill persons should be kept visibly clean on a routine basis. Surfaces that have been soiled, especially by feces or vomitus, should first be cleaned of visible material and then disinfected with an appropriate commercial germicidal product according to the manufacturer's instructions. Feces and vomitus collected during the cleaning procedure should be promptly disposed of in a manner that prevents transfer of this material to other surfaces or persons. Persons performing these tasks should wear appropriate protective barriers (e.g., utility gloves—and if splashing is anticipated, a mask or face shield and garments such as a uniform, jumpsuit, or gown to protect street clothing).

Minimize Contact Between Well and Ill Persons

When possible, ill persons should be separated from well persons until at least 2 days after resolution of symptoms. If nosocomial rotavirus is involved, this period should be longer—at least until the ill person's stool is negative by antigen detection, which may be greater than or equal to 1 week. In certain settings (e.g., camp, cruise ship, or nursing home), the clinic may function as a focus of transmission; persons with complaints of gastroenteritis should be seen by medical care personnel in the patient's living quarters, or at least in a separate area of the clinic.

Stop Renewal of Susceptible Population

In situations in which the epidemic is extended by periodic renewal of the susceptible population (e.g., camps and cruise ships), consideration may have to be given to interrupting this process until the outbreak has ended completely.

SPECIMEN COLLECTION DURING OUTBREAKS

Electron microscopy is necessary for complete viral diagnosis of an outbreak of gastroenteritis. Most of the electron microscopes in the United States are devoted to research or fee-related clinical diagnostic activity. Very few state laboratories have electron microscopes that can be used in the evaluation of outbreaks. Consequently, many state and local health departments submit outbreak specimens to CDC. Because of advances in the field of viral diagnostics, recommendations for specimen collection have changed substantially, and many investigators in the field may not be aware of these changes.

The following guidelines are designed to help outbreak investigators make the best use of CDC's viral laboratory facilities. Proper specimen collection is also critical for the diagnosis of bacterial and parasitic causes of gastroenteritis (see Appendix).

Guidelines for Collecting Specimens for Viral Diagnosis

Stool

- Collection in the first 48 hours. Presently, viral diagnosis of a stool sample can be made only when the level of excretion is approximately 1 million particles/ml. For many viruses, this level of excretion is present only during the first 2 days of illness, and occasionally during the third. If specimens are not collected during the first 2–3 days of illness, an agent is unlikely to be detected. Thus, appropriate specimens should be collected as soon as an outbreak occurs. Specimen collection should not await the results of epidemiologic and other investigations, since delay will almost certainly preclude a viral diagnosis. If information gathered subsequently indicates that a viral etiology is unlikely, the specimens can be discarded before the cost of testing is incurred.
- Ten diarrheal bulk specimens. Bulk samples (enough to fill a large stool cup) are preferred, and only those specimens loose enough to assume the shape of their containers are likely to yield positive results. Serial specimens from persons with acute, frequent, high-volume diarrhea are particularly useful. The smaller the specimen and the more formed the stool, the lower the diagnostic yield. Rectal swabs are of little or no value. Specimens from at least 10 ill persons should be collected to maximize the chance that a diagnosis can be made. (The diagnostic yield is low when specimens from less than 10 persons are submitted.)
- Storage at +4°C. Because freezing may destroy the characteristic viral morphology that permits a diagnosis by electron microscopy, specimens should be kept at +4°C.

Paired Serum Specimens (essential for diagnosis)

- Timing Acute: during the first week of symptoms
- Convalescent: third to sixth week
- Number 10 pairs from ill persons (the same persons submitting stool specimens) 10 pairs from well persons
- Quantity Adults: 10 ml
- Children: 3 ml
- Storage Tubes containing no anticoagulant (tubes with red tops) should be used for collection. Sera should be spun off and frozen. If a centrifuge is not available, a clot should be allowed to form, and the serum should be decanted and frozen. If this step cannot be taken, the whole blood should be refrigerated, not frozen.

Other Specimens

Viruses causing gastroenteritis cannot normally be detected in vomitus, water, food, or environmental samples. Although British researchers report electron microscope detection of virus in shellfish, no successful effort has yet been reported in the United States.

Consultation

At any time during the course of an outbreak, the Viral Gastroenteritis Section, REB, DVRD, CID (telephone 404-639-3577), is available for advice and assistance.

Since the viruses involved in most outbreaks of gastroenteritis reported to CDC cannot be cultivated, the antigen and antibody reagents used in diagnosis are not easily renewable. Thus, CDC cannot routinely screen persons and must limit use of these reagents. The following information would help determine the best use of laboratory resources:

- Setting of the outbreak (e.g., nursing home, restaurant)
- Date of onset of outbreak
- Number of persons exposed and number ill
- Population characteristics (e.g., elderly, children)
- Incubation period
- Duration of illness
- Symptoms
- Percent vomiting
- Percent with diarrhea
- Percent with bloody diarrhea
- Other (e.g., fever, myalgia, malaise)
- Adverse outcomes (e.g., hospitalizations, deaths)
- Suspected common source (e.g., shellfish, other food, food handler, water, other)
- Ongoing problems

Sending Specimens for Viral Diagnosis

If, after consultation, viral diagnostic services are considered to be useful, specimens may be shipped to the Viral Gastroenteritis Section, REB, DVRD, CID, following these guidelines:

- Each specimen should be labeled (waterproof) with a unique identifier firmly attached and should be accompanied by CDC Specimen Information Form 50.34.
- Stool specimens should be shipped as soon as they can be batched. Individual containers should be verified as leakproof and then enclosed in a plastic bag. The entire collection should be bagged in plastic and placed in a padded, insulated box with refrigerant packs.
- Frozen acute- and convalescent-phase serum samples should be batched and sent in a single shipment. Waterproof, padded, insulated boxes should be used, with dry ice added to maintain freezing. Whole blood samples should not be frozen, and refrigerant packs should be used instead of dry ice.

- Final notification should be made by telephone (404-639-3577) just before shipping.
- All shipments should be sent by overnight mail, due to arrive on a weekday, addressed to the Viral Gastroenteritis Section, REB, DVRD, CID, Mailstop G04, Centers for Disease Control, Atlanta, GA 30333.

REFERENCES: AS NUMBERED IN ORIGINAL PUBLICATION

 2. Ho M, Glass RI, Pinsky PF, et al. Diarrheal deaths in American children: are they preventable? JAMA 1988;260:3281–3285.
26. Hammond GW, Hannan C, Yeh T, Fischer K, Mauthe G, Straus SE. DNA hybridization for diagnosis of enteric adenovirus infection from directly spotted human fecal specimens. J Clin Microbiol 1987; 25:1881–1885.
52. Kaplan JE, Gary GW, Baron RC, et al. Epidemiology of Norwalk gastroenteritis and the role of Norwalk virus in outbreaks of acute nonbacterial gastroenteritis. Ann Intern Med 1982;96:756–761.
53. Yolken R, Leister F, Almeido-Hill J, Dubovi E, Reid R, Santosham M. Infantile gastroenteritis associated with excretion of pestivirus antigens. Lancet 1989;i:517–519.
57. Appleton H. Small round viruses: classification and role in food-borne infections. In: Bock G, Whelan J, eds. Novel diarrhoea viruses. (Ciba Foundation Symposium: 128). Chichester, UK: John Wiley & Sons, 1987:108–125.
64. Dennehy PH, Gauntlett DR, Tente WE. Comparison of nine commercial immunoassays for the detection of rotavirus in fecal samples. J Clin Microbiol 1988;26:1630–1634.
65. Thomas EE, Puterman ML, Kawano E, Curran M. Evaluation of seven immunoassays for detection of rotavirus in pediatric stool samples. J Clin Microbiol 1988;26:1189–1193.
66. Erdman DD, Gary GW, Anderson LJ. Development and evaluation of an IgM capture enzyme immunoassay for diagnosis of recent Norwalk virus infection. J Virol Meth 1989;24:57–66.
67. Erdman DD, Gary GW, Anderson LJ. Serum Immunoglobulin: a response to Norwalk virus infection. J Clin Microbiol 1989;27:1417–1418.
68. Glass RI, Monroe SS, Stine S, et al. Small round structured viruses: the Norwalk family of agents. In: Farthing MJG, ed. Viruses and the gut: Proceedings of the Ninth BSG-SK&F International Workshop. Welwyn Garden City, UK: Smith Kline & French Laboratories, 1988:87–90.
References 69 through 109 may be obtained from the Viral Gastroenteritis Section, REB, DVRD, CID, Mailstop G04, Centers for Disease Control, Atlanta, GA 30333.

APPENDIX

The following procedures [See Table 1, page 107] are recommended for use by state and local health departments for investigation of outbreaks. Instructions are summarized for each category of pathogens.

State public health laboratories can provide diagnostic services for most bacterial and parasitic pathogens. No specimens should be sent to CDC for diagnostic testing unless the specific program concerned has been consulted.

Reptile-Associated Salmonellosis—Selected States, 1994–1995

Original Citation: Reptile-Associated Salmonellosis—Selected States, 1994–1995. MMWR 1995;44(17):347–350.

RECOMMENDATIONS FOR PREVENTING TRANSMISSION OF SALMONELLA FROM REPTILES TO HUMANS

- Persons at increased risk for infection or serious complications of salmonellosis (e.g., pregnant women, children aged less than 5 years, and immunocompromised persons such as persons with AIDS) should avoid contact with reptiles.

- Reptiles should not be kept in child-care centers and may not be appropriate pets in households in which persons at increased risk for infection reside.
- Veterinarians and pet store owners should provide information to potential purchasers and owners of reptiles about the increased risk of acquiring salmonellosis from reptiles.
- Veterinarians and operators of pet stores should advise reptile owners always to wash their hands after handling reptiles and reptile cages.
- To prevent contamination of food-preparation areas (e.g., kitchens) and other selected sites, reptiles should be kept out of these areas in particular, kitchen sinks should not be used to bathe reptiles or to wash reptile dishes, cages, or aquariums.

Recommendations for Collection of Laboratory Specimens Associated with Outbreaks of Gastroenteritis

Original Citation: Recommendations for Collection of Laboratory Specimens Associated with Outbreaks of Gastroenteritis. MMWR 1990;39(RR-14):1–13.

New diagnostic laboratory techniques as well as modifications of standard ones have been used by investigators to identify viral, bacterial, and parasitic agents of outbreaks of gastroenteritis. Recently discovered causative agents associated with such outbreaks include the Norwalk-like agents, astrovirus, calicivirus, enteric adenovirus, enterohemorrhagic Escherichia coli, Cryptosporidium, and Isospora belli. Use of direct electron microscopy (EM), coupled with immunologic techniques (e.g., immune EM and enzyme immunoassays (EIAs)) and serologic studies, has enhanced understanding of viruses as a major cause of gastroenteritis. Bacteria and parasites continue to be recognized as important causes of diarrhea worldwide. Use of EIAs, tissue culture, molecular probes, and the polymerase chain reaction has improved the diagnosis of diarrhea caused by bacteria, and special concentrating and staining techniques have improved the process of detecting parasites such as Cryptosporidium and I. belli.

To ensure that these diagnostic advances can be used most effectively, earlier recommendations for collecting stool specimens must be updated. Because appropriate specimen-collection methods for viral, bacterial, and parasitic agents differ, the sections below are divided into guidelines by category of agent.

PROCEDURES FOR COLLECTING SPECIMENS
Stool

See Table 1

Table 1. General instructions for collection of stool specimens*

Instructions for collecting specimens	Type of agent to be tested for		
	Virus	Bacterium	Parasite
When to collect	Within 48–72 hours after onset of illness.	During period of active diarrhea (preferably as soon after onset of illness as possible).	Any time after onset of illness (preferably as soon after onset of illness as possible).
How much to collect	As much stool sample from each of 10 ill persons as possible (at least 10 cc each person); samples from 10 controls may also be submitted.	Two rectal swabs or swabs of fresh stool from each of 10 ill persons; samples from 10 controls may also be submitted.	A fresh stool sample from each of 10 ill persons; samples from 10 controls may also be submitted.
Method of collection	Place fresh stool specimens (liquid preferable), unmixed with urine, in clean, dry containers, (e.g., urine specimen cups).	For rectal swabs, moisten each of two swabs in Cary-Blair medium first, then insert sequentially 1–1.5 inches in rectum and gently rotate. Place both swabs into the same Cary-Blair medium tube. Break off top portions of swab sticks and discard.	Collect a bulk stool specimen, unmixed with urine, in a clean container. Place a portion of each stool sample into 10% formalin and polyvinyl alcohol preservatives at a ratio of 1 part stool to 3 parts preservative. Mix well.
Storage of specimen after collection	Immediately refrigerate at 4°C. DO NOT FREEZE if electron microscopy is anticipated.	Immediately refrigerate at 4°C if testing is to be done within 48 hours after collection; otherwise, freeze samples at −70°C.	Store at room temperature, or refrigerate at 4°C. DO NOT FREEZE.
Transportation	Keep refrigerated. Place bagged and sealed specimens on ice or with frozen refrigerant packs in an insulated box. Send by overnight mail. DO NOT FREEZE.	Refrigerate as directed for viral specimens. For frozen samples: place bagged and sealed samples on dry ice. Mail in insulated box by overnight mail.	Refrigerate as directed for viral specimens. For room-temperature samples: mail in water-proof containers. DO NOT FREEZE.

*Label each specimen container with a waterproof marker. Put samples in sealed, waterproof containers (e.g., plastic bags). Batch collection and send by overnight mail, scheduled to arrive at destination on a weekday or during business hours.

General Guidelines

Timing

Begin collecting stool specimens immediately after being notified of an outbreak, since delay may impede identification of the causative agent. To permit diagnosis of certain viral agents, specimens must be collected during the first 48 hours of illness.

Quantity

Collect diarrheal stool samples from at least 10 ill persons (assuming that at least that number are involved in the outbreak). For outbreaks thought to be of viral origin, collect large-volume stool specimens (at least a urine cupful).

Methods for Collection and Storage

Viruses

Place each diarrheal stool specimen, of as large a quantity as can be obtained (preferably, at least 10 cc), in a leak-proof, clean, dry container, and refrigerate at 4°C. Instructing patients to catch stool specimens in plastic kitchen wrap draped across the back half of the toilet under the toilet seat may facilitate collection of stool specimens. Do not freeze specimens if EM examination is anticipated.

Bacteria

Collect at least two rectal swabs or swabs of fresh stools from each patient and place swabs in refrigerated (i.e., chilled 1–2 hours before use) Cary-Blair transport medium. Collect specimens from persons who have not received antimicrobial therapy. When obtaining swabs from a patient, first moisten each rectal swab in the holding medium, insert the moistened swab into the rectum 1 to 1½ inches, rotate the swab gently, and then return the swab to the same tube of holding medium. Try to ensure that visible fecal material is present on each swab. After obtaining the two fecal swabs, insert both into the same tube of medium and push them to the bottom of the tube. Break off and discard the excess top portion of the swab sticks.

IMPORTANT: Refrigerate or freeze tubes after specimens are placed in them. If specimens will be examined within 48 hours after collection, they can be refrigerated; however, if specimens must be held longer than 48 hours, freeze them as soon as possible after they are collected. Although storage in an ultra-low freezer (−70°C) is preferable, storage in a home-type freezer (if it is properly set at −20°C) is acceptable for short periods.

Parasites

Mix fresh bulk-stool specimens thoroughly with each of two preservatives, 10% formalin and polyvinyl alcohol (PVA) fixative,* at a ratio of 1 part stool to 3 parts preservative. If there is a delay in obtaining the preservatives, refrigerate

---

*Preservatives are available in commercial kits.

untreated stool specimens at 4°C (do not freeze) for up to 48 hours. Once preserved, the specimens can be stored and transported at room temperature or refrigerated. Do not freeze.

Transportation (Specimen Handling)

Refrigerated Specimens

Enclose each specimen in a secure container (e.g., urine cup, Cary-Blair medium tube), to which has been affixed a waterproof label. Place this container in a waterproof bag with tissue, towels, or other blotting material to absorb any leakage.

Batch specimen containers, pack with ice or frozen refrigerant packs in an insulated box, and send by overnight mail scheduled to be delivered during business hours on a weekday, if possible. Submit a list of specimens and a CDC Identification Form 50.34 for each specimen.

Frozen Specimens (for Bacterial Testing Only)

So that they remain frozen, ship frozen specimens on dry ice. Use enough dry ice to keep the specimen frozen until it is received at the laboratory that will process it (i.e., enough dry ice to fill one-third to one-half of the shipping container). Do not allow glass tubes to be in direct contact with dry ice; place a layer of paper or other material between the tubes and the dry ice. To prevent excess exposure of specimens to carbon dioxide, tighten the screw caps on the Cary-Blair tubes and seal them with electrical tape, or seal the specimens in a plastic bag within the container of dry ice.

Serum

General Guidelines

Timing of Collection of Specimens

Submit two serum specimens (an acute-phase specimen and a convalescent-phase specimen) for each patient thought to have illness caused by viruses or bacteria. Obtain the acute-phase serum specimen as close to the time of onset of illness as possible (at most, within a week after onset of illness) and the convalescent-phase serum specimen 3–4 weeks after the onset of illness. If a viral agent is suspected, for optimal test results, specimens should be collected within 6 weeks after onset of illness.

Source(s) of Specimens

If possible, obtain paired serum specimens from the same 10 patients from whom stool samples were obtained. Ten paired serum specimens obtained from well persons can serve as control specimens in certain studies.

Methods for Collection and Storage

Collect blood specimens from adults (15 ml) and from children (3 ml) in tubes that do not contain anticoagulants (usually red-top tubes). Centrifuge the blood and send only the serum for analysis. If no centrifuge is available, store the blood specimens in a refrigerator until a clot has formed; then remove the serum and pipette it into an empty sterile tube (using a Pasteur pipette). Refrigerate the tubes of spun serum until they are shipped. Refrigerate, but do not freeze, tubes containing unspun serum.

Transportation

Ship serum specimens either refrigerated or frozen. If the clotting technique described above is used to obtain the serum, ship the specimens refrigerated so that they can be centrifuged before they are frozen. Specimens can be refrigerated by placing them in an insulated box with ice or frozen refrigerant packs. Frozen specimens can be kept frozen by shipping them on dry ice. Batch the specimens and send by overnight mail, scheduled to arrive at the laboratory during business hours on a weekday, if possible.

NOTE:

Certain specimens of food, water, or ice can be submitted for testing if they are epidemiologically implicated as the vehicle of the disease. However, because of the technical difficulties and the low yield associated with such studies, only send such specimens to CDC after staff in the appropriate laboratory have agreed. Refrigerate specimens for viral and parasitic diagnostic testing at 4 C, and freeze specimens for bacterial diagnostics at $-70°C$.

DETECTION OF PATHOGENS

Testing done at CDC is for research and/or outbreak situations. Contact the appropriate CDC staff member(s) to discuss any questions concerning outbreaks of gastroenteritis or methods of collecting specimens.

Viruses

General Guidelines

Some of the tests presently available are direct EM; immune EM; polyacrylamide gel electrophoresis; enzyme immune assays for rotavirus (groups A and B), enteric adenovirus, and astrovirus antigens; a serologic enzyme immune assay for Norwalk virus; and polymerase chain reaction for rotavirus serotyping. EIAs for calicivirus antigens and EIAs for astrovirus antibodies are being developed.

Stool

Many viruses—including rotaviruses, adenoviruses, astroviruses, caliciviruses, the Norwalk virus, and other small, round viruses—can be detected with EM. Because the electron microscope scans a field containing a millionth of a milliliter of stool, the specimen must contain at least a million particles per milliliter for one particle of virus to be detected. In order to assure that samples contain the highest concentration of virus possible, specimens must be collected as close to the onset of illness as possible, generally within the first 48–72 hours. Watery stool specimens are most likely to contain visible particles of virus.

Freezing may alter or obliterate the morphologic characteristics of some viruses; therefore, samples should be kept refrigerated at 4°C and should not be frozen if EM examination is anticipated. Because most enteric viruses (e.g., calicivirus, the Norwalk agents, and the non-group A rotaviruses) cannot be cultivated, reagents for diagnostic tests are limited. In fact, because human stool samples are the basic source of antigen and virus, the bulk collection of specimens is always encouraged. Proper collection and storage of large-volume specimens will facilitate EM examination and allow for concentration methods that enhance the likelihood of successful testing.

Serum

Antibodies to viruses usually begin to rise the first week after onset of illness, peak by the fourth week, and can fall by the sixth week (particularly for Norwalk agents). Acute-phase serum specimens should be collected in the first week of illness, and convalescent-phase serum specimens from the third to the fourth week after onset of illness (not later than the sixth week if the suspected pathogen is a Norwalk agent). Since many persons have preexisting antibodies to some of the viral agents, a single convalescent-phase serum sample is generally of little diagnostic value. At present, determination of the cause of outbreaks of viral gastroenteritis relies heavily on assays of serologic response; paired serum specimens should therefore be submitted for testing associated with all such outbreaks. A fourfold rise in specific antibody titer between acute- and convalescent-phase serum samples is accepted as diagnostic of a recent infection.

Bacteria

General Guidelines

Tests available for identification of organisms include isolation procedures for Salmonella, Shigella, Campylobacter, Vibrio, Yersinia enterocolitica, Aeromonas hydrophilia, Plesiomonas shigelloides, Bacillus cereus, Staphylococcus aureus, and Escherichia coli, as well as serodiagnostic assays for Salmonella typhi, Campylobacter, Vibrio cholerae, and E. coli 0157:H7. When no other pathogen is found, serotyping of E. coli recovered from ill persons and from appropriately chosen controls can identify previously unidentified E. coli pathogens. In addition, polymerase chain reaction for Shiga-like toxin-producing E. coli is presently being developed. Other diagnostic tests available are pathogenicity assays; ELISAs or DNA probes for detection of EPEC, EIEC, ETEC, and EHEC (including E. coli 0157:H7); and antimicrobial susceptibility testing, plasmid profiles, and other subtyping methods to determine the relatedness of enteric bacteria.

Stool

A pathogenic bacterium can be identified by isolating the organism in culture, by serotyping, or by identifying a characteristic marker for virulence. Fresh stool specimens should always be used when possible to ensure that fastidious organisms and toxins that decompose easily are detected before they degenerate. Expedient refrigeration of specimens is important since bacteria can easily be overgrown by competing organisms in stool specimens left at room temperature for greater than 4 hours. If testing must be delayed beyond 48 hours after the specimen is collected, the specimen should be frozen to retard the overgrowth of bacteria. Since most bacterial pathogens can be cultured from appropriately acquired rectal swab specimens, rectal swabs or swabs of fresh stools are preferred to bulk stool specimens. This method of collection also facilitates storage and transport.

Serum

Specific antibody testing may be possible for some bacterial enteric agents such as Shigella. As is true for viral infections, antibody titers to bacterial agents generally rise by the end of the first week after onset of illness and peak by 3–4 weeks. A fourfold rise in specific antibody titer is accepted as diagnostic of a recent infection.

Parasites

General Guidelines

Some tests available for formalin-preserved specimens include the formalin-ethyl acetate concentration, which is used for both helminths and protozoa, and the kinyoun carbol-fuchsin(modified acid-fast)-stained slide, which is used for Cryptosporidium. PVA-preserved specimens are used to prepare Trichrome-stained slides and examined for protozoa.

Stool

Parasites are usually detected and identified with microscopy of fresh or appropriately preserved stool specimen (although parasites can sometimes be grown on special media). Fresh specimens are needed for direct microscopy because trophozoites are fragile and may not survive environmental stress. The PVA and formalin fixatives preserve the morphology of cysts and trophozoites in stool specimens for diagnostic testing.

Serum

Unlike outbreaks of gastroenteritis due to bacteria or viruses, an outbreak of parasitic diarrheal illness can sometimes be identified with a convalescent-phase serum specimen only. However, it is sometimes necessary to have both acute and convalescent serum specimens to make a definitive diagnosis.

CDC CONTACTS FOR CONSULTATION

Viral Gastroenteritis Unit
Respiratory and Enteric Virus Branch
Division of Viral and Rickettsial Diseases
Center for Infectious Diseases

Centers for Disease Control
Mailstop G-04, SB47, Bldg. 7
Atlanta, GA 30333
(404) 639–3040
Food Borne and Diarrheal Diseases Branch
Division of Bacterial Diseases
Center for Infectious Diseases
Centers for Disease Control
Mailstop C-09
Bldg. 1, Rm. 5428
Atlanta, GA 30333
(404) 639–2206
Epidemiology Branch
Division of Parasitic Diseases
Center for Infectious Diseases
Centers for Disease Control
Mailstop F-13
Bldg. 23, Chamblee
Atlanta, GA 30333
(404) 488–4178

SELECTED BIBLIOGRAPHY

Balows A, Hausler Jr. WJ, Lennette EH, eds. Laboratory diagnosis of infectious diseases: principles and practice. 1st ed. New York: Springer-Verlag, Inc., 1988.

Benenson AS, ed. Control of communicable diseases in man. 14th ed. Washington, DC: American Public Health Association, 1985.

Ciba Foundation. Novel diarrhea viruses. In: Ciba foundation symposium. New York: John Wiley & Sons, Inc., 1987:128.

Cohen ML. Epidemiology of diarrheal disease: infectious diarrhea. Infect Dis Clin North Am 1988; 2(3):557–570.

Feigin RD, Cherry JD, eds. Gastrointestinal infections: textbook of pediatric infectious diseases. 2nd ed. Philadelphia: WB Saunders Co., 1987.

Guerrant RL. Gastrointestinal infections and food poisoning. In: Mandel GL, Douglas RG Jr, Bennet JE, eds. Principles and practice of infectious diseases. 2nd ed. New York: John Wiley & Sons, Inc., 1985:635–646.

Guerrant RL, Hughes JM. Nausea, vomiting, and non-inflammatory diarrhea. In: Mandell GL, Douglas RG Jr, Bennet JF, eds. Principles and practice of infectious diseases. 2nd ed. New York: John Wiley & Sons, Inc., 1985:646–655.

Hughes JM. Food poisoning. In: Mandell GL, Douglas RG Jr, Bennet JE, eds. Principles and practice of infectious diseases. 2nd ed. New York: John Wiley & Sons, Inc., 1985:680–691.

Kapikian AZ, Chanock RM. Viral gastroenteritis. In: Evans AS, ed. Viral infections of humans: epidemiology and control. 3rd ed. New York: Plenum Medical Book Co., 1989.

Manson-Bahr PEC, Bell DR. Diarrhea caused by protozoa. In: Manson's tropical diseases. 19th ed. London: Bailliere Tindall, 1987.

Penaranda ME, Cubitt WD, Sinarachatanant P, Taylor DN, Linkanonsakul S, Saif L, Glass RI. Group C rotavirus infections in patients with diarrhea in Thailand, Nepal, and England. J Infect Dis 1989;160(3):392–397.

Pickering LK, Cleary TG. Approach to patients with gastrointestinal infections and food poisoning. In: Feigin RD, Cherry JD, eds. Textbook of pediatric infectious diseases. 2nd ed. Philadelphia: WB Saunders Co., 1987:622–651.

Tanowitz HB, Weiss LM, Wittner M. Diagnosis and treatment of protozoan diarrheas. Am J Gastroenterol 1988;82(4):339–350.

Thorne GM. Diagnosis of infectious diarrheal diseases: infectious diarrhea. Infect Dis Clin North Am 1988;2(3):747–774.

TOPIC 9 / **EHRLICHIOSIS**

Human Granulocytic Ehrlichiosis

Original Citation: Human Granulocytic Ehrlichiosis—New York, 1995. MMWR 1995; 44(32):593–595.

Since 1986, two human tickborne diseases caused by Ehrlichia spp. have been recognized in the United States: human monocytic ehrlichiosis (HME), caused by E. chaffeensis, and human granulocytic ehrlichiosis (HGE), caused by an agent closely related to E. equi (1, 2).

EDITORIAL NOTE

Physicians evaluating patients with an acute febrile illness should consider ehrlichiosis in the differential diagnosis, particularly if the patient is leukopenic or thrombocytopenic, and should solicit a history of known or possible exposure to ticks. Empiric therapy with doxycycline antibiotics should be considered if the diagnosis of ehrlichiosis is suspected because delayed treatment while awaiting laboratory confirmation may increase the risk for adverse outcomes. The diagnosis can be confirmed through antibody assays and/or PCR. The agent that causes HGE has not been identified in cell culture, but tests for antibody to E. equi have been used to confirm the diagnosis. The sensitivity, specificity, and cross-reactivity of serologic assays for the two species are not well established. Because the geographic distribution of HME and HGE overlap, physicians should consider obtaining serologic tests for both E. equi and E. chaffeensis. PCR is a useful research tool but is not widely available for diagnostic purposes.

REFERENCES: AS NUMBERED IN ORIGINAL PUBLICATION

1. Dawson JE, Anderson BE, Fishbein DB, et al. Isolation and characterization of and Ehrlichia sp. from a patient diagnosed with human ehrlichiosis. J Clin Microbiol 1991;29:2741–2745.
2. Bakken JS, Dumler JS, Chen SM, Eckman MR, Van Etta LL, Walker DH. Human granulocytic ehrlichiosis in the upper midwest United States. JAMA 1994;272:212–218.

TOPIC 10 / **HANTAVIRUS**

Management of Patients with Suspected Viral Hemorrhagic Fever

Original Citation: Notice to Readers Update: Management of Patients with Suspected Viral Hemorrhagic Fever—United States, MMWR 1995;44(25):475–479.

This notice provides interim recommendations that update the 1988 guidelines for health-care settings in the United States. This update applies to four viruses that cause syndromes of VHF: Lassa, Marburg, Ebola, and Congo-Crimean hemorrhagic fever viruses; although the risk and/or mode of nosocomial transmission differs for each of these viruses, the limited data do not permit clear distinctions.

All suspected cases of infection with Ebola virus and other hemorrhagic fever viruses should be reported immediately to local and state health departments and to CDC (telephone [404] 639-1511; from 4:30 p.m. to 8 a.m., telephone [404] 639-2888). Specimens for virus-specific diagnostic tests should be sent to CDC as rapidly as possible according to instructions provided when contact is made. General information regarding Ebola virus infection is available through the CDC Ebola Hotline (telephone [800] 900-0681).

RECOMMENDATIONS

The following recommendations apply to patients who, within 3 weeks before onset of fever, have either (a) traveled in the specific local area of a country where VHF has recently occurred; (b) had direct contact with blood, other body fluids, secretions, or excretions of a person or animal with VHF; or (c) worked in a laboratory or animal facility that handles hemorrhagic fever viruses. The likelihood of acquiring VHF is considered extremely low in persons who do not meet any of these criteria. The cause of fever in persons who have traveled in areas where VHF is endemic is more likely to be a different infectious disease (e.g., malaria or typhoid fever); evaluation for and treatment of these other potentially serious infections should not be delayed.

1. Because most ill persons undergoing prehospital evaluation and transport are in the early stages of disease and would not be expected to have symptoms that increase the likelihood of contact with infectious body fluids (e.g., vomiting, diarrhea, or hemorrhage), universal precautions are generally sufficient (8). If a patient has respiratory symptoms (e.g., cough or rhinitis), face shields or surgical masks and eye protection (e.g., goggles or eyeglasses with side shields) should be worn by caregivers to prevent droplet contact (8). Blood, urine, feces, or vomitus, if present, should be handled as described in the following recommendations for hospitalized patients.

2. Patients in a hospital outpatient or inpatient setting should be placed in a private room. A negative pressure room is not required during the early stages of illness, but should be considered at the time of hospitalization to avoid the need for subsequent transfer of the patient. Nonessential staff and visitors should be restricted from entering the room. Caretakers should use barrier precautions to prevent skin or mucous membrane exposure to blood and other body fluids, secretions, and excretions. All persons entering the patient's room should wear gloves and gowns to prevent contact with items or environmental surfaces that may be soiled. In addition, face shields or surgical masks and eye protection (e.g., goggles or eyeglasses with side shields) should be worn by persons coming within approximately 3 feet of the patient to prevent contact with blood, other body fluids, secretions (including respiratory droplets), or excretions.

The need for additional barriers depends on the potential for fluid contact, as determined by the procedure performed and the presence of clinical symptoms that increase the likelihood of contact with body fluids from the patient (8). For example, if copious amounts of blood, other body fluids, vomit, or feces are present in the environment, leg and shoe coverings also may be needed. Before entering the hallway, all protective barriers should be removed and shoes that are soiled with body fluids should be cleaned and disinfected as described below (see recommendation 6). An anteroom for putting on and removing protective barriers and for storing supplies would be useful, if available (1).

3. For patients with suspected VHF who have a prominent cough, vomiting, diarrhea, or hemorrhage, additional precautions are indicated to prevent possible exposure to airborne particles that may contain virus. Patients with these symptoms should be placed in a negative-pressure room (9). Persons entering the room should wear personal protective respirators as recommended for care of patients with active tuberculosis (high efficiency particulate air [HEPA] respirators or more protective respirators) (9).

4. Measures to prevent percutaneous injuries associated with the use and disposal of needles and other sharp instruments should be undertaken as outlined in recommendations for universal precautions (8). If surgical or obstetric procedures are necessary, the state health department and CDC's National Center for Infectious Diseases, Hospital Infections Program (telephone [404] 639-6425) and Division of Viral and Rickettsial Diseases (telephone [404] 639-1511; from 4:30 p.m. to 8 a.m., telephone [404] 639-2888) should be consulted regarding appropriate precautions for these procedures.

5. Because of the potential risks associated with handling infectious materials, laboratory testing should be the minimum necessary for diagnostic evaluation and patient care. Clinical laboratory specimens should be obtained using precautions outlined above (see recommendations 1–4 above), placed in plastic bags that are sealed, then transported in clearly labeled, durable, leakproof containers directly to the specimen handling area of the laboratory. Care should be taken not to contaminate the external surfaces of the container. Laboratory staff should be alerted to the nature of the specimens, which should remain in the custody of a designated person until testing is done. Specimens in clinical laboratories should be handled in a class II biological safety cabinet following biosafety level 3 practices (10). Serum used in laboratory tests should be pretreated with polyethylene glycol p-tert-octylphenyl ether (Triton® X-100)*; treatment with 10 µL of 10% Triton® X-100 per 1 mL of serum for 1 hour reduces the titer of hemorrhagic fever viruses in serum, although 100% efficacy in inactivating these viruses should not be assumed. Blood smears (e.g., for malaria) are not infectious after fixation in solvents. Routine procedures can be used for automated analyzers; analyzers should be disinfected as recommended by the manufacturer or with a 500 parts per

---

*Use of trade names and commercial sources is for identification only and does not imply endorsement by the Public Health Service or the U.S. Department of Health and Human Services.

million solution of sodium hypochlorite (1:100 dilution of household bleach: 1/4 cup to 1 gallon water) after use. Virus isolation or cultivation must be done at biosafety level 4 (10). The CDC mobile isolation laboratory is no longer available (1).

6. Environmental surfaces or inanimate objects contaminated with blood, other body fluids, secretions, or excretions should be cleaned and disinfected using standard procedures (8). Disinfection can be accomplished using a U.S. Environmental Protection Agency (EPA)-registered hospital disinfectant or a 1:100 dilution of household bleach.

7. Soiled linens should be placed in clearly labeled leakproof bags at the site of use and transported directly to the decontamination area. Linens can be decontaminated in a gravity displacement autoclave or incinerated. Alternatively, linens can be laundered using a normal hot water cycle with bleach if universal precautions to prevent exposures are precisely followed (8) and linens are placed directly into washing machines without sorting.

8. There is no evidence for transmission of hemorrhagic fever viruses to humans or animals through exposure to contaminated sewage; the risk of such transmission would be expected to be extremely low with sewage treatment procedures in use in the United States. As an added precaution, however, measures should be taken to eliminate or reduce the infectivity of bulk blood, suctioned fluids, secretions, and excretions before disposal. These fluids should be either autoclaved, processed in a chemical toilet, or treated with several ounces of household bleach for greater than or equal to 5 minutes (e.g., in a bedpan or commode) before flushing or disposal in a drain connected to a sanitary sewer. Care should be taken to avoid splashing when disposing of these materials. Potentially infectious solid medical waste (e.g., contaminated needles, syringes, and tubing) should either be incinerated or be decontaminated by autoclaving or immersion in a suitable chemical germicide (i.e., an EPA-registered hospital disinfectant or a 1:100 dilution of household bleach), then handled according to existing local and state regulations for waste management.

9. If the patient dies, handling of the body should be minimal. The corpse should be wrapped in sealed leakproof material, not embalmed, and cremated or buried promptly in a sealed casket. If an autopsy is necessary, the state health department and CDC should be consulted regarding appropriate precautions (1).

10. Persons with percutaneous or mucocutaneous exposures to blood, body fluids, secretions, or excretions from a patient with suspected VHF should immediately wash the affected skin surfaces with soap and water. Application of an antiseptic solution or handwashing product may be considered also, although the efficacy of this supplemental measure is unknown. Mucous membranes (e.g., conjunctiva) should be irrigated with copious amounts of water or eyewash solution. Exposed persons should receive medical evaluation and follow-up management (1).

REFERENCES: AS NUMBERED IN ORIGINAL PUBLICATION

1. CDC. Management of patients with suspected viral hemorrhagic fever. MMWR 1988;37(no. S-3):1–15.
8. CDC. Guidelines for prevention of transmission of human immunodeficiency virus and hepatitis B virus to health-care and public safety workers. MMWR 1989;38:(no. S-6):1–37.
9. CDC. Guidelines for preventing the transmission of Mycobacterium tuberculosis in health-care facilities. MMWR 1994;43(no. RR-13):33–34, 71–81.

10. CDC/National Institutes of Health. Biosafety in microbiological and biomedical laboratories. 3rd ed. Atlanta: US Department of Health and Human Services, Public Health Service, 1993:DHHS publication no. (CDC)93–8395.

Hantavirus Infection: Interim Recommendations for Risk Reduction

Original Citation: Hantavirus Infection—Southwestern United States: Interim Recommendations for Risk Reduction. MMWR 1993;42(RR-11):1–13.

This report provides interim recommendations for prevention and control of hantavirus infections associated with rodents. It is based on principles of rodent and infection control and contains specific recommendations for reducing rodent shelter and food sources in and around the home, recommendations for eliminating rodents inside the home and preventing them from entering the home, precautions for preventing hantavirus infection while rodent-contaminated areas are being cleaned up, prevention measures for persons who have occupational exposure to wild rodents, and precautions for campers and hikers.

INTRODUCTION

The recently recognized hantavirus-associated disease among residents of the southwestern United States (1–4) and the identification of rodent reservoirs for the virus in the affected areas warrant recommendations to minimize the risk of exposure to rodents for both residents and visitors. While information is being gathered about the causative virus and its epidemiology, provisional recommendations can be made on the basis of knowledge about related hantaviruses. These recommendations are based on current understanding of the epidemiologic features of hantavirus infections in the Southwest; they will be periodically evaluated and modified as more information becomes available.

Rodents are the primary reservoir hosts of recognized hantaviruses. Each hantavirus appears to have preferential rodent hosts, but other small mammals can be infected as well (5, 6). Available data strongly suggest that the deer mouse (Peromyscus maniculatus) is the primary reservoir of the newly recognized hantavirus in the southwestern United States (1). Serologic evidence of infection has also been found in pion mice (P. truei), brush mice (P. boylii), and western chipmunks (Tamias spp.). P. maniculatus is highly adaptable and is found in different habitats, including human residences in rural and semi-rural areas, but generally not in urban centers.

Hantaviruses do not cause apparent illness in their reservoir hosts (7). Infected rodents shed virus in saliva, urine, and feces for many weeks, but the duration and period of maximum infectivity are unknown (8–11). The demonstrated presence of infectious virus in saliva of infected rodents and the marked sensitivity of these animals to hantaviruses following inoculation suggests that biting may be an important mode of transmission among rodents

(7). Human infection may occur when infective saliva or excreta are inhaled as aerosols produced directly from the animal. Persons visiting laboratories where infected rodents were housed have been infected after only a few minutes of exposure to animal holding areas (12). Transmission may also occur when dried materials contaminated by rodent excreta are disturbed, directly introduced into broken skin, introduced onto the conjunctivae, or, possibly, ingested in contaminated food or water. Persons have also become infected after being bitten by rodents (13, 14).

Arthropod vectors are not known to have a role in the transmission of hantaviruses (7, 12). Person-to-person transmission has not been associated with any of the previously identified hantaviruses (9) or with the recent outbreak in the Southwest. Cats and dogs are not known to be reservoir hosts of hantaviruses in the United States. However, these domestic animals may bring infected rodents into contact with humans.

Known hantavirus infections of humans occur primarily in adults and are associated with domestic, occupational, or leisure activities that bring humans into contact with infected rodents, usually in a rural setting. Patterns of seasonal occurrence differ, depending on the virus, species of rodent host, and patterns of human behavior (5, 7). Cases have been epidemiologically associated with the following situations:

- planting or harvesting field crops;
- occupying previously vacant cabins or other dwellings;
- cleaning barns and other outbuildings;
- disturbing rodent-infested areas while hiking or camping;
- inhabiting dwellings with indoor rodent populations;
- residing in or visiting areas in which the rodent population has shown an increase in density (15–17).

Hantaviruses have lipid envelopes that are susceptible to most disinfectants (e.g., dilute hypochlorite solutions, detergents, ethyl alcohol [70%], or most general-purpose household disinfectants) (18). How long these viruses survive after being shed in the environment is uncertain.

The reservoir hosts of the hantavirus in the southwestern United States also act as hosts for the bacterium Yersinia pestis, the etiologic agent of plague. Although fleas and other ectoparasites are not known to play a role in hantavirus epidemiology, rodent fleas transmit plague. Control of rodents without concurrent control of fleas may increase the risk of human plague as the rodent fleas seek an alternative food source. Eradicating the reservoir hosts of hantaviruses is neither feasible nor desirable. The best currently available approach for disease control and prevention is risk reduction through environmental hygiene practices that deter rodents from colonizing the home and work environment.

GENERAL HOUSEHOLD PRECAUTIONS IN AFFECTED AREAS

Although epidemiologic studies are being conducted to identify specific behaviors that may increase the risk for hantavirus infection in humans in the United States, rodent control in and around the home will continue to be the primary prevention strategy (Box 1 Table B1). CDC has issued recommendations for rodent-proofing urban and suburban dwellings and reducing rodent populations through habitat modification and sanitation (19, 20).

Table B1

Box 1. General precautions for residents of affected areas
Eliminate rodents and reduce the availability of food sources and nesting sites used by rodents inside the home.
— Follow the recommendations in the section on Eliminating Rodents Inside the Home.
— Keep food (including pet food) and water covered and stored in rodent-proof metal or thick plastic containers with tight-fitting lids.
— Store garbage inside homes in rodent-proof metal or thick plastic containers with tight-fitting lids.
— Wash dishes and cooking utensils immediately after use and remove all spilled food.
— Dispose of trash and clutter.
— Use spring-loaded rodent traps in the home continuously.
— As an adjunct to traps, use rodenticide with bait under a plywood or plastic shelter (covered bait station) on an ongoing basis inside the house.

Note: Environmental Protection Agency (EPA)-approved rodenticides are commercially available. Instructions on product use should always be followed. Products that are used outdoors should be specifically approved for exterior use. Any use of a rodenticide should be preceded by use of an insecticide to reduce the risk of plague transmission. Insecticide sprays or powders can be used in place of aerosols if they are appropriately labeled for flea control.

Prevent rodents from entering the home. Specific measures should be adapted to local circumstances.
— Use steel wool or cement to seal, screen, or otherwise cover all openings into the home that have a diameter greater than or equal to ¼ inch.
— Place metal roof flashing as a rodent barrier around the base of wooden, earthen, or adobe dwellings up to a height of 12 inches and buried in the soil to a depth of 6 inches.
— Place 3 inches of gravel under the base of homes or under mobile homes to discourage rodent burrowing.

Reduce rodent shelter and food sources within 100 feet of the home.
— Use raised cement foundations in new construction of sheds, barns, outbuildings, or woodpiles.
— When possible, place woodpiles 100 feet or more from the house, and elevate wood at least 12 inches off the ground.
— Store grains and animal feed in rodent-proof containers.
— Near buildings, remove food sources that might attract rodents, or store food and water in rodent-proof containers.
— Store hay on pallets, and use traps or rodenticide continuously to keep hay free of rodents.
— Do not leave pet food in feeding dishes.
— Dispose of garbage and trash in rodent-proof containers that are elevated at least 12 inches off the ground.
— Haul away trash, abandoned vehicles, discarded tires, and other items that may serve as rodent nesting sites.

- Cut grass, brush, and dense shrubbery within 100 feet of the home.
- Place spring-loaded rodent traps at likely spots for rodent shelter within 100 feet around the home, and use continuously.
- Use an EPA-registered rodenticide approved for outside use in covered bait stations at places likely to shelter rodents within 100 feet of the home.

NOTE: Follow the recommendations specified in the section on Clean-up of Rodent-Contaminated Areas if rodent nests are encountered while these measures are being carried out.

ELIMINATING RODENTS INSIDE THE HOME AND REDUCING RODENT ACCESS TO THE HOME

Rodent infestation can be determined by direct observation of animals or inferred from the presence of feces in closets or cabinets or on floors or from evidence that rodents have been gnawing at food. If rodent infestation is detected inside the home or outbuildings, rodent abatement measures should be completed (Box 2 Table B2). The directions in the section on Special Precautions should be followed if evidence of heavy rodent infestation (e.g., piles of feces or numerous dead animals) is present or if a structure is associated with a confirmed case of hantavirus disease.

Table B2

Box 2. Eliminating rodent infestation: Guidance for residents of affected areas

- Before rodent elimination work is begun, ventilate closed buildings or areas inside buildings by opening doors and windows for at least 30 minutes. Use an exhaust fan or cross ventilation if possible. Leave the area until the airing-out period is finished. This airing may help remove any aerosolized virus inside the closed-in structure.
- Second, seal, screen, or otherwise cover all openings into the home that have a diameter of greater than or equal to ¼ inch. Then set rodent traps inside the house, using peanut butter as bait. Use only spring-loaded traps that kill rodents.
- Next, treat the interior of the structure with an insecticide labeled for flea control; follow specific label instructions. Insecticide sprays or powders can be used in place of aerosols if they are appropriately labeled for flea control. Rodenticides may also be used while the interior is being treated, as outlined below.
- Remove captured rodents from the traps. Wear rubber or plastic gloves while handling rodents. Place the carcasses in a plastic bag containing a sufficient amount of a general-purpose household disinfectant to thoroughly wet the carcasses. Seal the bag and then dispose of it by burying in a 2- to 3-foot-deep hole or by burning. If burying or burning are not feasible, contact your local or state health department about other appropriate disposal methods. Rebait and reset all sprung traps.
- Before removing the gloves, wash gloved hands in a general household disinfectant and then in soap and water. A hypochlorite solution prepared by mixing 3 tablespoons of household bleach in 1 gallon of water may be used in place of a commercial disinfectant. When using the

chlorine solution, avoid spilling the mixture on clothing or other items
that may be damaged. Thoroughly wash hands with soap and water after
removing the gloves.
— Leave several baited spring-loaded traps inside the house at all times as
a further precaution against rodent reinfestation. Examine the traps
regularly. Disinfect traps no longer in use by washing in a general
household disinfectant or the hypochlorite solution. Disinfect and wash
gloves as described above, and wash hands thoroughly with soap and
water before beginning other activities.

NOTE: EPA-approved rodenticides are commercially available. Instructions on
product use should always be followed. Products that are used outdoors should
be specifically approved for exterior use. Any use of a rodenticide should be
preceded by use of an insecticide to reduce the risk of plague transmission. Insecticide sprays or powders can be used in place of aerosols if they are appropriately labeled for flea control.

CLEAN-UP OF RODENT-CONTAMINATED AREAS

Areas with evidence of rodent activity (e.g., dead rodents, rodent excreta)
should be thoroughly cleaned to reduce the likelihood of exposure to hantavirus-infected materials. Clean-up procedures must be performed in a manner that limits the potential for aerosolization of dirt or dust from all potentially contaminated surfaces and household goods (Box 3 Table B3).

Table B3

Box 3. Clean-up of rodent-contaminated areas: Guidance for residents of
affected areas
— Persons involved in the clean-up should wear rubber or plastic gloves.
— Spray dead rodents, rodent nests, droppings, or food or other items that
have been tainted by rodents with a general-purpose household disinfectant. Soak the material thoroughly, and place in a plastic bag. When
clean-up is complete (or when the bag is full), seal the bag, then place it
into a second plastic bag and seal. Dispose of the bagged material by
burying in a 2- to 3-foot-deep hole or by burning. If these alternatives
are not feasible, contact the local or state health department concerning
other appropriate disposal methods.
— After the above items have been removed, mop floors with a solution of
water, detergent, and disinfectant. Spray dirt floors with a disinfectant
solution. A second mopping or spraying of floors with a general-purpose
household disinfectant is optional. Carpets can be effectively disinfected
with household disinfectants or by commercial-grade steam cleaning or
shampooing. To avoid generating potentially infectious aerosols, do not
vacuum or sweep dry surfaces before mopping.
— Disinfect countertops, cabinets, drawers, and other durable surfaces by
washing them with a solution of detergent, water, and disinfectant, followed
by an optional wiping-down with a general-purpose household disinfectant.
— Rugs and upholstered furniture should be steam cleaned or shampooed.
If rodents have nested inside furniture and the nests are not accessible
for decontamination, the furniture should be removed and burned.

— Launder potentially contaminated bedding and clothing with hot water and detergent. (Use rubber or plastic gloves when handling the dirty laundry; then wash and disinfect the gloves as described in the section on Eliminating Rodents Inside the Home.) Machine-dry laundry on a high setting or hang it to air dry in the sun.

SPECIAL PRECAUTIONS FOR HOMES OF PERSONS WITH CONFIRMED HANTAVIRUS INFECTION OR BUILDINGS WITH HEAVY RODENT INFESTATIONS

Special precautions are indicated in the affected areas for cleaning homes or buildings with heavy rodent infestations (Box 4 Table B4). Persons conducting these activities should contact the responsible local, state, or federal public health agency for guidance. These precautions may also apply to vacant dwellings that have attracted numbers of rodents while unoccupied and to dwellings and other structures that have been occupied by persons with confirmed hantavirus infection. Workers who are either hired specifically to perform the clean-up or asked to do so as part of their work activities should receive a thorough orientation from the responsible health agency about hantavirus transmission and should be trained to perform the required activities safely.

Table B4

Box 4. Special precautions for clean-up in homes of persons with hantavirus infection or buildings with heavy rodent infestation

— A baseline serum sample, preferably drawn at the time these activities are initiated, should be available for all persons conducting the clean-up of homes or buildings with heavy rodent infestation. The serum sample should be stored at $-20°C$.

— Persons involved in the clean-up should wear coveralls (disposable if possible), rubber boots or disposable shoe covers, rubber or plastic gloves, protective goggles, and an appropriate respiratory protection device, such as a half-mask air-purifying (or negative-pressure) respirator with a high-efficiency particulate air (HEPA) filter or a powered air-purifying respirator (PAPR) with HEPA filters. Respirators (including positive-pressure types) are not considered protective if facial hair interferes with the face seal, since proper fit cannot be assured. Respirator practices should follow a comprehensive user program and be supervised by a knowledgeable person (21).

— Personal protective gear should be decontaminated upon removal at the end of the day. If the coveralls are not disposable, they should be laundered on site. If no laundry facilities are available, the coveralls should be immersed in liquid disinfectant until they can be washed.

— All potentially infective waste material (including respirator filters) from clean-up operations that cannot be burned or deep buried on site should be double bagged in appropriate plastic bags. The bagged material should then be labeled as infectious (if it is to be transported) and disposed of in accordance with local requirements for infectious waste.

— Workers who develop a febrile or respiratory illness within 45 days of the last potential exposure should immediately seek medical attention and inform the attending physician of the potential occupational risk of hantavirus infection. The physician should contact local health authorities promptly if hantavirus-associated illness is suspected. A blood sample should be obtained and forwarded with the baseline serum through the state health department to CDC for further hantavirus antibody testing.

PRECAUTIONS FOR WORKERS IN AFFECTED AREAS WHO ARE REGULARLY EXPOSED TO RODENTS

Persons who frequently handle or are exposed to rodents (e.g., mammalogists, pest-control workers) in the affected area are probably at higher risk for hantavirus infection than the general public because of their frequency of exposure. Therefore, enhanced precautions are warranted to protect them against hantavirus infection (Box 5 Table B5).

Table B5

Box 5. Precautions for workers in affected areas who are exposed to rodents

— A baseline serum sample, preferably drawn at the time of employment, should be available for all persons whose occupations involve frequent rodent contact. The serum sample should be stored at $-20°C$.

— Workers in potentially high-risk settings should be informed about the symptoms of the disease and be given detailed guidance on prevention measures.

— Workers who develop a febrile or respiratory illness within 45 days of the last potential exposure should immediately seek medical attention and inform the attending physician of the potential occupational risk of hantavirus infection. The physician should contact local health authorities promptly if hantavirus-associated illness is suspected. A blood sample should be obtained and forwarded with the baseline serum through the state health department to CDC for further hantavirus antibody testing.

— Workers should wear a half-face air-purifying (or negative-pressure) respirator or PAPR equipped with HEPA filters when removing rodents from traps or handling rodents in the affected area. Respirators (including positive-pressure types) are not considered protective if facial hair interferes with the face seal, since proper fit cannot be assured. Respirator use practices should be in accord with a comprehensive user program and should be supervised by a knowledgeable person (21).

— Workers should wear rubber or plastic gloves when handling rodents or handling traps containing rodents. Gloves should be washed and disinfected before removing them, as described above.

— Traps contaminated by rodent urine or feces or in which a rodent was captured should be disinfected with a commercial disinfectant or bleach solution. Dispose of dead rodents as described in the section on Eliminating Rodents Inside the Home.

— Persons removing organs or obtaining blood from rodents in affected areas should contact the Special Pathogens Branch, Division of Viral and Rickettsial Diseases, National Center for Infectious Diseases, Centers for Disease Control and Prevention, (telephone (404) 639-1115) for detailed safety precautions.

PRECAUTIONS FOR OTHER OCCUPATIONAL GROUPS WHO HAVE POTENTIAL RODENT CONTACT

Insufficient information is available at this time to allow general recommendations regarding risks or precautions for persons in the affected areas who work in occupations with unpredictable or incidental contact with rodents or their habitations. Examples of such occupations include telephone installers, maintenance workers, plumbers, electricians, and certain construction workers. Workers in these jobs may have to enter various buildings, crawl spaces, or other sites that may be rodent infested. Recommendations for such circumstances must be made on a case-by-case basis after the specific working environment has been assessed and state or local health departments have been consulted.

PRECAUTIONS FOR CAMPERS AND HIKERS IN THE AFFECTED AREAS

There is no evidence to suggest that travel into the affected areas should be restricted. Most usual tourist activities pose little or no risk that travelers will be exposed to rodents or their excreta. However, persons engaged in outdoor activities such as camping or hiking should take precautions to reduce the likelihood of their exposure to potentially infectious materials (Box 6 Table B6).

Table B6

Box 6. Reducing risk of hantavirus infection: Guidance for hikers and campers

- Avoid coming into contact with rodent and rodent burrows or disturbing dens (such as pack rat nests).
- Do not use cabins or other enclosed shelters that are rodent infested until they have been appropriately cleaned and disinfected.
- Do not pitch tents or place sleeping bags in areas in proximity to rodent feces or burrows or near possible rodent shelters (e.g., garbage dumps or woodpiles).
- If possible, do not sleep on the bare ground. Use a cot with the sleeping surface at least 12 inches above the ground. Use tents with floors.
- Keep food in rodent-proof containers.
- Promptly bury (or—preferably—burn followed by burying, when in accordance with local requirements) all garbage and trash, or discard in covered trash containers.
- Use only bottled water or water that has been disinfected by filtration, boiling, chlorination, or iodination for drinking, cooking, washing dishes, and brushing teeth.

CONCLUSION

The control and prevention recommendations in this report represent general measures to minimize the likelihood of human exposure to hantavirus-infected rodents in areas of the southwestern United States affected by the outbreak of hantavirus-associated respiratory illness. Many of the recommendations may not be applicable or necessary in unaffected locales.

REFERENCES: AS NUMBERED IN ORIGINAL PUBLICATION

1. CDC. Outbreak of acute illness—Southwestern United States, 1993. MMWR 1993;42;421–424.
2. CDC. Update: outbreak of hantavirus infection—Southwestern United States, 1993. MMWR 1993;42:477–479.
3. CDC. Update: outbreak of hantavirus infection—Southwestern United States, 1993. MMWR 1993;42:495–496.
4. CDC. Update: hantavirus infection—United States. MMWR 1993;42:517–519.
5. LeDuc JW. Epidemiology of Hantaan and related viruses. Lab Anim Sci 1987;37:413–418.
6. Childs JE, Glass GE, Korch GW, et al. The ecology and epizootiology of hantaviral infections in small mammal communities of Baltimore: a review and synthesis. Bull Soc Vector Ecol 1988;13:113–122.
7. McKee KT Jr, LeDuc JW, Peters CJ. Hantaviruses. In: Belshe RB, ed. Textbook of human virology. 2nd ed. St. Louis: Mosby Year Book, 1991:615–632.
8. Bogdanova SB, Gavrilovskaya IN, Boyko VA, et al. Persistent infection caused by hemorrhagic fever with renal syndrome in red mice (Clethrionomys glareolus), natural hosts of the virus. Mikrobiol Zh 1987;49:99–106.
9. Lee HW, French GR, Lee PW, et al. Observations on natural and laboratory infection of rodents with the etiologic agent of Korean hemorrhagic fever. Am J Trop Med Hyg 1981;30:477–482.
10. Lee HW, Lee PW, Baek LJ, et al. Intraspecific transmission of Hantaan virus, etiologic agent of Korean hemorrhagic fever, in the rodent Apodemus agrarius. Am J Trop Med Hyg 1981;30:1106–1112.
11. Yanagihara R, Amyx HC, Gajdusek DC. Experimental infection with Puumala virus, the etiologic agent of nephropathia epidemica, in bank voles (Clethrionomys glareolus). J Virol 1985;55:34–38.
12. Tsai TF. Hemorrhagic fever with renal syndrome: mode of transmission to humans. Lab Anim Sci 1987;37:428–430.
13. Dournon E, Moriniere B, Matheron S, et al. Hemorrhagic fever with renal syndrome after a wild rodent bite in Haute-Savoie and risk of exposure to Hantaan-like virus in a Paris laboratory. Lancet 1984;i:676–677.
14. Kawamata J, Yamanouchi T, Dohmae K, et al. Control of laboratory acquired hemorrhagic fever with renal syndrome (HFRS) in Japan. Lab Anim Sci 1987;37:431–436.
15. Gligic A, Obradovic M, Stojanovic R, et al. Epidemic hemorrhagic fever with renal syndrome in Yugoslavia, 1986. Am J Trop Med Hyg 1989;41:102–108.
16. Niklasson B, LeDuc JW. Epidemiology of nephropathia epidemica in Sweden. J Infect Dis 1987;269–276.
17. Xu ZY, Guo CS, Wu YL, Zhang XW, Liu K. Epidemiological studies of hemorrhagic fever with renal syndrome. Analysis of risk factors and mode of transmission. J Infect Dis 1985;152:137–144.
18. Prince HN, Prince DL, Prince RN. Principles of viral control and transmission. In: Block SS, ed. Disinfection, sterilization, and preservation, 4th ed. Philadelphia: Lea & Febiger, 1991:411–444.
19. Pratt HD, Brown RZ. Biological factors in domestic rodent control. Washington, DC: US Government Printing Office, DHEW Publication No. (CDC) 79–8144, 1979.
20. Scott HG, Borom MR. Rodent-borne disease control through rodent stoppage. Washington, DC: US Government Printing Office, DHEW Publication No. (CDC) 77–8343, 1977.
21. NIOSH. NIOSH guide to industrial respiratory protection. Cincinnati: National Institute for Occupational Safety and Health, DHHS (NIOSH) Publication No. 87–116, 1987.

TOPIC 11 / HAEMOPHILUS B

Recommendations for Use of Haemophilus b Conjugate Vaccines and a Combined Diphtheria, Tetanus, Pertussis, and Haemophilus b Vaccine

Original Citation: Recommendations for Use of Haemophilus b Conjugate Vaccines and a Combined Diphtheria, Tetanus, Pertussis, and Haemophilus b Vaccine. Recommendations of the Advisory Committee on Immunization Practices (ACIP). MMWR 1993;42(RR-13).

SUMMARY

These recommendations include information on two vaccines recently licensed for use among infants: Haemophilus b Conjugate Vaccine (PRP-T [ActHIB®, OmniHIB®]), manufactured by Pasteur Merieux Vaccins, and TETRAMUNE™, manufactured by Lederle Laboratories/Praxis Biologics. This statement also updates recommendations for use of other available Haemophilus b vaccines (PRP-D [ProHIBiT®]; HbOC [HibTITER®]; and PRP-OMP [PedvaxHIB®]) for infants and children.

INTRODUCTION

The incidence of Haemophilus influenzae type b (Hib) disease in the United States has declined since the mid-1980s (1). Before the introduction of effective vaccines, Hib was the leading cause of bacterial meningitis and other invasive bacterial disease among children less than 5 years of age; approximately one in 200 children developed invasive Hib disease before the age of 5 years. Nearly all infections occurred among children less than 5 years of age, and approximately two-thirds of all cases occurred among children less than 18 months of age. Meningitis occurred in approximately two-thirds of children with invasive Hib disease, resulting in hearing impairment or neurologic sequelae in 15%–30%. The case-fatality rate was 2%–5% (2).

In 1985, the first Hib vaccines were licensed for use in the United States. These vaccines contained purified polyribosylribitol phosphate (PRP) capsular material from type b strains. Antibody against PRP was shown to be the primary component of serum bactericidal activity against the organism. Although the vaccine was highly effective in trials in Finland among children greater than or equal to 18 months of age (3), postmarketing efficacy studies in the United States demonstrated variable efficacy (4, 5). PRP vaccines were ineffective in children less than 18 months of age because of the T-cell-independent nature of the immune response to PRP polysaccharide (3).

Conjugation of the PRP polysaccharide with protein carriers confers T-cell-dependent characteristics to the vaccine and substantially enhances the immunologic response to the PRP antigen. By 1989, Hib conjugate vaccines (PRP-D [ProHIBiT®], HbOC [HibTITER®], and PRP-OMP [PedvaxHIB®]) were licensed for use among children greater than or equal to 15 months of age. In late 1990, following two prospective studies, PRP-OMP (6) and HbOC (7) were licensed for use among infants. On the basis of findings establishing comparable immunogenicity, a third conjugate vaccine, PRP-T (ActHIB™, OmniHIB™) has now been licensed for use among infants. Specific characteristics of the four conjugate vaccines available for infants and children vary (e.g., the type of protein carrier, the size of the polysaccharide, and the chemical linkage between the polysaccharide and carrier) (Table 1).

Table 1. *Haemophilus influenzae* type b conjugate vaccines licensed for use among children

Vaccine	Trade name (manufacturer)	Polysaccharide	Linkage	Protein carrier
PRP-D	ProHIBiT® (Connaught)	Medium	6-carbon	Diphtheria toxoid
HbOC*	HibTITER® (Lederle-Praxis)	Small	None	CRM_{197} mutant *Corynebacterium diphtheriae* toxin protein
PRP-OMP	PedvaxHIB® (Merck Sharp and Dohme)	Medium	Thioether	*Neisseria meningitidis* outer membrane protein complex
PRP-T	ActHIB™ OmniHIB™ (Pasteur Mérieux Vaccins)	Large	6-carbon	Tetanus toxoid

*TETRAMUNE™ consists of HbOC and DTP vaccine (TRI-IMMUNOL®), manufactured by Lederle Laboratories/Praxis Biologics.

Current recommendations for universal vaccination of infants require parenteral administration of three different vaccines (diphtheria-tetanus-pertussis [DTP], Hib conjugate, and hepatitis B) during two or three different visits to a health-care provider. Combination vaccines were developed to reduce the number of injections at each visit. TETRAMUNE™ is the first licensed combination vaccine that provides protection against diphtheria, tetanus, pertussis, and Hib disease.

This statement (a) summarizes current immunogenicity and efficacy data regarding Hib conjugate vaccines, including PRP-T; (b) summarizes available information regarding the safety and immunogenicity of TETRAMUNE™; and (c) provides updated recommendations from the Advisory Committee on Immunization Practices (ACIP) for use of conjugate Hib vaccines and TETRAMUNE™ for infants and children.

HIB CONJUGATE VACCINES

Immunogenicity

Studies have been performed with all four Hib conjugate vaccines to determine immunogenicity in infants 2–6 months of age. Direct comparison of studies is complicated by differing vaccination and blood collection regimens and interlaboratory variation in assays for measurement of PRP antibody. Also, the precise level of antibody required for protection against invasive disease is not clearly established. However, a geometric mean titer (GMT) of 1 µg/mL 3 weeks postvaccination correlated with protection in studies following vaccination with unconjugated PRP vaccine and suggests long-term protection from invasive disease (8).

After three vaccinations at ages 2, 4, and 6 months, each of three Hib conjugate vaccines—HbOC, PRP-OMP, and PRP-T—produced protective levels of anticapsular antibody (9–13). One study reported comparative immunogenicity with PRP-OMP, HbOC, and PRP-T (12), and two other studies compared immunogenicity with all four conjugate vaccines (11, 13) (Table 2). In this age group, only PRP-OMP vaccine produced a substantial increase in antibody after one dose (12, 13). Antibody response among infants following a series of three infant vaccinations with PRP-D is limited (only 15%–45% of infants develop a GMT greater than or equal to 1 µg/mL after 3 doses) (11, 13, 14) and is lower than with HbOC, PRP-OMP, or PRP-T.

With each conjugate vaccine, antibody levels decline after administration of the primary series. Regardless of the conjugate vaccine used in the primary series for infants, booster vaccination of children greater than or equal to 12 months of age with any of the licensed conjugate vaccines will likely elicit an

Table 2. Immunogenicity of three *Haemophilus influenzae* type b vaccines among infants

Vaccine[†]	Study site	Geometric mean titer, µg/mL (% > 1 µg/mL)*			
		Before vaccination	After dose 1[§]	After dose 2	After dose 3
Study 1	Tennessee (11)				
PRP-D		0.07	—	0.08	0.28 (29)
PRP-OMP[¶]		0.11	0.83	0.84 (50)	1.14 (55)
HbOC		0.07	0.09	0.13	3.08 (75)
PRP-T		0.10	0.05	0.30	3.64 (83)
Study 2	Alaska (13)				
PRP-D		0.06 (4)	0.04 (2)	0.06 (11)	0.55 (45)
PRP-OMP[¶]		0.16 (14)	1.37 (57)	2.71 (79)	—
HbOC		0.15 (5)	0.07 (0)	0.59 (43)	13.70 (94)
PRP-T		0.18 (13)	0.06 (0)	0.32 (20)	2.46 (78)
Study 3	Minnesota/Missouri/				
PRP-OMP[¶]	Texas (12)	0.18	2.69 (80)	4.00 (85)	5.21 (88)
HbOC		0.17	0.11	0.45 (23)	6.31 (90)
PRP-T		0.25	0.19	1.25 (56)	6.37 (97)

*Measured by radioimmunoassay.

[†]In all studies, vaccine was administered at 2, 4, and 6 months of age.

[§]Antibody level after one dose includes data from only one of four data collection sites in Tennessee.

[¶]Current recommendations require only two doses of PRP-OMP in the primary series. For studies 1 and 3, three doses were administered.

—Data not available.

adequate response, as studies indicate that (a) unconjugated PRP (administered at 12–14 months of age) elicits a good booster response in infants who are administered PRP-OMP (15), HbOC (15, 16), or PRP-T (15, 16) during infancy; (b) PRP-D administered as a booster at age 15 months induces adequate immunologic response regardless of the Hib conjugate administered in the initial series (17); and (c) each conjugate vaccine demonstrates adequate immunogenicity when administered as a single vaccination to children greater than or equal to 15 months of age (18, 19).

Limited information is available regarding the interchangeability of different Hib vaccines for the primary series at 2, 4, and 6 months of age (Table 3). Preliminary findings from two studies suggest that the vaccination series consisting of PRP-OMP at 2 months, followed by either PRP-T (20, 21) or HbOC (20, 22) at 4 months and 6 months, induces adequate anti-PRP antibody response. The sequence HbOC, PRP-T, PRP-T was also immunogenic (20) after the complete primary series was administered. This information suggests that any combination of three doses of Hib conjugate vaccines licensed for use among infants will provide adequate protection.

The carrier proteins used in PRP-T, PRP-D, and HbOC (but not PRP-OMP) are derived from the toxoids used in DTP vaccine (Table 1). Limited data have indicated that prior or concurrent administration of DTP vaccine may enhance anti-PRP antibody response following vaccination with these Hib vaccines (23–26). It has been suggested that priming T-cells to the carrier proteins may be important for optimal antibody response to the conjugated vaccine. For infants, the immunogenicity of PRP-OMP (which has a carrier derived from the meningococcal outer membrane protein) appears to be unaffected by the absence of prior or concurrent DTP vaccination (24).

Efficacy

Efficacy studies of PRP-D, PRP-OMP, HbOC, and PRP-T vaccines administered to infants 2–6 months of age are summarized in this report (Table 4). Two randomized, double-blind trials evaluating PRP-T vaccine efficacy were discontinued in the United States in October 1990 after licensure was granted to HbOC and PRP-OMP vaccines. A third efficacy trial of PRP-T in England has recently been completed.

Efficacy of the PRP-D conjugate has varied with the age of the population studied. Postlicensure studies performed in the United States among children aged 15–60 months demonstrated point estimates of efficacy ranging from 74%–96%. Two studies have prospectively evaluated efficacy of PRP-D administered to children less than 12 months of age. In a trial in Finland involving 114,000 infants vaccinated at 3, 4, and 6 months of age, the point estimate of efficacy was 89% (95% confidence interval [CI] = 70–96) (27). In comparison, among Alaskan Natives vaccinated at ages 2, 4, and 6 months, the point estimate of efficacy was 35% (95% CI = −57–73) and not significantly different from zero (28).

Table 3. Summary of preliminary immunogenicity data using different Hib conjugate vaccine sequences among infants

Vaccine[†]	Study site	Sample size	Geometric mean titer, µg/mL*			
			Before vaccination	After dose 1	After dose 2	After dose 3
Study 1	Tennessee (22)					
O-H-H[§¶]		55	0.113	—	0.90	5.63
H-O-O[¶]		57	0.082	—	0.56	0.67
Study 2	Chicago (21)					
O-T-T		27	0.14	—	—	6.98
Study 3	California (20)					
O-H-H		10	0.10	3.68	5.84	16.4
O-H-H[¶]		23	0.09	0.48	2.72	12.7
H-T-T		24	0.16	0.11	3.13	11.1
O-T-T		28	0.06	2.42	6.10	12.3

*Measured by radioimmunoassay.
[†]In all studies, vaccine was administered at 2, 4, and 6 months of age.
[§]O = PRP-OMP, H = HbOC, T = PRP-T.
[¶]The manufacturer reported that immunogenicity conferred by PRP-OMP lots in these sequences was less than expected.
—Data not available.

Table 4. Efficacy of Hib conjugate vaccines among infants

Vaccine	Population	Design	Age at vaccination (mos)	% efficacy (95% CI*)
PRP-D	Finland (27)	Open, randomized	3, 4, 6	89 (70–96)
	Alaskan Natives (28)	Placebo-controlled, randomized	2, 4, 6	35 (57–73)
PRP-OMP	Navajo (6)	Placebo-controlled, randomized	2, 4	93 (53–98)[†] 100 (67–100)[§]
HbOC	California (7)	Open, partially randomized	2, 4, 6	100 (67–100)
	Finland (29)	Open	4, 6	97[¶]
PRP-T	California (30)	Controlled, randomized	2, 4, 6	**
	North Carolina (see text)	Placebo-controlled	2, 4, 6	**
	United Kingdom (31)	Open, controlled	2, 3, 4	‡
	Finland (32)	Historical controls	4, 6	‡

*Confidence interval.
[†]Includes cases that occurred before 18 months of age.
[§]Includes cases that occurred before 15 months of age.
[¶]Confidence intervals not reported.
**Studies evaluating efficacy of PRP-T vaccine in the United States were terminated before completion.
[‡]Point estimate and confidence intervals not reported.

PRP-OMP was shown to be 93%–100% efficacious in Navajo infants (a population at particularly high risk of disease) vaccinated at 2 and 4 months of age (6). Two studies have indicated a point estimate of efficacy of greater than or equal to 97% following the administration of two doses of HbOC (in Finland) (29) or three doses of vaccine (in the United States) (7) to infants.

Although the trials evaluating PRP-T vaccine efficacy among infants in the United States were terminated early, no cases of invasive Hib disease were reported among more than 6,200 vaccines at the time of termination (30; J.C. Parke, Carolinas Medical Center, unpublished data). In a trial in Great Britain, PRP-T was protective in infants vaccinated at ages 2, 3, and 4 months (31). Efficacy of PRP-T was also suggested in a nationwide immunization program that was implemented in Finland in January 1990. There were no reported cases of invasive Hib disease among more than 97,000 infants who received greater than or equal to 2 doses of PRP-T. Two children developed disease after one dose of vaccine (32).

In the United States, 30–50 cases of invasive Hib disease have been reported among children who had received appropriate vaccination with the Hib conjugate vaccine and therefore were expected to have had adequate levels of protective antibody (33–35). These cases may represent vaccine failure. Results of immunologic evaluation of children who had vaccine failure vary with the age of the child. In a study of children vaccinated with Hib conjugate vaccine at age greater than or equal to 15 months, subnormal immunoglobulin concentrations were present in approximately 40% of those who developed invasive Hib disease (33). However, in a separate study that evaluated fully vaccinated children less than 12 months of age who developed invasive Hib disease, only 9% had evidence of low immunoglobulin levels (34).

COMBINATION VACCINES

Tetramune™

On March 30, 1993, the Food and Drug Administration licensed TETRAMUNE™, a vaccine manufactured by Lederle Laboratories/Praxis Biologics by combining a licensed DTP vaccine (TRI-IMMUNOL®) and HbOC (HibTITER®). TETRA-MUNE™ contains 12.5 Lf of diphtheria toxoid, 5 Lf of tetanus toxoid, an estimated 4 protective units of pertussis vaccine, 10 μg of purified Hib polysaccharide, and approximately 25 μg of CRM197 protein. The single-dose volume is 0.5 mL to be administered intramuscularly.

Safety and Immunogenicity

The safety of TETRAMUNE™ vaccine was evaluated in a study of 6,497 infants in California who received doses at ages 2, 4, and 6 months, compared with 3,935 infants who received DTP (TRI-IMMUNOL®) and HbOC vaccines as separate concurrent injections (36; Lederle Laboratories/Praxis Biologics, unpublished data). Based on follow-up of a randomized subset of 1,411 infants (for whom 1,347 parents were interviewed), the risk for local and systemic reactions was similar for infants who received the combination product when compared with those who received two separate injections of DTP and HbOC. The infants who received the combination vaccine, however, experienced a higher likelihood of restless sleep following the second dose and greater than or equal to 1 inch of swelling at the injection site after administration of the first dose of the combination vaccine (Table 5).

Immunogenicity studies among infants who received TETRAMUNE™ at ages 2, 4, and 6 months (37; Lederle Laboratories/Praxis Biologics, unpub-

Table 5. Reactions following administration of TETRAMUNE™ compared with concurrent separate administration of DTP and HbOC vaccine among infants*†

Reaction	After dose 1		After dose 2		After dose 3	
	Combined (n = 585)	Separate§ (n = 550)	Combined (n = 540)	Separate (n = 430)	Combined (n = 470)	Separate (n = 380)
Local						
Redness	15.7	16.1	20.7	19.1	19.5	17.8
Redness ≥1 inch	4.9	3.0	1.8	1.6	1.5	0.8
Swelling	22.4	19.8	14.0	18.6	15.3	16.2
Swelling ≥1 inch	8.0¶	4.3	3.0	3.5	2.5	3.4
Tenderness	31.6	29.8	22.8	22.1	24.3	21.6
Tenderness ≥1 inch	9.6	6.6	6.0	5.2	5.4	3.8
Systemic	(n = 585)	(n = 570)	(n = 550)	(n = 450)	(n = 485)	(n = 395)
Perceived fever	38.0	35.6	39.7	38.4	40.0	38.3
Irritability	53.8	56.5	51.9	50.8	56.0	52.7
Restless sleep	19.9	24.1	32.0¶	26.1	31.1	32.0
Vomiting	1.7	2.6	1.8	2.2	2.1	2.0
Diarrhea	1.4	1.2	1.1	0.7	0.8	2.3
Loss of appetite	3.9	3.5	3.3	2.2	3.7	4.8
Other**	7.3	9.2	7.8	8.3	6.6	9.4

*Percentage of infants experiencing event within 24 hours of vaccination.
†From reference 36 and unpublished data from manufacturer.
§For the separate group, no attempt was made to sum reactions that occurred at both injection sites; reactions only to DTP site were counted.
¶$p < 0.05$, combined vs. separate vaccination groups.
**Rash, lethargy, congestion, runny nose/eyes, changes in bowel movement other than diarrhea, increased appetite/thirst, bruising/bleeding/hot at injection site.

lished data) indicated that antibody responses to Hib PRP, diphtheria, and tetanus toxins were comparable to or higher than those in persons who received separate, but concurrent administration of DTP and HbOC vaccines. Similarly, antibody responses to pertussis toxin, filamentous hemagglutinin, 69-kD outer-membrane protein (pertactin), and pertussis agglutinins were comparable to or higher than those following separate concurrent administration of DTP and HbOC vaccines (Table 6). Comparable immunogenicity results also were reported for children aged 15–18 months (who had received prior doses of DTP, but not Hib vaccine) following a dose of TETRAMUNE™ when compared with separate but concurrent administration of DTP and HbOC vaccines.

Table 6. Immunogenicity of TETRAMUNE™ versus separate injections of DTP and HbOC in infants*

Component	Geometric mean titer[†]		
	Combined (n = 189)	Separate (n = 189)	P-value[§]
HbOC (μg/mL)			
Pre	0.09	0.09	0.762
Post 1	0.12	0.10	0.002
Post 2	0.66	0.34	<0.001
Post 3	6.67	4.42	0.034
Diphtheria (IU/mL)			
Pre	0.04	0.05	0.624
Post 3	0.71	0.40	0.009
Tetanus (U/mL)			
Pre	0.45	0.50	0.404
Post 3	8.20	4.51	<0.001
Pertussis agglutinins (reciprocal dilution)			
Pre	6.53	4.69	0.121
Post 3	51.93	23.34	0.008
Pertussis toxin[†¶]			
Pre	1.09	1.80	
Post 3	85.92	17.60	0.001**
Pertactin (69K)[†¶]			
Pre	6.13	5.98	
Post 3	66.43	41.55	0.11**
FHA[†¶]			
Pre	3.97	4.73	
Post 3	2.32	0.79	0.0001**

*From reference 37 and unpublished data from manufacturer. Combined (DTP/HbOC) or separate (DTP and HbOC) vaccine administered at 2, 4, and 6 months of age.
[†]Antibody titers are measured in enzyme-linked immunosorbent assay units per mL unless otherwise indicated.
[§]Based on model controlling for treatment, study site, vaccine lot, age of infant, and baseline antibody level.
[¶]Subset of n = 52 for combined group; n = 34 for separate group.
**Calculated using a Wilcoxon 2-sample test.

Efficacy

No efficacy information is available for TETRAMUNE™, but the immuno-genicity information suggests TETRAMUNE™ will provide similar protection against Hib disease and diphtheria, tetanus, and pertussis as will the separate administration of HbOC or DTP vaccines.

Other combination vaccines

Published studies have evaluated the safety and immunogenicity of other vaccines that combine DTP (or DTaP [acellular pertussis component]) and Hib in the same formulation or the same syringe. However, none of these formulations (PRP-D-DTaP [38], HbOC-DTaP [39, 40], or PRP-T-DTP [41]) have been licensed for use. Two studies have shown a slight reduction in the immune response to pertussis when certain Hib vaccines were combined with DTP (42, 43), but the magnitude of the effect is unlikely to be clinically relevant.

Simultaneous vaccination

Large prelicensure and postlicensure studies have demonstrated the safety, immunogenicity, and efficacy of each of the licensed Hib conjugate vaccines administered to infants concurrently with DTP vaccine and oral polio vaccine (OPV) (6, 7, 9, 32) as well as the safety and immunogenicity of TETRAMUNE™ when administered concurrently with OPV in recommended schedules (36, 37). More limited data also support the safety and immunogenicity of Hib conjugate vaccines when administered simultaneously with hepatitis B vaccine to infants, and with DTP, OPV, measles, mumps, and rubella (MMR) and/or hepatitis B vaccine when administered at ages 12–18 months.

RECOMMENDATIONS FOR HIB VACCINATION

General

All infants should receive a conjugate Hib vaccine (separate or in combination with DTP (TETRAMUNE™), beginning at age 2 months (but not earlier than 6 weeks). If the first vaccination is delayed beyond age 6 months, the schedule of vaccination for previously unimmunized children should be followed (Table 7). When possible, the Hib conjugate vaccine used at the first vaccination should be used for all subsequent vaccinations in the primary series. When either Hib vaccines or TETRAMUNE™ is used, the vaccine should be administered intramuscularly using a separate syringe and administered at a separate site from any other concurrent vaccinations.

HbOC or PRP-T

Previously unvaccinated infants aged 2–6 months should receive three doses of vaccine administered 2 months apart, followed by a booster dose at age 12–15 months, at least 2 months after the last vaccination. Unvaccinated children ages 7–11 months should receive two doses of vaccine, 2 months apart, followed by a booster dose at age 12–18 months, at least 2 months after the last vaccination. Unvaccinated children ages 12–14 months should receive two

Table 7. Schedule for Hib conjugate vaccine administration among previously vaccinated children

Vaccine	Age at first vaccination (mos)	Primary series	Booster
HbOC/PRP-T*	2–6	3 doses, 2 mos apart	12–15 mos
	7–11	2 doses, 2 mos apart	12–18 mos
	12–14	1 dose	2 mos later
	15–59	1 dose	—
PRP-OMP	2–6	2 doses, 2 mos apart	12–15 mos
	7–11	2 doses, 2 mos apart	12–18 mos
	12–14	1 dose	2 mos later
	15–59	1 dose	—
PRP-D	15–59	1 dose	—

*TETRAMUNE™ may be administered by the same schedule for primary immunization as HbOC/PRP-T (when the series begins at 2–6 months of age). A booster dose of DTP or DTaP should be administered at 4–6 years of age, before kindergarten or elementary school. This booster is not necessary if the fourth vaccinating dose was administered after the fourth birthday. See ACIP statement for information on use of DTP and contraindications for use of pertussis vaccine (44).
—Not applicable.

doses of vaccine, at least 2 months apart. Any previously unvaccinated child aged 15–59 months should receive a single dose of vaccine.

PRP-OMP

Previously unvaccinated infants ages 2–6 months should receive two doses of vaccine administered at least 2 months apart. Although PRP-OMP induces a substantial antibody response after one dose, all children should receive all recommended doses of PRP-OMP. Because of the substantial antibody response after one dose, it may be advantageous to use PRP-OMP vaccine in populations that are known to be at increased risk for disease during early infancy (e.g., Alaskan Natives). A booster dose should be administered to all children at 12–15 months of age at least 2 months after the last vaccination. Unvaccinated children ages 7–11 months should receive two doses of vaccine, 2 months apart, followed by a booster dose at 12–18 months of age, at least 2 months after the last dose. Unvaccinated children ages 12–14 months should receive two doses of vaccine, 2 months apart. Any previously unvaccinated child 15–59 months of age should receive a single dose of vaccine.

PRP-D

One dose of PRP-D may be administered to unvaccinated children aged 15–59 months. This vaccine may be used as a booster dose at 12–18 months of age following a two- or three-dose primary series, regardless of the vaccine used in the primary series. This vaccine is not licensed for use among infants because of its limited immunogenicity and variable protective efficacy in this age group.

TETRAMUNE™

The combination vaccine TETRAMUNE™ may be used for routine vaccination of infants, beginning at age 2 months, to prevent diphtheria, tetanus, pertussis, and invasive Hib disease. Previously unvaccinated infants aged 2–6 months should receive three doses administered at least 2 months apart. An additional dose should be administered at 12–15 months of age, after at least a 6-month interval following the third dose. Alternatively, acellular DTP and Hib vaccine can be administered as separate injections at 12–15 months of age. Acellular DTP is preferred for doses four and five of the five-dose DTP series. For infants who begin both Hib and DTP vaccinations late (after 2 months of age), TETRAMUNE™ may be used for the first and second doses of the vaccine series. However, because delay in initiation of the DTP series does not reduce the number of required doses of DTP, additional doses of DTP without Hib are necessary to ensure that all four doses are administered. Infants ages 7–11 months who have not previously been vaccinated with DTP or Hib vaccines should receive two doses of TETRAMUNE™, administered at least 2 months apart, followed by a dose of DTP vaccine 4–8 weeks after the second dose of TETRAMUNE™. An additional dose of DTP and Hib vaccines should then be administered: DTP vaccine at least 6 months after the third immunizing dose against diphtheria, tetanus, and pertussis; and Hib vaccine at 12–18 months of age, at least 2 months after the last Hib dose.

TETRAMUNE™ may be used to complete an infant immunization series started with any Hib vaccine (licensed for use in this age group) and with any DTP vaccine if both vaccines are to be administered simultaneously. Completion of the primary series using the same Hib vaccine, however, is preferable. Conversely, any DTP vaccine may be used to complete a series initiated with TETRAMUNE™ (see the general ACIP statement on Diphtheria, Tetanus and Pertussis: Recommendations for Vaccine Use and Other Preventive Measures [44] for further information).

Other Considerations for Hib Vaccination

Other considerations for Hib vaccination are discussed in the following section:

1. Although an interval of 2 months between doses of Hib vaccine in the primary series is recommended, an interval of 1 month is acceptable, if necessary.
2. Unvaccinated children aged 15–59 months may be administered a single dose of any one of the four Hib conjugate vaccines or TETRAMUNE™ (if both Hib and DTP vaccines are indicated).
3. After the primary infant vaccination series is completed, any of the four licensed Hib conjugate vaccines (or TETRAMUNE™ if both Hib vaccine and DTP vaccine are indicated) may be used as a booster dose at age 12–15 months.
4. The primary vaccine series should preferably be completed with the same Hib conjugate vaccine. If, however, different vaccines are administered, a total of three doses of Hib conjugate vaccine is adequate. Any combination of Hib conjugate vaccines that is licensed for use among infants may be used to complete the primary series.
5. Infants born prematurely should be vaccinated according to the schedule recommended for other infants, beginning at age 2 months.
6. Hib conjugate vaccines may be administered simultaneously with DTP (or DTaP) vaccine, OPV, IPV, MMR, influenza, and hepatitis B vaccines. TETRAMUNE™ may be administered simultaneously with OPV, IPV, MMR, influenza, and hepatitis B vaccines.
7. Because natural infection does not always result in the development of protective anti-PRP antibody

levels (45), children less than 24 months of age who develop invasive Hib disease should receive Hib vaccine as recommended in the schedule. These children should be considered unimmunized, and vaccination should start as soon as possible during the convalescent phase of the illness.

8. Hib vaccine is immunogenic in patients with increased risk for invasive disease, such as those with sickle-cell disease (46), leukemia (47), human immunodeficiency virus (HIV) infection (48, 49), and in those who have had splenectomies (50). However, in persons with HIV infection, immunogenicity varies with stage of infection and degree of immunocompromise. Efficacy studies have not been performed in populations with increased risk of invasive disease (see the general ACIP statement on Use of Vaccines and Immune Globulins in Persons with Altered Immunocompetence [51]).

9. Children who attend day care are at increased risk for Hib disease. Therefore, efforts should be made to ensure that all day care attendees less than 5 years of age are fully vaccinated.

10. Rifampin chemoprophylaxis for household contacts of a person with invasive Hib disease is no longer indicated if all contacts ages less than 4 years are fully vaccinated against Hib disease. A child is considered fully immunized against Hib disease following (a) at least one dose of conjugate vaccine at greater than or equal to 15 months of age, (b) two doses of conjugate vaccine at 12–14 months of age, or (c) two or more doses of conjugate vaccine at less than 12 months of age, followed by a booster dose at greater than or equal to 12 months of age. In households with one or more infants less than 12 months of age (regardless of vaccination status) or with a child aged 1–3 years who is inadequately vaccinated, all household contacts should receive rifampin prophylaxis following a case of invasive Hib disease that occurs in any family member. The recommended dose is 20 mg/kg as a single daily dose (maximal daily dose 600 mg) for 4 days. Neonates (less than 1 month of age) should receive 10 mg/kg once daily for 4 days.

Adverse Reactions

Adverse reactions to each of the four Hib conjugate vaccines are generally uncommon. Swelling, redness, and/or pain have been reported in 5%–30% of recipients and usually resolve within 12–24 hours. Systemic reactions such as fever and irritability are infrequent. Available information on side effects and adverse reactions suggests that the risks for local and systemic events following TETRAMUNE™ administration are similar to those following concurrent administration of its individual component vaccines (i.e., DTP and Hib vaccines), and may be due largely to the pertussis component of the DTP vaccine (52).

Surveillance regarding the safety of TETRAMUNE™, PRP-T, and other Hib vaccines in large-scale use aids in the assessment of vaccine safety by identifying potential events that may warrant further study. The Vaccine Adverse Event Reporting System (VAERS) of the U.S. Department of Health and Human Services encourages reports of all serious adverse events that occur after receipt of any vaccine.* Invasive Hib disease is a reportable condition in 43 states. All health-care workers should report any case of invasive Hib disease to local and state health departments.

Contraindications and Precautions

Vaccination with a specific Hib conjugate vaccine is contraindicated in persons known to have experienced anaphylaxis following a prior dose of that vaccine. Vaccination should be delayed in children with moderate or severe illnesses. Minor illnesses (e.g., mild upper-respiratory infection) are not contraindications to vaccination.

Contraindications and precautions of the use of TETRAMUNE™ are the same as those for its individual component vaccines (i.e., DTP or Hib) (see the general ACIP statement on Diphtheria, Tetanus, and Pertussis: Recommendations for Vaccine Use and Other Preventive Measures [44] for more details on the use of vaccines containing DTP).

REFERENCES: AS NUMBERED IN ORIGINAL PUBLICATION

1. Adams WG, Deaver KA, Cochi SL, et al. Decline of childhood Haemophilus influenzae type b (Hib) disease in the Hib vaccine era. JAMA 1993;269:221–226.
2. Broome CV. Epidemiology of Haemophilus influenzae type b infections in the United States. Pediatr Infect Dis J 1987;6:779–782.
3. Peltola H, Kayhty H, Sivonen A, et al. Haemophilus influenzae type b capsular polysaccharide vaccine in children: a double-blind field study of 100,000 vaccinees 3 months to 5 years of age

*Questions about reporting requirements, completion of report forms, or requests for reporting forms should be directed to VAERS at 1-800-822-7967.

in Finland. Pediatrics 1977;60:730–737.

4. Ward JI, Broome CV, Harrison LH, Shinefield HR, Black SB. Haemophilus influenzae type b vaccines: lessons for the future. Pediatrics 1988;81:886–893.

5. Harrison LH, Broome CV, Hightower AW, et al. A day care-based study of the efficacy of Haemophilus b polysaccharide vaccine. JAMA 1988;260:1413–1418.

6. Santosham M, Wolff M, Reid R, et al. The efficacy in Navajo infants of a conjugate vaccine consisting of Haemophilus influenzae type b polysaccharide and Neisseria meningitidis outer-membrane protein complex. N Engl J Med 1991;324:1767–1772.

7. Black SB, Shinefield HR, Fireman B, et al. Efficacy in infancy of oligosaccharide conjugate Haemophilus influenzae type b (HbOC) vaccine in a United States population of 61,080 children. Pediatr Infect Dis J 1991;10:97–104.

8. Kayhty H, Peltola H, Karanko V, Makela PH. The protective level of serum antibodies to the capsular polysaccharide of Haemophilus influenzae type b. J Infect Dis 1983;147:1100.

9. Black SB, Shinefield HR, Lampert D, et al. Safety and immunogenicity of oligosaccharide conjugate Haemophilus influenzae type b (HbOC) vaccine in infancy. Pediatr Infect Dis J 1991;10:92–96.

10. Parke JC, Schneerson R, Reimer C, et al. Clinical and immunologic responses to Haemophilus influenzae type b-tetanus toxoid conjugate vaccine in infants injected at 3, 5, 7, and 18 months of age. J Pediatr 1991;118:184–190.

11. Decker MD, Edwards KM, Bradley R, Palmer P. Comparative trial in infants of four conjugate Haemophilus influenzae type b vaccines. J Pediatr 1992;120:184–189.

12. Granoff DM, Anderson EL, Osterholm MT, et al. Differences in the immunogenicity of three Haemophilus influenzae type b conjugate vaccines in infants. J Pediatr 1992;121:187–194.

13. Bulkow LR, Wainwright RB, Letson GW, Chang SJ, Ward JI. Comparative immunogenicity of four Haemophilus influenzae type b conjugate vaccines in Alaska Native infants. Pediatr Infect Dis J 1993;12:484–492.

14. Ward JI, Brenneman G, Lepow M, Lum M, Burkhart K, Chiu CY. Haemophilus influenzae type b anticapsular antibody responses to PRP-Pertussis and PRP-D vaccines in Alaska native infants. J Infect Dis 1988;158:719–723.

15. Granoff DM, Holmes SJ, Osterholm MT, et al. Induction of immunologic memory in infants primed with Haemophilus influenzae type b conjugate vaccines. J Infect Dis 1993;168:663–671.

16. Kayhty H, Eskola J, Peltola H, Saarinen L, Makela PH. High antibody response to booster doses of either Haemophilus influenzae capsular polysaccharide or conjugate vaccine after primary immunization with conjugate vaccines. J Infect Dis 1992;165(Suppl 1):S165–S166.

17. Decker MD, Edwards KM, Bradley R, Palmer P. Responses of children to booster immunization with their primary conjugate Haemophilus influenzae type b vaccine or with polyribosylribitol phosphate conjugated with diphtheria toxoid. J Pediatr 1993;122:410–413.

18. Turner RB, Cimino CO, Sullivan BJ. Prospective comparison of response of infants to three Haemophilus influenzae type b vaccines. Pediatr Infect Dis J 1991;10:108–112.

19. Holmes SJ, Murphy TV, Anderson RS, et al. Immunogenicity of four Haemophilus influenzae type b vaccines in 17- to 19-month-old children. J Pediatr 1991;118:364–371.

20. Greenberg DP, Lieberman JM, Marcy SM, et al. Safety and immunogenicity of mixed sequences of Haemophilus influenzae type B (HIB) conjugate vaccines in infants [Abstract #997]. Pediatr Res 1993;33:169A.

21. Daum RS, Milewski WM, Ballanco GA. Interchangeability of H. influenzae type B vaccines for the primary series ("mix and match")—a preliminary analysis [Abstract #976]. Pediatr Res 1993;33:166A.

22. Anderson EL, Decker MD, Edwards KM, Englund JA, Belshe RB. Interchangeability of conjugated Haemophilus influenzae type B (HIB) vaccines in infants [Abstract #493]. Pediatr Res 1993;33:85A.

23. Schneerson R, Robbins JB, Chu C, et al. Serum antibody responses of juvenile and infant rhesus monkeys injected with Haemophilus influenzae type b and pneumococcus type 6A capsular polysaccharide-protein conjugates. Infect Immun 1984;45:582–591.

24. Vella PA, Ellis RW. Immunogenicity of Haemophilus influenzae type b conjugate vaccines in infant rhesus monkeys. Pediatr Res 1991;29:10–13.

25. Granoff DM, Holmes SJ, Belshe RB, Anderson EL. The effect of carrier priming on the anticapsular (PRP) antibody responses to Haemophilus influenzae type b (Hib) conjugate vaccines [Abstract #994]. Pediatr Res 1993;33:169A.

26. Lieberman JM, Greenberg DP, Wong VK, et al. Does newborn immunization with diphtheria-tetanus toxoid (DT) prime for enhanced antibody responses to H. influenzae type B (HIB) conjugate vaccines? [Abstract #1028]. Pediatr Res 1993;33:174A.

27. Eskola J, Peltola H, Takala AK, et al. Efficacy of Haemophilus influenzae type b polysaccharide-diphtheria toxoid conjugate vaccine in infancy. N Engl J Med 1987;317:717–722.

28. Ward J, Brenneman G, Letson GW, Heyward WL. Alaska H. influenzae Vaccine Study Group. Limited efficacy of a H. influenzae type b conjugate vaccine in Alaska Native infants. N Engl J Med 1990;323:1381–1387.

29. Eskola J, Peltola H, Takala A, Palmgren J, Makela PH. Protective efficacy of the Haemophilus influenzae type b conjugate vaccine HbOC in Finnish infants [Abstract #60]. Thirtieth Interscience Conference on Antimicrobial Agents and Chemotherapy, Atlanta, Georgia, October 1990.

30. Vadheim CM, Greenberg DP, Partridge S, Jing J, Ward JI. Effectiveness and safety of an Haemophilus influenzae type b conjugate vaccine (PRP-T) in young infants. Pediatrics 1993; 92:272–279.

31. Booy R, Moxon ER, Macfarlane JA, Mayon-White RT, Slack MPE. Efficacy of Haemophilus influenzae type b conjugate vaccine in Oxford region. Lancet 1992;340:847.

32. Fritzell B, Plotkin S. Efficacy and safety of a Haemophilus influenzae type b capsular polysaccharide-tetanus protein conjugate vaccine. J Pediatr 1992;121:355–362.

33. Holmes SJ, Lucas AH, Osterholm MT, Froeschle JE, Granoff DM and the Collaborative Study Group. Immunoglobulin deficiency and idiotype expression in children developing Haemophilus influenzae type b disease after vaccination with conjugate vaccine. JAMA 1991; 266:1960–1965.

34. Holmes SJ, Osterholm MT, Zangwill KM, Wenger JD, Granoff DM, Vaccine Failure Group. Haemophilus influenzae type b disease in infants vaccinated with Hib conjugate vaccine at less than 12 months [Abstract #976]. Thirty-second Interscience Conference on Antimicrobial Agents and Chemotherapy, Anaheim, California, October 1992.

35. Frasch CE, Hiner EE, Gross TP. Haemophilus b disease after vaccination with Haemophilus b polysaccharide or conjugate vaccine. Am J Dis Child 1991;145:1379–1382.

36. Black S, Shinefield H, Hiatt R, Fireman B, Ray P, Lewis N. Safety of HDTP—a combined oligosaccharide conjugate (HbOC) Haemophilus influenzae type b (Hib) vaccine and DTP vaccine—in infancy [Abstract #932]. Pediatr Res 1992;31:158A.

37. Paradiso P, Hogerman D, Madore D, et al. Safety and immunogenicity in infants of a tetravalent vaccine composed of HbOC (HibTITER) and DTP (TRI-IMMUNOL) [Abstract #1028]. Pediatr Res 1992;31:174A.

38. Kovel A, Wald ER, Guerra N, Serdy C, Meschievitz CK. Safety and immunogenicity of acellular diphtheria-tetanus-pertussis and Haemophilus conjugate vaccines given in combination or at separate injection sites. J Pediatr 1992;120:84–87.

39. Shinefield H, Black S, Adelman T, Ensor K. Safety and immunogenicity of DTaP-HbOC—a combined oligosaccharide conjugate (HbOC, HibTITER) Haemophilus influenzae type b and acellular DTP vaccine (CTaP) in toddlers [Abstract #306]. Thirty-second Interscience Conference on Antimicrobial Agents and Chemotherapy, Anaheim, California, October 1992.

40. Paradiso P, Madore D, Hogerman D, Black S, Shinefield H. Immunogenicity of DTaP-HbOC in toddlers primed by DTP and HbOC as separate injections or DTP-HbOC combination vaccine [Abstract #307]. Interscience Conference on Antimicrobial Agents and Chemotherapy, Anaheim, California, October 1992.

41. Ferreccio C, Clemens J, Avendano A, et al. The clinical and immunologic response of Chilean infants to Haemophilus influenzae type b polysaccharide-tetanus protein conjugate vaccine coadministered in the same syringe with diphtheria-tetanus toxoids-pertussis vaccine at two, four, and six months of age. Pediatr Infect Dis J 1991;10:764–771.

42. Clemens JD, Ferreccio C, Levine MM, et al. Impact of Haemophilus influenzae type b polysaccharide-tetanus protein conjugate vaccine on responses to concurrently administered diphtheria-tetanus-pertussis vaccine. JAMA 1992;267:673–678.

43. Rothstein E, Bernstein M, Schiller K, et al. Safety and immunogenicity of PRP-D and DTP administered as a single injection [Abstract #1078]. Pediatr Res 1991;29:182A.

44. CDC. Diphtheria, tetanus, and pertussis: recommendations for vaccine use and other preventive measures. Recommendations of the Immunization Practices Advisory Committee (ACIP). MMWR 1991;40(No. RR-10):1–28.

45. Edmonson MB, Granoff DM, Barenkamp SJ, Chesney PJ. Outer membrane protein subtypes and investigation of recurrent Haemophilus influenzae type b disease. J Pediatr 1982;100: 202–208.
46. Frank AL, Labotka RJ, Rao S, et al. Haemophilus influenzae type b immunization of children with sickle cell diseases. Pediatrics 1988;82:571–575.
47. Feldman S, Gigliotti F, Shenep JL, Roberson PK, Lott L. Risk of Haemophilus influenzae type b disease in children with cancer and response of immunocompromised leukemic children to a conjugate vaccine. J Infect Dis 1990;161:926–931.
48. Steinhoff MC, Auerbach BS, Nelson K, et al. Antibody responses to Haemophilus influenzae type b vaccines in men with human immunodeficiency virus infection. N Engl J Med 1991;325: 1837–1842.
49. Janoff EN, Worel S, Douglas JM, et al. Natural immunity and response to conjugate vaccine for Haemophilus influenzae type b in men with HIV [Abstract #609]. Thirtieth Interscience Conference on Antimicrobial Agents and Chemotherapy, Atlanta, Georgia, October 1990.
50. Jakacki R, Luery N, McVerry P, Lange B. Haemophilus influenzae diphtheria protein conjugate immunization after therapy in splenectomized patients with Hodgkin Disease. Ann Intern Med 1990;112:143–144.
51. CDC. Recommendations of the Advisory Committee on Immunization Practices (ACIP): use of vaccines and immune globulins in persons with altered immunocompetence. MMWR 1993;42(No. RR-4):1–18.
52. Madore DV, Johnson CL, Phipps DC, et al. Safety and immunologic response to Haemophilus influenzae type b oligosaccharide CRM197 conjugate vaccine in 1- to 6-month-old infants. Pediatrics 1990;85:331–337.

TOPIC 12 / **HEPATITIS**

SUBTOPIC / VIRAL HEPATITIS

Protection Against Viral Hepatitis

Original Citation: Centers for Disease Control and Prevention. Protection Against Viral Hepatitis: Recommendations of the Immunization Practices Advisory Committee (ACIP). MMWR 1990;39(RR-2):1–26.

The following statement updates all previous recommendations on protection against viral hepatitis, including use of hepatitis B vaccine and hepatitis B immune globulin for prophylaxis of hepatitis B (MMWR 1985;34:313–324, 329–335, and MMWR 1987;36:353–366), universal screening of pregnant women to prevent perinatal hepatitis B transmission (MMWR 1988;37:341–346, 351), and use of immune globulin to prevent other types of viral hepatitis (MMWR 1985;34:313–324, 329–335).

INTRODUCTION

The term "viral hepatitis" is commonly used for several clinically similar diseases that are etiologically and epidemiologically distinct (1). Two of these, hepatitis A (formerly called infectious hepatitis) and hepatitis B (formerly called serum hepatitis), have been recognized as separate entities since the early 1940s and can be diagnosed with specific serologic tests. A third category, currently known as non-A, non-B hepatitis, includes two epidemiologically distinct types of hepatitis: parenterally transmitted and enterically transmitted non-A, non-B hepatitis. Parenterally transmitted non-A, non-B hepatitis is associated with both post-transfusion and sporadic cases of acute hepatitis and may be caused by at least two different agents. Part of the genome for one of these agents has recently been cloned, and a candidate serologic assay for antibody to this virus (proposed as hepatitis C virus) has been developed (2, 3). Enterically transmitted non-A, non-B hepatitis, which is spread by the fecal-oral route and is different from the types seen in the United

States, has been reported in parts of Asia, Africa, and Mexico (4). Another distinct type of hepatitis, delta hepatitis, is an infection dependent on the hepatitis B virus. It may occur as a coinfection with acute hepatitis B infection or as superinfection of a hepatitis B carrier (5).

HEPATITIS SURVEILLANCE

Approximately 28,500 cases of hepatitis A, 23,200 cases of hepatitis B, 2,620 cases of non-A, non-B hepatitis, and 2,470 cases of hepatitis type unspecified were reported in 1988 in the United States. Most cases of each type occur among young adults. Since reporting from many localities is incomplete, the actual number of hepatitis cases occurring annually is thought to be several times the reported number.

IMMUNE GLOBULINS

Immune globulins are important tools for preventing infection and disease before or after exposure to hepatitis viruses. Immune globulins used in medical practice are sterile solutions of antibodies (immunoglobulins) from human plasma. They are prepared by cold ethanol fractionation of large plasma pools and contain 10%–18% protein. In the United States, plasma is primarily obtained from paid donors. Only plasma shown to be free of hepatitis B surface antigen (HBsAg) and antibody to human immunodeficiency virus (HIV) is used to prepare immune globulins.

Immune globulin (IG) (formerly called immune serum globulin, ISG, or gamma globulin) produced in the United States contains antibodies against the hepatitis A virus (anti-HAV) and the HBsAg (anti-HBs). Hepatitis B immune globulin (HBIG) is an IG prepared from plasma containing high titers of anti-HBs.

There is no evidence that hepatitis B virus (HBV), HIV (the causative agent of acquired immunodeficiency syndrome (AIDS)), or other viruses have ever been transmitted by IG or HBIG commercially available in the United States (6). Since late April 1985, all plasma units for preparation of IGs have been screened for antibody to HIV, and reactive units are discarded. No instances of HIV infection or clinical illness have occurred that can be attributed to receiving IG or HBIG, including lots prepared before April 1985. Laboratory studies have shown that the margin of safety based on the removal of HIV infectivity by the fractionation process is extremely high (7). Some HBIG lots prepared before April 1985 have detectable HIV antibody. Shortly after being given HBIG, recipients have occasionally been noted to have low levels of passively acquired HIV antibody, but this reactivity does not persist (8).

Serious adverse effects from IGs administered as recommended have been rare. IGs prepared for intramuscular administration should be used for hepatitis prophylaxis. IGs prepared for intravenous administration to immunodeficient and other selected patients are not intended for hepatitis prophylaxis. IG and HBIG are not contraindicated for pregnant or lactating women.

HEPATITIS A

Hepatitis A is caused by the hepatitis A virus (HAV), a 27-nm ribonucleic acid (RNA) agent that is classified as a picornavirus. Patients with illness caused by HAV characteristically have abrupt onsets of symptoms including fever, malaise, anorexia, nausea, abdominal discomfort, dark urine, and jaundice. Severity is related to age. Among children, most infections are asymptomatic, and illness is usually not accompanied by jaundice. Most infected adults become symptomatically ill with jaundice. The case-fatality rate among reported cases is about 0.6%.

Hepatitis A is primarily transmitted by person-to-person contact, generally through fecal contamination and oral ingestion. Transmission is facilitated by poor personal hygiene, poor sanitation, and intimate (intrahousehold or sexual) contact. In recent years, cases of hepatitis A among intravenous drug users, most likely due to person-to-person contact, have been reported with increasing frequency (9). Common-source epidemics from contaminated food and water also occur. Sharing utensils or cigarettes or kissing is not believed to transmit the hepatitis A virus.

The incubation period of hepatitis A is 15–50 days (average 28). High concentrations of HAV (108 particles/g) are found in stool specimens from infected persons. Virus in the feces reaches its highest concentration late in the incubation period and early in the prodromal phase of illness, and it diminishes rapidly once jaundice appears. Greatest infectivity is during the 2-week period immediately before the onset of jaundice. Viremia probably occurs during the period that the virus is shed in feces. Virus has not been found in urine. A chronic carrier state with HAV in blood or feces has not been demonstrated. Transmission of HAV by blood transfusion has been reported but is uncommon (10).

The diagnosis of acute hepatitis A is confirmed by finding IgM anti-HAV in serum collected during the acute or early convalescent phase of the disease. IgG anti-HAV, which appears in the convalescent phase of the disease and remains detectable in serum thereafter, confers enduring protection against the disease. Commercial tests are available to detect IgM anti-HAV and total anti-HAV in serum.

Although the incidence of hepatitis A in the United States in the 1980s was lower than that in the 1970s, a 26% increase in incidence was observed between 1983 and 1988. It is still a common infection among older children and young adults. In 1988, 50% of reported cases of hepatitis in this country were attributable to hepatitis A.

Recommendations for IG Prophylaxis for Hepatitis A

Numerous field studies conducted in the past 4 decades confirm that IG given before exposure or during the incubation period of hepatitis A is protective against clinical illness (11–13). Its prophylactic value is greatest (80%–90%) when given early in the incubation period and declines thereafter (13). Recent tests have shown slightly decreased titers of anti-HAV in current IG lots compared with lots tested 8 years previously; however, no differences in IG efficacy have been noted.

Preexposure Prophylaxis

The major group for whom preexposure prophylaxis is recommended is international travelers. The risk of hepatitis A for U.S. citizens traveling abroad varies with living conditions, length of stay, and the incidence of hepatitis A infection in areas visited (14–16). In general, travelers to developed areas of North America, western Europe, Japan, Australia, and New Zealand are at no greater risk of infection than they would be in the United States. For travelers to developing countries, risk of infection increases with duration of travel and is highest for those who live in or visit rural areas, trek in back country, or frequently eat or drink in settings of poor sanitation. Nevertheless, recent studies have shown that many cases of travel-related hepatitis A occur in travelers with "standard" tourist itineraries, accommodations, and food and beverage consumption behaviors (16 and CDC unpublished data). In developing countries, travelers should minimize their exposure to hepatitis A and other enteric diseases by avoiding potentially contaminated water or food. Travelers should avoid drinking water (or beverages with ice) of unknown purity and eating uncooked shellfish or uncooked fruits or vegetables that they did not prepare.

IG is recommended for all susceptible travelers to developing countries (17). IG is especially important for persons who will be living in or visiting rural areas, eating or drinking in settings of poor or uncertain sanitation, or who will have close contact with local persons (especially young children) in settings with poor sanitary conditions. Persons who plan to reside in developing areas for long periods should receive IG regularly.

For travelers, a single dose of IG of 0.02 ml/kg of body weight is recommended if travel is for less than 3 months. For prolonged travel or residence in developing countries, 0.06 ml/kg should be given every 5 months. For persons who require repeated IG prophylaxis, screening for total anti-HAV before travel is useful to define susceptibility and eliminate unnecessary doses of IG for those who are immune. IG produced in developing countries may not meet the standards for purity required in most developed countries. Persons needing repeat doses overseas should use products that meet U.S. license requirements.

Postexposure Prophylaxis

Hepatitis A cannot be reliably diagnosed on clinical presentation alone, and serologic confirmation of index patients is recommended before contacts are treated. Serologic screening of contacts for anti-HAV before they are given IG is not recommended because screening is more costly than IG and would delay its administration.

For postexposure IG prophylaxis, a single intramuscular dose of 0.02 ml/kg is recommended. IG should be given as soon as possible after last exposure; giving IG more than 2 weeks after exposure is not indicated.

Specific recommendations for IG prophylaxis for hepatitis A depend on the nature of the HAV exposure.

1. Close personal contact. IG is recommended for all household and sexual contacts of persons with hepatitis A.
2. Day-care centers. Day-care facilities attended by children in diapers can be important settings for HAV transmission (18–20). IG should be administered to all staff and attendees of day-care centers or homes if (a) one or more children or employees are diagnosed as having hepatitis A, or (b) cases are recognized in two or more households of center attendees. When an outbreak (hepatitis cases in three or more families) occurs, IG should also be considered for members of households that have children (center attendees) in diapers. In centers not enrolling children in diapers, IG need only be given to classroom contacts of an index patient.
3. Schools. Contact at elementary and secondary schools is usually not an important means of transmitting hepatitis A. Routine administration of IG is not indicated for pupils and teachers in contact with a patient. However, when an epidemiologic investigation clearly shows the existence of a school- or classroom-centered outbreak, IG may be given to persons who have close contact with patients.
4. Institutions for custodial care. Living conditions in some institutions, such as prisons and facilities for the developmentally disabled, favor transmission of hepatitis A. When outbreaks occur, giving IG to residents and staff who have close contact with patients with hepatitis A may reduce the spread of disease. Depending on the epidemiologic circumstances, prophylaxis can be limited or can involve the entire institution.
5. Hospitals. Routine IG prophylaxis for hospital personnel is not indicated. Rather, sound hygienic practices should be emphasized. Staff education should point out the risk of exposure to hepatitis A and should emphasize precautions regarding direct contact with potentially infective materials (21).

    Outbreaks of hepatitis A occur occasionally among hospital staff, usually in association with an unsuspected index patient who is fecally incontinent. Large outbreaks have occurred from contact with infected infants in neonatal intensive care units (10). In outbreaks, prophylaxis of persons exposed to feces of infected patients may be indicated.
6. Offices and factories. Routine IG administration is not indicated under the usual office or factory conditions for persons exposed to a fellow worker with hepatitis A. Experience shows that casual contact in the work setting does not result in virus transmission.

7. Common-source exposure. IG use might be effective in preventing food-borne or waterborne hepatitis A if exposure is recognized in time. However, IG is not recommended for persons exposed to a common source of hepatitis infection after cases have begun to occur, since the 2-week period during which IG is effective will have been exceeded.

If a food handler is diagnosed as having hepatitis A, common-source transmission is possible but uncommon. IG should be administered to other food handlers but is usually not recommended for patrons (22). However, IG administration to patrons may be considered if all of the following conditions exist: (a) the infected person is directly involved in handling, without gloves, foods that will not be cooked before they are eaten, and (b) the hygienic practices of the food handler are deficient or the food handler has had diarrhea, and (c) patrons can be identified and treated within 2 weeks of exposure. Situations in which repeated exposures may have occurred, such as in institutional cafeterias, may warrant stronger consideration of IG use.

HEPATITIS B

Hepatitis B infection is caused by the hepatitis B virus (HBV), a 42-nm, double-shelled deoxyribonucleic acid (DNA) virus of the class hepadnaviridae. Several well-defined antigen-antibody systems are associated with HBV infection (Table 1). HBsAg is found on the surface of the virus and is also produced in excess amounts, circulating in blood as 22-nm spherical and tubular particles. HBsAg can be identified in serum 30–60 days after exposure to HBV and persists for variable periods. Anti-HBs develops after a resolved infection and is responsible for long-term immunity. Antibody to the core antigen (anti-HBc) develops in all HBV infections and persists indefinitely. IgM anti-HBc appears early in infection and persists for greater than or equal to 6 months. It is a reliable marker of acute or recent HBV infection. A third antigen, hepatitis B e antigen (HBeAg), may be detected in samples from persons with acute and chronic HBV infection. The presence of HBeAg correlates with viral replication and high infectivity. Antibody to HBeAg (anti-HBe) develops in most HBV infections and correlates with the loss of replicating virus and with lower infectivity.

The incubation period of hepatitis B is long (45–160 days; average = 120), and the onset of acute disease is generally insidious. Clinical symptoms and signs include anorexia, malaise, nausea, vomiting, abdominal pain, and jaundice. Extrahepatic manifestations of disease—such as skin rashes, arthralgias, and arthritis—can also occur. The case-fatality rate for reported cases is approximately 1.4%.

A variable proportion of individuals infected with HBV will become chronically infected with the virus. The HBV carrier is central to the epidemiology of HBV transmission. A carrier is defined as a person who is either HBsAg-positive on at least two occasions (at least 6 months apart) or who is HBsAg-positive and IgM anti-HBc negative when a single serum specimen is tested. Although the degree of infectivity is best correlated with HBeAg-positivity, any person positive for HBsAg is potentially infectious. The likelihood of becoming chronically infected with HBV varies inversely with the age at which infection occurs. HBV transmitted from HBsAg-positive mothers to their newborns results in HBV carriage for up to 90% of infants. Between 25% and 50% of children infected before 5 years of age become carriers, whereas only 6%–10% of acutely infected adults become carriers.

Carriers and persons with acute infection have the highest concentrations of HBV in blood and serous fluids. A lower concentration is present in other body fluids, such as saliva and semen. Transmission occurs via percutaneous or permucosal routes, and infective blood or body fluids can be introduced at birth, through sexual contact, or by contaminated needles. Infection can also occur in settings of continuous close personal contact (such as in households or among children in institutions for the developmentally disabled), presumably via inapparent or unnoticed contact of infective secretions with skin lesions or mucosal surfaces. Transmission of infection by transfusion of blood or blood products is rare because of routine screening of blood for HBsAg and because of current donor selection procedures. Transmission of HBV from infected health-care workers to patients is uncommon but has been documented during types of invasive procedures (e.g., oral and gynecologic surgery) (23, 24). HBsAg-positive health-care workers need not be restricted from patient contact unless they have been epidemiologically associated with HBV transmission. Rather, they should be educated about the potential mechanisms of HBV transmission. Adherence to aseptic techniques minimizes the risk of transmission. HBV is not transmitted via the fecal-oral route.

Table 1. Hepatitis nomenclature

	Abbreviation	Term	Definition/Comments
A. Hepatitis A	HAV	Hepatitis A virus	Etiologic agent of "infectious" hepatitis; a picornavirus; single serotype.
	Anti-HAV	Antibody to HAV	Detectable at onset of symptoms; lifetime persistence.
	IgM anti-HAV	IgM class antibody to HAV	Indicates recent infection with hepatitis A; detectable for 4–6 months after infection.
B. Hepatitis B	HBV	Hepatitis B virus	Etiologic agent of "serum" hepatitis; also known as Dane particle.
	HBsAg	Hepatitis B surface antigen	Surface antigen(s) of HBV detectable in large quantity in serum; several subtypes identified.
	HBeAg	Hepatitis B e antigen	Soluble antigen; correlates with HBV replication, high titer HBV in serum, and infectivity of serum.
	HBcAg	Hepatitis B core antigen	No commercial test available.
	Anti-HBs	Antibody to HBsAg	Indicates past infection with and immunity to HBV, passive antibody from HBIG, or immune response from HB vaccine.
	Anti-HBe	Antibody to HBeAg	Presence in serum of HBsAg carrier indicates lower titer of HBV.
	Anti-HBc	Antibody to HBcAg	Indicates prior infection with HBV at some undefined time.
	IgM anti-HBc	IgM class antibody to HBcAg	Indicates recent infection with HBV; detectable for 4–6 months after infection.
C. Delta hepatitis	HDV	Hepatitis D virus	Etiologic agent of delta hepatitis; can cause infection only in presence of HBV.
	HDAg	Delta antigen	Detectable in early acute delta infection.
	Anti-HDV	Antibody to delta antigen	Indicates present or past infection with delta virus.
D. Non-A, non-B hepatitis	PT-NANB	Parenterally transmitted	Diagnosis by exclusion. At least two candidate viruses, one of which has been proposed as hepatitis C virus; shares epidemiologic features with hepatitis B.
	ET-NANB	Enterically transmitted	Diagnosis by exclusion. Causes large epidemics in Asia, Africa, and Mexico; fecal-oral or waterborne.
E. Immune globulins	IG	Immune globulin (previously ISG, immune serum globulin, or gamma globulin)	Contains antibodies to HAV, low-titer antibodies to HBV.
	HBIG	Hepatitis B immune globulin	Contains high-titer antibodies to HBV.

Worldwide, HBV infection is a major cause of acute and chronic hepatitis, cirrhosis, and primary hepatocellular carcinoma. The frequency of HBV infection and patterns of transmission vary markedly in different parts of the world. In the United States, Western Europe, and Australia, it is a disease of low endemicity, with infection occurring primarily during adulthood and with only 0.2%–0.9% of the population being chronically infected. In contrast, HBV infection is highly endemic in China and Southeast Asia, most of Africa, most Pacific Islands, parts of the Middle East, and in the Amazon Basin. In these areas, most persons acquire infection at birth or during childhood, and 8%–15% of the population are chronically infected with HBV. In other parts of the world, HBV infection is moderately endemic, with 2%–7% of the population being HBV carriers. Prevention strategies for populations in which HBV infection is highly endemic are directed at vaccinating infants with hepatitis B vaccine, usually beginning at birth, to prevent both perinatal and childhood transmission of infection (25). Recommendations for hepatitis B prophylaxis in other areas should be designed to maximize the interruption of HBV transmission in accordance with local patterns of transmission. The recommendations that follow are intended for use in the United States.

Table 2. Prevalence of hepatitis B serologic markers in various population groups

Population group	Prevalence of serologic markers of HBV infection	
	HBsAg (%)	Any marker (%)
Immigrants/refugees from areas of high HBV endemicity	13	70–85
Alaskan Natives/Pacific Islanders	5–15	40–70
Clients in institutions for the developmentally disabled	10–20	35–80
Users of illicit parenteral drugs	7	60–80
Sexually active homosexual men	6	35–80
Household contacts of HBV carriers	3–6	30–60
Patients of hemodialysis units	3–10	20–80
Health-care workers—frequent blood contact	1–2	15–30
Prisoners (male)	1–8	10–80
Staff of institutions for the developmentally disabled	1	10–25
Heterosexuals with multiple partners	0.5	5–20
Health-care workers—no or infrequent blood contact	0.3	3–10
General population (NHANES II)*		
Blacks	0.9	14
Whites	0.2	3

*Second National Health and Nutrition Examination Survey (26).

Hepatitis B Virus Infection in the United States

Each year, an estimated 300,000 persons, primarily young adults, are infected with HBV. One-quarter become ill with jaundice, more than 10,000 patients require hospitalization, and an average of 250 die of fulminant disease. The United States currently contains an estimated pool of 750,000–1,000,000 infectious carriers. Approximately 25% of carriers develop chronic active hepatitis, which often progresses to cirrhosis. Furthermore, HBV carriers have a risk of developing primary liver cancer that is 12–300 times higher than that of other persons. An estimated 4,000 persons die each year from hepatitis B-related cirrhosis, and more than 800 die from hepatitis B-related liver cancer.

Serologic surveys demonstrate that, although HBV infection is uncommon among adults in the general population, it is highly prevalent in certain groups. Those at risk, based on the prevalence of serologic markers of infection, are described in Table 2. Persons born in areas of high HBV endemicity and their descendants remain at high risk of infection, as do certain populations in which HBV is highly endemic (Alaskan Natives and Pacific Islanders). Certain lifestyles (e.g., homosexual activity, intravenous drug abuse) result in early acquisition of HBV infection and high rates of infection. Persons who have heterosexual activity with multiple partners are at significant risk of infection. Inmates of prisons have a high prevalence of HBV markers, usually because of parenteral drug abuse before or during imprisonment. Patients in custodial institutions for the developmentally disabled are also at increased risk of having HBV infection. Household contacts and sexual partners of HBV carriers are at increased risk, as are hemodialysis patients and recipients of certain plasma-derived products that have not been inactivated (e.g., antihemophilic factor).

Those at occupational risk of HBV infection include medical and dental workers, related laboratory and support personnel, and public service employees who have contact with blood, as well as staff in institutions or classrooms for the mentally retarded.

Hepatitis B Prevention Strategies in the United States

The incidence of reported acute hepatitis B cases increased steadily over the past decade and reached a peak in 1985 (11.50 cases/105/year), despite the introduction of hepatitis B vaccine 3 years previously. Incidence decreased modestly (18%) by 1988, but still remains higher than a decade ago. This minimal impact of hepatitis B vaccine on disease incidence is attributable to several factors. The sources of infection for most cases include intravenous drug abuse (28%), heterosexual contact with infected persons or multiple partners (22%), and homosexual activity (9%). In addition, 30% of patients with Hepatitis B deny any of the recognized risk factors for infection.

The present strategy for hepatitis B prevention is to vaccinate those individuals at high risk of infection. Most persons receiving vaccine as a result of this strategy have been persons at risk of acquiring HBV infection through occupational exposure, a group that accounts for approximately 4% of cases. The major deterrents to vaccinating the other high-risk groups include their lack of knowledge about the risk of disease and its consequences, the lack of public sector programs, the cost of vaccine, and the inability to access most of the high-risk populations.

For vaccine to have an impact on the incidence of hepatitis B, a comprehensive strategy must be developed that will provide hepatitis B vaccination to persons before they engage in behaviors or occupations that place them at risk of infection. Universal HBsAg screening of pregnant women was recently recommended to prevent perinatal HBV transmission. The previous recommendations for selective screening failed to identify most HBsAg-positive pregnant women (27). As an alternative to high-risk-group vaccination, universal vaccination of infants and adolescents needs to be examined as a possible strategy to control the transmission of disease.

Hepatitis B Prophylaxis

Two types of products are available for prophylaxis against hepatitis B. Hepatitis B vaccines, first licensed in 1981, provide active immunization against HBV infection, and their use is recommended for both preexposure and postexposure prophylaxis. HBIG provides temporary, passive protection and is indicated only in certain postexposure settings.

HBIG

HBIG is prepared from plasma preselected to contain a high titer of anti-HBs. In the United States, HBIG has an anti-HBs titer of greater than 100,000 by radioimmunoassay (RIA). Human plasma from which HBIG is prepared is screened for antibodies to HIV; in addition, the Cohn fractionation process used to prepare this product inactivates and eliminates HIV from the final product. There is no evidence that the causative agent of AIDS (HIV) has been transmitted by HBIG (6).

Hepatitis B Vaccine

Two types of hepatitis B vaccines are currently licensed in the United States. Plasma-derived vaccine consists of a suspension of inactivated, alum-adsorbed, 22-nm, HBsAg particles that have been purified from human plasma by a combination of biophysical (ultracentrifugation) and biochemical procedures. Inactivation is a threefold process using 8M urea, pepsin at pH 2, and 1:4,000 formalin. These treatment steps have been shown to inactivate representatives of all classes of viruses found in human blood, including HIV (28). Plasma-derived vaccine is no longer being produced in the United States, and use is now limited to hemodialysis patients, other immunocompromised hosts, and persons with known allergy to yeast.

Currently licensed recombinant hepatitis B vaccines are produced by Saccharomyces cerevisiae (common baker's yeast), into which a plasmid containing the gene for the HBsAg has been inserted. Purified HBsAg is obtained by lysing the yeast cells and separating HBsAg from yeast components by biochemical and biophysical techniques. These vaccines contain more than 95% HBsAg protein. Yeast-derived protein constitutes no more than 5% of the final product.

Hepatitis B vaccines are packaged to contain 10–40 μg HBsAg protein/ml and are adsorbed with aluminum hydroxide (0.5 mg/ml). Thimerosal (1:20,000 concentration) is added as a preservative.

The recommended series of three intramuscular doses of hepatitis B vaccine induces an adequate antibody response* in greater than 90% of healthy adults and in greater than 95% of infants, children, and adolescents from birth through 19 years of age (29–31). The deltoid (arm) is the recommended site for hepatitis B vaccination of adults and children; immunogenicity of vaccine for adults is substantially lower when injections are given in the buttock (32). Larger vaccine doses (two to four times normal adult dose) or an increased number of doses (four doses) are required to induce protective antibody in a high proportion of hemodialysis patients and may also be necessary for other immunocompromised persons (such as those on immunosuppressive drugs or with HIV infection) (33, 34).

Field trials of the vaccines licensed in the United States have shown 80%–95% efficacy in preventing infection or clinical hepatitis among susceptible persons (31, 35). Protection against illness is virtually complete for persons who develop an adequate antibody response after vaccination. The duration of protection and need for booster doses are not yet fully defined. Between 30% and 50% of persons who develop adequate antibody after three doses of vaccine will lose detectable antibody within 7 years, but protection against viremic infection and clinical disease appears to persist (36–38). Immunogenicity and efficacy of the licensed vaccines for hemodialysis patients are much lower than in normal adults. Protection in this group may last only as long as adequate antibody levels persist (33).

Vaccine Usage

Primary vaccination comprises three intramuscular doses of vaccine, with the second and third doses given 1 and 6 months, respectively, after the first. Adults and older children should be given a full 1.0 ml divided by dose, while children less than 11 years of age should usually receive half (0.5 ml) this dose. See Table 3 for complete information on age-specific dosages of currently available vaccines. An alternative schedule of four doses of vaccine given at 0, 1, 2, and 12 months has been approved for one vaccine for postexposure prophylaxis or for more rapid induction of immunity. However, there is no clear evidence that this regimen provides greater protection than the standard three-dose series. Hepatitis B vaccine should be given only in the deltoid muscle for adults and children or in the anterolateral thigh muscle for infants and neonates.

For patients undergoing hemodialysis and for other immunosuppressed patients, higher vaccine doses or increased numbers of doses are required. A special formulation of one vaccine is now available for such persons (Table 3). Persons with HIV infection have an impaired response to hepatitis B vaccine. The immunogenicity of higher doses of vaccine is unknown for this group, and firm recommendations on dosage cannot be made at this time (34).

---

*An adequate antibody response is greater than or equal to 10 milliInternational Units (mIU)/ml, approximately equivalent to 10 sample ratio units (SRU) by RIA or positive by enzyme immunoassay (EIA), measured 1–6 months after completion of the vaccine series.

Table 3. Recommended doses and schedules of currently licensed HB vaccines

Group	Heptavax-B*,† Dose (μg)	(ml)	Recombivax HB* Dose (μg)	(ml)	Engerix-B*§ Dose (μg)	(ml)
Infants of HBV-carrier mothers	10	(0.5)	5	(0.5)	10	(0.5)
Other infants and children < 11 years	10	(0.5)	2.5	(0.25)	10	(0.5)
Children and adolescents 11–19 years	20	(1.0)	5	(0.5)	20	(1.0)
Adults > 19 years	20	(1.0)	10	(1.0)	20	(1.0)
Dialysis patients and other immunocompromised persons	40	(2.0)¶	40	(1.0)**	40	(2.0)¶,††

*Usual schedule: three doses at 0, 1, 6 months.
†Available only for hemodialysis and other immunocompromised patients and for persons with known allergy to yeast.
§Alternative schedule: four doses at 0, 1, 2, 12 months.
¶Two 1.0-ml doses given at different sites.
**Special formulation for dialysis patients.
††Four-dose schedule recommended at 0, 1, 2, 6 months.

Vaccine doses administered at longer intervals provide equally satisfactory protection, but optimal protection is not conferred until after the third dose. If the vaccine series is interrupted after the first dose, the second and third doses should be given separated by an interval of 3–5 months. Persons who are late for the third dose should be given this dose when convenient. Postvaccination testing is not considered necessary in either situation.

In one study, the response to vaccination by the standard schedule using one or two doses of one vaccine, followed by the remaining doses of a different vaccine, was comparable to the response to vaccination with a single vaccine. Moreover, because the immunogenicities of the available vaccines are similar, it is likely that responses in such situations will be comparable to those induced by any of the vaccines alone.

The immunogenicity of a series of three low doses (0.1 standard dose) of plasma-derived hepatitis B vaccine administered by the intradermal route has been assessed in several studies. The largest studies of adults show lower rates of developing adequate antibody (80%–90%) and twofold to fourfold lower antibody titers than with intramuscular vaccination with recommended doses (39 and CDC unpublished data). Data on immunogenicity of low doses of recombinant vaccines given intradermally are limited. At this time, intradermal vaccination of adults using low doses of vaccine should be done only under research protocol, with appropriate informed consent and with postvaccination testing to identify persons with inadequate response who would be eligible for revaccination. Intradermal vaccination is not recommended for infants or children.

All hepatitis B vaccines are inactivated (noninfective) products, and there is no evidence of interference with other simultaneously administered vaccines.

Data are not available on the safety of hepatitis B vaccines for the developing fetus. Because the vaccines contain only noninfectious HBsAg particles, there should be no risk to the fetus. In contrast, HBV infection of a pregnant woman may result in severe disease for the mother and chronic infection of the newborn. Therefore, pregnancy or lactation should not be considered a contraindication to the use of this vaccine for persons who are otherwise eligible.

Vaccine Storage and Shipment

Vaccine should be shipped and stored at 2°–8°C but not frozen. Freezing destroys the potency of the vaccine.

Side Effects and Adverse Reactions

The most common side effect observed following vaccination with each of the available vaccines has been soreness at the injection site. Postvaccination surveillance for 3 years after licensure of the plasma-derived vaccine showed an association of borderline significance between Guillain-Barré syndrome and receipt of the first vaccine dose (40). The rate of this occurrence was very low (0.5/100,000 vaccinees) and was more than compensated by disease prevented by the vaccine even if Guillain-Barré syndrome is a true side effect. Such postvaccination surveillance information is not available for the recombinant hepatitis B vaccines. Early concerns about safety of plasma-derived vaccine have proven to be unfounded, particularly the concern that infectious agents such as HIV present in the donor plasma pools might contaminate the final product.

Effect of Vaccination on Carriers and Immune Persons

Hepatitis B vaccine produces neither therapeutic nor adverse effects for HBV carriers (41). Vaccination of individuals who possess antibodies against HBV from a previous infection is not necessary but will not cause adverse effects. Such individuals will have a postvaccination increase in their anti-HBs levels. Passively acquired antibody, whether acquired from HBIG or IG administration or from the transplacental route, will not interfere with active immunization (42).

Prevaccination Serologic Testing for Susceptibility

The decision to test potential vaccine recipients for prior infection is primarily a cost-effectiveness issue and should be based on whether the costs of testing balance the costs of vaccine saved by not vaccinating individuals who have already been infected. Estimation of cost-effectiveness of testing depends on three variables: the cost of vaccination, the cost of testing for susceptibility, and the expected prevalence of immune individuals in the group.

Testing in groups with the highest risk of HBV infection (HBV marker prevalence greater than 20%, Table 2) is usually cost-effective unless testing costs are extremely high. Cost-effectiveness of screening may be marginal for groups at intermediate risk. For groups with a low expected prevalence of HBV serologic markers, such as health professionals in their training years, prevaccination testing is not cost-effective.

For routine testing, only one antibody test is necessary (either anti-HBc or anti-HBs). Anti-HBc identifies all previously infected persons, both carriers and those who are not carriers, but does not differentiate members of the two groups. Anti-HBs identifies persons previously infected, except for carriers. Neither test has a particular advantage for groups expected to have carrier rates of less than 2%, such as health-care workers. Anti-HBc may be preferred to avoid unnecessary vaccination of carriers for groups with higher carrier rates. If RIA is used to test for anti-HBs, a minimum of 10 sample ratio units should be used to designate immunity (2.1 is the usual designation of a positive test). If EIA is used, the positive level recommended by manufacturers is appropriate.

Postvaccination Testing for Serologic Response and Revaccination of Nonresponders

Hepatitis B vaccine, when given in the deltoid, produces protective antibody (anti-HBs) in greater than 90% of healthy persons. Testing for immunity after vaccination is not recommended routinely but is advised for persons whose subsequent management depends on knowing their immune status (such as dialysis patients and staff). Testing for immunity is also advised for persons for whom a suboptimal response may be anticipated, such as those who have received vaccine in the buttock, persons greater than or equal to 50 years of age, and persons known to have HIV infection. Postvaccination testing should also be considered for persons at occupational risk who may have needle-stick exposures necessitating postexposure prophylaxis. When necessary, postvaccination testing should be done between 1 and 6 months after completion of the vaccine series to provide definitive information on response to the vaccine.

Revaccination of persons who do not respond to the primary series (nonresponders) produces adequate antibody in 15%–25% after one additional dose and in 30%–50% after three additional doses when the primary vaccination has been given in the deltoid (36). For persons who did not respond to a primary vaccine series given in the buttock, data suggest that revaccination in the arm induces adequate antibody in greater than 75%. Revaccination with one or more additional doses should be considered for persons who fail to respond to vaccination in the deltoid and is recommended for those who have failed to respond to vaccination in the buttock.

Need for Vaccine Booster Doses

Available data show that vaccine-induced antibody levels decline steadily with time and that up to 50% of adult vaccinees who respond adequately to vaccine may have low or undetectable antibody levels by 7 years after vaccination. Nevertheless, both adults and children with declining antibody levels are still protected against hepatitis B disease. Current data also suggest excellent protection against disease for 5 years after vaccination among infants born to hepatitis B-carrier mothers. For adults and children with normal immune status, booster doses are not routinely recommended within 7 years after vaccination, nor is routine serologic testing to assess antibody levels necessary for vaccine recipients during this period. For infants born to hepatitis B-carrier mothers, booster doses are not necessary within 5 years after vaccination. The possible need for booster doses after longer intervals will be assessed as additional information becomes available.

For hemodialysis patients, for whom vaccine-induced protection is less complete and may persist only as long as antibody levels remain above 10 mIU/ml, the need for booster doses should be assessed by annual antibody testing, and booster doses should be given when antibody levels decline to less than 10 mIU/ml.

Groups Recommended for Preexposure Vaccination

Persons at substantial risk of HBV infection who are demonstrated or judged likely to be susceptible should be vaccinated. They include the following:

1. Persons with occupational risk. HBV infection is a major infectious occupational hazard for health-care and public-safety workers. The risk of acquiring HBV infection from occupational exposures is dependent on the frequency of percutaneous and permucosal exposures to blood or blood products. Any health-care or public-safety worker may be at risk for HBV exposure depending on the tasks that he or she performs. If those tasks involve contact with blood or blood-contaminated body fluids, such workers should be vaccinated. Vaccination should be considered for other workers depending on the nature of the task (43).

   Risks among health-care professionals vary during the training and working career of each individual but are often highest during the professional training period. For this reason, when possible, vaccination should be completed during training in schools of medicine, dentistry, nursing, laboratory technology, and other allied health professions before workers have their first contact with blood.

2. Clients and staff of institutions for the developmentally disabled. Susceptible clients in institutions for the developmentally disabled should be vaccinated. Staff who work closely with clients should also be vaccinated. The risk in institutional environments is associated not only with blood exposure but may also be consequent to bites and contact with skin lesions and other infective secretions. Susceptible clients and staff who live or work in smaller (group) residential settings with known HBV carriers should also receive hepatitis B vaccine. Clients discharged from residential institutions into community settings should be screened for HBsAg so that the community programs may take appropriate measures to prevent HBV transmission. These measures should include both environmental controls and appropriate use of vaccine.

   Staff of nonresidential day-care programs (e.g., schools, sheltered workshops for the developmentally disabled) attended by known HBV carriers have a risk of HBV infection comparable to that among health-care workers and therefore should be vaccinated (44). The risk of HBV infection for clients appears to be lower than the risk for staff. Vaccination of clients in day-care programs may be considered. Vaccination of classroom contacts is strongly encouraged if a classmate who is an HBV carrier behaves aggressively or has special medical problems that increase the risk of exposure to his/her blood or serous secretions.

3. Hemodialysis patients. Hepatitis B vaccination is recommended for susceptible hemodialysis patients. Although seroconversion rates and anti-HBs titers are lower than those for healthy persons, for those patients who do respond, hepatitis B vaccine will protect them from HBV infection and reduce the necessity for frequent serologic screening (45). Some studies have shown higher seroconversion rates and antibody titers for patients with uremia who were vaccinated before they required dialysis (46). Identification of patients for vaccination early in the course of their renal disease is encouraged.

4. Sexually active homosexual men. Susceptible sexually active homosexual men should be vaccinated regardless of their age or the duration of their homosexual practices. Persons should be vaccinated as soon as possible after their homosexual activity begins. Homosexual and bisexual men known to have HIV infection should be tested for anti-HBs response after completion of the vaccine series and should be counseled accordingly.

5. Users of illicit injectable drugs. All users of illicit injectable drugs who are susceptible to HBV should be vaccinated as early as possible after their drug abuse begins.

6. Recipients of certain blood products. Patients with clotting disorders who receive clotting-factor concentrates have an increased risk of HBV infection. Vaccination is recommended for these persons, and it should be initiated at the time their specific clotting disorder is identified. Prevaccination testing is recommended for patients who have already received multiple infusions of these products.

7. Household and sexual contacts of HBV carriers. Household contacts of HBV carriers are at high risk of HBV infection. Sexual contacts appear to be at greatest risk. When HBV carriers are identified through routine screening of donated blood, diagnostic testing in hospitals, prenatal screening, screening of refugees from certain areas, or other screening programs, they should be notified of their status. All household and sexual contacts should be tested and susceptible contacts vaccinated.

8. Adoptees from countries of high HBV endemicity. Families accepting orphans or unaccompanied minors from countries of high or intermediate HBV endemicity should have the children screened for HBsAg. If the children are HBsAg-positive, family members should be vaccinated (47).

9. Other contacts of HBV carriers. Persons in casual contact with carriers in settings such as schools and offices are at minimal risk of HBV infection, and vaccine is not routinely recommended for them. At child-care centers, HBV transmission between children or between children and staff has rarely been documented. Unless special circumstances exist, such as behavior problems (biting or scratching) or medical conditions (severe skin disease) that might facilitate transmission, vaccination of contacts of carriers in child care is not indicated.

10. Populations with high endemicity of HBV infection. In certain U.S. populations, including Alaskan Natives, Pacific Islanders, and refugees from HBV-endemic areas, HBV infection is highly endemic, and transmission occurs primarily during childhood. In such groups, universal hepatitis B vaccination of infants is recommended to prevent disease transmission during childhood. In addition, more extensive programs of "catch-up" childhood vaccination should be considered if resources are available.

    Immigrants and refugees from areas with highly endemic HBV disease (particularly Africa and eastern Asia) should be screened for HBV markers upon resettlement in the United States. If an HBV carrier is identified, all susceptible household contacts should be vaccinated. Even if no HBV carriers are found within a family, vaccination should be considered for susceptible children less than 7 years of age because of the high rate of interfamilial HBV infection that occurs among these children (48). Vaccination is recommended for all infants of women who were born in areas in which infection is highly endemic.

11. Inmates of long-term correctional facilities. The prison environment may provide a favorable setting for the transmission of HBV because of the use of illicit injectable drugs and because of male homosexual practices. Moreover, it provides an access point for vaccination of percutaneous drug abusers. Prison officials should consider undertaking screening and vaccination programs directed at inmates with histories of high-risk behaviors.

12. Sexually active heterosexual persons. Sexually active heterosexual persons with multiple sexual partners are at increased risk of HBV infection. Risk increases with increasing numbers of sexual partners. Vaccination is recommended for persons who are diagnosed as having recently acquired other sexually transmitted diseases, for prostitutes, and for persons who have a history of sexual activity with multiple partners in the previous 6 months.

13. International travelers. Vaccination should be considered for persons who plan to reside for more than 6 months in areas with high levels of endemic HBV and who will have close contact with the local population. Vaccination should also be considered for short-term travelers who are likely to have contact with blood from or sexual contact with residents of areas with high levels of endemic disease. Ideally, hepatitis B vaccination of travelers should begin at least 6 months before travel to allow for completion of the full vaccine series. Nevertheless, a partial series will offer some protection from HBV infection.

The alternative four-dose schedule may provide better protection during travel if the first three doses can be delivered before travel (second and third doses given 1 and 2 months, respectively, after first).

Postexposure Prophylaxis for Hepatitis B

Prophylactic treatment to prevent hepatitis B infection after exposure to HBV should be considered in the following situations: perinatal exposure of an infant born to an HBsAg-positive mother, accidental percutaneous or permucosal exposure to HBsAg-positive blood, sexual exposure to an HBsAg-positive person, and household exposure of an infant less than 12 months of age to a primary care giver who has acute hepatitis B.

Various studies have established the relative efficacies of HBIG and/or hepatitis B vaccine in different exposure situations. For an infant with perinatal exposure to an HBsAg-positive and HBeAg-positive mother, a regimen combining one dose of HBIG at birth with the hepatitis B vaccine series started soon after birth is 85%–95% effective in preventing development of the HBV carrier state (35, 49–51). Regimens involving either multiple doses of HBIG alone, or the vaccine series alone, have 70%–85% efficacy (52, 53).

For accidental percutaneous exposure, only regimens including HBIG and/or IG have been studied. A regimen of two doses of HBIG, one given after exposure and one a month later, is about 75% effective in preventing hepatitis B in this setting (54, 55). For sexual exposure, a single dose of HBIG is 75% effective if given within 2 weeks of last sexual exposure (56). The efficacy of IG for postexposure prophylaxis is uncertain. IG no longer has a role in postexposure prophylaxis of hepatitis B because of the availability of HBIG and the wider use of hepatitis B vaccine.

Recommendations on postexposure prophylaxis are based on available efficacy data and on the likelihood of future HBV exposure of the person requiring treatment. In all exposures, a regimen combining HBIG with hepatitis B vaccine will provide both short- and long-term protection, will be less costly than the two-dose HBIG treatment alone, and is the treatment of choice.

Perinatal Exposure and Recommendations

Transmission of HBV from mother to infant during the perinatal period represents one of the most efficient modes of HBV infection and often leads to severe long-term sequelae. Infants born to HBsAg-positive and HBeAg-positive mothers have a 70%–90% chance of acquiring perinatal HBV infection, and 85%–90% of infected infants will become chronic HBV carriers. Estimates are that greater than 25% of these carriers will die from primary hepatocellular carcinoma (PHC) or cirrhosis of the liver (57). Infants born to HBsAg-positive and HBeAg-negative mothers have a lower risk of acquiring perinatal infection; however, such infants have had acute disease, and fatal fulminant hepatitis has been reported (58, 59). Based on 1987 data in the United States, an estimated 18,000 births occur to HBsAg-positive women each year, resulting in approximately 4,000 infants who become chronic HBV carriers. Prenatal screening of all pregnant women identifies those who are HBsAg-positive and allows treatment of their newborns with HBIG and hepatitis B vaccine, a regimen that is 85%–95% effective in preventing the development of the HBV chronic carrier state. The following are perinatal recommendations:

1. All pregnant women should be routinely tested for HBsAg during an early prenatal visit in each pregnancy. This testing should be done at the same time that other routine prenatal screening tests are ordered. In special situations (e.g., when acute hepatitis is suspected, when a history of exposure to hepatitis has been reported, or when the mother has a particularly high-risk behavior, such as intravenous drug abuse), an additional HBsAg test can be ordered later in the pregnancy. No other HBV marker tests are necessary for the purpose of maternal screening, although HBsAg-positive mothers identified during screening may have HBV-related acute or chronic liver disease and should be evaluated by their physicians.

2. If a woman has not been screened prenatally or if test results are not available at the time of admission for delivery, HBsAg testing should be done at the time of admission, or as soon as possible thereafter. If the mother is identified as HBsAg-positive greater than 1 month after giving birth, the infant should be tested for HBsAg. If the results are negative, the infant should be given HBIG and hepatitis B vaccine.

3. Following all initial positive tests for HBsAg, a repeat test for HBsAg should be performed on the same specimen, followed by a confirmatory test using a neutralization assay. For women in labor who did not have HBsAg testing during pregnancy and who are found to be HBsAg-positive on first testing, initiation of treatment of their infants should not be delayed by more than 24 hours for repeat or confirmatory testing.

4. Infants born to HBsAg-positive mothers should receive HBIG (0.5 ml) intramuscularly once they are physiologically stable, preferably within 12 hours of birth (Table 4). Hepatitis B vaccine should be administered intramuscularly at the appropriate infant dose. The first dose should be given concurrently with HBIG but at a different site. If vaccine is not immediately available, the first dose should be given as soon as possible. Subsequent doses should be given as recommended for the specific vaccine. Testing infants for HBsAg and anti-HBs is recommended when they are 12–15 months of age to monitor the success or failure of therapy. If HBsAg is not detectable and anti-HBs is present, children can be consid-

Table 4. Hepatitis B virus postexposure recommendations

Exposure	HBIG		Vaccine	
	Dose	Recommended timing	Dose	Recommended timing
Perinatal	0.5 ml IM	Within 12 hours of birth	0.5 ml IM*	Within 12 hours of birth[†]
Sexual	0.06 ml/kg IM	Single dose within 14 days of last sexual contact	1.0 ml IM*	First dose at time of HBIG treatment[†]

*For appropriate age-specific doses of each vaccine, see Table 3.
[†]The first dose can be given the same time as the HBIG dose but in a different site; subsequent doses should be given as recommended for specific vaccine.

ered protected. Testing for anti-HBc is not useful, since maternal anti-HBc can persist for greater than 1 year. HBIG and hepatitis B vaccination do not interfere with routine childhood vaccinations. Breast-feeding poses no risk of HBV infection for infants who have begun prophylaxis.

5. Household members and sexual partners of HBV carriers identified through prenatal screening should be tested to determine susceptibility to HBV infection, and, if susceptible, should receive hepatitis B vaccine.

6. Obstetric and pediatric staff should be notified directly about HBsAg-positive mothers so that neonates can receive therapy without delay after birth and follow-up doses of vaccine can be given. Programs to coordinate the activities of persons providing prenatal care, hospital-based obstetrical services, and pediatric well-baby care must be established to assure proper follow-up and treatment both of infants born to HBsAg-positive mothers and of other susceptible household and sexual contacts.

7. In those populations under U.S. jurisdiction in which hepatitis B infection is highly endemic (including certain Alaskan Natives, Pacific Island groups, and refugees from highly endemic areas accepted for resettlement in the United States), universal vaccination of newborns with hepatitis B vaccine is the recommended strategy for hepatitis B control. HBsAg screening of mothers and use of HBIG for infants born to HBV-carrier mothers may be added to routine hepatitis B vaccination when practical, but screening and HBIG alone will not adequately protect children from HBV infection in endemic areas. In such areas, hepatitis B vaccine doses should be integrated into the childhood vaccination schedule. More extensive programs of childhood hepatitis B vaccination should be considered if resources are available.

Acute Exposure to Blood That Contains (or Might Contain) HBsAg

For accidental percutaneous (needle stick, laceration, or bite) or permucosal (ocular or mucous-membrane) exposure to blood, the decision to provide prophylaxis must include consideration of several factors: (a) whether the source of the blood is available, (b) the HBsAg status of the source, and (c) the hepatitis B vaccination and vaccine-response status of the exposed person. Such exposures usually affect persons for whom hepatitis B vaccine is recommended. For any exposure of a person not previously vaccinated, hepatitis B vaccination is recommended.

Following any such exposure, a blood sample should be obtained from the person who was the source of the exposure and should be tested for HBsAg. The hepatitis B vaccination status and anti-HBs response status (if known) of the exposed person should be reviewed. The outline below and Table 5 summarize prophylaxis for percutaneous or permucosal exposure to blood according to the HBsAg status of the source of exposure and the vaccination status and vaccine response of the exposed person.

For greatest effectiveness, passive prophylaxis with HBIG, when indicated, should be given as soon as possible after exposure (its value beyond 7 days after exposure is unclear).

1. Source of exposure HBsAg-positive
   a. Exposed person has not been vaccinated or has not completed vacci-

Table 5. Recommendations for hepatitis B prophylaxis following percutaneous or permucosal exposure

Exposed person	Treatment when source is found to be:		
	HBsAg-positive	HBsAg-negative	Source not tested or unknown
Unvaccinated	HBIG × 1* and initiate HB vaccine†	Initiate HB vaccine†	Initiate HB vaccine†
Previously vaccinated Known responder	Test exposed for anti-HBs 1. If adequate,§ no treatment 2. If inadequate, HB vaccine booster dose	No treatment	No treatment
Known nonresponder	HBIG × 2 or HBIG × 1 plus 1 dose HB vaccine	No treatment	If known high-risk source, *may treat as if source were HBsAg-positive*
Response unknown	Test exposed for anti-HBs 1. If inadequate,§ HBIG × 1 plus HB vaccine booster dose 2. If adequate, no treatment	No treatment	Test exposed for anti-HBs 1. If inadequate§, HB vaccine booster dose 2. If adequate, no treatment

*HBIG dose 0.06 ml/kg IM.
†HB vaccine dose—see Table 3.
§Adequate anti-HBs is ≥ 10 SRU by RIA or positive by EIA.

nation. Hepatitis B vaccination should be initiated. A single dose of HBIG (0.06 ml/kg) should be given as soon as possible after exposure and within 24 hours, if possible. The first dose of hepatitis B vaccine (Table 3) should be given intramuscularly at a separate site (deltoid for adults) and can be given simultaneously with HBIG or within 7 days of exposure. Subsequent doses should be given as recommended for the specific vaccine. If the exposed person has begun but not completed vaccination, one dose of HBIG should be given immediately, and vaccination should be completed as scheduled.

b. Exposed person has already been vaccinated against hepatitis B, and anti-HBs response status is known.

(1) If the exposed person is known to have had adequate response in the past, the anti-HBs level should be tested unless an adequate level has been demonstrated within the last 24 months. Although current data show that vaccine-induced protection does not

decrease as antibody level wanes, most experts consider the following approach to be prudent.

   (a) If anti-HBs level is adequate, no treatment is necessary.
   (b) If anti-HBs level is inadequate**, a booster dose of hepatitis B vaccine should be given.

   (2) If the exposed person is known not to have responded to the primary vaccine series, the exposed person should be given either a single dose of HBIG and a dose of hepatitis B vaccine as soon as possible after exposure, or two doses of HBIG (0.06 ml/kg), one given as soon as possible after exposure and the second 1 month later. The latter treatment is preferred for those who have failed to respond to at least four doses of vaccine.

   c. Exposed person has already been vaccinated against hepatitis B, and the anti-HBs response is unknown. The exposed person should be tested for anti-HBs.
      (1) If the exposed person has adequate antibody, no additional treatment is necessary.
      (2) If the exposed person has inadequate antibody on testing, one dose of HBIG (0.06 ml/kg) should be given immediately and a standard booster dose of vaccine (Table 3) given at a different site.

2.   Source of exposure known and HBsAg-negative
   a. Exposed person has not been vaccinated or has not completed vaccination. If unvaccinated, the exposed person should be given the first dose of hepatitis B vaccine within 7 days of exposure, and vaccination should be completed as recommended. If the exposed person has not completed vaccination, vaccination should be completed as scheduled.
   b. Exposed person has already been vaccinated against hepatitis B. No treatment is necessary.

3.   Source of exposure unknown or not available for testing
   a. Exposed person has not been vaccinated or has not completed vaccination. If unvaccinated, the exposed person should be given the first dose of hepatitis B vaccine within 7 days of exposure and vaccination completed as recommended. If the exposed person has not completed vaccination, vaccination should be completed as scheduled.
   b. Exposed person has already been vaccinated against hepatitis B, and anti-HBs response status is known.
      (1) If the exposed person is known to have had adequate response in the past, no treatment is necessary.
      (2) If the exposed person is known not to have responded to the vaccine, prophylaxis as described earlier in section l.b.ii. under "Source of exposure HBsAg-positive" may be considered if the source of the exposure is known to be at high risk of HBV infection.

**An adequate antibody level is greater than or equal to 10 milliInternational Units (mIU)/ml, approximately equivalent to 10 sample ratio units (SRU) by RIA or positive by EIA.

   c. Exposed person has already been vaccinated against hepatitis B, and
      the anti-HBs response is unknown. The exposed person should be tested
      for anti-HBs.
      (1) If the exposed person has adequate anti-HBs, no treatment is nec-
          essary.
      (2) If the exposed person has inadequate anti-HBs, a standard booster
          dose of vaccine should be given.

Sexual Partners of Persons with Acute HBV Infection

Sexual partners of HBsAg-positive persons are at increased risk of acquiring HBV infection, and HBIG has
been shown to be 75% effective in preventing such infections (56). Because data are limited, the period
after sexual exposure during which HBIG is effective is unknown, but extrapolation from other settings
makes it unlikely that this period would exceed 14 days. Before treatment, testing of sexual partners for
susceptibility is recommended if it does not delay treatment beyond 14 days after last exposure. Testing for
anti-HBc is the most efficient prescreening test to use in this population.

   All susceptible persons whose sexual partners have acute hepatitis B infection or whose sexual partners are discovered to be hepatitis B carriers should receive a single dose of HBIG (0.06 ml/kg) and should
begin the hepatitis B vaccine series if prophylaxis can be started within 14 days of the last sexual contact,
or if ongoing sexual contact with the infected person will occur. Giving the vaccine with HBIG may
improve the efficacy of postexposure treatment. The vaccine has the added advantage of conferring long-
lasting protection.

   An alternative treatment for persons who are not from a high-risk group for whom vaccine is routinely recommended and whose regular sexual partners have acute HBV infection is to give one dose of
HBIG (without vaccine) and retest the sexual partner for HBsAg 3 months later. No further treatment is
necessary if the sexual partner becomes HBsAg-negative. If the sexual partner remains HBsAg-positive, a
second dose of HBIG should be given and the hepatitis B vaccine series started.

Household Contacts of Persons with Acute HBV Infection

Since infants have close contact with primary care givers and they have a higher risk of becoming HBV carriers after acute HBV infection, prophylaxis of an infant less than 12 months of age with HBIG (0.5 ml)
and hepatitis B vaccine is indicated if the mother or primary care-giver has acute HBV infection.
Prophylaxis for other household contacts of persons with acute HBV infection is not indicated unless they
have had identifiable blood exposure to the index patient, such as by sharing toothbrushes or razors. Such
exposures should be treated similarly to sexual exposures. If the index patient becomes an HBV carrier,
all household contacts should be given hepatitis B vaccine.

DELTA HEPATITIS

The delta virus (also known as hepatitis D virus (HDV)) is a defective virus that may cause infection only
in the presence of active HBV infection. The HDV is a 35- to 37-nm viral particle, consisting of single-
stranded RNA (MW 500,000) and an internal protein antigen (delta antigen (HDAg)), coated with HBsAg
as the surface protein (5). Infection may occur as either coinfection with HBV or superinfection of an HBV
carrier, each of which usually causes an episode of clinical acute hepatitis. Coinfection usually resolves,
whereas superinfection frequently causes chronic HDV infection and chronic active hepatitis. Both types
of infection may cause fulminant hepatitis.

   HDV infection may be diagnosed by detecting HDAg in serum during early infection and by the
appearance of total or IgM-specific delta antibody (anti-HDV) during or after infection. A test for detection of total anti-HDV is commercially available. Other tests (HDAg, IgM anti-HDV) are available only in
research laboratories.

   Routes of transmission of HDV are similar to those of HBV. In the United States, HDV infection most
commonly affects persons at high risk of HBV infection, particularly parenteral drug abusers and persons
with hemophilia.

   Since HDV is dependent on HBV for replication, prevention of hepatitis B infection, either preexposure or postexposure, will suffice to prevent HDV infection for a person susceptible to hepatitis B.
Known episodes of perinatal, sexual, or percutaneous exposure to serum or exposure to persons known to
be positive for both HBV and HDV should be treated exactly as such exposures to HBV alone.

   Persons who are HBsAg carriers are at risk of HDV infection, especially if they participate in activities that put them at high risk of repeated exposure to HBV (parenteral drug abuse, male homosexual activity). However, at present no products are available that might prevent HDV infection in HBsAg carriers either before or after exposure.

NON-A, NON-B HEPATITIS

Parenterally Transmitted (PT) Non-A, Non-B Hepatitis

Parenterally transmitted non-A, non-B hepatitis accounts for 20%–40% of acute viral hepatitis in the United States and has epidemiologic characteristics similar to those of hepatitis B (60). Recently, a portion of the genome of a virus thought to be responsible for PT non-A, non-B hepatitis was cloned (2). A candidate serologic assay for antibody to this virus (proposed as hepatitis C virus) has been developed. This assay appears to detect a substantial number of persons with chronic infection and is being evaluated for screening potential blood donors (3). Although PT non-A, non-B hepatitis has traditionally been considered a transfusion-associated disease, most reported cases have not been associated with blood transfusion (61–64). Groups at high risk of acquiring this disease include transfusion recipients, parenteral drug users, and dialysis patients (62, 63). Health-care work that entails frequent contact with blood, personal contact with others who have had hepatitis in the past, and contact with infected persons within households have also been documented in some studies as risk factors for acquiring PT non-A, non-B hepatitis (63–65). However, the role of person-to-person contact in disease transmission has not been well defined, and the importance of sexual activity in the transmission of this type of hepatitis is unclear.

Multiple episodes of non-A, non-B hepatitis have been observed among the same individuals and may be due to different bloodborne agents. An average of 50% of patients who have acute PT non-A, non-B hepatitis infection later develop chronic hepatitis (66). Experimental studies of chimpanzees have confirmed the existence of a carrier state, which may be present in 1%–3% of the population (67, 68).

The risk and consequences of perinatal transmission of PT non-A, non-B hepatitis are not well defined. Only one small study has been published in which infants born of 12 women who had acute PT non-A, non-B hepatitis during pregnancy were followed. Six infants developed transient alanine aminotransferase (ALT) elevations at 4–8 weeks of age (69).

The results have been equivocal in several studies attempting to assess the value of prophylaxis with IGs against PT non-A, non-B hepatitis (70–72). For persons with percutaneous exposure to blood from a patient with PT non-A, non-B hepatitis, it may be reasonable to administer IG (0.06 ml/kg) as soon as possible after exposure. In other circumstances, no specific recommendations can be made.

Enterically Transmitted (ET) Non-A, Non-B Hepatitis

A distinct type of non-A, non-B hepatitis acquired by the fecal-oral route was first identified through investigations of large waterborne epidemics in developing countries. This ET non-A, non-B hepatitis, which has occurred in epidemics or sporadically in parts of Asia, North and West Africa, and Mexico, is serologically distinct from other known hepatitis viruses (4, 73). Young to middle-aged adults are most often affected, with an unusually high mortality among pregnant women. The disease has been transmitted to experimental animals, and candidate viruses have been identified; however, no serologic tests have yet been developed (74).

ET non-A, non-B hepatitis has not been recognized as an endemic disease in the United States or Western Europe, and it is unknown whether the causative agent is present in these areas. Cases have been documented, however, among persons returning from travel to countries in which this disease occurs (75).

Travelers to areas having ET non-A, non-B hepatitis may be at some risk of acquiring this disease by close contact with infected persons or by consuming contaminated food or water. There is no evidence that U.S.-manufactured IG will prevent this infection. As with hepatitis A and other enteric infections, the best means of preventing ET non-A, non-B hepatitis is avoiding potentially contaminated food or water.

REFERENCES

1. Francis DP, Maynard JE. The transmission and outcome of hepatitis A, B, and non-A, non-B: a review. Epidemiol Rev 1979;1:17–31.
2. Choo Q-L, Kuo G, Weiner AJ, et al. Isolation of a cDNA clone derived from a blood-borne non-A, non-B hepatitis genome. Science 1989;244:359–362.
3. Kuo G, Choo Q-L, Alter HJ, et al. An assay for circulating antibodies to a major etiologic virus of human non-A, non-B hepatitis. Science 1989;244:362–364.
4. Ramalingaswami V, Purcell RH. Waterborne non-A, non-B hepatitis. Lancet 1988;1:571–573.
5. Rizzetto M. The delta agent. Hepatology 1983;3:729–737.

6. CDC. Safety of therapeutic immune globulin preparations with respect to transmission of human T-lymphotropic virus type III/lymphadenopathy-associated virus infection. MMWR 1986;35:231–233.

7. Wells MA, Wittek AE, Epstein JS, et al. Inactivation and partition of human T-cell lymphotropic virus, type III, during ethanol fractionation of plasma. Transfusion 1986;26:210–213.

8. Tedder RS, Uttley A, Cheingsong-Popov R. Safety of immunoglobulin preparation containing anti-HTLV-III [Letter]. Lancet 1985;1:815.

9. CDC. Hepatitis A among drug abusers. MMWR 1988;37:297–300, 305.

10. Noble RC, Kane MA, Reeves SA, et al. Posttransfusion hepatitis A in a neonatal intensive care unit. JAMA 1984;252:2711–2715.

11. Kluge I. Gamma-globulin in the prevention of viral hepatitis: a study of the effect of medium-size doses. Acta Med Scand 1963;174:469–477.

12. Stokes J Jr, Neefe JR. Prevention and attenuation of infectious hepatitis by gamma globulin; preliminary note. JAMA 1945;127:144–145.

13. Mosley JW, Reisler DM, Brachott D, Roth D, Weiser J. Comparison of two lots of immune serum globulin for prophylaxis of infectious hepatitis. Am J Epidemiol 1968;87:539–550.

14. Woodson RD, Cahill KM. Viral hepatitis abroad. Incidence in Catholic missionaries. JAMA 1971;219:1191–1193.

15. Woodson RD, Clinton JJ. Hepatitis prophylaxis abroad. Effectiveness of immune serum globulin in protecting Peace Corps volunteers. JAMA 1969;209:1053–1058.

16. Steffen R, Rickenbach M, Wilhelm U, Helminger A, Schar M. Health problems after travel to developing countries. J Infect Dis 1987;156:84–91.

17. CDC. Health information for international travel 1989. Atlanta: CDC, 1989;HHS publication no. (CDC)89–8280.

18. Storch G, McFarland LM, Kelso K, Heilman CJ, Caraway CT. Viral hepatitis associated with day-care centers. JAMA 1979;242:1514–1518.

19. Hadler SC, Webster HM, Erben JJ, Swanson JE, Maynard JE. Hepatitis A in day-care centers. A community-wide assessment. N Engl J Med 1980;302:1222–1227.

20. Hadler SC, Erben JJ, Matthews D, Starko K, Francis DP, Maynard JE. Effect of immunoglobulin on hepatitis A in day care centers. JAMA 1983;249:48–53.

21. Favero MS, Maynard JE, Leger RT, Graham DR, Dixon RE. Guidelines for the care of patients hospitalized with viral hepatitis. Ann Intern Med 1979;91:872–876.

22. Carl M, Francis DP, Maynard JE. Food-borne hepatitis A: recommendations for control. J Infect Dis 1983;148:1133–1135.

23. Lettau LA, Smith JD, Williams D, et al. Transmission of hepatitis B with resultant restriction of surgical practice. JAMA 1986;255:934–937.

24. Kane MA, Lettau L. Transmission of HBV from dental personnel to patients. JADA 1985;110:634–636.

25. Maynard JE, Kane MA, Hadler SC. Global control of hepatitis B through vaccination: role of hepatitis B vaccine in the expanded programme on immunization. Rev Infect Dis 1989;11(S3):S574–S578.

26. McQuillan GM, Townsend TR, Fields HA, et al. Seroepidemiology of hepatitis B virus infection in the United States: 1976 to 1980. Am J Med 1989;87(3A):5S–10S.

27. CDC. Prevention of perinatal transmission of hepatitis B virus: prenatal screening of all pregnant women for hepatitis B surface antigen. MMWR 1988;37:341–346, 351.

28. Francis DP, Feorino PM, McDougal S, et al. The safety of hepatitis B vaccine: inactivation of the AIDS virus during routine vaccine manufacture. JAMA 1986;256:869–872.

29. Zajac BA, West DJ, McAleer WJ, Scolnick EM. Overview of clinical studies with hepatitis B vaccine made by recombinant DNA. J Infect 1986;13(Suppl A):39–45.

30. Andre FE, Safary A. Clinical experience with a yeast-derived hepatitis B vaccine. In: Zuckerman AJ, ed. Viral hepatitis and liver disease. New York: Alan R. Liss, 1988:1023–1030.

31. Szmuness W, Stevens CE, Harley EJ, et al. Hepatitis B vaccine: demonstration of efficacy in a controlled clinical trial in a high-risk population in the United States. N Engl J Med 1980;303:833–841.

32. CDC. Suboptimal response to hepatitis B vaccine given by injection into the buttock. MMWR 1985;34:105–113.

33. Stevens CE, Alter HJ, Taylor PE, et al. Hepatitis B vaccine in patients receiving hemodialysis. Immunogenicity and efficacy. N Engl J Med 1984;311:496–501.

34. Collier AC, Corey L, Murphy VL, Handsfield HH. Antibody to human immunodeficiency virus and suboptimal response to hepatitis B vaccination. Ann Intern Med 1988;109:101–105.

35. Stevens CE, Taylor PE, Tong MJ, et al. Yeast-recombinant hepatitis B vaccine: efficacy with hepatitis B immune globulin in prevention of perinatal hepatitis B virus transmission. JAMA 1987;257:2612–2616.

36. Hadler SC, Francis DP, Maynard JE, et al. Long-term immunogenicity and efficacy of hepatitis B vaccine in homosexual men. N Engl J Med 1986;315:209–214.

37. Wainwright RB, McMahon BJ, Bulkow LR, et al. Duration of immunogenicity and efficacy of hepatitis B vaccine in a Yupik Eskimo population. JAMA 1989;261:2362–2366.

38. Hadler SC. Are booster doses of hepatitis B vaccine necessary? Ann Intern Med 1988;109: 457–458.

39. Redfield RR, Innis BL, Scott RM, Cannon HG, Bancroft WH. Clinical evaluation of low-dose intradermally administered hepatitis B vaccine, a cost reduction strategy. JAMA 1985;254: 3203–3206.

40. Shaw FE, Graham DJ, Guess HA, et al. Postmarketing surveillance for neurologic adverse events reported after hepatitis B vaccination. Experience of the first three years. Am J Epidemiol 1988;127:337–352.

41. Dienstag JL, Stevens CE, Bhan AK, et al. Hepatitis B vaccine administered to chronic carriers of hepatitis B surface antigen. Ann Intern Med 1982;96:575–579.

42. Szmuness W, Stevens CE, Oleszko WR, et al. Passive-active immunization against hepatitis B: immunogenicity studies in adult Americans. Lancet 1981;1:575–577.

43. CDC. Guidelines for prevention of transmission of human immunodeficiency virus and hepatitis B virus to health-care and public-safety workers. MMWR 1989;38(no. S-6).

44. Breuer B, Friedman SM, Millner ES, et al. Transmission of hepatitis B in school contacts of retarded HBsAg carriers. JAMA 1985;254:3190–3195.

45. CDC. Routine screening for viral hepatitis in chronic hemodialysis centers. Hepatitis Surveillance Report No. 49. Atlanta: CDC, 1985:5–6.

46. Seaworth B, Drucker J, Starling J, Drucker R, Stevens C, Hamilton J. Hepatitis B vaccine in patients with chronic renal failure before dialysis. J Infect Dis 1988;157:332–337.

47. Hershow RC, Hadler SC, Kane MA. Adoption of children from countries with endemic hepatitis B: transmission risks and medical issues. Pediatr Infect Dis J 1987;6:431–437.

48. Franks AL, Berg CJ, Kane MA, et al. Hepatitis B virus infection among children born in the United States to Southeast Asian refugees. N Engl J Med 1989;321:1301–1305.

49. Beasley RP, Hwang L-Y, Lee GC, et al. Prevention of perinatally transmitted hepatitis B virus infections with hepatitis B immune globulin and hepatitis B vaccine. Lancet 1983;2:1099–1102.

50. Wong VCW, Ip HMH, Reesink HW, et al. Prevention of the HBsAg carrier state in newborn infants of mothers who are chronic carriers of HBsAg and HBeAg by administration of hepatitis-B vaccine and hepatitis-B immunoglobulin: double-blind randomised placebo-controlled study. Lancet 1984;1:921–926.

51. Stevens CE, Toy PT, Tong MJ, et al. Perinatal hepatitis B virus transmission in the United States: prevention by passive-active immunization. JAMA 1985;253:1740–1745.

52. Beasley RP, Hwang LY, Stevens CE, et al. Efficacy of hepatitis B immune globulin for prevention of perinatal transmission of the hepatitis B virus carrier state: final report of a randomized double-blind, placebo-controlled trial. Hepatology 1983;3:135–141.

53. Xu ZY, Liu CB, Francis DP, et al. Prevention of perinatal acquisition of hepatitis B virus carriage using vaccine: preliminary report of a randomized, double-blind placebo-controlled and comparative trial. Pediatrics 1985;76:713–718.

54. Seeff LB, Wright EC, Zimmerman HJ, et al. Type B hepatitis after needlestick exposure: prevention with hepatitis B immune globulin. Final report of the Veterans Administration Cooperative Study. Ann Intern Med 1978;88:285–293.

55. Grady GF, Lee VA, Prince AM, et al. Hepatitis B immune globulin for accidental exposures among medical personnel: final report of a multicenter controlled trial. J Infect Dis 1978;138:625–638.

56. Redeker AG, Mosley JW, Gocke DJ, McKee AP, Pollack W. Hepatitis B immune globulin as a prophylactic measure for spouses exposed to acute type B hepatitis. N Engl J Med 1975;293: 1055–1059.

57. Beasley RP, Hwang L-Y. Epidemiology of hepatocellular carcinoma. In: Vyas GN, Dienstag JL, Hoofnagle JH, eds. Viral hepatitis and liver disease. New York: Grune & Stratton, 1984: 209–224.

58. Sinatra FR, Shah P, Weissman JY, Thomas DW, Merritt RJ, Tong MJ. Perinatal transmitted acute icteric hepatitis B in infants born to hepatitis B surface antigen-positive and anti-hepatitis Be-positive carrier mothers. Pediatrics 1982;70:557–559.
59. Delaplane D, Yogev R, Crussi F, Schulman ST. Fatal hepatitis B in early infancy: the importance of identifying HBsAg-positive pregnant women and providing immunoprophylaxis to their newborns. Pediatrics 1983;72:176–180.
60. Alter MJ, Hadler SC, Francis DP, Maynard JE. The epidemiology of non-A, non-B hepatitis in the United States. In: Dodd RY, Barker LF, eds. Infection, immunity, and blood transfusion. New York: Alan R. Liss, 1985:71–79.
61. Alter HJ, Purcell RH, Holland PV, et al. Clinical and serological analysis of transfusion-associated hepatitis. Lancet 1975;2:838–841.
62. Dienstag JL. Non-A, non-B hepatitis. I. Recognition, epidemiology, and clinical features. Gastroenterology 1983;85:439–462.
63. Alter MJ, Gerety RJ, Smallwood LA, et al. Sporadic non-A, non-B hepatitis: frequency and epidemiology in an urban U.S. population. J Infect Dis 1982;145:886–893.
64. Alter MJ, Coleman PJ, Alexander WJ, et al., Importance of heterosexual activity in the transmission of hepatitis B and non-A, non-B hepatitis. JAMA 1989;262:1201–1205.
65. Guyer B, Bradley DW, Bryan JA, Maynard JE. Non-A, non-B hepatitis among participants in a plasmapheresis stimulation program. J Infect Dis 1979;139:634–640.
66. Dienstag JL, Alter HJ. Non-A, non-B hepatitis: evolving epidemiologic and clinical perspectives. Semin Liver Dis 1986;6:67–81.
67. Tabor E, Seeff LB, Gerety RJ. Chronic non-A, non-B hepatitis carrier state: transmissible agent documented in one patient over a six-year period. N Engl J Med 1980;303:140–143.
68. Aach RD, Szmuness W, Mosley JW, et al. Serum alanine aminotransferase of donors in relation to the risk of non-A, non-B hepatitis in recipients: the Transfusion-Transmitted Viruses Study. N Engl J Med 1981;304:989–994.
69. Tong MJ, Thursby M, Rakela J, et al. Studies on the maternal-infant transmission of the viruses which cause acute hepatitis. Gastroenterology 1981;80:999–1003.
References 70 through 75 may be obtained by writing to the Hepatitis Branch, Division of Viral and Rickettsial Diseases, Center for Infectious Diseases, Mailstop A33, Centers for Disease Control, Atlanta, Ga. 30333.

SUBTOPIC / HEPATITIS A

Licensure of Inactivated Hepatitis A Vaccine and Recommendations for Use Among International Travelers

Original Citation: Centers for Disease Control and Prevention. Notice to Readers Licensure of Inactivated Hepatitis A Vaccine and Recommendations for Use Among International Travelers MMWR 1995;44(29):559–560.

In February 1995, Havrix®*, an inactivated hepatitis A vaccine distributed by SmithKline Beecham Pharmaceuticals (Philadelphia, Pennsylvania) was licensed by the Food and Drug Administration for use in persons aged greater than or equal to 2 years to prevent hepatitis A virus (HAV) infection. The vaccine is licensed in adult and pediatric formulations, with different dosages and administration schedules Table 1 and should be

---

*Use of trade names and commercial sources is for identification only and does not imply endorsement by the Public Health Service or the U.S. Department of Health and Human Services.

Table 1. Recommended vaccination schedule for Havris® [a]

Age group (yrs)	Dose (EL.U.[+])	Volume (mL)	No. doses	Schedule (months) [&]
2–18	360	0.5	3	0, 1, 6–12
>18	1440	1.0	2	0, 6–12

[a]Inactivated hepatitis A vaccine distributed by SmithKline Beecham Pharmaceuticals (Philadelphia, Pennsylvania). Use of trade names and commercial sources is for identification only and does not imply endorsement by the Public Health Service or the U.S. Department of Health and Human Services.
[+]Enzyme-linked immunosorbent assay units.
[&]Zero months represent timing of the initial dose; subsequent numbers represent months after the initial dose.

administered by intramuscular injection into the deltoid muscle. Immunogenicity studies have indicated that virtually 100% of children, adolescents, and adults develop protective levels of antibody to hepatitis A virus (anti-HAV) after completing the vaccine series (1, 2). Based on a controlled clinical trial, the efficacy of two doses of vaccine (360 enzyme-linked immunosorbent assay units) administered 1 month apart in preventing hepatitis A in children was estimated to be 94% (95% confidence interval = 79%–99%) (3). Vaccine recipients have been followed for as long as 4 years and still have protective levels of anti-HAV. Kinetic models of antibody decline suggest that protective levels of anti-HAV could persist for at least 20 years (1, 4).

Hepatitis A vaccine can be administered simultaneously with other vaccines and toxoids—including hepatitis B, diphtheria, tetanus, oral typhoid, cholera, Japanese encephalitis, rabies, and yellow fever—without affecting immunogenicity or increasing the frequency of adverse events (5, 6). However, during simultaneous administration, the vaccines should be given at separate injection sites. When immune globulin (IG) is given concurrently with the first dose of vaccine, the proportion of persons who develop protective levels of anti-HAV is not affected, but antibody concentrations are lower. Because the final concentrations of anti-HAV are substantially higher than that considered to be protective, this reduced immunogenicity is not expected to be clinically important (7).

Vaccination of an immune person is not contraindicated and does not increase the risk for adverse effects. Prevaccination serologic testing may be indicated for adult travelers who probably have had prior HAV infection if the cost of testing is less than the cost of vaccination and if testing will not interfere with completion of the vaccine series. Such persons may include those aged greater than 40 years and those born in areas of the world with a high endemicity of HAV infection (see recommendations). Postvaccination testing for serologic response is not indicated.

The Advisory Committee on Immunization Practices (ACIP) offers the following interim recommendations for the use of inactivated hepatitis A vaccine among international travelers.

1. All susceptible persons traveling to or working in countries with intermediate or high HAV endemicity (countries other than Australia, Canada, Japan, New Zealand, and countries in Western Europe and Scandinavia) should be vaccinated with hepatitis A vaccine or receive IG before departure. Hepatitis A vaccine at the age-appropriate dose (Table 1) is preferred for persons who plan to travel repeatedly to or reside for long periods in these high-risk areas. IG is recommended for travelers aged less than 2 years.
2. After receiving the initial dose of hepatitis A vaccine, persons are considered to be protected by 4 weeks. For long-term protection, a second dose is needed 6–12 months later. For persons who will travel to high-risk areas less than 4 weeks after the initial vaccine dose, IG (0.02 mL per kg of body weight) should be administered simultaneously with the first dose of vaccine but at different injection sites.
3. Persons who are allergic to a vaccine component or otherwise elect not to receive vaccine should receive a single dose of IG (0.02 mL per kg of body weight), which provides effective protection against hepatitis A for up to 3 months. IG should be administered at 0.06 mL per kg of body weight and must be repeated if travel is greater than 5 months.

The complete ACIP recommendations for the prevention of hepatitis A will be published. Additional information about hepatitis A vaccine is available from CDC's Hepatitis Branch, Division of Viral and Rickettsial Diseases, National Center for Infectious Diseases, telephone (404)639-3048.

Reported By: Advisory Committee on Immunization Practices. Div of Viral and Rickettsial Diseases, National Center for Infectious Diseases, CDC.

REFERENCES: AS NUMBERED IN ORIGINAL PUBLICATION

1. Clemens R, Safary A, Hepburn A, Roche C, Stanbury WJ, Andre FE. Clinical experience with an inactivated hepatitis A vaccine. J Infect Dis 1995;171(Suppl 1):S44–S49.
2. Balcarek DB, Bagley MR, Pass RF, Schiff ER, Krause DS. Safety and immunogenicity of an inactivated hepatitis A vaccine in preschool children. J Infect Dis 1995;171(Suppl 1):S70–S72.
3. Innis BL, Snitbhan R, Kunasol P, et al. Protection against hepatitis A by an inactivated vaccine. JAMA 1994;271:1328–1334.
4. Ambrosch F, Widermann G, Andre FE, et al. Comparison of HAV antibodies induced by vaccination, passive immunization, and natural infection. In: Hollinger FB, Lemon SM, Margolis HS, eds. Viral hepatitis and liver disease. Baltimore: Williams and Wilkins, 1991:98–100.
5. Ambrosch F, Andre FE, Delem A, et al. Simultaneous vaccination against hepatitis A and B: results of a controlled study. Vaccine 1992;10(Suppl 1):S142–S145.
6. Kruppenbacher J, Bienzle U, Bock HL, Clemens R. Co-administration of an inactivated hepatitis A vaccine with other travelers vaccines: interference with the immune response [Abstract]. In: Proceedings of the 34th Interscience Conference on Antimicrobial Agents and Chemotherapy. Washington, DC: American Society of Microbiologists, 1994:256.
7. Wagner G, Lavanchy D, Darioli R, et al. Simultaneous active and passive immunization against hepatitis A studied in a population of travelers. Vaccine 1993;11:1027–1032.

SUBTOPIC / HEPATITIS B

Hepatitis B Prevention and Pregnancy

Original Citation: Hepatitis B Prevention and Pregnancy—U.S. Department of Health and Human Services, Public Health Service, Centers for Disease Control and Prevention, National Center for Infectious Diseases Division of Viral and Rickettsial Diseases, 1992.

WHAT IS HEPATITIS B?

Hepatitis B is a serious disease of the liver caused by hepatitis B virus, or HBV. All people, no matter how old they are or where they live, may be at risk for hepatitis B.

HBV attacks and destroys the liver, which is such an important organ that you cannot live without it.

Hepatitis B may cause

- Scarring (cirrhosis) of the liver
- Liver cancer
- Lifelong (chronic) HBV infection
- Liver failure
- Death

Why is Hepatitis B a Problem for Pregnant Women and Their Babies?

Pregnant women may have HBV in their blood without knowing it and can pass it on to their babies at birth. Many of these babies develop lifelong HBV infections and can pass the virus on to others throughout their lives. At first, babies may not look or feel sick, but as they grow up, they may have liver damage. About 25% of babies who develop lifelong HBV infections die of liver disease or liver cancer.

How Can You Get Hepatitis B?

HBV is spread from person to person by direct contact with infected blood or body fluids. Even small amounts of infected blood can cause infection.

HBV infection can be spread by

- An infected mother to her baby during birth
- Sharing needles for injecting drugs
- Having sex with an infected person

You are at increased risk for hepatitis B if

- You live in the same household with someone who has lifelong HBV infection
- You have a job that exposes you to human blood

If You Feel Healthy, Can You Still Have Hepatitis B?

Some people who have hepatitis B have no symptoms and may not know they are infected. Others who are infected with HBV never fully recover and carry the virus in their blood for the rest of their lives. These people are known as carriers, and they can infect other household and sexual contacts throughout their lives.

How Do You Find Out if You Have Hepatitis B?

Get a blood test at your clinic or doctor's office. If the test is positive, the doctor or nurse will tell you how to take care of yourself and how to prevent infecting your baby and others.

How Do You Protect Your Baby if Your Hepatitis B Blood Test Is Positive?

A safe vaccine has been used since 1982 to prevent hepatitis B. The vaccine is given in a series of three shots. If you have HBV infection, your baby will get the first shot within 12 hours of birth, along with another shot, hepatitis B immune globulin. The next two shots of hepatitis B vaccine will be given along with other baby shots. All other members of your household should get a blood test for hepatitis B. If the blood test is negative, hepatitis B vaccine should be given to the other household members.

Do You Need to Protect Your Baby if the Hepatitis B Blood Test Is Negative?

Hepatitis B vaccination is recommended for all infants to protect them from becoming infected with HBV. If your blood test for hepatitis B is negative, your baby will still receive the hepatitis B vaccine series with other baby shots, but will not need a shot of hepatitis B immune globulin. The baby may get the first shot either before leaving the hospital or with the first baby shots at the doctor's office or clinic. Ask your doctor or nurse when the next shots need to be given.

Protect Your Baby Against Hepatitis B

- Get a blood test
- Vaccinate your baby

For More Information on Hepatitis B and Pregnancy

Contact your local health department or call the CDC Hepatitis Hotline (404) 332-4555. Hepatitis Branch Division of Viral and Rickettsial Diseases, National Center for Infectious Diseases, Centers for Disease Control and Prevention, Atlanta, Georgia 30333.

Hepatitis B Virus: A Comprehensive Strategy for Eliminating Transmission in the United States Through Universal Childhood Vaccination

Original Citation: ACIP. Hepatitis B Virus: A Comprehensive Strategy for Eliminating Transmission in the United States Through Universal Childhood Vaccination: Recommendations of the Immunization Practices Advisory Committee (ACIP). MMWR 1991;40(RR-13):1–25.

The following statement updates all previous recommendations on protection against hepatitis B virus infection, including use of hepatitis B vaccine and hepatitis B immune globulin for prophylaxis against hepatitis B virus infection (MMWR 1985;34:313–324, 329–335, MMWR 1987;36:353–366, and MMWR 1990;39[No. RR-2]:8–19) and universal screening of pregnant women to prevent perinatal hepatitis B virus transmission (MMWR 1988;37:341–346, 351, and MMWR 1990;39[No. RR-2]:8–19). Recommendations concerning the prevention of other types of viral hepatitis are found in MMWR 1990;39(No. RR-2): 1–8, 22–26.

This document provides the rationale for a comprehensive strategy to eliminate transmission of hepatitis B virus in the United States. This prevention strategy includes making hepatitis B vaccine a part of routine vaccination schedules for all infants.

INTRODUCTION

The acute and chronic consequences of hepatitis B virus (HBV) infection are major health problems in the United States. The reported incidence of acute hepatitis B increased by 37% from 1979 to 1989, and an estimated 200,000–300,000 new infections occurred annually during the period 1980–1991. The estimated 1 million–1.25 million persons with chronic HBV infection in the United States are potentially infectious to others. In addition, many chronically infected persons are at risk of long-term sequelae, such as chronic liver disease and primary hepatocellular carcinoma; each year approximately 4,000–5,000 of these persons die from chronic liver disease (1).

Immunization with hepatitis B vaccine is the most effective means of preventing HBV infection and its consequences. In the United States, most infections occur among adults and adolescents (2, 3). The recommended strategy for preventing these infections has been the selective vaccination of persons with identified risk factors (1, 2). However, this strategy has not lowered the incidence of hepatitis B, primarily because vaccinating persons engaged in high-risk behaviors, life-styles, or occupations before they become infected generally has not been feasible. In addition, many infected persons have no identifiable source for their infections and thus cannot be targeted for vaccination (2).

Preventing HBV transmission during early childhood is important because of the high likelihood of chronic HBV infection and chronic liver disease that occurs when children less than 5 years of age become infected (3). Testing to identify pregnant women who are hepatitis B surface antigen (HBsAg)-positive and providing their infants with immunoprophylaxis effectively prevents HBV transmission during the perinatal period (4, 5). Integrating hepatitis B vaccine into childhood vaccination schedules in populations with high rates of childhood infection (e.g., Alaskan Natives and Pacific Islanders) has been shown to interrupt HBV transmission (6). This document provides the rationale for a comprehensive strategy to eliminate transmission of HBV and ultimately reduce the incidence of hepatitis B and hepatitis B-associated chronic liver disease in the United States. The recommendations for implementing this strategy include making hepatitis B vaccine a part of routine vaccination schedules for infants.

EPIDEMIOLOGY AND PREVENTION OF HEPATITIS B VIRUS INFECTION

Infections among Infants and Children

In the United States, children become infected with HBV through a variety of means. The risk of perinatal HBV infection among infants born to HBV-infected mothers ranges from 10% to 85%, depending on each mother's hepatitis B e antigen (HBeAg) status (3, 7, 8). Infants who become infected by perinatal transmission have a 90% risk of chronic infection, and up to 25% will die of chronic liver disease as adults (9). Even when not infected during the perinatal period, children of HBV-infected mothers remain at high risk of acquiring chronic HBV infection by person-to-person (horizontal) transmission during the first 5 years of life (10). More than 90% of these infections can be prevented if HBsAg-positive mothers are identified so that their infants can receive hepatitis B vaccine and hepatitis B immune globulin (HBIG) soon after birth (4, 5).

Because screening selected pregnant women for HBsAg has failed to identify a high proportion of HBV-infected mothers (11, 12), prenatal HBsAg testing of all pregnant women is now recommended (1, 13, 14). Universal prenatal testing would identify an estimated 22,000 HBsAg-positive women and could prevent at least 6,000 chronic HBV infections annually (3). Screening and vaccination programs for women and infants receiving care in the public sector have already been initiated through state immunization projects.

Horizontal transmission of HBV during the first 5 years of life occurs frequently in populations in which HBV infection is endemic. The risk of chronic infection is age dependent, ranging from 30% to 60% for children 1–5 years of age (15). Worldwide, it has been recommended that, in populations in which HBV infection is acquired during childhood, hepatitis B vaccine should be integrated into routine vaccination schedules for infants, usually as a part of the World Health Organization's Expanded Programme on Immunization (16). In the United States, racial/ethnic groups shown to have high rates of childhood HBV infection include Alaskan Natives (6, 17), Pacific Islanders (18), and infants of first-generation immigrant mothers from parts of the world where HBV infection is endemic, especially Asia (19, 20). Vaccination programs to prevent perinatal, childhood, and adult HBV infections among Alaskan Natives were begun in late 1982; as a result, the incidence of acute hepatitis B in this population has declined by over 99% (6). Hepatitis B vaccine was integrated into vaccination schedules for infants in American Samoa beginning in 1986 and by 1990 was incorporated into the schedules of the remaining Pacific Islands under U.S. jurisdiction.

Each year, approximately 150,000 infants are born to women who have immigrated to the United States from areas of the world where HBV infection is highly endemic (3). Children born to HBsAg-positive mothers can be identified through prenatal screening programs. However, children born to HBsAg-negative immigrant mothers are still at high risk of acquiring HBV infection, usually from other HBV carriers in their families or communities (3, 19, 20). Infections among these children can be prevented by making hepatitis B vaccine part of their routine infant vaccinations (1).

Infections among Adolescents and Adults

In the United States most persons with hepatitis B acquire the infection as adolescents or adults. Several specific modes of transmission have been identified, including sexual contact, especially among homosexual men and persons with multiple heterosexual partners; parenteral drug use; occupational exposures; household contact with a person who has an acute infection or with a chronic carrier; receipt of certain blood products; and hemodialysis. However, over one-third of patients with acute hepatitis B do not have readily identifiable risk factors (1, 2).

The rates of HBV infection differ significantly among various racial and ethnic groups (2, 21). For example, the prevalence of infection among adolescents and adults has been shown to be threefold to fourfold greater for blacks than for whites and to be associated with serologic evidence of previous infection with syphilis (21, 22).

Efforts to vaccinate persons in the major risk groups have had limited success. For example, programs directed at injecting drug users failed to motivate them to receive three doses of vaccine (CDC, unpublished data). Health-care providers are often not aware of groups at high risk of HBV infection and frequently do not identify candidates for vaccination during routine health-care visits (CDC, unpublished data). In addition, there has been limited vaccination of susceptible household and sexual contacts of HBsAg carriers identified in screening programs for blood donors (23). Hepatitis B vaccination of health-care workers appears to have resulted in a substantial decrease in the rate of disease in this group, but has had little effect on overall rates of hepatitis B (2). Moreover, to achieve widespread vaccination of persons at occupational risk, regulations have had to be developed to ensure implementation of vaccination programs (24).

Educational programs to reduce parenteral drug use and unprotected sexual activity are important components of the strategy to prevent infection with the human immunodeficiency virus (HIV), which causes acquired immunodeficiency syndrome. These programs appear to have reduced the risk of HBV infections among homosexual men but have not had an impact on hepatitis B attributable to parenteral drug use or heterosexual transmission (2). Educational efforts alone are not likely to fully eliminate the high-risk behaviors responsible for HBV transmission.

EPIDEMIOLOGY AND PREVENTION OF HEPATITIS DELTA VIRUS INFECTION

Hepatitis delta virus (HDV) is a defective virus that causes infection only in the presence of active HBV infection (25). HDV infection occurs as either coinfection with HBV or superinfection of an HBV carrier. Coinfection usually resolves; superinfection, however, frequently causes chronic HDV infection and chronic active hepatitis. Both types of infection may cause fulminant hepatitis.

Routes of transmission are similar to those of HBV. In the United States, HDV infection most commonly affects persons at high risk of HBV infection, particularly injecting drug users and persons receiving clotting factor concentrates (26). Preventing acute and chronic HBV infection of susceptible persons will also prevent HDV infection.

STRATEGY TO ELIMINATE HEPATITIS B VIRUS TRANSMISSION

A comprehensive strategy to prevent HBV infection, acute hepatitis B, and the sequelae of HBV infection in the United States must eliminate transmission that occurs during infancy and childhood, as well as during adolescence and adulthood. In the United States it has become evident that HBV transmission cannot be prevented through vaccinating only the groups at high risk of infection. No current medical treatment will reliably eliminate chronic HBV infection and thus eliminate the source of new infections in susceptible persons (27). Therefore, new infections can be prevented only by immunizing susceptible persons with hepatitis B vaccine. Routine visits for prenatal and well-child care can be used to target hepatitis B prevention. A comprehensive prevention strategy includes (a) prenatal testing of pregnant women for HBsAg to identify newborns who require immunoprophylaxis for the prevention of perinatal infection and to identify household contacts who should be vaccinated, (b) routine vaccination of children born to HBsAg-negative mothers, (c) vaccination of certain adolescents, and (d) vaccination of adults at high risk of infection. Infants and children can receive hepatitis B vaccine during routine health-care visits; no additional visits would be required. Costs include that of the vaccine and the incremental expense associated with delivering an additional vaccine during a scheduled health-care visit. Implementation of this immunization strategy would be greatly facilitated by the development and use of multiple-antigen vaccines (e.g., diphtheria-tetanus-pertussis [DTP]/hepatitis B, Haemophilus influenzae type b conjugate/ hepatitis B). These vaccines would reduce the number of injections received by the infant, reduce the cost of administration, and greatly facilitate widespread vaccine delivery.

Since most HBV infections occur among adults, disease control could be accelerated by vaccinating emerging at-risk populations, such as adolescents and susceptible contacts of chronic HBV carriers. The recommendation for universal infant vaccination neither precludes vaccinating adults identified to be at high risk of infection nor alters previous recommendations for postexposure prophylaxis for hepatitis B (1).

The reduction in acute hepatitis B and hepatitis B-associated chronic liver disease resulting from universal infant vaccination may not become apparent for a number of years. However, universal HBsAg screening of pregnant women to prevent perinatal HBV infection has been shown to be cost saving (28; CDC, unpublished data), and the estimated cost of universal hepatitis B vaccination for infants is less than the direct medical and work-loss costs associated with the estimated 5% lifetime risk of infection (CDC, unpublished data). Currently, the cost of an infant's dose of hepatitis B vaccine delivered in the public sector is about the same as each of the other childhood vaccinations. Vaccinating adolescents and adults is substantially more expensive because of the higher vaccine cost and the higher implementation costs of delivering vaccine to target populations. In the long term, universal infant vaccination would eliminate the need for vaccinating adolescents and high-risk adults.

PROPHYLAXIS AGAINST HEPATITIS B VIRUS INFECTION

Two types of products are available for prophylaxis against HBV infection. Hepatitis B vaccine, which provides long-term protection against HBV infection, is recommended for both preexposure and postexposure prophylaxis. HBIG provides temporary protection (i.e., 3–6 months) and is indicated only in certain postexposure settings.

Hepatitis B Immune Globulin

HBIG is prepared from plasma known to contain a high titer of antibody against HBsAg (anti-HBs). In the United States, HBIG has an anti-HBs titer of >100,000 by radioimmunoassay. The human plasma from which

HBIG is prepared is screened for antibodies to HIV; in addition, the process used to prepare HBIG inactivates and eliminates HIV from the final product. There is no evidence that HIV can be transmitted by HBIG (29, 30).

Hepatitis B Vaccine

Two types of hepatitis B vaccine have been licensed in the United States. One, which was manufactured from the plasma of chronically infected persons, is no longer produced in the United States. The currently available vaccines are produced by recombinant DNA technology. The recombinant vaccines are produced by using HBsAg synthesized by Saccharomyces cerevisiae (common bakers' yeast), into which a plasmid containing the gene for HBsAg has been inserted. Purified HBsAg is obtained by lysing the yeast cells and separating HBsAg from the yeast components by biochemical and biophysical techniques. Hepatitis B vaccines are packaged to contain 10–40 µg of HBsAg protein/mL after adsorption to aluminum hydroxide (0.5 mg/mL); thimerosal (1:20,000 concentration) is added as a preservative.

Routes and Sites of Administration

The recommended series of three intramuscular doses of hepatitis B vaccine induces a protective antibody response (anti-HBs ≥10 milli-international units [mIU]/mL) in >90% of healthy adults and in >95% of infants, children, and adolescents (31–33). Hepatitis B vaccine should be administered only in the deltoid muscle of adults and children or in the antero- lateral thigh muscle of neonates and infants; the immunogenicity of the vaccine for adults is substantially lower when injections are administered in the buttock (34). When hepatitis B vaccine is administered to infants at the same time as other vaccines, separate sites in the anterolateral thigh may be used for the multiple injections. This method is preferable to administering vaccine at sites such as the buttock or deltoid. Compared with three standard doses administered intramuscularly, three low doses of plasma-derived or recombinant vaccine administered intradermally to adults result in lower seroconversion rates (55%–81%) and lower final titers of anti-HBs (35–38), although four doses of plasma-derived vaccine administered intradermally have produced responses comparable with vaccine administered intramuscularly (39). Plasma-derived vaccine administered intradermally to infants and children does not induce an adequate antibody response (40). At this time, low-dose intradermal vaccination of adults should be performed only under research protocol with written informed consent. Persons who have been vaccinated intradermally should be tested for anti-HBs. Those with an inadequate response (anti-HBs <10 mIU/mL) should be revaccinated with three full doses of vaccine administered intramuscularly. Intradermal vaccination should not be used for infants or children.

Vaccination During Pregnancy

On the basis of limited experience, there is no apparent risk of adverse effects to developing fetuses when hepatitis B vaccine is administered to pregnant women (CDC, unpublished data). The vaccine contains noninfectious HBsAg particles and should cause no risk to the fetus. HBV infection affecting a pregnant woman may result in severe disease for the mother and chronic infection for the newborn. Therefore, neither pregnancy nor lactation should be considered a contraindication to vaccination of women.

Vaccine Usage

Preexposure Prophylaxis

Vaccination schedule and dose. The vaccination schedule most often used for adults and children has been three intramuscular injections, the second and third administered 1 and 6 months, respectively, after the first. An alternate schedule of four doses has been approved for one vaccine that would allow more rapid induction of immunity. However, for preexposure prophylaxis, there is no clear evidence that this regimen provides greater protection than that obtained with the standard three-dose schedule.

Each vaccine has been evaluated to determine the age-specific dose at which an optimum antibody response is achieved. The recommended dose varies by product and the recipient's age and, for infants, by the mother's HBsAg serologic status (Table 1). In general, the vaccine dose for children and adolescents is 50%–75% lower than that required for adults (Table 1).

Table 1. Recommended doses of currently licensed hepatitis B vaccines

Group	Recombivax HB*		Engerix-B*	
	Dose (μg)	(mL)	Dose (μg)	(mL)
Infants of HBsAg†-negative mothers and children < 11 years	2.5	(0.25)	10	(0.5)
Infants of HBsAg-positive mothers; prevention of perinatal infection	5	(0.5)	10	(0.5)
Children and adolescents 11–19 years	5	(0.5)	20	(1.0)
Adults ≥ 20 years	10	(1.0)	20	(1.0)
Dialysis patients and other immunocompromised persons	40	(1.0)§	40	(2.0)¶

*Both vaccines are routinely administered in a three-dose series. Engerix-B has also been licensed for a four-dose series administered at 0, 1, 2, and 12 months.
†HBsAg = Hepatitis B surface antigen.
§Special formulation.
¶Two 1.0-mL doses administered at one site, in a four-dose schedule at 0, 1, 2, and 6 months.

Incorporating hepatitis B vaccine into childhood vaccination schedules may require modifications of previously recommended schedules. However, a protective level of anti-HBs ($\geq$10 mIU/mL) was achieved when hepatitis B vaccine was administered in a variety of schedules, including those in which vaccination was begun soon after birth (5, 8, 41).

In a three-dose schedule, increasing the interval between the first and second doses of hepatitis B vaccine has little effect on immunogenicity or final antibody titer. The third dose confers optimal protection, acting as a booster dose. Longer intervals between the last two doses (4–12 months) result in higher final titers of anti-HBs (42, 43). Several studies have shown that the currently licensed vaccines produce high rates of seroconversion (>95%) and induce adequate levels of anti-HBs when administered to infants at birth, 2 months, and 6 months of age or at 2 months, 4 months, and 6 months of age (CDC, Merck Sharpe & Dohme, SmithKline Beecham, unpublished data). When the vaccine is administered in four doses at 0, 1, 2, and 12 months, the last dose is necessary to ensure the highest final antibody titer.

When hepatitis B vaccine has been administered at the same time as other vaccines, no interference with the antibody response of the other vaccines has been demonstrated (44).

If the vaccination series is interrupted after the first dose, the second dose should be administered as soon as possible. The second and third doses should be separated by an interval of at least 2 months. If only the third dose is delayed, it should be administered when convenient. The immune response when one or two doses of a vaccine produced by one manufacturer are followed by subsequent doses from a different manufacturer has been shown to be comparable with that resulting from a full course of vaccination with a single vaccine.

Larger vaccine doses or an increased number of doses are required to induce protective antibody in a high proportion of hemodialysis patients (45, 46) and may also be necessary for other immunocompromised persons (e.g., those who take immunosuppressive drugs or who are HIV positive), although few data are available concerning response to higher doses of vaccine by these patients (47).

Prevaccination testing for susceptibility. Susceptibility testing is not indicated for immunization programs for children or for most adolescents because of the low rate of HBV infection and the relatively low cost of vaccine. For adults, the decision to do prevaccination testing should include an analysis of cost effectiveness because of the higher cost of the vaccine. Testing for prior infection should be considered for adults in risk groups with high rates of HBV infection (e.g., injecting drug users, homosexual men, and household contacts of HBV carriers). The decision for testing should be based on whether the costs of testing balance the costs of vaccine saved by not vaccinating already-infected persons. Estimates of the cost effectiveness of testing depend on three variables: the cost of vaccination, the cost of testing for susceptibility, and the expected prevalence of immune persons. If susceptibility testing is being considered, careful attention should also be given to the likelihood of patient follow-up and vaccine delivery.

For routine testing, only one antibody test is necessary (antibody either to the core antigen [anti-HBc] or anti-HBs). Anti-HBc testing identifies all previously infected persons, including HBV carriers, but does not differentiate carriers and non-carriers. The presence of anti-HBs identifies previously infected persons, except for HBV carriers. Neither test has a particular advantage for groups expected to have HBV carrier rates <2%, such as health-care workers. Anti-HBc may be preferable so that unnecessary vaccination of HBV carriers can be avoided in groups with high carrier rates.

Postvaccination testing for serologic response. Such testing is not necessary after routine vaccination of infants, children, or adolescents. Testing for immunity is advised only for persons whose subsequent clinical management depends on knowledge of their immune status (e.g., infants born to HBsAg-positive mothers, dialysis patients and staff, and persons with HIV infection). Postvaccination testing should also be considered for persons at occupational risk who may have exposures from injuries with sharp instruments, because knowledge of their antibody response will aid in determining appropriate postexposure prophylaxis. When necessary, postvaccination testing should be performed from 1 to 6 months after completion of the vaccine series. Testing after immunoprophylaxis of infants born to HBsAg-positive mothers should be performed from 3 to 9 months after the completion of the vaccination series (see section on Postexposure prophylaxis).

Revaccination of nonresponders. When persons who do not respond to the primary vaccine series are revaccinated, 15%–25% produce an adequate antibody response after one additional dose and 30%–50% after three additional doses (48). Therefore, revaccination with one or more additional doses should be considered for persons who do not respond to vaccination initially.

Postexposure Prophylaxis

After a person has been exposed to HBV, appropriate immunoprophylactic treatment can effectively prevent infection. The mainstay of postexposure immunoprophylaxis is hepatitis B vaccine, but in some settings the addition of HBIG will provide some increase in protection. Table 2 provides a guide to recommended treatment for various HBV exposures.

Transmission of perinatal HBV infection can be effectively prevented if the HBsAg-positive mother is identified and if her infant receives appropriate immunoprophylaxis. Hepatitis B vaccination and one dose of HBIG, administered within 24 hours after birth, are 85%–95% effective in preventing both HBV infection and the chronic carrier state (4, 5, 8). Hepatitis B vaccine administered alone in either a three-dose or four-dose schedule (Table 1), beginning within 24 hours after birth, is 70%–95% effective in preventing perinatal HBV infections (8, 41). The infants of women admitted for delivery who have not had prenatal HBsAg testing pose problems in clinical management. Initiating hepatitis B vaccination at birth for infants born to these women will provide adequate postexposure prophylaxis if the mothers are indeed HBsAg positive. The few infections not prevented by either of these treatment regimens were most likely acquired in utero or may be due to very high levels of maternal HBV-DNA (49).

Serologic testing of infants who receive immunoprophylaxis to prevent perinatal infection should be considered as an aid in the long-term medical management of the few infants who become HBV carriers. Testing for anti-HBs and HBsAg at 9–15 months of age will determine the success of the therapy

Table 2. Guide to postexposure immunoprophylaxis for exposure to hepatitis B virus

Type of exposure	Immunoprophylaxis	Reference
Perinatal	Vaccination + HBIG	p. 178
Sexual—acute infection	HBIG ± Vaccination	Appendix*
Sexual—chronic carrier	Vaccination	p. 178
Household contact— chronic carrier	Vaccination	p. 178
Household contact— acute case	None unless known exposure	Appendix*
Household contact— acute case, known exposure	HBIG ± vaccination	Appendix*
Infant (<12 months)— acute case in primary care-giver	HBIG + vaccination	Appendix*
Inadvertent—percutaneous/ permucosal	Vaccination ± HBIG	Appendix*

HBIG = Hepatitis B immune globulin.
*See Appendix in original publication.

and, in the case of failure, will identify HBV carriers or infants who may require revaccination.

Recommendations for postexposure prophylaxis in circumstances other than the perinatal period (Table 2) have been addressed in a previous statement and are reprinted as Appendix A to this document [see Appendix in original publication].

Vaccine Efficacy and Booster Doses

Clinical trials of the hepatitis B vaccines licensed in the United States have shown that they are 80%–95% effective in preventing HBV infection and clinical hepatitis among susceptible children and adults (5, 33, 41, 50). If a protective antibody response develops after vaccination, vaccine recipients are virtually 100% protected against clinical illness. The duration of vaccine-induced immunity has been evaluated in long-term follow-up studies of both adults and children (48, 51). Only the plasma-derived hepatitis B vaccine has been evaluated because it has had the longest clinical use; however, on the basis of comparable immunogenicity and short-term efficacy, similar results would be expected with recombinant vaccines. The magnitude of the antibody response induced by the primary vaccination series is predictive of antibody persistence, and a logarithmic decline of antibody levels occurs over time. Among young adults (homosexual men and Alaskan Eskimos) who initially responded to a three-dose vaccine series, loss of detectable antibody has ranged from 13% to 60% after 9 years of follow-up. For children vaccinated after the first year of life, the rate of antibody decline has been lower than for adults (51). The peak antibody titers for infants are lower than those for children immunized after 12 months of age, but the rate of antibody decline is comparable with that observed for adults in the same population. Long-term studies of healthy adults and children indicate that immunologic memory remains intact for at least 9 years and confers protection against chronic HBV infection, even though anti-HBs levels may become low or decline below detectable levels (48, 51, 52). In these studies, the HBV infections were detected by the presence of anti-HBc. No episodes of clinical hepatitis were reported and HBsAg was not detected, although brief episodes of viremia may not have been detected because of infrequent testing. The mild, inapparent infections among persons who have been previously vaccinated should not produce the sequelae associated with chronic HBV infection and should provide lasting immunity. In general, follow-up studies of children vaccinated at birth to prevent perinatal HBV infection have shown that a continued high level of protection from chronic HBV infections persists at least 5 years (52, 53).

For children and adults whose immune status is normal, booster doses of vaccine are not recommended, nor is serologic testing to assess antibody levels necessary. The possible need for booster doses will be assessed as additional information becomes available. For hemodialysis patients, vaccine-induced protection may be less complete and may persist only as long as antibody levels are $\geq$10 mIU/mL. For these patients, the need for booster doses should be assessed by annual antibody testing, and a booster dose should be administered when antibody levels decline to <10 mIU/mL.

Vaccine Side Effects and Adverse Reactions

Hepatitis B vaccines have been shown to be safe when administered to both adults and children. Over 4 million adults have been vaccinated in the United States, and at least that many children have received hepatitis B vaccine worldwide.

Vaccine-associated Side Effects

Pain at the injection site (3%–29%) and a temperature greater than 37.7°C (1%–6%) have been among the most frequently reported side effects among adults and children receiving vaccine (5, 31–33, 50). In placebo-controlled studies, these side effects were reported no more frequently among vaccinees than among persons receiving a placebo (33, 50). Among children receiving both hepatitis B vaccine and DTP vaccine, these mild side effects have been observed no more frequently than among children receiving DTP vaccine alone.

Serious Adverse Events

In the United States, surveillance of adverse reactions has shown a possible association between Guillain-Barré syndrome (GBS) and receipt of the first dose of plasma-derived hepatitis B vaccine (54; CDC unpublished data). GBS was reported at a very low rate (0.5/100,000 vaccinees), no deaths were reported, and all reported cases were among adults. An estimated 2.5 million adults received one or more doses of recombinant hepatitis B vaccine during the period 1986–1990. Available data from reporting systems for adverse events do not indicate an association between receipt of recombinant vaccine and GBS (CDC, unpublished data).

Until recently, large-scale hepatitis B vaccination programs for infants (e.g., Taiwan, Alaska, and New Zealand) have primarily used plasma-derived hepatitis B vaccine. No association has been found between vaccination and the occurrence of severe adverse events, including seizures and GBS (55; B. McMahon and A. Milne, unpublished data). However, systematic surveillance for adverse reactions has been limited in these populations, and only a small number of children have received recombinant vaccine. Any presumed risk of adverse events possibly associated with hepatitis B vaccination must be balanced against the expected risk of acute and chronic liver disease associated with the current 5% lifetime risk of HBV infection in the United States. It is estimated that, for each U.S. birth cohort, 2,000–5,000 persons will die from HBV-related liver disease.

As hepatitis B vaccine is introduced for routine vaccination of infants, surveillance for vaccine-associated adverse events will continue to be an important part of the program in spite of the current record of safety. Any adverse event suspected to be associated with hepatitis B vaccination should be reported to the Vaccine Adverse Event Reporting System (VAERS). VAERS forms can be obtained by calling 1-800-822-7967.

RECOMMENDATIONS

Prevention of Perinatal Hepatitis B Virus Infection

1. All pregnant women should be routinely tested for HBsAg during an early prenatal visit in each pregnancy, preferably at the same time other routine prenatal laboratory testing is done. HBsAg testing should be repeated late in the pregnancy for women who are HBsAg negative but who are at high risk of HBV infection (e.g., injecting drug users, those with intercurrent sexually transmitted diseases) or who have had clinically apparent hepatitis. Tests for other HBV markers are not necessary for the purpose of maternal screening. However, HBsAg-positive women identified during screening may have HBV-related liver disease and should be evaluated (56).

2. Infants born to mothers who are HBsAg positive should receive the appropriate doses of hepatitis B vaccine (Table 1) and HBIG (0.5 mL) within 12 hours of birth. Both should be administered by intramuscular injection. Hepatitis B vaccine should be administered concurrently with HBIG but at a different site. Subsequent doses of vaccine should be administered according to the recommended schedule (Table 3).

3. Women admitted for delivery who have not had prenatal HBsAg testing should have blood drawn for testing. While test results are pending, the infant should receive hepatitis B vaccine within 12 hours of birth, in a dose appropriate for infants born to HBsAg-positive mothers (Table 1).

   a. If the mother is later found to be HBsAg positive, her infant should receive the additional protection of HBIG as soon as possible and within 7 days of birth, although the efficacy of HBIG administered after 48 hours of age is not known (57). If HBIG has not been administered, it is important that the infant receive the second dose of hepatitis B vaccine at 1 month and not later than 2 months of age because of the high risk of infection. The last dose should be administered at age 6 months (Table 3).*

---

* If a four-dose schedule is used (Table 1 and Table 3), the second and third doses should be administered at 1 and 2 months of age, respectively, and the fourth dose at 12–18 months of age.

Table 3. Recommended schedule of hepatitis B immunoprophylaxis to prevent perinatal transmission of hepatitis B virus infection

Infant born to mother known to be HBsAg* positive

Vaccine dose[†]	Age of infant
First	Birth (within 12 hours)
HBIG[§]	Birth (within 12 hours)
Second	1 month
Third	6 months[¶]

Infant born to mother not screened for HBsAg

Vaccine dose**	Age of infant
First	Birth (within 12 hours)
HBIG[§]	If mother is found to be HBsAg positive, administer dose to infant as soon as possible, not later than 1 week after birth
Second	1–2 months[††]
Third	6 months[¶]

*HBsAg = Hepatitis B surface antigen.
[†]See Table 1 for appropriate vaccine dose.
[§]Hepatitis B immune globulin (HBIG)-0.5 mL administered intramuscularly at a site different from that used for vaccine.
[¶]If four-dose schedule (Engerix-B) is used, the third dose is administered at 2 months of age and the fourth dose at 12–18 months.
**First dose = dose for infant of HBsAg-positive mother (see Table 1). If mother is found to be HBsAg positive, continue that dose; if mother is found to be HBsAg negative, use appropriate dose from Table 1.
[††]Infants of women who are HBsAg negative can be vaccinated at 2 months of age.

    b. If the mother is found to be HBsAg negative, her infant should continue to receive hepatitis B vaccine as part of his or her routine vaccinations (Table 3 and Table 4), in the dose appropriate for infants born to HBsAg-negative mothers (Table 1).

4. In populations in which screening pregnant women for HBsAg is not feasible, all infants should receive their first dose of hepatitis B vaccine within 12 hours of birth, their second dose at 1–2 months of age, and their third dose at 6 months of age as a part of their childhood vaccinations and well-child care (Table 3).

5. Household contacts and sex partners of HBsAg-positive women identified through prenatal screening should be vaccinated. The decision to do prevaccination testing of these contacts to determine susceptibility to HBV infection should be made according to the guidelines in the section "Prevaccination testing for susceptibility." Hepatitis B vaccine should be administered at the age-appropriate dose (Table 1) to those determined to be susceptible or judged likely to be susceptible to infection.

Universal Vaccination of Infants Born to HBsAg-Negative Mothers

1. Hepatitis B vaccination is recommended for all infants, regardless of the HBsAg status of the mother. Hepatitis B vaccine should be incorporated

Table 4. Recommended schedules of hepatitis B vaccination for infants born to HBsAg*-negative mothers

Hepatitis B vaccine	Age of infant
Option 1	
Dose 1	Birth—before hospital discharge
Dose 2	1–2 months[†]
Dose 3	6–18 months[†]
Option 2	
Dose 1	1–2 months[†]
Dose 2	4 months[†]
Dose 3	6–18 months[†]

*HBsAg = Hepatitis B surface antigen.
[†]Hepatitis B vaccine can be administered simultaneously with diphtheria-tetanus-pertussis, *Haemophilus influenzae* type b conjugate, measles-mumps-rubella, and oral polio vaccines at the same visit.

into vaccination schedules for children. The first dose can be administered during the newborn period, preferably before the infant is discharged from the hospital, but no later than when the infant is 2 months of age (Table 4). Because the highest titers of anti-HBs are achieved when the last two doses of vaccine are spaced at least 4 months apart, schedules that achieve this spacing may be preferable (Table 4). However, schedules with 2-month intervals between doses, which conform to schedules for other childhood vaccines, have been shown to produce a good antibody response (Table 4) and may be appropriate in populations in which it is difficult to ensure that infants will be brought back for all their vaccinations. The development of combination vaccines containing HBsAg may lead to other schedules that will allow optimal use of combined antigens.
  2. Special efforts should be made to ensure that high levels of hepatitis B vaccination are achieved in populations in which HBV infection occurs at high rates among children (Alaskan Natives, Pacific Islanders, and infants of immigrants from countries in which HBV is endemic).

Vaccination of Adolescents

All adolescents at high risk of infection because they are injecting drug users or have multiple sex partners (more than one partner/6 months) should receive hepatitis B vaccine. Widespread use of hepatitis B vaccine is encouraged. Because risk factors are often not identified directly among adolescents, universal hepatitis B vaccination of teenagers should be implemented in communities where injecting drug use, pregnancy among teenagers, and/or sexually transmitted diseases are common. Adolescents can be vaccinated in school-based clinics, community health centers, family planning clinics, clinics for the treatment of sexually transmitted diseases, and special adolescent clinics.

The 0-, 1-, and 6-month schedule is preferred for vaccinating adolescents with the age-appropriate dose of vaccine (Table 1). However, the choice of vaccination schedule should take into account the feasibility of delivering three doses of vaccine over a given period of time. The use of alternate schedules (e.g., 0, 2, and 4 months) may be advisable to achieve complete vaccination.

Vaccination of Selected High-Risk Groups

Efforts to vaccinate persons at high risk of HBV infection should follow the vaccine doses shown in Table 1. High-risk groups for whom vaccination is recommended include:

1. Persons with occupational risk. HBV infection is an occupational hazard for health-care workers and for public-safety workers who have exposure to blood in the workplace (24, 58). The risk of acquiring HBV infections from occupational exposures depends on the frequency of percutaneous and permucosal exposure to blood or blood-contaminated body fluids. Any health-care or public-safety worker may be at risk for HBV exposure, depending on the tasks he or she performs. Workers who perform tasks involving contact with blood or blood-contaminated body fluid should be vaccinated (24, 58, 59). For public-safety workers whose exposure to blood is infrequent, timely postexposure prophylaxis should be considered rather than routine preexposure vaccination.

   For persons in health-care fields, vaccination should be completed during training in schools of medicine, dentistry, nursing, laboratory technology, and other allied health professions, before trainees have their first contact with blood.

2. Clients and staff of institutions for the developmentally disabled. Susceptible clients in institutions for the developmentally disabled, as well as staff who work closely with clients, should be vaccinated. Susceptible clients and staff who live or work in smaller residential settings with known HBV carriers should also receive hepatitis B vaccine. Clients discharged from residential institutions into community programs should be screened for HBsAg so that appropriate measures can be taken to prevent HBV transmission. These measures should include both environmental controls and appropriate use of vaccine.

   Staff of nonresidential day-care programs for the developmentally disabled (e.g., schools, sheltered workshops) attended by known HBV carriers have a risk of infection comparable with that of health-care workers and therefore should be vaccinated (60). The risk of infection for other clients appears to be lower than the risk for staff. Vaccination of clients in day care programs may be considered. Vaccination of classroom contacts is strongly encouraged if a classmate who is an HBV carrier behaves aggressively or has special medical problems (e.g., exudative dermatitis, open skin lesions) that increase the risk of exposure to his or her blood or serous secretions.

3. Hemodialysis patients. Hepatitis B vaccination is recommended for susceptible hemodialysis patients. Vaccinating patients early in the course of their renal disease is encouraged because patients with uremia who are vaccinated before they require dialysis are more likely to respond to the vaccine (61). Although their seroconversion rates and anti-HBs titers are lower than those of healthy persons, patients who respond to vaccination will be protected from infection, and the need for frequent serologic testing will be reduced (62).

4. Recipients of certain blood products. Patients who receive clotting-factor concentrates have an increased risk of HBV infection and should be vaccinated as soon as their specific clotting disorder is identified. Prevaccination testing is recommended for patients who have already received multiple infusions of these products.

5. Household contacts and sex partners of HBV carriers. All household and sexual contacts of persons identified as HBsAg positive should be vaccinated. The decision to do prevaccination testing to determine susceptibility to HBV infection should be made according to the guidelines described earlier in the section "Prevaccination testing for susceptibility." Hepatitis B vaccine should be administered at the age-appropriate dose (Table 1) to those determined to be susceptible or judged likely to be susceptible to infection.

6. Adoptees from countries where HBV infection is endemic. Adopted or fostered orphans or unaccompanied minors from countries where HBV infection is endemic should be screened for HBsAg (3). If the children are HBsAg positive, other family members should be vaccinated (63).

7. International travelers. Vaccination should be considered for persons who plan to spend more than 6 months in areas with high rates of HBV infection and who will have close contact with the local population. Short-term travelers who are likely to have contact with blood (e.g., in a medical setting) or sexual contact with residents of areas with high or intermediate levels of endemic disease should be vaccinated. Vaccination should begin at least 6 months before travel to allow for completion of the full vaccine series, although a partial series will offer some protection. The alternate four-dose schedule (see Table 1) should provide protection if the first three doses can be delivered before departure.

8. Injecting drug users. All injecting drug users who are susceptible to HBV should be vaccinated as soon as their drug use begins. Because of the high rate of HBV infection in this population, prevaccination screening should be considered as outlined in the section "Prevaccination testing for susceptibility." Injecting drug users known to have HIV infection should be tested for anti-HBs response after completion of the vaccine series. Those who do not respond to vaccination should be counseled accordingly.

9. Sexually active homosexual and bisexual men. Susceptible sexually active homosexual and bisexual men should be vaccinated. Because of the high rate of HBV infection in this population, prevaccination screening should be considered as described in the section "Prevaccination testing for susceptibility." Men known to have HIV infection should be tested for anti-HBs response after completion of the vaccine series. Those who do not respond to vaccination should be counseled accordingly.

10. Sexually active heterosexual men and women. Vaccination is recommended for men and women who are diagnosed as having recently acquired other sexually transmitted diseases, for prostitutes, and for persons who have a history of sexual activity with more than one partner in the previous 6 months (2). Most patients seen in clinics for sexually transmitted diseases should be considered candidates for vaccination.

11. Inmates of long-term correctional facilities. Prison officials should consider undertaking screening and vaccination programs directed at inmates with histories of high-risk behaviors.

EVOLVING ISSUES IN HEPATITIS B IMMUNIZATION PROGRAMS

Hepatitis B vaccine has now been used extensively throughout the world and is currently being incorporated into the Expanded Programme on Immunization of the World Health Organization (16). New information, vaccines, and technology will have implications for this effort, and adjustments and changes are expected to occur over the years. Some of the issues that can be expected to be addressed in clinical and operational studies include the following:

1. In most developing countries with hepatitis B immunization programs, the first dose of vaccine is administered to all infants soon after birth to prevent perinatal infections; pregnant women are not screened for HBsAg; and HBIG is not used (8, 16, 45). The feasibility and effectiveness of incorporating this approach into the hepatitis B prevention strategy for the United States must be evaluated.
2. Booster doses of hepatitis B vaccine have not been recommended because of the persistence of protective efficacy 9 years after vaccination (48, 51). The duration of protective efficacy for adolescents who were vaccinated during infancy or childhood must be evaluated; the results will determine future recommendations concerning booster doses.
3. Flexible dosage schedules are required to effectively integrate hepatitis B vaccine into current and future immunization programs for infants. Schedules may change as optimum dosage and timing are studied and new information becomes available.
4. Multiple-antigen vaccines that incorporate HBsAg as one component are currently being evaluated. The routine use of these vaccines may alter childhood vaccination schedules or may result in the administration of additional doses of certain antigens. However, these vaccines should greatly facilitate vaccine delivery and minimize the number of injections.

REFERENCES

1. CDC. Protection against viral hepatitis: recommendations of the Immunization Practices Advisory Committee (ACIP). MMWR 1990;39:5–22.
2. Alter MJ, Hadler SC, Margolis HS, et al. The changing epidemiology of hepatitis B in the United States: need for alternative vaccination strategies. JAMA 1990;263:1218–1222.
3. Margolis HS, Alter MJ, Hadler SC. Hepatitis B: evolving epidemiology and implications for control. Semin Liver Dis 1991;11:84–92.
4. Stevens CE, Toy PT, Tong MJ, et al. Perinatal hepatitis B virus transmission in the United States: prevention by passive-active immunization. JAMA 1985;253:1740–1745.
5. Stevens CE, Taylor PE, Tong MJ, et al. Yeast-recombinant hepatitis B vaccine: efficacy with hepatitis B immune globulin in prevention of perinatal hepatitis B virus transmission. JAMA 1987;257:2612–2616.
6. McMahon BJ, Rhoades ER, Heyward WL, et al. A comprehensive programme to reduce the incidence of hepatitis B virus infection and its sequelae in Alaskan Natives. Lancet 1987;2:1134–1136.
7. Stevens CE, Neurath RA, Beasley RP, Szmuness W. HBeAg and anti-HBe detection by radioimmunoassay: correlation with vertical transmission of hepatitis B virus in Taiwan. J Med Virol 1979;3:237–241.
8. Xu Z-Y, Liu C-B, Francis DP, et al. Prevention of perinatal acquisition of hepatitis B virus carriage using vaccine: preliminary report of a randomized, double-blind placebo-controlled and comparative trial. Pediatrics 1985;76:713–718.
9. Beasley RP, Hwang L-Y. Epidemiology of hepatocellular carcinoma. In: Vyas GN, Dienstag JL, Hoofnagle JH, eds. Viral hepatitis and liver disease. New York: Grune & Stratton, 1984:209–224.
10. Beasley RP, Hwang L-Y. Postnatal infectivity of hepatitis B surface antigen-carrier mothers. J Infect Dis 1983;147:185–190.
11. Jonas MM, Schiff ER, O'Sullivan MJ, et al. Failure of the Centers for Disease Control criteria to identify hepatitis B infection in a large municipal obstetrical population. Ann Intern Med 1987;107:335–337.
12. Kumar ML, Dawson NV, McCullough AJ, et al. Should all pregnant women be screened for hepatitis B? Ann Intern Med 1987;107:273–277.
13. American Academy of Pediatrics. Hepatitis B. In: Peter G, Lepow ML, McCracken GH, Phillips CF, eds. Report of the Committee on Infectious Diseases. 22nd ed. Elk Grove Village, IL: American Academy of Pediatrics, 1991:238–255.
14. American Academy of Pediatrics and American College of Obsterics and Gynecology. Guidelines for prenatal care. 3rd ed. Elk Grove Village, IL: American Academy of Pediatrics, 1991 (in press).
15. McMahon BJ, Alward WLM, Hall DB, et al. Acute hepatitis B virus infection: relation of age to the clinical expression of disease and subsequent development of the carrier state. J Infect Dis 1985;151:599–603.
16. World Health Organization. Progress in the control of viral hepatitis: memorandum from a WHO meeting. Bull WHO 1988;66:443–455.
17. Schreeder MT, Bender TR, McMahon BJ, et al. Prevalence of hepatitis B in selected Alaskan Eskimo villages. Am J Epidemiol 1983;118:543–549.
18. Wong DC, Purcell RH, Rosen L. Prevalence of antibody to hepatitis A and hepatitis B viruses in selected populations of the South Pacific. Am J Epidemiol 1979;110:227–236.

19. Franks AL, Berg CJ, Kane MA, et al. Hepatitis B virus infection among children born in the United States to Southeast Asian refugees. N Engl J Med 1989;321:1301–1305.
20. Hurie MB, Mast EE, Davis JP. Horizontal transmission of hepatitis B virus infection to United States-born children of Hmong refugees. Pediatrics 1992;(in press).
21. McQuillan GM, Townsend TR, Fields HA, et al. The seroepidemiology of hepatitis B virus in the United States, 1976 to 1980. Am J Med 1989;87(Suppl 3A):5–10.
22. CDC. Racial differences in rates of hepatitis B virus infection—United States, 1976–1980. MMWR 1989; 38:818–821.
23. Moyer LA, Shapiro CN, Shulman G, Brugliera P. A survey of hepatitis B surface antigen positive blood donors: degree of understanding and action taken after notification. In: Hollinger FB, Lemon SM, Margolis HS, eds. Viral hepatitis and liver disease. Baltimore: Williams & Wilkins, 1991:728–729.
24. US Department of Labor, US Department of Health and Human Services. Joint Advisory Notice. Protection against exposure to hepatitis B virus (HBV) and human immunodeficiency virus (HIV). Federal Register 1987;52:41818-41824.
25. Rizzetto M. The delta agent. Hepatology 1983;3:729–737.
26. Hadler SC, Fields HA. Hepatitis delta virus. In: Belshe RB, ed. Textbook of human virology. St. Louis: Mosby Year Book, 1991:749–766.
27. Perrillo RP, Schiff ER, Davis FL, et al. A randomized, controlled trial of interferon alpha-2b alone and after prednisone withdrawal for the treatment of chronic hepatitis B. N Engl J Med 1990;323:295–301.
28. Arevalo JA, Washington E. Cost-effectiveness of prenatal screening and immunization for hepatitis B virus. JAMA 1988;259:365–369.
29. CDC. Safety of therapeutic immune globulin preparations with respect to transmission for human T-lymphotrophic virus type III/lymphadenopathy-associated virus infection. MMWR 1986;35: 231–233.
30. Wells MA, Wittek AE, Epstein JS, et al. Inactivation and partition of human T-cell lymphotrophic virus, type III, during ethanol fractionation of plasma. Transfusion 1986;26:210–213.
31. Zajac BA, West DJ, McAleer WJ, Scolnick EM. Overview of clinical studies with hepatitis B vaccine made by recombinant DNA. J Infect 1986;13(Suppl A):39–45.
32. Andre FE. Summary of safety and efficacy data on a yeast-derived hepatitis B vaccine. Am J Med 1989;87(Suppl 3A):14s–20s.
33. Szmuness W, Stevens CE, Harley EJ, et al. Hepatitis B vaccine: demonstration of efficacy in a controlled clinical trial in a high-risk population in the United States. N Engl J Med 1980;303:833–841.
34. Shaw FE Jr, Guess HA, Roets JM, et al. Effect of anatomic injection site, age, and smoking on the immune response to hepatitis B vaccination. Vaccine 1989;7:425–430.
35. Redfield RR, Innis BL, Scott RM, Cannon HG, Bancroft WH. Clinical evaluation of low-dose intradermally administered hepatitis B vaccine, a cost reduction strategy. JAMA 1985;254:3203–3206.
36. Coleman PJ, Shaw FE Jr, Serovich J, Hadler SC, Margolis HS. Intradermal hepatitis B vaccination in a large hospital employee population. Vaccine 1991;9:723–727.
37. Gonzalez ML, Usandizaga M, Alomar P, et al. Intradermal and intramuscular route for vaccination against hepatitis B. Vaccine 1990;8:402–405.
38. Lancaster D, Elam S, Kaiser AB. Immunogenicity of the intradermal route of hepatitis B vaccination with use of recombinant hepatitis B vaccine. Am J Infect Control 1989;17:126–129.
39. King JW, Taylor EM, Crow SD, et al. Comparison of the immunogenicity of hepatitis B vaccine administered intradermally and intramuscularly. Rev Infect Dis 1990;12:1035–1043.
40. Xu Z Y, Margolis HS. Determinants of hepatitis B vaccine efficacy and implications for vaccination strategies. Monogr Virol 1991;(in press).
41. Poovorawan Y, Sanpavat S, Pongpuniert W, Chumdermpadetsuk S, Sentrakul P, Safary A. Protective efficacy of a recombinant DNA hepatitis B vaccine in neonates of HBe antigen-positive mothers. JAMA 1989;261:3278–3281.
42. Jilg W, Schmidt M, Dienhardt F. Vaccination against hepatitis B: comparison of three different vaccination schedules. J Infect Dis 1989;160:766–769.
43. Hadler SC, Monzon MA, Lugo DR, Perez M. Effect of timing of hepatitis B vaccine dose on response to vaccine in Yucpa Indians. Vaccine 1989;7:106–110.
44. Coursaget P, Yvonnet B, Relyveld EH, Barres JL, Diop-Mar I, Chiron JP. Simultaneous administration of diphtheria-tetanus-pertussis-polio and hepatitis B vaccines in a simplified immunization program: Immune response to diphtheria toxoid, tetanus toxoid, pertussis and hepatitis B surface antigen. Infect Immun 1986;151:784–787.
45. Stevens CE, Alter HJ, Taylor PE, et al. Hepatitis B vaccine in patients receiving hemodialysis: immunogenicity and efficacy. N Engl J Med 1984;311:496–501.
46. Jilg W, Schmidt M, Weinel B, et al. Immunogenicity of recombinant hepatitis B vaccine in dialysis patients. J Hepatol 1986;3:190–195.
47. Collier AC, Corey L, Murphy VL, Handsfield HH. Antibody to human immunodeficiency virus (HIV) and suboptimal response to hepatitis B vaccination. Ann Intern Med 1988;109:101–105.
48. Hadler SC, Francis DP, Maynard JE, et al. Long-term immunogenicity and efficacy of hepatitis B vaccine in homosexual men. N Engl J Med 1986;315:209–214.

49. Lee S-D, Lo K-J, Wu J-C, et al. Prevention of maternal-infant hepatitis B virus transmission by immunization: role of serum hepatitis B virus DNA. Hepatology 1986;6:369–373.
50. Francis DP, Hadler SC, Thompson SE, et al. Prevention of hepatitis B with vaccine: report from the Centers for Disease Control multi-center efficacy trial among homosexual men. Ann Intern Med 1982;97:362–366.
51. Wainwright RB, McMahon BJ, Bulkow LR, et al. Duration of immunogenicity and efficacy of hepatitis B vaccine in a Yupik Eskimo population. JAMA 1989;261:2362–2366.
52. Lo K-J, Lee S-D, Tsai Y-T, et al. Long-term immunogenicity and efficacy of hepatitis B vaccine in infants born to HBeAg-positive HBsAg-carrier mothers. Hepatology 1988;8:1647–1650.
53. Hwang L-Y, Lee C-Y, Beasley RP. Five year follow-up of HBV vaccination with plasma-derived vaccine in neonates. Evaluation of immunogenicity and efficacy against perinatal transmission. In: Hollinger FB, Lemon SM, Margolis HS, eds. Viral hepatitis and liver disease. Baltimore: Williams & Wilkins, 1991: 759–761.
54. Shaw FE Jr, Graham DJ, Guess HA, et al. Postmarketing surveillance for neurologic adverse events reported after hepatitis B vaccination: experience of the first three years. Am J Epidemiol 1988;127:337–352.
55. Chen D-S. Control of hepatitis B in Asia: mass immunization program in Taiwan. In: Hollinger FB, Lemon SM, Margolis HS, eds. Viral hepatitis and liver disease. Baltimore: Williams & Wilkins, 1991:716–719.
56. CDC. Public Health Service inter-agency guidelines for screening donors of blood, plasma, organs, tissues and semen for evidence of hepatitis B and hepatitis C. MMWR 1991;40:5–6.
57. Beasley RP, Hwang L-Y, Stevens CE, et al. Efficacy of hepatitis B immune globulin for prevention of perinatal transmission of the hepatitis B virus carrier state: final report of a randomized double-blind, placebo-controlled trial. Hepatology 1983;3:135–141.
58. CDC. Guidelines for prevention of transmission of human immunodeficiency virus and hepatitis B virus to health-care and public-safety workers. MMWR 1989;38(Suppl 6):5–15.
59. Department of Labor. Occupational exposure to bloodborne pathogens: proposed rule and notice of hearing. Federal Register 1989;54:23042–23139.
60. Breuer B, Friedman SM, Millner ES, Kane MA, Snyder RH, Maynard JE. Transmission of hepatitis B virus in classroom contacts of mentally retarded carriers. JAMA 1985;254:3190–3195.
61. Seaworth B, Drucker J, Starling J, Drucker R, Stevens C, Hamilton J. Hepatitis B vaccines in patients with chronic renal failure before dialysis. J Infect Dis 1988;157:332–337.
62. Moyer LA, Alter MJ, Favero MS. Hemodialysis-associated hepatitis B: revised recommendations for serologic screening. Semin Dialysis 1990;3:201–204.
63. Hershow RC, Hadler SC, Kane MA. Adoption of children from countries with endemic hepatitis B: transmission risks and medical issues. Pediatr Infect Dis J 1987;6:431–437.

Hepatitis B Prevention

Original Citation: Hepatitis B Prevention—U.S. Department of Health and Human Services, Public Health Service, Center for Disease Control and Prevention, National Center for Infectious Diseases Division of Viral and Rickettsial Diseases, 1991.

HEPATITIS B PREVENTION

Hepatitis B is a serious public health problem that affects people of all ages in the United States and around the world. Each year, more than 240,000 persons get hepatitis B in the United States. The disease is caused by a highly infectious virus that attacks the liver. Hepatitis B virus infection can lead to severe illness, liver damage, and in some cases, death.

The best way to be protected from hepatitis B is to be vaccinated with hepatitis B vaccine, which has been proven safe and effective. Read this pamphlet to learn what hepatitis B is, what behaviors put you at risk, and how you can protect yourself against hepatitis B.

You May Be at Risk for Hepatitis B If You

- Have a job that exposes you to human blood.
- Live in the same house with someone who has lifelong hepatitis B virus infection.

- Inject drugs.
- Have sex with a person infected with hepatitis B virus.
- Have sex with more than one partner.
- Are a child whose parents were born in Southeast Asia, Africa, the Amazon Basin in South America, the Pacific Islands, or the Middle East.
- Are a patient or work in an institution for the developmentally disabled.
- Have hemophilia.
- Travel internationally to areas with a high prevalence of hepatitis B.

How Is Hepatitis B Virus Spread?

Hepatitis B virus is found in the blood and body fluids of persons with hepatitis B. Contact with even small amounts of infected blood can cause infection. You can get hepatitis B by direct contact with the blood or body fluids of an infected person, for example, by sharing needles or by having sex with an infected person. A baby can get hepatitis B from an infected mother during childbirth.

Can Hepatitis B Be Spread by Food?

Unlike hepatitis A, another form of hepatitis, hepatitis B is not spread through food or water. If you had hepatitis A, it is still possible to get hepatitis B. If you had hepatitis C, another form of hepatitis that can be spread by contact with blood, you can still get hepatitis B.

What Is the Hepatitis B Carrier State?

Some persons infected with hepatitis B virus never fully recover and carry the virus for the rest of their lives. These persons are known as carriers, and they can infect other household and sexual contacts throughout their lives. Among adults who have hepatitis B, 5% to 10% develop a lifelong infection; among children, the risk for lifelong infection is much higher. In the United States today, an estimated one million persons have life long hepatitis B virus infections.

What Are the Symptoms of Hepatitis B?

If you have hepatitis B, you may have:

- Yellowing of the skin or eyes.
- Loss of appetite, nausea, vomiting, fever.
- Extreme tiredness, stomach or joint pain.
- Feel very ill and be unable to work for weeks or even months.
- Have no symptoms and infect others without knowing it.

How Serious Is Hepatitis B?

Hepatitis B may cause:

- Serious liver problems, such as cirrhosis (scarring of the liver) and liver cancer.
- Lifelong hepatitis B virus infection.
- Liver failure and death.

What Are the Long-Term Effects of Hepatitis B?

Each year, approximately 5,000 persons in the United States die of cirrhosis of the liver related to hepatitis B, and another 1,500 die of liver cancer related to hepatitis B. Hepatitis B is the most common cause of liver cancer worldwide. Because these serious problems may not develop until many years after a person becomes infected with hepatitis B virus, those who have a lifelong infection should be evaluated periodically by a medical care provider.

Why Is Hepatitis B So Serious in Pregnant Women?

Pregnant women who are infected with hepatitis B virus frequently transmit the disease to their babies. Many of these babies develop lifelong infections, cirrhosis of the liver, and liver cancer. All pregnant women should be tested early in pregnancy to determine if they are infected with hepatitis B virus. If the blood test is positive, the baby should be vaccinated at birth and in the first year of life.

How Can Hepatitis B Be Prevented?

No cure is available for hepatitis B, so prevention is crucial. Vaccines can provide protection in 90% to 95% of healthy persons. The vaccine can be given safely to infants, children, and adults in three doses over a period of 6 months. For information about hepatitis B vaccine, visit your public health clinic or see your physician or public health nurse.

Who Should Be Vaccinated?

Preventing hepatitis B is important because of the high risk of lifelong infection leading to serious liver problems. The following persons should be vaccinated against hepatitis B:

- All babies, beginning at birth.
- Adolescents who have sex or inject drugs.
- Persons who engage in any of the high-risk behaviors listed in this pamphlet.
- Persons whose jobs expose them to human blood.

SUBTOPIC / HEPATITIS C

Outbreak of Hepatitis C Associated with Intravenous Immunoglobulin Administration

Original Citation: Outbreak of Hepatitis C Associated with Intravenous Immunoglobulin Administration—United States, October 1993–June 1994. MMWR 1994;43(28):505–509.

Chronic hepatitis develops in more than 60% of persons infected with HCV (3). Initial screening of these patients should include a test for ALT activity and an FDA-licensed enzyme immunoassay (EIA) for anti-HCV. All specimens repeatedly (two or more times) reactive for anti-HCV should be tested using an FDA-licensed supplemental anti-HCV assay to reduce the likelihood of false-positive EIA results.

Because some patients will have a prolonged interval between exposure and seroconversion to anti-HCV, patients who are anti-HCV-negative but have abnormal ALT levels should be retested for anti-HCV 3–6 months later. In most patients with normal immune status, seroconversion occurs within 6 months after infection (3, 4). However, approximately 10% of HCV-infected patients with normal immune status will be persistently negative for anti-HCV, even after prolonged follow-up (3). Persons with immunodeficiency disorders may be less likely to seroconvert or may have longer intervals between infection and seroconversion than persons with normal immune function.

Patients aged greater than or equal to 18 years with chronic hepatitis C (abnormal ALT levels for more than 6 months) should be evaluated for possible therapy with alpha interferon by a physician experienced in its use (5). Patients should be informed that the proportion of adults with chronic hepatitis C who sustain a long-term response to alpha interferon is low (approximately 20%). Although FDA has not licensed alpha interferon for patients aged less than 18 years, they can be considered for therapy if entered into an approved study protocol.

All patients with hepatitis C should be considered potentially infectious. However, because of limited data on the risk of household, sexual, and perinatal transmission and because testing cannot determine infectivity, PHS does not recommend substantial changes in behavior based on knowledge of infection status (1). PHS recommends that household articles such as toothbrushes and razors that could become contaminated with blood should not be shared, and cuts or skin lesions should be covered to prevent the spread of infectious secretions or blood (1). HCV transmission by sexual contact appears to occur, but this route of transmission is much less efficient than that for other blood-borne sexually transmitted diseases (3). Although anti-HCV-positive persons should be informed of the potential for sexual transmission, there are insufficient data to recommend changes in current sex practices for persons with one steady sex partner. To prevent many sexually transmitted diseases, including hepatitis and HIV infection, persons with multiple partners should follow safer sexual practices, including reducing the number of sex partners and using barriers (e.g., latex condoms) to prevent contact with body fluids. No evidence supports advising against pregnancy based on anti-HCV status or using any special treatments or precautions for pregnant women or their offspring.

REFERENCES: AS NUMBERED IN ORIGINAL PUBLICATION

1. CDC. Public Health Service inter-agency guidelines for screening donors of blood, plasma, organs, tissues, and semen for evidence of hepatitis B and hepatitis C. MMWR 1991;40(No. RR-4):6–17.
3. Alter MJ. The detection, transmission, and outcome of hepatitis C virus infection. Infect Agents Dis 1993;2:155–166.
4. Vallari DS, Jett BW, Alter HJ, Mimms LT, Holzman R, Shih JW. Serological markers of posttransfusion hepatitis C viral infection. J Clin Microbiol 1992;30:552–556.
5. Hoofnagle JH. Therapy of acute and chronic viral hepatitis. Adv Intern Med 1994;39:241–275.

Hepatitis C Prevention

Original Citation: Hepatitis C Prevention—U.S. Department of Health and Human Services, Public Health Service, Center for Disease Control and Prevention, National Center for Infectious Diseases, Division of Viral and Rickettsial Diseases, 1992.

What Is Hepatitis C?

Hepatitis C is a liver disease caused by hepatitis C virus (HCV), which is found in the blood of persons who have this disease. The infection is spread by behaviors involving contact with the blood of an infected person and by blood transfusions.

How Great Is the Risk for Hepatitis C?

About 40% of all persons who get hepatitis C do not know how they were infected with HCV. If you do not engage in any of the behaviors listed below, your risk for hepatitis C is probably low. However, if you are involved in any of these behaviors, your risk for hepatitis C could be very high.

You are at risk for hepatitis C if you:

- Have ever injected drugs
- Have a job that exposes you to human blood
- Are a hemodialysis patient
- Have ever received a blood transfusion

You may be at risk if you:

- Have multiple sex partners
- Live with a person who has hepatitis C

What Are the Symptoms of Hepatitis C?

If you have hepatitis C, you may have:

- Yellowing of the skin and eyes
- Loss of appetite
- Nausea and vomiting
- Fever
- Extreme fatigue
- Stomach pain

Some persons who are infected with HCV have no symptoms and can infect others without knowing it.

How Serious Is Hepatitis C?

In the United States, approximately 600 persons each year die of liver failure shortly after getting hepatitis C. About half of all persons who get hepatitis C never fully recover and can carry the virus for the rest of their lives. These persons have chronic (or lifelong) hepatitis C, and some may eventually develop cirrhosis (scarring) of the liver and liver failure.

How Is HCV Spread?

HCV is spread primarily by exposure to human blood. A person may get hepatitis C by sharing needles to inject drugs or through exposure to human blood in the workplace. Although the risk of getting hepatitis C from a blood transfusion still exists, this risk is very low because donated blood has been screened for HCV since May 1990.

Hepatitis C has been transmitted between sex partners and among household members; however, the degree of this risk is unknown.

There is no evidence that HCV is spread by sneezing, coughing, hugging, or other casual contact.

HCV cannot be spread by food or water.

A person who has had other types of viral hepatitis, such as hepatitis A or hepatitis B, can still get hepatitis C.

How Can You Find Out If You Have Hepatitis C?

A blood test is available for hepatitis C screening. The test shows if a person has been infected with HCV; however, it does not distinguish between recent and old infection. In addition, the test does not distinguish between persons who are infectious and those who have completely recovered and cannot pass the infection on to anyone else.

What If Your Test for Hepatitis C Is Positive?

If you have a positive test result and have risk factors for hepatitis C or have signs of liver disease, you probably have been infected with HCV. However, if you have no signs of liver disease and do not engage in high risk behaviors, your hepatitis C positive test result may be a "false positive." Contact your doctor to determine whether your hepatitis C test result is accurate and whether additional tests are needed.

What If You Have Hepatitis C?

If you have hepatitis C:

- Do not donate blood, plasma, body organs, other tissue, or sperm.
- Do not share toothbrushes, razors, or other items that could become contaminated with blood.
- Cover open sores or other breaks in your skin.

HCV may be spread by sexual contact with an infected person. To reduce the chances of spreading HCV by sexual contact, follow these "safer-sex" guidelines:

- Use latex condoms to prevent the exchange of body fluids.
- Have only one sex partner
- If you have multiple sex partners,
- Reduce the number of your sex partners to prevent others from getting infected
- Inform your sex partners about your illness

For More Information on Viral Hepatitis

Call CDC Hepatitis Hotline (404) 332-4555 or write Hepatitis Branch, Mailstop G37, Division of Viral and Rickettsial Diseases, National Center for Infectious Diseases, Centers for Disease Control and Prevention, Atlanta, Georgia 30333.

TOPIC 13 / **HISTOPLASMOSIS**

Recommendations for Protecting Workers from Histoplasma capsulatum: Exposure during Bat Guano Removal from a Church's Attic

Original Citation: Lenhart SW. Recommendations for Protecting Workers from Histoplasma capsulatum: exposure during bat guano removal from a church's attic. Appl Occup Environ Hyg 1994;9(4):230–236.

INTRODUCTION

The first corrective measure taken was screening of the major entry/exit locations. NIOSH was then contacted for guidance concerning a personal protective equipment recommendation to be followed by the employees of the insulation removal contractor.

Disinfection of soils contaminated with H. capsulatum has been tried with various chemicals. Formaldehyde has fungicidal properties, and it has been shown to be the most effective of the chemical agents tried based on the performance of pre- and post-treatment sampling for H. capsulatum (2). A 37 to 40 percent solution by weight (formalin) stabilized with 10 to 15 percent methanol has been the basic formulation used. For decontamination procedures outdoors, a 3 percent formalin solution has been found to be effective (24, 34, 35). However, exposures to formaldehyde during soil disinfection operations have been reported to cause adverse health effects among applicators. Workers at one site reported burning eyes and mucous membrane irritation (34), while workers at another site reported nausea with vomiting (35).

In addition to soil disinfection, formaldehyde has also been reported to be effective for disinfecting H. capsulatum-infected accumulations of bat droppings in the attics of buildings, using formalin concentrations of 3 (18) and 4 percent (22). Formaldehyde solutions should be used with caution since this chemical may cause adverse health effects following exposure via inhalation, ingestion, or dermal or eye contact (36). Mild to unpleasant eye irritation occurs at 2 to 10 ppm, and intolerable irritation (tissue damage possible) occurs at levels above 25 ppm (36). Workers exposed to 0.3 ppm of formaldehyde have reported symptoms of upper respiratory and acute bronchial irritation during a work shift (37). There have also been reports of primary skin irritation and allergic dermatitis as a result of skin contact with water solutions of formaldehyde. Although a threshold for the development of these skin conditions has not been clearly defined, it is estimated to be a water solution containing less than 5 percent formaldehyde (38). Based upon the results of laboratory tests which have demonstrated carcinogenic and mutagenic activity of formaldehyde in animals, NIOSH and Occupational Safety and Health Administration (OSHA) recommend that formaldehyde be handled in the workplace as a potential occupational carcinogen (39, 40). NIOSH recommends that occupational exposures to formaldehyde be controlled to the lowest feasible limit (39).

CONCLUSIONS AND RECOMMENDATIONS

The health risks associated with exposure to H. capsulatum were recommended to be communicated prior to the start of removal activities to each worker who might be exposed to bat droppings during the course of the project. Individuals with compromised cell-mediated immunity are at greater risk of clinical histoplasmosis should infection occur, so such workers should avoid exposure to all materials potentially contaminated with H. capsulatum.

To reduce the potential for aerosolization of both rock wool dust and bat dropping dust, spraying these materials with water was recommended. Then, the dampened materials were collected in heavy-duty trash bags, and immediately disposed of at a landfill. Because the water evaporated over the course of the removal operation, additional water was sprayed as needed. The addition of a surfactant (wetting agent), such as a small amount of detergent, to the water may have improved the dust suppression ability of the water alone. After removal of the bulky material, dust remaining in the attic was removed with an industrial vacuum cleaner equipped with a high-efficiency particulate air filter.

Workers were recommended to wear personal protective equipment while spraying water on the rock wool and bat droppings, and while collecting these materials in plastic bags. A NIOSH/MSHA-approved full-facepiece powered air-purifying respirator with high efficiency filters, disposable protective clothing with a hood, disposable latex gloves under cotton work gloves, and disposable shoe coverings was expected to provide adequate protection. Respirators were used in accordance with the regulations of OSHA (41) and the recommendations of NIOSH (42). Since the recommended ensemble of disposable personal protective equipment is more insulating than normal work clothing, sweat evaporation was anticipated to be impeded during removal activities. Therefore, precautions were taken during these activities to reduce the risk of heat stress-related illnesses, and removal activities were scheduled when temperatures in the attic were relatively cool.

Health risks are associated with exposures to even low air concentrations of formaldehyde (38). Therefore, alternative chemicals should be used to disinfect those materials for which removal is impractical, such as a large volume of contaminated soil. Household bleach is one possible alternative since it contains sodium hypochlorite, which has bactericidal and sporicidal properties. Household bleach also has the practical advantages of being readily available and less expensive than most other chemical bactericidal and sporicidal agents. However, a disadvantage of hypochlorites is that their activity is greatly reduced in the presence of organic matter (43). Because of the limited number of positive samples collected during this study, the effectiveness of bleach solutions to disinfect bat droppings containing H. capsulatum could not be evaluated. The effectiveness of bleach solutions or other disinfectants should be documented before their use is recommended for decontaminating environmental materials containing H. capsulatum.

REFERENCES: AS NUMBERED IN ORIGINAL PUBLICATION

2. Larsh, H.W. Histoplasmosis. In: DiSalvo AF, ed. Occupational mycoses. Philadelphia: Lea and Febiger, 1983:29–41.
18. Ajello L, Hosty TS, Palmer J. Bat Histoplasmosis in Alabama. Am J Trop Med Hyg 1967;16:329–331.
22. Bartlett PC, Vonbehren LA, Tewari RP, et al. Bats in the belfry: an outbreak of Histoplasmosis. Am J Public Health 1982;72:1369–1372.
24. Ajello L, Weeks RJ. Soil decontamination and other control measures. In: DiSalvo AF, ed. Occupational mycoses. Philadelphia: Lea and Febiger, 1983:229–238.
34. Tosh FE, Weeks RJ, Pfeiffer FR, et al. The use of formalin to kill Histoplasma capsulatum at an epidemic site. Am J Epidemiol 1967;85:259–265.
35. Bartlett PC, Weeks RJ, Ajello L. Decontamination of Histoplasma capsulatum-infested bird roost in Illinois. Arch Environ Health 1982;37:221–223.
36. National Institute for Occupational Safety and Health. Occupational Safety and Health Guidelines for Chemical Hazards. DHHS (NIOSH) Pub. No. 89–104, Supplement II-OHG. Cincinnati: NIOSH, 1988.
37. Alexandersson R, Kolmodin-Hedman B, Hedenstierna G. Exposure to formaldehyde: effects on pulmonary function. Arch Environ Health 1982;37:274–283.
38. American Conference of Governmental Industrial Hygienists. Notice of intended change—formaldehyde. Appl Occup Environ Hyg 1992;7:852–874.
39. NIOSH/OSHA. Current Intelligence Bulletin 34: Formaldehyde: evidence of carcinogenicity. DHHS (NIOSH) Publication No. 81–111. Cincinnati: NIOSH, 1980.
40. Occupational Safety and Health Administration. Occupational exposure to formaldehyde; final rule. Federal Register 57:22290 (codified at 29 CFR 1910.1048). Washington, DC: U.S. Government Printing Office, Office of the Federal Register, 1992.
41. Occupational Safety and Health Administration. Title 29, Code of Federal Regulations, Part 1910.134. Washington, DC: U.S. Government Printing Office, Office of the Federal Register, 1992.
42. Bollinger NJ, Schutz RH. NIOSH guide to industrial respiratory protection. DHHS (NIOSH) Publication No. 87–116. Cincinnati: NIOSH, 1987.
43. Russell AD. Chemical sporicidal and sporostatic agents. In: Block SS, ed. Disinfection, sterilization, and preservation. 4th ed. Philadelphia: Lea and Febiger, 1991:389.

EDITORIAL NOTE

Steve Lenhart is with the Hazard Evaluation and Technical Assistance Branch of NIOSH. More detailed information on this evaluation is contained in the Health Hazard Evaluation Report No. 92-0348-2361 available through NIOSH, Hazard Evaluation and Technical Assistance Branch, 4676 Columbia Parkway, Cincinnati, Ohio 45226; or by telephoning 1-800-35-NIOSH.

TOPIC 14 / HUMAN IMMUNODEFICIENCY VIRUS/ACQUIRED IMMUNODEFICIENCY SYNDROME

SUBTOPIC / TESTING, COUNSELING, AND EDUCATION

Recommendations for HIV Counseling and Voluntary Testing for Pregnant Women

Original Citation: Centers for Disease Control and Prevention. U.S. Public Health Service Recommendations for HIV Counseling and Voluntary Testing for Pregnant Women. MMWR 1995;44(RR-7):1–15.

Editor's Note: The information included here was based on an MMWR Recommendations and Reports (Vol. 44, RR-7) which summarized the recommendations of a U.S. Public Health Service Task Force. The original document also summarized background information on HIV infection and AIDS in women and children.

USE OF AZT TO PREVENT PERINATAL TRANSMISSION (ACTG 076): WORKSHOP ON IMPLICATIONS FOR TREATMENT, COUNSELING, AND HIV TESTING

Perinatal Transmission of HIV

HIV can be transmitted from an infected woman to her fetus or newborn during pregnancy, during labor and delivery, and during the postpartum period (through breast-feeding), although the percentage of infections transmitted during each of these intervals is not precisely known (7–9). Although transmission of HIV to a fetus can occur as early as the 8th week of gestation (7), data suggest that at least one half of perinatally transmitted infections from non-breast-feeding women occur shortly before or during the birth process (10–12). Breast-feeding may increase the rate of transmission by 10%–20% (9, 13, 14).

Several prospective studies have reported perinatal transmission rates ranging from 13% to 40% (15–19). Transmission rates may differ among studies depending on the prevalence of various factors that can influence the likelihood of transmission. Several maternal factors have been associated with an increased risk for transmission, including low CD4+ T-lymphocyte counts, high viral titer, advanced HIV disease, the presence of p24 antigen in serum, placental membrane inflammation, intrapartum events resulting in increased exposure of the fetus to maternal blood, breast-feeding, low vitamin A levels, premature rupture of membranes, and premature delivery (8, 11, 15, 20–23). Factors associated with a decreased rate of HIV transmission have included cesarean section delivery, the presence of maternal neutralizing antibodies, and maternal zidovudine therapy (11, 24–26).

HIV Prevention and Treatment Opportunities for Women and Infants

HIV counseling and testing for women of childbearing age offer important prevention opportunities for both uninfected and infected women and their infants. Such counseling is intended to (a) assist women in assessing their current or future risk for HIV infection; (b) initiate or reinforce HIV risk reduction behavior; and (c) allow for referral to other HIV prevention services (e.g., treatment for substance abuse and sexually transmitted diseases) when appropriate. For infected women, knowledge of their HIV infection status provides opportunities to (a) obtain early diagnosis and treatment for themselves and their infants, (b) make informed reproductive decisions, (c) use methods to reduce the risk for perinatal transmission, (d) receive information to prevent HIV transmission to others, and (e) obtain referral for psychological and social services, if needed. Interventions designed to reduce morbidity in HIV-infected persons require early diagnosis of HIV infection so that treatment can be initiated before the onset of opportunistic infections and disease progression. However, studies indicate that many HIV-infected persons do not know they are infected until late in the course of illness. A survey of persons diagnosed with AIDS between January 1990 and December 1992 indicated that 57% of the 2,081 men and 62% of the 360 women who participated in the survey gave illness as the primary reason for being tested for HIV infection; 36% of survey participants first tested positive within 2 months of their AIDS diagnosis (27).

Providing HIV counseling and testing services in gynecologic and prenatal and other obstetric settings presents an opportunity for early diagnosis of HIV infection because many young women frequently access the health-care system for obstetric- or gynecologic-related care. Clinics that provide prenatal and postnatal care, family planning clinics, sexually transmitted disease clinics, adolescent-health clinics, and other health-care facilities already provide a range of preventive services into which HIV education, counseling, and voluntary testing can be integrated. When provided appropriate access to ongoing care, HIV-infected women can be monitored for clinical and immunologic status and can be given preventive treatment and other recommended medical care and services (28). Diagnosis of HIV infection before or during pregnancy allows women to make informed decisions regarding prevention of perinatal transmission. Early in the HIV epidemic, strategies to prevent perinatal HIV transmission were limited to either avoiding pregnancy or avoiding breast-feeding (for women in the United States and other countries that have safe alternatives to breast milk). More recent strategies to prevent perinatal HIV transmission have focused on interrupting in utero and intrapartum transmission. Foremost among these strategies has been administration of ZDV to HIV-infected pregnant women and their newborns (1). Results from a multicenter, placebo-controlled clinical trial (the AIDS Clinical Trials Group [ACTG] protocol number 076) indicated that administration of ZDV to a selected group of HIV-infected women during pregnancy, labor, and delivery and to their newborns reduced the risk for perinatal HIV transmission by approximately two-thirds: 25.5% of infants born to mothers in the placebo group were infected, compared with

8.3% of those born to mothers in the ZDV group (1). The ZDV regimen caused minimal adverse effects among both mothers and infants; the only adverse effect after 18 months of follow-up was mild anemia in the infants that resolved without therapy. As a result of these findings, PHS issued recommendations regarding ZDV therapy to reduce the risk for perinatal HIV transmission (29). In addition, the Food and Drug Administration (FDA) has approved the use of ZDV for this therapy. Despite the substantial benefits and short-term safety of the ZDV regimen, however, the results of the trial present several unresolved issues, including (a) the long-term safety of the regimen for both mothers and infants, (b) ZDV's effectiveness in women who have different clinical characteristics (e.g., CD4+ T-lymphocyte count and previous ZDV use) than those who participated in the trial, and (c) the likelihood of the mother's adherence to the lengthy treatment regimen. The PHS recommendations for ZDV therapy emphasize that HIV-infected pregnant women should be informed of both benefits and potential risks when making decisions to receive such therapy. Discussions of treatment options should be noncoercive—the final decision to accept or reject ZDV treatment is the responsibility of the woman. Decisions concerning treatment can be complex and adherence to therapy, if accepted, can be difficult; therefore, good rapport and a trusting relationship should be established between the health-care provider and the HIV-infected woman.

Several other possible strategies to reduce the risk for perinatal HIV transmission are under study or are being planned (30); however, their efficacies have not yet been determined. These strategies include (a) administration of HIV hyperimmune globulin to infected pregnant women and their infants, (b) efforts to boost maternal and infant immune responses through vaccination, (c) virucidal cleansing of the birth canal before and during labor and delivery, (d) modified and shortened antiretroviral regimens, (e) cesarean section delivery, and (f) vitamin A supplementation. Knowledge of HIV infection status during pregnancy also allows for early identification of HIV-exposed infants, all of whom should be appropriately tested, monitored, and treated (28). Prompt identification and close monitoring of such children (particularly infants) is essential for optimal medical management (28, 31, 32). Approximately 10%–20% of perinatally infected children develop rapidly progressive disease and die by 24 months of age (33, 34). Pneumocystis carinii pneumonia (PCP) is the most common opportunistic infection in children who have AIDS and is often fatal. Because PCP occurs most commonly among perinatally infected children 3–6 months of age (35), effective prevention requires that children born to HIV-infected mothers be identified promptly, preferably through prenatal testing of their mothers, so that prophylactic therapy can be initiated as soon as possible. CDC and the National Pediatric & Family HIV Resource Center have published revised guidelines for prophylaxis against PCP in children that recommend that all children born to HIV-infected mothers be placed on prophylactic therapy at 4–6 weeks of age (32). Careful follow-up of these children to promptly diagnose other potentially treatable HIV-related conditions (e.g., severe bacterial infections or tuberculosis) can prevent morbidity and reduce the need for hospitalization (28). Infants born to HIV-infected women also require changes in their routine immunization regimens as early as 2 months of age (36).

Despite the potential benefits of HIV counseling and testing to both women and their infants, some persons have expressed concerns about the potential for negative effects resulting from widespread counseling and testing programs in prenatal and other settings. These concerns include the fear that (a) such programs could deter pregnant women from using prenatal-care services if testing is not perceived as voluntary and (b) women who have been tested but who choose not to learn their test results may be reluctant to return for further prenatal care. Other potential negative consequences following a diagnosis of HIV infection can include loss of confidentiality, job- or health-care-related discrimination and stigmatization, loss of relationships, domestic violence, and adverse psychological reactions. Although cases of discrimination against HIV-infected persons and loss of confidentiality have been documented (37), data concerning the frequency of these events for women are limited. Reported rates of abandonment, loss of relationships, severe psychological reactions, and domestic violence have ranged from 4% to 13% (38–41). Providing infected women with or referring them to psychological, social, or legal services may help minimize such potential risks and enable women to benefit from the many health advantages of early HIV diagnosis.

Counseling and Testing Strategies

Guidelines published in 1985 (42) regarding HIV counseling and testing of pregnant women recommended a targeted approach directed to women known to be at increased risk for HIV infection (e.g., injecting-drug users and women whose sex partners were HIV-infected or at risk for infection). However, several studies have indicated that counseling and testing strategies that offer testing only to those women who report risk factors fail to identify and offer services to many HIV-infected women (i.e., 50%–70% of infected women in some studies) (43–45). Women may be unaware of their risk for infection if they have unknowingly had sexual contact with an HIV-infected person (46). Other women may refuse testing to avoid the stigma often associated with high-risk sexual and injecting-drug-use behaviors.

Because of the advances in prevention and treatment of opportunistic infections for HIV-infected adults and children during the past 10 years, several professional organizations (47, 48) and others (49) have recommended a more widespread approach of offering HIV counseling and testing for pregnant women. This approach can be applied nationally to all pregnant women or to women in limited geographic areas based on the prevalence of HIV infection among childbearing women in those areas. However, a counseling and testing recommendation based on a prevalence threshold (e.g., one HIV-infected woman per 1,000 childbearing women) could delay or discourage implementation of counseling and testing services in areas (e.g., states) where prevalence data are inadequate, outdated, or unavailable, and would miss substantial numbers of HIV-infected pregnant women in areas with lower seroprevalence rates but high numbers of births (e.g., California). A prevalence-based approach also could lead to potentially discriminating testing practices, such as singling out a geographic area or racial/ethnic group. A universal approach of offering HIV counseling and testing to all pregnant women—regardless of the prevalence of HIV infection in their community or their risk for infection—provides a uniform policy that will reach HIV-infected pregnant women in all populations and geographic areas of the United States. Although this universal approach will necessitate increased resources (e.g., funding), effective implementation of HIV counseling and testing services for pregnant women and the ensuing medical interventions will reduce HIV-related morbidity in women and their infants and could ultimately reduce medical costs.

Counseling and testing policies also must address issues associated with provision of consent for testing. Data from universal, routine HIV counseling and voluntary testing programs in several areas indicate that high test-acceptance levels can be achieved without mandating testing (50–52). Mandatory testing may increase the potential for negative consequences of HIV testing and result in some women avoiding prenatal care altogether. In addition, mandatory testing may adversely affect the patient-provider relationship by placing the provider in an enforcing rather than facilitating role. Providers must act as facilitators to adequately assist women in making decisions regarding HIV testing and ZDV preventive therapy. Although few studies have addressed the issue of acceptance of HIV testing, higher levels of acceptance have been found in clinics where testing is voluntary but recommended by the health-care provider than in clinics that use a nondirective approach to HIV testing (i.e, patients are told the test is available, but testing is neither encouraged nor discouraged) (52).

Laboratory Testing Considerations

The HIV-1 testing algorithm recommended by PHS comprises initial screening with an FDA-licensed enzyme immunoassay (EIA) followed by confirmatory testing of repeatedly reactive EIAs with an FDA-licensed supplemental test (e.g., Western blot or immunofluorescence assay [IFA]) (53). Although each of these tests is highly sensitive and specific, the use of both EIA and supplementary tests further increases the accuracy of results.

Indeterminate Western blot results can be caused by either incomplete antibody response to HIV in sera from infected persons or non-specific reactions in sera from uninfected persons (54–56). Incomplete antibody responses that produce negative or indeterminate results on Western blot may occur in persons recently infected with HIV who are seroconverting, persons who have end-stage HIV disease, and perinatally exposed infants who are seroreverting (i.e., losing maternal antibody). In addition, non-specific reactions producing indeterminate results in uninfected persons have occurred more frequently among pregnant or parous women than among persons in other groups characterized by low HIV seroprevalence (55, 56). No large-scale studies to estimate the prevalence of indeterminate test results in pregnant women have been conducted. However, a survey testing more than 1 million neonatal dried-blood specimens for maternally acquired HIV-1 antibody indicated a relatively low rate of indeterminate Western blot results (i.e., <1 in every 4,000 specimens tested by EIA); overall, 1,044,944 EIAs and 2,845 Western blots were performed (56). IFA can be used to resolve an EIA-positive, Western blot-indeterminate sample. The FDA-licensed IFA kit is highly sensitive and specific and is less likely than Western blot to yield indeterminate results. Data from one study indicated that 211 of 234 Western blot-indeterminate samples were negative for HIV-1 antibody by IFA (57).

False-positive Western blot results (especially those with a majority of bands) are extremely uncommon. For example, in a study of >290,000 blood donors that used a sensitive culture technique, no false-positive Western blot results were detected (58). In a study of the frequency of false-positive diagnoses among military applicants from a low prevalence population (i.e., <1.5 infections per 1,000 population), one false-positive result among 135,187 persons tested was detected (59).

Incorrect HIV test results occur primarily because of specimen-handling errors, laboratory errors, or failure to follow the recommended testing algorithm. However, patients may report incorrect test results because they misunderstood previous test results or misperceive that they are infected (60). Although these occurrences are uncommon, increased testing of pregnant women will result in additional indeterminate, false-positive, and incorrect results. Because of (a) the significance of an HIV-positive test result for the mother and its impact on her reproductive decisions and (b) the potential toxicity of HIV therapeutic drugs for both the pregnant woman and her infant, HIV test results must be obtained and interpreted correctly. In some circumstances, correct interpretation may require consideration of not only additional or repeat testing, but also the woman's clinical condition and history of possible exposure to HIV. In addition to the standard antibody assays used for older children and adults, definitive diagnosis of HIV infection in infants requires the use of other assays (e.g., polymerase chain reaction [PCR] or virus culture). Virtually all infants born to HIV-infected mothers acquire maternal antibody and will test antibody positive for up to 18 months of age (61). Uninfected infants will gradually lose maternally derived antibody during this time, whereas infected infants generally remain antibody positive. Diagnosis of HIV infection in early infancy can be made on the basis of two or more positive assays (e.g., viral culture, PCR, or p24 antigen test) (62).

RECOMMENDATIONS

The following recommendations have been developed to provide guidance to health-care workers when educating women about HIV infection and the importance of early diagnosis of HIV. The recommendations are based on the advances made in treatment and prevention of HIV infection and stress the need for a universal counseling and voluntary testing program for pregnant women. These recommendations address (a) HIV-related information needed by infected and uninfected pregnant women for their own health and that of their infants, (b) laboratory considerations involved in HIV testing of this population, and (c) the importance of follow-up services for HIV-infected women, their infants, and other family members.

HIV Counseling and Voluntary Testing of Pregnant Women and Their Infants

- Health-care providers should ensure that all pregnant women are counseled and encouraged to be tested for HIV infection to allow women to know their infection status both for their own health and to reduce the risk for perinatal HIV transmission. Pretest HIV counseling of pregnant women should be done in accordance with previous guidelines for HIV counseling (63, 64). Such counseling should include information regarding the risk for HIV infection associated with sexual activity and injecting-drug use, the risk for transmission to the woman's infant if she is infected, and the availability of therapy to reduce this risk. HIV counseling, including any written materials, should be linguistically, culturally, educationally, and age appropriate for individual patients.
- HIV testing of pregnant women and their infants should be voluntary. Consent for testing should be obtained in accordance with prevailing legal requirements. Women who test positive for HIV or who refuse testing should not be (a) denied prenatal or other health-care services, (b) reported to child protective service agencies because of refusal to be tested or because of their HIV status, or (c) discriminated against in any other way (65).
- Health-care providers should counsel and offer HIV testing to women as early in pregnancy as possible so that informed and timely therapeutic and reproductive decisions can be made. Specific strategies and resources will be needed to communicate with women who may not obtain prenatal care because of homelessness, incarceration, undocumented citizenship status, drug or alcohol abuse, or other reasons.
- Uninfected pregnant women who continue to practice high-risk behaviors (e.g., injecting-drug use and unprotected sexual contact with an HIV-infected or high-risk partner) should be encouraged to avoid further exposure to HIV and to be retested for HIV in the third trimester of pregnancy (64).
- The prevalence of HIV infection may be higher in women who have not received prenatal care (66). These women should be assessed promptly for HIV infection. Such an assessment should include information regarding prior HIV testing, test results, and risk history. For women who are first identified as being HIV infected during labor and delivery, health-care providers should consider offering intrapartum and neonatal ZDV according to published recommendations (29). For women whose HIV infection status has not been determined, HIV counseling should be provided and HIV testing offered as soon as the mother's medical condition permits. However, involuntary HIV testing should never be substituted for counseling and voluntary testing.
- Some HIV-infected women do not receive prenatal care, choose not to be tested for HIV, or do not retain custody of their children. If a woman has not been tested for HIV, she should be informed of the benefits to her child's health of knowing her child's infection status and should be encouraged to allow the child to be tested. Counselors should ensure that the mother provides consent with the understanding that a positive HIV test for her child is indicative of infection in herself. For infants whose HIV infection status is unknown and who are in foster care, the person legally authorized to provide consent should be encouraged to allow the infant to be tested (with the

consent of the biologic mother, when possible) in accordance with the policies of the organization legally responsible for the child and with prevailing legal requirements for HIV testing.

- Pregnant women should be provided access to other HIV prevention and treatment services (e.g., drug-treatment and partner-notification services) as needed.

Interpretation of HIV Test Results

- HIV antibody testing should be performed according to the recommended algorithm, which includes the use of an EIA to test for antibody to HIV and confirmatory testing with an additional, more specific assay (e.g., Western blot or IFA) (53). All assays should be performed and conducted according to manufacturers' instructions and applicable state and federal laboratory guidelines.
- HIV infection (as indicated by the presence of antibody to HIV) is defined as a repeatedly reactive EIA and a positive confirmatory supplemental test. Confirmation or exclusion of HIV infection in a person with indeterminate test results should be made not only on the basis of HIV antibody test results, but with consideration of (a) the person's medical and behavioral history, (b) results from additional virologic and immunologic tests when performed, and (c) clinical follow-up. Uncertainties regarding HIV infection status, including laboratory test results, should be resolved before final decisions are made concerning pregnancy termination, ZDV therapy, or other interventions.
- Pregnant women who have repeatedly reactive EIA and indeterminate supplemental tests should be retested immediately for HIV antibody to distinguish between recent seroconversion and a negative test result. Additional tests (e.g., viral culture, PCR, or p24 antigen test) to diagnose or exclude HIV infection may be required for women whose test results remain indeterminate—especially women who have behavioral risk factors for HIV, have had recent exposure to HIV, or have clinical symptoms compatible with acute retroviral illness. In such situations, confirmation by an FDA-licensed IFA kit may be helpful because IFA is less likely to yield indeterminate results than Western blot.
- Women who have negative EIAs and those who have repeatedly reactive EIAs but negative supplemental tests should be considered uninfected.

Recommendations for HIV-Infected Pregnant Women

- HIV-infected pregnant women should receive counseling as previously recommended (64). Posttest HIV counseling should include an explanation of the clinical implications of a positive HIV antibody test result and the need for, benefit of, and means of access to HIV-related medical and other early intervention services. Such counseling should also include a discussion of the interaction between pregnancy and HIV infection (67), the risk for perinatal HIV transmission and ways to reduce this risk (29), and the prognosis for infants who become infected.
- HIV-infected pregnant women should be evaluated according to published recommendations to assess their need for antiretroviral therapy, antimicrobial prophylaxis, and treatment of other conditions (28, 68, 69). Although medical management of HIV infection is essentially the same for pregnant

and nonpregnant women, recommendations for treating a patient who has tuberculosis have been modified for pregnant women because of potential teratogenic effects of specific medications (e.g., streptomycin and pyrazinamide) (70). HIV-infected pregnant women should be evaluated to determine their need for psychological and social services.

- HIV-infected pregnant women should be provided information concerning ZDV therapy to reduce the risk for perinatal HIV transmission. This information should address the potential benefit and short-term safety of ZDV and the uncertainties regarding (a) long-term risks of such therapy and (b) effectiveness in women who have different clinical characteristics (e.g., CD4+ T-lymphocyte count and previous ZDV use) than women who participated in the trial. HIV-infected pregnant women should not be coerced into making decisions about ZDV therapy. These decisions should be made after consideration of both the benefits and potential risks of the regimen to the woman and her child. Therapy should be offered according to the appropriate regimen in published recommendations (29). A woman's decision not to accept treatment should not result in punitive action or denial of care.

- HIV-infected pregnant women should receive information about all reproductive options. Reproductive counseling should be nondirective. Healthcare providers should be aware of the complex issues that HIV-infected women must consider when making decisions about their reproductive options and should be supportive of any decision.

- To reduce the risk for HIV transmission to their infants, HIV-infected women should be advised against breastfeeding. Support services should be provided when necessary for use of appropriate breast-milk substitutes.

- To optimize medical management, positive and negative HIV test results should be available to a woman's health-care provider and included on both her and her infant's confidential medical records. After obtaining consent, maternal health-care providers should notify the pediatric-care providers of the impending birth of an HIV-exposed child, any anticipated complications, and whether ZDV should be administered after birth. If HIV is first diagnosed in the child, the child's health-care providers should discuss the implication of the child's diagnosis for the woman's health and assist the mother in obtaining care for herself. Providers are encouraged to build supportive health-care relationships that can facilitate the discussion of pertinent health information. Confidential HIV-related information should be disclosed or shared only in accordance with prevailing legal requirements.

- Counseling for HIV-infected pregnant women should include an assessment of the potential for negative effects resulting from HIV infection (e.g., discrimination, domestic violence, and psychological difficulties). For women who anticipate or experience such effects, counseling also should include (a) information on how to minimize these potential consequences, (b) assistance in identifying supportive persons within their own social network, and (c) referral to appropriate psychological, social, and legal services. In addition, HIV-infected women should be informed that discrimination based on HIV status or AIDS regarding matters such as housing, employment, state programs, and public accommodations (including physicians' offices and hospitals) is illegal (65).

- HIV-infected women should be encouraged to obtain HIV testing for any of their children born after they became infected or, if they do not know when they became infected, for children born after 1977. Older children (i.e., children >12 years of age) should be tested with informed consent of the parent and assent of the child. Women should be informed that the lack of signs and symptoms suggestive of HIV infection in older children may not indicate lack of HIV infection; some perinatally infected children can remain asymptomatic for several years.

Recommendations for Follow-Up of Infected Women and Perinatally Exposed Children

- Following pregnancy, HIV-infected women should be provided ongoing HIV-related medical care, including immune-function monitoring, antiretroviral therapy, and prophylaxis for and treatment of opportunistic infections and other HIV-related conditions (28, 68, 69). HIV-infected women should receive gynecologic care, including regular Pap smears, reproductive counseling, information on how to prevent sexual transmission of HIV, and treatment of gynecologic conditions according to published recommendations (28, 47, 71, 72).

- HIV-infected women (or the guardians of their children) should be informed of the importance of follow-up for their children. These children should receive follow-up care to determine their infection status, to initiate prophylactic therapy to prevent PCP, and, if infected, to determine the need for antiretroviral and other prophylactic therapy and to monitor disorders in growth and development, which often occur before 24 months of age (28, 31, 32, 73). HIV-infected children and other children living in households with HIV-infected persons should be vaccinated according to published recommendations for altered schedules (36).

- Because the identification of an HIV-infected mother also identifies a family that needs or will need medical and social services as her disease progresses, health-care providers should ensure that referrals to these services focus on the needs of the entire family.

REFERENCES: AS NUMBERED IN ORIGINAL PUBLICATION

1. Connor EM, Sperling RS, Gelber R, et al. Reduction of maternal-infant transmission of human immunodeficiency virus type 1 with zidovudine treatment. N Engl J Med 1994;331:1173–1180.
7. Lewis SH, Reynolds Kohler C, Fox HE, Nelson JA. HIV-1 in trophoblastic and villous Hofbauer cells, and haematological precursors in eight-week fetuses. Lancet 1990;335:565–568.
8. Mofenson LM, Wolinsky SM. Current insights regarding vertical transmission. In: Pizzo PA, Wilfert CM, eds. Pediatric AIDS: the challenge of HIV infection in infants, children, and adolescents. 2nd ed. Baltimore, MD: Williams & Wilkins, 1994:179–203.
9. Dunn DT, Newell ML, Ades AE, Peckham CS. Risk of human immunodeficiency virus type 1 transmission through breastfeeding. Lancet 1992;340:585–588.
10. Rogers MF, Ou C-Y, Rayfield M, et al. Use of the polymerase chain reaction for early detection of the proviral sequences of human immunodeficiency virus in infants born to seropositive mothers. N Engl J Med 1989;320:1649–1654.
11. Boyer PJ, Dillon M, Navaie M, et al. Factors predictive of maternal-fetal transmission of HIV-1: preliminary analysis of zidovudine given during pregnancy and/or delivery. JAMA 1994;271:1925–1930.
12. Rouzioux C, Costagliola D, Burgard M, et al. Timing of mother-to-child HIV-1 transmission depends on maternal status. AIDS 1993;7(Suppl 2):S49-S52.
13. St. Louis ME, Kalish M, Kamenga M, et al. The timing of perinatal HIV-1 transmission in an African setting [Abstract]. First National Conference on Human Retroviruses and Related Infections, Washington, DC, 1993.
14. Ekpini E, Wiktor SZ, Sibailly T, et al. Late postnatal mother-to-child HIV transmission in Abidjan, Cote d'Ivoire [Abstract]. Xth International Conference on AIDS, Yokohama, Japan, August 1994.
15. Ryder RW, Nsa W, Hassig SE, et al. Perinatal transmission of the human immunodeficiency virus type I to infants of seropositive women in Zaire. N Engl J Med 1989;320:1637–1642.

16. Blanche S, Rouzioux C, Moscato MG, et al. A prospective study of infants born to women seropositive for human immunodeficiency virus type 1. N Engl J Med 1989;320:1643–1648.
17. European Collaborative Study. Risk factors for mother-to-child transmission of HIV-1. Lancet 1992;339:1007–1012.
18. Gabiano C, Tovo P-A, de Martino M, et al. Mother-to-child transmission of human immunodeficiency virus type 1: risk of infection and correlates of transmission. Pediatrics 1992;90:369–374.
19. Dabis F, Msellati P, Dunn D, et al. Estimating the rate of mother-to-child transmission of HIV: report of a workshop on methodological issues—Ghent, Belgium, February 17–20, 1992. AIDS 1993;7:1139–1148.
20. St. Louis ME, Kamenga M, Brown C, et al. Risk for perinatal HIV-1 transmission according to maternal immunologic, virologic, and placental factors. JAMA 1993;269:2853–2859.
21. Burns DN, Landesman S, Muenz LR, et al. Cigarette smoking, premature rupture of membranes, and vertical transmission of HIV-1 among women with low CD4+ levels. J Acquir Immune Defic Syndr 1994;7:718–726.
22. Weisner B, Nachman S, Tropper P, et al. Quantitation of human immunodeficiency virus type 1 during pregnancy: relationship of viral titer to mother-to-child transmission and stability of viral load. Proc Natl Acad Sci USA 1994;91:8037–8041.
23. Semba RD, Miotti PG, Chiphangwi JD, et al. Maternal vitamin A deficiency and mother-to-child transmission of HIV-1. Lancet 1994;343:1593–1597.
24. Dunn DT, Newell ML, Mayaux MJ, et al. Mode of delivery and vertical transmission of HIV-1: a review of prospective studies. J Acquir Immune Defic Syndr 1994;7:1064–1066.
25. Scarlatti G, Albert J, Rossi P, et al. Mother-to-child transmission of human immunodeficiency virus type 1: correlation with neutralizing antibodies against primary isolates. J Infect Dis 1993;168:207–210.
26. Thomas PA, Weedon J, Krasinski K, et al. Maternal predictors of perinatal HIV transmission. Pediatr Infect Dis J 1994;13:489–495.
27. Wortley PM, Chu SY, Diaz T, et al. HIV testing patterns: where, why and when were persons with AIDS tested for HIV? AIDS 1995;9:487–492.
28. El-Sadr W, Oleske JM, Agins BD, et al. Evaluation and management of early HIV infection. Rockville, MD: US Department of Health and Human Services, Public Health Service, Agency for Health Care Policy and Research, January 1994. DHHS publication no. (AHCPR)94–0572. (Clinical Practice Guideline no. 7).
29. CDC. Recommendations of the U.S. Public Health Service Task Force on the use of zidovudine to reduce perinatal transmission of human immunodeficiency virus. MMWR 1994;43(No. RR-11).
30. Peckham CS, Newell M-L, eds. Measures to decrease the risk of mother-to-child transmission of HIV infection: highlights of a seminar meeting, January 11–13, 1993, London, UK. London: Colwood House Medical Publications, 1993.
31. Working Group on Antiretroviral Therapy: National Pediatric HIV Resource Center. Antiretroviral therapy and medical management of the human immunodeficiency virus-infected child. Pediatr Infect Dis J 1993;12:513–522.
32. CDC. 1995 Revised guidelines for prophylaxis against Pneumocystis carinii pneumonia for children infected with or perinatally exposed to human immunodeficiency virus. MMWR 1995;44(No. RR-4).
33. Blanche S, Mayaux M-J, Rouzioux C, et al. Relation of the course of HIV infection in children to the severity of the disease in their mothers at delivery. N Engl J Med 1994;330:308–312.
34. Byers B, Caldwell B, Oxtoby M, Pediatric Spectrum of Disease Project. Survival of children with perinatal HIV infection: evidence for two distinct populations [Abstract]. IXth International Conference on AIDS, Berlin, June 1993.
35. Simonds RJ, Oxtoby MJ, Caldwell MB, Gwinn ML, Rogers MF. Pneumocystis carinii pneumonia among U.S. children with perinatally acquired HIV infection. JAMA 1993;270:470–473.
36. ACIP. Recommendations of the Advisory Committee on Immunization Practices (ACIP): use of vaccines and immune globulins in persons with altered immunocompetence. MMWR 1993;42(No. RR-4).
37. New York City Commission on Human Rights (The AIDS Discrimination Division). Report on discrimination against people with AIDS and people perceived to have AIDS, January 1986-June 1987.
38. Moore J, Solomon L, Schoenbaum E, et al. Factors associated with stress and distress among HIV-infected and uninfected women [Abstract]. HIV Infection in Women Conference, Washington DC, February 1995.
39. Gielen A, O'Campo P, Faden R, Eke A. Women with HIV: disclosure, concerns, and experiences [Abstract]. HIV Infection in Women Conference, Washington DC, February 1995.
40. Perry SW, Jacobsberg LB, Fishman B, et al. Psychological responses to serological testing for HIV. AIDS 1990;4:145–152.
41. Brown GR, Rundell JR. A prospective study of psychiatric aspects of early HIV disease in women. Gen Hosp Psychiatry 1993;15:139–147.
42. CDC. Recommendations for assisting in the prevention of the perinatal transmission of human T-lymphotropic virus type III/lymphadenopathy-associated virus and acquired immunodeficiency syndrome. MMWR 1985;34:721–726, 731–732.
43. Barbacci MB, Dalabetta GA, Repke JT, et al. Human immunodeficiency virus infection in women attending an inner-city prenatal clinic: ineffectiveness of targeted screening. Sex Transm Dis 1990;Jul-Sept:122–126.

44. Fehrs LJ, Hill D, Kerndt PR, Rose TP, Henneman C. Targeted HIV screening at a Los Angeles prenatal/family planning health center. Am J Public Health 1991;81:619–622.
45. Lindsay MK, Adefris W, Peterson HB, et al. Determinants of acceptance of routine voluntary human immunodeficiency virus testing in an inner-city prenatal population. Obstet Gynecol 1989;78:678–680.
46. Ellerbrock TV, Lieb S, Harrington PE, et al. Heterosexually transmitted human immunodeficiency virus infection among pregnant women in a rural Florida community. N Engl J Med 1992;327: 1704–1709.
47. ACOG Technical Bulletin. Human immunodeficiency virus infections. June 1992:169.
48. Task Force on Pediatric AIDS. Perinatal human immunodeficiency virus (HIV) testing. Pediatrics 1992;89:791–794.
49. Hardy LM, ed. HIV screening of pregnant women and newborns. Washington, DC: National Academy Press, 1991.
50. Barbacci M, Repke JT, Chaisson RE. Routine prenatal screening for HIV infection. Lancet 1991; 337:709–711.
51. Lindsay MK, Peterson HB, Feng TI, Slade BA, Willis S, Klein L. Routine antepartum human immunodeficiency virus infection screening in an inner-city population. Obstet Gynecol 1989;74:289–294.
52. Cozen W, Mascola L, Enguidanos R, et al. Screening for HIV and hepatitis B virus in Los Angeles County prenatal clinics: a demonstration project. J Acquir Immune Defic Syndr 1993;6:95–98.
53. CDC. Public Health Service guidelines for counseling and antibody testing to prevent HIV infection and AIDS. MMWR 1987;36:509–515.
54. Celum CL, Coombs RW, Lafferty W, et al. Indeterminate human immunodeficiency virus type 1 Western blots: seroconversion risk, specificity of supplemental tests, and an algorithm for evaluation. J Infect Dis 1991;164:656–664.
55. Celum CL, Coombs RW, Jones JM, et al. Risk factors for repeatedly reactive HIV-1 EIA and indeterminate Western blots: a population-based case-control study. Arch Intern Med 1994;154:1129–1137.
56. Gwinn M, Redus MA, Granade TC. HIV-1 serologic test results for one million newborn dried-blood specimens: assay performance and implications for screening. J Acquir Immune Defic Syndr 1992;5:505–512.
57. Mucke H, Schinkinger M, Haushofer A, Fischer M, et al. Evaluation of a novel anti-HIV immunoflourescence assay in comparison with ELISA and Western blot. AIDS-Forschung 1990;191–199.
58. MacDonald KL, Jackson JB, Bowman RJ, et al. Performance characteristics of serologic tests for human immunodeficiency virus type 1 (HIV-1) antibody among Minnesota blood donors: public health and clinical implications. Ann Intern Med 1989;110:617–621.
59. Burke DS, Brundage JF, Redfield RR, et al. Measurement of the false positive rate in a screening program for human immunodeficiency virus infections. N Engl J Med 1988;319:961–964.
60. Sheon AR, Fox HE, Alexander G, et al. Misdiagnosed HIV infection in pregnant women: implications for clinical care. Public Health Rep 1994;109:694–699.
61. Rogers MF, Schochetman G, Hoff R. Advances in diagnosis of HIV infection in infants. In: Pizzo PA, Wilfert CM, eds. Pediatric AIDS: the challenge of HIV infection in infants, children, and adolescents. 2nd ed. Baltimore, MD: Williams & Wilkins, 1994:219–238.
62. CDC. 1994 Revised classification system for human immunodeficiency virus infection in children less than 13 years of age; Official authorized addenda—human immunodeficiency virus infection codes and official guidelines for coding and reporting ICD-9-CM. MMWR 1994;43(No. RR-12).
63. CDC. Recommendations for HIV testing services for inpatients and outpatients in acute-care hospital settings; and Technical guidance on HIV counseling. MMWR 1993;42(No. RR-2).
64. CDC. HIV counseling, testing, and referral: standards & guidelines. Atlanta, GA: US Department of Health & Human Services, Public Health Service, CDC, 1994.
65. Americans With Disabilities Act, 29 U.S.C. 706 and 42 U.S.C. 12101 et seq.
66. Lindsay MK, Feng TI, Peterson HB, Slade BA, Willis S, Klein L. Routine human immunodeficiency virus infection screening in unregistered and registered inner-city parturients. Obstet Gynecol 1991;77: 599–603.
67. Minkoff HL, Duerr A. Obstetric issues—relevance to women and children. In: Pizzo PA, Wilfert CM, eds. Pediatric AIDS: the challenge of HIV infection in infants, children, and adolescents. 2nd ed. Baltimore, MD: Williams & Wilkins, 1994:773–784.
68. Sande MA, Carpenter CCJ, Cobbs CG, et al. Antiretroviral therapy for adult HIV-infected patients: recommendations from a state-of-the-art conference. JAMA 1993;270:2583–2589.
69. CDC. Recommendations for prophylaxis against Pneumocystis carinii pneumonia for adults and adolescents infected with human immunodeficiency virus. MMWR 1992;41(No. RR-4).
70. CDC. Initial therapy for tuberculosis in the era of multidrug resistance: recommendations of the Advisory Council for the Elimination of Tuberculosis. MMWR 1993;42(No. RR-7).
71. CDC. 1993 Sexually transmitted diseases treatment guidelines. MMWR 1993;42(No. RR-14).
72. CDC. Update: barrier protection against HIV infection and other sexually transmitted diseases. MMWR 1993;42:589–591, 597.
73. Report of a Consensus Workshop, Siena, Italy, January 17–18, 1992. Early Diagnosis of HIV Infection in Infants. J Acquir Immune Defic Syndr 1992;5:1169–1178.

Recommendations for HIV Testing Services for Inpatients and Outpatients in Acute-Care Hospital Settings

Original Citation: Centers for Disease Control and Prevention. Recommendations for HIV Testing Services for Inpatients and Outpatients in Acute-Care Hospital Settings. MMWR 1993;42(RR-02).

Editor's Note: The information included here was based on an article which describes CDC recommendations for HIV counseling and testing of patients in acute care hospitals. The original article includes background information on HIV seroprevalence and on the number of HIV patients seen in acute care hospitals.

RECOMMENDATIONS

Voluntary and confidential HIV counseling and testing of patients in acute-care hospitals are useful for (a) assisting in differential diagnosis of medical conditions, (b) initiating early medical management of HIV infection, and (c) informing infected persons or persons at risk for infection about behaviors that can prevent HIV transmission.

To promote the appropriate use of HIV counseling and testing services, CDC recommends that acute-care facilities adopt the following guidelines*:

- Hospitals and associated clinics should encourage health-care providers to routinely ask patients about their risks for HIV infection and offer HIV counseling and voluntary testing services to patients at risk (1). Patients should give informed consent for testing in accordance with local laws.
- Hospitals and associated clinics should develop policies regarding provision of routine HIV counseling and voluntary testing services. Other health-care institutions such as drug treatment centers, mental health facilities, and private medical practitioners are also encouraged to consider offering these services. The decision to offer these services routinely may be based on the HIV seroprevalence in the patient population. This rate may be determined most directly by a representative sample of unlinked

---

* These guidelines are based in part on comments received by CDC at a meeting of consultants in Atlanta, Georgia, April 5–6, 1990. The consultants represented the American College of Emergency Physicians, American College of Obstetrics and Gynecology, American College of Orthopedic Surgery, American Hospital Association, American Medical Association, American Physicians for Human Rights, Association of State and Territorial Health Officers, Association of State and Territorial Public Health Laboratory Directors, Council of State and Territorial Epidemiologists, National Association of County Health Officers, National Association of Public Hospitals, National Institutes of Health, National Medical Association, Occupational Safety and Health Administration, and other technical experts. These Public Health Service recommendations may not reflect the views of all individual consultants or the organizations they represented.

anonymous specimens.** Alternatively, hospitals and other health-care providers may elect to use an indirect marker of HIV seroprevalence, such as the AIDS diagnosis rate (defined above).

- Hospitals with an HIV seroprevalence rate of at least 1% or an AIDS diagnosis rate greater than or equal to 1.0 per 1,000 discharges should strongly consider adopting a policy of offering HIV counseling and testing routinely to patients ages 15–54 years.
- HIV counseling and testing procedures in the acute-care setting should be structured to facilitate confidential, voluntary patient participation and should include (a) pretest information on the testing policies of the institution or physician and (b) basic information about the medical implications of the test, the patient's option to receive more information, and the documentation of informed consent.
- HIV counseling and testing should be offered in nonemergency settings in which patients are able to make an informed and voluntary decision regarding HIV testing. HIV counseling and testing for purposes other than immediate medical care should be deferred until a later time for persons who are too severely ill to understand the pretest information or give informed consent.
- Test results should be provided to the patient in a confidential manner and forwarded to state health departments in accordance with local law. Post-test counseling for infected patients and those at increased risk should be performed by trained health-care providers in accordance with existing CDC recommendations (1).
- Persons who decline HIV testing or who consent to testing and are HIV antibody positive must not be denied needed medical care or provided suboptimal care. HIV-infected persons should receive medical evaluation for HIV infection and specific therapies and prevention services as needed. If therapeutic and prevention services are not available, the acute-care facility or provider should establish an effective referral system to ensure that these services will be provided.
- Facilities offering HIV testing and counseling should take necessary steps to protect the confidentiality of test results. The ability of facilities to assure confidentiality of patients' test information and the public's confidence in that ability are crucial to efforts to increase the number of persons being counseled and tested for HIV infection. Moreover, to assure broad participation in counseling and testing programs, the public must be assured that persons found to be HIV positive will not be subject to discrimination (1).
- HIV testing programs must not be used as a substitute for universal precautions and other infection-control techniques.

THE ROLE OF HEALTH DEPARTMENTS

State and local health departments are a source for at least three forms of assistance for implementing these recommendations. First, state and local health

---

** To determine directly the rate of infection for a patient population, hospitals may consider conducting anonymous unlinked serologic surveys (i.e., testing of serum or plasma samples that were collected for other purposes and have had personal identifiers removed before testing). For guidelines regarding the conduct of blinded HIV serosurveys in hospitals, contact: Seroepidemiology Branch, Division of HIV/AIDS, Mailstop E-46, Centers for Disease Control and Prevention (CDC), Atlanta, Georgia, 30333.

departments can provide data to assist hospitals to determine their AIDS diagnosis rate. Second, state and local health departments can provide technical assistance and training for hospital staff responsible for HIV-related counseling and testing services in acute-care settings. Third, health departments can help hospitals by providing partner notification services for HIV-infected patients, as well as additional prevention services for uninfected patients who are at high risk for HIV infection. Effective and ongoing collaboration between acute-care providers and health departments will improve both prevention and treatment services for persons infected with HIV or at risk for HIV infection.

REFERENCES: AS NUMBERED IN ORIGINAL PUBLICATION

1. CDC. Public health service guidelines for counseling and antibody testing to prevent HIV infection and AIDS. MMWR 1987;36:509–515.

Technical Guidance on HIV Counseling

Original Citation: Centers for Disease Control and Prevention. Technical Guidance on HIV Counseling. MMWR 1993;42(RR-02).

Editor's Note: The information included here was based on an article which details technical guidance on the subject of HIV counseling and is based on a meeting of expert consultants. It also includes a general introduction to HIV counseling and testing.

RECOMMENDATIONS

HIV Prevention Messages

Counselors in programs that offer human immunodeficiency virus counseling and testing services (HIV-CTS) should take advantage of all available opportunities to provide clients with HIV-prevention messages.

Clients manifest varying degrees of acceptance of HIV CTS. Some clients are highly motivated to learn their HIV serostatus, while others may be wary or suspicious of suggestions that they learn their HIV serostatus. Still others may not perceive themselves to be at risk for HIV infection and consider the test unnecessary. Changing high-risk behavior is not an "all-or-nothing" process. Even after availing themselves of HIV-CTS, seronegative clients may continue to engage in behaviors that place them at risk for HIV infection.

Therefore, counselors should view all clinical encounters with clients as potential opportunities to provide and reinforce HIV-prevention messages. These messages should be clear and straight forward (e.g., "If you are not infected with HIV, you should take steps to make sure you stay that way, and, if you are already infected, early treatment can preserve your health by delaying the onset of illness.")

Client-Centered Counseling.

HIV counseling must be "client-centered."

To fulfill its public health functions, HIV counseling must be client-centered; i.e., tailored to the behaviors, circumstances, and special needs of the person being served. Risk-reduction messages must be personalized and realistic. Counseling should be:

- Culturally competent (i.e., program services provided in a style and format sensitive to cultural norms, values, and traditions that are endorsed by cultural leaders and accepted by the target population);
- Sensitive to issues of sexual identity;
- Developmentally appropriate (i.e., information and services provided at a level of comprehension that is consistent with the age and the learning skills of the person being served);
- Linguistically specific (i.e., information is presented in dialect and terminology consistent with the client's language and style of communication).

HIV counseling is not a lecture. An important aspect of HIV counseling is the counselor's ability to listen to the client in order to provide assistance and to determine specific prevention needs.

Although HIV counseling should adhere to minimal standards in terms of providing basic information, it should not become so routine that it is inflexible or unresponsive to particular client needs. Counselors should avoid providing information that is irrelevant to their clients and should avoid structuring counseling sessions on the basis of a data-collection instrument or form.

Client-Risk Assessment

HIV pretest counseling must include a personalized client-risk assessment.

A focused and tailored risk assessment is the foundation of HIV pretest counseling. Risk assessment is a process whereby the counselor helps the client to assess and take "ownership" of his/her risk for HIV infection. Client acceptance of risk is a critical component of this assessment. Risk assessment is not a counselor's passive appraisal of the client's behavior, such as checking off risks from a written list, but an interactive process between counselor and client. Risk assessment should be conducted in an empathic manner with special attention given to the ongoing behaviors and circumstances (e.g., sexual history, sexually transmitted disease [STD] history, drug use) that may continue to place the client at risk for HIV infection/transmission. For example, clients who are being counseled in STD clinics, where they have come for the treatment of a symptomatic STD (other than HIV), should be advised that their current infection demonstrates that they are at increased risk for HIV.

Because the risk-assessment process serves as the basis for assisting the client in formulating a plan to reduce risk, it is an essential component of all pretest counseling.

HIV Risk-Reduction Plan

HIV counseling should result in a personalized plan for the client to reduce the risk of HIV infection/transmission.

HIV counseling is more than providing routine information. Such counseling should also include the development of a personalized, negotiated HIV risk-reduction plan. This plan should be based on the client's skills, needs, and circumstances, and it must be consistent with the client's expressed or implied intentions to change behaviors. HIV counseling should not consist of the counselor "telling" the client what he/she needs to do to prevent HIV infection/transmission, but instead should outline a variety of specific options available to the client for reducing his/her own risk of HIV infection/transmission. The counselor should confirm with the client that the risk-reduction plan is realistic and feasible—otherwise, it is likely to fail.

When negotiating a personalized risk-reduction plan, counselors should be especially attentive to information provided by the client—especially information about past attempts at preventive behaviors that were unsuccessful (e.g., intentions to use condoms but failure to do so) and those which were successful. Identifying and discussing previous prevention failures help to ensure that the risk-reduction plan is realistic, attentive to the clients' prevention needs, and focused on actual barriers to safer behaviors. Identifying previous prevention successes (e.g., successful negotiation of condom use with a new sexual partner) offers the counselor the opportunity to reinforce and support positive prevention choices.

An interactive risk assessment and a personalized risk-reduction plan developed during pretest counseling ensure that clients receive adequate prevention information, even before they learn the results of their tests. Counselors can use the client's expectation of test results to facilitate the development of a personalized risk-reduction plan (e.g., "What do you expect your test results to be? Why? What will you do if you are HIV seropositive? Is there anything different you will do if you are HIV seronegative?").

Post-Test Counseling

Programs should take active steps to address the problem of failure to return for post-test counseling.

Not all clients who receive pretest HIV counseling and testing return for post-test counseling and test results. In 1991, 31 state and local health departments recorded HIV counseling and testing data in such a way that analysis of individual post-test counseling return rates was possible. These project areas reported an average 63% return rate for post-test counseling. However, this rate ranged from 41% to 86% and varied by age, sex, race/ethnicity, self-reported risk behavior, service-delivery site, and HIV serostatus. Analyses indicate that adolescents, blacks*, and clients served in family-planning clinics and STD clinics, have lower return rates for HIV post-test counseling (7).

HIV-CTS programs should be active in addressing the problem of failure to return for HIV post-test counseling. Program managers should determine if specific operational barriers exist that prevent clients from returning for HIV post-test counseling (e.g., excessive waiting time). Counselors should stress the importance

* CDC's National Center for Prevention Services recognizes that a variety of terms are used and preferred by different groups to describe race and ethnicity. Racial and ethnic terms used in this document reflect the way data are collected and reported by official health agencies.

of receiving post-test counseling and should identify it as a specific component of the personalized risk-reduction plan. HIV-CTS programs should give priority to contacting seropositive and high-risk seronegative clients who have not returned to learn their test results and have failed to receive post-test counseling.

As part of a comprehensive quality-assurance program, publicly funded counseling and testing programs must monitor: (a) blinded seroprevalence rates to assess the extent of client access and acceptance of recommended counseling, testing, referral, and partner-notification services (CTRPN); and (b) the rates at which clients return to receive HIV-antibody test results and post-test counseling.

When less than 50% of high-risk clients are receiving counseling and testing, or when low return rates (e.g., less than 80% for seropositives and less than 60% for high-risk seronegatives) are identified, documented "action steps" must be initiated to determine the reasons for such low rates and to resolve barriers to clients in accessing services, learning their test results, and obtaining counseling and referral services (6). Counselors should routinely assess whether clients require additional post-test counseling sessions.

Many HIV counselors have reported that some clients may require more than a single post-test counseling session. Seropositive clients are often disturbed by the realization that they have a life-threatening disease and often require additional counseling and support. Seronegative clients who are at increased risk for HIV infection or transmission may also require additional counseling to develop the skills needed to practice safer behaviors.

Although CDC does not require its funded programs to routinely provide repeated post-test counseling sessions, counselors and program managers should be aware that certain clients may require additional support and further counseling opportunities. If deemed appropriate, additional counseling should be provided on-site or through referral. In considering options for additional post-test counseling, program managers should work with local community-based organizations that might offer such services.

Programs should ensure that HIV CTS clients receive appropriate referrals.

Seronegative clients at continuing risk for HIV infection and HIV-infected clients often require additional primary and secondary HIV-prevention services that may not be available on-site. For example, clients, whose drug use continues to place them at risk for HIV infection should be referred for appropriate drug treatment. HIV-infected clients should be provided (on-site or through referral) with immune system monitoring and a medical evaluation to determine the need for anti-retroviral therapy and prophylaxis for Pneumocystis pneumonia. Facilitating referrals for these services, as well as for tuberculosis (TB) and STD care as needed, are important aspects of HIV post-test counseling.

Identifying appropriate referral sites (i.e., sites where appropriate services which meet acceptable standards of quality are offered in a timely manner) should not be the sole responsibility of the person performing HIV counseling. Program managers should take the lead in identifying referral sites and developing programmatic relations (e.g., contracts and memoranda of understanding) with those sites to facilitate needed client referrals.

Training and Counselor Feedback

Programs should provide training and counselor feedback to ensure the quality of HIV-CTS.

Counselors, as well as their supervisors, require adequate training in HIV-CTS. In addition to training on the scientific/public health aspects of HIV-CTS, training should address other relevant issues such as substance abuse, human sexuality, the process of behavior change, and the cultural perspectives of the clients being served.

Training for HIV counseling is not a one-time event—it should be an ongoing process. An important component of ongoing quality assurance and training for HIV counselors is routine, periodic observation during counseling sessions and subsequent feedback. When a trained supervisor is not available to perform this important function, routine observation should be done by trained peer counselors. Performance standards that define expectations for the content and delivery quality of counseling should be developed. (Note: observational supervision requires the consent of the client being counseled.)

CONCLUSION

Publicly funded HIV-CTS are a major component of the national HIV-prevention program (4). Further, national health promotion and disease prevention objectives for the year 2000 target increases in the proportion of HIV-infected persons who have been tested for HIV infection and the number of health-care facilities (e.g., family-planning clinics, TB clinics, drug-treatment centers, primary-care clinics) where counseling and testing is provided (8). These recommendations, which supplement existing guidelines (3), focus on the counseling portion of the HIV counseling and testing process—a cooperative endeavor that includes giving information and assisting the client in identifying his/her HIV-prevention needs, and in developing a strategy to address those needs (9). These guidelines stress the importance of ensuring that HIV counseling is empathic, a quality known to be important in other clinical encounters (10).

By ensuring that counseling is empathic and "client-centered," counselors will be able to develop a realistic appraisal of the client's level of risk and assess at which stage the client has reached in the behavior change process (11, 12). Assessing the client's state of behavior change is important since intentions to reduce/modify risky behavior or initiate/ increase healthy behavior will vary among clients. The "Stages of Behavior Change" model recognizes that persons usually pass through a series of steps before achieving consistently safe behavior—whether in terms of sexual or drug-use behavior (13, 14). These stages are: precontemplation (no intention to change one's behavior); contemplation (long-range intentions to change); ready for action (short-term intentions to change); action (attempts to change); maintenance (long-term consistent behavior change); and relapse (which can end the new behavior or restart the process) (11, 12, 14).

Assessing the client's stage of behavior change is necessary to ensure that prevention messages are individually relevant—a crucial consideration if HIV counseling is to effect behavior change. For instance, counseling messages that increase clients' intentions to reduce risky behaviors are different from those required to maintain safer behaviors and prevent relapse (15).

Cost-benefit analysis of HIV-CTRPN indicates that, even under conservative assumptions, CDC's expenditure on HIV-CTS results in a substantial net economic benefit to society (16). Program managers and staff must have realistic expectations about HIV counseling and testing programs. Although it is unlikely that a single episode of HIV counseling will result in the immediate and permanent adoption of safer behaviors (17), client-centered HIV counseling and attendant prevention services (i.e., referral and partner notification) do contribute to the initiation and maintenance of safer behaviors.

REFERENCES: AS NUMBERED IN ORIGINAL PUBLICATION

3. CDC. Public Health Service guidelines for counseling and antibody testing to prevent HIV infection and AIDS. MMWR 1987;36:509–515.
4. CDC. Publicly funded HIV counseling and testing—United States, 1991. MMWR 1992;41:613–617.
6. CDC. Cooperative agreements for human immunodeficiency virus (HIV) prevention projects, program announcement, and availability of funds for fiscal year 1993. Federal Register 1992;57:40675-40682.
7. Valdiserri RO, Moore M, Gerber AR, Campbell CH, Dillon BA, West GR. Return rates for HIV posttest counseling: implications for program efficacy. Public Health Rep 1993;108:12–18.
8. Public Health Service. Healthy people 2000:national health promotion and disease prevention objectives—full report, with commentary. Washington, DC: US Department of Health and Human Services, Public Health Service, 1991:DHHS publication no.(PHS)91–50212.
9. Davis H, Fallowfield L, eds. Counseling and communication in health care. New York: John Wiley and Sons, 1991:23–25.
10. Bellet PS, Maloney MJ. The importance of empathy as an interviewing skill in medicine. JAMA 1991;266(13):1831–1832.
11. Prochaska JO, DiClemente CC. Stages and processes of self-change of smoking: toward an integrative model of change. J Consulting Clin Psychol 1983;51:390–395.
12. Prochaska JO, DiClemente CC. Toward a comprehensive model of change. In: Miller W, Heather N, eds. Treating addictive behaviors. New York: Plenum Press, 1986:3–27.
13. Prochaska JO, DiClemente CC, Norcross JC. In search of how people change; applications to addictive behaviors. Am Psychol 1992;47(9):1102–1114.
14. O'Reilly KR, Higgins DL. AIDS community demonstration projects for HIV prevention among hard-to-reach groups. Public Health Rep 1991;106:714–720.
15. CDC. Patterns of sexual behavior change among homosexual/bisexual men—selected U.S. sites, 1987–1990. MMWR 1991;40:792–794.
16. Holtgrave DR, Valdiserri RO, Gerber AR, Hinman AR. HIV counseling, testing, referral, and partner notification services: a cost-benefit analysis. Arch Intern Med (in press).
17. Higgins DL, Galavotti C, O'Reilly KR, et al. Evidence for the effects of HIV antibody counseling and testing on risk behaviors. JAMA 1991;266:2419–2429.

Recommendations for Counseling Persons Infected with Human T-Lymphotrophic Virus, Types I and II

Original Citation: Centers for Disease Control and Prevention. Recommendations for Counseling Persons Infected with Human T-Lymphotrophic Virus, Types I and II*. MMWR 1993;42(RR-9);1–13.

* This report was previously published in Annals of Internal Medicine (Vol. 118, No. 6, March 15, 1993) and is printed here as a service to the MMWR readership.

Editor's Note: The information included here was based on an article which summarizes known information on human T-lymphotropic viruses, type I (HTLV-I) and type II (HTLV-II) and makes recommendations for counseling based on differing epidemiologies and disease associations. The introduction also summarizes information on serologic tests for HTLV-I and HTLV-II.

RECOMMENDATIONS FOR COUNSELING

In consideration of the information presented above, the following recommendations for counseling HTLV-seropositive persons have been issued. In instances in which viral typing is possible, counseling should be virus specific. As noted above, HTLV-I and HTLV-II are two different retroviruses with differing epidemiologies and disease associations. The specific recommendations for persons infected with HTLV-I or HTLV-II should therefore take these differences into account.

HTLV-I

Persons found to be seropositive for HTLV-I/II according to the USPHS criteria and positive for HTLV-I by additional testing should be informed that they are infected with HTLV-I. They should be told that HTLV-I is not the AIDS virus, that it does not cause AIDS, and that AIDS is caused by a different virus called HIV. They should be told that HTLV-I is a lifelong infection. They should be given information regarding modes and efficiency of transmission, disease associations, and the probability of developing disease.

In particular, persons infected with HTLV-I should be advised to:

• Share the information with their physician.
• Refrain from donating blood, semen, body organs, or other tissues.
• Refrain from sharing needles or syringes with anyone.
• Refrain from breast-feeding infants.
• Consider the use of latex condoms to prevent sexual transmission.

If the HTLV-I-positive person is in a mutually monogamous sexual relationship, testing of the sex partner should be recommended to help formulate specific counseling advice. If the sex partner is also positive, no further recommendations are indicated. If the sex partner is negative, the couple should be advised that the use of latex condoms can help prevent transmission of HTLV-I to the negative partner, male or female. Male-infected, female-non-infected couples desiring pregnancy should be made aware of the finite risk of sexual transmission of HTLV-I during attempts at pregnancy and of the small risk for vertical transmission from mother to infant unrelated to breast-feeding. Such couples might be advised to use latex condoms at all times except during the fertile period while they are attempting pregnancy. The use of latex condoms is strongly recommended for HTLV-I-positive persons with multiple sex partners or otherwise engaging in non-mutually monogamous sexual relationships. These persons should be reminded of the risk of acquiring other sexually transmitted infections, including HIV.

HTLV-II

Persons found to be seropositive for HTLV-I/II according to the USPHS criteria and positive for HTLV-II by additional testing should be informed that they are infected with HTLV-II. They should be told that HTLV-II is not the AIDS virus, that it does not cause AIDS, and that AIDS is caused by a different virus called HIV. They should be told that HTLV-II is a lifelong infection. They should be given information regarding possible modes of transmission and the lack of firm disease associations.

In particular, they should be advised to:

- Share the information with their physician.
- Refrain from donating blood, semen, body organs, or other tissues.
- Refrain from sharing drug needles or syringes with anyone.
- Refrain from breast-feeding infants. Although the risks of transmission of HTLV-II by breast-feeding and of disease from HTLV-II are unknown, the theoretical risk of transmission and disease, as for HTLV-I, makes it prudent to recommend that HTLV-II-infected mothers refrain from breast-feeding when and where safe nutritional alternatives exist.

Consider the use of barrier precautions to prevent sexual transmission. HTLV-II can be sexually transmitted, but the risks of disease are unknown. If the HTLV-II-positive person is in a mutually monogamous sexual relationship, testing of the sex partner should be recommended to help formulate specific counseling advice. If the sex partner is also positive, no further recommendations are indicated. If the sex partner is negative, the couple should be advised that the use of latex condoms can help prevent transmission of HTLV-II to the negative partner, male or female. The use of latex condoms is strongly recommended for HTLV-II-positive persons with multiple sex partners or otherwise engaging in non-mutually monogamous sexual relationships. These persons should be reminded of the risk of acquiring other sexually transmitted infections, including HIV.

HTLV-I/II.

Persons found to be seropositive for HTLV-I/II according to the USPHS criteria but without differentiation of their infection should be informed they are positive for HTLV-I/II and that they are likely infected with either HTLV-I or HTLV-II. Because of the differences in the epidemiologic and clinical correlates of HTLV-I and HTLV-II, an effort to type the infection should be made. If such efforts are unsuccessful, these HTLV-I/II seropositive persons should be given information regarding possible modes and efficiency of transmission of HTLV-I and HTLV-II, disease associations of HTLV-I, and the probability of developing disease. Specific counseling advice should be the same as for HTLV-I-infected persons (refer to HTLV-I section).

HTLV Indeterminate

Blood donors with serum specimens that are HTLV-indeterminate on two occasions at least 3 months apart should be advised that their specimens were reactive in a screening test for HTLV-I but that the results could not be confirmed by a second, more specific test. They should be reassured that "indeterminate" test results are only rarely caused by HTLV-I or HTLV-II infection. Persons testing "indeterminate" for HTLV-I/II on one occasion should be offered retesting to make sure they are not recently infected with HTLV-I or HTLV-II and in the process of seroconverting. If subsequent test results are the same, they should be reassured that they are unlikely to be infected with HTLV-I or HTLV-II.

HTLV False-Positive

Blood donors with serum specimens that are repeatably reactive by HTLV-I enzyme immunoassay but negative by Western immunoblot on two occasions should be advised that their HTLV-I screening test is falsely positive and that it could not be confirmed by a second, more specific test. They should be reassured that they are not infected with HTLV-I or HTLV-II.

Medical Follow-up

A periodic medical evaluation of HTLV-I- or HTLV-I/II-infected persons by a physician knowledgeable about these viruses is recommended. This evaluation might include a physical examination, including a neurologic examination, and a complete blood count with peripheral smear examination. Medical evaluation of HTLV-II-infected persons should be considered optional.

Testing for Antibodies to HIV Type 2 in the United States

Original Citation: Centers for Disease Control and Prevention. Testing for Antibodies to Human Immunodeficiency Virus Type 2 in the United States. MMWR 1992;41(RR-12):1–9.

Editor's Note: The information included here was based on an article which provides CDC recommendations for the diagnosis of HIV-1 and HIV-2 infections in persons being tested in settings other than blood centers and CDC/FDA guidelines for serologic testing with combination HIV-1/HIV-2 screening enzyme immunoassays (EIA's). Background information on testing materials, epidemiology and diagnosis of HIV-2 are given in the original article.

RECOMMENDATIONS FOR HIV-2 TESTING IN THE UNITED STATES

Indications for Testing for HIV-2 Infection

Because epidemiologic data indicate that the prevalence of HIV-2 in the United States is extremely low, CDC does not recommend routine testing for HIV-2 at U.S. HIV counseling and test sites or in settings other than blood centers. However, when HIV testing is to be performed, tests for antibodies to both HIV-1 and HIV-2 should be obtained if demographic or behavioral information suggests that HIV-2 infection might be present. Persons at risk for HIV-2 infection include:

- Sex partners of a person from a country where HIV-2 is endemic (this category includes persons originally from such countries).
- Sex partners of a person known to be infected with HIV-2.
- Persons who received a transfusion of blood or a nonsterile injection in a country where HIV-2 is endemic.
- Persons who shared needles with a person from a country where HIV-2 is endemic or with a person known to be infected with HIV-2.
- Children of women who have risk factors for HIV-2 infection or who are known to be infected with HIV-2.

Additionally, testing for HIV-2 is indicated when there is clinical evidence for or suspicion of HIV disease (such as an AIDS-associated opportunistic infection) in the absence of a positive test for antibodies to HIV-1 and in cases in which the HIV-1 Western blot exhibits the unusual indeterminate pattern of gag (p55, p24, or p17) plus pol (p66, p51, or p32) bands in the absence of env (gp160, gp120, or gp41) bands.

Other Considerations

The potential risk of HIV-2 infection in some populations (such as those described above) may justify routine HIV-2 testing for all persons for whom HIV-1 testing is warranted. The decision to implement routine HIV-2 testing requires consideration of the number of HIV-2-infected persons who would remain undiagnosed without routine HIV-2 testing compared with the problems and costs associated with its implementation. Because implementation of routine HIV-2 testing would increase the number of tests performed on some specimens and because confirmatory testing for HIV-2 would be limited to laboratories that perform nonlicensed HIV-2 supplemental tests, the maximum "turnaround" time required to complete HIV testing would increase for some specimens. At HIV counseling and test sites, clients might require an additional appointment after the routine post-test counseling session to receive HIV-2 test results and HIV-2 post-test counseling. Another factor to consider when routine HIV-2 testing is being contemplated is the predictive value of HIV-2 antibody screening tests in most U.S. populations. Given the extremely low prevalence of HIV-2 in the United States, very few persons who test positive by HIV-2 antibody screening tests will actually be HIV-2 infected. In addition, HIV-2 testing may identify persons with indeterminate HIV-2 test results that must be explained to the patient and appropriate follow-up initiated. Finally, implementation of routine HIV-2 testing would increase HIV testing costs, as HIV-1/HIV-2 combination EIAs are more expensive than HIV-1 EIAs, and testing with HIV-2 EIAs and supplemental tests would be required for some specimens.

GUIDELINES FOR SEROLOGIC TESTING WITH COMBINATION HIV-1/HIV-2 SCREENING EIAS

Laboratories that use a licensed combination HIV-1/HIV-2 screening test should follow the testing algorithm recommended by CDC and FDA (Figure 38.1). If a

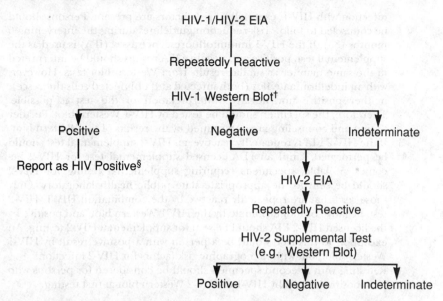

HIV-1/HIV-2 EIA

Repeatedly Reactive

HIV-1 Western Blot[†]

Positive — Negative — Indeterminate

Report as HIV Positive[§]

HIV-2 EIA

Repeatedly Reactive

HIV-2 Supplemental Test
(e.g., Western Blot)

Positive — Negative — Indeterminate

*HIV = Human immunodeficiency virus.
[†]An immunofluorescence assay (IFA) for HIV-1 antibodies has recently been licensed by the Food and Drug Administration and can be used instead of Western blot. Positive and negative IFA results should be interpreted in the same manner as similar results from Western blot tests. An indeterminate IFA should first be tested by HIV-1 Western blot and then as indicated by the Western blot results.
[§]Perform HIV-2 EIA only if there is an identified risk factor for HIV-2 infection.

Figure 38.1. Centers for Disease Control/Food and Drug Administration testing algortihm for use with combination HIV-1/HIV-2* enzyme immunoassays (EIAs).

combination test for HIV-1/HIV-2 is performed and is repeatedly reactive, additional, more specific testing is necessary to confirm the presence of antibodies either to HIV-1 or HIV-2 as follows:

1. A repeatedly reactive specimen determined by a combination HIV-1/HIV-2 EIA should be tested for antibodies to HIV-1 by a licensed Western blot or other licensed HIV-1 supplemental test. A positive HIV-1 Western blot confirms the presence of antibodies to HIV. Although this result does not always distinguish between antibodies to HIV-1 and HIV-2, further testing is not required for routine purposes. If the suspicion of HIV-2 infection (based on epidemiologic risk factors [see "Recommendations" section]) is high, additional testing for HIV-2 is indicated.

2. If the HIV-1 Western blot result is negative or indeterminate, an EIA for HIV-2 only (HIV-2 EIA) should be performed. If the HIV-1 Western blot is negative and HIV-2 EIA is not repeatedly reactive, the specimen should be considered negative for HIV antibodies. If the HIV-1 Western blot is indeterminate and the HIV-2 EIA is not repeatedly reactive, the specimen should be considered indeterminate and the person should be advised to have follow-up testing 6 months later to exclude the possibility of early

infection with HIV-1, especially if risk factors are present. Persons should be counseled to follow risk-reduction guidelines during the intervening 6 months (33). If the HIV-1 immunofluorescence assay (IFA) is used as the supplemental test, positive and negative IFA results should be interpreted in the same manner as similar results from Western blot tests. However, with an indeterminate IFA (both infected and uninfected cells fluoresce), neither positive nor negative interpretation of the test is possible. Therefore, the specimen should be tested by HIV-1 Western blot. Further testing and counseling are determined by the results of the Western blot.

3. If the HIV-2 EIA is repeatedly reactive, an HIV-2 supplemental test should be performed. Until an FDA-licensed supplemental test for HIV-2 becomes available, specimens requiring supplemental testing for HIV-2 should be sent to the appropriate state public health laboratory. Only those sera that are repeatedly reactive by the combination HIV-1/HIV-2 test, negative or indeterminate by the HIV-1 Western blot, and positive by the licensed HIV-2 EIA should be sent for supplemental HIV-2 testing. An exception to this rule would be a person with a positive result by HIV-1 Western blot, but with demographic risk factors for HIV-2 infection.

4. Retesting with a second specimen should be considered for persons who have positive results by HIV-1 or HIV-2 Western blot at first testing.

MEDICAL COUNSELING

Infection with either HIV-1 or HIV-2 can cause immunosuppression and the development of AIDS (34, 35). Although the period between infection and disease may be longer for persons with HIV-2 than for those with HIV-1 (36, 37), the modes of transmission and, therefore, preventive counseling are the same for persons with either virus. Furthermore, because data are limited regarding the effectiveness of antiviral therapy for HIV-2 infection, persons with a confirmed antibody test for HIV-2 should be managed similarly to persons with a confirmed antibody test for HIV-1. Additional testing to define the virus type is of epidemiologic importance and should be considered for persons with epidemiologic risk factors for infection with HIV-2.

Based on the epidemiology and prevalence of HIV-2 in the United States, CDC/FDA makes the following recommendations for notification of persons with repeatedly reactive combination screening tests for HIV-1/HIV-2.

1. If the HIV-1 Western blot is positive, the person should be considered to be HIV infected and counseled and managed as if infected with HIV-1. In infants, detection of antibodies soon after birth may indicate either infection or the presence of maternal HIV antibodies. Seropositive infants require additional follow-up to determine their HIV status.

2. If the HIV-1 Western blot is negative and HIV-2 EIA is not repeatedly reactive, the person should be informed that the test results for HIV infection are negative.

3. If an HIV-2 EIA is repeatedly reactive for a person with a negative or indeterminate HIV-1 Western blot, post-test counseling will depend on the results of the HIV-2 supplemental test. A person should not be diagnosed or counseled about HIV-2 infection on the basis of a repeatedly reactive HIV-2 EIA alone. in the absence of known epidemiologic risk factors for

HIV-2 infection, the vast majority of specimens from persons in the United States with a repeatedly reactive HIV-2 EIA and negative or indeterminate HIV-1 Western blot will represent false-positive results.

- If the HIV-2 supplemental test is negative, a person whose specimen was negative by HIV-1 Western blot, in the absence of recognized epidemiologic risk factors, should be considered to be uninfected with HIV and counseled accordingly. A person whose specimen was indeterminate by HIV-1 Western blot should be followed as previously recommended (38).
- If the HIV-2 supplemental test is positive, the person should be considered to be HIV infected and counseled and managed accordingly. The case should be reported to the state department of public health as presumptive HIV-2 infection.
- If the HIV-2 supplemental test is indeterminate, the person should have follow-up testing 6 months later to exclude the possibility of early infection with HIV-1 or HIV-2.

4. If an HIV-2 EIA is not repeatedly reactive for a person with an indeterminate HIV-1 Western blot, the person should be followed as previously recommended (38).

REFERENCES: AS NUMBERED IN ORIGINAL PUBLICATION

33. Jackson JB, Balfour HH Jr. Practical diagnostic testing for human immunodeficiency virus. Clin Microbiol Rev 1988;1:124–138.
34. Surgeon General's Report on Acquired Immune Deficiency Syndrome. JAMA 1986;256:2783–2789.
35. Clavel F, Mansinho K, Chamaret S, et al. Human immunodeficiency virus type 2 infection associated with AIDS in West Africa. N Engl J Med 1987;316:1180–1185.
36. Brun-Vezinet F, Rey MA, Katlama C, et al. Lymphadenopathy-associated virus type 2 in AIDS and AIDS-related complex. Lancet 1987;1:128–132.
37. Marlink R, Thior I, Dia MC, et al. Prospective study of the natural history of HIV-2 [Abstract Tu.C.104]. Presented at the VII International Conference on AIDS, Florence, June 18, 1991.
38. Pepin J, Morgan G, Dunn D, et al. HIV-2-induced immunosuppression among asymptomatic West African prostitutes: evidence that HIV-2 is pathogenic, but less so than HIV-1. AIDS 1991;5:1166–1172.

Guidelines for Effective School Health Education to Prevent the Spread of AIDS

Original Citation: Centers for Disease Control and Prevention. Guidelines for Effective School Health Education to Prevent the Spread of AIDS. MMWR 1988;37(S-2):1–14.

Editor's Note: The information included here was based on an article which summarizes guidelines to help school personnel and others plan, implement, and evaluate educational efforts to prevent AIDS. A list of organizations and individual consultants who helped develop the guidelines is included.

PLANNING AND IMPLEMENTING EFFECTIVE SCHOOL HEALTH EDUCATION ABOUT AIDS

The Nation's public and private schools have the capacity and responsibility to help assure that young people understand the nature of the AIDS epidemic and the specific actions they can take to prevent HIV infection, especially during their adolescence and young adulthood. The specific scope and content of

AIDS education in schools should be locally determined and should be consistent with parental and community values.

Because AIDS is a fatal disease and because educating young people about becoming infected through sexual contact can be controversial, school systems should obtain broad community participation to ensure that school health education policies and programs to prevent the spread of AIDS are locally determined and are consistent with community values.

The development of school district policies on AIDS education can be an important first step in developing an AIDS education program. In each community, representatives of the school board, parents, school administrators and faculty, school health services, local medical societies, the local health department, students, minority groups, religious organizations, and other relevant organizations can be involved in developing policies for school health education to prevent the spread of AIDS. The process of policy development can enable these representatives to resolve various perspectives and opinions, to establish a commitment for implementing and maintaining AIDS education programs, and to establish standards for AIDS education program activities and materials. Many communities already have school health councils that include representatives from the aforementioned groups. Such councils facilitate the development of a broad base of community expertise and input, and they enhance the coordination of various activities within the comprehensive school health program (6).

AIDS education programs should be developed to address the needs and the developmental levels of students and of school-age youth who do not attend school, and to address specific needs of minorities, persons for whom English is not the primary language, and persons with visual or hearing impairments or other learning disabilities. Plans for addressing students' questions or concerns about AIDS at the early elementary grades, as well as for providing effective school health education about AIDS at each grade from late elementary/middle school through junior high/senior high school, including educational materials to be used, should be reviewed by representatives of the school board, appropriate school administrators, teachers, and parents before being implemented.

Education about AIDS may be most appropriate and effective when carried out within a more comprehensive school health education program that establishes a foundation for understanding the relationships between personal behavior and health (7–9). For example, education about AIDS may be more effective when students at appropriate ages are more knowledgeable about sexually transmitted diseases, drug abuse, and community health. It may also have greater impact when they have opportunities to develop such qualities as decision-making and communication skills, resistance to persuasion, and a sense of self-efficacy and self-esteem. However, education about AIDS should be provided as rapidly as possible, even if it is taught initially as a separate subject.

State departments of education and health should work together to help local departments of education and health throughout the state collaboratively accomplish effective school health education about AIDS. Although all schools in a state should provide effective education about AIDS, priority should be given to areas with the highest reported incidence of AIDS cases.

PREPARATION OF EDUCATION PERSONNEL

A team of representatives including the local school board, parent-teachers associations, school administrators, school physicians, school nurses, teachers, educational support personnel, school counselors, and other relevant school personnel should receive general training about (a) the nature of the AIDS epidemic and means of controlling its spread, (b) the role of the school in providing education to prevent transmission of HIV, (c) methods and materials to accomplish effective programs of school health education about AIDS, and (d) school policies for students and staff who may be infected. In addition, a team of school personnel responsible for teaching about AIDS should receive more specific training about AIDS education. All school personnel, especially those who teach about AIDS, periodically should receive continuing education about AIDS to assure that they have the most current information about means of controlling the epidemic, including up-to-date information about the most effective health education interventions available. State and local departments of education and health, as well as colleges of education, should assure that such in-service training is made available to all schools in the state as soon as possible and that continuing in-service and pre-service training is subsequently provided. The local school board should assure that release time is provided to enable school personnel to receive such in-service training.

PROGRAMS TAUGHT BY QUALIFIED TEACHERS

In the elementary grades, students generally have one regular classroom teacher. In these grades, education about AIDS should be provided by the regular classroom teacher because that person ideally should be trained and experienced in child development, age-appropriate teaching methods, child health, and elementary health education methods and materials. In addition, the elementary teacher usually is sensitive to normal variations in child development and aptitudes within a class. In the secondary grades, students generally have a different teacher for each subject. In these grades, the secondary school health education teacher preferably should provide education about AIDS, because a qualified health education teacher will have training and experience in adolescent development, age-appropriate teaching methods, adolescent health, and secondary school health education methods and materials (including methods and materials for teaching about such topics as human sexuality, communicable diseases, and drug abuse). In secondary schools that do not have a qualified health education teacher, faculty with similar training and good rapport with students should be trained specifically to provide effective AIDS education.

PURPOSE OF EFFECTIVE EDUCATION ABOUT AIDS

The principal purpose of education about AIDS is to prevent HIV infection. The content of AIDS education should be developed with the active involvement of parents and should address the broad range of behavior exhibited by young people. Educational programs should assure that young people acquire the knowledge and skills they will need to adopt and maintain types of behavior that virtually eliminate their risk of becoming infected.

School systems should make programs available that will enable and encourage young people who have not engaged in sexual intercourse and who have not used illicit drugs to continue to—

- Abstain from sexual intercourse until they are ready to establish a mutually monogamous relationship within the context of marriage;
- Refrain from using or injecting illicit drugs.

For young people who have engaged in sexual intercourse or who have injected illicit drugs, school programs should enable and encourage them to—

- Stop engaging in sexual intercourse until they are ready to establish a mutually monogamous relationship within the context of marriage;
- To stop using or injecting illicit drugs.

Despite all efforts, some young people may remain unwilling to adopt behavior that would virtually eliminate their risk of becoming infected. Therefore, school systems, in consultation with parents and health officials, should provide AIDS education programs that address preventive types of behavior that should be practiced by persons with an increased risk of acquiring HIV infection. These include:

- Avoiding sexual intercourse with anyone who is known to be infected, who is at risk of being infected, or whose HIV infection status is not known;
- Using a latex condom with spermicide if they engage in sexual intercourse;
- Seeking treatment if addicted to illicit drugs;
- Not sharing needles or other injection equipment;
- Seeking HIV counseling and testing if HIV infection is suspected.

State and local education and health agencies should work together to assess the prevalence of these types of risk behavior, and their determinants, over time.

CONTENT

Although information about the biology of the AIDS virus, the signs and symptoms of AIDS, and the social and economic costs of the epidemic might be of interest, such information is not the essential knowledge that students must acquire in order to prevent becoming infected with HIV. Similarly, a single film, lecture, or school assembly about AIDS will not be sufficient to assure that students develop the complex understanding and skills they will need to avoid becoming infected.

Schools should assure that students receive at least the essential information about AIDS, as summarized in sequence in the following pages, for each of three grade-level ranges. The exact grades at which students receive this essential information should be determined locally, in accord with community and parental values, and thus may vary from community to community. Because essential information for students at higher grades requires an understanding of information essential for students at lower grades, secondary school personnel will need to assure that students understand basic concepts before teaching more advanced information. Schools simultaneously should assure that students have opportunities to learn about emotional and social factors that influence types of behavior associated with HIV transmission.

Early Elementary School

Education about AIDS for students in early elementary grades principally should be designed to allay excessive fears of the epidemic and of becoming infected.

AIDS is a disease that is causing some adults to get very sick, but it does not commonly affect children.

AIDS is very hard to get. You cannot get it just by being near or touching someone who has it.

Scientists all over the world are working hard to find a way to stop people from getting AIDS and to cure those who have it.

Late Elementary/Middle School

Education about AIDS for students in late elementary/middle school grades should be designed with consideration for the following information.

Viruses are living organisms too small to be seen by the unaided eye.

Viruses can be transmitted from an infected person to an uninfected person through various means.

Some viruses cause disease among people.

Persons who are infected with some viruses that cause disease may not have any signs or symptoms of disease.

AIDS (an abbreviation for acquired immunodeficiency syndrome) is caused by a virus that weakens the ability of infected individuals to fight off disease.

People who have AIDS often develop a rare type of severe pneumonia, a cancer called Kaposi's sarcoma, and certain other diseases that healthy people normally do not get.

About 1 to 1.5 million of the total population of approximately 240 million Americans currently are infected with the AIDS virus and consequently are capable of infecting others.

People who are infected with the AIDS virus live in every state in the United States and in most other countries of the world.

Infected people live in cities as well as in suburbs, small towns, and rural areas. Although most infected people are adults, teenagers can also become infected. Females as well as males are infected. People of every race are infected, including whites, blacks, Hispanics, Native Americans, and Asian/Pacific Islanders.

The AIDS virus can be transmitted by sexual contact with an infected person; by using needles and other injection equipment that an infected person has used; and from an infected mother to her infant before or during birth.

A small number of doctors, nurses, and other medical personnel have been infected when they were directly exposed to infected blood.

It sometimes takes several years after becoming infected with the AIDS virus before symptoms of the disease appear. Thus, people who are infected with the virus can infect other people—even though the people who transmit the infection do not feel or look sick.

Most infected people who develop symptoms of AIDS only live about 2 years after their symptoms are diagnosed.

The AIDS virus cannot be caught by touching someone who is infected, by being in the same room with an infected person, or by donating blood.

Junior High/Senior High School

Education about AIDS for students in junior high/senior high school grades should be developed and presented taking into consideration the following information.

The virus that causes AIDS, and other health problems, is called human immunodeficiency virus, or HIV.

The risk of becoming infected with HIV can be virtually eliminated by not engaging in sexual activities and by not using illegal intravenous drugs.

Sexual transmission of HIV is not a threat to those uninfected individuals who engage in mutually monogamous sexual relations.

HIV may be transmitted in any of the following ways: (a) by sexual contact with an infected person (penis/vagina, penis/rectum, mouth/vagina, mouth/ penis, mouth/ rectum); (b) by using needles or other injection equipment that an infected person has used; (c) from an infected mother to her infant before or during birth.

A small number of doctors, nurses, and other medical personnel have been infected when they were directly exposed to infected blood.

The following are at increased risk of having the virus that causes AIDS and consequently of being infectious: (a) persons with clinical or laboratory evidence of infection; (b) males who have had sexual intercourse with other males; (c) persons who have injected illegal drugs; (d) persons who have had numerous sexual partners, including male or female prostitutes; (e) persons who received blood clotting products before 1985; (f) sex partners of infected persons or persons at increased risk; and (g) infants born to infected mothers.

The risk of becoming infected is increased by having a sexual partner who is at increased risk of having contracted the AIDS virus (as identified previously), practicing sexual behavior that results in the exchange of body fluids (i.e., semen, vaginal secretions, blood), and using unsterile needles or paraphernalia to inject drugs.

Although no transmission from deep, open-mouth (i.e., "French") kissing has been documented, such kissing theoretically could transmit HIV from an infected to an uninfected person through direct exposure of mucous membranes to infected blood or saliva.

In the past, medical use of blood, such as transfusing blood and treating hemophiliacs with blood clotting products, has caused some people to become infected with HIV. However, since 1985 all donated blood has been tested to determine whether it is infected with HIV; moreover, all blood clotting products have been made from screened plasma and have been heated to destroy any HIV that might remain in the concentrate. Thus, the risk of becoming infected with HIV from blood transfusions and from blood clotting products is virtually eliminated. Cases of HIV infection caused by these medical uses of blood will continue to be diagnosed, however, among people who were infected by these means before 1985.

Persons who continue to engage in sexual intercourse with persons who are at increased risk or whose infection status is unknown should use a latex condom (not natural membrane) to reduce the likelihood of becoming infected. The latex condom must be applied properly and used from start to finish for every sexual act. Although a latex condom does not provide 100% protection—because it is possible for the condom to leak, break, or slip off—it provides the best protection for people who do not maintain a mutually monogamous relationship with an uninfected partner. Additional protection may be obtained by using spermicides that seem active against HIV and other sexually transmitted organisms in conjunction with condoms.

Behavior that prevents exposure to HIV also may prevent unintended pregnancies and exposure to the organisms that cause Chlamydia infection, gonorrhea, herpes, human papillomavirus, and syphilis.

Persons who believe they may be infected with the AIDS virus should take precautions not to infect others and to seek counseling and antibody testing to determine whether they are infected. If persons are not infected, counseling and testing can relieve unnecessary anxiety and reinforce the need to adopt or continue practices that reduce the risk of infection. If persons are infected, they should: (a) take precautions to protect sexual partners from becoming infected; (b) advise previous and current sexual or drug-use partners to receive counseling and testing; (c) take precautions against becoming pregnant; and (d) seek medical care and counseling about other medical problems that may result from a weakened immunologic system.

More detailed information about AIDS, including information about how to obtain counseling and testing for HIV, can be obtained by telephoning the AIDS National Hotline (toll free) at 800-342-2437; the Sexually Transmitted Diseases National Hotline (toll free) at 800-227-8922; or the appropriate state or local health department (the telephone number of which can be obtained by calling the local information operator).

CURRICULUM TIME AND RESOURCES

Schools should allocate sufficient personnel time and resources to assure that policies and programs are developed and implemented with appropriate community involvement, curricula are well-planned and sequential, teachers are well-trained, and up-to-date teaching methods and materials about AIDS are available. In addition, it is crucial that sufficient classroom time be provided at each grade level to assure that students acquire essential knowledge appropriate for that grade level, and have time to ask questions and discuss issues raised by the information presented.

PROGRAM ASSESSMENT

The criteria recommended in the foregoing "Guidelines for Effective School Health Education To Prevent the Spread of AIDS" are summarized in the following nine assessment criteria. Local school boards and administrators can assess the extent to which their programs are consistent with these guidelines by determining the extent to which their programs meet each point shown below. Personnel in state departments of education and health also can use these criteria to monitor the extent to which schools in the state are providing effective health education about AIDS.

1. To what extent are parents, teachers, students, and appropriate community representatives involved in developing, implementing, and assessing AIDS education policies and programs?
2. To what extent is the program included as an important part of a more comprehensive school health education program?
3. To what extent is the program taught by regular classroom teachers in elementary grades and by qualified health education teachers or other similarly trained personnel in secondary grades?
4. To what extent is the program designed to help students acquire essential knowledge to prevent HIV infection at each appropriate grade?
5. To what extent does the program describe the benefits of abstinence for young people and mutually monogamous relationships within the context of marriage for adults?
6. To what extent is the program designed to help teenage students avoid specific types of behavior that increase the risk of becoming infected with HIV?
7. To what extent is adequate training about AIDS provided for school administrators, teachers, nurses, and counselors—especially those who teach about AIDS?
8. To what extent are sufficient program development time, classroom time, and educational materials provided for education about AIDS?
9. To what extent are the processes and outcomes of AIDS education being monitored and periodically assessed?

REFERENCES: AS NUMBERED IN ORIGINAL PUBLICATION

6. Kolbe LJ, Iverson DC. Integrating school and community efforts to promote health: strategies, policies, and methods. Int J Health Educ 1983;2:40–47.
7. Noak M. Recommendations for school health education. Denver: Education Commission of the States, 1982.
8. Comprehensive school health education as defined by the national professional school health education organizations. J Sch Health 1984;54:312–315.
9. Allensworth D, Kolbe L, eds. The comprehensive school health program: exploring an expanded concept. J Sch Health 1987;57:402–476.

SUBTOPIC / PREVENTION

USPHS/IDSA Guidelines for the Prevention of Opportunistic Infections in Persons Infected with HIV: A Summary

Original Citation: Centers for Disease Control and Prevention. USPHS/IDSA Guidelines for the Prevention of Opportunistic Infections in Persons Infected with Human Immunodeficiency Virus: A Summary. MMWR 1995;44(RR-8):1–34.

Editor's Note: The information included here was based on an article which was published as an issue of MMWR recommendations and Reports (Vol. 44, No. RR-8) and is excerpted from a document developed by the USPHS/IDSA Working Group on the Prevention of Opportunistic Infections and published as a supplement to Clinical Infectious Diseases in August 1995. The original text also includes the background information on opportunistic infections in HIV infection and on the development of these recommendations.

Several factors were considered in developing these recommendations, including (a) the level of immunosuppression at which opportunistic disease is most likely to occur; (b) the incidence of disease; (c) the severity of disease in terms of morbidity, cost of care (including hospitalization), and mortality; (d) the feasibility, efficacy, and cost of the prevention measure; (e) the impact of the prevention measure on the quality of life; and (f) (for chemoprophylaxis recommendations) drug toxicities, drug interactions, and the potential for the development of drug resistance. Recommendations are rated according to the strength of the recommendation for or against use (letters A-E) and the quality of the evidence supporting the recommendation (Roman numerals I–III) (6) (Table 1, Table 2). When applying the letter ratings A–E to recommendations involving chemoprophylaxis, the strength of evidence and magnitude of clinical benefit were balanced against the toxicity, drug interactions, and cost of the chemoprophylactic regimen and the feasibility of alternative approaches such as early diagnosis and treatment of the opportunistic infection. Recommendations designated "A" are supported by evidence that is both statistically and clinically persuasive, are strongly recommended, should always be offered, and are considered standard care. Those designated "B" are recommended for consideration; such measures should generally be offered but should involve some discussion of the pros and cons between the provider and the patient. Measures designated "C" are considered optional, either because evidence of benefit is insufficient or because any proven benefit is minimal from the clinical standpoint and may not outweigh either the toxicity, drug interactions, or cost of the chemoprophylaxis or the feasibility of alternative approaches. Measures designated "D" should generally not be offered; those designated "E" are contraindicated. The Roman numeral ratings I–III refer to the quality of evidence that forms the basis for the recommendations regarding the use of a product or measure for preventing opportunistic infections in HIV-infected persons.

Applying this rating system to recommendations regarding prevention of exposure was complicated by the lack of information regarding the effectiveness of various counseling messages. Therefore, few "prevention of exposure" recommendations are rated "A"; many are considered optional (rating "C"). However, use of the rating system should facilitate understanding of the relative importance of the various prevention recommendations.

The prevention recommendations presented here differ from those previously published because they include strategies for preventing many opportunistic infections not previously discussed, particularly those associated with prevention of exposure. They also modify earlier recommendations. For ex-

Table 1. Categories reflecting the strength of each recommendation for or against the use of a product or measure for the prevention of opportunistic infection in HIV-infected persons

Category	Definition
A	Both strong evidence and substantial clinical benefit support a recommendation for use.
B	Moderate evidence—or strong evidence for only limited benefit—supports a recommendation for use.
C	Poor evidence supports a recommendation for or against use.
D	Moderate evidence supports a recommendation against use.
E	Good evidence supports a recommendation against use.

NOTE: Modified from Gross, et al. (10).

Table 2. Categories reflecting the quality of evidence forming the basis for recommendations regarding the use of a product or measure for the prevention of opportunistic infection in HIV-infected persons

Category	Definition
I	Evidence from at least one properly randomized, controlled trial
II	Evidence from at least one well-designed clinical trial without randomization, from cohort or case-controlled analytic studies (preferably from more than one center), or from multiple time-series studies or dramatic results from uncontrolled experiments
III	Evidence from opinions of respected authorities based on clinical experience, descriptive studies, or reports of expert committees

NOTE: Modified from Gross, et al. (10).

ample, for PCP prophylaxis for sulfa-intolerant patients, either dapsone or dapsone plus pyrimethamine are now recommended in preference to aerosolized pentamidine. For prophylaxis against initial episodes of disseminated MAC disease, the threshold of treatment has been lowered from 100 to 75 CD4+ T-lymphocytes/μL. Chemoprophylaxis against toxoplasmic encephalitis is now recommended.

In this report, the disease-specific recommendations are not listed in priority order. Health-care providers who manage and treat HIV-infected patients should consult the overview of the USPHS/IDSA guidelines, which addresses both the initial and follow-up evaluations of the HIV-infected patient (7). In addition to opportunistic infections addressed in the disease-specific recommendations, the overview of the guidelines briefly addresses other infections that occur with increased frequency in HIV-infected persons (e.g., syphilis, hepatitis B, and other sexually transmitted diseases). Sections on preventing opportunistic infections in children and in pregnant women are included. In this report, only the tables concerning drugs and doses in adults and children (Table 3a, Table 3b and Table 4a, Table 4b) and the summary of prevention of exposure recommendations (Table 5) have been excerpted from the overview. The approach to

Table 3a. Prophylaxis for first episode of opportunistic disease in HIV-infected adults and adolescents

Pathogen	Indication	Preventive regimens	
		First choice	Alternatives
I. Strongly recommended as standard of care			
Pneumocystis carinii*	CD4+ count of <200/μL or unexplained fever for ≥2 w OR oropharyngeal candidiasis	TMP-SMZ, 1 DS po q.d. (AI)	TMP-SMZ, 1 SS po q.d. (AI) or 1 DS po t.i.w. (AII); dapsone, 50 mg po b.i.d. or 100 mg po q.d., (AI); dapsone, 50 mg po q.d., PLUS pyrimethamine, 50 mg po q.w., PLUS leuco-vorin, 25 mg po q.w. (AI); dapsone, 200 mg po q.w., PLUS pyrimethamine, 75 mg po q.w., PLUS leucovorin, 25 mg po q.w. (AI); aerosolized pentamidine, 300 mg q.m. via Respirgard II nebulizer (AI)
Mycobacterium tuberculosis+ Isoniazid-sensitive	TST reaction of ≥5 mm OR prior positive TST result without treatment OR contact with case of active tuberculosis	Isoniazid, 300 mg po, PLUS pyridoxine, 50 mg po q.d. × 12 mo (AI); OR isoniazid, 900 mg po, PLUS pyridoxine, 50 mg po b.i.w. × 12 mo (BIII)	Rifampin, 600 mg po q.d. × 12 mo (BII)
Isoniazid-resistant	Same as above; high probability of exposure to isoniazid-resistant tuberculosis	Rifampin, 600 mg po q.d. × 12 mo (BII)	Rifabutin, 300 mg po q.d. × 12 mo (CIII)
Multidrug-resistant (isoniazid and rifampin)	Same as above; high probability of exposure to multidrug-resistant tuberculosis	Choice of drugs requires consultation with public health authorities	None

Table 3a.—continued

Pathogen	Indication	Preventive regimens	
		First choice	Alternatives
Toxoplasma gondii&	IgG antibody to Toxoplasma and CD4+ count of <100/µL	TMP-SMZ, 1 DS po q.d. (AII)	TMP-SMZ, 1 SS po q.d. OR 1 DS po t.i.w. (AII); dapsone, 50 mg po q.d. PLUS pyrimethamine, 50 mg po q.w., PLUS leucovorin, 25 mg po q.w. (AI)
II. Recommended for consideration in all patients			
Streptococcus pneumoniae@	All patients	Pneumococcal vaccine, 0.5 mL im × 1 (BIII)	None
Mycobacterium avium complex**	CD4+ count of <75/µL	Rifabutin, 300 mg po q.d. (BII)	Clarithromycin, 500 mg po b.i.d. (CIII); azithromycin, 500 mg po t.i.w. (CIII)
III. Not recommended for most patients; indicated for consideration ONLY in selected populations or patients			
Bacteria	Neutropenia	Granulocyte colony-stimulating factor 5–10 ug/kg sc q.d. × 2–4 w; OR granulocyte-macrophage colony-stimulating factor, 250 ug/m ((2)), i v over 2 h q.d. × 2–4 w (CIII)	None

Candida species	CD4+ count of <50/µL	Fluconazole, 100–200 mg po q.d. (CI)	Ketoconazole, 200 mg po q.d. (CIII)
Cryptococcus neoformans[++]	CD4+ count of <50/µL	Fluconazole, 100–200 mg po q.d. (BI)	Itraconazole, 200 mg po q.d. (CIII)
Histoplasma capsulatum[++]	CD4+ count of <50/µL, endemic geographic area	Itraconazole, 200 mg po q.d. (CIII)	Fluconazole, 200 mg po q.d. (CIII)
Coccidioides immitis[++]	CD4+ count of <50/µL, endemic geographic region	Fluconazole, 200 mg po q.d. (CIII)	Itraconazole, 200 mg po q.d. (CIII)
CMV[&&]	CD4+ count of <50/µL and CMV antibody positivity	Oral ganciclovir, 1 g po t.i.d. (CIII; only preliminary data available)	None
Unknown (herpesviruses?)[@@]	CD4+ count of <200/µL	Acyclovir, 800 mg po q.i.d. (CIII)	Acyclovir, 200 mg po t.i.d./q.i.d. (CIII)
IV. Recommended for consideration***			
Hepatitis B virus[@]	All susceptible (anti-HBc-negative) patients	Energix-B, 20 ug im × 3 (BII); OR Recombivax HB, 10 ug im × 3 (BI)	None
Influenza virus[@]	All patients (annually, before influenza season)	Whole or split virus, 0.5 mL im/y (BIII)	Rimantadine, 100 mg po b.i.d. (CIII); OR amantadine, 100 mg po b.i.d. (CIII)[+++]

NOTE: Not all of the recommended regimens reflect current Food and Drug Administration-approved labeling. Anti-HBc = antibody to hepatitis B core antigen; b.i.w. = twice weekly; CMV = cytomegalovirus; DS = double-strength tablet; q.m. = monthly; q.w. = weekly; ss = single-strength tablet; t.i.w. = three times weekly; TMP-SMZ = trimethoprim-sulfamethoxazole; and TST = tuberculin skin test. The Respigard II nebulizer is manufactured by Marquest, Englewood, CO; Energix-B by SmithKline Beecham, Rixensart, Belgium; and Recombivax HB by Merck & Co., West Point, PA. Letters and Roman numerals in parentheses after regimens indicate the strength of the recommendation and the quality of the evidence supporting it (see text).

*Patients receiving dapsone should be tested for glucose-6-phosphate dehydrogenase deficiency. A dosage of 50 mg q.d. is probably less effective than a dosage of 100 mg q.d. The efficacy of parenteral pentamidine (e.g., 4 mg/kg/q.m.) is uncertain. Inadequate data are available on the efficacy and safety of atovaquone or clindamycin/primaquine. Sulfadoxine/pyrimethamine (Fansidar, Roche Laboratories, Nutley, NJ) is rarely used because it can elicit severe hypersensitivity reactions. TMP-SMZ and dapsone/pyrimethamine (and possibly dapsone alone) appear to be protective against toxoplasmosis. TMP-SMZ may reduce the frequency of some bacterial infections. Patients receiving therapy for toxoplasmosis with sulfadiazine/pyrimethamine are protected against P. carinii pneumonia and do not need TMP-SMZ.

Table 3a.—*continued*

[+]Directly observed therapy is required for 900 mg of isonizid b.i.w.; isoniazid regimens should include pyridoxine to prevent peripheral neuropathy. Exposure to multidrug-resistant tuberculosis may require prophylaxis with two drugs; consult public health authorities. Possible regimens include pyrazinamide plus either ethambutol or a fluoroquinolone (16).

[&]Protection against T. gondii is provided by the preferred antipneumocystis regimens. Pyrimethamine alone probably provides little, if any, protection. Dapsone alone cannot be recommended on the basis of currently available data.

[@]Data are inadequate concerning clinical benefit of vaccines against S. pneumoniae, influenza virus, and hepatitis B virus in HIV-infected persons, although it is logical to assume that those patients who develop antibody responses will derive some protection. Some authorities are concerned that immunizations may stimulate the replication of HIV. Prophylaxis with TMP-SMZ may provide some clinical benefit by reducing the frequency of bacterial infections, but the prevalence of S. pneumoniae resistant to TMP-SMX is increasing. Hepatitis B vaccine has been recommended for all children and adolescents and for all adults with risk factors for hepatitis B infection. For additional information regarding vaccination against hepatitis B and vaccination and antiviral therapy against influenza, (17-19).

[**]Data on 500 mg of clarithromycin po b.i.d. have been presented but have not yet been thoroughly analyzed. Data on the efficacy and safety of azithromycin prophylaxis are not yet available.

[++]There may be a few unusual occupational or other circumstances under which prophylaxis should be considered; consult a specialist.

[&&]Data on oral ganciclovir are still being evaluated; the durability of its effect is unclear. Acyclovir is not protective against CMV.

[@@]Data regarding the efficacy of acyclovir for prolonging survival are controversial; if acyclovir is beneficial, the biologic basis for the effect and the optimal dose and timing of therapy are uncertain.

[***]These immunizations or chemoprophylactic regimens are not targeted against pathogens traditionally classified as opportunistic but should be considered for use in HIV-infected patients. While the use of those products is logical, their clinical efficacy has not been validated in this population.

[+++]During outbreaks of influenza A.

Table 3b. Prophylaxis for recurrence of opportunistic disease (after chemotherapy for acute disease) in HIV-infected adults and adolescents

Pathogen	Indication	Preventive regimens	
		First choice	Alternatives
I. Recommended for life as standard of care			
Pneumocystis carinii	Prior P. carinii pneumonia	TMP-SMZ, 1 DS po q.d. (AI)	TMP-SMZ, 1 SS po q.d. (AI) OR 1 DS po t.i.w. (AII); dapsone, 50 mg po b.i.d. OR 100 mg po q.d. (AI); dapsone, 50 mg po q.d., PLUS pyrimethamine, 50 mg po q.w., PLUS leucovorin, 25 mg po q.w. (AI); dapsone, 200 mg po q.w., PLUS pyrimethamine, 75 mg po q.w., PLUS leucovorin, 25 mg po q.w. (AI); aerosolized pentamidine, 300 mg q.m. via Respirgard II nebulizer (AI)
Toxoplasma gondii*	Prior toxoplasmic encephalitis	Sulfadiazine, 1.0–1.5 g po q6h, PLUS pyrimethamine, 25–75 mg po q.d., PLUS leucovorin, 10–25 mg po q.d.-q.i.d. (AII)	Clindamycin, 300–450 mg po q6-8h, PLUS pyrimethamine, 25–75 po q.d., PLUS leucovorin, 10–25 mg po q.d.-q.i.d. (AII)

Table 3b.—*continued*

Pathogen	Indication	Preventive regimens	
		First choice	Alternatives
Mycobacterium avium complex[+]	Documented disseminated disease	Clarithromycin, 500 mg po b.i.d., PLUS one or more of the following: ethambutol, 15 mg/kg po q.d.; clofazimine, 100 mg po q.d.; rifabutin, 300 mg po q.d.; ciprofloxacin, 500–750 mg po b.i.d. (BIII)	Azithromycin, 500 mg po q.d., PLUS one or more of the following: ethambutol, 15 mg/kg po q.d.; clofazimine, 100 mg po q.d.; rifabutin, 300 mg po q.d.; ciprofloxacin, 500–750 mg po b.i.d. (BIII)
Cytomegalovirus[&]	Prior end-organ disease	Ganciclovir, 5–6 mg/kg iv 5–7 d/w or 1,000 mg po t.i.d. (AI); OR foscarnet, 90–120 mg/kg iv q.d. (AI)	Sustained-release implants used investigationally
Cryptococcus neoformans	Documented disease	Fluconazole, 200 mg po q.d. (AI)	Itraconazole, 200 mg po q.d. (BIII); amphotericin B, 0.6–1.0 mg/kg iv q.w.-t.i.w. (AI)
Histoplasma capsulatum	Documented disease	Itraconazole, 200 mg po b.i.d. (AII)	Amphotericin B, 1.0 mg/kg iv q.w. (AI); fluconazole, 200–400 mg po q.d. (BIII)

Coccidioides immitis	Documented disease	Fluconazole, 200 mg po q.d. (AII)	Amphotericin B, 1.0 mg/kg iv q.w. (AI); itraconazole, 200 mg po b.i.d. (AII); ketoconazole, 400–800 mg po q.d. (BII)
Salmonella species (non-typhi)@	Bacteremia	Ciprofloxacin 500 mg po b.i.d. for several months (BII)	None
II. Recommended only if subsequent episodes are frequent or severe			
Herpes simplex virus	Frequent/severe recurrences	Acyclovir, 200 mg po t.i.d. OR 400 mg po b.i.d. (AI)	None
Candida species (oral, vaginal, or esophageal)	Frequent/severe recurrences	Fluconazole, 100–200 mg po q.d. (AI)	Ketoconazole, 200 mg po q.d. (BII); itraconazole, 100 mg po q.d. (BII); clotrimazole troche, 10 mg po 5×/d (BII); nystatin, 5×10 ((5)) U po 5×/d (CIII)

NOTE: Not all of the recommended regimens reflect current Food and Drug Administration-approved labeling. DS = double-strength tablet; q.m. = monthly; q.w. = weekly; SS = single-strength tablet; t.i.w. = three times weekly; and TMP-SMZ = trimethoprim-sulfamethoxazole. The Respirgard II nebulizer is manufactured by Marquest, Englewood, CO. Letters and Roman numerals in parentheses after regimens indicate the strength of the recommendation and the quality of the evidence supporting it (see text).

*Only pyrimethamine/sulfadiozine confers protection against P. carinii pneumonia.

+The long-term efficacy of any regimen is not well established. Many multiple-drug regimens are poorly tolerated. Drug interactions (e.g., those seen with clarithromycin/rifabutin) can be problematic. Rifabutin has been associated with uveitis, especially when given at daily doses of >300 mg or along with fluconazole or clarithromycin.

&Ganciclovir and foscarnet delay relapses by only modest intervals (often only 4–8 weeks). Ocular implants with sustained-release ganciclovir appear promising.

@Efficacious eradication of Salmonella has been demonstrated only for ciprofloxacin.

Table 4a. Prophylaxis for first episode of opportunistic disease in HIV-infected infants and children

Pathogen	Indication	Preventive regimens	
		First choice	Alternatives
I. Strongly recommended as standard of care			
Pneumocystis carinii*	All infants 1–4 mo old born to HIV-infected women; HIV-infected or HIV-indeterminate infants <12 mo old; HIV-infected children 1–5 y old with CD4+ count of <500/μL or CD4+ percentage of <15%; HIV-infected children 6–12 y old with CD4+ count of <200/μL or CD4+ percentage of <15%	TMP-SMZ, 150/750 mg/ m((2))/d in 2 divided doses po t.i.w. on consecutive days (AII); acceptable alternative schedules for same dosage (AII); single dose po t.i.w. on consecutive days, 2 divided doses po q.d., or 2 divided doses po t.i.w. on alternate days	Aerosolized pentamidine (children ≥5 y old), 300 mg q.m. via Respirgard II nebulizer (CIII); dapsone (children ≥1 mo old), 2 mg/kg (not to exceed 100 mg) po q.d. (CIII); iv pentamidine, 4 mg/kg every 2–4 w (CIII)
Mycobacterium tuberculosis			
Isoniazid-sensitive	TST reaction of ≥5 mm OR prior positive TST result without treatment OR contact with case of active tuberculosis	Isoniazid, 10–15 mg/kg (maximum, 300 mg) po or im q.d. × 12 mo OR 20–30 mg/kg (maximum, 900 mg) po b.i.w. × 12 mo (BIII)	Rifampin, 10–20 mg/kg (maximum, 600 mg) po or iv q.d. × 12 mo (BII)
Isoniazid-resistant	Same as above; high probability of exposure to isoniazid-resistant tuberculosis	Rifampin, 10–20 mg/kg (maximum, 600 mg) po or iv q.d. × 12 mo (BII)	Uncertain
Multidrug-resistant (isoniazid and rifampin)	Same as above; high probability of exposure to multidrug-resistant tuberculosis	Choice of drugs requires consultation with public health authorities	None

Pathogen	Indication	First choice	Alternatives
Varicella-zoster virus	Significant exposure to varicella with NO history of varicella	VZIG, 1 vial (1.25 mL)/10 kg (maximum, 5 vials) im, given ≤96 h after exposure, ideally within 48 h (AI) (Children routinely receiving IVIG should receive VZIG if the last dose of IVIG was given >14 d before exposure.)	None
Various pathogens	HIV exposure/infection	Immunizations**	None
II. Recommended for consideration in all patients			
Toxoplasma gondii+	IgG antibody to Toxoplasma with severe immunosuppression (CD4+ count of <100/µL) (Prophylaxis may be considered at higher CD4+ counts in the youngest infants, but no relevant data are available.)	TMP-SMZ, 150/750 mg/m((2))/d in 2 divided doses po t.i.w. on consecutive days (CIII); acceptable alternative schedules for same dosage (CIII): single dose po t.i.w. on consecutive days, 2 divided doses po q.d., or 2 divided doses po t.i.w. on alternate days	Dapsone (children ≥1 mo old), 2 mg/kg or 15 mg/m((2)) (maximum, 25 mg) po q.d., PLUS pyrimethamine, 1 mg/kg po q.d., PLUS leucovorin, 5 mg po every 3 d (CIII)
Mycobacterium avium complex	CD4+ count of <75/µL	Children 6–12 y old: rifabutin, 300 mg po q.d. (BI); children <6 y old: 5 mg/kg po q.d. when suspension is available (BI)	All ages: azithromycin, 7.5 mg/kg in 2 divided doses po q.d. (CIII); clarithromycin, 5–12 mg/kg po q.d. (CIII)
III. Not recommended for most patients; indicated for consideration ONLY in selected patients			
Invasive bacterial infections	Hypogammaglobulinemia	IVIG, 400 mg/kg q.m. (AI)	None

Table 4a.—_continued_

Pathogen	Indication	Preventive regimens	
		First choice	Alternatives
Candida species&	Severe immunosuppression	Nystatin (100,000 U/mL), 4–6 mL po q6h; or topical clotrimazole, 10 mg po 5×/d (CII)	Ketoconazole, 5–10 mg/kg po q12–24h (CI); fluconazole, 2–8 mg/kg po q.d. (CI)
Cryptococcus neoformans	Severe immunosuppression	Fluconazole, 2–8 mg/kg po q.d. (BI)	Itraconazole, 2–5 mg/kg po q12–24h (CIII)
Histoplasma capsulatum	Severe immunosuppression, endemic geographic area	Itraconazole, 2–5 mg/kg po q12–24h (CIII)	Fluconazole, 2–8 mg/kg po q.d. (CIII)
Coccidioides immitis	Severe immunosuppression, endemic geographic area	Fluconazole, 2–8 mg/kg po q.d. (CIII)	Itraconazole, 2–5 mg/kg po q12–24h (CIII)
CMV@	CD4+ count of <50/µL and CMV antibody positivity	Children 6–12 y old: oral ganciclovir under investigation	None
Influenza A virus	High risk of exposure (e.g., institutional outbreak)	Rimantadine or amantadine, 5 mg/kg q.d. (maximum, 150 mg) in 2 divided doses po for children <10 y old; for children ≥10 y old, 5 mg/kg up to 40 kg, then 200 mg in 2 divided doses po q.d.	None

NOTE: Not all of the recommended regimens reflect current Food and Drug Administration-approved labeling. b.i.w. = twice weekly; CMV = cytomegalovirus; IVIG = intravenous immune globulin; q.m = monthly; t.i.w. = three times weekly; TMP-SMZ = trimethoprim-sulfamethoxazole; and VZIG = varicella-zoster immune globulin. The Respirgard II nebulizer is manufactured by Marquest, Englewood, CO. Letters and Roman numerals in parentheses after regimens indicate the strength of the recommendation and the quality of the evidence supporting it (see text).
*The efficacy of parenteral pentamidine (e.g., 4 mg/kg q.m.) is controversial. TMP-SMZ and dapsone/pyrimethamine (and possibly dapsone alone) appear to be protective against toxoplasmosis, although relevant data have not been prospectively collected. Daily treatment with TMP-SMZ reduces the frequency of some bacterial infections. Patients receiving sulfadiazine/pyrimethamine for toxoplasmosis are protected against P. carinii pneumonia and do not need TMP-SMZ.

+Protection against T. gondii is provided by the preferred antipneumocystitis regimens. Dapsone alone cannot be recommended on the basis of currently available data. Pyrimethamine alone probably provides little, if any, protection.

&Ketoconazole and fluconazole are preferred for prophylaxis of esophagitis and severe mucocutaneous infection.

@Data on oral ganciclovir are still being evaluated; the durability of its effect is unclear. Acyclovir is not protective against CMV.

**The following immunization schedule for HIV-exposed/infected infants is strongly recommended as the standard of care:

Age (mo)	Immunization (dose)	Age (mo)	Immunization (dose)
Newborn	Hep B (1) [a]	7	Influenza (1) [e]
1	Hep B (2)	8	Influenza (2) [e]
2	DTP (1), Hib (1) [b]	12	Hib (3 or 4) [c], MMR [f]
3	EIPV (1) [b]	15	EIPV (3), DTaP (4) [g]
4	DTP (2), Hib (2) [b]	18	DTaP (4) [g]
5	EIPV (2) [b]	24	Pneumococcal, 23-valent [h]
6	DTP (3), Hib (3), Hep B (3) [b], [c], [d]		

NOTE: DTaP = diphtheria and tetanus toxoids with acellular pertussis; DTP = diphtheria-tetanus-pertussis; EIPV = enhanced inactivated polio vaccine; Hep B = hepatitis B; Hib = Haemophilus influenzae type b; and MMR = measles-mumps-rubella. This schedule differs from that recommended for immunization of immunocompetent children (20, 21) in the following ways: (i) EIPV replaces oral polio vaccine, and the first two doses of EIPV may be given at 3 and 5 months instead of 2 and 4 months; (ii) the second dose of Hep B vaccine is given at 1 month; and (iii) pneumococcal vaccine is recommended. This schedule is designed to deliver vaccine to HIV-infected children as early as possible and to limit the number of injections to two per visit.

[a] Infants born to mothers positive for hepatitis B surface antigen should receive hepatitis B immune globulin within 12 hours of birth in addition to Hep B vaccine (17).

[b] DTP and Hib vaccines are available together or separately. With the combined DTP-Hib vaccine, a single injection on each occasion is sufficient and can be given at 2, 4, and 6 months. Administration of EIPV as a second injection at 2 and 4 months can replace separate immunizations at 3 and 5 months.

[c] The need for a third dose of Hib vaccine depends on which formulation was used previously. Regardless of whether the primary series requires two or three doses, a booster dose is required at 12–15 months.

[d] If DTP and Hib are given as separate injections at 6 months, the third dose of Hep B vaccine may be postponed until the next visit.

[e] Primary immunization against influenza for children <9 years of age requires two doses of vaccine, the first of which can be given as early as 6 months of age (13, 18). Subsequent vaccination should be undertaken annually, before the influenza season.

[f] HIV-infected children should receive prophylactic immunoglobulin after exposure to measles, whether or not they have been vaccinated against measles.

[g] DTaP can be administered at either 15 or 18 months. Alternatively, a fourth dose of DTP can be given as early as 12 months.

[h] Some authorities recommend revaccination for HIV-infected children vaccinated ≥6 years previously (13).

Table 4b. Prophylaxis for recurrence of opportunistic disease (after chemotherapy for acute disease) in HIV-infected infants and children

Pathogen	Indication	Preventive regimens	
		First choice	Alternatives
I. Recommended for life as standard of care			
Pneumocystis carinii	Prior P. carinii pneumonia	TMP-SMZ, 150/750 mg/m((2))/d in 2 divided doses po t.i.w. on consecutive days (AI); acceptable alternative schedules for same dosage (AI); single dose po t.i.w. on consecutive days, 2 divided doses po q.d., or 2 divided doses po t.i.w. on alternate days	Aerosolized pentamidine (children ≥5 y old), 300 mg q.m. via Respirgard II nebulizer (AI); dapsone (children ≥1 mo old), 2 mg/kg (not to exceed 100 mg) po q.d. (CIII); iv pentamidine (4 mg/kg) every 2–4 w (CIII)
Toxoplasma gondii*	Prior toxoplasmic encephalitis	Sulfadiazine, 85–120 mg/kg in 2–4 divided doses po q.d. PLUS pyrimethamine, 1 mg/kg or 15 mg/m((2)) (maximum, 25 mg) po q.d., PLUS leucovorin, 5 mg po every 3 d (AII)	Clindamycin, 20–30 mg/kg in 4 divided doses po q.d., PLUS pyrimethamine, 1 mg/kg po q.d., PLUS leucovorin, 5 mg po every 3 d (AII)
Mycobacterium avium complex[+]	Prior disease	Clarithromycin, 30 mg/kg in 2 divided doses po q.d., PLUS at least one of the following: ethambutol, 15–25 mg/kg po q.d.; clofazimine, 50–100 mg po q.d.; rifabutin, 300 mg po q.d.; ciprofloxacin, 20–30 mg/kg in 2 divided doses po q.d. (CIII)	None

Pathogen	Indication	First choice	Alternative
Cryptococcus neoformans	Documented disease	Fluconazole, 2–8 mg/kg po q.d. (CIII)	Itraconazole, 2–5 mg/kg po q12–24h (CIII); amphotericin B, 0.5–1.5 mg/kg iv q.w.-t.i.w. (AI)
Histoplasma capsulatum	Documented disease	Itraconazole, 2–5 mg/kg po q12–48 h (CIII)	Fluconazole, 2–8 mg/kg po q.d. (CIII); amphotericin B, 1.0 mg/kg iv q.w. (AI)
Coccidioides immitis	Documented disease	Fluconazole, 2–8 mg/kg po q.d. (CIII)	Amphotericin B, 1.0 mg/kg iv q.w. (AI)
Cytomegalovirus&	Prior end-organ disease	Ganciclovir, 10 mg/kg in 2 divided doses iv q.d. for 1 w, then 5 mg/kg iv q.d.; OR foscarnet, 60–120 mg/kg iv q.d. (AI)	None
Salmonella species (non-typhi)@	Bacteremia	TMP/SMZ, 150/750 mg/m ((2)) in 2 divided doses po q.d. for several months (CIII)	Ampicillin, 50–100 mg in 4 divided doses po q.d. (CIII); chloramphenicol, 50–75 mg/kg in 4 divided doses po q.d. (CIII) (For children >6 y old, consider ciprofloxacin, 30 mg in 2 divided doses po q.d. (CIII)
II. Recommended only if subsequent episodes are frequent or severe			
Invasive bacterial infections	More than 2 infections in 1-yr period	IVIG, 400 mg/kg q.m. (AI)	TMP-SMZ 150/750 mg/m((2)) po q.d. (AI)
Herpes simplex virus	Frequent/severe recurrences	Acyclovir, 600–1,000 mg in 3–5 divided doses po q.d. (CIII)	

Table 4b.—*continued*

Pathogen	Indication	Preventive regimens	
		First choice	Alternatives
Candida species	Frequent/severe recurrences	Ketoconazole, 5–10 mg/kg po q12–24h; or fluconazole, 2–8 mg/kg po q.d. (BI)	

NOTE: Not all of the recommended regimens reflect current Food and Drug Administration-approved labeling. IVIG = intravenous immune globulin; q.m. = monthly; q.w. = weekly; t.i.w. = three times weekly; and TMP-SMZ = trimethoprim-sulfamethoxazole. The Respirgard II nebulizer is manufactured by Marquest, Englewood, CO. Letters and Roman numerals in parentheses after regimens indicate the strength of the recommendation and the quality of the evidence supporting it (see text).

*Only pyrimethamine/sulfadiazine confers protection against P. carinii pneumonia. Although the clindamycin/pyrimethamine regimen is an alternative for adults, it has not been tested in children. However, these drugs are safe and are used for other infections.

+Ciprofloxacin should not be given to children <6 years of age. Rifabutin (5 mg/kg po q.d.) may be given to children <6 years of age when a suspension becomes available.

&Oral ganciclovir has not been studied in children.

@Choice of drug should be determined by susceptibilities of the organism isolated.

Table 5. Advising patients about the avoidance of exposure to opportunistic pathogens

Sexual Exposures

1. Patients should use male latex condoms during every act of sexual intercourse to reduce the risk of exposure to cytomegalovirus, herpes simplex virus, and human papillomavirus, as well as to other sexually transmitted pathogens (AII). Use of latex condoms will also prevent the transmission of HIV to others.

2. Patients should avoid sexual practices that may result in oral exposure to feces (e.g., oral-anal contact) to reduce the risk of intestinal infections such as cryptosporidiosis, shigellosis, campylobacteriosis, amebiasis, giardiasis, and hepatitis A and B (BIII).

Environmental and Occupational Exposures

1. Certain activities or types of employment may increase the risk of exposure to tuberculosis (BIII). These include volunteer work or employment in health care facilities, correctional institutions, and shelters for the homeless as well as in other settings identified as high risk by local health authorities. Decisions about whether or not to continue with such activities should be made in conjunction with the health care provider and should take into account such factors as the patient's specific duties in the workplace, the prevalence of tuberculosis in the community, and the degree to which precautions designed to prevent the transmission of tuberculosis are taken in the workplace (BIII). These decisions will affect the frequency with which the patient should be screened for tuberculosis.

2. Child-care providers and parents of children in child-care facilities are at increased risk of acquiring CMV infection, cryptosporidiosis, and other infections (e.g., hepatitis A and giardiasis) from children. The risk of acquiring infection can be diminished by good hygienic practices, such as hand washing after fecal contact (e.g., during diaper changing) and after contact with urine or saliva (AII). All children in child-care facilities are also at increased risk of acquiring these same infections; parents and other caretakers of HIV-infected children should be advised of this risk (BIII).

3. Occupations involving contact with animals (e.g., veterinary work and employment in pet stores, farms, or slaughterhouses) may pose a risk of cryptosporidiosis, toxoplasmosis, salmonellosis, campylobacteriosis, or bartonella infection. However, the available data are insufficient to justify a recommendation against work in such settings.

4. Contact with young farm animals, especially animals with diarrhea, should be avoided to reduce the risk of cryptosporidiosis (BII).

5. Hand washing after gardening or other contact with soil may reduce the risk of cryptosporidiosis and toxoplasmosis (BIII).

6. In histoplasmosis-endemic areas, patients should avoid activities known to be associated with increased risk, including cleaning chicken coops, disturbing soil beneath bird-roosting sites, and exploring caves (CIII).

7. In coccidioidomycosis-endemic areas, when possible, patients should avoid activities associated with increased risk, including those involving extensive exposure to disturbed soil, as occurs at building excavation sites, on farms, or during dust storms (CIII).

Table 5.—_continued_

Pet-Related Exposures

Health care providers should advise HIV-infected persons of the potential risk posed by pet ownership. However, they should be sensitive to the possible psychological benefits of pet ownership and should not routinely advise HIV-infected persons to part with their pets (DIII). Specifically, providers should advise HIV-infected patients of the following.

General

1. Veterinary care should be sought when a pet develops diarrheal illness. If possible, HIV-infected persons should avoid contact with animals that have diarrhea (BIII). A fecal sample should be obtained from animals with diarrhea and examined for Cryptosporidium, Salmonella, and Campylobacter.

2. When obtaining a new pet, HIV-infected patients should avoid animals <6 months of age, especially those with diarrhea (BIII). Because the hygienic and sanitary conditions in pet breeding facilities, pet stores, and animal shelters are highly variable, the patient should exercise caution when obtaining a pet from these sources. Stray animals should be avoided. Animals <6 months of age, especially those with diarrhea, should be examined by a veterinarian for Cryptosporidium, Salmonella, and Campylobacter (BIII).

3. Patients should wash their hands after handling pets (especially before eating) and avoid contact with pets' feces to reduce the risk of cryptosporidiosis, salmonellosis, and campylobacteriosis (BIII). Hand washing by HIV-infected children should be supervised.

Cats

4. Patients should consider the potential risks of cat ownership because of the risks of toxoplasmosis and Bartonella infection, as well as enteric infection (CIII). Those who elect to obtain a cat should adopt or purchase an animal that is >1 year of age and in good health to reduce the risk of cryptosporidiosis, Bartonella infection, salmonellosis, and campylobacteriosis (BII).

5. Litter boxes should be cleaned daily, preferably by an HIV-negative, nonpregnant person; if the HIV-infected patient performs this task, he or she should wash hands thoroughly afterward to reduce the risk of toxoplasmosis (BIII).

6. Also to reduce the risk of toxoplasmosis, cats should be kept indoors, should not be allowed to hunt, and should not be fed raw or undercooked meat (BIII).

7. Although declawing is not generally advised, patients should avoid activities that may result in cat scratches or bites to reduce the risk of Bartonella infection (BII). Patients should also wash sites of cat scratches or bites promptly (CIII); and should not allow cats to lick open cuts or wounds (BIII).

8. Care of cats should include flea control, to reduce the risk of Bartonella infection (CIII).

9. Testing of cats for toxoplasmosis (EII) or Bartonella infection (DII) is not recommended.

Birds

10. Screening of healthy birds for Cryptococcus neoformans, Mycobacterium avium, or Histoplasma capsulatum is not recommended (DIII).

Other

11. Contact with reptiles (such as snakes, lizards, and turtles) should be avoided to reduce the risk of salmonellosis (BIII).
12. Gloves should be used during the cleaning of aquariums to reduce the risk of infection with Mycobacterium marinum (BIII).
13. Contact with exotic pets, such as nonhuman primates, should be avoided (CIII).

Food- and Water-Related Exposures

1. Raw or undercooked eggs (including foods that may contain raw eggs, such as some preparations of hollandaise sauce, Caesar and certain other salad dressings, and mayonnaise); raw or undercooked poultry, meat, seafood; and unpasteurized dairy products may contain enteric pathogens. Poultry and meat should be cooked until no longer pink in the middle (internal temperature, >165 degrees F). Produce should be washed thoroughly before being eaten (BIII).

2. Cross-contamination of foods should be avoided. Uncooked meats should not be allowed to come in contact with other foods; hands, cutting boards, counters, and knives and other utensils should be washed thoroughly after contact with uncooked foods (BIII).

3. Although the incidence of listeriosis is low, it is a serious disease that occurs unusually frequently among HIV-infected persons who are severely immunosuppressed. Some soft cheeses and some ready-to-eat foods (e.g., hot dogs and cold cuts from delicatessen counters) have been known to cause listeriosis. An HIV-infected person who is severely immunosuppressed and who wishes to reduce the risk of food-borne disease can prevent listeriosis by reheating these foods until they are steaming hot before eating (CIII).

4. Patients should not drink water directly from lakes or rivers because of the risk of cryptosporidiosis and giardiasis. Even accidental ingestion of lake or river water while swimming or engaging in other types of recreational activities carries this risk (BII).

5. During outbreaks or in other situations in which a community "boil-water" advisory is issued, boiling of water for 1 minute will eliminate the risk of cryptosporidiosis (AI). Use of submicron, personal-use water filters (home/office types) and/or drinking bottled water* may reduce the risk (CIII). Current data are inadequate to recommend that all HIV-infected persons boil or otherwise avoid drinking tap water in nonoutbreak settings. However, persons who wish to take independent action to reduce the risk of waterborne cryptosporidiosis may choose to take precautions similar to those recommended during outbreaks. Such decisions are best made in conjunction with the health care provider. Persons who opt for a personal-use filter or bottled water should be aware of the complexities involved in selecting the appropriate products, the lack of enforceable standards for destruction or removal of oocytes, the cost of the products, and the difficulty of using these products consistently.

Table 5.—_continued_

Travel-Related Exposures

1. Travel, particularly to developing countries, may carry significant risks for the exposure of HIV-infected persons to opportunistic pathogens, especially for patients who are severely immunosuppressed. Consultation with health care providers and/or with experts in travel medicine will help patients plan itineraries (BIII).

2. During travel to developing countries, HIV-infected persons are at even higher risk for food- and water-borne infections than they are in the United States. Foods and beverages—in particular, raw fruits and vegetables, raw or undercooked seafood or meat, tap water, ice made with tap water, unpasteurized milk and dairy products, and items purchased from street vendors—may be contaminated (AII). Items that are generally safe include steaming-hot foods, fruits that are peeled by the traveler, bottled (especially carbonated) beverages, hot coffee or tea, beer, wine, and water brought to a rolling boil for 1 minute (AII). Treatment of water with iodine or chlorine may not be as effective as boiling but can be used, perhaps in conjunction with filtration, when boiling is not practical (BIII).

3. Waterborne infections may result from the swallowing of water during recreational activities. To reduce the risk of cryptosporidiosis and giardiasis, patients should avoid swallowing water during swimming and should not swim in water that may be contaminated (e.g., with sewage or animal waste) (BII).

4. Antimicrobial prophylaxis for traveler's diarrhea is not recommended routinely for HIV-infected persons traveling to developing countries (DIII). Such preventive therapy can have adverse effects and can promote the emergence of drug-resistant organisms. Nonetheless, several studies (none involving an HIV-infected population) have shown that prophylaxis can reduce the risk of diarrhea among travelers. Under selected circumstances (e.g., those in which the risk of infection is very high and the period of travel brief), the provider and patient may weigh the potential risks and benefits and decide that antibiotic prophylaxis is warranted (CIII). For those individuals to whom prophylaxis is offered, fluoroquinolones, such as ciprofloxacin (500 mg q.d.) can be considered (BIII). Trimethoprim-sulfamethoxazole (TMP-SMZ) (one double-strength tablet daily) has also been shown to be effective, but resistance to this drug is now common in tropical areas. Persons already taking TMP-SMZ for prophylaxis against Pneumocystis carinii pneumonia (PCP) may gain some protection against traveler's diarrhea. For HIV-infected persons who are not already taking TMP-SMZ, the provider should use caution when prescribing this agent for prophylaxis of diarrhea because of the high rates of adverse reactions and the possible need for the agent for other purposes (e.g., PCP prophylaxis) in the future.

5. All HIV-infected travelers to developing countries should carry with them a sufficient supply of an antimicrobial agent to be taken as empirically should diarrhea develop (BIII). One appropriate regimen is 500 mg of ciprofloxacin b.i.d. for 3–7 days. Alternative antibiotics (e.g., TMP-SMZ) should be considered as empirical therapy for use by children and pregnant women (CIII). Travelers should consult a physician if their diarrhea is severe and does not respond to empiric therapy, if their stools contain blood, if fever is accompanied by shaking chills, or if dehydration develops. Antiperistaltic agents such as diphenoxylate and loperamide are used for the treatment of diarrhea; however, they should not be used by patients with high fever or with blood in the stool, and their use should be discontinued if symptoms persist beyond 48 hours (AII). These drugs are not recommended for children (DIII).

6. Travelers should be advised about other preventive measures appropriate for anticipated exposures, such as chemoprophylaxis for malaria, protection against arthropod vectors, treatment with immune globulin, and vaccination (AII). They should avoid direct contact of the skin with soil and sand (e.g., by wearing shoes and protective clothing and using towels on beaches) in areas where fecal contamination of soil is likely (BIII).

7. In general, live virus vaccines should be avoided (EII). An exception is measles vaccine, which is recommended for nonimmune persons. Inactivated (killed) poliovirus vaccine should be used instead of oral (live) poliovirus vaccine. Persons at risk for exposure to typhoid fever should be given inactivated parenteral typhoid vaccine instead of the live attenuated preparation. Yellow fever vaccine is a live virus vaccine with uncertain safety and efficacy in HIV-infected persons. Travelers with asymptomatic HIV infection who cannot avoid potential exposure to yellow fever should be offered the choice of vaccination. If travel to a zone with yellow fever is necessary and immunization is not performed, patients should be advised of the risk, instructed in methods for avoiding the bites of vector mosquitoes, and provided with a vaccination waiver letter.

8. In general, killed vaccines (e.g., diphtheria-tetanus, rabies, Japanese encephalitis vaccines) should be used for HIV-infected persons as they would be used for non-HIV-infected persons anticipating travel (BIII). Preparation for travel should include a review and updating of routine vaccinations, including diphtheria-tetanus for adults and all routine immunizations for children. The currently available cholera vaccine is not recommended for persons following the usual tourist itinerary, even if travel includes countries reporting cases of cholera (DII).

9. Travelers should be told about other area-specific risks and instructed in ways to reduce those risks (BIII). Geographically focal infections that pose a high risk to HIV-infected persons include visceral leishmaniasis (a protozoan infection transmitted by the sandfly) and several fungal infections (e.g., Penicillium marneffei infection, coccidioidomycosis, and histoplasmosis). Many tropical and developing areas have high rates of tuberculosis.

NOTE: Letters and Roman numerals in parentheses indicate the strength of the recommendation and the quality of the evidence supporting it (see text).
*See section on cryptosporidiosis in disease-specific recommendations for information on personal-use filters and bottled water.

preventing opportunistic infections and other infections commonly encountered in HIV-infected persons, as described in the overview, should be integrated with other aspects of HIV care, as described elsewhere (9).

PNEUMOCYSTIS CARINII PNEUMONIA

Prevention of Exposure

1. Although some authorities recommend that HIV-infected persons at risk for P. carinii pneumonia (PCP) not share a hospital room with a patient with PCP, data are insufficient to support this recommendation as standard practice (CIII).

Prevention of Disease

2. Adults and adolescents with HIV infection (including those who are pregnant) should receive chemoprophylaxis against PCP if they have a CD4+ lymphocyte count of <200/gmL (AI), unexplained fever (>100 degrees F) for greater than or equal to 2 weeks (AII), or a history of oropharyngeal candidiasis (AII).

Trimethoprim-sulfamethoxazole (TMP-SMZ) is the preferred prophylactic agent (AI). TMP-SMZ may confer cross-protection against toxoplasmosis (AII) and many bacterial infections (AII). For patients with an adverse reaction that is not life-threatening, treatment with TMP-SMZ should be continued if clinically feasible; for those who have discontinued such therapy, its reinstitution should be strongly considered (AII). Whether it is best to reintroduce the drug at the original dose or at a lower and gradually increasing dose or to try a desensitization regimen is unknown. If TMP-SMZ cannot be tolerated, alternative prophylactic regimens include dapsone (AI), dapsone plus pyrimethamine plus leucovorin (AI), and aerosolized pentamidine administered by the Respirgard II nebulizer (Marquest, Englewood, CO) (AI). Regimens including dapsone plus pyrimethamine are also protective against toxoplasmosis (AI) but not against most bacterial infections. Because data on their efficacy for PCP prophylaxis are insufficient, the following regimens generally cannot be recommended for this purpose: aerosolized pentamidine administered by other nebulization devices currently available in the United States, intermittently administered parenteral pentamidine, oral pyrimethamine/sulfadoxine, oral clindamycin plus primaquine, oral atovaquone, and intravenous trimetrexate. However, the use of these agents may be considered in unusual situations in which the recommended agents cannot be administered (CIII).

Prevention of Recurrence

3. Adults and adolescents with a history of PCP should receive chemoprophylaxis with the regimens indicated above to prevent recurrence (AI).

NOTES

PEDIATRIC NOTES

4. Children born to HIV-infected mothers should receive prophylaxis with TMP-SMZ beginning at 4–6 weeks of age (11) (AII). Prophylaxis should be discontinued for children who

are subsequently found not to be infected with HIV. HIV-infected children and children whose infection status remains unknown should continue to receive prophylaxis for the first year of life. The need for subsequent prophylaxis should be determined on the basis of age-specific CD4+ lymphocyte count thresholds (11, 12) (AII).

5. Children with a history of PCP should receive chemoprophylaxis as indicated above to prevent recurrence (AI).

NOTE REGARDING PREGNANCY

6. Chemoprophylaxis for PCP should be administered to pregnant women as to other adults and adolescents (AIII), although some providers, because of a general concern about administering drugs during the first trimester of pregnancy, may choose not to initiate such therapy until after the first trimester. Because of the increase in blood plasma volume and the reduced concentrations of drugs during pregnancy, the double-strength (DS) dose of TMP-SMZ (one DS tablet daily) should be used.

TOXOPLASMIC ENCEPHALITIS

Prevention of Exposure

1. HIV-infected persons should be tested for IgG antibody to Toxoplasma soon after the diagnosis of HIV infection to detect latent infection with Toxoplasma gondii (BIII).

2. All HIV-infected persons, but particularly those who lack IgG antibody to Toxoplasma, should be counseled about the various sources of toxoplasmic infection. They should be advised not to eat raw or undercooked meat, particularly undercooked pork, lamb, or venison (BIII). Specifically, meat should be cooked to an internal temperature of 150°F; meat cooked until no longer pink inside generally has an internal temperature of 165°F and therefore satisfies this requirement. HIV-infected persons should wash their hands after contact with raw meat and after gardening or other contact with soil; in addition, they should wash fruits and vegetables well before eating them raw (BIII). If the patient owns a cat, the litter box should be changed daily, preferably by an HIV-negative, nonpregnant person; alternatively, the patient should wash the hands thoroughly after changing the litter box (BIII). Patients should be encouraged to keep their cats inside and not to adopt or handle stray cats (BIII). Cats should be fed only canned or dried commercial food or well-cooked table food, not raw or undercooked meats (BIII). Patients need not be advised to part with their cats or to have their cats tested for toxoplasmosis (EII).

Prevention of Disease

3. Toxoplasma-seropositive patients with a CD4+ lymphocyte count of <100/gmL should receive prophylaxis against toxoplasmic encephalitis (TE) (AII). The doses of TMP-SMZ recommended for PCP prophylaxis appear to be effective against TE as well (AII). If patients cannot tolerate TMP-SMZ, the regimens including dapsone plus pyrimethamine that are recommended for PCP prophylaxis provide protection against TE (AI). Prophylactic monotherapy with dapsone, pyrimethamine, azithromycin, clarithromycin, or atovaquone cannot be recommended on the basis of current data (DII). Aerosolized pentamidine does not afford protection against TE (EI).

4. Toxoplasma-seronegative persons who are not taking a PCP prophylactic regimen known to be active against TE should be retested for IgG antibody

to Toxoplasma when their CD4+ lymphocyte count falls below 100/gmL to determine whether they have seroconverted and are therefore at risk for TE (CIII). Patients who have seroconverted should receive prophylaxis for TE as described above (AII).

Prevention of Recurrence

5. Patients who have had TE should receive lifelong suppressive therapy with drugs active against Toxoplasma to prevent relapse (AI). The combination of pyrimethamine plus sulfadiazine and leucovorin is highly effective for this purpose (AII). A commonly used regimen for patients who cannot tolerate sulfa drugs is pyrimethamine plus clindamycin (AII); however, only the combination of pyrimethamine plus sulfadiazine appears to provide protection against PCP as well (AII).

NOTES

PEDIATRIC NOTE

6. Current data are insufficient for the formulation of specific guidelines for children. The provider should consider the recommendations for adults; children >12 months of age who are seropositive for IgG antibody to Toxoplasma, have a CD4+ lymphocyte count of <100/μL, and are not already taking medication effective against Toxoplasma may be considered as candidates for chemoprophylaxis (CIII). Some providers would consider opting for chemoprophylaxis for very young children with higher CD4+ lymphocyte counts consistent with severe immunosuppression (12) and with evidence of toxoplasmic infection.

Notes Regarding Pregnancy

7. Because of the low incidence of TE during pregnancy and the possible risk associated with pyrimethamine treatment, chemoprophylaxis with pyrimethamine-containing regimens can reasonably be deferred until after pregnancy for women who are seropositive for IgG antibody to Toxoplasma (CIII). TMP-SMZ can be administered as described for prophylaxis of PCP. For prophylaxis of recurrent TE, pyrimethamine should be used with caution (CIII).

8. In rare cases, HIV-infected pregnant women with serological evidence of remote toxoplasmic infection have transmitted Toxoplasma to the fetus in utero. Pregnant HIV-infected women who have evidence of primary toxoplasmic infection or active toxoplasmosis (including TE) should be evaluated during pregnancy in consultation with appropriate specialists (CIII). Infants born to women with serological evidence of infections with HIV and Toxoplasma should be evaluated for congenital toxoplasmosis (CIII).

CRYPTOSPORIDIOSIS

Prevention of Exposure

1. HIV-infected persons should be educated and counseled about the many ways that Cryptosporidium can be transmitted. Modes of transmission include contact with infected adults and diaper-age children, contact with infected animals, consumption of contaminated drinking water, and contact with contaminated water during recreational activities (BIII).

2. HIV-infected persons should avoid contact with human and animal feces. They should be advised to wash their hands after contact with human feces (e.g., during diaper changing), after handling of pets, and after gardening or other contact with soil. HIV-infected persons should avoid sexual prac-

tices such as oral-anal intercourse that may result in oral exposure to feces (BIII).

3. HIV-infected persons should be advised that newborn and very young pets may pose a small risk of cryptosporidial infection, but they should not be advised to destroy or give away healthy pets. Persons contemplating the acquisition of a new pet should avoid bringing any animal with diarrhea into their households, should avoid purchasing a dog or cat <6 months of age, and should not adopt stray pets. HIV-infected persons who wish to assume the small risk of acquiring a puppy or kitten <6 months of age should request that their veterinarian examine the animal's stool for Cryptosporidium before they have contact with the animal (BIII).

4. HIV-infected persons should avoid exposure to calves and lambs and to premises where these animals are raised (BII).

5. HIV-infected persons should not drink water directly from lakes or rivers. Because water can be accidentally ingested, patients should be advised that swimming in lakes, rivers, or public swimming pools may put them at increased risk for infection (BII).

6. Several outbreaks of cryptosporidiosis have been linked to municipal water supplies. During outbreaks or in other situations in which a community "boil-water" advisory is issued, boiling of water for 1 minute will eliminate the risk of cryptosporidiosis (AI). Use of submicron personal-use water filters* (i.e., home/office types) and/or bottled water** (2) may reduce the risk (CIII). The magnitude of the risk of acquiring cryptosporidiosis from drinking water in a nonoutbreak setting is uncertain, and current data are inadequate to recommend that all HIV-infected persons boil or avoid drinking tap water in nonoutbreak settings. However, HIV-infected persons who wish to take independent action to reduce the risk of waterborne cryptosporidiosis may choose to take precautions similar to those recommended during outbreaks. Such decisions should be made in conjunction with health-care providers. Persons who opt for a personal-use filter or bottled water should be aware of the complexities involved in selecting appropriate products, the lack of enforceable standards for the destruction or removal of oocysts, the cost of the products, and the logistic difficulty of using these products consistently.

---

* Only filters capable of removing particles 1 μm in diameter and larger should be considered. Filters that provide the greatest assurance of oocyst removal include those that operate by reverse osmosis, those labeled as "absolute" 1-μm filters, and those labeled as meeting NSF (National Sanitation Foundation) standard no. 53 for "cyst removal." The "nominal" 1-μm filter rating is not standardized, and many filters in this category may not be capable of removing greater than or equal to 99% of oocysts.

** Sources of bottled water (wells, springs, municipal tap-water supplies, rivers, lakes) and methods for its disinfection vary; therefore, all brands should not be presumed to be free of cryptosporidial oocysts. Water from wells and springs is much less likely to be contaminated by oocysts than water from rivers or lakes. Treatment of bottled water by distillation or reverse osmosis ensures oocyst removal. Water passed through an "absolute" 1-μm filter or a filter labeled as meeting NSF standard no. 53 for "cyst removal" before bottling will provide nearly the same level of protection. Use of "nominal" 1-μm filters by bottlers as the only barrier to cryptosporidia may not result in the removal of greater than or equal to 99% of oocysts.

Prevention of Disease

7. No effective chemoprophylactic agents are available for cryptosporidiosis.

Prevention of Recurrence

8. No drug regimens are known to be effective in preventing the recurrence of cryptosporidiosis.

NOTE

PEDIATRIC NOTE

9. At present, no data indicate that formula-preparation practices for infants should be altered in an effort to prevent cryptosporidiosis (CIII).

MICROSPORIDIOSIS

Prevention of Exposure

1. Other than general attention to hand washing and other personal hygiene measures, no precautions to reduce exposure can be recommended at this time.

Prevention of Disease

2. No chemoprophylactic regimens are known to be effective in preventing microsporidiosis.

Prevention of Recurrence

3. No chemotherapeutic regimens are known to be effective in preventing the recurrence of microsporidiosis.

TUBERCULOSIS

Prevention of Exposure

1. HIV-infected persons should be advised that certain activities and occupations may increase the likelihood of exposure to tuberculosis (BIII). These include volunteer work or employment in health-care facilities, correctional institutions, and shelters for the homeless as well as in other settings identified as high risk by local health authorities. Decisions about whether to continue with activities in these settings should be made in conjunction with the health-care provider and should take into account such factors as the patient's specific duties in the workplace, the prevalence of tuberculosis in the community, and the degree to which precautions are taken to prevent the transmission of tuberculosis in the workplace (BIII). Whether or not the patient continues with such activities may affect the frequency with which screening for tuberculosis needs to be conducted.

Prevention of Disease

2. When HIV infection is first recognized, the patient should be screened by the Mantoux method with intermediate-strength (5-TU) PPD (AI). Routine evaluation for anergy is controversial; some experts recommend anergy testing for persons in settings where there is an increased risk of infection with Mycobacterium tuberculosis (i.e., in areas where the prevalence of such infection is >10%) (CIII).

3. All HIV-infected persons with a positive result in the tuberculin skin test (TST; greater than or equal to 5 mm of induration) should undergo chest radiography and clinical evaluation for the exclusion of active tuberculosis. HIV-infected individuals who have symptoms suggestive of tuberculosis should undergo chest radiography and clinical evaluation regardless of their TST status (AII).

4. All HIV-infected persons with a positive TST result who have no evidence of active tuberculosis and no history of treatment or prophylaxis for tuberculosis should receive 12 months of preventive chemotherapy with isoniazid (AI). Since HIV-infected persons are at risk for peripheral neuropathy, those receiving isoniazid should also receive pyridoxine (BIII). The decision to use alternative antimycobacterial agents for chemoprophylaxis should be based on the relative risk of exposure to resistant organisms and may require consultation with public health authorities (AII). The need for direct observation as a means of documenting compliance with chemoprophylaxis should be considered on an individual basis (BIII).

5. HIV-infected individuals who are close contacts of persons with infectious tuberculosis (i.e., acid-fast bacillary smear-positive pulmonary disease) should receive preventive therapy—regardless of TST results or prior courses of chemoprophylaxis—after active tuberculosis has been excluded (AII). Such persons should be tested with 5-TU PPD. If the TST result is initially negative, the individual should be evaluated again 3 months after the discontinuation of contact with the infectious source, and the information obtained should be considered in the course of decisions about whether chemoprophylaxis should continue (BIII).

6. TST-negative, HIV-infected persons from risk groups or geographic areas with a high prevalence of M. tuberculosis infection (>10%) may be at increased risk of tuberculosis. Some experts recommend preventive therapy for anergic individuals or perhaps for all persons in this category (CIII). However, the efficacy of preventive therapy in this group has not been demonstrated, and decisions concerning the use of chemoprophylaxis in these situations must be individualized.

7. Although the reliability of the TST may diminish as the CD4+ lymphocyte count declines, testing should be repeated at least annually for HIV-infected persons who are TST-negative on initial evaluation (BIII). In addition to documenting tuberculous infection, TST conversion in an HIV-infected person should alert health-care providers to the possibility of an infectious case in the environment and lead to notification of public health officials for investigation to identify a possible source case.

8. The administration of BCG vaccine to HIV-infected persons is contraindicated because of its potential to cause disseminated disease (EII).

Prevention of Recurrence

9. Chronic suppressive therapy for a patient who has successfully completed a recommended regimen of treatment for tuberculosis is not necessary (EII).

NOTES

PEDIATRIC NOTE

10. All infants born to HIV-infected mothers should have a TST (5-TU PPD) at 9–12 months of age (CIII). All children living in households with M. tuberculosis-infected (TST-

positive) persons should be evaluated for tuberculosis (13) (CIII); those exposed to a person with active tuberculosis should receive preventive therapy after active tuberculosis has been excluded (AII).

NOTE REGARDING PREGNANCY

11. HIV-infected pregnant women who have a positive TST result without evidence of active tuberculosis should receive standard chemoprophylaxis (AII). When possible, chest radiography should be undertaken and chemoprophylaxis should be initiated after the first trimester in order to avoid the critical period of major organogenesis. Preventive therapy with isoniazid should be accompanied by treatment with pyridoxine so that peripheral neuropathy does not develop. Alternative regimens (e.g., rifampin, rifabutin) should be used with caution during pregnancy.

DISSEMINATED INFECTION WITH MYCOBACTERIUM AVIUM COMPLEX

Prevention of Exposure

1. Organisms of the M. avium complex (MAC) are common in environmental sources such as food and water. Current information does not support specific recommendations regarding avoidance of exposure.

Prevention of Disease

2. Prophylaxis with rifabutin should be considered for HIV-infected adults and adolescents who have a CD4+ lymphocyte count of $<75/\mu L$, although some experts would wait until the count is $<50/\mu L$ (BII). Disseminated MAC disease should be ruled out (by a negative blood culture) before prophylaxis is initiated. Because treatment with rifabutin may result in the development of resistance to rifampin in individuals with active tuberculosis, the latter condition should be excluded before rifabutin prophylaxis is begun. Drug interactions, partial efficacy, and cost are among the other issues that should be considered in decisions about whether to institute prophylaxis for MAC disease. Data on the safety and efficacy of clarithromycin, azithromycin, and combinations of clarithromycin or azithromycin with rifabutin have not yet been reviewed sufficiently to warrant recommendations concerning these regimens.

3. Although the detection of MAC organisms in the respiratory or gastrointestinal tract may be predictive of the development of disseminated MAC infection, no data are available on the efficacy of prophylaxis with rifabutin or other drugs in patients with MAC organisms at these sites and a negative blood culture. Therefore, routine screening of respiratory or gastrointestinal specimens for MAC cannot be recommended at this time (DIII).

Prevention of Recurrence

4. Patients who are treated for disseminated MAC infection should continue to receive full therapeutic doses for life (BIII). The use of a macrolide, usually clarithromycin, is generally recommended in conjunction with at least one other drug, such as ethambutol, clofazimine, ciprofloxacin, or rifabutin.

NOTES

PEDIATRIC NOTE

5. HIV-infected children <12 years of age also develop disseminated MAC infections. Prophylaxis should be considered similar to that recommended for adults and adolescents (BI). For children 6–12 years of age, a CD4+ lymphocyte count of <75/μL is a reasonable threshold for the initiation of chemoprophylaxis. Some adjustment for age is necessary in the interpretation of CD4+ lymphocyte counts of children <6 years of age (12). No pediatric formulation of rifabutin is currently available, but a dosage of 5 mg/kg has been used in pharmacokinetic studies.

NOTE REGARDING PREGNANCY

6. Information is insufficient for recommendations concerning the use of rifabutin or clarithromycin during pregnancy.

BACTERIAL RESPIRATORY INFECTIONS

Prevention of Exposure

1. Because Streptococcus pneumoniae and Haemophilus influenzae are common in the community, there is no effective way to reduce exposure to these bacteria.

Prevention of Disease

2. As soon as possible after HIV infection is diagnosed, adults should receive a single dose of 23-valent polysaccharide pneumococcal vaccine (BIII). This recommendation is especially pertinent in light of the increasing incidence of invasive infections with drug-resistant strains of S. pneumoniae. Although the administration of protein-polysaccharide conjugate H. influenzae type b vaccine may be considered, data are insufficient to recommend the use of this vaccine in HIV-infected adults at this time.

3. TMP-SMZ, administered daily, may be effective in preventing serious bacterial respiratory infections (although not those caused by drug-resistant S. pneumoniae); this fact should be considered in the selection of an agent for PCP prophylaxis (AII). However, indiscriminate use of this drug (when not indicated for PCP prophylaxis or other specific reasons) may promote the development of resistant organisms.

4. An absolute neutrophil count that is depressed because of HIV disease or drug therapy may be increased by granulocyte colony-stimulating factor (G-CSF) or granulocyte-macrophage colony-stimulating factor (GM-CSF). However, data are insufficient for recommendations concerning the use of G-CSF or GM-CSF to prevent bacterial infections in HIV-infected patients with neutropenia.

Prevention of Recurrence

5. Some clinicians may choose to offer antibiotic chemoprophylaxis to HIV-infected patients with recurrent serious bacterial respiratory infections (BIII). TMP-SMZ, administered for PCP prophylaxis, is appropriate for drug-sensitive organisms.

6. All invasive pneumococcal isolates from HIV-infected patients should be tested for susceptibility to b-lactam antibiotics, and local patterns of resis-

tance should be considered in the choice of regimens for empirical treatment (AII). Invasive infections due to H. influenzae should be treated with regimens effective against b-lactamase-producing strains until drug susceptibilities are known (AII).

NOTES

PEDIATRIC NOTES

7. Children with HIV infection should receive H. influenzae type b vaccine in accordance with the guidelines of the Advisory Committee for Immunization Practices (14) and the American Academy of Pediatrics (13) (AII). Children >2 years of age should also receive 23-valent polysaccharide pneumococcal vaccine (BII).

8. To prevent serious bacterial infections in HIV-infected children with documented antibody deficiency, clinicians should use intravenous immunoglobulin (IVIG) (AI). The administration of IVIG should also be considered for HIV-infected children with recurrent serious bacterial infections (AI), but such treatment may not provide additional benefit to children receiving daily TMP-SMZ.

NOTE REGARDING PREGNANCY

9. Pneumococcal vaccine is not contraindicated during pregnancy.

BACTERIAL ENTERIC INFECTIONS

Prevention of Exposure

Food

1. Health-care providers should advise HIV-infected persons not to eat raw or undercooked eggs (including foods that may contain raw eggs—e.g., some preparations of hollandaise sauce, Caesar and other salad dressings, and mayonnaise); raw or undercooked poultry, meat, or seafood; or unpasteurized dairy products. Poultry and meat should be well cooked and should not be pink in the middle (internal temperature, >165°F). Produce should be thoroughly washed before being eaten (BIII).

2. Health-care providers should advise HIV-infected persons to avoid cross-contamination of foods. For example, uncooked meats should not come into contact with other foods, and hands, cutting boards, counters, and knives and other utensils should be washed thoroughly after contact with uncooked foods (BIII).

3. Health-care providers should advise HIV-infected persons that, although the incidence of listeriosis is low, it is a serious disease that occurs with unusually high frequency among HIV-infected persons who are severely immunosuppressed. Such persons may choose to avoid soft cheeses because some studies have shown an association between these foods and listeriosis. These studies have also documented an association between ready-to-eat foods (e.g., hot dogs and cold cuts from delicatessen counters) and listeriosis. An immunosuppressed, HIV-infected person who wishes to reduce the risk of food-borne disease as much as possible may choose to re-heat such foods until they are steaming hot before eating them (CIII).

Pets

4. When obtaining a new pet, HIV-infected persons should avoid young animals (<6 months of age), especially those with diarrhea (BIII).

5. HIV-infected persons should avoid contact with animals that have diarrhea (BIII). HIV-infected pet owners should seek veterinary care for animals with diarrheal illness, and a fecal sample from such animals should be examined for Cryptosporidium, Salmonella, and Campylobacter.
6. HIV-infected persons should wash their hands after handling pets (especially before eating) and should avoid contact with pets' feces (BIII).
7. HIV-infected persons should avoid contact with reptiles (such as snakes, lizards, and turtles) because of the risk of salmonellosis (BIII).

Travel

8. The risk of food- and waterborne infections among immunosuppressed, HIV-infected persons is magnified during travel to developing countries. Those who elect to travel to such countries should avoid foods and beverages that may be contaminated, particularly raw fruits and vegetables, raw or undercooked seafood or meat, tap water, ice made with tap water, unpasteurized milk and dairy products, and items sold by street vendors (AII). Foods and beverages that are generally safe include steaming-hot foods, fruits that are peeled by the traveler, bottled (especially carbonated) beverages, hot coffee and tea, beer, wine, and water brought to a rolling boil for 1 minute (AII). Treatment of water with iodine or chlorine may not be as effective as boiling but can be used when boiling is not practical (BIII).

Prevention of Disease

9. Prophylactic antimicrobial agents are not generally recommended for travelers (DIII). The effectiveness of these agents depends upon local antimicrobial-resistance patterns of gastrointestinal pathogens, which are seldom known. Moreover, these agents can elicit adverse reactions and can promote the emergence of resistant organisms. However, for HIV-infected travelers, antimicrobial prophylaxis may be considered, depending upon the level of immunosuppression and the region and duration of travel (CIII). The use of fluoroquinolones—such as ciprofloxacin (500 mg/d)—can be considered when prophylaxis is deemed necessary (BIII). As an alternative (e.g., for children, pregnant women, and persons already taking TMP-SMZ for PCP prophylaxis), TMP-SMZ may offer some protection against traveler's diarrhea (BIII). The risk of toxicity should be considered before treatment with TMP-SMZ is initiated solely because of travel.
10. Antimicrobial agents such as fluoroquinolones (e.g., 500 mg of ciprofloxacin b.i.d. for 3–7 days) should be given to patients before their departure, to be taken empirically should traveler's diarrhea develop (BIII). Alternative antibiotics for children and pregnant women should be discussed (CIII). Travelers should consult a physician if their diarrhea is severe and does not respond to empirical therapy, if their stools contain blood, if fever is accompanied by shaking chills, or if dehydration develops. Antiperistaltic agents such as diphenoxylate and loperamide can be used for the treatment of mild diarrhea. However, the use of these drugs should be discontinued if symptoms persist beyond 48 hours. Moreover, these agents should not be given to patients with high fever or with blood in the stool (AII).

11. Some experts recommend that HIV-infected persons with salmonella gastroenteritis receive antimicrobial therapy to prevent extraintestinal spread. However, no controlled study has demonstrated a beneficial effect of such treatment, and some studies of immunocompetent persons have suggested that antimicrobial therapy can lengthen the shedding period. The fluoroquinolones—primarily ciprofloxacin (750 mg b.i.d. for 14 days)—can be used when antimicrobial therapy is opted for (CIII).

Prevention of Recurrence

12. HIV-infected persons with salmonella septicemia require long-term therapy for the prevention of recurrence. The fluoroquinolones, primarily ciprofloxacin, are usually the drugs of choice for susceptible organisms (BII).

13. Household contacts of HIV-infected persons with salmonellosis or shigellosis should be evaluated for asymptomatic carriage of Salmonella or Shigella so that strict hygienic measures and/or antimicrobial therapy can be instituted and recurrent transmission to the HIV-infected person can be prevented (CIII).

NOTES

PEDIATRIC NOTES

14. Like HIV-infected adults, HIV-infected children should wash their hands after handling pets (especially before eating) and should avoid contact with pets' feces. Hand washing should be supervised (BIII).

15. HIV-exposed infants <3 months of age and all HIV-infected children with severe immunosuppression should receive treatment for salmonella gastroenteritis to prevent extraintestinal spread. Possible choices of antibiotics include TMP-SMZ, ampicillin, cefotaxime, ceftriaxone, or chloramphenicol; ciprofloxacin may be considered for the treatment of children >6 years of age (CIII).

16. HIV-infected children with salmonella septicemia require long-term therapy for the prevention of recurrence. TMP-SMZ is the drug of choice; ampicillin or chloramphenicol can be used if the organism is susceptible. Ciprofloxacin may be considered for the treatment of children >6 years of age (CIII).

17. Antiperistaltic drugs are not recommended for children (DIII).

Notes Regarding Pregnancy

18. Since both pregnancy and HIV infection confer a risk for listeriosis, pregnant HIV-infected women should pay particular attention to recommendations concerned with this disease (BII).

19. Fluoroquinolones should not be used during pregnancy. TMP-SMZ may offer some protection against traveler's diarrhea.

INFECTION WITH BARTONELLA (FORMERLY ROCHALIMAEA)

Prevention of Exposure

1. HIV-infected persons, particularly those who are severely immunosuppressed, are at unusually high risk of developing relatively severe disease due to Bartonella species. These individuals should consider the potential risks of cat ownership (CIII). Those who elect to acquire a cat should adopt or purchase an older animal (>1 year of age) that is in good health (BII).

2. Although declawing is not generally advised, HIV-infected persons should avoid rough play with cats and situations in which scratches are likely (BII). Any cat-associated wound should be washed promptly (CIII). HIV-infected persons should not allow cats to lick open cuts or wounds (BIII).
3. Care of cats should include flea control (CIII).
4. There is no evidence of benefit to cat or owner from routine culture or serological testing of the pet for Bartonella infection (DII).

Prevention of Disease

5. No data currently support chemoprophylaxis for Bartonella-associated disease (CIII).

Prevention of Recurrence

6. Relapse or reinfection with Bartonella has sometimes followed a course of primary treatment. Although no firm recommendation can be made regarding prophylaxis in this situation, long-term suppression of infection with erythromycin or doxycycline should be considered (CIII).

NOTE

PEDIATRIC NOTE

7. The risks of cat ownership for HIV-infected children who are severely immunocompromised should be discussed with parents/caretakers (CIII).

CANDIDIASIS
Prevention of Exposure

1. Candida organisms are common on mucosal surfaces and skin. No measures are available to reduce exposure to these fungi.

Prevention of Disease

2. Although data from a prospective controlled trial indicate that fluconazole can reduce the risk of mucosal (oropharyngeal, esophageal, and vaginal) candidiasis in patients with advanced HIV disease, routine primary prophylaxis is not recommended because of the effectiveness of therapy for acute disease, the low mortality associated with mucosal candidiasis, the potential for resistant Candida organisms to develop, the possibility of drug interactions, and the cost of prophylaxis (DII).

Prevention of Recurrence

3. Many experts do not recommend chronic prophylaxis of recurrent oropharyngeal or vulvovaginal candidiasis for the same reasons that they do not recommend primary prophylaxis. However, if recurrences are frequent or severe, intermittent or chronic administration of topical nystatin, topical clotrimazole, or an oral azole (ketoconazole, fluconazole, or itraconazole) may be considered (BI). Other factors that influence choices about such therapy include the impact of the recurrences on the patient's well-being and quality of life, the need for prophylaxis for other fungal infections, cost, toxicities, and drug interactions.

4. Adults or adolescents with a history of documented esophageal candidiasis, particularly multiple episodes, should be considered candidates for chronic suppressive therapy with fluconazole (BI).

NOTES

PEDIATRIC NOTES

5. Primary prophylaxis of candidiasis in HIV-infected infants is not indicated (DII).
6. Suppressive therapy with systemic azoles should be considered for infants with severe recurrent mucocutaneous candidiasis (BIII) and particularly for those with esophageal candidiasis (BI).

CRYPTOCOCCOSIS

Prevention of Exposure

1. Although HIV-infected persons cannot avoid exposure to Cryptococcus neoformans completely, avoiding sites that are likely to be heavily contaminated with C. neoformans (e.g., areas heavily contaminated with pigeon droppings) may reduce the risk of infection.

Prevention of Disease

2. Because of the low probability that the results will affect clinical decisions, routine testing of asymptomatic persons for serum cryptococcal antigen is not recommended (DIII).
3. Data from a prospective controlled trial indicate that fluconazole can reduce the frequency of cryptococcal disease among patients with advanced HIV disease; thus, physicians may wish to consider chemoprophylaxis for adult and adolescent patients with a CD4+ lymphocyte count of $<50/\mu L$ (BI). However, such prophylaxis should not be offered routinely because of the relative infrequency of cryptococcal disease, the possibility of drug interactions, the potential for development of resistance, and the cost of prophylaxis (DII). The need for prophylaxis or suppressive therapy for other fungal infections (e.g., candidiasis) should be considered in the course of decisions about prophylaxis for cryptococcosis.

Prevention of Recurrence

4. Patients who complete initial therapy for cryptococcosis should receive lifelong suppressive treatment with fluconazole (AI).

NOTES

PEDIATRIC NOTE

5. There are no data on which to base specific recommendations for children, but lifelong suppressive therapy with fluconazole after an episode of cryptococcosis is appropriate (CIII).

NOTE REGARDING PREGNANCY

6. Although treatment with fluconazole is indicated to prevent the recurrence of cryptococcosis, this drug should be used with caution in pregnant women (CIII). At high doses, fluconazole has been associated with both fetal death and increased rates of fetal abnormalities in rats.

HISTOPLASMOSIS

Prevention of Exposure

1. Although HIV-infected persons living in or visiting histoplasmosis-endemic areas cannot completely avoid exposure to Histoplasma capsulatum, they should avoid activities known to be associated with increased risk (e.g., cleaning chicken coops, disturbing soil beneath bird-roosting sites, and exploring caves) (CIII).

Prevention of Disease

2. Routine skin testing with histoplasmin in histoplasmosis-endemic areas is not predictive of disease and should not be performed (EII).
3. No recommendation can be made regarding chemoprophylaxis for HIV-infected persons in histoplasmosis-endemic areas or for histoplasmin-positive persons in nonendemic areas.

Prevention of Recurrence

4. Patients who complete initial therapy should receive lifelong suppressive treatment with itraconazole (AII).

NOTE

PEDIATRIC NOTE

5. Because primary histoplasmosis can lead to disseminated infection in children, HIV-infected children with histoplasmosis should receive suppressive therapy for life (CIII).

COCCIDIOIDOMYCOSIS

Prevention of Exposure

1. Although HIV-infected persons living in or visiting areas in which coccidioidomycosis is endemic cannot completely avoid exposure to Coccidioides immitis, they should, when possible, avoid activities associated with increased risk (e.g., those involving extensive exposure to disturbed soil as occurs at building excavation sites, on farms, or during dust storms) (CIII).

Prevention of Disease

2. Routine skin testing with coccidioidin (spherulin) in coccidioidomycosis-endemic areas is not predictive of disease and should not be performed (EII).
3. No recommendation can be made regarding routine chemoprophylaxis for HIV-infected individuals who live in coccidioidomycosis-endemic areas or for skin test-positive persons in nonendemic areas.

Prevention of Recurrence

4. Patients who complete initial therapy for coccidioidomycosis should receive lifelong systemic suppressive treatment (AII). Fluconazole is the preferred agent; alternative drugs include itraconazole, ketoconazole, and amphotericin B.

NOTE

PEDIATRIC NOTE

5. Although no specific data are available on coccidioidomycosis in HIV-infected children, it is reasonable to administer lifelong suppressive therapy after an acute episode of the disease (CIII).

CYTOMEGALOVIRUS DISEASE

Prevention of Exposure

1. HIV-infected persons who belong to risk groups with relatively low rates of seropositivity for cytomegalovirus (CMV) and who anticipate possible exposure to CMV (e.g., through blood transfusion or employment in a child-care facility) should be tested for antibody to CMV (BIII). These groups include patients who have not had male homosexual contact and those who are not injection drug users.

2. HIV-infected adolescents and adults should be advised that CMV is shed in semen, cervical secretions, and saliva and that latex condoms must always be used during sexual contact to reduce the risk of exposure to this virus and to other sexually transmitted pathogens (AII).

3. HIV-infected adults and adolescents who are child-care providers or parents of children in child-care facilities should be informed that they—like all children at these facilities—are at increased risk of acquiring CMV infection (BI). Parents and other care-takers of HIV-infected children should be advised of the increased risk to children at these centers (BIII). The risk of acquiring CMV infection can be diminished by good hygienic practices, such as hand washing (AII).

4. HIV-exposed infants and HIV-infected children, adolescents, and adults who are seronegative for CMV and require blood transfusion should receive only CMV antibody-negative or leukocyte-reduced cellular blood products in nonemergency situations (15) (BIII).

Prevention of Disease

5. Data on the efficacy and safety of oral ganciclovir have not yet been adequately reviewed; thus no recommendation concerning this drug can be made at this time. Acyclovir is not effective in preventing CMV disease (EII). Since no chemoprophylactic agent is currently available, the most important method for preventing severe CMV disease is recognition of the early manifestations of the disease. Early recognition of CMV retinitis is most likely when the patient has been educated on this topic and undergoes regular funduscopic examinations performed by a health-care provider (CIII). Patients should be made aware of the significance of increased "floaters" in the eye and should be advised to assess their visual acuity regularly by simple techniques such as reading newsprint (BIII).

Prevention of Recurrence

6. CMV disease is not cured with courses of the currently available antiviral agents ganciclovir and foscarnet. Chronic suppressive or maintenance therapy is indicated. The presently approved regimens include parenteral or oral ganciclovir or parenteral foscarnet (AI). In spite of maintenance

therapy, recurrences develop routinely and require reinstitution of high-dose induction therapy.

NOTE

PEDIATRIC NOTE

7. The recommendations for the prevention of CMV disease and of its recurrence apply to children as well as to adolescents and adults. However, oral ganciclovir has not been studied in children.

HERPES SIMPLEX VIRUS DISEASE

Prevention of Exposure

1. HIV-infected persons should use latex condoms during every act of sexual intercourse to reduce the risk of exposure to herpes simplex virus (HSV) and to other sexually transmitted pathogens (AII). They should specifically avoid sexual contact when herpetic lesions (genital or orolabial) are evident (AII).

Prevention of Disease

2. Prophylaxis of initial episodes of HSV disease is not recommended (DIII).***

Prevention of Recurrence

3. Because acute episodes of HSV infection can be treated successfully, chronic therapy with acyclovir is not required after lesions resolve. However, persons with frequent or severe recurrences can be given daily suppressive therapy with oral acyclovir (AI). Intravenous foscarnet can be used for the treatment of infection due to acyclovir-resistant isolates of HSV, which are routinely resistant to ganciclovir as well (AI).

NOTES

PEDIATRIC NOTE

4. The recommendations for the prevention of initial disease and recurrence apply to children as well as to adolescents and adults.

NOTE REGARDING PREGNANCY

5. The effectiveness of suppressive treatment with acyclovir in reducing the risk of perinatal HSV transmission has not been studied. Therefore, no relevant recommendation can be made.

VARICELLA-ZOSTER VIRUS INFECTION

Prevention of Exposure

1. HIV-infected children and adults who are susceptible to varicella-zoster virus (VZV)—i.e., those who have no history of chickenpox or are seroneg-

---

*** Controversy exists over the possible association of acyclovir therapy with prolonged survival of HIV-infected persons. Current data suggest that chronic acyclovir therapy may be considered but should not be standard practice (CIII).

ative for VZV—should avoid exposure to persons with chickenpox or shingles (AII).

Prevention of Disease

2. For the prophylaxis of chickenpox, HIV-infected children and adults who are susceptible to VZV should be given zoster immune globulin within 96 hours after close contact with a patient with chickenpox or shingles (AI). Data are lacking on the effectiveness of acyclovir for preventing chickenpox in HIV-infected children or adults.
3. No preventive measures are currently available for shingles.

Prevention of Recurrence

4. Recurrence of shingles is unusual, and no drug has been proven to prevent recurrence.

NOTE

NOTE REGARDING PREGNANCY

5. Zoster immune globulin is not contraindicated during pregnancy and should be given to VZV-susceptible pregnant women after exposure to VZV (AI).

HUMAN PAPILLOMAVIRUS INFECTION

Prevention of Exposure

1. HIV-infected persons should use latex condoms during every act of sexual intercourse to reduce the risk of exposure to human papillomavirus (HPV) as well as to other sexually transmitted pathogens (AII).

Prevention of Disease

HPV-Associated Genital Epithelial Cancers in HIV-Infected Women

2. HIV-infected women should have annual cervical Pap smears as part of their initial and routine gynecologic care. In accordance with the recommendation of the Agency for Health Care Policy and Research (9), a Pap smear should be obtained twice in the first year after diagnosis of HIV infection and, if the results are normal, annually thereafter (AII).
3. If an HIV-infected woman has a history of abnormal Pap smears, the caregiver may choose to monitor this individual with Pap smears every 6 months (BIII).
4. If the initial or follow-up Pap smear indicates inflammation with reactive squamous cellular changes, further management should be guided by diagnosis of the cause of the inflammation, and another Pap smear should be collected within 3 months (BIII). HIV-infected women with Pap smears showing only atypical cells of undetermined significance can be monitored with annual Pap smears (BIII).
5. Controversy exists concerning the management of HIV-infected women with low-grade squamous intraepithelial lesions (SIL) evident on the cervical Pap smear; the natural history of this finding in this population has not yet been well defined. Some experts would collect another Pap smear

within 3 months. If subsequent Pap smears again showed low-grade SIL, some of these authorities would refer the patient for colposcopic evaluation and biopsy (if indicated); while others would monitor compliant patients with repeat Pap smears at frequent intervals (e.g., every 3–6 months) (BIII). Other experts would refer all HIV-infected patients with low-grade SIL for colposcopy (BIII).

6. If a Pap smear indicates high-grade SIL or squamous cell carcinoma, the woman should be referred for colposcopic examination and, if indicated, colposcopically directed biopsy (AI).

HPV-Associated Anal Intraepithelial Neoplasia and Anal Cancer in HIV-Infected Men Who Have Sex with Men

7. Although the risks for anal intraepithelial neoplasia (AIN) and anal cancer are increased among HIV-infected men who have sex with men, the role of anal cytological screening and treatment of AIN in preventing anal cancer in these men is not well defined. Therefore, no recommendations can be made for periodic anal cytological screening for the detection and treatment of AIN.

Prevention of Recurrence

8. The risks for recurrence of SIL and cervical cancer after conventional therapy are increased among HIV-infected women. The prevention of illness associated with recurrence depends on careful follow-up of patients after treatment. Patients should be monitored with frequent cytological screening and, when indicated, with colposcopic examination for recurrent lesions (AI).

NOTE

PEDIATRIC NOTE

9. Newborns have been known to acquire laryngeal HPV from their mothers. No recommendations can currently be made to prevent such acquisition.

REFERENCES: AS NUMBERED IN ORIGINAL PUBLICATION

1. CDC. Estimates of HIV prevalence and projected AIDS cases: summary of a workshop, October 31—November 1, 1989. MMWR 1990;39:110–112, 117–119.
2. CDC. Projections of the number of persons diagnosed with AIDS and the number of immunosuppressed HIV-infected persons—United States, 1992–1994. MMWR 1992;41(No. RR-18):1–29.
3. CDC. Guidelines for prophylaxis against Pneumocystis carinii pneumonia for persons infected with human immunodeficiency virus. MMWR 1989;38(No. S-5):1–9.
4. CDC. Recommendations for prophylaxis against Pneumocystis carinii pneumonia for adults and adolescents infected with human immunodeficiency virus. MMWR 1992;41(No. RR-4): 1–11.
5. Masur H. Recommendations on prophylaxis and therapy for disseminated Mycobacterium avium complex disease in patients infected with the human immunodeficiency virus. N Engl J Med 1993;329: 898–904.
6. Kaplan JE, Masur H, Holmes KK, et al. USPHS/IDSA guidelines for the prevention of opportunistic infections in persons infected with human immunodeficiency virus: introduction. Clin Infect Dis 1995;21(Suppl 1):1–11.
7. Kaplan JE, Masur H, Holmes KK, et al. USPHS/IDSA guidelines for the prevention of opportunistic infections in persons infected with human immunodeficiency virus: an overview. Clin Infect Dis 1995;21(Suppl 1):12–31.
9. El-Sadr W, Oleske JM, Agins BD, et al. Evaluation and management of early HIV infection. Clinical practice guidelines no. 7. Rockville, MD: U.S. Department of Health and Human Services, 1994:AHCPR publication No. 94–0572.

10. Gross PA, Barrett TL, Dellinger P, et al. Purpose of quality standards for infectious diseases. Clin Infect Dis 1994;18.421.
11. CDC. 1995 revised guidelines for prophylaxis against Pneumocystis carinii pneumonia for children infected with or perinatally exposed to human immunodeficiency virus. MMWR 1995;44(No. RR-4):1–11.
12. CDC. 1994 revised classification system for human immunodeficiency virus infection in children less than 13 years of age. MMWR 1994;43(No. RR-12):1–10.
13. American Academy of Pediatrics. 1994 Red Book: report of the Committee on Infectious Diseases. 23rd ed. Elk Grove Village, IL: American Academy of Pediatrics, 1994:264, 279–280, 375, 496–497.
14. CDC. Recommendations of the Advisory Committee on Immunization Practices (ACIP): use of vaccines and immune globulins in persons with altered immunocompetence. MMWR 1993;42(No. RR-4):1–18.
15. D2.400 Standards for blood banks and transfusion services. 16th ed. Bethesda, MD: American Association of Blood Banks, 1994:12.
16. Castro, KG. Tuberculosis as an opportunistic disease in persons infected with human immunodeficiency virus. Clin Infect Dis 1995;21(Suppl 1):S66-S71.
17. CDC. Hepatitis B virus: a comprehensive strategy for eliminating transmission in the United States through universal childhood vaccination. MMWR 1991;40(No. RR-13):1–25.
18. CDC. Prevention and control of influenza: part I, vaccines. MMWR 1994;43(No. RR-9):1–13.
19. CDC. Prevention and control of influenza: part 2, antiviral agents. MMWR 1994;43(No. RR-15):1–10.
20. CDC. Recommended childhood immunization schedule—United States, January 1995. MMWR 1995;43:959–960.
21. Hall CB. The recommended childhood immunization schedule of the United States. American Academy of Pediatrics. Pediatrics 1995;95:135–137.

Guidelines for Preventing Transmission of HIV Through Transplantation of Human Tissue and Organs

Original Citation: Centers for Disease Control and Prevention. Guidelines for Preventing Transmission of Human Immunodeficiency Virus Through Transplantation of Human Tissue and Organs. MMWR 1994;43(RR-8):1–17.

Editor's Note: The information included here was based on an MMWR supplement which gives revised guidelines on the prevention of HIV transmission by transplantation of organs and tissues. The 1994 guidelines address issues such as donor screening, testing, and exclusionary criteria; quarantine of tissue from living donors; inactivation or elimination of infectious organisms in organs and tissues before transplantation; timely detection, reporting, and tracking of potentially infected tissues, organs, and recipients; and recall of stored tissues from donors found after donation to have been infected.

SUMMARY

Current Guidelines and Recommendations

Procedures for procurement and transplantation of organs and tissues are addressed by (a) federal laws, regulations, and guidelines; (b) state laws and regulations; and (c) voluntary industry standards. Several federal agencies either directly or indirectly regulate procurement and transplantation of organs and tissues. These activities range from the publication of guidelines that address the transmission of communicable diseases through transplantation to regulatory requirements for registration and premarket product licensure or approval (blood and certain other tissue products). The Health Resources and

Services Administration (HRSA), through the United Network for Organ Sharing (UNOS), administers the contract for OPTN as required by Section 372 of the Public Health Service Act and as amended [42 USC 274]. The contract covers specified solid organs (kidney, liver, heart, lung, and pancreas) but does not cover corneas, eyes, or other tissues. Technically, all UNOS policies are voluntary; however, HRSA is currently developing regulations dealing with OPTN membership and operation. Under a separate contract with HRSA, UNOS maintains a Scientific Registry for Transplant Recipients that includes information on all solid-organ transplant recipients (since October 1, 1987) from the date of transplantation until failure of the graft or death of the patient. In addition, HRSA informally conveys recommendations to organizations involved in procurement and transplantation of organs. Through OPTN and the Scientific Registry for Transplant Recipients, HRSA has the capacity to link organ donors and their recipients.

FDA regulates a limited number of specific tissues as either "biological products" or "medical devices." Examples of tissues include blood, dura mater, corneal lenticules, umbilical veins, nonautologous cultured skin, and heart valves. In addition, FDA has recently published regulations regarding behavioral screening and infectious-disease testing (HIV-1, HIV-2, hepatitis B virus, and hepatitis C virus) for donors of human tissue for transplantation (14). FDA also regulates certain agents and devices for processing bone marrow, although bone marrow transplants from unrelated donors are under the auspices of NHLBI.

NHLBI manages the federal contract for the National Marrow Donor Program. Two bone marrow donor registries currently exist: one independent registry and one registry managed through the NHLBI contractor. Each registry group has voluntary guidelines/standards that resemble blood-banking standards. Although federal regulations have not yet been promulgated, the current practice of bone marrow acquisition and transplantation includes procedures to reduce the risk of HIV transmission. NHLBI is preparing regulations that will set forth criteria, standards, and procedures for entities involved in bone marrow collection, processing, and transplantation. These entities include the National Marrow Donor Registry, individual donor centers, donor registries, marrow-collection centers, and marrow-transplant centers. The regulations will include donor-selection criteria to prevent the transmission of infectious diseases, including HIV infection.

Donor Screening

PHS has made recommendations for preventing HIV transmission through organ/tissue transplantation and artificial insemination (1–3, 15, 16). These recommendations include screening for behaviors that are associated with acquisition of HIV infection, a physical examination for signs and symptoms related to HIV infection, and laboratory screening for antibody to HIV. PHS has made no specific recommendations for donation and banking of human milk, although HIV-infected women in the United States are advised to avoid breast feeding their infants because of the risk of HIV transmission through breast milk (17). The Human Milk Banking Association of North America has issued guidelines for the establishment and operation of human milk banks (18). These guidelines state that all human milk donors should be screened according to the American Association of Blood Banks' standards for screening blood donors. All milk accepted for donation should be pasteurized unless the recipient's condition requires fresh-frozen milk, in which case the milk bank director should consult with the medical director and advisory board to approve the dispensing of microbiologically screened, fresh-frozen milk from suitable donors.

Since March 1985, the FDA has licensed a number of screening and supplemental tests for detection and confirmation of HIV antibody. All these tests are intended for use on either fresh or freezer-stored samples of serum or plasma. The FDA has not required manufacturers to submit data showing that HIV-1 antigen and antibody-detection kits produce accurate results when applied to postmortem blood samples. Postmortem blood samples are often hemolyzed, which may affect the specificity of screening assays for HIV antibody (19, 20).

The screening tests include enzyme immunoassays (EIAs), several of which are also approved for testing blood spots dried onto a specific filter paper, which may provide a method for storing samples. Rapid screening assays for HIV antibody that use a latex-agglutination or EIA (microparticle-based) format have also been approved for screening serum, plasma, or whole blood. A licensed EIA for detecting antibodies to HIV-2 is also commercially available, as are "combination tests" that simultaneously detect antibodies to HIV-1 and HIV-2 (21). FDA has also licensed one manufacturer to make and distribute a test for detection of HIV-1 p24 antigen for patient diagnosis and prognosis of HIV infection but not for screening blood donors. Western blot tests and an immunofluorescence assay for HIV-1 are approved for supplemental, more specific testing of serum, plasma, and whole-blood samples found reactive by HIV-1 antibody screening tests. No additional, more specific test is approved that confirms either antibodies to HIV-2 (21) or eluted, dried blood-spot results. The licensed p24-antigen test includes a neutralization procedure that is to be used for specific testing of samples with repeatedly reactive test results. Federal regulations already require that all donations of blood, blood components, and plasma intended for further processing into injectable products ("source plasma") be screened with a licensed test that detects HIV antibody. Since June 1992, PHS has also required that all blood and plasma donations be screened for HIV-2 antibody.

PHS has not recommended the use of the licensed HIV-1 p24-antigen assay for screening donated blood or source plasma, nor has the kit been approved for use in donor screening. This position is based on findings from several studies indicating that a blood donor with a positive test for antigen and a negative test for antibody is rare (22, 23). Such rarity is probably attributable to the effectiveness of the donor-qualification procedures, including donor education, voluntary exclusion, and antibody testing that together operate to prevent donation by persons at increased risk for HIV infection. Limited studies have been conducted to examine the use of the p24-antigen assay to screen organ/tissue donors (19, 20, 24). Among approximately 1,000 samples from HIV-1 antibody-negative donors, no donors had detectable HIV-1 p24 antigen.

Recipient Screening

Until recently, PHS had made no recommendations regarding routine testing of recipients of organs, tissues, semen, or donated human milk. However, in response to the July 18, 1991, report of the PHS Workgroup on Organ and Tissue Transplantation, HRSA asked UNOS to request that transplant centers implement an interim voluntary HIV-testing policy for organ recipients. HRSA has requested that recipients be tested for HIV-1 antibody immediately before transplantation and at 3, 6, and 12 months after transplantation. If HIV infection is diagnosed in an organ recipient, the results of the HIV test are reported by the transplant center to the Scientific Registry for Transplant Recipients and to the procuring OPO, in accordance with existing state laws. No comparable registry exists for recipients of tissues, semen, or donated human milk. However, the National Marrow Donor Program routinely tracks both donors and recipients of bone marrow for unrelated-donor transplants. This program reports no known seroconversions among either donors or recipients, although recipients are not routinely screened for HIV.

Routine testing of recipients after transplantation has several potential benefits. First, early identification of HIV infection in a recipient allows for early intervention before signs and symptoms develop. Both antiviral therapy to prevent progression to acquired immunodeficiency syndrome (AIDS) (25) and prophylactic therapy to prevent opportunistic infections (26, 27) have been recommended for HIV-infected patients, based on CD4+ T-lymphocyte levels. Second, early identification of HIV infection in a transplant recipient allows for early intervention to prevent further transmission from the recipient to sex or needle-sharing partners and to future offspring (through vertical transmission from mother to infant). Third, early identification of HIV infection in a recipient potentially identifies an infectious donor. Should further investigation indicate that the donor is the source of the HIV infection in the recipient, other recipients of tissue from that same donor can be notified and stored tissue can be retrieved, preventing further transmission through transplantation. Concern has been expressed that linking HIV infection in a transplant recipient to the transplantation may be difficult because many recipients may have also received blood or blood products or have other risk factors. However, identification of multiple HIV-infected recipients of tissue from the same donor strongly implicates the donor as the source of the HIV infection in the recipients. In addition, stored blood or lymphoid samples from the donor (when available) can be tested for the presence of virus to confirm the HIV-infection status of the donor (4).

Questions have been raised about whether transplant recipients who may be receiving immunosuppressive therapy to prevent rejection are capable of producing antibody against HIV if transmission occurs. Several reports now indicate that the HIV-antibody response is not delayed in transplant recipients receiving antirejection therapy, which primarily affects cellular immunity (4).

The additional costs of routine screening for HIV in recipients must be considered as well. The Institute of Medicine has estimated that laboratory costs are approximately $4 for a patient who tests negative and $35 for a patient who tests positive. (The latter cost includes the added expense of repeat EIAs and Western blot or other supplemental tests.) These costs may be underestimates, however. The time required for pretest and posttest counseling was estimated to be approximately 0.5–1.0 hour for an HIV-seronegative patient and 1.5–2.0 hours for an HIV-seropositive patient (28).

Inactivation of HIV in Tissues

Thorough donor screening is considered the most effective method for preventing HIV transmission through transplantation; however, the use of chemical or physical inactivating or sterilizing agents to reduce further the already low risk of transmission has been considered. If such agents are to be useful, they must either inactivate or eliminate the virus while maintaining the functional integrity of the tissue or organ. No mechanism for inactivating virus in whole organs currently exists. However, several agents have been suggested as possible disinfectants for tissues such as bone fragments (4). Pasteurization has been shown to inactivate HIV in human milk without substantially compromising nutritional and immunologic characteristics (29).

Although some physical and chemical agents have been shown to reduce the likelihood of isolating virus from treated solid tissues, conclusive evidence that those processes render solid tissue completely safe yet structurally intact is lacking. In the recent case of an HIV-infected donor who was antibody negative (4), tissues that had been processed in a variety of ways did not transmit HIV. These tissues included (a) lyophilized fascia lata, tendons, or ligaments; (b) dura mater that was lyophilized and irradiated with 3.0–3.4 Mrad of gamma radiation through a cobalt-60 source; (c) bone fragments that were treated with ethanol and lyophilized; and (d) one sample of fresh-frozen long bone with the marrow elements evacuated (4). However, because most of these tissues were relatively avascular, it is unclear whether the absence of HIV transmission was due to processing, avascularity, or both.

General Considerations

In developing guidelines for preventing HIV transmission from organ/tissue donors to recipients, several factors were considered: (a) differences between the screening of living, brain-dead, and cadaveric donors; (b) time constraints due to organ/tissue viability that may preclude performing certain screening procedures; (c) differences in the risk for HIV transmission from various organs and tissues; (d) differences between systems in place for procuring and distributing organs and tissues; (e) the effect of screening practices on the limited availability of organs and some tissues; and (f) the benefit of the transplant to the recipient (i.e., some transplants are lifesaving, whereas others are life enhancing).

Living donors can be interviewed about potential high-risk behavior, whereas deceased donors cannot. In the case of brain-dead or cadaveric donors, family members and others may be unable to provide an accurate risk history. Therefore, exclusion of potentially infected brain-dead or cadaveric donors relies even more heavily on laboratory screening and physical examinations than on interviews regarding high-risk behavior. Screening procedures that require more than 24 hours to complete may not be feasible for brain-dead or cadaveric donors of organs and certain tissues. Most tissues must be recovered and most organs must be recovered and transplanted shortly after cessation of circulatory function of the donor. Whereas some tissues can be stored for months, others must be transplanted within a few days after procurement. These time constraints may limit the ability to interview certain family members or significant life partners who are not nearby and may preclude the use of certain laboratory screening tests that cannot be performed within these time constraints.

The precise risk of HIV transmission from various tissues is not known, yet some organs and tissues clearly present a higher risk for HIV transmission than others (4). For example, studies indicate that the risk for transmission from an organ of an HIV-infected donor is nearly 100%. Fresh-frozen, unprocessed bone also appears to carry a high risk for transmission, particularly if marrow elements and adherent tissue are not removed. Relatively avascular solid tissue, some of which is also processed by using techniques that might inactivate HIV, appears to carry a lower risk for HIV transmission.

As noted earlier in these guidelines, there is considerable variability in the role of federal agencies regarding transplantation of organs and tissues and the procurement and distribution systems. Oversight for, existence of, and compliance with recommendations also vary between these systems. When organs and tissues are procured from a single donor, tracking systems must involve multiple distribution systems that may be difficult to link.

Donor-screening practices must also consider the already inadequate supply of most organs and tissues needed for transplantation. However, even though attempts should be made to ensure the highest level of safety, donor-screening practices should not unnecessarily exclude acceptable potential donors.

Those involved in developing guidelines should consider that some transplants are lifesaving (e.g., a heart transplant), whereas others are life enhancing. Some physicians may be willing to offer the patient a transplant of a lifesaving organ from a donor whose HIV risk status is questionable but would not use life-enhancing tissue from such a donor.

RECOMMENDATIONS

Donor Screening

1. All prospective living donors or next of kin or significant life partners accompanying brain-dead or cadaveric donors should be informed of the

general nature of the donor-evaluation process, including a review of medical and behavioral history, physical examination, and blood tests to exclude infectious agents that might be transmitted by organ or tissue transplant.

2. Prospective living donors or next of kin or significant life partners accompanying brain-dead or cadaveric donors should be informed about modes of transmission and risk factors for HIV infection, emphasizing that HIV can be transmitted via transplanted organs and tissues. They should be told that a negative test for HIV antibody does not guarantee that the donor is free of HIV infection because of the rare situation of donation after infection but before seroconversion. Therefore, organs and tissue must not be transplanted from persons who may have engaged in activities that placed them at increased risk for HIV infection. This information should be presented in simple language to ensure that the donor, next of kin, or significant life partner understands what is considered high-risk behavior and the importance of excluding persons who have engaged in this behavior. Persons soliciting the donation should not place undue pressure to donate on potential living donors and those persons providing permission for potential brain-dead or cadaveric donors who might otherwise decline to donate or give permission because of high-risk behavior.

3. To ascertain risk factors, all prospective living donors should be interviewed in a confidential and sensitive manner by a health-care professional competent to elicit information about behaviors that place persons at risk for HIV infection. Interviewers should ask direct questions about high-risk behavior.

4. For potential pediatric donors for whom maternal transmission of HIV is a consideration, the mother and, if possible, the father should be interviewed about behaviors that may have placed them at risk for acquiring HIV infection that could have been transmitted to their child.

5. Except where retrieval occurs by legal authorization, the next of kin or significant life partner of brain-dead or cadaveric donors should be interviewed in a confidential and sensitive manner by a health-care professional regarding potential HIV risk factors in the donor. Other family members, friends, and sex partners may also need to be interviewed, if available. When consent for removal of organs/tissue is required, at least the person signing the consent form should be interviewed. Other possible sources of information about behavioral risk factors may include hospital, police, and coroner's records, if available. When an interview is not performed, as allowed by legal authorization, the transplant surgeon should be fully informed that the donation was accepted, even though a direct interview with the next of kin or significant life partner was not performed.

6. If available, the medical records, including autopsy reports of all donors, should be reviewed for signs and symptoms associated with HIV infection and for evidence of high-risk behavior (e.g., male-to-male sexual contact, acquisition of sexually transmitted diseases, exchange of sex for money or drugs, injecting-drug use, or birth to a mother either at risk for or infected with HIV).

7. All prospective donors of organs, solid tissue, and semen should undergo a physical examination as close as possible before donation, with special at-

tention to physical signs of HIV disease and injecting-drug use. The extent of the physical examination should be determined by the responsible medical officials according to the context of organ/tissue donation. Human milk banks should obtain a release from the primary health-care provider certifying that the prospective donor is in good health and does not constitute a risk to potential recipients.

8. As with donors of blood and plasma, prospective living organ, tissue, semen, and milk donors found after careful screening to be acceptable donors should sign a consent statement indicating that they have reviewed and understand the information provided regarding the spread of HIV and have agreed not to donate should they be at potential risk for spreading HIV. The statement should also indicate that prospective donors understand that they must be tested for HIV as part of the donor-screening process and will be notified of positive results as specified by any existing state statutes, regulations, or guidelines. For acceptable brain-dead or cadaveric donors, procurement personnel should document that a careful attempt has been made to eliminate persons at high risk through available information, including interview of family members or significant life partners, physical examination, review of medical records, autopsy findings, and any other records that might provide information about high-risk behavior or possible HIV infection. For either type of donor, the statement should be included as part of a general checklist or donor evaluation form covering all important aspects of the donor evaluation and should be included in the transplant records or record of the procuring agency. All records generated by the interview should be kept confidential.

Donor Testing

1. For all prospective donors, a blood sample obtained before any transfusions were administered (during the current hospital admission for inpatients) should be collected as close to the time of retrieval of tissue as possible. Bone marrow donors must provide blood samples far enough in advance of marrow harvest to permit the tests to be performed and results reported before the recipient's preparative regimen (marrow ablation) is begun. Samples should be tested for antibodies to both HIV-1 and HIV-2 by using FDA-licensed tests. Separate tests or a combination test for HIV-1 and HIV-2 may be used. All antibody-screening tests should be performed by EIA unless the condition of the recipient or donor dictates the use of a more rapid screening assay.

2. Transfusions and infusion of other fluids to the prospective donor might produce false-negative results because of hemodilution. Efforts should be made to perform HIV-antibody testing on the most recent pretransfusion/infusion specimen for which identity and quality can be ensured. Specimens should not be drawn immediately downstream from an intravenous site to prevent dilution with intravenous fluids.

Posttransfusion/infusion specimens may be considered for testing after efforts to obtain a pretransfusion/infusion sample have been exhausted and posttransfusion/infusion samples have been assessed for evidence of dilution. The suitability of posttransfusion/infusion samples must consider (a) the volume of the material transfused as a percentage of the patient's total blood volume and (b) the amount of time between the last transfusion/infusion and the collection of the sample to be tested. An exchange of one total blood volume will reduce the concentration of an intravascular substance such as IgG to 35% of initial levels if there is no replacement from the extravascular space. More than 50% of total body IgG is extravascular, and reequilibration to normal levels of IgG should be nearly complete within 24 hours of a total blood volume exchange of albumin (30).

3. The HIV p24-antigen assay may identify a few of the rare donors who are HIV-infected, yet antibody-negative; however, studies examining the utility of this assay for screening organ/tissue donors are limited and currently do not allow a definitive recommendation on the use of this test (19, 24). The utility of other assays such as PCR, which are currently experimental, should be considered for evaluation as they become available for clinical use. Those institutions choosing to use the HIV-1 p24-antigen assay should be aware that in populations with low prevalence (e.g., organ/tissue donors), a large percentage of persons who test repeatedly reactive (without confirmation with the neutralization assay) will be false positive. Consideration should also be given to the potential problems with decreased specificity when the assay is used to test postmortem samples (19).

4. The testing algorithm for HIV-antibody assays should be performed as described in the package insert with an initial test and, if reactive, a retest on the same specimen. However, the time constraints of some situations may not accommodate the delay of repeat testing by EIA as described in the package insert. In such extreme cases of lifesaving organ transplantation, the sample should be set up in triplicate in the initial EIA. A repeatedly reactive result (positive screening test) is defined as reactivity above the test cutoff in two or more of the three assays. When testing by EIA is impractical, a more rapid licensed test should be performed in triplicate. Testing by the conventional algorithm should be performed as early as possible, even if it follows the procurement and/or transplant of the organs or tissues.

5. Results of HIV testing for organ/tissue donors should be handled confidentially, in accordance with general medical practices and applicable federal and state statutes, regulations, and guidelines.

6. Prospective living donors should be notified if they are found through the screening process to be HIV infected. Because of the possibility of sexual or parenteral transmission, the spouse or known sex partners of brain-dead or cadaveric donors should be notified in accordance with state law. All notifications should be handled in a manner congruent with current recommendations regarding counseling, testing, and partner notification (31, 32). Before the notification of these persons, transplant and procurement organizations should consult with their state health department concerning local notification policies. Also before notification, the repeatedly reactive screening assay should be confirmed with more specific supplemental tests. An aliquot of the original sample should be analyzed by using the following, more specific tests. For repeatedly reactive HIV-1 antibody EIAs, an HIV-1 Western blot or immunofluorescence assay should be per-

formed. For repeatedly reactive HIV-1 antigen assays (if performed), a neutralization procedure must be performed. For HIV-2, no licensed supplemental test is available; however, consideration may be given to the use of research assays such as Western blot, immunofluorescence, radioimmune precipitation, and synthetic peptide-based EIA. Arrangements for HIV-2 supplemental testing may need to be made with either the state or local health department. For repeatedly reactive combination HIV-1 and HIV-2 assays, the published testing algorithm should be followed (21). When the results of any supplemental tests are unclear, the use of research assays should be considered.

Notification of HIV-infected prospective living donors or spouses/known sex partners of cadaveric donors should be done in accordance with state law and in a confidential and sensitive manner by staff competent in counseling and discussing positive HIV results and their implications. If such staff are not available in the organ/tissue procurement organization, arrangements should be made with other organizations such as health departments or clinics to provide appropriate notification.

8. When it is possible to properly obtain and store samples, one or more of the following samples from the donor should be saved for at least 5 years after the expiration date of the tissue: dried blood spots, a frozen buffy coat, spleen cells, lymph node cells, bone marrow, and an aliquot of serum. These samples can be examined if subsequent information indicates that the donor may have donated during the period after infection but before antibody seroconversion.

9. Confirmed positive HIV test results in a prospective organ/tissue donor should be reported to state health agencies if required by state law or regulation.

Donor Exclusion Criteria

Regardless of their HIV antibody test results, persons who meet any of the criteria listed below should be excluded from donation of organs or tissues unless the risk to the recipient of not performing the transplant is deemed to be greater than the risk of HIV transmission and disease (e.g., emergent, life-threatening illness requiring transplantation when no other organs/tissues are available and no other lifesaving therapies exist). In such a case, informed consent regarding the possibility of HIV transmission should be obtained from the recipient.

Behavior/History Exclusionary Criteria

1. Men who have had sex with another man in the preceding 5 years.
2. Persons who report nonmedical intravenous, intramuscular, or subcutaneous injection of drugs in the preceding 5 years.
3. Persons with hemophilia or related clotting disorders who have received human-derived clotting factor concentrates
4. Men and women who have engaged in sex in exchange for money or drugs in the preceding 5 years.
5. Persons who have had sex in the preceding 12 months with any person described in items 1–4 above or with a person known or suspected to have HIV infection.

6. Persons who have been exposed in the preceding 12 months to known or suspected HIV-infected blood through percutaneous inoculation or through contact with an open wound, nonintact skin, or mucous membrane.
7. Inmates of correctional systems. (This exclusion is to address issues such as difficulties with informed consent and increased prevalence of HIV in this population.)

Specific Exclusionary Criteria for Pediatric Donors

1. Children meeting any of the exclusionary criteria listed above for adults should not be accepted as donors.
2. Children born to mothers with HIV infection or mothers who meet the behavioral or laboratory exclusionary criteria for adult donors (regardless of their HIV status) should not be accepted as donors unless HIV infection can be definitely excluded in the child as follows:

   Children greater than 18 months of age who are born to mothers with or at risk for HIV infection, who have not been breast fed within the last 12 months, and whose HIV antibody tests, physical examination, and review of medical records do not indicate evidence of HIV infection can be accepted as donors.

3. Children less than or equal to 18 months of age who are born to mothers with or at risk for HIV infection or who have been breast fed within the past 12 months should not be accepted as donors regardless of their HIV test results.

Laboratory and Other Medical Exclusionary Criteria

1. Persons who cannot be tested for HIV infection because of refusal, inadequate blood samples (e.g., hemodilution that could result in false-negative tests), or any other reasons.
2. Persons with a repeatedly reactive screening assay for HIV-1 or HIV-2 antibody regardless of the results of supplemental assays.
3. Persons whose history, physical examination, medical records, or autopsy reports reveal other evidence of HIV infection or high-risk behavior, such as a diagnosis of AIDS, unexplained weight loss, night sweats, blue or purple spots on the skin or mucous membranes typical of Kaposi's sarcoma, unexplained lymphadenopathy lasting greater than 1 month, unexplained temperature greater than 100.5°F (38.6°C) for greater than 10 days, unexplained persistent cough and shortness of breath, opportunistic infections, unexplained persistent diarrhea, male-to-male sexual contact, sexually transmitted diseases, or needle tracks or other signs of parenteral drug abuse.

Inactivation of HIV in Organs/Tissues

Definitive recommendations cannot yet be made regarding inactivation of HIV in organs and tissues because of lack of information about potentially effective inactivation measures. Research should continue in this area. Efforts to evaluate the effect of certain processing techniques on tissue sterility and quality should be expanded to include virologic studies for HIV. Thus, until more is known, it is prudent to process bone and bone fragments and carefully evacuate all marrow components from whole bone whenever feasible.

Quarantine

For semen donations and, when possible, for tissue donations from living donors, the collection should be placed in frozen quarantine and the donor retested for antibodies to HIV-1 and HIV-2 after 6 months (15). The quarantined material should be released only if the follow-up test results have been obtained and are negative.

Record Keeping for Tracking of Recipients and Tissues

1. Each establishment involved in the acquisition, processing, distribution, or storage of organs or tissues should have a graft identification system that allows the tracking of organs and tissues from the donor source to the recipient institution and vice versa. Furthermore, each establishment involved in the acquisition of organs or tissues from a single donor should have mechanisms in place to facilitate the communication between establishments for the purposes of tracking organs and tissues to recipients who should be notified if HIV transmission from donor source material is confirmed. Procurement, processing, distribution, and storage centers should keep accurate records of the distribution of each organ/tissue according to the donor identification number, tissue type and identifying number, and identifying information for the receiving center, along with dates of procurement and distribution. Records should be kept a minimum of 10 years after expiration of tissue.
2. The transplantation center, hospital, physician, or dentist should keep accurate records of all organs/tissues received and the disposition of each. These records must be separate from patients' medical records (e.g., in a log book) so that this information is easily obtainable should tracking be necessary. Recorded information should include the organ/tissue type; donor identification number; name of procurement or distribution center supplying the organ/tissue; recipient-identifying information; name of recipient's physician or dentist; and dates of (a) receipt by the center and (b) either transplantation to the recipient or further distribution.
3. The donor identification number and organ or tissue type should be recorded in the recipient's transplant/medical/dental record.

Testing and Reporting of Recipients

1. Health-care providers for transplant recipients and the recipients themselves should be aware of the small but potential risk of infections, including HIV, from transplanted organs and tissues. The recipient's informed consent to the transplant should include acknowledgment of the risks, including transmission of HIV and other infections.
2. Until the risk for HIV transmission from screened donors has been clarified, recipients of solid organs should be routinely advised to be tested for HIV immediately before transplantation and at 3 months following the transplant. Testing of recipients should be done with consent of the recip-

ient and should not be mandatory. Recipients of tissues other than solid organs do not require routine testing for HIV following receipt of the tissue from appropriately screened donors. Results of HIV testing of organ recipients should be collected and analyzed by the Scientific Registry for Transplant Recipients. (If data indicate no benefit from recipient testing, then this recommendation for recipient testing may be omitted in a revision of these guidelines.)

3. If a transplant recipient is found to be infected with HIV, the transplant center or health-care provider should, consistent with state law, immediately notify the state health department and the organization from which the tissue was obtained. HIV infection in a solid-organ recipient should also be reported to the Scientific Registry for Transplant Recipients.

Recall of Stored Tissue and Tracking of Recipients of Organs/Tissue from HIV-infected Donors

1. Upon being notified that an organ/tissue recipient is infected with HIV, the organ/tissue collection center, in collaboration with the state or local health department and with assistance from CDC, is responsible for determining as soon as possible whether the donor was HIV-infected. This is done by determining the HIV-infection status of other recipients of organs/tissues (particularly those recipients of organs and fresh-frozen bone) and by laboratory testing of stored donor material. Experimental diagnostic laboratory assays such as PCR may be useful in these situations and should be used when they become available.

2. If evidence suggests HIV infection in the donor either from testing of stored donor specimens or by finding HIV infection in other recipients, all other recipients of that donor's tissue or organs should be notified through their transplanting physician and informed of the likelihood of HIV exposure and advised to undergo HIV testing.

3. HIV-infected recipients should be counseled about their need for medical evaluation and about prevention of HIV transmission to others. They should also be advised to inform their sex or needle-sharing partners of their potential risk and need for HIV counseling and testing. HIV-infected women should be informed of the risk of transmission of HIV to their children born after the transplant and be advised to have these children evaluated and to avoid breast-feeding. Pregnant women should receive pregnancy counseling about HIV.

4. All stored organs/tissues from a donor found to be HIV-infected should be retrieved and quarantined immediately and either used only for research purposes or destroyed, except when the transplantation of an indispensable organ/tissue is necessary to save the patient's life.

REFERENCES: AS NUMBERED IN ORIGINAL PUBLICATION

1. CDC. Prevention of acquired immune deficiency syndrome (AIDS): report of inter-agency recommendations. MMWR 1983;32:101–103.
2. CDC. Provisional Public Health Service inter-agency recommendations for screening donated blood and plasma for antibody to the virus causing acquired immunodeficiency syndrome. MMWR 1985; 34:1–5.
3. CDC. Testing donors of organs, tissues, and semen for antibody to human T-lymphotropic virus type III/lymphadenopathy-associated virus. MMWR 1985;34:294.

4. Simonds RJ, Holmberg SD, Hurwitz RL, et al. Transmission of human immunodeficiency virus type 1 from a seronegative organ and tissue donor. N Engl J Med 1992;326:726–732.
14. Food and Drug Administration. Human tissue intended for transplantation. Federal Register 1993;58(236):65514-65521.
15. CDC. Semen banking, organ and tissue transplantation, and HIV antibody testing. MMWR 1988; 37:57–58, 63.
16. CDC. Transmission of HIV through bone transplantation: case report and public health recommendations. MMWR 1988;37:597–599.
17. CDC. Recommendations for assisting in the prevention of perinatal transmission of human T-lymphotropic virus type III/lymphadenopathy-associated virus and acquired immunodeficiency syndrome. MMWR 1985;34:721–732.
18. Human Milk Banking Association of North America, Inc. In: Arnold LDW, Tully MR, eds. Guidelines for the establishment and operation of a donor human milk bank. West Hartford, CT: Human Milk Banking Association of North America, Inc., 1994.
19. Pepose JS, Buerger DG, Paul DA, Quinn TC, Darragh TM, Donegan E. New developments in serologic screening of corneal donors for HIV-1 and hepatitis B virus infections. Ophthalmology 1992; 99:879–888.
20. Novick SL, Schrager JA, Nelson JA, Baskin BL. A comparison of two HBsAg and two HIV-1 (p24) antigen EIA test kits with hemolyzed cadaveric blood specimens. Tissue and Cell Report 1993;1:2–3.
21. CDC. Testing for antibodies to human immunodeficiency virus type 2 in the United States. MMWR 1992;41(No. RR-12):1–9.
22. Alter HJ, Epstein JS, Swenson SG, et al. Prevalence of human immunodeficiency virus type 1 p24 antigen in U.S. blood donors—an assessment of the efficacy of testing in donor screening. N Engl J Med 1990;323:1312–1317.
23. Busch MP, Taylor PE, Lenes BA, et al. Screening of selected male blood donors for p24 antigen of human immunodeficiency virus type 1. N Engl J Med 1990;323:1308–1312.
24. Callaway T, McCreedy B, Pruett T. Polymerase chain reaction for HIV screening of tissue donors [Abstract #02638 (S44)]. XIV International Congress of the Transplantation Society, Paris, France, August 16–21, 1992.
25. National Institute for Allergy and Infectious Diseases. State-of-the-art conference on azidothymidine therapy for early HIV infection. Am J Med 1990;89:335–344.
26. CDC. Recommendations for prophylaxis against Pneumocystis carinii pneumonia for adults and adolescents infected with human immunodeficiency virus. MMWR 1992;41(No. RR-4):1–11.
27. CDC. Guidelines for prophylaxis against Pneumocystis carinii pneumonia for children infected with human immunodeficiency virus. MMWR 1991;40(No. RR-2):1–13.
28. The Institute of Medicine. Cost estimates: early intervention for HIV infection. In: Hardy LM, ed. HIV screening of pregnant women and newborns. Washington, DC: National Academy Press, 1991:135–142.
29. Orloff SL, Wallingford JC, McDougal JS. Inactivation of human immunodeficiency virus type 1 in human milk: effects of intrinsic factors in human milk and of pasteurization. J Human Lactation 1993;9:13–17.
30. Chopek M, McCullough J. Protein and biochemical changes during plasma exchange. In: Berkman EM, Umlas J, eds. Therapeutic hemapheresis. Washington, DC: American Association of Blood Banks, 1980:13–52.
31. CDC. Technical guidance on HIV counseling. MMWR 1993;42(No. RR-2):8–17.
32. CDC. Public Health Service guidelines for counseling and antibody testing to prevent HIV infection and AIDS. MMWR 1987;36:509–515.

Barrier Protection Against HIV Infection and Other Sexually Transmitted Diseases

Original Citation: Update: Centers for Disease Control and Prevention. Barrier Protection Against HIV Infection and Other Sexually Transmitted Diseases. MMWR 1993;42(30):589–591, 597.

SUMMARY

Although refraining from intercourse with infected partners remains the most effective strategy for preventing human immunodeficiency virus

(HIV) infection and other sexually transmitted diseases (STDs), the Public Health Service also has recommended condom use as part of its strategy. Since CDC summarized the effectiveness of condom use in preventing HIV infection and other STDs in 1988 (1), additional information has become available, and the Food and Drug Administration has approved a polyurethane "female condom." This report updates laboratory and epidemiologic information regarding the effectiveness of condoms in preventing HIV infection and other STDs and the role of spermicides used adjunctively with condoms.

Two reviews summarizing the use of latex condoms among serodiscordant heterosexual couples (i.e., in which one partner is HIV positive and the other HIV negative) indicated that using latex condoms substantially reduces the risk for HIV transmission (2, 3). In addition, two subsequent studies of serodiscordant couples confirmed this finding and emphasized the importance of consistent (i.e., use of a condom with each act of intercourse) and correct condom use (4, 5). In one study of serodiscordant couples, none of 123 partners who used condoms consistently seroconverted; in comparison, 12 (10%) of 122 seronegative partners who used condoms inconsistently became infected (4). In another study of serodiscordant couples (with seronegative female partners of HIV-infected men), three (2%) of 171 consistent condom users seroconverted, compared with eight (15%) of 55 inconsistent condom users. When person-years at risk were considered, the rate for HIV transmission among couples reporting consistent condom use was 1.1 per 100 person-years of observation, compared with 9.7 among inconsistent users (5).

Condom use reduces the risk for gonorrhea, herpes simplex virus (HSV) infection, genital ulcers, and pelvic inflammatory disease (2). In addition, intact latex condoms provide a continuous mechanical barrier to HIV, HSV, hepatitis B virus (HBV), Chlamydia trachomatis, and Neisseria gonorrhoeae (2). A recent laboratory study (6) indicated that latex condoms are an effective mechanical barrier to fluid containing HIV-sized particles.

Three prospective studies in developed countries indicated that condoms are unlikely to break or slip during proper use. Reported breakage rates in the studies were 2% or less for vaginal or anal intercourse (2). One study reported complete slippage off the penis during intercourse for one (0.4%) of 237 condoms and complete slippage off the penis during withdrawal for one (0.4%) of 237 condoms (7).

Laboratory studies indicate that the female condom (Reality™*)—a lubricated polyurethane sheath with a ring on each end that is inserted into the vagina—is an effective mechanical barrier to viruses, including HIV. No clinical studies have been completed to define protection from HIV infection or

---

* Use of trade names is for identification only and does not imply endorsement by the Public Health Service or the U.S. Department of Health and Human Services.

other STDs. However, an evaluation of the female condom's effectiveness in pregnancy prevention was conducted during a 6-month period for 147 women in the United States. The estimated 12-month failure rate for pregnancy prevention among the 147 women was 26%. Of the 86 women who used this condom consistently and correctly, the estimated 12-month failure rate was 11%.

Laboratory studies indicate that nonoxynol-9, a nonionic surfactant used as a spermicide, inactivates HIV and other sexually transmitted pathogens. In a cohort study among women, vaginal use of nonoxynol-9 without condoms reduced risk for gonorrhea by 89%; in another cohort study among women, vaginal use of nonoxynol-9 without condoms reduced risk for gonorrhea by 24% and chlamydial infection by 22% (2). No reports indicate that nonoxynol-9 used alone without condoms is effective for preventing sexual transmission of HIV. Furthermore, one randomized controlled trial among prostitutes in Kenya found no protection against HIV infection with use of a vaginal sponge containing a high dose of nonoxynol-9 (2). No studies have shown that nonoxynol-9 used with a condom increases the protection provided by condom use alone against HIV infection.

EDITORIAL NOTE

This report indicates that latex condoms are highly effective for preventing HIV infection and other STDs when used consistently and correctly. Condom availability is essential in assuring consistent use. Men and women relying on condoms for prevention of HIV infection or other STDs should carry condoms or have them readily available.

Correct use of a latex condom requires (a) using a new condom with each act of intercourse; (b) carefully handling the condom to avoid damaging it with fingernails, teeth, or other sharp objects; (c) putting on the condom after the penis is erect and before any genital contact with the partner; (d) ensuring no air is trapped in the tip of the condom; (e) ensuring adequate lubrication during intercourse, possibly requiring use of exogenous lubricants; (f) using only water-based lubricants (e.g., K-Y Jelly™ or glycerine) with latex condoms (oil-based lubricants [e.g., petroleum jelly, shortening, mineral oil, massage oils, body lotions, or cooking oil] that can weaken latex should never be used); and (g) holding the condom firmly against the base of the penis during withdrawal and withdrawing while the penis is still erect to prevent slippage.

Condoms should be stored in a cool, dry place out of direct sunlight and should not be used after the expiration date. Condoms in damaged packages or condoms that show obvious signs of deterioration (e.g., brittleness, stickiness, or discoloration) should not be used regardless of their expiration date.

Natural-membrane condoms may not offer the same level of protection against sexually transmitted viruses as latex condoms. Unlike latex, natural-membrane condoms have naturally occurring pores that are small enough to prevent passage of sperm but large enough to allow passage of viruses in laboratory studies (2).

The effectiveness of spermicides in preventing HIV transmission is unknown. Spermicides used in the vagina may offer some protection against cervical gonorrhea and chlamydia. No data exist to indicate that condoms lubricated with spermicides are more effective than other lubricated condoms in protecting against the transmission of HIV infection and other STDs. Therefore, latex condoms with or without spermicides are recommended.

The most effective way to prevent sexual transmission of HIV infection and other STDs is to avoid sexual intercourse with an infected partner. If a person chooses to have sexual intercourse with a partner whose infection status is unknown or who is infected with HIV or other STDs, men should use a new latex condom with each act of intercourse. When a male condom cannot be used, couples should consider using a female condom.

Data from the 1988 National Survey of Family Growth underscore the importance of consistent and correct use of contraceptive methods in pregnancy prevention (8). For example, the typical failure rate during the first year of use was 8% for oral contraceptives, 15% for male condoms, and 26% for periodic abstinence. In comparison, persons who always abstain will have a zero failure rate, women who always use oral contraceptives will have a near-zero (0.1%) failure rate, and consistent male condom users will have a 2% failure rate (9). For prevention of HIV infection and STDs, as with pregnancy prevention, consistent and correct use is crucial. The determinants of proper condom use are complex and incompletely understood. Better understanding of both individual and societal factors will contribute to prevention efforts that support persons in reducing their risks for infection. Prevention messages must highlight the importance of consistent and correct condom use (10).

REFERENCES: AS NUMBERED IN ORIGINAL PUBLICATION

1. CDC. Condoms for prevention of sexually transmitted diseases. MMWR 1988;37:133–137.
2. Cates W, Stone KM. Family planning, sexually transmitted diseases, and contraceptive choice: a literature update. Fam Plann Perspect 1992;24:75–84.
3. Weller SC. A meta-analysis of condom effectiveness in reducing sexually transmitted HIV. Soc Sci Med 1993;1635–1644.
4. DeVincenzi I, European Study Group on Heterosexual Transmission of HIV. Heterosexual transmission of HIV in a European cohort of couples [Abstract no. WS-CO2–1]. Vol 1. IXth International Conference on AIDS/IVth STD World Congress. Berlin, June 9, 1993:83.
5. Saracco A, Musicco M, Nicolosi A, et al. Man-to-woman sexual transmission of HIV: longitudinal study of 343 steady partners of infected men. J Acquir Immune Defic Syndr 1993;6:497–502.
6. Carey RF, Herman WA, Retta SM, Rinaldi JE, Herman BA, Athey TW. Effectiveness of latex condoms as a barrier to human immunodeficiency virus-sized particles under conditions of simulated use. Sex Transm Dis 1992;19:230–234.
7. Trussell JE, Warner DL, Hatcher R. Condom performance during vaginal intercourse: comparison of Trojan-Enz™ and Tactylon™ condoms. Contraception 1992;45:11–19.
8. Jones EF, Forrest JD. Contraceptive failure rates based on the 1988 NSFG. Fam Plann Perspect 1992;24:12–19.
9. Trussell J, Hatcher RA, Cates W, Stewart FH, Kost K. Contraceptive failure in the United States: an update. Stud Fam Plann 1990;21:51–54.
10. Roper WL, Peterson HB, Curran JW. Commentary: condoms and HIV/STD prevention—clarifying the message. Am J Public Health 1993;83:501–503.

Improper Infection-Control Practices During Employee Vaccination Programs

Original Citation: Centers for Disease Control and Prevention. Improper Infection-Control Practices During Employee Vaccination Programs—District of Columbia and Pennsylvania, 1993. MMWR 1993;42(50):969–971.

Editor's Note: The information included here was based on an article which reports on several cases of the improper use of needles and syringes and contamination of multidose medication vials. It then gives guidance on the use of needles and syringes during parenteral injection.

The following infection-control principles are consistent with previous CDC recommendations and should be adhered to by health-care providers and all other persons who administer parenteral substances by injection (9, 10):

- A needle or syringe that previously has been used to inoculate a patient is considered contaminated and should not be used to aspirate medication or vaccine from a multidose vial if any of the contents of the vial will subsequently be administered to another patient.
- All hypodermic needles, as well as the lumens of syringes used to administer parenteral substances, should be sterile. Needles and syringes manufactured for single use only should be discarded and should not be reprocessed or reused on a different patient because the reprocessing method may not sterilize the internal surfaces and/or may alter the integrity of the device.
- Reusable needles and syringes should be cleaned and then sterilized by standard heat-based sterilization methods (e.g., steam autoclave or dry-air oven) between uses. Reprocessing of reusable needles and syringes by use of liquid chemical germicides cannot guarantee sterility and is not recommended.
- Used needles should never be recapped or otherwise manipulated using both hands or any other technique that involves directing the point of a needle toward any part of the body. Either a one-handed "scoop" technique or a mechanical device designed for holding the needle sheath should be used if recapping is necessary. Used needles and syringes should be disposed of in puncture-resistant containers located as close as practical to where the needles and syringes are used.

REFERENCES: AS NUMBERED IN ORIGINAL PUBLICATION

9. Garner JS, Favero MS. Guidelines for handwashing and hospital environmental control. Am J Infect Control 1986;14:110–126.
10. CDC. Recommendations for prevention of HIV transmission in health-care settings. MMWR 1987; 36(no. 2S).

Patient Exposures to HIV During Nuclear Medicine Procedures

Original Citation: Centers for Disease Control and Prevention. Patient Exposures to HIV During Nuclear Medicine Procedures. MMWR 1992;41(31):575–578.

Editor's Note: The information included here was based on an article in which three cases of inadvertent HIV infection from nuclear medicine procedures are cited leading to the following recommendations.

Institutions or clinics in which nuclear medicine procedures are performed should assess policies and procedures to assure routine adherence to the following recommendations:

- All health-care providers, including those who perform nuclear medicine procedures, should receive proper training and routine in-service education on proper infection-control procedures (5).
- Written infection-control policies and procedures specific for nuclear medicine should be promulgated, made accessible, and disseminated in departments where nuclear medicine procedures are performed. These policies should outline procedures to follow in the event of a potential emergency (e.g., an administration error).
- All doses and syringes should be examined for identification and radioassayed (i.e., radiation level checked) before injection (6).
- All syringes should be labeled with appropriate identifying information, including the patient's name and the pharmaceutical (6); a unique identification number should also be used.
- Consideration should be given to implementing a system to be used when administering biologic products (e.g., labeled cells) that is similar to the system used for administering blood. Such a system requires that two persons be present to cross-check all labeling of product to be injected, the prescription, and patient identification.
- Contaminated and used syringes should be disposed of safely and appropriately. Disposal containers for syringes should be located as close as practical to the location of syringe use (6, 7).
- All procedures should be documented; documentation should include, at a minimum, the date, name and amount of radiopharmaceutical, and route of administration (6). Ideally, the name or identifying information of the person administering the dose and the exact time of administration should be recorded either in the patient or departmental record.
- An administration error (e.g., administration involving the wrong patient or radiopharmaceutical) should be immediately reported to supervisory personnel and/or the physician in charge. Recommendations for the management of persons after a blood exposure in a health-care setting should be followed (7–9). All administration errors and narrowly avoided errors in administration should be carefully evaluated to determine whether additional precautions are necessary to prevent similar potential administration errors.

Careful adherence to these recommendations should minimize the risk of patient or health-care worker exposure to bloodborne pathogens during nuclear medicine procedures. Misadministrations, as defined by the NRC or by the equivalent state agency in states that have an agreement with the NRC to carry out similar functions, should be reported to the appropriate agency as required by law. In addition, to develop and evaluate additional measures for preventing bloodborne pathogen transmission in nuclear medicine departments and other health-care settings, CDC requests that incidents involving possible transmission of bloodborne pathogens to patients in a health-care setting be reported through local and state health departments to CDC's HIV Infections Branch, Hospital Infections Program, (telephone (404) 639-1547) or Hepatitis Branch, Division of Viral and Rickettsial Diseases (telephone (404) 639-3048).

REFERENCES: AS NUMBERED IN ORIGINAL PUBLICATION

5. Occupational Safety and Health Administration, US Department of Labor. Occupational exposure to bloodborne pathogens; final rule. Federal Register 1991;56:64004-64182.
6. Office of the Federal Register. Code of Federal Regulations—Energy. Part 35. Washington, DC: Office of the Federal Register, National Archives and Records Administration, 1992.
7. CDC. Recommendations for prevention of HIV transmission in health-care settings. MMWR 1987;36 (no. 2S):3S–18S.
8. CDC. Public Health Service statement on management of occupational exposure to human immunodeficiency virus, including considerations regarding zidovudine postexposure use. MMWR 1990; 39(no. RR-1).
9. CDC. Hepatitis B virus: a comprehensive strategy for eliminating transmission in the United States through universal childhood vaccination—recommendations of the Immunization Practices Advisory Committee (ACIP). MMWR 1991;40(no. RR-13):21–24.

Recommendations for Preventing Transmission of HIV and Hepatitis B Virus to Patients During Exposure-Prone Invasive Procedures

Original Citation: Centers for Disease Control and Prevention. Recommendations for Preventing Transmission of Human Immunodeficiency Virus and Hepatitis B Virus to Patients During Exposure-Prone Invasive Procedures. MMWR 1991;40(RR-08):1–9.

Editor's Note: The information included here was based on an article which contains recommendations for the prevention of HIV and HBV transmission during invasive procedures. The original document gives background on infection control practices, on transmission of HIV and HBV during invasive procedures, and discusses exposure-prone procedures.

RECOMMENDATIONS

Investigations of HIV and HBV transmission from health-care workers (HCWs) to patients indicate that, when HCWs adhere to recommended infection-control procedures, the risk of transmitting HBV from an infected HCW to a patient is small, and the risk of transmitting HIV is likely to be even smaller. However, the likelihood of exposure of the patient to an HCW's blood is greater for certain procedures designated as exposure-prone. To minimize the risk of HIV or HBV transmission, the following measures are recommended:

- All HCWs should adhere to universal precautions, including the appropriate use of hand washing, protective barriers, and care in the use and disposal of needles and other sharp instruments. HCWs who have exudative lesions or weeping dermatitis should refrain from all direct patient care and from handling patient-care equipment and devices used in performing invasive procedures until the condition resolves. HCWs should also comply with current guidelines for disinfection and sterilization of reusable devices used in invasive procedures.
- Currently available data provide no basis for recommendations to restrict the practice of HCWs infected with HIV or HBV who perform invasive procedures not identified as exposure-prone, provided the infected HCWs practice recommended surgical or dental technique and comply with universal precautions and current recommendations for sterilization/disinfection.
- Exposure-prone procedures should be identified by medical/surgical/dental organizations and institutions at which the procedures are performed.
- HCWs who perform exposure-prone procedures should know their HIV antibody status. HCWs who perform exposure-prone procedures and who do not have serologic evidence of immunity to HBV from vaccination or from previous infection should know their HBsAg status and, if that is positive, should also know their HBeAg status.
- HCWs who are infected with HIV or HBV (and are HBeAg positive) should not perform exposure-prone procedures unless they have sought counsel from an expert review panel and been advised under what circumstances, if any, they may continue to perform these procedures.* Such circumstances would include notifying prospective patients of the HCW's seropositivity before they undergo exposure-prone invasive procedures.
- Mandatory testing of HCWs for HIV antibody, HBsAg, or HBeAg is not recommended. The current assessment of the risk that infected HCWs will transmit HIV or HBV to patients during exposure-prone procedures does not support the diversion of resources that would be required to implement mandatory testing programs. Compliance by HCWs with recommendations can be increased through education, training, and appropriate confidentiality safeguards.

HCWS WHOSE PRACTICES ARE MODIFIED BECAUSE OF HIV OR HBV STATUS

HCWs whose practices are modified because of their HIV or HBV infection status should, whenever possible, be provided opportunities to continue appro-

---

* The review panel should include experts who represent a balanced perspective. Such experts might include all of the following: (a) the HCW's personal physician(s), (b) an infectious disease specialist with expertise in the epidemiology of HIV and HBV transmission, (c) a health professional with expertise in the procedures performed by the HCW, and (d) state or local public health official(s). If the HCW's practice is institutionally based, the expert review panel might also include a member of the infection-control committee, preferably a hospital epidemiologist. HCWs who perform exposure-prone procedures outside the hospital/institutional setting should seek advice from appropriate state and local public health officials regarding the review process. Panels must recognize the importance of confidentiality and the privacy rights of infected HCWs.

priate patient-care activities. Career counseling and job retraining should be encouraged to promote the continued use of the HCW's talents, knowledge, and skills. HCWs whose practices are modified because of HBV infection should be reevaluated periodically to determine whether their HBeAg status changes due to resolution of infection or as a result of treatment (44).

NOTIFICATION OF PATIENTS AND FOLLOW-UP STUDIES

The public health benefit of notification of patients who have had exposure-prone procedures performed by HCWs infected with HIV or positive for HBeAg should be considered on a case-by-case basis, taking into consideration an assessment of specific risks, confidentiality issues, and available resources. Carefully designed and implemented follow-up studies are necessary to determine more precisely the risk of transmission during such procedures. Decisions regarding notification and follow-up studies should be made in consultation with state and local public health officials.

ADDITIONAL NEEDS

- Clearer definition of the nature, frequency, and circumstances of blood contact between patients and HCWs during invasive procedures.
- Development and evaluation of new devices, protective barriers, and techniques that may prevent such blood contact without adversely affecting the quality of patient care.
- More information on the potential for HIV and HBV transmission through contaminated instruments.
- Improvements in sterilization and disinfection techniques for certain reusable equipment and devices.
- Identification of factors that may influence the likelihood of HIV or HBV transmission after exposure to HIV- or HBV-infected blood.

REFERENCE: AS NUMBERED IN ORIGINAL PUBLICATION

44. Perrillo RP, Schiff ER, Davis GL, et al. A randomized, controlled trial of interferon alpha-2b alone and after prednisone withdrawal for the treatment of chronic hepatitis B. N Engl J Med 1990;323:295–301.

APPENDIX

Definition of Invasive Procedure

An invasive procedure is defined as "surgical entry into tissues, cavities, or organs or repair of major traumatic injuries" associated with any of the following: "(a) an operating or delivery room, emergency department, or outpatient setting, including both physicians' and dentists' offices; (b) cardiac catheterization and angiographic procedures; (c) a vaginal or cesarean delivery or other invasive obstetric procedure during which bleeding may occur; or (d) the manipulation, cutting, or removal of any oral or perioral tissues, including tooth structure, during which bleeding occurs or the potential for bleeding exists."

Reprinted from: Centers for Disease Control. Recommendation for prevention of HIV transmission in health-care settings. MMWR 1987;36(Suppl. no. 2S):6S–7S.

Public Health Service Statement on Management of Occupational Exposure to HIV, Including Considerations Regarding Zidovudine Postexposure Use

Original Citation: Centers for Disease Control and Prevention. Public Health Service statement on management of occupational exposure to human immunodeficiency virus, including considerations regarding zidovudine postexposure use. MMWR 1990;39(RR-01):1–14.

Editor's Note: The information included here was based on an article giving Public Health Service (PHS) recommendations for postexposure management of workers who have occupational exposures that may place them at risk of acquiring HIV infection. Due to space limitations, background information on zidovudine and experience with zidovudine postexposure prophylaxis is not printed.

DEFINITION OF OCCUPATIONAL EXPOSURE

For purposes of this document, an occupational exposure (i.e., exposure that occurs during the performance of job duties) that may place a worker at risk of HIV infection is defined as a percutaneous injury (e.g., a needlestick or cut with a sharp object), contact of mucous membranes, or contact of skin (especially when the exposed skin is chapped, abraded, or afflicted with dermatitis or the contact is prolonged or involving an extensive area) with blood, tissues, or other body fluids to which universal precautions apply, including: (a) semen, vaginal secretions, or other body fluids contaminated with visible blood, because these substances have been implicated in the transmission of HIV infection (2); (b) cerebrospinal fluid, synovial fluid, pleural fluid, peritoneal fluid, pericardial fluid, and amniotic fluid, because the risk of transmission of HIV from these fluids has not yet been determined (2); and (c) laboratory specimens that contain HIV (e.g., suspensions of concentrated virus).

PHS RECOMMENDATIONS FOR MANAGEMENT OF PERSONS AFTER OCCUPATIONAL EXPOSURES THAT MAY PLACE THEM AT RISK OF ACQUIRING HIV INFECTION

Employers should make available to workers a system for promptly initiating evaluation, counseling, and follow-up after a reported occupational exposure that may place the worker at risk of acquiring HIV infection. Workers should be educated to report exposures immediately after they occur, because certain interventions that may be appropriate, e.g., prophylaxis against hepatitis B, must be initiated promptly to be effective (3, 8, 9). Workers who might reasonably be considered at risk of occupational exposure to HIV should be familiarized with the principles of postexposure management as part of job orientation and ongoing job training.

If an exposure occurs, the circumstances should be recorded in the worker's confidential medical record. Relevant information includes the following:

- Date and time of exposure
- Job duty being performed by worker at time of exposure
- Details of exposure, including amount of fluid or material, type of fluid or material, and severity of exposure (e.g., for a percutaneous exposure, depth of injury and whether fluid was injected; for a skin or mucous-membrane exposure, the extent and duration of contact and the condition of the skin, e.g., chapped, abraded, intact)
- Description of source of exposure—including, if known, whether the source material contained HIV or HBV
- Details about counseling, postexposure management, and follow-up

After an occupational exposure, both the exposed worker and the source individual should be evaluated to determine the possible need for the exposed worker to receive prophylaxis against hepatitis B according to previously published CDC recommendations (3, 8, 9). Because of the potentially severe consequences of hepatitis B virus infection, hepatitis B vaccine, which is both safe and highly effective (10), should be offered to any susceptible health-care worker who has an occupational exposure and has not previously been vaccinated with hepatitis B vaccine. Hepatitis B immune globulin may also be indicated, particularly if the source patient or material is found to be positive for hepatitis B surface antigen (HBsAg) (3, 8, 9).

In addition, the source individual should be informed of the incident and, if consent is obtained, tested for serologic evidence of HIV infection. If consent cannot be obtained (e.g., patient is unconscious), policies should be developed for testing source individuals in compliance with applicable state and local laws. Confidentiality of the source individual should be maintained at all times.

If the source individual has AIDS, is known to be HIV-seropositive, or refuses testing, the worker should be evaluated clinically and serologically for evidence of HIV infection as soon as possible after the exposure (baseline) and if seronegative, should be retested periodically for a minimum of 6 months after exposure (e.g., 6 weeks, 12 weeks, and 6 months after exposure) to determine whether HIV infection has occurred. The worker should be advised to report and seek medical evaluation for any acute illness that occurs during the follow-up period. Such illness, particularly if characterized by fever, rash, myalgia, fatigue, malaise, or lymphadenopathy, may be indicative of acute HIV infection, drug reaction, or another medical condition. During the follow-up period, especially the first 6–12 weeks after the exposure when most infected persons are expected to seroconvert, exposed workers should follow PHS recommendations for preventing transmission of HIV. These recommendations include refraining from blood, semen, or organ donation and abstaining from or using measures to prevent HIV transmission during sexual intercourse (11–14). In addition, in countries such as the United States where safe and effective alternatives to breast-feeding are available, exposed women should not breast-feed infants during the follow-up period in order to prevent the infant's possible exposure to HIV in breast milk. During all phases of follow-up, confidentiality of the worker should be protected.

If the source individual is HIV-seronegative and has no clinical manifestations of AIDS or HIV infection, no further HIV follow-up of the exposed worker is necessary unless epidemiologic evidence suggests that the source individual may have recently been exposed to HIV or if testing is desired by the worker or recommended by the health-care provider. In these instances, the guidelines may be followed as described above.

If the source individual cannot be identified, decisions regarding appropriate follow-up should be individualized, based on factors such as whether potential sources are likely to include a person at increased risk of HIV infection.

The employer should make serologic testing available to all workers who are concerned about possible infection with HIV through an occupational exposure. Appropriate psychological counseling may be indicated as well.

ZIDOVUDINE

Prophylaxis Schedules Currently Used After Occupational Exposure

Various regimens have been prescribed for zidovudine prophylaxis after occupational exposure. No data are available to enable investigators to determine the efficacy or compare the toxicity of these or other regimens. At the National Institutes of Health Clinical Center, workers who elect to receive zidovudine are treated with 200 mg every 4 hours (six times daily) for 6 weeks (6). At San Francisco General Hospital, workers who elect to receive zidovudine are treated with 200 mg every 4 hours (five times daily; no dose is given at 4:00 a.m.) for 4 weeks (6). Some clinicians have used an initial dose of 400 mg, and others have prescribed treatment courses ranging from 4 days to 4 months. At several institutions, attempts are made to begin prophylaxis within 1 hour after exposure for workers who elect to receive the drug.

DISCUSSION

Data from animal and human studies are inadequate to establish the efficacy or safety of zidovudine for prophylaxis after occupational exposure to HIV. However, some physicians believe that zidovudine should be offered as prophylaxis to persons after certain occupational exposures for the following reasons: the severity of the illness that may result from HIV infection, the documented antiviral effect of zidovudine in the treatment of persons with established HIV infection, the apparent reversibility of acute toxicity in persons taking zidovudine for a brief period, and the suggestion that in some animal studies, zidovudine postexposure may modify the course of some retroviral infections. Other physicians believe that zidovudine should not be recommended for uninfected persons after occupational exposures because of the lack of data demonstrating efficacy in postexposure prophylaxis, the limited data on toxicity in uninfected individuals, and the fact that zidovudine has been shown to be carcinogenic in rats and mice.

At this time, prophylaxis with zidovudine cannot be considered a necessary component of postexposure management. However, workers who might be at risk of occupational exposure to HIV should be informed, as part of job orientation and ongoing job training, of the considerations pertaining to the use of zidovudine for postexposure prophylaxis. The PHS recommends that if a physician decides to offer zidovudine to a worker after an exposure incident, that decision by the physician and the decision by the worker to take zidovudine should take into account the following considerations.

Considerations Regarding Use of Zidovudine After an Occupational Exposure

Risk of HIV Infection After Exposure

Evaluation of the risk of HIV infection after exposure should take into account existing knowledge from prospective studies of exposed workers, which demonstrate that on the average the risk of transmission of HIV per episode of percutaneous exposure (e.g., a needlestick or cut with a sharp object) to HIV-infected blood is approximately 0.4%. These studies also suggest that the risk of HIV transmission per episode of mucous-membrane or skin exposure to HIV-infected blood is less than that after a percutaneous exposure (7, 18–21). The risk of HIV transmission after occupational exposure to body fluids other than blood, for which universal precautions are recommended, is unknown. The risk of HIV infection for persons who take zidovudine postexposure prophylaxis cannot be determined at present because of the small number of persons studied.

Risk evaluation should also include an assessment of factors that may increase or decrease the probability of HIV transmission after an individual occupational exposure. These factors are not well understood, but include the likelihood that the source fluid contained HIV and probably also the concentration of HIV in the source fluid, the route of exposure, and the volume of fluid involved. For example, a percutaneous exposure to concentrated HIV in a research laboratory is probably more likely to result in transmission of infection than a similar exposure to HIV-infected blood in a clinical setting. A percutaneous exposure to HIV-infected blood is probably more likely to result in transmission than a mucous-membrane exposure to the same blood. Finally, an exposure to a larger quantity of HIV-infected blood, such as injection of several milliliters, is probably more likely to result in HIV transmission than an exposure to a smaller quantity of the same blood, such as in a needlestick exposure.

Interval Between Exposure and Initiation of Prophylaxis, if Given

Data from animal studies suggest that prophylaxis against certain retroviral infections other than HIV may be more effective when started within hours after exposure (22, 23). Because in vitro studies indicate that human HIV infection may be established in human lymphocytes within hours after exposure (24), and epidemiologic studies of exposed health-care workers indicate that acute retroviral illness may occur as early as 2 weeks after exposure (7), it appears that if the decision is made to use postexposure prophylaxis, prophylaxis should be initiated promptly.

Counseling and Informed Consent

If zidovudine prophylaxis is being considered, the worker should be counseled regarding (a) the theoretical rationale for postexposure prophylaxis, (b) the risk of occupationally acquired HIV infection due to the exposure, (c) the limitations of current knowledge of the efficacy of zidovudine when used as postexposure prophylaxis, (d) current knowledge of the toxicity of zidovudine (including the data from animal and human studies) and the limitations of this knowledge in predicting toxicity in uninfected individuals who take the drug after occupational exposures, and (e) the need for postexposure follow-up (including HIV serologic testing), regardless of whether zidovudine is taken. The worker should also be informed that there are diverse opinions among physicians regarding the use of zidovudine for postexposure prophylaxis, and the PHS cannot make a recommendation for or against the use of zidovudine for this purpose because of the limitations of current knowledge.

The duration of follow-up needed to detect evidence of HIV transmission or delayed toxicity among workers who take zidovudine is presently unknown. Workers taking zidovudine postexposure may require follow-up to detect HIV seroconversion for a longer period than that recommended for workers who do not take zidovudine. Regardless of the length of follow-up, mechanisms should be developed to permit workers taking zidovudine to be contacted if future information indicates the need for additional evaluation.

If a physician offers zidovudine as prophylaxis after an occupational exposure and the exposed worker elects to take the drug, the physician or other appropriate health-care provider should obtain written informed consent from the worker for the use of this drug. The consent document should reflect the information presented in the counseling session, as outlined above, emphasizing the need for follow-up medical evaluations and for precautions to prevent the transmission of HIV infection during the follow-up period, including refraining from blood, semen, or organ donation, refraining from breastfeeding, and either abstaining from sexual intercourse or using latex condoms during sexual intercourse, as discussed below.

Considerations regarding sexual intercourse for exposed workers taking zidovudine include (a) the possible risk of teratogenesis associated with zidovudine use, and (b) the risk of transmission of HIV to a sexual partner. The risk of teratogenesis among offspring of either men or women taking zidovudine is unknown. Therefore, men and women of reproductive age who are receiving zidovudine should abstain from, or use effective contraception during, sexual intercourse throughout the time zidovudine is being taken. In addition, to prevent HIV transmission to sexual partners, all exposed workers, including pregnant women, should abstain from, or use latex condoms during, sexual intercourse throughout the follow-up period.

REFERENCES: AS NUMBERED IN ORIGINAL PUBLICATION

2. CDC. Update: universal precautions for prevention of transmission of human immunodeficiency virus, hepatitis B virus, and other bloodborne pathogens in health-care settings. MMWR 1988;37:377–388.
3. CDC. Guidelines for prevention of transmission of human immunodeficiency virus and hepatitis B virus to health-care and public-safety workers. MMWR 1989;38(no. S-6).
6. Henderson DK, Gerberding JL. Prophylactic zidovudine after occupational exposure to the human immunodeficiency virus: an interim analysis. J Infect Dis 1989;160:321–327.
7. Marcus R, CDC Cooperative Needlestick Study Group. Surveillance of health-care workers exposed to blood from patients infected with the human immunodeficiency virus. N Engl J Med 1988;319:1118–1123.

8. CDC. Recommendations for protection against viral hepatitis: recommendations of the Immunization Practices Advisory Committee (ACIP). MMWR 1985;34:313–335.

9. CDC. Protection against viral hepatitis: recommendations of the Immunization Practices Advisory Committee (ACIP). MMWR 1990;(in press).

10. CDC. Update on hepatitis B prevention. MMWR 1987;36:353–366.

11. CDC. Public Health Service guidelines for counseling and antibody testing to prevent HIV infection and AIDS. MMWR 1987;36:509–515.

12. CDC. Additional recommendations to reduce sexual and drug abuse-related transmission of human T-lymphotropic virus type III/lymphadenopathy-associated virus. MMWR 1986;35:152–155.

13. CDC. Prevention of acquired immune deficiency syndrome (AIDS): report of inter-agency recommendations. MMWR 1983;32:101–103.

14. CDC. Provisional Public Health Service inter-agency recommendations for screening donated blood and plasma for antibody to the virus causing acquired immunodeficiency syndrome. MMWR 1985;34:1–5.

18. Henderson DK, Fahey BJ, Saah AJ, Schmitt JM, Lane HC. Longitudinal assessment of risk for occupational/nosocomial transmission of human immunodeficiency virus, type 1 in health care workers [Abstract]. In: Program and abstracts of the twenty-eighth Interscience Conference on Antimicrobial Agents and Chemotherapy (Los Angeles). Washington, DC: American Society for Microbiology, 1988:221.

19. Gerberding JL, Littell CG, Chambers HF, et al. Risk of occupational HIV transmission in intensively exposed health-care workers: follow-up [Abstract]. In: Program and abstracts of the twenty-eighth Interscience Conference on Antimicrobial Agents and Chemotherapy (Los Angeles). Washington, DC: American Society for Microbiology, 1988:169.

20. Elmslie K, Mulligan L, O'Shaughnessy M. National surveillance program: occupational exposure to human immunodeficiency virus (HIV-1) infection in Canada. V International Conference on AIDS. Montreal, June 4–9, 1989:148.

21. McEvoy M, Porter K, Mortimer P, Simmons N, Shanson D. Prospective study of clinical, laboratory, and ancillary staff with accidental exposures to blood or body fluids from patients infected with HIV. Br Med J 1987;294:1595–1597.

22. Ruprecht RM, O'Brien LG, Rossoni LD, Nusinoff-Lehrman S. Suppression of mouse viraemia and retroviral disease by 3'-azido-3'-deoxythymidine. Nature 1986;323:467–469.

23. Tavares L, Roneker C, Johnston K, Nusinoff-Lehrman S, de Noronha F. 3'-Azido-3'-deoxythymidine in feline leukemia virus-infected cats: a model for therapy and prophylaxis of AIDS. Cancer Res 1987; 47:3190–3194.

24. Sunyoung K, Byrn R, Groopman J, Baltimore D. Kinetics of HIV gene expression during the one-step multiplication of HIV [Abstract]. IV International Conference on AIDS. Book 1. Stockholm, June 12–16, 1988:119.

APPENDIX I

Results of Studies Conducted by the Burroughs-Wellcome Company of Zidovudine Carcinogenicity Involving Animals

In lifetime carcinogenicity bioassays, mice and rats were given various doses of zidovudine, up to the maximum tolerated doses, for most of their lifespans. Dose reductions were necessary for both species during the study because of the onset and persistence of drug-related anemia. Mice were treated initially with 30, 60, or 120 mg/kg/day; after 90 days, these doses were reduced to 20, 30, or 40 mg/kg/day, respectively. Rats were treated initially with 80, 220, or 600 mg/kg/day; after 90 days, the 600-mg/kg/day group was reduced to 450 mg/kg/day; and after 280 days, this group was further reduced to 300 mg/kg/day. Although anemia persisted at the reduced doses, drug treatment did not adversely affect survival in either species.

Among mice dosed for approximately 22 months, seven vaginal neoplasms occurred in 60 female animals at the highest dose. The earliest a tumor was discovered was after 19 months of continuous dosing; most tumors were discovered after 21 months of treatment. The tumors consisted of five nonmetastasizing squamous cell carcinomas and two benign tumors (one squamous cell papilloma and one squamous cell polyp). One benign vaginal tumor (squamous cell papilloma) was discovered in the middle-dose group after 22 months of treatment. In all instances, these lesions were discovered during histologic examination of tissues from animals that either died or were sacrificed, late in life from nontreatment-related causes, or sacrificed upon completion of lifetime dosing.

Among rats dosed for approximately 22 months, two nonmetastasizing vaginal squamous cell carcinomas were diagnosed on the basis of histologic examination of tissues from animals receiving the highest dose. These carcinomas were discovered after 20–22 months of dosing. No vaginal tumors occurred among rats given the middle or low dose.

No other drug-related tumors were observed among animals of either sex or of either species (Burroughs-Wellcome Company [letter to physicians], Dec. 5, 1989).

APPENDIX II

Studies of Zidovudine Prophylaxis Involving Animals

Studies of retrovirus infections other than HIV in mice and cats suggest that zidovudine may alter the course of some retroviral infections when given before or shortly after exposure to the virus. In one study, mice were injected with a large challenge inoculum (1 X 10((4)) plaque-forming units) of Rauscher murine leukemia virus (RMLV) and were given a 20-day course of zidovudine, at various doses, beginning 4 hours after inoculation. By day 69, all untreated mice had died of RMLV infection, whereas those treated with high doses of zidovudine had no clinical signs of infection and were not viremic. Both the protective effect of zidovudine and the incidence of zidovudine-induced bone marrow depression were greater with increasing doses (1).

In another study, cats were injected with a large challenge dose (2 X 10((3)) focus-inducing units) of Rickard feline leukemia virus (RFLV) and were given zidovudine at various doses and various intervals after inoculation. Of eight cats injected with RFLV and treated with a 6-week course of zidovudine beginning 1 hour after inoculation, none developed clinical evidence of RFLV disease, none had virus isolated from serum, and one had evidence of infection manifested by the development of neutralizing antibody within 3 months after treatment with zidovudine was stopped. In contrast, 11 of 12 untreated cats either became viremic or died of infection in the same period. When zidovudine prophylaxis was initiated 3 or 7 days after inoculation, a substantial proportion of animals in different dosage groups became viremic, developed neutralizing antibody, or both. All animals treated beginning 28 days after inoculation were viremic when zidovudine treatment was initiated (2).

Limited studies involving primates have not shown success in postexposure prophylaxis against simian immunodeficiency virus (SIV). In one study, macaque monkeys were inoculated with a small dose (10 TCID((50))) of a rapidly lethal variant of SIV (SMM/PBj-14) and later treated with zidovudine for 14 days. Of three animals whose treatment was begun 1 hour after inoculation, two developed infection, and one died. Of three animals treated within 24 hours, all developed infection, and two died. Of three animals treated within

72 hours, all developed infection, and two died. Of three control animals that were inoculated with the virus but not given zidovudine treatment, all developed infection, and two died (3). In another study of macaque monkeys, a 1-week course of zidovudine begun 8 hours before the animals were inoculated with SIV did not prevent viremia, but delayed its onset until 1–2 days after the zidovudine treatment was completed (4).

Finally, studies have been conducted by using the SCID-hu mouse model, an immunodeficient mouse with an immune system that has been reconstituted with transplanted human hematolymphoid organs susceptible to infection with HIV (5). Seventeen mice were treated with zidovudine for 24 hours before and for 2 weeks after intrathymic injection of a standard challenge dose of HIV (400–4,000 IU), the smallest dose causing infection in all animals. At 2 weeks after injection, none of the mice tested positive for HIV DNA by the polymerase chain reaction (PCR), although the presence of HIV RNA in some cells was detected by in situ hybridization. Four weeks after zidovudine was stopped, HIV DNA was detected by PCR in all 17 mice. In comparison, all of 40 mice not receiving zidovudine tested positive for HIV DNA by PCR 2 weeks after injection (6).

REFERENCES: AS NUMBERED IN ORIGINAL PUBLICATION

1. Ruprecht RM, O'Brien LG, Rossoni LD, Nusinoff-Lehrman S. Suppression of mouse viraemia and retroviral disease by 3'-azido-3'-deoxythymidine. Nature 1986;323:467–469.
2. Tavares L, Roneker C, Johnston K, Nusinoff-Lehrman S, de Noronha F. 3'-Azido-3'-deoxythymidine in feline leukemia virus-infected cats: a model for therapy and prophylaxis of AIDS. Cancer Res 1987;47:3190–3194.
3. McClure HM, Anderson DC, Fultz P, Ansari A, Brodie A, Lehrman A. Prophylactic effects of AZT following exposure of macaques to an acutely lethal variant of SIV (SIV/SMM/PBj-14) [Abstract]. V International Conference on AIDS. Montreal June 4–9, 1989;522.
4. Lundgren B, Hedstrom KG, Norrby E, Oberg B, Wahren B. Inhibition of early occurrence of antigen in SIV-infected macaques as a measurement of antiviral efficacy [Abstract]. Symposium on Nonhuman Primate Models for AIDS. November 1988.
5. Namikawa R, Kaneshima H, Lieberman M, Weissman IL, McCune JM. Infection of the SCID-hu mouse by HIV-1. Science 1988;242:1684–1686.
6. McCune JM, Namikawa R, Shih CC, Rabin L, Kaneshima H. 3'-Azido-3'-deoxythymidine suppresses HIV infection in SCID-hu mouse. Science 1990;(in press).

Guidelines for Prevention of Transmission of HIV and Hepatitis B Virus to Health-Care and Public-Safety Workers

Original Citation: Centers for Disease Control and Prevention. Guidelines for Prevention of Transmission of Human Immunodeficiency Virus and Hepatitis B Virus to Health-Care and Public-Safety Workers. MMWR 1989;38(No. S-6).

Editor's Note: The information included here was based on a report of recommendations for the prevention of HIV in public safety personnel as developed by the National Institute for Occupational Safety and Health in collaboration with the Center for Infectious Diseases. Background information on the transmission of hepatitis B and HIV to workers is not printed.

PRINCIPLES OF INFECTION CONTROL AND THEIR APPLICATION TO EMERGENCY AND PUBLIC-SAFETY WORKERS

General Infection Control

Within the health-care setting, general infection control procedures have been developed to minimize the risk of patient acquisition of infection from contact with contaminated devices, objects, or surfaces or of transmission of an infectious agent from health-care workers to patients (1–3). Such procedures also protect workers from the risk of becoming infected. General infection-control procedures are designed to prevent transmission of a wide range of microbiological agents and to provide a wide margin of safety in the varied situations encountered in the health-care environment.

General infection-control principles are applicable to other work environments where workers contact other individuals and where transmission of infectious agents may occur. The modes of transmission noted in the hospital and medical office environment are observed in the work situations of emergency and public-safety workers, as well. Therefore, the principles of infection control developed for hospital and other health-care settings are also applicable to these work situations. Use of general infection control measures, as adapted to the work environments of emergency and public-safety workers, is important to protect both workers and individuals with whom they work from a variety of infectious agents, not just HIV and HBV.

Because emergency and public-safety workers work in environments that provide inherently unpredictable risks of exposures, general infection-control procedures should be adapted to these work situations. Exposures are unpredictable, and protective measures may often be used in situations that do not appear to present risk. Emergency and public-safety workers perform their duties in the community under extremely variable conditions; thus, control measures that are simple and uniform across all situations have the greatest likelihood of worker compliance. Administrative procedures to ensure compliance also can be more readily developed than when procedures are complex and highly variable.

Universal Blood and Body Fluid Precautions to Prevent Occupational HIV and HBV Transmission

In 1985, CDC developed the strategy of "universal blood and body fluid precautions" to address concerns regarding transmission of HIV in the health-care setting (4). The concept, now referred to simply as "universal precautions" stresses that all patients should be assumed to be infectious for HIV and other blood-borne pathogens. In the hospital and other health-care setting, "universal precautions" should be followed when workers are exposed to blood, certain other body fluids (amniotic fluid, pericardial fluid, peritoneal fluid, pleural fluid, synovial fluid, cerebrospinal fluid, semen, and vaginal secretions), or any body fluid visibly contaminated with blood. Since HIV and HBV transmission has not been documented from exposure to other body fluids (feces, nasal secretions, sputum, sweat, tears, urine, and vomitus), "universal precautions" do not apply to these fluids. Universal precautions also do not apply to saliva, except in the dental setting, where saliva is likely to be contaminated with blood (7).

For the purpose of this document, human "exposure" is defined as contact with blood or other body fluids to which universal precautions apply through percutaneous inoculation or contact with an open wound, nonintact skin, or mucous membrane during the performance of normal job duties. An "exposed worker" is defined, for the purposes of this document, as an individual exposed, as described above, while performing normal job duties.

The unpredictable and emergent nature of exposures encountered by emergency and public-safety workers may make differentiation between hazardous body fluids and those which are not hazardous very difficult and often impossible. For example, poor lighting may limit the worker's ability to detect visible blood in vomitus or feces. Therefore, when emergency medical and public-safety workers encounter body fluids under uncontrolled, emergency circumstances in which differentiation between fluid types is difficult, if not impossible, they should treat all body fluids as potentially hazardous.

The application of the principles of universal precautions to the situations encountered by these workers results in the development of guidelines (listed below) for work practices, use of personal protective equipment, and other protective measures. To minimize the risks of acquiring HIV and HBV during performance of job duties, emergency and public-safety workers should be protected from exposure to blood and other body fluids as circumstances dictate. Protection can be achieved through adherence to work practices designed to minimize or eliminate exposure and through use of personal protective equipment (i.e., gloves, masks, and protective clothing), which provide a barrier between the worker and the exposure source. In some situations, redesign of selected aspects of the job through equipment modifications or environmental control can further reduce risk. These approaches to primary prevention should be used together to achieve maximal reduction of the risk of exposure.

If exposure of an individual worker occurs, medical management, consisting of collection of pertinent medical and occupational history, provision of treatment, and counseling regarding future work and personal behaviors, may reduce risk of developing disease as a result of the exposure episode (22). Following episodic (or continuous) exposure, decontamination and disinfection of the work environment, devices, equipment, and clothing or other forms of personal protective equipment can reduce subsequent risk of exposures. Proper disposal of contaminated waste has similar benefits.

EMPLOYER RESPONSIBILITIES

General

Detailed recommendations for employer responsibilities in protecting workers from acquisition of blood-borne diseases in the workplace have been published in the Department of Labor and Department of Health and Human Services Joint Advisory Notice and are summarized here (6). In developing programs to protect workers, employers should follow a series of steps: (a) classification of

Table 3. Summary of Task Categorization and Implications for Personal Protective Equipment

Joint Advisory Notice Category[1]	Nature of the Task/Activity	Personal protective equipment should be: Available?	Worn?
I.	Direct contact with blood or other body fluids to which universal precautions apply	Yes	Yes
II.	Activity performed without blood exposure but exposure may occur in emergency	Yes	No
III.	Task/activity does not entail predictable or unpredictable exposure to blood	No	No

[1]U.S. Department of Labor, U.S. Department of Health and Human Services. Joint advisory notice: protection against occupational exposure to hepatitis B virus (HBV) and human immunodeficiency virus (HIV) Washington, DC: US Department of Labor, US Department of Health and Human Services, 1987.

work activity, (b) development of standard operating procedures, (c) provision of training and education, (d) development of procedures to ensure and monitor compliance, and (e) workplace redesign. As a first step, every employer should classify work activities into one of three categories of potential exposure (Table 3). Employers should make protective equipment available to all workers when they are engaged in Category I or II activities. Employers should ensure that the appropriate protective equipment is used by workers when they perform Category I activities.

As a second step, employers should establish a detailed work practices program that includes standard operating procedures (SOPs) for all activities having the potential for exposure. Once these SOPs are developed, an initial and periodic worker education program to assure familiarity with work practices should be provided to potentially exposed workers. No worker should engage in such tasks or activities before receiving training pertaining to the SOPs, work practices, and protective equipment required for that task. Examples of personal protective equipment for the prehospital setting (defined as a setting where delivery of emergency health care takes place away from a hospital or other health-care setting) are provided in Table 4. (A curriculum for such training programs is being developed in conjunction with these guidelines and should be consulted for further information concerning such training programs.)

To facilitate and monitor compliance with SOPs, administrative procedures should be developed and records kept as described in the Joint Advisory Notice (6). Employers should monitor the workplace to ensure that required work practices are observed and that protective clothing and equipment are provided and properly used. The employer should maintain records documenting the administrative procedures used to classify job activities and copies of all SOPs for tasks or activities involving predictable or unpredictable exposure to blood or

Table 4. Examples of Recommended Personal Protective Equipment for Worker Protection Against HIV and HBV Transmission[1] in Prehospital[2] Settings

Task or Activity	Disposable Gloves	Gown	Mask[3]	Protective Eyewear
Bleeding control with spurting blood	Yes	Yes	Yes	Yes
Bleeding control with minimal bleeding	Yes	No	No	No
Emergency childbirth	Yes	Yes	Yes, if splashing is likely	Yes, if splashing is likely
Blood drawing	At certain times[4]	No	No	No
Starting an intravenous (IV) line	Yes	No	No	No
Endotracheal intubation, Esophageal obturator use	Yes	No	No, unless splashing is likely	No, unless splashing is likely
Oral/nasal suctioning, manually cleaning airway	Yes[5]	No	No, unless splashing is likely	No, unless splashing is likely
Handling and cleaning instruments with microbial contamination	Yes	No, unless soiling is likely	No	No
Measuring blood pressure	No	No	No	No
Measuring temperature	No	No	No	No
Giving an injection	No	No	No	No

[1]The examples provided in this table are based on application of universal precautions. Universal precautions are intended to supplement rather than replace recommendations for routine infection control, such as handwashing and using gloves to prevent gross microbial contamination of hands (e.g., contact with urine or feces).

[2]Defined as setting where delivery of emergency health care takes place away from a hospital or other health-care facility.

[3]Refers to protective masks to prevent exposure of mucous membranes to blood or other potentially contaminated body fluids. The use of resuscitation devices, some of which are also referred to as "masks," is discussed elsewhere in the original document.

[4]For clarification see Appendix A [of original publication].

[5]While not clearly necessary to prevent HIV or HBV transmission unless blood is present, gloves are recommended to prevent transmission of other agents (e.g., Herpes simplex).

other body fluids to which universal precautions apply. In addition, training records, indicating the dates of training sessions, the content of those training sessions along with the names of all persons conducting the training, and the names of all those receiving training should also be maintained.

Whenever possible, the employer should identify devices and other approaches to modifying the work environment which will reduce exposure risk. Such approaches are desirable, since they don't require individual worker action or management activity. For example, jails and correctional facilities should have classification procedures that require the segregation of offenders who indicate through their actions or words that they intend to attack correctional-facility staff with the intent of transmitting HIV or HBV.

Medical

In addition to the general responsibilities noted above, the employer has the specific responsibility to make available to the worker a program of medical management. This program is designed to provide for the reduction of risk of infection by HBV and for counseling workers concerning issues regarding HIV and HBV. These services should be provided by a licensed health professional. All phases of medical management and counseling should ensure that the confidentiality of the worker's and client's medical data is protected.

Hepatitis B Vaccination

All workers whose jobs involve participation in tasks or activities with exposure to blood or other body fluids to which universal precautions apply (as defined above) should be vaccinated with hepatitis B vaccine.

Management of Percutaneous Exposure to Blood and Other Infectious Body Fluids

Once an exposure has occurred (as defined above), a blood sample should be drawn after consent is obtained from the individual from whom exposure occurred and tested for hepatitis B surface antigen (HBsAg) and antibody to human immunodeficiency virus (HIV antibody). Local laws regarding consent for testing source individuals should be followed. Policies should be available for testing source individuals in situations where consent cannot be obtained (e.g., an unconscious patient). Testing of the source individual should be done at a location where appropriate pretest counseling is available; posttest counseling and referral for treatment should be provided. It is extremely important that all individuals who seek consultation for any HIV-related concerns receive counseling as outlined in the "Public Health Service Guidelines for Counseling and Antibody Testing to Prevent HIV Infection and AIDS" (22).

Hepatitis B Virus Postexposure Management

For an exposure to a source individual found to be positive for HBsAg, the worker who has not previously been given hepatitis B vaccine should receive the vaccine series. A single dose of hepatitis B immune globulin (HBIG) is also recommended, if this can be given within 7 days of exposure. For exposures from an HBsAg-positive source to workers who have previously received vaccine, the exposed worker should be tested for antibody to hepatitis B surface antigen (anti-HBs), and given one dose of vaccine and one dose of HBIG if the antibody level in the worker's blood sample is inadequate (i.e., 10 SRU by RIA, negative by EIA) (7).

If the source individual is negative for HBsAg and the worker has not been vaccinated, this opportunity should be taken to provide hepatitis B vaccination.

If the source individual refuses testing or he/she cannot be identified, the unvaccinated worker should receive the hepatitis B vaccine series. HBIG administration should be considered on an individual basis when the source individual is known or suspected to be at high risk of HBV infection. Management and treatment, if any, of previously vaccinated workers who receive an exposure from a source who refuses testing or is not identifiable should be individualized (7).

Human Immunodeficiency Virus Postexposure Management

For any exposure to a source individual who has AIDS, who is found to be positive for HIV infection (4), or who refuses testing, the worker should be counseled regarding the risk of infection and evaluated clinically and serologically for evidence of HIV infection as soon as possible after the exposure. In view of the evolving nature of HIV postexposure management, the health-care provider should be well informed of current PHS guidelines on this subject. The worker should be advised to report and seek medical evaluation for any acute febrile illness that occurs within 12 weeks after the exposure. Such an illness, particularly one characterized by fever, rash, or lymphadenopathy, may be indicative of recent HIV infection. Following the initial test at the time of exposure, seronegative workers should be retested 6 weeks, 12 weeks, and 6 months after exposure to determine whether transmission has occurred. During this follow-up period (especially the first 6–12 weeks after exposure, when most infected persons are expected to seroconvert), exposed workers should follow U.S. Public Health Service (PHS) recommendations for preventing transmission of HIV (22). These include refraining from blood donation and using appropriate protection during sexual intercourse (23).

During all phases of follow-up, it is vital that worker confidentiality be protected.

If the source individual was tested and found to be seronegative, baseline testing of the exposed worker with follow-up testing 12 weeks later may be performed if desired by the worker or recommended by the health-care provider.

If the source individual cannot be identified, decisions regarding appropriate follow-up should be individualized. Serologic testing should be made available by the employer to all workers who may be concerned they have been infected with HIV through an occupational exposure as defined above.

Management of Human Bites

On occasion, police and correctional-facility officers are intentionally bitten by suspects or prisoners. When such bites occur, routine medical and surgical therapy (including an assessment of tetanus vaccination status) should be implemented as soon as possible, since such bites frequently result in infection with organisms other than HIV and HBV. Victims of bites should be evaluated as described above for exposure to blood or other infectious body fluids.

Saliva of some persons infected with HBV has been shown to contain HBV-DNA at concentrations 1/1,000 to 1/10,000 of that found in the infected person's serum (5, 24). HbsAg-positive saliva has been shown to be infectious when injected into experimental animals and in human bite exposures (25–27). However, HBsAg-positive saliva has not been shown to be infectious when applied to oral mucous membranes in experimental primate studies (27) or through contamination of musical instruments or cardiopulmonary resuscitation dummies used by HBV carriers (28, 29). Epidemiologic studies of nonsexual household contacts of HIV-infected patients, including several small series in which HIV transmission failed to occur after bites or after percutaneous inoculation or contamination of cuts and open wounds with saliva from HIV-infected patients, suggest that the potential for salivary transmission of HIV is remote (5, 30–33). One case report from Germany has suggested the possibility of transmission of HIV in a household setting from an infected child to a sibling through a human bite (34). The bite did not break the skin or result in bleeding. Since the date of seroconversion to HIV was not known for either child in this case, evidence for the role of saliva in the transmission of virus is unclear (34).

Documentation of Exposure and Reporting

As part of the confidential medical record, the circumstances of exposure should be recorded. Relevant information includes the activity in which the worker was engaged at the time of exposure, the extent to which appropriate work practices and protective equipment were used, and a description of the source of exposure.

Employers have a responsibility under various federal and state laws and regulations to report occupational illnesses and injuries.

Existing programs in the National Institute for Occupational Safety and Health (NIOSH), Department of Health and Human Services; the Bureau of Labor Statistics, Department of Labor (DOL); and the Occupational Safety and Health Administration (DOL) receive such information for the purposes of surveillance and other objectives. Cases of infectious disease, including AIDS and HBV infection, are reported to the Centers for Disease Control through State health departments.

Management of HBV- or HIV-infected Workers

Transmission of HBV from health-care workers to patients has been documented. Such transmission has occurred during certain types of invasive procedures (e.g., oral and gynecologic surgery) in which health-care workers, when tested, had very high concentrations of HBV in their blood (at least 100 million infectious virus particles per milliliter, a concentration much higher than occurs with HIV infection), and the health-care workers sustained a puncture wound while performing invasive procedures or had exudative or weeping lesions or microlacerations that allowed virus to contaminate instruments or open wounds of patients (35, 36). A worker who is HBsAg positive and who has transmitted hepatitis B virus to another individual during the performance of his or her job duties should be excluded from the performance of those job duties which place other individuals at risk for acquisition of hepatitis B infection.

Workers with impaired immune systems resulting from HIV infection or other causes are at increased risk of acquiring or experiencing serious complications of infectious disease. Of particular concern is the risk of severe infection following exposure to other persons with infectious diseases that are easily transmitted if appropriate precautions are not taken (e.g., measles, varicella). Any worker with an impaired immune system should be counseled about the potential risk associated with providing health care to persons with any transmissible infection and should continue to follow existing recommendations for infection control to minimize risk of exposure to other infectious agents (2, 3). Recommendations of the Immunization Practices Advisory Committee (ACIP) and institutional policies concerning requirements for vaccinating workers with live-virus vaccines (e.g., measles, rubella) should also be considered.

The question of whether workers infected with HIV can adequately and safely be allowed to perform patient-care duties or whether their work assignments should be changed must be determined on an individual basis. These decisions should be made by the worker's personal physician(s) in conjunction with the employer's medical advisors.

Disinfection, Decontamination, and Disposal

As described in an earlier section, the only documented occupational risks of HIV and HBV infection are associated with parenteral (including open wound) and mucous membrane exposure to blood and other potentially infectious body fluids. Nevertheless, the precautions described below should be routinely followed.

Needle and Sharps Disposal

All workers should take precautions to prevent injuries caused by needles, scalpel blades, and other sharp instruments or devices during procedures; when cleaning used instruments; during disposal of used needles; and when handling sharp instruments after procedures. To prevent needlestick injuries, needles should not be recapped, purposely bent or broken by hand, removed from disposable syringes, or otherwise manipulated by hand. After they are used, disposable syringes and needles, scalpel blades, and other sharp items should be placed in puncture-resistant containers for disposal; the puncture-resistant containers should be located as close as practical to the use area (e.g., in the ambulance or, if sharps are carried to the scene of victim assistance from the ambulance, a small puncture-resistant container should be carried to the scene, as well). Reusable needles should be left on the syringe body and should be placed in a puncture-resistant container for transport to the reprocessing area.

Hand Washing

Hands and other skin surfaces should be washed immediately and thoroughly if contaminated with blood, other body fluids to which universal precautions apply, or potentially contaminated articles. Hands should always be washed after gloves are removed, even if the gloves appear to be intact. Hand washing should be completed using the appropriate facilities, such as utility or restroom sinks. Waterless antiseptic hand cleanser should be provided on responding units to use when hand-washing facilities are not available. When hand-washing facilities are available, wash hands with warm water and soap. When hand-washing facilities are not available, use a waterless antiseptic hand cleanser. The manufacturer's recommendations for the product should be followed.

Cleaning, Disinfecting, and Sterilizing

Table 5 presents the methods and applications for cleaning, disinfecting, and sterilizing equipment and surfaces in the prehospital setting. These methods also apply to housekeeping and other cleaning tasks. Previously issued guidelines for health-care workers contain more detailed descriptions (4).

Cleaning and Decontaminating Spills of Blood

All spills of blood and blood-contaminated fluids should be promptly cleaned up using an EPA-approved germicide or a 1:100 solution of household bleach in the following manner while wearing gloves. Visible material should first be removed with disposable towels or other appropriate means that will ensure against direct contact with blood.

If splashing is anticipated, protective eyewear should be worn along with an impervious gown or apron which provides an effective barrier to splashes. The area should then be decontaminated with an appropriate germicide. Hands should be washed following removal of gloves. Soiled cleaning equipment should be cleaned and decontaminated or placed in an appropriate container and disposed of according to agency policy.

Plastic bags should be available for removal of contaminated items from the site of the spill.

Shoes and boots can become contaminated with blood in certain instances. Where there is massive blood contamination on floors, the use of disposable impervious shoe coverings should be considered. Protective gloves should be worn to remove contaminated shoe coverings. The coverings and gloves should be disposed of in plastic bags. A plastic bag should be included in the crime scene kit or the car which is to be used for the disposal of contaminated items. Extra plastic bags should be stored in the police cruiser or emergency vehicle.

Laundry

Although soiled linen may be contaminated with pathogenic microorganisms, the risk of actual disease transmission is negligible. Rather than rigid procedures and specifications, hygienic storage and processing of clean and soiled linen are recommended. Laundry facilities and/or services should be made routinely available by the employer. Soiled linen should be handled as little as possible and with minimum agitation to prevent gross microbial contamination of the air and of persons handling the linen. All soiled linen should be bagged

Table 5. Reprocessing Methods for Equipment Used in the Prehospital[1] Health-Care Setting

Sterilization:	Destroys:	All forms of microbial life including high numbers of bacterial spores.
	Methods:	Steam under pressure (autoclave), gas (ethylene oxide), dry heat, or immersion in EPA-approved chemical "sterilant" for prolonged period of time, e.g., 6–10 hours or according to manufacturers' instructions. Note: liquid chemical "sterilants" should be used only on those instruments that are impossible to sterilize or disinfect with heat.
	Use:	For those instruments or devices that penetrate skin or contact normally sterile areas of the body, e.g., scalpels, needles, etc. Disposable invasive equipment eliminates the need to reprocess these types of items. When indicated, however, arrangements should be made with a health-care facility for reprocessing of reusable invasive instruments.
High-Level Disinfection:	Destroys:	All forms of microbial life except high numbers of bacterial spores.
	Methods:	Hot water pasteurization (80–100°C, 30 minutes) or exposure to an EPA-registered "sterilant" chemical as above, except for a short exposure time (10–45 minutes or as directed by the manufacturer).
	Use:	For reusable instruments or devices that come into contact with mucous membranes (e.g., laryngoscope blades, endotracheal tubes, etc.).
Intermediate-Level Disinfection:	Destroys:	Mycobacterium tuberculosis, vegetative bacteria, most viruses, and most fungi, but does not kill bacterial spores.
	Methods:	EPA-registered "hospital disinfectant" chemical germicides that have a label claim for tuberculocidal activity; commercially available hard-surface germicides or solutions containing at least 500 ppm free available chlorine (a 1:100 dilution of common household bleach—approximately ¼ cup bleach per gallon of tap water).
	Use:	For those surfaces that come into contact only with intact skin, e.g., stethoscopes, blood pressure cuffs, splints, etc., and have been visibly contaminated with blood or bloody body fluids. Surfaces must be precleaned of visible material before the germicidal chemical is applied for disinfection.

Table 5.—*continued*

Low-Level Disinfection:	Destroys:	Most bacteria, some viruses, some fungi, but not Mycobacterium tuberculosis or bacterial spores.
	Methods:	EPA-registered "hospital disinfectants" (no label claim for tuberculocidal activity).
	Use:	These agents are excellent cleaners and can be used for routine housekeeping or removal of soiling in the absence of visible blood contamination.
Environmental Disinfection:		Environmental surfaces which have become soiled should be cleaned and disinfected using any cleaner or disinfectant agent which is intended for environmental use. Such surfaces include floors, woodwork, ambulance seats, countertops, etc.
IMPORTANT:		To assure the effectiveness of any sterilization or disinfection process, equipment and instruments must first be thoroughly cleaned of all visible soil.

[1]Defined as setting where delivery of emergency health-care takes place prior to arrival at hospital or other health-care facility.

at the location where it was used. Linen soiled with blood should be placed and transported in bags that prevent leakage. Normal laundry cycles should be used according to the washer and detergent manufacturers' recommendations.

Decontamination and Laundering of Protective Clothing

Protective work clothing contaminated with blood or other body fluids to which universal precautions apply should be placed and transported in bags or containers that prevent leakage. Personnel involved in the bagging, transport, and laundering of contaminated clothing should wear gloves. Protective clothing and station and work uniforms should be washed and dried according to the manufacturer's instructions. Boots and leather goods may be brush-scrubbed with soap and hot water to remove contamination.

Infective Waste

The selection of procedures for disposal of infective waste is determined by the relative risk of disease transmission and application of local regulations, which vary widely. In all cases, local regulations should be consulted prior to disposal procedures and followed. Infective waste, in general, should either be incinerated or should be decontaminated before disposal in a sanitary landfill. Bulk blood, suctioned fluids, excretions, and secretions may be carefully poured down a drain connected to a sanitary sewer, where permitted. Sanitary sewers may also be used to dispose of other infectious wastes capable of being ground and flushed into the sewer, where permitted. Sharp items should be placed in puncture-proof containers and other blood-contaminated items should be placed in leak-proof plastic bags for transport to an appropriate disposal location.

Prior to the removal of protective equipment, personnel remaining on the scene after the patient has been cared for should carefully search for and remove contaminated materials. Debris should be disposed of as noted above.

FIRE AND EMERGENCY MEDICAL SERVICES

The guidelines that appear in this section apply to fire and emergency medical services. This includes structural fire fighters, paramedics, emergency medical technicians, and advanced life support personnel. Fire fighters often provide emergency medical services and therefore encounter the exposures common to paramedics and emergency medical technicians. Job duties are often performed in uncontrolled environments, which, due to a lack of time and other factors, do not allow for application of a complex decision-making process to the emergency at hand.

The general principles presented here have been developed from existing principles of occupational safety and health in conjunction with data from studies of health-care workers in hospital settings. The basic premise is that workers must be protected from exposure to blood and other potentially infectious body fluids in the course of their work activities. There is a paucity of data concerning the risks these worker groups face, however, which complicates development of control principles. Thus, the guidelines presented below are based on principles of prudent public health practice.

Fire and emergency medical service personnel are engaged in delivery of medical care in the prehospital setting. The following guidelines are intended to assist these personnel in making decisions concerning use of personal protective equipment and resuscitation equipment, as well as for decontamination, disinfection, and disposal procedures.

Personal Protective Equipment

Appropriate personal protective equipment should be made available routinely by the employer to reduce the risk of exposure as defined above. For many situations, the chance that the rescuer will be exposed to blood and other body fluids to which universal precautions apply can be determined in advance. Therefore, if the chances of being exposed to blood is high (e.g., CPR, IV insertion, trauma, delivering babies), the worker should put on protective attire before beginning patient care. Table 4 sets forth examples of recommendations for personal protective equipment in the prehospital setting; the list is not intended to be all-inclusive.

Gloves

Disposable gloves should be a standard component of emergency response equipment, and should be donned by all personnel prior to initiating any emergency patient care tasks involving exposure to blood or other body fluids to which universal precautions apply. Extra pairs should always be available. Considerations in the choice of disposable gloves should include dexterity, durability, fit, and the task being performed. Thus, there is no single type or thickness of glove appropriate for protection in all situations. For situations where large amounts of blood are likely to be encountered, it is important that gloves fit tightly at the wrist to prevent blood contamination of hands around the cuff. For multiple trauma victims, gloves should be changed between patient contacts, if the emergency situation allows. Greater personal protective equipment measures are indicated for situations where broken glass and sharp edges are likely to be encountered, such as extricating a person from an automobile wreck. Structural fire-fighting gloves that meet the Federal OSHA requirements for fire-fighters gloves (as contained in 29 CFR 1910.156 or National Fire Protection Association Standard 1973, Gloves for Structural Fire Fighters) should be worn in any situation where sharp or rough surfaces are likely to be encountered (37).

While wearing gloves, avoid handling personal items, such as combs and pens, that could become soiled or contaminated. Gloves that have become contaminated with blood or other body fluids to which universal precautions apply should be removed as soon as possible, taking care to avoid skin contact with the exterior surface. Contaminated gloves should be placed and transported in bags that prevent leakage and should be disposed of or, in the case of reusable gloves, cleaned and disinfected properly.

Masks, Eyewear, and Gowns

Masks, eyewear, and gowns should be present on all emergency vehicles that respond or potentially respond to medical emergencies or victim rescues. These protective barriers should be used in accordance with the level of exposure encountered. Minor lacerations or small amounts of blood do not merit the same extent of barrier use as required for exsanguinating victims or massive arterial bleeding. Management of the patient who is not bleeding, and who has no bloody body fluids present, should not routinely require use of barrier precautions. Masks and eyewear (e.g., safety glasses) should be worn together, or a faceshield should be used by all personnel prior to any situation where splashes of blood or other body fluids to which universal precautions apply are likely to occur. Gowns or aprons should be worn to protect clothing from splashes with blood. If large splashes or quantities of blood are present or anticipated, impervious gowns or aprons should be worn. An extra change of work clothing should be available at all times.

Resuscitation Equipment

No transmission of HBV or HIV infection during mouth-to-mouth resuscitation has been documented. However, because of the risk of salivary transmission of other infectious diseases (e.g., herpes simplex and Neisseria meningitidis) and the theoretical risk of HIV and HBV transmission during artificial ventilation of trauma victims, disposable airway equipment or resuscitation bags should be used. Disposable resuscitation equipment and devices should be used once and disposed of or, if reusable, thoroughly cleaned and disinfected after each use according to the manufacturer's recommendations.

Mechanical respiratory assist devices (e.g., bag-valve masks, oxygen demand valve resuscitators) should be available on all emergency vehicles and to all emergency response personnel that respond or potentially respond to medical emergencies or victim rescues. Pocket mouth-to-mouth resuscitation masks designed to isolate emergency response personnel (i.e., double lumen systems) from contact with victims' blood and blood-contaminated saliva, respiratory secretions, and vomitus should be provided to all personnel who provide or potentially provide emergency treatment.

LAW-ENFORCEMENT AND
CORRECTIONAL-FACILITY OFFICERS

Law-enforcement and correctional-facility officers may face the risk of exposure to blood during the conduct of their duties. For example, at the crime scene or during processing of suspects, law-enforcement officers may encounter blood-contaminated hypodermic needles or weapons, or be called upon to assist with body removal.

Correctional-facility officers may similarly be required to search prisoners or their cells for hypodermic needles or weapons, or subdue violent and combative inmates.

The following section presents information for reducing the risk of acquiring HIV and HBV infection by law-enforcement and correctional-facility officers as a consequence of carrying out their duties. However, there is an extremely diverse range of potential situations which may occur in the control of persons with unpredictable, violent, or psychotic behavior. Therefore, informed judgment of the individual officer is paramount when unusual circumstances or events arise. These recommendations should serve as an adjunct to rational decision making in those situations where specific guidelines do not exist, particularly where immediate action is required to preserve life or prevent significant injury.

The following guidelines are arranged into three sections: a section addressing concerns shared by both law-enforcement and correctional-facility officers, and two sections dealing separately with law-enforcement officers and correctional-facility officers, respectively. Table 4 contains selected examples of personal protective equipment that may be employed by law-enforcement and correctional-facility officers.

Law-Enforcement and Correctional-Facilities Considerations

Fights and Assaults

Law-enforcement and correctional-facility officers are exposed to a range of assaultive and disruptive behavior through which they may potentially become exposed to blood or other body fluids containing blood. Behaviors of particular concern are biting, attacks resulting in blood exposure, and attacks with sharp objects. Such behaviors may occur in a range of law-enforcement situations including arrests, routine interrogations, domestic disputes, and lockup operations, as well as in correctional-facility activities. Hand-to-hand combat may result in bleeding and may thus incur a greater chance for blood-to-blood exposure, which increases the chances for blood-borne disease transmission.

Whenever the possibility for exposure to blood or blood-contaminated body fluids exists, the appropriate protection should be worn, if feasible under the circumstances. In all cases, extreme caution must be used in dealing with the suspect or prisoner if there is any indication of assaultive or combative behavior. When blood is present and a suspect or an inmate is combative or threatening to staff, gloves should always be put on as soon as conditions permit. In case of blood contamination of clothing, an extra change of clothing should be available at all times.

Cardiopulmonary Resuscitation

Law-enforcement and correctional personnel are also concerned about infection with HIV and HBV through administration of cardiopulmonary resuscitation (CPR). Although there have been no documented cases of HIV transmission through this mechanism, the possibility of transmission of other infectious diseases exists. Therefore, agencies should make protective masks or airways available to officers and provide training in their proper use. Devices with one-way valves to prevent the patients' saliva or vomitus from entering the caregiver's mouth are preferable.

Law-Enforcement Considerations

Searches and Evidence Handling

Criminal justice personnel have potential risks of acquiring HBV or HIV infection through exposures which occur during searches and evidence handling. Penetrating injuries are known to occur, and puncture wounds or needle sticks in particular pose a hazard during searches of persons, vehicles, or cells, and during evidence handling. The following precautionary measures will help to reduce the risk of infection:

An officer should use great caution in searching the clothing of suspects. Individual discretion, based on the circumstances at hand, should determine if a suspect or prisoner should empty his own pockets or if the officer should use his own skills in determining the contents of a suspect's clothing.

A safe distance should always be maintained between the officer and the suspect.

Wear protective gloves if exposure to blood is likely to be encountered.

Wear protective gloves for all body cavity searches.

If cotton gloves are to be worn when working with evidence of potential latent fingerprint value at the crime scene, they can be worn over protective disposable gloves when exposure to blood may occur.

Always carry a flashlight, even during daylight shifts, to search hidden areas. Whenever possible, use long-handled mirrors and flashlights to search such areas (e.g., under car seats).

If searching a purse, carefully empty contents directly from purse, by turning it upside down over a table.

Use puncture-proof containers to store sharp instruments and clearly marked plastic bags to store other possibly contaminated items.

To avoid tearing gloves, use evidence tape instead of metal staples to seal evidence. Local procedures for evidence handling should be followed. In general, items should be air dried before sealing in plastic.

Not all types of gloves are suitable for conducting searches. Vinyl or latex rubber gloves provide little protection against sharp instruments, and they are not puncture-proof. There is a direct trade-off between level of protection and manipulability. In other words, the thicker the gloves, the more protection they provide, but the less effective they are in locating objects. Thus, there is no single type or thickness of glove appropriate for protection in all situations. Officers should select the type and thickness of glove which provides the best balance of protection and search efficiency.

Officers and crime scene technicians may confront unusual hazards, especially when the crime scene involves violent behavior, such as a homicide where large amounts of blood are present. Protective gloves should be available and worn in this setting. In addition, for very large spills, consideration should be given to other protective clothing, such as overalls, aprons, boots, or protective shoe covers. They should be changed if torn or soiled, and always removed prior to leaving the scene. While wearing gloves, avoid handling personal items, such as combs and pens, that could become soiled or contaminated. Face masks and eye protection or a face shield are required for laboratory and evidence technicians whose jobs which entail potential exposures to blood via a splash to the face, mouth, nose, or eyes. Airborne particles of dried blood may be generated when a stain is scraped. It is recommended that protective masks and eyewear or face shields be worn by laboratory or evidence technicians when removing the blood stain for laboratory analyses.

While processing the crime scene, personnel should be alert for the presence of sharp objects such as hypodermic needles, knives, razors, broken glass, nails, or other sharp objects.

Handling Deceased Persons and Body Removal

For detectives, investigators, evidence technicians, and others who may have to touch or remove a body, the response should be the same as for situations requiring CPR or first aid: wear gloves and cover all cuts and abrasions to create a barrier and carefully wash all exposed areas after any contact with blood. The precautions to be used with blood and deceased persons should also be used when handling amputated limbs, hands, or other body parts. Such procedures should be followed after contact with the blood of anyone, regardless of whether they are known or suspected to be infected with HIV or HBV.

Autopsies

Protective masks and eyewear (or face shields), laboratory coats, gloves, and waterproof aprons should be worn when performing or attending all autopsies. All autopsy material should be considered infectious for both HIV and HBV. Onlookers with an opportunity for exposure to blood splashes should be similarly protected. Instruments and surfaces contaminated during postmortem procedures should be decontaminated with an appropriate chemical germicide (4). Many laboratories have more detailed standard operating procedures for conducting autopsies; where available, these should be followed. More detailed recommendations for health-care workers in this setting have been published (4).

Forensic Laboratories

Blood from all individuals should be considered infective. To supplement other worksite precautions, the following precautions are recommended for workers in forensic laboratories.

1. All specimens of blood should be put in a well-constructed, appropriately labelled container with a secure lid to prevent leaking during transport. Care should be taken when collecting each specimen to avoid contaminating the outside of the container and of the laboratory form accompanying the specimen.

2. All persons processing blood specimens should wear gloves. Masks and protective eyewear or face shields should be worn if mucous-membrane contact with blood is anticipated (e.g., removing tops from vacuum tubes). Hands should be washed after completion of specimen processing.

3. For routine procedures, such as histologic and pathologic studies or microbiological culturing, a biological safety cabinet is not necessary. However, biological safety cabinets (Class I or II) should be used whenever procedures are conducted that have a high potential for generating droplets. These include activities such as blending, sonicating, and vigorous mixing.

4. Mechanical pipetting devices should be used for manipulating all liquids in the laboratory. Mouth pipetting must not be done.

5. Use of needles and syringes should be limited to situations in which there is no alternative, and the recommendations for preventing injuries with needles outlined under universal precautions should be followed.

6. Laboratory work surfaces should be cleaned of visible materials and then decontaminated with an appropriate chemical germicide after a spill of blood, semen, or blood-contaminated body fluid and when work activities are completed.

7. Contaminated materials used in laboratory tests should be decontaminated before reprocessing or be placed in bags and disposed of in accordance with institutional and local regulatory policies for disposal of infective waste.

8. Scientific equipment that has been contaminated with blood should be cleaned and then decontaminated before being repaired in the laboratory or transported to the manufacturer.

9. All persons should wash their hands after completing laboratory activities and should remove protective clothing before leaving the laboratory.

10. Area posting of warning signs should be considered to remind employees of continuing hazard of infectious disease transmission in the laboratory setting.

Correctional-Facility Considerations

Searches

Penetrating injuries are known to occur in the correctional-facility setting, and puncture wounds or needle sticks in particular pose a hazard during searches of prisoners or their cells. The following precautionary measures will help to reduce the risk of infection:

A correctional-facility officer should use great caution in searching the clothing of prisoners. Individual discretion, based on the circumstances at hand, should determine if a prisoner should empty his own pockets or if the officer should use his own skills in determining the contents of a prisoner's clothing.

A safe distance should always be maintained between the officer and the prisoner.

Always carry a flashlight, even during daylight shifts, to search hidden areas. Whenever possible, use long-handled mirrors and flashlights to search such areas (e.g., under commodes, bunks, and in vents in jail cells).

Wear protective gloves if exposure to blood is likely to be encountered.

Wear protective gloves for all body cavity searches.

Not all types of gloves are suitable for conducting searches. Vinyl or latex rubber gloves can provide little, if any, protection against sharp instruments, and they are not puncture-proof. There is a direct trade-off between level of protection and manipulability. In other words, the thicker the gloves, the more protection they provide, but the less effective they are in locating objects. Thus, there is no single type or thickness of glove appropriate for protection in all situations. Officers should select the type and thickness of glove which provides the best balance of protection and search efficiency.

Decontamination and Disposal

Prisoners may spit at officers and throw feces; sometimes these substances have been purposefully contaminated with blood. Although there are no documented cases of HIV or HBV transmission in this manner and transmission by this route would not be expected to occur, other diseases could be transmitted. These materials should be removed with a paper towel after donning gloves, and the area then decontaminated with an appropriate germicide. Following clean-up, soiled towels and gloves should be disposed of properly.

REFERENCES: AS NUMBERED IN ORIGINAL PUBLICATION

1. Garner JS, Favero MS. Guideline for handwashing and hospital environmental control, 1985. Atlanta: Public Health Service, Centers for Disease Control, 1985. HHS publication no. 99–1117.
2. Garner JS, Simmons BP. Guideline for isolation precautions in hospitals. Infect Control 1983;4(Suppl): 245–325.
3. Williams WW. Guideline for infection control in hospital personnel. Infect Control 1983;4(Suppl): 326–349.
4. Centers for Disease Control. Recommendations for prevention of HIV transmission in health-care settings. MMWR 1987;36(Suppl 2S).
5. Centers for Disease Control. Update: Universal precautions for prevention of transmission of human immunodeficiency virus, hepatitis B virus, and other bloodborne pathogens in health-care settings. MMWR 1988;37:377–382, 387–388.
6. U.S. Department of Labor, U.S. Department of Health and Human Services. Joint Advisory Notice: protection against occupational exposure to hepatitis B virus (HBV) and human immunodeficiency virus (HIV). Federal Register 1987;52:41818-41824.
7. Centers for Disease Control. Recommendations for protection against viral hepatitis. MMWR 1985; 34:313–324, 329–335.
22. Centers for Disease Control. Public Health Service guidelines for counseling and antibody testing to prevent HIV infection and AIDS. MMWR 1987;36:509–515.

23. Centers for Disease Control. Additional recommendations to reduce sexual and drug abuse-related transmission of human T-lymphotropic virus type III/lymphadenopathy-associated virus. MMWR 1986; 35:152–155.
24. Jenison SA, Lemon SM, Baker LN, Newbold JE. Quantitative analysis of hepatitis B virus DNA in saliva and semen of chronically infected homosexual men. J Infect Dis 1987;156:299–306.
25. Cancio-Bello TP, de Medina M, Shorey J, Valledor MD, Schiff ER. An institutional outbreak of hepatitis B related to a human biting carrier. J Infect Dis 1982;146:652–656.
26. MacQuarrie MB, Forghani B, Wolochow DA. Hepatitis B transmitted by a human bite. JAMA 1974;230:723–724.
27. Scott RM, Snitbhan R, Bancroft WH, Alter HJ, Tingpalapong M. Experimental transmission of hepatitis B virus by semen and saliva. J Infect Dis 1980;142:67–71.
28. Glaser JB, Nadler JP. Hepatitis B virus in a cardiopulmonary resuscitation training course: Risk of transmission from a surface antigen-positive participant. Arch Intern Med 1985;145:1653–1655.
29. Osterholm MT, Bravo ER, Crosson JT, et al. Lack of transmission of viral hepatitis type B after oral exposure to HBsAg-positive saliva. Br Med J 1979;2:1263–1264.
30. Lifson AR. Do alternate modes for transmission of human immunodeficiency virus exist? A review. JAMA 1988;259:1353–1356.
31. Friedland GH, Saltzman BR, Rogers MF, et al. Lack of transmission of HTLV-III/LAV infection to household contacts of patients with AIDS or AIDS-related complex with oral candidiasis. N Engl J Med 1986;314:344–349.
32. Curran JW, Jaffe HW, Hardy AM, et al. Epidemiology of HIV infection and AIDS in the United States. Science 1988;239:610–616.
33. Jason JM, McDougal JS, Dixon G, et al. HTLV-III/LAV antibody and immune status of household contacts and sexual partners of persons with hemophilia. JAMA 1986;255:212–215.
34. Wahn V, Kramer HH, Voit T, Brister HT, Scrampical B, Scheid A. Horizontal transmission of HIV infection between two siblings [Letter]. Lancet 1986;2:694.
35. Kane MA, Lettau LA. Transmission of HBV from dental personnel to patients. J Am Dent Assoc 1985;110:634–636.
36. Lettau LA, Smith JD, Williams D, et al. Transmission of hepatitis B virus with resultant restriction of surgical practice. JAMA 1986;255:934–937.
37. International Association of Fire Fighters. Guidelines to prevent transmission of communicable disease during emergency care for fire fighters, paramedics, and emergency medical technicians. New York: International Association of Fire Fighters, 1988.

Semen Banking, Organ and Tissue Transplantation, and HIV Antibody Testing

Original Citation: Centers for Disease Control and Prevention. Perspectives in Disease Prevention and Health Promotion: Semen Banking, Organ and Tissue Transplantation, and HIV Antibody Testing. MMWR 1988;37(4):57–58, 63.

The following recommendations regarding storage and use of semen were prepared by the Food and Drug Administration and the Centers for Disease Control with the endorsement of the American Association of Tissue Banks, the American Fertility Society, and the American College of Obstetricians and Gynecologists.

The Public Health Service published its initial recommendations regarding screening prospective donors of semen, organs, or tissues for the presence of antibody to human immunodeficiency virus (HIV) in 1985 (1). The role of donated semen in the transmission of HIV infection was confirmed later that year (2). In late 1986 and early 1987, transmission of acute viral hepatitis B resulting from artificial insemination with donated semen was reported (3, 4). In April of 1987, an allogenic skin graft was implicated in the transmission of HIV infection (5). A month later, a cadaveric organ donor was found positive for antibody to HIV after his organs were transplanted (6). Most recently, the House of Delegates of the American Medical Association, at its meeting held June 21–25, 1987, adopted a recommendation that testing for antibody to HIV be performed for all donors of blood, organs, or tissues intended for transplantation and for donors of semen or ova (7). Other professional organizations, such as the American Association of Tissue Banks and the American Fertility Society, have published standards and guidelines designed to prevent or minimize the possibility of transmitting disease through artificial insemination or allotransplants (8, 9).

Based on current knowledge, the following recommendations are made with respect to organ and tissue transplantation and artificial insemination:

Prospective donors of organs, tissues, and semen should be tested for antibody to HIV (1, 6). Tests for hospitalized donors should be run on a serum sample taken prior to the donor's receipt of any blood transfusions to avoid situations in which multiple transfusions might result in an antibody loss due to hemodilution (6). Organs and tissues from prospective donors found seropositive for HIV antibody should not be used except when the transplantation of an indispensable organ is necessary to save a patient's life.

In the past, fresh sperm has been routinely recommended for use in artificial insemination and may still be appropriate when semen is from a donor in a mutually monogamous marriage/relationship with the recipient. However, it is now considered prudent to freeze samples from all other donors and store them in that state for a minimum of 6 months. Before frozen semen is used for artificial insemination, a blood sample taken at the time the semen was collected and a second blood sample taken a minimum of 6 months later should be tested for HIV antibody. Responsible medical personnel must be certain that the blood samples are from the same donor, and the donor's identity must be assured. Frozen semen should be used only if both of the tests are negative. These special safeguards should be observed in addition to the preliminary precautions that the donor had (a) no history of risk factors for HIV infection and (b) a physical examination, properly documented by a licensed physician at the time of donation, that showed no obvious evidence of HIV infection.

The American Fertility Society has already modified its guidelines in accordance with these recommendations (10), and these revised guidelines have been accepted by the American College of Obstetricians and Gynecologists. The American Association of Tissue Banks is in the process of similarly revising its standards (personal communication).

REFERENCES: AS NUMBERED IN ORIGINAL PUBLICATION

1. Centers for Disease Control. Testing donors of organs, tissues, and semen for antibody to human T-lymphotropic virus type III/lymphadenopathy-associated virus. MMWR 1985;34:294.
2. Stewart GJ, Tyler JPP, Cunningham AL, et al. Transmission of human T-cell lymphotropic virus type III (HTLV-III) by artificial insemination by donor. Lancet 1985;2:581–584.
3. Mascola L, Guinan ME. Screening to reduce transmission of sexually transmitted diseases in semen used for artificial insemination. N Engl J Med 1986;314:1354–1359.
4. Berry WR, Gottesfeld RL, Alter HJ, Vierling JM. Transmission of hepatitis B virus by artificial insemination. JAMA 1987;257:1079–1081.
5. Clarke JA. HIV transmission and skin grafts [Letter]. Lancet 1987;1:983.
6. Centers for Disease Control. Human immunodeficiency virus infection transmitted from an organ donor screened for HIV antibody—North Carolina. MMWR 1987;36:306–308, 314–315.

7. American Medical Association. Prevention and control of acquired immunodeficiency syndrome: an interim report (Board of Trustees report YY). JAMA 1987;258:2097–2103.
8. American Association of Tissue Banks. Standards for tissue banking. Arlington, VA: American Association of Tissue Banks, 1987.
9. American Fertility Society. New guidelines for the use of semen donor insemination: 1986. Fertil Steril 1986;46(Suppl 2).
10. American Fertility Society. Revised new guidelines for the use of semen-donor insemination. Fertil Steril 1988;49:211.

Public Health Service Guidelines for Counseling and Antibody Testing to Prevent HIV Infection and AIDS

Original Citation: Centers for Disease Control and Prevention. Perspectives in Disease Prevention and Health Promotion Public Health Service Guidelines for Counseling and Antibody Testing to Prevent HIV Infection and AIDS. MMWR 1987;36(31):509–515.

Editor's Note: The information included here was based on guidelines on HIV Counseling and Testing developed from a series of meetings and conferences with public health professionals. The epidemiology of HIV and basics of HIV testing are explained in the original text.

GUIDELINES FOR COUNSELING AND TESTING FOR HIV ANTIBODY

These guidelines are based on public health considerations for HIV testing, including the principles of counseling before and after testing, confidentiality of personal information, and the understanding that a person may decline to be tested without being denied health care or other services, except where testing is required by law (5). Counseling before testing may not be practical when screening for HIV antibody is required. This is true for donors of blood, organs, and tissue; prisoners; and immigrants for whom testing is a Federal requirement as well as for persons admitted to state correctional institutions in states that require testing. When there is no counseling before testing, persons should be informed that testing for HIV antibody will be performed, that individual results will be kept confidential to the extent permitted by law, and that appropriate counseling will be offered. Individual counseling of those who are either HIV-antibody positive or at continuing risk for HIV infection is critical for reducing further transmission and for ensuring timely medical care.

Specific recommendations follow:

Persons Who May Have Sexually Transmitted Disease

All persons seeking treatment for a sexually transmitted disease, in all health-care settings including the offices of private physicians, should be routinely*counseled and tested for HIV antibody.

---

* "Routine counseling and testing" is defined as a policy to provide these services to all clients after informing them that testing will be done. Except where testing is required by law, individuals have the right to decline to be tested without being denied health-care or other services.

IV-Drug Abusers

All persons seeking treatment for IV-drug abuse or having a history of IV-drug abuse should be routinely counseled and tested for HIV antibody. Medical professionals in all health-care settings, including prison clinics, should seek a history of IV-drug abuse from patients and should be aware of its implications for HIV infection. In addition, state and local health policy makers should address the following issues:

Treatment programs for IV-drug abusers should be sufficiently available to allow persons seeking assistance to enter promptly and be encouraged to alter the behavior that places them and others at risk for HIV infection.

Outreach programs for IV-drug abusers should be undertaken to increase their knowledge of AIDS and of ways to prevent HIV infection, to encourage them to obtain counseling and testing for HIV antibody, and to persuade them to be treated for substance abuse.

Persons Who Consider Themselves At Risk

All persons who consider themselves at risk for HIV infection should be counseled and offered testing for HIV antibody.

Women of Childbearing Age

All women of childbearing age with identifiable risks for HIV infection should be routinely counseled and tested for HIV antibody, regardless of the health-care setting. Each encounter between a health-care provider and a woman at risk and/or her sexual partners is an opportunity to reach them with information and education about AIDS and prevention of HIV infection. Women are at risk for HIV infection if they:

Have used IV drugs.

Have engaged in prostitution.

Have had sexual partners who are infected or are at risk for infection because they are bisexual or are IV-drug abusers or hemophiliacs.

Are living in communities or were born in countries where there is a known or suspected high prevalence of infection among women.

Received a transfusion before blood was being screened for HIV antibody but after HIV infection occurred in the United States (e.g., between 1978 and 1985).

Educating and testing these women before they become pregnant allows them to avoid pregnancy and subsequent intrauterine perinatal infection of their infants (30%–50% of the infants born to HIV-infected women will also be infected).

All pregnant women at risk for HIV infection should be routinely counseled and tested for HIV antibody. Identifying pregnant women with HIV infection as early in pregnancy as possible is important for ensuring appropriate medical care for these women; for planning medical care for their infants; and for providing counseling on family planning, future pregnancies, and the risk of sexual transmission of HIV to others. All women who seek family planning services and who are at risk for HIV infection should be routinely counseled about AIDS and HIV infection and tested for HIV antibody. Decisions about the need for counseling and testing programs in a community should be based on the best available estimates of the prevalence of HIV infection and the demographic variables of infection.

Persons Planning Marriage

All persons considering marriage should be given information about AIDS, HIV infection, and the availability of counseling and testing for HIV antibody. Decisions about instituting routine or mandatory premarital testing for HIV antibody should take into account the prevalence of HIV infection in the area and/or population group as well as other factors and should be based upon the likely cost-effectiveness of such testing in preventing further spread of infection. Premarital testing in an area with a prevalence of HIV infection as low as 0.1% may be justified if reaching an infected person through testing can prevent subsequent transmission to the spouse or prevent pregnancy in a woman who is infected.

Persons Undergoing Medical Evaluation or Treatment

Testing for HIV antibody is a useful diagnostic tool for evaluating patients with selected clinical signs and symptoms such as generalized lymphadenopathy; unexplained dementia; chronic, unexplained fever or diarrhea; unexplained weight loss; or diseases such as tuberculosis as well as sexually transmitted diseases, generalized herpes, and chronic candidiasis.

Since persons infected with both HIV and the tubercle bacillus are at high risk for severe clinical tuberculosis, all patients with tuberculosis should be routinely counseled and tested for HIV antibody (6). Guidelines for managing patients with both HIV and tuberculous infection have been published (7). The risk of HIV infection from transfusions of blood or blood components from 1978–1985 was greatest for persons receiving large numbers of units of blood collected from areas with high incidences of AIDS. Persons who have this increased risk should be counseled about the potential risk of HIV infection and should be offered antibody testing (8).

Persons Admitted to Hospitals

Hospitals, in conjunction with state and local health departments, should periodically determine the prevalence of HIV infections in the age groups at highest risk for infection. Consideration should be given to routine testing in those age groups deemed to have a high prevalence of HIV infection.

Persons in Correctional Systems

Correctional systems should study the best means of implementing programs for counseling inmates about HIV infection and for testing them for such infection at admission and discharge from the system. In particular, they should examine the usefulness of these programs in preventing further transmission of HIV infection and the impact of the testing programs on both the inmates and the correctional system (9). Federal prisons have been instructed to test all prisoners when they enter and leave the prison system.

Prostitutes

Male and female prostitutes should be counseled and tested and made aware of the risks of HIV infection to themselves and others. Particularly prostitutes who are HIV-antibody positive should be instructed to discontinue the practice of prostitution. Local or state jurisdictions should adopt procedures to assure that these instructions are followed.

PARTNER NOTIFICATION/CONTACT TRACING

Sexual partners and those who share needles with HIV-infected persons are at risk for HIV infection and should be routinely counseled and tested for HIV antibody. Persons who are HIV-antibody positive should be instructed in how to notify their partners and to refer them for counseling and testing. If they are unwilling to notify their partners or if it cannot be assured that their partners will seek counseling, physicians or health department personnel should use confidential procedures to assure that the partners are notified.

Confidentiality and Antidiscrimination Considerations

The ability of health departments, hospitals, and other health-care providers and institutions to assure confidentiality of patient information and the public's confidence in that ability are crucial to efforts to increase the number of persons being counseled and tested for HIV infection. Moreover, to assure broad participation in the counseling and testing programs, it is of equal or greater importance that the public perceive that persons found to be positive will not be subject to inappropriate discrimination.

Every reasonable effort should be made to improve confidentiality of test results. The confidentiality of related records can be improved by a careful review of actual record-keeping practices and by assessing the degree to which these records can be protected under applicable state laws. State laws should be examined and strengthened when found necessary. Because of the wide scope of "need-to-know" situations, because of the possibility of inappropriate disclosures, and because of established authorization procedures for releasing records, it is recognized that there is no perfect solution to confidentiality problems in all situations. Whether disclosures of HIV-testing information are deliberate, inadvertent, or simply unavoidable, public health policy needs to carefully consider ways to reduce the harmful impact of such disclosures.

Public health prevention policy to reduce the transmission of HIV infection can be furthered by an expanded program of counseling and testing for HIV antibody, but the extent to which these programs are successful depends on the level of participation. Persons are more likely to participate in counseling and testing programs if they believe that they will not experience negative consequences in areas such as employment, school admission, housing, and medical services should they test positive. There is no known medical reason to avoid an infected person in these and ordinary social situations since the cumulative evidence is strong that HIV infection is not spread through casual contact. It is essential to the success of counseling and testing programs that persons who are tested for HIV are not subjected to inappropriate discrimination.

REFERENCES: AS NUMBERED IN ORIGINAL PUBLICATION

5. Bayer R, Levine C, Wolf SM. HIV antibody screening: an ethical framework for evaluating proposed programs. JAMA 1986;256:1768–1774.
6. CDC. Tuberculosis provisional data—United States, 1986. MMWR 1987;36:254–255.
7. CDC. Diagnosis and management of mycobacterial infection and disease in persons with human T-lymphotropic virus type III/lymphadenopathy-associated virus infection. MMWR 1986;35:448–452.
8. CDC. Human immunodeficiency virus infection in transfusion recipients and their family members. MMWR 1987;36:137–140.
9. Hammett TM. AIDS in correctional facilities: issues and options. 2nd ed. Washington, DC: U.S. Department of Justice, National Institute of Justice, 1987.

Recommendations for Prevention of HIV Transmission in Health-Care Settings

Original Citation: Centers for Disease Control and Prevention. Recommendations for Prevention of HIV Transmission in Health-Care Settings. MMWR 1987;36(SU-02):1.

Editor's Note: The information included here was based on an article which gives recommendations for the prevention of HIV transmission in health care settings. The epidemiology of AIDS in health care workers and the risk of acquiring HIV infection in health care workers is described in the original text.

PRECAUTIONS TO PREVENT TRANSMISSION OF HIV

Universal Precautions

Since medical history and examination cannot reliably identify all patients infected with HIV or other blood-borne pathogens, blood and body-fluid precautions should be consistently used for ALL patients. This approach, previously recommended by CDC (3, 4), and referred to as "universal blood and body-fluid precautions" or "universal precautions," should be used in the care of ALL patients, especially including those in emergency-care settings in which the risk of blood exposure is increased and the infection status of the patient is usually unknown (20).

1. All health-care workers should routinely use appropriate barrier precautions to prevent skin and mucous-membrane exposure when contact with blood or other body fluids of any patient is anticipated. Gloves should be worn for touching blood and body fluids, mucous membranes, or non-intact skin of all patients, for handling items or surfaces soiled with blood or body fluids, and for performing venipuncture and other vascular access procedures. Gloves should be changed after contact with each patient. Masks and protective eyewear or face shields should be worn during procedures that are likely to generate droplets of blood or other body fluids to

prevent exposure of mucous membranes of the mouth, nose, and eyes. Gowns or aprons should be worn during procedures that are likely to generate splashes of blood or other body fluids.

2. Hands and other skin surfaces should be washed immediately and thoroughly if contaminated with blood or other body fluids. Hands should be washed immediately after gloves are removed.

3. All health-care workers should take precautions to prevent injuries caused by needles, scalpels, and other sharp instruments or devices during procedures; when cleaning used instruments; during disposal of used needles; and when handling sharp instruments after procedures. To prevent needlestick injuries, needles should not be recapped, purposely bent or broken by hand, removed from disposable syringes, or otherwise manipulated by hand. After they are used, disposable syringes and needles, scalpel blades, and other sharp items should be placed in puncture-resistant containers for disposal; the puncture-resistant containers should be located as close as practical to the use area. Large-bore reusable needles should be placed in a puncture-resistant container for transport to the reprocessing area.

4. Although saliva has not been implicated in HIV transmission, to minimize the need for emergency mouth-to-mouth resuscitation, mouthpieces, resuscitation bags, or other ventilation devices should be available for use in areas in which the need for resuscitation is predictable.

5. Health-care workers who have exudative lesions or weeping dermatitis should refrain from all direct patient care and from handling patient-care equipment until the condition resolves.

6. Pregnant health-care workers are not known to be at greater risk of contracting HIV infection than health-care workers who are not pregnant; however, if a health-care worker develops HIV infection during pregnancy, the infant is at risk of infection resulting from perinatal transmission. Because of this risk, pregnant health-care workers should be especially familiar with and strictly adhere to precautions to minimize the risk of HIV transmission.

Implementation of universal blood and body-fluid precautions for ALL patients eliminates the need for use of the isolation category of "Blood and Body Fluid Precautions" previously recommended by CDC (7) for patients known or suspected to be infected with blood-borne pathogens. Isolation precautions (e.g., enteric, "AFB" [7]) should be used as necessary if associated conditions, such as infectious diarrhea or tuberculosis, are diagnosed or suspected.

Precautions for Invasive Procedures

In this document, an invasive procedure is defined as surgical entry into tissues, cavities, or organs or repair of major traumatic injuries (a) in an operating or delivery room, emergency department, or outpatient setting, including both physicians' and dentists' offices; (b) cardiac catheterization and angiographic procedures; (c) a vaginal or cesarean delivery or other invasive obstetric procedure during which bleeding may occur; or (d) the manipulation, cutting, or removal of any oral or perioral tissues, including tooth structure, during which bleeding occurs or the potential for bleeding exists. The universal blood and body-fluid precautions listed above, combined with the precautions listed below, should be the minimum precautions for ALL such invasive procedures.

1. All health-care workers who participate in invasive procedures must routinely use appropriate barrier precautions to prevent skin and mucous-membrane contact with blood and other body fluids of all patients. Gloves and surgical masks must be worn for all invasive procedures. Protective eyewear or face shields should be worn for procedures that commonly result in the generation of droplets, splashing of blood or other body fluids, or the generation of bone chips. Gowns or aprons made of materials that provide an effective barrier should be worn during invasive procedures that are likely to result in the splashing of blood or other body fluids. All health-care workers who perform or assist in vaginal or cesarean deliveries should wear gloves and gowns when handling the placenta or the infant until blood and amniotic fluid have been removed from the infant's skin and should wear gloves during post-delivery care of the umbilical cord.

2. If a glove is torn or a needlestick or other injury occurs, the glove should be removed and a new glove used as promptly as patient safety permits; the needle or instrument involved in the incident should also be removed from the sterile field.

Precautions for Dentistry*

Blood, saliva, and gingival fluid from ALL dental patients should be considered infective. Special emphasis should be placed on the following precautions for preventing transmission of blood-borne pathogens in dental practice in both institutional and non-institutional settings.

1. In addition to wearing gloves for contact with oral mucous membranes of all patients, all dental workers should wear surgical masks and protective eyewear or chin-length plastic face shields during dental procedures in which splashing or spattering of blood, saliva, or gingival fluids is likely. Rubber dams, high-speed evacuation and proper patient positioning, when appropriate, should be utilized to minimize generation of droplets and spatter.

2. Handpieces should be sterilized after use with each patient, since blood, saliva, or gingival fluid of patients may be aspirated into the handpiece or waterline. Handpieces that cannot be sterilized should at least be flushed, the outside surface cleaned and wiped with a suitable chemical germicide, and then rinsed. Handpieces should be flushed at the beginning of the day and after use with each patient. Manufacturers' recommendations should be followed for use and maintenance of waterlines and check valves and for flushing of handpieces. The same precautions should be used for ultrasonic scalers and air/water syringes.

3. Blood and saliva should be thoroughly and carefully cleaned from material that has been used in the mouth (e.g., impression materials, bite registration), especially before polishing and grinding intra-oral devices. Contaminated materials, impressions, and intra-oral devices should also be cleaned and disinfected before being handled in the dental laboratory and before they are placed in the patient's mouth. Because of the increasing va-

---

* General infection-control precautions are more specifically addressed in previous recommendations for infection-control practices for dentistry (8).

riety of dental materials used intra-orally, dental workers should consult with manufacturers as to the stability of specific materials when using disinfection procedures.

4. Dental equipment and surfaces that are difficult to disinfect (e.g., light handles or X-ray-unit heads) and that may become contaminated should be wrapped with impervious-backed paper, aluminum foil, or clear plastic wrap. The coverings should be removed and discarded, and clean coverings should be put in place after use with each patient.

Precautions for Autopsies or Morticians' Services

In addition to the universal blood and body-fluid precautions listed above, the following precautions should be used by persons performing postmortem procedures:

1. All persons performing or assisting in postmortem procedures should wear gloves, masks, protective eyewear, gowns, and waterproof aprons.
2. Instruments and surfaces contaminated during postmortem procedures should be decontaminated with an appropriate chemical germicide.

Precautions for Dialysis

Patients with end-stage renal disease who are undergoing maintenance dialysis and who have HIV infection can be dialyzed in hospital-based or free-standing dialysis units using conventional infection-control precautions (21). Universal blood and body-fluid precautions should be used when dialyzing ALL patients.

Strategies for disinfecting the dialysis fluid pathways of the hemodialysis machine are targeted to control bacterial contamination and generally consist of using 500–750 parts per million (ppm) of sodium hypochlorite (household bleach) for 30–40 minutes or 1.5%–2.0% formaldehyde overnight. In addition, several chemical germicides formulated to disinfect dialysis machines are commercially available. None of these protocols or procedures need to be changed for dialyzing patients infected with HIV.

Patients infected with HIV can be dialyzed by either hemodialysis or peritoneal dialysis and do not need to be isolated from other patients. The type of dialysis treatment (i.e., hemodialysis or peritoneal dialysis) should be based on the needs of the patient. The dialyzer may be discarded after each use. Alternatively, centers that reuse dialyzers—i.e. a specific single-use dialyzer is issued to a specific patient, removed, cleaned, disinfected, and reused several times on the same patient only—may include HIV-infected patients in the dialyzer-reuse program. An individual dialyzer must never be used on more than one patient.

Precautions for Laboratories**

Blood and other body fluids from ALL patients should be considered infective. To supplement the universal blood and body-fluid precautions listed above, the

---

** Additional precautions for research and industrial laboratories are addressed elsewhere (22, 23).

following precautions are recommended for health-care workers in clinical laboratories.

1. All specimens of blood and body fluids should be put in a well-constructed container with a secure lid to prevent leaking during transport. Care should be taken when collecting each specimen to avoid contaminating the outside of the container and of the laboratory form accompanying the specimen.

2. All persons processing blood and body-fluid specimens (e.g., removing tops from vacuum tubes) should wear gloves. Masks and protective eyewear should be worn if mucous-membrane contact with blood or body fluids is anticipated. Gloves should be changed and hands washed after completion of specimen processing.

3. For routine procedures, such as histologic and pathologic studies or microbiologic culturing, a biological safety cabinet is not necessary. However, biological safety cabinets (Class I or II) should be used whenever procedures are conducted that have a high potential for generating droplets. These include activities such as blending, sonicating, and vigorous mixing.

4. Mechanical pipetting devices should be used for manipulating all liquids in the laboratory. Mouth pipetting must not be done.

5. Use of needles and syringes should be limited to situations in which there is no alternative, and the recommendations for preventing injuries with needles outlined under universal precautions should be followed.

6. Laboratory work surfaces should be decontaminated with an appropriate chemical germicide after a spill of blood or other body fluids and when work activities are completed.

7. Contaminated materials used in laboratory tests should be decontaminated before reprocessing or be placed in bags and disposed of in accordance with institutional policies for disposal of infective waste (24).

8. Scientific equipment that has been contaminated with blood or other body fluids should be decontaminated and cleaned before being repaired in the laboratory or transported to the manufacturer.

9. All persons should wash their hands after completing laboratory activities and should remove protective clothing before leaving the laboratory.

Implementation of universal blood and body-fluid precautions for ALL patients eliminates the need for warning labels on specimens since blood and other body fluids from all patients should be considered infective.

ENVIRONMENTAL CONSIDERATIONS FOR HIV TRANSMISSION

No environmentally mediated mode of HIV transmission has been documented. Nevertheless, the precautions described below should be taken routinely in the care of ALL patients.

Sterilization and Disinfection

Standard sterilization and disinfection procedures for patient-care equipment currently recommended for use (25, 26) in a variety of healthcare settings—including hospitals, medical and dental clinics and offices, hemodialysis centers, emergency-care facilities, and long-term nursing-care facilities—are adequate to sterilize or disinfect instruments, devices, or other items contaminated with blood or other body fluids from persons infected with blood-borne pathogens including HIV (21, 23).

Instruments or devices that enter sterile tissue or the vascular system of any patient or through which blood flows should be sterilized before reuse. Devices or items that contact intact mucous membranes should be sterilized or receive high-level disinfection, a procedure that kills vegetative organisms and viruses but not necessarily large numbers of bacterial spores. Chemical germicides that are registered with the U.S. Environmental Protection Agency (EPA) as "sterilants" may be used either for sterilization or for high-level disinfection depending on contact time.

Contact lenses used in trial fittings should be disinfected after each fitting by using a hydrogen peroxide contact lens disinfecting system or, if compatible, with heat (78°C–80°C [172.4°F–176.0°F]) for 10 minutes.

Medical devices or instruments that require sterilization or disinfection should be thoroughly cleaned before being exposed to the germicide, and the manufacturer's instructions for the use of the germicide should be followed. Further, it is important that the manufacturer's specifications for compatibility of the medical device with chemical germicides be closely followed. Information on specific label claims of commercial germicides can be obtained by writing to the Disinfectants Branch, Office of Pesticides, Environmental Protection Agency, 401 M Street, SW, Washington, D.C. 20460.

Studies have shown that HIV is inactivated rapidly after being exposed to commonly used chemical germicides at concentrations that are much lower than used in practice (27–30). Embalming fluids are similar to the types of chemical germicides that have been tested and found to completely inactivate HIV. In addition to commercially available chemical germicides, a solution of sodium hypochlorite (household bleach) prepared daily is an inexpensive and effective germicide. Concentrations ranging from approximately 500 ppm (1:100 dilution of household bleach) sodium hypochlorite to 5,000 ppm (1:10 dilution of household bleach) are effective depending on the amount of organic material (e.g., blood, mucus) present on the surface to be cleaned and disinfected. Commercially available chemical germicides may be more compatible with certain medical devices that might be corroded by repeated exposure to sodium hypochlorite, especially to the 1:10 dilution.

Survival of HIV in the Environment

The most extensive study on the survival of HIV after drying involved greatly concentrated HIV samples, i.e., 10 million tissue-culture infectious doses per milliliter (31). This concentration is at least 100,000 times greater than that typically found in the blood or serum of patients with HIV infection. HIV was detectable by tissue-culture techniques 1–3 days after drying, but the rate of inactivation was rapid. Studies performed at CDC have also shown that drying HIV causes a rapid (within several hours) 1–2 log (90%–99%) reduction in HIV concentration. In tissue-culture fluid, cell-free HIV could be detected up to 15 days at room temperature, up to 11 days at 37°C (98.6°F), and up to 1 day if the HIV was cell-associated.

When considered in the context of environmental conditions in health-care facilities, these results do not require any changes in currently recommended sterilization, disinfection, or housekeeping strategies. When medical devices are contaminated with blood or other body fluids, existing recommendations include the cleaning of these instruments, followed by disinfection or sterilization, depending on the type of medical device. These protocols assume "worst-case" conditions of extreme virologic and microbiologic contamination, and whether viruses have been inactivated after drying plays no role in formulating these strategies. Consequently, no changes in published procedures for cleaning, disinfecting, or sterilizing need to be made.

Housekeeping

Environmental surfaces such as walls, floors, and other surfaces are not associated with transmission of infections to patients or health-care workers. Therefore, extraordinary attempts to disinfect or sterilize these environmental surfaces are not necessary. However, cleaning and removal of soil should be done routinely.

Cleaning schedules and methods vary according to the area of the hospital or institution, type of surface to be cleaned, and the amount and type of soil present. Horizontal surfaces (e.g., bedside tables and hard-surfaced flooring) in patient-care areas are usually cleaned on a regular basis, when soiling or spills occur, and when a patient is discharged. Cleaning of wails, blinds, and curtains is recommended only if they are visibly soiled. Disinfectant fogging is an unsatisfactory method of decontaminating air and surfaces and is not recommended.

Disinfectant-detergent formulations registered by EPA can be used for cleaning environmental surfaces, but the actual physical removal of microorganisms by scrubbing is probably at least as important as any antimicrobial effect of the cleaning agent used. Therefore, cost, safety, and acceptability by housekeepers can be the main criteria for selecting any such registered agent. The manufacturers' instructions for appropriate use should be followed.

Cleaning and Decontaminating Spills of Blood or Other Body Fluids

Chemical germicides that are approved for use as "hospital disinfectants" and are tuberculocidal when used at recommended dilutions can be used to decontaminate spills of blood and other body fluids. Strategies for decontaminating spills of blood and other body fluids in a patient-care setting are different than for spills of cultures or other materials in clinical, public health, or research laboratories. In patient-care areas, visible material should first be removed and then the area should be decontaminated. With large spills of cultured or concentrated infectious agents in the laboratory, the contaminated area should be flooded with a liquid germicide before cleaning, then decontaminated with fresh germicidal chemical. In both settings, gloves should be worn during the cleaning and decontaminating procedures.

Laundry

Although soiled linen has been identified as a source of large numbers of certain pathogenic microorganisms, the risk of actual disease transmission is negligible. Rather than rigid procedures and specifications, hygienic and common-sense storage and processing of clean and soiled linen are recommended (26). Soiled linen should be handled as little as possible and with minimum agitation to prevent gross microbial contamination of the air and of persons handling the linen. All soiled linen should be bagged at the location where it was used; it should not be sorted or rinsed in patient-care areas. Linen soiled with blood or body fluids should be placed and transported in bags that prevent leakage. If hot water is used, linen should be washed with detergent in water at least 71°C (160°F) for 25 minutes. If low-temperature (less than or equal to 70°C [158°F]) laundry cycles are used, chemicals suitable for low-temperature washing at proper use concentration should be used.

Infective Waste

There is no epidemiologic evidence to suggest that most hospital waste is any more infective than residential waste. Moreover, there is no epidemiologic evidence that hospital waste has caused disease in the community as a result of improper disposal. Therefore, identifying wastes for which special precautions are indicated is largely a matter of judgment about the relative risk of disease transmission. The most practical approach to the management of infective waste is to identify those wastes with the potential for causing infection during handling and disposal and for which some special precautions appear prudent. Hospital wastes for which special precautions appear prudent include microbiology laboratory waste, pathology waste, and blood specimens or blood products. While any item that has had contact with blood, exudates, or secretions may be potentially infective, it is not usually considered practical or necessary to treat all such waste as infective (23, 26). Infective waste, in general, should either be incinerated or should be autoclaved before disposal in a sanitary landfill. Bulk blood, suctioned fluids, excretions, and secretions may be carefully poured down a drain connected to a sanitary sewer. Sanitary sewers may also be used to dispose of other infectious wastes capable of being ground and flushed into the sewer.

IMPLEMENTATION OF RECOMMENDED PRECAUTIONS

Employers of health-care workers should ensure that policies exist for:

1. Initial orientation and continuing education and training of all health-care workers—including students and trainees—on the epidemiology, modes of transmission, and prevention of HIV and other blood-borne infections and the need for routine use of universal blood and body-fluid precautions for ALL patients.
2. Provision of equipment and supplies necessary to minimize the risk of infection with HIV and other blood-borne pathogens.
3. Monitoring adherence to recommended protective measures. When monitoring reveals a failure to follow recommended precautions, counseling, education, and/or re-training should be provided, and, if necessary, appropriate disciplinary action should be considered.

Professional associations and labor organizations, through continuing education efforts, should emphasize the need for health-care workers to follow recommended precautions.

SEROLOGIC TESTING FOR HIV INFECTION

Background

A person is identified as infected with HIV when a sequence of tests, starting with repeated enzyme immunoassays (EIA) and including a Western blot or similar, more specific assay, are repeatedly reactive. Persons infected with HIV usually develop antibody against the virus within 6–12 weeks after infection.

The sensitivity of the currently licensed EIA tests is at least 99% when they are performed under optimal laboratory conditions on serum specimens from persons infected for greater than or equal to 12 weeks. Optimal laboratory conditions include the use of reliable reagents, provision of continuing education of personnel, quality control of procedures, and participation in performance-evaluation programs. Given this performance, the probability of a false-negative test is remote except during the first several weeks after infection, before detectable antibody is present. The proportion of infected persons with a false-negative test attributed to absence of antibody in the early stages of infection is dependent on both the incidence and prevalence of HIV infection in a population.

The specificity of the currently licensed EIA tests is approximately 99% when repeatedly reactive tests are considered. Repeat testing of initially reactive specimens by EIA is required to reduce the likelihood of laboratory error. To increase further the specificity of serologic tests, laboratories must use a supplemental test, most often the Western blot, to validate repeatedly reactive EIA results. Under optimal laboratory conditions, the sensitivity of the Western blot test is comparable to or greater than that of a repeatedly reactive EIA, and the Western blot is highly specific when strict criteria are used to interpret the test results. The testing sequence of a repeatedly reactive EIA and a positive Western blot test is highly predictive of HIV infection, even in a population with a low prevalence of infection. If the Western blot test result is indeterminant, the testing sequence is considered equivocal for HIV infection. When this occurs, the Western blot test should be repeated on the same serum sample, and, if still indeterminant, the testing sequence should be repeated on a sample collected 3–6 months later. Use of other supplemental tests may aid in interpreting of results on samples that are persistently indeterminant by Western blot.

Testing of Patients

Previous CDC recommendations have emphasized the value of HIV serologic testing of patients for: (a) management of parenteral or mucous-membrane exposures of health-care workers, (b) patient diagnosis and management, and (c) counseling and serologic testing to prevent and control HIV transmission in the community. In addition, more recent recommendations have stated that hospitals, in conjunction with state and local health departments, should periodically determine the prevalence of HIV infection among patients from age groups at highest risk of infection (32).

Adherence to universal blood and body-fluid precautions recommended for the care of all patients will minimize the risk of transmission of HIV and other blood-borne pathogens from patients to health-care workers. The utility of routine HIV serologic testing of patients as an adjunct to universal precautions is unknown. Results of such testing may not be available in emergency or outpatient settings. In addition, some recently infected patients will not have detectable antibody to HIV.

Personnel in some hospitals have advocated serologic testing of patients in settings in which exposure of health-care workers to large amounts of patients' blood may be anticipated. Specific patients for whom serologic testing has been advocated include those undergoing major operative procedures and those undergoing treatment in critical-care units, especially if they have conditions involving uncontrolled bleeding. Decisions regarding the need to establish testing programs for patients should be made by physicians or individual institutions. In addition, when deemed appropriate, testing of individual patients may be performed on agreement between the patient and the physician providing care.

In addition to the universal precautions recommended for all patients, certain additional precautions for the care of HIV-infected patients undergoing major surgical operations have been proposed by personnel in some hospitals. For example, surgical procedures on an HIV-infected patient might be altered so that hand-to-hand passing of sharp instruments would be eliminated; stapling instruments rather than hand-suturing equipment might be used to perform tissue approximation; electrocautery devices rather than scalpels might be used as cutting instruments; and, even though uncomfortable, gowns that totally prevent seepage of blood onto the skin of members of the operative team might be worn. While such modifications might further minimize the risk of HIV infection for members of the operative team, some of these techniques could result in prolongation of operative time and could potentially have an adverse effect on the patient.

Testing programs, if developed, should include the following principles:

- Obtaining consent for testing.
- Informing patients of test results, and providing counseling for seropositive patients by properly trained persons.
- Assuring that confidentiality safeguards are in place to limit knowledge of test results to those directly involved in the care of infected patients or as required by law.
- Assuring that identification of infected patients will not result in denial of needed care or provision of suboptimal care.
- Evaluating prospectively (a) the efficacy of the program in reducing the incidence of parenteral, mucous-membrane, or significant cutaneous exposures of health-care workers to the blood or other body fluids of HIV-infected patients and (b) the effect of modified procedures on patients.

Testing of Health-care Workers

Although transmission of HIV from infected health-care workers to patients has not been reported, transmission during invasive procedures remains a possibility. Transmission of hepatitis B virus (HBV)—a blood-borne agent with a considerably greater potential for nosocomial spread—from health-care workers to patients has been documented. Such transmission has occurred in situations (e.g., oral and gynecologic surgery) in which health-care workers when tested had very high concentrations of HBV in their blood (at least 100 million infectious virus particles per milliliter, a concentration much higher than occurs with HIV infection), and the health-care workers sustained a puncture wound while performing invasive procedures or had exudative or weeping lesions or microlacerations that allowed virus to contaminate instruments or open wounds of patients (33, 34).

The hepatitis B experience indicates that only those health-care workers who perform certain types of invasive procedures have transmitted HBV to patients. Adherence to recommendations in this document will minimize the risk of transmission of HIV and other blood-borne pathogens from health-care workers to patients during invasive procedures. Since transmission of HIV from infected health-care workers performing invasive procedures to their patients has not been reported and would be expected to occur only very rarely, if at all, the utility of routine testing of such health-care workers to prevent transmission of HIV cannot be assessed. If consideration is given to developing a serologic testing program for health-care workers who perform invasive procedures, the frequency of testing, as well as the issues of consent, confidentiality, and consequences of test results—as previously outlined for testing programs for patients—must be addressed.

MANAGEMENT OF INFECTED HEALTH-CARE WORKERS

Health-care workers with impaired immune systems resulting from HIV infection or other causes are at increased risk of acquiring or experiencing serious complications of infectious disease. Of particular concern is the risk of severe infection following exposure to patients with infectious diseases that are easily transmitted if appropriate precautions are not taken (e.g., measles, varicella). Any health-care worker with an impaired immune system should be counseled about the potential risk associated with taking care of patients with any transmissible infection and should continue to follow existing recommendations for infection control to minimize risk of exposure to other infectious agents (7, 35). Recommendations of the Immunization Practices Advisory Committee (ACIP) and institutional policies concerning requirements for vaccinating health-care workers with live-virus vaccines (e.g., measles, rubella) should also be considered.

The question of whether workers infected with HIV—especially those who perform invasive procedures—can adequately and safely be allowed to perform patient-care duties or whether their work assignments should be changed must be determined on an individual basis. These decisions should be made by the health-care worker's personal physician(s) in conjunction with the medical directors and personnel health service staff of the employing institution or hospital.

MANAGEMENT OF EXPOSURES

If a health-care worker has a parenteral (e.g., needlestick or cut) or mucous-membrane (e.g., splash to the eye or mouth) exposure to blood or other body fluids or has a cutaneous exposure involving large amounts of blood or prolonged contact with blood—especially when the exposed skin is chapped, abraded, or afflicted with dermatitis—the source patient should be informed of the incident and tested for serologic evidence of HIV infection after consent is obtained. Policies should be developed for testing source patients in situations in which consent cannot be obtained (e.g., an unconscious patient).

If the source patient has AIDS, is positive for HIV antibody, or refuses the test, the health-care worker should be counseled regarding the risk of infection and evaluated clinically and serologically for evidence of HIV infection as soon as possible after the exposure. The health-care worker should be advised to report and seek medical evaluation for any acute febrile illness that occurs within 12 weeks after the exposure. Such an illness—particularly one characterized by fever, rash, or lymphadenopathy—may be indicative of recent HIV infection. Seronegative health-care workers should be retested 6 weeks post-exposure and on a periodic basis thereafter (e.g., 12 weeks and 6 months after exposure) to determine whether transmission has occurred. During this follow-up period, especially the first 6–12 weeks after exposure, when most infected persons are expected to seroconvert—exposed health-care workers should follow U.S. Public Health Service (PHS) recommendations for preventing transmission of HIV (36, 37).

No further follow-up of a health-care worker exposed to infection as described above is necessary if the source patient is seronegative unless the source patient is at high risk of HIV infection. In the latter case, a subsequent specimen (e.g., 12 weeks following exposure) may be obtained from the health-care worker for antibody testing. If the source patient cannot be identified, decisions regarding appropriate follow-up should be individualized. Serologic testing should be available to all health-care workers who are concerned that they may have been infected with HIV.

If a patient has a parenteral or mucous-membrane exposure to blood or other body fluid of a health-care worker, the patient should be informed of the incident, and the same procedure outlined above for management of exposures should be followed for both the source health-care worker and the exposed patient.

REFERENCES: AS NUMBERED IN ORIGINAL PUBLICATION

3. CDC. Recommendations for preventing transmission of infection with human T-lymphotropic virus type III/lymphadenopathy-associated virus in the workplace. MMWR 1985;34:681–686, 691–695.
4. CDC. Recommendations for preventing transmission of infection with human T-lymphotropic virus type III/lymphadenopathy-associated virus during invasive procedures. MMWR 1986;35:221–223.
7. Garner JS, Simmons BP. Guideline for isolation precautions in hospitals. Infect Control 1983;4 (Suppl):245–325.
8. CDC. Recommended infection control practices for dentistry. MMWR 1986;35:237–242.
20. Baker JL, Kelen GD, Sivertson KT, Quinn TC. Unsuspected human immunodeficiency virus in critically ill emergency patients. JAMA 1987;257:2609–2611.
21. Favero MS. Dialysis-associated diseases and their control. In: Bennett JV, Brachman PS, eds. Hospital infections. Boston: Little, Brown and Company, 1985:267–284.
22. Richardson JH, Barkley WE, eds. Biosafety in microbiological and biomedical laboratories, 1984. Washington, DC: U.S. Department of Health and Human Services, Public Health Service, HHS publication no. (CDC) 84–8395.
23. CDC. Human T-lymphotropic virus type III/lymphadenopathy-associated virus: agent summary statement. MMWR 1986;35:540–542, 547–549.

24. Environmental Protection Agency. EPA guide for infectious waste management. Washington, DC: U.S. Environmental Protection Agency, May 1986 (Publication no. EPA/530-SW-86–014).

25. Favero MS. Sterilization, disinfection, and antisepsis in the hospital. In: Manual of clinical microbiology. 4th ed. Washington, DC: American Society for Microbiology, 1985:129–137.

26. Garner JS, Favero MS. Guideline for handwashing and hospital environmental control, 1985. Atlanta: Public Health Service, Centers for Disease Control, 1985: HHS publication no. 99–1117.

27. Spire B, Montagnier L, Barre-Sinoussi F, Chermann JC. Inactivation of lymphadenopathy associated virus by chemical disinfectants. Lancet 1984;2:899–901.

28. Martin LS, McDougal JS, Loskoski SL. Disinfection and inactivation of the human T lymphotropic virus type III/lymphadenopathy-associated virus. J Infect Dis 1985;152:400–403.

29. McDougal JS, Martin LS, Cort SP, et al. Thermal inactivation of the acquired immunodeficiency syndrome virus-III/lymphadenopathy-associated virus, with special reference to antihemophilic factor. J Clin Invest 1985;76:875–877.

30. Spire B, Barre-Sinoussi F, Dormont D, Montagnier L, Chermann JC. Inactivation of lymphadenopathy-associated virus by heat, gamma rays, and ultraviolet light. Lancet 1985;1:188–189.

31. Resnik L, Veren K, Salahuddin SZ, Tondreau S, Markham PD. Stability and inactivation of HTLV-III/LAV under clinical and laboratory environments. JAMA 1986;255:1887–1891.

32. CDC. Public Health Service (PHS) guidelines for counseling and antibody testing to prevent HIV infection and AIDS. MMWR 1987;3:509–515.

33. Kane MA, Lettau LA. Transmission of HBV from dental personnel to patients. J Am Dent Assoc 1985;110:634–636.

34. Lettau LA, Smith JD, Williams D, et. al. Transmission of hepatitis B with resultant restriction of surgical practice. JAMA 1986;255:934–937.

35. Williams WW. Guideline for infection control in hospital personnel. Infect Control 1983;4(Suppl): 326–349.

36. CDC. Prevention of acquired immune deficiency syndrome (AIDS): report of inter-agency recommendations. MMWR 1983;32:101–103.

37. CDC. Provisional Public Health Service inter-agency recommendations for screening donated blood and plasma for antibody to the virus causing acquired immunodeficiency syndrome. MMWR 1985;34:1–5.

Recommendations for Preventing Transmission of Infection with Human T-Lymphotropic Virus Type III/ Lymphadenopathy-Associated Virus in the Workplace

Original Citation: Centers for Disease Control. Recommendations for Preventing Transmission of Infection with Human T-Lymphotropic Virus Type III/Lymphadenopathy-Associated Virus in the Workplace. MMWR 1985;34(45):682–686, 691–695.

Editor's Note: In the original article, the epidemiology of HIV infection and hepatitis B infection were explained in detail. The risk of transmission of HIV from patients to health care workers and from health care workers to patients is explored.

TRANSMISSION FROM PATIENTS TO HEALTH-CARE WORKERS

Precautions to Prevent Acquisition of HTLV-III/LAV Infection by Health-Care Workers in the Workplace

These precautions represent prudent practices that apply to preventing transmission of HTLV-III/LAV and other bloodborne infections and should be used routinely (18).

1. Sharp items (needles, scalpel blades, and other sharp instruments) should be considered as potentially infective and be handled with extraordinary care to prevent accidental injuries.

2. Disposable syringes and needles, scalpel blades, and other sharp items should be placed into puncture-resistant containers located as close as practical to the area in which they were used. To prevent needlestick injuries, needles should not be recapped, purposefully bent, broken, removed from disposable syringes, or otherwise manipulated by hand.

3. When the possibility of exposure to blood or other body fluids exists, routinely recommended precautions should be followed. The anticipated exposure may require gloves alone, as in handling items soiled with blood or equipment contaminated with blood or other body fluids, or may also require gowns, masks, and eye-coverings when performing procedures involving more extensive contact with blood or potentially infective body fluids, as in some dental or endoscopic procedures or postmortem examinations. Hands should be washed thoroughly and immediately if they accidentally become contaminated with blood.

4. To minimize the need for emergency mouth-to-mouth resuscitation, mouth pieces, resuscitation bags, or other ventilation devices should be strategically located and available for use in areas where the need for resuscitation is predictable.

5. Pregnant health-care workers (HCWs) are not known to be at greater risk of contracting HTLV-III/LAV infections than HCWs who are not pregnant; however, if a HCW develops HTLV-III/LAV infection during pregnancy, the infant is at increased risk of infection resulting from perinatal transmission. Because of this risk, pregnant HCWs should be especially familiar with precautions for the preventing HTLV-III/LAV transmission (19).

Precautions for HCWs during Home Care of Persons Infected with HTLV-III/LAV

Persons infected with HTLV-III/LAV can be safely cared for in home environments. Studies of family members of patients infected with HTLV-III/LAV have found no evidence of HTLV-III/LAV transmission to adults who were not sexual contacts of the infected patients or to children who were not at risk for perinatal transmission (3). HCWs providing home care face the same risk of transmission of infection as HCWs in hospitals and other health-care settings, especially if there are needlesticks or other parenteral or mucous membrane exposures to blood or other body fluids.

When providing health-care service in the home to persons infected with HTLV-III/LAV, measures similar to those used in hospitals are appropriate. As in the hospital, needles should not be recapped, purposefully bent, broken, removed from disposable syringes, or otherwise manipulated by hand. Needles and other sharp items should be placed into puncture-resistant containers and disposed of in accordance with local regulations for solid waste. Blood and other body fluids can be flushed down the toilet. Other items for disposal that are contaminated with blood or other body fluids that cannot be flushed down the toilet should be wrapped securely in a plastic bag that is impervious and sturdy (not easily penetrated). It should be placed in a second bag before being discarded in a manner consistent with local regulations for solid waste disposal. Spills of blood or other body fluids should be cleaned with soap and water or a household detergent. As in the hospital, individuals cleaning up such spills should wear disposable gloves. A disinfectant solution or a freshly prepared solution of sodium hypochlorite (household bleach, see below) should be used to wipe the area after cleaning.

Precautions for Providers of Prehospital Emergency Health-Care

Providers of prehospital emergency health-care include the following: paramedics, emergency medical technicians, law enforcement personnel, firefighters, lifeguards, and others whose job might require them to provide first-response medical care. The risk of transmission of infection, including HTLV-III/LAV infection, from infected persons to providers of prehospital emergency health care should be no higher than that for HCWs providing emergency care in the hospital if appropriate precautions are taken to prevent exposure to blood or other body fluids.

Providers of prehospital emergency health care should follow the precautions outlined above for other HCWs. No transmission of HBV infection during mouth-to-mouth resuscitation has been documented. However, because of the theoretical risk of salivary transmission of HTLV-III/LAV during mouth-to-mouth resuscitation, special attention should be given to the use of disposable airway equipment or resuscitation bags and the wearing of gloves when in contact with blood or other body fluids. Resuscitation equipment and devices known or suspected to be contaminated with blood or other body fluids should be used once and disposed of or be thoroughly cleaned and disinfected after each use.

Management of Parenteral and Mucous Membrane Exposures of HCWs

If a HCW has a parenteral (e.g., needlestick or cut) or mucous membrane (e.g., splash to the eye or mouth) exposure to blood or other body fluids, the source patient should be assessed clinically and epidemiologically to determine the likelihood of HTLV-III/LAV infection. If the assessment suggests that infection may exist, the patient should be informed of the incident and requested to consent to serologic testing for evidence of HTLV-III/LAV infection. If the source patient has AIDS or other evidence of HTLV-III/LAV infection, declines testing, or has a positive test, the HCW should be evaluated clinically and serologically for evidence of HTLV-III/LAV infection as soon as possible after the exposure, and, if seronegative, retested after 6 weeks and on a periodic basis thereafter (e.g., 3, 6, and 12 months following exposure) to determine if transmission has occurred. During this follow-up period, especially the first 6–12 weeks, when most infected persons are expected to seroconvert, exposed HCWs should receive counseling about the risk of infection and follow U.S. Public Health Service (PHS) recommendations for preventing transmission of AIDS (20, 21). If the source patient is seronegative and has no other evidence of HTLV-III/LAV infection, no further follow-up of the HCW is necessary. If the source patient cannot be identified, decisions regarding appropriate follow-up should be individualized based on the type of exposure and the likelihood that the source patient was infected.

Serologic Testing of Patients

Routine serologic testing of all patients for antibody to HTLV-III/LAV is not recommended to prevent transmission of HTLV-III/LAV infection in the workplace. Results of such testing are unlikely to further reduce the risk of transmission, which, even with documented needlesticks, is already extremely low. Furthermore, the risk of needlestick and other parenteral exposures could be reduced by emphasizing and more consistently implementing routinely recommended infection-control precautions (e.g., not recapping needles). Moreover, results of routine serologic testing would not be available for emergency cases and patients with short lengths of stay, and additional tests to determine whether a positive test was a true or false positive would be required in populations with low prevalence of infection. However, this recommendation is based only on considerations of occupational risks and should not be construed as a recommendation against other uses of the serologic test, such as for diagnosis or to facilitate medical management of patients. Since the experience with infected patients varies substantially among hospitals (75% of all AIDS cases have been reported by only 280 of the more than 6,000 acute-care hospitals in the United States), some hospitals in certain geographic areas may deem it appropriate to initiate serologic testing of patients.

TRANSMISSION FROM HEALTH-CARE WORKERS TO PATIENTS

Precautions to Prevent Transmission of HTLV-III/LAV Infection From HCWs to Patients

These precautions apply to all HCWs, regardless of whether they perform invasive procedures: (a) All HCWs should wear gloves for direct contact with mucous membranes or nonintact skin of all patients and (b) HCWs who have exudative lesions or weeping dermatitis should refrain from all direct patient care and from handling patient-care equipment until the condition resolves.

Management of Parenteral and Mucous Membrane Exposures of Patients

If a patient has a parenteral or mucous membrane exposure to blood or other body fluids of a HCW, the patient should be informed of the incident and the same procedure outlined above for exposures of HCWs to patients should be followed for both the source HCW and the potentially exposed patient. Management of this type of exposure will be addressed in more detail in the recommendations for HCWs who perform invasive procedures.

Serologic Testing of HCWs

Routine serologic testing of HCWs who do not perform invasive procedures (including providers of home and prehospital emergency care) is not recommended to prevent transmission of HTLV-III/LAV infection. The risk of transmission is extremely low and can be further minimized when routinely recommended infection-control precautions are followed. However, serologic testing should be available to HCWs who may wish to know their HTLV-III/LAV infection status. Whether indications exist for serologic testing of HCWs who perform invasive procedures is currently being considered.

Risk of Occupational Acquisition of Other Infectious Diseases by HCWs Infected With HTLV-III/LAV

HCWs who are known to be infected with HTLV-III/LAV and who have defective immune systems are at increased risk of acquiring or experiencing serious complications of other infectious diseases. Of particular concern is the risk of severe infection following exposure to patients with infectious diseases that are easily transmitted if appropriate precautions are not taken (e.g., tuberculosis). HCWs infected with HTLV-III/LAV should be counseled about the potential risk associated with taking care of patients with transmissible infections and should continue to follow existing recommendations for infection control to minimize their risk of exposure to other infectious agents (18, 19). The HCWs' personal physician(s), in conjunction with their institutions' personnel health services or medical directors, should determine on an individual basis whether the infected HCWs can adequately and safely perform patient-care duties and suggest changes in work assignments, if indicated. In making this determination, recommendations of the Immunization Practices Advisory Committee and institutional policies concerning requirements for vaccinating HCWs with live-virus vaccines should also be considered.

STERILIZATION, DISINFECTION, HOUSEKEEPING, AND WASTE DISPOSAL TO PREVENT TRANSMISSION OF HTLV-III/LAV

Sterilization and disinfection procedures currently recommended for use (22, 23) in health-care and dental facilities are adequate to sterilize or disinfect instruments, devices, or other items contaminated with the blood or other body fluids from individuals infected with HTLV-III/LAV. Instruments or other nondisposable items that enter normally sterile tissue or the vascular system or through which blood flows should be sterilized before reuse. Surgical instruments used on all patients should be decontaminated after use rather than just rinsed with water. Decontamination can be accomplished by machine or by hand cleaning by trained personnel wearing appropriate protective attire (24) and using appropriate chemical germicides. Instruments or other nondisposable items that touch intact mucous membranes should receive high-level disinfection.

Several liquid chemical germicides commonly used in laboratories and health-care facilities have been shown to kill HTLV-III/LAV at concentrations much lower then are used in practice (25). When decontaminating instruments or medical devices, chemical germicides that are registered with and approved by the U.S. Environmental Protection Agency (EPA) as "sterilants" can be used either for sterilization or for high-level disinfection depending on contact time; germicides that are approved for use as "hospital disinfectants'" and are mycobactericidal when used at appropriate dilutions can also be used for high-level disinfection of devices and instruments. Germicides that are mycobactericidal are preferred because mycobacteria represent one of the most resistant groups of microorganisms; therefore, germicides that are effective against mycobacteria are also effective against other bacterial and viral pathogenies. When chemical germicides are used, instruments or devices to be sterilized or disinfected should be thoroughly cleaned before exposure to the germicide, and the manufacturer's instructions for use of the germicide should be followed.

Laundry and dishwashing cycles commonly used in hospitals are adequate to decontaminate linens, dishes, glassware, and utensils. When cleaning environmental surfaces, housekeeping procedures commonly used in hospitals are adequate; surfaces exposed to blood and body fluids should be cleaned with a detergent followed by decontamination using an EPA-approved hospital disinfectant that is mycobactericidal. Individuals cleaning up such spills should wear disposable gloves. Information on specific label claims of commercial germicides can be obtained by writing to the Disinfectants Branch, Office of Pesticides, Environmental Protection Agency, 401 M Street SW, Washington, DC 20460.

In addition to hospital disinfectants, a freshly prepared solution of sodium hypochlorite (household bleach) is an inexpensive and very effective germicide (25). Concentrations ranging from 5,000 ppm (a 1:10 dilution of household bleach) to 500 ppm (a 1:100 dilution) sodium hypochlorite are effective, depending on the amount of organic material (e.g., blood, mucus, etc.) present on the surface to be cleaned and disinfected.

Sharp items should be considered as potentially infective and should be handled and disposed of with extraordinary care to prevent accidental injuries. Other potentially infective waste should be contained and transported in clearly identified impervious plastic bags. If the outside of the bag is contaminated with blood or other body fluids, a second outer bag should be used. Recommended practices for disposal of infective waste (23) are adequate for disposal of waste contaminated by HTLV-III/LAV. Blood and other body fluids may be carefully poured down a drain connected to a sanitary sewer.

CONSIDERATIONS RELEVANT TO OTHER WORKERS

Personal-Service Workers

Personal-service workers (PSWs) are defined as individuals whose occupations involve close personal contact with clients (e.g., hairdressers, barbers, estheticians, cosmetologists, manicurists, pedicurists, massage therapists). PSWs whose services (tattooing, ear piercing, acupuncture, etc.) require needles or other instruments that penetrate the skin should follow precautions indicated for HCWs. Although there is no evidence of transmission of HTLV-III/LAV from clients to PSWs, from PSWs to clients, or between clients of PSWs, a risk of transmission would exist from PSWs to clients and vice versa in situations where there is both (a) trauma to one of the individuals that would provide a portal of entry for the virus and (b) access of blood or serous fluid from one infected person to the open tissue of the other, as could occur if either sustained a cut. A risk of transmission from client to client exists when instruments contaminated with blood are not sterilized or disinfected between clients. However, HBV transmission has been documented only rarely in acupuncture, ear piercing, and tattoo establishments and never in other personal-service settings, indicating that any risk for HTLV-III/LAV transmission in personal-service settings must be extremely low.

All PSWs should be educated about transmission of bloodborne infections, including HTLV-III/LAV and HBV. Such education should emphasize principles of good hygiene, antisepsis, and disinfection. This education can be accomplished by national or state professional organizations, with assistance from state and local health departments, using lectures at meetings or self-instructional materials. Licensure requirements should include evidence of such education. Instruments that are intended to penetrate the skin (e.g., tattooing and acupuncture needles, ear piercing devices) should be used once and disposed of or be thoroughly cleaned and sterilized after each use using procedures recommended for use in health-care institutions. Instruments not intended to penetrate the skin but which may become contaminated with blood (e.g., razors), should be used for only one client and be disposed of or thoroughly cleaned and disinfected after use using procedures recommended for use in health-care institutions. Any PSW with exudative lesions or weeping dermatitis, regardless of HTLV-III/LAV infection status, should refrain from direct contact with clients until the condition resolves. PSWs known to be infected with HTLV-III/LAV need not be restricted from work unless they have evidence of other infections or illnesses for which any PSW should also be restricted.

Routine serologic testing of PSWs for antibody to HTLV-III/LAV is not recommended to prevent transmission from PSWs to clients.

Food-Service Workers

Food-service workers (FSWs) are defined as individuals whose occupations involve the preparation or serving of food or beverages (e.g., cooks, caterers, servers, waiters, bartenders, airline attendants). All epidemiologic and laboratory evidence indicates that bloodborne and sexually transmitted infections are not transmitted during the preparation or serving of food or beverages, and no instances of HBV or HTLV-III/LAV transmission have been documented in this setting.

All FSWs should follow recommended standards and practices of good personal hygiene and food sanitation (26). All FSWs should exercise care to avoid injury to hands when preparing food. Should such an injury occur, both aesthetic and sanitary considerations would dictate that food contaminated with blood be discarded. FSWs known to be infected with HTLV-III/LAV need not be restricted from work unless they have evidence of other infection or illness for which any FSW should also be restricted.

Routine serologic testing of FSWs for antibody to HTLV-III/LAV is not recommended to prevent disease transmission from FSWs to consumers.

Other Workers Sharing the Same Work Environment

No known risk of transmission to co-workers, clients, or consumers exists from HTLV-III/LAV-infected workers in other settings (e.g., office, schools, factories, construction sites). This infection is spread by sexual contact with infected persons, injection of contaminated blood or blood products, and by perinatal transmission. Workers known to be infected with HTLV-III/LAV should not be restricted from work solely based on this finding. Moreover, they should not be restricted from using telephones, office equipment, toilets, showers, eating facilities, and water fountains. Equipment contaminated with blood or other body fluids of any worker, regardless of HTLV-III/LAV infection status, should be cleaned with soap and water or a detergent. A disinfectant solution or a fresh solution of sodium hypochlorite (household bleach, see above) should be used to wipe the area after cleaning.

OTHER ISSUES IN THE WORKPLACE

The information and recommendations contained in this document do not address all the potential issues that may have to be considered when making specific employment decisions for persons with HTLV-III/LAV infection. The diagnosis of HTLV-III/LAV infection may evoke unwarranted fear and suspicion in some co-workers. Other issues that may be considered include the need for confidentiality, applicable federal, state, or local laws governing occupational safety and health, civil rights of employees, workers' compensation laws, provisions of collective bargaining agreements, confidentiality of medical records, informed consent, employee and patient privacy rights, and employee right-to-know statutes.

REFERENCES: AS NUMBERED IN ORIGINAL PUBLICATION

 3. CDC. Education and foster care of children infected with human T-lymphotropic virus type III/lymphadenopathy-associated virus. MMWR 1985;34:517–521.
18. Garner JS, Simmons BP. Guideline for isolation precautions in hospitals. Infect Control 1983;4:245–325.
19. Williams WW. Guideline for infection control in hospital personnel. Infect Control 1983;4:326–349.
20. CDC. Prevention of acquired immune deficiency syndrome (AIDS): report of inter-agency recommendations. MMWR 1983;32:101–103.
21. CDC. Provisional Public Health Service inter-agency recommendations for screening donated blood and plasma for antibody to the virus causing acquired immunodeficiency syndrome. MMWR 1985:34:1–5.
22. Favero MS. Sterilization, disinfection, and antisepsis in the hospital. In: Manual of clinical microbiology. 4th ed. Washington, DC: American Society for Microbiology, 1985:129–137.
23. Garner JS, Favero MS. Guideline for handwashing and hospital environmental control, 1985. Atlanta: Centers for Disease Control, 1985: Publication no. 99–1117.
24. Kneedler JA, Dodge GH. Perioperative patient care. Boston: Blackwell Scientific Publications, 1983: 210–211.
25. Martin LS, McDougal JS, Loskoski SL. Disinfection and inactivation of the human T-lymphotropic virus type III/lymphadenopathy-associated virus. J Infect Dis 1985:152:400–403.
26. Food Service Sanitation Manual 1976. DHEW publication no. (FDA) 78–2081. First printing June 1978.

Universal Precautions for Prevention of Transmission of HIV, Hepatitis B Virus, and Other Bloodborne Pathogens in Health-Care Settings

Original Citation: Centers for Disease Control and Prevention. Perspectives in Disease Prevention and Health Promotion Update: Universal Precautions for Prevention of Transmission of Human Immunodeficiency Virus, Hepatitis B Virus, and Other Bloodborne Pathogens in Health-care Settings. MMWR 1988;37(24):377–388.

BODY FLUIDS TO WHICH UNIVERSAL PRECAUTIONS APPLY

Universal precautions apply to blood and to other body fluids containing visible blood. Occupational transmission of HIV and HBV to health-care workers by blood is documented (4, 5). Blood is the single most important source of HIV, HBV, and other bloodborne pathogens in the occupational setting. Infection control efforts for HIV, HBV, and other bloodborne pathogens must focus on preventing exposures to blood as well as on delivery of HBV immunization.

Universal precautions also apply to semen and vaginal secretions. Although both of these fluids have been implicated in the sexual transmission of HIV and HBV, they have not been implicated in occupational transmission from patient to health-care worker. This observation is not unexpected, since exposure to semen in the usual health-care setting is limited, and the routine practice of wearing gloves for performing vaginal examinations protects health-care workers from exposure to potentially infectious vaginal secretions.

Universal precautions also apply to tissues and to the following fluids: cerebrospinal fluid (CSF), synovial fluid, pleural fluid, peritoneal fluid, pericardial fluid, and amniotic fluid. The risk of transmission of HIV and HBV from these fluids is unknown; epidemiologic studies in the health-care and community setting are currently inadequate to assess the potential risk to health-care workers from occupational exposures to them. However, HIV has been isolated from CSF, synovial, and amniotic fluid (6–8), and HBsAg has been detected in synovial fluid, amniotic fluid, and peritoneal fluid (9–11). One case of HIV transmission was reported after a percutaneous exposure to bloody pleural fluid obtained by needle aspiration (12). Whereas aseptic procedures used to obtain these fluids for diagnostic or therapeutic purposes protect health-care workers from skin exposures, they cannot prevent penetrating injuries due to contaminated needles or other sharp instruments.

BODY FLUIDS TO WHICH UNIVERSAL PRECAUTIONS DO NOT APPLY

Universal precautions do not apply to feces, nasal secretions, sputum, sweat, tears, urine, and vomitus unless they contain visible blood. The risk of transmission of HIV and HBV from these fluids and materials is extremely low or nonexistent. HIV has been isolated and HBsAg has been demonstrated in some of these fluids; however, epidemiologic studies in the health-care and community setting have not implicated these fluids or materials in the transmission of HIV and HBV infections (13, 14). Some of the above fluids and excretions represent a potential source for nosocomial and community-acquired infections with other pathogens, and recommendations for preventing the transmission of nonbloodborne pathogens have been published (2).

PRECAUTIONS FOR OTHER BODY FLUIDS IN SPECIAL SETTINGS

Human breast milk has been implicated in perinatal transmission of HIV, and HBsAg has been found in the milk of mothers infected with HBV (10, 13). However, occupational exposure to human breast milk has not been implicated in the transmission of HIV nor HBV infection to health-care workers. Moreover, the health-care worker will not have the same type of intensive exposure to breast milk as the nursing neonate. Whereas universal precautions do not apply to human breast milk, gloves may be worn by health-care workers in situations where exposures to breast milk might be frequent, for example, in breast milk banking.

Saliva of some persons infected with HBV has been shown to contain HBV-DNA at concentrations 1/1,000 to 1/10,000 of that found in the infected person's serum (15). HBsAg-positive saliva has been shown to be infectious when injected into experimental animals and in human bite exposures (16–18). However, HBsAg-positive saliva has not been shown to be infectious when applied to oral mucous membranes in experimental primate studies (18) or through contamination of musical instruments or cardiopulmonary resuscitation dummies used by HBV carriers (19, 20). Epidemiologic studies of nonsexual household contacts of HIV-infected patients, including several small series in which HIV transmission failed to occur after bites or after percutaneous inoculation or contamination of cuts and open wounds with saliva from HIV-infected patients, suggest that the potential for salivary transmission of HIV is remote (5, 13, 14, 21, 22). One case report from Germany has suggested the possibility of transmission of HIV in a household setting from an infected child to a sibling through a human bite (23). The bite did not break the skin or result in bleeding. Since the date of seroconversion to HIV was not known for either child in this case, evidence for the role of saliva in the transmission of virus is unclear (23). Another case report suggested the possibility of transmission of HIV from husband to wife by contact with saliva during kissing (24). However, follow-up studies did not confirm HIV infection in the wife (21).

Universal Precautions Do Not Apply to Saliva. General infection control practices already in existence—including the use of gloves for digital examination of mucous membranes and endotracheal suctioning, and handwashing after exposure to saliva—should further minimize the minute risk, if any, for salivary transmission of HIV and HBV (1, 25). Gloves need not be worn when feeding patients and when wiping saliva from skin.

Special precautions, however, are recommended for dentistry (1). Occupationally acquired infection with HBV in dental workers has been documented (4), and two possible cases of occupationally acquired HIV infection involving dentists have been reported (5, 26). During dental procedures, contamination of saliva with blood is predictable, trauma to health-care workers' hands is common, and blood spattering may occur. Infection control precautions for dentistry minimize the potential for nonintact skin and mucous membrane contact of dental health-care workers to blood-contaminated saliva of patients. In addition, the use of gloves for oral examinations and treatment in the dental setting may also protect the patient's oral mucous membranes from exposures to blood, which may occur from breaks in the skin of dental workers' hands.

USE OF PROTECTIVE BARRIERS

Protective barriers reduce the risk of exposure of the health-care worker's skin or mucous membranes to potentially infective materials. For universal precautions, protective barriers reduce the risk of exposure to blood, body fluids containing visible blood, and other fluids to which universal precautions apply. Examples of protective barriers include gloves, gowns, masks, and protective eyewear. Gloves should reduce the incidence of contamination of hands, but they cannot prevent penetrating injuries due to needles or other sharp instruments. Masks and protective eyewear or face shields should reduce the incidence of contamination of mucous membranes of the mouth, nose, and eyes.

Universal precautions are intended to supplement rather than replace recommendations for routine infection control, such as handwashing and using gloves to prevent gross microbial contamination of hands (27). Because specifying the types of barriers needed for every possible clinical situation is impractical, some judgment must be exercised.

The risk of nosocomial transmission of HIV, HBV, and other bloodborne pathogens can be minimized if health-care workers use the following general guidelines:*

1. Take care to prevent injuries when using needles, scalpels, and other sharp instruments or devices; when handling sharp instruments after procedures; when cleaning used instruments; and when disposing of used needles. Do not recap used needles by hand; do not remove used needles from disposable syringes by hand; and do not bend, break, or otherwise manipulate used needles by hand. Place used disposable syringes and needles, scalpel blades, and other sharp items in puncture-resistant containers for disposal. Locate the puncture-resistant containers as close to the use area as is practical.

---

* The August 1987 publication should be consulted for general information and specific recommendations not addressed in this update. Copies of this report and of the MMWR supplement entitled Recommendations for Prevention of HIV Transmission in Health-Care Settings published in August 1987 are available through the National AIDS Information Clearinghouse, P.O. Box 6003, Rockville, MD 20850.

2. Use protective barriers to prevent exposure to blood, body fluids containing visible blood, and other fluids to which universal precautions apply. The type of protective barrier(s) should be appropriate for the procedure being performed and the type of exposure anticipated.

3. Immediately and thoroughly wash hands and other skin surfaces that are contaminated with blood, body fluids containing visible blood, or other body fluids to which universal precautions apply.

GLOVE USE FOR PHLEBOTOMY

Gloves should reduce the incidence of blood contamination of hands during phlebotomy (drawing blood samples), but they cannot prevent penetrating injuries caused by needles or other sharp instruments. The likelihood of hand contamination with blood containing HIV, HBV, or other bloodborne pathogens during phlebotomy depends on several factors: (a) the skill and technique of the health-care worker, (b) the frequency with which the health-care worker performs the procedure (other factors being equal, the cumulative risk of blood exposure is higher for a health-care worker who performs more procedures), (c) whether the procedure occurs in a routine or emergency situation (where blood contact may be more likely), and (d) the prevalence of infection with bloodborne pathogens in the patient population. The likelihood of infection after skin exposure to blood containing HIV or HBV will depend on the concentration of virus (viral concentration is much higher for hepatitis B than for HIV), the duration of contact, the presence of skin lesions on the hands of the health-care worker, and—for HBV—the immune status of the health-care worker. Although not accurately quantified, the risk of HIV infection following intact skin contact with infective blood is certainly much less than the 0.5% risk following percutaneous needlestick exposures (5). In universal precautions, all blood is assumed to be potentially infective for bloodborne pathogens, but in certain settings (e.g., volunteer blood-donation centers) the prevalence of infection with some bloodborne pathogens (e.g., HIV, HBV) is known to be very low. Some institutions have relaxed recommendations for using gloves for phlebotomy procedures by skilled phlebotomists in settings where the prevalence of bloodborne pathogens is known to be very low.

Institutions that judge that routine gloving for all phlebotomies is not necessary should periodically reevaluate their policy. Gloves should always be available to health-care workers who wish to use them for phlebotomy. In addition, the following general guidelines apply:

1. Use gloves for performing phlebotomy when the health-care worker has cuts, scratches, or other breaks in his/her skin.

2. Use gloves in situations where the health-care worker judges that hand contamination with blood may occur, for example, when performing phlebotomy on an uncooperative patient.

3. Use gloves for performing finger and/or heel sticks on infants and children.

4. Use gloves when persons are receiving training in phlebotomy.

SELECTION OF GLOVES

The Center for Devices and Radiological Health, FDA, has responsibility for regulating the medical glove industry. Medical gloves include those marketed as sterile surgical or nonsterile examination gloves made of vinyl or latex. General purpose utility ("rubber") gloves are also used in the health-care setting, but they are not regulated by FDA since they are not promoted for medical use. There are no reported differences in barrier effectiveness between intact latex and intact vinyl used to manufacture gloves. Thus, the type of gloves selected should be appropriate for the task being performed.

The following general guidelines are recommended:

1. Use sterile gloves for procedures involving contact with normally sterile areas of the body.
2. Use examination gloves for procedures involving contact with mucous membranes, unless otherwise indicated, and for other patient care or diagnostic procedures that do not require the use of sterile gloves.
3. Change gloves between patient contacts.
4. Do not wash or disinfect surgical or examination gloves for reuse. Washing with surfactants may cause "wicking," i.e., the enhanced penetration of liquids through undetected holes in the glove. Disinfecting agents may cause deterioration.
5. Use general-purpose utility gloves (e.g., rubber household gloves) for housekeeping chores involving potential blood contact and for instrument cleaning and decontamination procedures. Utility gloves may be decontaminated and reused but should be discarded if they are peeling, cracked, or discolored, or if they have punctures, tears, or other evidence of deterioration.

WASTE MANAGEMENT

Universal precautions are not intended to change waste management programs previously recommended by CDC for health-care settings (1). Policies for defining, collecting, storing, decontaminating, and disposing of infective waste are generally determined by institutions in accordance with state and local regulations. Information regarding waste management regulations in health-care settings may be obtained from state or local health departments or agencies responsible for waste management.

EDITORIAL NOTE

Implementation of universal precautions does not eliminate the need for other category or disease-specific isolation precautions, such as enteric precautions for infectious diarrhea or isolation for pulmonary tuberculosis (1, 2). In addition to universal precautions, detailed precautions have been developed for the following procedures and/or settings in which prolonged or intensive exposures to blood occur: invasive procedures, dentistry, autopsies or morticians' services, dialysis, and the clinical laboratory. These detailed precautions are found in the August 21, 1987, "Recommendations for Prevention of HIV Transmission in

Health-care Settings" (1). In addition, specific precautions have been developed for research laboratories (28).

REFERENCES: AS NUMBERED IN ORIGINAL PUBLICATION

1. Centers for Disease Control. Recommendations for prevention of HIV transmission in health-care settings. MMWR 1987;36(Suppl no. 2S).
2. Garner JS, Simmons BP. Guideline for isolation precautions in hospitals. Infect Control 1983:4; 245–325.
4. Department of Labor, Department of Health and Human Services. Joint advisory notice: protection against occupational exposure to hepatitis B virus (HBV) and human immunodeficiency virus (HIV). Washington, DC: US Department of Labor, US Department of Health and Human Services, 1987.
5. Centers for Disease Control. Update: acquired immunodeficiency syndrome and human immunodeficiency virus infection among health-care workers. MMWR 1988;37:229–234, 239.
6. Hollander H, Levy JA. Neurologic abnormalities and recovery of human immunodeficiency virus from cerebrospinal fluid. Ann Intern Med 1987;106:692–695.
7. Wirthrington RH, Cornes P, Harris JRW, et al. Isolation of human immunodeficiency virus from synovial fluid of a patient with reactive arthritis. Br Med J 1987;294:484.
8. Mundy DC, Schinazi RF, Gerber AR, Nahmias AJ, Randall HW. Human immunodeficiency virus isolated from amniotic fluid. Lancet 1987;2:459–460.
9. Onion DK, Crumpacker CS, Gilliland BC. Arthritis of hepatitis associated with Australia antigen. Ann Intern Med 1971;75:29–33.
10. Lee AKY, Ip HMH, Wong VCW. Mechanisms of maternal-fetal transmission of hepatitis B virus. J Infect Dis 1978;138:668–671.
11. Bond WW, Petersen NJ, Gravelle CR, Favero MS. Hepatitis B virus in peritoneal dialysis fluid: a potential hazard. Dialysis Transplant 1982;11:592–600.
12. Oskenhendler E, Harzic M, Le Roux J-M, Rabian C, Clauvel JP. HIV infection with seroconversion after a superficial needlestick injury to the finger [Letter]. N Engl J Med 1986;315:582.
13. Lifson AR. Do alternate modes for transmission of human immunodeficiency virus exist? A review. JAMA 1988;259:1353–1356.
14. Friedland GH, Saltzman BR, Rogers MF, et al. Lack of transmission of HTLV-III/LAV infection to household contacts of patients with AIDS or AIDS-related complex with oral candidiasis. N Engl J Med 1986;314:344–349.
15. Jenison SA, Lemon SM, Baker LN, Newbold JE. Quantitative analysis of hepatitis B virus DNA in saliva and semen of chronically infected homosexual men. J Infect Dis 1987;156:299–306.
16. Cancio-Bello TP, de Medina M, Shorey J, Valledor MD, Schiff ER. An institutional outbreak of hepatitis B related to a human biting carrier. J Infect Dis 1982;146:652–656.
17. MacQuarrie MB, Forghani B, Wolochow DA. Hepatitis B transmitted by a human bite. JAMA 1974;230:723–724.
18. Scott RM, Snitbhan R, Bancroft WH, Alter HJ, Tingpalapong M. Experimental transmission of hepatitis B virus by semen and saliva. J Infect Dis 1980;142:67–71.
19. Glaser JB, Nadler JP. Hepatitis B virus in a cardiopulmonary resuscitation training course: Risk of transmission from a surface antigen-positive participant. Arch Intern Med 1985;145:1653–1655.
20. Osterholm MT, Bravo ER, Crosson JT, et al. Lack of transmission of viral hepatitis type B after oral exposure to HBsAg-positive saliva. Br Med J 1979;2:1263–1264.
21. Curran JW, Jaffe HW, Hardy AM, et al. Epidemiology of HIV infection and AIDS in the United States. Science 1988;239:610–616.
22. Jason JM, McDougal JS, Dixon G, et al. HTLV-III/LAV antibody and immune status of household contacts and sexual partners of persons with hemophilia. JAMA 1986;255:212–215.
23. Wahn V, Kramer HH, Voit T, Bruster HT, Scrampical B, Scheid A. Horizontal transmission of HIV infection between two siblings [Letter]. Lancet 1986;2:694.
24. Salahuddin SZ, Groopman JE, Markham PD, et al. HTLV-III in symptom-free seronegative persons. Lancet 1984;2:1418–1420.
25. Simmons BP, Wong ES. Guideline for prevention of nosocomial pneumonia. Atlanta: U.S. Department of Health and Human Services, Public Health Service, Centers for Disease Control, 1982.
26. Klein RS, Phelan JA, Freeman K, et al. Low occupational risk of human immunodeficiency virus infection among dental professionals. N Engl J Med 1988;318:86–90.
27. Garner JS, Favero MS. Guideline for handwashing and hospital environmental control, 1985. Atlanta: U.S. Department of Health and Human Services, Public Health Service, Centers for Disease Control, 1985: HHS publication no. 99–1117.
28. Centers for Disease Control. 1988 Agent summary statement for human immunodeficiency virus and report on laboratory-acquired infection with human immunodeficiency virus. MMWR 1988;37(Suppl no. S4):1S-22S.

SUBTOPIC / CASE DEFINITION, PROPHYLAXIS, AND TREATMENT

Zidovudine for the Prevention of HIV Transmission from Mother to Infant

Original Citation: Centers for Disease Control. Zidovudine for the prevention of HIV transmission from mother to infant. MMWR 1994;43(16):285–287.

Editor's Note: The information included here was based on an MMWR article which summarizes preliminary results from a randomized, multicenter, double-blinded clinical trial of zidovudine (ZDV) to prevent HIV transmission from mothers to infants.

Worldwide, perinatal (i.e., mother to infant) transmission accounts for most human immunodeficiency virus (HIV) infections among children; in the United States, of the approximately 7000 infants born to HIV-infected mothers each year, 1000–2000 are HIV-infected (1). Strategies for reducing perinatally acquired HIV infection have included preventing HIV infection among women and, for HIV-infected women, avoiding pregnancy or refraining from breast-feeding their infants (2). On February 21, 1994, the National Institutes of Health's National Institute of Allergy and Infectious Diseases (NIAID) and National Institute of Child Health and Human Development (NICHD) announced preliminary results from a randomized, multicenter, double-blinded clinical trial of zidovudine (ZDV) to prevent HIV transmission from mothers to their infants (AIDS Clinical Trials Group [ACTG] protocol 076). This report summarizes the interim results of that trial, which indicate effectiveness of ZDV for prevention of perinatal transmission. The study was initiated in April 1991 by the Pediatric ACTG of NIAID in collaboration with NICHD and the National Institute of Health and Medical Research (INSERM) and the National Agency of Research on AIDS (ANRS), France. Eligible participants were HIV-infected pregnant women who had received no antiretroviral treatment during their current pregnancy, had no clinical indications for maternal antepartum antiretroviral therapy in the judgment of their health-care provider, and who had a CD4+ T-lymphocyte count greater than 200/μL at time of entry into the study. Enrolled women were randomized to receive either a ZDV or placebo regimen. The ZDV regimen included antepartum ZDV (100 mg given orally five times daily) initiated at 14–34 weeks' gestation and continued for the remainder of the pregnancy; intravenous ZDV during labor (administered intravenously as a loading dose of 2 mg per kg body weight given over 1 hour, followed by continuous infusion of 1 mg per kg body weight per hour until delivery); and oral administration of ZDV to the newborn (ZDV syrup at 2 mg per kg body weight per dose given every 6 hours) for the first 6 weeks of life, beginning 8–12 hours after birth (see Table B1). The placebo regimen was given on the same schedule. Blood specimens were obtained for HIV culture from all

Table B1. Eligibility Criteria and Zidovudine Regimen for HIV-Infected Pregnant Women and Their Infants Participating in AIDS Clinical Trials Group Protocol 076

Patient Eligibility

    Has not received antiretroviral treatment during current pregnancy

    Has no clinical indications for maternal and antepartum antiretroviral therapy in the judgment of her health-care provider

    Has a CD4+ T-lymphocyte count greater than 200/μL at initial assessment

Zidovudine Regimen

    Oral administration of 100 mg zidovudine (ZDV) five times daily, initiated at 14–34 weeks' gestation and continued for the remainder of the pregnancy

    During labor, intravenous administration of ZDV in a loading dose of 2 mg per kg body weight given over 1 hour, followed by continuous infusion of 1 mg per kg body weight per hour until delivery

    Oral administration of ZDV to the newborn (ZDV syrup at 2 mg per kg body weight per dose given every 6 hours) for the first 6 weeks of life, beginning 8–12 hours after birth

---

infants at birth and at ages 12, 24, and 78 weeks. A positive viral culture was considered indicative of HIV infection. Infants also were tested for HIV antibody at ages 15 and 18 months.

Based on analysis of data for 364 births through December 1993, ZDV therapy was associated with a 67.5% reduction in the risk for HIV transmission; the estimated rates of transmission were 25.5% (95% confidence interval [CI] = 18.3%–33.7%) among the 184 children in the group receiving the placebo regimen compared with 8.3% (95% CI = 3.8%–13.8%) among the 180 children in the group receiving ZDV (Kaplan-Meier estimate at age 18 months; p = 0.00006). Although the ZDV regimen was well tolerated by mothers and infants, hemoglobin levels were lower for infants in the ZDV group (mean decrease in hemoglobin was less than 1 g/dL); however, this problem resolved without therapy following completion of ZDV treatment. The incidence of reported side effects was similar among mothers and infants between the two randomized groups.

Based on these interim findings, NIAID accepted the recommendation of an independent data and safety monitoring board to terminate enrollment into the trial and to offer ZDV to women in the group who had received the placebo but had not yet delivered and to their infants aged less than 6 weeks. An NIAID Clinical Trials Alert summarizing the trial is available by calling (800) 874-2572.

EDITORIAL NOTE

This clinical trial demonstrated efficacy of ZDV in reducing perinatal HIV transmission when administered to HIV-infected women meeting the study's eligibility criteria (see Table B1). However, these findings are subject to at least four limitations. First, the study did not assess the efficacy of ZDV among women with CD4+ T-lymphocyte counts less than or equal to 200 cells/μL or among women who had previously used ZDV for extended periods and who may be infected with ZDV-resistant strains of HIV. Second, this trial could not assess the relative or independent contributions of the antepartum treatment, intrapartum treatment, or treatment of the infant; therefore, the efficacy and side effects of ZDV regimens restricted to only one or two of these treatment periods is unknown. Third, the study did not evaluate the risk or benefit of ZDV use in the first trimester. Finally, the study has not yet provided information about long-term side effects for infants and mothers treated with ZDV, including infants who did not become infected with HIV; however, long-term follow-up of infants and mothers is being conducted to monitor for possible late side effects.

Based on the findings of ACTG protocol 076, the Public Health Service (PHS) provides the following interim recommendations:* (a) all health-care workers providing care to pregnant women and women of childbearing age should be informed of the results of ACTG protocol 076; (b) HIV-infected pregnant women meeting the protocol eligibility criteria should be informed of the potential benefits but unknown long-term risks of ZDV therapy as administered in ACTG protocol 076, and decisions to use ZDV for prevention of perinatal transmission should be made in consultation with their health-care providers (see Table B1); (c) health-care providers should inform their patients that this ZDV regimen substantially reduced, but did not eliminate, the risk for HIV infection among the infants; and (d) until the potential risk for teratogenicity and other complications from ZDV therapy given in the first trimester can be assessed, ZDV therapy only for the purpose of reducing the risk for perinatal transmission should not be instituted earlier than the 14th week of gestation. PHS is developing further recommendations for the uses of ZDV for HIV-infected pregnant women whose clinical indications differ from the ACTG protocol 076 eligibility criteria and for counseling and HIV-antibody testing for women of childbearing age. The international Antiretroviral Pregnancy Registry, sponsored by Burroughs Wellcome Co. (Research Triangle Park, North Carolina)** and Hoffmann-LaRoche Foundation, Inc. (Nutley, New Jersey),** is collecting observational, nonexperimental data on exposure to ZDV and dideoxycytidine (ddC) during pregnancy. Women who have been treated with either of these drugs at any time during pregnancy for any duration are eligible for registry enrollment. Patients can be enrolled by contacting the registry, telephone (800) 722-9292, extension 8465; fax (919) 315-8981.

REFERENCES: AS NUMBERED IN ORIGINAL PUBLICATION

1. CDC. National HIV serosurveillance summary: results through 1991. Vol 3. Atlanta: U.S. Department of Health and Human Services, Public Health Service, 1994.
2. CDC. Recommendations for assisting in the prevention of perinatal transmission of human T-lymphotropic virus type III/lymphadenopathy-associated virus and acquired immunodeficiency syndrome. MMWR 1985;34:721–726,731–732.

---

* These recommendations do not reflect current Food and Drug Administration-approved labeling for ZDV.

** Use of trade names and commercial sources is for identification only and does not imply endorsement by the Public Health Service or the U.S. Department of Health and Human Services.

Recommendations on the Use of Zidovudine to Reduce Perinatal Transmission of HIV

Original Citation: Centers for Disease Control. Recommendations of the United States Public Health Service Task Force on the Use of Zidovudine to Reduce Perinatal Transmission of HIV. MMWR 1994;43(RR-11):1–20.

Original Authors: Prepared by Lynne Mofenson, M.D., James Balsey, M.D., Ph.D. in collaboration with Robert J. Simonds, M.D., Martha F. Rogers, M.D., Robin R. Moseley, M.A.T.

Editor's Note: The information included here was based on an MMWR report which provides recommendations for the use of ZDV to reduce perinatal transmission and for medical monitoring of pregnant women and infants receiving this therapy. The recommendations are based on the results of AIDS Clinical Trials Group Protocol 076 which demonstrated that ZDV administered to a selected group of HIV-infected pregnant women and their infants can reduce the risk of perinatal HIV transmission by approximately two-thirds. The original article gives a detailed summary of the clinical trial, ACTG Protocol 076. The article also summarizes the epidemiology of HIV infections in children and women.

On June 6, 1994, the U.S. Public Health Service convened a workshop in Bethesda, Maryland, to develop recommendations for the use of zidovudine to reduce the risk for perinatal transmission of human immunodeficiency virus (HIV). The recent results of AIDS Clinical Trials Group Protocol 076, a controlled clinical trial sponsored by the National Institutes of Health in collaboration with the National Institute of Health and Medical Research and the National Agency of Research on AIDS in France, indicate that zidovudine administered to a selected group of HIV-infected women and their infants can reduce the risk for perinatal transmission of HIV by approximately two-thirds. The implications of these results for use of zidovudine in HIV-infected pregnant women and neonates were discussed at the workshop.

POTENTIAL LONG-TERM ADVERSE EFFECTS OF ZDV ADMINISTERED DURING PREGNANCY

The long-term effects of ZDV treatment during pregnancy solely to reduce perinatal transmission or of fetal and neonatal exposure to ZDV are not known. ZDV is a nucleoside analog that inhibits HIV replication by interfering with HIV RNA-dependent DNA polymerase. ZDV triphosphate also can inhibit human cellular DNA polymerases, but only at concentrations much higher than those required to inhibit HIV polymerase. However, gamma DNA polymerase, which is required for mitochondrial replication, may be inhibited by ZDV at concentrations nearer to those that can be achieved in vivo.

Concerns related to the potential long-term toxicity of nucleoside analogs include potential mutagenic and carcinogenic effects, possible effects on tissues with high mitochondrial content (such as hepatic and cardiac tissue), possible teratogenicity, and possible effects on the reproductive system.

ZDV has been shown to be a mutagen in vitro, and, in a mammalian in vitro cell transformation assay, ZDV was positive at concentrations of greater than or equal to 0.5 μg/mL (8). Noninvasive squamous epithelial vaginal tumors were produced after 19–21 months of continuous dosing in 12% of mice administered a dosage equivalent to three times the estimated human exposure at the recommended therapeutic dosage. Similar findings were observed in 3% of rats that received 24 times the recommended therapeutic dosage. Carcinogenicity studies in rodents, however, may not be predictive of human experience.

In humans, an increased incidence of non-Hodgkin's lymphoma has been reported in HIV-infected men receiving ZDV, but this increase probably reflects longer survival despite severe immunodeficiency rather than a direct effect of ZDV (9). The potential for carcinogenesis should be further assessed through continued follow-up of children who were exposed to ZDV in utero.

Myopathy and cardiomyopathy have been associated with ZDV therapy. In an individual patient, the effects secondary to ZDV are often difficult to distinguish from those of HIV infection. A prospective study of HIV-infected children demonstrated no effect of ZDV therapy on cardiac function (10).

Reproductivity/fertility studies in animals have demonstrated no adverse effects of ZDV on either the fertility of male or female rats or the reproductive capacity of their offspring (11). ZDV administered to mice early in gestation was associated with an embryotoxic effect and fetal resorptions; however, ZDV administered at or beyond midgestation had no detectable effect on the fetus (12, 13).

ZDV is assigned pregnancy category C status by the Food and Drug Administration (FDA).* Most studies of ZDV administered to pregnant animals have not demonstrated teratogenicity. In one study, pregnant rats were administered toxic doses of ZDV during organogenesis (i.e., equivalent to approximately 50 times the recommended daily clinical dose, based on relative body surface areas); developmental malformations and skeletal abnormalities were observed in 12% of fetuses (14).

In humans, observational studies involving small numbers of subjects have demonstrated no apparent association of fetal malformations with antenatal ZDV use (15–19). In ACTG Protocol 076, the incidence of congenital malfor-

---

* FDA pregnancy categories are: A, in which adequate and well-controlled studies of pregnant women fail to demonstrate a risk to the fetus during the first trimester of pregnancy (and there is no evidence of a risk during later trimesters); B, in which animal reproduction studies fail to demonstrate a risk to the fetus and adequate and well-controlled studies of pregnant women have not been conducted; C, in which safety in human pregnancies has not been determined, animal studies are either positive for fetal risk or have not been conducted, and the drug should not be used unless the potential benefit outweighs the potential risk to the fetus; D, in which there is positive evidence of human fetal risk based on adverse reaction data from investigational or marketing experiences, but the potential benefits from the use of the drug in pregnant women may be acceptable despite its potential risks; and X, in which studies in animals or reports of adverse reactions have indicated that the risk associated with the use of the drug for pregnant women clearly outweighs any possible benefit.

mations was similar for ZDV and placebo recipients. However, because ZDV was not administered until after 14 weeks of gestation in this study, the potential teratogenicity of ZDV administered during the first trimester cannot be assessed. Similarly, in a recent report from the Antiretroviral Pregnancy Registry maintained by the Wellcome Foundation and Hoffman LaRoche in conjunction with CDC, no increase in the risk of congenital abnormalities above that expected for all pregnancies was observed among infants born to 121 prospectively registered HIV-infected women who received ZDV during pregnancy, nor was there any unusual pattern of birth defects (20).

Use of ZDV during pregnancy could be associated with the development of ZDV-resistant virus, which may lessen the drug's therapeutic benefit for the woman when it is needed for her own health. However, patients with early-stage HIV disease rarely develop ZDV-resistant strains before they have received 18–24 months of continuous therapy (21). After discontinuation of ZDV therapy, an increase in ZDV-susceptible isolates has been observed in some patients who had ZDV-resistant isolates while they were receiving ZDV, although resistance to ZDV has been reported to persist for more than a year after therapy was discontinued (22, 23). Because the development of ZDV-resistant viral strains secondary to transient ZDV use during pregnancy is a theoretical concern, considerations for the woman's future health-care should include the availability of alternative drugs for treatment of HIV infection.

GENERAL PRINCIPLES REGARDING TREATMENT RECOMMENDATIONS

The following treatment recommendations have been formulated to provide a basis for discussion between the woman and her health-care provider about the use of ZDV to reduce perinatal transmission. HIV-infected women should be informed of the substantial benefit and short-term safety of ZDV administered during pregnancy and the neonatal period observed in ACTG Protocol 076. However, they also must be informed that the long-term risks of ZDV therapy to themselves and their children are unknown. A woman's decision to use ZDV to reduce the risk for HIV transmission to her infant should be based on a balance of the benefits and potential risks of the regimen to herself and to her child.

Discussion of treatment options should be noncoercive, and the final decision to accept or reject ZDV treatment recommended for herself and her child is the right and responsibility of the woman. A decision not to accept treatment should not result in punitive action or denial of care, nor should ZDV be denied to a woman who decides to receive the regimen. Various circumstances that commonly occur in clinical practice are described and the factors influencing treatment considerations are highlighted in the following discussion (Table B3). All potential clinical situations cannot be enumerated, and, in many cases, definitive evidence upon which to base a recommendation is not currently available. Therefore, each pregnant woman and her health-care provider must consider the potential benefits, unknown long-term effects, and gaps in knowledge relating to her clinical situation. Furthermore, health-caregivers and institutions should provide culturally, linguistically, and educa-

Table B1. Eligibility criteria for HIV-infected pregnant women participating in AIDS Clinical Trials Group Protocol 076

- Pregnancy at 14–34 weeks of gestation.
- No antiretroviral therapy during the current pregnancy.
- No clinical indications for antenatal antiretroviral therapy.
- CD4+ T-lymphocyte count greater than or equal to 200 cells/μL at the time of entry into the study.

Table B3. Summary: Clinical situations and recommendations for use of zidovudine* to reduce perinatal HIV transmission

I.   Pregnant HIV-infected women with CD4+ T-lymphocyte counts greater than or equal to 200/μL who are at 14–34 weeks of gestation and who have no clinical indications for ZDV and no history of extensive (greater than 6 months) prior antiretroviral therapy.

     Recommendation:
     The health-care provider should recommend the full ACTG Protocol 076 regimen to all HIV-infected pregnant women in this category. This recommendation should be presented to the pregnant woman in the context of a risk-benefit discussion: a reduced risk of transmission can be expected, but the long-term adverse consequences of the regimen are not known. The decision about this regimen should be made by the woman after discussion with her health-care provider.

II. Pregnant HIV-infected women who are at greater than 34 weeks of gestation, who have no history of extensive (greater than 6 months) prior antiretroviral therapy, and who do not require ZDV for their own health.

     Recommendation:
     The health-care provider should recommend the full ACTG Protocol 076 regimen in the context of a risk-benefit discussion with the pregnant woman. The woman should be informed that ZDV therapy may be less effective than that observed in ACTG Protocol 076, because the regimen is being initiated late in the third trimester.

III. Pregnant HIV-infected women with CD4+ T-lymphocyte counts less than 200/μL who are at 14–34 weeks of gestation, who have no other clinical indications for ZDV, and who have no history of extensive (greater than 6 months) prior anti-retroviral therapy.

     Recommendation:
     The health-care provider should recommend initiation of antenatal ZDV therapy to the woman for her own health benefit. The intrapartum and neonatal components of the ACTG Protocol 076 regimen should be recommended until further information becomes available. This recommendation should be presented in the context of a risk-benefit discussion with the pregnant woman.

IV. Pregnant HIV-infected women who have a history of extensive (greater than 6 months) ZDV therapy and/or other antiretroviral therapy before pregnancy.

Table B3.—*continued*

Recommendation:
Because data are insufficient to extrapolate the potential efficacy of the ACTG Protocol 076 regimen for this population of women, the health-care provider should consider recommending the ACTG Protocol 076 regimen on a case-by-case basis after a discussion of the risks and benefits with the pregnant woman. Issues to be discussed include her clinical and immunologic stability on ZDV therapy, the likelihood she is infected with a ZDV-resistant HIV strain, and, if relevant, the reasons for her current use of an alternative antiretroviral agent (e.g., lack of response to or intolerance of ZDV therapy). Consultation with experts in HIV infection may be warranted. The healthcare provider should make the ACTG Protocol 076 regimen available to the woman, although its effectiveness may vary depending on her clinical status.

V. Pregnant HIV-infected women who have not received antepartum anti-retroviral therapy and who are in labor.

Recommendation:
For women with HIV infection who are in labor and who have not received the antepartum component of the ACTG Protocol 076 regimen (either because of lack of prenatal care or because they did not wish to receive antepartum therapy), the health-care provider should discuss the benefits and potential risks of the intrapartum and neonatal components of the ACTG Protocol 076 regimen and offer ZDV therapy when the clinical situation permits.

VI. Infants who are born to HIV-infected women who have received no intrapartum ZDV therapy.

Recommendation:
If the clinical situation permits and if ZDV therapy can be initiated within 24 hours of birth, the health-care provider should offer the ACTG Protocol 076 postpartum component of 6 weeks of neonatal ZDV therapy for the infant in the context of a risk-benefit discussion with the mother. Data from animal prophylaxis studies indicate that, if ZDV is administered, therapy should be initiated as soon as possible (within hours) after delivery. If therapy cannot begin until the infant is greater than 24 hours of age and the mother did not receive therapy during labor, no data support offering therapy to the infant.

---

*These recommendations do not represent approval by the Food and Drug Administration (FDA) or approved labeling for the particular product or indications in question.

tionally appropriate information and counseling to the HIV-infected woman so that she can make informed decisions.

CLINICAL SITUATIONS AND RECOMMENDATIONS FOR USE OF ZDV TO REDUCE PERINATAL TRANSMISSION

Clinical Situation Meeting the Entry Criteria for ACTG Protocol 076

Pregnant HIV-infected women with CD4+ T-lymphocyte counts greater than or equal to $200/\mu L$ who are at 14–34 weeks of gestation and who have no clinical indications for ZDV and no history of extensive (greater than 6 months) prior antiretroviral therapy.

Discussion

The results of ACTG Protocol 076 are directly applicable only to women who meet the entry criteria for the study (Table B1). The data from that study indicate that the complete ACTG Protocol 076 ZDV regimen will likely reduce the risk for perinatal transmission by about two-thirds.

Because this study was randomized and placebo controlled, entry was restricted to women who had no clinical indications for ZDV use for their own health and who had CD4+ T-lymphocyte counts greater than or equal to $200/\mu L$. Prior ZDV use during the current pregnancy resulted in exclusion from the study. Few women (4%) had received ZDV before the current pregnancy, and most of that therapy was of limited duration.

Women were not enrolled either before the 14th week or after the 34th week of gestation. The rationale for exclusion before 14 weeks of gestation was to preclude ZDV exposure during fetal organogenesis. The 34-week limit allowed most women to receive several weeks of ZDV before delivery to allow time for a decrease in maternal viral load (a presumed important determinant of transmission risk).

Although ZDV was successful in reducing perinatal transmission, the study regimen did not completely prevent it. The possible reasons for transmission to these infected infants are being evaluated but have not yet been identified. Several case reports also have described perinatal transmission despite the initiation of ZDV therapy during pregnancy (24–27).

Although long-term toxicity to infants is unknown, this risk must be weighed against the decreased risk for transmission of an infection associated with substantial risk of death. Currently, there is no way to predict if an individual pregnancy will be associated with HIV transmission; therefore, each fetus must be considered to have an estimated 25% risk of a life-threatening infection. Because ZDV therapy reduced the rate of transmission by two-thirds (from 25.5% to 8.3%), any long-term toxicity related to ZDV would have to be severe (e.g., malignancy or profound developmental delay) and relatively common among ZDV-exposed infants to outweigh the substantial benefit.

Recommendation

The health-care provider should recommend the full ACTG Protocol 076 regimen to all HIV-infected pregnant women in this category. This recommendation should be presented to the pregnant woman in the context of a risk-benefit discussion: a reduced risk of transmission can be expected, but the long-term adverse consequences of the regimen are not known. The decision about this regimen should be made by the woman after discussion with her health-care provider.

Clinical Situations Not Meeting the Study Entry Criteria

Information about the benefit and short-term risks of ZDV therapy is applicable from this trial only for women who meet the entry criteria of the study. Recommendations about use of the ZDV regimen for women whose clinical conditions differ from the ACTG Protocol 076 eligibility criteria were derived from consensus interpretation of available scientific data.

Pregnant HIV-Infected Women Who Are at Greater than 34 Weeks of Gestation

Pregnant HIV-infected women who are at greater than 34 weeks of gestation, who have no history of extensive (greater than 6 months) prior antiretroviral therapy, and who do not require ZDV for their own health.

Discussion

This patient population has clinical characteristics similar to those of women enrolled in ACTG Protocol 076; the major difference is gestational age at which ZDV therapy would begin. Therefore, the ZDV regimen for these women would differ from the ACTG Protocol 076 regimen only in duration of antenatal therapy. As much as 50%–70% of perinatal transmission may occur close to or during delivery (28). Therefore, the ACTG Protocol 076 ZDV regimen may have some benefit when initiated at greater than 34 weeks of gestation, although the intervention is likely to decrease in effectiveness as the duration of antenatal ZDV administration is reduced. A study evaluating the effect of ZDV on quantitative p24 antigen levels indicates that maximal effect is observed after 8–16 weeks of therapy (29). A shorter duration of ZDV therapy may thus be associated with an effect on maternal viral load that is less than can be anticipated when ZDV is initiated before 34 weeks of gestation. Both potential risks and benefits for the woman and her infant may decrease the closer to delivery that the ZDV regimen is initiated. Further clinical trials should be designed to assess the efficacy of interventions that are initiated late in the third trimester for preventing perinatal transmission.

Recommendation

The health-care provider should recommend the full ACTG Protocol 076 regimen in the context of a risk-benefit discussion with the pregnant woman. The woman should be informed that ZDV therapy may be less effective than that observed in ACTG Protocol 076, because the regimen is being initiated late in the third trimester.

Pregnant HIV-Infected Women with CD4+ T-Lymphocyte Counts Less Than 200 μL

Pregnant HIV-infected women with CD4+ T-lymphocyte counts less than 200/μL who are at 14–34 weeks of gestation, who have no other clinical indications for ZDV, and who have no history of extensive (greater than 6 months) prior antiretroviral therapy.

Discussion

Women in this group meet the current standard of care for ZDV treatment of HIV infection for their own benefit (30, 31); therefore, administration of ZDV during pregnancy for these women provides direct benefit to them as well as potential benefit to their infants. The risk for HIV transmission to the infants of HIV- infected pregnant women with low CD4+ T-lymphocytes or percent of total lymphocytes ranges from 22% to 60% (32–38). Viral load has been shown to increase as CD4+ T-lymphocyte count decreases (39); thus, baseline viral loads can be expected to be high among the women in this group.

Although viral replication and resultant capacity for mutations in this group are high, preexisting ZDV-resistant viral strains are unlikely to be present because these women have had little or no exposure to ZDV. Therefore, ZDV therapy can be expected to result in an acute reduction in maternal viral load analogous to that observed in women who have CD4+ T-lymphocyte counts greater than or equal to 200/μL. Additionally, the mother's CD4+ T-lympho-cyte count would not be expected to affect ZDV levels or toxicity in the infant after administration of ZDV during labor and the first 6 weeks of life. Hence, maternal CD4+ T-lymphocyte count should not affect the potential utility of neonatal levels of systemic ZDV for reducing intrapartum transmission.

Although this population of pregnant women was not studied in ACTG Protocol 076, addition of the intrapartum and neonatal components of the ACTG Protocol 076 ZDV regimen to antenatal maternal therapy may reduce the risk for HIV transmission. However, the magnitude of the effect of ZDV on reducing the transmission rate in this group may not be the same as that demonstrated in ACTG Protocol 076 for women with CD4+ T-lymphocyte counts greater than or equal to 200. Further clinical trials should assess the util-ity of interventions in this group of women. Because ZDV therapy is clinically indicated for these women for their own health, the additional risk of the re-mainder of the ACTG Protocol 076 regimen is the discomfort to the woman of another intravenous infusion during labor and the possible effects of the addi-tional 6 weeks of ZDV exposure for the infant.

Recommendation

The health-care provider should recommend initiation of antenatal ZDV ther-apy to the woman for her own health benefit (31). The intrapartum and neonatal components of the ACTG Protocol 076 regimen should be recom-mended until further information becomes available. This recommendation should be presented in the context of a risk-benefit discussion with the preg-nant woman.

Pregnant HIV-Infected Women Who Have a History of Extensive (Greater than 6 Months) ZDV Therapy and/or Other Antiretroviral Therapy Before Pregnancy

Discussion

Women who have received extensive prior ZDV therapy may be infected with viral strains with reduced susceptibility to ZDV. These resistant strains of HIV can be transmitted from mother to fetus; however, the frequency with which such transmission occurs is unknown.

Resistant virus appears to emerge more quickly if therapy is initiated at later stages of HIV disease (21). The appearance of mutations associated with ZDV resistance follows a temporal pattern, and the level of in vitro resistance is proportional to the number of mutations in the reverse transcriptase-coding region of HIV (40). Phenotypically and genotypically diverse HIV populations can coexist in patients who are receiving ZDV therapy. In one study, ZDV-resistant strains appeared earlier during ZDV therapy in patients with advanced HIV disease than in patients whose ZDV therapy was initiated at an early stage of the disease. After 12 months of ZDV therapy, viral isolates from 89% of patients with late-stage disease and 31% of those with early-stage disease were resistant (21). However, isolates from only 33% of late-stage patients demonstrate high-level resistance (defined as a 100-fold decrease in susceptibility [41]). Resistant virus also was more likely to be isolated from patients who had low CD4+ T-lymphocyte counts when therapy was initiated: 1-year estimated rates of resistance in patients with baseline CD4+ T-lymphocyte counts of greater than 400, 100–400, and less than 100 cells/μL were 27%, 41%, and 89%, respectively. In patients with advanced disease, high-level resistance develops after 6–18 months of therapy. However, in patients with early-stage disease, high-level resistance appears to be delayed until after 24 months of therapy (22). Therefore, ZDV-resistant strains are likely to be more common in women with advanced disease who have received prolonged therapy. ZDV-resistant viral strains also may be more common in persons receiving alternative antiretroviral agents because their disease progressed while they were receiving ZDV therapy. There is controversy regarding the association of clinical disease progression during ZDV therapy with the development of ZDV resistance and regarding whether resistance persists when therapy is changed to an alternative antiretroviral agent (41). Some studies involving small numbers of children have indicated that in vitro susceptibility to ZDV is correlated with clinical outcome, suggesting that ZDV-resistant isolates are associated with diminished efficacy of ZDV and more rapid clinical progression (42, 43). However, at least one study indicated that disease progression may be associated more closely with the development of syncytia-inducing viral phenotype than with resistance to ZDV (44). Change to alternative antiretroviral therapy has been associated with reversal of ZDV resistance in some studies, but resistance has been reported to persist for considerable periods of time after discontinuation of ZDV (23, 45). The prevalence of ZDV-resistant viral strains in women who are receiving alternative antiretroviral agents because of disease progression has not been defined.

The capability of ZDV to reduce HIV transmission may be decreased for mothers in whom ZDV-resistant strains predominate, particularly if the strains have high-level resistance; however, this assumption is not yet supported by data. Further clinical trials to evaluate alternative approaches for such women are needed.

Recommendation

Because data are insufficient to extrapolate the potential efficacy of the ACTG Protocol 076 regimen for this population of women, the health-care provider should consider recommending the ACTG Protocol 076 regimen on a case-by-case basis after a discussion of the risks and benefits with the pregnant woman.

Issues to be discussed include her clinical and immunologic stability on ZDV therapy, the likelihood that she is infected with a ZDV-resistant HIV strain, and, if relevant, the reasons for her current use of an alternative antiretroviral agent (e.g., lack of response to or intolerance of ZDV therapy). Consultation with experts in HIV infection may be warranted. The health-care provider should make the ACTG Protocol 076 regimen available to the woman, although its effectiveness may vary depending on her clinical status.

Pregnant HIV-Infected Women Who Have Not Received Antepartum Antiretroviral Therapy and Who Are in Labor

Discussion

Data from studies in humans are insufficient to evaluate the potential effectiveness of ZDV in this situation. Because the mother's exposure to ZDV would be brief, such therapy can be expected to have no effect on the level of maternal virus in blood or genital secretions. However, because of the intravenous loading dose and continuous infusion of ZDV during labor, the infant will be born with circulating levels of ZDV similar to those of infants whose mothers have received antenatal as well as intrapartum ZDV. ZDV may have some utility for this group of patients—regardless of whether the pregnancy is at term or preterm—because the presence of systemic levels of ZDV in the infant before or shortly after HIV exposure through contact with the mother's blood and genital secretions during delivery may help prevent intrapartum transmission.

The intravenous route was chosen for drug dosing during labor in ACTG Protocol 076 because continuous intravenous infusion of drug after an initial loading dose results in predictable levels of ZDV in the mother. Under optimal circumstances, these maternal levels provide a substantial fetal blood level during birth, when the infant is presumed to be exposed extensively to HIV through contact with the mother's blood and genital secretions. Because gastric emptying is delayed during labor, the absorption of orally administered drugs is unpredictable (46). Therefore, oral administration of ZDV during labor might produce widely variable systemic levels in the mother and infant. Oral ZDV administered intrapartum cannot be assumed to be equivalent to the intravenous intrapartum ZDV component used in ACTG Protocol 076. Further studies are needed to characterize the pharmacokinetics of oral ZDV during labor. Intrapartum ZDV cannot prevent the substantial number of infections that occur before labor (26). Therefore, ZDV administered only during labor and to the newborn may not be effective. Because the mother would receive ZDV only during labor, her risk for developing resistant virus or ZDV toxicity would be minimal. The primary risk is that associated with an intravenous catheter. The risk to the infant would be limited to the potential toxicity associated with transfer of drug from the maternal intrapartum infusion and with 6 weeks of oral ZDV therapy, without in utero exposure to the drug. The effect of neonatal ZDV treatment in ameliorating disease progression in infected infants is unknown. Clinical trials should be designed to address the efficacy of antiretroviral therapy in this situation.

Recommendation

For women with HIV infection who are in labor and who have not received the antepartum component of the ACTG Protocol 076 regimen (either because of lack of prenatal care or because they did not wish to receive antepartum therapy), the health-care provider should discuss the benefits and potential risks of the intrapartum and neonatal components of the ACTG Protocol 076 regimen and offer ZDV therapy when the clinical situation permits.

Infants Who Are Born to HIV-Infected Women Who Have Received No intrapartum ZDV Therapy

Discussion

Infants whose mothers have not received ZDV during late pregnancy and/or labor will not have circulating ZDV levels during birth, a period of presumed viral exposure. Data are insufficient to allow assessment of the potential efficacy of postexposure prophylaxis with ZDV in this situation. Studies of postexposure prophylaxis of retroviral infection with ZDV in animal models have yielded inconclusive results. Additionally, studies involving animal models should be interpreted with caution: many of these studies have involved non-human retroviruses that may have different pathogenic mechanisms from those of HIV, used methods of viral inoculation that are not relevant to perinatal transmission (e.g., intrathymic injection), and/or used a massive inoculum of virus (47).

The limited data from animal studies indicate that if ZDV is to have any effect as postexposure prophylaxis, prompt administration (within hours) is important, and that even with early initiation of ZDV, such prophylaxis may not be protective. In a SCID-hu mouse model of HIV infection (an immune-deficient model reconstituted with human cells), a time-dependent suppression of HIV replication was observed with ZDV prophylaxis (48). When ZDV was administered within 2 hours of viral inoculation, viral replication was not detectable at 2 weeks after inoculation in all treated animals; when ZDV was administered 2–36 hours after inoculation, rates of viral detection at 2 weeks increased in proportion to increasing time since ZDV was administered; and when ZDV was administered 48 hours after inoculation, virus was detectable in all animals (48). Therefore, whether the effect of ZDV therapy is prevention or suppression of infection cannot be established. In several animal model systems, ZDV administration was observed only to suppress or ameliorate retroviral infection (49–51).

At least 13 reports have described the failure of prophylactic ZDV to prevent HIV infection in humans following exposure to HIV-infected blood, even though the drug was administered promptly after exposure (52). Although these anecdotal reports do not establish that ZDV therapy is ineffective as postexposure prophylaxis, its efficacy can be expected to be lower in this situation than with the full regimen. Further studies are needed to evaluate whether a therapy administered only during the neonatal period can effectively prevent perinatal transmission.

Recommendation

If the clinical situation permits and if ZDV therapy can be initiated within 24 hours of birth, the health-care provider should offer the ACTG Protocol 076 postpartum component of 6 weeks of neonatal ZDV therapy for the infant in the context of a risk-benefit discussion with the mother. Data from animal prophylaxis studies indicate that, if ZDV is administered, therapy should be initiated as soon as possible (within hours) after delivery. If therapy cannot begin until the infant is greater than 24 hours of age and the mother did not receive therapy during labor, no data support offering therapy to the infant.

RECOMMENDATIONS FOR MONITORING THE ZDV REGIMEN FOR MOTHERS AND INFANTS

Women and their children should receive care together in a family-centered setting. Care should be coordinated between gynecologic, pediatric, internal medicine, infectious disease, and other health-care specialists to ensure that both mother and child receive appropriate medical follow-up. A comprehensive program of support services is necessary to ensure that both mother and child continue to receive health-care.

Maternal Monitoring

HIV-infected pregnant women should be monitored in accordance with previously published guidelines (31, 53). Monitoring during pregnancy should include monthly assessment for ZDV-associated hematologic and liver chemistry abnormalities. Indications of toxicity that might require interrupting or stopping the dose of ZDV include (a) hemoglobin less than 8 gm/dL, (b) absolute neutrophil count less than 750 cells/μL, or (c) AST (SGOT) or ALT (SGPT) greater than five times the upper limit of normal. CD4+ T-lymphocyte counts should be monitored to determine if prophylaxis for opportunistic infections, such as Pneumocystis carinii pneumonia (PCP), should be initiated. Pregnant HIV-infected women with CD4+ T-lymphocyte counts less than 200 cells/μL should receive appropriate PCP prophylaxis. If the CD4+ T-lymphocyte count is less than 600 cells/μL, the evaluation should be repeated each trimester. CD4+ T-lymphocyte counts should be measured at 6 weeks and 6 months postpartum to evaluate if antiretroviral therapy is indicated.

Fetal Monitoring

Antepartum testing, including sonographic and nonstress testing and intrapartum fetal monitoring, should be performed only as clinically indicated, not specifically because the patient is being treated with ZDV during pregnancy.

Infant Monitoring

A complete blood count and differential should be performed at birth as a baseline evaluation. Repeat measurements of hemoglobin are recommended at 6 and 12 weeks of age. ZDV should be administered with caution to infants born with severe anemia (hemoglobin less than 8 gm/dL), and treatment of the anemia and intensive monitoring are warranted if the drug is administered.

Previously published guidelines contain recommendations for diagnosing HIV infection in infants and for initiating PCP prophylaxis and antiretroviral therapy for those who are infected (53–55). The potential efficacy of ZDV therapy for HIV-infected children who require antiretroviral therapy and who received ZDV in utero and during early infancy has not been determined. A specialist in pediatric HIV infection may be consulted if therapy is necessary for infected children whose mothers received ZDV during pregnancy. Further research is needed to describe the response to therapy and progression of disease in such infants.

POTENTIAL LONG-TERM EFFECTS OF ZDV THERAPY FOR MOTHERS AND INFANTS AND RECOMMENDATIONS FOR FOLLOW-UP

Discussion

Observational data about the pregnancy outcomes of women who receive ZDV during pregnancy are being collected through the Antiretroviral Pregnancy Registry. The purpose of the registry is to provide surveillance for possible teratogenicity among infants born to women who received ZDV during pregnancy. Health-care providers can register such patients by calling the registry at (800) 722-9292, extension 8465, in the United States or (919) 315-8465 outside the United States. Written reports are available from Antiretroviral Pregnancy Registry, P.O. Box 12700, Research Triangle Park, NC 27709.

Concerns about the potential long-term adverse effects among women include development of ZDV-resistant virus when ZDV therapy is used intermittently to reduce perinatal transmission, particularly during more than one pregnancy, and the potential effect such resistance could have on disease progression for the woman. Although results of studies have demonstrated an association between emergence of ZDV resistance and total duration of ZDV exposure, none of the study designs has specifically addressed the effect of intermittent therapy on development of resistance. Continued follow-up of the women who participated in ACTG Protocol 076 and of their infants is planned. A protocol to provide prospective evaluation of the health of the women enrolled in ACTG Protocol 076 is being designed by the Women's Health Committee of the ACTG. This protocol will evaluate virologic, immunologic, and clinical parameters among participating women.

Data are insufficient to address any effect that exposure to ZDV in utero might have on risk for neoplasia or organ system toxicities. ACTG Protocol 219 is an ongoing study designed to provide prospective evaluation for children who have been exposed through ACTG protocols to antiretroviral agents in utero or to HIV vaccines until they are 21 years of age. This protocol will provide intensive evaluation of multiple organ system functions, neuropsychologic testing, and quality of life. Information about the potential long-term effects of the complete or partial ACTG Protocol 076 ZDV regimen on women and children receiving the regimen outside a clinical trial protocol also may be provided from evaluation of federally funded and other prospective studies of HIV-infected women and their infants.

Recommendation

Additional efforts are required to characterize the long-term effects of the ACTG Protocol 076 ZDV regimen on women and children. The specific issues of viral resistance and disease progression should be addressed among women who receive ZDV during pregnancy solely to reduce perinatal HIV transmission. Monitoring for these HIV-infected women should include Pap smears and gynecologic examinations as recommended in previously published guidelines (56), as well as an assessment of the patient's future needs for family planning consultation and services.

Long-term follow-up of both uninfected and infected infants born to mothers receiving ZDV during pregnancy is important. Assessment of organ system toxicities, neurodevelopment, pubertal development, reproductive capacity, and development of neoplasms should be emphasized. Special studies will need to be developed to address these specific concerns, and innovative methods and support systems should be designed to assist in follow-up of these women and their children.

CONCLUSION

The decision by an HIV-infected pregnant woman to use ZDV to reduce the risk for perinatal transmission requires a complex balance of individual benefits and risks that is best accomplished through discussions with her health-care provider. Such discussions should be noncoercive, linguistically and culturally appropriate, and tailored to the patient's educational level.

The recommendations in this report have been developed for use in the United States. Although perinatal transmission of HIV infection is an international problem, alternative strategies may be appropriate in other countries (57). The policy and practice in other countries may differ from these recommendations and depend on local considerations, such as availability of ZDV, access to facilities for intravenous infusion during labor, and alternative interventions that may be under evaluation. These recommendations have been developed in response to the urgent need to provide guidance to women and health-care providers in the United States about the use of ZDV to reduce the risk for perinatal HIV transmission and about the possible adverse outcomes of such ZDV treatment. They have been formulated on the basis of the available data from ACTG Protocol 076 and current information regarding factors associated with transmission. The information on which these recommendations are based is incomplete, and additional information is needed to optimize use of ZDV for this purpose. The decision to use the ACTG Protocol 076 regimen for preventing perinatal transmission of HIV requires weighing the benefits and potential risks to the HIV-infected woman and her child despite numerous uncertainties. Further research is a high priority and should include (a) clarification of long-term risks of the ZDV regimen to the woman and/or her child, (b) elucidation of the reasons for transmission despite use of the ZDV regimen, (c) delineation of the relative efficacy of the various components of the ACTG Protocol 076 ZDV regimen for reducing transmission, (d) evaluation of the efficacy of the regimen in women whose characteristics differ from those enrolled in ACTG Protocol 076, and (e) evaluation of other interventions for preventing perinatal transmission. As further information becomes available, these recommendations may need to be modified. In addition, appropriate methods and materials should be developed for communicating treatment options, risks, and benefits to women and health-care providers so that they can make informed decisions about treatment.

REFERENCES: AS NUMBERED IN ORIGINAL PUBLICATION

8. Kaplan EL, Meier P. Nonparametric estimation from incomplete observations. J Am Stat Assoc 1958;53:457–481.
9. Ayers KM. Preclinical toxicology of zidovudine: an overview. Am J Med 1988;85(Suppl 2A):186–188.
10. McLeod GX, Hammer SM. Zidovudine: five years later. Ann Intern Med 1992;117:487–501.
11. Lipschutz SE, Orav EJ, Sanders SP, Hale AR, McIntosh K, Colan SD. Cardiac structure and function in children with human immunodeficiency virus infection treated with zidovudine. N Engl J Med 1992;327:1260–1265.
12. Physicians' desk reference. 48th ed. Montvale, NJ: Medical Economics Data Production Company, 1994:742–749.
13. Toltzis P, Marx CM, Kleinman N, Levine EM, Schmidt EV. Zidovudine-associated embryonic toxicity in mice. J Infect Dis 1991;163:1212–1218.
14. Toltzis P, Mourton T, Magnuson T. Effect of zidovudine on preimplantation murine embryos. Antimicrob Agents Chemother 1993;37:1610–1613.
15. Comprehensive information for investigators: retrovir (July 1993). Available from Burroughs Wellcome Company, Research Triangle Park, NC.
16. Sperling RS, Stratton P, O'Sullivan MJ, et al. A survey of zidovudine use in pregnant women with human immunodeficiency virus infection. N Engl J Med 1992;326:857–861.
17. O'Sullivan MJ, Boyer PJJ, Scott GB, et al. The pharmacokinetics and safety of zidovudine in the third trimester of pregnancy for women infected with human immunodeficiency virus and their infants: phase I ACTG study (protocol 082). Am J Obstet Gynecol 1993;168:1510–1516.
18. Watts DH, Brown ZA, Tartaglione T, et al. Pharmacokinetic disposition of zidovudine during pregnancy. J Infect Dis 1991;163:226–232.
19. Ferrazin A, de Maria A, Gotta C, et al. Zidovudine therapy of HIV-1 infection during pregnancy: assessment of the effect on the newborns. J Acquir Immune Defic Syndr 1993;6:376–379.
20. Boyer PJJ, Dillon M, Navaie M, et al. Factors predictive of maternal-fetal transmission of HIV-1: preliminary analysis of zidovudine (ZDV) given during pregnancy and/or delivery. JAMA 1994;271:1925–1930.
21. CDC. Birth outcomes following zidovudine therapy in pregnant women. MMWR 1994;43:409, 415–416.
22. Richman DD, Grimes JM, Lagakos SW. Effect of stage of disease and drug dose on zidovudine susceptibilities of isolates of human immunodeficiency virus. J Acquir Immune Defic Syndr 1990;3:743–746.
23. Hirsch MS, D'Aquila RT. Therapy for human immunodeficiency virus infection. N Engl J Med 1993;328:1686–1695.
24. Smith MS, Koerber KL, Pagano JS. Long-term persistence of zidovudine resistance mutations in plasma isolates from human immunodeficiency virus type 1 of dideoxyinosine-treated patients removed from zidovudine therapy. J Infect Dis 1994;169:184–188.
25. Chavanet P, Diquet B, Waldner A, Portier H. Perinatal pharmacokinetics of zidovudine [Letter]. N Engl J Med 1989;321:1548–1549.
26. Lyman WD, Tankaka KE, Kress Y, Rubinstein A, Soeiro R. Zidovudine concentrations in human fetal tissue: implications for perinatal AIDS [Letter]. Lancet 1990;335;1280–1281.
27. Bernard N, Boulley AM, Perol R, Rouzioux C, Colau JC. Failure of zidovudine prophylaxis after exposure to HIV-1 [Letter]. N Engl J Med 1990;323:916.
28. Barzilai A, Sperling RS, Hyatt AC, et al. Mother to child transmission of human immunodeficiency virus I infection despite zidovudine therapy from 18 weeks gestation. Pediatr Infect Dis J 1990;9:931–933.
29. Mofenson LM, Wolinsky SM. Vertical transmission of HIV. Part C: current insights regarding vertical transmission. In: Pizzo PA, Wilfert CM, eds. Pediatric AIDS: the challenge of HIV infection in infants, children, and adolescents. 2nd ed. Baltimore MD: Williams & Wilkins, 1994:179–203.
30. De Gruttola V, Beckett LA, Coombs RW, et al. Serum p24 antigen level as an intermediate end point in clinical trials of zidovudine in people infected with human immunodeficiency virus type 1. J Infect Dis 1994;169:713–721.
31. Sande MA, Carpenter CCJ, Cobbs G, et al. Antiretroviral therapy for adult HIV-infected patients—recommendations from a state-of-the-art conference. JAMA 1993;270:2583–2589.
32. Sperling RS, Stratton P, Obstetric Gynecologic Working Group of the AIDS Clinical Trials Group of the National Institute of Allergy and Infectious Diseases. Treatment options for human immunodeficiency virus-infected pregnant women. Obstet Gynecol 1992;79:443–448.
33. St. Louis ME, Kamenga M, Brown C, et al. Risk for perinatal HIV-1 transmission according to maternal immunologic, virologic and placental factors. JAMA 1993;269:2853–2859.
34. European Collaborative Study. Risk factors for mother-to-child transmission of HIV-1. Lancet 1992; 339:1007–1012.

35. Ryder RW, Nsa W, Hassig SE, et al. Perinatal transmission of the human immunodeficiency virus type 1 to infants of seropositive women in Zaire. N Engl J Med 1989;320:1637–1642.
36. Burns DN, Landesman S, Muenz LR, et al. Cigarette smoking, premature rupture of membranes and vertical transmission of HIV-1 among women with low CD4+ levels. J Acquir Immune Defic Syndr 1994;7:718–726.
37. Tibaldi C, Ziarati N, Salassa B, D'Ambrosio R, Sinicco A. Asymptomatic women at high risk of vertical HIV-1 transmission to their fetuses. Br J Obstet Gynecol 1993;100:334–337.
38. Bulterys M, Chao A, Dushimimana A, et al. Multiple sexual partners and mother-to-child transmission of HIV-1. AIDS 1993;7:1639–1645.
39. Pitt J, Landy A, McIntosh K, et al. Prenatal maternal circulating leukocyte HIV predisposes to HIV culture positivity in their infants: progress from a North American cohort [Abstract 598] In: Program and Abstracts of the 32nd Interscience Conference on Antimicrobial Agents and Chemotherapy. Anaheim, CA: American Society for Microbiology, 1992.
40. Yerly S, Chamot E, Hirschel B, Perrin LH. Quantitation of human immunodeficiency virus provirus and circulating virus: relationship with immunologic parameters. J Infect Dis 1992;166:269–276.
41. Boucher CAB, O'Sullivan E, Mulder JW, et al. Ordered appearance of zidovudine resistance mutations during treatment of 18 human immunodeficiency virus-positive subjects. J Infect Dis 1992;165:105–110.
42. Erice A, Balfour HH. Resistance of human immunodeficiency virus type 1 to antiretroviral agents: a review. Clin Infect Dis 1994;18:149–156.
43. Tudor-Williams G, St. Clair MH, McKinney RE, et al. HIV-1 sensitivity to zidovudine and clinical outcome in children. Lancet 1992;339:15–19.
44. Ogino MT, Dankner WM, Spector SA. Development and significance of zidovudine resistance in children infected with human immunodeficiency virus. J Pediatr 1993;123:1–8.
45. St. Clair MH, Hartigan PM, Andrews JC, et al. Zidovudine resistance, syncytium-inducing phenotype and HIV disease progression in a case-control study. J Acquir Immune Defic Syndr 1993;6:891–897.
46. Boucher CAB, Van Leeuwen R, Kellam P, et al. Effects of discontinuation of zidovudine treatment on zidovudine sensitivity of human immunodeficiency virus type 1 isolates. Antimicrob Agents Chemother 1993;37:1525–1530.
47. Davison JS, Davison MC, Hay DM. Gastric emptying time in late pregnancy and labour. J Obstet Gynaecol Br Commonw 1970;77:37.
48. Gerberding JL, Henderson DK. Management of occupational exposures to bloodborne pathogens: hepatitis B virus, hepatitis C virus, and human immunodeficiency virus. Clin Infect Dis 1992;14:1179–1185.
49. Shih CC, Kaneshima H, Rabin L, et al. Postexposure prophylaxis with zidovudine suppresses human immunodeficiency virus type I infection in SCID-hu mice in a time-dependent manner. J Infect Dis 1991;163:625–67.
50. Morrey JD, Okleberry KM, Sidwell RW. Early-initiated zidovudine therapy prevents disease but not low levels of persistent retrovirus in mice. J Acquir Immune Defic Syndr 1991;4:506–512.
51. Hayes KA, Lafrado LJ, Erickson JG, Marr JM, Mathes LE. Prophylactic ZDV therapy prevents early viremia and lymphocyte decline but not primary infection in feline immunodeficiency virus-inoculated cats. J Acquir Immune Defic Syndr 1993;6:127–134.
52. McCune JM, Namikawa R, Shih CC, Rabin L, Kaneshima H. Suppression of HIV-infection in AZT-treated SCID-hu mice. Science 1990;247:564–566.
53. Tokars JI, Marcus R, Culver DH, et al. Surveillance of HIV infection and zidovudine use among health care workers after occupational exposure to HIV-infected blood. Ann Intern Med 1993;118:913–919.
54. El-Sadr W, Oleske JM, Agins BD, et al. Evaluation and management of early HIV infection. Clinical practice guideline no. 7. AHCPR publication no. 94–0572. Rockville, MD: Agency for Health Care Policy and Research, Public Health Service, US Department of Health and Human Services, January 1994.
55. Working Group on Antiretroviral Therapy: National Pediatric HIV Resource Center. Antiretroviral therapy and medical management of the human immunodeficiency virus-infected child. Pediatr Infect Dis J 1993;12:513–522.
56. CDC. Guidelines for prophylaxis against Pneumocystis carinii pneumonia for children infected with human immunodeficiency virus. MMWR 1991;40(No. RR-2).
57. CDC. 1993 Sexually transmitted diseases treatment guidelines. MMWR 1993;42(No. RR-14).

1994 Revised Classification System for HIV Infection in Children Less Than 13 Years of Age

Original Citation: Centers for Disease Control and Prevention. 1994 Revised classification system for human immunodeficiency virus infection in children less than 13 years of age. MMWR 1994;43(RR-12):1–10

Editor's Note: The information included here was based on an MMWR Report which resulted from a Public Health Service Working Group on a revised pediatric HIV classification system. Omited here, but included on companion CD-ROM, is Table 1, describing categories N, A, B, and C.

DIAGNOSING HIV INFECTION IN CHILDREN

Diagnosis of HIV infection in children born to HIV-infected mothers (Box 1 Table B1) is complicated by the presence of maternal anti-HIV IgG antibody, which crosses the placenta to the fetus. Virtually all these children are HIV-antibody positive at birth, although only 15%–30% are actually infected. In uninfected children, this antibody usually becomes undetectable by 9 months of age but occasionally remains detectable until 18 months of age. Therefore, standard anti-HIV IgG antibody tests cannot be used to indicate reliably a child's infection status before 18 months of age (3). Polymerase chain reaction (PCR) and virus culture are probably the most sensitive and specific assays for detecting HIV infection in children born to infected mothers (4–6). Use of these assays can identify approximately 30%–50% of infected infants at birth and nearly 100% of infected infants by 3–6 months of age (7).

The standard p24-antigen assay is less sensitive than either virus culture or PCR, especially when anti-HIV antibody levels are high, because it fails to detect immune-complexed p24-antigen (8). However, modification of the p24-antigen assay to dissociate immune complexes has increased its sensitivity in diagnosing HIV infection among children exposed to HIV (9). Other laboratory assays (e.g., anti-HIV IgA and ELISPOT/in vitro antibody production [IVAP]) have not been included in the algorithm for determining infection status because they are not commonly used. In addition, they are less sensitive than both PCR or virus culture. However, clinicians who determine a child's antiretroviral therapy on the basis of such assays may use them to classify the child as being infected.

Some children develop severe clinical conditions resulting from HIV infection before their infection status has been sufficiently established. For the purposes of classification, a child meeting the criteria for AIDS in the 1987 case definition (10) should be considered HIV-infected—even in the absence of definitive laboratory assays.

Children born to mothers with HIV infection are defined as seroreverters (SRs) and are considered uninfected with HIV if they (a) become HIV-antibody negative after 6 months of age, (b) have no other laboratory evidence of HIV infection, and (c) have not met the AIDS surveillance case definition criteria (Box 1 Table B1). Sufficient data are not available to conclusively define a child who is uninfected on the basis of viral detection tests. However, in certain situations (e.g., clinical trials), negative viral detection tests may be used presumptively to exclude infection.

IMMUNOLOGIC CATEGORIES

The three immunologic categories (Table 2) were established to categorize children by the severity of immunosuppression attributable to HIV infection. CD4+ T-lymphocyte depletion is a major consequence of HIV infection and is respon-

Table B1. BOX 1. Diagnosis of human immunodeficiency virus (HIV) infection in children*

DIAGNOSIS: HIV INFECTED

(a) A child <18 months of age who is known to be HIV seropositive or born to an HIV-infected mother and:
- has positive results on two separate determinations (excluding cord blood)
  from one or more of the following HIV detection tests:
  —HIV culture,
  —HIV polymerase chain reaction,
  —HIV antigen (p24),
  or
- meets criteria for acquired immunodeficiency syndrome (AIDS) diagnosis based on the 1987 AIDS surveillance case definition (10).

(b) A child ≥18 months of age born to an HIV-infected mother or any child infected by blood, blood products, or other known modes of transmission (e.g., sexual contact) who:
- is HIV-antibody positive by repeatedly reactive enzyme immunoassay (EIA) and confirmatory test (e.g., Western blot or immunofluorescence assay (IFA));
  or
- meets any of the criteria in (a) above.

DIAGNOSIS: PERINATALLY EXPOSED (PREFIX E)

A child who does not meet the criteria above who:
- is HIV seropositive by EIA and confirmatory test (e.g., Western blot or IFA) and is <18 months of age at the time of test;
  or
- has unknown antibody status, but was born to a mother known to be infected with HIV.

DIAGNOSIS: SEROREVERTER (SR)

A child who is born to an HIV-infected mother and who:
- has been documented as HIV-antibody negative (i.e., two or more negative EIA tests performed at 6–18 months of age or one negative EIA test after 18 months of age);
  and
- has had no other laboratory evidence of infection (has not had two positive viral detection tests, if performed);
  and
- has not had an AIDS-defining condition.

*This definition of HIV infection replaces the definition published in the 1987 AIDS surveillance case definition (10).

sible for many of the severe manifestations of HIV infection in adults. For this reason, CD4+ counts are used in the adult HIV classification system (11). However, several findings complicate the use of CD4+ counts for assessing immunosuppression resulting from HIV infection in children. Normal CD4+

TABLE 2. Immunologic categories based on age-specific CD4+ T-lymphocyte counts and percent of total lymphocytes

	Age of child					
	<12 mos		1–5 yrs		6–12 yrs	
Immunologic category	μL	(%)	μL	(%)	μL	(%)
1: No evidence of suppression	≥1,500	(≥25)	≥1,000	(≥25)	(≥500	(≥25)
2: Evidence of moderate suppression	750–1,499	(15–24)	500–999	(15–24)	200–499	(15–24)
3: Severe suppression	<750	(<15)	<500	(<15)	<200	(<15)

counts are higher in infants and young children than in adults and decline over the first few years of life (12–16). In addition, children may develop opportunistic infections at higher CD4+ levels than adults (17–19). Although insufficient data exist to correlate CD4+ levels with disease progression at all age groups, low age-specific CD4+ counts appear to correlate with conditions associated with immunosuppression in children (12, 17, 20, 21). Therefore, despite these complications, classification based on age-specific CD4+ levels appears to be useful for describing the immunologic status of HIV-infected children.

Fewer data are available on age-specific values for CD4+ T-lymphocyte percent of total lymphocytes than for absolute counts. However, the CD4+ T-lymphocyte percent has less measurement variability than the absolute count (22). To establish the age-specific values of CD4+ percent that correlate with the CD4+ count thresholds, CDC compiled data from selected clinical projects in the United States and Europe. The data included greater than 9,000 CD4+ counts, with the corresponding CD4+ percent determinations, from both HIV-infected and uninfected children less than 13 years of age. Nonparametric regression modeling was used to establish the CD4+ percent boundaries that best correlated with the CD4+ count boundaries in the classification system.

The immunologic category classification (Table 2) is based on either the CD4+ T-lymphocyte count or the CD4+ percent of total lymphocytes. If both the CD4+ count and the CD4+ percent indicate different classification categories, the child should be classified into the more severe category. Repeated or follow-up CD4+ values that result in a change in classification should be confirmed by a second determination. Values thought to be in error should not be used. A child should not be reclassified to a less severe category regardless of subsequent CD4+ determinations.

CLINICAL CATEGORIES

Children infected with HIV or perinatally exposed to HIV may be classified into one of four mutually exclusive clinical categories based on signs, symptoms, or diagnoses related to HIV infection (Box 2 Table B2). As with the immunologic categories, the clinical categories have been defined to provide a staging classification (e.g., the prognosis for children in the second category would be less favorable than for those in the first category).

Category N, not symptomatic, includes children with no signs or symptoms considered to be the result of HIV infection or with only one of the conditions listed in Category A, mildly symptomatic. Category N was separated from Category A partly because of the substantial amount of time that can elapse before a child manifests the signs or symptoms defined in Category B, moderately symptomatic. Also, more staging information can be obtained during this early stage of disease by separating Categories N and A. In addition, for children who have uncertain HIV-infection status (prefix E), Categories N and A may help to distinguish those children who are more likely to be infected with HIV (23) (i.e., children in Category EA may be more likely to be infected than children in Category EN).

Category B includes all children with signs and symptoms thought to be caused by HIV infection but not specifically outlined under Category A or Category C, severely symptomatic. The conditions listed in Box 2 Table B2 are examples only; any other HIV-related condition not included in Category A or C should be included in Category B. Anemia, thrombocytopenia, and lymphopenia have defined thresholds in the new classification system (23). Category C includes all AIDS-defining conditions except lymphoid interstitial pneumonitis (LIP) (Box 3 Table B3). Several reports indicate that the prognosis for children with LIP is substantially better than that for children who have other AIDS-defining conditions (21, 24, 25). Thus, LIP has been separated from the other AIDS-defining conditions in Category C and placed in Category B.

Signs and symptoms related to causes other than HIV infection (e.g., inflammatory or drug-related causes) should not be used to classify children. For example, a child with drug-related hepatitis or anemia should not be classified in Category B solely because these conditions may be associated with HIV infection. In contrast, a child with anemia or hepatitis should be classified in Category B when the condition is thought to be related to HIV infection. The criteria for diagnosing some conditions and determining whether a child's signs, symptoms, or diagnoses are related to HIV infection may not be clear in all cases, and therefore may require judgment of the clinicians and researchers using the classification system.

Categories in the 1987 pediatric HIV classification system can be translated into categories in the 1994 system in most cases (Box 4 Table B4). Class P-0 is now designated by the prefix "E," and Class P-1 is now Class N. Children previously classified as P-2A are now classified in more than one category, reflecting the different prognoses for children with different conditions included in the P-2A category (e.g., children who have wasting syndrome have a worse prognosis than those who have lymphadenopathy).

Table B2. BOX 2. Clinical categories for children with human immunodeficiency virus (HIV) infection

CATEGORY N: NOT SYMPTOMATIC

Children who have no signs or symptoms considered to be the result of HIV infection or who have only one of the conditions listed in Category A.

CATEGORY A: MILDLY SYMPTOMATIC

Children with two or more of the conditions listed below but none of the conditions listed in Categories B and C.
  Lymphadenopathy (≥0.5 cm at more than two sites; bilateral = one site)
  Hepatomegaly
  Splenomegaly
  Dermatitis
  Parotitis
  Recurrent or persistent upper respiratory infection, sinusitis, or otitis media

CATEGORY B: MODERATELY SYMPTOMATIC

Children who have symptomatic conditions other than those listed for Category A or C that are attributed to HIV infection. Examples of conditions in clinical Category B include but are not limited to:
  Anemia (<8 gm/dL), neutropenia (<1,000/mm^3), or thrombocytopenia
    (<100,000/mm^3) persisting ≥30 days
  Bacterial meningitis, pneumonia, or sepsis (single episode)
  Candidiasis, oropharyngeal (thrush), persisting (>2 months) in children >6
    months of age
  Cardiomyopathy
  Cytomegalovirus infection, with onset before 1 month of age
  Diarrhea, recurrent or chronic
  Hepatitis
  Herpes simplex virus (HSV) stomatitis, recurrent (more than two episodes
    within 1 year)
  HSV bronchitis, pneumonitis, or esophagitis with onset before 1 month of age
  Herpes zoster (shingles) involving at least two distinct episodes or more
    than one dermatome
  Leiomyosarcoma
  Lymphoid interstitial pneumonia (LIP) or pulmonary lymphoid hyperplasia
    complex
  Nephropathy
  Nocardiosis
  Persistent fever (lasting >1 month)
  Toxoplasmosis, onset before 1 month of age
  Varicella, disseminated (complicated chickenpox)

CATEGORY C: SEVERELY SYMPTOMATIC

Children who have any condition listed in the 1987 surveillance case definition for acquired immunodeficiency syndrome (10), with the exception of LIP (Box 3).

Table B3. BOX 3. Conditions included in clinical Category C for children infected with human immunodeficiency virus (HIV)

CATEGORY C: SEVERELY SYMPTOMATIC*

Serious bacterial infections, multiple or recurrent (i.e., any combination of at least two culture-confirmed infections within a 2-year period), of the following types: septicemia, pneumonia, meningitis, bone or joint infection, or abscess of an internal organ or body cavity (excluding otitis media, superficial skin or mucosal abscesses, and indwelling catheter-related infections)

Candidiasis, esophageal or pulmonary (bronchi, trachea, lungs)

Coccidioidomycosis, disseminated (at site other than or in addition to lungs or cervical or hilar lymph nodes)

Cryptococcosis, extrapulmonary

Cryptosporidiosis or isosporiasis with diarrhea persisting >1 month

Cytomegalovirus disease with onset of symptoms at age >1 months (at a site other than liver, spleen, or lymph nodes)

Encephalopathy (at least one of the following progressive findings present for at least 2 months in the absence of a concurrent illness other than HIV infection that could explain the findings): (a) failure to attain or loss of developmental milestones or loss of intellectual ability, verified by standard development scale or neuropsychological tests; (b) impaired brain growth or acquired microcephaly demonstrated by head circumference measurements or brain atrophy demonstrated by computerized tomography or magnetic resonance imaging (serial imaging is required for children <2 years of age); (c) acquired symmetric motor deficit manifested by two or more of the following: paresis, pathologic reflexes, ataxia, or gait disturbance

Herpes simplex virus infection causing a mucocutaneous ulcer that persists for >1 month; or bronchitis, pneumonitis, or esophagitis for any duration affecting a child >1 month of age

Histoplasmosis, disseminated (at a site other than or in addition to lungs or cervical or hilar lymph nodes)

Kaposi's sarcoma

Lymphoma, primary, in brain

Lymphoma, small, noncleaved cell (Burkitt's), or immunoblastic or large cell lymphoma of B-cell or unknown immunologic phenotype

Mycobacterium tuberculosis, disseminated or extrapulmonary

Mycobacterium, other species or unidentified species, disseminated (at a site other than or in addition to lungs, skin, or cervical or hilar lymph nodes)

Mycobacterium avium complex of Mycobacterium kanasasii, disseminated (at site other than or in addition to lungs, skin, or cervical or hilar lymph nodes)

Pneumocystis carinii pneumonia

Progressive multifocal leukoencephalopathy

Salmonella (nontyphoid) septicemia, recurrent

Toxoplasmosis of the brain with onset at >1 month of age

Wasting syndrome in the absence of a concurrent illness other than HIV infection that could explain the following findings: (a) persistent weight loss >10% of baseline OR (b) downward crossing of at least two of the following percentile lines on the weight-for-age chart (e.g., 95th, 75th, 50th, 25th, 5th) in a child ≥1 year of age OR (c) <5th percentile on weight-for-height chart on two consecutive measurements, ≥30 days apart PLUS (a) chronic diarrhea (i.e., at least two loose stools per day for >30 days) OR (b) documented fever (for ≥30 days, intermittent or constant)

*See the 1987 AIDS surveillance case definition (10) for diagnosis criteria.

Table B4. BOX 4. Comparison of the 1987 and 1994 pediatric human immunodeficiency virus classification systems

1987 Classification	1994 Classification
P-0	Prefix "E"
P-1	N
P-2A	A, B, and C
P-2B	C
P-2C	B
P-2D1	C
P-2D2	C
P-2D3	B
P-2E1	C
P-2E2	B
P-2F	B

EFFECT ON THE AIDS SURVEILLANCE CASE DEFINITION FOR CHILDREN

Because the classification system is used in conjunction with the AIDS case definition, the 1994 revision provided an opportunity to update certain features of the 1987 AIDS surveillance case definition for children less than 13 years of age (10). Although LIP is in Category B under the new pediatric HIV classification system, it will continue to be reportable to state and local health departments (along with the conditions in Category C) as an AIDS-defining condition in children. Two changes in the definitions for other conditions are summarized in the following bulletted text:

- The new definitions for HIV encephalopathy and HIV wasting syndrome reflect increased knowledge of these conditions in children and replace the definitions published in the 1987 AIDS surveillance case definition for children. The definition of HIV en-cephalopathy follows the recommendations of the American Academy of Neurology AIDS Task Force (26). Because this condition is complex, diagnosis may require neurologic consultation.
- The new definition of HIV infection (Box 1 Table B1) replaces the definition for laboratory evidence of HIV infection in children used in the 1987 pediatric AIDS case definition. For children with an AIDS-defining condition that requires laboratory evidence of HIV infection, a single positive HIV-detection test (i.e., HIV culture, HIV PCR, or HIV antigen [p24]) is sufficient for a reportable AIDS diagnosis if the diagnosis is confirmed by a clinician.

REFERENCES: AS NUMBERED IN ORIGINAL PUBLICATION

3. Simpson BJ, Andiman WA. Difficulties in assigning human immunodeficiency virus-1 infection and seroreversion status in a cohort of HIV-exposed children using serologic criteria established by the CDC and Prevention. Pediatrics 1994;93:840–842.
4. Krivine A, Firtion G, Cao L, Francoual C, Henrion R, Lebon P. HIV replication during the first weeks of life. Lancet 1992;339:1187–1189.
5. Rogers MF, Ou C-Y, Rayfield M, et al. Use of the polymerase chain reaction for early detection of the proviral sequences of human immunode- ficiency virus in infants born to seropositive mothers. N Engl J Med 1989;320:1649–1654.
6. Burgard M, Mayaux M-J, Blanche S, et al. The use of viral culture and p24 antigen testing to diagnose human immunodeficiency virus infection in neonates. N Engl J Med 1992;327:1192–1197.

7. Anonymous. Report of a consensus workshop, Siena, Italy, January 17–18, 1992: early diagnosis of HIV infection in infants. J Acquir Immune Defic Syndr 1992;5:1169–1178.
8. Rogers M, Ou C, Kilbourne B, Schochetman G. Advances and problems in the diagnosis of human immunodeficiency virus infection in infants. Pediatr Infect Dis J 1991;10:523–531.
9. Miles SA, Baldern E, Magpantay L, et al. Rapid serologic testing with immune-complex-dissociated HIV p24 antigen for early detection of HIV infection in neonates. N Engl J Med 1993;328:297–302.
10. CDC. Revision of the CDC surveillance case definition for acquired immunodeficiency syndrome. MMWR 1987;36(Suppl):1S-15S.
11. CDC. 1993 Revised classification system for HIV infection and expanded surveillance case definition for AIDS among adolescents and adults. MMWR 1993;41(No. RR-17).
12. Erkeller-Yuksel FM, Deneys V, Yuksel B, et al. Age-related changes in human blood lymphocyte sub-populations. J Pediatr 1992;120:216–222.
13. Denny T, Yogev R, Gelman R, et al. Lymphocyte subsets in healthy children during the first 5 years of life. JAMA 1992;267:1484–1488.
14. McKinney RE, Wilfert CM. Lymphocyte subsets in children younger than 2 years old: normal values in a population at risk for human immunodeficiency virus infection and diagnostic and prognostic application to infected children. Pediatr Infect Dis J 1992;11:639–644.
15. The European Collaborative Study. Age-related standards for T-lymphocyte subsets based on uninfected children born to human immunodeficiency virus-1-infected women. Pediatr Infect Dis J 1992; 11:1018–1026.
16. Waecker NJ, Ascher DP, Robb ML, et al. Age adjusted CD4+ lymphocyte parameters in HIV at risk uninfected children. Clin Infect Dis 1993;17:123–126.
17. Leibovitz E, Rigaud M, Pollack H, et al. Pneumocystis carinii pneumonia in infants infected with the human immunodeficiency virus with more than 450 CD4 T lymphocytes per cubic millimeter. N Engl J Med 1990;323:531–533.
18. Connor E, Bagarazzi M, McSherry G, et al. Clinical and laboratory correlates of Pneumocystis carinii pneumonia in children infected with HIV. JAMA 1991;265:1693–1697.
19. Kovacs A, Frederick T, Church J, et al. CD4 T-Lymphocyte counts and Pneumocystis carinii pneumonia in pediatric HIV infection. JAMA 1991;265:1698–1703.
20. Butler KM, Husson RN, Lewis LL, et al. CD4 status and p24 antigenemia: are they useful predictors of survival in HIV-infected children receiving antiretroviral therapy. Am J Dis Child 1992;146:932–936.
21. de Martino M, Tovo PA, Galli L, et al. Prognostic significance of immunologic changes in 675 infants perinatally exposed to human immunode-ficiency virus. J Pediatr 1991;119:702–709.
22. Raszka WV, Meyer GA, Waecker NJ, et al. Variability of serial absolute and percent CD4+ lymphocyte counts in healthy children born to HIV-1-infected parents. Lancet 1994;13:70–72.
23. Caldwell B, Oxtoby M, Rogers M. Proposed CDC pediatric HIV classification system: evaluation in an active surveillance system [Abstract]. IXth International Conference on AIDS, Berlin, June 7–11, 1993.
24. Tovo PA, deMartino M, Gabiano C, et al. Prognostic factors and survival in children with perinatal HIV-1 infection. Lancet 1992;339:1249–1253.
25. Blanche S, Tardieu M, Duliege AM, et al. Longitudinal study of 94 symptomatic infants with perinatally acquired human immunodeficiency virus infection. Am J Dis Child 1990;144:1210–1215.
26. Working Group of the American Academy of Neurology AIDS Task Force. Nomenclature and research case definitions for neurologic manifestations of human immunodeficiency virus-type 1 (HIV-1) infection. Neurology 1991;41:778–786

Medical Issues Related to Caring for HIV-infected Children

Original Citation: Simonds RJ, Chanock S. Medical issues related to caring for human immunodeficiency virus-infected children in and out of the home. Pediatr Infec Dis J 1993;12;845–852.

Original Authors: R.J. Simmons, MD, and Stephen Chanock, MD.

Editor's Note: The information included here, based on an article by CDC authors in a 1993 article in the Pediatric Infectious Disease Journal, provides guidance for the protection of HIV-infected children and their caretakers, family, and playmates. The original article includes information about HIV transmission including the presence of HIV in body fluids and the risk of HIV transmission.

PREVENTION OF HIV TRANSMISSION

Knowledge of the risk of transmission of HIV and other blood-borne pathogens led to the development of precautions to prevent percutaneous, mucous membrane and skin exposures to blood-borne pathogens, including HIV (49–51). The principles of universal precautions include the use of safe practices and appropriate barrier precautions when contact is anticipated with blood or with body fluids that may transmit blood borne pathogens (Table 3). The most likely of these to be present in child-care settings are blood and body fluids containing blood. Under universal precautions all patients are considered to be potentially infected with a blood-borne pathogen because the patient's infection status is often unknown.

Detailed recommendations regarding universal precautions have been published (49–51). The principles underlying universal precautions are applicable in health-care and other settings, such as schools, day-care centers, playing fields and the home.

To prevent percutaneous exposures to blood-borne pathogens, including HIV, injuries with needles or other sharp items contaminated with blood must be avoided. Strategies to avoid such injuries include handling needles and other sharp instruments safely (e.g., not recapping, bending or breaking needles; disposing of sharp items in puncture-resistant containers), using self-sheathing

---

Table 3. Universal precautions to prevent transmission of blood-borne pathogens

HAND WASHING IS NECESSARY AFTER PHYSICAL CONTACT WITH ALL PATIENTS

Body fluids to which universal precautions apply
- Blood
- Any body fluid containing visible blood
- Semen and vaginal secretions
- Body tissues
- Cerebrospinal, synovial, pleural, peritoneal, pericardial, amniotic fluid

Body fluids and procedures for which hand-washing is sufficient for preventing transmission of blood-borne pathogens (unless fluid contains blood)*
- Urine
- Stool
- Vomitus
- Tears
- Nasal secretions
- Oral secretions
- Diaper changing

Special precautions for other body fluids (see text)
- Breast milk
- Saliva

---

*Gloves may be required to prevent transmission of other pathogens.

needles or other mechanical devices shown to reduce the risk of injury to health care workers and limiting unnecessary use of needles. To prevent skin and mucous membrane exposures, appropriate barrier precautions should be used when contact with blood or other body fluids is anticipated. Gloves should be used for touching blood, body fluids for which universal precautions apply, mucous membranes and nonintact skin of all patients and for handling items soiled with blood or body fluids for which universal precautions apply (Table 3). Hands should be washed immediately after contact with blood and after removal of gloves. Masks, protective eyewear and gowns should be used when splashes to the face or body may be expected. Nondisposable instruments or devices that enter sterile tissue or through which blood flows should be sterilized after use; under no circumstances should needles, syringes or other such equipment be used for more than one person without being sterilized. Finally blood and blood-containing fluids spilled on environmental surfaces should be promptly removed and contaminated surfaces cleaned with bleach (diluted 1:10 to 1:100, depending on the amount of organic material present) or other Environmental Protection Agency-approved disinfectant; gloves should always be worn during cleaning and decontaminating procedures.

Although universal precautions do not apply to human breast milk or saliva, some precautions against exposure to these fluids may be necessary. Because breast feeding has been implicated in the transmission of HIV infection from mother to infant, the use of gloves should be considered in situations, such as milk banks, where exposure to human breast milk is extensive. Gloves should also be worn for contact with oral mucosa, for endotracheal auctioning and for other oropharyngeal procedures that involve exposure to blood-contaminated saliva. Gloves do not need to be worn when feeding a child with bottled formula or breast milk or cleaning oral secretions that do not contain visible blood. However, gloves should be worn when changing diapers that contain bloody stools and when handling other body fluids with visible blood. Gloves may also be necessary to prevent transmission of enteric and other pathogens, and of course hands should always be washed immediately after handling any body fluid, whether or not gloves are worn.

Home

Children with HIV infection should be able to benefit from participation in all ordinary activities of home life. Safety and well-being can be enhanced by educating families of HIV-infected children about how HIV is transmitted. Such education should both emphasize ways to prevent transmission by minimizing contact with blood and other body fluids and promote ordinary family interactions by alleviating unfounded concerns about HIV transmission.

Four reports have suggested the possibility of HIV transmission during the provision of health care at home (52–55). With the increasing use of home parenteral therapy for HIV infection and other conditions, ensuring appropriate infection control practices in all homes in which such therapy is provided is essential (56, 57). In particular persons providing medical and nursing care in the home should receive training in infection control practices; have adequate supplies of gloves, needles and puncture-resistant containers; and take precautions to exclude young children from situations where exposure to blood or sharp objects is possible (e.g. during medical procedures performed on others). The puncture-resistant containers should be kept out of the reach of children.

Day-Care

No cases of HIV transmission in out-of home child-care settings have been reported. Furthermore the low risk of HIV transmission after household exposure to persons, including children, with HIV infection argues against a significant risk of HIV transmission through the types of contact that occur routinely in child-care settings. Therefore, the Centers for Disease Control and Prevention, the American Academy of Pediatrics and the American Public Health Association have recommended that children with HIV infection be allowed to attend child-care in most cases (58–60). Several considerations should be weighed when deciding about enrollment, including the child's propensity for aggressive biting, the child's likelihood of having uncontrollable bleeding episodes, the presence of oozing skin lesions that cannot be covered and the child's immune function. The child's physician should be directly involved with the decision about whether to enroll a child in day-care.

The confidentiality of children attending child-care must be protected to the greatest extent possible. A child's HIV status should be disclosed only with the informed consent of the parents or other legal guardians and then only to those who need such knowledge to care properly for the child. In general at least one staff member should be aware of the child's immunodeficiency so that potential exposures to blood-borne or other infections can be managed appropriately.

Because child-care settings may contain children who are unknowingly infected with HIV or other blood-borne infections, staff members should adopt routine procedures for handling blood and other body fluids of all children. They also should be diligent in recognizing and managing exposures of all children to such common childhood infections as varicella and such serious infections as tuberculosis. The staff should notify the local health department and parents of all children of any exposures to tuberculosis, measles or other reportable communicable disease. Children who are immunosuppressed because of HIV infection or other conditions may be particularly susceptible to infection with some pathogens (e.g., Cryptosporidium) and to serious illness if infected with others (e.g., respiratory syncytial virus, varicella. Salmonella). Staff should be alert to exposures to these types of infections and notify all parents if such an exposure occurs. Finally to prevent transmission of vaccine-preventable infections, immunizations should be current for all children attending day-care.

Toys should be kept clean and may be shared among all children. To prevent transmission of any pathogens, it has been recommended that toys that are mouthed routinely be cleaned and disinfected before being used by another child (60). Other toys should be cleaned and disinfected if they become contaminated by body fluids (e.g., blood, stool, vomitus).

To prevent the transmission of infections from childcare workers to children, work restrictions may be necessary for workers who have certain infections (60). Day-care center staff with HIV infection who adhere to infection control precautions may care for children unless they have conditions that would place them at increased risk of transmitting infection, such as pulmonary tuberculosis or open skin lesions that cannot be covered (60).

In some communities, day-care centers designed to meet the special medical. developmental and other needs of children with HIV infection may be available. These centers may afford a supportive environment for children with HIV infection but are not intended to be used to exclude these children from other day-care centers.

School

The well-publicized instances of discrimination against children with HIV infection at school are particularly unfortunate because they cause unnecessary pain and anguish for children and their families while propagating the unfounded notion that HIV is likely to be transmitted in schools. No cases of HIV transmission in school have been reported, and current epidemiologic data do not justify excluding children with HIV infection from school or isolating them in school to protect others. Children with HIV infection should be able to participate in all school activities with the same considerations as other children, to the extent that their health permits. Guidelines for the education of children with HIV infection (58–61) and for the development of school policies (62) have been published.

Like other children with special health needs, children with HIV injection benefit from educational programs that provide necessary medical services, such as management of emergencies and administration of medications. Moreover, a sound educational program can help create a more accepting environment for children with HIV infection. Evaluating each child's medical and educational needs on a case-by-case basis. with ongoing communication among the family, health care providers and school health staff. can optimize benefits to the child (63). All educational institutions should have a policy regarding students and staff who have HIV infection.

Until children with HIV infection are no longer stigmatized and discriminated against, confidentiality will remain an important issue. The right to privacy must always be protected in accordance with state and local law. The persons aware of the child's HIV infection should be limited to those who need such knowledge to care for the child. In most cases such persons include the school medical advisor, school nurse and teacher. Because the administration of HIV-related medications in school may compromise confidentiality, the infected child should be encouraged to self-administer medications, with the approval of the school nurse or medical advisor when possible. Children can use nearly all services for children with special needs without revealing their HIV status.

Because blood exposures from fights, unintentional injuries, nosebleeds, shed teeth, menstruation and other causes may occur at school, all schools should be prepared to handle blood and blood-containing body fluids using the principles of universal precautions. Supplies of gloves, disposable towels and disinfectants should be readily available. All schools should institute policies for managing blood exposures, and all staff, including teachers, athletic coaches, cafeteria workers and maintenance workers, should be educated in infection control.

Athletics

Many children and adolescents enjoy sports; one-third of girls and one-half of boys in United States high schools participated on varsity or junior varsity teams in 1990 (64). Participation in some contact sports may increase a child's risk of exposure to blood: forceful contact with hard surfaces, equipment, or other players may result in laceration or abrasion; and close player-to-player contact may lead to direct exposure to another person's blood. Nonetheless the risk of HIV transmission during sports is probably very low. Despite the large number of persons participating in contact sports, only one case of HIV transmission attributed to sports has been reported worldwide (65). In this case transmission was reported to have resulted from a collision that produced lacerations with copious bleeding and exchange of blood during a soccer match, but other modes of transmission for the young man who became infected were not satisfactorily excluded (65, 66). An outbreak of hepatitis B virus transmission during contact sports has been reported among high school sumo wrestlers (67).

The American Academy of Pediatrics, the National Collegiate Athletic Association, the National Football League and the World Health Organization have published guidelines addressing HIV infection and sports (68–71). Athletes with HIV infection should be permitted to participate in competitive sports at all levels. However, because of the potential risk to the athlete's own health and the theoretical risk of HIV transmission to others during contact sports, athletes with HIV infection interested in participating in contact sports such as wrestling, boxing or football should be evaluated on a case-by-case basis. This evaluation should consider such factors as the likelihood of blood contact (e.g., intramural touch football vs. varsity tackle football), the athlete's propensity to bleed (e.g., thrombocytopenia) and the presence of skin lesions that cannot be covered during active sport. The American Academy of Pediatrics recommends that an HIV-infected athlete considering a sport such as football or wrestling should be informed of the theoretical risk of transmission to others and be encouraged to consider another sport (68). The athlete's physician should be directly involved in the decision regarding participation.

The right to privacy should be protected; an athlete's HIV status need not be revealed to other players. On the playing field contact by trainers and first aid providers with blood should be minimized by following appropriate infection control measures, including promptly cleaning blood from skin with soap and water and from surfaces such as wrestling mats with bleach solution diluted 1:10 to 1:100; immediately controlling bleeding by covering abrasions, lacerations or other lesions; using gloves or other barriers when attending to wounds; and avoiding reuse of sponges, water or other first aid items to care for injuries involving blood. Finally the leadership role enjoyed by many coaches may provide them the opportunity to educate athletes and others about the risk of HIV transmission through unprotected sex and through the sharing of needles or syringes used to inject anabolic steroids or other drugs (72, 73).

Management of Exposures

The United States Public Health Service has published detailed recommendations for managing occupational exposures to blood and body fluids that may contain HIV (74). Evaluation of an exposure should include determining the likelihood that the exposing fluid contains HIV, the volume of fluid and the route of exposure. If the source person is known to be infected with HIV or refuses testing, the exposed person should be evaluated for HIV infection as soon as possible and if seronegative should be retested periodically for a minimum of 6 months. During the follow-up period the exposed person should seek medical evaluation for any acute illness; refrain from blood, semen and organ donation; and take measures to prevent sexual transmission of HIV.

Blood or body fluid exposures also may occur in the home or in other nonoccupational settings (e.g., needlestick injury by family member providing home medical care). Although not specifically addressed in these recommendations, the management of nonoccupational exposures should be based on the same principles as that of occupational exposures, and access to information regarding postexposure management should be available to persons outside of medical centers (74).

REFERENCES: AS NUMBERED IN ORIGINAL PUBLICATION

49. Centers for Disease Control. Recommendations for prevention of HIV transmission in health-care settings. MMWR 1987;36(Suppl. 2S):1S-18S.
50. Centers for Disease Control. Update: universal precautions for prevention of transmission of human immunodeficiency virus, hepatitis B virus, and other bloodborne pathogens in healthcare settings. MMWR 1988;37:377–382, 387–388.
51. National Commission on AIDS. Preventing HIV transmission in health care settings. Washington, DC: 1992.
52. Grint P, McEvoy M. Two associated cases of the acquired immunodeficiency syndrome (AIDS). Communicable Disease Report 1985;42:4.
53. Centers for Disease Control. Apparent transmission of human T-lymphotrophic virus type III/lymphadenopathy-associated virus from a child to a mother providing health care. MMWR 1986:35:76–79.
54. Koenig RE. Gautier T, Levy JA. Unusual intrafamilial transmission of human immunodeficiency virus. Lancet 1986;2:627.
55. Centers for Disease Control. HIV infection in two brothers receiving intravenous therapy for hemophilia. MMWR 1992:41:228–231.
56. Centers for Disease Control. Caring for someone with AIDS. National AIDS information and education program. Atlanta: CDC, 1991.
57. Simmons B, Trusler M, Roccaforte J, Smoth P, Scott R. Infection control for home health. Infect Control Hosp Epidemiol 1990;11:362–370.
58. Centers for Disease Control. Education and foster care of children infected with human T-lymphotrophic virus type III/ lymphadenopathy-associated virus. MMWR 1985;34:517–521.
59. American Academy of Pediatrics Committee on Infectious Diseases. Health guidelines for the atten-

dance in day-care and foster care settings of children infected with human immunodeficiency virus. Pediatrics 1987;79:466–471.

60. American Public Health Association, American Academy Pediatrics. Caring for our children—national health and safety performance standards: guidelines for out-of-home child care programs. Elkgrove Village, IL: American Public Health Association, 1992:231–236.

61. American Academy of Pediatrics Task Force on Pediatric AIDS. Education of children with human immunodeficiency virus infection. Pediatrics 1991:88:645–648.

62. Fraser K. Someone at school has AIDS. Alexandria, VA: National Association of State Boards of Education, 1989:1–35.

63. Santelli JS, Birn AE, Linde J. School placement for human immunodeficiency virus-infected children: the Baltimore city experience. Pediatrics 1992;89:843–848.

64. Centers for Disease Control. Vigorous physical activity among high school students—United States, 1990. MMWR 1992;41:33–35.

65. Torre D, Sampietro C, Ferraro G, Zeroli C, Speranza F. Transmission of HIV-1 infection via sports injury. Lancet 1990;335:1105.

66. Lifson AR. Do alternate modes for transmission of human immunodeficiency exist? A review. JAMA 1988;259:1353–1356.

67. Kashiwagi S, Hayashi J, Ikematsu H. An outbreak of hepatitis B in members of a high school sumo wrestling club. JAMA 1982;248:213–214.

68. American Academy of Pediatrics, Committee on Sports Medicine and Fitness. Human immunodeficiency virus (acquired immunodeficiency syndrome (AIDS) virus) in the athletic setting. Pediatrics 1991;88:640–641.

69. National Collegiate Athletic Association. AIDS and intercollegiate athletics. NCAA sports medicine handbook. Overland Park, KS: National Collegiate Athletic Association, 1992.

70. National Football League. HIV/AIDS-related policies. New York: National Football League, 1992.

71. World Health Organization. Consensus statement from consultation on AIDS and sports. Geneva: World Health Organization, 1989.

72. Scott MJ, Scott MJ Jr. HIV infection associated with injections of anabolic steroids. JAMA 1989;262: 207–208.

73. Sklarek HM, Mantovani RP, Erens E, Heisler D, Niederman MS, Fein AM. AIDS in a bodybuilder using anabolic steroids. N Engl J Med 1984;311:1701.

74. Centers for Disease Control. Public Health Service statement on management of occupational exposure to human immunodeficiency virus, including considerations regarding zidovudine use. MMWR 1990;39(No. RR-1):1–14.

Recommendations on Prophylaxis and Therapy for Disseminated Mycobacterium avium Complex for Adults and Adolescents Diagnosed with HIV

Original Citation: Centers for Disease Control and Prevention. Recommendations on prophylaxis and therapy for disseminated Mycobacterium avium complex for adults and adolescents diagnosed with HIV. MMWR 1993;42(RR-9):14–20

Editor's Note: The information included here was based on an article which gives recommendations for the prevention of disseminated mycobacterium avium complex (MAC) based on a meeting of a U.S. Public Health Service Task Force on December 7–8, 1992. An initial summary outlines the epidemiology of MAC.

INDICATIONS FOR PROPHYLAXIS

Patients with HIV infection and less than 100 CD4+ T-lymphocytes/μL should be administered prophylaxis against MAC. Prophylaxis should be continued for the patient's lifetime unless multiple drug therapy for MAC becomes necessary because of the development of MAC disease.

Clinicians must weigh the potential benefits of MAC prophylaxis against the potential for toxicities and drug interactions, the cost, the potential to produce resistance in a community with a high rate of tuberculosis, and the possibility that the addition of another drug to the medical regimen may adversely affect patients' compliance with treatment. Because of these concerns, therefore, in some situations rifabutin prophylaxis should not be administered.

EVALUATION BEFORE BEGINNING PROPHYLAXIS

Before prophylaxis is administered, patients should be assessed to ensure that they do not have active disease due to MAC, M. tuberculosis, or any other mycobacterial species. This assessment may include a chest radiograph and tuberculin skin test.

Prophylactic Regimens

Rifabutin, 300 mg by mouth daily, is recommended for the patient's lifetime unless disseminated MAC develops, which would then require multiple drug therapy (4, 5). Although other drugs, such as azithromycin and clarithromycin, have laboratory and clinical activity against MAC, none has been shown in a prospective, controlled trial to be effective and safe for prophylaxis. Thus, in the absence of data, no other regimen can be recommended at this time.

The 300-mg dose of rifabutin has been well tolerated (4, 5). Adverse effects included neutropenia, thrombocytopenia, rash, and gastrointestinal disturbances.

DIAGNOSIS OF MAC

Disseminated MAC is most readily diagnosed by one positive blood culture (6). Blood cultures should be performed in patients with symptoms, signs, or laboratory abnormalities compatible with mycobacterium infection. Blood cultures are not routinely recommended for asymptomatic persons, even for those who have CD4+ T-lymphocyte counts less than 100 cells/μL.

THERAPY OF DISSEMINATED MAC

Although studies have not yet identified an optimal regimen or confirmed that any therapeutic regimen produces sustained clinical benefit for patients with disseminated MAC, the Task Force concluded that the available information indicated the need for treatment of disseminated MAC (7–14). The Public Health Service therefore recommends that regimens be based on the following principles:

- Treatment regimens outside a clinical trial should include at least two agents.
- Every regimen should contain either azithromycin or clarithromycin; many experts prefer ethambutol as a second drug. Many clinicians have added one

or more of the following as second, third, or fourth agents: clofazimine, rifabutin, rifampin, ciprofloxacin, and in some situations amikacin. Isoniazid and pyrazinamide are not effective for the therapy of MAC.

- Therapy should continue for the lifetime of the patient if clinical and microbiologic improvement is observed.

MONITORING PATIENTS RECEIVING THERAPY FOR DISSEMINATED MAC

- Clinical manifestations of disseminated MAC—such as fever, weight loss, and night sweats—should be monitored several times during the initial weeks of therapy. Microbiologic response, as assessed by blood culture every 4 weeks during initial therapy, can also be helpful in interpreting the efficacy of a therapeutic regimen.
- Most patients who ultimately respond show substantial clinical improvement in the first 4–6 weeks of therapy. Elimination of the organisms from blood cultures may take somewhat longer, often requiring 4–12 weeks.

RECOMMENDATIONS FOR HIV-INFECTED CHILDREN

HIV-infected children less than 12 years of age also develop disseminated MAC. Some age adjustment is necessary when clinicians interpret CD4+ T-lymphocyte counts in children less than 2 years of age. Diagnosis, therapy, and prophylaxis should follow recommendations similar to those for adolescents and adults.

REFERENCES: AS NUMBERED IN ORIGINAL PUBLICATION

4. Gordin F, Nightingale S, Wynne B, et al. Rifabutin monotherapy prevents or delays Mycobacterium avium complex bacteremia in patients with AIDS [Abstract no. B100]. In: Program and Abstracts of the VIII International Conference on AIDS/Third STD World Congress (Amsterdam). Amsterdam: Harvard University/Dutch Foundation, 1992.
5. Cameron W, Sparti P, Pietroski N, et al. Rifabutin therapy for the prevention of M. avium complex bacteremia in patients with AIDS and CD4 less than 200 [Abstract no. We54]. In: Program and Abstracts of the VIII International Conference on AIDS/Third STD World Congress (Amsterdam). Amsterdam: Harvard University/Dutch Foundation, 1992.
6. Evans KD, Nakasome AS, Sutherland PA, de la Maza LM, Peterson EM. Identification of Mycobacterium tuberculosis and Mycobacterium avium-M. intracellulare directly from primary BactecR cultures by using acridinium-ester labeled DNA probes. J Clin Microbiol 1992;30:2427–2431.
7. Kemper C, Havlir D, Haghighat D, et al. Effect of ethambutol, rifampin, or clofazimine, given singly, on Mycobacterium avium bacteremia in AIDS. VIII International Conference on AIDS: Amsterdam, The Netherlands, July 19–24, 1992:PoB 3087.
8. Chaisson RE, Benson CA, Dube M, et al. Clarithromycin therapy for disseminated Mycobacterium avium-complex (MAC) in AIDS. Abstracts of the 32nd Interscience Conference on Antimicrobial Agents and Chemotherapy, Anaheim, California, 1992;891.
9. Dautzenberg B, Truffot C, Legris S, et al. Activity of clarithromycin against Mycobacterium avium infection in patients with the acquired immune deficiency syndrome: a controlled clinical trial. Am Rev Respir Dis 1992;144:564–569.
10. Young LS, Wiviott L, Wu M, Kolononski P, Bolan R, Inderlied CB. Azithromycin for treatment of Mycobacterium avium-intracellulare complex infection in patients with AIDS. Lancet 1991;338:1107–1109.
11. Kemper CA, Meng TC, Nussbaum J, et al. Treatment of Mycobacterium avium complex bacteremia in AIDS with a four-drug oral regimen: rifampin, ethambutol, clofazimine and ciprofloxacin. Ann Intern Med 1992;116:466–472.
12. Agins BD, Berman DS, Spicehandler D, El-Sadr W, Simberkoff MS, Rahal J. Effect of combined therapy with ansamycin, clofazimine, ethambutol, and isoniazid for Mycobacterium avium infection in patients with AIDS. J Infect Dis 1989;159:784–787.
13. Hoy J, Mijch A, Sandland M, Grayson L, Lucas R, Dwyer B. Quadruple-drug therapy for Mycobacterium avium bacteremia in AIDS patients. J Infect Dis 1990;161:801–805.
14. Horsburgh CR, Havlik JA, Metchock BG, Thompson SE. Oral therapy of disseminated Mycobacterium avium complex infection in AIDS relieves symptoms and is well tolerated. Am Rev Respir Dis 1991;143:A115.

1993 Revised Classification System for HIV Infection and Expanded Surveillance Case Definition for AIDS Among Adolescents and Adults

Original Citation: Centers for Disease Control and Prevention. 1993 Revised classification system for HIV infection and expanded surveillance case definition for AIDS among adolescents and adults. MMWR 1992;41(RR-17).

Editor's Note: The information included here was based on an issue of MMWR Recommendations and Reports (Vol. 41, No. RR-17) which lists the complicated new case definitions of AIDS and HIV infection.

The revised CDC classification system for HIV-infected adolescents and adults* categorizes persons on the basis of clinical conditions associated with HIV infection and CD4+ T-lymphocyte counts. The system is based on three ranges of CD4+ T-lymphocyte counts and three clinical categories and is represented by a matrix of nine mutually exclusive categories. This system replaces the classification system published in 1986, which included only clinical disease criteria and which was developed before the widespread use of CD4+ T-cell testing (1).

CD4+ T-LYMPHOCYTE CATEGORIES

The three CD4+ T-lymphocyte categories are defined as follows:

- Category 1: greater than or equal to 500 cells/mL
- Category 2: 200–499 cells/μL
- Category 3: less than 200 cells/μL

These categories correspond to CD4+ T-lymphocyte counts per microliter of blood and guide clinical and therapeutic actions in the management of HIV-infected adolescents and adults (22–28). The revised HIV classification system also allows for the use of the percentage of CD4+ T-cells (Appendix A).

HIV-infected persons should be classified based on existing guidelines for the medical management of HIV-infected persons (22). Thus, the lowest accurate, but not necessarily the most recent, CD4+ T-lymphocyte count should be used for classification purposes.

CLINICAL CATEGORIES

The clinical categories of HIV infection are defined as follows:

---

*Criteria for HIV infection for persons ages greater than 13 years: (a) repeatedly reactive screening tests for HIV antibody (e.g., enzyme immunoassay) with specific antibody identified by the use of supplemental tests (e.g., Western blot, immunofluorescence assay); (b) direct identification of virus in host tissues by virus isolation; (c) HIV antigen detection; or (d) a positive result on any other highly specific licensed test for HIV.

Category A

Category A consists of one or more of the conditions listed below in an adolescent or adult (greater than or equal to 13 years) with documented HIV infection. Conditions listed in Categories B and C must not have occurred.

- Asymptomatic HIV infection
- Persistent generalized lymphadenopathy
- Acute (primary) HIV infection with accompanying illness or history of acute HIV infection (29, 30)

Category B

Category B consists of symptomatic conditions in an HIV-infected adolescent or adult that are not included among conditions listed in clinical Category C and that meet at least one of the following criteria: (a) the conditions are attributed to HIV infection or are indicative of a defect in cell-mediated immunity; or (b) the conditions are considered by physicians to have a clinical course or to require management that is complicated by HIV infection. Examples of conditions in clinical Category B include, but are not limited to:

- Bacillary angiomatosis
- Candidiasis, oropharyngeal (thrush)
- Candidiasis, vulvovaginal; persistent, frequent, or poorly responsive to therapy
- Cervical dysplasia (moderate or severe)/cervical carcinoma in situ
- Constitutional symptoms, such as fever (38.5°C) or diarrhea lasting greater than 1 month
- Hairy leukoplakia, oral
- Herpes zoster (shingles), involving at least two distinct episodes or more than one dermatome
- Idiopathic thrombocytopenic purpura
- Listeriosis
- Pelvic inflammatory disease, particularly if complicated by tubo-ovarian abscess
- Peripheral neuropathy

For classification purposes, Category B conditions take precedence over those in Category A. For example, someone previously treated for oral or persistent vaginal candidiasis (and who has not developed a Category C disease) but who is now asymptomatic should be classified in clinical Category B.

Category C

Category C includes the clinical conditions listed in the AIDS surveillance case definition (Appendix B). For classification purposes, once a Category C condition has occurred, the person will remain in Category C.

EXPANSION OF THE CDC SURVEILLANCE CASE DEFINITION FOR AIDS

In 1991, CDC, in collaboration with the Council of State and Territorial Epidemiologists (CSTE), proposed an expansion of the AIDS surveillance case definition. This proposal was made available for public comment in November

1991 and was discussed at an open meeting on September 2, 1992. Based on information presented and reviewed during the public comment period and at the open meeting, CDC, in collaboration with CSTE, has expanded the AIDS surveillance case definition to include all HIV-infected persons with CD4+ T-lymphocyte counts of less than 200 cells/μL or a CD4+ percentage of less than 14. In addition to retaining the 23 clinical conditions in the previous AIDS surveillance definition, the expanded definition includes pulmonary tuberculosis (TB), recurrent pneumonia, and invasive cervical cancer.** This expanded definition requires laboratory confirmation of HIV infection in persons with a CD4+ T-lymphocyte count of less than 200 cells/μL or with one of the added clinical conditions. This expanded definition for reporting cases to CDC becomes effective January 1, 1993.

In the revised HIV classification system, persons in subcategories A3, B3, and C3 meet the immunologic criteria of the surveillance case definition, and those persons with conditions in subcategories C1, C2, and C3 meet the clinical criteria for surveillance purposes. This revised HIV classification system should be used by state and territorial health departments that conduct HIV infection surveillance. Because AIDS surveillance data will continue to represent only a portion of the total morbidity caused by HIV, surveillance for HIV infection may be particularly useful in depicting the total impact of HIV on health-care and social services (42). More accurate reporting and analysis of CD4+ T-lymphocyte counts, together with HIV-related clinical conditions, should facilitate efforts to evaluate health-care and referral needs for persons with HIV infection and to project future needs for these services.

Uses of the HIV Classification System or AIDS Surveillance Case Definition

The revised HIV classification system and the AIDS surveillance case definition are intended for use in conducting public health surveillance. The CDC's AIDS surveillance case definition was not developed to determine whether statutory or other legal requirements for entitlement to Federal disability or other benefits are met. Consequently, this revised surveillance case definition does not alter the criteria used by the Social Security Administration in evaluating claims based on HIV infection under the Social Security Disability Insurance and Supplemental Security Income programs. Other organizations and agencies providing medical and social services should develop eligibility criteria appropriate to the services provided and local needs.

Confidentiality

Every effort should be made by health-care providers, laboratories, and public health agencies to protect the confidentiality of CD4+ T-lymphocyte test

---

** Diagnostic criteria for AIDS-defining conditions included in the expanded surveillance case definition are presented in Appendix C and Appendix D.

results, including the review of record-keeping practices in laboratories and health-care settings. Some states have considered additional means to assure the confidentiality of CD4+ T-lymphocyte test results. For example, a proposal in Oregon would allow health-care providers to send specimens to laboratories for CD4+ T-lymphocyte testing with a unique code for each person being tested. If the test result indicates a CD4+ T-lymphocyte count of less than 200 cells/μL, the health department would notify the health-care provider that an AIDS case report is required if the person is HIV infected, the CD4+ T-lymphocyte count is valid, and the case has not been previously reported. Informed consent for CD4+ T-lymphocyte testing should be obtained in accordance with local laws or regulations. CD4+ T-lymphocyte test results alone should not be used as a surrogate marker for HIV or AIDS. A low CD4+ T-lymphocyte count without a positive HIV test result will not be reportable since other conditions may result in a low CD4+ T-lymphocyte count. Health-care providers must ensure that persons who have a CD4+ T-lymphocyte count of less than 200/μL are HIV infected before initiating treatment for HIV disease or reporting those persons as cases of AIDS.

APPENDIX A

Equivalences for CD4+ T-lymphocyte Count and
Percentage of Total Lymphocytes

Compared with the absolute CD4+ T-lymphocyte count, the percentage of CD4+ T-cells of total lymphocytes (or CD4+ percentage) is less subject to variation on repeated measurements (18, 74). However, data correlating natural history of HIV infection with the CD4+ percentage have not been as consistently available as data on absolute CD4+ T-lymphocyte counts (14–16, 18, 19, 21, 31). Therefore, the revised classification system emphasizes the use of CD4+ T-lymphocyte counts but allows for the use of CD4+ percentages.

Equivalences were derived from analyses of more than 15,500 lymphocyte subset determinations from seven different sources: one multistate study of diseases in HIV-infected adolescents and adults (59) and six laboratories (two commercial, one research, and three university-based). The six laboratories are involved in proficiency testing programs for lymphocyte subset determinations. In the analyses, concordance was defined as the proportion of patients classified as having CD4+ T-lymphocyte counts in a particular range among patients with a given CD4+ percentage. A threshold value of the CD4+ percentage was calculated to obtain optimal concordance with each stratifying value of the CD4+ T-lymphocyte counts (i.e., less than 200/μL and greater than or equal to 500/μL). The thresholds for the CD4+ percentages that best correlated with a CD4+ T-lymphocyte count of less than 200/μL varied minimally among the seven data sources (range, 13%–14%; median, 13%; mean, 13.4%). The average concordance for a CD4+ percentage of less than 14 and a CD4+ T-lymphocyte count of less than 200/μL was 90.2%. The threshold for the CD4+ percentages most concordant with CD4+ T-lymphocyte counts of greater than or equal to 500/μL varied more widely among the seven data sources (range, 22.5%–35%; median, 29%; mean, 29.1%). This wide range of percentages optimally concordant with greater than or equal to 500/μL CD4+ T-lymphocytes makes the concordance at this stratifying value less certain. The average concordance for a CD4+ percentage of greater than or equal to 29 and a CD4+ T-lymphocyte count of greater than or equal to 500/μL was 85% (CDC, unpublished data). Clinicians and other practitioners must recognize that these suggested equivalences may not always correspond with values observed in individual patients.

APPENDIX B

Conditions Included in the 1993 AIDS Surveillance Case Definition

- Candidiasis of bronchi, trachea, or lungs
- Candidiasis, esophageal
- Cervical cancer, invasive***
- Coccidioidomycosis, disseminated or extrapulmonary
- Cryptococcosis, extrapulmonary
- Cryptosporidiosis, chronic intestinal (greater than 1 month's duration)
- Cytomegalovirus disease (other than liver, spleen, or nodes)
- Cytomegalovirus retinitis (with loss of vision)
- Encephalopathy, HIV-related
- Herpes simplex: chronic ulcer(s) (greater than 1 month's duration); or bronchitis, pneumonitis, or esophagitis
- Histoplasmosis, disseminated or extrapulmonary
- Isosporiasis, chronic intestinal (greater than 1 month's duration)
- Kaposi's sarcoma
- Lymphoma, Burkitt's (or equivalent term)
- Lymphoma, immunoblastic (or equivalent term)
- Lymphoma, primary, of brain
- Mycobacterium avium complex or M. kansasii, disseminated or extrapulmonary
- Mycobacterium tuberculosis, any site (pulmonary*** or extrapulmonary)
- Mycobacterium, other species or unidentified species, disseminated or extrapulmonary
- Pneumocystis carinii pneumonia
- Pneumonia, recurrent***
- Progressive multifocal leukoencephalopathy
- Salmonella septicemia, recurrent
- Toxoplasmosis of brain
- Wasting syndrome due to HIV

*** Added in the 1993 expansion of the AIDS surveillance case definition.

APPENDIX C

Definitive Diagnostic Methods for Diseases Indicative of AIDS

Cryptosporidiosis, Isosporiasis, Kaposi's sarcoma, Lymphoma, Pneumocystis carinii pneumonia, Progressive multifocal leukoencephalopathy, Toxoplasmosis, Cervical cancer

Microscopy (histology or cytology)

Candidiasis

Gross inspection by endoscopy or autopsy or by microscopy (histology or cytology) on a specimen obtained directly from the tissues affected (including scrapings from the mucosal surface), not from a culture

Coccidioidomycosis, Cryptococcosis, Cytomegalovirus, Herpes simplex virus, Histoplasmosis

Microscopy (histology or cytology), culture, or detection of antigen in a specimen obtained directly from the tissues affected or a fluid from those tissues

Tuberculosis, Other mycobacteriosis, Salmonellosis Culture

HIV Encephalopathy (Dementia)

Clinical findings of disabling cognitive or motor dysfunction interfering with occupation or activities of daily living, progressing over weeks to months, in the absence of a concurrent illness or condition other than HIV infection that could explain the findings. Methods to rule out such concurrent illness and conditions must include cerebrospinal fluid examination and either brain imaging (computed tomography or magnetic resonance) or autopsy.

HIV Wasting Syndrome

Findings of profound involuntary weight loss of greater than 10% of baseline body weight plus either chronic diarrhea (at least two loose stools per day for greater than or equal to 30 days), or chronic weakness and documented fever (for greater than or equal to 30 days, intermittent or constant) in the absence of a concurrent illness or condition other than HIV infection that could explain the findings (e.g., cancer, tuberculosis, cryptosporidiosis, or other specific enteritis).

Pneumonia, Recurrent

Recurrent (more than one episode in a 1-year period), acute (new x-ray evidence not present earlier) pneumonia diagnosed by both: (a) culture (or other organism-specific diagnostic method) obtained from a clinically reliable specimen of a pathogen that typically causes pneumonia (other than Pneumocystis carinii or Mycobacterium tuberculosis), and (b) radiologic evidence of pneumonia; cases that do not have laboratory confirmation of a causative organism for one of the episodes of pneumonia will be considered to be presumptively diagnosed.

APPENDIX D

Suggested Guidelines for Presumptive Diagnosis of Diseases Indicative of AIDS

Candidiasis of Esophagus

1. Recent onset of retrosternal pain on swallowing; AND
2. Oral candidiasis diagnosed by the gross appearance of white patches or plaques on an erythematous base or by the microscopic appearance of fungal mycelial filaments from a noncultured specimen scraped from the oral mucosa.

Cytomegalovirus retinitis

A characteristic appearance on serial ophthalmoscopic examinations (e.g., discrete patches of retinal whitening with distinct borders, spreading in a centrifugal manner along the paths of blood vessels, progressing over several months, and frequently associated with retinal vasculitis, hemorrhage, and necrosis). Resolution of active disease leaves retinal scarring and atrophy with retinal pigment epithelial mottling.

Mycobacteriosis

Microscopy of a specimen from stool or normally sterile body fluids or tissue from a site other than lungs, skin, or cervical or hilar lymph nodes that shows acid-fast bacilli of a species not identified by culture.

Kaposi's Sarcoma

A characteristic gross appearance of an erythematous or violaceous plaque-like lesion on skin or mucous membrane. (Note: Presumptive diagnosis of Kaposi's sarcoma should not be made by clinicians who have seen few cases of it.)

Pneumocystis carinii Pneumonia

1. A history of dyspnea on exertion or nonproductive cough of recent onset (within the past 3 months); AND
2. Chest x-ray evidence of diffuse bilateral interstitial infiltrates or evidence by gallium scan of diffuse bilateral pulmonary disease; AND
3. Arterial blood gas analysis showing an arterial $pO_{(2)}$ of less than 70 mm Hg or a low respiratory diffusing capacity (less than 80% of predicted values) or an increase in the alveolar-arterial oxygen tension gradient; AND
4. No evidence of a bacterial pneumonia.

Pneumonia, Recurrent

Recurrent (more than one episode in a 1-year period), acute (new symptoms, signs, or x-ray evidence not present earlier) pneumonia diagnosed on clinical or radiologic grounds by the patient's physician.

Toxoplasmosis of Brain

1. Recent onset of a focal neurologic abnormality consistent with intracranial disease or a reduced level of consciousness; AND
2. Evidence by brain imaging (computed tomography or nuclear magnetic resonance) of a lesion having a mass effect or the radiographic appearance of which is enhanced by injection of contrast medium; AND
3. Serum antibody to toxoplasmosis or successful response to therapy for toxoplasmosis.

Tuberculosis, Pulmonary

When bacteriologic confirmation is not available, other reports may be considered to be verified cases of pulmonary tuberculosis if the criteria of the Division of Tuberculosis Elimination, National Center for Prevention Services, CDC, are used. The criteria in use as of January 1, 1993, are available in MMWR 1990; 39(No. RR-13):39–40.

REFERENCES: AS NUMBERED IN ORIGINAL PUBLICATION

1. CDC. Classification system for human T-lymphotropic virus type III/lymphadenopathy-associated virus infections. MMWR 1986;35:334-339.
14. Goedert JJ, Biggar RJ, Melbye M, et al. Effect of T4 count and cofactors on the incidence of AIDS in homosexual men infected with human immunodeficiency virus. JAMA 1987;257:331–334.
15. Nicholson JKA, Spira TJ, Aloisio CH, et al. Serial determinations of HIV-1 titers in HIV-infected homosexual men: association of rising titers with CD4 T cell depletion and progression to AIDS. AIDS Res Hum Retroviruses 1989;5:205–215.
16. Lang W, Perkins H, Anderson RE, Royce R, Jewell N, Winkelstein W. Patterns of T lymphocyte changes with human immunodeficiency virus infection: from seroconversion to the development of AIDS. J Acquir Immune Defic Syndr 1989;2:63–69.
18. Taylor JM, Fahey JL, Detels R, Giorgi J. CD4 percentage, CD4 numbers, and CD4:CD8 ratio in HIV infection: which to choose and how to use. J Acquir Immune Defic Syndr 1989;2:114–124.
19. Masur H, Ognibene FP, Yarchoan R, et al. CD4 counts as predictors of opportunistic pneumonias in human immunodeficiency virus (HIV) infection. Ann Intern Med 1989;111:223–231.
21. Fernandez-Cruz E, Desco M, Garcia Montes M, Longo N, Gonzalez B, Zabay JM. Immunological and serological markers predictive of progression to AIDS in a cohort of HIV-infected drug users. AIDS 1990;4:987–994.
22. National Institutes of Health. State-of-the-art conference on azidothymidine therapy for early HIV infection. Am J Med 1990;89:335–344.
23. CDC. Guidelines for prophylaxis against Pneumocystis carinii pneumonia for persons infected with human immunodeficiency virus. MMWR 1992;41(No. RR-4):1–11.
24. Fischl MA, Richman DD, Hansen N, et al. The safety and efficacy of zidovudine (AZT) in the treatment of subjects with mildly symptomatic human immunodeficiency virus type 1 (HIV) infection: a double blind, placebo controlled trial. Ann Intern Med 1990;112:727–737.
25. Volberding PA, Lagakos SW, Koch MA, et al. Zidovudine in asymptomatic human immunodeficiency virus infection: a controlled trial in persons with fewer than 500 CD4-positive cells per cubic millimeter. N Engl J Med 1990;322:941.
26. Lagakos S, Fischl MA, Stein DS, Lim L, Volberding PA. Effects of zidovudine therapy in minority and other subpopulations with early HIV infection. JAMA 1991;266:2709–2712.
27. Easterbrook PJ, Keruly JC, Creagh-Kirk T, et al. Racial and ethnic differences in outcome in zidovudine-treated patients with advanced HIV disease. JAMA 1991;266:2713–2718.
28. Hamilton JD, Hartigan PM, Simberkoff MS, et al. A controlled trial of early versus late treatment with zidovudine in symptomatic human immunodeficiency virus infection. N Engl J Med 1992;326:437–443.
29. Ho DD, Sarngadharan MG, Resnick L, et al. Primary human T-lymphotropic virus type III infection. Ann Intern Med 1985;103:880–883.
30. Tindall B, Cooper DA. Primary HIV infection: host responses and intervention strategies. AIDS 1991;5:1–14.
31. Redfield RR, Wright DC, Tramont EC. The Walter Reed Staging Classification for HTLV-III/LAV infection. N Engl J Med 1986;314:131–132.
42. CDC. Surveillance for HIV infection—United States. MMWR 1990;39:853,859–861.
59. Farizo KM, Buehler JW, Chamberland ME, et al. Spectrum of disease in persons with human immunodeficiency virus infection in the United States. JAMA 1992;267:1798–1805.
74. Kessler HA, Landay A, Pottage JC, Benson CA. Absolute number versus percentage of T-helper lymphocytes in human immunodeficiency virus infection. J Infect Dis 1990;161:356–357.

Risk for Cervical Disease in HIV-Infected Women

Original Citation: Centers for Disease Control and Prevention. Epidemiologic notes and reports risk for cervical disease in HIV-infected women—New York City. MMWR 1990;39(47):846–849.

Editor's Note: The information included here was based on an article which summarizes findings from four studies which suggest an association between HIV infection and cervical disease in women. The article makes the recommendation that HIV-infected women should have a Pap smear annually.

In 1988, a consensus recommendation for cervical cancer screening was adopted by the American Cancer Society, the National Cancer Institute, the American College of Obstetricians and Gynecologists, the American Medical Association, the American Nurses' Association, the American Academy of Family Physicians, and the American Medical Women's Association (16). The recommendation suggests that all women who are or who have been sexually active or who have reached age 18 years should have an annual Pap test and pelvic examination. After a woman has had three or more consecutive satisfactory normal annual examinations, the Pap test may be performed less frequently at the discretion of her physician. Another advisory group, the U.S. Preventive Services Task Force, recommended in 1989 that Pap smears should begin with the onset of sexual activity and should be repeated every 1–3 years at the physician's discretion (17). The time interval between Pap tests recommended by the physician should be based on the presence of risk factors for cervical cancer. In accordance with these recommendations and information suggesting that HIV-infected women may be at increased risk for cervical disease, HIV-infected women should have a Pap smear annually.

REFERENCES: AS NUMBERED IN ORIGINAL PUBLICATION

16. Fink DJ. Change in American Cancer Society checkup guidelines for detection of cervical cancer. CA 1988;38:127–128.
17. US Department of Health and Human Services, Preventive Services Task Force. Screening for cervical cancer. In: Guide to clinical preventive services: an assessment of the effectiveness of 169 interventions. Baltimore: Williams and Wilkins, 1989:57–62.

Tuberculosis and HIV Infection

Original Citation: Centers for Disease Control and Prevention. Tuberculosis and human immunodeficiency virus infection: recommendations of the Advisory Committee for the Elimination of Tuberculosis (ACET). MMWR 1989;38(14):236–238, 243–250.

Editor's Note: The information included here was based on an article which gives the recommendations of the Advisory Committee for Elimination of Tuberculosis (ACET) for the diagnosis and treatment of tuberculosis in persons with HIV infection. Epidemiology and clinical features of tuberculosis are given in the original article but omitted here due to space.

DIAGNOSIS

These unusual clinical features emphasize the importance of considering a diagnosis of TB in persons with known or possible HIV infection and a diagnosis of HIV infection in persons with TB. Persons who provide care to HIV-infected persons must be informed of the frequently uncharacteristic presentation of TB in this group so that the diagnosis is not overlooked. Failure to diagnose and manage TB appropriately can result in the death of the patient and infection of contacts, including other patients and health-care personnel.

To establish the diagnosis, a variety of specimens, including respiratory secretions, bronchial washings, gastric lavage, lung tissue, pleural fluid, lymph node tissue, bone marrow, blood, urine, stool, brain biopsy, and cerebrospinal fluid, may need to be obtained for mycobacterial culture. Specimens must be examined microscopically, but the inability to demonstrate acid-fast bacilli and the absence of granuloma formation does not exclude the diagnosis of TB (4, 19).

A Mantoux tuberculin skin test with 5 tuberculin units (TU) of tuberculin purified protein derivative (PPD) should be administered as a diagnostic aid, although some persons with HIV infection may have falsely negative reactions because of immunosuppression (2, 3). The severity of immunosuppression and the development of AIDS is related to the duration of HIV infection. Furthermore, the proportion of HIV-infected persons with TB who have negative tuberculin skin test reactions is related to the length of time between the diagnoses of TB and AIDS. In Florida, the proportion of TB patients with positive tuberculin skin tests progressively decreased with decreasing time between the two diagnoses. All five patients in whom TB was diagnosed greater than or equal to 2 years before the diagnosis of AIDS had positive reactions when TB was diagnosed, 27 (63%) of 43 who had TB diagnosed 1–24 months before the AIDS diagnosis had positive reactions, and seven (33%) of 21 in whom TB was diagnosed simultaneously with or after AIDS had positive tuberculin reactions (CDC/Florida Department of Health and Rehabilitative Services, unpublished data). In New York City, of 23 AIDS patients known to have developed TB and for whom information on the size of the tuberculin reaction was available, seven had no induration, one had a 1–4-mm induration, two had a 5–9-mm induration, and 13 had a greater than or equal to 10-mm induration (CDC/New York City Department of Health, unpublished data). Because HIV infection causes immunosuppression and the risk for TB is high in persons with both tuberculous and HIV infection, as a general guideline, tuberculin reactions of greater than 5-mm induration should be considered indicative of tuberculous infection in an HIV-infected person.

TREATMENT

Anti-TB chemotherapy as described below should be started whenever acid-fast bacilli are seen in a specimen from the respiratory tract of a person with HIV infection or from a person at increased risk for HIV infection whose HIV-antibody status is unknown and who declines to be tested. Because it is impossible to distinguish TB from MAC disease by any criterion other than culture (which often takes several weeks), and because of the individual and public health implications of TB, it is important to treat such patients with a regimen that is effective against M. tuberculosis. As a general rule, persons with TB and HIV infection respond well to standard anti-TB drugs (2, 4, 19), but data on clinical and bacteriologic response in these patients are limited. Longitudinal studies will help clarify the long-term outcome of these patients.

To achieve cure, the treatment period may need to be longer than the standard regimens used for TB patients without HIV infection. When HIV infection is known or suspected, the recommended drugs and dosages for adults are isoniazid, 300 mg/day, and rifampin, 600 mg/day (or 450 mg for patients weighing less than or equal to 50 kg), and pyrazinamide, 20–30 mg/kg/day, during the first 2 months of therapy. Patients treated with rifampin who are on methadone should have the methadone dosage increased to avoid withdrawal symptoms resulting from the interaction between the two drugs (25). Ethambutol, 25 mg/kg/day, should be added to the initial treatment regimen for patients with CNS or disseminated TB or when isoniazid resistance is suspected. The continuation phase should always include at least isoniazid and rifampin. Drug susceptibility tests should be performed routinely, and the treatment regimen should be revised accordingly if resistance to any of the drugs in the regimen is found. Treatment should be continued for a minimum of 9 months and for at least 6 months beyond documented culture conversion as evidenced by three negative cultures. In the absence of definitive data on benefits and risks, some experts suggest that, in persons with concomitant tuberculous and HIV infections, isoniazid therapy should be continued for the person's lifetime (26). If either isoniazid or rifampin is not or cannot be included in the regimen, therapy should last a minimum of 18 months and for at least 12 months after culture conversion. After completion of therapy, patients should be followed closely, and bacteriologic examinations should be repeated if signs of TB recur.

Compliance with therapy is sometimes poor. Supervised, directly administered ambulatory therapy is successful in noncompliant patients (27) and should be initiated if noncompliance is anticipated or suspected.

Monitoring for symptoms of toxicity to anti-TB drugs may be difficult in persons with AIDS, who frequently have similar symptoms due to HIV infection, other drugs, or other conditions. At least one study has reported a higher incidence of adverse reactions to anti-TB drugs in AIDS patients (28).

CONTACT INVESTIGATION

Persons with pulmonary TB, including those with AIDS or HIV infection, are potentially infectious until a satisfactory clinical and bacteriologic response to therapy is achieved. All cases must be reported immediately to the local health department so that standard procedures for TB contact investigation can be followed (29).

In one investigation carried out by the New York City Department of Health, prevalence of tuberculin positivity (21%) among contacts of pulmonary TB patients who also had, or later developed, AIDS was not substantially different from that among contacts of comparable pulmonary TB patients with no diagnosis of AIDS (30%) (CDC/New York City Department of Health, unpublished data). It is not known how much of this high cumulative prevalence of infection represents transmission by these index patients and how much represents prior background prevalence, but these data indicate that TB patients with HIV infection must be considered potential transmitters of M. tuberculosis.

INFECTION CONTROL

Published recommendations for preventing transmission of HIV infection and tuberculous infection to health-care workers should be followed (30–34). Because health-care workers' risk of exposure to blood during tuberculin skin testing or injecting medication is low, wearing gloves during these procedures to prevent HIV transmission is not routinely recommended. However, used needles should not be recapped and should be disposed of according to published guidelines (31). Recommendations for glove use during drawing of blood (e.g., for liver-function testing) have been published (31); whether to use gloves routinely during phlebotomy requires consideration of several factors.

TB should be considered in the differential diagnosis of persons with HIV infection and unexplained pulmonary symptoms, and appropriate precautions should be followed. These precautions, termed AFB isolation, are most important during and immediately after procedures that may induce coughing, such as bronchoscopy, sputum collection, aerosol induction of sputum, and administration of aerosolized medications, such as pentamidine. In clinical situations where airborne exposure of staff or other patients is likely, such procedures should be carried out in rooms or booths with negative air pressure in relation to adjacent rooms or hallways and with air exhausted directly to the outside and away from intake sources. The number of air exchanges per hour in the room or booth should be sufficient to remove infectious organisms during the time between patients. Ultraviolet lights are also useful in killing airborne tubercle bacilli (33, 34). Special care should be taken to prevent inhalation of tubercle bacilli by HIV-infected persons.

Home health-care workers, hospice volunteers, paramedics, and others who care for persons with AIDS in areas where tuberculous infection is also prevalent should be aware of the symptoms of TB, the airborne nature of its transmission, and the appropriate precautions for their particular setting. Workers who have regular contact with TB patients should participate in a TB screening program (29, 33). Consultation on methods to reduce transmission of TB is available from state and local health department TB-control programs.

EXAMINING PERSONS WITH TB OR TUBERCULOUS INFECTION FOR HIV INFECTION

All persons with TB or tuberculous infection need to be assessed for HIV infection because the medical management of TB and tuberculous infection must be altered in the presence of HIV infection. TB patients who are infected with HIV may also develop Pneumocystis carinii pneumonia, cytomegalovirus pneumonitis, and other pulmonary manifestations of HIV infection as their immunosuppression progresses. Assessing these patients' responses to anti-TB therapy and evaluating new infiltrates may be especially difficult. Because the differential diagnosis and medical management of pulmonary infiltrates varies greatly between normal and immunosuppressed persons, knowledge of patients' HIV status is crucial for appropriate medical management. Providing these persons with the benefits of HIV education and counseling and providing the opportunity for HIV testing may enhance HIV prevention and control efforts. All persons with TB or tuberculous infection can benefit from receiving information about reducing their risk of acquiring or transmitting HIV infection. TB patients who are infected with HIV will also benefit by being monitored for early diagnosis of opportunistic infections and other manifestations of HIV infection. Previously published guidelines for counseling and testing and notification of sex partners and those who share needles with HIV-infected persons should be followed (35).

All patients diagnosed with TB should be offered counseling and HIV-antibody testing. Particular emphasis should be placed on offering counseling and HIV-antibody testing to persons with extrapulmonary TB and persons with TB in the age groups in which most HIV infections have been found. Although there are probably some geographic areas and population groups in which most persons with TB are not likely to have HIV infection, data on the prevalence of HIV infection among TB patients in the United States are too limited to be useful in defining such populations. Furthermore, even if such data were available, there is no assurance that these populations will remain free of HIV infection in the future. Monitoring the prevalence of HIV infection among persons with TB is one method for detecting the spread of HIV infection into new areas and population groups and of assuring the appropriate management of TB in the HIV-infected patient.

While the occurrence of clinical TB may be an indication of immunosuppression related to HIV infection, the presence of a positive tuberculin skin test in a person without clinical manifestations of disease does not imply a higher likelihood of HIV infection. Nevertheless, behaviors* that are associated with an increased risk or prevalence of HIV infection should be routinely sought in persons with positive tuberculin skin test reactions. If HIV infection is considered a possibility, counseling and HIV-antibody testing should be strongly encouraged. Because HIV infection is one of the strongest known risk factors for the progression of latent tuberculous infection to TB, the presence of HIV infection in a person with a positive tuberculin skin test is an indication for pre-

---

* Based on seroprevalence studies, behaviors that place a person at risk for HIV infection include IV-drug use and male homosexual contact. Other factors that increase the risk for HIV infection in adults include having received blood or clotting factor concentrate between 1978 and 1985 and having had sexual relations at any time since 1978 with (a) a person known to be infected with HIV or to have AIDS, (b) a man who has had sexual contact with another man, (c) prostitutes, (d) IVDUs, or (e) persons born in countries where most transmission of HIV is thought to occur through heterosexual sexual contact. Risk factors for HIV infection in infants and children include (a) parents, especially the mother, with HIV infection or any of the adult risk factors, and (b) receipt of blood or clotting factor concentrates between 1978 and 1985.

ventive therapy regardless of that person's age. Preventive therapy should be started only after excluding active pulmonary or extrapulmonary TB.

Persons with positive skin test reactions and factors that put them at high risk for HIV infection who decline to be tested for HIV antibody should also be considered at increased risk for developing TB. At this time, isoniazid preventive therapy should be considered for such persons on an individual basis. However, as more data become available on the prevalence of HIV infection among various population groups in different geographic areas, more definitive recommendations may be issued. Such persons should be followed closely; the patients' ability and willingness to participate in the follow-up are factors that influence the decision to provide isoniazid preventive therapy.

Some HIV-infected persons and persons who decline testing but are at high risk for HIV infection might be considered at increased risk of developing TB even if their tuberculin skin tests are negative. Thus, preventive therapy might be considered for those persons with clinical or laboratory evidence of severe immunosuppression who are from developing countries where the prevalence of tuberculous infection is very high, who have a history of close contact with an infected person, who previously have had a positive tuberculin skin test reaction, or who have a radiographic abnormality consistent with past TB.

EXAMINING HIV-INFECTED PERSONS (AND PERSONS AT RISK FOR HIV INFECTION) FOR THE PRESENCE OF TB AND TUBERCULOUS INFECTION

HIV-infected persons, with or without AIDS or other HIV-related disease, should be given a Mantoux skin test with 5 TU tuberculin, PPD. Although false-negative results may occur in these persons because of HIV-induced immunosuppression, positive tuberculin reactions are clinically meaningful. If the skin test reaction shows greater than or equal to 5-mm induration, a chest radiograph should be obtained, and the patient should be examined for evidence of extrapulmonary TB. If abnormalities are noted, additional diagnostic studies for TB should be undertaken. Persons with clinical AIDS or other HIV-related disease should receive a chest radiograph and be examined for evidence of extrapulmonary TB, regardless of the skin test reaction.

Some population groups may have a substantially higher prevalence of HIV infection than the total population (e.g., clients in drug-treatment programs and inmates of correctional institutions). Health-care providers should routinely provide tuberculin skin testing for persons in these settings even if counseling and HIV- antibody testing are not routinely offered or such testing is refused.

PREVENTIVE THERAPY FOR TUBERCULOUS INFECTION

Because preventive therapy with isoniazid reduces the incidence of TB in a variety of populations with tuberculous infection, any person, regardless of age, who is HIV-infected and who has a positive tuberculin skin test reaction (greater than or equal to 5-mm induration) should be offered isoniazid preventive therapy unless it is medically contraindicated. The recommended duration is a minimum of 12 months, but, analogous to considerations for the treatment of TB in AIDS patients (26), some experts have suggested prolongation of isoniazid preventive therapy beyond 12 months. Although it is not known whether isoniazid prevents TB in HIV-infected persons as effectively as in other groups, the usually positive response to standard chemotherapy in HIV-infected persons with TB suggests that isoniazid preventive therapy would also be effective. Because of the particularly high risk for TB in persons with both HIV and tuberculous infection, ensuring completion of at least 12 months of preventive therapy is crucial.

PREVENTION AND CONTROL OF TB IN DRUG-TREATMENT PROGRAMS FOR INTRAVENOUS DRUG-USERS

Intravenous drug-users (IVDUs) require special consideration because they are at high risk for tuberculous as well as HIV infection. Tuberculin skin test surveys among heroin addicts in New York City showed that the prevalence of tuberculous infection in this population was considerably higher than in the city-wide population, even after adjustment for age, race, and economic status (36). Even before the HIV epidemic, opiate-dependent patients in New York City had a higher prevalence of TB than did nondependent patients (37).

HIV infection among IVDUs is responsible for much of the HIV-associated increase in TB in New York City and New Jersey (4, 9). Matching TB and AIDS registries in New York City revealed that 57% of the patients with both TB and AIDS were IVDUs (9).

Isoniazid preventive therapy for tuberculin-positive IVDUs provides an opportunity to prevent many TB cases, especially in the setting of drug-treatment programs, where compliance issues can be addressed. Federal regulations require tuberculin skin testing of IVDUs before admission to a treatment program (38). The recommended technique is the intradermal (Mantoux) test with 5 TU tuberculin PPD. Given the substantial risk for TB in this group and the potential for its prevention, drug-treatment programs should perform a skin test and record the diameter of induration on each new enrollee and on others already enrolled who have not been previously tested. Persons with a tuberculin skin test of greater than or equal to 5-mm induration should be further evaluated for clinical TB and, if disease is present, treated according to current guidelines. Counseling and HIV-antibody testing should be carried out for all consenting persons with greater than or equal to 5-mm induration on their tuberculin skin test, all persons with a past or present history of IV-drug use, and their sex partners (35).

If there is no clinical, radiographic, or laboratory evidence of TB, isoniazid preventive therapy should be recommended for all HIV-infected persons regardless of age with a tuberculin reaction of greater than or equal to 5-mm induration. Isoniazid preventive therapy should also be recommended for all other IVDUs with a tuberculin reaction of greater than 10-mm induration regardless of age. The rationale for this recommendation is based on epidemiologic studies of HIV seroprevalence among IVDUs. Although in some geographic areas the seroprevalence of HIV is still low in IVDUs, this should not be considered a stable situation. Studies of previously collected blood samples from IVDUs indicate the potential for very rapid spread of the virus within the group. The prevalence of HIV infection among IVDUs in Manhattan, Edinburgh (Scotland), and Italy had increased to 40% 3–4 years after the virus was first introduced into the group (39). Consequently, TB and HIV prevention programs are urgently needed for IVDUs, even in areas where the current HIV seroprevalence is very low. To ensure compliance, isoniazid therapy should preferably be fully supervised and administered (daily or on a twice-weekly basis) by the drug-treatment program staff, if possible at the same time the person is seen for treatment of IV-drug abuse. Patients who discontinue treatment before completing at least 6 months of uninterrupted preventive therapy should be restarted on preventive therapy after reenrollment into the treatment program. Drug-treatment programs should work closely with health department TB programs in their jurisdictions for assistance in carrying out these screening and prevention recommendations.

BCG VACCINATION OF HIV-INFECTED PERSONS

The benefits and risks of BCG vaccination of HIV-infected persons remain largely undocumented. However, disseminated M. bovis (BCG) disease was reported in one person with AIDS and Kaposi's sarcoma who was given a BCG vaccination, presumably to "stimulate" his immune system (40). The ACET agrees with the recommendation of the World Health Organization that BCG should not be administered to persons with HIV infection in countries where the risk of infection is low, such as in the United States (41).

REFERENCES: AS NUMBERED IN ORIGINAL PUBLICATION

2. Pitchenik AE, Cole C, Russell BW, Fischl MA, Spira TJ, Snider DE Jr. Tuberculosis, atypical mycobacteriosis, and the acquired immunodeficiency syndrome among Haitian and non-Haitian patients in south Florida. Ann Intern Med 1984;101:641–645.
3. Maayan S, Wormser GP, Hewlett D, et al. Acquired immunodeficiency syndrome (AIDS) in an economically disadvantaged population. Arch Intern Med 1985;145:1607–1612.
4. Sunderam G, McDonald RJ, Maniatis T, Oleske J, Kapila R, Reichman LB. Tuberculosis as a manifestation of the acquired immunodeficiency syndrome (AIDS). JAMA 1986;256:362–366.
9. CDC. Tuberculosis and acquired immunodeficiency syndrome—New York City. MMWR 1987;36:785–790, 795.
19. Louie E, Rice LB, Holzman RS. Tuberculosis in non-Haitian patients with acquired immunodeficiency syndrome. Chest 1986;90:542–545.
25. Kreek MJ, Garfield JW, Gutjahr CL, Giusti LM. Rifampin-induced methadone withdrawal. N Engl J Med 1976;294:1104–1106.
26. Iseman MD. Is standard chemotherapy adequate in tuberculosis patients infected with the HIV [Editorial]? Am Rev Respir Dis 1987;136:1326.
27. McDonald RJ, Memon AM, Reichman LB. Successful supervised ambulatory management of tuberculosis treatment failures. Ann Intern Med 1982;96:297–302.
28. Chaisson RE, Schecter GF, Theuer CP, Rutherford GW, Echenberg DF, Hopewell PC. Tuberculosis in patients with the acquired immunodeficiency syndrome: clinical features, response to therapy, and survival. Am Rev Respir Dis 1987;136:570–574.
29. American Thoracic Society/CDC. Control of tuberculosis. Am Rev Respir Dis 1983;128:336–342.
30. CDC. Recommendations for prevention of HIV transmission in health-care settings. MMWR 1987;36(Suppl 2S):1S–18S.
31. CDC. Update: universal precautions for prevention of transmission of human immunodeficiency virus, hepatitis B virus, and other bloodborne pathogens in health-care settings. MMWR 1988;37:377–382, 387–388.
32. Garner JS, Simmons BP. Guideline for isolation precautions in hospitals. Infect Control 1983;4:245–325.
33. CDC. Guidelines for prevention of TB transmission in hospitals. Atlanta: U.S. Department of Health and Human Services, Public Health Service, 1982:HHS publication no. (CDC)82–8371.
34. Riley RL. Airborne infection. Am J Med 1974;57:466–474.

35. CDC. Public Health Service guidelines for counseling and antibody testing to prevent HIV infection and AIDS. MMWR 1987;36:509–515.
36. Chaves AD. The problem of tuberculosis in selected populations. In: Status of immunization in tuberculosis in 1971. Bethesda, MD: U.S. Department of Health, Education, and Welfare, Public Health Service, National Institutes of Health, 1972:DHEW publication no. (NIH)72–68 (Fogarty International Center proceedings no. 14).
37. Reichman LB, Felton CP, Edsall JR. Drug dependence, a possible new risk factor for tuberculosis disease. Arch Intern Med 1979;139:337–339.
38. Food and Drug Administration/National Institute on Drug Abuse. Methadone in maintenance and detoxification; joint proposed revision of conditions for use; proposed rule. Federal Register 1987;52:37046-37061 (21 CFR Part 291).
39. Des Jarlais D, Hunt DE. AIDS and intravenous drug use. Washington, DC: U.S. Department of Justice, National Institute of Justice. AIDS Bull 1988(Feb):1–6.
40. CDC. Disseminated Mycobacterium bovis infection from BCG vaccination of a patient with acquired immunodeficiency syndrome. MMWR 1985;34:227–228.
41. World Health Organization. Special programme on AIDS and expanded programme on immunization—joint statement: consultation on human immunodeficiency virus (HIV) and routine childhood immunization. Wkly Epidemiol Rec 1987;62:297–309.

TOPIC 15 / **IMMUNIZATIONS—GENERAL RECOMMENDATIONS**

Recommended Childhood Immunization Schedule, 1995

Original Citation: Centers for Disease Control and Prevention. Recommended childhood immunization schedule—United States, 1995. MMWR 1995;44(RR-5);1–9.

Original Authors: Jacqueline S. Gindler, MD, Stephen C. Hadler, MD, Peter M. Strebel, MBChB, MPH, John C. Watson, MD, MPH

SUMMARY

The need for a single childhood immunization schedule prompted the unification of previous vaccine recommendations made by the American Academy of Pediatrics (AAP) and the Advisory Committee on Immunization Practices (ACIP). In addition to presenting the newly recommended schedule for the administration of vaccines during childhood, this report addresses the previous differences between the AAP and ACIP childhood vaccination schedules and the rationale for changing previous recommendations.

OPV

Recommendation

Because immune response is not affected by administering the third dose of OPV at as early as 6 months of age, and because earlier scheduling can ensure a higher rate of completion of the OPV primary series at a younger age, the third dose of OPV should be administered routinely at 6 months of age. Vaccination at as late as 18 months of age remains an acceptable alternative.

MMR

Recommendation

The slightly lower response to the first dose of measles vaccine when administered at 12 months of age compared with administration at 15 months of age has limited clinical importance because a second dose of MMR is recommended routinely for all children, enhancing the likelihood of seroconversion among children who do not respond to the first dose. In addition, earlier scheduling of the first dose of measles vaccine can improve vaccination coverage. In 1994, both AAP and ACIP recommended administration of the first dose of MMR vaccine at 12–15 months of age (2, 8); this schedule is still recommended.

Because response to the second dose is high when administered to children in either age group (CDC, unpublished data), and because state-specific laws govern the administration of the second dose of MMR, the second dose of MMR can be administered at either 4–6 years of age or 11–12 years of age.

HEPATITIS B

Recommendation

The routine hepatitis B vaccination series should begin at birth, with the second dose administered at 2 months of age, for infants whose mothers are hepatitis B surface antigen (HBsAg) negative. Acceptable ranges are from birth through 2 months of age for the first dose and from 1 through 4 months of age for the second dose, provided that at least 1 month elapses between these doses. The third dose should be administered at 6–18 months of age. Limited available data suggest an augmented response when the third dose is administered after 12 months of age (Merck Research Laboratories, unpublished data, 1994). Infants of HBsAg-positive mothers should receive the first dose of vaccine at birth (along with immunoprophylaxis with hepatitis B immune globulin); the second dose at 1 month of age; and the third dose at 6 months of age.

DIPHTHERIA AND TETANUS TOXOIDS AND PERTUSSIS VACCINE (DTP)

Recommendation

The current schedule for DTP vaccination is still recommended—including the option that the fourth dose may be administered at as early as 12 months of age if 6 months elapse after the third dose. Thus, the fourth dose of DTP can be scheduled with other vaccines that are administered at 12–18 months of age. DTaP currently is licensed for use only as the fourth and/or fifth dose of the DTP series for children greater than or equal to 15 months of age (2, 6).

TETANUS AND DIPHTHERIA TOXOIDS, ADSORBED, FOR ADULT USE (TD)

Recommendation

The booster dose of Td should be administered at 11–12 years of age, although vaccination at 14–16 years of age is an acceptable alternative. The earlier scheduling of this dose at 11–12 years of age encourages a routine preadolescent preventive care visit. During this visit, the practitioner should also administer a second dose of measles-containing vaccine to those persons who have not already received this dose and should ensure that children who previously have not received hepatitis B vaccine begin the vaccination series. Adolescent hepatitis B vaccination currently is recommended by AAP (2); ACIP will issue a similar recommendation. A routine visit at 11–12 years of age also will facilitate administration of other needed vaccines to adolescents.

SIMULTANEOUS ADMINISTRATION OF MULTIPLE VACCINES

Simultaneous administration of vaccines has been recommended through the administration of combined vaccines (e.g., DTP vaccine, trivalent OPV, and MMR vaccine) or administration of multiple vaccines at different sites or by different routes (e.g., simultaneous administration of DTP, OPV, and Hib). Several studies have examined the safety and immunogenicity of simultaneously administered MMR and Hib (24, 25); DTP, OPV, and MMR (26, 27); DTP, OPV, and Hib (25, 28); hepatitis B, DTP, and OPV (29–31); and hepatitis B and MMR (Merck Research Laboratories, unpublished data, 1993). Hepatitis B vaccine, the vaccine most recently licensed for use among infants, has been shown to be safe and effective when administered from birth through 15 months of age with other routinely recommended childhood vaccines (D. Greenberg, personal communication, 1994) (32). The available safety and immunogenicity data for vaccines currently recommended by ACIP and AAP have been reviewed recently (33). Although data are limited concerning the simultaneous administration of the entire recommended vaccine series (i.e., DTP, OPV, MMR, and Hib vaccines, with or without hepatitis B vaccine), data from numerous studies have indicated no interference between routinely recommended childhood vaccines (either live, attenuated or killed) (33). These findings support the simultaneous use of all vaccines as recommended.

CONCLUSION

The development of a unified childhood immunization schedule approved by ACIP, AAP, and AAFP represents the beginning of a process that will ensure continued collaboration among the recommending groups, the pharmaceutical manufacturing industry, and FDA to maintain and work toward further simplification of a unified schedule. The recommended childhood immunization schedule will be updated and published annually. Since the development of these recommendations in January 1995, FDA has licensed varicella zoster virus vaccine for use among susceptible persons greater than or equal to 12 months of age. The ACIP will publish recommendations for this new vaccine, and these recommendations will be incorporated into the 1996 Recommended Childhood Immunization Schedule.

REFERENCES: AS NUMBERED IN ORIGINAL PUBLICATION

2. American Academy of Pediatrics. Active and passive immunization. In: Peter G, ed. 1994 Red Book: report of the Committee on Infectious Diseases. 23rd ed. Elk Grove Village, IL: American Academy of Pediatrics, 1994:1–67.
6. ACIP. Pertussis vaccination: acellular pertussis vaccine for reinforcing and booster use—supplementary ACIP statement: recommendations of the Advisory Committee on Immunization Practices. MMWR 1992;41(No. RR-1):1–10.
8. ACIP. General recommendations on immunization: recommendations of the Advisory Committee on Immunization Practices (ACIP). MMWR 1994;43(No. RR-1):1–38.
24. Steinhoff MC, Thomas ML, Dannelfelser S, O'Donovan C. Immunogenicity of H. influenzae type B-CRM197 conjugate vaccine (HbOC) given simultaneously with routine childhood immunizations. Pediatr Res 1990;27:184A.

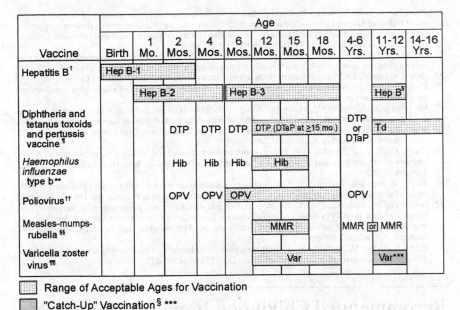

					Age						
Vaccine	Birth	1 Mo.	2 Mos.	4 Mos.	6 Mos.	12 Mos.	15 Mos.	18 Mos.	4-6 Yrs.	11-12 Yrs.	14-16 Yrs.
Hepatitis B[†]	Hep B-1										
		Hep B-2			Hep B-3					Hep B[§]	
Diphtheria and tetanus toxoids and pertussis vaccine[¶]			DTP	DTP	DTP	DTP (DTaP at ≥15 mo.)			DTP or DTaP	Td	
Haemophilus influenzae type b[**]			Hib	Hib	Hib	Hib					
Poliovirus[††]			OPV	OPV	OPV				OPV		
Measles-mumps-rubella[§§]						MMR				MMR or MMR	
Varicella zoster virus[¶¶]						Var				Var[***]	

░ Range of Acceptable Ages for Vaccination

▓ "Catch-Up" Vaccination[§ ***]

*Vaccines are listed under the routinely recommended ages.
†**Infants born to hepatitis B surface antigen (HBsAg)-negative mothers** should receive 2.5 µg of Recombivax HB® (Merck & Co.) or 10 µg of Engerix-B® (SmithKline Beecham). The second dose should be administered ≥1 month after the first dose. **Infants born to HBsAg-positive mothers** should receive 0.5 mL hepatitis B immune globulin (HBIG) within 12 hours of birth, and either 5 µg of Recombivax HB® or 10 µg of Engerix-B® at a separate site. The second dose is recommended at age 1–2 months and the third dose at age 6 months. **Infants born to mothers whose HBsAg status is unknown** should receive either 5 µg of Recombivax HB® or 10 µg of Engerix-B® within 12 hours of birth. The second dose of vaccine is recommended at age 1 month and the third dose at age 6 months.
§Adolescents who have not received three doses of hepatitis B vaccine should initiate or complete the series at age 11–12 years. The second dose should be administered at least 1 month after the first dose, and the third dose should be administered at least 4 months after the first dose and at least 2 months after the second dose.
¶The fourth dose of diphtheria and tetanus toxoids and pertussis vaccine (DTP) may be administered at age 12 months, if at least 6 months have elapsed since the third dose of DTP. Diphtheria and tetanus toxoids and acellular pertussic vaccine (DTaP) is licensed for the fourth and/or fifth vaccine dose(s) for children aged ≥15 months and may be preferred for these doses in this age group. Tetanus and diphtheria toxoids, adsorbed, for adult use (Td) is recommended at age 11–12 years if at least 5 years have elapsed since the last dose of DTP, DTaP, or diphtheria and tetanus toxoids, absorbed, for pediatric use (DT).
**Three *Haemophilus influenzae* type b (Hib) conjugate vaccines are licensed for infant use. If PedvaxHIB® (Merck & Co.) *Haemophilus* b conjugate vaccine (Meningococcal Protein Conjugate) (PRP-OMP) is administered at ages 2 and 4 months, a dose at 6 months is not required. After completing the primary series, any Hib conjugate vaccine may be used as a booster.
††Oral poliovirus vaccine (OPV) is recommended for routine infant vaccination. Inactivated poliovirus vaccine (IPV) is recommended for persons—or household contacts of persons—with a congenital or acquired immune deficiency disease or an altered immune status resulting from disease or immunosuppressive therapy, and is an acceptable alternative for other persons. The primary three-dose series for IPV should be given with a minimum interval of 4 weeks between the first and second doses and 6 months between the second and third doses.
§§The second dose of measles-mumps-rubella vaccine (MMR) is routinely recommended at 4–6 years or at age 11–12 years but may be administered at any visit provided at least 1 month has elapsed since receipt of the first dose.
¶¶Varicella zoster virus vaccine (Var) can be administered to susceptible children any time after age 12 months.
***Unvaccinated children who lack a reliable history of chickenpox should be vaccinated at age 11–12 years.

Source: Advisory Committee on Immunization Practices, American Academy of Pediatrics, and American Academy of Family Physicians.

Figure 1. Recommended childhood vaccination schedule—United States, January–June 1996.

25. Dashefsky B, Wald E, Guerra N, Byers C. Safety, tolerability, and immunogenicity of concurrent administration of Haemophilus influenzae type b conjugate vaccine (meningococcal protein conjugate) with either measles-mumps-rubella vaccine or diphtheria-tetanus-pertussis and oral poliovirus vaccines in 14- to 23-month old infants. Pediatrics 1990;85(Suppl):682–689.
26. Deforest A, Long SS, Lischner HW, et al. Simultaneous administration of measles-mumps-rubella vaccine with booster doses of diphtheria-tetanus-pertussis and poliovirus vaccines. Pediatrics 1988;81:237–246.
27. Berger R, Just M. Lack of interference between vaccines [Letter]. Pediatr Infect Dis J 1983;2:172.
28. Booy R, Moxon ER, MacFarlane JA, Mayon-White RT, Slack MPE. Efficacy of Haemophilus influenzae type B conjugate vaccine in Oxford Region [Letter]. Lancet 1992;340:847.
29. Greenberg DP, Vadheim SM, Marcy SM, Wong V, Margolis H, Ward JI. Safety and immunogenicity of two recombinant hepatitis B vaccines given to 5000 infants as part of routine immunization at 2, 4, and 6 months of age. In: Program and abstracts of the 31st Interscience Conference on Antimicrobial Agents and Chemotherapy. Chicago: ICAAC, 1991.
30. Huang LM, Lee CY, Hsu CY, et al. Effect of monovalent measles and trivalent measles-mumps-rubella vaccines at various ages and concurrent administration with hepatitis B vaccine. Pediatr Infect Dis J 1990;9:461–465.
31. Barone P, Mauro L, Leonardi S, et al. Simultaneous administration of HB recombinant vaccine with diphtheria and tetanus toxoid and oral polio vaccine: a pilot study. Acta Paediatr Jpn 1991;33:455–458.
32. Greenberg DP, Vadheim CM, Marcy SM, et al. Comparative safety and immunogenicity of two recombinant Hepatitis B (HBV) vaccines given to infants at 2, 4, and 6 months of age [Abstract]. In: Program and abstracts of the 32nd Interscience Conference on Antimicrobial Agents and Chemotherapy. Anaheim, CA: ICAAC, 1992:264.
33. King GE, Hadler SC. Simultaneous administration of childhood vaccines: an important public health policy that is safe and efficacious. Pediatr Infect Dis J 1994;13:394–407.

Recommended Childhood Immunization Schedule,1996

Original Citation: Centers for Disease Control and Prevention. Recommended childhood immunization schedule—United States, January–June 1996. MMWR 1996;44(51 & 52):940–943.

RECOMMENDED CHILDHOOD IMMUNIZATION SCHEDULE, 1996

This notice presents the recommended childhood immunization schedule for January–June 1996 (Fig. 1) to incorporate licensure of varicella zoster virus vaccine (Var) and recommendations for adolescent hepatitis B vaccination. OPV remains the recommended vaccine for routine polio vaccination in the United States. IPV is recommended for persons with compromised immune systems and their household contacts and is an acceptable alternative for other persons. ACIP is developing recommendations for expanded use of IPV in the United States.

Format Changes

A column has been added to the figure for age 1 month to indicate the second dose of hepatitis B vaccine may be given to infants as early as age 1 month. Shaded bars indicate ages at which adolescents should receive "catch-up" vaccinations if they have not received vaccinations before and, for chickenpox, lack a reliable history of the disease.

Vaccine Recommendations Changes

Hepatitis B, Infant

Because of the availability of different formulations of hepatitis B vaccine, doses are presented in micrograms rather than volumes. In addition, the footnote includes recommendations for vaccination of infants born to mothers whose hepatitis B surface antigen status is unknown.

Hepatitis B, Adolescent

A bar has been added to indicate that the three-dose series of hepatitis B vaccine should be initiated or completed for adolescents aged 11–12 years who have not previously received three doses of hepatitis B vaccine.

Poliovirus

A footnote has been added to indicate that, although oral poliovirus vaccine (OPV) is recommended for routine vaccination, inactivated poliovirus vaccine (IPV) is indicated for certain persons (i.e., those with a compromised immune system and their household contacts) and continues to be an acceptable alternative for other persons. The schedule for IPV is included in the footnote.

Measles-Mumps-Rubella Vaccine

The footnote has been changed to indicate that although the second dose of measles-mumps-rubella vaccine is routinely administered at age 4–6 years or at age 11–12 years, it may be administered at any visit if at least 1 month has elapsed since receipt of the first dose.

Var

Var was licensed in March 1995 and has been added to the schedule. This vaccine is recommended for all children at age 12–18 months. The footnote indicates that it may be administered to susceptible persons any time after age 12 months, and that it should be given at age 11–12 years to previously unvaccinated persons lacking a reliable history of chickenpox.

General Recommendations on Immunization

Original Citation: Centers for Disease Control and Prevention. General recommendations on immunization recommendations of the Advisory Committee on Immunization Practices (ACIP). MMWR 1994;43(RR-01):1–38.

Original Authors: John C. Watson, MD, MPH, Charles W. LeBaron, MD, Sonja S. Hutchins, MD, MPH, Stephen C. Hadler, MD, Walter W. Williams, MD, MPH.

DEFINITIONS

Immunobiologic

Immunobiologics include antigenic substances, such as vaccines and toxoids, or antibody-containing preparations, such as globulins and antitoxins, from human or animal donors. These products are used for active or passive immunization or therapy. The following are examples of immunobiologics:

Vaccine

A suspension of live (usually attenuated) or inactivated microorganisms (e.g., bacteria, viruses, or rickettsiae) or fractions thereof administered to induce immunity and prevent infectious disease or its sequelae. Some vaccines contain highly defined antigens (e.g., the polysaccharide of Haemophilus influenzae type b or the surface antigen of hepatitis B); others have antigens that are complex or incompletely defined (e.g., killed Bordetella pertussis or live attenuated viruses). For a list of licensed vaccines, see Table 1.

Table 1. Licensed vaccines and toxoids available in the United States, by type and recommended routes of administration

Vaccine	Type	Route
Adenovirus*	Live virus	Oral
Anthrax†	Inactivated bacteria	Subcutaneous
Bacillus of Calmette and Guérin (BCG)	Live bacteria	Intradermal/percutaneous
Cholera	Inactivated bacteria	Subcutaneous or intradermal§
Diphtheria-tetanus-pertussis (DTP)	Toxoids and inactivated whole bacteria	Intramuscular
DTP-*Haemophilus influenzae* type b conjugate (DTP-Hib)	Toxoids, inactivated whole bacteria, and bacterial polysaccharide conjugated to protein	Intramuscular
Diphtheria-tetanus-acellular pertussis (DTaP)	Toxoids and inactivated bacterial components	Intramuscular
Hepatitis B	Inactive viral antigen	Intramuscular
Haemophilus influenzae type b conjugate (Hib)¶	Bacterial polysaccharide conjugated to protein	Intramuscular
Influenza	Inactivated virus or viral components	Intramuscular
Japanese encephalitis	Inactivated virus	Subcutaneous
Measles	Live virus	Subcutaneous
Measles-mumps-rubella (MMR)	Live virus	Subcutaneous
Meningococcal	Bacterial polysaccharides of serotypes A/C/Y/W-135	Subcutaneous
Mumps	Live virus	Subcutaneous
Pertussis†	Inactivated whole bacteria	Intramuscular
Plague	Inactivated bacteria	Intramuscular
Pneumococcal	Bacterial polysaccharides of 23 pneumococcal types	Intramuscular or subcutaneous
Poliovirus vaccine, inactivated (IPV)	Inactivated viruses of all 3 serotypes	Subcutaneous
Poliovirus vaccine, oral (OPV)	Live viruses of all 3 serotypes	Oral
Rabies	Inactivated virus	Intramuscular or intradermal**
Rubella	Live virus	Subcutaneous
Tetanus	Inactivated toxin (toxoid)	Intramuscular‡
Tetanus-diphtheria (Td or DT)§§	Inactivated toxins (toxoids)	Intramuscular‡
Typhoid (parenteral)	Inactivated bacteria	Subcutaneous¶¶
(Ty21a oral)	Live bacteria	Oral
Varicella***	Live virus	Subcutaneous
Yellow fever	Live virus	Subcutaneous

*Available only to the U.S. Armed Forces.

†Distributed by the Division of Biologic Products, Michigan Department of Public Health.

§The intradermal dose is lower than the subcutaneous dose.

¶The recommended schedule for infants depends on the vaccine manufacturer; consult the package insert and ACIP recommendations for specific products.

The intradermal dose of rabies vaccine, human diploid cell (HDCV), is lower than the intramuscular dose and is used only for preexposure vaccination. **Rabies vaccine, adsorbed (RVA) should not be used intradermally.

‡Preparations with adjuvants should be administered intramuscularly.

Table 1.—*continued*

§§Td-tetanus and diphtheria toxoids for use among persons ≥7 years of age. Td contains the same amount of tetanus toxoid as DTP or DT, but contains a smaller dose of diphtheria toxoid. DT-tetanus and diphtheria toxoids for use among children <7 years of age.

¶¶Booster doses may be administered intradermally unless vaccine that is acetone-killed and dried is used.

***A live, attenuated varicella vaccine is currently under consideration for licensure. This vaccine may be available for use through a special study protocol to any physician requesting it for certain pediatric patients with acute lymphocytic leukemia. Additional information about eligibility criteria and vaccine administration is available from the Varivax Coordinating Center; telephone: (215) 283-0897 (4).

Toxoid

A modified bacterial toxin that has been made nontoxic, but retains the ability to stimulate the formation of antitoxin. For a list of licensed toxoids, see Table 1.

Immune Globulin (IG)

A sterile solution containing antibodies from human blood. It is obtained by cold ethanol fractionation of large pools of blood plasma and contains 15%–18% protein. Intended for intramuscular administration, IG is primarily indicated for routine maintenance of immunity of certain immunodeficient persons and for passive immunization against measles and hepatitis A. IG does not transmit hepatitis B virus, human immunodeficiency virus (HIV), or other infectious diseases. For a list of immune globulins, see Table 2.

Table 2. Immune globulins and antitoxins* available in the United States, by type of antibodies and indications for use

Immunobiologic	Type	Indication(s)
Botulinum antitoxin	Specific equine antibodies	Treatment of botulism
Cytomegalovirus immune globulin, intravenous (CMV-IGIV)	Specific human antibodies	Prophylaxis for bone marrow and kidney transplant recipients
Diphtheria antitoxin	Specific equine antibodies	Treatment of respiratory diphtheria
Immune globulin (IG)	Pooled human antibodies	Hepatitis A pre- and postexposure prophylaxis; measles post-exposure prophylaxis
Immune globulin, intravenous (IGIV)	Pooled human antibodies	Replacement therapy for antibody deficiency disorders; immune thrombocytopenic purpura (ITP); hypogammaglobulinemia in chronic lymphocytic leukemia; Kawasaki disease
Hepatitis B immune globulin (HBIG)	Specific human antibodies	Hepatitis B postexposure prophylaxis
Rabies immune globulin† (HRIG)	Specific human antibodies	Rabies postexposure management of persons not previously immunized with rabies vaccine
Tetanus immune globulin (TIG)	Specific human antibodies	Tetanus treatment; postexposure prophylaxis of persons not adequately immunized with tetanus toxoid
Vaccinia immune globulin (VIG)	Specific human antibodies	Treatment of eczema vaccinatum, vaccinia necrosum, and ocular vaccinia

Table 2.—*continued*

Immunobiologic	Type	Indication(s)
Varicella zoster immune globulin (VZIG)	Specific human antibodies	Post-exposure prophylaxis of susceptible immunocompromised persons, certain susceptible pregnant women, and perinatally exposed newborn infants

* Immune globulin preparations and antitoxins are administered intramuscularly unless otherwise indicated.
†HRIG is administered around the wounds in addition to the intramuscular injection.

Intravenous immune globulin (IGIV)

A product derived from blood plasma from a donor pool similar to the IG pool, but prepared so it is suitable for intravenous use. IGIV does not transmit infectious diseases. It is primarily used for replacement therapy in primary antibody-deficiency disorders, for the treatment of Kawasaki disease, immune thrombocytopenic purpura, hypogammaglobulinemia in chronic lymphocytic leukemia, and some cases of HIV infection. For a list of intravenous immune globulins, see Table 2.

Specific Immune Globulin

Special preparations obtained from blood plasma from donor pools preselected for a high antibody content against a specific antigen (e.g., hepatitis B immune globulin, varicella-zoster immune globulin, rabies immune globulin, tetanus immune globulin, vaccinia immune globulin, and cytomegalovirus immune globulin). Like IG and IGIV, these preparations do not transmit infectious diseases. For a list of specific immune globulins, see Table 2.

Antitoxin

A solution of antibodies (e.g., diphtheria antitoxin and botulinum antitoxin) derived from the serum of animals immunized with specific antigens. Antitoxins are used to confer passive immunity and for treatment. For a list of antitoxins, see Table 2.

Vaccination and Immunization

Vaccination and vaccine derive from vaccinia, the virus once used as smallpox vaccine. Thus, vaccination originally meant inoculation with vaccinia virus to make a person immune to smallpox. Vaccination currently denotes the physical act of administering any vaccine or toxoid.

Immunization is a more inclusive term denoting the process of inducing or providing immunity artificially by administering an immunobiologic. Immunization can be active or passive.

Active immunization is the production of antibody or other immune responses through the administration of a vaccine or toxoid. Passive immunization means the provision of temporary immunity by the administration of preformed antibodies. Three types of immunobiologics are administered for passive immunization: (a) pooled human IG or IGIV, (b) specific immune globulin preparations, and (c) antitoxins.

Although persons often use vaccination and immunization interchangeably in reference to active immunization, the terms are not synonymous because the administration of an immunobiologic cannot be automatically equated with the development of adequate immunity.

SUMMARY

This revision of the General Recommendations on Immunization updates the 1989 statement (1). Changes in the immunization schedule for infants and children include recommendations that the third dose of oral polio vaccine be administered routinely at 6 months of age rather than at age 15 months and that measles-mumps-rubella vaccine be administered routinely to all children at 12–15 months of age. Other updated or new sections include (a) a listing of vaccines and other immunobiologics available in the United States by type and recommended routes, advice on the proper storage and handling of immuno-biologics, a section on the recommended routes for administration of vaccines, and discussion of the use of jet injectors; b) revisions in the guidelines for spacing administration of immune globulin preparations and live virus vaccines, a discussion of vaccine interactions and recommendations for the simultaneous administration of multiple vaccines, a section on the interchangeability of vaccines from different manufacturers, and a discussion of hypersensitivity to vaccine components; (c) a discussion of vaccination during pregnancy, a section on breast-feeding and vaccination, recommendations for the vaccination of premature infants, and updated schedules for immunizing infants and children (including recommendations for the use of Haemophilus influenzae type b conjugate vaccines); (d) sections on the immunization of hemophiliacs and immunocompromised persons; (e) discussion of the Standards for Pediatric Immunization Practices (including a new table of contraindications and precautions to vaccination), information on the National Vaccine Injury Compensation Program, the Vaccine Adverse Events Reporting System, and Vaccine Information Pamphlets; and (f) guidelines for vaccinating persons without documentation of immunization, a section on vaccinations received outside the United States, and a section on reporting of vaccine-preventable diseases. These recommendations are based on information available before publishing and are not comprehensive for each vaccine. The most recent Advisory Committee on Immunization Practices (ACIP) recommendations for each specific vaccine should be consulted for more details.

Additional copies of this document and other ACIP statements can be purchased from Superintendent of Documents, U.S. Government Printing Office, Washington, DC 20202-9325. Telephone: (202) 783-3238

INTRODUCTION

Recommendations for vaccinating infants, children, and adults are based on characteristics of immunobiologics, scientific knowledge about the principles of active and passive immunization and the epidemiology of diseases, and judgments by public health officials and specialists in clinical and preventive medicine. Benefits and risks are associated with the use of all immunobiologics: no vaccine is completely safe or completely effective. Benefits of vaccination range from partial to complete protection against the consequences of infection, ranging from asymptomatic or mild infection to severe consequences, such as paralysis or death. Risks of vaccination range from common, minor, and inconvenient side effects to rare, severe, and life-threatening conditions. Thus, recommendations for immunization practices balance scientific evidence of benefits, costs, and risks to achieve optimal levels of protection against infectious disease. These recommendations describe this balance and attempt to minimize risk by providing information regarding dose, route, and spacing of immunobiologics and delineating situations that warrant precautions or contraindicate the use of these immunobiologics. These recommendations are for use only in the United States because vaccines and epidemiologic circumstances often differ in other countries. Individual circumstances may warrant deviations from these recommendations. The relative balance of benefits and risks can change as diseases are controlled or eradicated. For example, because smallpox has been eradicated throughout the world, the risk of complications associated with smallpox vaccine (vaccinia virus) now outweighs any theoretical risk of contracting smallpox or related viruses for the general population. Consequently, smallpox vaccine is no longer recommended routinely for civilians or most military personnel. Smallpox vaccine is now recommended only for selected laboratory and health-care workers with certain defined exposures to these viruses (2).

IMMUNOBIOLOGICS

The specific nature and content of immunobiologics can differ. When immunobiologics against the same infectious agents are produced by different manufacturers, active and inert ingredients in the various products are not always the same. Practitioners are urged to become familiar with the constituents of the products they use.

Suspending Fluids

These may be sterile water, saline, or complex fluids containing protein or other constituents derived from the medium or biologic system in which the vaccine is produced (e.g., serum proteins, egg antigens, and cell-culture-derived antigens).

Preservatives, Stabilizers, Antibiotics

These components of vaccines, antitoxins, and globulins are used to inhibit or prevent bacterial growth in viral cultures or the final product, or to stabilize the antigens or antibodies. Allergic reactions can occur if the recipient is sensitive to one of these additives (e.g., mercurials {thimerosal}, phenols, albumin, glycine, and neomycin).

Adjuvants

Many antigens evoke suboptimal immunologic responses. Efforts to enhance immunogenicity include mixing antigens with a variety of substances or adjuvants (e.g., aluminum adjuvants such as aluminum phosphate or aluminum hydroxide).

Storage and Handling of Immunobiologics

Failure to adhere to recommended specifications for storage and handling of immunobiologics can make these products impotent (3). Recommendations included in a product's package inserts, including reconstitution of vaccines, should be followed closely to assure maximum potency of vaccines. Vaccine quality is the shared responsibility of all parties from the time the vaccine is manufactured until administration. In general, all vaccines should be inspected and monitored to assure that the cold chain has been maintained during shipment and storage. Vaccines should be stored at recommended temperatures immediately upon receipt. Certain vaccines, such as oral polio vaccine (OPV) and yellow fever vaccine, are very sensitive to increased temperature. Other vaccines are sensitive to freezing, including diphtheria and tetanus toxoids and pertussis vaccine, adsorbed (DTP), diphtheria and tetanus toxoids and acellular pertussis vaccine, adsorbed (DTaP), diphtheria and tetanus toxoids for pediatric use (DT), tetanus and diphtheria toxoids for adult use (Td), inactivated poliovirus vaccine (IPV), Haemophilus influenzae type b conjugate vaccine (Hib), hepatitis B vaccine, pneumococcal vaccine, and influenza vaccine. Mishandled vaccine may not be easily distinguished from potent vaccine. When in doubt about the appropriate handling of a vaccine, contact the manufacturer.

ADMINISTRATION OF VACCINES

General Instructions

Persons administering vaccines should take the necessary precautions to minimize risk for spreading disease. They should be adequately immunized against hepatitis B, measles, mumps, rubella, and influenza. Tetanus and diphtheria toxoids are recommended for all persons. Hands should be washed before each new patient is seen. Gloves are not required when administering vaccinations, unless the persons who administer the vaccine will come into contact with potentially infectious body fluids or have open lesions on their hands. Syringes and needles used for injections must be sterile and preferably disposable to minimize the risk of contamination. A separate needle and syringe should be used for each injection. Different vaccines should not be mixed in the same syringe unless specifically licensed for such use.* Disposable needles and syringes should be discarded in labeled, puncture-proof containers to prevent inadvertent needlestick injury or reuse.

Routes of administration are recommended for each immunobiologic (Table 1). To avoid unnecessary local or systemic effects and to ensure optimal efficacy, the practitioner should not deviate from the recommended routes. Injectable immunobiologics should be administered where there is little likelihood of local, neural, vascular, or tissue injury. In general, vaccines containing adjuvants should be injected into the muscle mass; when administered subcutaneously or intradermally they can cause local irritation, induration, skin discoloration, inflammation, and granuloma formation. Before the vaccine is expelled into the body, the needle should be inserted into the injection site and the syringe plunger should be pulled back—if blood appears in the needle hub, the needle should be withdrawn and a new site selected. The process should be repeated until no blood appears.

Subcutaneous Injections

Subcutaneous injections are usually administered into the thigh of infants and in the deltoid area of older children and adults. A ⅝- to ¾-inch, 23- to 25-gauge needle should be inserted into the tissues below the dermal layer of the skin.

Intramuscular Injections

The preferred sites for intramuscular injections are the anterolateral aspect of the upper thigh and the deltoid muscle of the upper arm. The buttock should not be used routinely for active vaccination of infants, children, or adults because of the potential risk of injury to the sciatic nerve (5). In addition, injection into the buttock has been associated with decreased immunogenicity of hepatitis B and rabies vaccines in adults, presumably because of inadvertent subcutaneous injection or injection into deep fat tissue (6). If the buttock is used for passive immunization when large volumes are to be injected or multiple doses are necessary (e.g., large doses of immune globulin [IG]), the central region should be avoided; only the upper, outer quadrant should be used, and the needle should be directed anteriorly (i.e., not inferiorly or perpendicular to the skin) to minimize the possibility of involvement with the sciatic nerve (7).

For all intramuscular injections, the needle should be long enough to reach the muscle mass and prevent vaccine from seeping into subcutaneous tis-

*The only vaccines currently licensed to be mixed in the same syringe by the person administering the vaccine are PRP-T Haemophilus influenzae type b conjugate vaccine, lyophilized, which can be reconstituted with DTP vaccine produced by Connaught. This PRP-T/DTP combination was licensed by the FDA on November 18, 1993.

sue, but not so long as to endanger underlying neurovascular structures or bone. Vaccinators should be familiar with the structural anatomy of the area into which they are injecting vaccine. An individual decision on needle size and site of injection must be made for each person based on age, the volume of the material to be administered, the size of the muscle, and the depth below the muscle surface into which the material is to be injected.

Infants (Less than 12 Months of Age)

Among most infants, the anterolateral aspect of the thigh provides the largest muscle mass and is therefore the recommended site. However, the deltoid can also be used with the thigh; for example, when multiple vaccines must be administered at the same visit. In most cases, a ⅝- to 1-inch, 22- to 25-gauge needle is sufficient to penetrate muscle in the thigh of a 4-month-old infant. The free hand should bunch the muscle, and the needle should be directed inferiorly along the long axis of the leg at an angle appropriate to reach the muscle while avoiding nearby neurovascular structures and bone.

Toddlers and Older Children

The deltoid may be used if the muscle mass is adequate. The needle size can range from 22- to 25-gauge and from ⅝ to ¼ inches, based on the size of the muscle. As with infants, the anterolateral thigh may be used, but the needle should be longer—generally ranging from ⅞ to ¼ inches.

Adults

The deltoid is recommended for routine intramuscular vaccination among adults, particularly for hepatitis B vaccine. The suggested needle size is 1 to 1½ inches and 20- to 25-gauge.

Intradermal Injections

Intradermal injections are generally administered on the volar surface of the forearm, except for human diploid cell rabies vaccine (HDCV) for which reactions are less severe when administered in the deltoid area. With the bevel facing upwards, a ⅜- to ¾-inch, 25- or 27-gauge needle can be inserted into the epidermis at an angle parallel to the long axis of the forearm. The needle should be inserted so the entire bevel penetrates the skin and the injected solution raises a small bleb. Because of the small amounts of antigen used in intradermal injections, care must be taken not to inject the vaccine subcutaneously because it can result in a suboptimal immunologic response.

Multiple Vaccinations

If more than one vaccine preparation is administered or if vaccine and an immune globulin preparation are administered simultaneously, it is preferable to administer each at a different anatomic site. It is also preferable to avoid administering two intramuscular injections in the same limb, especially if DTP is one of the products administered. However, if more than one injection must be administered in a single limb, the thigh is usually the preferred site because of the greater muscle mass; the injections should be sufficiently separated (i.e., 1–2 inches apart) so that any local reactions are unlikely to overlap (8, 9).

Jet Injectors

Jet injectors that use the same nozzle tip to vaccinate more than one person (multiple-use nozzle jet injectors) have been used worldwide since 1952 to administer vaccines when many persons must be vaccinated with the same vaccine within a short time period. These jet injectors have been generally considered safe and effective for delivering vaccine if used properly by trained personnel; the safety and efficacy of vaccine administered by these jet injectors are considered comparable to vaccine administered by needle and syringe.

The multiple-use nozzle jet injector most widely used in the United States (Ped-o-Jet) has never been implicated in transmission of bloodborne diseases. However, the report of an outbreak of hepatitis B virus (HBV) transmission following use of one type of multiple-use nozzle jet injector in a weight loss clinic and laboratory studies in which blood contamination of jet injectors has been simulated have caused concern that the use of multiple-use nozzle jet injectors may pose a potential hazard of bloodborne-disease transmission to vaccine recipients (10). This potential risk for disease transmission would exist if the jet injector nozzle became contaminated with blood during an injection and was not properly cleaned and disinfected before subsequent injections. The potential risk of bloodborne-disease transmission would be greater when vaccinating persons at increased risk for bloodborne diseases such as HBV or human immunodeficiency virus (HIV) infection because of behavioral or other risk factors (11, 12).

Multiple-use nozzle jet injectors can be used in certain situations in which large numbers of persons must be rapidly vaccinated with the same vaccine, the use of needles and syringes is not practical, and state and/or local health authorities judge that the public health benefit from the use of the jet injector outweighs the small potential risk of bloodborne-disease transmission. This potential risk can be minimized by training health-care workers before the vaccine campaign on the proper use of jet injectors and by changing the injector tip or removing the jet injector from use if there is evidence of contamination with blood or other body fluids. In addition, mathematical and animal models suggest that the potential risk for bloodborne-disease transmission can be substantially reduced by swabbing the stationary injector tip with alcohol or acetone after each injection. It is advisable to consult sources experienced in the use of jet injectors (e.g., state or local health departments) before beginning a vaccination program in which these injectors will be used. Manufacturer's directions for use and maintenance of the jet injector devices should be followed closely.

Newer models of jet injectors that employ single-use disposable nozzle tips should not pose a potential risk of bloodborne disease transmission if used appropriately.

Regurgitated Oral Vaccine

Infants may sometimes fail to swallow oral preparations (e.g., oral poliovirus vaccine [OPV]) after administration. If, in the judgment of the person administering the vaccine, a substantial amount of vaccine is spit out, regurgitated, or vomited shortly after administration (i.e., within 5–10 minutes), another dose can be administered at the same visit. If this repeat dose is not retained, neither dose should be counted, and the vaccine should be re-administered at the next visit.

Non-Standard Vaccination Practices

The recommendations on route, site, and dosages of immunobiologics are derived from theoretical considerations, experimental trials, and clinical experience. The Advisory Committee on Immunization Practices (ACIP) strongly discourages any variations from the recommended route, site, volume, or number of doses of any vaccine.

Varying from the recommended route and site can result in (a) inadequate protection (e.g., when hepatitis B vaccine is administered in the gluteal area rather than the deltoid muscle or when vaccines are administered intradermally rather than intramuscularly) and (b) increased risk for reactions (e.g., when DTP is administered subcutaneously rather than intramuscularly). Administration of volumes smaller than those recommended, such as split doses, can result in inadequate protection. Use of larger than the recommended dose can be hazardous because of excessive local or systemic concentrations of antigens or other vaccine constituents. The use of multiple reduced doses that together equal a full immunizing dose or the use of smaller divided doses is not endorsed or recommended. The serologic response, clinical efficacy, and frequency and severity of adverse reactions with such schedules have not been adequately studied. Any vaccination using less than the standard dose or a nonstandard route or site of administration should not be counted, and the person should be revaccinated according to age. If a medically documented concern exists that revaccination may result in an increased risk of adverse effects because of repeated prior exposure from nonstandard vaccinations, immunity to most relevant antigens can be tested serologically to assess the need for revaccination.

AGE AT WHICH IMMUNOBIOLOGICS ARE ADMINISTERED

Recommendations for the age at which vaccines are administered (Table 3, Table 4, and Table 5) are influenced by several factors: age-specific risks of disease, age-specific risks of complications, ability of persons of a given age to respond to the vaccine(s), and potential interference with the immune response by passively transferred maternal antibody. In general, vaccines are recommended for the youngest age group at risk for developing the disease whose members are known to develop an adequate antibody response to vaccination.

SPACING OF IMMUNOBIOLOGICS

Interval Between Multiple Doses of Same Antigen

Some products require administration of more than one dose for development of an adequate antibody response. In addition, some products require periodic reinforcement or booster doses to maintain protection. In recommending the ages and intervals for multiple doses, the ACIP considers risks from disease and the need to induce or maintain satisfactory protection (Table 3, Table 4, and Table 5).

Longer-than-recommended intervals between doses do not reduce final antibody concentrations. Therefore, an interruption in the immunization schedule does not require reinstitution of the entire series of an immunobiologic or the addition of extra doses.

However, administering doses of a vaccine or toxoid at less than the recommended minimum intervals may decrease the antibody response and therefore should be avoided. Doses administered at less than the recommended minimum intervals should not be considered part of a primary series.

Some vaccines produce increased rates of local or systemic reactions in certain recipients when administered too frequently (e.g., adult Td, pediatric DT, tetanus toxoid, and rabies vaccines). Such reactions are thought to result from the formation of antigen-antibody complexes. Good recordkeeping, maintaining careful patient histories, and adherence to recommended schedules can decrease the incidence of such reactions without sacrificing immunity.

Table 3. Recommended schedule for routine active vaccination of infants and children*

Vaccine	At birth (before hospital discharge)	1–2 months	2 months†	4 months	6 months	6–18 months	12–15 months	15 months	4–6 years (before school entry)
Diphtheria-tetanus-pertussis§			DTP	DTP	DTP			DTaP/DTP¶	DTaP/DTP¶
Polio, live oral			OPV	OPV	OPV**				OPV
Measles-mumps-rubella							MMR		MMR‡
Haemophilus influenzae type b conjugate HbOC/PRP-T§,§§			Hib	Hib	Hib		Hib¶¶		
PRP-OMP§§			Hib	Hib			Hib¶¶		
Hepatitis B*** Option 1	HepB	HepB†††				HepB†††			
Option 2		HepB†††		HepB†††		HepB†††			

*See Table 4 for the recommended immunization schedule for infants and children up to their seventh birthday who do not begin the vaccination series at the recommended times or who are >1 month behind in the immunization schedule.

†Can be administered as early as 6 weeks of age.

§Two DTP and Hib combination vaccines are available (DTP/HbOC [TETRAMUNE™]; and PRP-T [ActHIB™, OmniHIB™] which can be reconstituted with DTP vaccine produced by Connaught).

¶This dose of DTP can be administered as early as 12 months of age provided that the interval since the previous dose of DTP is at least 6 months. *Diphtheria and tetanus toxoids and acellular pertussis vaccine (DTaP) is currently recommended only for use as the fourth and/or fifth doses of the DTP series among children aged 15 months through 6 years (before the seventh birthday).* Some experts prefer to administer these vaccines at 18 months of age.

*****The American Academy of Pediatrics (AAP) recommends this dose of vaccine at 6–18 months of age.

‡The AAP recommends that two doses of MMR should be administered by 12 years of age with the second dose being administered preferentially at entry to middle school or junior high school.

§§HbOC: [HibTITER®] (Lederle Praxis). PRP-T: [ActHIB™, OmniHIB™] (Pasteur Merieux). PRP-OMP: [PedvaxHIB®] (Merck, Sharp, and Dohme). A DTP/Hib combination vaccine can be used in place of HbOC/PRP-T.

¶¶After the primary infant Hib conjugate vaccine series is completed, any of the licensed Hib conjugate vaccines may be used as a booster dose at age 12–15 months.

***For use among infants born to HBsAg-negative mothers. The first dose should be administered during the newborn period, preferably before hospital discharge, but no later than age 2 months. Premature infants of HBsAg-negative mothers should receive the first dose of the hepatitis B vaccine series at the time of hospital discharge or when the other routine childhood vaccines are initiated. (All infants born to HBsAg-positive mothers should receive immunoprophylaxis for hepatitis B as soon as possible after birth.)

†††Hepatitis B vaccine can be administered simultaneously at the same visit with DTP (or DTaP), OPV, Hib, and/or MMR.

Table 4. Recommended accelerated immunization schedule for infants and children <7 years of age who start the series late* or who are >1 month behind in the immunization schedule[†] (i.e., children for whom compliance with scheduled return visits cannot be assured)

Timing	Vaccine(s)	Comments
First visit (≥4 mos of age)	DPT[§], OPV, Hib[¶,§], Hepatitis B, MMR (should be given as soon as child is age 12–15 mos)	All vaccines should be administered simultaneously at the appropriate visit.
Second visit (1 month after first visit)	DPT[§], Hib[¶,§], Hepatitis B	
Third visit (1 month after second visit)	DPT, OPV, HIB[¶,§]	
Fourth visit (6 weeks after third visit)	OPV	
Fifth visit (≥6 mos after third visit)	DTaP[§] or DTP, Hib[¶,§], Hepatitis B	
Additional visits (Age 4–6 yrs)	DTaP[§] or DTP, OPV, MMR	Preferably at or before school entry.
(Age 14–16 yrs)	Td	Repeat every 10 yrs throughout life.

DTP	Diphtheria-tetanus-pertussis
DTaP	Diphtheria-tetanus-acellular pertussis
Hib	Haemophilus influenzae type b conjugate
MMR	Measles-mumps-rubella
OPV	Poliovirus vaccine, live oral, trivalent
Td	Tetanus and diphtheria toxoids (for use among persons ≥7 years of age

*If initiated in the first year of life, administer DTP doses 1, 2, and 3 and OPV doses 1, 2, and 3 according to this schedule; administer MMR when the child reaches 12–15 months of age.
[†]See individual ACIP recommendations for detailed information on specific vaccines.
[§]Two DTP and Hib combination vaccines are available (DTP/HbOC [TETRAMUNE™]; and PRP-T (ActHIB™, OmniHIB™] which can be reconstituted with DTP vaccine produced by Connaught). DTaP preparations are currently recommended only for use as the fourth and/or fifth doses of the DTP series among children 15 months through 6 years of age (before the seventh birthday). DTP and DTaP should not be used on or after the seventh birthday.
[¶]The recommended schedule varies by vaccine manufacturer. For information specific to the vaccine being used, consult the package insert the ACIP recommendations. Children beginning the Hib vaccine series at age 2–6 months should receive a primary series of three doses of HbOC [HibTITER®] (Lederle-Praxis), PRP-T [ActHIB™, OmniHIB™] (Pasteur Merieux; SmithKline Beecham; Connaught), or a licensed DTP-Hib combination vaccine; or two doses of PRP-OMP (PedvaxHIB®) (Merck, Sharp, and Dohme). An additional booster dose of any licensed Hib conjugate vaccine should be administered at 12–15 months of age **and** at least 2 months after the previous dose. Children beginning the Hib vaccine series at 7–11 months of age should receive a primary series of two doses of an HbOC, PRP-T, PRP-OMP-containing vaccine. An additional booster dose of any licensed Hib conjugate vaccine should be administered at 12–18 months of age **and** at least 2 months after the previous dose. Children beginning the Hib vaccine series at ages 12–14 months should receive a primary series of one dose of an HbOC, PRP-T, or PRP-OMP-containing vaccine. An additional booster dose of any licensed Hib conjugate vaccine should be administered 2 months after the previous dose. Children beginning the Hib vaccine series at ages 15–59 months should receive one dose of any licensed Hib vaccine. Hib vaccine should not be administered after the fifth birthday except for special circumstances as noted in the specific ACIP recommendations for the use of Hib vaccine.

Table 5. Recommended immunization schedule for persons ≥7 years of age not vaccinated at the recommended time in early infancy*

Timing	Vaccine(s)	Comments
First visit	Td[†], OPV[§] MMR[¶], and Hepatitis B**	Primary poliovirus vaccination is not routinely recommended for persons ≥18 years of age.
Second visit (6–8 weeks after first visit)	Td, OPV, MMR[††,¶], Hepatitis B**	
Third visit (6 months after second visit)	Td, OPV, Hepatitis B**	
Additional visits	Td	Repeat every 10 years throughout life.

MMR	Measles-mumps-rubella
OPV	Poliovirus vaccine, live oral, trivalent
Td	Tetanus and diphtheria toxoids (for use among persons ≥7 years of age)

*See individual ACIP recommendations for details.
†The DTP and DTaP doses administered to children <7 years of age who remain incompletely vaccinated at age ≥7 years should be counted as prior exposure to tetanus and diphtheria toxoids (e.g., a child who previously received two doses of DTP needs only one dose of Td to complete a primary series of tetanus and diphtheria).
§When polio vaccine is administered to previously unvaccinated persons ≥18 years of age, inactivated poliovirus vaccine (IPV) is preferred. For the immunization schedule for IPV, see specific ACIP statement on the use of polio vaccine.
¶Persons born before 1957 can generally be considered immune to measles and mumps and need not be vaccinated. Rubella (or MMR) vaccine can be administered to persons of any age, particularly to nonpregnant women of childbearing age.
**Hepatitis B vaccine, recombinant. Selected high-risk groups for whom vaccination is recommended include persons with occupational risk, such as health-care and public-safety workers who have occupational exposure to blood, clients and staff of institutions for the developmentally disabled, hemodialysis patients, recipients of certain blood products (e.g., clotting factor concentrates), household contacts and sex partners of hepatitis B virus carriers, injecting drug users, sexually active homosexual and bisexual men, certain sexually active heterosexual men and women, inmates of long-term correctional facilities, certain international travelers, and families of HBsAg-positive adoptees from countries where HBV infection is endemic. Because risk factors are often not identified directly among adolescents, universal hepatitis B vaccination of teenagers should be implemented in communities where injecting drug use, pregnancy among teenagers, and/or sexually transmitted diseases are common.
‡The ACIP recommends a second dose of measles-containing vaccine (preferably MMR to assure immunity to mumps and rubella) for certain groups. Children with no documentation of live measles vaccination after the first birthday should receive two doses of live measles-containing vaccine not less than 1 month apart. In addition, the following persons born in 1957 or later should have documentation of measles immunity (i.e., two doses of measles-containing vaccine [at least one of which being MMR], physician-diagnosed measles, or laboratory evidence of measles immunity): (a) those entering post-high school educational settings; (b) those beginning employment in health-care settings who will have direct patient contact; and (c) travelers to areas with endemic measles.

Simultaneous Administration

Experimental evidence and extensive clinical experience have strengthened the scientific basis for administering certain vaccines simultaneously (13–16). Many of the commonly used vaccines can safely and effectively be administered simultaneously (i.e., on the same day, not at the same anatomic site). Simultaneous administration is important in certain situations, including (a) imminent exposure to several infectious diseases, (b) preparation for foreign travel, and (c) uncertainty that the person will return for further doses of vaccine.

Killed Vaccines

In general, inactivated vaccines can be administered simultaneously at separate sites. However, when vaccines commonly associated with local or systemic reactions (e.g., cholera, parenteral typhoid, and plague) are administered simultaneously, the reactions might be accentuated. When feasible, it is preferable to administer these vaccines on separate occasions.

Live Vaccines

The simultaneous administration of the most widely used live and inactivated vaccines has not resulted in impaired antibody responses or increased rates of adverse reactions. Administration of combined measles-mumps-rubella (MMR) vaccine yields results similar to administration of individual measles, mumps, and rubella vaccines at different sites. Therefore, there is no medical basis for administering these vaccines separately for routine vaccination instead of the preferred MMR combined vaccine.

Concern has been raised that oral live attenuated typhoid (Ty21a) vaccine theoretically might interfere with the immune response to OPV when OPV is administered simultaneously or soon after live oral typhoid vaccine (17). However, no published data exist to support this theory. Therefore, if OPV and oral live typhoid vaccine are needed at the same time (e.g., when international travel is undertaken on short notice), both vaccines may be administered simultaneously or at any interval before or after each other.

Routine Childhood Vaccines

Simultaneous administration of all indicated vaccines is important in childhood vaccination programs because it increases the probability that a child will be fully immunized at the appropriate age. During a recent measles outbreak, one study indicated that about one third of measles cases among unvaccinated preschool children could have been prevented if MMR had been administered at the same time another vaccine had been received (18).

The simultaneous administration of routine childhood vaccines does not interfere with the immune response to these vaccines. When administered at the same time and at separate sites, DTP, OPV, and MMR have produced seroconversion rates and rates of side effects similar to those observed when the vaccines are administered separately (13). Simultaneous vaccination of infants with DTP, OPV (or IPV), and either Hib vaccine or hepatitis B vaccine has resulted in acceptable response to all antigens (14–16). Routine simultaneous administration of DTP (or DTaP), OPV (or IPV), Hib vaccine, MMR, and hepatitis B vaccine is encouraged for children who are the recommended age to receive these vaccines and for whom no specific contraindications exist at the time of the visit, unless, in the judgment of the provider, complete vaccination of the child will not be compromised by administering different vaccines at different visits. Simultaneous administration is particularly important if the child might not return for subsequent vaccinations. Administration of MMR and Hib vaccine at 12–15 months of age, followed by DTP (or DTaP, if indicated) at age 18 months remains an acceptable alternative for children with caregivers known to be compliant with other health-care recommendations and who are likely to return for future visits; hepatitis B vaccine can be administered at either of these two visits. DTaP may be used instead of DTP only for the fourth and fifth dose for children 15 months of age through 6 years (i.e., before the seventh birthday). Individual vaccines should not be mixed in the same syringe unless they are licensed for mixing by the U.S. Food and Drug Administration (FDA).*

---

*The only vaccines currently licensed to be mixed in the same syringe by the person administering the vaccine are PRP-T Haemophilus influenzae type b conjugate vaccine, lyophilized, which can be reconstituted with DTP vaccine produced by Connaught. This PRP-T/DTP combination was licensed by the FDA on November 18, 1993.

Other Vaccines

The simultaneous administration of pneumococcal polysaccharide vaccine and whole-virus influenza vaccine elicits a satisfactory antibody response without increasing the incidence or severity of adverse reactions in adults (19). Simultaneous administration of pneumococcal vaccine and split-virus influenza vaccine can be expected to yield satisfactory results in both children and adults.

Hepatitis B vaccine administered with yellow fever vaccine is as safe and efficacious as when these vaccines are administered separately (20). Measles and yellow fever vaccines have been administered together safely and with full efficacy of each of the components (21).

The antibody response of yellow fever and cholera vaccines is decreased if administered simultaneously or within a short time of each other. If possible, yellow fever and cholera vaccinations should be separated by at least 3 weeks. If time constraints exist and both vaccines are necessary, the injections can be administered simultaneously or within a 3-week period with the understanding that antibody response may not be optimal. Yellow fever vaccine is required by many countries and is highly effective in protecting against a disease with substantial mortality and for which no therapy exists. The currently used cholera vaccine provides limited protection of brief duration; few indications exist for its use.

Antimalarials and Vaccination

The antimalarial mefloquine (Lariam®) could potentially affect the immune response to oral live attenuated typhoid (Ty21a) vaccine if both are taken simultaneously (17, 22, 23). To minimize this effect, it may be prudent to administer Ty21a typhoid vaccine at least 24 hours before or after a dose of mefloquine. Because chloroquine phosphate (and possibly other structurally related antimalarials such as mefloquine) may interfere with the antibody response to HDCV when HDCV is administered by the intradermal dose/route, HDCV should not be administered by the intradermal dose/route when chloroquine, mefloquine, or other structurally related antimalarials are used (24–26).

Nonsimultaneous Administration

Inactivated vaccines generally do not interfere with the immune response to other inactivated vaccines or to live vaccines except in certain instances (e.g., yellow fever and cholera vaccines). In general, an inactivated vaccine can be administered either simultaneously or at any time before or after a different inactivated vaccine or live vaccine. However, limited data have indicated that prior or concurrent administration of DTP vaccine may enhance anti-PRP antibody response following vaccination with certain Haemophilus influenzae type b conjugate vaccines (i.e., PRP-T, PRP-D, and HbOC) (27–29). For infants, the immunogenicity of PRP-OMP appears to be unaffected by the absence of prior or concurrent DTP vaccination (28, 30).

Theoretically, the immune response to one live-virus vaccine might be impaired if administered within 30 days of another live-virus vaccine; however no evidence exists for currently available vaccines to support this concern (31). Whenever possible, live-virus vaccines administered on different days should be administered at least 30 days apart (Table 6). However, OPV and MMR vaccines can be administered at any time before, with, or after each other, if indicated. Live-virus vaccines can interfere with the response to a tuberculin test (32–34). Tuberculin testing, if otherwise indicated, can be done either on the same day that live-virus vaccines are administered or 4–6 weeks later.

Immune Globulin/Live Vaccines

OPV and yellow fever vaccines can be administered at any time before, with, or after the administration of immune globulin or specific immune globulins (e.g., hepatitis B immune globulin [HBIG] and rabies immune globulin [RIG]) (Table 7) (35). The concurrent administration of immune globulin should not interfere with the immune response to oral Ty21a typhoid vaccine.

Table 6. Guidelines for spacing the administration of live and killed antigens

Antigen combination	Recommended minimum interval between doses
≥2 Killed antigens doses.*	None. May be administered simultaneously or at any interval between
Killed and live antigens	None. May be administered simultaneously or at any interval between doses.[†]
≥2 Live antigens	4-Week minimum interval if not administered simultaneously.[§] However, oral polio vaccine can be administered at any time before, with, or after measles-mumps-rubella, if indicated.

*If possible, vaccines associated with local or systemic side effects (e.g., cholera, parenteral typhoid, and plague vaccines) should be administered on separate occasions to avoid accentuated reactions.
[†]Cholera vaccine with yellow fever vaccine is the exception. If time permits, these antigens should not be administered simultaneously, and at least 3 weeks should elapse between administration of yellow fever vaccine and cholera vaccine. If the vaccines must be administered simultaneously or within 3 weeks of each other, the antibody response may not be optimal.
[§]If oral live typhoid vaccine is indicated (e.g., for international travel undertaken on short notice), it can be administered before, simultaneously with, or after OPV.

Previous recommendations, based on data from persons who received low doses of immune globulin, have stated that MMR and its individual component vaccines can be administered as early as 6 weeks to 3 months after administration of immune globulin (1, 36). However, recent evidence suggests that high doses of immune globulin can inhibit the immune response to measles vaccine for more than 3 months (37, 38). Administration of immune globulin can also inhibit the response to rubella vaccine (37). The effect of immune globulin preparations on the response to mumps and varicella vaccines is unknown, but commercial immune globulin preparations contain antibodies to these viruses.

Blood (e.g., whole blood, packed red blood cells, and plasma) and other antibody-containing blood products (e.g., immune globulin; specific immune globulins; and immune globulin, intravenous [IGIV]) can diminish the immune response to MMR or its individual component vaccines. Therefore, after an immune globulin preparation is received, these vaccines should not be administered before the recommended interval (Table 7 and Table 8). However, the postpartum vaccination of rubella-susceptible women with rubella or MMR vaccine should not be delayed because anti-Rho(D) IG (human) or any other blood product was received during the last trimester of pregnancy or at delivery. These women should be vaccinated immediately after delivery and, if possible, tested at least 3 months later to ensure immunity to rubella and, if necessary, to measles.

If administration of an immune globulin preparation becomes necessary because of imminent exposure to disease, MMR or its component vaccines can be administered simultaneously with the immune globulin preparation, although vaccine-induced immunity might be compromised. The vaccine should be administered at a site remote from that chosen for the immune globulin inoculation. Unless serologic testing indicates that specific antibodies have been produced, vaccination should be repeated after the recommended interval (Table 7 and Table 8).

If administration of an immune globulin preparation becomes necessary after MMR or its individual component vaccines have been administered, in-

Table 7. Guidelines for spacing the administration of immune globulin preparations* and vaccines

Immunobiologic combination	Simultaneous administration		Nonsimultaneous administration		
		Recommended minimum interval between doses	Immunobiologic administered		Recommended minimum interval between doses
			First	Second	
Immune globulin and killed antigen	None. May be given simultaneously at different sites or at any time between doses.		Immune globulin	Killed antigen	None
			Killed antigen	Immune globulin	None
Immune globulin and live antigen	Should generally not be administered simultaneously.[†] If simultaneous administration of measles-mumps-rubella [MMR], measles-rubella, and monovalent measles vaccine is unavoidable, administer at different sites and revaccinate or test for seroconversion after the recommended interval (Table 8).		Immune globulin	Live antigen	Dose related.[†§]
			Live antigen	Immune globulin	2 weeks

*Blood products containing large amounts of immune globulin (such as serum immune, globulin, specific immune globulins [e.g., TIG and HBIG], intravenous immune globulin [IGIV], whole blood, packed red cells, plasma, and platelet products).

[†]Oral polio virus, yellow fever, and oral typhoid (Ty21a) vaccines are exceptions to these recommendations. These vaccines may be administered at any time before, after, or simultaneously with an immune globulin-containing product without substantially decreasing the antibody response (35).

[§]The duration of interference of immune globulin preparations with the immune response to the measles component of the MMR, measles-rubella, and monovalent measles vaccine is dose-related (Table 8).

Table 8. Suggested intervals between administration of immune globulin preparations for various indications and vaccines containing live measles virus*

Indication	Dose (including mg IgG/kg)	Suggested interval before measles vaccination (months)
Tetanus (TIG)	250 units (10 mg IgG/kg)IM	3
Hepatitis A (IG)		
Contact prophylaxis	0.02 mL/kg (3.3 mg IgG/kg) IM	3
International travel	0.06 mL/kg (10 mg IgG/kg) IM	3
Hepatitis B prophylaxis (HBIG)	0.06 mL/kg (10 mg IgG/kg) IM	3
Rabies prophylaxis (HRIG)	20 IU/kg (22 mg IgG/kg) IM	4
Varicella prophylaxis (VZIG)	125 units/10 kg (20–40 mg IgG/kg) IM (Maximum 625 units)	5
Measles prophylaxis (IG)		
Normal contact	0.25 mL/kg (40 mg IgG/kg) IM	5
Immunocompromised contact	0.50 mL/kg (80 mg IgG/kg) IM	6
Blood transfusion		
Red blood cells (RBCs), washed	10 mL/kg (negligible IgG/kg) IV	0
RBCs, adenine-saline added	10 mL/kg (10 mg IgG/kg) IV	3
Packed RBCs (Hct 65%)[†]	10 mL/kg (60 mg IgG/kg) IV	6
Whole blood (Hct 35–50%)[†]	10 mL/kg (80–100 mg IgG/kg) IV	6
Plasma/platelet products	10 mL/kg (160 mg IgG/kg) IV	7
Replacement of humoral immune deficiencies	300–400 mg/kg IV[§] (as IGIV)	8
Treatment of:		
ITP[¶]	400 mg/kg IV (as IGIV)	8
ITP[¶]	1000 mg/kg IV (as IGIV)	10
Kawasaki disease	2 grams/kg IV (as IGIV)	11

*This table is not intended for determining the correct indications and dosage for the use of immune globulin preparations. Unvaccinated persons may not be fully protected against measles during the entire suggested interval and additional doses of immune globulin and/or measles vaccine may be indicated following measles exposure. The concentration of measles antibody in a particular immune globulin preparation can vary by lot. The rate of antibody clearance following receipt of an immune globulin preparation can also vary. The recommended intervals are extrapolated from an estimated half-life of 30 days for passively acquired antibody and an observed interference with the immune response to measles vaccine for 5 months following a dose of 80 mg IgG/kg (37).

†Assumes a serum IgG concentration of 16 mg/mL.

§Measles vaccination is recommended for children with HIV infection but is contraindicated in patients with congenital disorders of the immune system.

¶Immune (formally, idiopathic) thrombocytopenic purpura.

terference can occur. Usually, vaccine virus replication and stimulation of immunity will occur 1–2 weeks after vaccination. Thus, if the interval between administration of any of these vaccines and subsequent administration of an immune globulin preparation is less than 14 days, vaccination should be repeated after the recommended interval (Table 7 and Table 8), unless serologic testing indicates that antibodies were produced.

Killed Vaccines

Immune globulin preparations interact less with inactivated vaccines and toxoids than with live vaccines (39). Therefore, administration of inactivated vaccines and toxoids either simultaneously with or at any interval before or after receipt of immune globulins should not substantially impair the development of a protective antibody response. The vaccine or toxoid and immune globulin preparation should be administered at different sites using the standard recommended dose of corresponding vaccine. Increasing the vaccine dose volume or number of vaccinations is not indicated or recommended.

Interchangeability of Vaccines from Different Manufacturers

When at least one dose of a hepatitis B vaccine produced by one manufacturer is followed by subsequent doses from a different manufacturer, the immune response has been shown to be comparable with that resulting from a full course of vaccination with a single vaccine (11, 40).

Both HDCV and rabies vaccine, adsorbed (RVA) are considered equally efficacious and safe and, when used as licensed and recommended, are considered interchangeable during the vaccine series. RVA should not be used intradermally. The full 1.0-mL dose of either product, administered by intramuscular injection, can be used for both preexposure and postexposure prophylaxis (25).

When administered according to their licensed indications, different diphtheria and tetanus toxoids and pertussis vaccines as single antigens or various combinations, as well as the live and inactivated polio vaccines, also can be used interchangeably. However, published data supporting this recommendation are generally limited (41).

Currently licensed Haemophilus influenzae type b conjugate vaccines have been shown to induce different temporal patterns of immunologic response in infants (42). Limited data suggest that infants who receive sequential doses of different vaccines produce a satisfactory antibody response after a complete primary series (43–45). The primary vaccine series should be completed with the same Hib vaccine, if feasible. However, if different vaccines are administered, a total of three doses of Hib vaccine is considered adequate for the primary series among infants, and any combination of Hib conjugate vaccines licensed for use among infants (i.e., PRP-OMP, PRP-T, HbOC, and combination DTP-Hib vaccines) may be used to complete the primary series. Any of the licensed conjugate vaccines can be used for the recommended booster dose at 12–18 months of age (Table 3 and Table 4).

HYPERSENSITIVITY TO VACCINE COMPONENTS

Vaccine components can cause allergic reactions in some recipients. These reactions can be local or systemic and can include mild to severe anaphylaxis or anaphylactic-like responses (e.g., generalized urticaria or hives, wheezing, swelling of the mouth and throat, difficulty breathing, hypotension, and shock). The responsible vaccine components can derive from (a) vaccine antigen, (b) animal protein, (c) antibiotics, (d) preservatives, and (e) stabilizers.

The most common animal protein allergen is egg protein found in vaccines prepared using embryonated chicken eggs (e.g., influenza and yellow fever vaccines) or chicken embryo cell cultures (e.g., measles and mumps vaccines). Ordinarily, persons who are able to eat eggs or egg products safely can receive these vaccines; persons with histories of anaphylactic or anaphylactic-like allergy to eggs or egg proteins should not. Asking persons if they can eat eggs without adverse effects is a reasonable way to determine who might be at risk for allergic reactions from receiving measles, mumps, yellow fever, and influenza vaccines. Protocols requiring caution have been developed for testing and vaccinating with measles, mumps, and MMR vaccines those persons with anaphylactic reactions to egg ingestion (46–49). A regimen for administering influenza vaccine to children with egg hypersensitivity and severe asthma has also been developed (50). Rubella vaccine is grown in human diploid cell cultures and can safely be administered to persons with histories of severe allergy to eggs or egg proteins.

Some vaccines contain trace amounts of antibiotics (e.g., neomycin) to which patients may be hypersensitive. The information provided in the vaccine package insert should be carefully reviewed before deciding if the uncommon patient with such hypersensitivity should receive the vaccine(s). No currently recommended vaccine contains penicillin or penicillin derivatives.

MMR and its individual component vaccines contain trace amounts of neomycin. Although the amount present is less than would usually be used for the skin test to determine hypersensitivity, persons who have experienced anaphylactic reactions to neomycin should not receive these vaccines. Most often, neomycin allergy is a contact dermatitis—a manifestation of a delayed-type (cell-mediated) immune response—rather than anaphylaxis. A history of delayed-type reactions to neomycin is not a contraindication for these vaccines.

Certain parenteral bacterial vaccines such as cholera, DTP, plague, and typhoid are frequently associated with local or systemic adverse effects, such as redness, soreness, and fever. These reactions are difficult to link with a specific sensitivity to vaccine components and appear to be toxic rather than hypersensitive. Urticarial or anaphylactic reactions in DTP, DT, Td, or tetanus toxoid recipients have been reported rarely. When these reactions are reported, appropriate skin tests can be performed to determine sensitivity to tetanus toxoid before its use is discontinued (51). Alternatively, serologic testing to determine immunity to tetanus can be performed to evaluate the need for a booster dose of tetanus toxoid.

Exposure to vaccines containing the preservative thimerosal (e.g., DTP, DTaP, DT, Td, Hib, hepatitis B, influenza, and Japanese encephalitis) can lead to induction of hypersensitivity. However, most patients do not develop reactions to thimerosal given as a component of vaccines even when patch or intradermal tests for thimerosal indicate hypersensitivity. Hypersensitivity to thimerosal usually consists of local delayed-type hypersensitivity reactions (52, 53).

VACCINATION OF PRETERM INFANTS

Infants born prematurely, regardless of birth weight, should be vaccinated at the same chronological age and according to the same schedule and precautions as full-term infants and children (Table 3 and Table 4). Birth weight and size generally are not factors in deciding whether to postpone routine vaccination of a clinically stable premature infant (54–56). The full recommended dose of each vaccine should be used. Divided or reduced doses are not recommended (57). To prevent the theoretical risk of poliovirus transmission in the hospital, the administration of OPV should be deferred until discharge.

Any premature infant born to a hepatitis B surface antigen (HBsAg)-positive mother should receive immunoprophylaxis with hepatitis B vaccine and HBIG beginning at or shortly after birth. For premature infants of HBsAg-negative mothers, the optimal timing of hepatitis B vaccination has not been determined. Some studies suggest that decreased seroconversion rates might occur in some premature infants with low birth weights (i.e., less than 2000 grams) following administration of hepatitis B vaccine at birth (58). Such low birth weight premature infants of HBsAg-negative mothers should receive the hepatitis B vaccine series, which can be initiated at discharge from the nursery if the infant weighs at least 2000 grams or at 2 months of age along with DTP, OPV, and Hib vaccine.

BREAST-FEEDING AND VACCINATION

Neither killed nor live vaccines affect the safety of breast-feeding for mothers or infants. Breast-feeding does not adversely affect immunization and is not a contraindication for any vaccine. Breast-fed infants should be vaccinated according to routine recommended schedules (59–61).

Inactivated or killed vaccines do not multiply within the body. Therefore they should pose no special risk for mothers who are breast-feeding or for their infants. Although live vaccines do multiply within the mother's body, most have not been demonstrated to be excreted in breast milk. Although rubella vaccine virus may be transmitted in breast milk, the virus usually does not infect the infant, and if it does, the infection is well-tolerated. There is no contraindication for vaccinating breast-feeding mothers with yellow fever vaccine. Breast-feeding mothers can receive OPV without any interruption in the feeding schedule.

VACCINATION DURING PREGNANCY

Risk from vaccination during pregnancy is largely theoretical. The benefit of vaccination among pregnant women usually outweighs the potential risk when (a) the risk for disease exposure is high, (b) infection would pose a special risk to the mother or fetus, and (c) the vaccine is unlikely to cause harm.

Combined tetanus and diphtheria toxoids are the only immunobiologic agents routinely indicated for susceptible pregnant women. Previously vaccinated pregnant women who have not received a Td vaccination within the last 10 years should receive a booster dose. Pregnant women who are unimmunized or only partially immunized against tetanus should complete the primary series. Depending on when a woman seeks prenatal care and the required interval between doses, one or two doses of Td can be administered before delivery. Women for whom the vaccine is indicated but who have not completed the required three-dose series during pregnancy should be followed up after delivery to assure they receive the doses necessary for protection.

There is no convincing evidence of risk from vaccinating pregnant women with other inactivated virus or bacteria vaccines or toxoids. Hepatitis B vaccine is recommended for women at risk for hepatitis B infection, and influenza and pneumococcal vaccines are recommended for women at risk for infection and for complications of influenza and pneumococcal disease.

OPV can be administered to pregnant women who are at substantial risk of imminent exposure to natural infection (62). Although OPV is preferred, IPV may be considered if the complete vaccination series can be administered before the anticipated exposure. Pregnant women who must travel to areas where the risk for yellow fever is high should receive yellow fever vaccine. In these circumstances, the small theoretical risk from vaccination is far outweighed by the risk of yellow fever infection (21, 63). Known pregnancy is a contraindication for rubella, measles, and mumps vaccines. Although of theoretical concern, no cases of congenital rubella syndrome or abnormalities attributable to a rubella vaccine virus infection have been observed in infants born to susceptible mothers who received rubella vaccine during pregnancy.

Persons who receive measles, mumps, or rubella vaccines can shed these viruses but generally do not transmit them. These vaccines can be administered safely to the children of pregnant women. Although live polio virus is shed by persons recently vaccinated with OPV (particularly after the first dose), this vaccine can also be administered to the children of pregnant women because experience has not revealed any risk of polio vaccine virus to the fetus.

All pregnant women should be evaluated for immunity to rubella and tested for the presence of HBsAg. Women susceptible to rubella should be vaccinated immediately after delivery. A woman infected with HBV should be followed carefully to assure the infant receives HBIG and begins the hepatitis B vaccine series shortly after birth.

There is no known risk to the fetus from passive immunization of pregnant women with immune globulin preparations. Further information regarding immunization of pregnant women is available in the American College of Obstetricians and Gynecologists Technical Bulletin Number 160, October 1991. This publication is available from the American College of Obstetricians and Gynecologists, Attention: Resource Center, 409 12th Street SW, Washington, DC 20024-2188.

ALTERED IMMUNOCOMPETENCE

The ACIP statement on vaccinating immunocompromised persons summarizes recommendations regarding the efficacy, safety, and use of specific vaccines and immune globulin preparations for immunocompromised persons (64). ACIP statements on individual vaccines or immune globulins also contain additional information regarding these issues.

Severe immunosuppression can be the result of congenital immunodeficiency, HIV infection, leukemia, lymphoma, generalized malignancy or therapy with alkylating agents, antimetabolites, radiation, or large amounts of corticosteroids. Severe complications have followed vaccination with live, attenuated virus vaccines and live bacterial vaccines among immunocompromised patients (65–71). In general, these patients should not receive live vaccines except in certain circumstances that are noted below. In addition, OPV should not be administered to any household contact of a severely immunocompromised person. If polio immunization is indicated for immunocompromised patients, their household members, or other close contacts, IPV should be administered. MMR vaccine is not contraindicated in the close contacts of immunocompromised patients. The degree to which a person is immunocompromised should be determined by a physician.

Limited studies of MMR vaccination in HIV-infected patients have not documented serious or unusual adverse events. Because measles may cause severe illness in persons with HIV infection, MMR vaccine is recommended for all asymptomatic HIV-infected persons and should be considered for all symptomatic HIV-infected persons. HIV-infected persons on regular IGIV therapy may not respond to MMR or its individual component vaccines because of the continued presence of passively acquired antibody. However, because of the potential benefit, measles vaccination should be considered approximately 2 weeks before the next monthly dose of IGIV (if not otherwise contraindicated), although an optimal immune response is unlikely to occur. Unless serologic testing indicates that specific antibodies have been produced, vaccination should be repeated (if not otherwise contraindicated) after the recommended interval (Table 8).

An additional dose of IGIV should be considered for persons on routine IGIV therapy who are exposed to measles greater than or equal to 3 weeks after administration of a standard dose (100–400 mg/kg) of IGIV.

Killed or inactivated vaccines can be administered to all immunocompromised patients, although response to such vaccines may be suboptimal. All such childhood vaccines are recommended for immunocompromised persons in usual doses and schedules; in addition, certain vaccines such as pneumococcal vaccine or Hib vaccine are recommended specifically for certain groups of immunocompromised patients, including those with functional or anatomic asplenia.

Vaccination during chemotherapy or radiation therapy should be avoided because antibody response is poor. Patients vaccinated while on immunosuppressive therapy or in the 2 weeks before starting therapy should be considered unimmunized and should be revaccinated at least 3 months after therapy is discontinued. Patients with leukemia in remission whose chemotherapy has been terminated for 3 months may receive live-virus vaccines.

The exact amount of systemically absorbed corticosteroids and the duration of administration needed to suppress the immune system of an otherwise healthy child are not well defined. Most experts agree that steroid therapy usually does not contraindicate administration of live virus vaccine when it is short term (i.e., less than 2 weeks); low to moderate dose; long-term, alternate-day treatment with short-acting preparations; maintenance physiologic doses (replacement therapy); or administered topically (skin or eyes), by aerosol, or by intra-articular, bursal, or tendon injection (64). Although of recent theoretical concern, no evidence of increased severe reactions to live vaccines has been reported among persons receiving steroid therapy by aerosol, and such therapy is not in itself a reason to delay vaccination. The immunosuppressive effects of steroid treatment vary, but many clinicians consider a dose equivalent to either 2 mg/kg of body weight or a total of 20 mg per day of prednisone as sufficiently immunosuppressive to raise concern about the safety of vaccination with live virus vaccines (64). Corticosteroids used in greater than physiologic doses also can reduce the immune response to vaccines. Physicians should wait at least 3 months after discontinuation of therapy before administering a live-virus vaccine to patients who have received high systemically absorbed doses of corticosteroids for greater than or equal to 2 weeks.

VACCINATION OF PERSONS WITH HEMOPHILIA

Persons with bleeding disorders such as hemophilia have an increased risk of acquiring hepatitis B and at least the same risk as the general population of acquiring other vaccine-preventable diseases. However, because of the risk of hematomas, intramuscular injections are often avoided among persons with bleeding disorders by using the subcutaneous or intradermal routes for vaccines that are normally administered by the intramuscular route. Hepatitis B vaccine administered intramuscularly to 153 hemophiliacs using a 23-gauge needle, followed by steady pressure to the site for 1 to 2 minutes, has resulted in a 4% bruising rate with no patients requiring factor supplementation (72). Whether an antigen that produces more local reactions, such as pertussis, would produce an equally low rate of bruising is unknown.

When hepatitis B or any other intramuscular vaccine is indicated for a patient with a bleeding disorder, it should be administered intramuscularly if, in the opinion of a physician familiar with the patient's bleeding risk, the vaccine can be administered with reasonable safety by this route. If the patient receives antihemophilia or other similar therapy, intramuscular vaccination can be scheduled shortly after such therapy is administered. A fine needle (less than or equal to 23-gauge) can be used for the vaccination and firm pressure applied to the site (without rubbing) for at least 2 minutes. The patient or family should be instructed concerning the risk of hematoma from the injection.

MISCONCEPTIONS CONCERNING TRUE CONTRAINDICATIONS AND PRECAUTIONS TO VACCINATION

Some health-care providers inappropriately consider certain conditions or circumstances to be true contraindications or precautions to vaccination. This misconception results in missed opportunities to administer needed vaccines. Likewise, providers may fail to understand what constitutes a true contraindication or precaution and may administer a vaccine when it should be withheld. This practice can result in an increased risk of an adverse reaction to the vaccine.

Standards for Pediatric Immunization Practice

National standards for pediatric immunization practices have been established and include true contraindications and precautions to vaccination (Table 9) (73). True contraindications, applicable to all vaccines, include a history of anaphylactic or anaphylactic-like reactions to the vaccine or a vaccine constituent (unless the recipient has been desensitized) and the presence of a moderate or severe illness with or without a fever. Except as noted previously, severely immunocompromised persons should not receive live vaccines. Persons who developed an encephalopathy within 7 days of administration of a previous dose of DTP or DTaP should not receive further doses of DTP or DTaP. Persons infected with HIV, with household contacts infected with HIV, or with known altered immunodeficiency should receive IPV rather than OPV. Because of the theoretical risk to the fetus, women known to be pregnant should not receive MMR.

Table 9. Guide to contraindications and precautions to vaccinations*

True contraindications and precautions	Not contraindications (vaccines may be administered)
General for all vaccines (DTP/DTaP, OPV, IPV, MMR, Hib, Hepatitis B)	

Contraindications
  Anaphylactic reaction to a vaccine contraindicates further doses of that vaccine
	Not contraindications
	  Mild to moderate local reaction (soreness, redness, swelling) following a dose of an injectable antigen

Anaphylactic reaction to a vaccine constituent contraindicates the use of vaccines containing that substance	Mild acute illness with or without low-grade fever
Moderate or severe illnesses with or without a fever	Current antimicrobial therapy
	Convalescent phase of illnesses
	Prematurity (same dosage and indications as for normal, full-term infants)
	Recent exposure to an infectious disease
	History of penicillin or other nonspecific allergies or family history of such allergies
DTP/DTaP	

Contraindications
  Encephalopathy within 7 days of administration of previous dose of DTP
	Not contraindications
	  Temperature of <40.5° C (105° F) following a previous dose of DTP

Precautions[†] Fever of ≥40.5°C (105°F) within 48 hrs after vaccination with a prior dose of DTP	Family history of convulsions[§]
Collapse or shocklike state (hypotonic-hyporesponsive episode) within 48 hrs of receiving a prior dose of DTP	Family history of sudden infant death syndrome Family history of an adverse event following DTP administration
Seizures within 3 days of receiving a prior dose of DTP[§]	
Persistent, inconsolable crying lasting ≥3 hrs within 48 hrs of receiving a prior dose of DTP	

Table 9.—*continued*

OPV[1]

Contraindications	Not contraindications
Infection with HIV or a household contact with HIV	Breast-feeding
Known altered immunodeficiency (hematologic and solid tumors; congenital immunodeficiency; and long-term immunosuppressive therapy)	Current antimicrobial therapy
	Diarrhea
Immunodeficient household contact	

Precaution[†]
Pregnancy

IPV

Contraindication
Anaphylactic reaction to neomycin or streptomycin

Precaution[†]
Pregnancy

MMR[1]

Contraindications	Not contraindications
Anaphylactic reactions to egg ingestion and to neomycin[**]	Tuberculosis or positive PPD skin test
	Simultaneous TB skin testing[‡]
Pregnancy	
	Breast-feeding
Known altered immunodeficiency (hematologic and solid tumors; congenital immunodeficiency; and long-term immunosuppressive therapy)	Pregnancy of mother of recipient
	Immunodeficient family member or household contact
Precaution[†]	
Recent immune globulin administration (see Table 8)	Infection with HIV
	Nonanaphylactic reactions to eggs or neomycin

Hib

Contraindication	Not a contraindication
None identified	History of Hib disease

Hepatitis B

Contraindication	Not a contraindication
Anaphylactic reaction to common baker's yeast	Pregnancy

*This information is based on the recommendations of the Advisory Committee on Immunization Practices (ACIP) and those of the Committee on Infectious Diseases (Red Book Committee) of the American Academy of Pediatrics (AAP). Sometimes these recommendations vary from those contained in the manufacturer's package inserts. For more detailed information, providers should consult the published recommendations of the ACIP, AAP, and the manufacturer's package inserts.

†The events or conditions listed as precautions, although not contraindications, should be carefully reviewed. The benefits and risks of administering a specific vaccine to an individual under the circumstances should be considered. If the risks are believed to outweigh the benefits, the vaccination should be withheld; if the benefits are believed to outweigh the risks (for example, during an outbreak or foreign travel), the vaccination should be administered. Whether and when to administer DTP to children with proven or suspected underlying neurologic disorders should be decided on an individual basis. It is prudent on theoretical grounds to avoid vaccinating pregnant women. However, if immediate protection against poliomyelitis

is needed, OPV is preferred, although IPV may be considered if full vaccination can be completed before the anticipated imminent exposure.

§Acetaminophen given before administering DTP and thereafter every 4 hours for 24 hours should be considered for children with a personal or family history of convulsions in siblings or parents.

¶No data exist to substantiate the theoretical risk of a suboptimal immune response from the administration of OPV and MMR within 30 days of each other.

**Persons with a history of anaphylactic reactions following egg ingestion should be vaccinated only with caution. Protocols have been developed for vaccinating such persons and should be consulted. [J Pediatr 1983;102:196–199, J Pediatr 1988;113:504–506.]

‡Measles vaccination may temporarily suppress tuberculin reactivity. If testing can not be done the day of MMR vaccination, the test should be postponed for 4–6 weeks.

Certain conditions are considered precautions rather than true contraindications for vaccination. When faced with these conditions, some providers may elect to administer vaccine if they believe that the benefits outweigh the risks for the patient. For example, caution should be exercised in vaccinating a child with DTP who, within 48 hours of receipt of a prior dose of DTP, developed fever greater than or equal to 40.5°C (105°F); had persistent, inconsolable crying for greater than or equal to 3 hours; collapsed or developed a shock-like state; or had a seizure within 3 days of receiving the previous dose of DTP.

Conditions often inappropriately regarded as contraindications to vaccination are also noted (Table 9). Among the most important are diarrhea and minor upper-respiratory illnesses with or without fever, mild to moderate local reactions to a previous dose of vaccine, current antimicrobial therapy, and the convalescent phase of an acute illness. Diarrhea is not a contraindication to OPV.

Febrile Illness

The decision to administer or delay vaccination because of a current or recent febrile illness depends on the severity of symptoms and on the etiology of the disease.

All vaccines can be administered to persons with minor illness such as diarrhea, mild upper-respiratory infection with or without low-grade fever, or other low-grade febrile illness. Studies suggest that failure to vaccinate children with minor illness can seriously impede vaccination efforts (74–76). Among persons whose compliance with medical care cannot be assured, it is particularly important to take every opportunity to provide appropriate vaccinations.

Most studies from developed and developing countries support the safety and efficacy of vaccinating persons who have mild illness (77–79). One large ongoing study in the United States has indicated that more than 97% of children with mild illnesses develop measles antibody after vaccination (80). Only one study has reported a somewhat lower rate of seroconversion (79%) to the measles component of MMR vaccine among children with minor, afebrile upper-respiratory infection (81). Therefore, vaccination should not be delayed because of the presence of mild respiratory illness or other illness with or without fever.

Persons with moderate or severe febrile illness should be vaccinated as soon as they have recovered from the acute phase of the illness. This precaution avoids superimposing adverse effects of the vaccine on the underlying illness or mistakenly attributing a manifestation of the underlying illness to the vaccine.

Routine physical examinations and measuring temperatures are not prerequisites for vaccinating infants and children who appear to be healthy. Asking the parent or guardian if the child is ill and then postponing vaccination for those with moderate to severe illness, or proceeding with vaccination if no contraindications exist, are appropriate procedures in childhood immunization programs.

REPORTING OF ADVERSE EVENTS FOLLOWING VACCINATION

Modern vaccines are safe and effective. However, some adverse events have been reported following the administration of all vaccines. These events range from frequent, minor, local reactions to extremely rare, severe, systemic illness, such as paralysis associated with OPV. It is often impossible to establish evidence for cause-and-effect relationships on the basis of case reports alone because temporal association alone does not necessarily indicate causation. Unless the syndrome following vaccination is clinically or pathologically distinctive, more detailed epidemiologic studies to compare the incidence rates of the event in vaccinees with the incidence rates among unvaccinated persons may be necessary. Reporting of serious adverse events is extremely important to stimulate studies to confirm a causal association and to study risk factors for adverse events. More complete information on adverse reactions to a specific vaccine may be found in the ACIP recommendations for that vaccine.

Health-care providers are required to report selected events occurring after vaccination to the Vaccine Adverse Events Reporting System (VAERS). Persons other than health-care workers can also report adverse events to VAERS. Adverse events other than those that must be reported or that occur after administration of other vaccines, especially events that are serious or unusual, should also be reported to VAERS regardless of whether the provider thinks they are causally associated. VAERS forms and instructions are available in the FDA Drug Bulletin and the Physicians' Desk Reference, or by calling the 24-hour VAERS information recording at 1–800-822-7967.

VACCINE INJURY COMPENSATION

The National Vaccine Injury Compensation Program, established by the National Childhood Vaccine Injury Act of 1986, is a system under which compensation can be paid on behalf of a person who was injured or died as a result of receiving a vaccine. The program, which became effective on October 1, 1988, is intended as an alternative to civil litigation under the traditional tort system in that negligence need not be proven.

The law establishing the program also created a vaccine injury table, which lists the vaccines covered by the program and the injuries, disabilities, illnesses, and conditions (including death) for which compensation may be paid. The table also defines the period of time during which the first symptom or substantial aggravation of the injury must appear. Persons may be compensated for an injury listed in the established table or one that can be demonstrated to result from administration of a listed vaccine. Injuries following administration of vaccines not listed in the legislation authorizing the program are not eligible for compensation through the program. Additional information about the program is available from: National Vaccine Injury Compensation Program Health Resources and Services Administration Parklawn Building, Room 8–05 5600 Fishers Lane Rockville, MD 20857; Telephone: (800) 338-2382 (24-hour recording).

Persons wishing to file a claim for vaccine injury should call or write to: U.S. Court of Federal Claims 717 Madison Place, NW, Washington, DC 20005; Telephone: (202) 219-9657

PATIENT INFORMATION

Parents, guardians, legal representatives, and adolescent and adult patients should be informed about the benefits and risks of vaccine in understandable language. Opportunity for questions and answers should be provided before each vaccination.

Vaccine Information Pamphlets

The National Childhood Vaccine Injury Act (NCVIA) requires that vaccine information materials be developed for each vaccine covered by the Act (DTP or component antigens, MMR or component antigens, IPV, and OPV). The resulting Vaccine Information Pamphlets must be used by all public and private providers of vaccines, although private providers may elect to develop their own materials. Such materials must contain the specific, detailed elements required by law. Copies of these pamphlets are available from individual providers and from state health authorities responsible for immunization (82).

Important Information Statements

CDC has developed Important Information Statements for the vaccines not covered by the NCVIA. These statements must be used in public health clinics and other settings where federally purchased vaccines are used. Copies can be obtained from state health authorities responsible for immunization. The use of similar statements in the private sector is encouraged.

IMMUNIZATION RECORDS

Provider Records

Documentation of patient vaccinations helps ensure that persons in need of vaccine receive it and that adequately vaccinated patients are not overimmunized, increasing the risk for hypersensitivity (e.g., tetanus toxoid hypersensitivity). Serologic test results for vaccine-preventable diseases (such as those for rubella screening) as well as documented episodes of adverse events also should be recorded in the permanent medical record of the vaccine recipient.

Health-care providers who administer one or more of the vaccines covered by NVICP are required to ensure that the permanent medical record of the recipient (or a permanent office log or file) states the date the vaccine was administered, the vaccine manufacturer, the vaccine lot number, and the name, address, and title of the person administering the vaccine. The term health-care provider is defined as any licensed health-care professional, organization, or institution, whether private or public (including federal, state, and local departments and agencies), under whose authority a specified vaccine is administered. The ACIP recommends that the above information be kept for all vaccines and not only for those required by the National Vaccine Injury Act.

Patient's Personal Record

Official immunization cards have been adopted by every state and the District of Columbia to encourage uniformity of records and to facilitate the assessment of immunization status by schools and child care centers. The records are also important tools in immunization education programs aimed at increasing parental and patient awareness of the need for vaccines. A permanent immunization record card should be established for each newborn infant and maintained by the parent. In many states, these cards are distributed to new mothers before discharge from the hospital. Some states are developing computerized immunization record systems.

Persons Without Documentation of Vaccinations

Health-care providers frequently encounter persons who have no adequate documentation of vaccinations. Although vaccinations should not be postponed if records cannot be found, an attempt to locate missing records should be made by contacting previous health-care providers. If records cannot be located, such persons should be considered susceptible and should be started on the age-appropriate immunization schedule (Table 4 and Table 5). The following guidelines are recommended:

- MMR, OPV (or IPV, if indicated), Hib, hepatitis B, and influenza vaccines can be administered because no adverse effects of repeated vaccination have been demonstrated with these vaccines.
- Persons who develop a serious adverse reaction after administration of DTP, DTaP, DT, Td, or tetanus toxoid should be individually assessed before the administration of further doses of these vaccines (see the ACIP recommendations for use of diphtheria, tetanus, and pertussis vaccines) (14, 83, 84).
- Pneumococcal vaccine should be administered, if indicated. In most studies, local reactions in adults after revaccination were similar compared with initial vaccination (see the ACIP recommendations for the use of Pneumococcal Polysaccharide Vaccine for further details) (85).

Acceptability of Vaccinations Received Outside the United States

The acceptability of vaccines received in other countries for meeting vaccination requirements in the United States depends on vaccine potency, adequate documentation of receipt of the vaccine, and the vaccination schedule used. Although problems with vaccine potency have occasionally been detected (most notably with tetanus toxoid and OPV), the majority of vaccine used worldwide is from reliable local or international manufacturers. It is reasonable to assume that vaccine received in other countries was of adequate potency.

Thus, the acceptability of vaccinations received outside the United States depends primarily on whether receipt of the vaccine was adequately documented and whether the immunization schedule (i.e., age at vaccination and spacing of vaccine doses) was comparable with that recommended in the United States (Table 3, Table 4, Table 5, and Table 10). The following recommendations are derived from current immunization guidelines in the United States. They are based on minimum acceptable standards and may not represent optimal recommended ages and intervals.

Table 10. Minimum age for initial vaccination and minimum interval between vaccine doses, by type of vaccine

Vaccine	Minimum age for first dose*	Minimum interval from dose 1 to 2*	Minimum interval from dose 2 to 3*	Minimum interval from dose 3 to 4*
DTP (DT)†	6 weeks	4 weeks	4 weeks	6 months
Combined DTP-Hib	6 weeks	1 month	1 month	6 months
DTaP*	15 months			6 months
Hib (primary series)				
HbOC	6 weeks	1 month	1 month	¶
PRP-T	6 weeks	1 month	1 month	¶
PRP-OMP	6 weeks	1 month	¶	
OPV	6 weeks§	6 weeks	6 weeks	
IPV**	6 weeks	4 weeks	6 months‡	
MMR	12 months§§	1 month		
Hepatitis B	birth	1 month	2 months¶¶	

Table 10.—*continued*

DTP	Diphtheria-tetanus-pertussis
DTaP	Diphtheria-tetanus-acellular pertussis
Hib	*Haemophilus influenza* type b conjugate
IPV	Inactivated poliovirus vaccine
MMR	Measles-mumps-rubella
OPV	Live oral polio vaccine

*These minimum acceptable ages and intervals may not correspond with the optimal recommended ages and intervals for vaccination. See tables 3–5 for the current recommended routine and accelerated vaccination schedules.

†DTaP can be used in place of the fourth (and fifth) dose of DTP for children who are at least 15 months of age. Children who have received all four primary vaccination doses before their fourth birthday should receive a fifth dose of DTP (DT) or DTaP at 4–6 years of age before entering kindergarten or elementary school **and** at least 6 months after the fourth dose. The total number of doses of diphtheria and tetanus toxoids should not exceed six each before the seventh birthday (14).

§The American Academy of pediatrics permits DTP and OPV to be administered as early as 4 weeks of age in areas with high endemicity and during outbreaks.

¶The booster dose of Hib vaccine which is recommended following the primary vaccination series should be administered no earlier than 12 months of age **and** at least 2 months after the previous dose of Hib vaccine (Tables 3 and 4).

**See text to differentiate conventional inactivated poliovirus vaccine from enhanced-potency IPV.

‡For unvaccinated adults at increased risk of exposure to piliovirus with <3 months but >2 months available before protection is needed, three doses of IPV should be administered at least 1 month apart.

§§Although the age for measles vaccination may be as young as 6 months in outbreak areas where cases are occurring in children <1 year of age, children initially vaccinated before the first birthday should be revaccinated at 12–15 months of age and an additional dose of vaccine should be administered at the time of school entry or according to local policy. Doses of MMR or other measles-containing vaccines should be separated by at least 1 month.

¶¶This final dose is recommended no earlier than 4 months of age.

Only doses of vaccine with written documentation of the date of receipt should be accepted as valid. Self-reported doses of vaccine without written documentation should not be accepted.

Because childhood vaccination schedules vary in different countries, the age at vaccination and the spacing of doses may differ from that recommended in the United States. The age at vaccination is particularly important for measles vaccine. In most developing countries, measles vaccine is administered at 9 months of age when seroconversion rates are lower than at ages 12–15 months. For this reason, children vaccinated against measles before their first birthday should be revaccinated at 12–15 months of age and again, depending on state or local policy, upon entry to primary, middle, or junior high school. Doses of MMR or other measles-containing vaccines should be separated by at least 1 month. Combined MMR vaccine is preferred. Children who received monovalent measles vaccine rather than MMR on or after their first birthday also should receive a primary dose of mumps and rubella vaccines.

In most countries, including the United States, the first of three regularly scheduled doses of OPV is administered at 6 weeks of age at the same time as DTP vaccine. However, in polio-endemic countries, an extra dose of OPV is often administered at birth or at less than or equal to 2 weeks of age. For acceptability in the United States, doses of OPV and IPV administered at greater than or equal to 6 weeks (42 days) of age can be counted as a valid part of the vaccination series. For the primary vaccination series, each of the three doses of OPV should have been separated by a minimum of 6 weeks (42 days). If enhanced-potency IPV (available in the United States beginning in 1988) was received, the first two doses should have been separated by at least 4 weeks with at least 6 months between the second and third dose. If conventional inactivated poliovirus vaccine (available in the United States until 1988 and still used routinely in some countries [e.g., the Netherlands]) was used for the primary series, the first three doses should have been separated by at least 4 weeks with at least 6 months between the third and fourth dose. If both OPV and an inactivated poliovirus vaccine were received, the primary vaccination series should consist of a combined total of four doses of polio vaccine, unless the use of enhanced potency IPV can be verified. If OPV and enhanced-potency IPV were received, the primary series consists of a combined total of three doses of polio vaccine. Any dose of polio vaccine administered at the above recommended minimum intervals can be considered valid. Because the recommended polio vaccination schedule in many countries differs from that used in the United States, persons vaccinated outside the United States may need one or more additional doses of OPV (or enhanced-potency IPV) to meet current immunization guidelines in the United States.

Any dose of DTP vaccine or Hib vaccine administered at greater than or equal to 6 weeks of age can be considered valid. The "booster" dose of Hib vaccine should not have been administered before age 12 months. The first three doses of DTP vaccine should have been separated by a minimum of 4 weeks, and the fourth dose should have been administered no less than 6 months after the third dose. Doses of Hib vaccine in the primary series should have been administered no less than 1 month apart. The booster dose of Hib vaccine should have been administered at least 2 months after the previous dose.

The first dose of hepatitis B vaccine can be administered as early as at birth and should have been separated from the second dose by at least 1 month. The final (third or fourth) dose should have been administered no sooner than 4 months of age and at least 2 months after the previous dose, although an interval of at least 4 months is preferable.

Any dose of vaccine administered at the recommended minimum intervals can be considered valid. Intervals longer than those recommended do not affect antibody titers and may be counted. Immunization requirements for school entry vary by state. Specific state requirements should be consulted if vaccinations have been administered by schedules substantially different from those routinely recommended in the United States.

VACCINE PROGRAMS

The best way to reduce vaccine-preventable diseases is to have a highly immune population. Universal immunization is an important part of good health care and should be accomplished through routine and intensive programs carried out in physicians' offices and in public-health clinics. Programs should be established and maintained in all communities with the goal to ensure vaccination of all children at the recommended age. In addition, appropriate vaccinations should be available for all adults.

Providers should strive to adhere to the Standards for Pediatric Immunization Practices (74). These Standards define appropriate immunization practices for both the public and private sectors. The Standards provide guidance on how to make immunization services more conducive to the needs of children through implementation of practices which will result in eliminating barriers to vaccination. These include practices aimed at eliminating unnecessary prerequisites for receiving vaccines, eliminating missed opportunities to vaccinate, improving procedures to assess a child's need for vaccines, enhancing knowledge about vaccinations among both parents and providers, and improving the management and reporting of adverse events. In addition, the Standards address the importance of tracking systems and the use of audits to monitor clinic/office immunization coverage levels among clients. The Standards are the goal to which all providers should strive to attain appropriate vaccination of all children.

Standards of practice have also been published to increase vaccination levels among adults (86). All adults should complete a primary series of tetanus and diphtheria toxoids and receive a booster dose every 10 years. Persons greater than or equal to 65 years of age and all adults with medical conditions that place them at risk for pneumococcal disease or serious complications of influenza should receive pneumococcal polysaccharide vaccine and annual injections of influenza vaccine. Adult immunization programs should also provide MMR vaccine whenever possible to anyone susceptible to measles, mumps, or rubella. Persons born after 1956 who are attending college (or other post-high school educational institutions), who are newly employed in situations that place them at high risk for measles transmission (e.g., health-care facilities), or who are traveling to areas with endemic measles, should have documentation of having received two doses of live MMR on or after their first birthday or other evidence of immunity. All other young adults in this age group should have documentation of a single dose of live MMR vaccine on or after their first birthday or have other evidence of immunity. Use of MMR causes no harm if the vaccinee is already immune to one or more of its components and its use ensures that the vaccinee has been immunized against three different diseases. In addition, widespread use of hepatitis B vaccine is encouraged for all persons who are or may be at increased risk (e.g., adolescents and adults who are either in a high-risk group or reside in areas with high rates of injecting drug use, teenage pregnancy, and/or sexually transmitted disease).

Every visit to a health-care provider is an opportunity to update a patient's immunization status with needed vaccines. Official health agencies should take necessary steps, including developing and enforcing school immunization requirements, to assure that students at all grade levels (including college students) and those in child care centers are protected against vaccine-preventable diseases. Agencies should also encourage institutions such as hospitals and long-term-care facilities to adopt policies regarding the appropriate vaccination of patients, residents, and employees.

Dates of vaccination (day, month, and year) should be recorded on institutional immunization records, such as those kept in schools and child care centers. This will facilitate assessments that a primary vaccine series has been completed according to an appropriate schedule and that needed boosters have been obtained at the correct time.

The ACIP recommends the use of "tickler" or recall systems by all health-care providers. Such systems should also be used by health-care providers who treat adults to ensure that at-risk persons receive influenza vaccine annually and that other vaccinations, such as Td, are administered as needed.

REPORTING VACCINE-PREVENTABLE DISEASES

Public health officials depend on the prompt reporting of vaccine-preventable diseases to local or state health departments by health-care providers to effectively monitor the occurrence of vaccine-preventable diseases for prevention and control efforts.

Nearly all vaccine-preventable diseases in the United States are notifiable; individual cases should be reported to local or state health departments. State health departments report these diseases each week to CDC. The local and state health departments and CDC use these surveillance data to determine whether outbreaks or other unusual events are occurring and to evaluate prevention and control strategies. In addition, CDC uses these data to evaluate the impact of national policies, practices, and strategies for vaccine programs.

SOURCES OF VACCINE INFORMATION

In addition to these general recommendations, other sources are available that contain specific and updated vaccine information. These sources include the following:

Official Vaccine Package Circulars

Manufacturer-provided product-specific information approved by the FDA with each vaccine. Some of these materials are reproduced in the Physician's Desk Reference (PDR).

Morbidity and Mortality Weekly Report (MMWR)

Published weekly by CDC, MMWR contains regular and special ACIP recommendations on vaccine use and statements of vaccine policy as they are developed and reports of specific disease activity. Subscriptions are available through Superintendent of Documents, U.S. Government Printing Office, Washington, DC 20402-9235; Telephone: (202) 783-3238. Also available through MMS Publications, C.S.P.O. Box 9120, Waltham, MA 02254-9120;Telephone: (800) 843-6356.

Health Information for International Travel

This booklet is published annually by CDC as a guide to national requirements and contains recommendations for specific immunizations and health practices for travel to foreign countries. Purchase from the Superintendent of Documents (address above).

Advisory Memoranda

Published as needed by CDC, these memoranda advise international travelers or persons who provide information to travelers about specific outbreaks of communicable diseases abroad. They include health information for prevention and specific recommendations for immunization. Memoranda and/or placement on mailing list are available from: Travelers' Health Section, Division of Quarantine MS-E03, National Center for Prevention Services (NCPS), CDC, Atlanta, GA 30333. The Division of Quarantine also maintains a 24-hour Travelers' Health Hotline voice information system that can be reached by dialing: (404) 332-4559.

The Report of the Committee on Infectious Diseases of the American Academy of Pediatrics (Red Book)

This report, which contains recommendations on all licensed vaccines, is updated every 2–3 years—most recently in 1991. The next revision will be published in May 1994. Policy changes for individual recommendations for immunization practices are published as needed by the American Academy of Pediatrics in the journal Pediatrics. They are available from the American Academy of Pediatrics, Publications Division, 141 Northwest Point Boulevard, P.O. Box 927, Elk Grove Village, IL 60009-0927; Telephone: (708) 228-5005.

Control of Communicable Diseases in Man

This manual is published by the American Public Health Association every 5 years—most recently in 1990 (15th ed.). The manual contains information about infectious diseases, their occurrence worldwide, diagnoses and therapy, and up-to-date recommendations on isolation and other control measures for each disease presented. It is available from the American Public Health Association, 1015 Fifteenth Street NW, Washington, DC 20005; Telephone: (202) 789-5600.

Guide for Adult Immunization (1990)

Produced by the American College of Physicians for physicians caring for adults, this guide emphasizes use of vaccines in healthy adults and adults with specific disease problems. It is available from Subscriber Services, American College of Physicians, Independence Mall West, Sixth Street at Race, Philadelphia, PA 19106-1572; Telephone: (215) 351-2600 or (800) 523-1546. (A new edition should be published within 1994.)

Technical bulletins of the American College of Obstetricians and Gynecologists

These bulletins contain important information on immunization of pregnant women and are updated periodically. They are available from the American College of Obstetricians and Gynecologists, Attention: Resource Center, 409 12th Street SW, Washington, DC 20024-2188.

State and Many Local Health Departments

These departments frequently provide technical advice, printed information on vaccines and immunization schedules, posters, and other educational materials.

National Immunization Program, CDC

This program maintains a 24-hour voice information hotline that provides technical advice on vaccine recommendations, disease outbreak control, and sources of immunobiologics. In addition, a course on the epidemiology, prevention, and control of vaccine preventable diseases is offered each year in Atlanta and in various states. For further information, contact CDC, National Immunization Program, Atlanta, GA 30333; Telephone: (404) 332-4553.

REFERENCES

1. CDC. General recommendations on immunization: recommendations of the Immunization Practices Advisory Committee (ACIP). MMWR 1989;38:205–214, 219–227.
2. CDC. Vaccinia (smallpox) vaccine: recommendations of the Immunization Practices Advisory Committee. MMWR 1991;40(No. RR-14):1–10.
3. U.S. Department of Health and Human Services, Public Health Service, CDC. Vaccine management: recommendations for handling and storage of selected biologicals. March 1991.
4. CDC. Change in source of information: availability of varicella vaccine for children with acute lymphocytic leukemia. MMWR 1993;42:499.
5. Gilles FH, French JH. Postinjection sciatic nerve palsies in infants and children. J Pediatr 1961;58: 195–204.
6. Shaw FE Jr, Guess HA, Roets JM, et al. Effect of anatomic injection site, age, and smoking on the immune response to hepatitis B vaccination. Vaccine 1989;7:425–430.
7. Bergeson PS, Singer SA, Kaplan AM. Intramuscular injections in children. Pediatrics 1982;70:944–948.
8. Scheifele D, Bjornson G, Barreto L, Meekison W, Guasparini R. Controlled Trial of Haemophilus influenzae type B diphtheria, tetanus and pertussis vaccines, in 18-month-old children, including comparison of arm versus thigh injection. Vaccine 1992;10:455–460.
9. Ipp MM, Gold R, Goldback M, et al. Adverse reactions to diphtheria, tetanus, pertussis-polio vaccination at 18 months of age: effect of injection site and needle length. Pediatrics 1989;83:679–682.
10. Canter J, Mackay K, Good LS, et al. An outbreak of hepatitis B associated with jet injections in a weight reduction clinic. Arch Intern Med 1990;150:1923–1927.
11. CDC. Hepatitis B virus: a comprehensive strategy for eliminating transmission in the United States through universal childhood vaccination. Recommendations of the Immunization Practices Advisory Committee (ACIP). MMWR 1991;40(No. RR-13):1–25.
12. CDC. Publicly funded HIV counseling and testing—United States, 1991. MMWR 1992;41:613–617.
13. Deforest A, Long SS, Lischner HW, et al. Simultaneous administration of measles-mumps-rubella vaccine with booster doses of diphtheria-tetanus-pertussis and poliovirus vaccines. Pediatrics 1988;81:237–246.
14. CDC. Diphtheria, tetanus, and pertussis: recommendations for vaccine use and other preventive measures. Immunization Practices Advisory Committee (ACIP). MMWR 1991;40(No. RR-10):1–28.
15. Dashefsky B, Wald E, Guerra N, Byers C. Safety, tolerability, and immunogenicity of concurrent administration of Haemophilus influenzae type B conjugate vaccine (meningococcal protein conjugate) with either measles-mumps-rubella vaccine or diphtheria-tetanus-pertussis and oral poliovirus vaccines in 14- to 23-month-old infants. Pediatrics 1990;85(Suppl):682–689.
16. Giammanco G, LiVolti S, Mauro L. Immune response to simultaneous administration of a recombinant DNA hepatitis B vaccine and multiple compulsory vaccines in infancy. Vaccine 1991;9:747–750.

17. Cryz SJ. Post-marketing experience with live oral Ty21a vaccine [Letter]. Lancet 1993;341:49–50.
18. Hutchins SS, Escolan J, Markowitz LE, et al. Measles outbreak among unvaccinated preschool-age children: opportunities missed by health care providers to administer measles vaccine. Pediatrics 1989;83:369–374.
19. DeStefano F, Goodman RA, Noble GR, et al. Simultaneous administration of influenza and pneumococcal vaccines. JAMA 1982;247:2551–2554.
20. Yvonnet B, Coursaget P, Deubel V, et al. Simultaneous administration of hepatitis B and yellow fever vaccinations. Bull WHO 1986;19:307–311.
21. CDC. Yellow fever vaccine: recommendations of the Immunization Practices Advisory Committee (ACIP). MMWR 1990;39(No. RR-6):1–6.
22. Ambrosch F, Hirschl A, Kollaritsch H, et al. Immunologic investigations with oral live typhoid vaccine Ty21a strain. In: Steffen R, Lobel HO, Bradley DJ, eds. Travel Medicine: Proceedings of the First Conference on International Travel Medicine. Berlin: Springer-Verlag, 1989:248–253.
23. Horowitz H, Carbonaro CA. Inhibition of the Salmonella typhi oral vaccine strain Ty21a, by mefloquine and chloroquine. J Infect Dis 1992;166:1462–1464.
24. Pappaioanou M, Fishbein DB, Dreeson DW, et al. Antibody response to pre-exposure human diploid-cell rabies vaccine given concurrently with chloroquine. N Engl J Med 1986;314:280–284.
25. CDC. Rabies prevention—1991: recommendations of the Immunization Practices Advisory Committee (ACIP). MMWR 1991;40(No. RR-3):1–19.
26. Bernard KW, Fishbein DB, Miller KD, et al. Pre-exposure rabies immunization with human diploid cell vaccine: decreased antibody responses in persons immunized in developing countries. Am J Trop Med Hyg 1985;34:633–647.
27. Schneerson R, Robbins JB, Chu C, et.al. Serum antibody responses of juvenile and infant rhesus monkeys injected with Haemophilus influenzae type b and pneumococcus type 6A capsular polysaccharide-protein conjugates. Infect Immun 1984;45:582–591.
28. Vella PA, Ellis RW. Immunogenicity of Haemophilus influenzae type b conjugate vaccines in infant rhesus monkeys. Pediatr Res 1991;29:10–13.
29. Granoff DM, Rathore MH, Holmes SJ, Granoff PD, Lucas AH. Effect of immunity to the carrier protein on antibody responses to Haemophilus influenzae type b conjugate vaccines. Vaccine 1993;11:S46-S51.
30. CDC. Recommendations for use of Haemophilus b conjugate vaccines and a combined diphtheria, tetanus, pertussis, and Haemphilus b vaccine. MMWR 1993;42(No. RR-13):1–15.
31. Petralli JK, Merigan TC, Wilbur JR. Action of endogenous interferon against vaccinia infection in children. Lancet 1965;2:401–405.
32. Starr S, Berkovich S. The effects of measles, gamma globulin modified measles and vaccine measles on the tuberculin test. N Engl J Med 1964;270:386–391.
33. Brickman HF, Beaudry PH, Marks MI. The timing of tuberculin tests in relation to immunization with live viral vaccines. Pediatrics 1975;55:392–396.
34. Berkovich S, Starr S. Effects of live type 1 poliovirus vaccine and other viruses on the tuberculin test. N Engl J Med 1966;274:67–72.
35. Kaplan JE, Nelson DB, Schonberger LB, et al. The effect of immune globulin on the response to trivalent oral poliovirus and yellow fever vaccinations. Bull WHO 1984;62:585–590.
36. CDC. Measles prevention: recommendations of the Immunization Practices Advisory Committee. MMWR 1989;38(S-9):1–18.
37. Siber GR, Werner BC, Halsey NA. Interference of immune globulin with measles and rubella immunization. J Pediatr 1993;122:204–211.
38. Mason W, Takahashi M, Schneider T. Persisting passively acquired measles antibody following gamma globulin therapy for Kawasaki disease and response to live virus vaccination. Presented at the 32nd meeting of the Interscience Conference on Antimicrobial Agents and Chemotherapy, Abstract 311. Los Angeles, October 1992.
39. Siber GR, Snydman DR. Use of immune globulin in the prevention and treatment of infections. In: Remington J, Swartz M, eds. Current clinical topics in infectious diseases. Vol 12. Oxford: Blackwell Scientific, 1992.
40. Bush LM, Moonsammy GI, Boscia JA. Evaluation of initiating a hepatitis B vaccination schedule with one vaccine and completing it with another. Vaccine 1991;9:807–809.
41. Faden H, Modlin JF, Thoms ML, McBean AM, Ferdon MB, Ogra PL. Comparative evaluation of immunization with live attenuated and enhanced-potency inactivated trivalent poliovirus vaccines in childhood: systemic and local immune responses. J Infect Dis 1990;162:1291–1297.
42. Granoff DM, Anderson EL, Osterholm MT, et al. Differences in the immunogenicity of three Haemophilus influenzae type b conjugate vaccines in infants. J Pediatr 1992;121:187–194.
43. Greenberg DP, Leiberman JM, Marcy SM, et al. Safety and immunogenicity of mixed sequences of Haemophilus influenzae type B (HIB) conjugate vaccines in infants [Abstract #997]. Pediatr Res 1993; 33:169A.
44. Daum RS, Milewski WM, Ballanco GA. Interchangeability of H. influenzae type B vaccines for the primary series ("mix and match")—a preliminary analysis [Abstract #976]. Pediatr Res 1993;33:166A.
45. Anderson EL, Decker MD, Edwards KM, Englund JA, Belshe RB. Interchangeability of conjugated

Haemophilus influenzae type B (HIB) vaccines in infants [Abstract #493]. Pediatr Res 1993;33:85A.
46. Peter G, Lepow ML, McCracken GH Jr, Phillips CF, eds. 1991 Redbook—Report of the Committee on Infectious Diseases. American Academy of Pediatrics, 1991.
47. Lavi S, Zimmerman B, Koren G, Gold R. Administration of measles, mumps, and rubella virus vaccine (live) to egg-allergic children. JAMA 1990;263:269–271.
48. Greenberg MA, Birx DL. Safe administration of mumps-measles-rubella vaccine in egg-allergic children. J Pediatr 1988;13:504–506.
49. Herman JJ, Radin R, Schneiderman R. Allergic reactions to measles (rubeola) vaccine in patients hypersensitive to egg protein. J Pediatr 1983;102:196–199.
50. Murphy KR, Strunk RC. Safe administration of influenza vaccine in asthmatic children hypersensitive to egg proteins. J Pediatr 1985;106:931–933.
51. Jacobs RL, Lowe RS, Lanier BQ. Adverse reactions to tetanus toxoid. JAMA 1982;247:40–42.
52. Kirkland LR. Ocular sensitivity to thimerosal: a problem with hepatitis vaccine? South Med J 1990;83:497–499.
53. Aberer W. Vaccination despite thimerosal sensitivity. Contact Dermatitis 1991;24:6–10.
54. Bernbaum JC, Daft A, Anolik R, et al. Response of preterm infants to diphtheria-tetanus-pertussis immunizations. J Pediatr 1985;107:184–188.
55. Koblin BA, Townsend TR, Munoz A, Onorato I, Wilson M, Polk BF. Response of preterm infants to diphtheria-tetanus-pertussis vaccine. Pediatr Infect Dis J 1988;7:704–711.
56. Smolen P, Bland R, Heiligenstein E, Lawless MR, Dillard R, Abramson J. Antibody response to oral polio vaccine in premature infants. J Pediatr 1983;103:917–919.
57. Bernbaum J, Daft A, Samuelson J, Polin RA. Half-dose immunization for diphtheria, tetanus, pertussis: response of pre-term infants. Pediatrics 1989;83:471–476.
58. Lau YL, Tam AYC, Ng KW, et al. Response of preterm infants to hepatitis B vaccine. J Pediatr 1992;121:962–965.
59. Kim-Farley R, Brink E, Orenstein W, Bart K. Vaccination and breast-feeding [Letter]. JAMA 1982;248:2451–2452.
60. Patriarca PA, Wright PF, John TJ. Factors affecting the immunogenicity of oral polio vaccine in developing countries: review. Rev Infect Dis 1991;13:926–939.
61. Hahn-Zoric M, Fulconis F, Minoli I, et al. Antibody response to parenteral and oral vaccines are impaired by conventional and low-protein formulas as compared to breast-feeding. ACTA Paediatr Scand 1990;79:1137–1142.
62. CDC. Poliomyelitis prevention: enhanced-potency inactivated poliomyelitis vaccine—supplementary statement. MMWR 1987;36:795–798.
63. Tsai TF, Paul R, Lynberg MC, Letson GW. Congenital yellow fever virus infection after immunization in pregnancy. J Infect Dis 1993;168:1520–1523.
64. CDC. Recommendations of the Advisory Committee on Immunization Practices (ACIP): use of vaccines and immune globulins in persons with altered immunocompetence. MMWR 1993;42(No. RR-4):1–18.
65. Sixby JW. Routine immunization of the immunocompromised child. Adv Pediatr Infect Dis 1987;2:79–114.
66. Wright PF, Hatch MH, Kasselberg AG, et al. Vaccine-associated poliomyelitis in a child with sex-linked agammaglobulinemia. J Pediatr 1977;91:408–412.
67. Wyatt HV. Poliomyelitis in hypogammaglobulinemics. J Infect Dis 1973;128:802–806.
68. Davis LE, Bodian D, Price D, et al. Chronic progressive poliomyelitis secondary to vaccination of an immunodeficient child. N Engl J Med 1977;297:241–245.
69. CDC. Disseminated mycobacterium bovis infection from BCG vaccination of a patient with acquired immunodeficiency syndrome. MMWR 1985;34:227–228.
70. Ninane J, Grymonprez A, Burtonboy G, et al. Disseminated BCG in HIV infection. Arch Dis Child 1988;63:1268–1269.
71. Redfield RR, Wright DC, James WD, et al. Disseminated vaccinia in a military recruit with human immunodeficiency virus (HIV) disease. N Engl J Med 1987;316:673–676.
72. Evans DIK, Shaw, A. Safety of intramuscular injection of hepatitis B vaccine in haemophiliacs. Br Med J 1990;300:1694–1695.
73. CDC. Standards for pediatric immunization practices recommended by the National Vaccine Advisory Committee. MMWR 1993;42:1–13.
74. Wald ER, Dashefsky B, Byers C, et al. Frequency and severity of infections in day care. J Pediatr 1988;112:540–546.
75. Lewis T, Osborn LM, Lewis K, et al. Influence of parental knowledge and opinions on 12-month diphtheria, tetanus, and pertussis vaccination rates. Am J Dis Child 1988;142:283–286.
76. Farizo KM, Stehr-Green PA, Markowitz LE, Patriarca PA. Vaccination levels and missed opportunities for measles vaccination: a record audit in a public pediatric clinic. Pediatrics 1992;89:589–592.
77. Halsey NA, Boulos R, Mode F, et al. Response to measles vaccine in Haitian infants 6 to 12 months old. Influence of maternal antibodies, malnutrition, and concurrent illnesses. N Engl J Med 1985;313:544–549.

78. Ndikuyeze A, Munoz A, Stewart S, et al. Immunogenicity and safety of measles vaccine in ill African children. Int J Epidemiol 1988;17:448–455.
79. Lindegren ML, Reynolds S, Atkinson W, Davis A, Falter K, Patriarca P. Adverse events following measles vaccination of ill preschool-aged children [Abstract 270]. Abstracts of the 1991 Interscience Conference on Antimicrobial Agents and Chemotherapy (ICAAC), 1991:144.
80. Atkinson W, Markowitz L, Baughman A, et al. Serologic response to measles vaccination among ill children [Abstract 422]. Abstracts of the 1992 Interscience Conference on Antimicrobial Agents and Chemotherapy, 1992:181.
81. Krober MS, Stracener LE, Bass JW. Decreased antibody measles antibody response after measles-mumps-rubella vaccine in infants with colds. JAMA 1991;265:2095–2096.
82. CDC. Publication of vaccine information pamphlets. MMWR 1991;40:726–727.
83. CDC. Pertussis vaccination: acellular pertussis vaccine for reinforcing and booster use—supplementary ACIP statement: recommendations of the Immunization Practices Advisory Committee (ACIP). MMWR 1992;41(No. RR-1):1–10.
84. CDC. Pertussis vaccination: acellular pertussis vaccine for the fourth and fifth doses of the DTP series: update to the supplementary ACIP statement: recommendations of the Advisory Committee on Immunization Practices. MMWR 1992;41(No. RR-15):1–5.
85. CDC. Pneumococcal polysaccharide vaccine: recommendations of the Immunization Practices Advisory Committee. MMWR 1989;38:64–68, 73–76.
86. CDC. The public health burden of vaccine preventable diseases among adults: standards for adult immunization practice. MMWR 1990;39:725–729.

Update on Adult Immunization

Original Citation: Centers for Disease Control and Prevention. Update on adult immunization: recommendations of the Immunization Practices Advisory Committee (ACIP). MMWR 1991; 40(RR-12):1–52.

SUMMARY

This statement on adult immunization is a supplement to the "General Recommendations on Immunization" of the Immunization Practices Advisory Committee (ACIP) (1) and updates the previous supplement published in September 1984. This statement presents an overview on immunization for adults and makes specific immunization recommendations. The statement provides information on vaccine-preventable diseases; indications for use of vaccines, toxoids, and immune globulins recommended for adults; and specific side effects, adverse reactions, precautions, and contraindications associated with use of these immunobiologics. It also gives immunization recommendations for adults in specific age groups and for those who have special immunization requirements because of occupation, life-style, travel, environmental situations, and health status.

This statement is a compendium of ACIP recommendations and will not be updated regularly. The ACIP periodically reviews individual immunization statements that are published in the MMWR. The reader must use the detailed, up-to-date individual statements in conjunction with this compendium to keep abreast of current information. A list of the current ACIP recommendations for specific diseases and vaccines can be found in Appendix 1.

INTRODUCTION

General Considerations

Immunization policies have primarily been directed towards vaccinating infants, children, and adolescents. Although vaccination is routine in pediatric practice, it is not commonplace in the practice of physicians who treat adults.

The widespread implementation of childhood vaccination programs has substantially reduced the occurrence of many vaccine-preventable diseases. However, successful childhood vaccination alone will not eliminate specific disease problems. A substantial proportion of the remaining morbidity and mortality from vaccine-preventable diseases presently occurs among older adolescents and adults. Persons who escaped natural infection or were not vaccinated with toxoids or vaccines against diphtheria, tetanus, measles, mumps, rubella, and poliomyelitis may be at risk of these diseases and their complications. Many factors have influenced the use of vaccines among adults, including lack of awareness of safe vaccines and vaccine-preventable health burdens, unfounded concerns about adverse reactions, and missed opportunities by health-care providers to vaccinate adults during office, clinic, or hospital visits. To improve adult immunization levels, the National Coalition for Adult Immunization (NCAI) was formed in 1988. The coalition consists of professional, private, public, and voluntary organizations with the common goal of improving vaccine use among adults by educating health-care providers and patients. A listing of member organizations is provided in Appendix 2.

To reduce further the unnecessary occurrence of these vaccine-preventable diseases, health-care providers for older adolescents and adults should provide vaccinations as a routine part of their practice. In addition, the epidemiology of other vaccine-preventable diseases (e.g., hepatitis B, rabies, influenza, and pneumococcal disease) indicates that persons in certain age, occupational, environmental, and life-style groups and those with special health problems are at increased risk of these illnesses and should be vaccinated. Travelers to some countries may also be at increased risk of exposure to vaccine-preventable illnesses. Finally, foreign students, immigrants, and refugees may be susceptible to these diseases.

A systematic approach to vaccination is necessary to ensure that every adult is appropriately protected against vaccine-preventable diseases. Every visit by an adult to a health-care provider should be an opportunity to provide this protection. However, several factors need to be considered before any patient is vaccinated. These include the susceptibility of the patient, the risk of exposure to the disease, the risk from the disease, and the benefits and risks of the immunizing agent.

Physicians should maintain detailed records containing information about each person's previous vaccinations. The National Childhood Vaccine Injury Act of 1986 (NCVIA) requires physicians and other health-care providers who administer vaccines to maintain permanent vaccination records and to report occurrences of certain adverse events specified in the Act for all vaccines containing measles, mumps, rubella, poliomyelitis, diphtheria, tetanus, and pertussis antigens for all patients, adults as well as children (Table 1). Ideally, information for all vaccines and toxoids should be recorded. Information should also include the person's history of vaccine-preventable illnesses, occupation, and life-style. Vaccines and toxoids administered at appropriate ages and intervals should be documented in writing.

Table 1. On the basis of The National Childhood Vaccine Injury Act of 1986 (NCVIA), the vaccines and toxoids, adverse events, and intervals from vaccination to onset of adverse event required for reporting or compensation, United States

		Interval from vaccination to onset of event	
Vaccine/toxoid*	Adverse event	For reporting[†]	For compensation[§]
DTP, P, DTP/ Poliovirus combined	A. Anaphylaxis or anaphylactic shock	24 hours	24 hours
	B. Encephalopathy (or encephalitis)[¶]	7 days	3 days
	C. Shock-collapse or hypotonic-hyporesponsive collapse**	7 days	3 days
	D. Residual seizure disorder[‡]	[‡]	3 days
	E. Any acute complication or sequela (including death) of above events	No limit	Not applicable
	F. Events described as contraindications to additional doses of vaccine (see manufacturer's package insert)[§§]	(See package insert)[§§]	
Measles, Mumps, and Rubella; DT, Td, T	A. Anaphylaxis or anaphylactic shock	24 hours	24 hours
	B. Encephalopathy (or enceophalitis)[¶]	15 days (for measles, mumps, and rubella vaccines); 7 days (for DT, Td, and T)	15 days for measles, mumps, and rubella vaccine; 3 days (for DT, Td, and T)
	C. Residual seizure disorder[‡]	[‡]	15 days (for measles, mumps, or rubella vaccine); 3 days for DT, Td, or T)
	D. Any acute complication or sequela (including death) of above events	No limit	

Table 1. —*continued*

Vaccine/toxoid*	Adverse event	Interval from vaccination to onset of event	
		For reporting[†]	For compensation[§]
	E. Events described as contraindications to additional doses of vaccine (see manufacturer's package insert)[§§]	(See package insert)[§§]	
OPV	A. Paralytic poliomyelitis in a nonimmunodeficient recipient	30 days	30 days
	in an immunodeficient recipient	6 months	6 months
	in a vaccine-associated community case	No limit	Not applicable
	B. Any acute complication or sequela (including death) of above events	No limit	Not applicable
	C. Events described as contraindications to additional doses of vaccine (see manufacturer's package insert)[§§]	(See package insert)[§§]	
Inactivated Polio Vaccine	A. Anaphylaxis or anaphylactic shock	24 hours	24 hours
	B. Any acute complication or sequela (including death) of above events	No limit	Not applicable
	C. Events described as contraindications to additional doses of vaccine (see manufacturer's package insert)[§§]	(See package insert)[§§]	

*The vaccine/toxoid abbreviations are defined, in alphabetical order, as follows: DT = Diphtheria and tetanus toxoids, adsorbed; DTP = Diphtheria and tetanus toxoids and pertussis vaccine, adsorbed (pediatric); OPV = Oral poliovirus vaccine, live, trivalent; P = Pertussis vaccine; T = Tetanus toxoid, adsorbed; and Td = Tetanus and diphtheria toxoids, adsorbed (for adult use).

[†]Adverse events that are required by NCVIA to be reported to Vaccine Adverse Events Reporting System (VAERS) if their onset is within the indicated interval after vaccination.

[§]Adverse events that may be compensable under NCVIA if the onset is within this interval after vaccination.

[¶]*Encephalopathy* means any significant acquired abnormality of, injury to, or impairment of function of the brain. Among the frequent manifestations of encephalopathy are focal and diffuse neurologic signs, increased intracranial pressure, or changes lasting at least 6 hours in level of consciousness, with or without convulsions. The neurologic signs and symptoms of encephalopathy may be temporary with complete recovery or may result in various degrees of permanent impairment. Signs and symptoms such as high-pitched and unusual screaming, persistent inconsolable crying, and bulging fontanel are compatible with an encephalopathy, but in and of themselves are not conclusive evidence of encephalopathy. Encephalopathy usually can be documented by slow wave activity on an electroencephalogram.

[**] *Shock-collapse* or *hypotonic-hyporesponsive collapse* may include signs or symptoms such as decrease or loss of muscle tone, paralysis (partial or complete), hemiplegia, hemiparesis, loss of color or turning pale white or blue, unresponsiveness to environmental stimuli, depression of or loss of consciousness, prolonged sleeping with difficulty being aroused, or cardiovascular or respiratory arrest.

[‡]*Residual seizure disorder* may have occurred if no other seizure or convulsion unaccompanied by fever or accompanied by a fever of <102°F occurred before the first seizure or convulsion after the administration of the vaccine involved, and if, in the case of measles-, mumps-, or rubella-containing vaccines, the first seizure or convulsion occurred within 15 days after vaccination, or, in the case of any other vaccine, the first seizure or convulsion occurred within 3 days after vaccination, and, if two or more seizures or convulsions unaccompanied by fever or accompanied by a fever of <102°F occurred within 1 year after vaccination. The terms *seizure* and *convulsion* include grand mal, petit mal, absence, myoclonic, tonic-clonic, and focal motor seizures and signs.

[§§]Refer to the CONTRAINDICATION section of the manufacturer's package insert for each vaccine/toxoid.

Attention to factors such as military service and age may help to determine whether vaccines or toxoids are advisable for an individual. Persons who have served in the military can be considered to have been vaccinated against measles, rubella, tetanus, diphtheria, and polio. However, the practitioner should be aware that policies of the different branches of the military have varied over time and among the branches. After being administered any immunobiologic, the patient should be given written documentation of its receipt and information about which vaccines or toxoids will be needed in the future. For this purpose, a vaccination record such as the suggested form found in Appendix 3 should be used routinely.

The patient or responsible person (e.g., guardian) should be given information on the risks of immunobiologics as well as their major benefits in preventing disease, both among individuals and in the community. No formal, legally acceptable statement has been universally adopted for the private medical sector. The NCVIA requires development and use of materials providing vaccine information for all covered vaccines. All physicians must give those materials, when available, to prospective vaccinees. However, CDC has developed "Important Information Statements" for use with vaccines purchased through federal contracts. (Many of these will be replaced by "Vaccine Information Pamphlets" in April 1992.) Practitioners may wish to consider these or similar materials for patients. Examples of Important Information Statements can be obtained from state and many local health departments. Forms are not available for all vaccines, however, especially those of limited use. Regardless, the ACIP recommends that health-care providers allow ample opportunity for questions before each vaccination.

Modern immunobiologics are extremely safe and effective, but not completely so. Adverse events have been reported after administration of all immunobiologics. These adverse events range from frequent, minor, local reactions to extremely rare, severe systemic illness, such as paralysis associated with oral poliovirus vaccine, live, trivalent (OPV). Cause-and-effect relationships frequently cannot be established when adverse events occur after vaccination, because temporal association alone does not necessarily indicate causation. All temporally associated events severe enough to require the recipient to seek medical attention should be evaluated and reported in detail to the Vaccine Adverse Event Reporting System (VAERS) in order to improve knowledge about adverse reactions. (See "Requirements for Permanent Vaccination Records and Reporting of Adverse Events" section.)

General vaccination considerations and recommendations are found in the ACIP statement "General Recommendations on Immunization" (1). The following recommendations apply to persons in the indicated groups. For more detailed information on immunobiologics—including indications, side effects, adverse reactions, precautions, contraindications, dosages, and routes of administration—providers should refer to the tables and appendices at the back of this supplement. Also, package inserts for the individual products should be consulted as necessary. Appendix 4 provides a list of vaccines, toxoids, and immune globulins available in the United States as of March 1, 1991.

Reference can also be made to the Guide for Adult Immunization (2), published by the American College of Physicians, and to the recommendations of the U.S. Preventive Services Task Force (3).

Age Groups

The following text and Table 2 summarize the vaccines and toxoids recommended for most adults, by specific age groups. Table 3 summarizes the vaccines and toxoids recommended for normal infants and children. Refer to the section "Vaccine-Preventable Diseases and Their Immunobiologics" for other essential information.

Adults 18-24 Years Old

All young adults should complete a primary series of diphtheria and tetanus toxoids if they have not done so during childhood. A primary series for adults is three doses of preparations containing diphtheria and tetanus toxoids; the first two doses should be given at least 4 weeks apart and the third dose, 6–12 months after the second. Those who have completed a primary series should receive a booster dose every 10 years. Doses need not be repeated when the series schedule is delayed. The combined tetanus and diphtheria toxoids, adsorbed (for adult use) (Td), should be used. Persons with unknown or uncer-

Table 2. Vaccines and toxoids* recommended for adults, by age groups, United States

Age group (years)	Vaccine/toxoid					
	Td[†]	Measles	Mumps	Rubella	Influenza	Pneumococcal Polysaccharide
18–24	X	X	X	X		
25–64	X	X[§]	X[§]	X		
≥65	X				X	X

*Refer also to sections in text on specific vaccines or toxoids for indications, contraindications, precautions, dosages, side effects, adverse reactions, and special considerations.
[†]Td = Tetanus and diphtheria toxoids, adsorbed (for adult use), which is a combined preparation containing <2 flocculation units of diphtheria toxoid.
[§]Indicated for persons born after 1956.

Table 3. Recommended schedule of vaccinations for all children

2 months	4 months	6 months	12 months	15 months	4–6 years (before beginning school)
DTP	DTP	DTP		DTP*	DTP
Polio	Polio			Polio*	Polio
				MMR[†]	MMR[§]
HbCV:					
Option 1[¶]	HbCV	HbCV		HbCV	
Option 2[¶]	HbCV		HbCV		

	At birth (before hospital discharge)	1–2 months	4 months	6–18 months
HBv:				
Option 1	HBv	HBv**		HBv**
Option 2		HBv**	HBv**	HBv**

DTP: Diphtheria, Tetanus, and Pertussis Vaccine
Polio: Live Oral Polio Vaccine drops (OPV) or Killed (Inactivated) Polio Vaccine shots (IPV)
MMR: Measles, Mumps, and Rubella Vaccine
HbCV: Haemophilus influenzae type b Conjugate Vaccine
HBv: Hepatitis B vaccine
*Many experts recommend these vaccines at 18 months.
[†]In some areas this dose of MMR vaccine may be administered at 12 months.
[§]Many experts recommend this dose of MMR vaccine be administered at entry into middle school or junior high school.
[¶]HbCV vaccine is administered in either a 4-dose schedule (1) or a 3-dose schedule (2), depending on the type of vaccine used.
**HBv can be administered at the same time as DTP and/or HbCV.

tain histories of receiving diphtheria or tetanus toxoids should be considered unvaccinated and should receive a full three-dose primary series of Td.

Young adults should be immune to measles, rubella, and mumps. In 1989, as a result of outbreaks of measles in school and college settings, new recommendations were made to implement a routine two-dose schedule for measles-mumps-rubella vaccine, live (MMR). The schedule will usually be implemented gradually, one age group at a time, beginning with entry into kindergarten or first grade. Some areas of the country may implement the second dose of MMR at an older age (e.g., entry into middle school or junior high school). Young adults who are attending college (or other post-high school educational institutions) or who are newly employed in situations that place them at high risk of measles transmission (e.g., health-care facilities) should have documentation of having received two doses of live MMR on or after their first birthday or other evidence of immunity. Persons born after 1956 who are traveling to areas endemic with measles should be given two doses of live MMR. All other young adults in this age group should have documentation of a single dose of live MMR on or after their first birthday, documentation of physician-diagnosed disease, or laboratory evidence of immunity. Eventually, all persons in this age group will require two doses of measles vaccine. However, until the new recommendations are fully implemented, a single dose on or after the first birthday will be sufficient evidence of immunity for most persons.

During outbreaks of measles, all persons at risk should have evidence of immunity to measles. Acceptable evidence of measles immunity consists of documentation of two doses of a live measles vaccine (preferably MMR), given at least 1 month apart after the first birthday; documentation of physician-diagnosed measles; or laboratory evidence of immunity to measles. During outbreaks of mumps and rubella, all persons at risk should have evidence of immunity to mumps and rubella. Acceptable evidence of mumps/rubella immunity consists of documentation of at least one dose of live mumps- and/or rubella-containing vaccine (preferably MMR), laboratory evidence of immunity, or physician-diagnosed mumps. Physician diagnosis is not adequate evidence of immunity against rubella.

Persons vaccinated with killed-measles-virus vaccine (available in the United States from 1963 until 1967) or with a measles vaccine of unknown type should receive two doses of live-measles-virus vaccine at least 1 month apart to prevent measles disease or atypical measles syndrome—if exposed to wild measles virus. Persons are considered immune to rubella only if they have a record of vaccination with rubella vaccine on or after their first birthday or laboratory evidence of immunity. MMR is the vaccine of choice if recipients are likely to be susceptible to more than one of the three diseases. Persons lacking adequate documentation should be vaccinated.

Adults 25–64 Years Old

All adults 25–64 years of age should have completed a primary series of diphtheria and tetanus toxoids. If needed, a primary series for adults is three doses of preparations containing diphtheria and tetanus toxoids—the first two doses given at least 4 weeks apart and the third dose given 6–12 months after the second. Those who have completed a primary series should receive a booster dose every 10 years. To enhance protection against both diseases, Td should be used. Persons with unknown or uncertain histories of receiving diphtheria or tetanus toxoids should be considered unvaccinated and should receive a full three-dose primary series of Td.

All adults born in 1957 or later who do not have a medical contraindication should receive one dose of measles vaccine unless they have a dated record of vaccination with at least one dose of live measles vaccine on or after their first birthday, documentation of physician-diagnosed disease, or laboratory evidence of immunity. Serologic studies of hospital workers indicate that up to 9.3% of persons born before 1957 were not immune to measles (4, 5). In addition, of all measles cases reported to the CDC from 1985 through 1990, 3.7% occurred among persons born before 1957. These data suggest that most persons born before 1957 can be considered immune to measles and do not need to be vaccinated. However, 97 (29%) of 341 health-care workers who had measles in the period 1985–1989 were born before 1957 (6). Therefore, because health-care workers are at particularly high risk of measles and a small proportion born before 1957 will be susceptible, vaccine should be offered to such persons if there is reason to believe that they may be susceptible.

Some adults, such as college students, persons working in health-care facilities, and international travelers, are at increased risk of measles. Such persons should have evidence of two doses of live measles vaccine or other evidence of measles immunity, if born in 1957 or later. Although most adults are likely to have been infected naturally with mumps, mumps vaccine should be given to adults who are considered susceptible. Persons born in 1957 or later can be considered immune if they have evidence of one dose of live mumps vaccine or other evidence of mumps immunity.

Unless proof of vaccination with rubella vaccine or laboratory evidence of immunity is available, rubella vaccine is recommended for adults, especially women of childbearing age. The vaccine of choice is MMR if recipients are likely to be susceptible to more than one of these three diseases.

Adults Greater than or Equal to 65 Years Old

All older adults should have completed a primary series of diphtheria and tetanus toxoids. If needed, a primary series for adults is three doses of preparations containing diphtheria and tetanus toxoids; the first two doses should be given at least 4 weeks apart and the third dose 6–12 months after the second. Those who have completed a primary series should receive a booster dose every 10 years. Td should be used to provide protection against both diseases. Persons with unknown or uncertain histories of receiving diphtheria or tetanus toxoids should be considered unvaccinated and should receive a full three-dose primary series of Td.

All older adults should receive influenza vaccine annually. They should also receive a single dose of pneumococcal polysaccharide vaccine. Revaccination should be strongly considered greater than or equal to 6 years after the first dose for those at highest risk of (a) fatal pneumococcal disease (such as asplenic patients) or (b) rapid decline in antibody levels (e.g., transplant recipients or those with chronic renal failure or nephrotic syndrome).

Special Occupations

Persons in specific occupations may be at increased risk of exposure to certain vaccine-preventable illnesses. Such persons may need selected vaccines and toxoids in addition to those routinely recommended for their age group. Table 4 provides a summary of immunobiologics recommended for various special occupational groups. The reader is referred to the section on "Vaccine-Preventable Diseases and Their Immunobiologics" for other essential information.

Table 4. Immunobiologics* recommended for special occupations, life-styles, environmental circumstances, travel, foreign students, immigrants, and refugees, United States

Indication	Immunobiologic
Occupation	
Hospital, laboratory, and other health-care personnel	Hepatitis B
	Influenza
	Measles
	Rubella
	Mumps
	Polio
Public-safety personnel	Hepatitis B
	Influenza
Staff of institutions for the developmentally disabled	Hepatitis B
Veterinarians and animal handlers	Rabies
	Plague
Selected field workers (those who come into contact with possibly infected animals)	Plague
	Rabies
Selected occupations (those who work with imported animal hides, furs, wool, animal hair, and bristles)	Anthrax
Life-styles	
Homosexual males	Hepatitis B
Injecting drug users	Hepatitis B
Heterosexual persons with multiple sexual partners or recently acquired sexually transmitted disease	Hepatitis B
Environmental situation	
Inmates of long-term correctional facilities	Hepatitis B
Residents of institutions for the developmentally disabled	Hepatitis B
Household contacts of HBV carriers	Hepatitis B
Homeless persons	Tetanus/diphtheria
	Measles
	Mumps
	Rubella
	Influenza
	Pneumococcal polysaccharide
Travel[†]	Measles
	Mumps
	Rubella
	Polio
	Influenza
	Hepatitis B
	Rabies
	Meningococcal polysaccharide
	Tetanus/diphtheria[§]
	Yellow fever
	Typhoid
	Cholera
	Plague[¶]
	Immune globulin[**]

Table 4.—*continued*

Indication	Immunobiologic
Foreign students, immigrants, and refugees	Measles
	Rubella
	Diphtheria
	Tetanus
	Mumps
	Hepatitis B

*Refer also to sections in text on specific immunobiologics for use by specific risk groups, details on indications, contraindications, precautions, dosages, side effects, and adverse reactions, and special considerations. Unless specifically contraindicated, the vaccines or toxoids recommended for adults are also indicated. Table 2 shows vaccines and toxoids appropriate for most adults by age.
†Vaccines needed for travelers will vary depending on individual itineraries; travelers should refer to *Health Information for International Travelers* for more detailed information.
§If not received within 10 years.
¶In or during travel to areas with enzootic or epidemic plague in which exposure to rodents cannot be prevented.
**For Hepatitis A prophylaxis.

Health- and Public-Safety-Related Occupations

Because of their contact with patients or infectious material from patients, many health-care workers (e.g., physicians, nurses, dental professionals, medical and nursing students, laboratory technicians, and administrative staff) and public-safety workers (e.g., police, emergency medical personnel, firefighters) are at risk for exposure to and possible transmission of vaccine-preventable diseases. Optimal use of immunizing agents will not only safeguard the health of workers but also will protect patients from becoming infected. A consistent program of vaccinations could eliminate the problem of having susceptible health-care workers in hospitals and health departments (with the attendant risks to other workers and patients). The CDC publication "Immunization Recommendations for Health-Care Workers" (7) and the section below discuss this subject in detail.

Hepatitis B virus (HBV) infection is a major occupational hazard for health-care and public-safety workers. The risk of acquiring HBV infection from occupational exposures depends on the frequency of percutaneous and permucosal exposures to blood or blood products. Any health-care or public-safety worker may be at risk for HBV exposure, depending on the tasks that he or she performs. If those tasks involve contact with blood or blood-contaminated body fluids, workers should be vaccinated. Vaccination should be considered for other workers, depending on their exposure to blood and/or bodily fluids. Selected staff of institutions for the developmentally disabled may be at increased risk of HBV infection because of exposure to human bites and contact with skin lesions, saliva, and other potentially infected secretions in addition to blood. The Occupational Safety and Health Administration, Department of Labor, is developing regulations that will require employers who have employees at risk of occupational exposure to hepatitis B to offer these employees hepatitis B (HB) vaccine at the employer's expense. These regulations are expected to accelerate and broaden the use of HB vaccine among health-care workers and to assure efforts to prevent this occupational disease.

Among health-care personnel with frequent exposure to blood, the prevalence of serologic evidence of HBV infection ranges between approximately 15% and 30%. In contrast, the prevalence in the general population averages 5%. The cost-effectiveness of serologic screening to detect susceptible individuals among health-care personnel depends on the prevalence of infection and the costs of testing and of the HB vaccine. Each institution must decide whether serologic screening is cost effective. Vaccination of persons who already have antibodies to HBV has not been shown to cause adverse effects. HB vaccine provides protection against HBV for greater than or equal to 7 years after vaccination; booster doses are not recommended during this interval. The need for later booster doses will be assessed as additional information becomes available.

Influenza vaccination is recommended yearly for physicians, nurses, and other personnel in hospital, chronic-care, and outpatient-care settings who have contact with high-risk patients in all age groups. Those who provide essential community services (e.g., public-safety workers) may consider receiving the vaccine also. Vaccination should reduce the possibility of transmitting influenza from health-care workers to patients and reduce health-care workers' risk of illness and absenteeism due to influenza.

Transmission of rubella in health facilities (e.g., hospitals, physicians' or dentists' offices, and clinics) can disrupt hospital or office routines and cause considerable expense. Although no cases of congenital rubella syndrome (CRS) have been reported in association with rubella transmission in health facilities, therapeutic abortions have been sought by pregnant staff members after rubella infection (8). To prevent such situations, all medical, dental, laboratory, and other support health personnel, both male and female, who might be at risk of exposure to patients infected with rubella or who might have contact with pregnant patients should be vaccinated. Rubella vaccine is recommended for all such personnel unless they have either proof of vaccination with rubella vaccine on or after their first birthday or laboratory evidence of immunity. The vaccine of choice is MMR if recipients are likely to be susceptible to measles and/or mumps as well as to rubella.

Measles and mumps transmission in health facilities can also be disruptive and costly. To prevent such situations, all new employees in health-care facilities who were born in 1957 or later who may have direct patient contact should be vaccinated. Such persons can be considered immune only if they have documentation of having received two doses of live measles vaccine and at least one dose of live mumps vaccine on or after their first birthday, a record of physician-diagnosed measles or mumps, or laboratory evidence of immunity. Institutions may wish to extend this requirement to all employees, not only beginning ones. If recipients are likely to be susceptible to rubella as well as to measles and mumps, MMR is the vaccine of choice. Adults born before 1957 can be considered immune to both measles and mumps because these infections were virtually universal before the availability of measles and mumps vaccines. However, because serologic studies of hospital workers indicate that up to 9.3% of those born before 1957 were not immune to measles (4, 5) and because 97 (29%) of 341 health-care workers who had measles in the period 1985–1989 in medical facilities were born before 1957 (6), health facilities should consider requiring at least one dose of measles vaccine for older employees who are at risk of occupational exposure to measles and do not have proof of immunity to this disease.

Poliovirus vaccine is not routinely recommended for persons older than high-school age (greater than or equal to 18 years old). However, hospital personnel who have close contact with patients who may be excreting wild polioviruses and laboratory personnel who handle specimens that may contain wild polioviruses should have completed a primary series of poliovirus vaccine. For personnel who do not have proof of having completed a primary series, completion with enhanced potency inactivated poliovirus vaccine (eIPV) is recommended. This vaccine is preferred because adults have a slightly increased risk of vaccine-associated paralysis after receiving OPV. In addition, because vaccine polioviruses may be excreted by OPV recipients for greater than or equal to 30 days, the use of OPV increases the risk of acquiring vaccine-associated paralytic poliomyelitis among susceptible immunocompromised OPV recipients and/or their close contacts.

Smallpox (vaccinia) vaccination is indicated only for laboratory workers involved with orthopox viruses and certain health-care workers involved in clinical trials of vaccinia recombinant vaccines. When indicated, smallpox (vaccinia) vaccination should be given at least every 10 years.

Plague vaccine is indicated for laboratory personnel working with Yersinia pestis possibly resistant to antimicrobial agents and for persons performing aerosol experiments with Y. pestis.

Anthrax vaccine is indicated for laboratory personnel working with Bacillus anthracis.

Preexposure rabies vaccination is indicated for laboratory workers directly involved with testing or isolating rabies virus.

Veterinarians and Animal Handlers

Veterinarians and animal handlers are at risk of rabies exposure because of occupational contact with domestic and wild animals. They should receive preexposure prophylaxis with human diploid cell rabies vaccine (HDCV). Preexposure vaccination against rabies does NOT eliminate the need for additional therapy after exposure to rabies. Preexposure vaccination does, however, simplify postexposure therapy by eliminating the need for human rabies immune globulin (HRIG) and by decreasing the number of postexposure doses of vaccine needed. Persons at continued risk of frequent exposure should receive a booster dose of HDCV every 2 years or have their serum tested for rabies antibody every 2 years; if the titer is inadequate (<5 by the rapid fluorescent-focus inhibition test), they should receive a booster dose.

Plague vaccine should be considered in the western United States for veterinarians and their assistants who may be exposed to bubonic or pneumonic infection in animals, particularly domestic cats.

Selected Field Personnel

Plague vaccine is indicated for field personnel who cannot avoid regular exposure to potentially plague-infected wild rodents and rabbits and their fleas.

Preexposure rabies vaccine prophylaxis should be considered for field personnel who are likely to have contact with potentially rabid dogs, cats, skunks, raccoons, bats, or other wildlife species.

Selected Occupations

Anthrax vaccine is indicated for individuals who come in contact in the workplace with imported animal hides, furs, bonemeal, wool, animal hair (especially goat hair), and bristles.

Sewage workers, as all other adults, should be adequately vaccinated against diphtheria and tetanus. Sewage workers are not at increased risk of polio, typhoid fever, or hepatitis A; poliovirus and typhoid vaccines and immune globulin (IG) are not routinely recommended for them.

Life-Styles

Various life-styles may increase the risk of exposure to certain vaccine-preventable illnesses. Persons with these life-styles may require vaccines in addition to those routinely recommended for their age group. Table 4 provides a summary of the vaccines recommended.

Homosexually Active Males

Homosexually active males are at high risk of HBV as well as human immunodeficiency virus (HIV) infection. Between 35% and 80% have serologic evidence of HBV infection. Susceptible homosexual males should be vaccinated with HB vaccine as early as possible after they begin homosexual activity because 10%–20% can be expected to acquire HBV infection each year. Because of the high prevalence of infection, serologic screening of homosexual males before vaccination may be cost effective regardless of age or length of homosexual activity. Homosexual men known to have HIV infection should be tested for antibody to hepatitis B surface antigen (HBsAg) 1–6 months after completing the vaccine series (HB vaccine is less effective among HIV-infected persons than among similar persons without HIV infection). Revaccination with one or more doses should be considered if the level of antibody to HBsAg (anti-HBs) is <10 milli-international units [mIU]/milliliter (mL).

Injecting Drug Users

Injecting drug users are at high risk of HBV as well as HIV infection. Serologic evidence of HBV infection has been found in 60%–80% of these individuals. Efforts should be made to vaccinate susceptible users with HB vaccine as early as possible after their drug use begins, because 10%–20% can be expected to acquire HBV infection each year. Because of the high prevalence of infection, serologic screening of injecting drug users before vaccination to avoid unnecessary vaccination is cost effective. Injecting drug users with known HIV infection should be tested for antibody to HBsAg 1–6 months after completion of the vaccine series; revaccination with one or more doses should be considered if their anti-HBs level is <10 mIU/mL.

Drug users are also at increased risk of tetanus; their tetanus vaccination status should therefore be kept up to date with Td.

Heterosexually Active Persons

Heterosexually active persons with multiple sex partners are at increased risk of HBV infection. Vaccination is recommended for persons who are diagnosed to have other sexually transmitted diseases, for male or female prostitutes, and for persons who have had sexual activity with multiple partners during the previous 6 months.

Environmental Situations

Certain environments may place an individual at increased risk of vaccine-preventable diseases. Table 4 summarizes additional vaccines recommended for persons in selected environments. The section on "Vaccine-Preventable Diseases and Their Immunobiologics" contains other essential information.

Inmates of Long-Term Correctional Facilities

Serologic evidence of HBV infection has been found among 10%–80% of male prisoners. Although the frequency of transmission during imprisonment has not been clearly documented, the environment of long-term correctional facilities may be associated with a high risk of transmission of HBV infection because of the likelihood of homosexual behavior and of injecting drug use. In selected long-term institutional settings, prison officials may elect to undertake serologic HBV screening and vaccination programs.

Measles and rubella outbreaks have been documented in long-term correctional facilities. All inmates of such facilities should be vaccinated against measles and rubella. If recipients are likely to be susceptible to mumps as well as to measles and rubella, MMR is the vaccine of choice.

All inmates of such facilities greater than or equal to 65 years of age and those with high-risk conditions, including HIV infection, should receive yearly influenza vaccination. Pneumococcal vaccination within the past 6 years should also be documented.

Residents of Institutions for the Developmentally Disabled

Institutions for the developmentally disabled provide a setting conducive to the transmission of HBV infection through human bites and contact with residents' blood, skin lesions, saliva, and other potentially infectious secretions. Serologic evidence of HBV infection has been found among 35%–80% of residents of such institutions. Persons newly admitted to these institutions should be vaccinated as soon as possible. For current residents, screening and vaccination of susceptible residents is recommended. Because of the high prevalence of infection, serologic screening before vaccination of those already institutionalized may be cost effective; however, screening of new admissions very likely will not be. Residents of group homes, foster homes, and similar settings who have household contact with an HBV carrier should also be vaccinated.

Many of the residents of these institutions have chronic medical conditions that put them at risk for complications from influenza illness; therefore, all residents should receive influenza vaccine yearly.

Household Contacts of HBV Carriers

Household contacts of HBV carriers are at high risk of infection. When HBV carriers are identified through routine screening of donated blood, prenatal screening, or other screening programs, the carriers should be notified of their status. All household contacts should be tested and susceptible contacts vaccinated.

Homeless Persons

There are limited data on vaccine-preventable diseases among the homeless. However, such persons will need completed vaccinations for tetanus, diphtheria, measles, mumps, rubella, influenza, and pneumococcal disease. Also, some will be at risk for HBV infection and some will require tuberculin skin testing. The vaccination status of homeless persons should be assessed whenever they are seen in any medical setting.

Travel

The risk of acquiring illness during international travel depends on the areas to be visited and the extent to which the traveler is likely to be exposed to diseases. When considering travel, people often seek advice regarding vaccination from health-care personnel. This provides a good opportunity to review the person's vaccination status and to administer primary series or booster doses, if needed.

In most countries, measles, mumps, and rubella remain uncontrolled. Therefore, the risk of acquiring these diseases while traveling outside the United States is greater than the risk incurred within the United States. Approximately 61% of imported measles cases reported for 1985–1989 occurred among citizens returning to the United States (CDC, unpublished data). To minimize diseases imported by U.S. citizens, all persons traveling abroad should be immune to measles. Consideration should be given to providing a dose of measles vaccine to persons born in or after 1957 who travel abroad, who have not previously received two doses of measles vaccine, and who do not have other evidence of measles immunity (e.g., physician-diagnosed measles or laboratory evidence of measles immunity). If recipients are likely to be susceptible to mumps or rubella in addition to measles, MMR is the vaccine of choice. Travelers, particularly women of childbearing ages, should be immune to rubella before leaving the United States.

In developed countries such as Japan, Canada, Australia, New Zealand, and European countries, the risk of acquiring other vaccine-preventable diseases such as poliomyelitis, diphtheria, and tetanus is usually no greater than the risk incurred while traveling in the United States. In contrast, travelers to developing countries are at increased risk of exposure to many infections, including wild polioviruses and diphtheria. Accordingly, such travelers should be immune to poliomyelitis and diphtheria in particular.

For protection against poliomyelitis, unvaccinated adults should receive at least two doses of eIPV 1 month apart, preferably a complete primary series, before traveling to a developing country or any country with endemic polio; eIPV is preferred because the risk of vaccine-associated paralysis is slightly higher for adults than for children. If travel plans do not permit this interval, a single dose of either OPV or eIPV is recommended. For adults previously incompletely vaccinated with OPV or inactivated poliovirus vaccine (IPV), the remaining doses of either vaccine required for completion of the primary series should be given, regardless of the interval since the last dose or the type of vaccine previously received. Travelers to developing countries who have previously completed a primary series of OPV should receive a single supplementary dose of OPV. Those who have previously received a primary series of IPV should receive a single supplementary dose of either OPV or eIPV. The need for further doses of either vaccine has not been established.

Persons whose age or health status places them at increased risk of complications from influenza illness and who are planning travel to the tropics at any time of year or the southern hemisphere during April through September should review their influenza vaccination history. If not vaccinated during the previous fall or winter, such persons should consider influenza vaccination before travel. Persons in the high-risk categories should be especially encouraged to receive the most currently available vaccine. Persons at high risk given the previous season's vaccine in preparation for travel should be revaccinated in the fall or winter with the current vaccine and therefore may receive two doses of influenza vaccine within 1 year.

Selective vaccination of travelers with vaccines against yellow fever, cholera, typhoid, plague, meningococcal disease, rabies, or HBV infection, or administration of IG to prevent hepatitis A, is recommended on the basis of known or perceived disease-specific risks in the country or countries to be visited and the type and duration of travel within a country. For cholera and yellow fever, vaccination requirements may have been established by the country to be visited. Countries currently reporting yellow fever, cholera, and plague are identified biweekly in the "Summary of Health Information for International Travel."* Information on known or possibly infected areas is published annually in "Health Information for International Travel,"* which also lists specific requirements for cholera and yellow fever vaccinations for each country. All state health departments and many county and city health departments receive both publications. They may also be obtained by calling CDC Information Services at 404–639-1819. For entry into countries requiring yellow fever or cholera vaccination, travelers must have an International Certificate of Vaccination validated by an appropriate authority. State or local health departments can provide the addresses of persons or centers able to validate certificates.

---

*Published by CDC's National Center for Prevention Services, Division of Quarantine, 1600 Clifton Road, NE, Atlanta, Georgia 30333.

Additional information on specific vaccine-preventable illnesses that a traveler might encounter is provided in the sections describing specific vaccines.

Foreign Students, Immigrants, and Refugees

In many countries, children and adolescents are not routinely vaccinated against diphtheria, tetanus, measles, mumps, rubella, and poliomyelitis. As a result, persons entering the United States as college or postgraduate students, immigrants, or refugees may be susceptible to one or more of these diseases.

Refugees from areas of high HBV endemicity (e.g., Southeast Asia) should be screened for HBsAg and anti-HBs. Susceptible household and sexual contacts of HBsAg carriers should receive HB vaccine.

Unless foreign students, immigrants, and refugees can provide a vaccination record documenting the receipt of recommended vaccines or toxoids at appropriate ages and intervals or laboratory evidence of immunity, they should receive the appropriate vaccines for their age, as noted in the "Age Groups" section and in Table 2.

Special Health Status

Some vaccines may be contraindicated for persons with certain health problems; other vaccines may be indicated because of an underlying health condition. Table 5 provides a summary of immunobiologics indicated or contraindicated for persons with selected health problems.

Table 5. Vaccines and toxoids* indicated or specifically contraindicated for situations involving special health status, United States

Health situation	Vaccine/toxoid	
	Indicated	Contraindicated
Pregnancy	Tetanus/diphtheria	Live-virus vaccines
Immunocompromised[†]	Influenza Pneumococcal polysaccharide Haemophilus influenzae type b[§]	Live-virus vaccines Bacille Calmette-Guerin Oral typhoid
Splenic dysfunction or anatomic asplenia	Pneumococcal polysaccharide Influenza Meningococcal polysaccharide Haemophilus influenzae type b[§]	
Hemodialysis or transplant recipients	Hepatitis B[¶] Influenza Pneumococcal polysaccharide	
Deficiencies of factors VIII or IX	Hepatitis B	
Chronic alcoholism	Pneumococcal polysaccharide	
Diabetes and other high-risk diseases	Influenza Pneumococcal polysaccharide	

*Refer also to sections in text on specific vaccines or toxoids for details on indications, contraindications, precautions, dosages, side effects and adverse reactions, and special considerations. Unless specifically contraindicated, the vaccines and toxoids recommended for adults are also indicated. See Table 2 for vaccines and toxoids appropriate for most adults, by age.
†Recommendations specific to persons infected with human immunodeficiency virus are listed in Table 6.
§May be considered.
¶These patients will need a higher dose or an increased number of doses; see "Hemodialysis and Transplantation" section in text.

Pregnancy

When any vaccine or toxoid is to be given during pregnancy, delaying until the second or third trimester, when possible, is a reasonable precaution to minimize concern about possible teratogenicity.

Pregnant women not vaccinated previously against tetanus and diphtheria should receive two doses of Td, properly spaced. Those who have previously received one or two doses of tetanus or diphtheria toxoid should complete their primary series during pregnancy. A primary series is three doses of preparations containing diphtheria and tetanus toxoids, with the first two doses given at least 4 weeks apart and the third dose given 6–12 months after the second. Pregnant women who have completed a primary series should receive a booster dose of Td if greater than or equal to 10 years have elapsed since their last dose.

Because of a theoretical risk to the developing fetus, live-virus vaccines usually should not be given to pregnant women or to those likely to become pregnant within 3 months. If, however, immediate protection against poliomyelitis or yellow fever is needed because of imminent exposure, OPV or yellow fever vaccine may be given. If the only reason to vaccinate a pregnant woman with yellow fever vaccine is an international travel requirement, efforts should be made to obtain a waiver letter. The ACIP strongly recommends that rubella vaccine be administered in the postpartum period to women not known to be immune, preferably before discharge from the hospital.

Data are not available on the safety of HB vaccines for the developing fetus. Because the vaccines contain only noninfectious HBsAg particles, the fetus should not be at risk. In contrast, HBV infection in a pregnant woman may result in severe disease for the mother and chronic infection of the newborn. Therefore, pregnancy or lactation should not be considered a contraindication to the use of this vaccine for persons who are otherwise eligible. Prenatal screening of all pregnant women for HBsAg is recommended. Such screening identifies those who are HBsAg positive and allows treatment of their newborns with hepatitis B immune globulin (HBIG) and HB vaccine, a regimen that is 85%-95% effective in preventing the development of chronic carriage of the HBV.

Pregnant women who have other medical conditions that increase their risks for complications from influenza should be vaccinated; the vaccine is considered safe for pregnant women. Administering the vaccine after the first trimester is a reasonable precaution to minimize any concern over the theoretical risk of teratogenicity. However, it is undesirable to delay vaccinating pregnant women who have high-risk conditions and who will still be in the first trimester of pregnancy when the influenza season begins.

The safety of pneumococcal vaccine for pregnant women has not been evaluated. Ideally, women at high risk of pneumococcal disease should be vaccinated before pregnancy.

Information about immunobiologics and vaccine-preventable diseases during pregnancy is summarized in Appendix 5.

Conditions that Compromise the Immune System

Persons receiving immunosuppressive therapies or with conditions that compromise their immune responses (e.g., leukemia, lymphoma, generalized malignancy, and HIV infection) should receive annual influenza vaccinations with the currently formulated vaccine. Persons with these conditions have been associated with increased risk of pneumococcal disease or its complications and should receive a single dose of pneumococcal polysaccharide vaccine; revaccination should be considered 6 years after the first dose. Haemophilus influenzae type b (Hib) conjugate vaccine (HbCV) is of unproven benefit in immunocompromised persons but may be considered for those with anatomic or functional asplenia or HIV infection. The effectiveness of these vaccines among such persons may be limited, but the risk of disease is substantial and adverse reactions are minimal.

Bacille Calmette-Guerin (BCG), oral typhoid vaccine, or live-virus vaccines should not be given to persons who are immunocompromised as a result of immune deficiency diseases, leukemia, lymphoma, or generalized malignancy or who are immunosuppressed as a result of therapy with corticosteroids, alkylating drugs, antimetabolites, or radiation. However, susceptible patients with leukemia in remission who have not had chemotherapy for at least 3 months may receive live-virus vaccines. The exact interval between discontinuing immunosuppressives and regaining the ability to respond to individual vaccines is not known. Estimates of experts vary from 3 months to 1 year (9). In addition, persons with asymptomatic HIV infection should be vaccinated against measles, mumps, and rubella. Such vaccination should be considered for persons with symptomatic HIV infection because of the danger of serious or fatal measles and the accumulating evidence of the safety of administering MMR to these patients (Table 6).

Table 6. Recommendations for routine vaccination of HIV-infected persons*, United States

	HIV infection	
Vaccine/toxoid[†]	Known asymptomatic	Symptomatic
DTP/TD	yes	yes
OPV	no	no
eIPV[§]	yes	yes
MMR	yes	yes[¶]
HbCV**	yes	yes
Pneumococcal	yes	yes
Influenza	yes[¶]	yes

*Appropriate for human immunodeficiency virus (HIV)-infected children and adults.
[†]The vaccine/toxoid abbreviations are defined as follows: DTP = Diphtheria and tetanus toxoids and pertussis vaccine, adsorbed (pediatric); Td = Tetanus and diphtheria toxoids, adsorbed (for adult use); OPV = Oral poliovirus vaccine; eIPV = Enhanced-potency inactivated poliovirus vaccine; MMR = Measles, mumps, and rubella vaccine; HbCV = Haemophilus influenzae type b conjugate vaccine; and Pneumococcal = Pneumococcal polysaccharide vaccine.
[§]For adults ≥18 years of age, use only if indicated. (See text.)
[¶]Should be considered.
**May be considered for HIV-infected adults (see "Special Health Status: Conditions that Compromise the Immune System" in text).

Short-term (<2-week) corticosteroid therapy, topical steroid therapy (e.g., nasal or skin), and intra-articular, bursal, or tendon injections with corticosteroids should not be immunosuppressive and do not contraindicate vaccination with live-virus vaccines. Vaccination should be avoided if systemic immunosuppressive levels are achieved by topical application.

Vaccines given to immunocompromised patients cannot be assumed to be as effective as when given to normal individuals. When available, postvaccination antibody titrations can be done, but, in the absence of specific antibody information, appropriate immune globulins should be considered for exposures to vaccine-preventable diseases, as discussed in the "Immune Globulins" section.

Hemodialysis and Transplantation

Persons receiving hemodialysis have been at high risk of infection with HBV, although environmental control measures have reduced this risk during the past decade. Nationwide, an estimated 15% of hemodialysis patients have serologic evidence of HBV infection, and routine serologic screening of hemodialysis patients is currently recommended. Susceptible patients who will soon require or are currently receiving long-term hemodialysis should receive three doses of HB vaccine as soon as possible. Larger doses (two to four times those for healthy adults) and/or increased numbers of doses are recommended for these patients because of lower vaccine immunogenicity. The individual manufacturer's vaccine package inserts should be inspected to learn the proper dosages of each vaccine. Postvaccination screening to demonstrate antibody to HBsAg is recommended in this group. Approximately 60% of hemodialysis patients who receive recommended doses of HB vaccine develop protective antibodies against HBV. Revaccination with one or more additional doses should be considered for persons who do not respond to vaccination. In hemodialysis patients, protection lasts only as long as anti-HBs levels remain >10 mIU/mL. Such patients should be tested for anti-HBs annually and revaccinated when anti-HBs declines below this level.

Because renal transplant recipients and persons with chronic renal disease are at increased risk of adverse consequences (including transplant rejection) from infections of the lower respiratory tract, these persons should receive annual influenza vaccination with the current formulated vaccine. Because these patients are also at increased risk of developing pneumococcal infection and experiencing more severe pneumococcal disease, they should receive pneumococcal polysaccharide vaccine.

Splenic Dysfunction or Anatomic Asplenia

Persons with splenic dysfunction or anatomic asplenia are at increased risk of contracting fatal pneumococcal bacteremia and should receive pneumococcal polysaccharide vaccine. They are also at risk for meningococcal bacteremia and should receive meningococcal polysaccharide vaccine. The theoretical increased risk for invasive Hib disease suggests that such persons may be considered for HbCV. Persons scheduled for elective splenectomy should receive both pneumococcal and meningococcal polysaccharide vaccines at least 2 weeks before the operation.

Factor VIII and IX Deficiencies

Patients with clotting disorders who receive factor VIII or IX concentrates have an increased risk of HBV infection. Such patients without serologic markers for hepatitis B should be vaccinated against hepatitis B before receiving any blood products. To avoid hemorrhagic complications, vaccination should be given subcutaneously (SC), rather than intramuscularly (IM) as in the nonhemophilic patient. Prevaccination serologic screening for HBV markers is recommended for patients who have already received multiple infusions of these products.

Chronic Alcoholism

Persons with chronic alcoholism may be at increased risk of contracting a pneumococcal infection or having a more severe pneumococcal illness. Such persons, especially those with cirrhosis, should receive pneumococcal polysaccharide vaccine.

High-Risk Diseases

Persons with disease conditions that increase the risk of adverse consequences from lower-respiratory-tract infections should receive annual influenza vaccination with the current formulated vaccine. These conditions include the following: acquired or congenital heart disease with actual or potentially altered circulatory dynamics; any chronic disorder or condition that compromises pulmonary function; diabetes mellitus or other metabolic diseases that increase the likelihood that infections will be more severe; chronic renal disease with azotemia or nephrotic syndrome; and chronic hemoglobinopathies, such as sickle cell disease.

Some chronic illnesses (e.g., chronic pulmonary disease, congestive heart failure, diabetes mellitus) predispose individuals to an increased risk of pneumococcal illness or its complications. Such persons should receive pneumococcal polysaccharide vaccine.

REQUIREMENTS FOR PERMANENT VACCINATION RECORDS AND REPORTING ADVERSE EVENTS

NCVIA requires physicians and other health-care providers who administer vaccines to maintain permanent vaccination records and to report occurrences of certain adverse events specified in the Act (Table 1). The vaccines and toxoids to which these requirements apply are measles, mumps, and rubella single-antigen vaccines and combination vaccines (MMR, measles, rubella vaccine, live [MR]); diphtheria and tetanus toxoids, adsorbed (pediatric) (DT); Td; tetanus toxoid, adsorbed (T); OPV; IPV; diphtheria and tetanus toxoids and pertussis vaccine, adsorbed (pediatric) (DTP); and pertussis vaccine (P).

Requirements for Recording

All health-care providers who administer one or more of these vaccines or toxoids are required to ensure that the recipient's permanent medical record (or a permanent office log or file) states the date the vaccine was administered, the vaccine manufacturer, the vaccine lot number, the name, the address, and the title of the person administering the vaccine. The term health-care provider is defined as any licensed health-care professional, organization, or institution, whether private or public (including federal, state, and local departments and agencies), under whose authority a specified vaccine is administered.

Requirements for Reporting Adverse Events

Health-care providers are required to report selected events occurring after vaccination to the Vaccine Adverse Events Reporting System (VAERS).

Reportable adverse events are shown in Table 1 and include events described in the vaccine manufacturer's package insert as contraindications to receiving additional doses of vaccine.

Adverse events other than those listed on Table 1 or occurring after administration of other vaccines, especially events that are serious or unusual, can also be reported to VAERS. VAERS forms and instructions are available in the "FDA Drug Bulletin" (Food and Drug Administration) and the "Physicians' Desk Reference" or by calling VAERS at 1-800-822-7967.

Vaccine Injury Compensation

The National Vaccine Injury Compensation Program is a system under which compensation can be paid on behalf of an individual who died or was injured as a result of being given a vaccine. The program is intended as an alternative to civil litigation under the traditional torts system in that negligence need not be proven. The program was created by NCVIA and became effective on October 1, 1988.

The law established a vaccine injury table (Table 1), which lists the vaccines covered by the program as well as the injuries, disabilities, illnesses, and conditions (including death) for which compensation may be paid. The program also sets out the period of time during which the first symptom or significant aggravation of the injury must appear. This period often differs from that required for reporting. Persons may be compensated for an injury listed in Table 1 or one that can be demonstrated to result from administration of a listed vaccine. Additional information about the program is available from Administrator, National Vaccine Injury Compensation Program, Health Resources and Services Administration, 6001 Montrose Road, Room 702, Rockville, MD 20852, Telephone: (301) 443-6593.

Persons wishing to file a claim for a vaccine injury should call or write to: U.S. Claims Court, 717 Madison Place, NW, Washington, D.C. 20005, Telephone: (202) 633-7257.

VACCINE-PREVENTABLE DISEASES AND THEIR IMMUNOBIOLOGICS

Vaccines, toxoids, and immune globulins are available for use in preventing many diseases. These diseases and their specific immunobiologics are presented in this section. For each immunobiologic, the dosage, route of delivery, indications for use, side effects, adverse reactions, precautions, and contraindications are described here. These are also summarized in Table 7.

Toxoids

Diphtheria

The occurrence of diphtheria has decreased dramatically in the United States, largely because of the widespread use of diphtheria toxoid. Only 11 cases of respiratory diphtheria were reported in the period 1985–1989. Seven of these 11 cases occurred among adults greater than or equal to 20 years of age, and three among adults greater than or equal to 60 years of age. Diphtheria occurs primarily among unvaccinated or inadequately vaccinated individuals. Limited serosurveys done since 1977 indicate that 22%–62% of adults 18–39 years of age and 41%–84% of those greater than or equal to 60 years of age lack protective levels of circulating antitoxin against diphtheria (10–13).

Diphtheria Toxoid

Complete and appropriately timed vaccination is at least 85% effective in preventing diphtheria. The combined preparation Td is recommended for use among adults because a large proportion of them lack protective levels of circulating antibody against tetanus (10–13). Furthermore, Td contains much less diphtheria toxoid than other diphtheria toxoid-containing products, and, as a result, reactions to the diphtheria component are less likely. Vaccination with any diphtheria toxoid does not, however, prevent or eliminate carriage of Corynebacterium diphtheriae.

Toxoid Indications

All adults lacking a completed primary series of diphtheria and tetanus toxoids should complete the series with Td. A primary series for adults is three doses of preparations containing diphtheria and tetanus toxoids, with the first two doses given at least 4 weeks apart and the third dose given 6–12 months after the sec-

Table 7. Immunobiologics* and schedules for adults (≥18 years of age)*† , United States

Immunobiologic generic name	Primary schedule and booster(s)	Indications	Major precautions and contraindications§	Special considerations
TOXOIDS				
Tetanus/diphtheria toxoid, adsorbed (for adult use) (Td)	Two doses intramuscularly (IM) 4 weeks apart; third doses 6–12 months after second dose. Booster every 10 years.	All adults.	Except in the first trimester, pregnancy is not a contraindication. History a neurologic reaction or immediate hypersensitivity reaction following a previous dose. History of severe local (Arthus-type) reaction following previous dose. Such individuals should not be given further routine or emergency doses of Td for 10 years.	Tetanus prophylaxis in wound management. (See text and Table 8.)
LIVE-VIRUS VACCINES Measles vaccine, live	One dose subcutaneously (SC); second dose at least 1 month later, at entry into college or post-high school education, beginning medical facility employment, or before traveling. Susceptible travelers should receive one dose.	All adults born after 1956 without documentation of live vaccine on or after first birthday, physician-diagnosed measles, or laboratory evidence of immunity; persons born	Pregnancy; immunocompromised persons¶; history of anaphylactic reactions following egg ingestion or receipt of neomycin. (See text.)	MMR is the vaccine of choice if recipients are likely to be susceptible to rubella and/or mumps as well as to measles. Persons vaccinated between 1963 and

Vaccine	Dose/Schedule	Indications	Contraindications	Comments
(measles, continued)		before 1957 are generally considered immune.		1967 with a killed measles vaccine alone, killed vaccine followed by live vaccine, or with a vaccine of unknown type should be revaccinated with live measles virus vaccine. MMR is the vaccine of choice if recipients are likely to be susceptible to measles and rubella as well as to mumps.
Mumps vaccine, live	One dose SC; no booster.	All adults believed to be susceptible can be vaccinated. Adults born before 1957 can be considered immune.	Pregnancy; immunocompromised persons[1]; history of anaphylactic reaction following egg ingestion. (See text.)	
Rubella vaccine, live	One dose SC; no booster.	Indicated for adults, both male and female, lacking documentation of live vaccine on or after first birthday or laboratory evidence of immunity, particularly young adults who work or congregate in places such as hospitals,	Pregnancy; immunocompromised persons[1]; history of anaphylactic reaction following receipt of neomycin.	Women pregnant when vaccinated or who become pregnant within 3 months of vaccination should be counseled on the theoretical risks to the fetus. The risk of rubella vaccine-associated malformations in

Table 7.—*continued*

Immunobiologic generic name	Primary schedule and booster(s)	Indications	Major precautions and contraindications	Special considerations
		colleges, and military, as well as susceptible travelers.		these women is so small as to be negligible. MMR is the vaccine of choice if recipients are likely to be susceptible to measles or mumps as well as to rubella.
Smallpox vaccine (vaccinia virus)	THERE ARE NO INDICATIONS FOR THE USE OF SMALLPOX VACCINE IN THE GENERAL CIVILIAN POPULATION.			Laboratory workers working with orthopox viruses or health-care workers involved in clinical trials of vaccinia-recombinant vaccines.
Yellow fever attenuated virus, live (17D strain)	One dose SC 10 days to 10 years before travel; booster every 10 years.	Selected persons traveling or living in areas where yellow fever infection exists.	Although specific information is not available concerning adverse effects on the developing fetus, it is prudent on theoretical grounds to avoid vaccinating a pregnant	Some countries require a valid International Certificate of Vaccination showing receipt of vaccine. If the only reason to vaccinate

Vaccine	Primary schedule and booster(s)	Indications	Contraindications and precautions	Special considerations
		woman unless she must travel where the risk of yellow fever is high.	Immunocompromised persons[1]; history of hypersensitivity to egg ingestion.	a pregnant woman is an international requirement, efforts should be made to obtain a waiver letter (see text).
LIVE-VIRUS AND INACTIVATED-VIRUS VACCINES Polio vaccines; Enhanced potency inactivated polio-virus vaccine (eIPV) Oral poliovirus vaccine, live (OPV)	eIPV preferred for primary vaccination; two doses SC 4 weeks apart; a third dose 6–12 months after second; for adults with a completed primary series and for whom a booster is indicated, either OPV or eIPV can be administered. If immediate protection is needed, OPV is recommended.	Persons traveling to areas where wild poliovirus is epidemic or endemic. Certain health-care personnel. (See text for recommendations for incompletely vaccinated adults and adults in households of children to be immunized.)	Although there is no convincing evidence documenting adverse effects of either OPV or eIPV on the pregnant woman or developing fetus, it is prudent on theoretical grounds to avoid vaccinating pregnant women. However, if immediate protection against poliomyelitis is needed, OPV is recommended. OPV should not be given to immunocompromised individuals or to persons with known or possibly immunocompromised family members.[1] eIPV is recommended in such situations.	Although a protective immune response to eIPV in the immunocompromised person cannot be assured, the vaccine is safe, and some protection may result from its administration.

Table 7.—*continued*

Immunobiologic generic name	Primary schedule and booster(s)	Indications	Major precautions and contraindications	Special considerations
INACTIVATED-VIRUS VACCINES				
Hepatitis B (HB) inactivated-virus vaccine	Two doses IM 4 weeks apart; third dose 5 months after second; booster doses not necessary within 7 years of primary series. Alternate schedule for one vaccine: three doses IM 4 weeks apart; fourth dose 10 months after the third.	Adults at increased risk of occupational, environmental, social, or family exposure.	Data are not available on the safety of the vaccine for the developing fetus. Because the vaccine contains only non-infectious HBsAg particles, the risk should be negligible. Pregnancy should *not* be considered a vaccine contraindication if the woman is otherwise eligible.	The vaccine produces neither therapeutic nor adverse effects on HBV-infected persons. Prevaccination serologic screening for susceptibility before vaccination may or may not be cost effective depending on costs of vaccination and testing and on the prevalence of immune persons in the group.
Influenza vaccine (inactivated whole-virus and split-virus) vaccine	Annual vaccination with current vaccine. Either whole- or split-virus vaccine may be used.	Adults with high-risk conditions, residents of nursing homes or other chronic-care facilities, medical-care personnel, or	History of anaphylactic hypersensitivity to egg ingestion.	No evidence exists of maternal or fetal risk when vaccine is administered in pregnancy because of an underlying high-risk condition

Immunobiologic	Primary schedule and booster(s)	Indications	Precautions and contraindications
		healthy persons ≥65 years.	in a pregnant woman. However, it is reasonable to wait until the second or third trimester, if possible, before vaccination. Complete preexposure prophylaxis does not eliminate the need for additional therapy with rabies vaccine after a rabies exposure. The decision for postexposure use of HDCV depends on the species of biting animal, the circumstances of biting incident, and the type of exposure (e.g., bite, saliva contamination of wound). The type of and schedule
Human diploid cell rabies vaccine (HDCV) inactivated, whole-virion), rabies vaccine, adsorbed (RVA)	Preexposure prophylaxis: two doses 1 week apart; third dose 3 weeks after second. If exposure continues, booster doses every 2 years, or an antibody titer determined and a booster dose administered if titer is inadequate (<5). Postexposure prophylaxis: All postexposure treatment should begin with soap and water. 1. Persons who have (a) previously received postexposure prophylaxis with HDCV, (b) received recommended IM preexposure series of HDCV, (c) received recommended ID	Veterinarians, animal handlers, certain laboratory workers, and persons living in or visiting countries for >1 month where rabies is a constant threat.	If there is substantial risk of exposure to rabies, preexposure vaccination may be indicated during pregnancy. Corticosteroids and immunosuppressive agents can interfere with the development of active immunity; history of anaphylactic or Type III hypersensitivity reaction to previous dose of HDCV. (See text.)

Table 7.—*continued*

Immunobiologic generic name	Primary schedule and booster(s)	Indications	Major precautions and contraindications	Special considerations
	preexposure series of HDCV in the United States, or (d) have a previously documented rabies antibody titer considered adequate: two doses of HDCV, 1.0 mL IM, one each on days 0 and 3. 2. Persons not previously immunized as above: HRIG 20 IU/kg body weight, half infiltrated at bite site if possible; remainder IM; and five doses of HDCV, 1.0 mL IM one each on days 0, 3, 7, 14, 28.			for postexposure prophylaxis depends upon the person's previous rabies vaccination status, or the result of a previous or current serologic test for rabies antibody. For postexposure prophylaxis, HDCV should always be administered IM, *not* ID.
INACTIVATED BACTERIA VACCINES				
Cholera vaccine	Two 0.5-mL doses SC or IM or two 0.2-mL doses ID 1 week to 1 month apart; booster doses (0.5 mL IM or 0.2 mL ID) every 6 months.	Travelers to countries requiring evidence of cholera vaccination for entry.	No specific information on vaccine safety during pregnancy. Use in pregnancy should reflect actual increased risk. Persons who have had severe local or systemic reactions to a previous dose.	One dose generally satisfies International Health Regulations. Some countries may require evidence of a complete primary series or a booster dose given within 6

Vaccine	Dosage and route	Indications	Contraindications and precautions	Comments
				months before arrival. Vaccination should not be considered an alternative to continued careful selection of foods and water.
Haemophilus influenzae type b conjugate vaccine (HbCV)	Dosage for adults has not been determined.	May be considered for adults at highest theoretical risk e.g., those with anatomic or functional asplenia or HIV infection).	No specific information on vaccine safety during pregnancy.	No efficacy data available for adults; not indicated for adult contacts of children with invasive disease.
Meningococcal polysaccharide vaccine tetravalent A, C, W135, and Y)	One dose in volume and by route specified by manufacturer; need for boosters unknown.	Travelers visiting areas of a country that are recognized as having epidemic meningococcal disease.	Pregnancy unless there is substantial risk of infection.	
Plague vaccine	Three IM doses; first dose 1.0 mL; second dose 0.2 mL 1 month later; third dose 0.2 mL 5 months after second; booster doses 0.2 mL) at 1- to 2-year intervals if exposure continues.	Selected travelers to countries reporting cases, or in which avoidance of rodents and fleas is impossible; all laboratory and field personnel working with Yersinia pestis organisms possibly resistant to antimicrobials;	Pregnancy, unless there is substantial and unavoidable risk of exposure; persons with known hypersensitivity to any of the vaccine constituents (see manufacturer's label); patients who have had severe local or systemic reactions to a previous dose.	Prophylactic antibiotics may be recommended for definite exposure whether or not the exposed person has been vaccinated.

Table 7.—*continued*

Immunobiologic generic name	Primary schedule and booster(s)	Indications	Major precautions and contraindications	Special considerations
		those engaged in *Y. pestis* aerosal experiments or in field operations in areas with enzootic plague where regular exposure to potentially infected wild rodents, rabbits, or their fleas cannot be prevented.		
Pneumococcal polysaccharide vaccine (23 valent).	One dose; revaccination recommended for those at highest risk ≥6 years after the first dose.	Adults who are at increased risk of pneumococcal disease and its complications because of underlying health conditions; older adults, especially those ≥65 years of age who are healthy.	The safety of vaccine for pregnant women has not been evaluated; it should not be given during pregnancy unless the risk of infection is high. Previous recipients of any type of pneumococcal polysaccharide vaccine who are at highest risk of fatal infection or antibody loss may be revaccinated ≥6 years after the first dose. (See text.)	

INACTIVATED BACTERIA AND LIVE-BACTERIA VACCINES

	Dosage	Indications	Contraindications/Precautions	Comments
Typhoid vaccine, SC and oral	Two 0.5-mL doses SC 4 or more weeks apart, booster 0.5 mL SC or 0.1 mL ID every 3 years if exposure continues. Four oral doses on alternate days. The manufacturer recommends revaccination with the entire four-dose series every 5 years.	Travelers to areas where there is a recognized risk of exposure to typhoid.	Severe local or systemic reaction to a previous dose. Acetone-killed and -dried vaccines should not be administered ID.	Vaccination should not be considered an alternative to continued careful selection of foods and water.

LIVE-BACTERIA VACCINE

	Dosage	Indications	Contraindications/Precautions	Comments
Bacille Calmette-Guerin vaccine (BCG)	One dose ID or percutaneously. (See package label.)	For children only, who have prolonged close contact with untreated or ineffectively treated active tuberculosis patients; groups with excessive rates of new infection in which other control measures have not been successful.	Pregnancy, unless there is unavoidable exposure to infective tuberculosis; immunocompromised patients.[1]	In the United States, tuberculosis-control efforts are directed towards early identification and treatment of cases, and preventive therapy with isoniazid.

IMMUNE GLOBULINS

	Dosage	Indications	Contraindications/Precautions	Comments
Cytomegalovirus immune globulin (intravenous)	Bone marrow transplant recipients: 1.0 g/kg weekly; kidney transplant recipients: 150 mg/kg initially, then 50–100 mg/kg every 2 weeks.	As prophylaxis for bone marrow and kidney transplant recipients.		Prophylaxis must be continued for 3–4 months to be effective.

Table 7.—continued

Immunobiologic generic name	Primary schedule and booster(s)	Indications	Major precautions and contraindications	Special considerations
Immune globulin (IG)	Hepatitis A prophylaxis: *Preexposure:* one IM dose of 0.02 mL/kg for anticipated risk of 2–3 months; IM dose of 0.06 mL/kg for anticipated risk of 5 months; repeat appropriate dose at above intervals if exposure continues.	Nonimmune persons traveling to developing countries		For travelers, IG is not an alternative to continued careful selection of foods and water. Frequent travelers should be tested for hepatitis A antibody. IG is not indicated for persons with antibody to hepatitis A.
	Postexposure: one IM dose of 0.02 mL/kg administered within 2 weeks of exposure.	Household and sexual contacts of persons with hepatitis A; staff, attendees, and parents of diapered attendees in day care center outbreaks.		
	Measles prophylaxis: 0.25 mL/kg IM (maximum 15 mL) administered within 6 days after exposure.	Exposed susceptible contacts of measles cases.	IG should *not* be used to control measles.	IG administered within 6 days after exposure can prevent or modify measles. Recipients

of IG for measles prophylaxis should receive live measles vaccine 3 months later.

Hepatitis B immune globulin (HBIG)	0.06 mL/kg IM as soon as possible after exposure (with HB vaccine started at a different site); a second dose of HBIG should be administered 1 month later (percutaneous/mucous-membrane exposure) or 3 months later (sexual exposure) if the HB vaccine series has not been started. (See text.)	Following percutaneous or mucous-membrane exposure to blood known to be HBsAgpositive (within 7 days); following sexual exposure to a person with acute HBV or an HBV carrier (within 14 days).
Tetanus immune globulin (TIG)	250 U IM.	Part of the management of nonclean, nonminor wound in a person with unknown tetanus toxoid status, with less than two previous doses or with two previous doses and a wound more than 24 hours old.

Table 7.—continued

Immunobiologic generic name	Primary schedule and booster(s)	Indications	Major precautions and contraindications	Special considerations
Rabies immune globulin, human (HRIG)	20 IU/kg, up to half infiltrated around wound; remainder IM.	Part of management of rabies exposure in persons lacking a history of recommended preexposure or postexposure propylaxis with HDCV.		Although preferable to administer the first dose of vaccine, can be administered up to the eighth day after the first dose of vaccine.
Vaccinia immune globulin	0.6 mL/kg in divided doses over 24–36 hours; may be repeated every 2–3 days until no new lesions appear.	Treatment of eczema vaccinatum, vaccinia necrosum, and ocular vaccinia.		Of no benefit for postvaccination encephalitis.
Varicella-zoster immune globulin (VZIG)	Persons >50 kg: 125 U/10 kg IM; persons >50 kg: 625 U**	Immunocompromised patients known or likely to be susceptible with close and prolonged exposure to a household contact case or to an infectious hospital staff member		

or hospital roommate.

*Refer also to sections of text on specific vaccines or toxoids for further details on indications, contraindications, precautions, dosages, side effects and adverse reactions, and special considerations. Refer also to individual ACIP statements (see list of published ACIP statements, Appendix 2). Several other vaccines, toxoids, and immune globulins are licensed and available. These are noted in Appendix 3. In addition, the following antitoxins are licensed and available: (a) botulism antitoxin, trivalent equine (ABE) (distributed by CDC only), and (b) tetanus antitoxin (equine).

†Several vaccines and toxoids are in "Investigational New Drug" (IND) status and available only through the U.S. Army Research Institute for Infectious Diseases (telephone 301-663-2403). These are: (a) eastern equine encephalitis vaccine (EEE), (b) western equine encephalitis vaccine (WEE), (c) Venezuelan equine encephalitis vaccine (VEE), and (d) tularemia vaccine. Pentavalent (ABCDE) botulinum toxoid is available only through CDC's Drug Service.

‡When any vaccine or toxoid is indicated during pregnancy, waiting until the second or the third trimester, when possible, is a reasonable precaution that minimizes concern about teratogenicity.

¶Persons immunocompromised because of immune deficiency diseases, HIV infection (who should primarily not receive OPV and yellow fever vaccines) (see text), leukemia, lymphoma, or generalized malignancy or immunosuppressed as a result of therapy with corticosteroids, alkylating drugs, antimetabolites, or radiation.

**Some persons have recommended 125 U/10 kg regardless of total body weight.

ond. All adults for whom greater than or equal to 10 years have elapsed since completion of their primary series or since their last booster dose should receive a dose of Td. Thereafter, a booster dose of Td should be administered every 10 years. There is no need to repeat doses if the schedule for the primary series or booster doses is delayed.

Tetanus

The occurrence of tetanus has decreased dramatically, largely because of the widespread use of tetanus toxoid. Nevertheless, the number of cases remained relatively constant from 1986 through 1989, during which 48–64 cases were reported annually. Tetanus occurs almost exclusively among unvaccinated or inadequately vaccinated persons. Immune pregnant women transfer temporary protection against tetanus to their infants through transplacental maternal antibody.

In the period 1982–1989, persons greater than or equal to 20 years of age accounted for 95% of the 513 reported tetanus cases for which patient ages were known; persons greater than or equal to 60 years of age accounted for 59%. The age distribution of persons who died from tetanus was similar. Serosurveys done since 1977 indicate that 6%–11% of adults 18–39 years of age and 49%–66% of those greater than or equal to 60 years of age lack protective levels of circulating antitoxin against tetanus (10–13). Although surveys of emergency rooms suggest that only 1%–6% of all persons who receive medical care for injuries that can lead to tetanus receive inadequate prophylaxis (14), in 1987–1988, 81% of the people who developed tetanus after an acute injury and sought medical care did not receive adequate prophylaxis as recommended by the ACIP (14).

Tetanus Toxoid

Complete and appropriately timed vaccination is nearly 100% effective in preventing tetanus. Td is the preferred preparation for active tetanus immunization of adults because a large proportion of them also lack protective levels of circulating antitoxin against diphtheria (10–13).

Toxoid Indications

All adults lacking a complete primary series of diphtheria and tetanus toxoids should complete the series with Td. A primary series for adults is three doses of preparations containing tetanus and diphtheria toxoids, with the first two doses given at least 4 weeks apart and the third dose given 6–12 months after the second. Persons who have served in the military can be considered to have received a primary series of diphtheria and tetanus toxoids. The practitioner should be aware that policies of the different branches of the military have varied among themselves and over time. All adults for whom greater than or equal to 10 years have elapsed since completion of their primary series or since their last booster dose should receive a booster dose of Td. Thereafter, a booster dose of Td should be administered every 10 years. Doses need not be repeated if the primary schedule for the series or booster doses is delayed.

The recommended pediatric schedule for DTP includes a booster dose at age 4–6 years. The first Td booster is recommended at age 14–16 years (10 years after the dose at age 4–6 years). One means of ensuring that persons continue to receive boosters every 10 years is to vaccinate persons routinely at mid-decade ages (e.g., 25 years of age, 35 years of age).

For wound management, the need for active immunization, with or without passive immunization, depends on the condition of the wound and the patient's vaccination history. A summary of the indications for active and passive immunization is provided in Table 8. Only rarely have cases of tetanus occurred among persons with a documented primary series of toxoid injections.

Evidence indicates that complete primary vaccination with tetanus toxoid provides long-lasting protection (greater than or equal to 10 years among most recipients). Consequently, after complete primary tetanus vaccination, boosters are recommended at 10-year intervals. For clean and minor wounds occurring during the 10-year interval, no additional booster is recommended. For other wounds, a booster is appropriate if the patient has not received tetanus toxoid within the preceding 5 years. Antitoxin antibodies develop rapidly in persons who have previously received at least two doses of tetanus toxoid.

Persons who have not completed a full primary series of injections or whose vaccination status is unknown or uncertain may require tetanus toxoid and passive immunization at the time of wound cleaning and debridement. Ascertaining the interval since the most recent toxoid dose is not sufficient. A careful attempt should be made to determine whether a patient has previously

Table 8. Summary guide to tetanus prophylaxis* in routine wound management, United States

	Clean, minor wounds		All other wounds[†]	
	Td[§]	TIG[¶]	Td[§]	TIG
Uncertain or <3	Yes	No	Yes	Yes
>3**	No[‡]	No	No[§§]	No

*Refer also to text on specific vaccines or toxoids for contraindications, precautions, dosages, side effects, adverse reactions, and special considerations. Important details are in the text and in the ACIP recommendations on diphtheria, tetanus, and pertussis (DTP) (MMWR 1991:40[RR-10]).

[†]Such as, but not limited to: wounds contaminated with dirt, feces, and saliva; puncture wounds; avulsions; and wounds resulting from missiles, crushing, burns, and frostbite.

[§]Td = Tetanus and diphtheria toxoids, adsorbed (for adult use). For children <7 years old, DTP (DT, if pertussis vaccine is contraindicated) is preferred to tetanus toxoid alone. For persons ≥7 years old, Td is preferred to tetanus toxoid alone.

[¶]TIG = Tetanus immune globulin.

**If only three doses of fluid toxoid have been received, a fourth dose of toxoid, preferably an adsorbed toxoid, should be given.

[‡]Yes, >10 years since last dose.

[§§]Yes, >5 years since last dose. (More frequent boosters are not needed and can accentuate side effects.)

completed primary vaccination and, if not, how many doses have been given. Persons with unknown or uncertain previous vaccination histories should be considered to have had no previous tetanus toxoid doses.

In managing the wounds of adults, Td is the preferred preparation for active tetanus immunization. This toxoid preparation is also used to enhance protection against diphtheria, because a large proportion of adults are susceptible. Thus, if advantage is taken of visits for care of acute health problems, such as for wound management, some patients who otherwise would remain susceptible can be protected against both diseases. Primary vaccination should ultimately be completed for persons documented to have received fewer than the recommended number of doses, including doses given as part of wound management.

If passive immunization is needed, human tetanus immune globulin (TIG) is the product of choice. The currently recommended prophylactic dose of TIG for wounds of average severity is 250 units IM. When T or Td and TIG are given concurrently, separate syringes and separate sites should be used. Most experts consider the use of adsorbed toxoid mandatory in this situation.

Toxoid Side Effects and Adverse Reactions

Local reactions (usually erythema and induration, with or without tenderness) can occur after Td is administered. Fever and other systemic symptoms are less common.

Arthus-type hypersensitivity reactions, characterized by severe local reactions starting 2–8 hours after an injection and often associated with fever and malaise, may occur, particularly among persons who have received multiple boosters of tetanus toxoid, adsorbed (T).

Rarely, severe systemic reactions, such as generalized urticaria, anaphylaxis, or neurologic complications, have been reported after administration of tetanus and diphtheria toxoids. Peripheral neuropathy has been reported rarely after administration of T, although a causal relationship has not been established.

Toxoid Precautions and Contraindications

Although no evidence suggests that diphtheria and tetanus toxoids are teratogenic, waiting until the second trimester of pregnancy to administer Td is a reasonable precaution.

A history of a neurologic reaction or a severe hypersensitivity reaction (e.g., generalized urticaria or anaphylaxis) after a previous dose is a contraindication to diphtheria and tetanus toxoids. Local side effects alone do not preclude continued use. If a prior systemic reaction suggests allergic hypersensitivity, appropriate skin testing to document immediate hypersensitivity may be useful before T vaccination is discontinued. Protocols exist for using both Td and single-antigen tetanus toxoids for skin testing (15). Mild, nonspecific skin-test reactivity to T toxoid is common. Most vaccinees develop a delayed but inconsequential cutaneous hypersensitivity to the toxoid.

Persons experiencing severe Arthus-type hypersensitivity reactions to a dose of T usually have very high serum tetanus antitoxin levels and should not be given even emergency booster doses of Td more frequently than every 10 years.

If a contraindication to using preparations containing T exists in a person who has not completed a primary immunizing course of T and other than a clean minor wound is sustained, only passive immunization should be given using TIG.

Although a minor illness, such as a mild upper respiratory infection, should not be cause for postponing vaccination, a severe febrile illness is reason to defer routine vaccination.

Live-Virus Vaccines

Measles

Before the introduction of measles vaccine in 1963, approximately 500,000 cases of measles and 500 measles-associated deaths were reported annually in the United States. Because of the widespread use of measles vaccine, the number of reported measles cases decreased to an all-time low of 1,497 in 1983. From 1984 through 1988, the annual number of reported measles cases averaged 3,600, which represents <1% of the cases reported annually in the pre-vaccine era. In 1989 and 1990, a substantial increase in cases was reported, primarily because of a large number of outbreaks among unvaccinated preschool-age children and vaccinated high-school and college-age students. The 27,786 cases provisionally reported in 1990 represent the largest number of cases reported in any year since 1978. Measles cases were reported from 49 states and the District of Columbia. Adults greater than or equal to 20 years of age accounted for 22% of cases, of which 67% were not appropriately vaccinated (unvaccinated with vaccine indicated). Twenty-five percent of these adults with measles required greater than or equal to 1 day of hospitalization. A provisional total of 130 measles-associated deaths was reported in 1989 and 1990; 36 (28%) of these were persons greater than or equal to 20 years of age. At least 267 measles outbreaks were reported; 17 (6%) occurred on college campuses. Two percent of reported cases were among college students or were epidemiologically linked to campus outbreaks.

Encephalitis or death follows measles disease in approximately one case per 1,000. Aside from infants, the risk of encephalitis is greatest among adult patients.

Measles illness during pregnancy increases rates of spontaneous abortion, premature labor, and low birth weight for infants. Although cases of congenital malformation after measles infection during pregnancy have been reported, no specific syndrome has been demonstrated.

Measles Vaccine

Measles vaccine produces a mild or inapparent noncommunicable infection. A single subcutaneously administered dose of live measles vaccine provides durable protection against measles illness for greater than or equal to 95% of susceptible children vaccinated at greater than or equal to 15 months, extending probably for their lifetime. The vaccine of choice is MMR.

Vaccine Indications

All adults born in 1957 or later who do not have a medical contraindication should receive one dose of measles vaccine unless they have a dated record of vaccination with at least one dose of live measles vaccine on or after their first birthday, documentation of physician-diagnosed disease, or laboratory evidence of immunity. Most persons born before 1957 can be considered immune and do not need vaccination. Of all measles cases reported to CDC from 1985 through 1990, 96.3% occurred among persons born in 1957 or later. However, because a small proportion will be susceptible, vaccine should be offered to such individuals, particularly health-care workers, if there is reason to believe that they may be susceptible. Serologic studies of hospital workers indicate that up to 9.3% of persons born before 1957 were not immune to measles (4, 5). Ninety-seven (29%) of 341 health-care workers who developed measles in the period 1985–1989 were born before 1957 (6).

As noted above, a single dose of live measles vaccine given on or after the first birthday can be expected to provide long-lasting immunity to measles in at least 95% of recipients. In most situations, a high rate of vaccination resulting in 95% of the population being immune is sufficient to prevent transmission of measles. However, in some circumstances, 5% susceptibility provides enough nonimmune persons to sustain transmission of measles. This situation occurs most commonly in school and college settings, where large numbers of young adults congregate. Other circumstances in which transmission may occur despite high levels of immunity are in hospitals and other health-care facilities and among persons traveling in places where measles is endemic. In these situations, assuring high levels of immunity to measles among vaccinees by providing a second dose of measles vaccine is desirable. The two-dose schedule is expected to provide protection to most persons who do not respond to their initial vaccination.

Entrants into colleges, universities, and other institutions of post-high school education as well as employees in health-care facilities who do not have evidence of immunity to measles (documented physician-diagnosed measles or laboratory evidence of immunity) should be required to provide documentation of two doses of measles vaccine on or after their first birthday. Use of MMR is preferred for both vaccine doses to assure immunity to all three viruses. Individuals who have no documentation of ever having received any doses of measles vaccine and who do not have other evidence of measles immunity should be given one dose of measles vaccine on entry into college or when beginning employment; they should be revaccinated with a second dose not less than 1 month later. If feasible, colleges and health-care facilities may wish to extend this requirement to all students and employees.

During outbreaks of measles in schools, colleges, or health-care facilities, all persons born in 1957 or later who cannot provide evidence of receiving two doses of measles vaccine or other evidence of measles immunity should receive one dose of measles-containing vaccine. Those persons should receive their second dose of vaccine not less than 1 month later. Because some medical personnel who have acquired measles in medical facilities were born before 1957, vaccination of older employees who may have occupational exposure to measles should also be considered during outbreaks.

An estimated 600,000–900,000 persons in the United States received killed measles vaccine in the period 1963–1967. Individuals who received killed measles vaccine, killed measles vaccine followed within 3 months by live measles vaccine, measles vaccine of unknown type in the period 1963–1967, or vaccine before their first birthday should be considered unvaccinated and should receive at least one dose of live measles vaccine. If these persons are beginning college or other post-high school education or beginning employment in a medical setting, they should receive two doses of measles vaccine at least 1 month apart, as described above.

Because the risk of acquiring measles outside the United States is greater than the risk incurred in the United States, travelers should be immune to measles before leaving the United States. Consideration should be given to providing a dose of measles vaccine to persons born during or after 1957 who travel abroad, who have not previously received two doses of measles vaccine, and who do not have other evidence of measles immunity.

Young adults who are exposed to measles and who have no or uncertain documentation of live measles vaccination on or after their first birthday, no record of physician-diagnosed measles, and no laboratory evidence of immunity should be vaccinated within 72 hours after exposure; vaccination is most likely to be protective during that time. If the exposure did not result in infection, the vaccine should induce protection against subsequent measles infection. An acceptable alternative is to use immune globulin (IG), which can prevent or modify infection if administered within 6 days after exposure. This alternative is principally indicated when measles vaccine is contraindicated. IG should not be used in an attempt to control measles outbreaks. The recommended dose of IG is 0.25 mL/kg IM, not to exceed 15 mL. Live measles vaccine should be given 3 months after IG is administered, by which time the passive measles antibodies should have disappeared. Because postexposure vaccination or administration of IG is not completely effective, medical personnel should be removed from patient contact 5–21 days after exposure.

Vaccine side effects and adverse reactions. A temperature of greater than or equal to 103°F (39.4°C) may develop among approximately 5%–15% of vaccinees, usually beginning between the fifth and twelfth days after vaccination; fever usually lasts 1–2 days and, rarely, up to 5 days.

Rashes have been reported among approximately 5% of vaccinees. Encephalitis after measles vaccination is extremely rare, and its incidence cannot be discerned from the background incidence rate of encephalitis of an unknown etiology. The incidence of postvaccination encephalitis is much lower than the incidence after natural measles.

Reactions after live measles vaccination occur among 4%–55% of prior recipients of killed measles vaccine. The reactions are generally mild, consisting of a local reaction with or without a low-grade fever of 1–2 days duration. Such reactions can be fairly severe but are milder than atypical measles syndrome, an illness that may affect prior recipients of killed measles vaccine who are exposed to natural measles.

No evidence suggests increased risk from live measles vaccination among persons who are already immune to measles as a result of either previous vaccination or natural disease.

Vaccine Precautions and Contraindications

Vaccination should not be postponed because of a minor illness, such as a mild upper-respiratory infection. However, vaccination of persons with severe febrile illnesses should be postponed until recovery. Vaccine should be given 14 days before—or deferred for at least 6 weeks and preferably 3 months after—a person has received IG, whole blood, or other blood products containing antibody.

Because of a theoretical risk to the developing fetus, measles vaccine should not be given to pregnant women.

Measles vaccine also should not be given to persons who are immunocompromised as a result of immune deficiency diseases, leukemia, lymphoma, or generalized malignancy or who are immunosuppressed as a result of therapy with corticosteroids, alkylating drugs, antimetabolites, or radiation. However, persons with leukemia who are in remission and have not received chemotherapy for at least 3 months and HIV-infected persons should be vaccinated against measles, if considered susceptible. (See "Conditions that Compromise the Immune System" and Table 5 and Table 6.)

No evidence suggests that live measles vaccine exacerbates tuberculosis. If tuberculin skin testing is needed, the testing should be done on the day of vaccination and read 48–72 hours later. A recent vaccinee should wait 4–6 weeks after receiving measles vaccine before a tuberculin skin test is administered, because measles vaccination may temporarily suppress tuberculin reactivity.

Persons with a history of any sign or symptom of an anaphylactic reaction (e.g., hives, swelling of the mouth and throat, difficulty breathing, hypotension, or shock) after ingestion of eggs or receipt of neomycin should be given measles vaccine only with extreme caution. Protocols have been developed for vaccinating such persons (16). Persons with reactions that are not anaphylactic are not at increased risk and can be vaccinated.

Mumps

The reported occurrence of mumps cases in the United States has decreased steadily since the introduction of live mumps vaccine. In 1985, a record low of 2,982 cases was reported; this number represented a 98% decline from the 185,691 cases reported in 1967, the year live mumps vaccine was licensed. However, reported cases increased to 7,790 in 1986, followed by 12,848 cases in

1987. In 1988, 1989, and 1990, totals of 4,866, 5,712, and 5,075 cases, respectively, were reported. Largely because of expense, mumps vaccine was not recommended by the ACIP for routine use until 1977, which led to the development of a relatively underimmunized cohort of teenagers and young adults (17). Data from the U.S. Immunization Survey suggest that only approximately 50% of persons of college age in 1986 had received mumps vaccine. In 1989, 38% of reported mumps cases for whom age was known occurred among persons greater than or equal to 15 years of age, compared with 12% in 1977.

Although mumps disease is generally self limiting, meningeal signs may appear in up to 15% of cases, and orchitis in 20%–30% of clinical cases among postpubertal males. Sterility is a rare sequela of mumps orchitis among males. Unilateral sensorineural deafness occurs at a rate of one case per 20,000 cases of mumps.

Mumps Vaccine

Live mumps vaccine has been available since 1967. A single dose of live mumps vaccine administered SC provides protective and long-lasting levels of antibody in >90% of recipients. Clinical vaccine efficacy reports range between 75% and 95%. If recipients are likely to be susceptible to measles and/or rubella as well as to mumps, MMR is the vaccine of choice.

Vaccine Indications

Mumps vaccine is indicated for all adults believed to be susceptible. Persons should be considered susceptible to mumps unless they have documentation of physician-diagnosed mumps, adequate immunization with live mumps vaccine on or after their first birthday, or laboratory evidence of immunity. Most adults born before 1957 are likely to have been infected naturally and can be considered immune, even if they did not have clinically recognizable mumps disease. Killed mumps vaccine was available from 1950 until 1978. Persons who received killed mumps vaccine might benefit from vaccination with live mumps vaccine. Revaccination with MMR is recommended under certain circumstances for measles (see "Measles" section) and may also be important for mumps because recent studies have shown that mumps can occur in highly vaccinated populations. Persons who are unsure of their mumps disease/vaccination history should be vaccinated.

Vaccine Side Effects and Adverse Reactions

Parotitis and fever after vaccination have been reported rarely. Allergic reactions including rash, pruritus, and purpura have been associated temporally with mumps vaccination but are uncommon, usually mild, and of brief duration. The frequency of reported central nervous system (CNS) dysfunction after mumps vaccination is not greater than the observed background incidence rate in the general population.

Because of the recommendation to use MMR for revaccination against measles, many persons will receive two doses of live mumps vaccine. No evidence suggests an increased risk from live mumps vaccination among persons who are already immune to mumps as a result of either previous vaccination or natural disease.

Vaccine precautions and contraindications. Vaccine should be given at least 14 days before, or deferred for at least 6 weeks—and preferably 3 months—after a person has received IG, whole blood, or other blood products containing antibody.

Because of the theoretical risk of fetal harm after administration of a live-virus vaccine to a pregnant woman, avoiding administering mumps vaccine to pregnant women is prudent.

Mumps vaccine should not be given to persons who are immunocompromised as a result of immune deficiency diseases, leukemia, lymphoma, or generalized malignancy or to persons who are immunosuppressed as a result of therapy with corticosteroids, alkylating drugs, antimetabolites, or radiation. Mumps vaccine should be given to asymptomatic HIV-infected individuals and may be considered for those who are symptomatic. (See "Conditions that Compromise the Immune System" and Table 5 and Table 6.) Persons with a history of any sign or symptom of an anaphylactic reaction (e.g., hives, swelling of the mouth and throat, difficulty breathing, hypotension, or shock) after ingestion of eggs or receipt of neomycin should be vaccinated only with extreme caution. Protocols have been developed for vaccinating persons with severe egg allergy (16). Persons with reactions that are not anaphylactic are not at increased risk and can be vaccinated.

Rubella

Preventing fetal infection and consequent CRS are the objectives of rubella immunization. Fetal infection occurring during the first trimester of pregnancy can lead to CRS in up to 80% of fetuses. Also, fetal death because of miscarriage or therapeutic abortion after maternal rubella disease or exposure during the first trimester continues to occur frequently.

The number of reported rubella cases has decreased steadily from >56,000 cases in 1969, the year rubella vaccine was licensed, to 225 cases in 1988. Until the mid-1970s, the strategy was to vaccinate all children; this strategy dramatically reduced the incidence of rubella but had less impact on older age groups, resulting in an increased proportion of cases in adolescents and adults. During the period 1976–1979, >70% of the reported rubella cases occurred among persons greater than or equal to 15 years of age. During 1980 to 1990, this percentage varied widely, reaching a low of 38% in 1988. However, a fivefold increase in rubella incidence occurred between 1988 and 1990. Provisional data indicate that incidence rose sharply among persons greater than or equal to 15 years of age to approximately 57% of 931 cases (with known age) in 1990. A cluster of at least 11 CRS cases among infants born in 1990 was reported to the National CRS Registry. Increased efforts to increase delivery of vaccine to college-age and older persons have led to the current decline in the incidence rates for these age groups. However, an estimated 6%–11% of young adults remain susceptible to rubella, and limited outbreaks continue to be reported in universities, colleges, and places of employment—notably hospitals.

Vaccination of young children has prevented widespread epidemics of rubella and of CRS and eventually will lead to the elimination of CRS as vaccinated cohorts enter the childbearing age. However, increased efforts to ensure that all adults, particularly women of childbearing age, are vaccinated will hasten the elimination of rubella and CRS in the United States. Additional aids to eliminate rubella and CRS include achieving and maintaining high vaccination levels, maintaining vigorous surveillance, and practicing aggressive outbreak control.

Rubella Vaccine

A single SC-administered dose of live, attenuated rubella vaccine provides long-term (probably lifetime) immunity among approximately 95% of vaccinees. Moreover, there has been no identified transmission of vaccine virus in studies of >1,200 susceptible household contacts of vaccinees and in >20 years of experience with live rubella vaccine. If recipients are likely to be susceptible to measles and/or mumps as well as to rubella, MMR is the vaccine of choice.

Vaccine Indications

Rubella vaccine is recommended for adults, particularly females, unless proof of immunity is available (i.e., documented rubella vaccination on or after the first birthday or positive results from a serologic test) or unless the vaccine is specifically contraindicated. In particular, nonpregnant susceptible women of childbearing age should be provided rubella vaccination (a) during routine internal medicine and gynecologic outpatient care, (b) during routine care in a family planning clinic, (c) after premarital screening, (d) before discharge from a hospital for any reason, and (e) after childbirth or abortion. Ideally, any contact with the health-care system should be used as an opportunity to vaccinate susceptible women. Also, evidence of rubella immunity should be required for all persons in colleges and universities. Health-care programs in workplaces and in other places where women of childbearing age congregate should ensure that the vaccination status of every employee is evaluated and that rubella vaccination is made available. All hospital personnel (male and female) who might be at risk of exposure to patients infected with rubella or who might have contact with pregnant patients or personnel should be immune to rubella. Consideration should be given to making rubella immunity a condition for employment. Finally, since the risk of acquiring rubella while traveling outside the United States is greater than the risk incurred within the United States, all women travelers, particularly those of childbearing age, should be immune before leaving the United States.

Vaccine Side Effects and Adverse Reactions

Up to 25% of susceptible postpubertal female vaccinees in large-scale field trials have had arthralgia after vaccination; arthritis signs and symptoms occur transiently among 10% of recipients. Arthralgia and transient arthritis occur more frequently and tend to be more severe among susceptible women than among seropositive women and children. When joint symptoms or other types of pain and paresthesias do occur, they usually begin 1–3 weeks after vaccination, persist from 1 day to 3 weeks, and rarely recur. Adults with joint problems usually have not had to disrupt work activities. Sporadic cases of persistent joint symptoms among susceptible vaccinees, primarily adult women, have been reported. Although one group of investigators has reported the frequency of chronic joint symptoms and signs among adult women to be as high as 5%–11% (18, 19), other data from the United States and experience from other countries that use the RA 27/3 strain suggest that such phenomena are rare. In comparative studies, the frequency of chronic joint complaints is substantially higher after natural infection than after vaccination (19). Complaints of transient peripheral neuritis, such as paresthesias and pain in the arms and legs, have occurred very rarely and only among susceptible vaccinees; these symptoms rarely persist.

Because a two-dose schedule of MMR is being implemented in the United States, some persons will receive two doses of rubella vaccine. There is no conclusive evidence of any increased risk of the reactions described above for persons who are already immune when vaccinated.

Vaccine Precautions and Contraindications

Rubella vaccine should be given at least 14 days before administration of IG or deferred for at least 6 weeks—and preferably 3 months—after administration. On the other hand, previous administration of whole blood or other blood products containing antibody (e.g., human anti-Rho [D] IG) does not interfere with an immune response and is not a contraindication to postpartum vaccination. However, in this situation, serologic testing should be done 6–8 weeks after vaccination to assure that seroconversion has occurred.

Rubella vaccine should not be given to pregnant women or to those likely to become pregnant within 3 months after receiving the vaccine. Through 1988, CDC monitored prospectively 305 susceptible pregnant women who had received rubella vaccine within 3 months before or after conception and carried their pregnancies to term. Ninety-four received Cendehill or HPV-77, 210 received RA 27/3, and one received an unknown strain of vaccine. None of the infants had malformations compatible with CRS. The ACIP believes that the risk of vaccine-associated malformation is so small as to be negligible. Although a final decision must rest with the individual patient and her physician, the ACIP believes that rubella vaccination during pregnancy should not ordinarily be a reason to recommend interruption of pregnancy.

Because of the theoretical risk to the fetus, reasonable precautions should be taken before women of childbearing age are vaccinated. These precautions include (a) asking women if they are pregnant, (b) excluding those who say they are, and (c) explaining the theoretical risks of the vaccine to the others and counseling them not to become pregnant for 3 months after vaccination. If a pregnant woman is vaccinated or if a woman becomes pregnant within 3 months after vaccination, she should be counseled on the theoretical risks to the fetus.

Rubella vaccine should not be given to persons who are immunocompromised as a result of immune deficiency diseases, leukemia, lymphoma, or generalized malignancy or who are immunosuppressed as a result of therapy with corticosteroids, alkylating drugs, antimetabolites, or radiation. HIV infection is an exception; rubella vaccine should be given to asymptomatic HIV-infected persons and may be considered for those who are symptomatic. (See "Conditions that Compromise the Immune System" and Table 5 and Table 6.)

Rubella vaccine is prepared in human diploid cell cultures and has rarely been reported to be associated with allergic reactions. The vaccine does contain trace amounts of neomycin to which patients may be allergic. Persons with a history of any sign or symptom of an anaphylactic reaction (e.g., hives, swelling of the mouth and throat, difficulty breathing, hypotension, or shock) after receipt of neomycin should not receive rubella vaccine. Persons with reactions to neomycin that are not anaphylactic are not at increased risk and can be vaccinated. Rubella vaccine does not contain penicillin.

Smallpox (Vaccinia)

In May 1980, the World Health Organization (WHO) declared the world free of smallpox (vaccinia). A smallpox vaccination certificate is not required by any country as a condition of entry for international travelers. In May 1983, the distribution of vaccine for civilian use in the United States was discontinued.

Vaccine Indications

Only laboratory personnel working with orthopox viruses and certain health-care workers involved in clinical trials of vaccinia recombinant vaccines may need to be given smallpox vaccine. Otherwise, there are no indications for its use in civilian populations.

No evidence suggests that smallpox vaccination has therapeutic value in the treatment of recurrent herpes simplex infection, warts, or any other disease. Smallpox vaccine should never be used therapeutically for these or any other conditions.

When indicated, smallpox vaccination should be given every 10 years. For advice on vaccine administration and contraindications, contact the CDC Drug Service, Building 1, Room 1259, CDC, Atlanta, GA 30333, telephone: 404–639-3356, or the Division of Immunization, CDC Mailstop (E05), Atlanta, GA 30333, telephone: 404-639-1870.

Varicella Zoster

Most adults (85%–95%) with negative or unknown histories of varicella (chickenpox) are likely to be immune. Primary varicella can be more severe among adults than it is among normal (immunocompetent) children; however, the risk of serious complications among normal adults is substantially less than it is among those who are immunocompromised. Live, attenuated varicella-zoster vaccine may be licensed for use in normal children in the near future. Its potential use among adults, particularly health-care workers, has not been defined.

Yellow Fever

Cases of yellow fever are reported only from Africa and South America. Two forms of yellow fever—urban and jungle—are distinguishable epidemiologically. Clinically and etiologically, the two forms are identical.

Urban yellow fever is an epidemic viral disease transmitted from infected to susceptible persons by the Aedes aegypti mosquito. In areas where the Ae. aegypti mosquito has been eliminated or suppressed, urban yellow fever has disappeared. However, periodic reinfestations of some countries in Central and South America have occurred in recent years, and other countries remain infested. In West Africa, an Ae. aegypti-transmitted epidemic involving an urban population occurred as recently as 1987.

Jungle yellow fever is an enzootic viral disease transmitted among nonhuman hosts by a variety of mosquito vectors. Only in forested areas of South America and forest-savannah zones of tropical Africa has it been observed, but it occasionally extends into Central America and the island of Trinidad. In South America, 100–300 cases are recognized annually, mainly among persons with occupational exposure in forested areas; the disease is, however, believed to be greatly underreported. In Africa, sporadic endemic cases and epidemics that affect thousands of persons are spread by forest mosquito vectors. The cycle of jungle yellow fever may be active but unrecognized in forested areas of countries within the endemic yellow fever zone (Fig. 66.1).

Yellow Fever Vaccine

The yellow fever vaccine available in the United States is an attenuated, live-virus vaccine prepared from the 17D strain of virus grown in chick embryos.

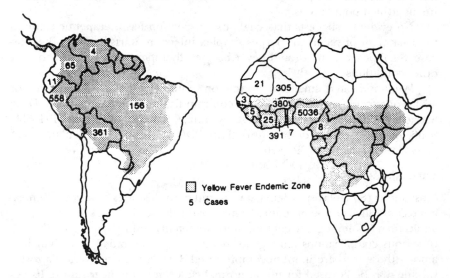

Figure 66.1. Yellow fever endemic zones in Americas and Africa and number of yellow fever cases reported to World Health Organization, 1980–1987.

Immunity is induced by a single SC injection of 0.5 mL of reconstituted vaccine and persists for >10 years.

Yellow fever vaccines must be approved by WHO and administered at an approved Yellow Fever Vaccination Center. Centers can be identified by contacting state and local health departments. Vaccinees should have an International Certificate of Vaccination filled out, dated, signed, and validated with the stamp of the center where the vaccine is given. Vaccine must be received 10 days to 10 years before travel for the certificate to be valid.

Vaccine Indications

Vaccination is recommended for persons traveling or living in areas in which yellow fever infection occurs—currently parts of Africa and Central and South America. Information on known or probably infected areas is published annually in "Health Information for International Travel." Countries currently reporting yellow fever are noted biweekly in "Summary of Health Information for International Travel" (see earlier). All state health departments and many county and city health departments receive these publications. The actual areas of yellow fever activity far exceed the zones officially reported to be infected. Vaccination is also recommended for laboratory personnel who might be exposed to virulent yellow fever virus.

Booster doses are needed at 10-year intervals.

Some countries, especially in Africa, require evidence of vaccination from all entering travelers. Other countries may waive the requirements for travelers coming from noninfected areas and staying <2 weeks. Some countries require a traveler, even if only in transit, to have a valid certificate if the traveler has visited any country thought to harbor yellow fever virus. Requirements of individual countries may change, and the most current information is published biweekly in "Summary of Health Information for International Travel" and summarized annually in "Health Information for International Travel" (see earlier).

Vaccine Side Effects and Adverse Reactions

Reactions to 17D yellow fever vaccine are generally mild. From 2% to 5% of vaccinees have mild headache, myalgia, low-grade fever, or other minor symptoms 5–10 days after vaccination. Fewer than 0.2% curtail regular activities. Immediate hypersensitivity reactions, characterized by rash, urticaria, and/or asthma, are extremely uncommon and occur principally among persons with a history of egg allergy. Although >34 million doses of vaccines have been distributed, only two cases of encephalitis temporally associated with vaccinations have been reported in the United States; in one fatal case, 17D virus was isolated from the brain.

Vaccine Precautions and Contraindications

Yellow fever vaccine should not be given to persons who are immunocompromised as a result of immune deficiency diseases (including symptomatic HIV infection), leukemia, lymphoma, or generalized malignancy, or to persons who are immunosuppressed as a result of therapy with corticosteroids, alkylating drugs, antimetabolites, or radiation. (See "Conditions that Compromise the Immune System.") Persons who have asymptomatic HIV infection and who cannot avoid potential exposure to yellow fever virus should be offered the choice of vaccination.

Although specific information is not available on adverse effects of yellow fever vaccine on the developing fetus, avoiding vaccination of pregnant women and advising that they postpone travel to areas where yellow fever occurs until after delivery seems prudent. Pregnant women who must travel to areas in which the risk of yellow fever is high should be vaccinated. The risk of yellow fever infection far outweighs the small theoretical risk to mother and fetus from vaccination in such circumstances. However, if international travel regulations constitute the only reason to vaccinate a pregnant woman or a patient hypersensitive to eggs, efforts should be made to obtain a letter of waiver from a physician clearly stating the contraindication to vaccination. Ideally, this letter should be written on letterhead stationery and bear the stamp used by health departments and official immunization centers to validate the International Certificates of Vaccination. Under these conditions, travelers should obtain specific, authoritative advice from the country or countries they plan to visit. The countries' embassies or consulates may be contacted and a letter substantiating the waiver of requirements should be obtained.

Because live yellow fever vaccine is produced in chick embryos, persons with a history of any signs or symptoms of an anaphylactic reaction (e.g., hives, swelling of the mouth and throat, difficulty breathing, hypotension, or shock) after eating eggs should not receive yellow fever vaccine. If vaccination of an individual with a questionable history of egg hypersensitivity is considered essential because of a high risk of exposure, an intradermal (ID) test dose may be administered under close medical supervision. Specific directions for skin testing are found in the package insert.

Some data have indicated that persons given yellow fever and cholera vaccines simultaneously or 1–3 weeks apart had lower than normal antibody responses to both vaccines. Unless there are time constraints, cholera and yellow fever vaccines should be administered at a minimum interval of 3 weeks. If the vaccines cannot be administered at least 3 weeks apart, they can be administered simultaneously or at any time within the 3-week interval.

Yellow fever vaccine may be given simultaneously with measles, BCG, or hepatitis B vaccines, as well as with IG.

Both Live-Virus and Inactivated-Virus Vaccines

Poliomyelitis

The risk of poliomyelitis is very small in the United States; however, epidemics could occur if the high immunity level of the general population is not maintained by vaccinating children routinely or if wild poliovirus is introduced into susceptible populations in communities with low immunization levels. In the United States, inapparent infection with wild poliovirus strains no longer contributes significantly to establishing or maintaining immunity. Most adults are already immune.

Poliovirus Vaccines

Two types of poliovirus vaccines are currently licensed in the United States: OPV and eIPV. A primary vaccination series with either vaccine produces immunity to all three types of poliovirus in >95% of recipients. The primary series of OPV consists of three doses: two doses given 6–8 weeks apart and a third dose given at least 6 weeks and customarily 12 months after the second. The primary series for eIPV consists of three doses: two doses each given 4–8 weeks apart and a third dose given 6–12 months after the second. A primary vaccine series need not be given to adults living in the United States who have not had a primary series as children. However, for adults who have not had a primary series and who are at greater risk of exposure than the general population to wild polioviruses because of foreign travel or health occupation, eIPV is preferred because the risk of OPV-associated paralysis is slightly higher among adults than among children. Poliovirus vaccine is not routinely recommended for persons older than high school age (greater than or equal to 18 years old).

Vaccine Indications

Travelers to areas where wild poliovirus is epidemic or endemic should have completed a primary series of poliovirus vaccine. For previously unvaccinated adults, eIPV is indicated. However, if <4 weeks is available before protection is needed, a single dose of OPV or eIPV is recommended. Travelers who have previously received less than a full primary course of OPV or IPV should be given the remaining required doses of either vaccine, regardless of the interval since the last dose and the type of vaccine previously received. Travelers to developing countries who have previously completed a primary series of OPV should receive a single dose of OPV. Those who have previously received a primary series of IPV should receive a dose of either OPV or eIPV. The need for further doses of either vaccine has not been established.

Health-care personnel in close contact with patients who may be excreting wild polioviruses and laboratory personnel handling specimens that may contain wild polioviruses should have completed a primary series of poliovirus vaccine. Because of the slightly increased risk to adults of vaccine-associated paralysis after OPV administration, eIPV is indicated; also, virus may be shed after receipt of OPV vaccine and may inadvertently expose susceptible immunocompromised contacts to live vaccine virus.

Vaccine Adverse Reactions

Inactivated poliovirus vaccine.   No serious side effects of currently available eIPV have been documented. Because eIPV contains trace amounts of streptomycin and neomycin, hypersensitivity reactions are possible among persons sensitive to these antibiotics. Persons with signs and symptoms of an anaphylactic reaction (e.g., hives, swelling of mouth and throat, difficulty breathing, hypotension, or shock) after receipt of streptomycin or neomycin should not receive eIPV. Persons with reactions that are not anaphylactic are not at increased risk and may be vaccinated.

Oral poliovirus vaccine.   In rare instances, administration of OPV has been associated with paralysis among healthy recipients and their contacts. Although the risk of vaccine-associated paralytic poliomyelitis is extremely small for immunologically normal vaccinees (approximately one case per 1.4 million first doses distributed and one case per 41.5 million subsequent doses) and for their susceptible immunologically normal household contacts (approximately one case per 1.9 million first doses distributed and one case per 13.8 million subsequent doses), vaccinees should be informed of this risk (20).

Vaccine Precautions and Contraindications

Inactivated poliovirus vaccine.   No convincing evidence of adverse effects of eIPV for the pregnant woman or developing fetus exists; regardless, theoretically vaccination of pregnant women should be avoided. However, if immediate protection against poliomyelitis is needed, OPV, not eIPV, is recommended.

Oral poliovirus vaccine.   Unlike other live-virus vaccines that are administered parenterally, OPV is administered orally. IG and other antibody-containing blood products do not appear to interfere with the immune response to OPV.

OPV should not be administered to persons who are or may be immunocompromised as a result of immune deficiency diseases, HIV infection, leukemia, lymphoma, or generalized malignancy or to persons who are or may be immunosuppressed as a result of therapy with corticosteroids, alkylating drugs, antimetabolites, or radiation. (See "Conditions that Compromise the Immune System.") If polio vaccination is indicated for immunosuppressed patients, their household members, or other close contacts, these persons should be given eIPV rather than OPV. Although OPV has not been harmful when administered to asymptomatic HIV-infected children, eIPV is the vaccine of choice if the patient is known or suspected to be infected. The use of eIPV not only eliminates any theoretical risk to the vaccinee but also prevents the possibility of vaccine virus spread to immunocompromised close contacts. Although a protective immune response cannot be assured in the immunocompromised patient, some protection may be provided.

OPV should not be used for vaccinating household contacts of patients immunocompromised as a result of immune deficiency disease, HIV infection, leukemia, lymphoma, or generalized malignancy or for vaccinating patients immunosuppressed as a result of therapy with corticosteroids, alkylating drugs, antimetabolites, or radiation. If protection is indicated, eIPV should be used for vaccinating household contacts of such patients. OPV should not be given to anyone in a family with a known family history of immunodeficiency until the immune status of all family members is documented.

When children in the household receive OPV, adults who are not adequately vaccinated against poliomyelitis are at a very small risk of contracting OPV-associated paralytic poliomyelitis. Because of the overriding importance of ensuring prompt and complete vaccination of the child and the extreme rarity of OPV-associated disease in contacts of vaccinees, the ACIP recommends the administration of OPV to a child, regardless of the poliovirus-vaccine status of adult household contacts. This is the standard practice in the United States. The responsible adult should be informed of the small risk involved and of the precautions to be taken, such as hand washing after changing a diaper. An acceptable alternative, if there is strong assurance that ultimate, full vaccination of the child will not be jeopardized or unduly delayed, is to vaccinate adults with eIPV or OPV, as appropriate to their immunity status, before giving OPV to the child.

Inactivated-Virus Vaccines

Hepatitis B Virus Infection

The estimated lifetime risk of acquiring HBV infection in the United States is approximately 5% for the population as a whole but may approach 100% for the highest risk groups. Annually, an estimated 300,000 HBV infections occur in the United States, leading to approximately 10,000 hospitalizations and 250 deaths due to fulminant hepatitis B.

In 1988, 89% of HBV cases for which the patient's age was known occurred among persons greater than or equal to 20 years of age. Between 6% and 10% of adults with HBV infection become carriers. The United States currently has 750,000–1,000,000 carriers. Chronic active hepatitis occurs among an estimated 25% of carriers. Each year in the United States, approximately 4,000 persons die of HBV-related cirrhosis and 800 of HBV-related liver cancer.

Hepatitis B Vaccine

Two types of HB vaccines are currently licensed in the United States. Plasma-derived HB vaccine consists of a suspension of inactivated, alum-adsorbed 22-nm HBsAg particles that have been purified from human plasma. Although still available, plasma-derived vaccine is no longer being produced in the United States. Currently licensed recombinant HB vaccines are produced by Saccharomyces cerevisiae (common baker's yeast), into which a plasmid containing the gene for the HBsAg has been inserted. These vaccines contain >95% HBsAg protein.

Dosages of vaccines vary with manufacturer and age of the recipient. Package inserts should be consulted for proper dosages. Both types of vaccines are given as three-dose series, with the first two doses given 1 month apart, and the third dose 5 months after the second. An alternative schedule for one vaccine, with three doses 1 month apart followed by a fourth dose 12 months after the first, has been approved for postexposure prophylaxis or for more rapid induction of immunity. However, no clear evidence that this regimen offers greater protection than the standard schedule exists. Duration of protection from HB vaccines is at least 7 years among healthy adults; the possible need for booster doses will be assessed as further information becomes available.

Because the prevalence of HBV infection varies widely among various population groups, serologic screening to detect susceptible individuals before vaccination may or may not be cost effective. Cost-effectiveness depends on the known or expected prevalence of immune individuals in the target population, the cost of screening, and the cost of HB vaccine. Postvaccination testing for immunity is not recommended routinely but is advised for persons whose subsequent management depends on knowing their immune status (dialysis patients and staff) and for those in whom suboptimal response is anticipated (persons with HIV infection and those who have received vaccine in the buttock). When indicated, such testing should be done within 1–6 months after completing vaccination. Postvaccination testing should also be considered for health-care workers at risk of needlestick exposures. If such testing demonstrates an antibody level <10 mIU/mL, revaccination with one or more doses should be considered.

Vaccine Indications

Vaccination is recommended for adults at increased risk of occupational, social, family, environmental, or illness-related exposure to HBV. These include homosexual males, injecting drug users, heterosexual persons with multiple partners or other sexually transmitted diseases, household and sexual contacts of HBV carriers, workers in health-related and public-safety occupations requiring frequent exposure to blood, residents and staff of institutions for the developmentally disabled, hemodialysis patients, recipients of factor VIII or IX concentrates, and morticians and their assistants. Inmates in some long-term correctional facilities may also be candidates for vaccination.

Vaccination should also be considered for persons who plan to reside for >6 months in areas with high levels of endemic HBV and who will have close contact with the local population and for travelers intending a short stay who are likely to have contact with blood from or sexual contact with residents of areas with high levels of endemic disease (particularly areas of eastern Asia and sub-Saharan Africa). Such persons should allow 6 months before travel to complete the HB vaccine primary series. The alternative four-dose schedule may offer better protection if three doses can be given before travel.

HB vaccine is intended primarily for preexposure prophylaxis; however, it has been recommended for postexposure use in certain situations, particularly for nonimmune persons who belong to a high-risk group for whom preexposure administration of vaccine is recommended (21). HB vaccine, in combination with HBIG, provides sustained protective levels of antibody and obviates the need for a second dose of HBIG in such exposures. Therefore, a normal series of HB vaccine, combined with a single dose (0.06 mL/kg or 5 mL for adults) of HBIG given at a different site, is recommended for postexposure prophylaxis of nonimmune (and previously unvaccinated) health workers after accidental percutaneous or mucous-membrane exposure to blood containing HBsAg, and after all sexual exposure to HBsAg-positive persons if the first dose of vaccine can be administered within 14 days of sexual exposure or if sexual contact with the infected person will continue.

Vaccine Side Effects and Adverse Reactions

The most common side effect observed after vaccination with each of the available vaccines has been soreness at the injection site. Postvaccination surveillance for 3 years after licensure of the plasma-derived vaccine showed an association of borderline significance between Guillain-Barré syndrome (GBS) and receipt of the first vaccine dose (22). The rate of this occurrence was very low (0.5/100,000 vaccinees), and, even if a true side effect, was more than compensated for by disease prevented by the vaccine. Such postvaccination surveillance information is not available for the recombinant HB vaccines. Early concerns about safety of plasma-derived vaccine, particularly the concern that infectious agents such as HIV present in the donor plasma pools might contaminate the final product, have proved to be unfounded.

Vaccine Precautions and Contraindications

Pregnancy should not be considered a contraindication to vaccinating women who are otherwise candidates for receiving HB vaccine. Although data are not available on the safety of the vaccine for the developing fetus, HB vaccine contains only noninfectious HBsAg particles and should pose no risk to the fetus. In contrast, HBV infection in a pregnant woman may result in a severe disease for the mother and chronic infection for the newborn.

Influenza

Influenza viruses have continually demonstrated the ability to cause major epidemics of respiratory disease. High attack rates of acute illness and the frequent occurrence of lower respiratory tract complications usually result in dramatic rises in visits to physicians' offices and hospital emergency rooms. Furthermore, influenza frequently infects individuals who, because of their age or underlying health status, are poorly able to cope with the disease and often require medical attention, including hospitalization. Such persons are considered, medically, to be at "high risk" in epidemics. In one recent study, for example, rates of hospitalization for adults with high-risk medical conditions increased during major epidemics by approximately twofold to fivefold in different age groups, reaching a maximum rate of about 800/100,000 population.

Influenza epidemics cause excess mortality that is attributable not only to influenza pneumonia but also to cardiopulmonary disease. Nineteen times in the period 1957–1986 epidemics have been associated with greater than or equal to 10,000 excess deaths. Approximately 80%–90% of the excess deaths attributed to pneumonia and influenza were among persons greater than or equal to 65 years of age during major epidemics.

Influenza has its greatest impact when new strains appear against which most of the population lacks immunity. In these circumstances (e.g., 1957 and 1968), pandemics occur. During pandemics, one-fourth or more of the U.S. population has been affected over a period of 2–3 months.

Because the proportion of elderly persons in the United States is increasing and because age and its associated chronic diseases are risk factors for severe influenza illness, the toll of influenza may also increase unless control measures are used more vigorously than in the past.

Influenza Vaccine

Influenza A viruses are classified into subtypes on the basis of two antigens: hemagglutinin (H) and neuraminidase (N). Three subtypes of hemagglutinin (H1, H2, H3) and two subtypes of neuraminidases (N1, N2) are recognized among influenza A viruses that have caused widespread human disease. Immunity to these antigens, especially hemagglutinin, reduces the likelihood of infection and the severity of disease if a person does become infected. However, sufficient antigenic variation (antigenic drift) within the same subtype over time may exist, so that infection or vaccination with one strain may not induce immunity to distantly related strains of the same subtype. Although influenza B viruses have shown much more antigenic stability than influenza A viruses, antigenic variation does occur. As a consequence, the antigenic characteristics of current strains provide the basis for selecting virus strains to be included in the vaccine for a given year.

The potency of present vaccines is such that nearly all vaccinated young adults develop hemagglutination-inhibition antibody titers that usually protect them against infection by strains like those in the vaccine, and often by related variants that emerge. The elderly, the very young, and patients with certain chronic diseases may develop lower antibody titers after vaccination than do young adults. Under these circumstances, influenza vaccine may be more effective in preventing lower-respiratory-tract involvement or other complications of influenza than in preventing upper-respiratory-tract involvement. Influenza vaccine will not prevent primary illnesses caused by other respiratory pathogens.

Vaccine Indications

Use of inactivated influenza vaccine is the single most important measure in preventing and attenuating influenza infection. Since 1963, annual vaccination against influenza has been recommended for individuals at high risk of lower-respiratory-tract complications and death after influenza infection (i.e., the elderly and persons with chronic disorders of the cardiovascular, pulmonary, and/or renal systems; metabolic diseases; severe anemia; and/or compromised immune function, including HIV infection). These groups have been identified primarily by review of death certificate data, supported by hospital-based or population-based studies. Within each broadly defined high-risk category, however, some persons are more likely than others to suffer severe complications from influenza infection.

Among nursing-home residents, chronic diseases and other debilitating conditions are common, and influenza can often be spread explosively, with attack rates as high as 60% and case-fatality ratios greater than or equal to 30%.

Medical personnel, while working, may transmit influenza infections to their high-risk patients while they themselves are incubating an infection, undergoing a subclinical infection, or having mild symptoms. Nosocomial outbreaks of influenza have been reported. The potential for introducing influenza to a high-risk group, such as patients with severely compromised cardiopulmonary or immune systems or infants in neonatal intensive care units, should be reduced by targeted vaccination programs of medical personnel.

On the basis of these observations, the previous, broadly defined high-risk adult groups have been assigned further priority for receiving vaccine so that special efforts can be directed at providing vaccine to those who may derive the greatest benefit.

Groups at increased risk for influenza-related complications. To maximize protection of high-risk persons, both the persons at risk and their close contacts should be targeted for organized vaccination programs. These include the following:

1. Persons greater than or equal to 65 years of age.
2. Residents of nursing homes and other chronic-care facilities housing patients of any age with chronic medical conditions.
3. Adults and children with chronic disorders of the pulmonary or cardiovascular systems, including children with asthma.
4. Adults and children who have required regular medical follow-up or hospitalization during the preceding year because of chronic metabolic diseases (including diabetes mellitus), renal dysfunction, hemoglobinopathies, or immunosuppression (including immunosuppression caused by medications).
5. Children and teenagers (ages 6 months–18 years) who are receiving long-term aspirin therapy and therefore may be at risk of developing Reye syndrome after an influenza infection.

Groups potentially capable of transmitting influenza to high-risk persons. Care-givers of or household members attending high-risk persons can transmit influenza infections to them while they themselves are undergoing subclinical or symptomatic infection. Some high-risk persons (e.g., the elderly, transplant recipients, or persons with acquired immunodeficiency syndrome [AIDS]) can have relatively low antibody responses to influenza vaccine. Efforts to protect them against influenza may be improved by reducing the chances that their care providers may expose them to influenza. Therefore, the following groups should be vaccinated:

1. Physicians, nurses, and other personnel in hospital and outpatient-care settings who have contact with high-risk patients in all age groups, including infants.
2. Employees of nursing homes and chronic-care facilities who have contact with patients or residents.
3. Providers of home care to high-risk persons (e.g., visiting nurses, volunteer workers).
4. Household members (including children) of high-risk persons.

In addition, influenza vaccine may be offered to persons who provide essential community service, to any adult who wishes to reduce the likelihood of an influenza infection, to the elderly, or to those with high-risk conditions who travel to areas with active influenza disease.

Vaccination of other groups.   Pregnant women who have other medical conditions that increase their risks for complications from influenza should be vaccinated, as the vaccine is considered safe for pregnant women. Administering the vaccine after the first trimester is a reasonable precaution to minimize any concern over the theoretical risk of teratogenicity. However, delaying vaccination of pregnant women who have high-risk conditions and who will still be in the first trimester of pregnancy when the influenza season begins is undesirable.

Little information exists on the frequency and severity of influenza illness among HIV-infected persons, but recent reports suggest that symptoms may be prolonged and the risk of complications increased for this high-risk group. Therefore, vaccination is a prudent precaution and will result in protective antibody levels among many recipients. However, the antibody response to vaccine may be low in persons with advanced HIV-related illnesses. A booster dose of vaccine has not improved the immune response for these individuals.

Strategies for implementing influenza vaccine recommendations.   Effective programs for giving influenza vaccine are needed in nursing homes and other chronic-care facilities, in physicians' offices, and in hospital settings. Residents of nursing homes and chronic-care facilities should receive routine annual vaccinations. Other adult high-priority groups should receive influenza vaccine at the time of regular medical follow-ups in the autumn or should be notified to come in specifically to receive the vaccine. Patients with high-risk conditions who are hospitalized during the autumn should be considered for influenza vaccine before being discharged from the hospital. The target groups for receiving influenza and pneumococcal polysaccharide vaccine overlap considerably. These vaccines can be given at the same time at different sites without an increase in side effects or compromise in immunogenicity; however, influenza vaccine is given annually, whereas pneumococcal polysaccharide vaccine is not given more often than every 6 years to adults.

Amantadine hydrochloride, an antiviral drug, can prevent influenza A or be used therapeutically to reduce symptoms of influenza A infections. It is not a substitute for vaccine. Specific circumstances in which amantadine prophylaxis is recommended are described in the ACIP recommendations on prevention and control of influenza. (See Appendix 1.)

Vaccine Side Effects and Adverse Reactions

Vaccines used in recent years have been associated with infrequent reactions. Local redness or induration for 1 or 2 days at the site of injection has reportedly developed among fewer than one-third of vaccinees.

Systemic reactions have been of two types. First, malaise, myalgia, and other systemic symptoms of toxicity, although infrequent, most often affect those who have had no experience with the influenza virus antigens contained in the vaccine. These reactions, which begin 6–12 hours after vaccination and persist 1–2 days, are usually attributed to the influenza antigens (even though the virus is inactivated) and constitute most of the systemic side effects of influenza vaccination.

Second, immediate, presumably allergic responses, such as flare and wheal or various respiratory tract symptoms of hypersensitivity, occur extremely rarely after influenza vaccination. These symptoms probably result from sensitivity to some vaccine component—most likely residual egg protein. Although current influenza vaccines contain only a small quantity of egg protein, vaccine can induce hypersensitivity reactions on rare occasions. Unlike the 1976 swine influenza vaccine, vaccines used subsequently have not been clearly associated with an increased frequency of Guillain-Barré syndrome.

Vaccine Precautions and Contraindications

Persons with a history of any signs or symptoms of an anaphylactic reaction (e.g., hives, swelling of the mouth and throat, difficulty breathing, hypotension, or shock) after eating eggs should not be given inactivated influenza vaccine.

Persons with acute febrile illnesses normally should not be vaccinated until their symptoms have abated.

Rabies

Although rabies rarely affects humans in the United States, approximately 18,000 persons receive rabies vaccine every year for postexposure prophylaxis, and an additional 10,000 persons receive preexposure prophylaxis. The likelihood of human exposure to rabies from domestic animals has decreased greatly in recent years. In every year since 1976, >85% of all reported cases of animal rabies have been among wild animals, the most important source of possible infection for humans in the United States. However, for persons traveling overseas to developing countries with endemic rabies, the dog remains the animal most likely to transmit the disease.

Rabies Vaccine

Two inactivated rabies vaccines are currently licensed for preexposure and postexposure prophylaxis in the United States. HDCV is supplied in two forms: (a) for IM administration (single-dose vials containing lyophilized vaccine that is reconstituted in the vial with the accompanying diluent to a final volume of 1.0 mL just before administration), and (b) for ID administration (single-dose syringes containing lyophilized vaccine that is reconstituted in the syringe to a volume of 0.1 mL just before administration).

Rabies vaccine adsorbed (RVA), prepared from the Kissling strain of rabies virus adapted to fetal rhesus lung diploid cell culture, was licensed in 1988. Developed and distributed by the Biologics Products Program, Michigan Department of Public Health, RVA is currently available only to residents of the state of Michigan.

Rabies vaccine derived from human diploid cell developed in the United States (Wyeth-Ayerst Laboratories, WYVAC) was recalled from the market in 1985 and is no longer available.

Preexposure prophylaxis, consisting of three 1.0-mL injections of HDCV or RVA, should be given IM (deltoid), one each on days 0, 7, and 28. Alternatively, using the specially designed syringe, three 0.1-mL injections of HDCV (but not RVA) may be given ID in the deltoid on days 0, 7, and 21 or 28 (23). The proper postexposure rabies prophylaxis regimen depends on whether the person has had previous preexposure or postexposure prophylaxis. Persons who (a) have previously received postexposure prophylaxis with HDCV or RVA, (b) have received a three-dose IM preexposure regimen of HDCV or RVA, (c) have received a three-dose ID preexposure regimen of HDCV in the United States, or (d) have a previously documented adequate rabies titer should receive two 1-mL IM doses of HDCV—one dose each on days 0 and 3. Human rabies immune globulin (HRIG) is not recommended in these circumstances. Persons not meeting the above criteria should be treated with a single 20-IU/kg dose of HRIG and five 1-mL doses IM of HDCV—one each on days 0, 3, 7, 14, and 28. HRIG should be administered at the beginning of HDCV postexposure prophylaxis but can be given up to the eighth day after the first dose of HDCV was given. The HRIG dose should be divided. Up to half should infiltrate the area of the wound, if possible, and the rest should be administered IM, but never in the same site or in the same syringe as HDCV. Only IM administration of HDCV is indicated for postexposure prophylaxis. Among adults, only the deltoid area is acceptable for vaccine administration.

Vaccine Indications

Preexposure immunization should be considered for high-risk groups: animal handlers, certain laboratory workers and field personnel, and persons planning to spend more than 1 month in areas of countries where rabies is a constant threat. Persons whose vocations or avocations bring them into contact with potentially rabid animals, including skunks, raccoons, and bats, should also be considered for preexposure vaccination. Persons with continuing risk of exposure should receive a booster dose every 2 years, or they should have their serum tested for rabies antibody every 2 years and, if the titer is inadequate, receive a booster dose. If substantial risk of exposure to rabies exists, preexposure rabies prophylaxis may be indicated during pregnancy.

The decision to provide postexposure antirabies treatment should include the following considerations:

1. Type of exposure. Rabies is transmitted primarily by the bite of infected animals. Aerosols or the introduction of saliva or other potentially infectious material from a rabid animal into open cuts or wounds in the skin or via mucous membranes also may transmit rabies.
2. Species of biting animal. Carnivorous wild animals (especially skunks, raccoons, and foxes) and bats are most commonly infected with rabies in the United States. Elsewhere in the world, dogs, cats, carnivorous wildlife, and bats are the major vectors. The likelihood that domestic cats or dogs in the United States will be infected varies from region to region. Most rodents, such as squirrels, hamsters, guinea pigs, gerbils, rats and mice, and lagomorphs (including rabbits and hares) are rarely infected. However, woodchucks are an exception and have accounted for 70% of rabies cases among rodents reported to CDC between 1971 and 1988. The state or local health department should be consulted in cases of rodent bites before postexposure prophylaxis is initiated.
3. Circumstances of a biting incident. An unprovoked bite indicates a rabid animal more than a provoked bite.

Vaccine Side Effects and Adverse Reactions

Local reactions, such as pain, erythema, and swelling or itching at the injection site, are reported by up to 74% of recipients. Mild systemic reactions, such as headache, nausea, abdominal pain, muscle aches, and dizziness, are reported by between 5% and 40% of recipients. After primary vaccination, systemic allergic reactions ranging from hives to anaphylaxis occur among an estimated 11 of 10,000 vaccinees. After booster doses, mild immune-complex-like hypersensitivity reactions consisting of hives, itching, and angioedema occur 2–21 days later among approximately 6% of recipients and are the most frequently reported allergic reactions (24). Fewer than 1% of persons develop such reactions after primary administration of HDCV. Two cases of neurologic illness resembling GBS that resolved without sequelae in 12 weeks have been reported—as well as a number of different subacute central and peripheral nervous system disorders temporally associated with HDCV vaccine, but a causal relationship has not been established (25).

Vaccine Precautions and Contraindications

Corticosteroids and other immunosuppressive agents can interfere with the development of active immunity and should not be administered during preexposure therapy. When rabies postexposure prophylaxis is administered to persons known or suspected of being immunosuppressed or to those who are receiving steroids or immunosuppressive therapy, the serum should be tested to ensure an adequate rabies antibody response.

Chloroquine phosphate administered for malaria chemoprophylaxis and unidentified factors among persons living in developing countries may interfere with the antibody response to HDCV among persons traveling to developing countries (26). Among persons receiving preexposure prophylaxis and chloroquine in preparation for travel to an area in which rabies is enzootic, the administration of the 0.1-mL dose ID should be initiated at least 1 month before travel to allow the three-dose series to be completed before antimalarial prophylaxis begins. If this is not possible, the 1.0-mL dose should be administered IM.

If person experiences a possible anaphylactic reaction (e.g., hives, swelling of the mouth and throat, difficulty breathing, hypotension, or shock) after receiving HDCV, no further preexposure doses of HDCV should be given. In contrast, if a person needing postexposure therapy has had a previous anaphylactic reaction to HDCV or has such a reaction during the postexposure course, public health officials should be contacted to determine if HDCV therapy should continue. The person should receive the subsequent doses in an appropriate medical setting.

Inactivated-Bacteria Vaccines

Cholera

Cholera continues to be a health risk in Africa, Asia, and Latin America. Persons who follow the usual tourist itinerary and who use tourist accommodations in countries affected by cholera are at virtually no risk of infection. The traveler's best protection against cholera is avoiding food and water that might be contaminated.

Cholera Vaccine

The vaccine may be administered as a 0.5-mL dose SC or IM or as a 0.2-mL dose ID. Although a single dose of vaccine is sufficient for entry into most countries, some countries may require evidence of a complete primary series of two doses given 1 week to greater than or equal to 1 month apart, or a booster dose within 6 months before arrival.

The currently available cholera vaccine has been shown in field trials to be only approximately 50% effective in preventing clinical illness for a period of 3–6 months. The vaccine does not prevent transmission of infection. The risk of cholera to most U.S. travelers is so low that the vaccination is of dubious benefit. WHO no longer recommends cholera vaccination for travel to or from cholera-infected areas. However, some countries affected or threatened by cholera may require evidence of cholera vaccination as a condition of entry. Current information on cholera-vaccination requirements of individual countries is published annually in "Health Information for International Travel" (see earlier). All state health departments and many county and city health departments receive this publication. Travelers to countries with cholera-vaccination requirements should have an International Certificate of Vaccination completed, dated, signed, and validated, showing receipt of the vaccine 6 days–6 months before entry into the country. Most city, county, and state health departments can validate certificates. Failure to secure validation may cause travelers to be revaccinated or quarantined.

Vaccine Indications

Cholera vaccine is indicated for travelers to countries requiring evidence of cholera vaccination for entry. In addition, the complete primary series is suggested only for special high-risk groups that live in areas in which cholera is highly endemic under insanitary conditions. Boosters may be given every 6 months if required by a country.

Vaccine Side Effects and Adverse Reactions

Vaccination often results in 1–2 days of pain, erythema, and induration at the site of injection. The local reaction may be accompanied by fever, malaise, and headache. Serious reactions, including neurologic reactions, after cholera vaccination are extremely rare.

Vaccine Precautions and Contraindications

No specific information is available on the safety of cholera vaccine during pregnancy. Because cholera disease during pregnancy is a serious illness, whether to use cholera vaccine should be determined in individual circumstances based on the actual risk of disease and the probable benefits of the vaccine.

The only contraindication to cholera vaccine is a history of a severe reaction after a previous dose. Most governments will permit unvaccinated travelers to enter the country if they carry a physician's statement of medical contraindication. However, some countries may quarantine such unvaccinated persons or place them under surveillance if they come from areas with cholera. Some data have indicated that persons given yellow fever and cholera vaccines simultaneously or 1–3 weeks apart had lower than normal antibody responses to both vaccines. Unless there are time constraints, cholera and yellow fever vaccines should be administered at a minimal interval of 3 weeks. If the vaccines cannot be administered at least 3 weeks apart, they can be given simultaneously or anytime within the 3-week interval.

Haemophilus Influenzae Type b

Healthy adults are not at increased risk of invasive Hib disease. Over 85% of invasive H. influenzae cases occur among children <5 years of age (27). Among adults, invasive H. influenzae disease occurs primarily among persons with chronic pulmonary disease and underlying conditions that predispose to infections with encapsulated bacteria. Hib bacteria cause less than half the cases of invasive H. influenzae disease among adults. Nontypeable H. influenzae bacteria are a more common cause of invasive disease, such as pneumonia in adults, as well as of mucosal infections, such as otitis media and bronchitis.

Haemophilus Influenzae Type b Vaccine

The Hib vaccines available include three polysaccharide protein conjugate vaccines licensed during the period 1987–1989. The conjugate vaccines are known to be more immunogenic among children <2 years of age and among immunocompromised persons than the polysaccharide polyribosyl-ribitol-phosphate (PRP) vaccine, licensed in 1985. For this reason, this PRP vaccine is no longer being produced in the United States.

Vaccine Indications

No data documenting the efficacy of any Hib vaccine among children >5 years of age or adults exist. This includes those persons with underlying conditions (e.g., splenectomy, sickle cell disease, Hodgkin disease and other hematologic neoplasms, and immunosuppression) that predispose to infections with encapsulated bacteria. Studies suggest, however, good immunogenicity among patients with sickle cell disease (28) or leukemia (29) and among adults who have had splenectomies (30) or HIV infection (31, 32). Because of the theoretical risk to such patients, physicians may wish to consider use of HbCV among individuals with functional or anatomic asplenia or with HIV infection. Administering Hib vaccine to such patients is not contraindicated. One study reported 12 (100%) of 12 healthy adults and 20 (87%) of 23 patients who had undergone splenectomies responded with protective levels of antibody to conjugate vaccine, although the antibody levels were significantly lower among the splenectomized patients (30). Because healthy adults are not at risk for invasive Hib disease, routinely vaccinating health-care and day care workers who may come into close contact with children with invasive Hib disease is unnecessary.

Rifampin prophylaxis is recommended for all household and day care contacts of cases of invasive Hib disease, including children and adults, when there are any children <4 years of age (households) or <2 years of age (day care classrooms) in the exposed group. Although not at risk themselves, adults who have been exposed to a child with invasive Hib disease in a household or day care setting may be asymptomatic carriers of the organism and can transmit it to other susceptible children. Pregnant women should not receive rifampin, because its effect on the fetus has not been established and it is teratogenic among laboratory animals.

Vaccine Side Effects and Adverse Reactions

In one study of children 15–24 months of age, local reactions were noted for 12.5% of children receiving conjugate vaccine; moderate fever (temperature >39.0°C [>102.2°F]) occurred among 0.7% of children (33). In a study of 35 children >9 years of age and of adults who received conjugate vaccine (30) (23 of whom had had Hodgkin disease and had had surgical splenectomy), 3 (8.5%) of the 35 complained of systemic side effects: weakness, nausea and vertigo (1), myalgias (2), and fever (1).

Vaccine Precautions and Contraindications

The safety of HbCV for pregnant women has not been established. On theoretical grounds, avoiding vaccination of pregnant women unless there is a substantial risk of infection (e.g., anatomic or functional asplenia or HIV infection) is prudent.

Meningococcal Disease

Meningococcal disease is endemic throughout the world but may also occur in epidemics. Among U.S. civilians, meningococcal disease occurs primarily as single, isolated cases, or, infrequently, in small, localized clusters. One-third of all cases of meningococcal disease occur among patients greater than or equal to 20 years old. Serogroup B and C strains cause the majority of U.S. cases, with serogroups Y and W135 accounting for most of the rest.

Meningococcal Polysaccharide Vaccine

One meningococcal polysaccharide vaccine, a quadrivalent A, C, Y, and W135 vaccine, is available for use in the United States. The vaccine is given as a single dose and induces serogroup-specific immunity of unknown duration.

Vaccine Indications

Vaccine may be of benefit for travelers to areas with epidemic meningococcal disease. Vaccine may also be used in aborting and controlling outbreaks caused by serogroups represented in the vaccine. In addition, the ACIP recommends the vaccine for individuals with terminal complement component deficiencies and those with anatomic or functional asplenia. The need for booster doses has not been established.

Routine vaccination of U.S. civilians with meningococcal polysaccharide vaccine is not recommended because of the lack of availability of a group B vaccine and the low risk of infection in the United States.

Vaccine Side Effects and Adverse Reactions

Adverse reactions to meningococcal polysaccharide vaccine are infrequent and mild, consisting principally of localized erythema lasting 1–2 days.

Vaccine Precautions and Contraindications

The safety of meningococcal polysaccharide vaccine for pregnant women has not been established. On theoretical grounds, avoiding it unless there is a substantial risk of infection is prudent.

Plague

Plague is a natural infection of rodents and their fleas. In the United States, an average of 19 cases has been reported yearly between 1979 and 1988 among humans exposed in the western United States to infected animals (primarily rodents) and their fleas. Other countries currently reporting plague infections are noted in the biweekly publication "Summary of Health Information for International Travel" (see earlier). All state health departments and many county and city health departments receive this publication. A number of countries in Africa, Asia, and South America continue to report sporadic, epidemic, and epizootic infection. In most of these countries, the risk of exposure exists primarily in rural or semirural areas.

Plague Vaccine

A primary series of plague vaccine consists of three IM doses. The first dose, 1 mL, is followed in 4 weeks by a second dose of 0.2 mL. The third dose, also 0.2 mL, is administered 5 months after the second. The effectiveness of a primary series of plague vaccine has never been measured precisely. Field experience indicates that vaccination with plague vaccine reduces the incidence and severity of disease resulting from the bite of infected fleas. The degree of protection offered against primary pneumonic infection is unknown. Because plague vaccination may only ameliorate illness, prophylactic antibiotics may be indicated whenever a person, vaccinated or not, has a definite exposure.

Vaccine Indications

Vaccination is indicated for certain vocational groups. These include all laboratory and field personnel working with Y. pestis organisms that may be resistant to antimicrobials, persons engaged in aerosol experiments with Y. pestis, and field personnel engaged in operations in areas with enzootic or epidemic plague in which preventing exposure to rodents and fleas is impossible.

Vaccine may also be considered for travelers to areas known to have endemic plague, particularly if travel will not be limited to urban areas with tourist-hotel accommodations.

For persons with continuing exposure, two booster doses, each 0.1–0.2 mL, should be given approximately 6 months apart. Thereafter, booster doses at 1- to 2-year intervals should provide good protection.

Vaccine Side Effects and Adverse Reactions

For approximately 10% of recipients, primary vaccination may result in general malaise, headache, fever, mild lymphadenopathy, and/or erythema and induration at the injection site. These reactions occur more commonly with repeated injections. Sterile abscesses occur rarely. Sensitivity reactions, manifested by urticarial and asthmatic phenomena, have occasionally been reported.

Vaccine Precautions and Contraindications

Neither the safety nor the efficacy of vaccination with plague vaccine during pregnancy has been determined; therefore, it should not be used unless there is a substantial risk of infection.

Plague vaccine should not be administered to anyone with a known hypersensitivity to any of its constituents (beef protein, soy, casein, and phenol). Patients who have had severe local or systemic reactions to plague vaccine should not be revaccinated.

Pneumococcal Disease

Precise data on the occurrence of serious pneumococcal disease in the United States are not available; however, the annual incidence rate of pneumococcal bacteremia is estimated to be 15–19 cases/100,000 population for all persons, and 50 cases/100,000 for persons greater than or equal to 65 years old. The incidence of pneumococcal pneumonia, which causes a substantial number of deaths annually, can be three to five times that of the detected rates of bacteremia. Mortality from all pneumococcal disease, estimated at 40,000 deaths annually in the United States, is highest among patients who have bacteremia or meningitis, patients with underlying medical conditions, and older persons.

Patients with certain chronic conditions are at increased risk of pneumococcal infection and severe pneumococcal illness. Patients with chronic cardiovascular diseases, chronic pulmonary disease, diabetes mellitus, alcoholism, and cirrhosis have increased risk. Other patients at elevated risk include those with functional or anatomic asplenia (e.g., sickle cell disease or splenectomy), Hodgkin disease, lymphoma, multiple myeloma, chronic renal failure, nephrotic syndrome, and organ transplantation. Patients with AIDS are also at increased risk of pneumococcal disease, with an annual attack rate of pneumococcal bacteremia as high as 9.4/1,000/year (34). Recurrent pneumococcal meningitis may occur among patients with cerebrospinal fluid leakage that is complicating skull fractures or neurologic procedures.

Pneumococcal Polysaccharide Vaccine

The pneumococcal polysaccharide vaccine currently available contains purified capsular materials of the 23 types of S. pneumoniae responsible for 88% of recent bacteremic pneumococcal disease in the United States. Most healthy adults show a two-fold rise in type-specific antibody 2–3 weeks after administration of a single dose of vaccine. The titer of antibody that is protective against each serotype has not been determined.

The duration of vaccine-induced immunity is unknown. Studies of persistence of vaccine-induced antibody show elevated titers 5 years after vaccination among healthy adults.

Estimates of pneumococcal vaccine efficacy have varied widely in several studies. Studies based on CDC's pneumococcal surveillance system suggest an efficacy of 60%–64% for vaccine-type strains among patients with bacteremic disease. For all persons greater than or equal to 65 years of age, vaccine efficacy was 44%–61%. Three case-control studies that have emphasized complete assessment of vaccination status suggest a range of efficacy against pneumococcal bacteremia from 61% to 81%. Despite findings of varying efficacy, the data continue to support the use of the pneumococcal vaccine for certain well-defined groups at risk.

Patients who have received the earlier pneumococcal polysaccharide vaccine containing capsular material from only 14 types of Streptococcus pneumoniae should not be routinely revaccinated with the 23-valent pneumococcal polysaccharide vaccine, as the increased coverage is modest. However, revaccination should be strongly considered greater than or equal to 6 years after the first dose for those at highest risk of rapid decline in antibody levels (i.e., those with chronic renal failure, nephrotic syndrome, or transplanted organs) or of fatal pneumococcal infection (i.e., asplenic patients).

Vaccine Indications

Available data regarding vaccine efficacy support the broader use of pneumococcal polysaccharide vaccine in the United States. Vaccination is particularly recommended for the following groups:

1. Immunocompetent adults who are at increased risk of pneumococcal disease or its complications because of chronic illnesses (e.g., cardiovascular disease, pulmonary disease, diabetes mellitus, alcoholism, cirrhosis, or cerebrospinal fluid leaks) or who are greater than or equal to 65 years old.
2. Immunocompromised adults at increased risk of pneumococcal disease or its complications (e.g., persons with splenic dysfunction or anatomic asplenia, Hodgkin disease, lymphoma, multiple myeloma, chronic renal failure, nephrotic syndrome, or conditions such as organ transplantation associated with immunosuppression).
3. Adults with asymptomatic or symptomatic HIV infection.
4. Persons living in special environments or social settings with an identified increased risk of pneumococcal disease or its complications (e.g., certain Native American populations).

Programs for vaccine delivery in the recommended high-risk groups need to be developed further. Specifically, more effective programs are needed for giving vaccine in physicians' offices, hospitals, nursing homes, and other chronic-care facilities.

Two-thirds of persons with serious pneumococcal disease have been hospitalized within a 5-year period before the pneumococcal illness (35). Therefore, vaccine should be given to hospitalized patients in the high-risk groups before discharge in order to prevent future admissions for pneumococcal disease. Also, persons with chronic conditions who visit physicians frequently are probably at higher risk of pneumococcal infection than those who require infrequent visits. Office-based programs to identify and vaccinate patients requiring frequent medical care should help prevent pneumococcal illness. Furthermore, pneumococcal polysaccharide vaccine and influenza vaccine can be given at different sites at the same time without an increase in side effects (36).

Medicare has partially reimbursed the cost of pneumococcal polysaccharide vaccination since 1981. Hospitals may be reimbursed for pneumococcal vaccination of Medicare recipients independent of reimbursement based on systems of prospective payments.

Vaccine Side Effects and Adverse Reactions

About half the persons given pneumococcal polysaccharide vaccine experience mild side effects such as erythema and pain at the site of injection. Fever, myalgias, and severe local reactions have been reported by <1% of those given pneumococcal polysaccharide vaccine (37). Severe adverse effects such as anaphylactic reactions have rarely been reported—approximately five cases per million doses administered. A similar incidence of adverse events after primary vaccination and revaccination has been noted among adults when revaccination occurs >4 years after primary vaccination (Merck Sharp & Dohme, unpublished data).

When the interval between first and second doses was less than or equal to 13 months, local reactions were more severe (38); these reactions are thought to result from localized antigen-antibody reactions involving antibody induced by a previous vaccination. Until more information is available, revaccination should be given only to adults at highest risk of pneumococcal illness, as noted above in the "Vaccine Indications" section.

Vaccine Precautions and Contraindications

The safety of pneumococcal polysaccharide vaccine among pregnant women has not been evaluated. Women at high risk of pneumococcal disease ideally should be vaccinated before pregnancy.

Both Inactivated-Bacteria and Live-Bacteria Vaccines

Typhoid

The occurrence of typhoid fever remained constant in the period 1975–1989, with an average of 447 cases reported annually. During the period 1975–1989, 59% of cases for which the patient's age was known occurred among patients greater than or equal to 20 years of age. Approximately 69% of typhoid cases reported in the United States in 1984 were acquired by travelers to other countries.

Typhoid Vaccine

A primary series of two 0.5-mL doses of phenol-inactivated typhoid vaccine (given SC) 4 weeks apart has been shown to protect 51%–76% of recipients.

A live, attenuated oral typhoid vaccine was licensed in 1989. Its efficacy is approximately 67%, when taken as recommended (four doses on alternate days).

An acetone-killed and -dried typhoid vaccine is available only to the U.S. Armed Forces.

Vaccine Indications

Vaccination is indicated for travelers to areas where a recognized risk of exposure to typhoid exists, although no country requires typhoid immunization for entry. Vaccination is particularly recommended for travelers who will have prolonged exposure to potentially contaminated food and water in smaller villages or rural areas off the usual tourist routes. Further information to guide travelers about typhoid immunization is contained in the publication "Health Information for International Travel" (see earlier). Even after typhoid vaccination, food and water should be selected carefully in these areas. Two other groups for whom selective vaccination is indicated are persons with intimate exposure (i.e., continued household contact) to a documented typhoid carrier and workers in microbiology laboratories who frequently work with Salmonella typhi. Typhoid vaccination is not recommended in the United States for use in areas of natural disaster. Booster doses of the inactivated vaccine should be given at least every 3 years to persons with continued or repeated exposure; these may be administered SC (0.5 mL) or ID (0.1 mL). The optimal booster schedule for live, attenuated Ty21a oral vaccine has not been determined, although efficacy has been shown to persist for 5 years with a four-dose regimen. The manufacturer of Ty21a recommends revaccination with the entire four-dose series every 5 years. No experience with using live, attenuated oral vaccine as a booster among persons who were previously vaccinated with parenteral vaccine exists. The acetone-killed and -dried vaccine, available only to the U.S. Armed Forces, should not be given ID.

Vaccine Side Effects and Adverse Reactions

Inactivated typhoid vaccine given SC often results in 1–2 days of discomfort at the site of injection. The local reaction may be accompanied by fever, malaise, and headache.

Adverse reactions from the oral typhoid vaccine reported to the manufacturer occurred at a rate of <1/100,000 doses administered. Reactions reported consisted of nausea, abdominal cramps, vomiting, and skin rash or urticaria.

Vaccine Precautions and Contraindications

The only contraindication to inactivated typhoid vaccine is a history of a severe local or systemic reaction after a previous dose.

Oral typhoid vaccine is not recommended for children <6 years of age or immunocompromised persons, including those with asymptomatic HIV infection.

Live-Bacteria Vaccines

Tuberculosis

The number of tuberculosis cases in the United States has markedly declined since nationwide reporting began in 1953. Between 1972 and 1984, the annual incidence of tuberculosis declined from 15.8 cases/100,000 population to 9.4/100,000, a decrease of 41%. Since 1984, however, the number of cases reported and the case rate have increased. This increase is probably attributable to the occurrence of tuberculosis among persons with HIV infection. In 1989, approximately 92.2% of 23,485 reported cases with patient ages known occurred among persons greater than or equal to 20 years of age. The risk of infection with Mycobacterium tuberculosis is greatest for those who have repeated exposure to persons with unrecognized or untreated sputum-positive pulmonary tuberculosis. In the United States, efforts to control tuberculosis are directed toward early identification and treatment of cases, preventive therapy with isoniazid for infected persons at high risk of disease, and prevention of transmission to others.

Bacille Calmette-Guerin Vaccine

Although BCG is widely used in many areas of the world, results of a recent large-scale field trial in India have raised questions about its efficacy (39). BCG vaccines currently available in the United States differ from the products used in the published field trials, and their efficacy has not been demonstrated directly. In the United States, vaccines for ID and for percutaneous administration are licensed. (For percutaneous administration, one drop of vaccine is placed on the skin and introduced through the skin by multiple punctures with a bifurcated or other type of needle.) Vaccination should be only by the route indicated on the package labeling.

Vaccine Indications

In the United States, BCG vaccination is no longer recommended for health-care workers or other adults at high risk for acquiring TB infection. The only situations in which BCG might be considered are for children with negative tuberculin skin tests who fall into the following categories: (a) those who cannot be placed on isoniazid preventive therapy but who have continuous exposure to persons with active disease, (b) those with continuous exposure to patients with organisms resistant to isoniazid and rifampin, or (c) those belonging to groups with exceptionally high annual rates of new infection (i.e., >1% per year).

Vaccine Side Effects and Adverse Reactions

BCG has been associated with severe or prolonged ulceration at the vaccination site, regional adenitis, disseminated BCG infection, and osteitis. Severe ulceration and adenitis occur among approximately 1%–10% of vaccinees, although disseminated infections and osteitis are quite rare (1–10 per million doses).

Vaccine Precautions and Contraindications

Although no harmful effects of BCG on the fetus have been observed, avoiding vaccination during pregnancy unless there is immediate excessive risk of exposure to infective tuberculosis is prudent.

Because BCG is a live-bacteria vaccine, it should not be given to persons immunocompromised as a result of immune deficiency diseases (including HIV infection), leukemia, lymphoma, and generalized malignancy, or to persons immunosuppressed as a result of therapy with corticosteroids, alkylating drugs, antimetabolites, or radiation. (See "Conditions that Compromise the Immune System.")

Other Licensed Vaccines

Adenovirus and Adenovirus Vaccine

Adenovirus types 4 and 7 have frequently been the cause of outbreaks of acute, febrile respiratory tract disease among young adults during military training. Live, oral adenovirus vaccines for types 4 and 7 are available for vaccination of military populations. Use of the vaccines in other populations is not recommended.

Anthrax and Anthrax Vaccine

Anthrax is infrequently encountered. Anthrax vaccine is recommended only for individuals who come in contact in the workplace with imported animal hides, furs, bonemeal, wool, animal hair (especially goat hair), and bristles and for persons undertaking investigations involving Bacillus anthracis.

Primary vaccination consists of six SC 0.5-mL injections, the first three at 2-week intervals and the other three at 6-month intervals. Booster doses of 0.5-mL SC are recommended at 1-year intervals. The vaccine is only available from the Biologic Products Program, Michigan Department of Public Health. Details on reactions and vaccine contraindications are found in the package insert.

Immune Globulins

IG and specific immune globulins (i.e., HBIG, TIG, HRIG, and varicella-zoster immune globulin [VZIG]) are indicated to prevent or modify certain diseases in specific circumstances.

Cytomegalovirus Immune Globulin

This is a hyperimmune intravenous preparation that is effective in both prophylaxis (alone) and treatment (with ganciclovir) of cytomegalovirus (CMV) infections in bone marrow and kidney transplant recipients. When used as a prophylactic agent, CMV immune globulin has been used over a period of several months and does not diminish the frequency of CMV infections, but it does limit disease and reduce death rates.

Hepatitis B Immune Globulin

HBIG, alone or in combination with HB vaccine, is used for postexposure prophylaxis of HBV infection among persons who have not previously received HB vaccine or who are known not to have responded to the vaccine series. For percutaneous or mucous-membrane exposure to blood known to be HBsAg positive or from a bite by an HBV carrier, a single dose of HBIG (0.06 mL/kg or 5 mL for adults) should be administered as soon as possible and a series of three doses of HB vaccine begun within 1 week after exposure. Vaccine and HBIG may be administered simultaneously, but at different sites. For those who choose not to take HB vaccine, a second, identical dose of HBIG should be administered 1 month later.

After any percutaneous exposure to blood, serologic confirmation of the HBsAg status of the source patient should be obtained as soon as possible. If the source patient is HBsAg positive, the exposed person should immediately receive HBIG and HB vaccine according to the schedule above. The value of HBIG given beyond 7 days after exposure is unclear. For management of HBsAg-positive percutaneous exposure among persons who have previously received HB vaccine, the ACIP's Recommendations for "Protection of Viral Hepatitis" should be consulted (21) (Table 9).

Table 9. Recommendations for postexposure prophylaxis for percutaneous or permucosal exposure to hepatitis B, United States

Exposed person	Treatment when source is:		
	HBsAg* positive	HBsAg Negative	Source not tested or unknown
Unvaccinated	HBIG† 3 1§ and initiate HB¶ vaccine**	Initiate HB vaccine**	Initiate HB vaccine**
Previously vaccinated	Test exposed for anti-HBs‡	No treatment	No treatment
Known responder	1. If adequate,§§ no treatment 2. If inadequate, HB vaccine booster dose		
Known nonresponder	HBIG × 2 or HBIG × 1 plus 1 HB vaccine	No treatment	If known high-risk source, may treat as if source were HBsAg positive
Response unknown	Test exposed for anti-HBs 1. If inadequate,§§ HBIG × 1 plus HB vaccine booster dose 2. If adequate, no treatment	No treatment	Test exposed for anti-HBs 1. If inadequate,§§ HB vaccine booster dose 2. If adequate, no treatment

*HBsAg = Hepatitis B surface antigen.
†HBIG = Hepatitis B immune globulin.
§HBIG dose 0.06 mL/kg IM.
¶HB = Hepatitis B.
**For HB vaccine dose, see reference 21.
‡Antibody to hepatitis B surface antigen.
§§Adequate anti-HBs is 10 SRU by radioimmunoassay or positive by enzyme immunoassay.

All susceptible persons whose sex partners have acute HBV infection or whose sex partners are discovered to be HBsAg carriers should receive a single dose of HBIG (0.06 mL/kg) and should begin the HB vaccine series if prophylaxis can be started within 14 days of the last sexual contact or if ongoing sexual contact will occur. Administering the vaccine with HBIG may improve the efficacy of postexposure treatment; in addition, the vaccine has the advantage of conferring long-lasting protection. These recommendations, along with those for newborn infants exposed to HBsAg-carrier mothers, are listed in Table 10. An alternative treatment for persons who are not from a high-risk group for whom vaccine is routinely recommended and whose regular sex partners have acute HBV infection is to give one dose of HBIG within 14 days of exposure (without vaccine) and retest the sex partner for HBsAg 3 months later. No further treatment is necessary if the sex partner becomes HBsAg negative. If the sex partner remains HBsAg positive, a second dose of HBIG should be administered and the HBV vaccine series started.

Human Rabies Immune Globulin

Postexposure prophylaxis for rabies should always include HRIG with one exception: persons who have been previously vaccinated with the recommended preexposure or postexposure regimens of HDCV or have been vaccinated with other types of rabies vaccines and have a history of documented adequate rabies antibody titer should not receive HRIG (Table 7). The recommended dose of HRIG is 20 IU/kg body weight. If anatomically feasible, thoroughly infiltrate the area around the wound with up to half the dose of HRIG; the rest of the HRIG should be administered IM.

Immune Globulin for Intramuscular Use

IG is given IM for preexposure prophylaxis against hepatitis A to travelers areas where contact with potentially contaminated food and water is anticipated. For

Table 10. Recommendations for postexposure prophylaxis for perinatal and sexual exposure to hepatitis B, United States

| Exposure | HBIG* | | Vaccine | |
	Dose	Recommended timing	Dose	Recommended timing
Perinantal	0.5 mL IM[†]	Within 12 hours of birth	0.5 mL IM[†§]	Within 12 hours of birth[¶]
Sexual	0.06 mL/ kg IM[†]	Single dose within 14 days of last sexual contact	1.0 mL IM[†§]	First dose at time of HBIG* treatment[¶]

*HBIG = Hepatitis B immunoglobulin.
[†]IM = intramuscularly
[§]For appropriate age-specific doses of each vaccine, see reference 21.
[¶]The first dose can be administered the same time as the HBIG dose but at a different site; subsequent doses should be administered as recommended for specific vaccine.

travelers at risk for 2–3 months, a single IM dose of 0.02 mL/kg is recommended. For more prolonged travel, 0.06 mL/kg should be administered every 5 months. For persons whose travel repeatedly places them at risk for hepatitis A, testing for antibodies to hepatitis A is useful to identify those who are immune and to eliminate unnecessary doses of IG. IG is also indicated for postexposure prophylaxis for close household and sexual contacts of persons with hepatitis A, staff and attendees of day-care centers, household contacts of diapered children in day-care centers in which hepatitis A transmission is occurring, selected staff and clients of custodial institutions in which an outbreak is occurring, and co-workers of food handlers with hepatitis A. For such contacts, a single dose of 0.02 mL/kg of IG is recommended as soon as possible after exposure. IG is not effective unless given within 2 weeks after exposure.

IG can be used to prevent or modify measles disease in susceptible contacts of persons with measles, especially those for whom measles vaccine is contraindicated, if given within 6 days after exposure. The recommended dose is 0.25 mL/kg, or 0.5 mL/kg for immunocompromised persons (maximum dose = 15 mL in both situations). IG should not be used to control measles outbreaks.

Immune Globulin for Intravenous Use

IG modified for intravenous (IV) use may be administered to prevent acute infections among patients with defective antibody synthesis or, in unusual situations, as prophylaxis against hepatitis A or measles for patients for whom the IM preparation is contraindicated because of thrombocytopenia or disorders that can cause IM hemorrhage. However, no data are available about the efficacy of IG when administered IV in preventing either hepatitis A or measles. Because IG modified for IV use is made from a relatively small pool of donors, it may not contain antibodies to hepatitis A. ONLY IG MODIFIED FOR IV USE CAN BE GIVEN INTRAVENOUSLY. The IV dose is 100 mg/kg, administered slowly. The IV preparation is supplied in 50-mL vials containing 2.5 g of IG.

Tetanus Immune Globulin

TIG is indicated in tetanus prophylaxis as part of the management of wounds other than clean, minor wounds in persons (a) whose previous T toxoid vaccination status is unknown or uncertain or (b) who have received fewer than three previous T toxoid doses. The currently recommended prophylactic dose for wounds of average severity is 250 units (U) IM. Td should be administered at the same time but at a separate site.

A summary of the indications for active and passive immunization in the management of wounds is provided in Table 8.

Vaccinia Immune Globulin

Vaccinia immune globulin (VIG) is available only from CDC's Drug Service (404–639-3670) for the treatment of eczema vaccinatum, vaccinia necrosum, and ocular vaccinia developed as a result of smallpox vaccination. VIG is of no benefit in the treatment of postvaccination encephalitis. The recommended dose is 0.6 mL/kg IM to be administered as soon as possible after onset of symptoms. Because therapeutic doses of VIG can be quite large (e.g., 42 mL for a 70-

kg person), the doses should be divided over a 24- to 36-hour period. Doses may be repeated at the discretion of the attending physician, usually every 2–3 days, until no new lesions appear.

Varicella-Zoster Immune Globulin

Most persons with a clearly positive history of previous varicella are probably immune. Most adults (85%–95%) with negative or unknown histories of varicella disease (chickenpox) are likely to be immune. (Susceptibility rates for adults raised in some tropical areas, particularly remote areas, may be somewhat higher.) When available, serologic screening may be used to define susceptibility more precisely. Rates of complications and death for immunocompromised adults who contract varicella are likely to be substantially greater than for normal adults. After being carefully and individually evaluated, an immunocompromised patient who is believed to be susceptible and who has had significant exposure to varicella should receive VZIG to prevent complications.

Significant exposure to a person with varicella includes household contact, close contact indoors of >1 hour, sharing the same two- to four-bed hospital room, or prolonged, direct, face-to-face contact such as occurs with nurses or doctors who care for the patient.

Chickenpox can be more severe among adults than among normal children. The decision to administer VZIG to a normal adult should be made on an individual basis. The objective of VZIG use for normal adults is to modify rather than prevent illness in the hope of inducing lifelong immunity. When deciding whether to administer VZIG, the clinician should consider the patient's health status, the type of exposure, and the likelihood of previous infection. Adults who were older siblings in large families or whose children have had varicella are probably immune. If, after being carefully evaluated, a normal adult with substantial exposure to varicella is believed to be susceptible, VZIG may be administered. Pregnant women and potentially susceptible hospital personnel should be evaluated in the same way as other adults. Supplies of VZIG are limited, and indiscriminate administration of VZIG to normal adults would quickly exhaust supplies and prevent prophylaxis for known high-risk individuals. The cost of a five-vial adult dose is approximately $400.

VZIG, available through some American Red Cross distribution centers (Appendix 6), is supplied in vials containing 125 U. Although 125 U/10 kg of body weight up to a maximum of 625 U is considered likely to prevent or modify varicella among normal adults, higher doses may be necessary for the immunocompromised adult. However, the appropriate dose for immunocompromised adults has not been determined. VZIG should be administered IM as directed by the manufacturer. Although the duration of protection is unknown, the protection should probably last for at least one half-life of the IG, that is, approximately 3 weeks.

Immune Globulin Side Effects and Adverse Reactions

Serious adverse effects from immune globulins administered as recommended have been rare.

Immune Globulin Precautions and Contraindications

IG, if needed, is not contraindicated for pregnant women, Except for its IV preparation, IG is prepared for IM use and should not be given IV. The various preparations intended for IM use should not be given to patients with severe thrombocytopenia or other coagulation disorders that would ordinarily contraindicate IM injections, unless the expected benefits outweigh the risks.

Parenterally administered live-virus vaccines (e.g., MMR or other combinations) should be given at least 14 days before, or at least 6 weeks and preferably 3 months after, the administration of IG preparations. If an IG must be administered within 14 days after the administration of most live-virus vaccines, the vaccine should be administered again 3 months after the IG. If the interval between receipt of the vaccine and receipt of the IG is longer, the vaccine need not be readministered.

Preliminary data indicate that IG preparations do not interfere with the immune response to either OPV or yellow fever vaccine. No evidence suggests that HBV, HIV, or other viruses have ever been transmitted by the IG or HBIG that is commercially available in the United States (40). Since April 1985, all plasma units for preparation of all IG have been screened for antibody to HIV, and reactive units are discarded. No instance of HIV transmission or clinical illness consistent with HIV infection attributable to receiving IG or HBIG, including lots prepared before April 1985, has been observed. Laboratory studies have shown that the margin of safety based on the removal of HIV infectivity by the fractionation process is extremely high (41). Some HBIG lots prepared before April 1985 have detectable HIV antibody; low levels of passively acquired HIV antibody can occasionally be detected among recipients shortly after administration, but this reactivity does not persist (42).

REFERENCES

1. ACIP: Recommendations of the Immunization Practices Advisory Committee (ACIP). General recommendations on immunization. MMWR 1989;38:205–214, 219–227.
2. American College of Physicians Task Force on Adult Immunization and Infectious Diseases Society of America. Guide for adult immunization. 2nd ed. Philadelphia: American College of Physicians, 1990.
3. US Preventive Services Task Force. Guide to clinical preventive services: an assessment of the effectiveness of 169 interventions. Baltimore: Williams & Wilkins, 1989.
4. Braunstein H, Thomas S, Ito R. Immunity to measles in a large population of varying age: significance with respect to vaccination. Am J Dis Child 1990;144:296–298.
5. Smith E, Welch W, Berhow M, Wong VK. Measles susceptibility of hospital employees as determined by ELISA. Clin Res 1990;38:183A.
6. Atkinson WL, Markowitz LE, Adams NC, Seastrom GR. Transmission of measles in medical settings—United States, 1985–1989. Am J Med 1991(Suppl 3A):1S-5S.
7. CDC. Immunization recommendations for health-care workers. Atlanta: US Department of Health and Human Services, Public Health Service, 1989.
8. CDC. Rubella in hospitals—California. MMWR 1983;32:37–39.
9. American Academy of Pediatrics Committee on Infectious Diseases. Report of the Committee on Infectious Diseases. 22nd ed. Elk Grove Village, IL: American Academy of Pediatrics, 1991.
10. Weiss BP, Strassburg MA, Feeley JC. Tetanus and diphtheria immunity in an elderly population in Los Angeles County. Am J Public Health 1983;73:802–804.
11. Crossley K, Irvine P, Warren JB, Lee BK, Mead K. Tetanus and diphtheria immunity in urban Minnesota adults. JAMA 1979;242:2298–3000.

12. Ruben FL, Nagel J, Fireman P. Antitoxin responses in the elderly to tetanus-diphtheria (Td) immunization. Am J Epidemiol 1978;108:145–149.
13. Koblin BA, Townsend TR. Immunity to diphtheria and tetanus in inner-city women of childbearing age. Am J Public Health 1989;79:1297–1298.
14. CDC. Tetanus—United States, 1987 and 1988. MMWR 1990;39:37–41.
15. Jacobs RL, Lowe RS, Lanier BQ. Adverse reactions to tetanus toxoid. JAMA 1982;247:40–42.
16. Herman JJ, Radin R, Schneiderman R. Allergic reactions to measles (rubeola) vaccine in patients hypersensitive to egg protein. J Pediatr 1983;102:196–199.
17. Cochi SL, Preblud SR, Orenstein WA. Perspectives on the relative resurgence of mumps in the United States. Am J Dis Child 1988;142:499–507.
18. Tingle AJ, Yang T, Allen M, Kettyls GD, Larke RPB, Schulzer M. Prospective immunological assessment of arthritis induced by rubella vaccine. Infect Immun 1983;40:22–28.
19. Tingle AJ, Allen M, Petty RE, Kettyls GD, Chantler JK. Rubella-associated arthritis. I. Comparative study of joint manifestations associated with natural rubella infection and RA 27/3 rubella immunization. Ann Rheum Dis 1986;45:110–114.
20. Strebel PM, Sutter RW, Cochi SL, et al. Epidemiology of poliomyelitis in the US: One decade after the last reported case of indigenous wild virus-associated disease. Rev Infect Dis (in press).
21. CDC. Protection against viral hepatitis: recommendations of the Immunization Practices Advisory Committee (ACIP). MMWR 1990;39(RR-2):17–22.
22. Shaw FE Jr, Graham DJ, Guess HA, et al. Postmarketing surveillance for neurologic adverse events reported after hepatitis B vaccination: experience of the first three years. Am J Epidemiol 1988;127:337–352.
23. Turner GS, Nicholson KG, Tyrrell DAJ, Akoi FY. Evaluation of a human diploid cell strain rabies vaccine: final report of a three year study of pre-exposure immunization. J Hyg 1982;89:101–110.
24. CDC. Systemic allergic reactions following immunization with human diploid cell rabies vaccine. MMWR 1984;33:185–187.
25. Bernard KW, Smith PW, Kader FJ, Moran MJ. Neuroparalytic illness and human diploid cell rabies vaccine. JAMA 1982;248:3136–3138.
26. Pappaioanou M, Fishbein DB, Dreesen DW, et al. Antibody response to preexposure human diploid-cell rabies vaccines given concurrently with chloroquine. N Engl J Med 1986;314:280–284.
27. Ward J, Cochi S. Haemophilus influenzae vaccines. In: Plotkin SA, Mortimer EA Jr, eds. Vaccines. Philadelphia: WB Saunders, 1988:300–333.
28. Frank AL, Labotka RJ, Rao S, et al. Haemophilus influenzae type b immunization of children with sickle cell diseases. Pediatrics 1988;82:571–575.
29. Feldman S, Gigliotti F, Shenep JL, Roberson PK, Lott L. Risk of Haemophilus influenzae type b disease in children with cancer and response of immunocompromised leukemic children to a conjugate vaccine. J Infect Dis 1990;161:926–931.
30. Jakacki R, Luery N, McVerry P, Lange B. Haemophilus influenzae diphtheria protein conjugate immunization after therapy in splenectomized patients with Hodgkin disease. Ann Intern Med 1990;112:143–144.
31. Steinhoff MC, Auerbach BS, Nelson K, et al. Effect of protein conjugation on immune response of HIV-infected adults to H. influenzae type b (Hib) polysaccharide (PS) vaccine. In: Program and Abstracts of the Thirtieth Interscience Conference on Antimicrobial Agents and Chemotherapy. Atlanta: American Society for Microbiology, October 21–24, 1990.
32. Janoff EN, Worel S, Douglas JM, et al. Natural immunity and response to conjugate vaccine for Haemophilus influenzae type b in men with HIV. In: Program and Abstracts of the Thirtieth Interscience Conference on Antimicrobial Agents and Chemotherapy. Atlanta: American Society for Microbiology, October 21–24, 1990.
33. Berkowitz CD, Ward JI, Meier K, et al. Safety and immunogenicity of Haemophilus influenzae type b polysaccharide and polysaccharide diphtheria toxoid conjugate vaccines in children 15 to 24 months of age. J Pediatr 1987;110:509–514.
34. Redd SC, Rutherford GW III, Sande MA, et al. The role of human immunodeficiency virus infection in pneumococcal bacteremia in San Francisco residents. J Infect Dis 1990;162:1012–1017.
35. Fedson DS, Chiarello LA. Previous hospital care and pneumococcal bacteremia: importance for pneumococcal immunization. Arch Intern Med 1983;143:885–889.
36. DeStefano F, Goodman RA, Noble GR, McClary GD, Smith S J, Broome CV. Simultaneous administration of influenza and pneumococcal vaccines. JAMA 1982;247:2551–2554.

37. Semel JD, Seskind C. Severe febrile reaction to pneumococcal vaccine [Letter]. JAMA 1979; 241:1792.
38. Borgono JM, McLean AA, Vella PP, et al. Vaccination and revaccination with polyvalent pneumococcal polysaccharide vaccines in adults and infants. Proc Soc Exp Biol Med 1978;157:148–154.
39. Clemens JD, Chuong JJH, Feinstein AR. The BCG controversy: a methodological and statistical reappraisal. JAMA 1983;249:2362–2369.
40. CDC. Safety of therapeutic immune globulin preparations with respect to transmission to human T-lymphotrophic virus type III/lymphadenopathy-associated virus infection. MMWR 1986; 35:231–233.
41. Wells MA, Wittek AE, Epstein JS, et al. Inactivation and partition of human T-cell lymphotrophic virus, type III, during ethanol fractionation of plasma. Transfusion 1986;26:210–213.
42. Tedder RS, Uttley A, Cheingsong-Popov R. Safety of immunoglobulin preparation containing anti-HTLV-III [Letter]. Lancet 1985;1:815.

APPENDIX 1
Published ACIP Statements* Related to Specific Diseases and Immunobiologics Recommendations, as of September 1, 1991

Subject	MMWR Publication
General recommendations on immunizations	1989;38:205–14, 219–27
	Erratum: 1989;38:311
Bacille Calmette-Guerin	1988;37:663–4, 669–75
Cholera	1988;37:617–24
Diphtheria, tetanus, and pertussis	1991;40(No. RR-10):1–28
Haemophilus influenzae type b conjugate	1991;40(no. RR-1):1–7
Hepatitis, viral	1990;39 (No. RR-2):1–26
Human T-lymphotropic virus type III/ lymphadenopathy-associated virus, immunization of children with	1986;35:595–8, 603–6
Human immunodeficiency virus, immunization of children with (supplementary statement)	1988;37:181–6
Influenza†	1991;40(No. RR-6):1–15
Measles	1989;38:(No. S-9):1–18
Meningococcal polysaccharide	1985;34:255–9
Mumps	1989;38:388–92, 397–400
Plague	1982;31:301–4
Pneumococcal polysaccharide	1989;38:64–8, 73–6
Poliomyelitis	1982;31:22–6, 31–4
Poliomyelitis, enhanced potency inactivated vaccine	1987;36:795–8
Rabies	1991;40(No. RR-3):1–19
Rubella	1990;39(No. RR-15):1–18
Smallpox (Vaccinia)	1985;34:341–2
Typhoid	1990;39(No. RR-10):1–5
Yellow fever	1990;39(No. RR-6):1–6
Varicella-zoster (chickenpox) immune globulin	1984;33:84–90, 95–100

*The Immunization Practices Advisory Committee (ACIP) periodically reviews recommendations on vaccination and prophylaxis. When recommendations are revised, they are published individually in the MMWR.
†Each year influenza vaccine recommendations are reviewed and amended to reflect updated information on influenza activity in the United States for the preceding influenza season and to provide information on the vaccine available for the upcoming influenza season. These recommendations are published in the MMWR annually, usually in May or June.

APPENDIX 2
National Coalition of Adult Immunization
Member Organizations
(as of March 1, 1991)

American Academy of Family Physicians
American Academy of Otolaryngology—
Head and Neck Surgery
American Academy of Pediatrics
American Academy of Physician Assistants
American Association of Medical Colleges
American Association for World Health
American Association of Retired Persons
American College of Obstetricians and
Gynecologists
American College Health Association
American College of Physicians
American College of Preventive Medicine
American Council of Life Insurance
American Dental Association
American Geriatrics Society
American Group Practice Association
American Hepatitis Association
American Hospital Association
American Indian Health Care Association
American Liver Foundation
American Lung Association
American Medical Association
American Managed Care and Review
Association
American Medical Student Association
American Nurses' Association
American Podiatric Medical Association
American Public Health Association
American Social Health Association
American Society for Microbiology
American Society of Hospital Pharmacists
American Society of Internal Medicine
American Thoracic Society
Association of American Medical Colleges
Association of Practitioners in Infection
Control
Association of State and Territorial Health
Officials
Association of Teachers of Preventive
Medicine
Catholic Health Association
Centers for Disease Control
Conference of State and Territorial
Epidemiologists
Connaught Laboratories, Inc., A
Pasteur Merieux Company
Du Pont Pharmaceuticals
Federation of American Health Systems

Food and Drug Administration
Gray Panthers
Harvard Community Health Plan
Health Insurance Association of America
Infectious Diseases Society of America
Lederle-Praxis Biologicals, A Cyanamid
Business Unit
March of Dimes Birth Defects Foundation
Merck Sharp & Dohme
National AIDS Network
National Association of City and County
Health Officials
National Association of Hispanic Elderly
National Council of Community Hospitals
National Council for Education of Health
Professionals—Health Promotion
National Council of Senior Citizens
National Foundation for Infectious Diseases
National Health Council
National Institute of Allergy and Infectious
Diseases, National Institutes of Health
National Leadership Coalition of AIDS
Parke-Davis Division of Warner-Lambert
Company
Pharmaceutical Manufacturers Association
Phi Delta Chi Pharmacy Fraternity
Program for Appropriate Technology in Health
Retirement Advisors
Roche Laboratories, A Division of
Hoffmann-La Roche, Inc.
Sclavo, Inc.
Saint Louis Department of Health and
Hospitals
Service Employees International Union,
AFL-CIO, CLC
SmithKline Beecham Pharmaceuticals
Society of General Internal Medicine
Society of Hospital Epidemiologists of
America
E.R. Squibb and Sons, Inc.
State of Washington Division of Health
The Surgeon General, U.S. Public Health
Service
U.S. Conference of Local Health Officers
U.S. Department of Defense
United States Pharmacopeial Convention
Veterans Administration Medical Center,
Minneapolis
Wyeth-Ayerst Laboratories

APPENDIX 3
Suggested Immunization Record Form for Health-Care Provider

Name_____ Sex_____ Birth Date_____

Vaccine	Vaccine type	Date given Mo/Day/Yr	Vaccine lot #	Doctor or clinic	Date next dose due
Polio (OPV or eIPV)*					
Diphtheria Tetanus Pertussis (DTP or DT, Pediatric or Td [Adult])*					
Measles Mumps, Rubella, or Combinations*					
Influenza					
Pneumococcal Polysaccharide					
Hepatitis B					
Other vaccines or Immune Globulins*					
Tuberculin Test					

Notes:

*Specify type used.

APPENDIX 4
Immunobiologics Available, as of March 1, 1991, by Product Name and Manufacturer, with Manufacturers' Addresses and Telephone Numbers*

Immunobiologic	Manufacturer	Product name
Adenovirus vaccine	Wyeth-Ayerst Labs, Inc.	Adenovirus, Live, Oral, Type 4[†] Adenovirus, Live, Oral, Type 7[†]
Anthrax vaccine	Michigan Department of Public Health	Anthrax Vaccine, Absorbed[§]
BCG vaccine	Organon Teknika Corporation	BCG Vaccine
Cholera vaccine	Wyeth-Ayerst Labs, Inc.	Cholera Vaccine
Cytomegalovirus immune globulin	Massachusetts Public Health Biologic Labs	Cytomegalovirus Immune Globulin, Intravenous
Diphtheria and tetanus toxoids, adsorbed	Connaught Labs, Inc.	Diphtheria and Tetanus Toxoids, Adsorbed (Pediatric)
	Lederle Laboratories, Division of American Cyanamid Co.	Diphtheria and Tetanus Toxoids, Adsorbed (Purogeneted for Pediatric Use)
	Massachusetts Public Health Biologic Labs	Diphtheria and Tetanus Toxoids, Adsorbed (Pediatric)

APPENDIX 4—continued

Immunobiologic	Manufacturer	Product name
	Michigan Department of Public Health	Diphtheria and Tetanus Toxoids, Adsorbed (Pediatric)[§]
	Sclavo SpA[¶]	Diphtheria and Tetanus Toxoids, Adsorbed, USP (Pediatric)
	Wyeth-Ayerst Labs, Inc.	Diphtheria and Tetanus Toxoids, Adsorbed (For Pediatric Use)
Diphtheria and tetanus toxoids and pertussis vaccine, adsorbed	Connaught Labs, Inc.	Diphtheria and Tetanus Toxoids, and Pertussis Vaccine, Adsorbed
	Lederle Laboratories, Division of American Cyanamid Co.	Diphtheria and Tetanus Toxoids and Pertussis Vaccine, Adsorbed (Tri Immunol)
	Massachusetts Public Health Biologic Labs	Diphtheria and Tetanus Toxoids and Pertussis Vaccine, Adsorbed
	Michigan Department of Public Health	Diphtheria and Tetanus Toxoids and Pertussis Vaccine, Adsorbed[§]
Haemophilus influenzae type b vaccine (polysaccharide-conjugate)	Connaught Labs, Inc.	ProHIBit
	Lederle-Praxis Biologicals	HibTITER
	Merck Sharp & Dohme, Division of Merck & Co., Inc.	Pedvax-Hib
Hepatitis B Immune globulin	Merck Sharp & Dohme, Division of Merck & Co., Inc.	Hepatitis B Immune Globulin (Human) (MSD, HEP-B-GAMMAGEE)
	Cutter Biological, Division of Miles, Inc.	Hepatitis B Immune Globulin (HYPER-HEP)
	Abbott Laboratories	Hepatitis B Immune Globulin (Human) (H-BIG)
Hepatitis B vaccine (recombinant)	Merck Sharp & Dohme, Division of Merck & Co., Inc.	Recombivax HB
	SmithKline Beecham	Engerix B
Immune globulin	Armour Pharmaceutical Company	Immune Serum Globulin (Human) (GAMMAR; GAMMAR-IV)
	Central Laboratory Blood Transfusion Service, Swiss Red Cross	Immune Globulin Intravenous (SANDOGLOBULIN)
	Cutter Biological, Division of Miles, Inc.	Immune Globulin Intravenous [5% in 10% Maltose (GAMIMUNE)]
		Immune Globulin (Human), USP (GAMASTAN)
	Hyland Division Baxter Healthcare Corp.	Immune Globulin Intravenous (Human); (GAMMAGARD)
	Massachusetts Public Health Biologic Labs	Immune Serum Globulin (Human)
	Michigan Department of Public Health	Immune Serum Globulin (Human)[§]

APPENDIX 4—continued

Immunobiologic	Manufacturer	Product name
	New York Blood Ctr, Inc.	Immune Serum Globulin (Human)
Influenza vaccine	Connaught Labs, Inc.	Influenza Virus Vaccine (Zonal Purified) Whole Virion (FLUZONE)
	Connaught Labs, Inc.	Influenza Virus Vaccine (Zonal Purified) Split Virion (FLUZONE)
	Lederle Laboratories, Division of American Cyanamid Co.	Influenza Virus Vaccine (Split Virion [FLUIMUNE])
	Parke-Davis, Division of Warner-Lambert Co.	Influenza Virus Vaccine (Split Virion [FLUOGEN])
	Wyeth-Ayerst Labs, Inc.	Influenza Virus Vaccine, Subvirion Type
Measles, mumps, and rubella vaccine	Merck Sharp & Dohme, Division of Merck & Co., Inc.	Measles, Mumps, and Rubella Virus Vaccine, Live (MSD, MMR II)
Measles and rubella vaccine	Merck, Sharp & Dohme, Division of Merck & Co., Inc.	Measles and Rubella Virus Vaccine, Live (MSD, M-R-VAX II)
Measles vaccine	Merck Sharp & Dohme, Division of Merck & Co., Inc.	Measles Virus Vaccine, Live (Attenuated [MSD] ATTENUVAX)
Meningococcal polysaccharide vaccine A, C, Y, and W 135	Connaught Labs, Inc.	Meningococcal Polysaccharide Vaccine (MENOMUNE-A/C/Y/W-135)
Mumps vaccine	Merck Sharp & Dohme, Division of Merck & Co., Inc.	Mumps Virus Vaccine, Live (MSD, MUMPSVAX)
Pertussis vaccine, adsorbed	Michigan Department of Public Health	Pertussis Vaccine, Adsorbed
Plague vaccine	Cutter Biological, Division of Miles, Inc.	Plague Vaccine
Pneumococcal polysaccharide vaccine	Lederle Laboratories, Division of American Cyanamid Co.	Pneumococcal Vaccine, Polyvalent (PNU-IMUNE 23)
	Merck Sharp & Dohme Division of Merck & Co., Inc.	Pneumococcal Vaccine, Polyvalent (MSD, PNEUMOVAX 23)
Poliovirus vaccine inactivated	Connaught Labs, Inc.	Poliovax
Poliovirus vaccine, live, oral	Lederle Laboratories, Division of American Cyanamid Co.	Poliovirus Vaccine, Live, Oral Trivalent (ORIMUNE)
Rabies immune globulin	Cutter Biological, Division of Miles, Inc.	Rabies Immune Globulin (Human) (HYPERAB)
	Institut Merieux[**]	Rabies Immune Globulin (Human) (IMOGAMRABIES)
Rabies vaccine	Institut Merieux[**]	Rabies Vaccine (Human Diploid Cell [IMOVAX-RABIES], [IMOVAX-RABIES ID])
Rabies vaccine	Michigan Department of Public Health	Rabies Vaccine, Adsorbed[§]
Rubella vaccine	Merck Sharp & Dohme, Division of Merck & Co., Inc.	Rubella Virus Vaccine, Live (MSD, MERUVAX II)
Rubella and mumps vaccine	Merck Sharp & Dohme, Division of Merck & Co., Inc.	Rubella and Mumps Virus Vaccine, Live (MSD, BIAVAX II)

APPENDIX 4—*continued*

Immunobiologic	Manufacturer	Product name
Tetanus antitoxin	Sclavo, SpA[1]	Tetanus Antitoxin Purified, USP
Tetanus immune globulin	Cutter Biological, Division of Miles, Inc.	Tetanus Immune Globulin (Human) (HYPER-TET)
	Massachusetts Public Health Biologic Labs	Tetanus Immune Globulin (Human)
Tetanus and diphtheria toxoids, adsorbed	Connaught Labs, Inc.	Tetanus and Diphtheria Toxoids, Adsorbed (For Adult Use)
	Lederle Laboratories, Division of American Cyanamid Co.	Tetanus and Diphtheria Toxoids, Adsorbed (For Adult Use) (Purogenated Parenteral)
	Massachusetts Public Health Biologic Labs	Tetanus and Diphtheria Toxoids, Adsorbed (For Adult Use)
	Sclavo SpA[1]	Tetanus and Diphtheria Toxoids, Adsorbed, USP (Adult)
	Wyeth-Ayerst Labs, Inc.	Tetanus and Diphtheria Toxoids, Adsorbed (For Adult Use) (Aluminum Phosphate, Ultrafined)
Tetanus toxoid, adsorbed	Connaught Labs, Inc.	Tetanus Toxoid, Adsorbed
	Lederle Laboratories, Division of American Cyanamid Co.	Tetanus Toxoid, Adsorbed (Purogenated [Aluminum Phosphate Adsorbed])
	Massachusetts Public Health Biologic Labs	Tetanus Toxoid, Adsorbed
	Michigan Department of Public Health	Tetanus Toxoid, Adsorbed[§]
	Sclavo-SpA[1]	Tetanus Toxoid, Adsorbed, USP
	Wyeth-Ayerst Labs, Inc.	Tetanus Toxoid, Adsorbed (Aluminum Phosphate Adsorbed, Ultrafined)
Tetanus toxoid, fluid	Connaught Labs, Inc.	Tetanus Toxoid (Fluid)
	Lederle Laboratories, Division of American Cyanamid Co.	Tetanus Toxoid (Purogenated, Tetanus Toxoid Fluid)
	Sclavo SpA[1]	Tetanus Toxoid (Fluid)
	Wyeth-Ayerst Labs, Inc.	Tetanus Toxoid (Fluid, Purified, Ultrafined)
Typhoid vaccine	Wyeth-Ayerst Labs, Inc.	Typhoid Vaccine, U.S.P.
	Wyeth-Ayerst Labs, Inc.	Typhoid Vaccine[†] (Acetone-killed and -dried)
Typhoid vaccine, live, oral/Ty21A	Swiss Serum and Vaccine Institute	Vivotif Berna
Vaccinia immune globulin	None (CDC and Department of Defense stockpiles only)	Vaccinia Immune Globulin (Human)
Vaccinia vaccine	None (CDC stockpiles only)	Smallpox Vaccine

APPENDIX 4—*continued*

Immunobiologic	Manufacturer	Product name
Varicella-Zoster immune globulin	Massachusetts Public Health Biologic Labs	Varicella Zoster Immune Globulin (Human)‡
Yellow fever vaccine	Connaught Labs, Inc.	Yellow Fever Vaccine (Live, 17D Virus, YF-VAX)

*In the preparation of this appendix, every effort was made to assure its completeness and accuracy. This appendix was compiled from information obtained from manufacturers, the Division of Product Certification, Food and Drug Administration, and the Physicians' Desk Reference, 44th Edition, 1991, and, to the best of our knowledge, is an accurate and complete listing as of March 1, 1991. However, omissions and errors may have occurred inadvertently. This appendix is intended to be a resource and does not replace the provider's obligation to remain otherwise current on the availability of vaccines, toxoids, and immune globulins.

†Available only to the U.S. Armed Forces

§Outside Michigan, sold only to providers who will sign a "hold harmless" agreement.

¶Sclavo SpA products distributed in United States by Sclavo, Inc.

**Institut Merieux products distributed by Connaught Labs, Inc.

‡Varicella-zoster immune globulin is available from selected blood banks in various locations in the United States. Consult Appendix 6 for a listing.

Immunobiologics Manufacturers/Distributors

Manufacturer/Distributor	Telephone
1. Abbot Laboratories Abbott Park, IL 60064	(708) 937-6100 or (800) 323-9100, x131
2. Armour Pharmaceutical Company Kankakee, IL 60901	(815) 932-6771 or (800) 435-1852
3. Connaught Laboratories, Inc. Swiftwater, PA 19370	(717) 839-7189 or (800) 822-2463
4. Cutter Biological Division of Miles Laboratories, Inc. Berkeley, CA 94701	(415) 420-5177 (800) 288-8371
5. Hyland Division Baxter Healthcare Corporation Glendale, CA 91202	(800) 423-2090
6. Lederle Laboratories Division of American Cyanamid Co. Pearl River, NY 10965 Wayne, NJ 07470	(914) 732-5000 (201) 831-2000 (800) 533-3753
7. Lederle-Praxis Biologicals 30 Corporate Woods Suite 300 Rochester, NY 14623	(800) 526-7870
8. Massachusetts Public Health Biologic Laboratories Boston, MA 02130	(617) 522-3700
9. Merck Sharp & Dohme Division of Merck & Co., Inc. West Point, PA 19486	(215) 661-5000
10. Merieux Institute, Inc. Miami, FL 33169	(305) 593-9577 or (800) 327-2842
11. Michigan Department of Public Health Lansing, MI 48909	(517) 335-8119
12. New York Blood Center Blood Derivatives New York, NY 10021	(212) 570-3000 (800) 487-8751
13. Organon Teknika Corporation 5516 Nicholson Lane Kensington, MD 20895	(800) 323-6442

APPENDIX 4—*continued*

Immunobiologics Manufacturers/Distributors

Manufacturer/Distributor	Telephone
14. Parke-Davis Division of Warner-Lambert Co. Morris Plains, NJ 07950	(201) 540-2000
15. Sclavo, Inc. Wayne, NJ 07470	(201) 696-8300 or (800) 526-5260
16. Swiss Serum and Vaccine Institute Berna Products Coral Gables, FL	(305) 443-2900
17. SmithKline Beecham Philadelphia, PA 19101	(215) 751-4912
18. Wyeth-Ayerst Laboratories, Inc. Philadelphia, PA 19101	(215) 688-4400 or (800) 321-2304

APPENDIX 5
Use of Immunobiologics in Pregnancy*

Immunizing agent	Risk from disease to pregnant female	Risk from disease to fetus of neonate	Type of immunizing agent	Risk from immunizing agent to fetus	Indications for immunization during pregnancy	Dose schedule	Comments
LIVE-VIRUS VACCINES							
Measles	Significant morbidity, low mortality (not altered by pregnancy)	Significant increase in abortion rate; may cause malformation	Live, attenuated-virus vaccine	None confirmed	Contraindicated (See immune globulins)	One or two doses, depending on school/work status (see text)	Vaccination of susceptible women should be part of postpartum care
Mumps	Low morbidity and mortality (not altered by pregnancy)	Probable increased rate of abortion in first trimester. Questionable association of fibroelastosis in neonates	Live, attenuated-virus vaccine	None confirmed	Contraindicated	Single dose	
Rubella	Low morbidity and mortality (not altered by pregnancy)	High rate of abortion and congenital rubella syndrome	Live, attenuated-virus vaccine	None confirmed	Contraindicated	Single dose	Teratogenicity of vaccine is theoretical, not confirmed to date; vaccination of susceptible women should be part of postpartum care
Yellow fever	Significant morbidity and mortality (not altered by pregnancy)	Unknown	Live, attenuated-virus vaccine	Unknown	Contraindicated except if exposure risk is high	Single dose	Postponement of travel preferable to vaccination, if possible
TOXOIDS							
Tetanus-Diphtheria	Severe morbidity; tetanus mortality, 60%; diphtheria mortality, 10% (both of which are not altered by pregnancy)	Neonatal tetanus mortality, 60%	Combined tetanus-diphtheria toxoids preferred; adult tetanus-diphtheria formulation	None confirmed	Lack of primary series or no booster within past 10 years	Primary: two doses at 1- to 2-month interval with a third dose 6–12 months after the second. Booster: single dose every 10 years after	Updating of immune status should be part of antepartum care; unvaccinated women should be vaccinated,

Immunobiologic	Risk from disease to pregnant woman	Risk from disease to fetus or neonate	Type of immunizing agent	Risk from immunizing agent to fetus	Indications for immunization during pregnancy	Dose schedule	Comments
(continued from previous page)						completion of the primary series	preferably after first trimester
INACTIVATED-VIRUS AND LIVE-VIRUS VACCINES Poliomyelitis	No increased incidence in pregnancy but may be more severe if it does occur	Anoxic fetal damage reported; 50% mortality in neonatal disease	Live, attenuated-virus (OPV) and inactivated virus (eIPV) vaccine	None confirmed	Not routinely recommended for adults in United States, except persons at increased risk of exposure.	Primary: two doses of eIPV 4–8 weeks apart and a third dose 6–12 months after the second dose; two doses of OPV with a 6- to 8-week interval and a third dose at least 6 weeks later, customarily 8–12 months later	OPV indicated for susceptible pregnant women traveling in endemic areas or in other high-risk situations. No data on safety of eIPV in pregnancy.
INACTIVATED VIRUS VACCINES Hepatitis B	Possible increased severity during third trimester	Possible increase in abortion rate and prematurity; perinatal transmission may occur if mother is a chronic carrier or is acutely infected	Inactivated HB vaccine	None reported	Indications for prophylaxis not altered by pregnancy	1.0 mL intramuscularly at 0, 1, and 6 months	Infants born to HBsAg-positive mothers should receive 0.5 mL HBIG as soon as possible after birth, plus 0.5 mL HB vaccine within 1 week of birth. Vaccine should be repeated at 1 and 6 months
Influenza	Possible increase in mortality during epidemic of new antigenic strain	Possible increased abortion rate; no malformation confirmed	Inactivated type A and type B virus vaccines	None confirmed	Usually recommended only for patients with serious underlying diseases; public health authorities to be consulted for current recommendation	Consult with public health authorities because recommendations change each year	Criteria for vaccination of pregnant women same as for all adults

APPENDIX 5—continued

Immunizing agent	Risk from disease to pregnant female	Risk from disease to fetus or neonate	Type of immunizing agent	Risk from immunizing agent to fetus	Indications for immunization during pregnancy	Dose schedule	Comments
Rabies	Near 100% fatality (not altered by pregnancy)	Determined by maternal disease	Killed-virus vaccine	Unknown	Indications for prophylaxis not altered by pregnancy; each case considered individually	Public health authorities to be consulted for indications and dosage	
INACTIVATED-BACTERIA VACCINES							
Cholera	Significant morbidity and mortality; more severe during third trimester	Increased risk of fetal death during maternal illness occurring during third trimester	Killed-bacteria vaccine	Unknown	Only to meet international travel requirements	Two infections, 4–8 weeks apart	Vaccine of low efficacy
Meningococcus	No increased risk during pregnancy; no increase in severity of disease	Unknown	Killed-bacteria vaccine	No data available on use during pregnancy	Indications not altered by pregnancy; vaccination recommended only in unusual outbreak situations	Public health authorities to be consulted	
Plague	Significant morbidity and mortality (not altered by pregnancy)	Determined by maternal disease	Killed-bacteria vaccine	None reported	Very selective vaccination of exposed persons	Public health authorities to be consulted for indications and dosage	
Pneumococcus	No increased risk during pregnancy; no increase in severity of disease	Unknown	Polyvalent polysaccharide vaccine	No data available on use during pregnancy	Indications not altered by pregnancy; vaccine used only for persons at high risk	In adults one dose only, unless they are at highest risk of fatal infection or antibody loss; such persons may be revaccinated >6 years after the first dose (see text)	

Typhoid	Significant morbidity and mortality (not altered by pregnancy)	Unknown	Killed-bacteria vaccine; live, attenuated-bacteria vaccine	None confirmed	Not recommended routinely except for close, continued exposure or travel to areas where disease is endemic	Killed primary: two injections, 4 weeks apart; booster: single dose every 3 years; oral primary: four doses on alternate days; booster: four doses every 5 years
IMMUNE GLOBULINS Hepatitis A	Possible increased severity during third trimester	Possible increase in abortion rate and prematurity; possible transmission to neonate at delivery if mother is incubating the virus or is acutely ill at that time	Pooled immune globulin (IG)	None reported	Postexposure prophylaxis	0.02 mL/kg in one dose of IG
						IG should be given as soon as possible and within 2 weeks of exposure; infants born to mothers who are incubating the virus or are acutely ill at delivery should receive one dose of 0.5 mL as soon as possible after birth
Hepatitis B	Possible increased severity during third trimester	Possible increase in abortion rate and prematurity; perinatal transmission may occur if mother is a chronic carrier or is acutely infected; newborns are at risk of fulminant hepatitis or chronic carriage	Hepatitis B immune globulin (HBIG)	None reported	Postexposure prophylaxis	0.06 mL/kg or 5 mL immediately, plus HB vaccine series, when indicated
						Infants born to HBsAg-positive mothers should receive 0.5 mL HBIG as soon as possible after birth, plus 0.5 mL HB vaccine within 1 week of birth. Vaccine should be repeated at 1 and 6 months
Measles	Significant morbidity, low mortality (not altered by pregnancy)	Significant increase in abortion rate; may cause malformations	Pooled immune globulin (IG)	None reported	Postexposure prophylaxis	0.25 mL/kg in one dose of IG, up to 15 mL
						Unclear if IG prevents abortion; must be given within 6 days of exposure

APPENDIX 5—continued

Immunizing agent	Risk from disease to pregnant female	Risk from disease to fetus of neonate	Type of immunizing agent	Risk from immunizing agent to fetus	Indications for immunization during pregnancy	Dose schedule	Comments
Rabies	Near 100% fatality (not altered by pregnancy)	Determined by maternal disease	Human rabies immune globulin (HRIG)	None reported	Postexposure prophylaxis	20 IU/kg in one dose of HRIG	Used with rabies killed-virus vaccine
Tetanus	Severe morbidity; mortality, 60%	Neonatal tetanus mortality, 60%	Tetanus immune globulin (TIG)	None reported	Postexposure prophylaxis	250 U in one dose of TIG	Used with tetanus toxoid
Varicella	Possible increase in severe varicella pneumonia	Can cause neonatal varicella with increased mortality in neonatal period; very rarely causes congenital defects	Varicella-zoster immune globulin (VZIG)	None reported	Not routinely indicated in healthy pregnant women exposed to varicella	One vial per kilogram in one dose of VZIG, up to five vials	Primarily indicated for newborns of mothers who had varicella within five days before delivery or 48 hours after delivery. Approximately 90%–95% of adults are immune to varicella

*Modified from American College of Obstetricians and Gynecologists (ACOG). Immunization during pregnancy *ACOG Technical Bulletin #64.* Washington, DC: ACOG, 1982. This appendix describes methods and techniques of clinical practice that are currently acceptable and used by recognized authorities. However, it does not represent official policy or recommendations of the American College of Obstetricians and Gynecologists. Its publication should not be construed as excluding other acceptable methods of handling similar problems.

APPENDIX 6
Varicella-Zoster Immune Globulin Regional Distribution Centers and Service Areas

Service areas	Regional center and 24-hour telephone
United States and territories	
Alabama	American Red Cross
	Blood Services
	Alabama region
	(205) 322-5661
Alaska	(see Oregon)
Arizona	American Red Cross
	Blood Services
	Southern Arizona region
	(602) 623-0541
Arkansas	(see Missouri)
California, northern	American Red Cross
	Blood Services
	Central California region
	(408) 292-1626
California, southern	American Red Cross
	Blood Services
	L.A.-Orange County region
	(213) 739-5200
Colorado	(see New Mexico)
Connecticut	American Red Cross
	Blood Services
	Connecticut region
	(203) 678-2730
Delaware	(see Pennsylvania)
Florida	South Florida
	Blood Service
	(305) 326-8888
	American Red Cross
	Blood Services
	Mid-Florida region
	(904) 255-5444
Georgia	American Red Cross
	Blood Services
	Atlanta region
	(404) 881-9800
	(404) 881-6752 (night)
Hawaii	(see California, southern)
Idaho	American Red Cross
	Blood Services
	Snake River region
	(208) 342-4500
Illinois, northern	American Red Cross
	Blood Services
	Mid-America region
	(312) 440-2222
Illinois, southern	(see Missouri)
Indiana	American Red Cross
	Blood Services
	Fort Wayne region
	(219) 482-3781
Iowa	(see Wisconsin, S.E.)
Kansas	(see Missouri)
Kentucky	(see Missouri)
Louisiana	(see Texas [Gulf coast])
Maine	American Red Cross
	Blood Services
	Northeast-Portland
	(207) 775-2367

APPENDIX 6—*continued*

Service areas	Regional center and 24-hour telephone
Maryland	American Red Cross Blood Services (301) 764-4639 (also see Washington, DC)
Massachusetts	Massachusetts Public Health United States Biologics Laboratories (617) 522-3700
Michigan	American Red Cross Blood Services Southeastern Michigan region (313) 494-2715 American Red Cross Blood Services Wolverine region (313) 232-1176 American Red Cross Blood Services Great Lakes region (517) 484-7461
Minnesota	American Red Cross Blood Services St. Paul region (612) 291-6789 (612) 291-6767 (night)
Mississippi	(see Alabama)
Missouri	American Red Cross Blood Services (314) 658-2000 (314) 658-2136 (night)
Montana	(see Oregon)
Nebraska	American Red Cross Blood Services Midwest region (402) 341-2723
Nevada	(see California, northern)
New Hampshire	(see Vermont)
New Jersey, northern	(see Greater New York Blood Program)
New Jersey, southern	(see Pennsylvania)
New Mexico	United Blood Services (505) 247-9831
New York	The Greater New York Blood Program (212) 468-2106 (212) 570-3068 (night) American Red Cross Blood Services Northeastern New York region (518) 449-5020 (518) 462-7461 (518) 462-6964 (night) American Red Cross Blood Services Greater Buffalo Chapter (716) 886-6866 American Red Cross Blood Services Rochester region (716) 461-9800 American Red Cross Blood Services Syracuse region (315) 425-1647

APPENDIX 6—*continued*

Service areas	Regional center and 24-hour telephone
North Carolina	American Red Cross Blood Services Carolinas region (704) 376-1661
North Dakota	(see Wisconsin, S.E.)
Ohio	American Red Cross Blood Services Northern Ohio region (216) 781-1800 American Red Cross Central Ohio region (614) 253-7981
Oklahoma	(see Texas [Gulf Coast])
Oregon	American Red Cross Blood Services Pacific Northwest region (503) 243-5286
Pennsylvania	American Red Cross Blood Services Penn-Jersey region (215) 299-4126
Puerto Rico	American Red Cross Puerto Rico Blood Services (809) 759-7979
Rhode Island	Rhode Island Blood Center (401) 863-8368
South Carolina	American Red Cross Blood Services South Carolina region (803) 256-2301
South Dakota	(see Wisconsin, S.E.)
Tennessee	American Red Cross Nashville region (615) 327-1931, ext. 315
Texas	Gulf Coast Regional Blood Center (713) 791-6250 American Red Cross Blood Services Central Texas region (871) 776-8754 American Red Cross Blood Services Red River region (817) 322-8686
Utah	(see California, northern)
Vermont	American Red Cross Blood Services Vermont-New Hampshire region (802) 659-6400, ext 217
Virginia (also see Washington, DC)	American Red Cross Blood Services Tidewater region (804) 446-7709 Richmond Metropolitan Blood Service (804) 359-5100 American Red Cross Blood Services Appalachian region (703) 985-3595

APPENDIX 6—*continued*

Service areas	Regional center and 24-hour telephone
Washington	Puget Sound Blood Center (206) 292-6525
Washington, DC	American Red Cross Blood Services Washington region (202) 728-6426
West Virginia	(see Washington, DC)
Wisconsin	The Blood Center of S.E. Wisconsin (414) 933-5000 American Red Cross Blood Services Badger region (608) 255-0021
Wyoming	(see California, northern)
Other countries	
Canada	Canadian Red Cross Blood Transfusion Service National Office (416) 923-6692
Central and South America	South Florida Community Blood Center (305) 326-8888
All other countries	American Red Cross Blood Services Northeast region (617) 449-0773 American Red Cross Blood Services (617) 731-2130

TOPIC 16 / **INFLUENZA**

Prevention and Control of Influenza: Part I

Original Citation: Centers for Disease Control and Prevention. Prevention and Control of Influenza—Recommendations of the Advisory Committee on Immunization Practices. MMWR 1995;44(RR-3);1–22.

Original Authors: Nancy H. Arden, MN, Nancy J. Cox, PhD, Lawrence B. Schonberger, MD, MPH.

Editor's Note: ACIP changes its influenza recommendations annually. Be sure you have the latest version.

SUMMARY

These recommendations update information on the vaccine and antiviral agents available for controlling influenza during the 1995–96 influenza season (superseding MMWR 1994;43(No. RR-9):1–13 and MMWR 1994;43(No. RR-15):1–10). The principal changes include information about (a) the influenza virus strains included in the trivalent vaccine for 1995–96, (b) side effects and adverse reactions, and (c) the vaccination of pregnant women.

INTRODUCTION

Influenza A viruses are classified into subtypes on the basis of two surface antigens: hemagglutinin (H) and neuraminidase (N). Three subtypes of hemagglutinin (H1, H2, and H3) and two subtypes of neuraminidase (N1 and N2) are recognized among influenza A viruses that have caused widespread human disease. Immunity to these antigens—especially to the hemagglutinin—reduces the likelihood of infection and lessens the severity of disease if infection occurs. Infection with a virus of one subtype confers little or no protection against viruses of other subtypes. Furthermore, over time, antigenic variation (antigenic drift) within a subtype may be so marked that infection or vaccination with one strain may not induce immunity to distantly related strains of the same subtype. Although influenza B viruses have shown more antigenic stability than influenza A viruses, antigenic variation does occur. For these reasons, major epidemics of respiratory disease caused by new variants of influenza continue to occur. The antigenic characteristics of circulating strains provide the basis for selecting the virus strains included in each year's vaccine.

Typical influenza illness is characterized by abrupt onset of fever, myalgia, sore throat, and nonproductive cough. Unlike other common respiratory illnesses, influenza can cause severe malaise lasting several days. More severe illness can result if either primary influenza pneumonia or secondary bacterial pneumonia occurs. During influenza epidemics, high attack rates of acute illness result in both increased numbers of visits to physicians' offices, walk-in clinics, and emergency rooms and increased hospitalizations for management of lower respiratory tract complications. Elderly persons and persons with underlying health problems are at increased risk for complications of influenza. If they become ill with influenza, such members of high-risk groups (see Groups at Increased Risk for Influenza-Related Complications under Target Groups for Special Vaccination Programs) are more likely than the general population to require hospitalization. During major epidemics, hospitalization rates for persons at high risk may increase twofold to fivefold, depending on the age group. Previously healthy children and younger adults may also require hospitalization for influenza-related complications, but the relative increase in their hospitalization rates is less than for persons who belong to high-risk groups.

An increase in mortality further indicates the impact of influenza epidemics. Increased mortality results not only from influenza and pneumonia but also from cardiopulmonary and other chronic diseases that can be exacerbated by influenza. It is estimated that greater than 20,000 influenza-associated deaths occurred during each of 10 different U.S. epidemics from 1972–73 to 1990–91, and greater than 40,000 influenza-associated deaths occurred during each of three of these epidemics. More than 90% of the deaths attributed to pneumonia and influenza occurred among persons greater than or equal to 65 years of age.

Because the proportion of elderly persons in the U.S. population is increasing and because age and its associated chronic diseases are risk factors for severe influenza illness, the number of deaths from influenza can be expected to increase unless control measures are implemented more vigorously. The number of persons less than 65 years of age at increased risk for influenza-related complications is also increasing. Better survival rates for organ-transplant recipients, the success of neonatal intensive-care units, and better management of diseases such as cystic fibrosis and acquired immunodeficiency syndrome (AIDS) result in a higher survival rate for younger persons at high risk.

OPTIONS FOR THE CONTROL OF INFLUENZA

In the United States, two measures are available that can reduce the impact of influenza: immunoprophylaxis with inactivated (killed-virus) vaccine and chemoprophylaxis or therapy with an influenza-specific antiviral drug (amantadine or rimantadine). Vaccination of persons at high risk each year before the influenza season is currently the most effective measure for reducing the impact of influenza. Vaccination can be highly cost effective when it is (a) directed at persons who are most likely to experience complications or who are at increased risk for exposure and (b) administered to persons at high risk during hospitalizations or routine health-care visits before the influenza season, thus making special visits to physicians' offices or clinics unnecessary. When vaccine and epidemic strains of virus are well matched, achieving high vaccination rates among persons living in closed settings (e.g., nursing homes and other chronic-care facilities) can reduce the risk for outbreaks by inducing herd immunity.

INACTIVATED VACCINE FOR INFLUENZA A AND B

Each year's influenza vaccine contains three virus strains (usually two type A and one type B) representing the influenza viruses that are likely to circulate in the United States in the upcoming winter. The vaccine is made from highly purified, egg-grown viruses that have been made noninfectious (inactivated). Influenza vaccine rarely causes systemic or febrile reactions. Whole-virus, subvirion, and purified-surface-antigen preparations are available. To minimize febrile reactions, only subvirion or purified-surface-antigen preparations should be used for children; any of the preparations may be used for adults.

Most vaccinated children and young adults develop high postvaccination hemagglutination-inhibition antibody titers. These antibody titers are protective against illness caused by strains similar to those in the vaccine or the related variants that may emerge during outbreak periods. Elderly persons and persons with certain chronic diseases may develop lower postvaccination antibody titers than healthy young adults and thus may remain susceptible to influenza-related upper respiratory tract infection. However, even if such persons develop influenza illness despite vaccination, the vaccine can be effective in preventing lower respiratory tract involvement or other secondary complications, thereby reducing the risk for hospitalization and death.

The effectiveness of influenza vaccine in preventing or attenuating illness varies, depending primarily on the age and immunocompetence of the vaccine recipient and the degree of similarity between the virus strains included in the vaccine and those that circulate during the influenza season. When there is a good match between vaccine and circulating viruses, influenza vaccine has been shown to prevent illness in approximately 70% of healthy persons less than 65 years of age. In these circumstances, studies have also indicated that the effectiveness of influenza vaccine in preventing hospitalization for pneumonia and influenza among elderly persons living in settings other than nursing homes or similar chronic-care facilities ranges from 30%–70%.

Among elderly persons residing in nursing homes, influenza vaccine is most effective in preventing severe illness, secondary complications, and death. Studies of this population have indicated that the vaccine can be 50%–60% effective in preventing hospitalization and pneumonia and 80% effective in preventing death, even though efficacy in preventing influenza illness may often be in the range of 30%–40% among the frail elderly. Achieving a high rate of vaccination among nursing home residents can reduce the spread of infection in a facility, thus preventing disease through herd immunity.

RECOMMENDATIONS FOR THE USE OF INFLUENZA VACCINE

Influenza vaccine is strongly recommended for any person greater than or equal to 6 months of age who—because of age or underlying medical condition—is at increased risk for complications of influenza. Health-care workers and others (including household members) in close contact with persons in high-risk groups should also be vaccinated. In addition, influenza vaccine may be administered to any person who wishes to reduce the chance of becoming infected with influenza. The trivalent influenza vaccine prepared for the 1995–96 season will include A/Texas/36/91-like (H1N1), A/Johannesburg/33/94-like (H3N2), and B/Beijing/184/93-like hemagglutinin antigens. The actual influenza type B strain used by U.S. manufacturers is B/Harbin/07/94, which is antigenically equivalent to the B/Beijing/184/93 strain. Guidelines for the use of vaccine among certain patient populations follow. Dosage recommendations are also summarized (Table 1).

Table 1. Influenza Vaccine* Dosage, by Age Group—United States, 1995–96 Season

Age group	Product[+]	Dosage	No. of doses	Route[&]
6–35 mos	Split virus only	0.25 mL	1 or 2[@]	IM
3–8 yrs	Split virus only	0.50 mL	1 or 2[@]	IM
9–12 yrs	Split virus only	0.50 mL	1	IM
>12 yrs	Whole or split virus	0.50 mL	1	IM

*Contains 15 mg each of A/Texas/36/91-like (H1N1), A/Johannesburg/33/94-like (H3N2), and B/Beijing/184/93-like hemagglutinin antigens in each 0.5 mL. The actual influenza type B strain used by U.S. manufacturers is B/Harbin/07/94, which is antigenically equivalent to the B/Beijing/184/93 strain. Manufacturers include: Connaught Laboratories, Inc. (Fluzone® whole or split); Evans Medical Ltd. (distributed by Adams Laboratories, Inc.) (Fluviron™ purified surface antigen vaccine); Parke-Davis (Fluogen® split); and Wyeth-Ayerst Laboratories (Flushield™ split). For further product information call Connaught, (800) 822-2463; Adams, (800) 932-1950; Parke-Davis, (800) 223-0432; Wyeth-Ayerst, (800) FLU-SHIELD.
[+]Because of the lower potential for causing febrile reactions, only split-virus vaccines should be used for children. They may be labeled as "split," "subvirion," or "purified-surface-antigen" vaccine. Immunogenicity and side effects of split- and whole-virus vaccines are similar among adults when vaccines are administered at the recommended dosage.
[&]The recommended site of vaccination is the deltoid muscle for adults and older children. The preferred site for infants and young children is the anterolateral aspect of the thigh.
[@]Two doses administered at least 1 month apart are recommended for children <9 years of age who are receiving influenza vaccine for the first time.

　　Although the current influenza vaccine can contain one or more of the antigens administered in previous years, annual vaccination with the current vaccine is necessary because immunity declines in the year following vaccination. Because the 1995–96 vaccine differs from the 1994–95 vaccine, supplies of 1994–95 vaccine should not be administered to provide protection for the 1995–96 influenza season.

　　Two doses administered at least 1 month apart may be required for satisfactory antibody responses among previously unvaccinated children less than 9 years of age; however, studies of vaccines similar to those being used currently have indicated little or no improvement in antibody response when a second dose is administered to adults during the same season. During the past decade, data on influenza vaccine immunogenicity and side effects have been obtained for intramuscularly administered vaccine. Because recent influenza vaccines have not been adequately evaluated when administered by other routes, the intramuscular route is recommended. Adults and older children should be vaccinated in the deltoid muscle and infants and young children in the anterolateral aspect of the thigh.

TARGET GROUPS FOR SPECIAL VACCINATION PROGRAMS

To maximize protection of high-risk persons, they and their close contacts should be targeted for organized vaccination programs.

Groups at Increased Risk for Influenza-Related Complications

- Persons greater than or equal to 65 years of age
- Residents of nursing homes and other chronic-care facilities that house persons of any age with chronic medical conditions
- Adults and children with chronic disorders of the pulmonary or cardiovascular systems, including children with asthma
- Adults and children who have required regular medical follow-up or hospitalization during the preceding year because of chronic metabolic diseases (including diabetes mellitus), renal dysfunction, hemoglobinopathies, or immunosuppression (including immunosuppression caused by medications)
- Children and teenagers (6 months-18 years of age) who are receiving long-term aspirin therapy and therefore might be at risk for developing Reye syndrome after influenza

Groups that Can Transmit Influenza to Persons at High Risk

Persons who are clinically or subclinically infected and who care for or live with members of high-risk groups can transmit influenza virus to them. Some persons at high risk (e.g., the elderly, transplant recipients, and persons with AIDS) can have a low antibody response to influenza vaccine. Efforts to protect these members of high-risk groups against influenza might be improved by reducing the likelihood of influenza exposure from their caregivers. Therefore, the following groups should be vaccinated:

- Physicians, nurses, and other personnel in both hospital and outpatient-care settings;
- Employees of nursing homes and chronic-care facilities who have contact with patients or residents;
- Providers of home care to persons at high risk (e.g., visiting nurses and volunteer workers); and
- Household members (including children) of persons in high-risk groups.

VACCINATION OF OTHER GROUPS

General Population

Physicians should administer influenza vaccine to any person who wishes to reduce the likelihood of becoming ill with influenza. Persons who provide essential community services should be considered for vaccination to minimize disruption of essential activities during influenza outbreaks. Students or other persons in institutional settings (e.g., those who reside in dormitories) should be encouraged to receive vaccine to minimize the disruption of routine activities during epidemics.

Pregnant Women

Influenza-associated excess mortality among pregnant women has not been documented except during the pandemics of 1918–19 and 1957–58. However, additional case reports and limited studies suggest that women in the third trimester of pregnancy and early puerperium, including those women without underlying risk factors, might be at increased risk for serious complications from influenza. Health-care workers who provide care for pregnant women should consider administering influenza vaccine to all women who would be in the third trimester of pregnancy or early puerperium during the influenza season. Pregnant women who have medical conditions that increase their risk for complications from influenza should be vaccinated before the influenza season, regardless of the stage of pregnancy. Administration of influenza vaccine is considered safe at any stage of pregnancy.

Persons Infected with Human Immunodeficiency Virus (HIV)

Limited information exists regarding the frequency and severity of influenza illness among HIV-infected persons, but reports suggest that symptoms might be prolonged and the risk for complications increased for some HIV-infected persons. Because influenza can result in serious illness and complications, vaccination is a prudent precaution and will result in protective antibody levels in many recipients. However, the antibody response to vaccine can be low in persons with advanced HIV-related illnesses; a booster dose of vaccine does not improve the immune response for these persons.

Foreign Travelers

The risk for exposure to influenza during foreign travel varies, depending on season and destination. In the tropics, influenza can occur throughout the year; in the Southern Hemisphere, most activity occurs from April through September. Because of the short incubation period for influenza, exposure to the virus during travel can result in clinical illness that begins while traveling, an inconvenience or potential danger, especially for persons at increased risk for complications. Persons preparing to travel to the tropics at any time of year or to the Southern Hemisphere from April through September should review their influenza vaccination histories. If they were not vaccinated the previous fall or winter, they should consider influenza vaccination before travel. Persons in the high-risk categories should be especially encouraged to receive the most current vaccine. Persons at high risk who received the previous season's vaccine before travel should be revaccinated in the fall or winter with the current vaccine.

PERSONS WHO SHOULD NOT BE VACCINATED

Inactivated influenza vaccine should not be administered to persons known to have anaphylactic hypersensitivity to eggs or to other components of the influenza vaccine without first consulting a physician (see Side Effects and

Adverse Reactions). Use of an antiviral agent (i.e., amantadine or rimantadine) is an option for prevention of influenza A in such persons. However, persons who have a history of anaphylactic hypersensitivity to vaccine components but who are also at high risk for complications of influenza can benefit from vaccine after appropriate allergy evaluation and desensitization. Specific information about vaccine components can be found in package inserts for each manufacturer.

Adults with acute febrile illness usually should not be vaccinated until their symptoms have abated. However, minor illnesses with or without fever should not contraindicate the use of influenza vaccine, particularly among children with mild upper respiratory tract infection or allergic rhinitis.

SIDE EFFECTS AND ADVERSE REACTIONS

Because influenza vaccine contains only noninfectious viruses, it cannot cause influenza. Respiratory disease after vaccination represents coincidental illness unrelated to influenza vaccination. The most frequent side effect of vaccination reported by fewer than one third of vaccinees is soreness at the vaccination site that lasts for up to 2 days. In addition, two types of systemic reactions have occurred:

- Fever, malaise, myalgia, and other systemic symptoms occur infrequently and most often affect persons who have had no exposure to the influenza virus antigens in the vaccine (e.g., young children). These reactions begin 6–12 hours after vaccination and can persist for 1 or 2 days;
- Immediate—presumably allergic—reactions (e.g., hives, angioedema, allergic asthma, and systemic anaphylaxis) occur rarely after influenza vaccination. These reactions probably result from hypersensitivity to some vaccine component; the majority of reactions are most likely related to residual egg protein. Although current influenza vaccines contain only a small quantity of egg protein, this protein can induce immediate hypersensitivity reactions among persons who have severe egg allergy. Persons who have developed hives, have had swelling of the lips or tongue, or have experienced acute respiratory distress or collapse after eating eggs should consult a physician for appropriate evaluation to help determine if vaccine should be administered. Persons with documented immunoglobulin E (IgE)-mediated hypersensitivity to eggs—including those who have had occupational asthma or other allergic responses due to exposure to egg protein—might also be at increased risk for reactions from influenza vaccine, and similar consultation should be considered. The protocol for influenza vaccination developed by Murphy and Strunk may be considered for patients who have egg allergies and medical conditions that place them at increased risk for influenza-associated complications (Murphy and Strunk, 1985). Hypersensitivity reactions to any vaccine component can occur.

Although exposure to vaccines containing thimerosal can lead to induction of hypersensitivity, most patients do not develop reactions to thimerosal when administered as a component of vaccines—even when patch or intradermal tests for thimerosal indicate hypersensitivity. When reported, hypersensitivity to thimerosal has usually consisted of local, delayed-type hypersensitivity reactions.

Unlike the 1976 swine influenza vaccine, subsequent vaccines prepared from other virus strains have not been clearly associated with an increased frequency of Guillain-Barré syndrome (GBS). However, a precise estimate of risk is difficult to determine for a rare condition such as GBS, which has an annual background incidence of only one to two cases per 100,000 adult population. Among persons who received the swine influenza vaccine, the rate of GBS that exceeded the background rate was slightly less than one case per 100,000 vaccinations.

An investigation of GBS cases in 1990–91 indicated no overall increase in frequency of GBS among persons who were administered influenza vaccine; a slight increase in GBS cases among vaccinated persons might have occurred in the age group 18–64 years, but not among persons greater than or equal to 65 years of age. In contrast to the swine influenza vaccine, the epidemiologic features of the possible association of the 1990–91 vaccine with GBS were not as convincing. The rate of GBS cases after vaccination that was passively reported to the Vaccine Adverse Event Reporting System (VAERS) during 1993–94 was estimated to be approximately twice the average rate reported during other recent seasons (i.e., 1990–91, 1991–92, 1992–93 and 1994–95). The data currently available are not sufficient to determine whether this represents an actual risk. However, even if GBS were a true side effect, the very low estimated risk for GBS is less than that for severe influenza that could be prevented by vaccination.

Whereas the incidence of GBS in the general population is very low, persons with a history of GBS have a substantially greater likelihood of subsequently developing GBS than persons without such a history. Thus, the likelihood of coincidentally developing GBS after influenza vaccination is expected to be greater among persons with a history of GBS than among persons with no history of this syndrome. Whether influenza vaccination might be causally associated with this risk for recurrence is not known. Although it would seem prudent to avoid a subsequent influenza vaccination in a person known to have developed GBS within 6 weeks of a previous influenza vaccination, for most persons with a history of GBS who are at high risk for severe complications from influenza, the established benefits of influenza vaccination justify yearly immunization.

SIMULTANEOUS ADMINISTRATION OF OTHER VACCINES, INCLUDING CHILDHOOD VACCINES

The target groups for influenza and pneumococcal vaccination overlap considerably. For persons at high risk who have not previously been vaccinated with pneumococcal vaccine, health-care providers should strongly consider administering both pneumococcal and influenza vaccines concurrently. Both vaccines can be administered at the same time at different sites without increasing side effects. However, influenza vaccine is administered each year, whereas pneumococcal vaccine is not. Children at high risk for influenza-related complications can receive influenza vaccine at the same time they receive other routine vaccinations, including pertussis vaccine (DTP or DTaP). Because influenza vaccine can cause fever when administered to young children, DTaP might be preferable in those children greater than or equal to 15 months of age who are receiving the fourth or fifth dose of pertussis vaccine. DTaP is not licensed for the initial three-dose series of pertussis vaccine.

TIMING OF INFLUENZA VACCINATION ACTIVITIES

Beginning each September (when vaccine for the upcoming influenza season becomes available) persons at high risk who are seen by health-care providers for routine care or as a result of hospitalization should be offered influenza vaccine. Opportunities to vaccinate persons at high risk for complications of influenza should not be missed.

The optimal time for organized vaccination campaigns for persons in high-risk groups is usually the period from mid-October through mid-November. In the United States, influenza activity generally peaks between late December and early March. High levels of influenza activity infrequently occur in the contiguous 48 states before December. Administering vaccine too far in advance of the influenza season should be avoided in facilities such as nursing homes, because antibody levels might begin to decline within a few months of vaccination. Vaccination programs can be undertaken as soon as current vaccine is available if regional influenza activity is expected to begin earlier than December. Children less than 9 years of age who have not been vaccinated previously should receive two doses of vaccine at least 1 month apart to maximize the likelihood of a satisfactory antibody response to all three vaccine antigens. The second dose should be administered before December, if possible. Vaccine should be offered to both children and adults up to and even after influenza virus activity is documented in a community.

STRATEGIES FOR IMPLEMENTING INFLUENZA VACCINE RECOMMENDATIONS

Although rates of influenza vaccination have increased in recent years, surveys indicate that less than half of the high-risk population receives influenza vaccine each year. More effective strategies are needed for delivering vaccine to persons at high risk and to their health-care providers and household contacts.

Successful vaccination programs have combined education for health-care workers, publicity and education targeted toward potential recipients, a plan for identifying persons at high risk (usually by medical-record review), and efforts to remove administrative and financial barriers that prevent persons from receiving the vaccine. Persons for whom influenza vaccine is recommended can be identified and vaccinated in the settings described in the following paragraphs.

Outpatient Clinics and Physicians' Offices

Staff in physicians' offices, clinics, health-maintenance organizations, and employee health clinics should be instructed to identify and label the medical records of patients who should receive vaccine. Vaccine should be offered during visits beginning in September and throughout the influenza season. The offer of vaccine and its receipt or refusal should be documented in the medical record. Patients in high-risk groups who do not have regularly scheduled visits during the fall should be reminded by mail or telephone of the need for vaccine. If possible, arrangements should be made to provide vaccine with minimal waiting time and at the lowest possible cost.

Facilities Providing Episodic or Acute Care

Health-care providers in these settings (e.g., emergency rooms and walk-in clinics) should be familiar with influenza vaccine recommendations. They should offer vaccine to persons in high-risk groups or should provide written information on why, where, and how to obtain the vaccine. Written information should be available in language(s) appropriate for the population served by the facility.

Nursing Homes and Other Residential Long-Term-Care Facilities

Vaccination should be routinely provided to all residents of chronic-care facilities with the concurrence of attending physicians rather than by obtaining individual vaccination orders for each patient. Consent for vaccination should be obtained from the resident or a family member at the time of admission to the facility, and all residents should be vaccinated at one time, immediately preceding the influenza season. Residents admitted during the winter months after completion of the vaccination program should be vaccinated when they are admitted.

Acute-Care Hospitals

All persons greater than or equal to 65 years of age and younger persons (including children) with high-risk conditions who are hospitalized at any time from September through March should be offered and strongly encouraged to receive influenza vaccine before they are discharged. Household members and others with whom they will have contact should receive written information about why and where to obtain influenza vaccine.

Outpatient Facilities Providing Continuing Care to Patients at High Risk

All patients should be offered vaccine before the beginning of the influenza season. Patients admitted to such programs (e.g., hemodialysis centers, hospital specialty-care clinics, and outpatient rehabilitation programs) during the winter months after the earlier vaccination program has been conducted should be vaccinated at the time of admission. Household members should receive written information regarding the need for vaccination and the places to obtain influenza vaccine.

Visiting Nurses and Others Providing Home Care to Persons at High Risk

Nursing-care plans should identify patients in high-risk groups, and vaccine should be provided in the home if necessary. Caregivers and other persons in the household (including children) should be referred for vaccination.

Facilities Providing Services to Persons Greater than or Equal to 65 Years of Age

In these facilities (e.g., retirement communities and recreation centers), all unvaccinated residents/attendees should be offered vaccine on site before the influenza season. Education/publicity programs should also be provided; these programs should emphasize the need for influenza vaccine and provide specific information on how, where, and when to obtain it.

Clinics and Others Providing Health-Care for Travelers

Indications for influenza vaccination should be reviewed before travel, and vaccine should be offered if appropriate (see Foreign Travelers).

Health-Care Workers

Administrators of all health-care facilities should arrange for influenza vaccine to be offered to all personnel before the influenza season. Personnel should be provided with appropriate educational materials and strongly encouraged to receive vaccine. Particular emphasis should be placed on vaccination of persons who care for members of high-risk groups (e.g., staff of intensive-care units {including newborn intensive-care units}, staff of medical/ surgical units, and employees of nursing homes and chronic-care facilities). Using a mobile cart to take vaccine to hospital wards or other work sites and making vaccine available during night and weekend work shifts can enhance compliance, as can a follow-up campaign early in the course of a community outbreak.

ANTIVIRAL AGENTS FOR INFLUENZA A

The two antiviral agents with specific activity against influenza A viruses are amantadine hydrochloride and rimantadine hydrochloride. These chemically related drugs interfere with the replication cycle of type A (but not type B) influenza viruses. When administered prophylactically to healthy adults or children before and throughout the epidemic period, both drugs are approximately 70%–90% effective in preventing illness caused by naturally occurring strains of type A influenza viruses. Because antiviral agents taken prophylactically can prevent illness but not subclinical infection, some persons who take these drugs can still develop immune responses that will protect them when they are exposed to antigenically related viruses in later years.

In otherwise healthy adults, amantadine and rimantadine can reduce the severity and duration of signs and symptoms of influenza A illness when administered within 48 hours of illness onset. Studies evaluating the efficacy of treatment for children with either amantadine or rimantadine are limited. Amantadine was approved for treatment and prophylaxis of all influenza type A virus infections in 1976. Although few placebo-controlled studies were conducted to determine the efficacy of amantadine treatment among children prior to approval, amantadine is indicated for treatment and prophylaxis of adults and children greater than or equal to 1 year of age. Rimantadine was approved in 1993 for treatment and prophylaxis in adults but was approved only for prophylaxis in children. Further studies might provide the data needed to support future approval of rimantadine treatment in this age group.

As with all drugs, amantadine and rimantadine can cause adverse reactions in some persons. Such adverse reactions are rarely severe; however, for some categories of patients, severe adverse reactions are more likely to occur. Amantadine has been associated with a higher incidence of adverse central nervous system (CNS) reactions than rimantadine (see Considerations for Selecting Amantadine or Rimantadine for Chemoprophylaxis or Treatment).

RECOMMENDATIONS FOR THE USE OF AMANTADINE AND RIMANTADINE

Use as Prophylaxis

Chemoprophylaxis is not a substitute for vaccination. Recommendations for chemoprophylaxis are provided primarily to help health-care providers make decisions regarding persons who are at greatest risk for severe illness and complications if infected with influenza A virus. When amantadine or rimantadine is administered as prophylaxis, factors such as cost, compliance, and potential side effects should be considered when determining the period of prophylaxis. To be maximally effective as prophylaxis, the drug must be taken each day for the duration of influenza activity in the community. However, to be most cost effective, amantadine or rimantadine prophylaxis should be taken only during the period of peak influenza activity in a community.

Persons at High Risk Vaccinated after Influenza A Activity Has Begun

Persons at high risk can still be vaccinated after an outbreak of influenza A has begun in a community. However, the development of antibodies in adults after vaccination can take as long as 2 weeks, during which time chemoprophylaxis should be considered. Children who receive influenza vaccine for the first time can require as long as 6 weeks of prophylaxis (i.e., prophylaxis for 2 weeks after the second dose of vaccine has been received). Amantadine and rimantadine do not interfere with the antibody response to the vaccine.

Persons Providing Care to Those at High Risk

To reduce the spread of virus to persons at high risk, chemoprophylaxis may be considered during community outbreaks for (a) unvaccinated persons who have frequent contact with persons at high risk (e.g., household members, visiting nurses, and volunteer workers) and (b) unvaccinated employees of hospitals, clinics, and chronic-care facilities. For those persons who cannot be vaccinated, chemoprophylaxis during the period of peak influenza activity may be considered. For those persons who receive vaccine at a time when influenza A is present in the community, chemoprophylaxis can be administered for 2 weeks after vaccination. Prophylaxis should be considered for all employees, regardless of their vaccination status, if the outbreak is caused by a variant strain of influenza A that might not be controlled by the vaccine.

Persons Who Have Immune Deficiency

Chemoprophylaxis might be indicated for persons at high risk who are expected to have an inadequate antibody response to influenza vaccine. This category includes persons who have HIV infection, especially those who have advanced HIV disease. No data are available concerning possible interactions with other drugs used in the management of patients who have HIV infection. Such patients should be monitored closely if amantadine or rimantadine chemoprophylaxis is administered.

Persons for Whom Influenza Vaccine Is Contraindicated

Chemoprophylaxis throughout the influenza season or during peak influenza activity might be appropriate for persons at high risk who should not be vaccinated. Influenza vaccine may be contraindicated in persons who have severe anaphylactic hypersensitivity to egg protein or other vaccine components.

Other Persons

Amantadine or rimantadine also can be administered prophylactically to anyone who wishes to avoid influenza A illness. The health-care provider and patient should make this decision on an individual basis.

Use of Antivirals as Therapy

Amantadine and rimantadine can reduce the severity and shorten the duration of influenza A illness among healthy adults when administered within 48 hours of illness onset. Whether antiviral therapy will prevent complications of influenza type A among persons at high risk is unknown. Insufficient data exist to determine the efficacy of rimantadine treatment in children. Thus, rimantadine is currently approved only for prophylaxis in children, but it is not approved for treatment in this age group. Amantadine- and rimantadine-resistant influenza A viruses can emerge when either of these drugs is administered for treatment; amantadine-resistant strains are cross-resistant to rimantadine and vice versa. Both the frequency with which resistant viruses emerge and the extent of their transmission are unknown, but data indicate that amantadine- and rimantadine-resistant viruses are no more virulent or transmissible than amantadine- and rimantadine-sensitive viruses. The screening of naturally occurring epidemic strains of influenza type A has rarely detected amantadine- and rimantadine-resistant viruses. Resistant viruses have most frequently been isolated from persons taking one of these drugs as therapy for influenza A infection. Resistant viruses have been isolated from persons who live at home or in an institution where other residents are taking or have recently taken amantadine or rimantadine as therapy. Persons who have influenza-like illness should avoid contact with uninfected persons as much as possible, regardless of whether they are being treated with amantadine or rimantadine. Persons who have influenza type A infection and who are treated with either drug can shed amantadine- or rimantadine-sensitive viruses early in the course of treatment, but can later shed drug-resistant viruses, especially after 5–7 days of therapy. Such persons can benefit from therapy even when resistant viruses emerge; however, they also can transmit infection to other persons with whom they come in contact. Because of possible induction of amantadine or rimantadine resistance, treatment of persons who have influenza-like illness should be discontinued as soon as clinically warranted, generally after 3–5 days of treatment or within 24–48 hours after the disappearance of signs and symptoms. Laboratory isolation of influenza viruses obtained from persons who are receiving amantadine or rimantadine should be reported to CDC through state health departments, and the isolates should be saved for antiviral sensitivity testing.

Outbreak Control in Institutions

When confirmed or suspected outbreaks of influenza A occur in institutions that house persons at high risk, chemoprophylaxis should be started as early as possible to reduce the spread of the virus. Contingency planning is needed to ensure rapid administration of amantadine or rimantadine to residents. This planning should include preapproved medication orders or plans to obtain physicians' orders on short notice. When amantadine or rimantadine is used for outbreak control, the drug should be administered to all residents of the institution—regardless of whether they received influenza vaccine the previous fall. The drug should be continued for at least 2 weeks or until approximately 1 week after the end of the outbreak. The dose for each resident should be determined after consulting the dosage recommendations and precautions (see Considerations for Selecting Amantadine or Rimantadine for Chemoprophylaxis or Treatment) and the manufacturer's package insert. To reduce the spread of virus and to minimize disruption of patient care, chemoprophylaxis also can be offered to unvaccinated staff who provide care to persons at high risk. Prophylaxis should be considered for all employees, regardless of their vaccination status, if the outbreak is caused by a variant strain of influenza A that is not controlled by the vaccine.

Chemoprophylaxis also may be considered for controlling influenza A outbreaks in other closed or semi-closed settings (e.g., dormitories or other settings where persons live in close proximity). To reduce the spread of infection and the chances of prophylaxis failure due to transmission of drug-resistant virus, measures should be taken to reduce contact as much as possible between persons on chemoprophylaxis and those taking drug for treatment.

CONSIDERATIONS FOR SELECTING AMANTADINE OR RIMANTADINE FOR CHEMOPROPHYLAXIS OR TREATMENT

Side Effects/Toxicity

Despite the similarities between the two drugs, amantadine and rimantadine differ in their pharmacokinetic properties. More than 90% of amantadine is excreted unchanged, whereas approximately 75% of rimantadine is metabolized by the liver. However, both drugs and their metabolites are excreted by the kidney.

The pharmacokinetic differences between amantadine and rimantadine might explain differences in side effects. Although both drugs can cause CNS and gastrointestinal side effects when administered to young, healthy adults at equivalent dosages of 200 mg/day, the incidence of CNS side effects (e.g., nervousness, anxiety, difficulty concentrating, and lightheadedness) is higher among persons taking amantadine compared with those taking rimantadine. In a 6-week study of prophylaxis in healthy adults, approximately 6% of participants taking rimantadine at a dose of 200 mg/day experienced at least one CNS symptom, compared with approximately 14% of those taking the same dose of amantadine and 4% of those taking placebo. The incidence of gastrointestinal side effects (e.g., nausea and anorexia) is approximately 3% among persons taking either drug, compared with 1%–2% among persons receiving the placebo. Side effects associated with both drugs are usually mild and cease soon after discontinuing the drug. Side effects can diminish or disappear after the first week despite continued drug ingestion. However, serious side effects have been observed (e.g., marked behavioral changes, delirium, hallucinations, agitation, and seizures). These more severe side effects have been associated with high plasma drug concentrations and have been observed most often among persons who have renal insufficiency, seizure disorders, or certain psychiatric disorders and among elderly persons who have been taking amantadine as prophylaxis at a dose of 200 mg/day. Clinical observations and studies have indicated that lowering the dosage of amantadine among these persons reduces the incidence and severity of such side effects, and recommendations for reduced dosages for these groups of patients have been made. Because rimantadine has only recently been approved for marketing, its safety in certain patient populations (e.g., chronically ill and elderly persons) has been evaluated less frequently. Clinical trials of rimantadine have more commonly involved young, healthy persons.

Providers should review the package insert before using amantadine or rimantadine for any patient. The patient's age, weight, and renal function; the presence of other medical conditions; the indications for use of amantadine or rimantadine (i.e., prophylaxis or therapy); and the potential for interaction with other medications must be considered, and the dosage and duration of treatment must be adjusted appropriately. Modifications in dosage might be required for persons who have impaired renal or hepatic function, the elderly, children, and persons with a history of seizures. The following are guidelines for the use of amantadine and rimantadine in certain patient populations. Dosage recommendations are also summarized (Table 2).

Table 2. Recommend Dosage for Amantadine and Rimantadine Treatment and Prophylaxis

| Antiviral Agent | Age | | | |
	1–9 yrs	10–13 yrs	14–64 yrs	≥65 yrs
Amantadine*				
Treatment	5 mg/kg/day up to 150 mg[+] in two divided doses	100 mg twice daily[&]	100 mg twice daily	≤100 mg/day
Prophylaxis	5 mg/kg/day up to 150 mg[+] in two divided doses	100 mg twice daily[&]	100 mg twice daily	≤100 mg/day
Rimantadine[@]				
Treatment	NA	NA	100 mg twice daily	100 or 200[**] mg/day
Prophylaxis	5 mg/kg/day up to 150 mg[+] in two divided doses	100 mg twice daily[&]	100 mg twice daily	100 or 200[**] mg/day

NOTE: Amantadine manufacturers include: Dupont Pharma (Symmetrel®—syrup); Solvay Pharmaceuticals (Symadine™—capsule); Chase Pharmaceuticals and Invamed (Amatadine HCL—capsule); and Copley Pharmaceuticals, Barre National, and Mikart (Amantadine HCL—syrup). Rimantadine is manufactured by Forest Laboratories (Flumadine®—tablet and syrup).
*The drug package insert should be consulted for dosage recommendations for administering amantadine to persons with creatinine clearance ≤50 mL/min.
[+]5 mg/kg of amantadine or rimantadine syrup = 1 tsp/22 lbs.
[&]Children ≥10 years of age who weigh <40 kg should be administered amantadine or rimantadine at a dose of 5 mg/kg/day.
[@]A reduction in dose to 100 mg/day of rimantadine is recommended for persons who have severe hepatic dysfunction or those with creatinine clearance ≤10 mL/min. Other persons with less severe hepatic or renal dysfunction taking >100 mg/day of rimantadine should be observed closely, and the dosage should be reduced or the drug discontinued, if necessary.
[**]Elderly nursing-home residents should be administered only 100 mg/day of rimantadine. A reduction in dose to 100 mg/day should be considered for all persons ≥65 years of age if they experience possible side effects when taking 200 mg/day.
NA = Not applicable.

Persons Who Have Impaired Renal Function

Amantadine

Amantadine is excreted unchanged in the urine by glomerular filtration and tubular secretion. Thus, renal clearance of amantadine is reduced substantially in persons with renal insufficiency. A reduction in dosage is recommended for patients with creatinine clearance less than or equal to 50 mL/min. Guidelines for amantadine dosage based on creatinine clearance are found in the packet insert. However, because recommended dosages based on creatinine clearance might provide only an approximation of the optimal dose for a given patient, such persons should be observed carefully so that adverse reactions can be recognized promptly and either the dose can be further reduced or the drug can be discontinued, if necessary. Hemodialysis contributes little to drug clearance.

Rimantadine

The safety and pharmacokinetics of rimantadine among patients with renal insufficiency have been evaluated only after single-dose administration. Further studies are needed to determine the multiple-dose pharmacokinetics and the most appropriate dosages for these patients. In a single-dose study of patients with anuric renal failure, the apparent clearance of rimantadine was approximately 40% lower, and the elimination half-life was approximately 1.6-fold greater than that in healthy controls of the same age. Hemodialysis did not contribute to drug clearance. In studies among persons with less severe renal disease, drug clearance was also reduced, and plasma concentrations were higher compared with control patients without renal disease who were the same weight, age, and sex.

A reduction in dosage to 100 mg/day is recommended for persons with creatinine clearance less than or equal to 10 mL/min. Because of the potential for accumulation of rimantadine and its metabolites, patients with any degree of renal insufficiency, including elderly persons, should be monitored for adverse effects, and either the dosage should be reduced or the drug should be discontinued, if necessary.

Persons Greater than or Equal to 65 Years of Age

Amantadine

Because renal function declines with increasing age, the daily dose for persons greater than or equal to 65 years of age should not exceed 100 mg for prophylaxis or treatment. For some elderly persons, the dose should be further reduced. Studies suggest that because of their smaller average body size, elderly women are more likely than elderly men to experience side effects at a daily dose of 100 mg.

Rimantadine

The incidence and severity of CNS side effects among elderly persons appear to be substantially lower among those taking rimantadine at a dose of 200 mg/day compared with elderly persons taking the same dose of amantadine. However, when rimantadine has been administered at a dosage of 200 mg/day to chronically ill elderly persons, they have had a higher incidence of CNS and gastrointestinal symptoms than healthy, younger persons taking rimantadine at the same dosage. After long-term administration of rimantadine at a dosage of 200 mg/day, serum rimantadine concentrations among elderly nursing-home residents have been two to four times greater than those reported in younger adults.

The dosage of rimantadine should be reduced to 100 mg/day for treatment or prophylaxis of elderly nursing-home residents. Although further studies are needed to determine the optimal dose for other elderly persons, a reduction in dosage to 100 mg/day should be considered for all persons greater than or equal to 65 years of age if they experience signs and symptoms that might represent side effects when taking a dosage of 200 mg/day.

Persons Who Have Liver Disease

Amantadine

No increase in adverse reactions to amantadine has been observed among persons with liver disease.

Rimantadine

The safety and pharmacokinetics of rimantadine have only been evaluated after single-dose administration. In a study of persons with chronic liver disease (most with stabilized cirrhosis), no alterations were observed after a single dose. However, in persons with severe liver dysfunction, the apparent clearance of rimantadine was 50% lower than that reported for persons without liver disease. A dose reduction to 100 mg/day is recommended for persons with severe hepatic dysfunction.

Persons Who Have Seizure Disorders

Amantadine

An increased incidence of seizures has been reported in patients with a history of seizure disorders who have received amantadine. Patients with seizure disorders should be observed closely for possible increased seizure activity when taking amantadine.

Rimantadine

In clinical trials, seizures (or seizure-like activity) have been observed in a few persons with a history of seizures who were not receiving anticonvulsant medication while taking rimantadine. The extent to which rimantadine might increase the incidence of seizures among persons with seizure disorders has not been adequately evaluated, because such persons have usually been excluded from participating in clinical trials of rimantadine.

Children

Amantadine

The use of amantadine in children less than 1 year of age has not been adequately evaluated. The FDA-approved dosage for children 1–9 years of age is 4.4–8.8 mg/kg/day, not to exceed 150 mg/day. Although further studies to determine the optimal dosage for children are needed, physicians should consider prescribing only 5 mg/kg/day (not to exceed 150 mg/day) to reduce the risk for toxicity. The approved dosage for children greater than or equal to 10 years of age is 200 mg/day; however, for children weighing less than 40 kg, prescribing 5 mg/kg/day, regardless of age, is advisable.

Rimantadine

The use of rimantadine in children less than 1 year of age has not been adequately evaluated. In children 1–9 years of age, rimantadine should be administered in one or two divided doses at a dosage of 5 mg/kg/day, not to exceed 150 mg/day. The approved dosage for children greater than or equal to 10 years of age is 200 mg/day (100 mg twice a day); however, for children weighing less than 40 kg, prescribing 5 mg/kg/day, regardless of age, also is recommended.

Drug Interactions

Amantadine

Careful observation is advised when amantadine is administered concurrently with drugs that affect the CNS, especially CNS stimulants.

Rimantadine

No clinically significant interactions between rimantadine and other drugs have been identified. For more detailed information concerning potential drug interactions for either drug, the package insert should be consulted.

SOURCES OF INFORMATION ON INFLUENZA-CONTROL PROGRAMS

Information regarding influenza surveillance is available through the CDC Voice Information System (influenza update), telephone (404) 332-4551, or through the CDC Information Service on the Public Health Network electronic bulletin board. From October through May, the information is updated at least every other week. In addition, periodic updates about influenza are published in the weekly MMWR. State and local health departments should be consulted regarding availability of influenza vaccine, access to vaccination programs, and information about state or local influenza activity.

SELECTED BIBLIOGRAPHY

General

Douglas RG. Drug therapy: prophylaxis and treatment of influenza. N Engl J Med 1990;322:443–450.
Kendal AP, Patriarca PA, eds. Options for the control of influenza. New York: Alan R. Liss, 1986.
Kilbourne ED. Influenza. New York: Plenum Publishing, 1987.
Noble GR. Epidemiological and clinical aspects of influenza. In: Beare AS, ed. Basic and applied influenza research. Boca Raton, FL: CRC Press, 1982:11–50.

Surveillance, Morbidity, and Mortality

Barker WH. Excess pneumonia and influenza associated hospitalization during influenza epidemics in the United States, 1970–78. Am J Public Health 1986;76:761–765.
Barker WH, Mullooly JP. Impact of epidemic type A influenza in a defined adult population. Am J Epidemiol 1980;112:798–813.
Barker WH, Mullooly JP. Pneumonia and influenza deaths during epidemics: implications for prevention. Arch Intern Med 1982;142:85–89.
Baron RC, Dicker RC, Bussell KE, Herndon JL. Assessing trends in mortality in 121 U.S. cities, 1970–79, from all causes and from pneumonia and influenza. Public Health Rep 1988;103:120–128.
Couch RB, Kasel WP, Glezen TR, et al. Influenza: its control in persons and populations. J Infect Dis 1986;153:431–440.
Glezen WP. Serious morbidity and mortality associated with influenza epidemics. Epidemiol Rev 1982;4:25–44.
Glezen WP, Six HR, Frank AL, Taber LH, Perrotta DM, Decker M. Impact of epidemics upon communities and families. In: Kendal AP, Patriarca PA, eds. Options for the control of influenza. New York: Alan R. Liss, 1986:63–73.
Lui KJ, Kendal AP. Impact of influenza epidemics on mortality in the United States from October 1972 to May 1985. Am J Public Health 1987;77:712–716.
Mullooly JP, Barker WH, Nolan TF Jr. Risk of acute respiratory disease among pregnant women during influenza A epidemics. Public Health Rep 1986;101:205–211.
Perrotta DM, Decker M, Glezen WP. Acute respiratory disease hospitalizations as a measure of impact of epidemic influenza. Am J Epidemiol 1985;122:468–476.
Thacker SB. The persistence of influenza A in human populations. Epidemiol Rev 1986;8:129–42.

Vaccines

SAFETY, IMMUNOGENICITY, EFFICACY

ACIP. General recommendations on immunization. MMWR 1994;43(No. RR-1):1–38.

Arden NH, Patriarca PA, Kendal AP. Experiences in the use and efficacy of inactivated influenza vaccine in nursing homes. In: Kendal AP, Patriarca PA, eds. Options for the control of influenza. New York: Alan R. Liss, 1986:155–168.

Barker WH, Mullooly JP. Effectiveness of inactivated influenza vaccine among non-institutionalized elderly persons. In: Kendal AP, Patriarca PA, eds. Options for the control of influenza. New York: Alan R. Liss, 1986:169–182.

Beyer WEP, Palache AM, Baljet M, Masurel N. Antibody induction by influenza vaccines in the elderly: a review of the literature. Vaccine 1989;7:385–394.

Cate TR, Couch RB, Parker D, Baxter B. Reactogenicity, immunogenicity, and antibody persistence in adults given inactivated influenza virus vaccines—1978. Rev Infect Dis 1983;5:737–747.

CDC. Influenza vaccination levels in selected states—Behavioral Risk Factor Surveillance System, 1987. MMWR 1989;38:124,129–133.

Dowdle WR. Influenza immunoprophylaxis after 30 years' experience. In: Nayak DP, ed. Genetic variation among influenza viruses. New York: Academic Press, 1981:525–534.

Fedson DS, Wajda A, Nichol JP, et al. Clinical effectiveness of influenza vaccination in Manitoba. JAMA 1993;27(16):1956–1961.

Foster DA, Talsma AN, Furumoto-Dawson A, et al. Influenza vaccine effectiveness in preventing hospitalization for pneumonia in the elderly. Am J Epidemiol 1992;136:296–307.

Glezen WP, Glezen LS, Alcorn R. Trivalent, inactivated influenza virus vaccine in children with sickle cell disease. Am J Dis Child 1983;137:1095–1097.

Gross PA, Quinnan GV, Rodstein M, et al. Association of influenza immunization with reduction in mortality in an elderly population: a prospective study. Arch Intern Med 1988;148:562–565.

Gross PA, Weksler ME, Quinnan GV Jr, Douglas RG Jr, Gaerlan PF, Denning CR. Immunization of elderly people with two doses of influenza vaccine. J Clin Microbiol 1987;25:1763–1765.

Gruber WC, Taber LH, Glezen WP, et al. Live attenuated and inactivated influenza vaccine in school-aged children. Am J Dis Child 1990;144:595–600.

Helliwell BE, Drummond MF. The costs and benefits of preventing influenza in Ontario's elderly. Can J Public Health 1988;79:175–180.

La Montagne JR, Noble GR, Quinnan GV, et al. Summary of clinical trials of inactivated influenza vaccine—1978. Rev Infect Dis 1983;5:723–736.

Nichol KL, Margolis KL, Wuorenema J, Sternberg T. The efficacy and cost effectiveness of vaccination against influenza among elderly persons living in the community. N Engl J Med 1994;331(12): 778–784.

Patriarca PA, Weber JA, Parker RA, et al. Efficacy of influenza vaccine in nursing homes: reduction in illness and complications during an influenza A(H3N2) epidemic. JAMA 1985;253:1136–1139.

Quinnan GV, Schooley R, Dolin R, Ennis FA, Gross P, Gwaltney JM. Serologic responses and systemic reactions in adults after vaccination with monovalent A/USSR/77 and trivalent A/USSR/77, A/Texas/77, B/Hong Kong/72 influenza vaccines. Rev Infect Dis 1983;5:748–757.

Wright PF, Cherry JD, Foy HM, et al. Antigenicity and reactogenicity of influenza A/USSR/77 virus vaccine in children—a multicentered evaluation of dosage and safety. Rev Infect Dis 1983;5: 758–764.

SIDE EFFECTS, ADVERSE REACTIONS, INTERACTIONS

Aberer W. Vaccination despite thimerosal sensitivity. Contact Dermatitis 1991;24:6–10.

American Academy of Pediatrics Committee on Infectious Diseases. The Red Book: report of the Committee on Infectious Disease. 22nd ed. Elk Grove, IL: American Academy of Pediatrics, 1991.

Bierman CW, Shapiro GG, Pierson WE, Taylor JW, Foy HM, Fox JP. Safety of influenza vaccination in allergic children. J Infect Dis 1977;136:S652–S655.

Chen R, Kent J, Rhodes P, Simon P, Schonberger L. Investigation of a possible association between influenza vaccination and Guillain-Barré Syndrome in the United States, 1990–1991 [Abstract]. Post Marketing Surveillance 1992;6:5–6.

Govaet TME, Aretz K, Masurel N, et al. Adverse reactions to influenza vaccine in elderly people: a randomized double blind placebo controlled trial. Br Med J 1993;307:988–990.

Kaplan JE, Katona P, Hurwitz ES, Schonberger LB. Guillain-Barré syndrome in the United States, 1979–1980 and 1980–1981: lack of an association with influenza vaccination. JAMA 1982;248: 698–700.

Margolis KL, Nichol KL, Poland GA, et al. Frequency of adverse reactions to influenza vaccine in the elderly: a randomized, placebo-controlled trial. JAMA 1990;307:988–990.

Margolis KL, Poland GA, Nichol KL, et al. Frequency of adverse reactions after influenza vaccination. Am J Med 1990;88:27–30.

Murphy KR, Strunk RC. Safe administration of influenza vaccine in asthmatic children hypersensitive to egg proteins. J Pediatr 1985;106:931–933.

SIMULTANEOUS ADMINISTRATION OF OTHER VACCINES

ACIP. Recommendations of the ACIP: pneumococcal polysaccharide vaccine. MMWR 1989;38: 64–68, 73–76.

DeStefano F, Goodman RA, Noble GR, McClary GD, Smith J, Broome CV. Simultaneous administration of influenza and pneumococcal vaccines. JAMA 1982;247:2551–2554.

Peter G, ed. Summaries of infectious diseases: influenza. In: Report of the Committee on Infectious Diseases. 21st ed. Elk Grove Village, IL: American Academy of Pediatrics, 1988:243–251.

VACCINATION OF PERSONS INFECTED WITH HIV

Huang KL, Ruben FL, Rinaldo CR Jr, Kingsley L, Lyter DW, Ho M. Antibody responses after influenza and pneumococcal immunization in HIV-infected homosexual men. JAMA 1987;257: 2047–2050.

Miotti PG, Nelson KE, Dallabetta GA, Farzadegan H, Margolick J, Clements ML. The influence of HIV infection on antibody responses to a two-dose regimen of influenza vaccine. JAMA 1989;262:779–783.

Nelson KE, Clements ML, Miotti P, Cohn S, Polk BF. The influence of human immunodeficiency virus (HIV) infection on antibody responses to influenza vaccines. Ann Intern Med 1988;109: 383–388.

Safrin S, Rush JD, Mills J. Influenza in patients with human immunodeficiency virus infection. Chest 1990;98:33–37.

Thurn JR, Henry K. Influenza A pneumonitis in a patient infected with the human immunodeficiency virus (HIV). Chest 1989;95:807–810.

VACCINATION OF FOREIGN TRAVELERS

CDC. Update: influenza activity—worldwide and recommendations for influenza vaccine composition for the 1990–91 influenza season. MMWR 1990;39:293–296.

CDC. Acute respiratory illness among cruise-ship passengers—Asia. MMWR 1988;37:63–66.

Influenza in the Institutional Setting

Bean B, Rhame FS, Hughes RS, Weiler MD, Peterson LR, Gerding DN. Influenza B: hospital activity during a community epidemic. Diagn Microbiol Infect Dis 1983;1:177–183.

Gomolin IH, Leib HB, Arden NH, Sherman FT. Control of influenza outbreaks in the nursing home: guidelines for diagnosis and management. J Am Geriatr Soc 1995;43:71–74.

Pachucki CT, Walsh Pappas SA, Fuller GF, Krause SL, Lentino JR, Schaaff DM. Influenza A among hospital personnel and patients: implications for recognition, prevention, and control. Arch Intern Med 1989;149:77–80.

Strategies for Vaccination of High-risk Groups

Buffington J, Bell KM, LaForce FM, et al. A target-based model for increasing influenza immunizations in private practice. J Gen Intern Med 1991;6:204–209.

CDC. Arm with the facts: a guidebook for promotion of adult immunization. Atlanta: US Department of Health and Human Services, Public Health Service, 1987.

Fedson DS. Immunizations for health care workers and patients in hospitals. In: Wenzel RP, ed. Prevention and control of nosocomial infections. Baltimore, MD: Williams & Wilkins, 1987:116–174.

Fedson DS, Kessler HA. A hospital-based influenza immunization program, 1977–78. Am J Public Health 1983;73:442–445.

Margolis KL, Lofgren RP, Korn JE. Organizational strategies to improve influenza vaccine delivery: a standing order in a general medical clinic. Arch Intern Med 1988;148:2205–2207.

Nichol KL, Korn JE, Margolis KL, Poland GA, Petzel RA, Lofgren RP. Achieving the national health objective for influenza immunization: success of an institution-wide vaccination program. Am J Med 1990;89:156–160.

Nichol KL. Improving influenza vaccination rates for high-risk inpatients. Am J Med 1991;91:584–588.

Weingarten S, Riedinger M, Bolton LB, Miles P, Ault M. Barriers to influenza vaccine acceptance: a survey of physicians and nurses. Am J Infect Control 1989;17:202–207.

Williams WW, Garner JS. Personnel health services. In: Bennett JV, Brachman PS, eds. Hospital infections. 2nd ed. Boston: Little, Brown, and Company, 1986:17–38.

Williams WW, Hickson MA, Kane MA, Kendal AP, Spika JS, Hinman AR. Immunization policies and vaccine coverage among adults: the risk for missed opportunities. Ann Intern Med 1988;108: 616–625.

Diagnostic Methods

Harmon MW. Influenza viruses. In: Lennette EH, ed. Laboratory diagnosis of viral infections. 2nd ed. New York: Marcel Dekker Inc., 1992:515–534.

Ziegler T, Cox NJ. Influenza viruses. In: Murray PR et al., eds. Manual of Clinical Microbiology. 6th ed. Washington, DC. ASM Press, 1995:918–925

Antiviral Agents

Aoki FY, Sitar DS. Amantadine kinetics in healthy elderly men: implications for influenza prevention. Clin Pharmacol Ther 1985;37:137–144.

Aoki FY, Sitar DS. Clinical pharmacokinetics of amantadine hydrochloride. Clin Pharmacokinet 1988;14:35–51.

Atkinson WL, Arden NH, Patriarca PA, Leslie N, Lui KJ, Gohd R. Amantadine prophylaxis during an institutional outbreak of type A (H1N1) influenza. Arch Intern Med 1986;146:1751–1756.

Balfour HH Jr, Englund JA. Antiviral drugs in pediatrics. Am J Dis Child 1989;143:1307–1316.

Belshe RB, Burk B, Newman F, Cerruti RL, Sim IS. Resistance of influenza A virus to amantadine and rimantadine: results of one decade of surveillance. J Infect Dis 1989;159:430–435.

Dolin R, Reichman RC, Madore HP, Maynard R, Linton PN, Webber-Jones J. A controlled trial of amantadine and rimantadine in the prophylaxis of influenza A infection. N Engl J Med 1982; 307:580–583.

Douglas RG. Drug therapy: prophylaxis and treatment of influenza. N Engl J Med 1990;322: 443–450.

Hall CB, Dolin R, Gala CL, et al. Children with influenza A infection: treatment with rimantadine. Pediatrics 1987;80:275–282.

Hayden FG, Belshe RB, Clover RD, Hay AJ, Oakes MG, Soo W. Emergence and apparent transmission of rimantadine-resistant influenza A viruses in families. N Engl J Med 1989;321:1696–1702.

Hayden FG, Couch RB. Clinical and epidemiological importance of influenza A viruses resistant to amantadine and rimantadine. Rev Med Virol 1992;2:89–96.

Hayden FG, Hay AJ. Emergence and transmission of influenza A viruses resistant to amantadine and rimantadine. Curr Top Microbiol Immunol 1992;176:120–130.

Horadam VW, Sharp JG, Smilack JD, et al. Pharmacokinetics of amantadine hydrochloride in subjects with normal and impaired renal function. Ann Intern Med 1981;94:454–458.

Mast EE, Harmon MW, Gravenstein S, et al. Emergence and possible transmission of amantadine resistant viruses during nursing home outbreaks of influenza A(H3N2). Am J Epidemiol 1991;13:988–997.

Monto AS, Arden NH. Implications of viral resistance to amantadine in control of influenza A. Clin Infect Dis 1992;15:362–367.

Pettersson RF, Hellstrom PE, Penttinen K, et al. Evaluation of amantadine in the prophylaxis of influenza A (H1N1) virus infection: a controlled field trial among young adults and high-risk patients. J Infect Dis 1980;142:377–383.

Sears SD, Clements ML. Protective efficacy of low-dose amantadine in adults challenged with wild-type influenza A virus. Antimicrob Agents Chemother 1987;31:1470–1473.

Somani SK, Degelau J, Cooper SL, et al. Comparison of pharmacokinetic and safety profiles of amantadine 50- and 100-mg daily doses in elderly nursing home residents. Pharmacotherapy 1991;11:460–466.

Stange KC, Little DW, Blatnick B. Adverse reactions to amantadine prophylaxis of influenza in a retirement home. J Am Geriatr Soc 1991;39:700–705.

Tominack RL, Hayden FG. Rimantadine hydrochloride and amantadine hydrochloride use in influenza A virus infections. Infect Dis Clin North Am 1987;1:459–478.

Prevention and Control of Influenza: Part II, Antiviral Agents

Original Citation: ACIP. Prevention and control of influenza: Part II, Antiviral Agents. Recommendations of the Advisory Committee on Immunization Practices. MMWR 1994;43(RR-15):1–10.

Original Authors: Nancy H. Arden, MN, Nancy J. Cox, PhD, Lawrence B. Schonberger, MD, MPH

SUMMARY

These recommendations provide information about two antiviral agents: amantadine hydrochloride and rimantadine hydrochloride. These recommendations supersede MMWR 1992;41(No. RR-9). The primary changes include information about the recently licensed drug rimantadine, expanded information on the potential for adverse reactions to amantadine and rimantadine, and guidelines for the use of these drugs among certain persons.

INTRODUCTION

The two antiviral agents with specific activity against influenza A viruses are amantadine hydrochloride and rimantadine hydrochloride. These chemically related drugs interfere with the replication cycle of type A (but not type B) influenza viruses. When administered prophylactically to healthy adults or children before and throughout the epidemic period, both drugs are approximately 70%–90% effective in preventing illness caused by naturally occurring strains of type A influenza viruses. Because antiviral agents taken prophylactically may prevent illness but not subclinical infection, some persons who take these drugs may still develop immune responses that will protect them when they are exposed to antigenically related viruses in later years.

In otherwise healthy adults, amantadine and rimantadine can reduce the severity and duration of signs and symptoms of influenza A illness when administered within 48 hours of illness onset. Studies evaluating the efficacy of treatment for children with either amantadine or rimantadine are limited. Amantadine was approved for treatment and prophylaxis of all influenza type A virus infections in 1976. Although few placebo-controlled studies were conducted to determine the efficacy of amantadine treatment among children prior to approval, amantadine is indicated for treatment and prophylaxis of adults and children greater than or equal to 1 year of age. Rimantadine was approved in 1993 for treatment and prophylaxis in adults but was approved only for prophylaxis in children. Further studies may provide the data needed to support future approval of rimantadine treatment in this age group.

As with all drugs, amantadine and rimantadine may cause adverse reactions in some persons. Such adverse reactions are rarely severe; however, for some categories of patients, severe adverse reactions are more likely to occur. Amantadine has been associated with a higher incidence of adverse central nervous system (CNS) reactions than rimantadine (see Considerations for Selecting Amantadine or Rimantadine for Chemoprophylaxis or Treatment).

RECOMMENDATIONS FOR THE USE OF AMANTADINE AND RIMANTADINE

Use as Prophylaxis

Chemoprophylaxis is not a substitute for vaccination. Recommendations for chemoprophylaxis are provided primarily to help health-care providers make decisions regarding persons who are at greatest risk of severe illness and complications if infected with influenza A virus (i.e., persons at high risk). Groups at high risk for influenza-related complications include:

- Persons greater than or equal to 65 years of age;
- Residents of nursing homes and other chronic-care facilities that house persons of any age with chronic medical conditions;
- Adults and children with chronic disorders of the pulmonary or cardiovascular systems, including children with asthma;
- Adults and children who have required regular medical follow-up or hospitalization during the preceding year because of chronic metabolic diseases (including diabetes mellitus), renal dysfunction, hemoglobinopathies, or immunosuppression (including immunosuppression caused by medications); and
- Children and teenagers (6 months–18 years of age) who are receiving long-term aspirin therapy and therefore may be at risk for developing Eye syndrome after influenza.

When amantadine or rimantadine is administered as prophylaxis, factors such as cost, compliance, and potential side effects should be considered when determining the period of prophylaxis. To be maximally effective as prophylaxis, the drug must be taken each day for the duration of influenza activity in the community. However, to be most cost effective, amantadine or rimantadine prophylaxis should be taken only during the period of peak influenza activity in a community.

Persons at High Risk Vaccinated after Influenza A Activity Has Begun

Persons at high risk can still be vaccinated after an outbreak of influenza A has begun in a community. However, the development of antibodies in adults after vaccination can take as long as 2 weeks, during which time chemoprophylaxis should be considered. Children who receive influenza vaccine for the first time may require as long as 6 weeks of prophylaxis (i.e., prophylaxis for 2 weeks after the second dose of vaccine has been received). Amantadine and rimantadine do not interfere with the antibody response to the vaccine.

Persons Providing Care to Those at High Risk

To reduce the spread of virus to persons at high risk, chemoprophylaxis may be considered during community outbreaks for (a) unvaccinated persons who have frequent contact with persons at high risk (e.g., household members, visiting nurses, and volunteer workers) and (b) unvaccinated employees of hospitals, clinics, and chronic-care facilities. For those persons who cannot be vaccinated, chemoprophylaxis during the period of peak influenza activity may be considered. For those persons who receive vaccine at a time when influenza A is present in the community, chemoprophylaxis can be administered for 2 weeks after vaccination. Prophylaxis should be considered for all employees, regardless of their vaccination status, if the outbreak is caused by a variant strain of influenza A that may not be controlled by the vaccine.

Persons Who Have Immune Deficiency

Chemoprophylaxis may be indicated for persons at high risk who are expected to have an inadequate antibody response to influenza vaccine. This category includes persons with human immunodeficiency virus (HIV) infection, especially those with advanced HIV disease. No data are available on possible interactions with other drugs used in the management of patients with HIV infection. Such patients should be monitored closely if amantadine or rimantadine chemoprophylaxis is administered.

Persons for Whom Influenza Vaccine Is Contraindicated

Chemoprophylaxis throughout the influenza season or during peak influenza activity may be appropriate for persons at high risk who should not be vaccinated. Influenza vaccine may be contraindicated in persons with severe anaphylactic hypersensitivity to egg protein or other vaccine components.

Other Persons

Amantadine or rimantadine also can be administered prophylactically to anyone who wishes to avoid influenza A illness. The health-care provider and patient should make this decision on an individual basis.

Use of Antivirals as Therapy

Amantadine and rimantadine can reduce the severity and shorten the duration of influenza A illness among healthy adults when administered within 48 hours of illness onset. Whether antiviral therapy will prevent complications of influenza type A among high-risk persons is unknown. Insufficient data exist to determine the efficacy of rimantadine treatment in children. Thus, rimantadine is currently approved only for prophylaxis in children, but it is not approved for treatment in this age group.

Amantadine- and rimantadine-resistant influenza A viruses can emerge when either of these drugs is administered for treatment; amantadine-resistant strains are cross-resistant to rimantadine and vice versa. Both the frequency with which resistant viruses emerge and the extent of their transmission are unknown, but data indicate that amantadine- and rimantadine- resistant viruses are no more virulent or transmissible than amantadine- and rimantadine-sensitive viruses.

The screening of naturally occurring epidemic strains of influenza type A has rarely detected amantadine- and rimantadine-resistant viruses. Resistant viruses have most frequently been isolated from persons taking one of these drugs as therapy for influenza A infection. Resistant viruses have been isolated from persons who live at home or in an institution where other residents are taking or have recently taken amantadine or rimantadine as therapy. Persons who have influenza-like illness should avoid contact with uninfected persons as much as possible, regardless of whether they are being treated with amantadine or rimantadine. Persons who have influenza type A infection and who are treated with either drug may shed amantadine- or rimantadine-sensitive viruses early in the course of treatment, but may later shed drug-resistant viruses, especially after 5–7 days of therapy. Such persons can benefit from therapy even when resistant viruses emerge; however, they also can transmit infection to other persons with whom they come in contact. Because of possible induction of amantadine or rimantadine resistance, treatment of persons who have influenza-like illness should be discontinued as soon as clinically warranted, generally after 3–5 days of treatment or within 24–48 hours after the disappearance of signs and symptoms. Laboratory isolation of influenza viruses obtained from persons who are receiving amantadine or rimantadine should be reported to CDC through state health departments, and the isolates should be saved for antiviral sensitivity testing.

Outbreak Control in Institutions

When confirmed or suspected outbreaks of influenza A occur in institutions that house persons at high risk, chemoprophylaxis should be started as early as possible to reduce the spread of the virus. Contingency planning is needed to ensure rapid administration of amantadine or rimantadine to residents. This planning should include preapproved medication orders or plans to obtain physicians' orders on short notice. When amantadine or rimantadine is used for outbreak control, the drug should be administered to all residents of the institution—regardless of whether they received influenza vaccine the previous fall. The drug should be continued for at least 2 weeks or until approximately 1 week after the end of the outbreak. The dose for each resident should be determined after consulting the dosage recommendations and precautions (see Considerations for Selecting Amantadine or Rimantadine for Chemoprophylaxis or Treatment) and the manufacturer's package insert. To reduce the spread of virus and to minimize disruption of patient care, chemoprophylaxis also can be offered to unvaccinated staff who provide care to persons at high risk. Prophylaxis should be considered for all employees, regardless of their vaccination status, if the outbreak is caused by a variant strain of influenza A that is not controlled by the vaccine.

Chemoprophylaxis also may be considered for controlling influenza A outbreaks in other closed or semi-closed settings (e.g., dormitories or other settings where persons live in close proximity). To reduce the spread of infection and the chances of prophylaxis failure due to transmission of drug- resistant virus, measures should be taken to reduce contact as much as possible between persons on chemoprophylaxis and those taking drug for treatment.

CONSIDERATIONS FOR SELECTING AMANTADINE OR RIMANTADINE FOR CHEMOPROPHYLAXIS OR TREATMENT

Side Effects/Toxicity

Despite the similarities between the two drugs, amantadine and rimantadine differ in their pharmacokinetic properties. More than 90% of amantadine is excreted unchanged, whereas approximately 75% of rimantadine is metabolized by the liver. However, both drugs and their metabolites are excreted by the kidney.

The pharmacokinetic differences between amantadine and rimantadine may partially explain differences in side effects. Although both drugs can cause CNS and gastrointestinal side effects when administered to young, healthy adults at equivalent dosages of 200 mg/day, the incidence of CNS side effects (e.g., nervousness, anxiety, difficulty concentrating, and lightheadedness) is higher among persons taking amantadine compared with those taking rimantadine. In a 6-week study of prophylaxis in healthy adults, approximately 6% of participants taking rimantadine at a dose of 200 mg/day experienced at least one CNS symptom, compared with approximately 14% of those taking the same dose of amantadine and 4% of those taking placebo. The incidence of gastrointestinal side effects (e.g., nausea and anorexia) is approximately 3% in persons taking either drug, compared with 1%–2% of persons receiving the placebo. Side effects associated with both drugs are usually mild and cease soon after discontinuing the drug. Side effects may diminish or disappear after the first week despite continued drug ingestion. However, serious side effects have been observed (e.g., marked behavioral changes, delirium, hallucinations, agitation, and seizures). These more severe side effects have been associated with high plasma drug concentrations and have been observed most often among persons who have renal insufficiency, seizure disorders, or certain psychiatric disorders and among elderly persons who have been taking amantadine as prophylaxis at a dose of 200 mg/day. Clinical observations and studies have indicated that lowering the dosage of amantadine among these persons reduces the incidence and severity of such side effects, and recommendations for reduced dosages for these groups of patients have been made. Because rimantadine has only recently been approved for marketing, its safety in certain patient populations (e.g., chronically ill and elderly persons) has been evaluated less frequently. Clinical trials of rimantadine have more commonly involved young, healthy persons.

Providers should review the package insert before using amantadine or rimantadine for any patient. The patient's age, weight, renal function, other medications, presence of other medical conditions, and indications for use of amantadine or rimantadine (prophylaxis or therapy) must be considered, and the dosage and duration of treatment must be adjusted appropriately. Modifications in dosage may be required for persons who have impaired renal or hepatic function, the elderly, children, and persons with a history of seizures. The following are guidelines for the use of amantadine and rimantadine in certain patient populations. Dosage recommendations are also summarized (Table 1).

Table 1. Recommended dosage for amantadine and rimantadine treatment and prophylaxis

Antiviral	Age			
	1–9 yrs	10–13 yrs	14–64 yrs	≥65 years
Amantadine*				
Treatment	5 mg/kg/day	100 mg up to 150 mg[+]	100 mg twice daily[&]	≤100 mg/day twice daily in two divided doses
Prophylaxis	5 mg/kg/day	100 mg up to 150 mg[+]	100 mg twice daily[&]	≤100 mg/day twice daily in two divided doses
Rimantadine[@]				
Treatment	NA	NA	100 mg	100 or 200[**] mg/day twice daily
Prophylaxis	5 mg/kg/day	100 mg up to 150 mg[+]	100 mg twice daily	100 or 200[**] mg/day twice daily in two divided doses

NOTE: Amantadine manufacturers include: Dupont Pharma (Symmetrel®—syrup); Solvay Pharmaceuticals (Symadine™—capsule); Chase Pharmaceuticals and Invamed (Amatadine HCL—capsule). Rimantadine is manufactured by Forest Laboratories (Flumandine®—tablet and syrup).

*The drug package insert should be consulted for dosage recommendations for administering amantadine to persons with creatinine clearance ≤50 mL/min.

[+]5 mg/kg of amantadine or rimantadine syrup = 1 tsp/22 lbs.

[&]Children ≥10 years of age who weigh <40 kg should be administered amantadine or rimantadine at a dose of 5 mg/kg/day.

[@]A reduction in dose to 100 mg/day of rimantadine is recommended for persons who have severe hepatic dysfunction or those with creatinine clearance ≤10 mL/min. Other persons with less severe hepatic or renal dysfunction taking >100 mg/day should be observed closely, and the dosage should be reduced or the drug discontinued, if necessary.

[**]Elderly nursing-home residents should be administered only 100 mg/day of rimantadine. A reduction in dose to 100 mg/day should be considered for all persons ≥65 years of age if they experience possible side effects when taking 200 mg/day.

NA = Not applicable.

Persons Who Have Impaired Renal Function

Amantadine

Amantadine is excreted unchanged in the urine by glomerular filtration and tubular secretion. Thus, renal clearance of amantadine is reduced substantially in persons with renal insufficiency. A reduction in dosage is recommended for patients with creatinine clearance less than or equal to 50 mL/min. Guidelines for amantadine dosage based on creatinine clearance are found in the packet insert. However, because recommended dosages based on creatinine clearance may provide only an approximation of the optimal dose for a given patient, such persons should be observed carefully so that adverse reactions can be recognized promptly and either the dose can be further reduced or the drug can be discontinued, if necessary. Hemodialysis contributes little to drug clearance.

Rimantadine

The safety and pharmacokinetics of rimantadine among patients with renal insufficiency have been evaluated only after single-dose administration. Further studies are needed to determine the multiple-dose pharmacokinetics and the most appropriate dosages for these patients.

In a single-dose study of patients with anuric renal failure, the apparent clearance of rimantadine was approximately 40% lower, and the elimination half-life was approximately 1.6-fold greater than that in healthy controls of the same age. Hemodialysis did not contribute to drug clearance. In studies among persons with less severe renal disease, drug clearance was also reduced, and plasma concentrations were higher compared with control patients without renal disease who were the same weight, age, and sex.

A reduction in dosage to 100 mg/day is recommended for persons with creatinine clearance less than or equal to 10 mL/min. Because of the potential for accumulation of rimantadine and its metabolites, patients with any degree of renal insufficiency, including elderly persons, should be monitored for adverse effects, and either the dosage should be reduced or the drug should be discontinued, if necessary.

Persons Greater than or Equal to 65 Years of Age

Amantadine

Because renal function declines with increasing age, the daily dose for persons greater than or equal to 65 years of age should not exceed 100 mg for prophylaxis or treatment. For some elderly persons, the dose should be further reduced. Studies suggest that because of their smaller average body size, elderly women are more likely than elderly men to experience side effects at a daily dose of 100 mg.

Rimantadine

The incidence and severity of CNS side effects among elderly persons appear to be substantially lower among those taking rimantadine at a dose of 200 mg/day compared with elderly persons taking the same dose of amantadine. However, when rimantadine has been administered at a dosage of 200 mg/day to chronically ill elderly persons, they have had a higher incidence of CNS and gastrointestinal symptoms than healthy, younger persons taking rimantadine at the same dosage. After long-term administration of rimantadine at a dosage of 200 mg/day, serum rimantadine concentrations among elderly nursing-home residents have been two to four times greater than those reported in younger adults.

The dosage of rimantadine should be reduced to 100 mg/day for treatment or prophylaxis of elderly nursing-home residents. Although further studies are needed to determine the optimal dose for other elderly persons, a reduction in dosage to 100 mg/day should be considered for all persons greater than or equal to 65 years of age if they experience signs and symptoms that may represent side effects when taking a dosage of 200 mg/day.

Persons Who Have Liver Disease

Amantadine

No increase in adverse reactions to amantadine has been observed among persons with liver disease.

Rimantadine

The safety and pharmacokinetics of rimantadine have only been evaluated after single-dose administration. In a study of persons with chronic liver disease (most with stabilized cirrhosis), no alterations were observed after a single dose. However, in persons with severe liver dysfunction, the apparent clearance of rimantadine was 50% lower than that reported for persons without liver disease. A dose reduction to 100 mg/day is recommended for persons with severe hepatic dysfunction.

Persons Who Have Seizure Disorders

Amantadine

An increased incidence of seizures has been reported in patients with a history of seizure disorders who have received amantadine. Patients with seizure disorders should be observed closely for possible increased seizure activity when taking amantadine.

Rimantadine

In clinical trials, seizures (or seizure-like activity) have been observed in a few persons with a history of seizures who were not receiving anticonvulsant medication while taking rimantadine. The extent to which rimantadine may increase the incidence of seizures among persons with seizure disorders has not been adequately evaluated, because such persons have usually been excluded from participating in clinical trials of rimantadine.

Children

Amantadine

The use of amantadine in children less than 1 year of age has not been adequately evaluated. The FDA-approved dosage for children 1–9 years of age is 4.4–8.8 mg/kg/day, not to exceed 150 mg/day. Although further studies to determine the optimal dosage for children are needed, physicians should consider prescribing only 5 mg/kg/day (not to exceed 150 mg/day) to reduce the risk for toxicity. The approved dosage for children greater than or equal to 10 years of age is 200 mg/day; however, for children weighing less than 40 kg, prescribing 5 mg/kg/day, regardless of age, is advisable.

Rimantadine

The use of rimantadine in children less than 1 year of age has not been adequately evaluated. In children 1–9 years of age, rimantadine should be administered in one or two divided doses at a dosage of 5 mg/kg/day, not to exceed 150 mg/day. The approved dosage for children greater than or equal to 10 years of age is 200 mg/day (100 mg twice a day); however, for children weighing less than 40 kg, prescribing 5 mg/kg/day, regardless of age, also is recommended.

Drug Interactions

Amantadine

Careful observation is advised when amantadine is administered concurrently with drugs that affect the CNS, especially CNS stimulants.

Rimantadine

No clinically significant drug interactions have been identified. For more detailed information concerning potential drug interactions for either drug, the package insert should be consulted.

SOURCES OF INFORMATION ON INFLUENZA-CONTROL PROGRAMS

Information regarding influenza surveillance is available through the CDC Voice Information System (influenza update), telephone (404) 332-4551, or through the CDC Information Service on the Public Health Network electronic bulletin board. From October through May, the information is updated at least every other week. In addition, periodic updates about influenza are published in the weekly MMWR. State and local health departments should be consulted regarding availability of influenza vaccine, access to vaccination programs, and information about state or local influenza activity.

SELECTED BIBLIOGRAPHY

Aoki FY, Sitar DS. Amantadine kinetics in healthy elderly men: implications for influenza prevention. Clin Pharmacol Ther 1985;37:137–144.

Aoki FY, Sitar DS. Clinical pharmacokinetics of amantadine hydrochloride. Clin Pharmacokinet 1988;14: 35–51.

Atkinson WL, Arden NH, Patriarca PA, Leslie N, Lui KJ, Gohd R. Amantadine prophylaxis during an institutional outbreak of type A (H1N1) influenza. Arch Intern Med 1986;146:1751–1756.

Balfour HH Jr, Englund JA. Antiviral drugs in pediatrics. Am J Dis Child 1989;143:1307–1316.

Belshe RB, Burk B, Newman F, Cerruti RL, Sim IS. Resistance of influenza A virus to amantadine and rimantadine: results of one decade of surveillance. J Infect Dis 1989;159:430–435.

Dolin R, Reichman RC, Madore HP, Maynard R, Linton PN, Webber-Jones J. A controlled trial of amantadine and rimantadine in the prophylaxis of influenza A infection. N Engl J Med 1982;307:580–583.

Douglas RG. Drug therapy: prophylaxis and treatment of influenza. N Engl J Med 1990;322:443–450.

Hall CB, Dolin R, Gala CL, et al. Children with influenza A infection: treatment with rimantadine. Pediatrics 1987;80:275–282.

Hayden FG, Belshe RB, Clover RD, Hay AJ, Oakes MG, Soo W. Emergence and apparent transmission of rimantadine-resistant influenza A viruses in families. N Engl J Med 1989;321:1696–1702.

Hayden FG, Couch RB. Clinical and epidemiological importance of influenza A viruses resistant to amantadine and virus. Rev Med Virol 1992;2:89–96.

Hayden FG, Hay AJ. Emergence and transmission of influenza A viruses resistant to amantadine and rimantadine. Curr Top Microbiol Immunol 1992;176:120–130.

Horadam VW, Sharp JG, Smilack JD, et al. Pharmacokinetics of amantadine hydrochloride in subjects with normal and impaired renal function. Ann Intern Med 1981;94:454–458.

Mast EE, Harmon MW, Gravenstein S, et al. Emergence and possible transmission of amantadine-resistant viruses during nursing home outbreaks of influenza A(H3N2). Am J Epidemiol 1991;13:988–997.

Monto AS, Arden NH. Implications of viral resistance to amantadine in control of influenza A. Clin Infect Dis 1992;15:362–367.

Pettersson RF, Hellstrom PE, Penttinen K, et al. Evaluation of amantadine in the prophylaxis of influenza A (H1N1) virus infection: a controlled field trial among young adults and high-risk patients. J Infect Dis 1980;142:377–383.

Sears SD, Clements ML. Protective efficacy of low-dose amantadine in adults challenged with wild-type influenza A virus. Antimicrob Agents Chemother 1987;31:1470–1473.

Somani SK, Degelau J, Cooper SL, et al. Comparison of pharmacokinetic and safety profiles of amantadine 50- and 100-mg daily doses in elderly nursing home residents. Pharmacotherapy 1991;11:460–466.

Stange KC, Little DW, Blatnick B. Adverse reactions to amantadine prophylaxis of influenza in a retirement home. J Am Geriatr Soc 1991;39:700–705.

Tominack RL, Hayden FG. Rimantadine hydrochloride and amantadine hydrochloride use in influenza A virus infections. Infect Dis Clin North Am 1987;1:459–478.

TOPIC 17 / **LEPTOSPIROSIS**

Outbreak of Acute Febrile Illness and Pulmonary Hemorrhage

Original Citation: Centers for Disease Control and Prevention. Outbreak of acute febrile illness and pulmonary hemorrhage—Nicaragua, 1995. MMWR 1995;44(44):841–843.

Leptospirosis is a zoonotic disease of worldwide distribution, involving many wild and domestic animals (3). Human infection may result from indirect or direct exposure to infected urine, often through contaminated water or soil. The investigation in Nicaragua is examining the possibility that infection in humans resulted from exposure to water and soil contaminated by animal urine following recent heavy rainfall and flooding in that region.

The spectrum of leptospiral disease is broad and may include fever, headache, chills, myalgia, abdominal pain, and conjunctival suffusion; more severe manifestations include renal failure, jaundice, meningitis, hypotension, hemorrhage, and/or hemorrhagic pneumonitis (4). Severe pulmonary symptoms and pulmonary hemorrhage have not been characteristic of leptospirosis in the Western Hemisphere but have been associated with large outbreaks in Korea and China (5, 6). Clinical features of leptospirosis are similar to many other febrile illnesses; in the tropics, the differential diagnosis of such illnesses also may include dengue and malaria. Leptospirosis is diagnosed by isolation of leptospires from blood or cerebrospinal fluid during the acute illness and from urine greater than or equal to 10 days after the onset of symptoms or by documenting rising titers in serologic tests, such as the microagglutination test.

Penicillin is the antibiotic of choice for leptospirosis, and treatment should be initiated early in the course of illness (7). Alternatives are amoxicillin, ampicillin, doxycycline, and tetracycline. Supportive therapy is essential for managing dehydration, hypotension, hemorrhage, renal failure, and pulmonary involvement. For adults with short-term, high-risk exposure to leptospirosis, doxycycline provides effective prophylaxis when administered weekly in a single oral dose of 200 mg (8). Public health measures include controlling rodents, preventing contact with animal urine, wearing protective clothing (e.g., water-resistant boots) when exposure is likely, and avoiding swimming or wading in potentially contaminated water (i.e., with urine of infected animals).

REFERENCES: AS NUMBERED IN ORIGINAL PUBLICATION

3. Torten M, Marshall RB. Leptospirosis. In: Beran GW, ed. Handbook of zoonoses. Section A: bacterial, rickettsial, chlamydial, and mycotic. Boca Raton, FL: CRC Press, 1994:245–264.
4. Farr RW. Leptospirosis. Clin Infect Dis 1995;21:1–8.
5. Wang CN, Liu J, Chang TF, Cheng WJ, Luo MY, Hung AT. Studies on anicteric leptospirosis: I. Clinical manifestations and antibiotic therapy. Chinese Med J 1965;84:283–391.
6. Park SK, Lee SH, Rhee YK, et al. Leptospirosis in Chonbuk Province of Korea in 1987: a study of 93 patients. Am J Trop Med Hyg 1989;41:345–51.
7. Farrar WE. Leptospira species (Leptospirosis). In: Mandell GL, Bennett JE, Dolin R, eds. Principles and practice of infectious diseases. 4th ed. New York: Churchill Livingstone, 1995:2137–2141.
8. Takafuji ET, Kirkpatrick JW, Miller RN, et al. An efficacy trial of doxycycline chemoprophylaxis against leptospirosis. N Engl J Med 1984;310:497–500.

---

18 / LISTERIOSIS

Preventing Foodborne Illness: Listeriosis

Original Citation: Preventing foodborne illness: listeriosis. U.S. Department of Health and Human Services, Public Health Service, Centers for Disease Control and Prevention, Division of Bacterial and Mycotic Diseases, 1992.

PREVENTING FOODBORNE ILLNESS: LISTERIOSIS

Listeriosis, a serious infection caused by eating food contaminated with the bacterium Listeria monocytogenes, has recently become an important public health problem in the United States. The disease affects primarily pregnant women, newborns, and adults with weakened immune systems. It can be avoided by following a few simple recommendations.

How Great Is the Risk for Listeriosis?

In the United States, an estimated 1,850 persons become seriously ill with listeriosis each year. Of these, 425 die.

At increased risk are:

- Pregnant women. They are about 20 times more likely than other healthy adults to get listeriosis. About one-third of listeriosis cases happen during pregnancy.
- Newborns. Newborns rather than the pregnant women themselves suffer the serious effects of infection in pregnancy.
- Persons with weakened immune systems.
- Persons with cancer, diabetes, or kidney disease.
- Persons with AIDS. They are almost 300 times more likely to get listeriosis than people with normal immune systems.
- Persons who take glucocorticosteroid medications.
- The elderly.

Healthy adults and children occasionally get infected with Listeria, but they rarely become seriously ill.

How Does Listeria Get into Food?

Listeria monocytogenes is found in soil and water. Vegetables can become contaminated from the soil or from manure used as fertilizer. Animals can carry the bacterium without appearing ill and can contaminate foods of animal origin such as meats and dairy products. The bacterium has been found in a variety of raw foods, such as uncooked meats and vegetables, as well as in processed foods that become contaminated after processing, such as soft cheeses and cold cuts at the deli counter. Unpasteurized (raw) milk or foods made from unpasteurized milk may contain the bacterium.

Listeria is killed by pasteurization, and heating procedures used to prepare ready-to-eat processed meats should be sufficient to kill the bacterium; however, unless good manufacturing practices are followed, contamination can occur after processing.

How Do You Get Listeriosis?

You get listeriosis by eating food contaminated with Listeria. Babies can be born with listeriosis if their mothers eat contaminated food during pregnancy. Although healthy persons may consume contaminated foods without becoming ill, those at increased risk for infection can probably get listeriosis after eating food contaminated with even a few bacteria. Persons at risk can prevent Listeria infection by avoiding certain high-risk foods and by handling food properly.

How Do You Know If You Have Listeriosis?

A person with listeriosis usually has fever, muscle aches, and sometimes gastrointestinal symptoms such as nausea or diarrhea. If infection spreads to the nervous system, symptoms such as headache, stiff neck, confusion, loss of balance, or convulsions can occur.

Infected pregnant women may experience only a mild, flu-like illness; however, infection during pregnancy can lead to premature delivery, infection of the newborn, or even stillbirth.

There is no routine screening test for susceptibility to listeriosis during pregnancy, as there is for rubella and some other congenital infections. If you have symptoms such as fever or stiff neck, consult your doctor. A blood or spinal fluid test (to cultivate the bacteria) will show if you have listeriosis. During pregnancy, a blood test is the most reliable way to find out if your symptoms are due to listeriosis.

Can Listeriosis Be Prevented?

The general guidelines recommended for the prevention of listeriosis are similar to those used to help prevent other foodborne illnesses, such as salmonellosis.

How Can You Reduce Your Risk for Listeriosis?

General Recommendations

- Cook thoroughly raw food from animal sources, such as beef, pork, or poultry.
- Wash raw vegetables thoroughly before eating.
- Keep uncooked meats separate from vegetables and from cooked foods and ready-to-eat foods.
- Avoid raw (unpasteurized) milk or foods made from raw milk.
- Wash hands, knives, and cutting boards after handling uncooked foods.

Recommendations for Persons at High Risk, Such as Pregnant Women and Persons with Weakened Immune Systems

In addition to the recommendations listed above,

- Avoid soft cheeses such as feta, Brie, Camembert, blue-veined, and Mexican-style cheese. (Hard cheeses, processed cheeses, cream cheese, cottage cheese, or yogurt need not be avoided.)
- Cook until steaming hot left-over foods or ready-to-eat foods, such as hot dogs, before eating.
- Although the risk of listeriosis associated with foods from deli counters is relatively low, pregnant women and immunosuppressed persons may choose to avoid these foods or thoroughly reheat cold cuts before eating.

Can Listeriosis Be Treated?

When infection occurs during pregnancy, antibiotics given promptly to the pregnant woman can often prevent infection of the fetus or newborn. Babies with listeriosis receive the same antibiotics as adults, although a combination of antibiotics is often used until physicians are certain of the diagnosis. Even with prompt treatment, some infections result in death. This is particularly likely in the elderly and in persons with other serious medical problems.

What Is Being Done?

Government agencies and the food industry have taken steps to reduce contamination of food by the Listeria bacterium. The Food and Drug Administration and the U.S. Department of Agriculture monitor food regularly. When a processed food is found to be contaminated, food monitoring and plant inspection are intensified, and if necessary, the implicated food is recalled.

FURTHER INFORMATION ON LISTERIOSIS

Is available from the Division of Bacterial and Mycotic Diseases, National Center for Infectious Diseases, Centers for Disease Control and Prevention, 1600 Clifton Road, Mailstop C09, Atlanta, Georgia 30333.

TOPIC 19 / **LYME DISEASE**

Test Performance and Interpretation of Serologic Diagnosis of Lyme Disease

Original Citation: Centers for Disease Control and Prevention. Recommendations for test performance and interpretation from the Second National Conference on Serologic Diagnosis of Lyme Disease. MMWR 1995;44(31):590–591.

The Association of State and Territorial Public Health Laboratory Directors, CDC, the Food and Drug Administration, the National Institutes of Health, the Council of State and Territorial Epidemiologists, and the National Committee for Clinical Laboratory Standards cosponsored the Second National Conference on Serologic Diagnosis of Lyme Disease held October 27–29, 1994. Conference recommendations were grouped into four categories: (a) serologic test performance and interpretation, (b) quality-assurance practices, (c) new test evaluation and clearance, and (d) communication of developments in Lyme disease (LD) testing. This report represents recommendations for serologic test performance and interpretation, which included substantial changes in the recommended tests and their interpretation for the serodiagnosis of LD.

A two-test approach for active disease and for previous infection using a sensitive enzyme immunoassay (EIA) or immunofluorescent assay (IFA) followed by a Western immunoblot was the algorithm of choice. All specimens positive or equivocal by a sensitive EIA or IFA should be tested by a standardized Western immunoblot. Specimens negative by a sensitive EIA or IFA need not be tested further. When Western immunoblot is used during the first 4 weeks of disease onset (early LD), both immunoglobulin M (IgM) and immunoglobulin G (IgG) procedures should be performed. A positive IgM test result alone is not recommended for use in determining active disease in persons with illness greater than 1 month's duration because the likelihood of a false-positive test result for a current infection is high for these persons. If a patient with suspected early LD has a negative serology, serologic evidence of infection is best obtained by testing of paired acute- and convalescent-phase serum samples. Serum samples from persons with disseminated or late-stage LD almost always have a strong IgG response to Borrelia burgdorferi antigens.

It was recommended that an IgM immunoblot be considered positive it two of the following three bands are present: 24 kDa (OspC)*, 39 kDa (BmpA), and 41 kDa (Fla) (1). It was further recommended that an that IgG immunoblot be considered positive if five of the following 10 bands are present: 18 kDa, 21 kDa (OspC)*, 28 kDa, 30 kDa, 39 kDa (BmpA), 41 kDa(Fla), 45 kDa, 58 kDa (not GroEL), 66 kDa, and 93 kDa (2).

The details of both plenary sessions and the work group deliberations are included in the publication of the proceedings, which is available from the Association of State and territorial Public Health Laboratory Directors; telephone (202) 822-5227.

REFERENCES: AS NUMBERED IN ORIGINAL PUBLICATION

1. Engstrom SM, Shoop E, Johnson RC. Immunoblot interpretation criteria for serodiagnosis of early Lyme disease. J Clin Microbiol 1995;33:419–422.
2. Dressler F, Whelan JA, Reinhart BN, Steere AC. Western blotting in the serodiagnosis of Lyme disease. J Infect Dis 1993;167:392–400.

Lyme Disease: A Public Information Guide

Original Citation: Centers for Disease Control and Prevention. Lyme disease: a public information guide. Brochure.

SYMPTOMS AND SIGNS OF LYME DISEASE

Early Lyme Disease

The early stage of Lyme disease is usually marked by one or more of the following symptoms and signs:

- Fatigue.
- Chills and fever.
- Headache.
- Muscle and joint pain.
- Swollen lymph nodes.
- A characteristic skin rash, called erythema migrans.

Erythema migrans is a red circular patch that appears usually three days to one month after the bide of an infected tick at the site of the bite (Fig. 72.1). The patch then expands, often to a large size. Sometimes many patches appear, varying in shape, depending on their location. Common sites are the thigh. Groin, trunk, and the armpits. The center of the rash may clear as it enlarges, resulting in a "bulls-eye" appearance. The rash may be warm, but it usually is not painful. Not all rashes that occur at the site of a tick bite are due to Lyme disease, however. For example, an allergic reaction to tick saliva often occurs at the site of a tick bite. The resulting rash can be confused with the rash of Lyme

---

*The apparent molecular mass of OspC is dependent on the strain of B. Burgdorferi being tested. The 24 kDa and 21 kDa proteins referred to are the same.

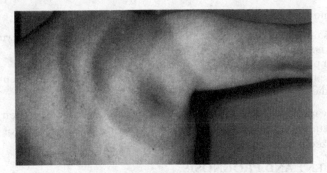

Figure 72.1. Erythema migrans.

disease. Allergic reactions to tick saliva usually occur within hours to a few days after the tick bite, usually do not expand, and disappear within a few days.

Late Lyme Disease

Some symptoms and signs of Lyme disease may not appear until weeks, months, or years after a tick bite:

- Arthritis is most likely to appear as brief bouts of pain and swelling, usually in one or more large joints, especially the knees.
- Nervous system abnormalities can include numbness, pain, Bell's palsy (paralysis of the facial muscles, usually on one side), and meningitis (fever, stiff neck, and severe headache).
- Less frequently, irregularities of the heart rhythm occur.
- In some persons the rash never forms; in some, the first and only sign of Lyme disease is arthritis, and in others, nervous system problems are the only evidence of Lyme disease.

LYME DISEASE AND PREGNANCY

In rare cases, Lyme disease acquired during pregnancy may lead to infection of the fetus and possibly to stillbirth, but adverse effects to the fetus have not been conclusively documented. The Centers for Disease Control and Prevention (CDC) maintains a registry of pregnant women with Lyme disease to advance the understanding of the effects of Lyme disease on the developing fetus.

DIAGNOSIS

Lyme disease is often difficult to diagnose because its symptoms and signs mimic those of many other diseases. The fever, muscle aches, and fatigue of Lyme disease can easily be mistaken for viral infections, such as influenza or infectious mononucleosis. Joint pain can be mistaken for other types of arthritis, such as rheumatoid arthritis, and neurologic signs can mimic those caused by other conditions, such as multiple sclerosis. At the same time, other types of arthritis or neurologic diseases can be misdiagnosed as Lyme disease.

Diagnosis of Lyme disease should take into account

- History of possible exposure to ticks, especially in areas where Lyme disease is known to occur.
- Symptoms and signs.
- The results of blood tests used to determine whether the patient has antibodies to Lyme disease bacteria.

These tests are most useful in later stages of illness, but even then they may give inaccurate results. Laboratory tests for Lyme disease have not yet been standardized nationally.

TREATMENT AND PROGNOSIS

Lyme disease is treated with antibiotics under the supervision of a physician. Several antibiotics are effective. Antibiotics usually are given by mouth but may be given intravenously in more severe cases. Patients treated in the early stages with antibiotics usually recover rapidly and completely. Most patients who are treated in later stages of the disease also respond well to antibiotics, and full recovery is the rule. In a few patients who are treated for Lyme disease, symptoms of persisting infection may continue or recur, making additional antibiotic treatment necessary. Varying degrees of permanent damage to joint or the nervous system can develop in patients with late chronic Lyme disease. Typically these are patients in whom Lyme disease was unrecognized in the early stages or for whom the initial treatment was unsuccessful. Rare deaths from Lyme disease have been reported.

PREVENTION

Tick Control

Removing leaves and clearing brush and tall grass around houses and at the edges of gardens may reduce the numbers of ticks that transmit Lyme disease. This is particularly important in the eastern United States, where most transmission of Lyme disease is thought to occur near the home.

Applying acaricides (chemicals that are toxic to ticks) to gardens, lawns, and the edge of woodlands near homes is being done in some areas, but questions remain regarding its effectiveness and environmental safety. Wide-area acaricide application should be supervised by a licensed professional pest control expert.

Reducing and managing deer populations in geographic areas where Lyme disease occurs may reduce tick abundance. Removing plants that attract deer and constructing physical barriers may help discourage deer from coming near homes.

Personal Protection from Tick Bites

The chances of being bitten by a tick can be decreased with a few precautions.

- Avoid tick-infested areas, especially in May, June, and July (many local health departments and park or extension services have information on the local distribution of ticks).
- Wear light-colored clothing so that ticks can be spotted more easily.
- Tuck pant legs into socks or boots and shirt into pants.

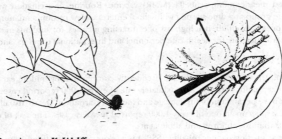

Drawings by K. Wolff

Figure 72.2. Removal of tick.

- Tape the area where pants and socks meet so that ticks cannot crawl under clothing.
- Spray insect repellent containing DEET on clothes and on exposed skin other than the face, or treat clothes (especially pants, socks, and shoes) with permethrin, which kills ticks on contact.
- Wear a hat and a long-sleeved shirt for added protection.
- Walk in the center of trails to avoid overhanging grass and brush.

After being outdoors, remove clothing and wash and dry it at a high temperature, inspect body carefully and remove attached ticks with tweezers, grasping the tick as close to the skin surface as possible and pulling straight back with a slow steady force; avoid crushing the tick's body (Fig. 72.2). In some areas, ticks (saved in a sealed container) can be submitted to the local health department for identification.

Preventive Antibiotic Treatment

Antibiotic treatment to prevent Lyme disease after a known tick bite may not be warranted. Physicians must determine whether the advantages of using antibiotics outweigh the disadvantages in any particular instance. If antibiotics are not used, physicians should alert patients to the symptoms of early Lyme disease and advise them to return for reevaluation if symptoms occur.

TOPIC 20 / **MEASLES**

Measles Prevention

Original Citation: ACIP. Measles prevention: recommendations of the Immunization Practices Advisory Committee. MMWR 1989;38(S-9):1–18.

These revised recommendations of the Immunization Practices Advisory Committee (ACIP) on Measles Prevention replace previous recommendations published in 1987 (1) and 1989 (2). The recommendations include a basic change in the routine childhood vaccination schedule from a one-dose to a two-dose schedule using combined measles-mumps-rubella (MMR) vaccine. Routine revaccination will generally be implemented one age group at a time starting with school enterers. New recommendations are also included for vaccination of preschool children at high risk of contracting measles, for students in colleges and other institutions of higher education, for health-care personnel and international travelers, and for outbreak control.

INTRODUCTION

Measles (rubeola) is often a severe disease, frequently complicated by middle ear infection or bronchopneumonia. Encephalitis occurs in approximately one of every 1,000 reported cases; survivors of this complication often have permanent brain damage and mental retardation. Death, usually from respiratory and neurologic causes, occurs in one of every 1,000 reported measles cases. The risk of death is greater for infants and adults than for children and adolescents.

Subacute sclerosing panencephalitis (SSPE) is a "slow virus" infection of the central nervous system associated with measles virus. Widespread use of measles vaccine has led to the virtual disappearance of SSPE from the United States (3).

Measles illness during pregnancy leads to increased rates of premature labor, spontaneous abortion, and low-birth-weight infants (4, 5). Whether measles infection in the first trimester of pregnancy is associated with an increased rate of congenital malformations is still unresolved.

Before measles vaccine was available, more than 400,000 measles cases were reported each year in the United States (6). However, since virtually all children acquired measles, the true number of cases probably exceeded 4 million per year (i.e., the entire birth cohort). Since 1963, when both an inactivated and a live attenuated vaccine (Edmonston B strain) were licensed for use in the United States, both the type of measles vaccine and the recommended age for measles vaccination have changed several times. After 1967 and 1975, the inactivated and the Edmonston B vaccine, respectively, were no longer distributed. A live, further attenuated vaccine (Schwarz strain) was first introduced in 1965, and a similar vaccine (Moraten strain) was licensed in 1968. These further attenuated vaccines cause fewer reactions than the Edmonston B vaccine, yet are equally effective. The Moraten vaccine is the vaccine used currently in the United States.

A single dose of live measles vaccine had been recommended since measles vaccine was first licensed (1). In 1963, the recommended age for vaccination was 9 months, but in 1965 it was changed to 12 months, and in 1976 it was changed to 15 months because of evidence demonstrating greater efficacy when children were vaccinated at these ages. Persons vaccinated before the first birthday needed to be revaccinated.

MEASLES EPIDEMIOLOGY AND ELIMINATION EFFORTS

Since vaccine licensure in 1963, the collaborative efforts of professional and voluntary medical and public health organizations in vaccination programs have resulted in a 99% reduction in the reported incidence of measles. During the late 1960s and early 1970s, the number of reported cases decreased to between 22,000 and 75,000 cases per year. Although incidence fell dramatically in all age groups, children less than 10 years of age showed the greatest decline, while older children had a slightly less dramatic decrease. As a result, the proportion of total cases occurring in different age groups changed. From 1984 to 1988, 58% of reported cases affected children greater than or equal to 10 years of age, compared with 10% during the period 1960 to 1964 (6).

In 1978, the Department of Health, Education, and Welfare initiated a Measles Elimination Program, with a goal to eliminate indigenous measles from the United States by October 1, 1982. The three components of this program have been (a) maintenance of high levels of immunity, (b) careful surveillance of disease, and (c) aggressive outbreak control. As a result of these efforts, the number of cases reported annually dropped from 26,871 in 1978 to an all-time low of 1,497 in 1983. The number of cases reported then increased until 1986 (6,282) cases (7). Reported cases decreased in 1987 and 1988 but rose again during the first 48 weeks of 1989, when more than 14,000 cases were reported. Measles cases are routinely reported by state and local health departments to the MMWR. The Division of Immunization, Center for Prevention Services, CDC, collects supplementary data on cases, including information on vaccination status (i.e., vaccinated or unvaccinated). Persons appropriately vaccinated for measles are those who have received a dose of live measles vaccine on or after their first birthday.

Unvaccinated persons with measles can be subclassified into three general groups: those for whom vaccine is not routinely indicated (e.g., those less than 16 months of age, born before 1957, with prior physician diagnosis of measles, or with medical contraindications), those for whom vaccination is difficult to achieve (e.g., non-U.S. citizens and persons exempted for religious or philosophic reasons), and those for whom vaccine is indicated (e.g., children greater than or equal to 16 months of age and children vaccinated before their first birthdays). From 1985 through 1988, information on vaccination status for 16,819 measles cases was collected by the Division of Immunization. Appropriately vaccinated persons accounted for 42%, and 92% of cases in this group occurred among persons greater than or equal to 5 years of age. In 26% of these cases, the patients were unvaccinated persons for whom vaccine was not routinely indicated or for whom vaccination was difficult to achieve. The remaining 32% were unvaccinated persons for whom vaccine was indicated. Forty-two percent of the persons in this latter group were children 16 months to 4 years of age.

In recent years, two major types of outbreaks have occurred in the United States: those among unvaccinated preschool-aged children, including those younger than the recommended age for vaccination (i.e., less than 15 months), and those among vaccinated school-aged children (8). In addition, particularly in 1989, a substantial number of cases occurred among students and personnel on college campuses. Large outbreaks occurred among unvaccinated preschool-aged children in several inner-city areas. In these outbreaks, of the cases that occurred among vaccine-eligible children 16 months-4 years of age, up to 88% of the children were unvaccinated. As many as 40% of cases occurred among children less than 16 months of age. In some of these areas, surveys indicate that 49%–65% of 2-year-olds had received measles vaccine (9). Among school-aged children, outbreaks have occurred in schools with vaccination levels of greater than 98%. These outbreaks have occurred in all parts of the country, including areas that had not reported measles for years. In general, attack rates in individual schools were low (1%–5%) and the calculated vaccine efficacy high. Most of the persons with measles in college outbreaks were also likely to have been vaccinated, although documentation of vaccination was often lacking. However, in many outbreaks, children vaccinated at 12–14 months of age had higher attack rates than those vaccinated at older ages (10). In a few outbreaks, older persons vaccinated in the more distant past were at increased risk for disease; this risk was independent of age at vaccination (11).

The goal of eliminating measles in the United States has not been reached primarily because of (a) failure to implement the current vaccination strategy, resulting in large numbers of unvaccinated preschool-age children in some areas, and (b) vaccine failure. A substantial number of cases occur among persons who previously have been vaccinated. Theoretically, vaccine failures may either be primary (i.e., an adequate response to vaccination never developed) or secondary (i.e., an adequate response initially developed, but immunity was lost over time). Some of the reported vaccine failures may be explained by the fact that a person's records incorrectly indicated appropriate vaccination. Measles vaccine is at least 95% effective for children vaccinated at greater than or equal to 15 months of age. However, efficacy may be slightly lower for persons vaccinated between 12 and 14 months of age, presumably because transplacental maternal antibody persists beyond the first birthday in some children and interferes with the response to vaccination. Also, secondary vaccine failure could occur after successful vaccination as a result of waning immunity, but the percentage of persons to whom this applies appears to be small (12, 13). Overall, the great majority of vaccinees appear to have long-term and probably life-long immunity. Nevertheless, further studies are needed to determine the duration of vaccine-induced immunity.

CHANGES IN MEASLES VACCINATION POLICY

The Committee reviewed current measles epidemiology and the measles elimination strategy and considered modifications. New recommendations were developed to help achieve the goal of measles elimination (Tables 1 and 2). A routine two-dose measles vaccination schedule now is recommended. This schedule is expected to provide protection to most persons who do not respond to their initial vaccination.

Table 1. 1989 Recommendations for measles vaccination

Routine childhood schedule, United States

Most areas	Two doses[*][†] first dose at 15 months second dose at 4–6 years (entry to kindergarten or first grade)[§]
High-risk areas[¶]	Two doses[*][†] first dose at 12 months second dose at 4–6 years (entry to kindergarten or first grade)[§]

Table 1.—*continued*

Colleges and other educational institutions post-high school	Documentation of receipt of two doses of measles vaccine after the first birthday[†] or other evidence of measles immunity[**]
Medical personnel beginning employment	Documentation of receipt of two doses of measles vaccine after the first birthday[†] or other evidence of measles immunity[**]

*Both doses should preferably be given as combined measles, mumps, rubella vaccine (MMR).

[†]No less than 1 month apart. If no documentation of any dose of vaccine, vaccine should be given at the time of school entry or employment and no less than 1 month later.

[§]Some areas may elect to administer the second dose at an older age or to multiple age groups (see "Age at Vaccination").

[¶]A county with more than five cases among preschool-aged children during each of the last 5 years, a county with a recent outbreak among unvaccinated preschool-aged children, or a county with a large inner-city urban population. These recommendations may be applied to an entire county or to identified risk areas within a county.

[**]Prior physician-diagnosed measles disease, laboratory evidence of measles immunity, or birth before 1957.

Table 2. Recommendations for measles outbreak control*

Outbreaks in preschool-aged children	Lower age for vaccination to as low as 6 months of age in outbreak area if cases are occurring in children <1 year of age[†].
Outbreaks in institutions: day-care centers, K–12th grades, colleges, and other institutions	Revaccination of all students and their siblings and of school personnel born in or after 1957 who do not have documentation of immunity to measles.[§]
Outbreaks in medical facilities	Revaccination of all medical workers born in or after 1957 who have direct patient contact and who do not have proof of immunity to measles.[§] Vaccination may also be considered for workers born before 1957.
	Susceptible personnel who have been exposed should be relieved from direct patient contact from the 5th to the 21st day after exposure (regardless of whether they received measles vaccine or IG) or— if they become ill—for 7 days after they develop rash.

*Mass revaccination of entire populations is not necessary. Revaccination should be limited to populations at risk, such as students attending institutions where cases occur.

[†]Children initially vaccinated before the first birthday should be revaccinated at 15 months of age. A second dose should be administered at the time of school entry or according to local policy.

[§]Documentation of physician-diagnosed measles disease, serologic evidence of immunity to measles, or documentation of receipt of two doses of measles vaccine on or after the first birthday.

The first dose is recommended at 15 months of age for children in most areas of the country but at 12 months of age for children in some areas with recurrent measles transmission. The second dose is recommended at the time a child enters school at kindergarten or first grade (see "Vaccine Usage"). Because programs to administer a second dose of measles vaccine at school entry to kindergarten or first grade will not have an immediate effect on the incidence of measles for school-aged children, programs also are recommended for outbreak control (see "Outbreak Control") and for the routine vaccination of students entering college (see "Special Situations"). When fully implemented, this schedule should lead to the elimination of measles among school-aged children and college students. It is expected to prevent the 35%–40% of cases affecting persons greater than or equal to 5 years of age who appear to be vaccine failures, and it may indirectly protect unvaccinated persons since the risk of exposure to measles will decrease. Outbreaks of measles in school settings are likely to cease, thus avoiding the substantial disruption of routine activities and the high cost of outbreak control. However, the overall goal of eliminating measles in the United States also requires more intensive efforts to vaccinate preschool children at the recommended ages, particularly children residing in inner cities.

All contacts with health-care providers in physicians' offices, clinics, emergency rooms, and hospitals are opportunities for evaluating the vaccination status of children, both patients and accompanying siblings, and for offering vaccine to those who need it. Unvaccinated children should not be rescheduled for vaccination; rather, they should be vaccinated immediately if no contraindication exists. Particular attention should be paid to offering simultaneous vaccination. No preschool child who needs MMR should be offered other vaccines without being offered MMR. Special efforts are also needed to educate and motivate parents to have such children vaccinated.

MEASLES VIRUS VACCINE

Live measles virus vaccine* used in the United States is prepared in chick-embryo-cell culture. It is available in monovalent (measles only) form and in two combinations: measles-rubella (MR) and measles-mumps-rubella (MMR) vaccines.** Measles vaccine produces an inapparent or mild, noncommunicable infection. Measles antibodies develop in at least 95% of susceptible children vaccinated at greater than or equal to 15 months of age. Although the titers of vaccine-induced antibodies are lower than those following natural disease, both serologic and epidemiologic evidence indicate that vaccine-induced protection appears to be long-lasting in most individuals.

Vaccine Shipment and Storage

The administration of improperly stored vaccine may fail to provide protection against measles. Although the current measles vaccine may be more thermostable than vaccine produced in the past, it should be stored at 2–8°C (35.6–46.4°F) or colder during storage. Vaccine must be shipped at 10°C (50°F) or colder and may be shipped on dry ice. It must be protected from light, which may inactivate the virus. Reconstituted vaccine must be stored in a refrigerator (not frozen) and discarded if not used within 8 hours.

---

*Official name: Measles Virus Vaccine, Live Attenuated.

**Available in the United States as Attenuvax (single antigen), M-R-Vax (measles-rubella) and M-M-R II (measles-mumps-rubella), from the Merck, Sharp and Dohme Co.

VACCINE USAGE

General Recommendations

All vaccines containing measles virus are recommended for routine use for children 15 months of age. Persons born in or after 1957 who lack documentation of measles immunity (see "Measles Immunity") are considered susceptible and should be vaccinated if there are no contraindications (see "Precautions and Contraindications"). All vaccinations should be documented in the patient's permanent medical record (14). A parental history of vaccination, by itself, is not considered adequate documentation. A physician should not provide an immunization record for a patient unless s/he has administered the vaccine or has seen a record that documents vaccination. Most persons born before 1957 are likely to have been naturally infected with measles virus and generally need not be considered susceptible; however, vaccination may be offered to these persons if there is reason to believe they may be susceptible.

Both doses of measles vaccine should be given as combined MMR vaccine when given on or after the first birthday. The combined vaccine is preferred to assure immunity to all three viruses. Mumps revaccination is particularly important. Recent studies have shown that mumps can occur in highly vaccinated populations, resulting in substantial numbers of cases among persons with histories of prior mumps vaccination. Although rubella vaccine failure has not been a major problem, the potential consequences of rubella vaccine failure are substantial (i.e., congenital rubella syndrome), and the use of MMR should provide an additional safeguard against such failures.

The most commonly used laboratory test for assessing immunity to measles has been the hemagglutination-inhibition (HI) test. Other more sensitive assays, such as the enzyme immuno-assay (EIA), are now being used by many laboratories. Persons with measles-specific antibody, detectable by any test, are considered immune. Routine serologic screening to determine measles immunity is not generally recommended, although it may be cost-effective in some situations (e.g., large prepaid medical programs). However, the test may not be widely available, and screening requires that tracking systems be established to assure that identified susceptibles return for vaccination. In addition, screening for antibodies for mumps and rubella would further decrease the cost-effectiveness of this strategy.

Dosage

Two doses of measles vaccine, generally given as MMR, are recommended for all children after the first birthday. The dose is 0.5 ml and should be given subcutaneously.

Age at Vaccination

Routine Childhood Immunization Schedule for Most Areas of the United States

The first dose of measles vaccine should be given when children are greater than or equal to 15 months of age. The second dose should routinely be given when children enter kindergarten or first grade (4–6 years of age).

The recommended time for the second dose is based primarily on administrative considerations. The current childhood immunization schedule recommends other vaccines (diphtheria and tetanus toxoids and pertussis vaccine (DTP) and oral poliovirus vaccine (OPV)) when children enter school; therefore, an additional provider visit for the second dose of measles vaccine is not necessary. In addition, most school authorities have systems at this grade level for identifying and tracking children with incomplete immunizations.

Because many of the vaccine failures in recent outbreaks of measles have occurred among 10- to 19-year-old children and adolescents, administering the second dose at the time of school entry may not achieve full impact on the incidence of measles for 5 to 15 years. For the impact to occur more rapidly, some localities may choose to give students the second dose at an older age (e.g., when they enter middle school or junior high school). In deciding when to administer the second dose, health officials should consider how they can best achieve a high vaccination rate since this is essential to assure maximum impact of a two-dose schedule. Some localities may want to provide a second dose to multiple age groups from kindergarten through 12th grade to achieve complete immunization of all school-aged children more rapidly.

Children who have received two doses of live measles vaccine on or after the first birthday (at least 1 month apart) do not need an additional dose when they enter school. Children who have no documentation of live measles vaccination when they enter school should be admitted after the first dose. A second dose should be given according to local policy, but no less than 1 month later. Routine childhood immunization schedule for areas with recurrent measles transmission

Initial vaccination with MMR at 12 months of age is recommended for children living in high-risk areas. This strategy assumes that the benefit of preventing measles cases between 12 and 15 months of age outweighs the slightly lower efficacy of the vaccine when given at this age. A high-risk area is defined as: (a) a county with more than five cases among preschool-aged children during each of the last 5 years, (b) a county with a recent outbreak among unvaccinated preschool-aged children, or (c) a county with a large inner-city urban population. These recommendations may be implemented for an entire county or only in defined high-risk areas.

Revaccination of Persons Vaccinated According to Earlier Recommendations

Previous Vaccination with Live Vaccine

Persons vaccinated with live measles vaccine before their first birthday should be considered unvaccinated. If they are entering kindergarten or first grade, college or other post-high school educational institutions (see "Special Situations"), or beginning employment in a medical facility (see "Special Situations") and cannot provide documentation of immunity to measles (see "Measles Immunity"), they should receive two doses of vaccine no less than 1 month apart.

Live attenuated Edmonston B vaccine (distributed from 1963–1975) was usually administered with immune globulin (IG) or high-titer measles immune globulin (MIG; no longer available in the United States). This vaccine, administered on or after the first birthday, is acceptable as an effective first dose of vaccine. A second dose should be administered as recommended above. However, if a further attenuated measles vaccine (i.e., Schwarz or Moraten) was given simultaneously with IG or MIG, the IG or MIG may have impaired the immune response to vaccination. Persons who received measles vaccine of unknown type or further attenuated measles vaccine accompanied by IG or MIG should be considered unvaccinated and should be given two doses of vaccine as outlined above.

Previous Vaccination with Inactivated Vaccine or Vaccine of Unknown Type

Inactivated (killed) measles vaccine was available in the United States only from 1963 to 1967 but was available through the early 1970s in some other countries. It was frequently given as a series of two or three injections. Some persons who received inactivated vaccine are at risk of developing severe atypical measles syndrome when exposed to the natural virus (15). Consequently, such persons should receive two doses of live vaccine separated by no less than 1 month. Persons vaccinated with inactivated vaccine followed within 3 months by live vaccine should be revaccinated with two doses of live vaccine. Revaccination is particularly important when the risk of exposure to natural measles virus is increased, as may occur during international travel.

A wide range (4%–55%) of recipients of inactivated measles vaccine who were later revaccinated with live measles vaccine have had reactions to the live vaccine (16). Most of these reactions have been mild, consisting of local swelling and erythema, with or without low-grade fever lasting 1–2 days. Rarely, more severe reactions, including prolonged high fevers and extensive local reactions, have been reported. However, recipients of inactivated measles vaccine are more likely to have serious illness when exposed to natural measles than when given live measles virus vaccine.

These same recommendations for revaccination apply to persons vaccinated between 1963 and 1967 with vaccine of unknown type, since they may have received inactivated vaccine. Since inactivated measles vaccine was not distributed in the United States after 1967, persons vaccinated after 1967 with a vaccine of unknown type need not be revaccinated routinely unless the original vaccination occurred before the first birthday or was accompanied by IG or MIG. However, such persons should receive a second dose if they are entering college, beginning employment in medical facilities, or planning international travel.

Measles Immunity

Persons are considered immune to measles if they (a) were born before 1957, (b) have documentation of physician-diagnosed measles, (c) have laboratory evidence of immunity to measles, or (d) have documentation of adequate vaccination. Eventually, adequate vaccination will be defined as receipt of one dose of live measles vaccine on or after the first birthday for children before they enter school and two doses of measles vaccine on or after the first birthday for children who are entering or have entered school.

For localities implementing the second dose for students at ages beyond school entry (e.g., entry to middle school or junior high school), acceptable evidence of immunity will be one dose at school entry and two doses for students older than the routine age of the second dose (see "Age at Vaccination").

Since most areas will implement the two-dose schedule one age group at a time, criteria for adequate vaccination will vary in the interim. For example, if the two-dose schedule is implemented in 1990, children in kindergarten or first grade will need to have documentation of two doses of measles vaccine after the first birthday to be considered adequately vaccinated. However, a single dose of vaccine will be acceptable evidence of adequate vaccination for children in higher grades. Two years later, children in kindergarten through second or third grade will need two doses of measles vaccine for acceptable evidence of adequate vaccination. Similar criteria would apply if the second-dose strategy is implemented at an older age (see "Age at Vaccination").

The interim vaccination criteria for adequate measles vaccination noted above apply to routine settings only. During outbreaks, all persons at risk and born in or after 1957 who are in kindergarten, first grade, or beyond will need two doses on or after the first birthday as evidence of adequate vaccination (see "Outbreak Control").

Individuals Exposed to Disease

Use of Vaccine

Exposure to measles is not a contraindication to vaccination. If live measles vaccine is given within 72 hours of measles exposure, it may provide some protection. This approach is preferable to using IG for persons greater than or equal to 12 months of age. If the exposure does not result in infection, vaccination should induce protection against subsequent measles infection.

Use of IG

IG can prevent or modify measles in a susceptible person if given within 6 days of exposure. The recommended dose of IG is 0.25 ml/kg (0.11 ml/lb) of body weight (maximum dose = 15 ml). IG may be especially indicated for susceptible household contacts of measles patients, particularly contacts less than 1 year of age, pregnant women, or immunocompromised persons, for whom the risk of complications is increased. The recommended dose of IG for immunocompromised persons is 0.5 ml/kg of body weight (maximum dose = 15 ml). Live measles vaccine should be given 3 months later (when passively acquired measles antibodies should have disappeared) if the individual is then at least 15 months old. IG should not be used to control measles outbreaks.

Special Situations

Recommendations for colleges and other institutions Colleges, technical schools, and other institutions for post-high school education should require documentation of two doses of live measles-containing vaccines, documentation of prior physician-diagnosed measles disease, or laboratory evidence of measles immunity before entry for all students born in or after 1957. Students who have no documentation of live measles vaccination or other evidence of measles immunity at the time of school entry should be admitted after receiving the first dose. A second dose should be given no less than 1 month later. Institutions may wish to extend this requirement to all classes.

Recommendations for Medical Facilities

Medical personnel are at higher risk for acquiring measles than the general population (17). Hospitals should require evidence of two live measles vaccinations, documentation of physician-diagnosed measles disease, or laboratory evidence of measles immunity for medical staff beginning employment who will have direct patient contact. Persons born in or after 1957 who have no documentation of vaccination or other evidence of measles immunity should be vaccinated at the time of employment and revaccinated no less than 1 month later. If resources are available, institutions may wish to extend this recommendation to all medical personnel, not just those beginning employment. Since some medical personnel who have acquired measles in medical facilities were born before 1957, institutions may consider requiring at least one dose of measles vaccine for older employees who are at risk of occupational exposure to measles.

Recommendations for International Travel

Persons traveling abroad should be immune to measles. The protection of young adults who have escaped measles disease and have not been vaccinated is especially important. Consideration should be given to providing a dose of measles vaccine to persons born in or after 1957 who travel abroad, who have not previously received two doses of measles vaccine, and who do not have other evidence of measles immunity (see "Measles Immunity"). The age for measles vaccination should be lowered for children traveling to areas in which measles is endemic or epidemic. Children 12–14 months of age should receive MMR vaccine before their departure. Children 6–11 months of age should receive a dose of monovalent measles vaccine before departure, although there is no specific contraindication to the use of MMR for this age group if monovalent measles vaccine is not available. Seroconversion rates observed for measles, mumps, and rubella antigens are significantly less among children vaccinated before the first birthday than among older children. Children who receive monovalent measles vaccine or MMR before their first birthday should be considered unvaccinated and should receive two doses of MMR at later ages. Whereas the optimal age for the first revaccination dose is 15 months, the age for revaccination may be as low as 12 months if the child remains in a high-risk area (see "Routine childhood immunization schedule for areas with recurrent measles transmission"). The second revaccination dose would normally be given when a child enters school or according to local policy.

Since virtually all infants less than 6 months of age will be protected by maternally derived antibodies, no additional protection against measles is necessary in this age group.

SIDE EFFECTS AND ADVERSE REACTIONS

More than 170 million doses of measles vaccine were distributed in the United States from 1963 through 1988. The vaccine has an excellent record of safety. From 5%–15% of vaccinees may develop a temperature of greater than or equal to 103°F (greater than or equal to 39.4°C) beginning 5–12 days after vaccination and usually lasting several days (18). Most persons with fever are otherwise asymptomatic. Transient rashes have been reported for approximately 5% of vaccinees. Central nervous system conditions, including encephalitis and encephalopathy, have been reported with a frequency of less than one per million doses administered. The incidence of encephalitis or encephalopathy after measles vaccination of healthy children is lower than the observed incidence of encephalitis of unknown etiology. This finding suggests that the reported severe neurologic disorders temporally associated with measles vaccination were not caused by the vaccine. These adverse events should be anticipated only in susceptible vaccinees and do not appear to be age-related. After revaccination, reactions should be expected to occur only among the small proportion of persons who failed to respond to the first dose.

Personal and Family History of Convulsions

As with the administration of any agent that can produce fever, some children may have a febrile seizure. Although children with a personal or family history of seizures are at increased risk for developing idiopathic epilepsy, febrile seizures following vaccinations do not in themselves increase the probability of subsequent epilepsy or other neurologic disorders. Most convulsions following measles vaccination are simple febrile seizures, and they affect children without known risk factors. An increased risk of these convulsions may occur among children with a prior history of convulsions or those with a history of convulsions in first-degree family members (i.e., siblings or parents) (19). Although the precise risk cannot be determined, it appears to be low.

In developing vaccination recommendations for these children, the Committee considered a number of factors, including risks from measles disease, the large proportion (5%–7%) of children with a personal or family history of convulsions, and the fact that convulsions following measles vaccine are uncommon and have not been associated with permanent brain damage. The Committee concluded that the benefits of vaccinating these children greatly outweigh the risks. They should be vaccinated just as children without such histories.

Because the period for developing vaccine-induced fever occurs approximately 5–12 days after vaccination, prevention of febrile seizures is difficult. Prophylaxis with antipyretics is one alternative, but these agents may not be effective if given after the onset of fever. They would have to be initiated before the expected onset of fever and continued for 5–7 days. However, parents should be alert to the occurrence of fever after vaccination and should treat their children appropriately. Children who are being treated with anticonvulsants should continue to take them after measles vaccination. Because protective levels of most currently available anticonvulsant drugs (e.g., phenobarbitol) are not achieved for some time after therapy is initiated, prophylactic use of these drugs does not seem feasible.

The parents of children who have either a personal or family history of seizures should be advised of the small increased risk of seizures following measles vaccination. In particular, they should be told in advance what to do in the unlikely event that a seizure occurs. The permanent medical record should document that the small risk of postimmunization seizures and the benefits of vaccination have been discussed.

Revaccination Risks

There is no evidence of increased risk from live measles vaccination in persons who are already immune to measles, as a result of either previous vaccination or natural disease.

PRECAUTIONS AND CONTRAINDICATIONS

Pregnancy

Live measles vaccine, when given as a component of MR or MMR, should not be given to women known to be pregnant or who are considering becoming pregnant within the next 3 months. Women who are given monovalent measles vaccine should not become pregnant for at least 30 days after vaccination. This precaution is based on the theoretical risk of fetal infection, although no evidence substantiates this theoretical risk. Considering the importance of protecting adolescents and young adults against measles, asking women if they are pregnant, excluding those who are, and explaining the theoretical risks to the others before vaccination are sufficient precautions.

Febrile Illness

The decision to administer or delay vaccination because of a current or recent febrile illness depends largely on the cause of the illness and the severity of symptoms. Minor illnesses, such as a mild upper-respiratory infection with or without low-grade fever, are not contraindications for vaccination. For persons whose compliance with medical care cannot be assured, every opportunity should be taken to provide appropriate vaccinations. Children with moderate or severe febrile illnesses can be vaccinated as soon as they have recovered. This wait avoids superimposing adverse effects of vaccination on the underlying illness or mistakenly attributing a manifestation of the underlying illness to the vaccine. Performing routine physical examinations or measuring temperatures are not prerequisites for vaccinating infants and children who appear to be in good health. Asking the parent or guardian if the child is ill, postponing vaccination for children with moderate or severe febrile illnesses, and vaccinating those without contraindications are appropriate procedures in childhood immunization programs.

Allergies

Hypersensitivity reactions following the administration of live measles vaccine are rare. Most of these reactions are minor and consist of a wheal and flare or urticaria at the injection site. More than 170 million doses of measles vaccine have been distributed in the United States, but only five reported cases of immediate allergic reactions have occurred among children who had histories of anaphylactic reactions to egg ingestion. These reactions could potentially have been life-threatening. Four children experienced difficulty in breathing, and one of these four had hypotension. Persons with a history of anaphylactic reactions (hives, swelling of the mouth and throat, difficulty in breathing, hypotension, and shock) following egg ingestion should be vaccinated only with extreme caution. Protocols have been developed for vaccinating such persons (20, 21). However, persons are not at increased risk if they have egg allergies that are not anaphylactic in nature; they can be vaccinated in the usual manner. Persons with allergies only to chickens or feathers are not at increased risk of reaction to measles vaccination. MMR vaccine and its component vaccines contain trace amounts of neomycin. Although the amount present is less than that usually used for a skin test to determine hypersensitivity, persons who have experienced anaphylactic reactions to neomycin should not be given these vaccines. Most often, neomycin allergy is manifested by contact dermatitis rather than anaphylaxis. A history of contact dermatitis to neomycin is not a contraindication to receiving measles vaccine. Live measles virus vaccine does not contain penicillin.

Recent Administration of IG

Vaccine virus replication and stimulation of immunity usually occurs 1–2 weeks after vaccination. When the live measles vaccine is given after IG or specific IG preparations, the vaccine virus might not replicate successfully, and the antibody response could be diminished. Measles vaccine should not be given for at least 6 weeks, and preferably for 3 months, after a person has been given IG, whole blood, or other antibody-containing blood products. If vaccine is given to a person who has received such products within the preceding 3 months, the dose should not be counted and the person should be revaccinated approximately 3 months later unless serologic testing indicates that measles-specific antibodies have been produced. For international travelers, measles vaccination should precede the administration of IG by at least 2 weeks to preclude interference with replication of the vaccine virus. If the interval between measles vaccination and subsequent administration of an IG preparation is less than 14 days, vaccination should be repeated 3 months later, unless serologic testing indicates that antibodies were produced.

Tuberculosis

Tuberculosis may be exacerbated by natural measles infection. Live measles virus vaccine has not been shown to have such an effect. Tuberculin skin testing is not a prerequisite for measles vaccination. If tuberculin testing is needed for other reasons, it can be done the day of vaccination. Otherwise, the test should be postponed for 4–6 weeks, since measles vaccination may temporarily suppress tuberculin reactivity.

Altered Immunocompetence

Replication of vaccine viruses can be enhanced in persons with immune-deficiency diseases and in persons with immunosuppression, as occurs with leukemia, lymphoma, generalized malignancy, or therapy with alkylating agents, antimetabolites, radiation, or large doses of corticosteroids. For this reason, patients with such conditions or therapies (except patients with symptomatic infection with human immunodeficiency virus (HIV); see below) should not be given live measles virus vaccine.

Patients with leukemia in remission who have not received chemotherapy for at least 3 months may receive live-virus vaccines. Short-term (less than 2 weeks), low- to moderate-dose systemic corticosteroid therapy, topical steroid therapy (e.g., nasal, skin), long-term alternate-day treatment with low to moderate doses of short-acting systemic steroids, and intra-articular, bursal, or tendon injection of corticosteroids are not immunosuppressive in their usual doses and do not contraindicate the administration of measles vaccine. The growing number of infants and preschoolers with HIV infection has directed special attention to the appropriate immunization of such children. Asymptomatic children do not need to be evaluated and tested for HIV infection before decisions concerning vaccination are made. Asymptomatic HIV-infected persons in need of MMR should receive it. MMR should be considered for all symptomatic HIV-infected children, including children with acquired immunodeficiency syndrome (AIDS), since measles disease in these children can be severe. Limited data on MMR vaccination among both asymptomatic and symptomatic HIV-infected children indicate that MMR has not been associated with severe or unusual adverse events, although antibody responses have been unpredictable (22–24).

The administration of high-dose intravenous immune globulin (IGIV) at regular intervals to HIV-infected children is being studied to determine whether it will prevent a variety of infections. MMR vaccine may be ineffective if it is administered to a child who has received IGIV during the preceding 3 months.

Management of Patients with Contraindications to Measles Vaccine

If immediate protection against measles is required for persons with contraindications to measles vaccination, passive immunization with IG, 0.25 ml/kg (0.11 ml/lb) of body weight (maximum dose = 15 ml), should be given as soon as possible after known exposure. Exposed symptomatic HIV-infected and other immunocompromised persons should receive IG regardless of their previous vaccination status; however, IG in usual doses may not be effective in such patients. For immunocompromised persons, the recommended dose is 0.5 ml/kg of body weight if IG is administered intramuscularly (maximum dose = 15 ml). This corresponds to a dose of protein of approximately 82.5 mg/kg (maximum dose = 2,475 mg). Intramuscular IG may not be needed if a patient with HIV infection is receiving 100–400 mg/kg IGIV at regular intervals and the last dose was given within 3 weeks of exposure to measles. Because the amounts of protein administered are similar, high-dose IGIV may be as effective as IG given intramuscularly. However, no data are available concerning the effectiveness of IGIV in preventing measles.

Simultaneous Administration of Vaccines

In general, simultaneous administration of the most widely used live and inactivated vaccines does not impair antibody responses or increase rates of adverse reactions (25). The administration of MMR vaccine yields results similar to the administration of individual measles, mumps, and rubella vaccines at different sites or at different times.

There are equivalent antibody responses and no clinically significant increases in the frequency of adverse events when DTP, MMR, and OPV or inactivated poliovirus vaccine (IPV) are administered either simultaneously at different sites or at separate times. Routine simultaneous administration of MMR, DTP, and OPV (or IPV) is recommended for all children greater than or equal to 15 months of age who are eligible to receive these vaccines. Vaccination with MMR at 15 months followed by DTP, OPV (or IPV), and Haemophilus influenzae b conjugate vaccine (HbCV) at 18 months remains an acceptable alternative for children with caregivers known to be generally compliant with other health-care recommendations. No data are available on the concomitant administration of HbCV or H. influenzae b polysaccharide vaccine (HbPV) and OPV and MMR vaccine. If the child might not be brought back for future vaccinations, the simultaneous administration of all vaccines (including DTP, OPV, MMR, and HbCV or HbPV) is recommended, as appropriate to the recipient's age and previous vaccination status.

OUTBREAK CONTROL

All reports of suspected measles cases should be investigated promptly. A measles outbreak exists in a community whenever one case of measles is confirmed. Once this occurs, preventing the dissemination of measles depends on the prompt vaccination of susceptible persons. Control activities should not be delayed for laboratory results on suspected cases. Persons who cannot readily provide documentation of measles immunity (see "Measles Immunity") should be vaccinated or excluded from the setting (e.g., school). Documentation of vaccination is adequate only if the date of vaccination is provided. Almost all persons who are excluded from an outbreak area because they lack documentation of immunity quickly comply with vaccination requirements. Persons who have been exempted from measles vaccination for medical, religious, or other reasons should be excluded from the outbreak area until at least 2 weeks after the onset of rash in the last case of measles.

School-Based Outbreaks

During outbreaks in day-care centers; elementary, middle, junior, and senior high schools; and colleges and other institutions of higher education, a program of revaccination with MMR vaccine is recommended in the affected schools. Consideration should be given to revaccination in unaffected schools that may be at risk of measles transmission. Revaccination should include all students and their siblings and all school personnel born in or after 1957 who cannot provide documentation that they received two doses of measles-containing vaccine on or after their first birthday or other evidence of measles immunity (see "Measles Immunity"). Persons revaccinated, as well as unvaccinated persons receiving their first dose as part of the outbreak control program, may be immediately readmitted to school. Mass revaccination of entire communities is not necessary.

Quarantine

Imposing quarantine measures for outbreak control is both difficult and disruptive to schools and other organizations. Under special circumstances restriction of an event might be warranted; however, such action is not recommended as a routine measure for outbreak control.

Outbreaks Among Preschool-aged Children

The risk of complications from measles is high among infants less than 1 year of age. Therefore, considering the benefits and risks, vaccination with monovalent measles vaccine is recommended for infants as young as 6 months of age when exposure to natural measles is considered likely. MMR may be administered to children before the first birthday if monovalent measles vaccine is not readily available. Children vaccinated before the first birthday should be revaccinated when they are 15 months old and when they enter school to ensure adequate protection (see "General Recommendations").

Medical Settings

If an outbreak occurs in the areas served by a hospital or within a hospital, all employees with direct patient contact who were born in or after 1957 who cannot provide documentation that they received two doses of measles vaccine on or after their first birthday or other evidence of immunity to measles (see "Measles Immunity") should receive a dose of measles vaccine. Since some medical personnel who have acquired measles in medical facilities were born before 1957, vaccination of older employees who may have occupational exposure to measles should also be considered during outbreaks. Susceptible personnel who have been exposed should be relieved from direct patient contact from the fifth to the 21st day after exposure regardless of whether they received vaccine or IG after the exposure. Personnel who become ill should be relieved from patient contact for 7 days after they develop rash.

DISEASE SURVEILLANCE AND REPORTING OF ADVERSE EVENTS

Disease Surveillance

As the incidence of measles declines in the United States, aggressive surveillance becomes increasingly important. Effective surveillance can delineate inadequate levels of protection, define groups needing special attention, and assess the effectiveness of control activities.

Known or suspected measles cases should be reported immediately to local health departments. Serologic confirmation should be attempted for every suspected case of measles that cannot be linked to a confirmed case. Reporting of suspected cases and implementation of outbreak-control activities should not be delayed pending laboratory results.

The traditional serologic diagnosis of measles requires a significant rise in antibody titer between acute- and convalescent-phase sera. However, the diagnosis can also be made by demonstrating the presence of IgM antibody in a single specimen. Correct interpretation of serologic data depends upon the proper timing of specimen collection in relation to rash onset. This timing is especially important for interpreting negative IgM results, since IgM antibody peaks approximately 10 days after rash onset and is usually undetectable 30 days after rash onset.

Asymptomatic reinfection can occur in persons who have previously developed antibodies, whether from vaccination or from natural disease. Symptomatic reinfections are rare. These reinfections have been accompanied by rises in measles antibody titers.

Reporting of Adverse Events

The National Childhood Vaccine Injury Act of 1986 requires physicians and other health care providers who administer vaccines to maintain permanent immunization records and to report occurrences of adverse events specified in the Act (14). These adverse events, as well as other adverse events that require medical attention, must be reported to the U.S. Department of Health and Human Services. Although there eventually will be one system for reporting adverse events following immunizations, two separate systems currently exist. The appropriate reporting method depends on the source of funding used to purchase the vaccine. If a vaccine was purchased with public funds, adverse events should be reported to the appropriate local, county, or state health department. The state health department submits its report to CDC. If vaccine was purchased with private money, adverse events should be reported directly to the Food and Drug Administration.

REFERENCES

1. ACIP. Measles prevention. MMWR 1987;36:409–418, 423–425.
2. ACIP. Measles prevention: supplementary statement. MMWR 1989;38:11–14.
3. Bloch AB, Orenstein WA, Stetler HC, et al. Health impact of measles vaccination in the United States. Pediatrics 1985;76:524–532.
4. Siegel M, Fuerst HT. Low birth weight and maternal virus diseases: a prospective study of rubella, measles, mumps, chickenpox, and hepatitis. JAMA 1966;197:680–684.
5. Jespersen CS, Littauer J, Sagild U. Measles as a cause of fetal defects. Acta Paediatr Scand 1977;66:367–372.
6. CDC. Measles surveillance report No. 11, 1977–1981. September 1982.
7. CDC. Measles—United States, 1987. MMWR 1988;37:527–531.
8. Markowitz L, Preblud SR, Orenstein WA, et al. Patterns of transmission in measles outbreaks in the United States, 1985–1986. N Engl J Med 1989;320:75–81.
9. CDC. Measles—Dade County, Florida. MMWR 1987;36:45–48.
10. Orenstein WA, Markowitz LE, Preblud SR, et al. Appropriate age for measles vaccination in the United States. Dev Biol Stand 1986;65:13–21.
11. CDC. Measles, United States—1988. MMWR 1989;38:601–605.
12. Mathias RG, Meeklson WG, Arcand TA, et al. The role of secondary vaccine failures in measles outbreaks. Am J Public Health 1989;79:474–478.
13. Zhuji Measles Vaccine Study Group. Epidemiologic examination of immunity period of measles vaccine. Chin Med J 1987;67:19–22.
14. CDC. National Childhood Vaccine Injury Act: requirements for permanent vaccination records and for reporting of selected events after vaccination. MMWR 1988;37:197–200.
15. Annunziato D, Kaplan MH, Hall WW, et al. Atypical measles syndrome: pathologic and serologic findings. Pediatr 1982;70:203–209.
16. Krause PJ, Cherry JD, Naiditch MJ, et al. Revaccination of previous recipients of killed measles vaccine: clinical and immunologic studies. J Pediatr 1978;93:565–571.
17. Davis R, Orenstein WA, Frank JA, et al. Transmission of measles in medical settings. JAMA 1986;255:1295–1298.
18. Peltola H, Heinonen O. Frequency of true adverse reactions to Measles-Mumps-Rubella Vaccine. Lancet 1986;1:939–942.
19. CDC. Adverse events following immunization. Surveillance Report No. 3, 1985–1986, Issued February 1989.
20. Herman JJ, Radin R, Schneiderman R. Allergic reactions to measles (rubeola) vaccine in patients hypersensitive to egg protein. J Pediatric 1983;102:196–199.
21. Greenberg MA, Birx DL. Safe administration of mumps-measles-rubella vaccine in egg-allergic children. J Pediatr 1988;113:504–506.
22. Krasinski K, Borkowsky W. Measles and measles immunity in children infected with human immunodeficiency virus. JAMA 1989;261:2512–2516.
23. McLaughlin P, Thomas PA, Onorato I, et al. Use of live virus vaccine in HIV-infected children; a retrospective survey. Pediatrics 1988;82:229–223.
24. ACIP. Immunization of children infected with human immunodeficiency virus—supplementary ACIP statement. MMWR 1988;37:181–183.
25. Deforest A, Long SS, Lischner HW, et al. Simultaneous administration of measles-mumps-rubella vaccine with booster doses of diphtheria-tetanus-pertussis and poliovirus vaccines. Pediatrics 1988;81:237–246.

TOPIC 21 / **MENINGOCOCCOSIS**

Meningococcal Vaccines

Original Citation: ACIP. Meningococcal vaccines: recommendation of the Immunization Practices Advisory Committee (ACIP). MMWR 1985;34(18):255–259.

INTRODUCTION

A polysaccharide vaccine against disease caused by Neisseria meningitidis serogroups A, C, Y, and W-135 is currently licensed in the United States. This statement updates the previous statement (MMWR 1978;27:327–329), summarizes available information on the vaccine, and offers guidelines for its use in the civilian population of the United States.

MENINGOCOCCAL DISEASE

N. meningitidis causes both endemic and epidemic disease, principally meningitis and meningococcemia. It is the second most common cause of bacterial meningitis in the United States (approximately 20% of all cases), affecting an estimated 3,000–4,000 people each year. The case-fatality rate is approximately 10% for meningococcal meningitis and 20% for meningococcemia, despite therapy with antimicrobial agents, such as penicillin, to which all strains remain highly sensitive.

No major epidemic of meningococcal disease has occurred in the United States since 1946, although localized community outbreaks have been reported. The incidence of endemic meningococcal disease peaks in the late winter to early spring. Attack rates are highest among children aged 6–12 months and then steadily decline; by age 5 years, the incidence approximates that for adults. Serogroup B, for which a vaccine is not yet available, accounts for 50%–55% of all cases; serogroup C, for 20%–25%; and serogroup W-135, for 15%. Serogroups Y (10%) and A (1%–2%) account for nearly all remaining cases. Serogroup W-135 has emerged as a major cause of disease only since 1975 (1). While serogroup A causes only a small proportion of endemic disease in the United States, it is the most common cause of epidemics elsewhere. Less commonly, serogroups C and B can also cause epidemic disease.

People with certain chronic conditions appear to be at increased risk of developing meningococcal infection. Meningococcal disease is particularly common among individuals with component deficiencies in the final common complement pathway (C3, C5-C9), many of whom experience multiple episodes of infection (2). Asplenic persons seem also to be at increased risk of developing meningococcal disease and experience particularly severe infections (3). It is uncertain whether individuals with other diseases associated with immunosuppression are at higher risk of acquiring meningococcal disease, as they are for disease caused by other encapsulated bacteria. In the past, new military recruits were at especially high risk, particularly for serogroup C disease; however, since routine vaccination of recruits with the bivalent A/C vaccine began in 1971, disease caused by those serogroups has been uncommon. Military recruits currently receive the A,C,Y,W-135 vaccine.

MENINGOCOCCAL POLYSACCHARIDE VACCINES

The recently licensed quadrivalent A,C,Y,W-135 vaccine (Menomune®—A/C/Y/W-135, manufactured by Squibb-Connaught) is the formulation currently available in the United States. The vaccine consists of 50 μg each of the respective purified bacterial capsular polysaccharides.

Vaccine Efficacy

Numerous studies have demonstrated the immunogenicity and clinical efficacy of the A and C vaccines. The serogroup A polysaccharide induces antibody in some children as young as 3 months of age, although a response comparable to that seen in adults is not achieved until 4 or 5 years of age; the serogroup C component does not induce a good antibody response before age 18–24 months (4, 5). The serogroup A vaccine has been shown to have a clinical efficacy of 85%–95% and to be of use in controlling epidemics. A similar level of clinical efficacy has been demonstrated for the serogroup C vaccine, both in American military recruits and in an epidemic. The group Y and W-135 polysaccharides have been shown to be safe and immunogenic in adults (6–9) and in children over 2 years of age; clinical protection has not been demonstrated directly, but is assumed, based on the production of bactericidal antibody, which for group C has been correlated with clinical protection. The antibody responses to each of the four polysaccharides in the quadrivalent vaccine are serogroup-specific and independent.

Duration of Efficacy

Antibodies against the group A and C polysaccharides decline markedly over the first 3 years following a single dose of vaccine (5, 10–13). This antibody decline is more rapid in infants and young children than in adults. Similarly, while vaccine-induced clinical protection probably persists in schoolchildren and adults for at least 3 years, a recent study in Africa has demonstrated a marked decline in the efficacy of the group A vaccine in young children over time. In this study, efficacy declined from greater than 90% to less than 10% over 3 years in those under 4 years of age at the time of vaccination; in older children, efficacy was still 67% 3 years after vaccination (14).

RECOMMENDATIONS FOR VACCINE USE

Routine vaccination of civilians with meningococcal polysaccharide vaccine is not recommended for the following reasons: (a) the risk of infection in the United States is low; (b) a vaccine against serogroup B, the major cause of meningococcal disease in the United States, is not yet available; and (c) much of the meningococcal disease in the United States occurs among children too young to benefit from the vaccine. However, the vaccine has been shown to be of use in aborting outbreaks due to serogroups represented in the vaccine and should be used in their control. In an outbreak, the serogroup should be determined and the population at risk delineated by neighborhood, school, dormitory, or other reasonable boundary. Although endemic disease is very uncommon above age 5 years, older children, adolescents, and young adults constitute a higher proportion of cases during epidemics and may warrant vaccination during an outbreak (15).

Routine immunization with the quadrivalent vaccine is recommended for particular high-risk groups, including individuals with terminal complement component deficiencies and those with anatomic or functional asplenia. Persons splenectomized because of trauma or nonlymphoid tumors and those with inherited complement deficiencies have acceptable antibody responses to meningococcal vaccine, although clinical efficacy has not been documented (2, 16). It should be recognized that such individuals frequently have preexisting antibody against N. meningitidis and may not be protected by vaccination.

Vaccination with the A-C vaccine may benefit some travelers to countries recognized as having hyperendemic or epidemic disease and Americans living in these areas, particularly those who will have prolonged contact with the local populace. One area of the world recognized as having recurrent epidemics of meningococcal disease is the part of sub-Saharan Africa known as the "meningitis belt," which extends from Mauritania in the west to Ethiopia in the east. Epidemics have been recognized in other parts of the world, and updated information can be obtained from travelers' clinics, state health departments, and CDC.

Primary Immunization

For both adults and children, vaccine is administered subcutaneously as a single 0.5-ml dose. The vaccine can be given at the same time as other immunizations, if needed. Good antibody levels are achieved within 10–14 days after vaccination.

PRECAUTIONS AND CONTRAINDICATIONS

Reactions

Adverse reactions to meningococcal vaccine are mild and infrequent, consisting principally of localized erythema lasting 1–2 days. Up to 2% of young children develop fever transiently after vaccination (13).

Pregnancy

On theoretical grounds, it is prudent not to immunize pregnant women unless there is a substantial risk of infection. However, evaluation of the vaccine in pregnant women during an epidemic in Brazil demonstrated no adverse effects. Further, antibody studies in these women showed good antibody levels in maternal and cord blood following vaccination during any trimester; antibody levels in the infants declined over the first few months and did not affect their subsequent response to immunization (17).

REVACCINATION

Revaccination may be indicated for individuals at high risk of infection, particularly children who were first immunized under 4 years of age; such children should be considered for revaccination after 2 or 3 years if they remain at high risk. The need for revaccination in older children and adults remains unknown.

PROSPECTS FOR FUTURE MENINGOCOCCAL VACCINES

Work is continuing on a serogroup B meningococcal vaccine, as well as on improved A and C vaccines. Candidate vaccines include capsular polysaccharides complexed with meningococcal outer-membrane proteins or covalently linked to carrier proteins. Clinical efficacy data for these vaccines are not available.

ANTIMICROBIAL CHEMOPROPHYLAXIS

Antimicrobial chemoprophylaxis of intimate contacts remains the chief preventive measure in sporadic cases of N. meningitidis disease in the United States. Intimate contacts include (a) household members, (b) day-care-center contacts, and (c) anyone directly exposed to the patient's oral secretions, such as through mouth-to-mouth resuscitation or kissing. The attack rate for household contacts is 0.3%–1%, 300-1000 times the rate in the general population.

Unless the causative organism is known to be sensitive to sulfadiazine, the drug of choice is rifampin, given twice daily for 2 days (600 mg every 12 hours to adults; 10 mg/kg every 12 hours to children 1 month of age or older; 5 mg/kg every 12 hours to children under 1 month of age). Rifampin has been shown to be 90% effective in eradicating nasopharyngeal carriage. No serious adverse effects have been noted. However, rifampin prophylaxis is not recommended for pregnant women, as the drug is feratogenic in laboratory animals. Also, as well as turning urine orange, rifampin is excreted in tears, resulting in staining of contact lenses; thus, they should not be used during the course of therapy.

Because systemic antimicrobial therapy of meningococcal disease does not reliably eradicate nasopharyngeal carriage of N. meningitidis, it is also important to give chemoprophylaxis to the index patient before discharge from the hospital (18).

Nasopharyngeal cultures are not helpful in determining who warrants chemoprophylaxis and unnecessarily delay institution of the preventive measure.

REFERENCES

1. Band JD, Chamberland ME, Platt T, Weaver RE, Thornsberry C, Fraser DW. Trends in meningococcal disease in the United States, 1975–1980. J Infect Dis 1983;148:754–758.

2. Ross SC, Densen P. Complement deficiency states and infection: epidemiology, pathogenesis and consequences of neisserial and other infections in an immune deficiency. Medicine 1984;63:243–273.

3. Francke EL, Neu HC. Postsplenectomy infection. Surg Clin North Am 1981;61:135–155.

4. Peltola H, Kayhty H, Kuronen T, Haque N, Sarna S, Makela PH. Meningococcus group A vaccine in children three months to five years of age. Adverse reactions and immunogenicity related to endotoxin content and molecular weight of the polysaccharide. J Pediatr 1978;92:818–822.

5. Gold R, Lepow ML, Goldschneider I, Draper TF, Gotschlich EC. Kinetics of antibody production to group A and group C meningococcal polysaccharide vaccines administered during the first six years of life: prospects for routine immunization of infants and children. J Infect Dis 1979;140:690–697.

10. Artenstein MS. Meningococcal infections: 5. Duration of polysaccharide-vaccine-induced antibody. Bull WHO 1971;45:291–293.

11. Lepow ML, Goldschneider I, Gold R, Randolph M, Gotschlich EC. Persistence of antibody following immunization of children with groups A and C meningococcal polysaccharide vaccines. Pediatrics 1977;60:673–680.

12. Greenwood BM, Whittle HC, Bradley AK, Fayet MT, Gilles HM. The duration of the antibody response to meningococcal vaccination in an African village. Trans R Soc Trop Med Hyg 1980;74:756–760.

13. Kayhty H, Karanko V, Peltola H, Sarna S, Makela PH. Serum antibodies to capsular polysaccharide vaccine of group A Neisseria meningitidis followed for three years in infants and children. J Infect Dis 1980;142:861–868.

14. CDC. Unpublished data.

15. Peltola H. Meningococcal disease: still with us. Rev Infect Dis 1983;5:71–91.

16. Ruben FL, Hankins WA, Zeigler Z, et al. Antibody responses to meningococcal polysaccharide vaccine in adults without a spleen. Am J Med 1984;76:115–121.

17. McCormick JB, Gusmao HH, Nakamura S, et al. Antibody response to serogroup A and C meningococcal polysaccharide vaccines in infants born of mothers vaccinated during pregnancy. J Clin Invest 1980;65:1141–1144.

18. Abramson JS, Spika JS. Persistence of Neisseria meningitidis in the upper respiratory tract after intravenous antibiotic therapy for systemic meningococcal disease. J Infect Dis 1985;151:370–371.

TOPIC 22 / **MUMPS**

Mumps Prevention

Original Citation: ACIP. Mumps prevention: recommendations of the Immunization Practices Advisory Committee Mumps Prevention. MMWR 1989;38(22):388–392, 397–400.

This revised Immunization Practices Advisory Committee (ACIP) recommendation on mumps vaccine updates the 1982 recommendation (1). Changes include: a discussion of the evolving epidemiologic characteristics of mumps, introduction of a cutoff of 1957 as the oldest birth cohort for which mumps vaccination is routinely recommended, and more aggressive outbreak-control measures. Although there are no major changes in vaccination strategy, these revised recommendations place a greater emphasis on vaccinating susceptible adolescents and young adults.

INTRODUCTION

Mumps Disease

Mumps disease is generally self-limited, but it may be moderately debilitating. Naturally acquired mumps infection, including the estimated 30% of infections that are subclinical, confers long-lasting immunity.

Among the reported mumps-associated complications, strong epidemiologic and laboratory evidence for an association with meningoencephalitis, deafness, and orchitis has been reported (2). Meningeal signs appear in up to 15% of cases. Reported rates of mumps encephalitis range as high as five cases per 1000 reported mumps cases. Permanent sequelae are rare, but the reported encephalitis case-fatality rate has averaged 1.4%. Although overall mortality is low, death due to mumps infection is much more likely to occur in adults; about half of mumps-associated deaths have been in persons greater than or equal to 20 years old (2). Sensorineural deafness is one of the most serious of the rare complications involving the central nervous system (CNS). It occurs with an estimated frequency of 0.5–5.0 per 100,000 reported mumps cases. Orchitis (usually unilateral) has been reported as a complication in 20%–30% of clinical mumps cases in postpubertal males (3). Some testicular atrophy occurs in about 35% of cases of mumps orchitis, but sterility rarely occurs. Symptomatic involvement of other organs has been observed less frequently. There are limited experimental, clinical, and epidemiologic data that suggest permanent pancreatic damage may result from injury caused by direct viral invasion. Further research is needed to determine whether mumps infection contributes to the pathogenesis of diabetes mellitus. Mumps infection during the first trimester of pregnancy may increase the rate of spontaneous abortion (reported to be as high as 27%). There is no evidence that mumps during pregnancy causes congenital malformations.

Epidemiology

Following the introduction of the live mumps virus vaccine in 1967 and recommendation of its routine use in 1977, the incidence rate of reported mumps cases decreased steadily in the United States. In 1985, a record low of 2982 cases was reported, representing a 98% decline from the 185,691 cases reported in 1967. However, between 1985 and 1987, a relative resurgence of mumps occurred, with 7790 cases reported in 1986 and 12,848 cases in 1987 (4). During this 3-year period, the annual reported incidence rate rose almost fivefold, from 1.1 cases per 100,000 population to 5.2 cases per 100,000 population. In 1988, a provisional total of 4730 cases was reported, representing a 62% decrease from 1987.

As in the prevaccine era, the majority of reported mumps cases still occur in school-aged children (5–14 years of age). Almost 60% of reported cases occurred in this population between 1985 and 1987, compared with an average of 75% of reported cases between 1967 and 1971, the first 5-year period postlicensure. However, for the first time since mumps became a reportable disease, the reported peak incidence rate shifted from 5–9-year-olds to older age groups for two consecutive years (1986 and 1987). Persons greater than or equal to 15 years of age accounted for more than one-third of the reported total between 1985 and 1987; in 1967–1971, an average of only 8% of reported cases occurred among this population. Although reported mumps incidence increased in all age groups from 1985 to 1987, the most dramatic increases were among 10–14-year-olds (almost a sevenfold increase) and 15–19-year-olds (more than an eightfold increase).

The increased occurrence of mumps in susceptible adolescents and young adults has been demonstrated in several recent outbreaks in high schools and on college campuses (5, 6) and in occupational settings (7). Nonetheless, despite this age shift in reported mumps, the overall reported risk of disease in persons 10–14 and greater than or equal to 15 years of age is still lower than that in the prevaccine and early postvaccine era.

Consistent with previous findings (8), reported incidence rates are lower in states with comprehensive school immunization laws. The District of Columbia and 14 states that routinely reported mumps cases in 1987 had comprehensive laws that require proof of immunity against mumps for school attendance from kindergarten through grade 12 (K–12). In these 15 areas, the incidence rate in 1987 was 1.1 mumps cases per 100,000 population. In contrast, among the other states that routinely reported mumps cases in 1987, mumps incidence was highest in the 14 states without requirements for mumps vaccination (11.5 cases per 100,000 population), and intermediate (6.2 cases per 100,000 population) in the 18 states with partial vaccination requirements for school attendance (i.e., those that include some children but do not comprehensively include K–12). Furthermore, the shift in age-specific risk noted above occurred only in states without comprehensive K–12 school vaccination requirements.

Both the shift in risk to older persons and the relative resurgence of reported mumps activity noted in recent years are attributable to the relatively underimmunized cohort of children born between 1967 and 1977 (9). There is no evidence of waning immunity in vaccinated persons. During 1967–1977, the risk of exposure to mumps declined rapidly even though vaccination of children against mumps was only gradually being accepted as a routine practice. Simultaneously, mumps vaccine coverage did not reach levels greater than 50% in any age group until 1976 (5–9-year-olds); in persons 15–19 years old, vaccine coverage did not reach these levels until 1983. This lag in coverage relative to measles and rubella vaccines reflects the lack of an ACIP recommendation for routine mumps vaccine until 1977 and the lack of emphasis in

ACIP recommendations on vaccination beyond toddler age until 1980. These facts and the observed shift in risk to older persons in states without comprehensive mumps immunization school laws provide further evidence that a failure to vaccinate, rather than vaccine failure, is primarily responsible for the recently observed changes in mumps occurrence.

MUMPS VIRUS VACCINE

A killed mumps virus vaccine was licensed for use in the United States from 1950 through 1978. This vaccine induced antibody, but the immunity was transient. The number of doses of killed mumps vaccine administered between licensure of live attenuated mumps vaccine in 1967 until 1978 is unknown but appears to have been limited.

Mumps virus vaccine* is prepared in chick-embryo cell culture. More than 84 million doses were distributed in the United States from its introduction in December 1967 through 1988. The vaccine produces a subclinical, noncommunicable infection with very few side effects. Mumps vaccine is available both in monovalent (mumps only) form and in combinations: mumps-rubella and measles-mumps-rubella (MMR) vaccines.

The vaccine is approximately 95% efficacious in preventing mumps disease (10, 11); greater than 97% of persons known to be susceptible to mumps develop measurable antibody following vaccination (12). Vaccine-induced antibody is protective and long-lasting (13, 14), although of considerably lower titer than antibody resulting from natural infection (12). The duration of vaccine-induced immunity is unknown, but serologic and epidemiologic data collected during 20 years of live vaccine use indicate both the persistence of antibody and continuing protection against infection. Estimates of clinical vaccine efficacy ranging from 75% to 95% have been calculated from data collected in outbreak settings using different epidemiologic study designs (8, 15).

Vaccine Shipment and Storage

Administration of improperly stored vaccine may fail to protect against mumps. During storage before reconstitution, mumps vaccine must be kept at 2–8°C (35.6–46.4°F) or colder. It must also be protected from light, which may inactivate the virus. Vaccine must be shipped at 10°C (50°F) or colder and may be shipped on dry ice. After reconstitution, the vaccine should be stored in a dark place at 2–8°C (35.6–46.4°F) and discarded if not used within 8 hours.

VACCINE USAGE

(See also the current ACIP statement, "General Recommendations on Immunization" (16).)

General Recommendations

Susceptible children, adolescents, and adults should be vaccinated against mumps, unless vaccination is contraindicated. Mumps vaccine is of particular value for children approaching puberty and for adolescents and adults who have not had mumps. MMR vaccine is the vaccine of choice for routine administration and should be used in all situations where recipients are also likely to be susceptible to measles and/or rubella. The favorable benefit-cost ratio for routine mumps immunization is more marked when vaccine is administered as MMR (17). Persons should be considered susceptible to mumps unless they have documentation of (a) physician-diagnosed mumps, (b) adequate immunization with live mumps virus vaccine on or after their first birthday, or (c) laboratory evidence of immunity. Because live mumps vaccine was not used routinely before 1977 and because the peak age-specific incidence was in 5–9-year-olds before the vaccine was introduced, most persons born before 1957 are likely to

---

* Official name: Mumps Virus Vaccine, Live.

have been infected naturally between 1957 and 1977. Therefore, they generally may be considered to be immune, even if they may not have had clinically recognizable mumps disease. However, this cutoff date for susceptibility is arbitrary. Although outbreak-control efforts should be focused on persons born after 1956, these recommendations do not preclude vaccination of possibly susceptible persons born before 1957 who may be exposed in outbreak settings.

Persons who are unsure of their mumps disease history and/or mumps vaccination history should be vaccinated. There is no evidence that persons who have previously either received mumps vaccine or had mumps are at any increased risk of local or systemic reactions from receiving live mumps vaccine. Testing for susceptibility before vaccination, especially among adolescents and young adults, is not necessary. In addition to the expense, some tests (e.g., mumps skin test and the complement-fixation antibody test) may be unreliable, and tests with established reliability (neutralization, enzyme immunoassay, and radial hemolysis antibody tests) are not readily available.

Dosage

A single dose of vaccine in the volume specified by the manufacturer should be administered subcutaneously. While not recommended routinely, intramuscular vaccination is effective and safe.

Age

Live mumps virus vaccine is recommended at any age on or after the first birthday for all susceptible persons, unless a contraindication exists. Under routine circumstances, mumps vaccine should be given in combination with measles and rubella vaccines as MMR, following the currently recommended schedule for administration of measles vaccine. It should not be administered to infants less than 12 months old because persisting maternal antibody might interfere with seroconversion. To insure immunity, all persons vaccinated before the first birthday should be revaccinated on or after the first birthday.

Persons Exposed to Mumps

Use of Vaccine

When given after exposure to mumps, live mumps virus vaccine may not provide protection. However, if the exposure did not result in infection, vaccine should induce protection against infection from subsequent exposures. There is no evidence that the risk of vaccine-associated adverse events increases if vaccine is administered to persons incubating disease.

Use of Immune Globulin

Immune globulin (IG) has not been demonstrated to be of established value in postexposure prophylaxis and is not recommended. Mumps immune globulin has not been shown to be effective and is no longer available or licensed for use in the United States.

Adverse Effects of Vaccine Use

In field trials before licensure, illnesses did not occur more often in vaccinees than in unvaccinated controls (18). Reports of illnesses following mumps vaccination have mainly been episodes of parotitis and low-grade fever. Allergic reactions including rash, pruritus, and purpura have been temporally associated with mumps vaccination but are uncommon and usually mild and of brief duration. The reported occurrence of encephalitis within 30 days of receipt of a mumps-containing vaccine (0.4 per million doses) is not greater than the observed background incidence rate of CNS dysfunction in the normal population. Other manifestations of CNS involvement, such as febrile seizures and deafness, have also been infrequently reported. Complete recovery is usual. Reports of nervous system illness following mumps vaccination do not necessarily denote an etiologic relationship between the illness and the vaccine.

Contraindications to Vaccine Use

Pregnancy

Although mumps vaccine virus has been shown to infect the placenta and fetus (19), there is no evidence that it causes congenital malformations in humans. However, because of the theoretical risk of fetal damage, it is prudent to avoid giving live virus vaccine to pregnant women. Vaccinated women should avoid pregnancy for 3 months after vaccination. Routine precautions for vaccinating postpubertal women include asking if they are or may be pregnant, excluding those who say they are, and explaining the theoretical risk to those who plan to receive the vaccine. Vaccination during pregnancy should not be considered an indication for termination of pregnancy. However, the final decision about interruption of pregnancy must rest with the individual patient and her physician.

Severe Febrile Illness

Vaccine administration should not be postponed because of minor or intercurrent febrile illnesses, such as mild upper respiratory infections. However, vaccination of persons with severe febrile illnesses should generally be deferred until they have recovered.

Allergies

Because live mumps vaccine is produced in chick-embryo cell culture, persons with a history of anaphylactic reactions (hives, swelling of the mouth and throat, difficulty breathing, hypotension, or shock) after egg ingestion should be vaccinated only with caution using published protocols (20, 21). Known allergic children should not leave the vaccination site for 20 minutes. Evidence indicates that persons are not at increased risk if they have egg allergies that are not anaphylactic in nature. Such persons may be vaccinated in the usual manner. There is no evidence to indicate that persons with allergies to chickens or feathers are at increased risk of reaction to the vaccine.

Since mumps vaccine contains trace amounts of neomycin (25 μg), persons who have experienced anaphylactic reactions to topically or systemically administered neomycin should not receive mumps vaccine. Most often, neomycin allergy is manifested as a contact dermatitis, which is a delayed-type (cell-mediated) immune response, rather than anaphylaxis. In such persons, the adverse reaction, if any, to 25 μg of neomycin in the vaccine would be an erythematous, pruritic nodule or papule at 48–96 hours. A history of contact dermatitis to neomycin is not a contraindication to receiving mumps vaccine. Live mumps virus vaccine does not contain penicillin.

Recent IG Injection

Passively acquired antibody can interfere with the response to live, attenuated-virus vaccines. Therefore, mumps vaccine should be given at least 2 weeks before the administration of IG or deferred until approximately 3 months after the administration of IG.

Altered Immunity

In theory, replication of the mumps vaccine virus may be potentiated in patients with immune deficiency diseases and by the suppressed immune responses that occur with leukemia, lymphoma, or generalized malignancy or with therapy with corticosteroids, alkylating drugs, antimetabolites, or radiation. In general, patients with such conditions should not be given live mumps virus vaccine. Because vaccinated persons do not transmit mumps vaccine virus, the risk of mumps exposure for those patients may be reduced by vaccinating their close susceptible contacts.

An exception to these general recommendations is in children infected with human immunodeficiency virus (HIV); all asymptomatic HIV-infected children should receive MMR at 15 months of age (22). If measles vaccine is administered to symptomatic HIV-infected children, the combination MMR vaccine is generally preferred (23).

Patients with leukemia in remission whose chemotherapy has been terminated for at least 3 months may also receive live mumps virus vaccine. Short-term (less than 2 weeks' duration) corticosteroid therapy, topical steroid therapy (e.g., nasal, skin), and intraarticular, bursal, or tendon injection with corticosteroids do not contraindicate mumps vaccine administration. However, mumps vaccine should be avoided if systemic immunosuppressive levels are reached by prolonged, extensive, topical application.

Other

There is no known association between mumps vaccination and pancreatic damage or subsequent development of diabetes mellitus (24).

MUMPS CONTROL

The principal strategy to prevent mumps is to achieve and maintain high immunization levels, primarily in infants and young children. Universal immunization as a part of good health care should be routinely carried out in physicians' offices and public health clinics. Programs aimed at vaccinating children with MMR should be established and maintained in all communities. In addition, all other persons thought to be susceptible should be vaccinated unless otherwise contraindicated. This is especially important for adolescents and young adults in light of the recently observed increase in risk of disease in these populations.

Because access to some population subgroups is limited, the ACIP recommends taking maximal advantage of clinic visits to vaccinate susceptible persons greater than or equal to 15 months of age by administering MMR, diphtheria-tetanus-pertussis (DTP), and oral polio vaccine (OPV) simultaneously if all are needed. Health agencies should take necessary steps, including the development, adoption, and enforcement of comprehensive immunization requirements, to ensure that all persons in schools at all grade levels and in day-care settings are protected against mumps. Similar requirements should be considered for colleges, as recommended by the American College Health Association (25), and selected places of employment where persons in this age cohort are likely to be concentrated or where the consequences of disease spread may be more severe (e.g., medical-care settings).

In determining means to control mumps outbreaks, exclusion of susceptible students from affected schools and schools judged by local public health authorities to be at risk for transmission should be considered. Such exclusion should be an effective means of terminating school outbreaks and quickly increasing rates of immunization. Excluded students can be readmitted immediately after vaccination. Pupils who have been exempted from mumps vaccination because of medical, religious, or other reasons should be excluded until at least 26 days after the onset of parotitis in the last person with mumps in the affected school. Experience with outbreak control for other vaccine-preventable diseases indicates that almost all students who are excluded from the outbreak area because they lack evidence of immunity quickly comply with requirements and can be readmitted to school.

MUMPS DISEASE SURVEILLANCE AND REPORTING OF ADVERSE EVENTS

There is a continuing need to improve the reporting of mumps cases and complications and to document the duration of vaccine effectiveness. Thus, for areas in which mumps is a reportable disease, all suspected cases of mumps should be reported to local or state health officials.

The National Childhood Vaccine Injury Compensation Program established by the National Childhood Vaccine Injury Compensation Act of 1986 requires physicians and other health-care providers who administer vaccines to maintain permanent immunization records and to report occurrences of certain adverse events to the U.S. Department of Health and Human Services. Recording and reporting requirements took effect on March 21, 1988. Reportable adverse events include those listed in the Act for mumps (26) and events specified in the manufacturer's vaccine package insert as contraindications to further doses of mumps vaccine.

Although there eventually will be one system for reporting adverse events following immunizations, two separate systems currently exist. The appropriate reporting method currently depends on the source of funding used to purchase the vaccine (26). Events that occur after receipt of a vaccine purchased with public (federal, state, and/or local government) funds must be reported by the administering health provider to the appropriate local, county, or state health department. The state health department completes and submits the correct forms to CDC. Reportable events that follow administration of vaccines purchased with private money are reported by the health-care provider directly to the Food and Drug Administration.

RECOMMENDATIONS FOR INTERNATIONAL TRAVEL

Mumps is still endemic throughout most of the world. While vaccination against mumps is not a requirement for entry into any country, susceptible children, adolescents, and adults would benefit by being vaccinated with a single dose of vaccine (usually as MMR), unless contraindicated, before beginning travel. Because of concern about inadequate seroconversion due to persisting maternal antibodies and because the risk of serious disease from mumps infection is relatively low, persons less than 12 months of age need not be given mumps vaccine before travel.

REFERENCES

1. ACIP. Mumps vaccine. MMWR 1982;31:617–620, 625.
2. CDC. Mumps surveillance, January 1977-December 1982. Atlanta: US Department of Health and Human Services, Public Health Service, 1984.
3. Philip RN, Reinhard KR, Lackman DB. Observations on a mumps epidemic in a "virgin" population. Am J Hyg 1959;69:91–111.
4. CDC. Mumps—United States, 1985–1988. MMWR 1989;38:101–105.
5. Sosin DM, Cochi SL, Gunn RA, Jennings CE, Preblud SR. The changing epidemiology of mumps and its impact on university campuses. Pediatrics 1989 (in press).

6. Wharton M, Cochi SL, Hutcheson RH, Bistowish JM, Schaffner W. A large outbreak of mumps in the postvaccine era. J Infect Dis 1988;158:1253–1260.

7. Kaplan KM, Marder DC, Cochi SL, Preblud SR. Mumps in the workplace: further evidence of the changing epidemiology of a childhood vaccine-preventable disease. JAMA 1988;260:1434–1438.

8. Chaiken BP, Williams NM, Preblud SR, Parkin W, Altman R. The effect of a school entry law on mumps activity in a school district. JAMA 1987;257:2455–2458.

9. Cochi SL, Preblud SR, Orenstein WA. Perspectives on the relative resurgence of mumps in the United States. Am J Dis Child 1988;142:499–507.

10. Hilleman MR, Weibel RE, Buynak EB, Stokes J Jr, Whitman JE Jr. Live, attenuated mumps virus vaccine: 4. Protective efficacy as measured in a field evaluation. N Engl J Med 1967;276: 252–258.

11. Sugg WC, Finger JA, Levine RH, Pagano JS. Field evaluation of live virus mumps vaccine. J Pediatr 1968;72:461–466.

12. Weibel RE, Stokes J Jr, Buynak EB, Whitman JE Jr, Hilleman MR. Live, attenuated mumps virus vaccine: 3. Clinical and serologic aspects in a field evaluation. N Engl J Med 1967;276:245–251.

13. Weibel RE, Buynak EB, McLean AA, Hilleman MR. Follow-up surveillance for antibody in human subjects following live attenuated measles, mumps, and rubella virus vaccines. Proc Soc Exp Biol Med 1979;162:328–332.

14. Weibel RE, Buynak EB, McLean AA, Roehm RR, Hilleman MR. Persistence of antibody in human subjects for 7 to 10 years following administration of combined live attenuated measles, mumps, and rubella virus vaccines. Proc Soc Exp Biol Med 1980;165:260–263.

15. Kim-Farley R, Bart S, Stetler H, et al. Clinical mumps vaccine efficacy. Am J Epidemiol 1985; 121:593–597.

16. ACIP. General recommendations on immunization. MMWR 1989;38:205–214, 219–227.

17. Koplan JP, Preblud SR. A benefit-cost analysis of mumps vaccine. Am J Dis Child 1982;136:362–364.

18. Hilleman MR, Buynak EB, Weibel RE, Stokes J Jr. Live, attenuated mumps-virus vaccine. N Engl J Med 1968;278:227–232.

19. Yamauchi T, Wilson C, St. Geme JW Jr. Transmission of live, attenuated mumps virus to the human placenta. N Engl J Med 1974;290:710–712.

20. Herman JJ, Radin R, Schneiderman R. Allergic reactions to measles (rubeola) vaccine in patients hypersensitive to egg protein. J Pediatr 1983;102:196–199.

21. Greenberg MA, Birx DL. Safe administration of mumps-measles-rubella vaccine in egg-allergic children. J Pediatr 1988;113:504–506.

22. ACIP. Immunization of children infected with human T-lymphotrophic virus type III/lymphadenopathy-associated virus. MMWR 1986;35:595–598, 603–606.

23. ACIP. Immunization of children infected with human immunodeficiency virus—supplementary ACIP statement. MMWR 1988;37:181–183.

24. Sinaniotis CA, Daskalopoulou E, Lapatsanis P, Doxiadis S. Diabetes mellitus after mumps vaccination [Letter]. Arch Dis Child 1975;50:749–750.

25. American College Health Association. Position statement on immunization policy. J Am Coll Health 1983;32:7–8.

26. CDC. National Childhood Vaccine Injury Act: requirements for permanent vaccination records and for reporting of selected events after vaccination. MMWR 1988;37:197–200.

TOPIC 23 / **PNEUMOCOCCOSIS**

Pneumococcal Polysaccharide Vaccine

Original Citation: ACIP. Pneumococcal polysaccharide vaccine, recommendations of the Immunization Practices Advisory Committee. MMWR 1989;38(5):64–68, 73–76.

These recommendations update the last statement by the Immunization Practices Advisory Committee (ACIP) on pneumococcal polysaccharide vaccine (MMWR 1984;33:273–276, 281) and include new information regarding (a) vaccine efficacy, (b) use in persons with human immunodeficiency virus (HIV) infection and in other groups at increased risk of pneumococcal disease, and (c) guidelines for revaccination.

INTRODUCTION

Disease caused by Streptococcus pneumoniae (pneumococcus) remains an important cause of morbidity and mortality in the United States, particularly in the very young, the elderly, and persons with certain high-risk conditions. Pneumococcal pneumonia accounts for 10%–25% of all pneumonias and an estimated 40, 000 deaths annually (1). Although no recent data from the United States exist, in the United Kingdom pneumococcal infections may account for 34% of pneumonias in adults who require hospitalization (2). The best estimates of the incidence of serious pneumococcal disease in the United States are based on surveys and community-based studies of pneumococcal bacteremia. Recent studies suggest annual rates of bacteremia of 15–19/100,000 for all persons, 50/100,000 for persons greater than or equal to 65 years old, and 160/100,000 for children less than or equal to 2 years old (3, 4). These rates are 2–3 times those previously documented in the United States. The overall rate for pneumococcal bacteremia in some Native American populations can be six times the rate of the general population (5). The incidence of pneumococcal pneumonia can be 3–5 times that of the detected rates of bacteremia. The estimated incidence of pneumococcal meningitis is 1–2/100,000 persons.

Mortality from pneumococcal disease is highest in patients with bacteremia or meningitis, patients with underlying medical conditions, and older persons. In some high-risk patients, mortality has been reported to be greater than 40% for bacteremic disease and 55% for meningitis, despite appropriate antimicrobial therapy. Over 90% of pneumococci remain very sensitive to penicillin.

In addition to the very young and persons greater than or equal to 65 years old, patients with certain chronic conditions are at increased risk of developing pneumococcal infection and severe pneumococcal illness. Patients with chronic cardiovascular diseases, chronic pulmonary disease, diabetes mellitus, alcoholism, and cirrhosis are generally immunocompetent but have increased risk. Other patients at greater risk because of decreased responsiveness to polysaccharide antigens or more rapid decline in serum antibody include those with functional or anatomic asplenia (e.g., sickle cell disease or splenectomy), Hodgkin's disease, lymphoma, multiple myeloma, chronic renal failure, nephrotic syndrome, and organ transplantation. In a recent population-based study, all persons 55–64 years old with pneumococcal bacteremia had at least one of these chronic conditions (4). Studies indicate that patients with acquired immunodeficiency syndrome (AIDS) are also at increased risk of pneumococcal disease, with an annual attack rate of pneumococcal pneumonia as high as 17.9/1000 (6–8). This observation is consistent with the B-cell dysfunction noted in patients with AIDS (9, 10). Recurrent pneumococcal meningitis may occur in patients with cerebrospinal fluid leakage complicating skull fractures or neurologic procedures.

PNEUMOCOCCAL POLYSACCHARIDE VACCINE

The current pneumococcal vaccine (Pneumovax 23, Merck Sharp & Dohme, and Pnu-Imune 23, Lederle Laboratories) is composed of purified capsular polysaccharide antigens of 23 types of S. pneumoniae (Danish types 1, 2, 3, 4, 5, 6B, 7F, 8, 9N, 9V, 10A, 11A, 12F, 14, 15B, 17F, 18C, 19F, 19A, 20, 22F, 23F, 33F). It was licensed in the United States in 1983, replacing a 14-valent vaccine licensed in 1977. Each vaccine dose (0.5 mL) contains 25 mg of each polysaccharide antigen. The 23 capsular types in the vaccine cause 88% of the bacteremic pneumococcal disease in the United States. In addition, studies of the human antibody response indicate that cross-reactivity occurs for several types (e.g., 6A and 6B) that cause an additional 8% of bacteremic disease (11).

Most healthy adults, including the elderly, show a twofold or greater rise in type-specific antibody, as measured by radioimmunoassay, within 2–3 weeks of vaccination. Similar antibody responses have been reported in patients with alcoholic cirrhosis and diabetes mellitus requiring insulin. In immunocompromised patients, the response to vaccination may be less. In children less than 2 years old, antibody response to most capsular types is generally poor. In addition, response to some important pediatric pneumococcal types (e.g., 6A and 14) is decreased in children less than 5 years old (12, 13).

Following vaccination of healthy adults with polyvalent pneumococcal vaccine, antibody levels for most pneumococcal vaccine types remain elevated at least 5 years; in some persons, they fall to prevaccination levels within 10 years (14, 15). A more rapid decline in antibody levels may occur in children. In children who have undergone splenectomy following trauma and in those with sickle cell disease, antibody titers for some types can fall to prevaccination levels 3–5 years after vaccination (16, 17). Similar rates of decline can occur in children with nephrotic syndrome (18).

Patients with AIDS have been shown to have an impaired antibody response to pneumococcal vaccine (10, 19). However, asymptomatic HIV-infected men or those with persistent generalized lymphadenopathy respond to the 23-valent pneumococcal vaccine (20).

VACCINE EFFICACY

In the 1970s, pneumococcal vaccine was shown to reduce significantly the occurrence of pneumonia in young, healthy populations in South Africa and Papua New Guinea, where incidence of pneumonia is high (21, 22). It was also demonstrated to protect against systemic pneumococcal infection in hyposplenic patients in the United States (23). Since then, studies have attempted to assess vaccine efficacy in other U.S. populations (24–30; CDC, unpublished data) (Table 1). A prospective, ongoing case-control study in Connecticut has shown an overall protective efficacy of 61% against pneumococcal bacteremia caused by vaccine- and vaccine-related serotypes. The protective efficacy was 60% for patients with alcoholism or chronic pulmonary, cardiac, or renal disease and 64% for patients greater than or equal to 55 years old without other high-risk chronic conditions (25, 26). In another multicenter case-control study, vaccine efficacy in immunocompetent persons greater than or equal to 55 years old was 70% (27). A smaller case-control study of veterans failed to show efficacy in preventing pneumococcal bacteremia (28), but determination of the vaccination status was judged to be inadequate and the selection of controls was considered to be potentially biased.

Studies based on CDC's pneumococcal surveillance system suggest an efficacy of 60%–64% for vaccine-type strains in patients with bacteremic disease. For all persons greater than or equal to 65 years of age (including persons with chronic heart disease, pulmonary disease, or diabetes mellitus), vaccine efficacy was 44%–61% (29; CDC, unpublished data). In addition, estimates of vaccine efficacy for serologically related types were 29%–66% (29). Limited data suggest that clinical efficacy may decline greater than or equal to6 years after vaccination (CDC, unpublished data).

A randomized, double-blind, placebo-controlled trial among high-risk veterans showed no vaccine efficacy against pneumococcal pneumonia or bronchitis (30); however, case definitions used were judged to have uncertain specificity. In addition, this study had only a 6% ability to detect a vaccine efficacy of 65% for pneumococcal bacteremia (31). In contrast, a French clinical trial found pneumococcal vaccine to be 77% effective in reducing the incidence of pneumonia in nursing home residents (32).

Despite conflicting findings, the data continue to support the use of the pneumococcal vaccine for certain well-defined groups at risk.

Table 1. Clinical effectiveness of pneumococcal vaccination in U.S. populations

Location	Method	No. persons	Type infection	Vaccine efficacy (%)	95% C.I.
Connecticut (25, 26)	Case-control*	543 cases 543 controls	VT[+], VT-related	61	42, 73
Philadelphia (27)	Case-control*	122 cases 244 controls	All serotypes	70	37, 86
Denver (28)	Case-control*	89 cases 89 controls	All serotypes	−21	−221, 55
CDC-1 (29)	Epidemiologic*	249 vaccinated 1638 unvaccinated	VT	64	47, 76
CDC-2 (unpublished)	Epidemiologic*	240 vaccinated 1527 unvaccinated	VT	60	45, 70
VA cooperative study (30)	Randomized controlled trial§	1145 vaccinated 1150 controls	All serotypes VT	−34[¶] −19[¶]	−119, 18[¶] −164, 47[¶]

*Only patients with isolates from normally sterile body sites were included.
[†]Vaccine-type pneumococcal infection.
[§]Pneumococcal pneumonia and bronchitis were diagnosed primarily by culture of respiratory secretions.
[¶]Values calculated from the published data.

RECOMMENDATIONS FOR VACCINE USE

Adults

1. Immunocompetent adults who are at increased risk of pneumococcal disease or its complications because of chronic illnesses (e.g., cardiovascular disease, pulmonary disease, diabetes mellitus, alcoholism, cirrhosis, or cerebrospinal fluid leaks) or who are greater than or equal to 65 years old.
2. Immunocompromised adults at increased risk of pneumococcal disease or its complications (e.g., persons with splenic dysfunction or anatomic asplenia, Hodgkin's disease, lymphoma, multiple myeloma, chronic renal failure, nephrotic syndrome, or conditions such as organ transplantation associated with immunosuppression).
3. Adults with asymptomatic or symptomatic HIV infection.

Children

1. Children greater than or equal to 2 years old with chronic illnesses specifically associated with increased risk of pneumococcal disease or its complications (e.g., anatomic or functional asplenia (including sickle cell disease), nephrotic syndrome, cerebrospinal fluid leaks, and conditions associated with immunosuppression).
2. Children greater than or equal to 2 years old with asymptomatic or symptomatic HIV infection.
3. The currently available 23-valent vaccine is not indicated for patients having only recurrent upper respiratory tract disease, including otitis media and sinusitis.

Special Groups

Persons living in special environments or social settings with an identified increased risk of pneumococcal disease or its complications (e.g., certain Native American populations).

ADVERSE REACTIONS

Approximately 50% of persons given pneumococcal vaccine develop mild side effects, such as erythema and pain at the injection site. Fever, myalgia, and severe local reactions have been reported in less than 1% of those vaccinated. Severe systemic reactions, such as anaphylaxis, rarely have been reported.

PRECAUTIONS

The safety of pneumococcal vaccine for pregnant women has not been evaluated. Ideally, women at high risk of pneumococcal disease should be vaccinated before pregnancy.

TIMING OF VACCINATION

When elective splenectomy is being considered, pneumococcal vaccine should be given at least 2 weeks before the operation, if possible. Similarly, for planning cancer chemotherapy or immunosuppressive therapy, as in patients who undergo organ transplantation, the interval between vaccination and initiation of chemotherapy or immunosuppression should also be at least 2 weeks.

REVACCINATION

In one study, local reactions after revaccination in adults were more severe than after initial vaccination when the interval between vaccinations was 13 months (33) (Table 2). Reports of revaccination after longer intervals in children and adults, including a large group of elderly persons revaccinated at least 4 years after primary vaccination, suggest a similar incidence of such reactions after primary vaccination and revaccination (unpublished data; 17, 34–38).

Table 2. Reactions to revaccination with pneumococcal vaccine

| Study | Vaccinees | | | Revaccination period | Reactions |
	Condition	Age	No.		
Borgono, et al. 1978 (33)	Normal	Adults	7	13 mos	Increase in local reactions
Carlson, et al. 1979 (34)	Normal	21–62 yrs	23	12–18 mos	Increase in local reactions
Rigau-Perez, et al. 1983 (35)	Sickle cell disease	≥3 yrs	28	28–35 mos	No increase in reactions compared with primary vaccination
Lawrence, et al. 1983 (36)	Normal	2–5 yrs	52	35 mos (mean)	Increase in local reactions
Mufson, et al. 1984 (37)	Normal	23–40 yrs	12	24–48 mos	No increase in reactions compared with primary vaccination
Weintrub, et al. 1984 (17)	Sickle cell disease	10–27 yrs	17	8–9 yrs	No "serious" local reactions
Kaplan, et al. 1986 (38)	Sickle cell disease	4–23 yrs	86	37–53 mos	Four "severe" reactions*

*Severe reaction was defined as presence of local pain, redness, swelling, and axillary temperature <100°F (37.8°C); two patients aged 21 and 23 years had temperatures of 102°F (38.9°C).

Without more information, persons who received the 14-valent pneumococcal vaccine should not be routinely revaccinated with the 23-valent vaccine, as increased coverage is modest and duration of protection is not well defined. However, revaccination with the 23-valent vaccine should be strongly considered for persons who received the 14-valent vaccine if they are at highest risk of fatal pneumococcal infection (e.g., asplenic patients). Revaccination should also be considered for adults at highest risk who received the 23-valent vaccine greater than or equal to 6 years before and for those shown to have rapid decline in pneumococcal antibody levels (e.g., patients with nephrotic syndrome, renal failure, or transplant recipients). Revaccination after 3–5 years should be considered for children with nephrotic syndrome, asplenia, or sickle cell anemia who would be less than or equal to 10 years old at revaccination.

STRATEGIES FOR VACCINE DELIVERY

Recommendations for pneumococcal vaccination have been made by the ACIP, the American Academy of Pediatrics, the American College of Physicians, and the American Academy of Family Physicians. Recent analysis indicates that pneumococcal vaccination of elderly persons is cost-effective (39). The vaccine is targeted for approximately 27 million persons aged greater than or equal to 65 years and 21 million persons aged less than 65 years with high-risk conditions (1). Despite Medicare reimbursement for costs of the vaccine and its administration, which began in 1981, annual use of pneumococcal vaccine has not increased above levels observed in earlier years (40) (Fig. 1). In 1985, less than 10% of the 48 million persons considered to be at increased risk of serious pneumococcal infection were estimated to have ever received pneumococcal vaccine (1).

Opportunities to vaccinate high-risk persons are missed both at time of hospital discharge and dur-

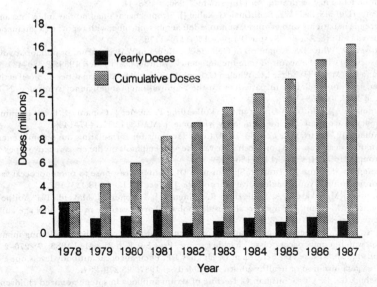

Figure 1. Pneumococcal vaccine distribution—United States 1978–1987. (Data for 1978–1985 were obtained from reference 40. Data for 1986 and 1987 were obtained from Lederle Laboratories and Merck Sharp & Dohme (net doses distributed).)

ing visits to clinicians' offices. Two-thirds or more of patients with serious pneumococcal disease had been hospitalized at least once within 5 years before their pneumococcal illness, yet few had received pneumococcal vaccine (40). More effective programs for vaccine delivery are needed, including offering pneumococcal vaccine in hospitals (at the time of discharge), clinicians' offices, nursing homes, and other chronic-care facilities. Many patients who receive pneumococcal vaccine should also be immunized with influenza vaccine (41), which can be given simultaneously at a different site. In contrast to pneumococcal vaccine, influenza vaccine is given annually.

VACCINE DEVELOPMENT

A more immunogenic pneumococcal vaccine preparation is needed, particularly for children less than 2 years old. The development of a protein-polysaccharide conjugate vaccine for selected capsular types holds promise.

REFERENCES

1. Williams WW, Hickson MA, Kane MA, Kendal AP, Spika JS, Hinman AR. Immunization policies and vaccine coverage among adults: the risk for missed opportunities. Ann Intern Med 1988; 108:616–625.
2. Research Committee of the British Thoracic Society and the Public Health Laboratory Service. Community-acquired pneumonia in adults in British hospitals in 1982–1983: a survey of aetiology, mortality, prognostic factors and outcome. Quart J Med 1987;62:195–220.
3. Istre GR, Tarpay M, Anderson M, Pryor A, Welch D, Pneumococcus Study Group. Invasive disease due to Streptococcus pneumoniae in an area with a high rate of relative penicillin resistance. J Infect Dis 1987;156:732–735.
4. Breiman RF, Navarro VJ, Darden PM, Darby CP, Spika JS. Streptococcus pneumoniae bacteremia in residents of Charleston County, South Carolina, a decade later [Abstract]. In: Program and Abstracts of the 28th Interscience Conference on Antimicrobial Agents and Chemotherapy. Washington, DC: American Society for Microbiology, 1988:343.
5. Davidson M, Schraer CD, Parkinson AJ, et al. Invasive pneumococcal disease in an Alaska Native population, 1980 through 1986. JAMA 1989;261:715–718.
6. Polsky B, Gold JWM, Whimbey E, et al. Bacterial pneumonia in patients with the acquired immunodeficiency syndrome. Ann Intern Med 1986;104:38–41.
7. Simberkoff MS, Sadr WE, Schiffman G, Rahal JJ. Streptococcus pneumoniae infections and bacteremia in patients with acquired immune deficiency syndrome, with report of a pneumococcal vaccine failure. Am Rev Respir Dis 1984;130:1174–1176.
8. Stover DE, White DA, Romano PA, Gellene RA, Robeson WA. Spectrum of pulmonary diseases associated with the acquired immune deficiency syndrome. Am J Med 1985;78:429–437.
9. Lane CH, Masur H, Edgar LC, Whalen G, Rook AH, Fauci AS. Abnormalities of B-cell activation and immunoregulation in patients with the acquired immunodeficiency syndrome. N Engl J Med 1983;309:453–458.
10. Ammann AJ, Schiffman G, Abrams D, Volberding P, Ziegler J, Conant M. B-cell immunodeficiency in acquired immune deficiency syndrome. JAMA 1984;251:1447–1449.
11. Robbins JB, Austrian R, Lee C-J, et al. Considerations for formulating the second-generation pneumococcal capsular polysaccharide vaccine with emphasis on the cross-reactive types within groups. J Infect Dis 1983;148:1136–1159.
12. Douglas RM, Paton JC, Duncan SJ, Hansman DJ. Antibody response to pneumococcal vaccination in children younger than five years of age. J Infect Dis 1983;148:131–137.
13. Leinonen M, Sakkinen A, Kalliokoski R, Luotenen J, Timonen M, Makelda PH. Antibody response to 14-valent pneumococcal capsular polysaccharide vaccine in pre-school age children. Pediatr Infect Dis 1986;5:39–44.
14. Mufson MA, Krause HE, Schiffman G. Long-term persistence of antibody following immunization with pneumococcal polysaccharide vaccine. Proc Soc Exp Biol Med 1983;173:270–275.
15. Mufson MA, Krause HE, Schiffman G, Hughey DF. Pneumococcal antibody levels one decade after immunization of healthy adults. Am J Med Sci 1987;293:279–284.
16. Giebink GS, Le CT, Schiffman G. Decline of serum antibody in splenectomized children after vaccination with pneumococcal capsular polysaccharides. J Pediatr 1984;105:576–584.
17. Weintrub PS, Schiffman G, Addiego JE Jr, et al. Long-term follow-up and booster immunization

with polyvalent pneumococcal polysaccharide in patients with sickle cell anemia. J Pediatr 1984;105:261–263.

18. Spika JS, Halsey NA, Le CT, et al. Decline of vaccine-induced antipneumococcal antibody in children with nephrotic syndrome. Am J Kidney Dis 1986;7:466–470.

19. Ballet J-J, Sulcebe G, Couderc L-J, et al. Impaired anti-pneumococcal antibody response in patients with AIDS-related persistent generalized lymphadenopathy. Clin Exp Immunol 1987;68:479–487.

20. Huang K-L, Ruben FL, Rinaldo CR Jr, Kingsley L, Lyter DW, Ho M. Antibody responses after influenza and pneumococcal immunization in HIV-infected homosexual men. JAMA 1987;257:2047–2050.

21. Austrian R, Douglas RM, Schiffman G, et al. Prevention of pneumococcal pneumonia by vaccination. Trans Assoc Am Physicians 1976;89:184–194.

22. Riley ID, Tarr PI, Andrews M, et al. Immunisation with a polyvalent pneumococcal vaccine: reduction of adult respiratory mortality in a New Guinea Highlands community. Lancet 1977;1:1338–1341.

23. Ammann AJ, Addiego J, Wara DW, Lubin B, Smith WB, Mentzer WC. Polyvalent pneumococcal-polysaccharide immunization of patients with sickle-cell anemia and patients with splenectomy. N Engl J Med 1977;297:897–900.

24. Austrian R. Surveillance of pneumococcal infection for field trials of polyvalent pneumococcal vaccines. Bethesda, MD: National Institutes of Health, National Institute of Allergy and Infectious Diseases, 1980:report no. DAB-VDP-12–84.

25. Shapiro ED, Clemens JD. A controlled evaluation of the protective efficacy of pneumococcal vaccine for patients at high risk of serious pneumococcal infections. Ann Intern Med 1984;101:325–330.

26. Shapiro ED, Austrian R, Adair RK, Clemens JD. The protective efficacy of pneumococcal vaccine [Abstract]. Clin Res 1988;36:470A.

27. Sims RV, Steinmann WC, McConville JH, King LR, Zwick WC, Schwartz JS. The clinical effectiveness of pneumococcal vaccine in the elderly. Ann Intern Med 1988;108:653–657.

28. Forrester HL, Jahnigen DW, LaForce FM. Inefficacy of pneumococcal vaccine in a high-risk population. Am J Med 1987;83:425–430.

29. Bolan G, Broome CV, Facklam RR, Plikaytis BD, Fraser DW, Schlech WF III. Pneumococcal vaccine efficacy in selected populations in the United States. Ann Intern Med 1986;104:1–6.

30. Simberkoff MS, Cross AP, Al-Ibrahim M, et al. Efficacy of pneumococcal vaccine in high-risk patients: results of a Veterans Administration cooperative study. N Engl J Med 1986;315:1318–1327.

31. Shapiro ED. Pneumococcal vaccine failure [Letter]. N Engl J Med 1987;316:1272–1273.

32. Gaillat J, Zmirou D, Mallaret MR, et al. Essai clinique du vaccin antipneumococcique chez des personnes agees vivant en institution. Rev Epidemiol Sante Publique 1985;33:437–444.

33. Borgono JM, McLean AA, Vella PP, et al. Vaccination and revaccination with polyvalent pneumococcal polysaccharide vaccines in adults and infants. Proc Soc Exper Biol Med 1978;157:148–154.

34. Carlson AJ, Davidson WL, McLean AA, et al. Pneumococcal vaccine: dose, revaccination, and coadministration with influenza vaccine. Proc Soc Exper Biol Med 1979;161:558–563.

35. Rigau-Perez JG, Overturf GD, Chan LS, Weiss J, Powars D. Reactions to booster pneumococcal vaccination in patients with sickle cell disease. Pediatr Infect Dis 1983;2:199–202.

36. Lawrence EM, Edwards KM, Schiffman G, Thompson JM, Vaughn WK, Wright PF. Pneumococcal vaccine in normal children. Am J Dis Child 1983;137:846–850.

37. Mufson MA, Krause HE, Schiffman G. Reactivity and antibody responses of volunteers given two or three doses of pneumococcal vaccine. Proc Soc Exper Biol Med 1984;177:220–225.

38. Kaplan J, Sarnaik S, Schiffman G. Revaccination with polyvalent pneumococcal vaccine in children with sickle cell anemia. Am J Pediatr Hematol Oncol 1986;8:80–82.

39. Sisk JE, Riegelman RK. Cost effectiveness of vaccination against pneumococcal pneumonia: an update. Ann Intern Med 1986;104:79–86.

40. Fedson DS. Influenza and pneumococcal immunization strategies for physicians. Chest 1987;91:436–443.

41. ACIP. Prevention and control of influenza. MMWR 1988;37:361–364, 369–373.

TOPIC 24 / **PARVOVIRUS B19**

Risks Associated with Human Parvovirus B19 Infection

Original Citation: Centers for Disease Control and Prevention. Current Trends Risks Associated with Human Parvovirus B19 Infection. MMWR 1989;38(6);81–88, 93–97.

Human Parvovirus B19 was discovered in England in 1975 in serum specimens from healthy blood donors (1). Since its discovery, B19 has been shown to be the causative agent of erythema infectiosum (EI) (also known as fifth disease) and is the primary etiologic agent of TAC in patients with chronic hemolytic anemias (2–4). B19 has also been associated with fetal death (both spontaneous abortions and stillbirths), acute arthralgias and arthritis, and chronic anemia in immunodeficient patients (5–14).

PREVENTION OF INFECTION

Risk Groups

Although B19 infection usually produces a mild, self-limited illness, three groups of persons are at risk for serious complications of infection: (a) persons with chronic hemolytic anemias, (b) persons with congenital or acquired immunodeficiencies, and (c) pregnant women. Since infection in these persons can lead to substantial morbidity and some mortality, consideration should be given to preventing or ameliorating disease.

Immunization Active

There is no vaccine to prevent B19, but a recently developed cell line that expresses B19 capsid proteins as noninfectious viruslike particles has been proposed as a source of antigen for development of a candidate vaccine (62).

Passive

No studies have been conducted to determine whether preexposure or postexposure prophylaxis with commercially available immune globulin (IG) preparations would prevent infection or modify the course of illness during community outbreaks. Routine prophylaxis with IG cannot be recommended at this time.

Health-Care Settings

Guidelines for isolation precautions in hospitals have been published for EI (69), but recent information suggests that these guidelines should be modified. Most patients with EI are past their period of infectiousness and do not present a risk for further transmission; thus isolation precautions are not indicated. However, there is risk for nosocomial transmission of B19 from patients with TAC and from immunodeficient patients with chronic B19 infection. These patients should be considered infectious and placed on isolation precautions for the duration of their illness or until the infection has been cleared. Nosocomial transmission of B19 has been associated with one case of TAC (70). Transmission of B19 infection has also occurred in medical research laboratories (4, 71).

Patients with TAC or chronic B19 infection should be admitted to private rooms. Persons in close contact with the patients should wear masks. Gloves should be worn by persons likely to touch infective material such as respiratory secretions, and gowns should be worn when soiling is anticipated (contact isolation) (69). Hands should be washed after the patient or potentially contaminated articles are touched and before care is provided to another patient. B19-infected patients may share a room with another B19-infected patient unless sharing is contraindicated by another infection or condition.

Health-care workers should be advised that they are at risk of B19 infection after exposure in the hospital or in the community and that there may be a risk for further transmission to patients. Routine infection-control practices should minimize the risk of transmission. Personnel who may be pregnant or who might become pregnant should know about potential risks to the fetus from B19 infection and about preventive measures that may reduce those risks.

Homes, Schools, and Workplaces

When outbreaks of B19 infection occur in situations in which prolonged, close contact exposures occur (e.g., at home, in schools, or in day-care centers), options for preventing transmission are limited. The greatest risk of transmitting the virus occurs before symptoms of EI develop; therefore, transmission cannot be prevented by identifying and excluding persons with EI. The efficacy of decontaminating toys and environmental surfaces to decrease B19 transmission has not been studied. The efficacy of handwashing to decrease B19 transmission has not been studied either, but handwashing is recommended as a practical and probably effective measure.

When outbreaks occur, parents of school-aged children and employees should be advised about the risk of transmitting and acquiring infection and about who is at risk for serious complications. Persons who wish to obtain additional information about risks and management of B19 exposures should be referred to their health-care provider and state or local health officials.

The decision to try to decrease any person's risk of infection by avoiding a workplace or school environment in which an EI outbreak is occurring should be made by the person after discussions with family members, health-care providers, public health officials, and employers or school officials. A policy to routinely exclude members of high-risk groups is not recommended.

PATIENT MANAGEMENT

Patients with Chronic Hemolytic Anemia

The exposed patient with chronic hemolytic anemia should be managed by alerting the patient or his/her parents or guardians about the exposure, the symptoms and signs associated with TAC (pallor, weakness, and lethargy), and the need to consult a physician immediately if symptoms or signs of TAC develop. Management of the patient with TAC is based on treating symptoms of the associated anemia and may require blood transfusion.

Patients with Congenital and Acquired Immunodeficiencies

The exposed patient with a congenital or acquired immunodeficiency should be managed by advising the patient or his/her parents or guardians about the exposure and the possibility that B19 infection may lead to chronic anemia. The physician should consider B19 infection in the differential diagnosis of chronic anemia in this group of patients, especially if there is an outbreak of EI in the community. In several patients with acute lymphocytic leukemia, the administration of IG resulted in disappearance of viremia and improvement in red cell indices (10). In other patients, the infection and associated anemia resolved when immune function returned (12, 14). The role of IG in the treatment of these patients needs further study.

Pregnant Women

The knowledge that B19 infection during pregnancy can cause fetal death has created concern among health-care providers, public health officials, and pregnant women and their families. In managing exposed pregnant women, risks should be considered in the context of other risks to the pregnancy and the risks associated with intervention. For women with a documented infection, maternal serum α-fetoprotein levels and diagnostic ultrasound examinations have been used to identify adversely affected fetuses, but the sensitivity and specificity of these tests, their appropriate timing, and the risks and benefits of their use in managing infected pregnant women have not yet been determined (39, 41). Interpretation of the ultrasound is difficult early in pregnancy and should be supervised by a physician experienced in diagnosing fetal abnormalities. Intrauterine blood transfusion (IBT) has been proposed as treatment for the fetus with B19-induced severe anemia. However, IBT is a high-risk, specialized procedure of unproven benefit in this situation and cannot be recommended for routine treatment of B19-related hydrops fetalis (72).

AVAILABILITY OF DIAGNOSTIC TESTING AT CDC

Diagnostic testing is available at only a few sites, primarily research laboratories; increasing the availability of diagnostic testing is a public health priority. The Division of Viral Diseases, Center for Infectious Diseases, CDC, can accept a limited number of specimens for B19 diagnostic testing. At this time, CDC is accepting specimens through state health departments from patients with TAC, immunodeficient patients with chronic anemia, pregnant women exposed to B19 or with symptoms suggestive of B19 infection, and cases of nonimmune fetal hydrops possibly related to B19 infection, and not accepting specimens for routine antibody testing. Physicians can arrange testing at CDC by consulting their state health department.

REFERENCES: AS NUMBERED IN ORIGINAL PUBLICATION

1. Cossart YE, Field AM, Cant B, Widdows D. Parvovirus-like particles in human sera. Lancet 1975;1:72–73.
2. Anderson MJ, Jones SE, Fisher-Hoch SP, et al. Human parvovirus, the cause of erythema infectiosum (fifth disease) [Letter]? Lancet 1983;1:1378.
3. Anderson MJ, Lewis E, Kidd IM, Hall SM, Cohen BJ. An outbreak of erythema infectiosum associated with human parvovirus infection. J Hyg (Lond) 1984;93:85–93.
4. Pattison JR, Jones SE, Hodgson J, et al. Parvovirus infections and hypoplastic crisis in sickle-cell anaemia [Letter]. Lancet 1981;1:664–665.
5. Knott PD, Welply GAC, Anderson MJ. Serologically proved intrauterine infection with parvovirus. Br Med J 1984;289:1660.
6. Brown T, Anand A, Ritchie LD, Clewley JP, Reid TMS. Intrauterine parvovirus infection associated with hydrops fetalis [Letter]. Lancet 1984;2:1033–1034.
7. White DG, Woolf AD, Mortimer PP, Cohen BJ, Blake DR, Bacon PA. Human parvovirus arthropathy. Lancet 1985;1:419–421.
8. Reid DM, Reid TMS, Brown T, Rennie JAN, Eastmond CJ. Human parvovirus-associated arthritis: a clinical and laboratory description. Lancet 1985;1:422–425.
9. Van Horn DK, Mortimer PP, Young N, Hanson GR. Human parvovirus-associated red cell aplasia in the absence of underlying hemolytic anemia. Am J Pediatr Hematol Oncol 1986;8:235–239.
10. Kurtzman GJ, Ozawa K, Cohen B, Hanson G, Oseas R, Young NS. Chronic bone marrow failure due to persistent B19 parvovirus infection. N Engl J Med 1987;317:287–294.
11. Davidson JE, Gibson B, Gibson A, Evans TJ. Parvovirus infection, leukaemia, and immunodeficiency [Letter]. Lancet 1989;1:102.
12. Smith MA, Shah NR, Lobel JS, Cera PJ, Gary GW, Anderson LJ. Severe anemia caused by human parvovirus in a leukemia patient on maintenance chemotherapy. Clin Pediatr 1988;27:383–386.
13. Kurtzman GJ, Cohen B, Meyers P, Amunullah A, Young NS. Persistent B19 parvovirus infection as a cause of severe chronic anaemia in children with acute lymphocytic leukaemia. Lancet 1988;2:1159–1162.
14. Coulombel L, Morinet F, Mielot F, Tchernia G. Parvovirus infection, leukaemia, and immunodeficiency [Letter]. Lancet 1989;1:101–102.
39. Carrington D, Gilmore DH, Whittle MJ, et al. Maternal serum alpha-fetoprotein—a marker of fetal aplastic crisis during intrauterine human parvovirus infection. Lancet 1987;1:433–435.
41. Anand A, Gray ES, Brown T, Clewley JP, Cohen BJ. Human parvovirus infection in pregnancy and hydrops fetalis. N Engl J Med 1987;316:183–186.
62. Kajigaya S, Fujita S, Ozawa K, et al. A cell line that expresses B19 parvovirus structural proteins and produces empty capsids [Abstract no. 86]. Blood 1988;72(Suppl 1).
69. Garner JS, Simmons BP. Guideline for isolation precautions in hospitals. Infect Control 1983; 4(Suppl):245–325.
70. Evans JPM, Rossiter MA, Kumaran TO, Marsh GW, Mortimer PP. Human parvovirus aplasia: case due to cross infection in a ward. Br Med J 1984;288:681.
71. Cohen BJ, Courouce AM, Schwarz TF, Okochi K, Kurtzman GJ. Laboratory infection with parvovirus B19 [Letter]. J Clin Pathol 1988;41:1027–1028.
72. Schwarz TF, Roggendorf M, Hottentrager B, et al. Human parvovirus B19 infection in pregnancy [Letter]. Lancet 1988;2:566–567.

TOPIC 25 / **PLAGUE**

Human Plague

Original Citation: Centers for Disease Control and Prevention. International notes: human plague—India, 1994. MMWR 1994;43(38):689–691.

EDITORIAL NOTE

Plague is caused by infection with Yersinia pestis, a bacterium carried by rodents and transmitted by fleas commonly found in parts of Asia, Africa, and

North and South America (1, 2). Sporadic human cases associated with epizootics in wild rodents occur annually in the western United States (3); however, no pneumonic plague cases resulting from person-to-person spread have been reported in the United States since 1924 (1).

Travelers to plague-endemic countries are at low risk for infection with Y. pestis. To reduce risk, travelers should avoid areas with recently reported human plague cases. Persons who must travel to these areas should (a) avoid rat-infested areas—especially areas where dead rats have been observed; (b) apply insect repellents to ankles and legs, and apply repellents and insecticides to clothing and outer bedding as directed by the manufacturer; (c) avoid handling dead or sick animals; and (d) if the risk for exposure is high, take prophylactic antibiotics. For adults, the preferred antibiotic for prophylaxis is tetracycline or doxycycline, and for children aged less than or equal to 8 years, sulfonamides (2). Because maximal antibody responses from plague vaccine require administration of multiple doses over several months, plague vaccine is not recommended for immediate protection during outbreaks.

International travelers should be advised to report immediately to a physician any febrile illness beginning within 7 days after leaving endemic areas. Although imported cases are expected to be rare, physicians should be alert for evidence of plague in persons who have traveled to plague-endemic areas and who developed a febrile illness within 7 days after leaving the area. All suspected plague patients should be hospitalized and isolated, specimens should be obtained from patients for laboratory diagnosis, chest roentgenogram should be performed, and antibiotic therapy should be promptly initiated. For all suspected cases, appropriate diagnostic specimens include blood for culture and serum antibodies; for suspected pneumonic cases, sputum samples; and for suspected bubonic cases, aspirates from affected lymph nodes. Streptomycin is the preferred drug for treatment of plague, but gentamicin, tetracyclines, and chloramphenicol also are effective (2, 7). Prompt treatment can reduce overall plague mortality from 60%–100% to 10%–15%.

Prophylactic antibiotic treatment should be administered to all persons who have had face-to-face contact or who have occupied a closed space with a person with pneumonic plague. Household contacts of bubonic plague patients also should receive prophylactic antibiotic treatment.

Suspected human plague cases in international travelers should be reported through state and local health departments to CDC's Division of Quarantine, National Center for Prevention Services, telephone (404) 639-8107 or (404) 639-2888 (nights, Sundays, and holidays). Specimens for confirmatory testing can be submitted through state health departments to CDC. Inquiries about the availability of streptomycin should be directed to Pfizer, Inc.,* telephone (800) 254-4445. Additional information about plague is avail-

---

* Use of trade names and commercial sources is for identification only and does not imply endorsement by the Public Health Service or the U.S. Department of Health and Human Services.

able to physicians and the general public from the CDC Voice Information System, telephone (404) 332-4555, and to physicians and laboratory personnel from CDC's Division of Vector-Borne Infectious Diseases, National Center for Infectious Diseases, telephone (303) 221-6453.

REFERENCES: AS NUMBERED IN ORIGINAL PUBLICATION

1. Barnes AM. Surveillance and control of bubonic plague in the United States. In: Edwards MA, McDonnel U, eds. Animal disease in relation to conservation. New York: Academy Press, 1982:237–270.
2. Poland JD. Plague. In: Hoeprich PD, Jordan MC, eds. Infectious diseases. Grand Rapids, Michigan: JB Lippincott, 1989:1296–1306.
3. CDC. Human plague—United States, 1993–1994. MMWR 43:242–246.
7. Medical Economics Data Production Company. Physicians' desk reference. 48th ed. Montvale, New Jersey: Medical Economics Data Production Company, 1994:1610–1611.

Plague Vaccine

Original Citation: ACIP. Plague vaccine: recommendations of the Immunization Practices Advisory Committee (ACIP). MMWR 1982;31(22):301–304.

SUMMARY

These revised ACIP recommendations on plague vaccine represent an update of the previous recommendations (MMWR 1978;27:255–258) to include current information and practices.

INTRODUCTION

Plague is a natural infection of rodents and their ectoparasites and occurs in many parts of the world, including the western United States. In this country, a few human cases develop each year following exposure to infected wild rodents or their fleas and, less commonly, to other infected wild animals (bobcats, coyotes, rabbits) and domestic animals (cats, dogs). Epidemic plague may result when domestic rat populations and their fleas become infected. Recently, the areas of the most intensive epidemic and epizootic infection have been some countries in Africa, Asia, and South America.

General Recommendations

Because human plague is rare in most parts of the world, there is no need to vaccinate persons other than those at particularly high risk of exposure. Routine vaccination is not necessary for persons living in areas with enzootic plague such as the western United States. It is not indicated for most travelers to countries reporting cases,* particularly if their travel is limited to urban areas with modern hotel accommodations.

Many plague patients in the western United States are infected as a direct result of wild-rodent plague in the immediate vicinity of their homes. Recommended risk-reduction measures include eliminating wild-rodent harborage and food sources near homes, ridding pet dogs and cats of fleas at least weekly, and avoiding direct contact with sick or dead rodents.

In most countries of Africa, Asia, and South America where plague is reported, the risk of exposure exists primarily in rural mountainous or upland areas. Following natural disasters and at times when regular sanitary practices are interrupted, plague can extend from its usual areas of endemicity into urban centers. Rarely, pneumonic plague has been reported in conjunction with outbreaks of bubonic plague, and tourist travel to areas with reported cases of plague should be avoided.

Routine bacteriologic precautions, including the use of a biological safety cabinet to isolate procedures that may produce aerosols, are sufficient to prevent accidental infection with plague among clinical laboratory workers. Few laboratory-associated cases have ever been reported, and these almost exclusively

---

* For a current listing, consult the most recent issue of the World Health Organization's Weekly Epidemiological Record; current information is also available from the Quarantine Division, Center for Prevention Services, Centers for Disease Control, Atlanta, Georgia 30333.

occurred at plague research laboratories or involved unusual exposures. Vaccination of clinical laboratory workers is not indicated.

Ecologists and other field workers who might come in contact with wild animals and their ectoparasites in areas where plague has been known to occur should be made aware of the potential risks of plague and told how to minimize direct contact with potentially infective animals and their tissues or parasites. These precautionary measures are generally sufficient to prevent infection.

PLAGUE VACCINE

Plague vaccines** have been used since the late 19th century, but their effectiveness has never been measured precisely. Field experience indicates that vaccination with plague vaccine reduces the incidence and severity of disease resulting from the bite of infected fleas. The degree of protection afforded against primary pneumonic infection is not known. Persons exposed to plague patients who have pneumonia or to Yersinia pestis*** aerosols in the laboratory should be given a 7- to 10-day course of antimicrobic therapy regardless of vaccination history. Recommended antimicrobials include tetracyclines, chloramphenicol, or streptomycin.

The plague vaccine licensed for use in the United States is prepared from Y. pestis organisms grown in artificial media, inactivated with formaldehyde, and preserved in 0.5% phenol. The vaccine contains trace amounts of beef-heart extract, yeast extract, agar, and peptones and peptides of soya and casein.

Serum antibody to Fraction I capsular antigen, as measured by the passive hemagglutination (PHA) test, is correlated with resistance to Y. pestis infection in experimental animals. A comparable correlation between PHA titer and immunity probably occurs in humans.

Following the primary series of 3 injections, about 7% of individuals do not produce PHA antibody, and a few fail to develop a titer of 128, the level correlated with immunity in experimental animals. PHA titers should be determined for individuals who have an unusually high risk of infection or who have a history of serious reactions to the vaccine in order to govern the frequency of booster doses. Such testing can be arranged through state health departments. Since plague vaccination may only ameliorate illness, whenever a vaccinated person has a definite exposure, prophylactic antibiotics may be indicated whether or not an antibody response has been demonstrated.

Vaccine Recipients

Vaccination is recommended for:

1. All laboratory and field personnel who are working with Y. pestis organisms resistant to antimicrobics,
2. Persons engaged in aerosol experiments with Y. pestis, and
3. Persons engaged in field operations in areas with enzootic plague where preventing exposure is not possible (such as some disaster areas).

Selective plague vaccination should be considered for:

1. Laboratory personnel regularly working with Y. pestis or plague-infected rodents,
2. Workers (for example, Peace Corps volunteers and agricultural advisors) who reside in rural areas with enzootic or epidemic plague where avoidance of rodents and fleas is impossible, and
3. Persons whose vocation brings them into regular contact with wild rodents or rabbits in areas with enzootic plague.

Primary Vaccination

All injections should be given intramuscularly.

** Official name: Plague Vaccine

*** The designation Yersinia pestis is used advisedly since there is reportedly a recommendation by the International Committee on Systematic Bacteriology to reclassify this organism as Yersinia pseudotuberculosis ssp. pestis (WHO. Weekly Epidemiological Record 1981;56:399).

Adults and Children Greater than or Equal to 11 Years Old

The primary series consists of 3 doses of vaccine. The first dose, 1.0 ml, is followed by the second dose, 0.2 ml, 4 weeks later. The third dose, 0.2 ml, is administered 6 months after the first dose. If an accelerated schedule is essential, 3 doses of 0.5 ml each, administered at least 1 week apart, may be given. The efficacy of this schedule has not been determined.

Children less than or Equal to 10 Years Old

The primary series is also 3 doses of vaccine, but the doses are smaller (Table 1). The intervals between injections are the same as for adults.

Booster Doses

When needed because of continuing exposure, 3 booster doses should be given at approximately 6-month intervals. Thereafter, antibody levels decline slowly and booster doses at 1- to 2-year intervals, depending on the degree of continuing exposure, should provide good protection.

The recommended booster dosages for children and adults are the same as the second and third doses in the primary series. However, if serious side effects to the vaccine occur, their severity may be reduced by using half the usual dose. The primary series need never be repeated for booster doses to be effective (Table 1).

Table 1. Plague vaccine doses (in milliliters), by age group (in years), for primary and booster vaccinations*

Dose number	<1	1–4	5–10	>10
1	0.2	0.4	0.6	1.0
2 & 3	0.04	0.04	0.12	0.2
Boosters[†]	0.02–0.04	0.04–0.08	0.06–0.12	0.1–0.2

*Important details are in the text.

†Smaller dose volume may be used if severe side effects are expected.

SIDE EFFECTS OF VACCINE

Primary vaccination may result in general malaise, headache, fever, mild lymphadenopathy, and erythema and induration at the injection site in about 10% of recipients. These reactions occur more commonly with repeated injections. Sterile abscesses occur rarely. Rare cases of sensitivity reactions manifested by urticarial and asthmatic phenomena have been reported.

PRECAUTIONS AND CONTRAINDICATIONS

Plague vaccine should not be administered to anyone with a known hypersensitivity to any of the constituents, such as beef protein, soya, casein, and phenol. Patients who have had severe local or systemic reactions to plague vaccine should not be revaccinated.

The safety or efficacy of vaccination with plague vaccine during pregnancy has not been determined, and therefore it should not be used unless there is a substantial risk of infection.

SELECTED BIBLIOGRAPHY

Bartelloni PJ, Marshall JD Jr, Cavanaugh DC. Clinical Serological responses toplaque vaccine. USP Mills Med 1973;138:720–722.

Burmeister RW, Tigertt WD, Overhold EL. Laboratory-acquired pneumonic plague. Ann Intern
    Med 1962;56:789–800.
Cavanaugh DC, Elisberg BL, Llewellyn CH, et al. Plague immunization. V. Indirect evidence for the
    efficacy of plague vaccine. J Infect Dis 1974;129(Suppl):S37-S40.
Chen TH, Meyer KF. An evaluation of Pasteurella pestis fraction-1-specific antibody for the confir-
    mation of plague infections. Bull WHO 1966;34:911–918.
Marshall JD Jr, Bartelloni PJ, Cavanaugh DC, et al. Plague immunization. II. Relation of adverse
    clinical reactions to multiple immunizations with killed virus. J Infect Dis 1974;129(Suppl):S19-
    S25.
Marshall JD Jr, Cavanaugh DC, Bartelloni PJ, et al. Plague immunization. III. Serologic response to
    multiple inoculations of vaccine. J Infect Dis 1974;129(Suppl):S26-S29.
Meyer KF. Effectiveness of live or killed plague vaccines in man. Bull WHO 1970;42:653–666.

TOPIC 26 / **POLIO**

Limited Supplies of Inactivated Poliovirus Vaccine

Original Citation: Centers for Disease Control and Prevention. Limited supplies of inactivated poliovirus vaccine—United States. MMWR 1994;43(32):595–596.

Editor's Note: The Advisory Committee on Immunization Practices has voted unanimously to recommend
the introduction of inactivated polio vaccine (IPV) into the U.S. schedule of routine immunizations.
However, the details of this policy change will not be worked out until later in 1996. Until that time, the current OPV-only regimen remains the CDC-recommended schedule for routine immunizations.

There is a shortage of inactivated poliovirus vaccine (IPV) in the United States.
The Food and Drug Administration (FDA), the manufacturers (Pasteur Merieux Serums & Vaccines,
S.A. [Lyon, France] [IPOL™]*, and Connaught Laboratories, Limited [Willowdale, Ontario, Canada]
[POLIOVAX™]), and the distributor, Connaught Laboratories, Inc. (Swiftwater, Pennsylvania), are work-
ing to resolve the shortage.

Until IPV becomes readily available, CDC recommends that its use be restricted to (a) never-vaccinated persons aged greater than 18 years who are at
risk for exposure to wild poliovirus (e.g., who will be traveling to areas in which
poliomyelitis is endemic), and (b) persons for whom oral polio vaccine (OPV)
is contraindicated (i.e., persons diagnosed with or living in a household with a
person with a congenital or acquired immune deficiency). Inadequately or
fully vaccinated adults who have previously received IPV or OPV and need poliovirus vaccine can be given OPV (1, 2). OPV continues to be recommended
routinely for all children, except as noted above.

If supplies are not available locally, poliovirus vaccination of persons for
whom OPV is contraindicated should be delayed until IPV becomes available.

---

* Use of trade names and commercial sources is for identification only and does not imply endorsement by the Public Health Service or the U.S. Department of Health and Human Services.

Because no case of polio resulting from indigenously transmitted wild poliovirus has been reported in the United States since 1979, postponing vaccination for these persons until IPV is available is not likely to pose a risk to those persons. Unvaccinated adults who may be exposed to wild poliovirus during travel to polio-endemic areas and cannot obtain IPV should consider vaccination with OPV but should be informed that the risk for vaccine-associated paralytic polio is slightly higher in adults than in children (1, 2). Otherwise, these persons should avoid activities or travel that might result in exposure to wild poliovirus.

Information about obtaining IPV for high-risk persons is available from the distributor, Connaught Laboratories, Inc., telephone (800) 822-2463. MMWR will provide updated information when the shortage is alleviated.

REFERENCES

1. ACIP. Poliomyelitis prevention. MMWR 1982;31:22–26, 31–34.
2. ACIP. Poliomyelitis prevention: enhanced-potency inactivated poliomyelitis vaccine—supplementary statement. MMWR 1987;36:795–798.

Polio Prevention

Original Citation: ACIP. Poliomyelitis prevention. MMWR 1982;31(3):22–26, 31–34.

This revised ACIP recommendation on poliomyelitis prevention addresses issues important in poliomyelitis control in the United States today. Specifically, situations that constitute increased risk are defined, and alternatives for protection are outlined. Recommendations for immunization of adults are presented, clarifying the role of inactivated polio vaccine in immunizing adults. These recommendations also address the problems of interrupted immunization schedules and completion of primary immunization. Oral polio vaccine remains the vaccine of choice for primary immunization of children.

INTRODUCTION

Poliovirus vaccines, used widely since 1955, have dramatically reduced the incidence of poliomyelitis in the United States. The annual number of reported cases of paralytic disease declined from more than 18,000 in 1954 to an average annual number of less than 13 in 1973–1980. The risk of poliomyelitis is generally very small in the United States today, but epidemics are likely to occur if the immunity of the population is not maintained by immunizing children beginning in the first year of life. Small outbreaks have occurred in 1970, 1972, and 1979 as a result of introduction of virus into susceptible populations in communities with low immunization levels.

As a result of the Childhood Immunization Initiative efforts 1977–1979, immunization levels in children are now higher than ever before. The School Enterer Assessments in kindergarten and first-grade levels have indicated that the percentage of these children who have completed primary vaccination against poliomyelitis reached 95% in the 1980–1981 school year. Immunization levels in preschool children and in those who are in higher grades may be substantially lower than the levels at school entry. Laboratory surveillance of enteroviruses shows that the circulation of wild polioviruses has diminished markedly. Inapparent infection with wild strains no longer contributes significantly to establishing or maintaining immunity, making universal vaccination of infants and children even more important.

POLIOVIRUS VACCINES

Two types of poliovirus vaccines are currently licensed in the United States: Oral Polio Vaccine (OPV)* and Inactivated Polio Vaccine (IPV).**

---

* Official name: Poliovirus, Live, Oral, Trivalent.

** Official name: Poliomyelitis Vaccine.

Oral Polio Vaccine (OPV)

Within several years after it was licensed in the United States in 1963, trivalent OPV, the live attenuated vaccine combining all 3 strains of poliovirus, almost totally supplanted the individual monovalent OPV antigens used earlier. Full primary vaccination with OPV will produce long-lasting immunity to all 3 poliovirus types in more than 95% of recipients. Most recipients are protected after a single dose.

OPV consistently induces intestinal immunity that provides resistance to reinfection with polioviruses. Administration of OPV may interfere with simultaneous infection by wild polioviruses, a property which is of special value in epidemic-control campaigns. In rare instances (once in approximately 3.2 million doses distributed), OPV has been associated with paralytic disease in vaccine recipients or their close contacts. In the 12-year period 1969–1980, approximately 290 million doses of OPV were distributed, and 92 cases of paralysis associated with vaccine were reported. Twenty-five cases of paralysis occurred in otherwise healthy vaccine recipients, 55 cases in healthy close contacts of vaccine recipients, and 12 cases in persons (recipients or contacts) with immune-deficiency conditions.

Inactivated Polio Vaccine (IPV)

Licensed in 1955, IPV has been used extensively in this country and many other parts of the world. It is given by subcutaneous injection. Where extensively used, IPV has brought about a great reduction in paralytic poliomyelitis cases. Approximately 428 million doses have been administered in the United States, mostly before 1962. Although IPV has not been widely used in this country for more than a decade, a Canadian product licensed for use in the United States is now available.

It is generally accepted that primary vaccination with 4 doses of IPV produces immunity to all 3 poliovirus types in more than 95% of recipients. Additional experience with the IPV product available since 1968 is necessary to establish whether the duration of immunity is comparable to that induced by OPV. Experience in other countries forms the basis for the present recommendations on booster doses.

There is considerable evidence from epidemiologic studies that immunizing with IPV diminishes circulation of wild poliovirus in the community, although it is known that persons vaccinated with IPV can subsequently be infected with and excrete in feces either wild strains or attenuated vaccine virus strains. No paralytic reactions to IPV are known to have occurred since the 1955 cluster of poliomyelitis cases caused by vaccine that contained live polioviruses that had escaped inactivation. Serious adverse reactions are not anticipated with the current IPV product.

An improved IPV product with higher potency has been developed in Europe. Studies in Africa and Europe have revealed essentially 100% seroconversion following 2 doses. Duration of protection is under study. Preliminary studies are now under way in a US. population to compare this product with OPV.

ROUTINE IMMUNIZATION

Rationale for Choice of Vaccine

Although IPV and OPV are both effective in preventing poliomyelitis. OPV is the vaccine of choice for primary immunization of children in the United States when the benefits and risks for the entire population are considered. OPV is preferred because it induces intestinal immunity, is simple to administer, is well accepted by patients, results in immunization of some contacts of vaccinated persons, and has a record of having essentially eliminated disease associated with wild polioviruses in this country. The choice of OPV as the preferred polio vaccine in the United States has also been made by the Committee on Infectious Diseases of the American Academy of Pediatrics (1) and a special expert committee of the Institute of Medicine, National Academy of Sciences (2).

Some poliomyelitis experts contend that greater use of IPV in the United States for routine vaccination would provide continued control of naturally occurring poliovirus infections and simultaneously reduce the problem of OPV-associated disease. They argue that there is no substantial evidence that OPV and currently available IPV differ in their ability to protect individuals from disease. They question the public health significance of higher levels of gastrointestinal immunity achieved with OPV, and they question whether the transmission of vaccine virus to close contacts contributes substantially to the level of immunity achieved in the community.

Some countries successfully prevent poliomyelitis with IPV. However, because of many differences between these countries and the United States, particularly with respect to risks of exposure to wild polioviruses and the ability to achieve and maintain very high vaccination rates in the population, their experiences with IPV may not be directly applicable here.

Prospective vaccinees or their parents should be made aware of the polio vaccines available and the reasons why recommendations are made for giving specific vaccines at particular ages and under certain circumstances. Furthermore, the benefits and risks of the vaccines for individuals and the community should be stated so that vaccination is carried out among persons who are fully informed.

RECOMMENDATIONS FOR INFANTS, CHILDREN, AND ADOLESCENTS

Primary Immunization (Table 1)

Table 1. Routine poliomyelitis immunization schedule summary, 1981*

Dose	OPV age/interval	IPV age/interval
Primary 1	Initial visit, preferably 6–12 weeks of age	Initial visit, preferably 6–12 weeks of age
Primary 2	Interval of 6–8 weeks	Interval of 4–8 weeks
Primary 3	Interval of ≥6 weeks customarily 8–12 months	Interval of 4–8 weeks
Primary 4		Interval of 6–12 months
Supplementary	4–6 years of age[+] (school entry)	4–6 years of age[+] (school entry)
Additional supplementary		Interval of every 5 years[&]

*Important details are in the text.

[+]If the third primary dose of OPV is administered on or after the fourth birthday, a fourth (supplementary) dose is not required. If the fourth primary dose of IPV is administered on or after the fourth birthday, a fifth (supplementary) dose is not required at school entry.

[&]Supplementary doses are recommended every 5 years after the last dose until the 18th birthday or unless a complete primary series of OPV has been completed.

OPV

For infants, children, and adolescents through secondary school age (generally up to age 18) the primary series of OPV consists of 3 doses. In infancy the primary series is integrated with DTP vaccination, and the first dose is commonly given at 6–12 weeks of age. At all ages the first 2 doses should be separated by at least 6, and preferably 8, weeks. The third dose is given at least 6 weeks, customarily 8–12 months, after the second dose. In high-risk areas, an additional dose of OPV is often given within the first 6 months of life. Breast feeding does not interfere with successful immunization.

IPV

The primary series consists of 4 doses of vaccine; volume and route of injection are specified by the manufacturer. In infancy, the primary schedule is usually integrated with DTP vaccination, as with OPV. Three doses can be given at 4- to 8-week intervals; the fourth dose should follow 6–12 months after the third.

All children should complete primary immunization before entering school, preferably with all OPV or all IPV. If, however, a combination of IPV and OPV is used, a total of 4 doses constitutes a primary series.

Supplementary Immunization

OPV

Before entering school, all children who previously received primary immunization with OPV (3 doses) in early childhood should be given a fourth dose. However, if the third primary dose is administered on or after the fourth birthday, a fourth (supplementary) dose is not required. The additional dose will increase the likelihood of complete immunity in the small percentage of children who have not previously developed serum antibodies to all 3 types of polioviruses. The need for supplementary doses after 4 doses of OPV has not been established, but children considered to be at increased risk of exposure to poliovirus (as noted below under RECOMMENDATIONS FOR ADULTS) may be given a single additional dose of OPV.

IPV

Before entering school, all children who previously received primary immunization with either IPV alone or a combination of IPV and OPV (a total of 4 doses) in early childhood should be given at least 1 dose of OPV or 1 additional dose of IPV. However, if the fourth primary dose is administered on or after the fourth birthday, a fifth (supplementary) dose is not required at school entry. Use of a primary series of OPV would eliminate the need for subsequent booster doses of IPV. Children who received primary immunization with IPV should obtain a booster dose of IPV every 5 years until the age of 18 years, unless a primary series of OPV is given. The need for such supplementary doses after the 5 basic doses of the currently available IPV product has not been firmly established. Further experience may lead to alteration of this recommendation.

Children Incompletely Immunized

Polio vaccination status should be reevaluated periodically, and those who are inadequately protected should complete their immunizations.

OPV

To help assure seroconversion to all 3 serotypes of poliovirus, completion of the primary series of 3 doses of OPV is recommended. Time intervals between doses longer than those recommended for routine primary immunization do not necessitate additional doses of vaccine. Individuals who received only 1 dose of each of the monovalent OPVs in the past should receive 2 doses of trivalent OPV at least 6 weeks apart. One dose of each monovalent OPV (poliovirus types 1, 2, and 3) is at least equivalent to 1 dose of trivalent OPV.

IPV

Regulations for vaccine licensure adopted since 1968 require a higher potency IPV than was previously manufactured. Four doses of IPV administered after 1968 are considered a complete primary series. As with OPV, time intervals between doses longer than those recommended for routine primary immunization do not necessitate additional doses. Incompletely immunized children who are at increased risk of exposure to poliovirus (as noted below under RECOMMENDATIONS FOR ADULTS) should be given the remaining required dose or, if time is a limiting factor, at least a single dose of OPV.

RECOMMENDATIONS FOR ADULTS

Routine primary poliovirus vaccination of adults (generally those 18 years old or older) residing in the United States is not necessary. Most adults are already immune and also have a very small risk of exposure to poliomyelitis in the United States. Immunization is recommended for certain adults who are at greater risk of exposure to wild polioviruses than the general population, including:

1. Travelers to areas or countries where poliomyelitis is epidemic or endemic;
2. Members of communities or specific population groups with disease caused by wild polioviruses;
3. Laboratory workers handling specimens which may contain polioviruses;
4. Health-care workers in close contact with patients who may be excreting polioviruses.

For individuals in the above categories, polio vaccination is recommended as detailed below.

Unvaccinated Adults

For adults at increased risk of exposure to poliomyelitis, primary immunization with IPV is recommended whenever this is feasible. IPV is preferred because the risk of vaccine-associated paralysis following OPV is slightly higher in adults than in children. Three doses should be given at intervals of 1–2 months; a fourth dose should follow 6–12 months after the third.

In circumstances where time will not allow at least 3 doses of IPV to be given before protection is required, the following alternatives are recommended:

1. If less than 8, but more than 4, weeks are available before protection is needed, 2 doses of IPV should be given at least 4 weeks apart.
2. If less than 4 weeks are available before protection is needed, a single dose of OPV is recommended. In both instances, the remaining doses of vaccine should be given later at the recommended intervals, if the person remains at increased risk.

Incompletely Immunized Adults

Adults who are at increased risk of exposure to poliomyelitis and who have previously received less than a full primary course of OPV or IPV should be given the remaining required doses of either vaccine regardless of the interval since the last dose and the type of vaccine previously received.

Adults Previously Given a Complete Primary Course of OPV or IPV

Adults who are at increased risk of exposure to poliomyelitis and who have previously completed a primary course of OPV may be given another dose of OPV. The need for further supplementary doses has not been established. Those adults who previously completed a primary course of IPV may be given a dose of either IPV or OPV. If IPV is used exclusively, additional doses may be given every 5 years, but their need also has not been established.

UNIMMUNIZED OR INADEQUATELY IMMUNIZED ADULTS IN HOUSEHOLDS IN WHICH CHILDREN ARE TO BE GIVEN OPV

Adults who have not been adequately immunized against poliomyelitis with OPV or IPV are at a very small risk of developing OPV-associated paralytic poliomyelitis when children in the household are given OPV. About 4 such cases have occurred annually among contacts since 1969, during which time about 24 million doses of OPV were distributed yearly. (See ADVERSE REACTIONS.)

Because of the overriding importance of ensuring prompt and complete immunization of the child and the extreme rarity of OPV-associated disease in contacts, the Committee recommends the administration of OPV to a child regardless of the poliovirus-vaccine status of adult household contacts. This is the usual practice in the United States. The responsible adult should be informed of the small risk involved. An acceptable alternative, if there is strong assurance that ultimate, full immunization of the child will not be jeopardized or unduly delayed, is to immunize adults according to the schedule outlined above before giving OPV to the child.

PRECAUTIONS AND CONTRAINDICATIONS

Pregnancy

Although there is no convincing evidence documenting adverse effects of either OPV or IPV on the pregnant woman or developing fetus, it is prudent on theoretical grounds to avoid vaccinating pregnant women. However, if immediate protection against poliomyelitis is needed, OPV is recommended.

Immunodeficiency

Patients with immune-deficiency diseases, such as combined immunodeficiency. hypogammaglobulinemia and agammaglobulinemia, should not be given OPV because of their substantially increased risk of vaccine-associated disease. Furthermore, patients with altered immune states due to diseases such as leukemia, lymphoma, or generalized malignancy, or with immune systems compromised by therapy with corticosteroids, alkylating drugs, antimetabolites, or radiation should not receive OPV because of the theoretical risk of paralytic disease. OPV should not be used for immunizing immunodeficient patients and their household contacts; IPV is recommended. Many immunosuppressed patients will be immune to polioviruses by virtue of previous immunization or exposure to wild-type virus at a time when they were immunologically competent. Although these persons should not receive OPV, their risk of paralytic disease is thought to be less than that of naturally immunodeficient individuals. Although a protective immune response to IPV in the immunodeficient patient cannot be assured, the vaccine is safe and some protection may result from its administration. If OPV is inadvertently administered to a household-type contact of an immunodeficient patient, close contact between the patient and the recipient of OPV should be avoided for approximately 1 month after vaccination. This is the period of maximum excretion of vaccine virus. Because of the possibility of immunodeficiency in other children born to a family in which there has been 1 such case, OPV should not be given to a member of a household in which there is a family history of immunodeficiency until the immune status of the recipient and other children in the family is documented.

ADVERSE REACTIONS

OPV

In rare instances, administration of OPV has been associated with paralysis in healthy recipients and their contacts. Other than efforts to identify persons with immune-deficiency conditions, no procedures are currently available for identifying persons likely to experience such adverse reactions. Although the risk of vaccine-associated paralysis is extremely small for vaccinees and their susceptible, close, personal contacts, they should be informed of this risk.

IPV

No serious side effects of currently available IPV have been documented. Since IPV contains trace amounts streptomycin and neomycin, there is a possibility of hypersensitivity reactions in individuals sensitive to these antibiotics.

CASE INVESTIGATION AND EPIDEMIC CONTROL

Each suspected case of poliomyelitis should prompt an immediate epidemiologic investigation, including an active search for other cases. If evidence implicates wild poliovirus and there is a possibility of transmission, a vaccination plan designed to contain spread should be developed. If evidence implicates vaccine-derived poliovirus, no vaccination plan need be developed, as no outbreaks associated with vaccine virus have been documented to date. Within an epidemic area, OPV should be provided for all persons over 6 weeks of age who have not been completely immunized or whose immunization status is unknown, with the exceptions noted above under Immunodeficiency.

This recommendation supersedes the recommendation on poliomyelitis published in MMWR 1979;28:510–520.

REFERENCES

1. American Academy of Pediatrics. Report of the Committee on Infectious Diseases. 18th ed. Evanston, Illinois: AAP, 1977.
2. Nightingale E. Recommendations for a national policy on poliomyelitis vaccination. N Engl J Med 1977;297:249–253.

SELECTED BIBLIOGRAPHY

CDC. Poliomyelitis surveillance summary 1979. Atlanta: CDC, 1981.
Fite-Wassilak SG. Hinman AR. Is there a need for "catch-up" pollo vaccination preadolescence? JAMA 1981;246:1239.
Hardy GE, Hopkins CC, Linnenman CC Jr, et al. Trivalent oral poliovirus vaccine: a comparison of two infant immunization schedules. Pediatrics 1970;45:444–448.
International symposium on reassessment of inactivated poliomyelitis vaccine, Bilthoven 1980. Develop Biol Standard 47 (S. Karger, Basel 1981).
Krugman S, Katz SL. Childhood immunization procedures. JAMA 1977;237:2228–2230.
Mayer TR, Balfour HH. Prevalence of poliovirus neutralizing antibodies in young adult women. JAMA 1981;246:1207–1209.
Nightingale E. Recommendations for a national policy on poliomyelitis vaccination. N Engl J Med 1977;297:249–253.
Salk J, Salk D. Control of influenza and poliomyelitis with killed virus vaccines. Science 1977;195:834–847.
Sanders DY, Cramblett HG. Antibody titers to polloviruses in patients ten years after immunization with Sabin vaccine. J Pediatr 1974;84:406–408.
Schonberger LB, McGowan JE, Gregg MB. Vaccine-associated poliomyelitis in the United States, 1961–1972. Am J Edipemiol 1976;104:202–211.
World Health Organization. The relation between acute persisting spinal paralysis and poliomyelitis vaccine (oral): results of a WHO enquiry. Bull WHO 1976;53:319–331.

Polio Prevention: Supplementary Statement

Original Citation: ACIP. Poliomyelitis prevention: enhanced potency inactivated poliomyelitis vaccine—supplementary statement. MMWR 1987; 36(48): 795–798.

The supplementary statement provides information on and recommendations for the use of inactivated poliovirus vaccine (IPV) of enhanced potency.*** The Immunization Practices Advisory Committee (ACIP) believes that, in the United States, polio immunization should rely primarily on oral poliovirus vaccine (OPV), with selected use of enhanced-potency IPV as specified in this document. However, this subject should be reviewed on a continuing basis, and an extensive review of polio vaccines and potential vaccine policies will take place during 1988. General recommendations on poliomyelitis prevention, including the use of and schedules for OPV, are found in the current ACIP recommendations (1).

Introduction

Conventional IPV

IPV was introduced in the United States in 1955 and was used widely until OPV became available during the period 1961–1964. Thereafter, the use of IPV rapidly declined to a level of less than 1% of all polio vaccine distributed annually in the United States.

In recent U.S. studies, three doses of IPV administered in the first year of life produced antibodies to poliovirus serotypes 1, 2, and 3 in 87%, 97%, and 95% of recipients, respectively. More than 99% of children completing the four-dose primary series by 18 months of age produced antibodies to all three serotypes (2).

Enhanced-Potency IPV

A method of producing a more potent IPV with greater antigenic content was developed in 1978 and led to the newly licensed IPV, which is produced in human diploid cells (3). Results of studies from several countries have indicated that a reduced number of doses of IPV produced with this technique can immunize children satisfactorily (4–6). A clinical trial of two preparations of enhanced-potency IPV was completed in the United States in 1984 (7). Children received three doses of one of the enhanced-potency IPVs at 2, 4, and 18 months of age. In spite of the presence of maternal antibodies in the majority of the infants at the time of the first dose, 99%–100% of the children were seropositive for all three poliovirus types at 6 months of age (2 months after their second dose). The percentage of seropositive children did not rise or fall significantly during the 14-month period following the second dose, a result that confirms that seroconversion had occurred in almost all children. Furthermore, geometric mean titers increased 5- to 10-fold following both the second and third doses. Conclusive studies are not yet available concerning antibody persistence following three doses of the enhanced-potency IPV to be made available in the United States. However, unpublished studies of an IPV with lower antigen content have shown 100% seropositivity 5 years after the third dose (2). The effect of enhanced-potency IPV on the circulation of poliovirus in a community has not yet been determined, but it is likely to be at least as good as that seen with conventional IPV. In a recent study of poliovirus excretion following type 1 vaccine-virus challenge after the third dose of enhanced-potency IPV, the decrease in excretion was at least as great as that after conventional IPV, but still significantly less than that found after three doses of OPV (8).

Vaccine Usage

Indications

Persons with a congenital immune deficiency disease, such as agammmaglobulinemia; an acquired immune deficiency disease, such as acquired immunodeficiency syndrome (AIDS); or an altered immune status as a result of other diseases or immunosuppressive therapy are at increased risk for paralysis associated with OPV. Therefore, if polio immunization is indicated, these persons and their household members and other close contacts should receive IPV rather than OPV. Although a protective immune response following receipt of enhanced-potency IPV cannot be assured, some protection may

***Poliovirus Vaccine Inactivated, which is manufactured by Connaught Laboratories Ltd., will be distributed by Connaught Laboratories Inc. beginning in March 1988.

be provided to the immunocompromised patient. Available data on children previously diagnosed with asymptomatic human immunodeficiency virus (HIV) infection do not suggest that they are at increased risk of adverse consequences from OPV. However, for such persons, use of IPV rather than OPV is prudent since family members may be immunocompromised because of AIDS or HIV infection and may be at increased risk for paralysis from contact with an OPV virus. Routine primary poliovirus vaccination of adults (generally those 18 years of age or older) residing in the United States is not recommended. Adults at increased risk of exposure to either vaccine or wild poliovirus (1) should receive polio vaccination in accordance with the schedule prescribed later.

In households where polio vaccine is to be administered to immunologically normal children, ACIP recommends giving OPV regardless of the poliovirus-vaccine status of adult household contacts (1). The overall risk of vaccine-associated paralytic disease in immunologically normal contacts of OPV recipients is one case per 5.5 million doses of OPV distributed (9). As an alternative, adult contacts can first complete their primary series of polio vaccine as detailed in the schedule below, if there is strong assurance that subsequent immunization of the child will not be jeopardized or unduly delayed.

Schedules

The primary series for enhanced-potency IPV consists of three 0.5-mL doses administered subcutaneously. The interval between the first two doses should be at least 4 weeks, but preferably 8 weeks. The third dose should follow in at least 6 months, but preferably nearer to 12 months. A primary series can be started as early as 6 weeks of age, but preferably at 2 months of age. Although studies have not been conducted, young children should receive the third dose along with diphtheria, tetanus, pertussis vaccine (DTP) and measles, mumps, rubella vaccine (MMR) at 15 months of age, if possible.

A primary series of polio vaccine usually consists of enhanced-potency IPV alone or OPV alone. However, a combination of both vaccines totalling three doses and separated by appropriate intervals constitutes a primary series. If enhanced-potency IPV is administered to persons with a previously incomplete series of conventional IPV, a final total of four doses of polio vaccine is necessary for a primary series.

All children who received a primary series of enhanced-potency IPV or of a combination of polio vaccines should be given a booster dose before entering school, unless the final dose of the primary series was administered on or after the fourth birthday. The need for routinely administering additional doses is unknown at this time.

For unvaccinated adults at increased risk of exposure to poliovirus, a primary series of enhanced-potency IPV is recommended. While the responses of adults to a primary series have not been studied, the recommended schedule for adults is two doses given at a 1- to 2-month interval and a third dose given 6 to 12 months later. If less than 3 months but more than 2 months are available before protection is needed, three doses of enhanced-potency IPV should be given at least 1 month apart. Likewise, if only 1 to 2 months are available, two doses of enhanced-potency IPV should be given at least 1 month apart. If less than 1 month is available, a single dose of either OPV or enhanced-potency IPV is recommended.

Adults who are at increased risk of exposure and have had (a) at least one dose of OPV, (b) fewer than three doses of conventional IPV, or (c) a combination of conventional IPV and OPV totalling fewer than three doses should receive at least one dose of OPV or enhanced-potency IPV. Additional doses needed to complete a primary series should be given if time permits.

Adults who are at increased risk of exposure and who have previously completed a primary series with any one or combination of polio vaccines can be given a dose of OPV or enhanced-potency IPV.

Side Effects and Adverse Reactions

Available data indicate that the rate of adverse reactions in the kidney cells of monkeys receiving enhanced-potency IPV are low and that the reactions are not different from those following administration of a placebo. The recently licensed human diploid cell-derived vaccine was not compared to a placebo. Rates of local adverse events following its use are similar to rates found in controlled studies using vaccine derived from the kidney cells of monkeys. There is no evidence that conventional IPV causes any serious side effects. Consequently, serious side effects are not expected to occur with enhanced-potency IPV. This conclusion can be confirmed only with postmarketing surveillance. Parents of children receiving the vaccine, older vaccine recipients, and health-care providers are encouraged to report all adverse events occurring within 4 weeks of receipt of enhanced-potency IPV to the manufacturer and to local or state health departments. The information will be forwarded to the appropriate federal agency.****

Precautions and Contraindications

Vaccine administration should not be postponed because of minor illnesses, such as mild upper-respiratory infections. Generally, however, persons with severe febrile illnesses should not be vaccinated until they have recovered. The enhanced-potency IPV may contain trace amounts of streptomycin and neomycin. Persons who have had anaphylactic reactions to topically or systemically administered streptomycin and neomycin should not receive enhanced-potency IPV.

There is no convincing evidence documenting adverse effects of conventional IPV on the pregnant woman or developing fetus. Data on adverse events following use of enhanced-potency IPV are not available. On theoretical grounds, it is prudent to avoid vaccinating pregnant women. However, if a pregnant woman needs immediate protection against poliomyelitis, OPV is recommended.

REFERENCES

1. Immunization Practices Advisory Committee. Poliomyelitis prevention. MMWR 1982;31:22–26, 31–34.
2. Bernier RH. Improved inactivated poliovirus vaccine: an update. Ped Infect Dis 1986;5:289–292.
3. von Seefried A, Chun JH, Grant JA, Letvenuk L, Pearson EW. Inactivated poliovirus vaccine and test development at Connaught Laboratories Ltd. Rev Infect Dis 1984;6(Suppl 2):S345-S349.
4. van Wezel AL, van Steenis G, Hannik CA, Cohen H. New approach to the production of concentrated and purified inactivated polio and rabies tissue culture vaccines. Dev Biol Stand 1978; 41:159–168.

**** Center for Biologics Evaluation and Research, Food and Drug Administration, or the Centers for Disease Control.

5. Salk J, Stoeckel P, van Wezel AL, Lapinleimu K, van Steenis G. Antigen content of inactivated poliovirus vaccine for use in a one- or two-dose regimen. Ann Clin Res 1982;14:204–212.
6. Simoes EA, Padmini B, Steinhoff MC, Jadhav M, John TJ. Antibody response of infants to two doses of inactivated poliovirus vaccine of enhanced potency. Am J Dis Child 1985;139:977–980.
7. McBean AM, Thoms ML, Johnson RH, et al. A comparison of the serologic responses to oral and injectable trivalent poliovirus vaccines. Rev Infect Dis 1984;6(Suppl 2):S552–S555.
8. Onorato I, Modlin J, Bernier R, McBean M, Thoms ML. Intestinal immunity induced by enhanced-potency inactivated polio vaccine and oral polio vaccine [Abstract]. In: Program and abstracts of the Interscience Conference on Antimicrobial Agents and Chemotherapy. Washington, DC: American Society for Microbiology, 1987.
9. Nkowane BM, Wassilak SGF, Orenstein WA, et al. Vaccine-associated paralytic poliomyelitis— United States: 1973 through 1984. JAMA 1987;257:1335–1340.

TOPIC 27 / **RABIES**

Compendium of Animal Rabies Control

Original Citation: 1995 National Association of State Public Health Veterinarians, Inc. Compendium of animal rabies control. MMWR 1995;44(RR-2).

Original Authors: Suzanne R. Jenkins, VMD, MPH, Keith A. Clark, DVM, PhD, John G. Debbie, MS, DVM, Russell J. Martin, DVM, PHM, Grayson B. Miller Jr., MD, F.T. Satalowich, DVM, MSPH, Faye E. Sorhage, VMD, MPH.

The purpose of this Compendium is to provide rabies information to veterinarians, public health officials, and others concerned with rabies control. These recommendations serve as the basis for animal rabies-control programs throughout the United States and also facilitate standardization of procedures among jurisdictions, thereby contributing to an effective national rabies-control program. This document is reviewed annually and revised as necessary. Recommendations for immunization procedures are contained in Part I; all animal rabies vaccines licensed by the U.S. Department of Agriculture (USDA) and marketed in the United States are listed in Part II; Part III details the principles of rabies control.

PART I: RECOMMENDATIONS FOR IMMUNIZATION PROCEDURES

Vaccine Administration

All animal rabies vaccines should be restricted to use by, or under the direct supervision of, a veterinarian.

Vaccine Selection

In comprehensive rabies-control programs, only vaccines with a 3-year duration of immunity should be used. This procedure constitutes the most effective method of increasing the proportion of immunized dogs and cats in any population. (See Part II.)

Route of Inoculation

All vaccines must be administered in accordance with either the specifications of the product label or the package insert. If administered intramuscularly, vaccine must be administered at one site in the thigh.

Wildlife Vaccination

Parenteral vaccination of captive wildlife is not recommended because the efficacy of rabies vaccines in such animals has not been established and no vaccine is licensed for wildlife. For this reason and because virus-shedding periods are unknown, bats and wild or exotic carnivores should not be kept as pets. Zoos or research institutions may establish vaccination programs that attempt to protect valuable animals, but these programs should not be in lieu of appropriate public health activities that protect humans. The use of licensed oral vaccines for the mass immunization of wildlife should be considered in selected situations, with the approval of the state agency responsible for animal rabies control.

Accidental Human Exposure to Vaccine

Accidental inoculation may occur during administration of animal rabies vaccine. Such exposure to inactivated vaccines constitutes no risk for acquiring rabies.

Identification of Vaccinated Animals

All agencies and veterinarians should adopt the standard tag system. This practice will aid persons who administer local, state, national, and international rabies control procedures. Animal license tags should be distinguishable in shape and color from rabies tags.

Anodized aluminum rabies tags should be no less than 0.064 inches in thickness.

Rabies Tags

Rabies Certificate

All agencies and veterinarians should use the NASPHV form #51, Rabies Vaccination Certificate, which can be obtained from vaccine manufacturers. Computer-generated forms containing the same information are acceptable.

PART II: VACCINES MARKETED IN THE UNITED STATES AND NASPHV RECOMMENDATIONS

Table 1.

PART III: RABIES CONTROL

Principles of Rabies Control

Human Rabies Prevention

Rabies in humans can be prevented either by eliminating exposures to rabid animals or by providing exposed persons with prompt local treatment of

Table 1. Vaccines Marketed in the United States and NASPHV Recommendations

Product name	Produced by	Marketed by	For use in	Dosage (mL)	Age at primary vaccination*	Booster recommended	Route of inoculation
A. Inactivated							
TRIMUNE	Fort Dodge License No. 112	Fort Dodge	Dogs	1	3 mos&	Triennially	IM+
			Cats	1	1 yr later	Triennially	IM
ANNUMUNE	Fort Dodge License No. 112	Fort Dodge	Dogs	1	3 mos	Annually	IM
			Cats	1	3 mos	Annually	IM
DURA-RAB 1	ImmunoVet License No. 302-A	ImmunoVet, Vedco, Inc.	Dogs	1	3 mos	Annually	IM
			Cats	1	3 mos	Annually	IM
DURA-RAB 3	ImmunoVet License No. 302-A	ImmunoVet, Vedco, Inc.	Dogs	1	3 mos&	Triennially	IM
			Cats	1	1 yr later	Triennially	IM
RABCINE 3	ImmunoVet License No. 302-A	SmithKline Beecham Animal Health	Dogs	1	3 mos&	Triennially	IM
			Cats	1	1 yr later	Triennially	IM
ENDURALL-K	SmithKline Beecham License No. 189	SmithKline Beecham Animal Health	Dogs	1	3 mos	Annually	IM
			Cats	1	3 mos	Annually	IM
ENDURALL-P	SmithKline Beecham License No. 189	SmithKline Beecham Animal Health	Dogs	1	3 mos	Annually	IM or SQ&
			Cats	1	3 mos	Annually	SQ
RABGUARD-TC	SmithKline Beecham License No. 189	SmithKline Beecham Animal Health	Dogs	1	3 mos&	Triennially	IM
			Cats	1	1 yr later	Triennially	IM
			Sheep	1	3 mos	Annually	IM
			Cattle	1	3 mos	Annually	IM
			Horses	1	3 mos	Annually	IM
DEFENSOR	SmithKline Beecham License No. 189	SmithKline Beecham Animal Health	Dogs	1	3 mos&	Triennially	IM or SQ
			Cats	1	1 yr later	Triennially	SQ
			Sheep	2	3 mos	Annually	IM
			Cattle	2	3 mos	Annually	IM
RABDOMUN	SmithKline Beecham License No. 189	Mallinckrodt Veterinary, Inc.	Dogs	1	3 mos&	Triennially	IM or SQ
			Cats	1	1 yr later	Triennially	SQ
			Sheep	2	3 mos	Annually	IM
			Cattle	2	3 mos	Annually	IM

Table 1.—continued

Product name	Produced by	Marketed by	For use in	Dosage (mL)	Age at primary vaccination*	Booster recommended	Route of inoculation
RABDOMUN-1	SmithKline Beecham License No. 189	Mallinckrodt Veterinary, Inc.	Dogs	1	3 mos	Annually	IM or SQ
			Cats	1	3 mos	Annually	SQ
SENTRYRAB-1	SmithKline Beecham License No. 225	Synbiotics Corp.	Dogs	1	3 mos	Annually	IM
			Cats	1	3 mos	Annually	IM
CYTORAB	Coopers Animal Health, Inc., License No. 107	Coopers Animal Health, Inc.	Dogs	1	3 mos	Annually	IM
			Cats	1	3 mos	Annually	IM
TRIRAB	Coopers Animal Health, Inc., License No. 107	Coopers Animal Health, Inc.	Dogs	1	3 mos& / 1 yr later	Triennially	IM
EPIRAB	Coopers Animal Health, Inc., License No. 107	Coopers Animal Health, Inc.	Cats	1	3 mos	Annually	IM
			Dogs	1	3 mos&	Triennially	IM
			Cats	1	1 yr later	Triennially	IM
RABVAC 1	Solvay Animal Health, Inc., License No. 195-A	Solvay Animal Health, Inc.	Dogs	1	3 mos	Annually	IM or SQ
			Cats	1	3 mos	Annually	IM or SQ
RABVAC 3	Solvay Animal Health, Inc., License No. 195-A	Solvay Animal Health, Inc.	Dogs	1	3 mos&	Triennially	IM or SQ
			Cats	1	1 yr later	Triennially	IM or SQ
			Horses	2	3 mos	Annually	IM
PRORAB 1	Intervet, Inc. License No. 286	Intervet, Inc.	Dogs	1	3 mos	Annually	IM or SQ
			Cats	1	3 mos	Annually	IM or SQ
			Sheep	2	3 mos	Annually	IM
RM IMRAB 1	Rhone Merieux, Inc. License No. 298	Rhone Merieux, Inc.	Dogs	1	3 mos	Annually	IM or SQ
			Cats	1	3 mos	Annually	IM or SQ
RM IMRAB BOVINE PLUS	Rhone Merieux, Inc. License No. 298	Rhone Merieux, Inc.	Cattle	2	3 mos	Annually	IM or SQ
			Horses	2	3 mos	Annually	IM or SQ
			Sheep	2	3 mos	Triennially	IM or SQ

Product	Manufacturer	Animal	Number of doses	Age/schedule	Booster	Route
RM IMRAB 3	Rhone Merieux, Inc. License No. 298	Dogs	1	3 mos&, 1 yr later	Triennially	IM or SQ
		Cats	1	3 mos&, 1 yr later	Triennially	IM or SQ
		Sheep	2	3 mos	Triennially	IM or SQ
		Cattle	2	3 mos	Annually	IM or SQ
		Horses	2	3 mos	Annually	IM or SQ
		Ferrets	1	3 mos	Annually	SQ
B. Combination (inactivated rabies)						
ECLIPSE 3 KP-R	Solvay Animal Health, Inc., License No. 195-A	Cats	1	3 mos	Annually	IM
ECLIPSE 4 KP-R	Solvay Animal Health, Inc., License No. 195-A	Cats	1	3 mos	Annually	IM
CYTORAB RCP	Coopers Animal Health, Inc., License No. 107	Cats	1	3 mos	Annually	IM
FEL-O-VAX PCT-R	Fort Dodge License No. 112	Cats	1	3 mos&, 1 yr later	Triennially	IM
RM FELINE 4+ IMRAB 3	Rhone Merieux, Inc. License No. 298	Cats	1	3 mos&, 1 yr later	Triennially	SQ
RM FELINE 3+ IMRAB 3	Rhone Merieux, Inc. License No. 298	Cats	1	3 mos&, 1 yr later	Triennially	SQ
RM EQUINE POTOMAVAC + IMRAB	Rhone Merieux, Inc. License No. 298	Horses	1	3 mos	Annually	IM

* ≥3 months of age and revaccinated 1 year later.
+ Intramuscularly.
& Subcutaneously.

wounds combined with appropriate passive and active immunization. Both the rationale for recommending preexposure and postexposure rabies prophylaxis and details of their administration can be found in the current recommendations of the Advisory Committee on Immunization Practices (ACIP) of the Public Health Service (PHS). These recommendations are available from state health departments, along with information concerning the current local and regional status of animal rabies and the availability of human rabies biologics.

Rabies in Domestic Animals

Local governments should initiate and maintain effective programs to ensure vaccination of all dogs and cats and to remove strays and unwanted animals. Such procedures in the United States have reduced laboratory-confirmed rabies cases in dogs from 6,949 in 1947 to 130 in 1993. Because more rabies cases are reported annually involving cats than dogs, vaccination of cats should be required. The recommended vaccination procedures and the licensed animal vaccines are specified in Parts I and II of the Compendium.

Rabies in Wildlife

The control of rabies among wildlife reservoirs is difficult. Selective population reduction may be useful in some situations, but the success of such procedures depends on the circumstances surrounding each rabies outbreak. (See Control Methods in Wildlife.)

Control Methods in Domestic and Confined Animals

Preexposure Vaccination and Management

Animal rabies vaccines should be administered only by, or under the direct supervision of, a veterinarian. This is the only way to ensure that a responsible person can be held accountable to assure the public that an animal has been properly vaccinated. Within 1 month after primary vaccination, a peak rabies antibody titer is reached and the animal can be considered immunized. An animal is currently vaccinated and is considered immunized if it was vaccinated at least 30 days previously and if all vaccinations have been administered in accordance with this Compendium. Regardless of the age at initial vaccination, a second vaccination should be given 1 year later. (See Parts I and II for recommended vaccines and procedures.)

Dogs and Cats

All dogs and cats should be vaccinated against rabies at 3 months of age and revaccinated in accordance with Part II of this Compendium.

Ferrets

Ferrets can be vaccinated against rabies at 3 months of age and revaccinated in accordance with Part II of this Compendium.

Livestock

It is neither economically feasible nor justified from a public health standpoint to vaccinate all livestock against rabies. However, consideration should be given to the vaccination of livestock, especially animals that are particularly valuable and/or might have frequent contact with humans, in areas where rabies is epizootic in terrestrial animals.

Other Animals

Wild. No rabies vaccine is licensed for use in wild animals. Because of the risk for rabies among wild animals (especially raccoons, skunks, coyotes, foxes, and bats), the American Veterinary Medical Association (AVMA), the National Association of State Public Health Veterinarians, Inc. (NASPHV), and the Council of State and Territorial Epidemiologists (CSTE) recommend the enactment of state laws prohibiting the importation, distribution, relocation, or keeping of wild animals and wild animals that are crossbred to domestic dogs and cats as pets.

Maintained in Exhibits and in Zoological Parks. Captive animals that are not completely excluded from all contact with rabies vectors can become infected. Moreover, wild animals can be incubating rabies when initially captured; therefore, wild-caught animals susceptible to rabies should be quarantined for a minimum of 180 days before exhibition. Persons (e.g., employees) who work with animals at such facilities should receive preexposure rabies immunization. The use of preexposure or postexposure rabies immunizations of persons who work with animals at such facilities might reduce the need for euthanasia of captive animals.

Stray Animals. Stray dogs and cats should be removed from the community, especially in areas where rabies is epizootic. Local health departments and animal control officials can enforce the removal of strays more effectively if owners either confine their animals or keep them on leash. Strays should be impounded for at least 3 days to determine if human exposure has occurred and to give owners sufficient time to reclaim animals.

Quarantine

International

CDC regulates the importation of dogs and cats into the United States, but current PHS regulations* governing the importation of such animals are insufficient to prevent the introduction of rabid animals into the country. All dogs and cats imported from countries with enzootic rabies should be currently vaccinated against rabies as recommended in this Compendium. Appropriate public health officials of the state of destination should be notified within 72 hours of any unvaccinated dog or cat imported into their jurisdiction. The conditional admission of such animals into the United States is subject to state and

---

* 42 CFR No. 71.51.

local laws governing rabies. Failure to comply with these requirements should be reported promptly to the Division of Quarantine, CDC (404) 639-8107.

Interstate

Before interstate movement, dogs and cats should be currently vaccinated against rabies in accordance with the Compendium's recommendations. (See B.1. Preexposure Vaccination and Management.) Animals in transit should be accompanied by a currently valid NASPHV Form #51, Rabies Vaccination Certificate.

Adjunct Procedures

Methods or procedures that enhance rabies control include the following:

1. Licensure. Registration or licensure of all dogs and cats can be used to aid in rabies control. A fee is frequently charged for such licensure, and revenues collected are used to maintain rabies or animal control programs. Vaccination is an essential prerequisite to licensure.
2. Canvassing of Area. House-to-house canvassing by animal control personnel facilitates enforcement of vaccination and licensure requirements.
3. Citations. Citations are legal summonses issued to owners for violations, including the failure to vaccinate or license their animals. The authority for officers to issue citations should be an integral part of each animal control program.
4. Animal Control. All communities should incorporate stray animal control, leash laws, and training of personnel in their programs.

Postexposure Management

Any animal bitten or scratched by a wild, carnivorous mammal (or a bat) not available for testing should be regarded as having been exposed to rabies.

Dogs and Cats

Unvaccinated dogs and cats exposed to a rabid animal should be euthanized immediately. If the owner is unwilling to do this, the animal should be placed in strict isolation for 6 months and vaccinated 1 month before being released. Dogs and cats that are currently vaccinated should be revaccinated immediately, kept under the owner's control, and observed for 45 days.

Livestock

All species of livestock are susceptible to rabies; cattle and horses are among the most frequently infected of all domestic animals. Livestock that is exposed to a rabid animal and is currently vaccinated with a vaccine approved by USDA for that species should be revaccinated immediately and observed for 45 days. Unvaccinated livestock should be slaughtered immediately. If the owner is unwilling to do this, the animal should be kept under close observation for 6 months.

The following are recommendations for owners of unvaccinated livestock exposed to rabid animals:

1. If the animal is slaughtered within 7 days of being bitten, its tissues may be eaten without risk of infection, provided liberal portions of the exposed

area are discarded. Federal meat inspectors must reject for slaughter any animal known to have been exposed to rabies within 8 months.

2. Neither tissues nor milk from a rabid animal should be used for human or animal consumption. However, because pasteurization temperatures will inactivate rabies virus, drinking pasteurized milk or eating cooked meat does not constitute a rabies exposure.

3. It is rare to have more than one rabid animal in a herd or to have herbivore-to-herbivore transmission; therefore; it may not be necessary to restrict the rest of the herd if a single animal has been exposed to or infected by rabies.

4. Other Animals. Other animals bitten by a rabid animal should be euthanized immediately. Such animals currently vaccinated with a vaccine approved by USDA for that species can be revaccinated immediately and placed in strict isolation for at least 90 days.

Management of Animals That Bite Humans

A healthy dog or cat that bites a person should be confined and observed for 10 days; it is recommended that rabies vaccine not be administered during the observation period. Such animals should be evaluated by a veterinarian at the first sign of illness during confinement. Any illness in the animal should be reported immediately to the local health department. If signs suggestive of rabies develop, the animal should be humanely killed, its head removed, and the head shipped under refrigeration for examination by a qualified laboratory designated by the local or state health department. Any stray or unwanted dog or cat that bites a person may be humanely killed immediately and the head submitted as described above for rabies examination. Other biting animals that might have exposed a person to rabies should be reported immediately to the local health department. Prior vaccination of an animal may not preclude the necessity for euthanasia and testing if the period of virus shedding is unknown for that species. Management of animals other than dogs and cats depends on the species, the circumstances of the bite, and the epidemiology of rabies in the area.

Control Methods in Wildlife

The public should be warned not to handle wildlife. Wild mammals (as well as the offspring of wild species cross-bred with domestic dogs and cats) that bite or otherwise expose humans, pets, or livestock to rabies should be considered for euthanasia and rabies examination. A person bitten by any wild mammal should immediately report the incident to a physician who can evaluate the need for antirabies treatment.**

Terrestrial Mammals

Continuous and persistent government-funded programs for trapping or poisoning wildlife are not cost effective in reducing wildlife rabies reservoirs on a

---

** Centers for Disease Control and Prevention. Rabies Prevention—United States, 1991. MMWR 1991;40(No. RR-3):1–19.

statewide basis. However, limited control in high-contact areas (e.g., picnic grounds, camps, or suburban areas) might be indicated for the removal of selected high-risk species of wildlife. The state wildlife agency and state health department should be consulted for coordination of any proposed population reduction programs.

Bats

Indigenous rabid bats have been reported from every state except Alaska and Hawaii and, since 1951, have been associated with at least 21 human deaths in the United States. However, it is neither feasible nor desirable to control rabies in bats through programs to reduce bat populations. Bats should be excluded from houses and surrounding structures to prevent direct association with humans. Such structures should then be made bat-proof by sealing entrances used by bats.

Mass Treatment of Humans Exposed to Rabies

Original Citation: Centers for Disease Control and Prevention. Mass treatment of humans exposed to rabies—New Hampshire, 1994. MMWR 1995;44(26):484–486.

EDITORIAL NOTE

CDC recommends implementation of four measures to minimize the number of exposed persons and the costs associated with exposures to persons. First, to facilitate efforts to investigate incidents of rabies associated with pet stores, pet stores should keep adequate records (e.g., health certificates, animal source identification, and complete sales receipts). Second, to prevent the exposure to, or the transmission of, rabies and other zoonotic diseases—as well as injuries such as bites and scratches—animals should be kept and displayed separate from customers or at least confined to a discrete area within the store. Third, because feral animals are less likely to have been vaccinated and more likely to have been in contact with wildlife disease reservoirs, acquisition and sale of these animals should be monitored closely. Finally, prompt and standardized assessment of exposure by public health officials should help minimize the number of persons who unnecessarily receive rabies postexposure treatment. The rabies virus is transmitted only when introduced into open wounds or mucous membranes through a bite or direct saliva contact. Other forms of contact (e.g., petting a rabid animal or contact with blood, urine, or feces of a rabid animal) do not constitute an exposure and are not indications for prophylaxis (1). Skillful interviewing is essential to assess individual exposures, especially when the potential exposure occurred some time ago or in another family member (e.g., a young child).

REFERENCE:

1. ACIP. Rabies prevention—United States, 1991: recommendations of the Immunization Practices Advisory Committee (ACIP). MMWR 1991;40(RR-3).

Rabies Prevention

Original Citation: ACIP. Rabies prevention—United States, 1991. Recommendations of the Immunization Practices Advisory Committee (ACIP). MMWR 1991;40(RR-03):1–19.

These revised recommendations of the Immunization Practices Advisory Committee (ACIP) on rabies prevention update the previous recommendations (MMWR 1984;33:393–402, 407–408) to reflect the current status of rabies and antirabies biologics in the United States.*

INTRODUCTION

Following the marked decrease of rabies cases among domestic animals in the United States in the 1940s and 1950s, indigenously acquired rabies among humans decreased to fewer than two cases per year in the 1960s and 1970s and fewer than one case per year during the 1980s (1). In 1950, for example, 4,979 cases of rabies were reported among dogs and 18 were reported among human populations; in 1989, 160 cases were reported among dogs and one was reported among humans. Thus, the likelihood of human exposure to a rabid domestic animal has decreased greatly; however, the many possible exposures that result from frequent contact between domestic dogs and humans continue to be the basis of most antirabies treatments (2).

Rabies among wild animals—especially skunks, raccoons, and bats—has become more prevalent since the 1950s, accounting for greater than 85% of all reported cases of animal rabies every year since 1976 (1). Rabies among animals occurs throughout the continental United States; only Hawaii remains consistently rabies-free. Wild animals now constitute the most important potential source of infection for both humans and domestic animals in the United States. In much of the rest of the world, including most of Asia, Africa, and Latin America, the dog remains the major species with rabies and the major source of rabies among humans. Nine of the 13 human rabies deaths reported to CDC from 1980 through 1990 appear to have been related to exposure to rabid animals outside of the United States (3–9). Although rabies among humans is rare in the United States, every year approximately 18,000 persons receive rabies preexposure prophylaxis and an additional 10,000 receive postexposure prophylaxis. Appropriate management of persons possibly exposed to rabies depends on the interpretation of the risk of infection. Decisions about management must be made immediately. All available methods of systemic prophylactic treatment are complicated by occasional adverse reactions, but these are rarely severe (10–14).

Data on the efficacy of active and passive rabies immunization have come from both human and animal studies. Evidence from laboratory and field experience in many areas of the world indicates that postexposure prophylaxis combining local wound treatment, passive immunization, and vaccination is uniformly effective when appropriately applied (15–20). However, rabies has occasionally developed among humans when key elements of the rabies postexposure prophylaxis treatment regimens were omitted or incorrectly administered (see Postexposure Treatment Outside the United States).

RABIES IMMUNIZING PRODUCTS

There are two types of rabies immunizing products:

1. Rabies vaccines induce an active immune response that includes the production of neutralizing antibodies. This antibody response requires approximately 7–10 days to develop and usually persists for greater than or equal to 2 years.
2. Rabies immune globulins (RIG) provide rapid, passive immune. protection that persists for only a short time (half-life of approximately 21 days) (21, 22). In almost all postexposure prophylaxis regimens, both products should be used concurrently.

*For assistance with problems or questions about rabies prophylaxis, contact your local or state health department. If local or state health department personnel are unavailable, call the Division of Viral and Rickettsial Diseases, Center for Infectious Diseases, CDC ((404) 639-1075 during working hours or (404) 639-2888 nights, weekends, and holidays).

Rabies Immunizing Products, United States, 1991

Human Rabies Vaccine
  Rabies Vaccine, Human Diploid Cell (HDCV)
    Intramuscular   Imovax® Rabies
    Intradermal   Imovax® Rabies I.D.
  Rabies Vaccine Adsorbed (RVA)
Rabies Immune Globulin (RIG)
  Rabies Immune Globulin, Human (HRIG):   Hyperab®
                                           Imogam® Rabies

Vaccines Licensed for Use in the United States

Two inactivated rabies vaccines are currently licensed for preexposure and post-exposure prophylaxis in the United States.

Rabies Vaccine, Human Diploid Cell (HDCV)

HDCV is prepared from the Pitman-Moore strain of rabies virus grown in MRC-5 human diploid cell culture and concentrated by ultrafiltration (23). The vaccine is inactivated with betapropiolactone (18) and is supplied in forms for:

1. Intramuscular (IM) administration, a single-dose vial containing lyophilized vaccine (Pasteur-Merieux Serum et Vaccins, Imovax® Rabies, distributed by Connaught Laboratories, Inc., Phone: 800-VACCINE) that is reconstituted in the vial with the accompanying diluent to a final volume of 1.0 mL just before administration.
2. Intradermal (ID) administration, a single-dose syringe. containing lyophilized vaccine (Pasteur-Merieux Serum et Vaccins, Imovax® Rabies I.D., distributed by Connaught Laboratories, Inc.) that is reconstituted in the syringe to a volume of 0.1 mL just before administration (24).

    A human diploid cell-derived rabies vaccine developed in the United States (Wyeth Laboratories, Wyvac®) was recalled by the manufacturer from the market in 1985 and is no longer available (25).

Rabies Vaccine, Adsorbed (RVA)

RVA (Michigan Department of Public Health) was licensed on March 19, 1988; it was developed and is currently distributed by the Biologics Products Program, Michigan Department of Public Health. The vaccine is prepared from the Kissling strain of Challenge Virus Standard (CVS) rabies virus adapted to fetal rhesus lung diploid cell culture (26–32). The vaccine virus is inactivated with betapropiolactone and concentrated by adsorption to aluminum phosphate. Because RVA is adsorbed to aluminum phosphate, it is liquid rather than lyophilized. RVA is currently available only from the Biologics Products Program, Michigan Department of Public Health. Phone: (517) 335-8050.

    Both types of rabies vaccines are considered equally efficacious and safe when used as indicated. The full 1.0-mL dose of either product can be used for both preexposure and postexposure prophylaxis. Only the Imovax® Rabies

I.D. vaccine (HDCV) has been evaluated by the ID dose/route for preexposure vaccination (33–36); the antibody response and side effects after ID administration of RVA have not been studied (24). Therefore, RVA should not be used intradermally.

Rabies Immune Globulins Licensed for Use in the United States

HRIG (Cutter Biological (a division of Miles Inc.), Hyperab®; and Pasteur-Merieux Serum et Vaccins, Imogam® Rabies, distributed by Connaught Laboratories, Inc.) is an antirabies gamma globulin concentrated by cold ethanol fractionation from plasma of hyperimmunized human donors. Rabies neutralizing antibody content, standardized to contain 150 international units (IU) per mL, is supplied in 2-mL (300 IU) and 10-mL (1,500 IU) vials for pediatric and adult use, respectively.

Both HRIG preparations are considered equally efficacious and safe when used as described in this document.

POSTEXPOSURE PROPHYLAXIS: RATIONALE FOR TREATMENT

Physicians should evaluate each possible exposure to rabies and if necessary consult with local or state public health officials regarding the need for rabies prophylaxis (Table 1). In the United States, the following factors should be considered before specific antirabies treatment is initiated.

Table 1. Rabies postexposure prophylaxis guide, United States, 1991

Animal type	Evaluation and disposition of animal	Postexposure prophylaxis recommendations
Dogs and cats	Healthy and available for 10 days observation	Should not begin prophylaxis unless animal develops symptoms of rabies*
	Rabid or suspected rabid	Immediate vaccination
	Unknown (escaped)	Consult public health officials
Skunks, raccoons, bats, foxes, and most other carnivores; woodchucks	Regarded as rabid unless geographic area is known to be free of rabies or until animal proven negative by laboratory tests†	Immediate vaccination
Livestock, rodents, and lagomorphs (rabbits and hares)	Consider individually	Consult public health officials. Bites of squirrels, hamsters, guinea pigs, gerbils, chipmunks, rats, mice, other rodents, rabbits, and hares almost never require antirabies treatment

*During the 10-day holding period, begin treatment with HRIG and HDCV or RVA at first sign of rabies in a dog or cat that has bitten someone. The symptomatic animal should be killed immediately and tested.

†The animal should be killed and tested as soon as possible. Holding for observation is not recommended. Discontinue vaccine if immunofluorescence test results of the animal are negative.

Type of Exposure

Rabies is transmitted only when the virus is introduced into open cuts or wounds in skin or mucous membranes. If there has been no exposure (as described in this section), postexposure treatment is not necessary. The likelihood of rabies infection varies with the nature and extent of exposure. Two categories of exposure (bite and nonbite) should be considered.

Bite

Any penetration of the skin by teeth constitutes a bite exposure. Bites to the face and hands carry the highest risk, but the site of the bite should not influence the decision to begin treatment (17).

Nonbite

Scratches, abrasions, open wounds, or mucous membranes contaminated with saliva or other potentially infectious material (such as brain tissue) from a rabid animal constitute nonbite exposures. If the material containing the virus is dry, the virus can be considered noninfectious.

Other contact by itself, such as petting a rabid animal and contact with the blood, urine, or feces (e.g., guano) of a rabid animal, does not constitute an exposure and is not an indication for prophylaxis.

Although occasional reports of transmission by nonbite exposure suggest that such exposures constitute sufficient reason to initiate postexposure prophylaxis under some circumstances, nonbite exposures rarely cause rabies (37). The nonbite exposures of highest risk appear to be exposures to large amounts of aerosolized rabies virus, organs (i.e., corneas) transplanted from patients who died of rabies, and scratches by rabid animals. Two cases of rabies have been attributed to airborne exposures in laboratories, and two cases of rabies have been attributed to probable airborne exposures in a bat-infested cave in Texas (38, 39).

The only documented cases of rabies caused by human-to-human transmission occurred among six recipients of transplanted corneas. Investigations revealed each of the donors had died of an illness compatible with or proven to be rabies (40–43). The six cases occurred in four countries: Thailand (two cases), India (two cases), the United States (one case), and France (one case). Stringent guidelines for acceptance of donor corneas have reduced this risk.

Apart from corneal transplants, bite and nonbite exposures inflicted by infected humans could theoretically transmit rabies, but no such cases have been documented (44). Adherence to respiratory precautions will minimize the risk of airborne exposure (45).

Animal Rabies Epidemiology and Evaluation of Involved Species

Wild Animals

Carnivorous wild animals (especially skunks, raccoons, and foxes) and bats are the animals most often infected with rabies and the cause of most indigenous cases of human rabies in the United States since 1960 (1). All bites by wild carnivores and bats must be considered possible exposures to the disease. Postexposure prophylaxis should be initiated when patients are exposed to wild carnivores unless (a) the exposure occurred in a part of the continental United States known to be free of terrestrial rabies and the results of immunofluorescence antibody testing will be available within 48 hours or (b) the animal has already been tested and shown not to be rabid. If treatment has been initiated and subsequent immunofluorescence testing shows that the exposing animal was not rabid, treatment can be discontinued.

Signs of rabies among carnivorous wild animals cannot be interpreted reliably; therefore, any such animal that bites or scratches a person should be killed at once (without unnecessary damage to the head) and the brain submitted for rabies testing. If the results of testing are negative by immunofluorescence, the saliva can be assumed to contain no virus, and the person bitten does not require treatment.

If the biting animal is a particularly rare or valuable specimen and the risk of rabies small, public health authorities may choose to administer postexposure treatment to the bite victim in lieu of killing the animal for rabies testing (46). Such animals should be quarantined for 30 days.

Rodents (such as squirrels, hamsters, guinea pigs, gerbils, chipmunks, rats, and mice) and lagomorphs (including rabbits and hares) are almost never found to be infected with rabies and have not been known to cause rabies among humans in the United States. However, from 1971 through 1988, woodchucks accounted for 70% of the 179 cases of rabies among rodents reported to CDC (47). In all cases involving rodents, the state or local health department should be consulted before a decision is made to initiate postexposure antirabies prophylaxis.

Exotic pets (including ferrets) and domestic animals crossbred with wild animals are considered wild animals by the National Association of State Public Health Veterinarians (NASPHV) and the Conference of State and Territorial Epidemiologists (CSTE) because they may be highly susceptible to rabies and could transmit the disease. Because the period of rabies virus shedding in these animals is unknown, these animals should be killed and tested rather than confined and observed when they bite humans (46). Wild animals (skunks, raccoons, and bats) and wild animals crossbred with dogs should not be kept as pets (46).

Domestic Animals

The likelihood that a domestic animal is infected with rabies varies by region; hence, the need for postexposure prophylaxis also varies. In the continental United States, rabies among dogs is reported most commonly along the U.S.-Mexico border and sporadically from the areas of the United States with enzootic wildlife rabies, especially the Midwest. During most of the 1980s in the United States, more cats than dogs were reported rabid; the majority of these cases were associated with the mid-Atlantic epizootic of rabies among raccoons. The large number of rabies-infected cats may be attributed to fewer cat vaccination laws, fewer leash laws, and the roaming habits of cats. Cattle tend to be most often exposed to rabies via rabid skunks.

In areas where canine rabies is not enzootic (including virtually all of the United States and its territories), a healthy domestic dog or cat that bites a person should be confined and observed for 10 days. Any illness in the animal during confinement or before release should be evaluated by a veterinarian and reported immediately to the local health department. If signs suggestive of rabies develop, the animal should be humanely killed and its head removed and shipped, under refrigeration, for examination by a qualified laboratory. Any stray or unwanted dog or cat that bites a person should be killed immediately and the head submitted as described for rabies examination (46).

In most developing countries of Asia, Africa, and Central and South America, dogs are the major vector of rabies; exposures to dogs in such countries represent a special threat. Travelers to these countries should be aware that greater than 50% of the rabies cases among humans in the United States result from exposure to dogs outside the United States. Although dogs are the main reservoir of rabies in these countries, the epizootiology of the disease among animals differs sufficiently by region or country to warrant the evaluation of all animal bites. Exposures to dogs in canine rabies-enzootic areas outside the United States carry a high risk; some authorities therefore recommend that postexposure rabies treatment be initiated immediately after such exposures. Treatment can be discontinued if the dog or cat remains healthy during the 10-day observation period.

Circumstances of Biting Incident and Vaccination Status of Exposing Animal

An unprovoked attack by a domestic animal is more likely than a provoked attack to indicate that the animal is rabid. Bites inflicted on a person attempting to feed or handle an apparently healthy animal should generally be regarded as provoked.

A fully vaccinated dog or cat is unlikely to become infected with rabies, although rare cases have been reported (48). In a nationwide study of rabies among dogs and cats in 1988, only one dog and two cats that were vaccinated contracted rabies (49). All three of these animals had received only single doses of vaccine; no documented vaccine failures occurred among dogs or cats that had received two vaccinations.

POSTEXPOSURE PROPHYLAXIS: LOCAL TREATMENT OF WOUNDS AND VACCINATION

The essential components of rabies postexposure prophylaxis are local wound treatment and the administration, in most instances, of both HRIG and vaccine (Table 2). Persons who have been bitten by animals suspected or proven rabid should begin treatment within 24 hours. However, there have been instances when the decision to begin treatment was not made until many months after the exposure because of a delay in recognition that an exposure had occurred and awareness that incubation periods of greater than 1 year have been reported.

Table 2. Rabies postexposure prophylaxis schedule, United States, 1991

Vaccination status	Treatment	Regimen*
Not previously vaccinated	Local wound cleansing	All postexposure treatment should begin with immediate thorough cleansing of all wounds with soap and water.
	HRIG	20 IU/kg body weight. If anatomically feasible, up to one-half the dose should be infiltrated around the wound(s) and the rest should be administered IM in the gluteal area. HRIG should not be administered in the same syringe or into the same anatomical site as vaccine. Because HRIG may partially suppress active production of antibody, no more than the recommended dose should be given.
	Vaccine	HDCV or RVA, 1.0 mL, IM (deltoid area[†]), one each on days 0, 3, 7, 14 and 28.
Previously vaccinated[§]	Local wound cleansing	All postexposure treatment should begin with immediate thorough cleansing of all wounds with soap and water.
	HRIG	HRIG should not be administered.
	Vaccine	HDCV or RVA, 1.0 mL, IM (deltoid area[†]), one each on days 0 and 3.

*These regimens are applicable for all age groups, including children.

[†]The deltoid area is the only acceptable site of vaccination for adults and older children. For younger children, the outer aspect of the thigh may be used. Vaccine should never be administered in the gluteal area.

[§]Any person with a history of preexposure vaccination with HDCV or RVA; prior postexposure prophylaxis with HDCV or RVA; or previous vaccination with any other type of rabies vaccine and a documented history of antibody response to the prior vaccination.

In 1977, the World Health Organization (WHO) recommended a regimen of RIG and six doses of HDCV over a 90-day period. This recommendation was based on studies in Germany and Iran (16, 20). When used this way, the vaccine was found to be safe and effective in protecting persons bitten by proven rabid animals and induced an excellent antibody response in all recipients (16). Studies conducted in the United States by CDC have shown that a regimen of one dose of HRIG and five doses of HDCV over a 28-day period was safe and induced an excellent antibody response in all recipients (15).

Local Treatment of Wounds

Immediate and thorough washing of all bite wounds and scratches with soap and water is an important measure for preventing rabies. In studies of animals, simple local wound cleansing has been shown to reduce markedly the likelihood of rabies (50, 51). Tetanus prophylaxis and measures to control bacterial infection should be given as indicated. The decision to suture large wounds should take into account cosmetic factors and the potential for bacterial infections.

Immunization

Vaccine Usage

Two rabies vaccines are currently available in the United States; either is administered in conjunction with HRIG at the beginning of postexposure therapy. A regimen of five 1-mL doses of HDCV or RVA should be given intramuscularly. The first dose of the five-dose course should be given as soon as possible after exposure. Additional doses should be given on days 3, 7, 14, and 28 after the first vaccination. For adults, the vaccine should always be administered IM in the deltoid area. For children, the anterolateral aspect of the thigh is also acceptable. The gluteal area should never be used for HDCV or RVA injections, since administration in this area results in lower neutralizing antibody titers (52).

Postexposure antirabies vaccination should always include administration of both passive antibody and vaccine, with the exception of persons who have previously received complete vaccination regimens (preexposure or postexposure) with a cell culture vaccine, or persons who have been vaccinated with other types of vaccines and have had documented rabies antibody titers. These persons should receive only vaccine (see Postexposure Therapy of Previously Vaccinated Persons). The combination of HRIG (local and systemic) and vaccine is recommended for both bite and nonbite exposures (see Postexposure Prophylaxis: Rationale for Treatment), regardless of the interval between exposure and initiation of treatment.

Because the antibody response after the recommended postexposure vaccination regimen with HDCV or RVA has been satisfactory, routine postvaccination serologic testing is not recommended. Serologic testing is only indicated in unusual instances, as when the patient is known to be immunosuppressed. The state health department may be contacted for recommendations on this matter.

HRIG Usage

HRIG is administered only once (i.e., at the beginning of antirabies prophylaxis) to provide immediate antibodies until the patient responds to HDCV or RVA by actively producing antibodies. If HRIG was not given when vaccination was begun, it can be given through the seventh day after administration of the first dose of vaccine. Beyond the seventh day, HRIG is not indicated since an antibody response to cell culture vaccine is presumed to have occurred. The recommended dose of HRIG is 20 IU/kg. This formula is applicable for all age groups, including children. If anatomically feasible, up to one-half the dose of HRIG should be thoroughly infiltrated in the area around the wound and the rest should be administered intramuscularly in the gluteal area. HRIG should never be administered in the same syringe or into the same anatomical site as vaccine. Because HRIG may partially suppress active production of antibody, no more than the recommended dose should be given (53).

VACCINATION AND SEROLOGIC TESTING

The effectiveness of rabies vaccines is primarily measured by their ability to protect persons exposed to rabies. HDCV has been used effectively with HRIG or equine antirabies serum (ARS) worldwide to treat persons bitten by various rabid animals (15, 16). An estimated one million people worldwide have received rabies postexposure prophylaxis with HDCV since its introduction 12 years ago (54).

In studies of animals, antibody titers have been shown to be markers of protection. Antibody titers will vary with time since the last vaccination. Differences among laboratories that test blood samples may also influence the results.

Serologic Response Shortly After Vaccination

All persons tested at CDC 2–4 weeks after completion of preexposure and postexposure rabies prophylaxis according to ACIP guidelines have demonstrated an antibody response to rabies (15, 55, 56). Therefore, it is not necessary to test serum samples from patients completing preexposure or postexposure prophylaxis to document seroconversion unless the person is immunosuppressed (see Precautions and Contraindications). If titers are obtained, specimens collected 2–4 weeks after preexposure or postexposure prophylaxis should completely neutralize challenge virus at a 1:25 serum dilution by the rapid fluorescent focus inhibition test (RFFIT). (This dilution is approximately equivalent to the minimum titer of 0.5 IU recommended by the WHO.)

Serologic Response and Preexposure Booster Doses of Vaccine

Two years after primary preexposure vaccination, a 1:5 serum dilution will fail to neutralize challenge virus completely (by RFFIT) among 2%–7% of persons who received the three-dose preexposure series intramuscularly and 5%–17% of persons who received the three-dose series intradermally (57). If the titer falls below 1:5, a preexposure booster dose of vaccine is recommended for a person at continuous or frequent risk (Table 3) of exposure to rabies. The following guidelines are recommended for determining when serum testing should be performed after primary preexposure vaccination:

1. A person in the continuous risk category (Table 3) should have a serum sample tested for rabies antibody every 6 months (58).
2. A person in the frequent risk category (Table 3) should have a serum sample tested for rabies antibody every 2 years.

State or local health departments may provide the names and addresses of laboratories performing rabies serologic testing.

Table 3. Rabies preexposure prophylaxis guide, United States, 1991

Risk category	Nature of risk	Typical populations	Preexposure recommendations
Continuous	Virus present continuously, often in high concentrations. Aerosol, mucous membrane, bite, or nonbite exposure. Specific exposures may go unrecognized.	Rabies research lab worker;* rabies biologics production workers.	Primary course. Serologic testing every 6 months; booster vaccination when antibody level falls below acceptable level.†
Frequent	Exposure usually episodic, with source recognized, but exposure may also be unrecognized. Aerosol, mucous membrane, bite, or nonbite exposure.	Rabies diagnostic lab workers,* spelunkers, veterinarians and staff, and animal-control and wildlife workers in rabies enzootic areas. Travelers visiting foreign areas of enzootic rabies for more than 30 days.	Primary course. Serologic testing or booster vaccination every 2 years.†
Infrequent (greater than population at large)	Exposure nearly always episodic with source recognized. Mucous membrane, bite, or nonbite exposure.	Veterinarians and animal-control and wildlife workers in areas of low rabies enzooticity. Veterinary students.	Primary course; no serologic testing or booster vaccination.
Rare (population at large)	Exposures always episodic. Mucous membrane, or bite with source unrecognized.	U.S. population at large, including persons in rabies epizootic areas.	No vaccination necessary.

*Judgment of relative risk and extra monitoring of vaccination status of laboratory workers is the responsibility of the laboratory supervisor (58).

†Minimum acceptable antibody level is complete virus neutralization at a 1:5 serum dilution by RFFIT. Booster dose should be administered if the titer falls below this level.

POSTEXPOSURE TREATMENT OUTSIDE THE UNITED STATES

U.S. citizens and residents who are exposed to rabies while traveling outside the United States in countries where rabies is endemic may sometimes receive postexposure therapy with regimens or biologics that are not used in the United States. The following information is provided to familiarize physicians with some of the regimens used more widely abroad. These schedules have not been submitted for approval by the Food and Drug Administration (FDA) for use in the United States. If postexposure treatment is begun outside the United States using one of these regimens or biologics of nerve tissue origin, it may be necessary to provide additional treatment when the patient reaches the United States. State or local health departments should be contacted for specific advice in such cases.

Modifications to the postexposure vaccine regimen approved for use in the United States have been made to reduce the cost of postexposure prophylaxis and hasten the development of active immunity (59). Costs are reduced primarily by substituting various schedules of ID injections (0.1 mL each) of HDCV (or newer tissue culture-derived rabies vaccines for humans) for IM injection of HDCV. Two such regimens are efficacious among persons bitten by rabid animals (60). One of these regimens consists of 0.1-mL ID doses of HDCV given at eight different sites (deltoid, suprascapular, thigh, and abdominal wall) on day 0; four ID 0.1-mL doses given at four sites on day 7 (deltoid, thigh); and one ID 0.1-mL dose given in the deltoid on both day 28 and 91. Another ID regimen shown to be efficacious and now widely used in Thailand employs Purified VERO Cell Rabies Vaccine (Pasteur-Merieux), with 0.1-mL doses given at two different sites on days 0, 3, and 7, followed by one 0.1-mL booster on days 30 and 90 (61).

Strategies designed to hasten the development of active immunity have concentrated on administering more IM or ID doses at the time postexposure prophylaxis is initiated with fewer doses thereafter (62). The most extensively evaluated regimen in this category, developed in Yugoslavia, has been the 2–1–1 regimen (two 1.0-mL IM doses on day 0, and one each on days 7 and 21) (63–65). However, when using HRIG in conjunction with this schedule, there may be some suppression of the neutralizing antibody response (65).

Purified antirabies sera of equine origin (Sclavo; Pasteur-Merieux; Swiss Serum and Vaccine Institute, Bern) have been used effectively in developing countries where HRIG may not be available. The incidence of adverse reactions has been low (0.8%–6.0%) and most of those that occurred were minor (66–68).

Although no postexposure vaccine failures have occurred in the United States during the 10 years that HDCV has been licensed, seven persons have contracted rabies after receiving postexposure treatment with both HRIG and HDCV outside the United States. An additional six persons have contracted the disease after receiving postexposure prophylaxis with other cell culture-derived vaccines and HRIG or ARS. However, in each of these cases, there was some deviation from the recommended postexposure treatment protocol (69–71).

Specifically, patients who contracted rabies after postexposure prophylaxis did not have their wounds cleansed with soap and water or other antiviral agents, did not receive their rabies vaccine injections in the deltoid area (i.e., vaccine was administered in the gluteal area), or did not receive passive vaccination around the wound site.

PREEXPOSURE VACCINATION AND POSTEXPOSURE THERAPY OF PREVIOUSLY VACCINATED PERSONS

Preexposure vaccination should be offered to persons among high-risk groups, such as veterinarians, animal handlers, certain laboratory workers, and persons spending time (e.g., 1 month) in foreign countries where canine rabies is endemic. Other persons whose activities bring them into frequent contact with rabies virus or potentially rabid dogs, cats, skunks, raccoons, bats, or other species at risk of having rabies should also be considered for preexposure prophylaxis.

Preexposure prophylaxis is given for several reasons. First, it may provide protection to persons with inapparent exposures to rabies. Second, it may protect persons whose postexposure therapy might be delayed. Finally, although preexposure vaccination does not eliminate the need for additional therapy after a rabies exposure, it simplifies therapy by eliminating the need for HRIG and decreasing the number of doses of vaccine needed—a point of particular importance for persons at high risk of being exposed to rabies in areas where immunizing products may not be available or where they may carry a high risk of adverse reactions.

Primary Preexposure Vaccination

Intramuscular Primary Vaccination

Three 1.0-mL injections of HDCV or RVA should be given intramuscularly (deltoid area), one each on days 0, 7, and 21 or 28 (Table 4). In a study in the United States, greater than 1,000 persons received HDCV according to this regimen. Antibody was demonstrated in serum samples of all subjects when tested by the RF-FIT. Other studies have produced comparable results (33, 56, 72, 73).

Table 4. Rabies preexposure prophylaxis schedule, United States, 1991

Type of vaccination	Route	Regimen
Primary	IM	HDCV or RVA, 1.0 mL (deltoid area), one each on days 0, 7, and 21 or 28
	ID	HDCV, 0.1 mL, one each on days 0, 7, and 21 or 28
Booster*	IM	HDCV or RVA, 1.0 mL (deltoid area), day 0 only
	ID	HDCV, 0.1 mL, day 0 only

*Administration of routine booster dose of vaccine depends on exposure risk category as noted in Table 3.

Intradermal Primary Vaccination

A regimen of three 0.1-mL doses of HDCV, one each on days 0, 7, and 21 or 28 (10, 33, 34, 36, 72, 73), is also used for preexposure vaccination (Table 4). The ID dose/route has been recommended previously by the ACIP as an alternative to the 1.0-mL IM dose/route for rabies preexposure prophylaxis with HDCV (24, 74). Pasteur-Merieux developed a syringe containing a single dose of lyophilized HDCV (Imovax® Rabies I.D.) that is reconstituted in the syringe just before administration. The syringe is designed to deliver 0.1 mL of HDCV reliably and was approved by the FDA in 1986 (24). The 0.1-mL ID doses, given in the area over the deltoid (lateral aspect of the upper arm) on days 0, 7, and 21 or 28, are used for primary preexposure vaccination. One 0.1-mL ID dose is used for booster vaccination (see Table 3). The 1.0-mL vial is not approved for multi-dose ID use. RVA should not be given by the ID dose/route (26).

Chloroquine phosphate (administered for malaria chemoprophylaxis) interferes with the antibody response to HDCV (75). Accordingly, HDCV should not be administered by the ID dose/route to persons traveling to malaria-endemic countries while the person is receiving chloroquine (76). The IM dose/route of preexposure prophylaxis provides a sufficient margin of safety in this situation (76). For persons who will be receiving both rabies preexposure prophylaxis and chloroquine in preparation for travel to a rabies-enzootic area, the ID dose/route should be initiated at least 1 month before travel to allow for completion of the full three-dose vaccine series before antimalarial prophylaxis begins. If this schedule is not possible, the IM dose/route should be used. Although interference with the immune response to rabies vaccine by other antimalarials structurally related to chloroquine (e.g., mefloquine) has not been evaluated, it would seem prudent to follow similar precautions for persons receiving these drugs.

Booster Vaccination

Preexposure Booster Doses of Vaccine

Persons who work with live rabies virus in research laboratories or vaccine production facilities (continuous risk category; see Table 3) are at the highest risk of inapparent exposures. Such persons should have a serum sample tested for rabies antibody every 6 months (Table 4). Booster doses (IM or ID) of vaccine should be given to maintain a serum titer corresponding to at least complete neutralization at a 1:5 serum dilution by the RFFIT. The frequent risk category includes other laboratory workers, such as those doing rabies diagnostic testing, spelunkers, veterinarians and staff, animal-control and wildlife officers in areas where animal rabies is epizootic, and international travelers living or visiting (for greater than 30 days) in areas where canine rabies is endemic. Persons among this group should have a serum sample tested for rabies antibody every 2 years and, if the titer is less than complete neutralization at a 1:5 serum dilution by the RFFIT, should have a booster dose of vaccine. Alternatively, a booster can be administered in lieu of a titer determination. Veterinarians and animal control and wildlife officers working in areas of low rabies enzooticity (infrequent exposure group) do not require routine preexposure booster doses of HDCV or RVA after completion of primary preexposure vaccination (Table 3).

Postexposure Therapy of Previously Vaccinated Persons

If exposed to rabies, persons previously vaccinated should receive two IM doses (1.0 mL each) of vaccine, one immediately and one 3 days later. Previously vaccinated refers to persons who have received one of the recommended preexposure or postexposure regimens of HDCV or RVA, or those who received another vaccine and had a documented rabies antibody titer. HRIG is unnecessary and should not be given in these cases because an anamnestic antibody response will follow the administration of a booster regardless of the prebooster antibody titer (77).

Preexposure Vaccination and Serologic Testing

Because the antibody response after these recommended preexposure prophylaxis vaccine regimens has been satisfactory, serologic testing is not necessary except for persons suspected of being immunosuppressed. Patients who are immunosuppressed by disease or medications should postpone preexposure vaccinations. Immunosuppressed persons who are at risk of rabies exposure should be vaccinated and their antibody titers checked.

UNINTENTIONAL INOCULATION WITH MODIFIED LIVE RABIES VIRUS

Veterinary personnel may be inadvertently exposed to attenuated rabies virus while administering modified live rabies virus (MLV) vaccines to animals. Although there have been no reported rabies cases among humans resulting from exposure to needle sticks or sprays with licensed MLV vaccines, vaccine-induced rabies has occurred among animals given these vaccines. Absolute assurance of a lack of risk for humans, therefore, cannot be given. The best evidence for low risk is the absence of recognized cases of vaccine-associated disease among humans despite frequent inadvertent exposures.

MLV animal vaccines that are currently available are made with one attenuated strain of rabies virus: high egg passage (HEP) Flury strain. The HEP Flury strain has been used in animal vaccines for more than 25 years without evidence of associated disease among humans; therefore, postexposure treatment is not recommended following exposure to this type of vaccine by needle sticks or sprays.

Because the data are insufficient to assess the true risk associated with any of the MLV vaccines, preexposure vaccination and periodic boosters are recommended for all persons whose activities either bring them into contact with potentially rabid animals or who frequently handle attenuated animal rabies vaccine.

ADVERSE REACTIONS

Human Diploid Cell Rabies Vaccine and Rabies Vaccine Adsorbed

Reactions after vaccination with HDCV and RVA are less serious and common than with previously available vaccines (78, 79). In studies using a three-dose postexposure regimen of HDCV, local reactions, such as pain, erythema, and swelling or itching at the injection site, have been reported among 30%–74% of recipients. Systemic reactions, such as headache, nausea, abdominal pain, muscle aches, and dizziness have been reported among 5%–40% of recipients. Three cases of neurologic illness resembling Guillain-Barre syndrome that resolved without sequelae in 12 weeks have been reported (10, 80, 81). In addition, a few other subacute central and peripheral nervous system disorders have been temporally associated with HDCV vaccine, but a causal relationship has not been established (82).

An immune complex-like reaction occurs among approximately 6% of persons receiving booster doses of HDCV (11, 12) 2–21 days after administration of the booster dose. These patients develop a generalized urticaria, sometimes accompanied by arthralgia, arthritis, angioedema, nausea, vomiting, fever, and malaise. In no cases have the illnesses been life-threatening. This reaction occurs much less frequently among persons receiving primary vaccination.

The reaction has been associated with the presence of betapropiolactone-altered human serum albumin in the HDCV and the development of immunoglobulin E (IgE) antibodies to this allergen (83, 84). Among persons who have received their primary vaccination series with HDCV, administration of boosters with a purified HDCV produced in Canada (Connaught Laboratories Ltd., Rabies Vaccine Inactivated (Diploid Cell Origin)-Dried) does not appear to be associated with this reaction (57). This vaccine is not yet licensed in the United States.

Vaccines and Immune Globulins Used in Other Countries

Many developing countries use inactivated nerve tissue vaccines made from the brains of adult animals or suckling mice. Nerve tissue vaccine (NTV) is reported to induce neuroparalytic reactions among approximately 1 per 200 to 1 per 2,000 vaccinees; suckling mouse brain vaccine (SMBV) causes reactions in among approximately 1 per 8,000 (17).

Human Rabies Immune Globulins

Local pain and low-grade fever may follow receipt of HRIG. Although not reported specifically for HRIG, angioneurotic edema, nephrotic syndrome, and anaphylaxis have been reported after injection of immune globulin (IG). These reactions occur so rarely that a causal relationship between IG and these reactions is not clear.

There is no evidence that hepatitis B virus (HBV), human immunodeficiency virus (HIV, the causative agent of Acquired Immunodeficiency Syndrome (AIDS)), or other viruses have ever been transmitted by commercially available HRIG in the United States.

Management of Adverse Reactions

Once initiated, rabies prophylaxis should not be interrupted or discontinued because of local or mild systemic adverse reactions to rabies vaccine. Usually such reactions can be successfully managed with anti-inflammatory and antipyretic agents (e.g., aspirin).

When a person with a history of serious hypersensitivity to rabies vaccine must be revaccinated, antihistamines may be given. Epinephrine should be readily available to counteract anaphylactic reactions, and the person should be observed carefully immediately after vaccination.

Although serious systemic, anaphylactic, or neuroparalytic reactions are rare during and after the administration of rabies vaccines, such reactions pose a serious dilemma for the attending physician (11). A patient's risk of acquiring rabies must be carefully considered before deciding to discontinue vaccination. Advice and assistance on the management of serious adverse reactions for persons receiving rabies vaccines may be sought from the state health department or CDC.

All serious systemic, neuroparalytic, or anaphylactic reactions to HDCV should be reported immediately to Connaught Laboratories, Inc., Swiftwater, PA 18370. Phone: (800) VACCINE or (717) 839-7187. Serious reactions after the administration of RVA should be reported immediately to Coordinating Physicians, Bureau of Laboratories and Epidemiological Services, Michigan Department of Public Health, P. O. Box 30035, 3500 N. Logan, Lansing, MI 48909. Phone: (517) 335-8050.

PRECAUTIONS AND CONTRAINDICATIONS

Immunosuppression

Corticosteroids, other immunosuppressive agents, antimalarials, and immunosuppressive illnesses can interfere with the development of active immunity after vaccination and may predispose the patient to rabies (75, 85). Preexposure prophylaxis should be administered to such persons with the awareness that the immune response may be inadequate (see Intradermal Primary Vaccination). Immunosuppressive agents should not be administered during postexposure therapy unless essential for the treatment of other conditions. When rabies postexposure prophylaxis is administered to persons receiving steroids or other immunosuppressive therapy, it is especially important that a serum sample be tested for rabies antibody to ensure that an acceptable antibody response has developed (see Vaccination and Serologic Testing).

Pregnancy

Because of the potential consequences of inadequately treated rabies exposure, and because there is no indication that fetal abnormalities have been associated with rabies vaccination, pregnancy is not considered a contraindication to postexposure prophylaxis (86). If there is substantial risk of exposure to rabies, preexposure prophylaxis may also be indicated during pregnancy.

Allergies

Persons who have a history of serious hypersensitivity to rabies vaccine should be revaccinated with caution (see Management of Adverse Reactions).

REFERENCES

1. Reid-Sanden FL, Dobbins JG, Smith JS, Fishbein DB. Rabies surveillance, United States during 1989. J Am Vet Med Assoc 1990;197:1571–1583.
2. Helmick CG. The epidemiology of human rabies postexposure prophylaxis, 1980–1981. JAMA 1983;250:1990–1996.
3. CDC. Human rabies diagnosed 2 months postmortem—Texas. MMWR 1985;34:700, 705–707.
4. CDC. Human rabies acquired outside the United States. MMWR 1985;34:235–236.
5. CDC. Human rabies—California, 1987. MMWR 1988;37:305–308.
6. CDC. Human rabies—Oregon, 1989. MMWR 1989;38:335–337.
7. CDC. Human rabies—Texas. MMWR 1984;33:469–470.
8. CDC. Imported human rabies. MMWR 1983;32:78–80, 85–86.
9. CDC. Human rabies acquired outside the United States from a dog bite. MMWR 1981;30: 537–540.
10. Bernard KW, Smith PW, Kader FJ, Moran MJ. Neuroparalytic illness and human diploid cell rabies vaccine. JAMA 1982;248:3136–3138.
11. CDC. Systemic allergic reactions following immunization with human diploid cell rabies vaccine. MMWR 1984;33:185–187.
12. Dreesen DW, Bernard KW, Parker RA, Deutsch AJ, Brown J. Immune complex-like disease in 23 persons following a booster dose of rabies human diploid cell vaccine. Vaccine 1986;4:45–49.
13. Aoki FY, Tyrrell DA, Hill LE. Immunogenicity and acceptability of a human diploid-cell culture rabies vaccine in volunteers. Lancet 1975;1:660–662.
14. Cox JH, Schneider LG. Prophylactic immunization of humans against rabies by intradermal inoculation of human diploid cell culture vaccine. J Clin Microbiol 1976;3:96–101.
15. Anderson LJ, Sikes RK, Langkop CW, et al. Postexposure trial of a human diploid cell strain rabies vaccine. J Infect Dis 1980;142:133–138.
16. Bahmanyar M, Fayaz A, Nour-Salehi S, Mohammadi M, Koprowski H. Successful protection of humans exposed to rabies infection. Postexposure treatment with the new human diploid cell rabies vaccine and antirabies serum. JAMA 1976;236:2751–2754.
17. Hattwick MAW. Human rabies. Public Health Rev 1974;3:229–274.
18. Wiktor TJ, Plotkin SA, Koprowski H. Development and clinical trials of the new human rabies vaccine of tissue culture (human diploid cell) origin. Dev Biol Stand 1978;40:3–9.
19. World Health Organization. WHO expert committee on rabies. WHO Tech Rep Ser 1984;709: 1–104.
20. Kuwert EK, Werner J, Marcus I, Cabasso VJ. Immunization against rabies with rabies immune globulin, human (RIGH) and a human diploid cell strain (HDCS) rabies vaccine. J Biol Stand 1978;6:211–219.
21. Winkler WG, Schmidt RC, Sikes RK. Evaluation of human rabies immune globulin and homologous and heterologous antibody. J Immunol 1969;102:1314–1321.
22. Cabasso VJ, Loofbourow JC, Roby RE, Anuskiewicz W. Rabies immune globulin of human origin: preparation and dosage determination in non-exposed volunteer subjects. Bull WHO 1971;45:303–315.
23. Wiktor TJ, Sokol F, Kuwert E, Koprowski H. Immunogenicity of concentrated and purified rabies vaccine of tissue culture origin. Proc Soc Exp Biol Med 1969;131:799–805.
24. CDC. Rabies prevention: supplementary statement on the preexposure use of human diploid cell rabies vaccine by the intradermal route. MMWR 1986;35:767–768.

25. CDC. Rabies postexposure prophylaxis with human diploid cell rabies vaccine: lower neutralizing antibody titers with Wyeth vaccine. MMWR 1985;34:90–92.

26. CDC. Rabies vaccine, adsorbed: a new rabies vaccine for use in humans. MMWR 1988;37: 217–218, 223.

27. Burgoyne GH, Kajiya KD, Brown DW, Mitchell JR. Rhesus diploid rabies vaccine (adsorbed): a new rabies vaccine using FRhL-2 cells. J Infect Dis 1985;152:204–210.

28. Levenbook IS, Elisberg BL, Driscoll BF. Rhesus diploid rabies vaccine (adsorbed): neurological safety in guinea pigs and Lewis rats. Vaccine 1986;4:225–227.

29. Berlin BS, Goswick C. Rapidity of booster response to rabies vaccine produced in cell culture [Letter]. J Infect Dis 1984;150:785.

30. Berlin BS, Mitchell JR, Burgoyne GH, Brown WE, Goswick C. Rhesus diploid rabies vaccine (adsorbed), a new rabies vaccine. II. Results of clinical studies simulating prophylactic therapy for rabies exposure. JAMA 1983;249:2663–2665.

31. Berlin BS, Mitchell JR, Burgoyne GH, et al. Rhesus diploid rabies vaccine (adsorbed), a new rabies vaccine. Results of initial clinical studies of preexposure vaccination. JAMA 1982;247: 1726–1728.

32. Berlin BS. Rabies vaccine adsorbed: neutralizing antibody titers after three-dose pre-exposure vaccination. Am J Public Health 1990;80:476–477.

33. Nicholson KG, Turner GS, Aoki FY. Immunization with a human diploid cell strain of rabies virus vaccine: two-year results. J Infect Dis 1978;137:783–788.

34. Bernard KW, Roberts MA, Sumner J, et al. Human diploid cell rabies vaccine. Effectiveness of immunization with small intradermal or subcutaneous doses. JAMA 1982;247:1138–1142.

35. Bernard KW, Mallonee J, Wright JC, et al. Preexposure immunization with intradermal human diploid cell rabies vaccine. Risks and benefits of primary and booster vaccination. JAMA 1987;257:1059–1063.

36. Fishbein DB, Pacer RE, Holmes DF, Ley AB, Yager P, Tong TC. Rabies preexposure prophylaxis with human diploid cell rabies vaccine: a dose-response study. J Infect Dis 1987;156:50–55.

37. Afshar A. A review of non-bite transmission of rabies virus infection. Br Vet J 1979;135:142–148.

38. Winkler WG, Fashinell TR, Leffingwell L, Howard P, Conomy P. Airborne rabies transmission in a laboratory worker. JAMA 1973;226:1219–1221.

39. CDC. Rabies in a laboratory worker—New York. MMWR 1977;26:183–184.

40. CDC. Human-to-human transmission of rabies via corneal transplant—Thailand. MMWR 1981; 30:473–474.

41. Gode GR, Bhide NK. Two rabies deaths after corneal grafts from one donor [Letter]. Lancet 1988;2:791.

42. CDC. Human-to-human transmission of rabies via a corneal transplant—France. MMWR 1980; 29:25–26.

43. Houff SA, Burton RC, Wilson RW, et al. Human-to-human transmission of rabies virus by corneal transplant. N Engl J Med 1979;300:603–604.

44. Helmick CG, Tauxe RV, Vernon AA. Is there a risk to contacts of patients with rabies? Rev Infect Dis 1987;9:511–518.

45. Garner JS, Simmons BP. Guidelines for isolation precautions in hospitals. Infect Cont 1983; 4(Suppl):245–325.

46. National Association of State Public Health Veterinarians. Compendium of animal rabies control. J Am Vet Med Assoc 1990;196:36–39.

47. Fishbein DB, Belotto AJ, Pacer RE, et al. Rabies in rodents and lagomorphs in the United States, 1971–1984: increased cases in the woodchuck (Marmota monax) in mid-Atlantic states. J Wildl Dis 1986;22:151–155.

48. CDC. Imported dog and cat rabies—New Hampshire, California. MMWR 1988;37:559–560.

49. Eng TR, Fishbein DB. Epidemiologic factors, clinical findings, and vaccination status of rabies in cats and dogs in the United States in 1988. J Am Vet Med Assoc 1990;197:201–209.

50. Dean DJ, Baer GM. Studies on the local treatment of rabies infected wounds. Bull WHO 1963; 28:477–486.

51. Kaplan MM, Cohen D, Koprowski H, Dean D, Ferrigan L. Studies on the local treatment of wounds for the prevention of rabies. Bull WHO 1962;26:765–775.

52. Fishbein DB, Sawyer LA, Reid-Sanden FL, Weir EH. Administration of human diploid-cell rabies vaccine in the gluteal area [Letter]. N Engl J Med 1988;318:124–125.

53. Helmick CG, Johnstone C, Sumner J, Winkler WG, Fager S. A clinical study of Merieux human rabies immune globulin. J Biol Stand 1982;10:357–367.
54. Roumiantzeff M. The present status of rabies vaccine development and clinical experience with rabies vaccine. Southeast Asian J Trop Med Public Health 1988;19:549–561.
55. Kuwert EK, Marcus I, Werner J, et al. Post-exposure use of human diploid cell culture rabies vaccine. Dev Biol Stand 1976;37:273–286.
56. CDC. Recommendation of the Immunization Practices Advisory Committee (ACIP). Supplementary statement on pre-exposure rabies prophylaxis by the intradermal route. MMWR 1982;31:279–280, 285.
57. Fishbein DB, Dreesen DW, Holmes DF, et al. Human diploid cell rabies vaccine purified by zonal centrifugation: a controlled study of antibody response and side effects following primary and booster pre-exposure immunization. Vaccine 1990;7:437–442.
58. Richardson JH, Barkley WE, eds. Biosafety in Microbiological and Biomedical Laboratories. 2nd ed. Washington, DC: U.S. Government Printing Office, 1988. HHS Publication No. (NIH) 88–8395.
59. Nicholson KG. Rabies. Lancet 1990;335:1201–1205.
60. Warrell MJ, Nicholson KG, Warrell DA, et al. Economical multiple-site intradermal immunisation with human diploid-cell-strain vaccine is effective for post-exposure rabies prophylaxis. Lancet 1985;1:1059–1062.
61. Chutivongse S, Wilde H, Supich C, Baer GM, Fishbein DB. Postexposure prophylaxis for rabies with antiserum and intradermal vaccination. Lancet 1990;335:896–898.
62. Anderson LJ, Baer GM, Smith JS, Winkler WG, Holman RC. Rapid antibody response to human diploid rabies vaccine. Am J Epidemiol 1981;113:270–275.
63. Vodopija I, Sureau P, Lafon M, et al. An evaluation of second generation tissue culture rabies vaccines for use in man: a four-vaccine comparative immunogenicity study using a pre-exposure vaccination schedule and an abbreviated 2-1-1 postexposure schedule. Vaccine 1986; 4:245–248.
64. Vodopija I, Sureau P, Smerdel S, et al. Comparative study of two human diploid rabies vaccines administered with antirabies globulin. Vaccine 1988;6:489–490.
65. Vodopija I, Sureau P, Smerdel S, et al. Interaction of rabies vaccine with human rabies immunoglobulin and reliability of a 2-1-1 schedule application for postexposure treatment. Vaccine 1988;6:283–286.
66. Wilde H, Chomchey P, Prakongsri S, Punyaratabandhu P. Safety of equine rabies immune globulin [Letter]. Lancet 1987;2:1275.
67. Wilde H, Chomchey P, Prakongsri S, Punyaratabandhu P, Chutivongse S. Adverse effects of equine rabies immune globulin. Vaccine 1989;7;10–11.
68. Wilde H, Chomchey P, Punyaratabandhu P. Purified equine rabies immune globulin; a safe and affordable alternative to human rabies immune globulin (experience with 3156 patients). Bull WHO (in press).
69. CDC. Human rabies despite treatment with rabies immune globulin and human diploid cell rabies vaccine—Thailand. MMWR 1987;36:759–760, 765.
70. Shill M, Baynes RD, Miller SD. Fatal rabies encephalitis despite appropriate post-exposure prophylaxis. A case report. N Engl J Med 1987;316:1257–1258.
71. Wilde H, Choomkasien P, Hemachudha T, Supich C, Chutivongse S. Failure of rabies postexposure treatment in Thailand. Vaccine 1989;7:49–52.
72. Turner GS, Nicholson KG, Tyrrell DA, Aoki FY. Evaluation of a human diploid cell strain rabies vaccine: final report of a three year study of pre-exposure immunization. J Hyg (Lond) 1982;89:101–110.
73. Cabasso VJ, Dobkin MB, Roby RE, Hammar AH. Antibody response to a human diploid cell rabies vaccine. Appl Microbiol 1974;27:553–561.
74. CDC. Rabies prevention—United States, 1984. MMWR 1984;33:393–402, 407–408.
75. Pappaioanou M, Fishbein DB, Dreesen DW, et al. Antibody response to preexposure human diploid-cell rabies vaccine given concurrently with chloroquine. N Engl J Med 1986;314: 280–284.
76. Bernard KW, Fishbein DB, Miller KD, et al. Pre-exposure rabies immunization with human diploid cell vaccine: decreased antibody responses in persons immunized in developing countries. Am J Trop Med Hyg 1985;34:633–647.

77. Fishbein DB, Bernard KW, Miller KD, et al. The early kinetics of the neutralizing antibody response after booster immunizations with human diploid cell rabies vaccine. Am J Trop Med Hyg 1986;35:663–670.

78. Rubin RH, Hattwick MA, Jones S, Gregg MB, Schwartz VD. Adverse reactions to duck embryo rabies vaccine. Range and incidence. Ann Intern Med 1973;78:643–649.

79. Corey L, Hattwick MA, Baer GM, Smith JS. Serum neutralizing antibody after rabies postexposure prophylaxis. Ann Intern Med 1976;85:170–176.

80. Boe E, Nylan H. Guillain-Barré syndrome after vaccination with human diploid cell rabies vaccine. Scand J Infect Dis 1980;12:231–232.

81. Knittel T, Ramadori G, Mayet WJ, Lohr H, Meyer zum Buschenfelde KH. Guillain-Barré syndrome and human diploid cell rabies vaccine [Letter]. Lancet 1989;1:1334–1335.

82. Tornatore CS, Richert JR. CNS demyelination associated with diploid cell rabies vaccine [Letter]. Lancet 1990;335:1346–1347.

83. Anderson MC, Baer H, Frazier DJ, Quinnan GV. The role of specific IgE and beta-propiolactone in reactions resulting from booster doses of human diploid cell rabies vaccine. J Allergy Clin Immunol 1987;80:861–868.

84. Swanson MC, Rosanoff E, Gurwith M, Deitch M, Schnurrenberger P, Reed CE. IgE and IgG antibodies to beta-propiolactone and human serum albumin associated with urticarial reactions to rabies vaccine. J Infect Dis 1987;155:909–913.

85. Enright JB. The effects of corticosteroids on rabies in mice. Can J Microbiol 1974;16:667.

86. Varner MW, McGuinness GA, Galask RP. Rabies vaccination in pregnancy. Am J Obstet Gynecol 1982;143:717–718.

TOPIC 28 / SEXUALLY TRANSMITTED DISEASES

Guidelines for Health Education and Risk Reduction Activities

Original Citation: Centers for Disease Control and Prevention. Guidelines for health education and risk reduction activities. National Center for Prevention Services, Division of Sexually Transmitted Diseases/HIV Prevention, 1995.

Editor's Note: Please refer to the complete publication, Guidelines for Health Education and Risk Reduction Activities, for a comprehensive overview of sexually transmitted disease (STD)/HIV health education program considerations.

HEALTH EDUCATION AND RISK REDUCTION ACTIVITIES

Individual and Group Interventions

Health education and risk reduction activities are targeted to reach persons at increased risk of becoming infected with HIV or, if already infected, of transmitting the virus to others. The goal of health education and risk reduction programs is to reduce the risk of these events occurring. Activities should be directed to persons whose behaviors or personal circumstances place them at risk. Street and community outreach, risk reduction counseling, prevention case management, and community-level intervention have been identified as successful health education and risk reduction activities.

Street and Community Outreach

Street and community outreach can be described as an activity conducted outside a more traditional, institutional health care setting for the purposes of providing direct health education and risk reduction services or referrals. However, before conducting any outreach activity in a community, an agency must define the specific population to be served and determine their general needs. Based on this definition and determination, an agency can then decide appropriately where to conduct intervention efforts. Street and community outreach may be conducted anywhere from a street corner to a pool hall, from a parish hall to a school room. To determine the setting, an agency need only decide that the setting is easily, readily, and regularly accessed by the designated client population.

Outreach demonstrates an agency's willingness to go to the community rather than wait for the community to come to it. Often, agencies enlist and train peer educators to conduct the outreach activities. It is recommended that the content of the outreach activity be contingent upon the setting. The nature of activity varies in scope and intensity; the activity is best determined before an outreach team or individual educator goes out. Yet, flexibility is also very important. Remember, everything is not appropriate everywhere, all of the time. A street corner may be an appropriate place to conduct a brief HIV risk assessment, but it is not an appropriate place to conduct HIV counseling and testing.

While street and community outreach can be complementary service components of a single agency, some agencies, based on needs assessment findings and staff capacity, may choose to provide one service and not the other. Street outreach and community outreach can also be "standalone" pieces.

Street Outreach

Street outreach commonly involves outreach specialists moving throughout a particular neighborhood or community to deliver risk reduction information and materials. The outreach specialist may set up an HIV/AIDS information table on a street corner. They may supply bleach to injecting drug users at shooting galleries and condoms to commercial sex workers and their customers at the hotels or locations that they frequent. The fundamental principle of street outreach is that the outreach specialist establishes face-to-face contact with the client to provide HIV/AIDS risk reduction information and services.

Effective street outreach staff:

- Know the target group's language.
- Have basic training and experience in health education.
- Are sensitive to community norms, values, cultural beliefs, and traditions.
- Have a shared identity with the population served, stemming from shared common personal experiences with the group.
- Are trusted by the group they serve.
- Act as role models to the clients they serve.
- Advocate for the population served.

- Act as liaisons between the community and the agency.
- Are informed about community resources and use them.

Street outreach is not simply moving standard agency operations out onto the sidewalk. A number of specific issues are unique to the delivery of services through this type of outreach and must be considered before instituting a program of street outreach. These matters are usually addressed in an agency's street outreach program plan and include the following:

- Regular contact among educators, outreach specialists, and supervisors.
- Observation of potential outreach areas to determine the locations, times of day, and the day of the week that are most productive for reaching the population to be served.
- A written and comprehensive field safety protocol that is regularly updated (Table 1).
- Establishment of and adherence to regular and consistent schedules of activities, including times and locations (Table 2).
- A mechanism for measuring the use of referral services.

Table 1. Field safety protocol

Field safety protocols are based on program activities and are intended to provide the staff and peer educators with guidance regarding their professional behavior.

— Carry picture identification (I.D.) at all times that includes name of the organization, name of the project, your name, and the purpose for your presence.

— Work in pairs and always know where your partner is.

— Establish a mechanism to keep your supervisor aware of your location and activities (e.g., carry a beeper, call telephone mailbox at a specified time).

— Establish contact with local police precincts in the area. Leave copy of I.D. with the commander. If appropriate for your program, maintain relations with the police; introduce the program and staff.

— Have contingency plans for worst case scenarios and share them with your partner.

— Make sure you have made contact with and have permission from a key person in the community before entering the setting in which you will conduct the intervention (e.g., shooting galleries, crack houses, or local high schools).

— Leave the area if tension or violence is observed or perceived.

— Avoid controversy and debate with clients and program participants.

— When you start your job as a peer educator in the field, get a TB skin test; you should be re-tested periodically thereafter.

— Be aware of weather conditions and be prepared for natural occurrences.

— Design and adhere to a schedule for outreach or peer education.

— Avoid drinking alcoholic beverages and buying, receiving, or sampling drugs while conducting outreach or peer education.

- Creation and maintenance of a positive relationship between the agency and the local law enforcement authorities.
- Identification and development of collaborative relationships with gate-keepers (key informants) in the community.
- Activities for building and earning the trust and respect of the community.
- Descriptions of skills-building exercises relevant to stated program objectives.
- Establishment of mechanisms for maintaining client confidentiality.

Table 2. Example of Weekly Outreach Schedule

	8 AM–12 noon	1–5 PM	6–8 PM
MONDAY	No activity	No activity	No activity
TUESDAY	Office Staff meeting	Homeless shelter IDU outreach	Methadone clinic Client presentation
WEDNESDAY	STD clinic waiting room	City park IDU outreach	No activity
THURSDAY	Office Paperwork and data analysis	Street work 10th and Vine IDU outreach	No activity
FRIDAY	Office Materials development	Motel alley Sex worker/IDU outreach	Shooting gallery outreach
SATURDAY	No activity	City park IDU outreach	Street work 10th and Vine IDU outreach
SUNDAY	No activity	No activity	No activity

Community Outreach: Workshops and Presentations

Workshops and presentations are typical activities of community outreach. Because they usually follow lecture formats, they can be highly structured health education and risk reduction intervention efforts. While they supply important opportunities to disseminate HIV/AIDS prevention information, their impact on behavior change is limited because they are usually single-encounter experiences. Although they provide crucial technical information that raises awareness and increases knowledge and may be a critical first step in the change process, the information alone is usually inadequate to sustain behavior change.

To maximize their benefit, workshops and presentations should be planned carefully with knowledge goals and objectives specified before the individual sessions. To the extent possible, presenters should be informed about the setting where the workshop or presentation will take place, as well as the composition and knowledge level of the anticipated audience. The following are examples of issues the presenter might consider before conducting a presentation or workshop:

- Where will the workshop or presentation be held?
- What is the age range of the participants/audience?
- What is the language(s) of the participants/audience?
- What audiovisual equipment is available?

A well-planned, detailed outline, which allows flexibility, can prove useful and beneficial to the presenter and the participants/audience. Such an outline helps keep the presentation on track and focused. If a pretest evaluation is to be used, an outline can ensure that all relevant material will be covered in the lecture.

In a workshop or presentation, audience participation is to be strongly encouraged. Time must be allotted, usually at the end of the presentation, for a question and answer session. However, some questions may be so pressing, or some participants so persistent, that the presenter will have to address some questions and concerns during the presentation. The presenter should answer the questions succinctly and return to the original order of the presentation.

To increase the number of workshops and presentations they are able to provide, some agencies will elect to develop speaker's bureaus to augment their paid staff. Recruitment, training, and retention of volunteers present complex programmatic questions and are not to be undertaken lightly. Several references related to volunteers are provided at the end of this document and should be reviewed carefully.

A more detailed list of important points to consider for workshops and presentations is contained in Appendix C. The points below are relevant to agencies providing workshops and presentations either by paid staff or by volunteers in a speaker's bureaus. Effective presenters:

- Possess organizational and public speaking skills.
- Are well informed and comfortable talking about the subject.
- Ensure that the presentation is linguistically appropriate for the audience.
- Elicit and encourage audience participation.
- Are adaptable to logistics and audience needs.
- Are non-judgmental.
- Assess the nature of questions to make appropriate responses, i.e., whether better answered in private.
- Seek accurate answers to difficult questions and provide information in a timely manner.

A few items specifically needed in a Community Outreach Program Plan are listed below.

- A comprehensive workshop/presentation curriculum. (See Appendix C.)
- Assurance that curricula provide for discussion of related issues.
- Detailed workshop/presentation outlines.
- Logistical guidance for workshops/presentations (e.g., time and location, room arrangement, number of participants, number of facilitators).
- Methods to assure that the audience is informed about workshop/ presentation goals and objectives and that discussion of subject matter is facilitated.
- Descriptions of skills-building exercises relevant to stated program objectives.

- Training in the operation of audiovisual equipment and the use of diverse forms of audiovisual equipment.

Recruitment of staff with organizational and public speaking skills.

Peer Educators

Agencies that provide street and community outreach will frequently engage peer educators to conduct intervention activities. Peer education implies a role-model method of education in which trained, self-identified members of the client population provide HIV/AIDS education to their behavioral peers. This method provides an opportunity for individuals to perceive themselves as empowered by helping persons in their communities and social networks, thus supporting their own health enhancing practices. At the same time, the use of peer educators sustains intervention efforts in the community long after the professional service providers are gone.

Effective peer educators:

- Have a shared identity with the targeted community or group.
- Are within the same age range as the targeted community or group.
- Speak the same "language" as the community or group.
- Are familiar with the group's cultural nuances and are able to convey these norms and values to the agency.
- Act as an advocate, serving as a liaison between the agency and the targeted community or group.

Peer education can be very powerful, if it is applied appropriately. The peer educator not only teaches a desired risk reduction practice but s/he also models it. Peer educators demonstrate behaviors that can influence the community norms in order to promote HIV/AIDS risk reduction within their networks. They are better able to inspire and encourage their peers to adopt health seeking behaviors because they are able to share common weaknesses, strengths, and experiences.

Agencies often recruit and train peer educators from among their client populations. However, not everyone is an educator. The model client does not necessarily make the model teacher, no matter how consistently s/he practices HIV/AIDS risk reduction or is liked by agency staff. Peer educators should be instinctive communicators. They should be empathetic and non-judgmental. They should also be committed to client confidentiality.

Peer educators will not replace an agency's professional health educators, but they can complement the intervention team and enhance intervention efforts. Peer educators may act as support group leaders or street outreach volunteers who distribute materials to friends. They may be members of an agency's speaker's bureau and give workshop presentations.

They may run shooting galleries, keeping bleach and clean water readily available to other intravenous drug users (IDUs). They may be at-risk adolescents who model responsible sexual behaviors. The role of the peer educator is determined by the intervention need of the client population and the skill of the peer educator.

Although some agencies will hire peer educators as paid staff, others will not. As in the case of speaker's bureaus, engaging volunteer peer educators also involves issues of volunteer recruitment, training, and retention. Several references in the list of publications included at the end of this document provide more information on this issue. In addition to the core elements identified for health education and risk reduction activities, an effective peer education program plan contains the following:

- A written and comprehensive field safety protocol (Table 1).
- Establishment of and adherence to regular and consistent schedules of activities, including times and locations (Table 2).
- A description of skills-building exercises relevant to the stated program objectives.

Risk Reduction Counseling

The purpose of risk reduction counseling is to provide counseling and health education interventions to persons who are at high risk for HIV infection. The interventions promote and reinforce safe behavior. The participants may range from a single individual to couples, families, groups, or entire communities.

Risk reduction counseling is interactive. Such counseling assists clients in building the skills and abilities to implement behavior change. These programs offer training in the interpersonal skills needed to negotiate and sustain appropriate behavior changes. For example, sessions could concentrate on delaying the initiation of sexual activity, on methods for avoiding unsafe sex and negotiating safer sex, and on techniques to avoid sharing injecting drug paraphernalia. Risk reduction may be implemented in a variety of formats. The interventions may take the form of role plays, safer sex games, small group discussion, individual counseling, or group counseling.

Effective risk reduction counseling sessions:

- Emphasize confidentiality.
- Begin with an assessment of the specific HIV/STD prevention needs of the client(s).
- Identify, with the group or individual, the appropriate goals/ objectives (e.g., condom use negotiation skills for female sex partners of IDUs).
- Use skills-building exercises designed to meet the specific needs of the client(s).
- Include negotiations with the client(s) on suggestions and recommendations for changing and sustaining behavior change as appropriate to their situation.
- Enable/motivate participants to initiate/maintain behavior change independently.
- Enhance abilities of the participant(s) to access appropriate services (e.g., referrals to drug treatment).

Risk Reduction Program Plans

An effective risk reduction program plan includes the following:

- Protocols and procedures specific to each activity and logistical check lists for implementation.

- Development of innovative behavior modification strategies.
- Provision for regular updates in techniques for skills building.
- Provisions for updates on client-focused approaches to risk reduction activities.
- Provision for updates in techniques for increasing facilitators' skills in managing group or one-on-one dynamics.

Conducting Groups

Groups can provide significant informational and therapeutic HIV risk reduction interventions to individuals who are ready to initiate and/or maintain specific health promoting behaviors. Groups are usually formed around common issues or problems. Some groups, originally established to provide information and skills training, may evolve into support groups, which encourage maintenance of newly acquired behaviors. Utilizing groups suggests a systems approach to intervention. Groups provide access to social networks that enable and reinforce health enhancing behavior change through peer modeling and peer support.

Although open-ended groups (e.g., support groups) may have less structure than the more close-ended kinds of groups (e.g., educational or skills-building), both types should have clearly defined goals/objectives and specifically defined processes. The structure of a group should be determined based upon the needs of the members.

At times, the open-ended group with its open enrollment and extended life is more suited to members' needs. By being open-ended, potential members are able to drop in when they need to and thus avoid the wait for new groups to form. This type of group is likely to appeal to the individual whose commitment to the group's process is initially limited. In the open-ended group, members determine their own topic of discussion at each meeting. For this reason, an open-ended model, that encourages drop-ins, is perhaps less amenable to instructional sessions which usually need to build on information presented at earlier meetings. The open model, because of its unpredictable structure and enrollment, may be more amenable to process evaluation (i.e., percentage of agency's clients attending a determined number of sessions).

The close-ended model will have a defined lifespan and is also likely to set membership limits. The closed group allows for important continuity and facilitating the development of trust among members, as they get to know each other over time. Members can expect the same individuals to be present each week, which can aid in building significant, supportive relationships. The closed group model is more suitable to the establishment of client-specific outcome objectives that can be monitored over time (i.e., self-reported reduction in number of sex partners at the end of 8 weeks of group attendance).

There are significant advantages to both open and closed models, and determination of which model to employ is based on the needs of an agency's clients and on an agency's capacity to implement the model. Whatever the model selected, the size of the group is an important consideration. Group facilitation is not crowd control. Smaller groups can be more manageable and result in enhanced group dynamics.

Group facilitators or instructors may be peers or professionals; in some instances, they may be both. They should be skilled at promoting effective group dynamics, encouraging reticent members to speak up and guiding the dominant ones. Skilled facilitators and instructors are astute observers. They not only listen to what is being said, but they also note nonverbal cues. Good observation skills are especially critical for support or therapeutic group facilitators. Skilled facilitators and instructors are able to see changes in body language, hear sighs, and catch subtle changes in facial expressions.

Groups are a naturally occurring phenomenon. People come together for a variety of reasons and left to themselves, they will develop informal but powerful supportive networks. Proactive HIV risk reduction programs can tap into this resource and enhance program effectiveness.

HIV Prevention Case Management

HIV Prevention Case Management (PCM) is a one-on-one client service designed to assist both uninfected persons and those living with HIV. PCM provides intensive, individualized support and prevention counseling to assist persons to remain seronegative or to reduce the risk for HIV transmission to others by those who are seropositive. PCM is intended for persons who are having or who are likely to have difficulty initiating and sustaining safer behavior. The client's participation is always voluntary, and services are provided with the client's informed consent.

Prevention Case Management involves the assessment of HIV risk behavior and the assessment of other psychosocial and health service needs in order to provide risk reduction counseling and to assure psychosocial and medical referrals, such as housing, drug treatment, and other health and social services. PCM provides an ongoing, sustained relationship with the client in order to assure multiple-session HIV risk reduction counseling and access to service referrals. PCM should not duplicate Ryan White CARE Act case management services for persons living with HIV.

Case managers work with clients to assess their HIV risk and psychosocial and medical needs, develop a plan for meeting those needs, facilitate the implementation of the PCM plan through referral and follow-up, provide ongoing HIV risk-reduction counseling, and advocate on behalf of the client to obtain services. HIV Prevention Case Management creates bridges to assist clients in obtaining services with which they are unfamiliar or that pose special barriers to access. Clients are active participants in developing their PCM plan for risk reduction. Prevention Case Management may be carried out in a variety of settings, including the client's home, a community-based organization's office or storefront, clinics, or institutional settings.

Referral services may include HIV counseling and testing services (CT), psychosocial assessment and care, other HIV health education and risk reduction programs, medical evaluation and treatment, legal assistance, substance abuse treatment, crisis intervention, and housing and food assistance. Additionally, HIV PCM services should assist the client in obtaining STD prevention and treatment services, women's health services, TB testing and treatment, and other primary health care services. A strong relationship with STD clinics, TB testing sites, HIV counseling and testing clinics, and other health service agencies may be extremely beneficial to successfully recruiting persons at high risk who are appropriate for this type of intervention. PCM services are not intended as substitutes for medical case management, extended social services, or long-term psychological care.

The case manager needs a thorough knowledge of available community social and medical services as well as HIV prevention, treatment, and related services. This includes specific knowledge of the scope of services available, the protocol for accessing these services, and contact persons working with local agencies. Case managers are usually skilled in providing individual or couples' HIV risk-reduction counseling on an ongoing basis. Case managers usually have an academic background or special training in psychosocial assessment and counseling (e.g., social work, drug and alcohol treatment counseling, nursing, health education). Prevention Case Management supervisors need the academic training and/or experience to adequately develop PCM protocols, case documentation, and policies. The following provides further information on counseling and testing issues: HIV Counseling, Testing, and Referral: Standards and Guidelines, U.S. Department of Health and Human Services, Public Health Service, Centers for Disease Control and Prevention, May 1994.

Staff Characteristics of the Prevention Case Manager

Effective case managers are:

- Non-judgmental in addressing the needs of the client.
- Empathetic and critical listeners.
- Skilled in dispute mediation.
- Skilled in individual and relationship counseling.
- Skilled in conducting a thorough behavioral risk assessment and psychosocial assessment at client intake and skilled in developing an individualized case plan.
- Comfortable working in the home environments of their clients as well as in street settings, if necessary.
- Continually concerned about the protection of the client's rights, including confidentiality, and always respectful of guidelines in the agency protocol document.
- Sensitive to the client's ability to read literature and comprehend oral presentations.
- Responsive to the financial resources of clients in regard to case planning and referrals. Additionally, case managers:
- Maintain communication with case managers from other agencies working with the client to assure a coordinated treatment plan.
- Identify resources and services for the client and assist them in accessing service needs.
- Take into account and provide for cognitive impairments that may be related to the health status of the client.
- Reinforce behavioral change accomplished by the client at all opportunities.

- Troubleshoot episodes of client's unsafe behavior and relapse to identify barriers to practicing safer behavior and provide support and skills-building counseling.
- Establish a rapport with clients and maintain open communication with them and their partner(s).
- Act as an advocate in gaining access to services for clients.

Characteristics of the Prevention Case Management Program Plan:

- Includes specific, measurable, realistic, and time-phased program objectives.
- Assures that all services in the plan conform to agency policies and local, state, and Federal laws (for example, confidentiality of information).
- Assures the development of a written, formal PCM protocol for service delivery.
- Provides for the development of specific, measurable, realistic, and time-phased objectives in each client's case plan.
- Provides for regular meetings with each client to assess changing needs, monitor progress, and revise the service plan accordingly.
- Assures that each case manager negotiates a risk reduction plan with the client, referring to the plan at each session in order to assess progress.
- Assures the development and use of a comprehensive HIV risk assessment instrument to assess the behavioral variables influencing the client's risk taking.
- Assures the development and use of a comprehensive psychosocial assessment instrument to assess psychosocial and medical service needs of the client as well as financial resources, language preferences, barriers to accessing these services, etc.
- Assures that prevention case managers and their supervisors meet frequently for case presentations and supervision.
- Defines collaboration with other local service providers through memoranda of agreement and regular meetings between agencies to facilitate access to other social and health services as well as to discuss and coordinate treatment plans for individual clients.
- Assures that the memoranda of understanding among agencies are periodically updated, accurately reflecting collaborative activities.
- Assures that the assessment of progress in meeting the case plan is communicated to the client for review and comment.
- Assures that case records include documentation that acknowledges voluntary client participation and mutually satisfactory case plans.
- Assures that an updated written or computerized database of service referrals and a system for documenting successful referrals are maintained.
- Assures that regularly scheduled staff meetings are held to discuss challenges, successes, and barriers encountered by case managers; adequate time must be allocated for staff to share concerns, frustrations, grief, and other emotions experienced through the close work with persons at risk or with persons living with HIV.

PCM staff training plans usually include the following:

- Staff training in established PCM protocols, agency policies, and referral mechanisms.
- Periodic training addressing the local services available for client referral.

- Skills training to improve the HIV risk reduction counseling provided to clients.
- Training that addresses how to effectively intervene with clients who are in extreme states, such as persons who are combative, in emotional crisis, mentally ill, or under the influence of drugs and/or alcohol.

Community Level Intervention

Community Level Intervention combines community organization and social marketing—a strategy that takes a systems approach. Its foundation is an assumption that individuals make up large and small social networks or systems. Within these social networks or systems, individuals acquire information, form attitudes, and develop beliefs. Also, within these networks, individuals acquire skills and practice behaviors.

The fundamental program goal of Community Level Intervention is to influence specific behaviors by using social networks to consistently deliver HIV risk reduction interventions. Although the intervention strategy is community-based, Community Level Interventions target specific populations—not simply the community in general. The client populations have identified shared risk behaviors for HIV infection and also may be defined by race, ethnicity, gender, or sexual orientation.

In order to influence norms that support HIV risk reduction behavior, Community Level Interventions are directed at the population, rather than at the individual. The primary goal of these interventions is to improve health status by promoting healthy behaviors and changing those factors that negatively affect the health of a community's residents. A specific intervention may take the form of persuasive behavior change messages, or it may be a skills-building effort. Whatever its form, an intervention achieves reduced HIV risk by changing group norms to improve or enhance the quality of health for members of the client population. These norms may relate to condom use, contraceptive use, or needle-sharing. They may also focus on diagnosis and treatment of sexually transmitted diseases or HIV.

It takes time to change social norms. Social norms cannot be changed quickly or at the same rate that knowledge acquisition or skills development can occur. Change occurs as a result of sustained, consistent intervention efforts over time. The intervention must be implemented thoroughly throughout the social networks. A firm grounding in behavioral theory is essential to the development and implementation of Community Level Interventions.

Community-based needs assessment is critical to the development and implementation of Community Level Interventions. This phase is important for identifying and describing structural, environmental, behavioral, and psychological facilitators and barriers to HIV risk reduction. To successfully conduct this intervention, a program must identify the sources for and patterns of communication within a social network. Peer networks must be defined and described.

Note: Community Level Intervention is referred to as Community Intervention Programs in Program Announcement #300.

The following questions should be considered in designing community level interventions:

- Who are the gatekeepers to the client population?
- What are the important points of access?
- What are the appropriate and relevant risk-reduction messages, methods, and materials?
- What are the linguistic and literacy needs of the client population? A needs assessment should yield this vital information.

For further reading on the developmental steps of Community Level Intervention, see Cooperative Agreement for Human Immunodeficiency Virus (HIV) Prevention Projects Program Announcement and Notice of Availability of Funds for Fiscal Year 1993.

A variety of methods exists for collecting the answers to these questions. It is recommended that programs select the method that is most appropriate for their professional orientation (e.g., social work, health education). Whatever method is chosen, it is critical that the formative activity be community-based and as collaborative as possible with the client population.

The information gathered during the formative phase provides the foundation on which an effective program can be built. Completing this activity should result in culturally competent, developmentally appropriate, linguistically specific, and sexual-identity-sensitive interventions that promote HIV risk reduction.

Members of existing and relevant social networks can be enlisted to deliver the interventions. Other peer networks may also be created and mobilized to provide intervention services. This, of course, means volunteer recruitment and management. Community Level Intervention strategies offer opportunities for peers to acquire skills in HIV risk reduction and, in turn, reinforce these abilities when the peers become the teachers of these same skills to others.

In this manner, Community Level Interventions become community-owned and operated; thus, they are more likely to be sustained by the community when the program activity is completed. Social norms changed in this way are likely to have a long-lasting and effective impact upon HIV risk reduction.

APPENDIX A
Street Outreach Activity Report

MSM's Client   Group 4/22/92 Date

Southside Location   __ A.M. X P.M. __ Evening

35_____ Total # of Contacts   AMR/JAV Team

Demographics of Contacts
30 # Male   5 # Female

21 # African American   9 # Latino   1 # White   2 # Native American

2 # Asian/Pacific Islander   0 Other

Materials Distributed To Individuals   Referrals for Services

105 # of Condoms Distributed   3 # STD Clinic

2 # of Bleach Kits Distributed   __ # HIV C/T Site

APPENDIX A—*continued*

Materials Distributed To Individuals	Referrals for Services
35 # of Safer Sex Kits Distributed	0 # TB Clinic
29 # of Brochures Distributed	3 # Drug Treatment
1 # of Other poster	0 # Family Planning

Materials Drop-off Sites

Type of Site:	Materials Distributed:
Al's Place (bar)	100 condoms, 200 brochures, 1 poster
Midtown Adult Book Store	200 condoms, 200 safer sex cards
St. Mary's Homeless Shelter	2 posters, 100 condoms, 50 bleach kits
Hair Unlimited (beauty shop)	100 condoms, 50 brochures, 2 posters

---

APPENDIX B
Quality Assurance
Program Assessment Form
Street and Community Outreach

OUTREACH SPECIALIST: _____

REVIEWER: _____

DATE: _____

DIRECTIONS: Check the appropriate columns to indicate degree to which the outreach specialist met criteria:

EXCELLENT indicates that performance met criteria beyond fully successful.

FULLY SUCCESSFUL indicates performance met criteria successfully.

NEEDS ATTN indicates performance needs supervisory guidance to meet criteria.

N/A indicates this criteria did not apply to this situation.

Check only within and not between the boxes. If undecided, use "comments" section to clarify.

Excellent	Fully Successful	Needs Attn	N/A

STAFF

☐	☐	☐	☐	1. Staff respects client's privacy and confidentiality at all times.
☐	☐	☐	☐	2. Staff is trained and experienced in health education.
☐	☐	☐	☐	3. Staff is sensitive to community norms, values, cultural beliefs, and traditions.
☐	☐	☐	☐	4. Staff advocates for the population served.
☐	☐	☐	☐	5. Staff acts as liaison between the community and agency.
☐	☐	☐	☐	6. Staff is representative of the population served.
☐	☐	☐	☐	7. Staff is informed about community resources and is able to use them.

COMMENTS

PROGRAM

☐	☐	☐	☐	1. Program proposes realistic, measurable, and attainable goals and objectives.
☐	☐	☐	☐	2. Program identifies specific methodologies and activities to achieve stated goals and objectives.
☐	☐	☐	☐	3. Program defines target population by geographic locale, risk behavior(s), gender, sexual orientation, and race and ethnicity.

☐ ☐ ☐ ☐   4. Program ensures adequate supplies of appropriate and relevant risk-reduction materials before conducting outreach activities (e.g., pamphlets, condoms, bleach, sexual responsibility kits).

☐ ☐ ☐ ☐   5. Program includes observation of potential outreach areas to determine the locations, times of day, and the day of the week that are most productive for reaching the population to be served.

☐ ☐ ☐ ☐   6. Program has regular and consistent hours for outreach activities.

☐ ☐ ☐ ☐   7. Program facilitates professional development of program staff.

☐ ☐ ☐ ☐   8. Program has a comprehensive and written field safety protocol.

☐ ☐ ☐ ☐   9. Program has a written policy and personnel procedures to address stress, burn-out, and relapse among staff.

☐ ☐ ☐ ☐   10. Program has written procedures for the referral of clients to appropriate services outside the agency.

☐ ☐ ☐ ☐   11. Program has long-range plans for the continuation of services.

☐ ☐ ☐ ☐   12. Program establishes and maintains a relationship between the agency and other local authorities.

☐ ☐ ☐ ☐   13. Program identifies and develops collaborative relationships with relevant gatekeepers (key informants) to the target population.

☐ ☐ ☐ ☐   14. Program coordinates intervention services with identified gate-keepers.

COMMENTS:

EVALUATION

☐ ☐ ☐ ☐   1. Evaluation plan includes process evaluation measures.

☐ ☐ ☐ ☐   2. Evaluation plan has consistent, accurate data collection procedures.

☐ ☐ ☐ ☐   3. Evaluation plan includes staff supervision, observation, and feedback on a regularly scheduled basis.

☐ ☐ ☐ ☐   4. Evaluation plan provides findings for program modifications, as appropriate.

COMMENTS:

TRAINING

☐ ☐ ☐ ☐   1. Training plan defines staff roles, duties, and responsibilities.

☐ ☐ ☐ ☐   2. Training plan includes staff orientation to the agency (organization) and the community served.

☐ ☐ ☐ ☐   3. Training plan includes ongoing staff professional development.

☐ ☐ ☐ ☐   4. Training plan uses role play, observation, and feedback.

COMMENTS:

APPENDIX C
Quality Assurance
Program Assessment Form—Community Educator

TOPIC: _____ EDUCATOR: _____

GROUP (TYPE & SIZE): _____ REVIEWER: _____

DATE: _____ TIME: _____ PROGRAM LENGTH: _____

DIRECTIONS: Check the appropriate columns to indicate degree to which the educator met performance criteria:

APPENDIX C—*continued*

WELL—would indicate met criteria well.

ADEQUATELY—would indicate met criteria adequately.

NEEDS ATTN—needs attention and supervisory guidance to meet criteria.

N/A—would indicate this criteria did not apply to this situation.

Check only within and not between the boxes. If undecided, use "comments" section to clarify.

WELL	ADEQUATELY	NEEDS ATTN	N/A

INTRODUCTIONS

☐ ☐ ☐ ☐ 1. Introduces self by name and title.

☐ ☐ ☐ ☐ 2. Introduces others as appropriate.

☐ ☐ ☐ ☐ 3. Clearly states purpose, goals, and objectives for session.

☐ ☐ ☐ ☐ 4. Starts program at or within 10 minutes after starting time.

☐ ☐ ☐ ☐ 5. Attends to participants' physical comfort.

COMMENTS:

CONTENT

☐ ☐ ☐ ☐ 1. Selects program content relevant to agency goals and audience needs.

☐ ☐ ☐ ☐ 2. Imparts factual information.

☐ ☐ ☐ ☐ 3. Displays confidence in knowledge of material.

☐ ☐ ☐ ☐ 4. Provides background and supporting evidence to substantiate facts stated by participants and by self.

☐ ☐ ☐ ☐ 5. Organizes activities and information in clear manner.

COMMENTS:

PROFESSIONAL PRESENCE

☐ ☐ ☐ ☐ 1. Dresses in a manner that doesn't detract from aims of presentation.

☐ ☐ ☐ ☐ 2. Remembers and uses names of people, as appropriate.

☐ ☐ ☐ ☐ 3. Is tactful when discussing controversial topics.

☐ ☐ ☐ ☐ 4. Imparts attitudes and information consistent with agency goals and policy.

☐ ☐ ☐ ☐ 5. Avoids careless use of slang words.

☐ ☐ ☐ ☐ 6. Uses grammatically correct English.

☐ ☐ ☐ ☐ 7. Handles unexpected or difficult questions with minimal display of embarrassment or confusion.

☐ ☐ ☐ ☐ 8. Makes positive and tactful corrective statements.

☐ ☐ ☐ ☐ 9. Acknowledges contrary viewpoints.

COMMENTS:

STRUCTURE

☐ ☐ ☐ ☐ 1. Focuses attention on topic with films, pre-test, or other motivational techniques.

☐ ☐ ☐ ☐ 2. Selects teaching methods geared to audience and content (i.e., brainstorm, lectures, etc.).

☐ ☐ ☐ ☐ 3. Selects teaching materials that enhance lesson plan.

APPENDIX C—continued

☐ ☐ ☐ ☐ 4. Allows sufficient time for activities.

☐ ☐ ☐ ☐ 5. Modifies teaching plan as indicated by audience response.

☐ ☐ ☐ ☐ 6. Keeps session on track, sticks to the point.

☐ ☐ ☐ ☐ 7. Creates opportunities for questions, comments, clarifications, and expression of opinions and feelings (elicits and pauses, etc.).

COMMENTS:

PROCESS SKILLS

☐ ☐ ☐ ☐ 1. Uses descriptive and reinforcing gestures.

☐ ☐ ☐ ☐ 2. Maintains eye contact with entire audience.

☐ ☐ ☐ ☐ 3. Adapts vocabulary level to understanding of group.

☐ ☐ ☐ ☐ 4. Enunciates and projects voice clearly.

☐ ☐ ☐ ☐ 5. Sets stage for activities and materials.

☐ ☐ ☐ ☐ 6. Explains materials used.

☐ ☐ ☐ ☐ 7. Demonstrates knowledge and skill in operating a.v. Equipment.

☐ ☐ ☐ ☐ 8. Uses illustrative examples.

☐ ☐ ☐ ☐ 9. Encourage all participants to be involved in activities.

☐ ☐ ☐ ☐ 10. Avoids lags in flow of presentation.

☐ ☐ ☐ ☐ 11. Acknowledges and accepts statements of feelings and experiences of others.

☐ ☐ ☐ ☐ 12. Listens actively.

☐ ☐ ☐ ☐ 13. Affirms information accurately.

☐ ☐ ☐ ☐ 14. Restates/clarifies/emphasizes participants' comments and questions.

COMMENTS:

CONCLUSION

☐ ☐ ☐ ☐ 1. Summarizes major program points.

☐ ☐ ☐ ☐ 2. Reviews program objectives before concluding.

☐ ☐ ☐ ☐ 3. Helps group identify further human or material resources.

☐ ☐ ☐ ☐ 4. Remains available for individuals to approach them after the program.

☐ ☐ ☐ ☐ 5. Uses a tool to assess participants' satisfaction with program and program impact.

COMMENTS:

COMMENTS ON CONCLUSIONS:

AUDIENCE RESPONSE TO SPEAKER:

OVERALL SUGGESTIONS AND REMARKS:

SPEAKER'S COMMENTS AND SIGNATURE:

APPENDIX D
Quality Assurance
Program Assessment Form—Support Group Facilitator

TITLE: _____   FACILITATOR: _____

REVIEWER: _____

DATE: _____

DIRECTIONS: Check the appropriate columns to indicate degree to which the facilitator met performance criteria:

    EXCELLENT indicates that performance met criteria beyond fully successful.

    FULLY SUCCESSFUL indicates performance met criteria successfully.

    NEEDS ATTN indicates performance needs supervisory guidance to meet criteria.

    N/A indicates this criteria did not apply to this situation.

Check only within and not between the boxes. If undecided, use "comments" section to clarify.

EXCELLENT	FULLY SUCCESSFUL	NEEDS ATTN	N/A

INTRODUCTIONS

☐	☐	☐	☐	1. Introduces self by name and title.
☐	☐	☐	☐	2. Facilitates introductions and stresses confidentiality among group members.
☐	☐	☐	☐	3. Clearly states purpose, goals, objectives, and ground rules for session.
☐	☐	☐	☐	4. Allows members to share their expectations from the group.
☐	☐	☐	☐	5. Starts group at or within 10 minutes after starting time.
☐	☐	☐	☐	6. Attends to group members' physical comfort.
☐	☐	☐	☐	7. Makes required administrative announcements.

COMMENTS:

GROUP FACILITATION

☐	☐	☐	☐	1. Assures maintenance of group structure and schedule by promoting adherence to rules and guidelines.
☐	☐	☐	☐	2. Guides members through group processes, e.g., group dynamics.
☐	☐	☐	☐	3. Asks open-ended questions.
☐	☐	☐	☐	4. Maintains focus of discussion.
☐	☐	☐	☐	5. Synthesizes and abstracts pertinent information.
☐	☐	☐	☐	6. Creates opportunities for questions, comments, clarifications, and expressions of opinions and feelings.

APPENDIX D—*continued*

☐ ☐ ☐ ☐   7. Makes appropriate referrals and interventions, as needed.

☐ ☐ ☐ ☐   8. Provides members with education materials and information to substantiate discussion.

COMMENTS:

PROFESSIONAL PRESENCE

☐ ☐ ☐ ☐   1. Dresses in suitable attire.

☐ ☐ ☐ ☐   2. Remembers and uses names of group members, as appropriate.

☐ ☐ ☐ ☐   3. Is tactful when discussing controversial topics.

☐ ☐ ☐ ☐   4. Imparts attitudes and information consistent with agency goals and policy.

☐ ☐ ☐ ☐   5. Avoids careless or inappropriate use of slang words.

☐ ☐ ☐ ☐   6. Handles unexpected or difficult disclosures with minimal display of value judgement, embarrassment, or confusion.

☐ ☐ ☐ ☐   7. Makes positive and tactful corrective statements.

☐ ☐ ☐ ☐   8. Acknowledges contrary viewpoints.

COMMENTS:

PROCESS SKILLS

☐ ☐ ☐ ☐   1. Uses descriptive and reinforcing gestures.

☐ ☐ ☐ ☐   2. Maintains eye contact with group members.

☐ ☐ ☐ ☐   3. Speaks in vernacular that is germane to group.

☐ ☐ ☐ ☐   4. Clearly enunciates and projects voice.

☐ ☐ ☐ ☐   5. Sets stage for group session.

☐ ☐ ☐ ☐   6. Encourages all group members to be involved in activities.

☐ ☐ ☐ ☐   7. Listens actively.

COMMENTS:

CONCLUSION

☐ ☐ ☐ ☐   1. Brings group to closure in a tactful manner.

☐ ☐ ☐ ☐   2. Summarizes group session.

☐ ☐ ☐ ☐   3. Reviews session objectives with group members.

☐ ☐ ☐ ☐   4. Helps group identify further human or material resources.

☐ ☐ ☐ ☐   5. Remains available for group members' questions and comments after the session.

☐ ☐ ☐ ☐   6. Uses a tool to assess participants' satisfaction with session and group impact.

COMMENTS:

COMMENTS ON CONCLUSION:

GROUP RESPONSE TO FACILITATOR:

OVERALL SUGGESTIONS AND REMARKS:

FACILITATOR'S COMMENTS AND SIGNATURE:

APPENDIX E
Quality Assurance
Material Review Checklist

TITLE: _____ AUTHOR: _____

REVIEWER: _____

DATE: _____

DIRECTIONS: Check the appropriate columns to indicate degree to which the author met criteria:

EXCELLENT indicates that performance met criteria beyond fully successful.

FULLY SUCCESSFUL indicates performance met criteria successfully.

NEEDS ATTN indicates performance needs supervisory guidance to meet criteria.

N/A indicates this criteria did not apply to this situation.

Check only within and not between the boxes. If undecided, use "comments" section to clarify.

EXCELLENT　　　　FULLY SUCCESSFUL　　　　NEEDS ATTN　　　　N/A

MATERIAL REVIEW CHECKLIST

☐　☐　☐　☐　1. Material is clearly introduced and states the purpose of the text to the reader.

☐　☐　☐　☐　2. Major points of text are summarized at the end.

☐　☐　☐　☐　3. Materials are brief, concise, and in the language or dialect of the target audience.

☐　☐　☐　☐　4. Materials are written at the educational and reading level of the target audience. Avoids jargon and technical phrases.

☐　☐　☐　☐　5. Materials use language and terms with which the target audience is comfortable.

☐　☐　☐　☐　6. Use active verbs and short, simple sentences, with one concept per sentence in short paragraphs.

☐　☐　☐　☐　7. Materials avoid or define difficult words and concepts. Examples are used to clarify.

☐　☐　☐　☐　8. Use terms consistently (e.g., "HIV" and "AIDS virus" are not used interchangeably).

☐　☐　☐　☐　9. Materials are straightforward and clear. (Do not use abbreviations, acronyms, euphemisms, symbolism, statistics, or anything else that could cause confusion.)

☐ ☐ ☐ ☐   10. Text uses line drawings if illustrations are included.

☐ ☐ ☐ ☐   11. Illustration of anatomy shows position of organs within the whole body (gives relative size and location reference).

☐ ☐ ☐ ☐   12. Text uses lists, bullets, or illustrations instead of long discussions. Visuals (overheads, slides) are used to emphasize key points.

☐ ☐ ☐ ☐   13. Text is underlined, boldfaced, or "boxed" for reinforcement.

COMMENTS:

MATERIAL REVIEW CHECKLIST

☐ ☐ ☐ ☐   14. The text dispels myths, uses acceptable channels, refers to value systems for reasons to change behavior or adopt a new perspective.

☐ ☐ ☐ ☐   15. Materials provide a call for action.

☐ ☐ ☐ ☐   16. The text illustrates manual skills from audience perspective.

☐ ☐ ☐ ☐   17. The text provides reasons for changing behavior.

☐ ☐ ☐ ☐   18. Materials provide current and accurate medical information.

☐ ☐ ☐ ☐   19. Materials do not contain sexual preference or racial, gender, or ethnic bias.

☐ ☐ ☐ ☐   20. Text offers alternative behaviors to the one(s) that put a person at risk.

☐ ☐ ☐ ☐   21. Realistic and relevant examples are given.

☐ ☐ ☐ ☐   22. The format of the text is not visually distracting:

☐ ☐ ☐ ☐   a. Small type (less than 10 point) is not used.

☐ ☐ ☐ ☐   b. Sentences are neither too short nor too long.

☐ ☐ ☐ ☐   c. Text does not contain larger blocks of print.

☐ ☐ ☐ ☐   d. Right margins are justified.

☐ ☐ ☐ ☐   e. Only photographs that are reproducible are included.*

☐ ☐ ☐ ☐   f. Only professional—quality drawings are included.

☐ ☐ ☐ ☐   g. Technical diagrams are avoided.

☐ ☐ ☐ ☐   23. Graphics are immediately identifiable, relevant, and simple. They reinforce the text.

COMMENTS:

*Note: A written release should be obtained from all persons pictured. The release should clearly state permission to use the photograph and the conditions for use.

APPENDIX F
HIV Prevention Case Management (PCM) Checklist

Develop a quality assurance plan that:

- Establishes a minimal level of service delivery and identifies methods to monitor service delivery.
- Identifies and assesses evidence of the quality and quantity of all services provided through the PCM program.
- Reviews PCM protocols periodically for adequacy and relevancy and is revised accordingly.
- Reviews intake and case management documents for accuracy and compliance with program protocol.
- Examines the documentation of case termination and transfer.
- Ensures regular, periodic audits of case files by the supervisor.
- Provides for a mechanism to respond to discrepancies in performance identified by the supervisor.

APPENDIX G
Example

"Cleaning Your Needles" Pamphlet

OBJECTIVE:	Demonstrate and remind.
WHO:	The designated audience is out-of-treatment IDUs.
WHAT:	The specific message is "clean your needles with bleach."
WHERE:	In their "copping" area (e.g., 10th and Vine).
HOW:	Outreach specialists initiate conversation with people in the area, identify IDUs, provide instruction on needle cleaning, supply IDUs with bleach kits and a brief pamphlet, "Cleaning Your Needles" (illustrating the needle cleaning process) as a reminder of the instruction.
EVALUATION:	Process: Outreach specialists keep track of the number of hours spent at outreach locations, the number and demographics of people spoken to, and the number of people who took bleach kits and pamphlets. Outreach specialists observe whether people keep or discard pamphlets.

"Teens and AIDS" Video

OBJECTIVE:	Inform, demonstrate, and remind.
WHO:	Sexually active teens.
WHAT:	The message is condom use and negotiation skills.
WHEN:	Early afternoon (after school).
WHERE:	Neighborhood community center.
HOW:	Outreach worker:

- shows video portraying situations where sex is being considered and the parties negotiate condom use;
- leads discussion to personalize negotiation;
- facilities role play by participants;
- demonstrates proper care and use of condoms and has participants practice on a model;
- supplies pamphlets outlining negotiation strategies and other pamphlets illustrating condom use as reminders or references.

EVALUATION: Process: Outreach worker documents how many presentations are done, how many teens attend, group demographics, the number of pamphlets distributed.

Prevention and Management of Chlamydia trachomatis

Original Citation: Centers for Disease Control. Recommendations for the prevention and management of Chlamydia trachomatis infections. MMWR 1993;42(No. RR-12).

Editor's Note: This article provides guidance for establishing screening programs for the prevention of C. trachomatis reproductive tract disease and for integrating relevant messages into behavioral risk reduction programs. Please refer to the entire publication for more information about the epidemiology and pathogenesis of C. trachomatis, and screening tests. Approaches to the prevention of C. trachomatis infection and the related biotechnology are evolving rapidly.

INTRODUCTION

Chlamydia trachomatis infections are common in sexually active adolescents and young adults in the United States (CDC, unpublished review). More than 4 million chlamydial infections occur annually (2, 3). Infection by this organism is insidious—symptoms are absent or minor among most infected women and many men. This large group of asymptomatic and infectious persons sustains transmission within a community. In addition, these persons are at risk for acute illness and serious long-term sequelae. The direct and indirect costs of chlamydial illness exceed $2.4 billion annually (2–4).

Until recently, chlamydia prevention and patient care were impeded by the lack of suitable laboratory tests for screening and diagnosis. Such tests are now available. Through education, screening, partner referral, and proper patient care, public health workers and health-care practitioners can combine efforts to decrease the morbidity and costs resulting from this infection.

PREVENTION STRATEGIES

The principal goal of chlamydia prevention strategies is to prevent both overt and silent chlamydia salpingitis and its sequelae. Other goals include the prevention of perinatal and postpartum infection and other adverse consequences of chlamydial infection.

General Approach

The prevention of chlamydia salpingitis, pregnancy-related complications, and other chlamydial illnesses requires that chlamydia prevention programs include both primary and secondary prevention strategies.

Primary Prevention Strategies

Primary prevention strategies are efforts to prevent chlamydial infection. Primary prevention of chlamydia can be accomplished in two general ways.

- Behavioral changes that reduce the risk of acquiring or transmitting infection should be promoted (e.g., delaying age at first intercourse, decreasing the number of sex partners, partner selection, and the use of barrier contraception [condoms]). Efforts to effect behavioral changes are not specific to chlamydia prevention but are also critical components in preventing sexual transmission of the human immunodeficiency virus (HIV) and other sexually transmitted diseases (STDs) (45, 115–117).
- Identify and treat persons with genital chlamydial infection before they infect their sex partners, and for pregnant women before they infect their babies. Efforts to detect chlamydial infection are essential to chlamydia prevention. Identifying and treating chlamydial infections require active screening and referral of sex partners of infected persons, since infections among women and men are usually asymptomatic.

Secondary Prevention Strategies

Secondary prevention strategies are efforts to prevent complications among persons infected with chlamydia. The most important complication to be prevented is salpingitis and its potential sequelae (i.e., ectopic pregnancy, tubal infertility, and chronic pelvic pain). Secondary prevention of chlamydia salpingitis can be accomplished by (a) screening women to identify and treat asymptomatic chlamydial infection; (b) treating the female partners of men with infection; (c) recognizing clinical conditions such as mucopurulent cervicitis (MPC) and the urethral syndrome, and then applying or using appropriate chlamydia diagnostic tests and treatment, as appropriate.

Target Population

Chlamydial infection is especially prevalent among adolescents. Furthermore, PID occurs more commonly after chlamydial infection among adolescent females than among older women (42). Therefore, chlamydia prevention efforts should be directed toward young women.

All sexually active adolescents and young adults are at high risk for chlamydia; the infection is broadly distributed geographically and socioeconomically. Therefore, chlamydia prevention programs should target all sexually active adolescents and young adults. All private and public health-care providers should be involved in these prevention efforts.

Specific Strategies

Specific strategies for the prevention of chlamydia are grouped into two categories. Those categories are: (a) community-based strategies, and (b) health-care provider strategies.

Community-Based Strategies

Since the prevalence of chlamydia is consistently high among adolescents and young adults regardless of socioeconomic status, race, or geographic location, prevention efforts should be implemented community-wide.

Public Awareness

Community-based strategies should increase public awareness of chlamydia, its consequences, and the availability and importance of diagnosis and treatment. Groups at high risk for chlamydial infection and the persons who educate and care for them (e.g., parents, teachers, and health-care providers) must be informed about the high rate of genital chlamydial infection and its sequelae among sexually active adolescents and young adults.

HIV/STD Risk Reduction Programs

Programs designed to reduce the risk of sexual transmission of HIV and other STDs by means of behavioral changes should emphasize the especially high risk of chlamydial infection. In addition, chlamydial infection may be a sentinel for unsafe sexual practices. Concern about chlamydia may provide additional motivation for persons to delay initiation of sexual activity, limit the number of sex partners, avoid sex partners at increased risk for STDs, and use condoms.

Schools

Because of their access to adolescents, educators have an important role to play in chlamydia prevention programs. Chlamydia-specific material should be integrated into educational curricula that address HIV and other STDs. In addition, school programs should assist students in developing the social and behavioral skills needed to avoid chlamydial infection, HIV, and other STDs.

Although most school health education curricula address HIV, fewer discuss other STDs (including chlamydia). Information that should be provided through school health education programs are listed below:

- Rates of chlamydial infection among adolescents
- Adverse consequences of chlamydia (e.g., PID and infertility)
- Symptoms and signs of chlamydial infection (and other STDs)
- Asymptomatic infection
- Treatment for sex partners
- Where and how to obtain health care (including locations, telephone numbers [e.g., STD hot-line number], costs, and issues of confidentiality)

Some schools may offer more than classroom instruction (e.g., access to health-care for infected persons and screening programs to identify asymptomatic chlamydial infection). Personnel in school-based clinics that perform pelvic examinations should use the opportunity to test for chlamydial infection. However, tests also are needed to identify asymptomatic males (e.g., by screening urine collected during sports physical examinations or other health-screening programs). The leukocyte esterase test (LET) of urine is one possible method for testing males, but the accuracy of the test requires additional evaluation (118). Such approaches to identifying and treating young men with asymptomatic chlamydial infection may prove important since these persons may account for most of the transmission of chlamydia to young women.

Out-of-School Adolescents

The prevalence of chlamydia may be even greater among adolescents who have dropped out of school. Therefore, organizations serving these adolescents (e.g., Job Corps, vocational training centers, detention centers, community-based recreational programs) should offer health care that addresses chlamydial infection as part of STD/HIV risk reduction programs.

Health-Care Provider Strategies

Reducing the high prevalence of chlamydial infection requires that health-care providers be aware of the high prevalence of chlamydia and recognize chlamydial illness, screen asymptomatic patients, arrange for the treatment of sex partners, and counsel all sexually active patients about the risks of STD infections. Medical providers should be trained to recognize and manage the following conditions that may be caused by chlamydia: MPC, PID, urethral syndrome (women), and urethritis and epididymitis (men).

Screening

The screening of women for chlamydial infection is a critical component in a chlamydia prevention program since many women are asymptomatic, and the infection may persist for extended periods of time. Many women of reproductive age undergo pelvic examination during visits for routine health-care or because of illness. During these examinations, specimens can be obtained for chlamydia screening tests.

Female patients of adolescent-care providers, women undergoing induced abortion, women attending STD clinics, and women in detention facilities should be screened for chlamydial infection. Screening of these women is important because (a) many are adolescents or young adults, (b) they are at high risk for salpingitis, and (c) they or their partners are likely to transmit infection.

Chlamydia screening at family planning and prenatal care clinics is particularly cost-effective because of the large number of sexually active young women who undergo pelvic examinations.

Providers such as family physicians, internists, obstetricians-gynecologists, and pediatricians who provide care for sexually active young women also should implement chlamydia screening programs—although a lower volume of such patients may increase the cost of testing. The following criteria can help identify women who should be tested for chlamydia:

- Women with MPC
- Sexually active women less than 20 years of age
- Women 20–24 years of age who meet either of the following criteria, or women greater than 24 years of age who meet both criteria—inconsistent use of barrier contraception, or new or more than one sex partner during the last 3 months.

Patient selection criteria should be evaluated periodically. Although the incidence of chlamydial infection among all women previously tested for chlamydia is unknown, the incidence of chlamydial infection among previously infected adolescent females has been as high as 39% (118). Because of the high incidence of chlamydial infection among sexually active adolescent females, recommendations for the frequency of testing are listed below:

- Women less than 20 years of age should be tested when undergoing a pelvic examination, unless sexual activity since the last test for chlamydia has been limited to a single, mutually monogamous partner.

- All other women who meet the suggested screening criteria (listed above) should be tested for chlamydia annually.

Although young men infrequently seek routine health care, medical providers should use such opportunities to evaluate them for asymptomatic chlamydial infection.

Treatment of Sex Partners

Treatment of sex partners of infected persons is an important strategy for reaching large numbers of men and women with asymptomatic chlamydial infection. Also, if partners are not treated, reinfection may occur. In addition, treating the male partners of infected women is critical since this is the principal way to eliminate asymptomatic infection among males. If chlamydia screening is widely implemented, the number of infected women identified may exceed the capacity of some public health systems to notify, evaluate, and treat partners. Therefore, health department personnel should assist health-care providers in developing cooperative approaches to refer partners for treatment. Where possible, health-care providers who treat female patients for chlamydia should offer examination and treatment services for the patients' male sex partner(s), or should arrange the appropriate referral of such partners.

Risk Reduction Counseling

In addition to screening, treatment, and referral of sex partners(s) of persons with chlamydial infection, health-care providers should:

- Educate sexually active patients regarding HIV and other STDs
- Assess the patients' risk factors for infection
- Offer at-risk patients advice about behavior changes to reduce the risk of infection
- Encourage the use of condoms

Preventing Chlamydial Infection During Pregnancy

To prevent maternal postnatal complications and chlamydial infection among infants, pregnant women should be screened for chlamydia during the third trimester, so that treatment, if needed, will be completed before delivery (see Primary Prevention Strategies). The screening criteria already discussed can identify those at higher risk for infection. Screening during the first trimester prevents transmission of the infection and adverse effects of chlamydia during the pregnancy. However, the evidence for adverse effects during pregnancy is minimal. If screening is performed only during the first trimester, a longer period exists for infection before delivery.

Infants with chlamydial infections respond readily to treatment; morbidity can be limited by the early diagnosis and systematic treatment of infants who have conjunctivitis and pneumonia caused by chlamydial infection (secondary prevention strategies). Further, the mothers of infants diagnosed with chlamydial infection and the sex partner(s) of those mothers should be evaluated and treated.

LABORATORY TESTING

Diagnostic test manufacturers have introduced a variety of nonculture tests for chlamydia. Because nonculture tests do not require strict handling of specimens, they are easier to perform and less expensive than culture tests; consequently the numbers of laboratories and health-care providers offering chlamydia testing have increased. The expanded use of nonculture tests is a cornerstone of chlamydia prevention strategies.

Although nonculture tests have advantages that make them more suitable than cell culture tests for widespread screening programs, nonculture tests also have limitations. In particular, nonculture tests are less specific than culture tests and may produce false-positive results. All positive nonculture results should be interpreted as presumptive infection until verified by culture or other nonculture test. The decision to treat and perform additional tests should be based on the specific clinical situation.

The test methodologies discussed in these recommendations are for the detection of Chlamydia trachomatis—not other chlamydia species (e.g., C. psittaci and C. pneumoniae). A number of commercial products for the detection of C. trachomatis are available; however, most information relating to the performance of most of these products is the manufacturers' data. When possible, health-care providers and laboratory staff should compare a potential nonculture test's performance with that of an appropriate standard in their own laboratory.

Specimens for Screening

The proper collection and handling of specimens are important in all the methods used to identify chlamydia. Even diagnostic tests with the highest performance ratings cannot produce accurate results when specimens submitted to the laboratory are improperly collected. Clinicians require training and periodic assessment to maintain proper technique.

Because chlamydia are obligate intracellular organisms that infect the columnar epithelium, the objective of specimen collection procedures is to obtain columnar epithelial cells from the endocervix or the urethra. The following recommendations for specimen collection apply to all screening tests.

PATIENT CARE: AN EXPANDED ROLE FOR THE USE OF CHLAMYDIA TESTS

The Chlamydia trachomatis infections policy guidelines published in 1985 (1) emphasized the need to include treatment for chlamydia in regimens for patients whose diagnoses were strongly associated with

chlamydial infection. The increasing availability of accurate and economical chlamydia tests permits widespread screening of asymptomatic
persons, but also suggests that chlamydia treatment for symptomatic patients and the referral of sex partners in the absence of testing, a key
strategy in past guidelines, should be discouraged. These tests should be
used to diagnose chlamydia for patients with symptoms or signs suggestive of chlamydial infection even if therapy is administered and partners
are referred before test results are available. A specific chlamydia diagnosis should facilitate sex partner referral since a positive chlamydia test
result indicates that the patient's infection is sexually transmitted. A specific diagnosis may also facilitate medical care for patients who do not
respond as expected to initial chlamydia therapy.

Some providers do not have resources to screen asymptomatic patients for chlamydia and to also test patients whose conditions warrant
presumptive treatment and partner referral. If presumptive treatment
of patients with symptoms or signs of chlamydia without testing is
elected, efforts must be made to ensure the treatment of partners.

Although the benefits of chlamydia tests for screening and diagnosis justify their use, the potential for adverse consequences must also be
recognized and steps taken to minimize them. The adverse consequences for infected patients and their sex partners, including disease
complications and transmission of chlamydial infection, may occur if
chlamydia treatment is delayed while waiting for test results or if treatment is withheld because of a false-negative test result. Adverse consequences also may occur if uninfected patients and their sex partners are
treated unnecessarily because the chlamydia test result is unavailable or
false-positive. The adverse consequences of treating uninfected persons
are more likely to be psychosocial, resulting from the misdiagnosis of a
sexually transmitted infection; adverse effects of the antibiotic used to
treat chlamydia are relatively uncommon and mild.

These adverse consequences can be avoided by (a) treating patients
who are symptomatic or have a substantially increased risk of chlamydial
infection and treating their sex partners for chlamydia without waiting
for chlamydia test results, and (b) arranging for a second test to verify
an initial positive screening test result for patients and their sex partners
who are susceptible to the adverse psychosocial consequences of having
a false diagnosis of an STD.

Presumptive Diagnosis of Chlamydial Infection

Several conditions—NGU, PID, epididymitis, and gonococcal infection—
are consistently associated with an increased prevalence of chlamydial infection among patients and their sex partners (Table 2). Patients with
these illnesses require immediate treatment to relieve symptoms and/or
to prevent complications. Treatment for these conditions should include
an antibiotic regimen for chlamydia. Sex partners of infected patients

Table 2. Conditions warranting a presumptive diagnosis of chlamydial infection

Condition	Chlamydia prevalence (%)*	
	Patients	Partners
NGU (heterosexual men)	30–40	10–43
PID	8–54	36
Epididymitis (men <35 years of age)	50	10–43+
Gonococcal infection		
Men	5–30	40
Women	25–50	Unknown

*Unpublished review of literature.

+Expected to approximate or exceed prevalence for partners of men with NGU.

NOTE: Chlamydia may be a relatively uncommon cause of NGU or PID in some patient care settings. In such settings, immediate treatment, including an antibiotic regimen for chlamydia is warranted, but clinicians may refer sex partners contingent upon a positive test result for C. trachomatis or N. gonorrhoeae.

should be evaluated and treated for chlamydia without waiting for the patient's test results.

Immediate chlamydia treatment of MPC is warranted by an increased prevalence of chlamydia among women with this condition in most patient care settings. However, immediate chlamydia treatment of MPC or urethral syndrome among females or proctitis among homosexual males—and the referral of sex partners of patients with any of these conditions before obtaining a microbiologic diagnosis—may not always be warranted (Table 3). Chlamydia risk factors (e.g., age less than 25 years, having new or multiple sex partners) and the likelihood of compliance with follow-up visits should be considered when deciding whether to defer chlamydia treatment and referral of sex partners until chlamydia test results are available. Whenever possible, these decisions should be based on local estimates of chlamydia prevalence.

Table 3. Conditions that may not warrant a presumptive diagnosis of chlamydial infection

Condition	Chlamydia prevalence (%)*	
	Patients	Partners
MPC	9–51	2–27+
Proctitis (homosexual males)	8–16	Unknown
Acute urethral syndrome	13–63	Unknown

*Unpublished review of literature.

+Lower value is the product of lowest reported prevalence among women with MPC multiplied by lowest reported prevalence among partners of women with chlamydia; highest value is the product of the highest reported prevalence among women with MPC and the highest reported prevalence among partners of women with chlamydia.

Chlamydia Tests for Patients Who Are Treated Presumptively

Even if a patient with a presumptive diagnosis of chlamydial infection will be treated and counseled to refer partners before test results are known, chlamydia tests should be performed:

- Ensuring appropriate medical care, particularly if symptoms persist,
- Facilitating counseling of the patient
- Providing firm grounds for partner notification
- Improving compliance

Limited resources may require health-care providers to decide between performing chlamydia tests for patients who would be treated for chlamydia because of symptoms or signs and patients who are asymptomatic and would not otherwise receive chlamydia treatment. If the health-care provider elects to provide presumptive treatment for patients with symptoms or signs—but without chlamydia testing—efforts must be made to ensure treating the sex partners of patients.

Screening Women for Chlamydial Infection

Screening of women for chlamydial infection is a principal element of a chlamydia prevention program (see Health-care Provider Strategies). The decision to provide treatment for patients whose screening results are positive and to evaluate and treat their sex partners depends upon the patient's risk for a sexually transmitted infection and the potential for adverse psychosocial consequences. A positive second chlamydia test strongly supports the validity of a positive screening test; a negative second test following a positive second test does not rule out chlamydial infection.

Verification of the initial positive chlamydia test result should be obtained for persons who have a positive nonculture chlamydia test and who are at low risk for infection (e.g., involved in a monogamous relationship, have no history of sexually transmitted infection, member of low-prevalence [less than 5%] patient populations) or for whom a misdiagnosis of chlamydial infection could lead to social/psychological distress. If verification of the initial positive chlamydia test result is indicated, these patients and their sex partners should be treated while waiting for the results of the supplementary test. The health-care provider should postpone treatment and partner referral only if the likelihood and adverse consequences of a false-positive test outweigh the risks of transmission and disease progression. Risk factors for chlamydial infection and the probability that the patient will return for follow-up visits should also be considered. (see Nonculture Chlamydia Tests and Clinician-Laboratory Protocols for Verifying Positive Tests).

Physical Examination of Sex Partners

Female partners of males with chlamydial infection should be referred for examination, chlamydia testing, and treatment. The examination and testing of female partners is recommended because (a) sensitive tests are available, and a positive test result may lead to additional partners who are likely to be infected; (b) women can be asymptomatic but, when examined, have signs of PID, which requires more intensive therapy; and (c) women may be asymptomatically infected with other STDs. However, information is needed on the rates of PID and other STDs among female partners of infected men.

Male sex partners of females with chlamydial infections should be evaluated for symptoms of chlamydia and other sexually transmitted infections and for allergy to the treatment drug. A physical examination of male sex partners should be encouraged, but an examination is less important than treatment.

The examination and testing of asymptomatic male partners are recommended because (a) a positive test result may lead to the treatment of additional partners who are likely to be infected, (b) men can be asymptomatically infected with other STDs, and (c) male partners may be allergic to the treatment drug. However, chlamydia tests for asymptomatic males are insensitive. Further, low rates of other STDs among asymptomatic male partners of women with chlamydial infection have been demonstrated in limited studies. Also, many males do not have readily identifiable sources of medical care for STDs and so may be unlikely to be evaluated by a clinician even if asked to do so by a sex partner. For some male partners of women with chlamydial infection, therefore, it may be reasonable for the woman's clinician to evaluate the male partner even if, in the case of providers who do not offer health-care services for men, this means evaluation without a physical examination. Although approaches to evaluating male partners without a physical examination have not been adequately studied, evaluation of the male partner could be performed at the clinician's office or possibly by telephone. Before prescribing treatment without an examination, the clinician should determine that the male partner does not have symptoms suggestive of another STD and is not allergic to the treatment drug.

Exposure Periods

For women with chlamydial infections and for asymptomatically infected men, health-care providers should treat all sex partners with whom patients have ongoing sexual relations and all other partners with whom patients have had sexual exposures within 60 days before the date of the patient's examination/test.

For males with symptomatic chlamydial infection, the 30-day period is sufficient to detect person(s) who probably transmitted the infection to the index patient, as well as recent sex partners who may have been exposed to the infection by the patient.

For males and females with asymptomatic infections, a longer exposure period helps to identify additional infected partners. These extended periods, however, have received insufficient evaluation to support specific recommendations. If no sexual exposure has occurred within the specified exposure periods, the most recent sex partner is presumed to be at increased risk for chlamydial infection and should be evaluated.

Responsibility for Referral of Sex Partners

Health-care providers should inform infected patients that they must have their sex partners evaluated and treated. Health-care providers or health departments should ensure the notification, evaluation, and treatment of the sex partners of patients with chlamydial infection. Partner referral can be performed by patients (patient referral) or by providers (provider referral). Patients who do comply with partner referral notify their sex partners of their exposure and encourage them to be examined and treated. Provider referrals require that third parties (e.g., health department personnel) assume responsibility for notifying sex partners of their exposure and providing evaluation and treatment.

Provider referral of partners—including field follow-up by health department staff—is cost effective (155). However, because of the high prevalence of chlamydial infection among some populations and the limited number of health department outreach workers, patient referrals remain the only method of referral available to most clinicians.

The responsibility for evaluating the sex partners of persons with chlamydial infection is often unclear and is a major reason partners remain untreated. This is a particular problem for male partners of females with chlamydial infection; male partners (who are often asymptomatic) may be reluctant to visit an STD clinic. Health-care providers who treat women with chlamydial infection should assist in making arrangements for the evaluation and treatment of male partner(s). Health departments can assist health-care providers in developing effective referral systems.

Clinician-Laboratory Protocols for Verifying Positive Tests

Clinician-laboratory protocols for chlamydia testing are necessary to maximize the benefits of testing for chlamydia while minimizing adverse consequences and cost. These protocols should address which initial and supplementary tests the laboratory will perform, how clinicians should request these tests, and what specimens the clinicians should collect and submit to the laboratory during the patient's initial and follow-up visits. State and local health departments should facilitate the collaboration between health-care providers and laboratories that is necessary to develop suitable testing protocols (See Nonculture Chlamydia Tests).

When developing clinician-laboratory protocols for chlamydia testing, the prevalence of chlamydial infection in the patient population should be considered. In settings with a high prevalence of infection (e.g., false-positive test results account for a small proportion of total positive test results), initial positive test results might only be verified if requested by the clinician on the basis of an assessment of a patient's risk for infection and the potential adverse effects of a false-positive result. In settings with a low prevalence of infection (e.g., false-positive test results account for a substantial proportion of total positive test results), an additional test for verification should be performed on all patients whose screening test results are positive.

Three alternative testing protocols are suitable for supplementary testing. With the first protocol, a test system is chosen that permits performing the supplementary test on the residual material from the initial specimen. With the second protocol, a test system is chosen in which the supplementary test is performed on a second specimen. The clinician routinely obtains the second specimen at the same time as the initial specimen and submits both specimens to the laboratory; the supplementary test is performed on the second specimen if the initial test is positive and verification is required. With the third protocol, the laboratory reports a positive result from the initial test to the clinician who arranges the patient's return visit for treatment and then obtains a second specimen for a supplemental test. In most settings, one of the first two protocols is preferable since they do not require a return visit to collect an additional specimen. The choice of supplementary test systems and related protocols is difficult because insufficient information is available regarding their comparative performance and cost.

ANTIMICROBIAL REGIMENS

Recommendations for the treatment of genital chlamydial infections have been published (146, 156). Two new antimicrobials approved by the FDA for the treatment of chlamydia—ofloxacin and azithromycin—offer the clinician additional therapeutic choices. A substantial advantage of azithromycin, in comparison with all other therapies, is that a single dose is effective; this antimicrobial may prove most useful in situations in which compliance with a 7-day regimen of another antimicrobial cannot be ensured. In view of the high efficacy of tetracycline and doxycycline, cost also should be considered when selecting a treatment regimen.

The recommended treatment regimens for uncomplicated urethral, endocervical, or rectal chlamydial infections among adults are listed below:

- Doxycycline 100 mg orally 2 times a day for 7 days, or
- Azithromycin 1 gm orally in a single dose

NOTE: Doxycycline and azithromycin are not recommended for use during pregnancy.

Alternative Treatment Regimens

Alternative treatment regimens for uncomplicated urethral, endocervical, or rectal chlamydial infections among adults are listed below:

- Ofloxacin 300 mg orally 2 times a day for 7 days, or
- Erythromycin base 500 mg orally 4 times a day for 7 days, or
- Erythromycin ethylsuccinate 800 mg orally 4 times a day for 7 days, or
- Sulfisoxazole 500 mg orally 4 times a day for 10 days

NOTE: Ofloxacin is not recommended for treating adolescents less than or equal to 17 years of age nor for pregnant women. The efficacy of sulfisoxazole is inferior to other regimens.

The recommended treatment regimen for chlamydial infection during pregnancy is stated below:

- Erythromycin base 500 mg orally 4 times a day for 7 days

If this regimen cannot be tolerated, the following regimens are recommended:

- Erythromycin base 250 mg orally 4 times a day for 14 days, or
- Erythromycin ethylsuccinate 800 mg orally 4 times a day for 7 days, or
- Erythromycin ethylsuccinate 400 mg orally 4 times a day for 14 days

If the patient cannot tolerate erythromycin, the following regimen is recommended:

- Amoxicillin 500 mg orally 3 times a day for 7–10 days

NOTE: Erythromycin estolate is contraindicated during pregnancy, since drug-related hepatotoxicity can result.

For the treatment of complicated chlamydial infection, chlamydia-associated conditions, and chlamydial infection among infants or children, see the 1993 Sexually Transmitted Diseases Treatment Guidelines (146) for the treatment of adults, and the American Academy of Pediatrics Report of the Committee on Infectious Diseases (157) for the treatment of infants and children.

Follow-up of Patients Treated for Chlamydial Infection

Treatment failure, indicated by positive cultures 7–14 days after therapy, is uncommon after successful completion of a greater than or equal to 7 day regimen of tetracycline or doxycycline; failure rates of 0%–3% have been reported for males and 0%–8% for females (156, 158). However, in one study of adolescents followed up to 24 months after therapy for chlamydial infection, rates of infection were 39% (118). Whether these infections are reinfections or cases of latent, unsuccessfully treated chlamydial infection is unknown. Further, some studies suggest that women with chlamydial infections are at increased risk for subsequent infection.

Although routine test-of-cure visits during the immediate post-treatment period are not recommended, health-care providers should consider retesting females infected with chlamydia weeks to months after initial therapy (see Nonculture Chlamydia Tests).

REFERENCES: AS NUMBERED IN ORIGINAL PUBLICATION

2. Washington AE, Johnson RE, Sanders LL, Barnes RC, Alexander ER. Incidence of Chlamydia trachomatis infections in the United States using reported Neisseria gonorrhoeae as a surrogate. In: Oriel D, Ridgway G, Schachter J, Taylor-Robinson D, Ward M, eds. Chlamydia infections: proceedings of the sixth international symposium on human Chlamydial infections. Cambridge: Cambridge University Press, 1986:487–490.
3. Washington AE, Johnson RE, Sanders LL Jr. Chlamydia trachomatis infections in the United States. What are they costing us? JAMA 1987;257:2070–2072.
4. Washington AE, Katz P. Cost of and payment source for pelvic inflammatory disease. Trends and projections, 1983 through 2000. JAMA 1991;266:2565–2569.
42. Westrom L, Svensson L, Wolner-Hanssen P, Mardh P-A. Chlamydial and gonococcal infections in a defined population of women. Scand J Infect Dis 1982;32(Suppl):157–162.
45. CDC. Policy guidelines for the prevention and management of pelvic inflammatory disease (PID). MMWR 1991;40(RR-5):1–25.
115. CDC. Guidelines for AIDS prevention program operations. Center for Prevention Services, Public Health Service, U.S. Department of Health and Human Services, 1987.
116. CDC. AIDS: Information/education plan to prevent and control AIDS in the United States. Washington, DC: Public Health Service, U.S. Department of Health and Human Services, 1987.
117. CDC. Guidelines for effective school health education to prevent the spread of AIDS. MMWR 1988;37(S-2):1–14.
118. Jones RB. Treatment of Chlamydia trachomatis infections of the urogenital tract. In: Bowie WR, Caldwell HD, Jones RP, et al, eds. Chlamydial infections: proceedings of the seventh international symposium on human chlamydial infections. Cambridge: Cambridge University Press, 1990:509–518.
146. CDC. Sexually transmitted diseases treatment guidelines, 1993. MMWR 1993;(in press).
155. Katz BP, Danos CS, Quinn TS, Caine V, Jones RB. Efficiency and cost-effectiveness of field follow-up for patients with Chlamydia trachomatis infection in a sexually transmitted diseases clinic. Sex Transm Dis 1988;15:11–16.
156. Toomey KE, Barnes RC. Treatment of Chlamydia trachomatis genital infection. Rev Infect Dis 1990;12:S645–S655.
157. Committee on Infectious Diseases American Academy of Pediatrics. Chlamydia trachomatis. In: Peter G, Lepow ML, McCracken GH Jr., Phillips CF, eds. Report of the Committee on Infectious Diseases 1991. 22nd ed. Elk Grove Village, IL: American Academy of Pediatrics, 1991.
158. Sanders LL, Harrison HR, Washington AE. Treatment of sexually transmitted chlamydial infections. JAMA 1986;255:1750–1756.

1993 Sexually Transmitted Diseases Treatment Guidelines

Original Citation: Centers for Disease Control and Prevention. 1993 Sexually transmitted diseases treatment guidelines. MMWR 1993;42(RR-14).

PREVENTION METHODS
Condoms

When used consistently and correctly, condoms are very effective in preventing a variety of sexually transmitted diseases (STDs), including HIV infection. Multiple cohort studies, including those of serodiscordant couples, have demonstrated a strong protective effect of condom use against HIV infection. Condoms are regulated as medical devices and subject to random sampling and testing by the Food and Drug Administration (FDA). Each latex condom manufactured in the United States is tested electronically for holes before packaging. Condom breakage rates during use are low in the United States (less than or equal to 2 per 100 condoms tested). Condom failure usually results from inconsistent or incorrect use rather than condom breakage.

Patients should be advised that condoms must be used consistently and correctly to be effective in preventing STDs. Patients should also be instructed in the correct use of condoms. The following recommendations ensure the proper use of condoms:

- Use a new condom with each act of intercourse.
- Carefully handle the condom to avoid damaging it with fingernails, teeth, or other sharp objects.
- Put the condom on after the penis is erect and before any genital contact with the partner.
- Ensure that no air is trapped in the tip of the condom.
- Ensure that there is adequate lubrication during intercourse, possibly requiring the use of exogenous lubricants.
- Use only water-based lubricants (e.g., K-Y Jelly™ or glycerine) with latex condoms (oil-based lubricants [e.g., petroleum jelly, shortening, mineral oil, massage oils, body lotions, or cooking oil] that can weaken latex should never be used).
- Hold the condom firmly against the base of the penis during withdrawal, and withdraw while the penis is still erect to prevent slippage.

Condoms and Spermicides

The effectiveness of spermicides in preventing HIV transmission is unknown. No data exist to indicate that condoms lubricated with spermicides are more effective than other lubricated condoms in protecting against the transmission of HIV infection and other STDs. Therefore, latex condoms with or without spermicides are recommended.

Female Condoms

Laboratory studies indicate that the female condom (Reality™)—a lubricated polyurethane sheath with a ring on each end that is inserted into the vagina—is an effective mechanical barrier to viruses, including HIV. Aside from a small study of trichomoniasis, no clinical studies have been completed to evaluate protection from HIV infection or other STDs. However, an evaluation of the female condom's effectiveness in pregnancy prevention was conducted during a 6-month period for 147 women in the United States. The estimated 12-month failure rate for pregnancy prevention among the 147 women was 26%.

Vaginal Spermicides, Sponges, Diaphragms

As demonstrated in several cohort studies, vaginal spermicides (i.e., film, gel, suppositories; contraceptive foam has not been studied) used alone without condoms reduce the risk for cervical gonorrhea and chlamydia, but protection against HIV infection has not been established in human studies. The vaginal contraceptive sponge protects against cervical gonorrhea and chlamydia, but increases the risk for candidiasis as evidenced by cohort studies. Diaphragm use has been demonstrated to protect against cervical gonorrhea, chlamydia, and trichomoniasis, but only in case-control and cross-sectional studies; no cohort studies have been performed. Gonorrhea and chlamydia among women usually involve the cervix as a portal of entry, whereas other STD pathogens (including HIV) may infect women through the vagina or vulva, as well as the cervix. Protection of women against HIV infection should not be assumed from the use of vaginal spermicides, vaginal sponges, or diaphragms. The role of spermicides, sponges, and diaphragms for preventing STDs among men has not been studied.

Nonbarrier Contraception, Surgical Sterilization, Hysterectomy

Women who are not at risk for pregnancy may incorrectly perceive themselves to be at no risk for STDs, including HIV infection. Nonbarrier contraceptive methods offer no protection against HIV or other STDs. Women using hormonal contraception (oral contraceptives, Norplant™, Depo-Provera™), who have been surgically sterilized or who have had hysterectomies should be counseled regarding the use of condoms and the risk for STDs, including HIV infection.

Injection Drug Users

Prevention messages appropriate for injection drug users are the following:

- Enroll or continue in a drug treatment program.
- Do not, under any circumstances, use injection equipment (needles, syringes) that has been used by another person.
- Persons who continue to use injection equipment that has been used by other persons should first clean the equipment with bleach and water. (Disinfecting with bleach does not sterilize the equipment and does not guarantee that HIV is inactivated. However, thoroughly and consistently cleaning injection equipment with bleach should reduce the rate of HIV transmission when equipment is shared.)

HIV Prevention Counseling

During pretest counseling, the clinician should conduct a personalized risk assessment, explain the meaning of positive and negative test results, ask for informed consent for the HIV test, and help the person to develop a realistic, personalized risk reduction plan.

During posttest counseling, the clinician should inform the patient of the results, review the meaning of the results, and reinforce prevention messages. If the patient is HIV positive, posttest counseling should include referral for follow-up medical services and for social and psychological services, if needed. HIV-seronegative persons at continuing risk for HIV infection also may benefit from referral for additional counseling and prevention services.

HIV counseling is considered to be an important HIV-prevention strategy, although its efficacy in reducing risk behavior is still under evaluation. By ensuring that counseling is empathic and "client-centered," clinicians will be able to develop a realistic appraisal of the person's risk and help him or her to develop a specific and realistic HIV-prevention plan (2).

Partner Notification and Management of Sex Partners

Patients with STDs should ensure that their sex partners, including those without symptoms, are referred for evaluation. Providers should be prepared to assist in that effort. In most circumstances, partners of patients with STDs should be examined. When a diagnosis of a treatable STD is considered likely, appropriate antibiotics should be administered even though there may be no clinical signs of infection and before laboratory test results are available. In most states, the local or state health department can assist in notifying the partners of patients with selected STDs, especially HIV, syphilis, gonorrhea, and chlamydia.

Breaking the chain of transmission is crucial to STD control. For treatable STDs, further transmission and reinfection can be prevented by referral of sex partners for diagnosis, treatment, and counseling. The following two strategies are used for partner notification: (a) patient referral (index patients notify their partners), and (b) provider referral (partners named by infected patients are notified and counseled by health department staff). When a physician refers an infected person to a local or state health department, trained professionals may interview the patient to obtain names and locating information about all of his or her sex partners. Every health department protects the privacy of patients in partner notification activities. Because of the advantage of confidentiality, many patients prefer that public health officials notify partners.

If a patient with HIV infection refuses to notify partners while continuing to place them at risk, the physician has an ethical and legal responsibility to inform persons that they are at risk of HIV infection. This duty-to-warn may be most applicable to primary care physicians, who often have knowledge about a patient's social and familial relationships. The decision to invoke the duty-to-warn measure should be a last resort—applicable only in cases in which all efforts to persuade the patient to disclose positive test results to those who need to know have failed.

Although compelling ethical, theoretical, and public health reasons exist to undertake partner notification, the efficacy of partner notification as an STD prevention strategy is under evaluation, and its effectiveness may be disease-specific.

Clinical guidelines for sex partner management and recommendations for partner notification for specific STDs are included for each STD addressed in this report.

Reporting and Confidentiality

The accurate identification and timely reporting of STDs form an integral part of successful disease control. Reporting assists local health authorities in identifying sex partners who may be infected. Reporting also is important for assessing morbidity trends. STD/HIV and acquired immunodeficiency syndrome (AIDS) cases should be reported in accordance with local statutory requirements and in a timely manner.

Syphilis, gonorrhea, and AIDS are reportable diseases in every state. The requirements for reporting other STDs and asymptomatic HIV infection differ from state to state, and clinicians should be familiar with local STD reporting requirements.

Reporting may be provider- and/or laboratory-based. Clinicians who are unsure of local reporting requirements should seek advice from local health departments or state STD programs. STD and HIV reports are held in strictest confidence and in many jurisdictions are protected by statute from subpoena. Further, before any follow-up of a positive STD test is conducted by program representatives, these persons consult with the patient's health-care provider to verify the diagnosis and treatment.

SPECIAL POPULATIONS

Pregnant Women

The following screening tests are recommended for pregnant women:

- A serologic test for syphilis
- A serologic test for hepatitis B surface antigen (HBsAg)
- A test for Neisseria gonorrhoeae
- A test for Chlamydia trachomatis
- A test for HIV infection Patients with risk factors for HIV or with a high-risk sex partner should be tested for HIV infection.

Other Issues

- In the absence of lesions during the third trimester, routine serial cultures for herpes simplex virus (HSV) are not indicated for women with a history of recurrent genital herpes. However, obtaining cultures from such women at the time of delivery may be useful in guiding neonatal management. "Prophylactic" caesarean section is not indicated for women who do not have active genital lesions at the time of delivery.
- The presence of genital warts is not considered an indication for caesarean section.

Adolescents

All adolescents in the United States can consent to the confidential diagnosis and treatment of STDs. Medical care for these conditions can be provided to adolescents without parental consent or knowledge. Furthermore, in many states adolescents can consent to HIV counseling and testing.

Children

Management of children with STDs requires close cooperation between the clinician, laboratory, and child-protection authorities. Investigations, when indicated, should be initiated promptly. Some diseases, such as gonorrhea, syphilis, and chlamydia, if acquired after the neonatal period, are almost 100% indicative of sexual contact. For other diseases, such as HPV infection and vaginitis, the association with sexual contact is not as clear (see Sexual Assault and STDs).

HIV INFECTION AND EARLY INTERVENTION

For the purpose of these recommendations, early intervention for HIV is defined as care for persons infected with HIV who are without symptoms. However, recently detected HIV infection may not have been recently acquired. Persons newly diagnosed with HIV may be at many different stages of the infection. Therefore, early intervention also involves assuming the responsibility for coordinating care and for arranging access to resources necessary to meet the medical, psychological, and social needs of persons with more advanced HIV infection.

Diagnostic Testing for HIV-1 and HIV-2

Specific recommendations for the diagnostic testing of HIV are listed below:

- Informed consent must be obtained before an HIV test is performed. Some states require written consent. See HIV Prevention Counseling for a discussion of pretest and posttest counseling.
- Positive screening tests for HIV antibody must be confirmed by a more specific confirmatory test (either the Western blot assay or indirect immunofluorescence assay [IFA]) before being considered definitive for confirming HIV infection.
- Persons with positive HIV tests must receive medical and psychosocial evaluation and monitoring services, or be referred for these services.

The prevalence of HIV-2 in the United States is extremely low, and CDC does not recommend routine testing for HIV-2 in settings other than blood centers, unless demographic or behavioral information suggests that HIV-2 infection might be present. Those at risk for HIV-2 infection include persons from a country in which HIV-2 is endemic or the sex partners of such persons. (As of July 1992, HIV-2 was endemic in parts of West Africa and an increased prevalence of HIV-2 had been reported in Angola, France, Mozambique, and Portugal.) Additionally, testing for HIV-2 should be conducted when there is clinical evidence or suspicion of HIV disease in the absence of a positive test for antibodies to HIV-1 (6).

Counseling for Patients with HIV Infection

- Persons who test positive for HIV antibody should be counseled by a person who is able to discuss the medical, psychological, and social implications of HIV infection.
- Appropriate social support and psychological resources should be available, either on site or through referral, to assist patients in coping with emotional distress.
- Persons who continue to be at risk for transmitting HIV should receive assistance in changing or avoiding behaviors that can transmit infection to others.

Initial Evaluation and Planning for Care

- Identification of patients in need of immediate medical care (e.g., patients with symptomatic HIV infection or emotional crisis) and of those in need of antiretroviral therapy or prophylaxis for opportunistic infections (e.g., PCP).
- Evaluation for the presence of diseases associated with HIV, such as TB and STDs.
- Administration of recommended vaccinations.
- Case management or referral for case management.
- Counseling (see Counseling for Patients with HIV Infection).
- A detailed history, including sexual history, substance abuse history, and a review of systems for specific HIV-related symptoms.
- A physical examination; for females, this examination should include a gynecologic examination.
- For females, testing for N. gonorrhoeae, C. trachomatis, a Papanicolaou (Pap) smear, and wet mount examination of vaginal secretions.
- A syphilis serology.
- A CD4+ T-lymphocyte analysis.
- Complete blood and platelet counts.
- A purified protein derivative (PPD) tuberculin skin test by the Mantoux method and anergy testing with two delayed-type hypersensitivity (DTH) antigens (Candida, mumps, or tetanus toxoid) administered by the Mantoux method or a multipuncture device.
- A thorough psychosocial evaluation, including ascertainment of behavioral factors indicating risk for transmitting HIV and elucidation of information about any partners who should be notified about possible exposure to HIV.

Preventive Therapy for TB

Studies conducted among persons with and without HIV infection have suggested that HIV infection can depress tuberculin reactions before signs and symptoms of HIV infection develop. Cutaneous anergy (defined as skin test response of less than or equal to 3 mm to all DTH antigens) may be present among greater than or equal to 10% of asymptomatic persons with CD4+ counts greater than 500 cells/μL, and among greater than 60% of persons with CD4+ counts less than 200.

HIV-positive persons with a PPD reaction greater than or equal to 5 mm induration are considered to be infected with M. tuberculosis and should be evaluated for preventive treatment with isoniazid after active TB has been excluded. Anergic persons whose risk for tuberculous infection is estimated to be greater than or equal to 10%, based on available prevalence data, also should be considered for preventive therapy. For further details regarding evaluation of patients for TB, refer to Purified Protein Derivative (PPD-tuberculin anergy) and HIV Infection: Guidelines for Anergy Testing and Management of Anergic Persons at Risk of Tuberculosis (7).

The preliminary results from a randomized clinical trial suggest that treatment with isoniazid is effective for preventing active TB among HIV-infected persons. The usual regimen is isoniazid 10 mg/kg daily, up to a maximum adult dose of 300 mg daily. Twelve months of isoniazid preventive treatment is recommended for persons with HIV infection. For further details regarding preventive therapy for TB, refer to The Use of Preventive Therapy for Tuberculous Infection in the United States (8) and Management of Persons Exposed to Multidrug-Resistant Tuberculosis (9).

Recommended Immunizations for Adults and Adolescents

- Pneumococcal vaccination and an annual influenza vaccination should be administered.
- Persons at increased risk for acquiring HBV and who lack evidence of immunity may receive a three-dose schedule of hepatitis B vaccine, with postvaccination serologic testing between 1 and 6 months after the vaccination series.

Recommendations for vaccinating HIV-infected persons are based on expert opinions and consensus of the Advisory Committee on Immunization Practices (ACIP). No clinical data exist to document the efficacy of inactivated vaccines among HIV-infected persons, and pneumococcal vaccine failures have been reported. However, the use of inactivated vaccines may be beneficial for persons with HIV infection and there is no evidence that they are harmful. Immunogenicity studies have suggested a generally poorer response among HIV-infected persons, with higher response rates among asymptomatic persons than among those with advanced HIV disease.

Current evidence indicates that HIV infection does not increase susceptibility to HBV, nor does it increase the severity of clinical disease. The presence of HIV infection is not an indication for hepatitis B vaccine, but HIV-infected persons are at increased risk for becoming chronic carriers after hepatitis B infection. Because the routes of transmission of HBV parallel those of HIV, efforts to modify risky behaviors must be the primary focus of prevention efforts. However, vaccine should be administered to HIV-infected patients who continue to have a high likelihood for HBV exposure.

Persons with HIV infection also are at increased risk for invasive Haemophilus influenzae type B (Hib) disease and for complications from measles. Immunization against Hib and measles should be considered for asymptomatic HIV-infected persons who may have an increased risk for exposure to these infections (10).

Follow-Up Evaluation

- An interim history and physical examination;
- A complete blood count, platelet count, and lymphocyte subset analysis;
- Re-evaluation of psychosocial status and behavioral factors indicating risk for transmitting HIV.

To follow CD4+ measurements, providers should use the same laboratory and, optimally, obtain each specimen at the same time each day. When unexpected or discrepant results are obtained or when major treatment decisions are to be made, health-care providers should consider repeating the CD4+ measurement after at least 1 week.

More frequent laboratory monitoring, every 3–4 months, is indicated if CD4+ results indicate a patient is close to a point when a clinical intervention may be indicated.

Continuing Management of Patients with Early HIV Infection

Providing comprehensive, continuing management of patients with early HIV infection can include additional diagnostic studies (e.g., chest x-ray, serum chemistry, antibody testing for toxoplasmosis and hepatitis B), antiretroviral therapy and monitoring, and PCP prophylaxis. Treatment of HIV infection and prophylaxis against opportunistic infections continue to evolve rapidly. This treatment should be undertaken in consultation with physicians who are familiar with the care of persons with HIV infection. The complete therapeutic management of HIV infection is beyond the scope of this document.

Antiretroviral Therapy

The optimal time for initiating antiretroviral therapy has not yet been established. Zidovudine (ZDV) at a dose of 500 mg/day (100 mg orally every 4 hours while the patient is awake) has been recommended for symptomatic persons with less than 500 CD4+ T-cells/μL, and for asymptomatic persons with less than 300 CD4+ T-cells/μL. This recommendation is based on results of short-term follow-up in three randomized clinical trials demonstrating that the initiation of ZDV therapy delays progression to advanced disease. Evidence for improved long-term survival after early treatment is less conclusive. The effects of ZDV may be transient, possibly because of the development of viral resistance or other factors. Sequential or combination therapy with other antiretroviral agents could be more efficacious.

Whether other daily dosages, dose schedules, or dosages based on body weight would result in greater therapeutic benefit or few side effects is not known. Providers should work with patients to design a treatment strategy that is both clinically sound and appropriate for each individual patient's needs, priorities, and circumstances. An initial dose of 600 mg in divided doses has been recommended by a panel of experts convened by the National Institute of Allergy and Infectious Diseases (NIAID). Preliminary data suggest ZDV can yield therapeutic results when the dosing interval is increased to 8 hours, and at doses of 200 mg three times daily. Antiretroviral efficacy is diminished at doses less than 300 mg/day, and it has been suggested that higher oral doses may be required to achieve effective levels in the central nervous system.

There are no data to support the use of antiretroviral drugs other than ZDV as initial therapy. Didanosine (DDI) is recommended for persons who are intolerant of ZDV or who experience progression of symptoms despite ZDV. Two 100 mg tablets of DDI are recommended every 12 hours for persons who weigh greater than or equal to 60 kg; the recommended dose for adults less than 60 kg is one 100 mg tablet and one 25 mg tablet every 12 hours. Two tablets are recommended at each dose so that adequate buffering is provided to prevent gastric acid degradation of the drug.

Benefits have been reported from other antiretroviral regimens, including treatment with combinations of ZDV, DDC (dideoxycytidine [zalcitabine]), and DDI, or switching therapy to DDI after long-term therapy with ZDV. Experience with these alternatives is insufficient to serve as a basis for recommendations. Providers managing patients who are taking antiretroviral therapy should be familiar with evidence being developed in several clinical trials. Current information is available from the NIAID AIDS Clinical Trials Information Service, 1–800-TRI-ALSA.

Side effects that are serious (e.g., anemia, cytopenia, pancreatitis, and peripheral neuropathy) and uncomfortable (e.g., nausea, vomiting, headaches, and insomnia) are common during antiretroviral therapy. Although hematologic toxicity from ZDV is less common with the lower doses recommended, approximately 2% of patients who receive 500 mg/day manifest severe anemia by the 18th month of treatment—most within the 3rd through 8th month of treatment. Careful hematologic monitoring of patients receiving ZDV is recommended.

PCP Prophylaxis

Adults and adolescents with less than 200 CD4+ T-cells/μL or with constitutional symptoms, such as thrush or unexplained fever greater than 100°F for greater than or equal to 2 weeks, and any patient with a previous episode of PCP should receive PCP prophylaxis. Prophylaxis should be continued for the lifetime of the patient.

Based upon evidence from randomized controlled clinical trials, the Public Health Service Task Force on Antipneumocystis Prophylaxis has recommended the following regimens for PCP prophylaxis among adults and adolescents:

- Oral trimethoprim-sulfamethoxazole (TMP-SMX) at a dose of one double-strength tablet (800 mg SMX and 160 mg TMP) orally once a day.
- For patients unable to tolerate TMP-SMX: aerosol pentamidine administered by either the Respirgard II nebulizer regimen (300 mg once a month) or the Fisoneb nebulizer (initial loading regimen of five 60 mg doses during a 2-week period, followed by a 60 mg dose every 2 weeks).

The efficacy of alternatives for patients unable to tolerate TMP-SMX, including dapsone 100 mg orally once a day and sulfa desensitization, has not been studied extensively (11).

Management of Sex Partners

- Persons who are HIV-positive should be encouraged to notify their partners and to refer them for counseling and testing. Providers should assist in this process, if desired by the patient, either directly or through referral to health department partner notification programs.
- If patients are unwilling to notify their partners or if it cannot be assured that their partners will seek counseling, physicians or health department personnel should use confidential procedures to assure that the partners are notified.

SPECIAL CONSIDERATIONS

Pregnancy

Women who are HIV-infected should be specifically informed about the risk for perinatal infection. Current evidence indicates that 15%–39% of infants born to HIV-infected mothers are infected with HIV, and the virus also can be transmitted from an infected mother by breast-feeding. Pregnancy among HIV-infected patients does not appear to increase maternal morbidity or mortality.

Women should be counseled about their options regarding pregnancy. The objective of counseling is to provide HIV-infected women with current information for making reproductive decisions, analogous to the model used in genetic counseling. Contraceptive, prenatal, and abortion services should be available on site or by referral.

Minimal information is available on the use of ZDV or other antiretroviral drugs during pregnancy. Trials to evaluate its efficacy in preventing perinatal transmission and its safety during pregnancy are being conducted. A case series of 43 pregnant women has been published; dosages of ZDV ranged from 300 to 1,200 mg/day. ZDV was well tolerated and there were no malformations among the newborns in this series. Although this observation is encouraging, this series of negative case reports cannot be used to infer that ZDV is not teratogenic.

Burroughs Wellcome Co. and Hoffmann-LaRoche, Inc., in cooperation with CDC, maintain a registry to assess the effects of the use of ZDV and DDC during pregnancy. Women who receive either ZDV or DDC during pregnancy should be reported to this registry (1–800-722-9292, ext. 58465).

HIV Infection Among Infants and Children

Infants and young children with HIV infection differ from adults and adolescents with respect to the diagnosis, clinical presentation, and management of HIV disease. For example, total lymphocytes and absolute CD4+ cell counts are much higher in infants and children than in healthy adults and are age dependent. Specific indications and dosages for both antiretroviral and prophylactic therapy have been developed for children (12). Other modifications must be made in health services that are recommended for infants and children, such as avoiding vaccination with live oral polio vaccine when a child (or close household contact) is infected with HIV.

State laws differ regarding consent of minor persons (less than 18 years of age) for HIV counseling and testing, evaluation, treatment services, and participation in clinical trials. Although most adolescents receive adult doses of antiretroviral and prophylactic therapy, there are no data on modification of these dosages during puberty. Management of infants, children, and adolescents—who are known or suspected to be infected with HIV requires referral to, or close consultation with, physicians familiar with the manifestations and treatment of pediatric HIV infection.

DISEASES CHARACTERIZED BY GENITAL ULCERS
Management of the Patient with Genital Ulcers

In the United States, most patients with genital ulcers have genital herpes, syphilis, or chancroid. The relative frequency of each varies by geographic area and patient population, but in most areas of the United States genital herpes is the most common of these diseases. More than one of these diseases may be present among at least 3%–10% of patients with genital ulcers. Each disease has been associated with an increased risk for HIV infection.

A diagnosis based only on history and physical examination is often inaccurate. Therefore, evaluation of all persons with genital ulcers should include a serologic test for syphilis and possibly other tests. Although ideally all of these tests should be conducted for each patient with a genital ulcer, use of such tests (other than a serologic test for syphilis) may be based on test availability and clinical or epidemiologic suspicion. Specific tests for the evaluation of genital ulcers are listed below:

- Darkfield examination or direct immunofluorescence test for Treponema pallidum,
- Culture or antigen test for HSV, and
- Culture for Haemophilus ducreyi.

HIV testing should be considered in the management of patients with genital ulcers, especially for those with syphilis or chancroid.

A health-care provider often must treat a patient before test results are available (even after complete testing, at least one-quarter of patients with genital ulcers have no laboratory-confirmed diagnosis). In that circumstance, the clinician should treat for the diagnosis considered most likely. Many experts recommend treatment for both chancroid and syphilis if the diagnosis is unclear or if the patient resides in a community in which chancroid morbidity is notable (especially when diagnostic capabilities for chancroid and syphilis are not ideal).

Chancroid

Chancroid is endemic in many areas of the United States and also occurs in discrete outbreaks. Chancroid has been well-established as a cofactor for HIV transmission and a high rate of HIV infection among patients with chancroid has been reported in the United States and in other countries. As many as 10% of patients with chancroid may be coinfected with T. pallidum or HSV.

Definitive diagnosis of chancroid requires identification of H. ducreyi on special culture media that are not commercially available; even using these media, sensitivity is no higher than 80% and is usually lower. A probable diagnosis, for both clinical and surveillance purposes, may be made if the person has one or more painful genital ulcers, and (a) no evidence of T. pallidum infection by darkfield examination of ulcer exudate or by a serologic test for syphilis performed at least 7 days after onset of ulcers, and (b) either the clinical presentation of the ulcer(s) is not typical of disease caused by HSV or the HSV test results are negative. The combination of a painful ulcer with tender inguinal adenopathy (which occurs among one-third of patients) is suggestive of chancroid, and when accompanied by suppurative inguinal adenopathy is almost pathognomonic.

Treatment

Successful treatment cures infection, resolves clinical symptoms, and prevents transmission to others. In extensive cases, scarring may result despite successful therapy.

Recommended Regimens

Azithromycin 1 g orally in a single dose or Ceftriaxone 250 mg intramuscularly (IM) in a single dose or Erythromycin base 500 mg orally 4 times a day for 7 days.

All three regimens are effective for the treatment of chancroid among patients without HIV infection. Azithromycin and ceftriaxone offer the advantage of single-dose therapy. Antimicrobial resistance to ceftriaxone and azithromycin has not been reported. Although two isolates resistant to erythromycin were reported from Asia a decade ago, similar isolates have not been reported.

Other Management Considerations

Patients should be tested for HIV infection at the time of diagnosis. Patients also should be tested 3 months later for both syphilis and HIV, if initial results are negative.

Follow-Up

Patients should be re-examined 3–7 days after initiation of therapy. If treatment is successful, ulcers improve symptomatically within 3 days and improve objectively within 7 days after therapy. If no clinical improvement is evident, the clinician must consider whether (a) the diagnosis is correct, (b) coinfection with another STD agent exists, (c) the patient is infected with HIV, (d) treatment was not taken as instructed, or (e) the H. ducreyi strain causing infection is resistant to the prescribed antimicrobial.

The time required for complete healing is related to the size of the ulcer; large ulcers may require greater than or equal to 2 weeks. Clinical resolution of fluctuant lymphadenopathy is slower than that of ulcers and may require needle aspiration through adjacent intact skin—even during successful therapy.

Management of Sex Partners

Persons who had sexual contact with a patient who has chancroid within the 10 days before onset of the patient's symptoms should be examined and treated. The examination and treatment should be administered even in the absence of symptoms.

Special Considerations

PREGNANCY

The safety of azithromycin for pregnant and lactating women has not been established. Ciprofloxacin is contraindicated during pregnancy. No adverse effects of chancroid on pregnancy outcome or on the fetus have been reported.

HIV INFECTION

Patients coinfected with HIV should be closely monitored. These patients may require courses of therapy longer than those recommended in this report. Healing may be slower among HIV-infected persons and treatment failures do occur, especially after shorter-course treatment regimens. Since data on therapeutic efficacy with the recommended ceftriaxone and azithromycin regimens among patients infected with HIV are limited, those regimens should be used among persons known to be infected with HIV only if follow-up can be assured. Some experts suggest using the erythromycin 7-day regimen for treating HIV-infected persons.

Genital Herpes Simplex Virus Infections

Genital herpes is a viral disease that may be recurrent and has no cure. Two serotypes of HSV have been identified: HSV-1 and HSV-2; most cases of genital herpes are caused by HSV-2. On the basis of serologic studies, approximately 30 million persons in the United States may have genital HSV infection.

Most infected persons never recognize signs suggestive of genital herpes; some will have symptoms shortly after infection and then never again. A minority of the total infected U.S. population will have recurrent episodes of genital lesions. Some cases of first clinical episode genital herpes are manifested by extensive disease that requires hospitalization. Many cases of genital herpes are acquired from persons who do not know that they have a genital infection with HSV or who were asymptomatic at the time of the sexual contact.

Randomized trials show that systemic acyclovir provides partial control of the symptoms and signs of herpes episodes when used to treat first clinical episodes, or when used as suppressive therapy. However, acyclovir neither eradicates latent virus nor affects subsequent risk, frequency, or severity of recurrences after administration of the drug is discontinued. Topical therapy with acyclovir is substantially less effective than the oral drug and its use is discouraged. Episodes of HSV infection among HIV-infected patients may require more aggressive therapy. Immunocompromised persons may have prolonged episodes with extensive disease. For these persons, infections caused by acyclovir-resistant strains require selection of alternate antiviral agents.

First Clinical Episode of Genital Herpes

Recommended Regimen

Acyclovir 200 mg orally 5 times a day for 7–10 days or until clinical resolution is attained.

First Clinical Episode of Herpes Proctitis

Recommended Regimen

Acyclovir 400 mg orally 5 times a day for 10 days or until clinical resolution is attained.

Recurrent Episodes

When treatment is instituted during the prodrome or within 2 days of onset of lesions, some patients with recurrent disease experience limited benefit from therapy. However, since early treatment can seldom be administered, most immunocompetent patients with recurrent disease do not benefit from acyclovir treatment, and it is not generally recommended.

Recommended Regimen

Acyclovir 200 mg orally 5 times a day for 5 days, or Acyclovir 400 mg orally 3 times a day for 5 days, or Acyclovir 800 mg orally 2 times a day for 5 days.

Daily Suppressive Therapy

Daily suppressive therapy reduces the frequency of HSV recurrences by at least 75% among patients with frequent recurrences (i.e., six or more recurrences per year). Suppressive treatment with oral acyclovir does not totally eliminate symptomatic or asymptomatic viral shedding or the potential for transmission. Safety and efficacy have been documented among persons receiving daily therapy for as long as 5 years. Acyclovir-resistant strains of HSV have been isolated from some persons receiving suppressive therapy, but these strains have not been associated with treatment failure among immunocompetent patients. After 1 year of continuous suppressive therapy, acyclovir should be discontinued to allow assessment of the patient's rate of recurrent episodes.

Recommended Regimen

Acyclovir 400 mg orally 2 times a day.

Alternative Regimen

Acyclovir 200 mg orally 3–5 times a day.

The goal of the alternative regimen is to identify for each patient the lowest dose that provides relief from frequently recurring symptoms.

Severe Disease

Intravenous (IV) therapy should be provided for patients with severe disease or complications necessitating hospitalization (e.g., disseminated infection that includes encephalitis, pneumonitis, or hepatitis).

Recommended Regimen

Acyclovir 5–10 mg/kg body weight IV every 8 hours for 5–7 days or until clinical resolution is attained.

Other Management Considerations

Other considerations for managing patients with genital HSV infection are as follows:

- Patients should be advised to abstain from sexual activity while lesions are present.
- Patients with genital herpes should be told about the natural history of the disease, with emphasis on the potential for recurrent episodes, asymptomatic viral shedding, and sexual transmission. Sexual transmission of HSV has been documented to occur during periods without evidence of lesions. Many cases are transmitted during such asymptomatic periods.
- The use of condoms should be encouraged during all sexual exposures. The risk for neonatal infection should be explained to all patients—male and female—with genital herpes. Women of childbearing age who have genital herpes should be advised to inform health-care providers who care for them during pregnancy about their HSV infection.

Management of Sex Partners

Sex partners of patients who have genital herpes are likely to benefit from evaluation and counseling. Symptomatic sex partners should be managed in the same manner as any patient with genital lesions. However, the majority of persons with genital HSV infection do not have a history of typical genital lesions. These asymptomatic persons may benefit from evaluation and counseling; thus, even asymptomatic partners should be queried about histories of typical and atypical genital lesions and encouraged to examine themselves for lesions in the future.

Commercially available HSV type-specific antibody tests have not demonstrated adequate performance characteristics; their use is not currently recommended. Sensitive and specific type-specific serum antibody assays now utilized in research settings might contribute to future intervention strategies. Should tests with adequate sensitivity and specificity become commercially available, it might be possible to accurately identify asymptomatic persons infected with HSV-2, to focus counseling on how to detect lesions by self-examination, and to reduce the risk for transmission to sex partners.

Special Considerations

ALLERGY, INTOLERANCE, OR ADVERSE REACTIONS

Effective alternatives to therapy with acyclovir are not available.

HIV INFECTION

Lesions caused by HSV are relatively common among patients infected with HIV. Intermittent or suppressive therapy with oral acyclovir may be needed.

The acyclovir dosage for HIV-infected persons is controversial, but experience strongly suggests that immunocompromised patients benefit from increased dosage. Regimens such as 400 mg orally 3 to 5 times a day, as used for other immunocompromised persons, have been found useful. Therapy should be continued until clinical resolution is attained.

For severe disease, IV acyclovir therapy may be required. If lesions persist among patients undergoing acyclovir treatment, resistance to acyclovir should be suspected. These patients should be managed in consultation with an expert. For severe disease because of proven or suspected acyclovir-resistant strains, hospitalization should be considered. Foscarnet, 40 mg/kg body weight IV every 8 hours until clinical resolution is attained, appears to be the best available treatment.

PREGNANCY

The safety of systemic acyclovir therapy among pregnant women has not been established. Burroughs Wellcome Co., in cooperation with CDC, maintains a registry to assess the effects of the use of acyclovir during pregnancy. Women who receive acyclovir during pregnancy should be reported to this registry (1–800-722-9292, ext. 58465).

Current registry findings do not indicate an increase in the number of birth defects identified among the prospective reports when compared with those expected in the general population. Moreover, no consistent pattern of abnormalities emerges among retrospective reports. These findings provide some assurance in counseling women who have had inadvertent prenatal exposure to acyclovir. However, accumulated case histories comprise a sample of insufficient size for reaching reliable and definitive conclusions regarding the risks of acyclovir treatment to pregnant women and to their fetuses.

In the presence of life-threatening maternal HSV infection (e.g., disseminated infection that includes encephalitis, pneumonitis, or hepatitis), acyclovir administered IV is indicated. Among pregnant women without life-threatening disease, systemic acyclovir should not be used to treat recurrences nor should it be used as suppressive therapy near-term (or at other times during pregnancy) to prevent reactivation.

PERINATAL INFECTIONS

Most mothers of infants who acquire neonatal herpes lack histories of clinically evident genital herpes. The risk for transmission to the neonate from an infected mother appears highest among women with first episode genital herpes near the time of delivery, and is low (less than or equal to 3%) among women with recurrent herpes. The results of viral cultures during pregnancy do not predict viral shedding at the time of delivery, and such cultures are not routinely indicated.

At the onset of labor, all women should be carefully questioned about symptoms of genital herpes and should be examined. Women without symptoms or signs of genital herpes infection (or prodrome) may deliver their babies vaginally. Among women who have a history of genital herpes, or who have a sex partner with genital herpes, cultures of the birth canal at delivery may aid in decisions relating to neonatal management.

Infants delivered through an infected birth canal (proven by virus isolation or presumed by observation of lesions) should be followed carefully, including virus cultures obtained 24–48 hours after birth. Available data do not support the routine use of acyclovir as anticipatory treatment for asymptomatic infants delivered through an infected birth canal. Treatment should be reserved for infants who develop evidence of clinical disease and for those with positive postpartum cultures.

All infants with evidence of neonatal herpes should be treated with systemic acyclovir or vidarabine; refer to the Report of the Committee on Infectious Diseases, American Academy of Pediatrics (13). For ease of administration and to lower toxicity, acyclovir (30 mg/kg/day for 10–14 days) is the preferred drug. The care of these infants should be managed in consultation with an expert.

Lymphogranuloma Venereum

Lymphogranuloma venereum (LGV), a rare disease in the United States, is caused by serovars L1, L2, or L3 of C. trachomatis. The most common clinical manifestation of LGV among heterosexuals is tender inguinal lymphadenopathy that is most commonly unilateral. Women and homosexually active men may have proctocolitis or inflammatory involvement of perirectal or perianal lymphatic tissues resulting in fistulas and strictures. When patients seek care, most no longer have the self-limited genital ulcer that sometimes occurs at the site of inoculation. The diagnosis is usually made serologically and by exclusion of other causes of inguinal lymphadenopathy or genital ulcers.

Treatment

Treatment cures infection and prevents ongoing tissue damage, although tissue reaction can result in scarring. Buboes may require aspiration or incision and drainage through intact skin. Doxycycline is the preferred treatment.

Recommended Regimen

Doxycycline 100 mg orally 2 times a day for 21 days.

Alternative Regimens

Erythromycin 500 mg orally 4 times a day for 21 days or Sulfisoxazole 500 mg orally 4 times a day for 21 days or equivalent sulfonamide course.

Follow-Up

Patients should be followed clinically until signs and symptoms have resolved.

Management of Sex Partners

Persons who have had sexual contact with a patient who has LGV within the 30 days before onset of the patient's symptoms should be examined, tested for urethral or cervical chlamydial infection, and treated.

Special Considerations

PREGNANCY

Pregnant and lactating women should be treated with the erythromycin regimen.

HIV INFECTION

Persons with HIV infection and LGV should be treated following the regimens previously cited.

Syphilis

General Principles

Background

Diagnostic considerations and use of serologic tests. Darkfield examinations and direct fluorescent antibody tests of lesion exudate or tissue are the definitive methods for diagnosing early syphilis. Presumptive diagnosis is possible with the use of two types of serologic tests for syphilis: (a) nontreponemal (e.g., Venereal Disease Research Laboratory [VDRL] and RPR, and (b) treponemal (e.g., fluorescent treponemal antibody absorbed [FTA-ABS] and microhemag-glutination assay for antibody to T. pallidum [MHA-TP]). The use of one type of test alone is not sufficient for diagnosis. Nontreponemal test antibody titers usually correlate with disease activity, and results should be reported quantitatively. A fourfold change in titer, equivalent to a change of two dilutions (e.g., from 1:16 to 1:4, or from 1:8 to 1:32), is necessary to demonstrate a substantial difference between two nontreponemal test results that were obtained using the same serologic test. A patient who has a reactive treponemal test usually will have a reactive test for a lifetime, regardless of treatment or disease activity (15%–25% of patients treated during the primary stage may revert to being serologically nonreactive after 2–3 years). Treponemal test antibody titers correlate poorly with disease activity and should not be used to assess response to treatment.

Sequential serologic tests should be performed using the same testing method (e.g., VDRL or RPR) by the same laboratory. The VDRL and RPR are equally valid, but quantitative results from the two tests cannot be directly compared because RPR titers are often slightly higher than VDRL titers.

Abnormal results of serologic testing (unusually high, unusually low, and fluctuating titers) have been observed among HIV-infected patients. For such patients, use of other tests (e.g., biopsy and direct microscopy) should be considered. However, serologic tests appear to be accurate and reliable for the diagnosis of syphilis and for evaluation of treatment response for the vast majority of HIV-infected patients.

Treatment

Parenteral penicillin G is the preferred drug for treatment of all stages of syphilis. The preparation(s) used (i.e., benzathine, aqueous procaine, or aqueous crystalline), the dosage, and the length of treatment depend on the stage and clinical manifestations of disease.

Parenteral penicillin G is the only therapy with documented efficacy for neurosyphilis or for syphilis during pregnancy. Patients with neurosyphilis and pregnant women with syphilis in any stage who report penicillin allergy should almost always be treated with penicillin, after desensitization, if necessary. Skin testing for penicillin allergy may be useful for some patients and in some settings (see Management of the Patient With a History of Penicillin Allergy). However, minor determinants needed for penicillin skin testing are not available commercially.

Management of Sex Partners

Sexual transmission of T. pallidum occurs only when mucocutaneous syphilitic lesions are present; such manifestations are uncommon after the first year of infection. However, persons sexually exposed to a patient with syphilis in any stage should be evaluated clinically and serologically according to the following recommendations:

- Persons who were exposed to a patient with primary, secondary, or latent (duration less than 1 year) syphilis within the preceding 90 days might be infected even if seronegative, and therefore should be treated presumptively.
- Persons who were sexually exposed to a patient with primary, secondary, or latent (duration less than 1 year) syphilis greater than 90 days before examination should be treated presumptively if serologic test results are not available immediately, and the opportunity for follow-up is uncertain.
- For purposes of partner notification and presumptive treatment of exposed sex partners, patients who have syphilis of unknown duration and who have high nontreponemal serologic test titers (greater than or equal to 1:32) may be considered to be infected with early syphilis.
- Long-term sex partners of patients with late syphilis should be evaluated clinically and serologically for syphilis.

The time periods before treatment used for identifying at-risk sex partners are 3 months plus duration of symptoms for primary syphilis, 6 months plus duration of symptoms for secondary syphilis, and 1 year for early latent syphilis.

Primary and Secondary Syphilis

Treatment

Four decades of experience indicate that parenteral penicillin G is effective in achieving local cure (healing of lesions and prevention of sexual transmission) and in preventing late sequelae. However, no adequately conducted comparative trials have been performed to guide the selection of an optimal penicillin regimen (i.e., dose, duration, and preparation). Substantially fewer data on nonpenicillin regimens are available.

Recommended regimen for adults. Nonallergic patients with primary or secondary syphilis should be treated with the following regimen: Benzathine penicillin G, 2.4 million units IM in a single dose.

NOTE: Recommendations for treating pregnant women and HIV-infected persons for syphilis are discussed in separate sections.

Recommended regimen for children. After the newborn period, children diagnosed with syphilis should have a CSF examination to exclude a diagnosis of neurosyphilis, and birth and maternal medical records should be reviewed to assess whether the child has congenital or acquired syphilis (see Congenital Syphilis). Children with acquired primary or secondary syphilis should be evaluated (including consultation with child-protection services) and treated using the following pediatric regimen (see Sexual Assault or Abuse of Children): Benzathine penicillin G, 50,000 units/kg IM, up to the adult dose of 2.4 million units in a single dose.

OTHER MANAGEMENT CONSIDERATIONS

All patients with syphilis should be tested for HIV. In areas with high HIV prevalence, patients with primary syphilis should be retested for HIV after 3 months.

Patients who have syphilis and who also have symptoms or signs suggesting neurologic disease (e.g., meningitis) or ophthalmic disease (e.g., uveitis) should be fully evaluated for neurosyphilis and syphilitic eye disease (including CSF analysis and ocular slit-lamp examination). Such patients should be treated appropriately according to the results of this evaluation.

Invasion of CSF by T. pallidum with accompanying CSF abnormalities is common among adults who have primary or secondary syphilis. However, few patients develop neurosyphilis after treatment with the regimens described in this report. Therefore, unless clinical signs or symptoms of neurologic involvement are present (e.g., auditory, cranial nerve, meningeal, or ophthalmic manifestations), lumbar puncture is not recommended for routine evaluation of patients with primary or secondary syphilis.

FOLLOW-UP

Treatment failures can occur with any regimen. However, assessing response to treatment is often difficult, and no definitive criteria for cure or failure exist. Serologic test titers may decline more slowly among patients with a prior syphilis infection. Patients should be re-examined clinically and serologically at 3 months and again at 6 months.

Patients with signs or symptoms that persist or recur or who have a sustained fourfold increase in nontreponemal test titer compared with either the baseline titer or to a subsequent result, can be considered to have failed treatment or to be reinfected. These patients should be re-treated after evaluation for HIV infection. Unless reinfection is likely, lumbar puncture also should be performed.

Failure of nontreponemal test titers to decline fourfold by 3 months after therapy for primary or secondary syphilis identifies persons at risk for treatment failure. Those persons should be evaluated for HIV infection. Optimal management of such patients is unclear if they are HIV negative. At a minimum, these patients should have additional clinical and serologic follow-up. If further follow-up cannot be assured, retreatment is recommended. Some experts recommend CSF examination in such situations.

When patients are re-treated, most experts recommend re-treatment with three weekly injections of benzathine penicillin G 2.4 million units IM, unless CSF examination indicates that neurosyphilis is present.

MANAGEMENT OF SEX PARTNERS

Refer to General Principles, Management of Sex Partners.

SPECIAL CONSIDERATIONS

Penicillin allergy

Nonpregnant penicillin-allergic patients who have primary or secondary syphilis should be treated with the following regimen: Doxycycline 100 mg orally 2 times a day for 2 weeks or Tetracycline 500 mg orally 4 times a day for 2 weeks.

There is less clinical experience with doxycycline than with tetracycline, but compliance is likely to be better with doxycycline. Therapy for a patient who cannot tolerate either doxycycline or tetracycline should be based upon whether the patient's compliance with the therapy regimen and with follow-up examinations can be assured.

For nonpregnant patients whose compliance with therapy and follow-up can be assured, an alternative regimen is erythromycin 500 mg orally 4 times a day for 2 weeks. Various ceftriaxone regimens also may be considered.

Patients whose compliance with therapy or follow-up cannot be assured should be desensitized, if necessary, and treated with penicillin. Skin testing for penicillin allergy may be useful in some situations (see Management of the Patient With a History of Penicillin Allergy).

Erythromycin is less effective than other recommended regimens. Data on ceftriaxone are limited, and experience has been too brief to permit identification of late failures. Optimal dose and duration have not been established for ceftriaxone, but regimens that provide 8–10 days of treponemicidal levels in the blood should be used. Single dose ceftriaxone therapy is not effective for treating syphilis.

Pregnancy

Pregnant patients who are allergic to penicillin should be treated with penicillin, after desensitization, if necessary (see Management of the Patient With a History of Penicillin Allergy and Syphilis During Pregnancy).

HIV infection

Refer to Syphilis Among HIV-Infected Patients.

Latent Syphilis

Latent syphilis is defined as those periods after infection with T. pallidum when patients are seroreactive, but show no other evidence of disease. Patients who have latent syphilis and who have acquired syphilis within the preceding year are classified as having early latent syphilis. Patients can be demonstrated to have acquired syphilis within the preceding year on the basis of documented seroconversion, a fourfold or greater increase in titer of a nontreponemal serologic test, history of symptoms of primary or secondary syphilis, or if they had a sex partner with primary, secondary, or latent syphilis (documented independently as duration less than 1 year). Nearly all others have latent syphilis of unknown duration and should be managed as if they had late latent syphilis.

Treatment

Treatment of latent syphilis is intended to prevent occurrence or progression of late complications. Although clinical experience supports belief in the effectiveness of penicillin in achieving those goals, limited evidence is available for guidance in choosing specific regimens. There is very little evidence to support the use of nonpenicillin regimens.

Recommended regimens for adults.   These regimens are for nonallergic patients with normal CSF examination (if performed).

> Early Latent Syphilis—Benzathine penicillin G, 2.4 million units IM in a single dose.
> Late Latent Syphilis or Latent Syphilis of Unknown Duration—Benzathine penicillin G, 7.2 million units total, administered as 3 doses of 2.4 million units IM each, at 1-week intervals.

Recommended regimens for children.   After the newborn period, children diagnosed with syphilis should have a CSF examination to exclude neurosyphilis, and birth and maternal medical records should be reviewed to assess whether the child has congenital or acquired syphilis (see Congenital Syphilis). Older children with acquired latent syphilis should be evaluated as described for adults and treated using the following pediatric regimens (see Sexual Assault or Abuse of Children). These regimens are for nonallergic children who have acquired syphilis and who have had a normal CSF examination.

Early Latent Syphilis—Benzathine penicillin G, 50,000 units/kg IM, up to the adult dose of 2.4 million units in a single dose.

Late Latent Syphilis or Latent Syphilis of Unknown Duration—Benzathine penicillin G, 50,000 units/kg IM, up to the adult dose of 2.4 million units, for three total doses (total 150,000 units/kg up to adult total dose of 7.2 million units).

OTHER MANAGEMENT CONSIDERATIONS

All patients with latent syphilis should be evaluated clinically for evidence of tertiary disease (e.g., aortitis, neurosyphilis, gumma, and iritis). Recommended therapy for patients with latent syphilis may not be optimal therapy for the persons with asymptomatic neurosyphilis. However, the yield from CSF examination, in terms of newly diagnosed cases of neurosyphilis, is low.

Patients with any one of the criteria listed below should have a CSF examination before treatment:

- Neurologic or ophthalmic signs or symptoms;
- Other evidence of active syphilis (e.g., aortitis, gumma, iritis);
- Treatment failure;
- HIV infection;
- Serum nontreponemal titer greater than or equal to 1:32, unless duration of infection is known to be less than 1 year; or
- Nonpenicillin therapy planned, unless duration of infection is known to be less than 1 year.
- If dictated by circumstances and patient preferences, CSF examination may be performed for persons who do not meet the criteria listed above. If a CSF examination is performed and the results show abnormalities consistent with CNS syphilis, the patient should be treated for neurosyphilis (see Neurosyphilis).
- All syphilis patients should be tested for HIV.

FOLLOW-UP

Quantitative nontreponemal serologic tests should be repeated at 6 months and again at 12 months. Limited data are available to guide evaluation of the response to therapy for a patient with latent syphilis. If titers increase fourfold, or if an initially high titer (greater than or equal to 1:32) fails to decline at least fourfold (two dilutions) within 12–24 months, or if the patient develops signs or symptoms attributable to syphilis, the patient should be evaluated for neurosyphilis and re-treated appropriately.

MANAGEMENT OF SEX PARTNERS

Refer to General Principles, Management of Sex Partners.

SPECIAL CONSIDERATIONS

Penicillin allergy

For patients who have latent syphilis and who are allergic to penicillin, nonpenicillin therapy should be used only after CSF examination has excluded neurosyphilis. Nonpregnant, penicillin-allergic patients should be treated with the following regimens.

Doxycycline 100 mg orally 2 times a day or Tetracycline 500 mg orally 4 times a day.

Both drugs are administered for 2 weeks if duration of infection is known to have been less than 1 year; otherwise, for 4 weeks.

Pregnancy

Pregnant patients who are allergic to penicillin should be treated with penicillin, after desensitization, if necessary (see Management of the Patient With a History of Penicillin Allergy and Syphilis During Pregnancy).

HIV infection

Refer to Syphilis Among HIV-Infected Patients.

Late Syphilis

Late (tertiary) syphilis refers to patients with gumma and patients with cardiovascular syphilis, but not to neurosyphilis. Nonallergic patients without evidence of neurosyphilis should be treated with the following regimen.

Recommended Regimen

Benzathine penicillin G, 7.2 million units total, administered as 3 doses of 2.4 million units IM, at 1-week intervals.

OTHER MANAGEMENT CONSIDERATIONS

Patients with symptomatic late syphilis should undergo CSF examination before therapy. Some experts treat all patients who have cardiovascular syphilis with a neurosyphilis regimen. The complete management of patients with cardiovascular or gummatous syphilis is beyond the scope of these guidelines. These patients should be managed in consultation with experts.

FOLLOW-UP

There is minimal evidence regarding follow-up of patients infected with late syphilis. Clinical response depends partly on the nature of the lesions.

MANAGEMENT OF SEX PARTNERS

Refer to General Principles, Management of Sex Partners.

SPECIAL CONSIDERATIONS

Penicillin allergy

Patients allergic to penicillin should be treated according to treatment regimens recommended for late latent syphilis.

Pregnancy

Pregnant patients who are allergic to penicillin should be treated with penicillin, after desensitization, if necessary (see Management of the Patient With a History of Penicillin Allergy and Syphilis During Pregnancy).

HIV infection

Refer to Syphilis Among HIV-Infected Patients.

Neurosyphilis

Treatment

Central nervous system disease can occur during any stage of syphilis. A patient with clinical evidence of neurologic involvement (e.g., ophthalmic or auditory symptoms, cranial nerve palsies) with syphilis warrants a CSF examination. Although four decades of experience have confirmed the effectiveness of penicillin, the evidence to guide the choice of the best regimen is limited.

Syphilitic eye disease is frequently associated with neurosyphilis, and patients with this disease should be treated according to neurosyphilis treatment recommendations. CSF examination should be performed on all such patients to identify those patients with CSF abnormalities who should have follow-up CSF examinations to assess response to treatment.

Patients who have neurosyphilis or syphilitic eye disease (e.g., uveitis, neuroretinitis, or optic neuritis) and who are not allergic to penicillin should be treated with the following regimen.

Recommended regimen. 12–24 million units aqueous crystalline penicillin G daily, administered as 2–4 million units IV every 4 hours, for 10–14 days.

If compliance with therapy can be assured, patients may be treated with the following alternative regimen.

Alternative regimen. 2.4 million units procaine penicillin IM daily, plus probenecid 500 mg orally 4 times a day, both for 10–14 days.

The durations of these regimens are shorter than that of the regimen used for late syphilis in the absence of neurosyphilis. Therefore, some experts administer benzathine penicillin, 2.4 million units IM after completion of these neurosyphilis treatment regimens to provide a comparable total duration of therapy.

OTHER MANAGEMENT CONSIDERATIONS

Other considerations in the management of the patient with neurosyphilis are the following:

• All patients with syphilis should be tested for HIV.
• Many experts recommend treating patients with evidence of auditory disease caused by syphilis in the same manner as for neurosyphilis, regardless of the findings on CSF examination.

FOLLOW-UP

If CSF pleocytosis was present initially, CSF examination should be repeated every 6 months until the cell count is normal. Follow-up CSF examinations also may be used to evaluate changes in the VDRL-CSF or CSF protein in response to therapy, though changes in these two parameters are slower and persistent abnormalities are of less certain importance. If the cell count has not decreased at 6 months, or if the CSF is not entirely normal by 2 years, re-treatment should be considered.

MANAGEMENT OF SEX PARTNERS

Refer to General Principles, Management of Sex Partners.

SPECIAL CONSIDERATIONS

Penicillin allergy

No data have been collected systematically for evaluation of therapeutic alternatives to penicillin for treatment of neurosyphilis. Therefore, patients who report being allergic to penicillin should be treated with penicillin, after desensitization if necessary, or should be managed in consultation with an expert. In some situations, skin testing to confirm penicillin
allergy may be useful (see Management of the Patient With a History of Penicillin Allergy).

Pregnancy

Pregnant patients who are allergic to penicillin should be treated with penicillin, after desensitization if necessary (see Syphilis During Pregnancy).

HIV infection

Refer to Syphilis Among HIV-Infected Patients.

Syphilis Among HIV-Infected Patients

Diagnostic Considerations

Unusual serologic responses have been observed among HIV-infected
persons who also have syphilis. Most reports involved serologic titers that
were higher than expected, but false-negative serologic test results or delayed appearance of seroreactivity have also been reported. Nevertheless,
both treponemal and nontreponemal serologic tests for syphilis are accurate for the majority of patients with syphilis and HIV coinfection.

When clinical findings suggest that syphilis is present, but serologic
tests are nonreactive or confusing, it may be helpful to perform such alternative tests as biopsy of a lesion, darkfield examination, or direct fluorescent antibody staining of lesion material.

Neurosyphilis should be considered in the differential diagnosis of
neurologic disease among HIV-infected persons.

Treatment

Although adequate research-based evidence is not available, published
case reports and expert opinion suggest that HIV-infected patients with
early syphilis are at increased risk for neurologic complications and
have higher rates of treatment failure with currently recommended regimens. The magnitude of these risks, although not precisely defined, is
probably small. No treatment regimens have been demonstrated to be
more effective in preventing development of neurosyphilis than those
recommended for patients without HIV infection. Careful follow-up after therapy is essential.

Primary and Secondary Syphilis Among HIV-Infected Patients

Treatment

Treatment with benzathine penicillin G 2.4 million units IM, as for patients without HIV infection, is recommended. Some experts recom-

mend additional treatments, such as multiple doses of benzathine penicillin G as suggested for late syphilis, or other supplemental antibiotics
in addition to benzathine penicillin G 2.4 million units IM.

OTHER MANAGEMENT CONSIDERATIONS

CSF abnormalities are common among HIV-infected patients who have primary or
secondary syphilis, but these abnormalities are of unknown prognostic significance.
Most HIV-infected patients respond appropriately to currently recommended penicillin therapy; however, some experts recommend CSF examination before therapy
and modification of treatment accordingly.

FOLLOW-UP

Patients should be evaluated clinically and serologically for treatment failure at 1 month
and at 2, 3, 6, 9, and 12 months after therapy. Although of unproven benefit, some experts recommend performing CSF examination after therapy (i.e., at 6 months).

　　HIV-infected patients who meet the criteria for treatment failure should undergo CSF examination and be retreated just as for patients without HIV infection.
CSF examination and re-treatment also should be strongly considered for patients in
whom the suggested fourfold decrease in nontreponemal test titer does not occur
within 3 months for primary or secondary syphilis. Most experts would re-treat patients with benzathine penicillin G 7.2 million units (as 3 weekly doses of 2.4 million
units each) if the CSF examination is normal.

SPECIAL CONSIDERATIONS

Penicillin allergy

Penicillin regimens should be used to treat HIV-infected patients in all stages of syphilis. Skin
testing to confirm penicillin allergy may be used (see Management of the Patient With a
History of Penicillin Allergy), but data on the utility of that approach among immunocompromised patients are inadequate. Patients may be desensitized, then treated with penicillin.

Latent Syphilis Among HIV-Infected Patients

Diagnostic Considerations

Patients who have both latent syphilis (regardless of apparent duration)
and HIV infection should undergo CSF examination before treatment.

Treatment

A patient with latent syphilis, HIV infection, and a normal CSF examination can be treated with benzathine penicillin G 7.2 million units (as
3 weekly doses of 2.4 million units each).

Special Considerations
Penicillin allergy

Penicillin regimens should be used to treat all stages of syphilis among HIV-infected patients.
Skin testing to confirm penicillin allergy may be used (see Management of the Patient With a
History of Penicillin Allergy), but data on the utility of that approach in immunocompromised
patients are inadequate. Patients may be desensitized, then treated with penicillin.

Syphilis During Pregnancy

All women should be screened serologically for syphilis during the early
stages of pregnancy. In populations in which utilization of prenatal care

is not optimal, RPR-card test screening and treatment, if that test is re-active, should be performed at the time a pregnancy is diagnosed. In communities and populations with high syphilis prevalence or for patients at high risk, serologic testing should be repeated during the third trimester and again at delivery. (Some states mandate screening at delivery for all women.) Any woman who delivers a stillborn infant after 20 weeks gestation should be tested for syphilis. No infant should leave the hospital without the serologic status of the infant's mother having been determined at least once during pregnancy.

Diagnostic Considerations

Seropositive pregnant women should be considered infected unless treatment history is clearly documented in a medical or health department record and sequential serologic antibody titers have appropriately declined.

Treatment

Penicillin is effective for preventing transmission to fetuses and for treating established infection among fetuses. Evidence is insufficient, however, to determine whether the specific, recommended penicillin regimens are optimal.

Recommended regimens. Treatment during pregnancy should be the penicillin regimen appropriate for the woman's stage of syphilis. Some experts recommend additional therapy (e.g., a second dose of benzathine penicillin 2.4 million units IM) 1 week after the initial dose, particularly for those women in the third trimester of pregnancy and for women who have secondary syphilis during pregnancy.

OTHER MANAGEMENT CONSIDERATIONS

Women who are treated for syphilis during the second half of pregnancy are at risk for premature labor or fetal distress, or both, if their treatment precipitates the Jarisch-Herxheimer reaction. These women should be advised to seek medical attention following treatment if they notice any change in fetal movements or if they have contractions. Stillbirth is a rare complication of treatment; however, since therapy is necessary to prevent further fetal damage, that concern should not delay treatment. All patients with syphilis should be tested for HIV.

FOLLOW-UP

Serologic titers should be checked monthly until adequacy of treatment has been assured. The antibody response should be appropriate for the stage of disease.

MANAGEMENT OF SEX PARTNERS

Refer to General Principles, Management of Sex Partners.

SPECIAL CONSIDERATIONS

Penicillin allergy

There are no proven alternatives to penicillin. A pregnant woman with a history of penicillin allergy should be treated with penicillin, after desensitization, if necessary. Skin testing may be helpful for some patients and in some settings (see Management of the Patient With a History of Penicillin Allergy). Tetracycline and doxycycline are contraindicated during pregnancy. Erythromycin should not be used because it cannot be relied upon to cure an infected fetus.

Congenital Syphilis

Diagnostic Considerations

Infants should be evaluated for congenital syphilis if they were born to seropositive (nontreponemal test confirmed by treponemal test) women who meet the following criteria:

- Have untreated syphilis;* or
- Were treated for syphilis during pregnancy with erythromycin; or
- Were treated for syphilis less than 1 month before delivery; or
- Were treated for syphilis during pregnancy with the appropriate penicillin regimen, but nontreponemal antibody titers did not decrease sufficiently after therapy to indicate an adequate response (greater than or equal to fourfold decrease); or
- Do not have a well-documented history of treatment for syphilis; or
- Were treated appropriately before pregnancy but had insufficient serologic follow-up to assure that they had responded appropriately to treatment and are not currently infected (greater than or equal to fourfold decrease for patients treated for early syphilis; stable or declining titers less than or equal to 1:4 for other patients).

No infant should leave the hospital without the serologic status of the infant's mother having been documented at least once during pregnancy. Serologic testing also should be performed at delivery in communities and populations at risk for congenital syphilis. Serologic tests can be nonreactive among infants infected late during their mother's pregnancy.

Evaluation of the Infant

The clinical and laboratory evaluation of infants born to women described above should include the following:

- A thorough physical examination for evidence of congenital syphilis;
- A quantitative nontreponemal serologic test for syphilis performed on the infant's sera (not on cord blood);
- CSF analysis for cells, protein, and VDRL;
- Long bone x-rays;
- Other tests as clinically indicated (e.g., chest x-ray, complete blood count, differential and platelet count, liver function tests);
- For infants who have no evidence of congenital syphilis on the above evaluation, determination of presence of specific antitreponemal IgM antibody by a testing method recognized by CDC as having either provisional or standard status;

---

*A woman treated with a regimen other than those recommended for treatment of syphilis (for pregnant women or otherwise) in these guidelines should be considered untreated.

- Pathologic examination of the placenta or amniotic cord using specific fluorescent antitreponemal antibody staining.

Treatment

Therapy decisions. Infants should be treated for presumed congenital syphilis if they were born to mothers who, at delivery, had untreated syphilis or who had evidence of relapse or reinfection after treatment (see Congenital Syphilis, Diagnostic Considerations). Additional criteria for presumptively treating infants with congenital syphilis are as follows:

- Physical evidence of active disease;
- X-ray evidence of active disease;
- A reactive VDRL-CSF or, for infants born to seroreactive mothers, an abnormal** CSF white blood cell count or protein, regardless of CSF serology;
- A serum quantitative nontreponemal serologic titer that is at least fourfold greater than the mother's titer***;
- Specific antitreponemal IgM antibody detected by a testing method that has been given provisional or standard status by CDC;
- If they meet the previously cited criteria for "Who Should Be Evaluated," but have not been fully evaluated (see Congenital Syphilis, Diagnostic Considerations).

NOTE: Infants with clinically evident congenital syphilis should have an ophthalmologic examination.

Recommended regimens. Aqueous crystalline penicillin G, 100,000–150,000 units/kg/day (administered as 50,000 units/kg IV every 12 hours during the first 7 days of life and every 8 hours thereafter) for 10–14 days, or Procaine penicillin G, 50,000 units/kg IM daily in a single dose for 10–14 days.

If more than 1 day of therapy is missed, the entire course should be restarted. An infant whose complete evaluation was normal and whose mother was (a) treated for syphilis during pregnancy with erythromycin, or (b) treated for syphilis less than 1 month before delivery, or (c) treated with an appropriate regimen before or during pregnancy but did not yet have an adequate serologic response should be treated with benzathine penicillin G, 50,000 units/kg IM in a single dose. In some

---

**In the immediate newborn period, interpretation of CSF test results may be difficult; normal values vary with gestational age and are higher in preterm infants. Other causes of elevated values also should be considered when an infant is being evaluated for congenital syphilis. Though values as high as 25 white blood cells (WBC)/mm³ and 150 mg protein/dL occur among normal neonates, some experts recommend that lower values (5 WBC/mm³ and 40 mg/dL) be considered the upper limits of normal. The infant should be treated if test results cannot exclude infection.

***The absence of a fourfold greater titer for an infant cannot be used as evidence against congenital syphilis.

cases, infants with a normal complete evaluation for whom follow-up can be assured can be followed closely without treatment.

Treatment of Older Infants and Children with Congenital Syphilis

After the newborn period, children diagnosed with syphilis should have a CSF examination to exclude neurosyphilis and records should be reviewed to assess whether the child has congenital or acquired syphilis (see Primary and Secondary Syphilis and Latent Syphilis). Any child who is thought to have congenital syphilis (or who has neurologic involvement) should be treated with aqueous crystalline penicillin G, 200,000–300,000 units/kg/day IV or IM (administered as 50,000 units/kg every 4–6 hours) for 10–14 days.

FOLLOW-UP

A seroreactive infant (or an infant whose mother was seroreactive at delivery) who is not treated for congenital syphilis during the perinatal period should receive careful follow-up examinations at 1 month and at 2, 3, 6, and 12 months after therapy. Nontreponemal antibody titers should decline by 3 months of age and should be nonreactive by 6 months of age if the infant was not infected and the titers were the result of passive transfer of antibody from the mother. If these titers are found to be stable or increasing, the child should be re-evaluated, including CSF examination, and fully treated. Passively transferred treponemal antibodies may be present for as long as 1 year. If they are present greater than 1 year, the infant should be re-evaluated and treated for congenital syphilis.

Treated infants also should be followed every 2–3 months to assure that nontreponemal antibody titers decline; these infants should have become nonreactive by 6 months of age (response may be slower for infants treated after the neonatal period). Treponemal tests should not be used to evaluate response to treatment because test results can remain positive despite effective therapy if the child was infected. Infants with CSF pleocytosis should undergo CSF examination every 6 months, or until the cell count is normal. If the cell count is still abnormal after 2 years, or if a downward trend is not present at each examination, the child should be re-treated. The VDRL-CSF also should be checked at 6 months; if still reactive, the infant should be re-treated.

Follow-up of children treated for congenital syphilis after the newborn period should be the same as that prescribed for congenital syphilis among neonates.

SPECIAL CONSIDERATIONS

Penicillin allergy

Children who require treatment for syphilis after the newborn period, but who have a history of penicillin allergy, should be treated with penicillin after desensitization, if necessary. Skin testing may be helpful in some patients and settings (see Management of the Patient With a History of Penicillin Allergy).

HIV infection

Mothers of infants with congenital syphilis should be tested for HIV. Infants born to mothers who have HIV infection should be referred for evaluation and appropriate follow-up.

No data exist to suggest that infants with congenital syphilis whose mothers are coinfected with HIV require different evaluation, therapy, or follow-up for syphilis than is recommended for all infants.

Management of the Patient With a History of Penicillin Allergy

No proven alternatives to penicillin are available for treating neurosyphilis, congenital syphilis, or syphilis among pregnant women. Penicillin also is recommended for use, whenever possible, with HIV-infected patients. Unfortunately, 3%–10% of the adult population in the United States have experienced urticaria, angioedema, or anaphylaxis (upper airway obstruction, bronchospasm, or hypotension) with penicillin therapy. Re-administration of penicillin can cause severe immediate reactions among these patients. Because anaphylactic reactions to penicillin can be fatal, every effort should be made to avoid administering penicillin to penicillin-allergic patients, unless the anaphylactic sensitivity has been removed by acute desensitization.

However, only approximately 10% of persons who report a history of severe allergic reactions to penicillin are still allergic. With the passage of time after an allergic reaction to penicillin, most persons who have experienced a severe reaction stop expressing penicillin-specific IgE. These persons can be treated safely with penicillin. Many studies have found that skin testing with the major and minor determinants can reliably identify persons at high risk for penicillin reactions. Although these reagents are easily generated and have been available in academic centers for greater than 30 years, currently only penicilloyl-poly-L-lysine (Pre-Pen, the major determinant) and penicillin G are available commercially. Experts estimate that testing with only the major determinant and penicillin G detects 90%–97% of the currently allergic patients. However, because skin testing without the minor determinants would still miss 3%–10% of allergic patients, and serious or fatal reactions can occur among these minor determinant positive patients, experts suggest caution when the full battery of skin test reagents listed in the table is not available.

RECOMMENDATIONS

If the full battery of skin-test reagents is available, including the major and minor determinants (see Penicillin Allergy Skin Testing), patients who report a history of penicillin reaction and are skin-test negative can receive conventional penicillin therapy. Skin-test positive patients should be desensitized.

If the full battery of skin-test reagents, including the minor determinants, is not available, the patient should be skin tested using penicilloyl (the major determinant, Pre-Pen) and penicillin G. Those with positive tests should be desensitized. Some experts believe that persons with negative tests, in that situation, should be regarded as probably allergic and should be desensitized. Others suggest that those with negative skin tests can be test-dosed gradually with oral penicillin in a monitored setting in which treatment for anaphylactic reaction is possible.

PENICILLIN ALLERGY SKIN TESTING

Patients at high risk for anaphylaxis (i.e., a history of penicillin-related anaphylaxis, asthma or other diseases that would make anaphylaxis more dangerous, or therapy with beta-adrenergic blocking agents) should be tested with 100-fold dilutions of the full-strength skin-test reagents before testing with full-strength reagents. In these situations, patients should be tested in a monitored setting in which treatment for an anaphylactic reaction is possible. If possible, the patient should not have taken antihistamines (e.g., chlorpheniramine maleate or terfenadine during the past 24 hours, diphenhydramine HCl or hydroxyzine during the past 4 days, or astemizole during the past 3 weeks).

REAGENTS (ADAPTED FROM BEALL [14])[#]

Major determinant

- Benzylpenicilloyl poly-L-lysine (Pre-Pen [Taylor Pharmacal Company, Decatur, Illinois]) (6 × 10–5M).

[#] Reprinted with permission from G.N. Beall in Annals of Internal Medicine.

Minor determinant precursors[##]
- Benzylpenicillin G (10–2M, 3.3 mg/mL, 6000 U/mL),
- Benzylpenicilloate (10–2M, 3.3 mg/mL),
- Benzylpenilloate (or penicilloyl propylamine) (10–2M, 3.3 mg/mL).

Positive control
- Commercial histamine for epicutaneous skin testing (1 mg/mL).

Negative control
- Diluent used to dissolve other reagents, usually phenol saline.

Procedures
Dilute the antigens 100-fold for preliminary testing if the patient has had a life-threatening reaction, or 10-fold if the patient has had another type of immediate, generalized reaction within the past year.

Epicutaneous (prick) tests. Duplicate drops of skin-test reagent are placed on the volar surface of the forearm. The underlying epidermis is pierced with a 26-gauge needle without drawing blood.

An epicutaneous test is positive if the average wheal diameter after 15 minutes is 4 mm larger than that of negative controls; otherwise, the test is negative. The histamine controls should be positive to assure that results are not falsely negative because of the effect of antihistaminic drugs.

Intradermal test. If epicutaneous tests are negative, duplicate 0.02 mL intradermal injections of negative control and antigen solutions are made into the volar surface of the forearm using a 26- or 27-gauge needle on a syringe. The crossed diameters of the wheals induced by the injections should be recorded.

An intradermal test is positive if the average wheal diameter 15 minutes after injection is 2 mm or larger than the initial wheal size and also is at least 2 mm larger than the negative controls. Otherwise, the tests are negative.

DESENSITIZATION
Patients who have a positive skin test to one of the penicillin determinants can be desensitized. This is a straightforward, relatively safe procedure that can be done orally or IV. Although the two approaches have not been compared, oral desensitization is thought to be safer, simpler, and easier. Patients should be desensitized in a hospital setting because serious IgE-mediated allergic reactions, although unlikely, can occur. Desensitization can usually be completed in about 4 hours, after which the first dose of penicillin is given Table 1 (see original publication). STD programs should have a referral center where patients with positive skin tests can be desensitized. After desensitization, patients must be maintained on penicillin continuously for the duration of the course of therapy.

DISEASES CHARACTERIZED BY URETHRITIS AND CERVICITIS
Management of the Patient with Urethritis

Urethritis, or inflammation of the urethra, is caused by an infection characterized by the discharge of mucoid or purulent material and by burning during urination. However, asymptomatic infections are com-

---

[##] Aged penicillin is not an adequate source of minor determinants. Penicillin G should be freshly prepared or should come from a fresh-frozen source.

mon. The two bacterial agents primarily responsible for urethritis among men are N. gonorrhoeae and C. trachomatis. Testing to determine the specific diagnosis is recommended because both of these infections are reportable to state health departments and because with a specific diagnosis, treatment compliance may be better and the likelihood of partner notification may be improved. If diagnostic tools (e.g., Gram stain and microscope) are unavailable, health-care providers should treat patients for both infections. The added expense of treating a person with nongonococcal urethritis (NGU) for both infections also should encourage the health-care provider to make a specific diagnosis. (See Nongonococcal Urethritis, Chlamydial Infections, and Gonococcal Infections.)

Nongonococcal Urethritis

NGU, or inflammation of the urethra not caused by gonococcal infection, is characterized by a mucoid or purulent urethral discharge. In the presence or absence of a discharge, NGU may be diagnosed by greater than or equal to 5 polymorphonuclear leukocytes per oil immersion field on a smear of an intraurethral swab specimen. Increasingly, the leukocyte esterase test (LET) is being used to screen urine from asymptomatic males for evidence of urethritis (either gonococcal or nongonococcal). The diagnosis of urethritis among males tested with LET .should be confirmed with a Gram-stained smear of a urethral swab specimen. C. trachomatis is the most frequent cause of NGU (23%–55% of cases); however, prevalence varies among age groups, with lower prevalence found among older men. Ureaplasma urealyticum causes 20%–40% of cases, and Trichomonas vaginalis 2%–5%. HSV is occasionally responsible for cases of NGU. The etiology of the remaining cases of NGU is unknown.

Complications of NGU among men infected with C. trachomatis include epididymitis and Reiter's syndrome. Female sex partners of men who have NGU are at risk for chlamydial infection and associated complications.

Recommended Regimen

Doxycycline 100 mg orally 2 times a day for 7 days.###

Alternative Regimens

Erythromycin base 500 mg orally 4 times a day for 7 days or Erythromycin ethylsuccinate 800 mg orally 4 times a day for 7 days.

If a patient cannot tolerate high-dose erythromycin schedules, one of the following regimens may be used: Erythromycin base 250 mg orally

---

Azithromycin 1 g in a single dose, according to manufacturer's data, is equivalent to doxycycline. However, this study has not been published in a peer-reviewed journal. For a discussion comparing azithromycin and doxycycline, refer to Chlamydial Infections.

4 times a day for 14 days or Erythromycin ethylsuccinate 400 mg orally 4 times a day for 14 days.

Treatment with the recommended regimen has been demonstrated in most cases to result in alleviation of symptoms and in microbiologic cure of infection. If the etiologic organism is susceptible to the antimicrobial agent used, sequelae specific to that organism will be prevented, as will further transmission; this is especially important for cases of NGU caused by C. trachomatis.

Follow-Up

Patients should be instructed to return for evaluation if symptoms persist or recur after completion of therapy. Patients with persistent or recurrent urethritis should be retreated with the initial regimen if they failed to comply with the treatment regimen or if they were re-exposed to an untreated sex partner. Otherwise, a wet mount examination and culture of an intraurethral swab specimen for T. vaginalis should be performed; if negative, the patient should be retreated with an alternative regimen extended to 14 days (e.g., erythromycin base 500 mg orally 4 times a day for 14 days). The use of alternative regimens ensures treatment of possible tetracycline-resistant U. urealyticum.

Effective regimens have not been identified for treating patients who experience persistent symptoms or frequent recurrences following treatment with doxycycline and erythromycin. Urologic examinations do not usually reveal a specific etiology. Such patients should be assured that, although they have persistent or frequently recurring urethritis, the condition is not known to cause complications among them or their sex partners and is not known to be sexually transmitted. However, men exposed to a new sex partner should be re-evaluated. Symptoms alone, without documentation of signs or laboratory evidence of urethral inflammation, are not a sufficient basis for re-treatment.

Management of Sex Partners

Patients should be instructed to refer sex partners for evaluation and treatment. Since exposure intervals have received limited evaluation, the following recommendations are somewhat arbitrary. Sex partners of symptomatic patients should be evaluated and treated if their last sexual contact with the index patient was within 30 days of onset of symptoms. If the index patient is asymptomatic, sex partners whose last sexual contact with the index patient was within 60 days of diagnosis should be evaluated and treated. If the patient's last sexual intercourse preceded the time intervals previously described, the most recent sex partner should be treated. A specific diagnosis may facilitate partner referral and partner cooperation. Therefore, testing for both gonorrhea and chlamydia is encouraged.

Patients should be instructed to abstain from sexual intercourse until patient and partners are cured. In the absence of microbiologic test-of-cure, this means when therapy is completed and patient and partners are without symptoms or signs.

Special Considerations

HIV INFECTION

Persons with HIV infection and NGU should receive the same treatment as patients without HIV infection.

Management of the Patient With Mucopurulent Cervicitis

Mucopurulent cervicitis (MPC) is characterized by a yellow endocervical exudate visible in the endocervical canal or in an endocervical swab specimen. Some experts also make the diagnosis on the basis of an increased number of polymorphonuclear leukocytes on cervical Gram stain. The condition is asymptomatic among many women, but some may experience an abnormal vaginal discharge and abnormal vaginal bleeding (e.g., following intercourse). The condition can be caused by C. trachomatis or N. gonorrhoeae, although in most cases neither organism can be isolated. Patients with MPC should have cervical specimens tested for C. trachomatis and cultured for N. gonorrhoeae. MPC is not a sensitive predictor of infection; however, most women with C. trachomatis or N. gonorrhoeae do not have MPC.

Treatment

The results of tests for C. trachomatis or N. gonorrhoeae should determine the need for treatment, unless the likelihood of infection with either organism is high or unless the patient is unlikely to return for treatment. Treatment for MPC should include the following:

- Treatment for gonorrhea and chlamydia in patient populations with high prevalence of both infections, such as patients seen at many STD clinics.
- Treatment for chlamydia only, if the prevalence of N. gonorrhoeae is low but the likelihood of chlamydia is substantial.
- Await test results if the prevalence of both infections are low and if compliance with a recommendation for a return visit is likely.

Follow-Up

Follow-up should be as recommended for the infections for which the woman is being treated.

Management of Sex Partners

Management of sex partners of women with MPC should be appropriate for the STD (C. trachomatis or N. gonorrhoeae) identified. Partners should be notified, examined, and treated on the basis of test results. However, partners of patients who are treated presumptively should receive the same treatment as the index patient.

Special Considerations

HIV INFECTION

Persons with HIV infection and MPC should receive the same treatment as patients without HIV infection.

Chlamydial Infections

Chlamydial genital infection is common among adolescents and young adults in the United States. Asymptomatic infection is common among both men and women. Testing sexually active adolescent girls for chlamydial infection should be routine during gynecologic examination, even if symptoms are not present. Screening of young adult women 20–24 years of age also is suggested, particularly for those who do not consistently use barrier contraceptives and who have new or multiple partners. Periodic surveys of chlamydial prevalence among these groups should be conducted to confirm the validity of using these recommendations in specific clinical settings.

Chlamydial Infections Among Adolescents and Adults

The following recommended treatment regimens or the alternative regimens relieve symptoms and cure infection. Among women, several important sequelae may result from C. trachomatis infection, the most serious among them being PID, ectopic pregnancy, and infertility. Some women with apparently uncomplicated cervical infection already have subclinical upper reproductive tract infection. Treatment of cervical infection is believed to reduce the likelihood of sequelae, although few studies have demonstrated that antimicrobial therapy reduces the risk of subsequent ascending infections or decreases the incidence of long-term complications of tubal infertility and ectopic pregnancy.

Treatment of infected patients prevents transmission to sex partners, and for infected pregnant women may prevent transmission of C. trachomatis to infants during birth. Treatment of sex partners will help to prevent re-infection of the index patient and infection of other partners.

Because of the high prevalence of coinfection with C. trachomatis among patients with gonococcal infection, presumptive treatment for chlamydia of patients being treated for gonorrhea is appropriate, particularly if no diagnostic test for C. trachomatis infection will be performed (see Gonococcal Infections).

Recommended Regimens

Doxycycline 100 mg orally 2 times a day for 7 days, or Azithromycin 1 g orally in a single dose.

Alternative Regimens

Ofloxacin 300 mg orally 2 times a day for 7 days or Erythromycin base 500 mg orally 4 times a day for 7 days or Erythromycin ethylsuccinate 800 mg orally 4 times a day for 7 days or Sulfisoxazole 500 mg orally 4 times a day for 10 days (inferior efficacy to other regimens).

Doxycycline and azithromycin appear similar in efficacy and toxicity; however, the safety and efficacy of azithromycin for persons less than or equal to 15 years of age have not been established. Doxycycline has a longer history of extensive use, safety, efficacy, and the advantage of low cost. Azithromycin has the advantage of single-dose administration. Ofloxacin is similar in efficacy to doxycycline and azithromycin, but is more expensive than doxycycline, cannot be used during pregnancy or with persons less than or equal to 17 years of age, and offers no advantage in dosing. Ofloxacin is the only quinolone with proven efficacy against chlamydial infection. Sulfisoxazole is the least desirable treatment because of inferior efficacy.

Follow-Up

Patients do not need to be retested for chlamydia after completing treatment with doxycycline or azithromycin unless symptoms persist or re-infection is suspected.

Retesting may be considered 3 weeks after completion of treatment with erythromycin, sulfisoxazole, or amoxicillin. This is usually unnecessary if the patient was treated with doxycycline, azithromycin, or ofloxacin. The validity of chlamydial culture testing performed at less than 3 weeks following completion of therapy among patients failing therapy has not been established. False-negative results may occur because of small numbers of chlamydial organisms. In addition, nonculture tests conducted at less than 3 weeks following completion of therapy for patients successfully treated may sometimes be false-positive because of the continued excretion of dead organisms.

Some studies have demonstrated high rates of infection among women retested several months following treatment, presumably because of reinfection. Rescreening women several months following treatment may be an effective strategy for detecting further morbidity in some populations.

Management of Sex Partners

Patients should be instructed to refer their sex partners for evaluation and treatment. Because exposure intervals have received limited evaluation, the following recommendations are somewhat arbitrary. Sex partners of symptomatic patients with C. trachomatis should be evaluated and treated for chlamydia if their last sexual contact with the index patient was within 30 days of onset of the index patient's symptoms. If the index patient is asymptomatic, sex partners whose last sexual contact with the index patient was within 60 days of diagnosis should be evaluated and treated. Healthcare providers should treat the last sex partner even if last sexual intercourse took place before the foregoing time intervals.

Patients should be instructed to avoid sex until they and their partners are cured. In the absence of microbiologic test-of-cure, this means until therapy is completed and patient and partner(s) are without symptoms.

Special Considerations

PREGNANCY

Doxycycline and ofloxacin are contraindicated for pregnant women, and sulfisoxazole is contraindicated for women during pregnancy near-term and for women who are nursing. The safety and efficacy of azithromycin among pregnant and lactating women have not been established. Repeat testing, preferably by culture, after completing therapy with the following regimens is recommended because there are few data regarding the effectiveness of these regimens, and the frequent gastrointestinal side effects of erythromycin may discourage a patient from complying with the prescribed treatment.

Recommended regimen for pregnant women

Erythromycin base 500 mg orally 4 times a day for 7 days.

Alternative regimens for pregnant women

Erythromycin base 250 mg orally 4 times a day for 14 days or Erythromycin ethylsuccinate 800 mg orally 4 times a day for 7 days or Erythromycin ethylsuccinate 400 mg orally 4 times a day for 14 days or if erythromycin cannot be tolerated:

Amoxicillin 500 mg orally 3 times a day for 7–10 days.

NOTE: Erythromycin estolate is contraindicated during pregnancy because of drug-related hepatotoxicity. Few data exist concerning the efficacy of amoxicillin.

HIV INFECTION

Persons with HIV infection and chlamydial infection should receive the same treatment as patients without HIV infection.

Chlamydial Infections Among Infants

Prenatal screening of pregnant women can prevent chlamydial infection among neonates. Pregnant women less than 25 years of age and those with new or multiple sex partners should, in particular, be targeted for screening. Periodic surveys of chlamydial prevalence can be conducted to confirm the validity of using these recommendations in specific clinical settings.

C. trachomatis infection of neonates results from perinatal exposure to the mother's infected cervix. The prevalence of C. trachomatis infection generally exceeds 5% among pregnant women, regardless of race/ethnicity or socioeconomic status. Neonatal ocular prophylaxis with silver nitrate solution or antibiotic ointments is ineffective in preventing perinatal transmission of chlamydial infection from mother to infant. However, ocular prophylaxis with those agents does prevent gonococcal ophthalmia and should be continued for that reason (see Prevention of Ophthalmia Neonatorum).

Initial C. trachomatis perinatal infection involves mucous membranes of the eye, oropharynx, urogenital tract, and rectum. C. trachomatis infection among neonates can most often be recognized because of conjunctivitis developing 5–12 days after birth. Chlamydia is the most frequent identifiable infectious cause of ophthalmia neonatorum. C. trachomatis also is a common cause of subacute, afebrile pneumonia with onset from 1 to 3 months of age. Asymptomatic infections of the oropharynx, genital tract, and rectum among neonates also occur.

Ophthalmia Neonatorum Caused by C. trachomatis

A chlamydial etiology should be considered for all infants with conjunctivitis through 30 days of age.

Diagnostic considerations. Sensitive and specific methods to diagnose chlamydial ophthalmia for the neonate include isolation by tissue culture and nonculture tests, direct fluorescent antibody tests, and immunoassays. Giemsa-stained smears are specific for C. trachomatis, but are not sensitive. Specimens must contain conjunctival cells, not exudate alone. Specimens for culture isolation and nonculture tests should be obtained from the everted eyelid using a dacron-tipped swab or the swab specified by the manufacturer's test kit. A specific diagnosis of C. trachomatis infection confirms the need for chlamydial treatment not only for the neonate, but also for the mother and her sex partner(s). Ocular exudate from infants being evaluated for chlamydial conjunctivitis should also be tested for N. gonorrhoeae.

Recommended Regimen

Erythromycin 50 mg/kg/day orally divided into 4 doses for 10–14 days.

Topical antibiotic therapy alone is inadequate for treatment of chlamydial infection and is unnecessary when systemic treatment is undertaken.

Follow-Up

The possibility of chlamydial pneumonia should be considered. The efficacy of erythromycin treatment is approximately 80%; a second course of therapy may be required. Follow-up of infants to determine resolution is recommended.

Management of Mothers and Their Sex Partners

The mothers of infants who have chlamydial infection and the mother's sex partners should be evaluated and treated following the treatment recommendations for adults with chlamydial infections (see Chlamydial Infections Among Adolescents and Adults).

Infant Pneumonia Caused by C. trachomatis

Characteristic signs of chlamydial pneumonia among infants include a repetitive staccato cough with tachypnea, and hyperinflation and bilateral diffuse infiltrates on a chest roentgenogram. Wheezing is rare, and infants are typically afebrile. Peripheral eosinophilia, documented in a complete blood count, is sometimes observed among infants with chlamydial pneumonia. Because variation from this clinical presentation is common, initial treatment and diagnostic tests should encompass C. trachomatis for all infants 1–3 months of age who have possible pneumonia.

Diagnostic Considerations

Specimens should be collected from the nasopharynx for chlamydial testing. Tissue culture remains the definitive standard for chlamydial pneumonia; nonculture tests can be used with the knowledge that nonculture tests of nasopharyngeal specimens produce lower sensitivity and specificity than nonculture tests of ocular specimens. Tracheal aspirates and lung biopsy specimens, if collected, should be tested for C. trachomatis.

The microimmunofluorescence test for C. trachomatis antibody is useful but not widely available. An acute IgM antibody titer greater than or equal to 1:32 is strongly suggestive of C. trachomatis pneumonia.

Because of the delay in obtaining test results for chlamydia, inclusion of an agent active against C. trachomatis in the antibiotic regimen must frequently be decided on the basis of the clinical and radiologic findings. Conducting tests for chlamydial infection is worthwhile, not only to assist in the management of an infant's illness, but also to determine the need for treatment of the mother and her sex partners.

Recommended Regimen

Erythromycin 50 mg/kg/day orally divided into 4 doses for 10–14 days.

FOLLOW-UP

The effectiveness of erythromycin treatment is approximately 80%; a second course of therapy may be required. Follow-up of infants is recommended to determine that the pneumonia has resolved. Some infants with chlamydial pneumonia have had abnormal pulmonary function tests later in childhood.

MANAGEMENT OF MOTHERS AND THEIR SEX PARTNERS

Mothers of infants who have chlamydial infection and the mother's sex partners should be evaluated and treated according to the recommended treatment of adults with chlamydial infections (see Chlamydial Infections Among Adolescents and Adults).

Infants Born to Mothers Who Have Chlamydial Infection

Infants born to mothers who have untreated chlamydia are at high risk for infection and should be evaluated and treated as for infants with ophthalmia neonatorum caused by C. trachomatis.

Chlamydial Infections Among Children

Sexual abuse must be considered a cause of chlamydial infection among preadolescent children, although perinatally transmitted C. trachomatis infection of the nasopharynx, urogenital tract, and rectum may persist beyond 1 year (see Sexual Assault or Abuse of Children). Because of the potential for a criminal investigation and legal proceedings for sexual abuse, diagnosis of C. trachomatis among preadolescent children requires the high specificity provided by isolation in cell culture. The cultures should be confirmed by microscopic identification of the characteristic intracytoplasmic inclusions, preferably by fluorescein-conjugated monoclonal antibodies specific for C. trachomatis.

Diagnostic Considerations

Nonculture chlamydia tests should not be used because of the possibility of false-positive test results. With respiratory tract specimens, false-positive test results can occur because of cross-reaction of test reagents with Chlamydia pneumoniae; with genital and anal specimens, false-positive test results occur because of cross-reaction with fecal flora.

Recommended Regimen

Children who weigh less than 45 kg. Erythromycin 50 mg/kg/day divided into four doses for 10–14 days.

NOTE: The effectiveness of erythromycin treatment is approximately 80%; a second course of therapy may be required.

Children who weigh greater than or equal to 45 kg but who are less than 8 years of age. Use the same treatment regimens for these children as the adult regimens of erythromycin (see Chlamydial Infections Among Adolescents and Adults).

Children greater than or equal to 8 years of age. Use the same treatment regimens for these children as the adult regimens of doxycycline or tetracycline (see Chlamydial Infections Among Adolescents and

Adults). Adult regimens of azithromycin also may be considered for adolescents.

OTHER MANAGEMENT CONSIDERATIONS

See Sexual Assault or Abuse of Children.

FOLLOW-UP

Follow-up cultures are necessary to ensure that treatment has been effective.

Gonococcal Infections

Gonococcal Infections Among Adolescents and Adults

An estimated 1 million new infections with N. gonorrhoeae occur in the United States each year. Most infections among men produce symptoms that cause the person to seek curative treatment soon enough to prevent serious sequelae—but not soon enough to prevent transmission to others. Many infections among women do not produce recognizable symptoms until complications such as PID have occurred. PID, whether symptomatic or asymptomatic, can cause tubal scarring leading to infertility or ectopic pregnancy. Because gonococcal infections among women are often asymptomatic, a primary measure for controlling gonorrhea in the United States has been the screening of high-risk women.

Uncomplicated Gonococcal Infections

Recommended Regimens

Ceftriaxone 125 mg IM in a single dose or Cefixime 400 mg orally in a single dose or Ciprofloxacin 500 mg orally in a single dose or Ofloxacin 400 mg orally in a single dose
PLUS
A regimen effective against possible coinfection with C. trachomatis, such as doxycycline 100 mg orally 2 times a day for 7 days.

Many antibiotics are safe and effective for treating gonorrhea, eradicating N. gonorrhoeae, ending the possibility of further transmission, relieving symptoms, and reducing the chances of sequelae.

Selection of a treatment regimen for N. gonorrhoeae infection requires consideration of the anatomic site of infection, resistance of N. gonorrhoeae strains to antimicrobials, the possibility of concurrent infection with C. trachomatis, and the side effects and costs of the various treatment regimens.

Because coinfection with C. trachomatis is common, persons treated for gonorrhea should be treated presumptively with a regimen that is effective against C. trachomatis (see Chlamydial Infections).

Most experts agree that other regimens recommended for the treatment of C. trachomatis infection are also likely to be satisfactory for the treatment of co-infection (see Chlamydial Infections). However, studies have not been conducted to investigate possible interactions between other treatments for N. gonorrhoeae and C. trachomatis, including interactions influencing the effectiveness and side effects of cotreatment.

In clinical trials, these recommended regimens cured greater than 95% of anal and genital infections; any of the regimens may be used for uncomplicated anal or genital infection. Published studies indicate that ceftriaxone 125 mg and ciprofloxacin 500 mg can cure greater than or equal to 90% of pharyngeal infections. If pharyngeal infection is a concern, one of these two regimens should be used.

Ceftriaxone in a single dose of either 125 mg or 250 mg provides sustained, high bactericidal levels in the blood. Extensive clinical experience indicates that both doses are safe and effective for the treatment of uncomplicated gonorrhea at all sites. In the past, the 250 mg dose has been recommended on the supposition that the routine use of a higher dose may forestall the development of resistance. However, on the basis of ceftriaxone's activity against N. gonorrhoeae, its pharmacokinetics, and the results in clinical trials of doses as low as 62.5 mg, the 125 mg dose appears to have a therapeutic reserve at least as large as that of other accepted treatment regimens. No ceftriaxone-resistant strains of N. gonorrhoeae have been reported. The drawbacks of ceftriaxone are that it is expensive, currently unavailable in vials of less than 250 mg, and must be administered by injection. Some health-care providers believe that the discomfort of the injection may be reduced by using 1% lidocaine solution as a diluent. Ceftriaxone also may abort incubating syphilis, a concern when gonorrhea treatment is not accompanied by a 7-day course of doxycycline or erythromycin for the presumptive treatment of chlamydia.

Cefixime has an antimicrobial spectrum similar to that of ceftriaxone, but the 400 mg oral dose does not provide as high nor as sustained a bactericidal level as does 125 mg of ceftriaxone. Cefixime appears to be effective against pharyngeal gonococcal infection, but few patients with pharyngeal infection have been included in studies. No gonococcal strains resistant to cefixime have been reported. The advantage of cefixime is that it can be administered orally. It is not known if the 400 mg dose can cure incubating syphilis.

Ciprofloxacin at a dose of 500 mg provides sustained bactericidal levels in the blood. Clinical trials have demonstrated that both 250 mg and 500 mg doses are safe and effective for the treatment of uncomplicated gonorrhea at all sites. Most clinical experience in the United States has been with the 500 mg dose. Ciprofloxacin can be administered orally and is less expensive than ceftriaxone. No resistance has been reported in the United States, but strains with decreased susceptibility to some quinolones are becoming common in Asia and have been reported in North America. The 500 mg dose is recommended, rather than the 250 mg dose, because of the trend toward decreasing susceptibility to quinolones and because of rare reports of treatment failure. Quinolones are contraindicated for pregnant or nursing women and for persons less than or equal to 17 years of age on the basis of information from animal studies. Quinolones are not active against T. pallidum.

Ofloxacin is active against N. gonorrhoeae, has favorable pharmacokinetics, and the 400 mg dose has been effective for the treatment of uncomplicated anal and genital gonorrhea. In published studies a 400 mg dose cured 22 (88%) of 25 pharyngeal infections.

ALTERNATIVE REGIMENS

- Spectinomycin 2 g IM in a single dose. Spectinomycin has the disadvantages of being injectable, expensive, inactive against T. pallidum, and relatively ineffective against pharyngeal gonorrhea. In addition, resistant strains have been reported in the United States. However, spectinomycin remains useful for the treatment of patients who can tolerate neither cephalosporins nor quinolones.
- Injectable cephalosporin regimens other than ceftriaxone 125 mg that have demonstrated efficacy against uncomplicated anal or genital gonococcal infections include these injectable cephalosporins: ceftizoxime 500 mg IM in a single dose; cefotaxime 500 mg IM in a single dose; cefotetan 1 g IM in a single dose; and cefoxitin 2 g IM in a single dose.

None of these injectable cephalosporins offers any advantage compared with ceftriaxone, and there is less clinical experience with them for the treatment of uncomplicated gonorrhea. Of these four regimens, ceftizoxime 500 mg appears to be the most effective according to cumulative experience in published clinical trials.

- Oral cephalosporin regimens other than cefixime 400 mg include cefuroxime axetil 1 g orally in a single dose and cefpodoxime proxetil 200 mg orally in a single dose. These two regimens have anti-gonococcal activity and pharmacokinetics less favorable than the 400 mg cefixime regimen, and there is less clinical experience with them in the treatment of gonorrhea. They have not been very effective against pharyngeal infections among the few patients studied.
- Quinolone regimens other than ciprofloxacin 500 mg and ofloxacin 400 mg include enoxacin 400 mg orally in a single dose; lomefloxacin 400 mg orally in a single dose; and norfloxacin 800 mg orally in a single dose. They appear to be safe and effective for the treatment of uncomplicated gonorrhea, but none appears to offer any advantage over ciprofloxacin at a dose of 500 mg or ofloxacin at 400 mg.
- Enoxacin and norfloxacin are active against N. gonorrhoeae, have favorable pharmacokinetics, and have been effective in clinical trials, but there is minimal experience with their use in the United States. Lomefloxacin is effective against N. gonorrhoeae and has very favorable pharmacokinetics, but there are few published clinical studies to support its use for the treatment of gonorrhea, and there is little experience with its use in the United States.

Many other antimicrobials are active against N. gonorrhoeae. These guidelines are not intended to be a comprehensive list of all effective treatment regimens.

OTHER MANAGEMENT CONSIDERATIONS

Persons treated for gonorrhea should be screened for syphilis by serology when gonorrhea is first detected. Gonorrhea treatment regimens that include ceftriaxone or a 7-day course of either doxycycline or erythromycin may cure incubating syphilis, but few data relevant to this topic are available.

FOLLOW-UP

Persons who have uncomplicated gonorrhea and who are treated with any of the regimens in these guidelines need not return for a test-of-cure. Those persons with symptoms persisting after treatment should be evaluated by culture for N. gonorrhoeae, and any gonococci isolated should be tested for antimicrobial susceptibility. Infections detected after treatment with one of the recommended regimens more commonly occur because of reinfection rather than treatment failure, indicating a need for improved sex partner referral and patient education. Persistent urethritis, cervicitis, or proctitis also may be caused by C. trachomatis and other organisms.

MANAGEMENT OF SEX PARTNERS

Patients should be instructed to refer sex partners for evaluation and treatment. Sex partners of symptomatic patients who have N. gonorrhoeae infection should be evaluated and treated for N. gonorrhoeae and C. trachomatis infections, if their last sexual contact with the patient was within 30 days of onset of the patient's symptoms. If the index patient is asymptomatic, sex partners whose last sexual contact with the patient was within 60 days of diagnosis should be evaluated and treated. Health-care providers should treat the most recent sex partner, if last sexual intercourse took place before those time periods.

Patients should be instructed to avoid sexual intercourse until patient and partner(s) are cured. In the absence of microbiologic test-of-cure, this means until therapy is completed and patient and partner(s) are without symptoms.

SPECIAL CONSIDERATIONS
Allergy, intolerance, or adverse reactions

Persons who cannot tolerate cephalosporins should, in general, be treated with quinolones. Those who can take neither cephalosporins nor quinolones should be treated with spectinomycin, except for those patients who are suspected or known to have pharyngeal infection. For pharyngeal infections among persons who can tolerate neither a cephalosporin nor quinolones, some studies suggest that trimethoprim/ sulfamethoxazole may be effective at a dose of 720 mg trimethoprim/3,600 mg sulfamethoxazole orally once a day for 5 days.

Pregnancy

Pregnant women should not be treated with quinolones or tetracyclines. Those infected with N. gonorrhoeae should be treated with a recommended or alternate cephalosporin. Women who cannot tolerate a cephalosporin should be administered a single dose of 2 g of spectinomycin IM. Erythromycin is the recommended treatment for presumptive or diagnosed C. trachomatis infection during pregnancy (see Chlamydial Infections).

HIV infection

Persons with HIV infection and gonococcal infection should receive the same treatment as persons not infected with HIV.

Gonococcal Conjunctivitis

Only one North American study of the treatment of gonococcal conjunctivitis among adults has been published in recent years. In that study, 12 of 12 patients responded favorably to a single 1 g IM injection of ceftriaxone. The recommendations that follow reflect the opinions of expert consultants.

Treatment

Recommended regimen. A single, 1 g dose of ceftriaxone should be administered IM, and the infected eye should be lavaged with saline solution once.

As for uncomplicated infections, patients should be instructed to refer sex partner(s) for evaluation and treatment (see Uncomplicated Gonococcal Infections, Management of Sex Partners).

Disseminated Gonococcal Infection

Disseminated gonococcal infection (DGI) results from gonococcal bacteremia, often resulting in petechial or pustular acral skin lesions, asymmetrical arthralgias, tenosynovitis or septic arthritis—and is occasionally complicated by hepatitis and, rarely, by endocarditis or meningitis. Strains of N. gonorrhoeae that cause DGI tend to cause little genital inflammation. These strains have become uncommon in the United States during the past decade.

No North American studies of the treatment of DGI have been published recently. The recommendations that follow reflect the opinions of expert consultants.

Treatment

Hospitalization is recommended for initial therapy, especially for patients who cannot be relied on to comply with treatment, for those for whom the diagnosis is uncertain, and for those who have purulent synovial effusions or other complications. Patients should be examined for clinical evidence of endocarditis and meningitis. Patients treated for DGI should be treated presumptively for concurrent C. trachomatis infection.

Recommended initial regimen: Ceftriaxone 1 g IM or IV every 24 hours.

Alternative initial regimens: Cefotaxime 1 g IV every 8 hours or Ceftizoxime 1 g IV every 8 hours or for persons allergic to lactam drugs: Spectinomycin 2 g IM every 12 hours.

All regimens should be continued for 24–48 hours after improvement begins; then therapy may be switched to one of the following regimens to complete a full week of antimicrobial therapy: Cefixime 400 mg orally 2 times a day or Ciprofloxacin 500 mg orally 2 times a day.

NOTE: Ciprofloxacin is contraindicated for children, adolescents less than or equal to 17 years of age, and pregnant and lactating women.

Gonococcal infection is often asymptomatic in sex partners of patients with DGI. As for uncomplicated infections, patients should be instructed to refer sex partner(s) for evaluation and treatment (see Uncomplicated Gonococcal Infections, Management of Sex Partners).

Gonococcal Meningitis and Endocarditis

Recommended Initial Regimen

1–2 g of ceftriaxone IV every 12 hours.

Therapy for meningitis should be continued for 10–14 days and for endocarditis for at least 4 weeks. Treatment of complicated DGI should be undertaken in consultation with an expert.

MANAGEMENT OF SEX PARTNERS

As for uncomplicated infections, patients should be instructed to refer sex partners for evaluation and treatment (see Uncomplicated Gonococcal Infections, Management of Sex Partners).

Gonococcal Infections Among Infants

Gonococcal infection among neonates usually results from peripartum exposure to infected cervical exudate of the mother. Gonococcal infection among neonates is usually an acute illness beginning 2–5 days after birth. The incidence of N. gonorrhoeae among neonates varies in U.S. communities, depends on the prevalence of infection among pregnant women, on whether pregnant women are screened for gonorrhea, and on whether newborns receive ophthalmia prophylaxis. The prevalence of infection is less than 1% in most prenatal patient populations, but may be higher in some settings.

Of greatest concern are complications of ophthalmia neonatorum and sepsis, including arthritis and meningitis. Less serious manifestations at sites of infection include rhinitis, vaginitis, urethritis, and inflammation at sites of intrauterine fetal monitoring.

Ophthalmia Neonatorum Caused by N. gonorrhoeae

In most patient populations in the United States, C. trachomatis and nonsexually transmitted agents are more common causes of neonatal conjunctivitis than N. gonorrhoeae. However, N. gonorrhoeae is especially important because gonococcal ophthalmia may result in perforation of the globe and in blindness.

Diagnostic Considerations

Infants at high risk for gonococcal ophthalmia in the United States are those who do not receive ophthalmia prophylaxis, whose mothers have had no prenatal care, or whose mothers have a history of STDs or substance abuse. The presence of typical Gram-negative diplococci in a Gram-stained smear of conjunctival exudate suggests a diagnosis of N. gonorrhoeae conjunctivitis. Such patients should be treated presumptively for gonorrhea after obtaining appropriate cultures for N. gonorrhoeae; appropriate chlamydial testing should be done simultaneously. The decision not to treat presumptively for N. gonorrhoeae among patients without evidence of gonococci on a Gram-stained smear of conjunctival exudate, or among patients for whom a Gram-stained smear cannot be performed, must be made on a case-by-case basis after considering the previously described risk factors.

A specimen of conjunctival exudate also should be cultured for isolation of N. gonorrhoeae, since culture is needed for definitive microbiologic identification and for antibiotic susceptibility testing. Such definitive testing is required because of the public health and social consequences for the infant and mother that may result from the diagnosis of gonococcal ophthalmia. Moraxella catarrhalis and other Neisseria species are uncommon causes of neonatal conjunctivitis that can mimic N. gonorrhoeae on Gram-stained smear. To differentiate N. gonorrhoeae from M. catarrhalis and other Neisseria species, the laboratory should be instructed to perform confirmatory tests on any colonies that meet presumptive criteria for N. gonorrhoeae.

Recommended Regimen

Ceftriaxone 25–50 mg/kg IV or IM in a single dose, not to exceed 125 mg.

NOTE: Topical antibiotic therapy alone is inadequate and is unnecessary if systemic treatment is administered.

OTHER MANAGEMENT CONSIDERATIONS

Simultaneous infection with C. trachomatis has been reported and should be considered for patients who do not respond satisfactorily. The mother and infant should be tested for chlamydial infection at the same time that gonorrhea testing is done (see Ophthalmia Neonatorum Caused by C. trachomatis). Ceftriaxone should be administered cautiously among infants with elevated bilirubin levels, especially premature infants.

FOLLOW-UP

Infants should be admitted to the hospital and evaluated for signs of disseminated infection (e.g., sepsis, arthritis, and meningitis). One dose of ceftriaxone is adequate for gonococcal conjunctivitis, but many pediatricians prefer to maintain infants on antibiotics until cultures are negative at 48–72 hours. The decision on duration of therapy should be made with input from experienced physicians.

MANAGEMENT OF MOTHERS AND THEIR SEX PARTNERS

The mothers of infants with gonococcal infection and their sex partners should be evaluated and treated following the recommendations for treatment of gonococcal infections in adults (see Gonococcal Infections Among Adolescents and Adults).

Disseminated Gonococcal Infection Among Infants

Sepsis, arthritis, meningitis, or any combination thereof are rare complications of neonatal gonococcal infection. Gonococcal scalp abscesses also may develop as a result of fetal monitoring. Detection of gonococcal infection among neonates who have sepsis, arthritis, meningitis, or scalp abscesses requires cultures of blood, CSF, and joint aspirate on chocolate agar. Cultures of specimens from the conjunctiva, vagina, oropharynx, and rectum onto gonococcal selective medium are useful to identify sites of primary infection, especially if inflammation is present. Positive Gram-stained smears of exudate, CSF, or joint aspirate provide a presumptive basis for initiating treatment for N. gonorrhoeae. Diagnoses based on positive Gram-stained smears or presumptive isolation by cultures should be confirmed with definitive tests on culture isolates.

Recommended Regimen

Ceftriaxone 25–50 mg/kg/day IV or IM in a single daily dose for 7 days, with a duration of 10–14 days, if meningitis is documented; or Cefotaxime 25 mg/kg IV or IM every 12 hours for 7 days, with a duration of 10–14 days, if meningitis is documented.

Prophylactic Treatment for Infants Whose Mothers Have Gonococcal Infection

Infants born to mothers who have untreated gonorrhea are at high risk for infection.

Recommended regimen in the absence of signs of gonococcal infection. Ceftriaxone 25–50 mg/kg IV or IM, not to exceed 125 mg, in a single dose.

OTHER MANAGEMENT CONSIDERATIONS

If simultaneous infection with C. trachomatis has been reported, mother and infant should be tested for chlamydial infection.

FOLLOW-UP

Follow-up examination is not required.

MANAGEMENT OF MOTHERS AND THEIR SEX PARTNERS

The mothers of infants with gonococcal infection and the mother's sex partners should be evaluated and treated following the recommendations for treatment of gonococcal infections among adults (see Gonococcal Infections).

Gonococcal Infections Among Children

After the neonatal period, sexual abuse is the most common cause of gonococcal infection among preadolescent children (see Sexual Assault or Abuse of Children). Vaginitis is the most common manifestation of gonococcal infection among preadolescent children. PID following vaginal infection appears to be less common than among adults. Among sexually-abused children, anorectal and pharyngeal infections with N. gonorrhoeae are common and are frequently asymptomatic.

Diagnostic Considerations

Because of the potential medical/legal use of the test results for N. gonorrhoeae among children, only standard culture systems for the isolation of N. gonorrhoeae should be used to diagnose N. gonorrhoeae for these children. Nonculture gonococcal tests, including Gram-stained smear, DNA probes, or EIA tests should not be used; none of these tests have been approved by the FDA for use in the oropharynx, rectum, or genital tract of children. Specimens from the vagina, urethra, pharynx, or rectum should be streaked onto selective media for isolation of N. gonorrhoeae. All presumptive isolates of N. gonorrhoeae should be confirmed by at least two tests that involve different principles, e.g., biochemical, enzyme substrate, or serologic. Isolates should be preserved to permit additional or repeated analysis.

Recommended Regimen for Children

Children who weigh greater than 45 kg.   Children who weigh greater than or equal to 45 kg should be administered the same treatment regimens as those recommended for adults (see Gonococcal Infections).

Children who weigh less than 45 kg.   The following treatment recommendations are for children with uncomplicated gonococcal vulvovaginitis, cervicitis, urethritis, pharyngitis, or proctitis.

Ceftriaxone 125 mg IM in a single dose.

Alternative regimen: Spectinomycin 40 mg/kg (maximum 2 g) IM in a single dose.

Children who weigh less than 45 kg and who have bacteremia, arthritis, or meningitis.   Recommended regimen: Ceftriaxone 50 mg/kg (maximum 1 g) IM or IV in a single dose daily for 7 days.

NOTE: For meningitis, increase the duration of treatment to 10–14 days and the maximum dose to 2 g.

FOLLOW-UP

Follow-up cultures of specimens from infected sites are necessary to ensure that treatment has been effective.

OTHER MANAGEMENT CONSIDERATIONS

Only parenteral cephalosporins are recommended for use among children. Ceftriaxone is approved for all gonococcal indications among children; cefotaxime is approved for gonococcal ophthalmia only. Oral cephalosporins (cefixime, cefuroxime axetil, cefpodoxime) have not received adequate evaluation in the treatment of gonococcal infections among pediatric patients to recommend their use. The pharmacokinetic activity of these drugs among adults cannot be extrapolated to children.

All children with gonococcal infections should be evaluated for coinfection with syphilis and C. trachomatis. For a discussion of issues regarding sexual assault, refer to Sexual Assault or Abuse of Children.

Ophthalmia Neonatorum Prophylaxis

Instillation of a prophylactic agent into the eyes of all newborn infants is recommended to prevent gonococcal ophthalmia neonatorum and is required by law in most states. Although all the regimens that follow effectively prevent gonococcal eye disease, their efficacy in preventing chlamydial eye disease is not clear. Furthermore, they do not eliminate nasopharyngeal colonization with C. trachomatis. Treatment of gonococcal and chlamydial infections among pregnant women is the best method for preventing neonatal gonococcal and chlamydial disease. However, ocular prophylaxis should continue because it can prevent gonococcal ophthalmia and, in some populations, greater than 10% of pregnant women may receive no prenatal care.

Prophylaxis

Recommended preparations.   Silver nitrate (1%) aqueous solution in a single application or Erythromycin (0.5%) ophthalmic ointment in a single application or Tetracycline ophthalmic ointment (1%) in a single application.

One of the above preparations should be instilled into the eyes of every neonate as soon as possible after delivery. If prophylaxis is delayed (i.e., not administered in the delivery room), hospitals should establish a monitoring system to see that all infants receive prophylaxis. All infants should be administered ocular prophylaxis, whether delivery is vaginal or caesarian. Single-use tubes or ampules are preferable to multiple-use tubes. Bacitracin is not effective.

DISEASES CHARACTERIZED BY VAGINAL DISCHARGE
Management of the Patient with Vaginitis

Vaginitis is characterized by a vaginal discharge (usually) or vulvar itching and irritation; a vaginal odor may be present. The three common diseases characterized by vaginitis include trichomoniasis (caused by T. vaginalis), BV (caused by a replacement of the normal vaginal flora by an overgrowth of anaerobic microorganisms and Gardnerella vaginalis), and candidiasis (usually caused by Candida albicans). MPC caused by C. trachomatis or N. gonorrhoeae may uncommonly cause a vaginal discharge. Although vulvovaginal candidiasis is not usually transmitted sexually, it is included here because it is a common infection among women being evaluated for STDs.

The diagnosis of vaginitis is made by pH and microscopic examination of fresh samples of the discharge. The pH of the vaginal secretions can be determined by narrow-range pH paper for the elevated pH (greater than 4.5) typical of BV or trichomoniasis. One way to examine the discharge is to dilute a sample in 1–2 drops of 0.9% normal saline solution on one slide and 10% potassium hydroxide (KOH) solution on a second slide. An amine odor detected immediately after applying KOH suggests either BV or trichomoniasis. A cover slip is placed on each slide and they are examined under a microscope at low- and high-dry power. The motile T. vaginalis or the clue cells of BV are usually easily identified in the saline specimen. The yeast or pseudohyphae of Candida species are more easily identified in the KOH specimen. The presence of objective signs of vulvar inflammation in the absence of vaginal pathogens, along with a minimal amount of discharge, suggests the possibility of mechanical or chemical irritation of the vulva. Culture for T. vaginalis or Candida species is more sensitive than microscopic examination, but the specificity of culture for Candida species to diagnose vaginitis is less clear. Laboratory testing fails to identify a cause among a substantial minority of women.

Bacterial Vaginosis

BV is a clinical syndrome resulting from replacement of the normal H_2O_2-producing Lactobacillus spp in the vagina with high concentrations of anaerobic bacteria (e.g., Bacteroides spp, Mobiluncus spp), G. vaginalis, and Mycoplasma hominis. This condition is the most prevalent cause of vaginal discharge or malodor. However, half the women who meet clinical criteria for BV have no symptoms. The cause of the microbial alteration is not fully understood. Although BV is associated with sexual activity in that women who have never been sexually active are rarely affected and acquisition of BV is associated with having multiple sex partners, BV is not considered exclusively an STD. Treatment of the male sex partner has not been found beneficial in preventing the recurrence of BV.

Diagnostic Considerations

BV may be diagnosed by the use of clinical or Gram stain criteria. Clinical criteria require three of the following symptoms or signs:

- A homogeneous, white, noninflammatory discharge that adheres to the vaginal walls;
- The presence of clue cells on microscopic examination;
- pH of vaginal fluid greater than 4.5;
- A fishy odor of vaginal discharge before or after addition of 10% KOH (whiff test).

When Gram stain is used, determining the relative concentration of the bacterial morphotypes characteristic of the altered flora of BV is an acceptable laboratory method for diagnosing BV. Culture of G. vaginalis is not recommended as a diagnostic tool because it is not specific. G. vaginalis can be isolated from vaginal cultures among half of normal women.

Treatment

The principal goal of therapy is to relieve vaginal symptoms and signs. Therefore, only women with symptomatic disease require treatment. Because male sex partners of women with BV are not symptomatic, and because treatment of male partners has not been shown to alter either the clinical course of BV in women during treatment or the relapse/reinfection rate, preventing transmission to men is not a goal of therapy.

Many bacterial flora characterizing BV have been recovered from the endometrium or salpinx of women with PID. BV has been associated with endometritis, PID, or vaginal cuff cellulitis following invasive procedures such as endometrial biopsy, hysterectomy, hysterosalpingography, placement of IUD, caesarian section, or uterine curettage. A randomized controlled trial found that treatment of BV with metronidazole substantially reduced post-abortion PID. Based on these data, it may be reasonable to consider treatment of BV (symptomatic or asymptomatic) before performing surgical abortion procedures. However, more data are needed to consider treatment of asymptomatic patients with BV when performing other invasive procedures.

Recommended Regimen

Metronidazole 500 mg orally 2 times a day for 7 days. NOTE: Patients should be advised to avoid using alcohol during treatment with metronidazole and for 24 hours thereafter.

Alternative Regimens

Metronidazole 2 g orally in a single dose.

The following alternative regimens have been effective in clinical trials, although experience with these regimens is limited.

Clindamycin cream, 2%, one full applicator (5 g) intravaginally at bedtime for 7 days; or Metronidazole gel, 0.75%, one full applicator (5 g) intravaginally, 2 times a day for 5 days; or Clindamycin 300 mg orally 2 times a day for 7 days.

Oral metronidazole has been shown in numerous studies to be efficacious for the treatment of BV, resulting in relief of symptoms and improvement in clinical course and flora disturbances. Based on efficacy data from four randomized-controlled trials, the overall cure rates are 95% for the 7-day regimen and 84% for the 2 g single-dose regimen.

Some health-care providers remain concerned about the possibility of metronidazole mutagenicity, which has been suggested by experiments on animals using extremely high and prolonged doses. However, there is no evidence for mutagenicity in humans. Some health-care providers prefer the intravaginal route because of lack of systemic side effects such as mild-to-moderate gastrointestinal upset and unpleasant taste (mean peak serum concentrations of metronidazole following intravaginal administration are less than 2% those of standard 500 mg oral doses and mean bioavailability of clindamycin cream is about 4%).

Follow-Up

Follow-up visits are not necessary if symptoms resolve. Recurrence of BV is common. The alternative treatment regimens suitable for BV treatment may be used for treatment of recurrent disease. No long-term maintenance regimen with any therapeutic agent is currently available.

Management of Sex Partners

Treatment of sex partners in clinical trials has not influenced the woman's response to therapy, nor has it influenced the relapse or recurrence rate. Therefore, routine treatment of sex partners is not recommended.

Special Considerations

Allergy or Intolerance to the Recommended Therapy Clindamycin cream is preferred in case of allergy or intolerance to metronidazole. Metronidazole gel can be considered for patients who do not tolerate systemic metronidazole, but patients allergic to oral metronidazole should not be administered metronidazole vaginally.

PREGNANCY

Because metronidazole is contraindicated during the first trimester of pregnancy, clindamycin vaginal cream is the preferred treatment for BV during the first trimester of pregnancy (clindamycin cream is recommended instead of oral clindamycin because of the general desire to limit the exposure of the fetus to medication). During the second and third trimesters of pregnancy, oral metronidazole can be used, although the vaginal metronidazole gel or clindamycin cream may be preferable.

BV has been associated with adverse outcomes of pregnancy (e.g., premature rupture of the membranes, preterm labor, preterm delivery), and the organisms found in increased concentration in BV are also commonly present in postpartum or post-caesarean endometritis. Whether treatment of BV among pregnant women would reduce the risk of adverse pregnancy outcomes is unknown; randomized controlled trials have not been conducted.

HIV INFECTION

Persons with HIV and BV should receive the same treatment as persons without HIV.

Trichomoniasis

Trichomoniasis is caused by the protozoan T. vaginalis. The majority of men infected with T. vaginalis are asymptomatic, but many women are symptomatic. Among women, T. vaginalis typically causes a diffuse, malodorous, yellow-green discharge with vulvar irritation. There is recent evidence of a possible relationship between vaginal trichomoniasis and adverse pregnancy outcomes, particularly premature rupture of the membranes and preterm delivery.

Recommended Regimen: Metronidazole 2 g orally in a single dose.

Alternative Regimen: Metronidazole 500 mg twice daily for 7 days.

Only metronidazole is available in the United States for the treatment of trichomoniasis. In randomized clinical trials, both of the recommended metronidazole regimens have resulted in cure rates of approximately 95%. Treatment of the patient and sex partner results in relief of symptoms, microbiologic cure, and reduction of transmission. Metronidazole gel has been approved for the treatment of BV but it has not been studied for the treatment of trichomoniasis. Earlier preparations of metronidazole for topical vaginal therapy demonstrated low efficacy against trichomoniasis.

Follow-Up

Follow-up is unnecessary for men and for women who become asymptomatic after treatment.

Infections by strains of T. vaginalis with diminished susceptibility to metronidazole occur. However, most of these organisms respond to higher doses of metronidazole. If failure occurs with either regimen, the patient should be retreated with metronidazole 500 mg 2 times a day for 7 days. If repeated failure occurs, the patient should be treated with a single 2 g dose of metronidazole once daily for 3–5 days.

Patients with culture-documented infection who do not respond to the regimens described in this report and in whom reinfection has been excluded, should be managed in consultation with an expert. Evaluation of such cases should include determination of the susceptibility of T. vaginalis to metronidazole.

Management of Sex Partners

Sex partners should be treated. Patients should be instructed to avoid sex until patient and partner(s) are cured. In the absence of microbiologic test-of-cure, this means when therapy has been completed and patient and partner(s) are without symptoms.

Special Considerations

ALLERGY, INTOLERANCE, OR ADVERSE REACTIONS

Effective alternatives to therapy with metronidazole are not available.

PREGNANCY

The use of metronidazole is contraindicated in the first trimester of pregnancy. Patients may be treated after the first trimester with 2 g of metronidazole in a single dose.

HIV INFECTION

Persons with HIV infection and trichomoniasis should receive the same treatment as persons without HIV.

Vulvovaginal Candidiasis

Vulvovaginal candidiasis (VVC) is caused by C. albicans or, occasionally, by other Candida spp, Torulopsis sp, or other yeasts. An estimated 75% of women will experience at least one episode of VVC during their lifetime, and 40%–45% will experience two or more episodes. A small percentage of women (probably less than 5%) experience recurrent VVC (RVVC). Typical symptoms of VVC include pruritus and vaginal discharge. Other symptoms may include vaginal soreness, vulvar burning, dyspareunia, and external dysuria. None of these symptoms is specific for VVC. VVC usually is not sexually acquired or transmitted.

Diagnostic Considerations

A diagnosis of Candida vaginitis is suggested clinically by pruritus in the vulvar area together with erythema of the vagina or vulva; a white discharge may occur. The diagnosis can be made when a woman has signs and symptoms of vaginitis, and when a wet preparation or Gram stain of vaginal discharge demonstrates yeasts or pseudohyphae, or when a culture or other test yields a positive result for a yeast species. Vaginitis solely because of Candida infection is associated with a normal vaginal pH (less than or equal to 4.5). Use of 10% KOH in wet preparations improves the visualization of yeast and mycelia by disrupting cellular material that may obscure the yeast or pseudohyphae. Identifying Candida in the absence of symptoms should not lead to treatment, because approximately 10%–20% of women normally harbor Candida spp and other yeasts in the vagina. VVC may be present concurrently with STDs.

Treatment

Topical formulations provide effective treatment for VVC. The topically applied azole drugs are more effective than nystatin. Treatment with azoles results in relief of symptoms and negative cultures among 80%–90% of patients after therapy is completed.

Recommended Regimens

The following intravaginal formulations are recommended for the treatment of VVC. Butoconazole 2% cream 5 g intravaginally for 3 days@; or Clotrimazole 1% cream 5 g intravaginally for 7–14 days@@; or Clotrimazole 100 mg vaginal tablet for 7 days@@; or Clotrimazole 100 mg vaginal tablet, two tablets for 3 days; or Clotrimazole 500 mg vaginal tablet, one tablet single application; or Miconazole 2% cream 5 g intravaginally for 7 days@@@; or Miconazole 200 mg vaginal suppository, one suppository for 3 days@; or Miconazole 100 mg vaginal suppository, one suppository for 7 days@@@; or Tioconazole 6.5% ointment 5 g intravaginally in a single application@; or Terconazole 0.4% cream 5 g intravaginally for 7 days; or Terconazole 0.8% cream 5 g intravaginally for 3 days; or Terconazole 80 mg suppository, 1 suppository for 3 days.@

Although information is not conclusive, single-dose treatments should probably be reserved for cases of uncomplicated mild-to-moderate VVC. Multi-day regimens (3- and 7-day) are the preferred treatment for severe or complicated VVC.

Preparations for intravaginal administration of both miconazole and clotrimazole are now available over-the-counter (OTC [nonprescription]), and women with VVC can choose one of those preparations. The duration for treatment with either preparation is 7 days. Self-medication with OTC preparations should be advised only for women who have been diagnosed previously with VVC and who experience a recurrence of the same symptoms. Any woman whose symptoms persist after using an OTC preparation or who experiences a recurrence of symptoms within 2 months should seek medical care.

ALTERNATIVE REGIMENS

Several trials have demonstrated that oral azole agents such as fluconazole, ketoconazole, and itraconazole may be as effective as topical agents. The optimum dose and duration of oral therapy have not been established, but a range of 1–5 days of treatment, depending on the agent, has been effective in clinical trials. The ease of administration of oral agents is an advantage over topical therapies. However, the potential for toxicity associated with using a systemic drug, particularly ketoconazole, must be considered. No oral agent is approved currently by the FDA for the treatment of acute VVC.

Follow-Up

Patients should be instructed to return for follow-up visits only if symptoms persist or recur. Women who experience three or more episodes of VVC per year should be evaluated for predisposing conditions (see Recurrent Vulvovaginal Candidiasis).

@ These creams and suppositories are oil-based and may weaken latex condoms and diaphragms. Refer to product labeling for further information.

@@ Over-the-counter (OTC) preparations.

@@@ The 1988 Bethesda System for Reporting Cervical/Vaginal Cytologic Diagnoses introduced the new terms low-grade squamous intraepithelial lesion (SIL) and high-grade SIL. Low-grade SIL encompasses cellular changes associated with HPV and mild dysplasia/cervical intraepithelial neoplasia 1 (CIN 1). High grade SIL includes moderate dysplasia/CIN 2, severe dysplasia/CIN 3, and carcinoma in situ (CIS)/(CIN 3 (16)).

Management of Sex Partners

VVC is not acquired through sexual intercourse; treatment of sex partners has not been demonstrated to reduce the frequency of recurrences. Therefore, routine notification or treatment of sex partners is not warranted. A minority of male sex partners may have balanitis, which is characterized by erythematous areas on the glans in conjunction with pruritus or irritation. These partners may benefit from treatment with topical antifungal agents to relieve symptoms.

Special Considerations

ALLERGY OR INTOLERANCE TO THE RECOMMENDED THERAPY

Topical agents are usually free of systemic side effects, although local burning or irritation may occur. Oral agents occasionally cause nausea, abdominal pain, and headaches. Therapy with the oral azoles has been associated rarely with abnormal elevations of liver enzymes. Hepatotoxicity secondary to ketoconazole therapy has been estimated to appear in 1:10,000 to 1:15,000 exposed persons. Clinically important interactions may occur when these oral agents are administered with other drugs, including terfenadine, rifampin, astemizole, phenytoin, cyclosporin A, coumarin-like agents, or oral hypoglycemic agents.

PREGNANCY

VVC is common during pregnancy. Only topical azole therapies should be used for the treatment of pregnant women. The most effective treatments that have been studied for pregnant women are clotrimazole, miconazole, butoconazole, and terconazole. Many experts recommend 7 days of therapy during pregnancy.

HIV INFECTION

Acute VVC occurs frequently among women with HIV infection and may be more severe for these women than for other women. However, insufficient information exists to determine the optimal management of VVC in HIV-infected women. Until such information becomes available, women with HIV infection and acute VVC should be treated following the same regimens as for women without HIV infection.

Recurrent Vulvovaginal Candidiasis

RVVC, usually defined as three or more episodes of symptomatic VVC annually, affects a small proportion of women (probably less than 5%). The natural history and pathogenesis of RVVC are poorly understood. Risk factors for RVVC include diabetes mellitus, immunosuppression, broad spectrum antibiotic use, corticosteroid use, and HIV infection, although the majority of women with RVVC have no apparent predisposing conditions. Clinical trials addressing the management of RVVC have involved continuing therapy between episodes.

Treatment

The optimal treatment for RVVC has not been established. Ketoconazole 100 mg orally, once daily for up to 6 months reduces the frequency of episodes of RVVC. Current studies are evaluating weekly intravaginal administration of clotrimazole, as well as oral therapy with itraconazole and fluconazole, in the treatment of RVVC. All cases of RVVC should be confirmed by culture before maintenance therapy is initiated.

Although patients with RVVC should be evaluated for predisposing conditions, routinely performing HIV testing for women with RVVC who do not have HIV risk factors is unwarranted.

Follow-Up

Patients who are receiving treatment for RVVC should receive regular follow-up to monitor the effectiveness of therapy and the occurrence of side effects.

Management of Sex Partners

Treatment of sex partners does not prevent recurrences, and routine therapy is not warranted. However, partners with symptomatic balanitis or penile dermatitis should be treated with a topical agent.

Special Considerations

HIV INFECTION

Insufficient information exists to determine the optimal management of RVVC among HIV-infected women. Until such information becomes available, management should be the same as for other women with RVVC.

PELVIC INFLAMMATORY DISEASE

PID comprises a spectrum of inflammatory disorders of the upper genital tract among women and may include any combination of endometritis, salpingitis, tubo-ovarian abscess, and pelvic peritonitis. Sexually transmitted organisms, especially N. gonorrhoeae and C. trachomatis, are implicated in the majority of cases; however, microorganisms that can be part of the vaginal flora, such as anaerobes, G. vaginalis, H. influenzae, enteric Gram-negative rods, and Streptococcus agalactiae also can cause PID. Some experts also believe that M. hominis and U. urealyticum are etiologic agents of PID.

Diagnostic Considerations

Because of the wide variation in many symptoms and signs among women with this condition, a clinical diagnosis of acute PID is difficult. Many women with PID exhibit subtle or mild symptoms that are not readily recognized as PID. Consequently, delay in diagnosis and effective treatment probably contributes to inflammatory sequelae in the upper reproductive tract. Laparoscopy can be used to obtain a more accurate diagnosis of salpingitis and a more complete bacteriologic diagnosis. However, this diagnostic tool is often neither readily available for acute cases nor easily justifiable when symptoms are mild or vague. Moreover, laparoscopy will not detect endometritis and may not detect subtle inflammation of the fallopian tubes. Consequently, the diagnosis of PID is usually made on the basis of clinical findings.

The clinical diagnosis of acute PID is also imprecise. Data indicate that a clinical diagnosis of symptomatic PID has a positive predictive value (PPV) for salpingitis of 65%–90% when compared with laparoscopy as the standard. The PPV of a clinical diagnosis of acute PID varies depending on epidemiologic characteristics and the clinical set-ting, with higher PPV among sexually active young (especially teenage) women and among patients attending STD clinics or from settings with high rates of gonorrhea or chlamydia. In all settings, however, no single historical, physical, or laboratory finding is both sensitive and specific for the diagnosis of acute PID (i.e., can be used both to detect all cases of PID and to exclude all women without PID). Combinations of diag-nostic findings that improve either sensitivity (detect more women who have PID) or specificity (exclude more women who do not have PID) do so only at the expense of the other. For example, requiring two or more findings excludes more women without PID but also reduces the num-ber of women with PID who are detected.

Many episodes of PID go unrecognized. Although some women may have asymptomatic PID, others are undiagnosed because the patient or the health-care provider fails to recognize the implications of mild or nonspecific symptoms or signs, such as abnormal bleeding, dyspareu-nia, or vaginal discharge ("atypical PID"). Because of the difficulty of di-agnosis and the potential for damage to the reproductive health of women even by apparently mild or atypical PID, experts recommend that providers maintain a low threshold of diagnosis for PID. Even so, the long-term outcome of early treatment of women with asymptomatic or atypical PID on important clinical outcomes is unknown. The follow-ing recommendations for diagnosing PID are intended to help health-care providers recognize when PID should be suspected and when they need to obtain additional information to increase diagnostic certainty. These recommendations are based in part on the fact that diagnosis and management of other common causes of lower abdominal pain (e.g., ectopic pregnancy, acute appendicitis, and functional pain) are unlikely to be impaired by initiating empiric antimicrobial therapy for PID.

Minimum Criteria

Empiric treatment of PID should be instituted on the basis of the pres-ence of all of the following three minimum clinical criteria for pelvic inflammation and in the absence of an established cause other than PID:

- Lower abdominal tenderness,
- Adnexal tenderness, and
- Cervical motion tenderness.

Additional Criteria

For women with severe clinical signs, more elaborate diagnostic evalua-tion is warranted because incorrect diagnosis and management may cause unnecessary morbidity. These additional criteria may be used to increase the specificity of the diagnosis.

Listed below are the routine criteria for diagnosing PID:

- Oral temperature greater than 38.3°C,
- Abnormal cervical or vaginal discharge,
- Elevated erythrocyte sedimentation rate,
- Elevated C-reactive protein,
- Laboratory documentation of cervical infection with N. gonorrhoeae or C. trachomatis.

Listed below are the elaborate criteria for diagnosing PID:

- Histopathologic evidence of endometritis on endometrial biopsy,
- Tubo-ovarian abscess on sonography or other radiologic tests,
- Laparoscopic abnormalities consistent with PID.

Although initial treatment decisions can be made before bacteriologic diagnosis of C. trachomatis or N. gonorrhoeae infection, such a diagnosis emphasizes the need to treat sex partners.

Treatment

PID therapy regimens must provide empiric, broad-spectrum coverage of likely pathogens. Antimicrobial coverage should include N. gonorrhoeae, C. trachomatis, Gram-negative facultative bacteria, anaerobes, and streptococci. Although several antimicrobial regimens have proven effective in achieving clinical and microbiologic cure in randomized clinical trials with short-term follow-up, few studies have been done to assess and compare elimination of infection of the endometrium and fallopian tubes, or the incidence of long-term complications such as tubal infertility and ectopic pregnancy.

No single therapeutic regimen has been established for persons with PID. When selecting a treatment regimen, health-care providers should consider availability, cost, patient acceptance, and regional differences in antimicrobial susceptibility of the likely pathogens.

Many experts recommend that all patients with PID be hospitalized so that supervised treatment with parenteral antibiotics can be initiated. Hospitalization is especially recommended when the following criteria are met:

- The diagnosis is uncertain, and surgical emergencies such as appendicitis and ectopic pregnancy cannot be excluded,
- Pelvic abscess is suspected,
- The patient is pregnant,
- The patient is an adolescent (among adolescents, compliance with therapy is unpredictable),
- The patient has HIV infection,
- Severe illness or nausea and vomiting preclude outpatient management,
- The patient is unable to follow or tolerate an outpatient regimen,
- The patient has failed to respond clinically to outpatient therapy,
- Clinical follow-up within 72 hours of starting antibiotic treatment cannot be arranged.

Inpatient Treatment

Experts have experience with both of the following regimens. Also, there are multiple randomized trials demonstrating the efficacy of each regimen.

Regimen A. Cefoxitin 2 g IV every 6 hours or cefotetan 2 g IV every 12 hours, PLUS Doxycycline 100 mg IV or orally every 12 hours.

NOTE: This regimen should be continued for at least 48 hours after the patient demonstrates substantial clinical improvement, after which doxycycline 100 mg orally 2 times a day should be continued for a total of 14 days. Doxycycline administered orally has bioavailability similar to that of the IV formulation and may be administered if normal gastrointestinal function is present.

Clinical data are limited for other second- or third-generation cephalosporins (e.g., ceftizoxime, cefotaxime, and ceftriaxone), which might replace cefoxitin or cefotetan, although many authorities believe they also are effective therapy for PID. However, they are less active than cefoxitin or cefotetan against anaerobic bacteria.

Regimen B. Clindamycin 900 mg IV every 8 hours, PLUS Gentamicin loading dose IV or IM (2 mg/kg of body weight) followed by a maintenance dose (1.5 mg/kg) every 8 hours. NOTE: This regimen should be continued for at least 48 hours after the patient demonstrates substantial clinical improvement, then followed with doxycycline 100 mg orally 2 times a day or clindamycin 450 mg orally 4 times a day to complete a total of 14 days of therapy. When tubo-ovarian abscess is present, many health-care providers use clindamycin for continued therapy rather than doxycycline, because it provides more effective anaerobic coverage. Clindamycin administered intravenously appears to be effective against C. trachomatis infection; however, the effectiveness of oral clindamycin against C. trachomatis has not been determined.

Alternative inpatient regimens. Limited data support the use of other inpatient regimens, but two regimens have undergone at least one clinical trial and have broad-spectrum coverage. Ampicillin/sulbactam plus doxycycline has good anaerobic coverage and appears to be effective for patients with a tubo-ovarian abscess. Intravenous ofloxacin has been studied as a single agent. A regimen of ofloxacin plus either clindamycin or metronidazole provides broad-spectrum coverage. Evidence is insufficient to support the use of any single agent regimen for inpatient treatment of PID.

Outpatient Treatment

Clinical trials of outpatient regimens have provided little information regarding intermediate and long-term outcomes. The following regimens provide coverage against the common etiologic agents of PID, but evidence from clinical trials supporting their use is limited. The second regimen provides broader coverage against anaerobic organisms but costs substantially more than the other regimen. Patients who do not respond to outpatient therapy within 72 hours should be hospitalized to confirm the diagnosis and to receive parenteral therapy.

Regimen A: Cefoxitin 2 g IM plus probenecid, 1 g orally in a single dose concurrently, or ceftriaxone 250 mg IM or other parenteral third-generation cephalosporin (e.g., ceftizoxime or cefotaxime), PLUS Doxycycline 100 mg orally 2 times a day for 14 days.

Regimen B: Ofloxacin 400 mg orally 2 times a day for 14 days, PLUS Either clindamycin 450 mg orally 4 times a day, or metronidazole 500 mg orally 2 times a day for 14 days.

Clinical trials have demonstrated that the cefoxitin regimen is effective in obtaining short-term clinical response. Fewer data support the use of ceftriaxone or other third-generation cephalosporins, but, based on their similarities to cefoxitin, they also are considered effective. No data exist regarding the use of oral cephalosporins for the treatment of PID.

Ofloxacin is effective against both N. gonorrhoeae and C. trachomatis. One clinical trial demonstrated the effectiveness of oral ofloxacin in obtaining short-term clinical response with PID. Despite results of this trial, there is concern related to ofloxacin's lack of anaerobic coverage; the addition of clindamycin or metronidazole provides this coverage. Clindamycin, but not metronidazole, further enhances the Gram-positive coverage of the regimen.

Alternative outpatient regimens. Information regarding other outpatient regimens is limited. The combination of amoxicillin/clavulanic acid plus doxycycline was effective in obtaining short-term clinical response in one clinical trial, but many of the patients had to discontinue the regimen because of gastrointestinal symptoms.

Follow-Up

Hospitalized patients receiving IV therapy should show substantial clinical improvement (e.g., defervescence, reduction in direct or rebound abdominal tenderness, and reduction in uterine, adnexal, and cervical motion tenderness) within 3–5 days of initiation of therapy. Patients who do not demonstrate improvement within this time period usually require further diagnostic workup or surgical intervention, or both.

If the provider elects to prescribe outpatient therapy, follow-up examination should be performed within 72 hours, using the criteria for clinical improvement previously described.

Because of the risk for persistent infection, particularly with C. trachomatis, patients should have a microbiologic re-examination 7–10 days after completing therapy. Some experts also recommend rescreening for C. trachomatis and N. gonorrhoeae 4–6 weeks after completing therapy.

Management of Sex Partners

Evaluation and treatment of sex partners of women who have PID is imperative because of the risk for re-infection and the high likelihood of urethral gonococcal or chlamydial infection of the partner.

Since nonculture, and perhaps culture, tests for C. trachomatis and N. gonorrhoeae are thought to be insensitive among asymptomatic men, sex partners should be treated empirically with regimens effective against both of these infections—regardless of the apparent etiology of PID or pathogens isolated from the infected woman.

Even in clinical settings in which only women are seen, special arrangements should be made to provide care for male sex partners of women with PID. When this is not feasible, health-care providers should ensure that sex partners are appropriately referred for treatment.

Special Considerations

PREGNANCY

Pregnant women with suspected PID should be hospitalized and treated with parenteral antibiotics.

HIV INFECTION

Differences in the clinical manifestations of PID between HIV-infected women and noninfected women have not been described clearly. However, in one study, HIV-infected women with PID tended to have a leukopenia or a lesser leukocytosis than women who were not HIV-infected, and they were more likely to require surgical intervention. HIV-infected women who develop PID should be managed aggressively. Hospitalization and inpatient therapy with one of the IV antimicrobial regimens described in this report is recommended.

EPIDIDYMITIS

Among men less than 35 years of age, epididymitis is most often caused by N. gonorrhoeae or C. trachomatis. Epididymitis caused by sexually transmitted Escherichia coli infection also occurs among homosexual men who are the insertive partners during anal intercourse. Sexually transmitted epididymitis is usually accompanied by urethritis, which is often asymptomatic. Nonsexually transmitted epididymitis associated with urinary tract infections caused by Gram-negative enteric organisms is more common among men greater than 35 years of age, and among men who have recently undergone urinary tract instrumentation or surgery.

Diagnostic Considerations

Men with epididymitis typically have unilateral testicular pain and tenderness; palpable swelling of the epididymis is usually present. Testicular torsion, a surgical emergency, should be considered in all cases but is more frequent among adolescents. Emergency testing for torsion may be indicated when the onset of pain is sudden, pain is severe, or test results available during the initial visit do not permit a diagnosis of urethritis or urinary tract infection. The evaluation of men for epididymitis should include the following procedures:

- A Gram-stained smear of urethral exudate or intraurethral swab specimen for N. gonorrhoeae and for NGU (greater than or equal to 5 polymorphonuclear leukocytes per oil immersion field),
- A culture of urethral exudate or intraurethral swab specimen for N. gonorrhoeae,

- A test of an intraurethral swab specimen for C. trachomatis,
- Culture and Gram-stained smear of uncentrifuged urine for Gram-negative bacteria.

Treatment

Empiric therapy is indicated before culture results are available. Treatment of epididymitis caused by C. trachomatis or N. gonorrhoeae will result in microbiologic cure of infection, improve signs and symptoms, and prevent transmission to others.

Patients with suspected sexually transmitted epididymitis should be treated with an antimicrobial regimen effective against C. trachomatis and N. gonorrhoeae; confirmation of these agents by testing will assist in partner notification efforts, but current tests for C. trachomatis are not sufficiently sensitive to exclude infection with that agent.

Recommended Regimen

Ceftriaxone 250 mg IM in a single dose and Doxycycline 100 mg orally 2 times a day for 10 days.

The effect of substituting the 125 mg dose of ceftriaxone recommended for treatment of uncomplicated N. gonorrhoeae, or the azithromycin regimen recommended for treatment of C. trachomatis, is unknown.

As an adjunct to therapy, bed rest and scrotal elevation are recommended until fever and local inflammation have subsided.

Alternative Regimen

Ofloxacin 300 mg orally 2 times a day for 10 days. RX = NOTE: Ofloxacin is contraindicated for persons less than or equal to 17 years of age.

FOLLOW-UP

Failure to improve within 3 days requires re-evaluation of both the diagnosis and therapy, and consideration of hospitalization. Swelling and tenderness that persist after completing antimicrobial therapy should be evaluated for testicular cancer and tuberculous or fungal epididymitis.

MANAGEMENT OF SEX PARTNERS

Patients with epididymitis that is known or suspected to be caused by N. gonorrhoeae or C. trachomatis should be instructed to refer sex partners for evaluation and treatment. Sex partners of these patients should be referred if their contact with the index patient was within 30 days of onset of symptoms.

Patients should be instructed to avoid sexual intercourse until patient and partner(s) are cured. In the absence of microbiologic test-of-cure, this means until therapy is completed and patient and partner(s) are without symptoms.

SPECIAL CONSIDERATIONS

HIV Infection

Persons with HIV infection and uncomplicated epididymitis should receive the same treatment as persons without HIV. Fungal and mycobacterial causes of epididymitis are more common, however, among patients who are immunocompromised.

HUMAN PAPILLOMAVIRUS INFECTION
Genital Warts

Exophytic genital and anal warts are benign growths most commonly caused by HPV types 6 or 11. Other types that may be present in the anogenital region (e.g., types 16, 18, 31, 33, and 35) have been strongly associated with genital dysplasia and carcinoma. These types are usually associated with subclinical infection, but occasionally are found in exophytic warts.

Treatment

The goal of treatment is removal of exophytic warts and the amelioration of signs and symptoms—not the eradication of HPV. No therapy has been shown to eradicate HPV. HPV has been identified in adjacent tissue after laser treatment of HPV-associated cervical intraepithelial neoplasia and after attempts to eliminate subclinical HPV by extensive laser vaporization of the anogenital area.

Genital warts are generally benign growths that cause minor or no symptoms aside from their cosmetic appearance. Treatment of external genital warts is not likely to influence the development of cervical cancer. A multitude of randomized clinical trials and other treatment studies have demonstrated that currently available therapeutic methods are 22%–94% effective in clearing external exophytic genital warts, and that recurrence rates are high (usually at least 25% within 3 months) with all modalities. Several well-designed studies have indicated that treatment is more successful for genital warts that are small and that have been present less than 1 year. No studies have assessed if treatment of exophytic warts reduces transmission of HPV. Many experts speculate that exophytic warts may be more infectious than subclinical infection, and therefore, the risk for transmission might be reduced by "debulking" genital warts. Most experts agree that recurrences of genital warts more commonly result from reactivation of subclinical infection than reinfection by a sex partner. The effect of treatment on the natural history of HPV is unknown. If left untreated, genital warts may resolve on their own, remain unchanged, or grow. In placebo-controlled studies, genital warts have cleared spontaneously without treatment in 20%–30% of patients within 3 months.

Regimens

Treatment of genital warts should be guided by the preference of the patient. Expensive therapies, toxic therapies, and procedures that result in scarring should be avoided. A specific treatment regimen should be chosen with consideration given to anatomic site, size, and number of warts as well as the expense, efficacy, convenience, and potential for adverse effects. Extensive or refractory disease should be referred to an expert.

Carbon dioxide laser and conventional surgery are useful in the management of extensive warts, particularly for those patients who have not responded to other regimens; these alternatives are not appropriate for treatment of limited lesions. One randomized trial of laser therapy indicated efficacy of 43%, with recurrence among 95% of patients. A randomized trial of surgical excision demonstrated efficacy of 93%, with recurrences among 29% of patients. These therapies and more cost-effective treatments do not eliminate HPV infection.

Interferon therapy is not recommended because of its cost and its association with a high frequency of adverse side effects, and efficacy is no greater than that of other available therapies. Two randomized trials established systemic interferon alpha to be no more effective than placebo. Efficacy of interferon injected directly into genital warts (intralesional therapy) during two randomized trials was 44%–61%, with recurrences among none to 67% of patients.

Therapy with 5-fluorouracil cream has not been evaluated in controlled studies, frequently causes local irritation, and is not recommended for the treatment of genital warts.

External Genital/Perianal Warts

Cryotherapy with liquid nitrogen or cryoprobe. or Podofilox 0.5% solution for self-treatment (genital warts only). Patients may apply podofilox with a cotton swab to warts twice daily for 3 days, followed by 4 days of no therapy. This cycle may be repeated as necessary for a total of 4 cycles. Total wart area treated should not exceed 10 cm^2, and total volume of podofilox should not exceed 0.5 mL per day. The health-care provider should demonstrate the proper application technique and identify which warts should be treated. If possible, the health-care provider should apply the initial treatment to demonstrate the proper application technique and identify which warts should be treated. The use of podofilox is contraindicated during pregnancy.
OR

Podophyllin 10%–25%, in compound tincture of benzoin. To avoid the possibility of problems with systemic absorption and toxicity, some experts recommend that application be limited to less than or equal to 0.5 mL or less than or equal to 10 cm^2 per session. Thoroughly wash off in 1–4 hours. Repeat weekly if necessary. If warts persist after six applications, other therapeutic methods should be considered. The use of podophyllin is contraindicated during pregnancy.
OR

Trichloroacetic acid (TCA) 80%–90%. Apply only to warts; powder with talc or sodium bicarbonate (baking soda) to remove unreacted acid. Repeat weekly if necessary. If warts persist after six applications, other therapies should be considered.
OR

Electrodesiccation or electrocautery. Electrodesiccation and electrocautery are contraindicated for patients with cardiac pacemakers or for lesions proximal to the anal verge.

Cryotherapy is relatively inexpensive, does not require anesthesia, and does not result in scarring if performed properly. Special equipment is required, and most patients experience moderate pain during and after the procedure. Efficacy during four randomized trials was 63%–88%, with recurrences among 21%–39% of patients.

Therapy with 0.5% podofilox solution is relatively inexpensive, simple to use, safe, and is self-applied by patients at home. Unlike podophyllin, podofilox is a pure compound with a stable shelf-life and does not need to be washed off. Most patients experience mild/moderate pain or local irritation after treatment. Heavily keratinized warts may not respond as well as those on moist mucosal surfaces. To apply the podofilox solution safely and effectively, the patient must be able to see and reach the warts easily. Efficacy during five recent randomized trials was 45%–88%, with recurrences among 33%–60% of patients.

Podophyllin therapy is relatively inexpensive, simple to use, and safe. Compared with other available therapies, a larger number of treatments may be required. Most patients experience mild to moderate pain or local irritation after treatment. Heavily keratinized warts may not respond as well as those on moist mucosal surfaces. Efficacy in four recent randomized trials was 32%–79%, with recurrences among 27%–65% of patients.

Few data on the efficacy of TCA are available. One randomized trial among men demonstrated 81% efficacy and recurrence among 36% of patients; the frequency of adverse reactions was similar to that seen with the use of cryotherapy. One study among women showed efficacy and frequency of patient discomfort to be similar to podophyllin. No data on the efficacy of bichloracetic acid are available.

Few data on the efficacy of electrodesiccation are available. One randomized trial of electrodesiccation demonstrated an efficacy of 94%, with recurrences among 22% of patients; another randomized trial of diathermocoagulation demonstrated an efficacy of 35%. Local anesthesia is required, and patient discomfort is usually moderate.

Cervical Warts

For women with (exophytic) cervical warts, dysplasia must be excluded before treatment is begun. Management should be carried out in consultation with an expert.

Vaginal Warts

Cryotherapy with liquid nitrogen. The use of a cryoprobe in the vagina is not recommended because of the risk for vaginal perforation and fistula formation.
OR

TCA 80%–90%. Apply only to warts; powder with talc or sodium bicarbonate (baking soda) to remove unreacted acid. Repeat weekly as necessary. If warts persist after six applications, other therapeutic methods should be considered.

OR

Podophyllin 10%–25% in compound tincture of benzoin. Apply to the treatment area, which must be dry before removing the speculum. Treat less than or equal to 2 cm² per session. Repeat application at weekly intervals. Because of concern about potential systemic absorption, some experts caution against vaginal application of podophyllin. The use of podophyllin is contraindicated during pregnancy.

Urethral Meatus Warts

Cryotherapy with liquid nitrogen.

OR

Podophyllin 10%–25% in compound tincture of benzoin. The treatment area must be dry before contact with normal mucosa. Podophyllin must be washed off in 1–2 hours. Repeat weekly if necessary. If warts persist after six applications, other therapeutic methods should be considered. The use of podophyllin is contraindicated during pregnancy.

Anal Warts

Cryotherapy with liquid nitrogen.

OR

TCA 80%–90%. Apply only to warts; powder with talc or sodium bicarbonate (baking soda) to remove unreacted acid. Repeat weekly if necessary. If warts persist after six applications, other therapeutic methods should be considered.

OR

Surgical removal.

NOTE: Management of warts on rectal mucosa should be referred to an expert.

Oral Warts

Cryotherapy with liquid nitrogen

OR

Electrodesiccation or electrocautery

OR

Surgical removal.

FOLLOW-UP

After warts have responded to therapy, follow-up is not necessary. Annual cytologic screening is recommended for women with or without genital warts. The presence of genital warts is not an indication for colposcopy.

MANAGEMENT OF SEX PARTNERS

Examination of sex partners is not necessary for management of genital warts because the role of reinfection is probably minimal. Many sex partners have obvious exophytic warts and may desire treatment; also, partners may benefit from counseling. Patients with exophytic anogenital warts should be made aware that they are contagious to uninfected sex partners. The majority of partners, however, are probably already subclinically infected with HPV, even if they do not have visible warts. No practical screening tests for subclinical infection are available. Even after removal of warts, patients may harbor HPV in surrounding normal tissue, as may persons without exophytic warts. The use of condoms may reduce transmission to partners likely to be uninfected, such as new partners; however, the period of communicability is unknown. Experts speculate that HPV infection may persist throughout a patient's lifetime in a dormant state and become infectious intermittently. Whether patients with subclinical HPV infection are as contagious as patients with exophytic warts is unknown.

SPECIAL CONSIDERATIONS

Pregnancy

The use of podophyllin and podofilox are contraindicated during pregnancy. Genital papillary lesions have a tendency to proliferate and to become friable during pregnancy. Many experts advocate removal of visible warts during pregnancy.

HPV types 6 and 11 can cause laryngeal papillomatosis among infants. The route of transmission (transplacental, birth canal, or postnatal) is unknown, and laryngeal papillomatosis has occurred among infants delivered by caesarean section. Hence, the preventive value of caesarean delivery is unknown. Caesarean delivery must not be performed solely to prevent transmission of HPV infection to the newborn. However, in rare instances, caesarean delivery may be indicated for women with genital warts if the pelvic outlet is obstructed or if vaginal delivery would result in excessive bleeding.

HIV Infection

Persons infected with HIV may not respond to therapy for HPV as well as persons without HIV.

Subclinical Genital HPV Infection (Without Exophytic Warts)

Subclinical genital HPV infection is much more common than exophytic warts among both men and women. Infection is often indirectly diagnosed on the cervix by Pap smear, colposcopy, or biopsy and on the penis, vulva, and other genital skin by the appearance of white areas after application of acetic acid. Acetowhitening is not a specific test for HPV infection, and false-positive tests are common. Definitive diagnosis of HPV infection relies on detection of viral nucleic acid (DNA or RNA) or capsid proteins. Pap smear diagnosis of HPV generally does not correlate well with detection of HPV DNA in cervical cells. Cell changes attributed to HPV in the cervix are similar to those of mild dysplasia and often regress spontaneously without treatment. Tests for the detection of several types of HPV DNA in cells scraped from the cervix are now widely available, but the clinical utility of these tests for managing patients is not known. Management decisions should not be made on the basis of HPV DNA tests. Screening for subclinical genital HPV infection using DNA tests or acetic acid is not recommended.

Treatment

In the absence of coexistent dysplasia, treatment is not recommended for subclinical genital HPV infection diagnosed by Pap smear, colposcopy, biopsy, acetic acid soaking of genital skin or mucous membranes, or the detection of HPV nucleic acids (DNA or RNA) or capsid antigen, because diagnosis often is questionable and no therapy has been demonstrated to eradicate infection. HPV has been demonstrated in adjacent tissue after laser treatment of HPV-associated dysplasia and after attempts to eliminate subclinical HPV by extensive laser vaporization of the anogenital area of men and women.

In the presence of coexistent dysplasia, management should be based on the grade of dysplasia.

Management of Sex Partners

Examination of sex partners is not necessary. The majority of partners are probably already infected subclinically with HPV. No practical screening tests for subclinical infection are available. The use of condoms may reduce transmission to partners likely to be uninfected, such as new partners; however, the period of communicability is unknown. Experts speculate that HPV infection may persist throughout a patient's lifetime in a dormant state and become infectious intermittently. Whether patients with subclinical HPV infection are as contagious as patients with exophytic warts is unknown.

CERVICAL CANCER SCREENING FOR WOMEN WHO ATTEND STD CLINICS OR WHO HAVE A HISTORY OF STDS

Women who have a history of STDs are at increased risk for cervical cancer, and women attending STD clinics may have additional characteristics that place them at even higher risk. Prevalence studies have found that precursor lesions for cervical cancer occur approximately five times more often among women attending STD clinics than among women attending family planning clinics.

The Pap smear (cervical smear) is an effective and relatively low-cost screening test for invasive cervical cancer and squamous intraepithelial lesions (SIL)[+], the precursors of cervical cancer. The screening guidelines of both the American College of Obstetricians and Gynecologists and the American Cancer Society recommend annual Pap smears for sexually active women. Although these guidelines take the position that Pap smears can be obtained less frequently in some situations, women who attend STD clinics or who have a history of STDs should be screened annually because of their increased risk for cervical cancer. Moreover, reports from STD clinics indicate that many women do not understand the purpose or importance of Pap smears, and many women who have had a pelvic examination believe they have had a Pap smear when they actually have not.

[+] A woman treated with a regimen other than those recommended for treatment of syphilis (for pregnant women or otherwise) in these guidelines should be considered untreated.

Recommendations

Whenever a woman has a pelvic examination for STD screening, the health-care provider should inquire about the result of her last Pap smear and should discuss the following information with the patient:

- Purpose and importance of the Pap smear,
- Whether a Pap smear was obtained during the clinic visit,
- Need for a Pap smear each year,
- Names of local providers or referral clinics that can obtain Pap smears and adequately follow up results (if a Pap smear was not obtained during this examination).

If a woman has not had a Pap smear during the previous 12 months, a Pap smear should be obtained as part of the routine pelvic examination in most situations. Health-care providers should be aware that, after a pelvic examination, many women may believe they have had a Pap smear when they actually have not, and therefore may report they have had a recent Pap smear.

In STD clinics, a Pap smear should be obtained during the routine clinical evaluation of women who have not had a documented normal smear within the past 12 months.

A woman may benefit from receiving printed information about Pap smears and a report containing a statement that a Pap smear was obtained during her clinic visit. Whenever possible, a copy of the Pap smear result should be sent to the patient for her records.

FOLLOW-UP

If a Pap smear shows severe inflammation with reactive cellular changes, the woman should be advised to have another Pap smear within 3 months. If possible, underlying infection should be treated before the repeat Pap smear is obtained.

If a Pap smear shows either SIL (or equivalent) or atypical squamous cells of undetermined significance (ASCUS), the woman should be notified promptly and appropriate follow-up initiated.

Appropriate follow-up of Pap smears showing a high-grade SIL (or equivalent) on Pap smears should always include referral to a health-care provider who has the capacity to provide a colposcopic examination of the lower genital tract and, if indicated, colposcopically directed biopsies. Because clinical follow-up of abnormal Pap smears with colposcopy and biopsy is beyond the scope of many public clinics, including most STD clinics, in most situations women with Pap smears demonstrating these abnormalities will need to be referred to other local providers or clinics. Women with either a low-grade SIL or ASCUS also need similar follow-up, although some experts believe that, in some situations, a repeat Pap smear may be a satisfactory alternative to referral for colposcopy and biopsy.

OTHER MANAGEMENT CONSIDERATIONS

Other considerations in performing Pap smears are the following:

- The Pap smear is not an effective screening test for STDs;
- If a woman is menstruating, a Pap smear should be postponed and the woman should be advised to have a Pap smear at the earliest opportunity;
- If a woman has an obvious severe cervicitis, the Pap smear may be deferred until after antibiotic therapy has been completed to obtain an optimum smear;

- A woman with external genital warts does not require Pap smears more frequently than a woman without warts, unless otherwise indicated.

SPECIAL CONSIDERATIONS

Pregnancy

Women who are pregnant should have a Pap smear as part of routine prenatal care. A cytobrush may be used for obtaining Pap smears from pregnant women, although care should be taken not to disrupt the mucous plug.

HIV Infection

Recent studies have documented an increased prevalence of SIL among women infected with HIV. Also, HIV may hasten the progression of precursor lesions to invasive cervical cancer; however, evidence supporting such a progression is limited. The following provisional recommendations for Pap smear screening among HIV-infected women are based partially on consultation with experts in the care and management of cervical cancer and HIV infection among women.

These provisional recommendations may be altered in the future as more information regarding cervical disease among HIV-infected women becomes available:

- Women who are HIV-infected should be advised to have a comprehensive gynecologic examination, including a Pap smear, as part of their initial medical evaluation.
- If initial Pap smear results are within normal limits, at least one additional Pap smear should be obtained in approximately 6 months to rule out the possibility of false-negative results on the initial Pap smear. If the repeat Pap smear is normal, HIV-infected women should be advised to have a Pap smear obtained annually.
- If the initial or follow-up Pap smear shows severe inflammation with reactive squamous cellular changes, another Pap smear should be collected within 3 months.
- If the initial or follow-up Pap smear shows SIL (or equivalent) or ASCUS, the woman should be referred for a colposcopic examination of the lower genital tract and, if indicated, colposcopically directed biopsies. HIV infection is not an indication for colposcopy among women with normal Pap smears.

HEPATITIS B

Hepatitis B is a common STD. Sexual transmission accounts for an estimated one-third to two-thirds of the estimated 200,000 to 300,000 new HBV infections that occurred annually in the United States during the past 10 years. Of persons infected as adults, 6%–10% become chronic HBV carriers. These persons are capable of transmitting HBV to others and are at risk for developing fatal complications. HBV leads to an estimated 5,000 deaths annually in the United States from cirrhosis of the liver and hepatocellular carcinoma.

The risk of perinatal HBV infection among infants born to HBV-infected mothers ranges from 10% to 85%, depending on the mother's hepatitis B e antigen status. Infected newborns usually become HBV carriers and are at high risk for developing chronic liver disease.

Prevention

Infection of both adults and neonates can be readily prevented with a safe and effective vaccine that has been used in the United States for more than 10 years. Universal vaccination of newborns is now recommended (17). The use of hepatitis B immune globulin (HBIG) combined with vaccination can prevent infection among persons exposed sexually to HBV if administered within 14 days of exposure.

Vaccination Eligibility

Persons known to be at high risk for acquiring HBV (e.g., persons with multiple sex partners, sex partners of HBV carriers, or injecting drug users) should be advised of their risk for HBV infection (as well as HIV infection) and the means to reduce their risk (i.e., exclusivity in sexual relationships, use of condoms, avoidance of nonsterile drug injection equipment, and HBV vaccination).

Selected high-risk groups for which HBV vaccination is recommended by the ACIP include the following persons:

- Sexually active homosexual and bisexual men,
- Men and women diagnosed as having recently acquired another STD,
- Persons who have had more than one sex partner in the preceding 6 months.

Such persons should be vaccinated unless they are immune to HBV as a result of past infection or vaccination. Refer to Hepatitis B Virus: A Comprehensive Strategy for Eliminating Transmission in the United States Through Universal Child Vaccination, Recommendations of the Advisory Committee on Immunization Practices (ACIP) (17).

Screening for Antibody Versus Vaccination Without Screening

The prevalence of past HBV infection among sexually active homosexual men and among injecting drug users is high. Serologic screening for evidence of past infection before vaccinating members of these groups may be cost-effective, depending on the relative costs of laboratory testing and vaccine. Among those attending STD clinics, it may be cost-effective to screen older persons for past infection. During a recent study of 2,000 STD clinic patients who accepted HBV vaccination, 28% of those greater than or equal to 25 years of age had evidence of past infection, whereas only 7% of persons less than 25 years of age had evidence of past infection. Past infection with HBV can be detected with a serologic test for antibody to the hepatitis B core antigen (anti-HBc). Immunity can be demonstrated by a test for antibody to the hepatitis B surface antigen (anti-HBs). The HBV carrier state can be detected by a test for HBsAg. If only a test for anti-HBc is used to screen for susceptibility to infection, persons immune because of prior vaccination will be falsely classified as susceptible. If only a test for anti-HBs is used, carriers will be falsely classified as susceptible.

Vaccination Schedules

The usual vaccination schedule is three doses of vaccine at 0, 1, and 6 months. An alternative schedule of 0, 1, 2, and 12 months also has been approved for one vaccine. The dose is 1 mL for adults, which must be administered IM in the deltoid—not in a buttock. For persons 11–19 years of age, the dose is either 0.5 or 1 mL, depending on the manufacturer of the vaccine.

Management of Persons Exposed to HBV

Susceptible persons exposed to HBV through sexual contact with a person who has acute or chronic HBV infection should receive postexposure prophylaxis with 0.06 mL/kg of HBIG in a single IM dose within 14 days of their last exposure; early administration may be more effective. HBIG administration should be followed by the standard three-dose immunization series with HBV vaccine beginning at the time of HBIG administration.

SPECIAL CONSIDERATIONS
Pregnancy
Pregnancy is not a contraindication to HBV or HBIG vaccine administration.

HIV Infection
Among HIV-infected persons, HBV infection is more likely to lead to chronic HBV carriage. HIV infection also impairs the response to HBV vaccine. Therefore, HIV-infected persons who are vaccinated should be tested for anti-HBs 1–2 months after the third vaccine dose. Revaccination with one or more doses should be considered for those who do not respond to vaccination initially. Those who do not respond to additional doses should be advised that they may remain susceptible.

PROCTITIS, PROCTOCOLITIS, AND ENTERITIS

Sexually transmitted gastrointestinal syndromes include proctitis, proctocolitis, and enteritis. Proctitis occurs predominantly among persons who participate in anal intercourse, and enteritis occurs among those whose sexual practices include oral-fecal contact. Proctocolitis may be acquired by either route depending on the pathogen. Evaluation should include appropriate diagnostic procedures, such as anoscopy or sigmoidoscopy, stool examination, and culture.

Proctitis is an inflammation limited to the rectum (the distal 10–12 cm) that is associated with anorectal pain, tenesmus, and rectal discharge. N. gonorrhoeae, C. trachomatis (including LGV serovars), T. pallidum, and HSV are the most common sexually transmitted pathogens involved. Among patients coinfected with HIV, herpes proctitis may be especially severe.

Proctocolitis is associated with symptoms of proctitis plus diarrhea and/or abdominal cramps and inflammation of the colonic mucosa extending to 12 cm. Pathogenic organisms include Campylobacter spp, Shigella spp, Entamoeba histolytica, and, rarely, C. trachomatis (LGV serovars). CMV or other opportunistic agents may be involved among immunosuppressed patients with HIV infection.

Enteritis usually results in diarrhea and abdominal cramping without signs of proctitis or proctocolitis. In otherwise healthy patients, Giardia lamblia is most commonly implicated. Among patients with HIV infection, other infections that are not generally sexually transmitted may occur, including CMV, Mycobacterium avium-intracellulare, Salmonella spp, Cryptosporidium, Microsporidium, and Isospora. Multiple stool examinations may be necessary to detect Giardia, and special stool preparations are required to diagnose cryptosporidiosis and microsporidiosis. Additionally, enteritis may be a primary effect of HIV infection.

When laboratory diagnostic capabilities are available, treatment should be based on the specific diagnosis. Diagnostic and treatment recommendations for all enteric infections are beyond the scope of these guidelines.

Treatment

Acute proctitis of recent onset among persons who have recently practiced receptive anal intercourse is most often sexually transmitted. Such patients should be examined by anoscopy and should be evaluated for infection with HSV, N. gonorrhoeae, C. trachomatis, and T. pallidum. If anorectal pus is found on examination, or if polymorphonuclear leukocytes are found on a Gram-stained smear of anorectal secretions, the following therapy may be prescribed pending results of further laboratory tests.

Recommended Regimen

Ceftriaxone 125 mg IM (or another agent effective against anal and genital gonorrhea) and Doxycycline 100 mg orally 2 times a day for 7 days. NOTE: For patients with herpes proctitis, refer to Genital Herpes Simplex Virus Infections.

FOLLOW-UP

Follow-up should be based on specific etiology and severity of clinical symptoms. Reinfection may be difficult to distinguish from treatment failure.

MANAGEMENT OF SEX PARTNERS

Partners of patients with sexually transmitted enteric infections should be evaluated for any diseases diagnosed in the index patient.

ECTOPARASITIC INFECTIONS
Pediculosis Pubis

Patients with pediculosis pubis (pubic lice) usually seek medical attention because of pruritus. Commonly, they also notice lice on pubic hair.

Recommended Regimens

Lindane 1% shampoo applied for 4 minutes and then thoroughly washed off (not recommended for pregnant or lactating women or for children less than 2 years of age) or Permethrin 1% creme rinse applied to affected areas and washed off after 10 minutes or Pyrethrins with piperonyl butoxide applied to the affected area and washed off after 10 minutes.

The lindane regimen remains the least expensive therapy; toxicity (as indicated by seizure and aplastic anemia) has not been reported when treatment is limited to the recommended 4-minute period. Permethrin has less potential for toxicity in the event of inappropriate use.

Other Management Considerations

The recommended regimens should not be applied to the eyes. Pediculosis of the eyelashes should be treated by applying occlusive ophthalmic ointment to the eyelid margins two times a day for 10 days.

Bedding and clothing should be decontaminated (machine washed or machine dried using heat cycle or dry-cleaned) or removed from body contact for at least 72 hours. Fumigation of living areas is not necessary.

Follow-Up

Patients should be evaluated after 1 week if symptoms persist. Re-treatment may be necessary if lice are found or if eggs are observed at the hair-skin junction. Patients who are not responding to one of the recommended regimens should be retreated with an alternative regimen.

Management of Sex Partners

Sex partners within the last month should be treated.

Special Considerations

PREGNANCY

Pregnant and lactating women should be treated with permethrin or pyrethrins with piperonyl butoxide.

HIV INFECTION

Persons with HIV infection and pediculosis pubis should receive the same treatment as those without HIV infection.

Scabies

The predominant symptom of scabies is pruritus. For pruritus to occur, sensitization to Sarcoptes scabiei must occur. Among persons with their first infection, sensitization takes several weeks to develop, while pruritus may occur within 24 hours after reinfestation. Scabies among adults may be sexually transmitted, although scabies among children is usually not sexually transmitted.

Recommended Regimen

Permethrin cream (5%) applied to all areas of the body from the neck down and washed off after 8–14 hours, or Lindane (1%) 1 oz. of lotion or 30 g of cream applied thinly to all areas of the body from the neck down and washed off thoroughly after 8 hours. NOTE: Lindane should not be used following a bath, and it should not be used by persons with extensive dermatitis, pregnant or lactating women, and children less than 2 years of age.

Alternative Regimen

Crotamiton (10%) applied to the entire body from the neck down, nightly for 2 consecutive nights, and washed off 24 hours after the second application.

Permethrin is effective and safe but costs more than lindane. Lindane is effective in most areas of the country, but lindane resistance has been reported in some areas of the world, including parts of the United States. Seizures have occurred when lindane was applied after a bath or used by patients with extensive dermatitis. Aplastic anemia following lindane use also has been reported.

Other Management Considerations

Bedding and clothing should be decontaminated (machine washed or machine dried using hot cycle or dry-cleaned) or removed from body contact for at least 72 hours. Fumigation of living areas is not necessary.

Follow-Up

Pruritus may persist for several weeks. Some experts recommend re-treatment after 1 week for patients who are still symptomatic; other experts recommend re-treatment only if live mites can be observed. Patients who are not responding to the recommended treatment should be retreated with an alternative regimen.

Management of Sex Partners

Both sexual and close personal or household contacts within the last month should be examined and treated.

Special Considerations

PREGNANT WOMEN, INFANTS, AND YOUNG CHILDREN

Infants, young children, and pregnant and lactating women should not be treated with lindane. They may be treated with permethrin or crotamiton regimens.

HIV INFECTION

Persons with HIV infection and uncomplicated scabies should receive the same treatment as persons without HIV infection. Persons with HIV infection and others who are immunosuppressed are at increased risk for Norwegian scabies, a disseminated dermatologic infection. Such patients should be managed in consultation with an expert.

SEXUAL ASSAULT AND STDS
Adults and Adolescents

Recommendations in this report are limited to the identification and treatment of sexually transmitted infections and conditions commonly identified in the management of such infections. The documentation of findings and collection of specimens for forensic purposes and the management of potential pregnancy or physical and psychological trauma are beyond the scope of these recommendations. Among sexually active adults, the identification of sexually transmitted infections following assault is usually more important for the psychological and medical management of the patient than for legal purposes, if the infection could have been acquired before the assault.

Trichomoniasis, chlamydia, gonorrhea, and BV appear to be the infections most commonly diagnosed among women following sexual assault. Since the prevalence of these conditions is substantial among sexually active women, their presence (post-assault) does not necessarily signify acquisition during the assault. Chlamydial and gonococcal infection among females are of special concern because of the possibility of ascending infection.

Evaluation for Sexually Transmitted Infections

Initial Examination

An initial examination should include the following procedures:

- Cultures for N. gonorrhoeae and C. trachomatis from specimens collected from any sites of penetration or attempted penetration.
- If chlamydial culture is not available, nonculture tests for chlamydia are an acceptable substitute, although false-negative test results are more common with nonculture tests and false-positive test results may occur. If a nonculture test is used, a positive test result should be verified with a second test based on a different diagnostic principle or with a blocking antibody or competitive probe procedure.
- Wet mount and culture of a vaginal swab specimen for T. vaginalis infection. If vaginal discharge or malodor is evident, the wet mount should also be examined for evidence of BV and yeast infection.
- Collection of a serum sample to be preserved for subsequent analysis if follow-up serologic tests are positive (see Follow-Up Examination 12 Weeks after Assault).

Follow-Up Examination 2 Weeks after Assault

Examination for sexually transmitted infections should be repeated 2 weeks after the assault. Because infectious agents acquired through assault may not have produced sufficient concentrations of organisms to result in positive tests at the initial examination, culture and wet mount tests should be repeated at the 2-week visit unless prophylactic treatment has already been provided.

Follow-Up Examination 12 Weeks after Assault

Serologic tests for syphilis and HIV infection should be performed 12 weeks after the assault. If positive, testing of the sera collected at the initial examination will assist in determining whether the infection antedated the assault.

Prophylaxis

Although not all experts agree, most patients probably benefit from prophylaxis because (a) follow-up of patients who have been sexually assaulted can be difficult, and (b) patients may be reassured if offered treatment or prophylaxis for possible infection. The following prophylactic measures address the more common micro-organisms:

- HBV vaccination (see HEPATITIS B).
- Antimicrobial therapy: empiric regimen for chlamydial, gonococcal, and trichomonal infections and for BV.

Recommended Regimen

Ceftriaxone 125 mg IM in a single dose
PLUS
Metronidazole 2 g orally in a single dose
PLUS
Doxycycline 100 mg orally 2 times a day for 7 days.
NOTE: For patients requiring alternative treatments, see the appropriate sections of this report addressing those agents.

Other Management Considerations

At the initial examination and, as indicated, at follow-up examinations, patients should be counseled regarding the following:

- Symptoms of STDs and the need for immediate examination if symptoms occur, and
- Use of condoms for sexual intercourse until STD prophylactic treatment is completed.

Risk for Acquiring HIV Infection

Although HIV-antibody seroconversion has been reported among persons whose only known risk factor was sexual assault or sexual abuse, the risk for acquiring HIV infection through sexual assault is minimal in most instances. Although the overall rate of transmission of HIV from an HIV-infected person during a single act of heterosexual intercourse is thought to be low (less than 1%), this risk depends on many factors. Prophylactic treatment for HIV is not known to be effective and is not generally recommended in this situation. However, all persons should be offered HIV counseling and testing after the assault.

Raising the issue of the potential for HIV infection during the initial medical evaluation may add to the acute psychological stress the patient may be experiencing because of the assault. An alternative is to address the issue at the 2-week follow-up appointment when the patient may be better able to receive this information and give informed consent for HIV testing. All persons electing to be tested for HIV should receive pretest and posttest counseling.

Sexual Assault or Abuse of Children

Recommendations in this report are limited to the identification and treatment of sexually transmitted infections. Management of the psychosocial and legal aspects of the sexual assault or abuse of children are important, but are beyond the scope of these recommendations.

The identification of sexually transmissible agents among children beyond the neonatal period suggests sexual abuse. However, there are exceptions; for example, rectal or genital infection with C. trachomatis among young children may be the result of perinatally acquired infection and may persist for as long as 3 years. In addition, BV and genital mycoplasmas have been identified among children who have been abused and among those who have not been abused. A finding of genital warts, although suggestive of assault, is not specific for sexual abuse without other evidence. When the only evidence of sexual abuse is the isolation of an organism or the detection of antibodies to a sexually transmissible agent, findings should be confirmed and the implications carefully considered.

Evaluation for Sexually Transmitted Infections

Examinations of children for sexual assault or abuse should be conducted so as to minimize trauma to the child. The decision to evaluate the child for STDs must be made on an individual basis. Situations involving a high risk for STDs and a strong indication for testing include the following:

- A suspected offender is known to have an STD or to be at high risk for STDs (e.g., multiple partners or past history of STD),
- The child has symptoms or signs of an STD,
- There is a high STD prevalence in the community.

Obtaining the indicated specimens requires skill to avoid psychological and physical trauma to the child. The clinical manifestations of some sexually transmitted infections are different among children when compared with adults. Examinations and specimen collection should be conducted by practitioners who have experience and training in the evaluation of abused or assaulted children.

A principal purpose of the examination is to obtain evidence of an infection that is likely to have been sexually transmitted. However, because of the legal and psychosocial consequences of a false-positive diagnosis, only tests with high specificities should be used. Additional cost and time are justified to obtain such tests.

The scheduling of examinations should depend on the history of assault or abuse. If initial exposure is recent, infectious agents acquired through the exposure may not have produced sufficient concentrations of organisms to result in positive tests. A follow-up visit approximately 2 weeks after the last sexual exposure should include a repeat physical examination and collection of additional specimens. To allow sufficient time for antibody to develop, another follow-up visit approximately 12 weeks after the last sexual exposure also is necessary to collect sera. A single examination may be sufficient if the child was abused for an extended period of time, or if the last suspected episode of abuse took place some time before the child received the medical evaluation.

The following recommendation for scheduling examinations is a general guide. The exact timing and nature of follow-up contacts should be determined on an individual basis and should be considerate of the patient's psychological and social needs. Compliance with follow-up appointments may be improved when law enforcement personnel or child protective services are involved.

Initial and 2-Week Examinations

During the initial examination and 2-week follow-up examination (if indicated), the following should be performed:

- Cultures for N. gonorrhoeae specimens collected from the pharynx and anus in both sexes, the vagina in girls, and the urethra in boys. Cervical specimens are not recommended for prepubertal girls. For boys, a meatal specimen of urethral discharge is an adequate substitute for an intraurethral swab specimen when discharge is present. Only standard culture systems for the isolation of N. gonorrhoeae should be used. All presumptive isolates of N. gonorrhoeae should be confirmed by at least two tests that involve different principles (e.g., biochemical, enzyme substrate, or serologic methods). Isolates should be preserved in case additional or repeated testing is needed.
- Cultures for C. trachomatis from specimens collected from the anus in both sexes and from the vagina in girls. Limited information suggests that the likelihood of recovering chlamydia from the urethra of prepubertal boys is too low to justify the trauma involved in obtaining an intraurethral specimen. A urethral specimen should be obtained if urethral discharge is present. Pharyngeal specimens for C. trachomatis also are not recommended for either sex because the yield is low, perinatally acquired infection may persist beyond infancy, and culture systems in some laboratories do not distinguish between C. trachomatis and C. pneumoniae.

Only standard culture systems for the isolation of C. trachomatis should be used. The isolation of C. trachomatis should be confirmed by microscopic identification of inclusions by staining with fluorescein-conjugated monoclonal antibody specific for C. trachomatis. Isolates should be preserved. Nonculture tests for chlamydia are not sufficiently specific for use in circumstances involving possible child abuse or assault.

- Culture and wet mount of a vaginal swab specimen for T. vaginalis infection. The presence of clue cells in the wet mount suggests BV among children with vaginal discharge. The significance of clue cells or other indicators of BV as an indicator of sexual exposure is unclear. The clinical significance of clue cells or other indicators of BV in the absence of vaginal discharge also is not clear.
- Collection of a serum sample to be preserved for subsequent analysis if follow-up serologic tests are positive. If the last sexual exposure occurred greater than 8 weeks before the initial examination, sera should be tested immediately for antibody to sexually transmitted agents. Agents for which suitable tests are available include T. pallidum, HIV, and HBV. The choice of agents for serologic tests should be made on a case-by-case basis (see Examination 12 Weeks After Assault).

Examination 12 Weeks after Assault

An examination approximately 12 weeks after the last suspected sexual exposure is recommended to allow time for antibodies to infectious agents to develop. Serologic tests for the agents listed below should be considered:

- T. pallidum,
- HIV,
- HBV.

The prevalence of these infections varies greatly among communities, and depends upon whether risk factors are known to be present in the abuser or assailant. Also, results of HBV tests must be interpreted carefully, because HBV may be transmitted by nonsexual modes as well as sexually. The choice of tests must be made on a case-by-case basis.

Presumptive Treatment

There are few data upon which to establish the risk of a child's acquiring a sexually transmitted infection as a result of sexual abuse. The risk is believed to be low in most circumstances, although documentation to support this position is inadequate.

Presumptive treatment for children who have been sexually assaulted or abused is not widely recommended because girls appear to be at lower risk for ascending infection than adolescent or adult women, and regular follow-up can usually be assured. However, some children or their parents or guardians may be very concerned about the possibility of contracting an STD, even if the risk is perceived by the health-care practitioner to be low. Addressing patient concerns may be an appropriate indication for presumptive treatment in some settings.

Reporting

Every state, the District of Columbia, Puerto Rico, Guam, the Virgin Islands, and American Samoa have laws that require the reporting of child abuse. The exact requirements vary from state to state but, generally, if there is reasonable cause to suspect child abuse, it must be reported. Health-care providers should contact their state or local child protective service agency about child abuse reporting requirements in their areas.

REFERENCES: AS NUMBERED IN ORIGINAL PUBLICATION

2. CDC. Technical guidance on HIV counseling. MMWR 1993;42(RR-2):8–17.
6. CDC. Testing for antibodies to human immunodeficiency virus type 2 in the United States. MMWR 1992;41(RR-12):1–9.
7. CDC. Purified protein derivative (PPD-tuberculin anergy) and HIV infection: guidelines for anergy testing and management of anergic persons at risk of tuberculosis. MMWR 1991;40(RR-5):27–33.
8. CDC. The use of preventive therapy for tuberculous infection in the United States. MMWR 1990;39(RR-8):6–8.
9. CDC. Management of persons exposed to multidrug-resistant tuberculosis. MMWR 1992; 41(RR-11):59–71.
10. Recommendations of the Advisory Committee on Immunization Practices (ACIP). Use of vaccines and immune globulins in persons with altered immunocompetence. MMWR 1993; 42(RR-4):1–18.
11. CDC. Recommendations for prophylaxis against Pneumocystis carinii pneumonia for adults and adolescents infected with human immunodeficiency virus. MMWR 1992;41(RR-4):1–11.
12. CDC. Guidelines for prophylaxis against Pneumocystis carinii pneumonia for children infected with human immunodeficiency virus. MMWR 1991;40(RR-2):1–13.

13. Committee on Infectious Diseases, American Academy of Pediatrics. Report of the Committee on Infectious Diseases, 22nd edition, 1991.
14. Beall GN. Penicillins. In: Saxon A, moderator. Immediate hypersensitivity reactions to beta lactam antibiotics. Ann Intern Med 1987;107:204–215.
16. National Cancer Institute Workshop. The 1988 Bethesda System for reporting cervical/vaginal cytological diagnoses. JAMA 1989;262:931–934.
17. CDC. Hepatitis B virus: a comprehensive strategy for eliminating transmission in the United States through universal childhood vaccination. Recommendations of the Advisory Committee on Immunization Practices (ACIP). MMWR 1991;40(RR-13):1–25.

TOPIC 29 / **TUBERCULOSIS**

SUBTOPIC / PREVENTION

The Use of Preventive Therapy for Tuberculous Infection in the United States

Original Citation: Centers for Disease Control and Prevention. The use of preventive therapy for tuberculous infection in the United States. Recommendations of the Advisory Committee for Elimination of Tuberculosis. MMWR 1990;39(RR-8):9–12.

Editor's Note: The information included here was based on an MMWR Reports and Recommendations (Vol. 39, RR-8) which gives the recommendations of the Advisory Committee for Elimination of Tuberculosis (ACET) to increase effective application of preventive therapy for tuberculosis. Background information was included in the original article but omitted here due to space considerations.

RECOMMENDATIONS

The main purpose of preventive therapy is to prevent latent (asymptomatic) infection from progressing to clinical disease (9). Such therapy also is used to prevent initial infection and to prevent recurrence of past disease.

Although the number of persons in the United States who are asymptomatically infected with Mycobacterium tuberculosis is not known, projections based on previous data range from 10 million to 15 million (CDC, unpublished data). Estimates are that greater than 90% of current tuberculosis cases occur from this large pool of previously infected persons. Unless preventive therapy is more effectively applied to reduce this reservoir of infection, hundreds of thousands of new tuberculosis cases and tens of thousands of deaths can be expected over the next few decades.

High-Risk Groups

Certain groups within the infected population are at greater risk than others and should receive high priority for preventive therapy. In the United States, persons with any of the following six risk factors should be considered candidates for preventive therapy, regardless of age, if they have not previously been treated:

Persons with human immunodeficiency virus (HIV) infection (greater than or equal to 5 mm)* and persons with risk factors for HIV infection whose HIV infection status is unknown but who are suspected of having HIV infection.

Close contacts of persons with newly diagnosed infectious tuberculosis (greater than or equal to 5 mm). In addition, tuberculin-negative (less than 5 mm) children and adolescents who have been close contacts of infectious persons within the past 3 months are candidates for preventive therapy until a repeat tuberculin skin test is done 12 weeks after contact with the infectious source.

Recent converters, as indicated by a tuberculin skin test (greater than or equal to 10 mm increase within a 2-year period for those less than 35 years old; greater than or equal to 15 mm increase for those greater than or equal to 35 years of age). Persons with abnormal chest radiographs that show fibrotic lesions likely to represent old healed tuberculosis (greater than or equal to 5 mm).

Intravenous drug users known to be HIV-seronegative (greater than or equal to 10 mm).

Persons with medical conditions that have been reported to increase the risk of tuberculosis (greater than or equal to 10 mm).

In addition, in the absence of any of the above risk factors, persons less than 35 years of age in the following high-incidence groups are appropriate candidates for preventive therapy if their reaction to a tuberculin skin test is greater than or equal to 10 mm:

Foreign-born persons from high-prevalence countries.

Medically underserved low-income populations, including high-risk racial or ethnic minority populations, especially blacks, Hispanics, and Native Americans.

Residents of facilities for long-term care (e.g., correctional institutions, nursing homes, and mental institutions).

In addition to the groups listed above, public health officials should be alert for other high-risk populations in their communities. For example, through a review of cases reported in the community over several years, health officials may use geographic or sociodemographic factors to identify groups that should be targeted for intervention. Screening and preventive therapy programs should be initiated and promoted within these populations based on an analysis of cases and infection in the community. To the extent possible, members of high-risk groups and their health-care providers should be involved in the design, implementation, and evaluation of these programs. Staff of facilities in which an individual with disease would pose a risk to large numbers of susceptible persons (e.g., correctional institutions, nursing homes, mental institutions, other health-care facilities,

---

*The criterion for a positive reaction to a skin test (in millimeters of induration) for each group is given in parentheses and is based on data cited in references 11–13.

schools, and child-care facilities) may also be considered for preventive therapy if their tuberculin reaction is greater than or equal to 10 mm induration.

Preventive Therapy

The usual preventive therapy regimen is isoniazid (10 mg/kg daily for children, up to a maximum adult dose of 300 mg daily). The recommended duration of isoniazid preventive treatment varies from 6 to 12 months of continuous therapy (9). Twelve months of therapy is recommended for persons with HIV infection and persons with stable abnormal chest radiographs consistent with past tuberculosis. The other groups should receive a minimum of 6 continuous months of therapy.

To ensure that persons in high-risk groups comply with therapy, healthcare personnel should, if necessary, directly observe the therapy. Isoniazid can be given twice weekly in a dose of 15 mg/kg (up to 900 mg) when therapy must be directly observed and resources are inadequate for daily therapy. Recommendations of the ACET are summarized in Table 1.

Table 1. Criteria for determining need for preventive therapy for persons with positive tuberculin reactions, by category and age group

	Age group (yrs)	
Category	<35	≥35
With risk factor[a]	Treat at all ages if reaction to 5TU purified protein derivative (PPD) ≥10 mm (or ≥5 mm and patient is recent contact, HIV-infected, *or* has radiographic evidence of old TB).	
No risk factor High-incidence group[b]	Treat if PPD ≥10 mm	Do not treat
No risk factor Low-incidence group	Treat if PPD ≥15 mm[c]	Do not treat

[a]Risk factors include HIV infection, recent contact with infectious person, recent skin-test conversion, abnormal chest radiograph, intravenous drug abuse, and certain medical risk factors (see text).

[b]High-incidence groups include foreign-born persons, medically underserved low-income populations, and residents of long-term-care facilities.

[c]Lower or higher cut points may be used for identifying positive reactions, depending upon the relative prevalence of Mycobacterium tuberculosis infection and nonspecific cross-reactivity in the population.

Patients should be thoroughly educated and should be monitored monthly, in person, by appropriately trained personnel. Isoniazid preventive therapy should not be prescribed if monthly monitoring cannot be done. Some data indicate that black and Hispanic women, especially postpartum, may be at greater risk of serious or fatal adverse reactions and, therefore, should be closely monitored (14–16). Reducing the risk of adverse reactions, even when this risk is low, is as important as providing the benefits of preventive therapy. Additional details on preventive therapy have been published (9).

REFERENCES: AS NUMBERED IN ORIGINAL PUBLICATION

9. American Thoracic Society/CDC. Treatment of tuberculosis and tuberculosis infection in adults and children. Am Rev Respir Dis 1986;134:355–363.
11. Narain R, Chandrasekhar P, Naganna K. A fresh look at the definition of tuberculous infection and new infection. Ind J Med Res 1976;64:336–357.
12. Stead WW, To T. The significance of the tuberculin skin test in elderly persons. Ann Intern Med 1987;107:837–842.
13. Bass JB, Sanders RV, Kirkpatrick MB. Choosing an appropriate cutting point for conversion in annual tuberculin skin testing. Am Rev Respir Dis 1985;132:379–381.
14. Kopanoff DE, Snider DE, Caras GJ. Isoniazid related hepatitis. Am Rev Respir Dis 1978;117:991–1001.
15. Franks AL, Binkin NJ, Snider DE, Rokaw WM, Becker S. Isoniazid hepatitis among pregnant and post-partum Hispanic patients. Public Health Rep 1989;104:151–155.
16. Moulding TS, Redeker AG, Kanel GC. Twenty isoniazid-associated deaths in one state. Am Rev Respir Dis 1989;140:700–705.

Transmission of Multidrug-Resistant Mycobacterium Tuberculosis During a Long Airplane Trip

Original Citation: Kenyon TA, Valway SE, Ihle WW, Onorato IM, Castro KG. Transmission of multidrug-resistant mycobacterium tuberculosis during a long airplane trip. N Engl J Med 1996;334(15):933–938.

Original Authors: Thomas A. Kenyon MD, MPH, Sarah E. Valway, DMD, MPH, Walter W. Ihle, MPA, Ida M. Onorato, MD, Kenneth G. Castro, MD.

Table 4 shows suggested criteria and procedures for the notification of contacts that were distributed nationally to airline companies, state health departments, and tuberculosis-control programs in March 1995. The decision to notify passengers and crew members potentially exposed to tuberculosis should be guided by three criteria: the flight duration, the infectiousness of the index patient (e.g., whether he or she has smear-positive, cavitary pulmonary tuberculosis or laryngeal tuberculosis and whether there has been documented transmission to contacts), and seating proximity to the index patient, depending on the aircraft design (2). In cases in which the airline is informed first, it should provide the name of the passenger's physician to the state health department in the state where the patient resides or is being treated for tuberculosis so that the health department can make a determination of infectiousness. Applying these criteria to instances of exposure to tuberculosis on aircraft will make it easier to decide when to inform those who may potentially benefit from preventive therapy, while averting the expenditure of resources in circumstances in which the transmission of M. tuberculosis is highly unlikely.

Table 4. Suggested criteria and procedures for notifying passengers and flight crews after exposure to tuberculosis on commercial aircraft

1. When a health department determines that a passenger with tuberculosis was probably infectious at the time of a flight (2), it should consult the airline company to verify that the person with tuberculosis was on the flight in question and to ascertain the duration of the flight.

2. Health departments and airline medical consultants may consider limiting notification to flights longer than eight hours. Health departments may consider notification after shorter flights when patients are considered to be particularly infectious, such as those with laryngeal tuberculosis, which has been reported to result in transmission after only five hours of classroom exposure (22).

3. Depending on the design of the aircraft, notification of only the passengers seated in the same cabin area as the person with tuberculosis, and the crew working there, may be adequate. Collaboration between the health department and the airline is essential in determining who should be notified and how notification will occur.

4. The airline should notify passengers and flight crews in writing, in cooperation with the health department.

REFERENCES AS NUMBERED IN ORIGINAL PUBLICATION

2. Exposure of passengers and flight crew to Mycobacterium tuberculosis on commercial aircraft. 1992–1995. MMWR 1995;44:137–140.
22. Braden CR, Valway SE, Onorato IM, et al. Infectiousness of a university student with laryngeal and cavitary tuberculosis. Clin Infect Dis 1995;21:565–570.

Prevention and Control of Tuberculosis in U.S. Communities with At-Risk Minority Populations

Original Citation: Centers for Disease Control and Prevention. Prevention and control of tuberculosis in U.S. communities with at-risk minority populations: recommendations of the Advisory Council for the Elimination of Tuberculosis and Prevention and control of tuberculosis among homeless persons: recommendations of the Advisory Council for the Elimination of Tuberculosis. MMWR 1992;41(RR-5):1.

SUMMARY

Tuberculosis (TB) is an increasing public health problem in the United States, particularly among racial/ethnic minorities. In 1990, the number of reported TB cases increased 9.4% compared with 1989 and 15.5% compared with 1984. In 1990, almost 70% of all TB cases and 86% of those among children ages less than 15 years occurred among racial/ethnic minorities. Compared with non-Hispanic whites, the 1990 TB case rate was notably higher for racial/ethnic minorities.

Adverse social and economic factors, the human immunodeficiency virus epidemic, and immigration of persons with tuberculous infection are contributing factors to the increase in TB cases. Other contributing factors include physician nonadherence in prescribing recommended treatment regimens and patient nonadherence in following prescribed recommended treatment regimens.

To eliminate TB in U.S. communities with at-risk racial/ethnic minorities, the Advisory Council for the Elimination of Tuberculosis* recommends (a) initiating public awareness campaigns to alert these communities about the increasing TB problems; (b) training and educating public and private health-care providers in the skills needed to relate effectively to the at-risk communities being served, and empowering at-risk populations with knowledge and other resources needed to influence the TB programs directed toward their communities; (c) building coalitions to help design and implement intensified community TB prevention and control efforts; (d) intensifying the screening of at-risk populations for TB and tuberculous infection and providing appropriate treatment and preventive therapy; (e) increasing the speed and completeness with which all health-care providers report confirmed and suspected TB cases to appropriate health departments; and (f) improving the availability and quality of TB health-care services in socioeconomically disadvantaged areas.

INTRODUCTION

A national plan for the elimination of tuberculosis (TB) in the United States has specified three basic steps: (a) more effective use of existing tools and technology; (b) the development of new diagnostic, treatment, and prevention tools; and (c) rapid introduction of new technology and tools (1). Providing TB screening and preventive interventions to high-risk populations is the plan's top priority. Implementation of these intervention programs among U.S. racial/ethnic minority populations is of great urgency because TB has become epidemic among some racial/ethnic groups. For example, in 1990, almost 70% of all reported TB cases occurred among racial/ ethnic minorities. Among children ages less than 15 years, 85.9% of reported TB cases occurred among racial/ethnic minorities.

This document is a blueprint for the many agencies and organizations that must work together to plan, develop, and implement effective strategies to eliminate TB in racial/ethnic minority population groups and high-risk geographic areas. The Advisory Council for the Elimination of Tuberculosis urges that resources be directed to areas where the disease has shifted into clearly identifiable geographic enclaves, and where the disease disproportionately affects socioeconomically disadvantaged racial/ethnic minorities.

BACKGROUND

Magnitude and Extent of Problem

Ongoing analyses of TB morbidity data in the United States continue to identify the magnitude and extent of the TB problem among U.S. racial / ethnic minorities. The number of reported TB cases in the United States decreased from 84,304 in 1953 (when uniform national reporting of TB was initiated) to 22,255 in 1984—a reduction of 73.6%. In the same period, the annual risk of TB decreased from a case rate of 53.0/100,000 population to 9.4/100,000—a reduction of 82.3%. From 1953 through 1984, the number of reported TB cases declined by an average of almost 5% per year.

Since 1984, the TB morbidity trend has changed. In 1990, 25,701 cases were reported for a case rate of 10.3/100,000 population; this represents a 9.4% increase over the cases reported in 1989 and is 15.5% higher than the number of cases reported in 1984. When the trend for 1953 through 1984 was used to calculate expected cases, 28,000 more cases were reported than expected from 1985 through 1990.

From 1985 through 1990, Miami, Atlanta, San Francisco, Newark, Tampa, and New York City consistently ranked among the 10 cities with populations greater than 250,000 with the highest TB rates. In 1990, the TB rates for these six cities ranged from 38/100,000 in Tampa to 68.3/100,000 in Newark. Certain sociodemographic and geographic pockets, such as Central Harlem in New York City, have rates approaching or exceeding 300/100,000 population. From 1985 through 1990, increases in TB cases occurred among non-Hispanic blacks, Hispanics, and Asians/Pacific Islanders, while decreases occurred among non-Hispanic whites and American Indians/Alaskan Natives. Increases in TB cases among non-Hispanic blacks were largest in the 5-to 14-year-old and 25- to 44-year-old groups (41.1% and 55.1%, respectively). Among Hispanics, the largest increases were also in the 5- to 14-year-old and 25- to 44-year-old groups (102.6% and 76.7%, respectively). Of the 25,701 cases of TB reported in the United States in 1990, 17,814 (69.3%) occurred among racial/ethnic minorities, 7,836 cases (30.5%) occurred among non-Hispanic whites, and 51 cases (0.2%) were in persons whose race/ethnicity was not noted. The risk of TB (compared with the case rate of 4.2/100,000 population among non-Hispanic whites) was 9.9 times higher for Asians/Pacific

---

*The Advisory Council for the Elimination of Tuberculosis recognizes that a variety of terms are used and preferred by different groups to describe race and ethnicity. Racial and ethnic terms used throughout the document reflect the way data are collected and reported by official health agencies.

Islanders, 7.9 times higher for non-Hispanic blacks, 5.1 times higher for Hispanics, and 4.5 times higher for American Indians/Alaskan Natives.

There is evidence that the human immunodeficiency virus (HIV) epidemic is a major factor associated with the recent increase in TB cases. Immunosuppression resulting from HIV infection allows persons with latent tuberculous infection and newly infected persons to progress rapidly to clinical disease. Because the prevalence of latent tuberculous infection is higher among racial/ethnic minorities than among non-Hispanic whites, clinical TB is likely to be more common among HIV-infected minority populations than among HIV-infected non-Hispanic whites. In addition to the HIV epidemic, persons immigrating from countries with a high incidence of TB also appear to be contributing to increases in TB cases. From 1986 through 1990, the number of TB cases among the foreign-born increased from 4,925 to 6,262 and the percentage of total cases among foreign-born persons increased from 21.6% to 24.4%.

Because of HIV infection and immigration, increasing rates of clinical TB among persons of childbearing/child-rearing age in racial/ethnic populations place the less than or equal to 14-year-old group in affected racial/ethnic minority populations at greater risk of being exposed to and becoming infected with TB. This may explain the recent increase in TB cases in this age group. Other factors that may contribute to increases include social and economic factors such as substance abuse, limited access to available and acceptable health care, poverty, substandard housing, and homelessness. The role of each of these factors, if any, cannot be quantified, but they are major components in the complex circumstances that make more difficult the prevention and control of TB among disadvantaged groups in our society. Multiple-drug-resistant (MDR) TB is an emerging problem. MDR TB is associated with (a) immigration of persons from countries with a high incidence of resistant TB, (b) inappropriate treatment regimens prescribed by private- and public-sector physicians, and (c) patients who do not comply with appropriately prescribed treatment regimens.

Case Prevention Potential for High-Risk Areas and Groups

Of the 25,701 cases reported in 1990, 8,381 occurred among persons ages less than 35 years. Cases in this age group are considered potentially preventable by administration of preventive therapy to infected persons who have not yet developed disease. Eighty-five percent of potentially preventable cases occurred among racial/ethnic minorities.

A large proportion of potentially preventable cases are distributed among a few geographic locations. Of the 3,436 cases among non-Hispanic blacks ages less than 35 years, 70.3% (2,414) occurred in 53 counties that reported 10 or more such cases. Of the 2,412 cases among Hispanics ages less than 35 years, 79.8% (1,924) occurred in 40 counties that reported 10 or more such cases. Of the 1,139 cases among Asians/Pacific Islanders ages less than 35 years, 55.3% (630) occurred in 19 counties that reported 10 or more such cases. Of the 121 cases among American Indians/Alaskan Natives ages less than 35 years, 12.4% (15) occurred in one county that reported 10 or more such cases.

During 1990, 79.7% of the potentially preventable TB cases among racial/ethnic minorities were reported by 106 counties that reported 10 or more such cases. This represents 3.4% of the nation's 3,138 counties. These counties are located primarily in the Southeastern states, along the East and West coasts, and in Texas. Representatives and health-care providers from at-risk communities, appropriate government agencies, and interested organizations should work collectively with these counties to intensify TB elimination efforts.

RECOMMENDATIONS

Public Awareness Campaigns

Individuals in at-risk population groups, including local leaders, are often unaware of the extent of the TB problem in their communities and the potential for preventing infection. Public awareness campaigns can provide essential information.

1. A public awareness campaign should be initiated by national, state, and local organizations to alert communities at high risk for TB about the increasing TB threat and to the potential for eliminating the disease.
2. At the national level, this campaign should be designed and supported by CDC, the American Lung Association/American Thoracic Society (ALA/ATS), the American Public Health Association, and other national

organizations that support or provide services to high-risk population groups.

3. At the state and local levels, health departments should collect and analyze epidemiologic data to identify local communities and population groups with high incidences so that TB prevention activities and public awareness campaigns can be appropriately directed. Local public awareness campaigns should be focused toward community members, health-care providers, and religious, social, economic, and other influential organizations. Awareness campaigns should be designed and supported by health departments and ALA/ATS affiliates working with recognized community leaders, organizations, and health-care providers.

4. The media (print, radio, and television) should be effectively utilized to disseminate information about TB prevention and related elimination efforts:
   a. Local community, minority, and ethnic media (newspapers, magazines, newsletters, radio, and television) should deliver the information to the general public, high-risk communities, and at-risk population groups.
   b. Messages should be disseminated through national and community-based organizations such as churches and forums focused on economic, medical, political, and social activities.

5. National and local TB awareness programs should be supported by the availability of convenient and high-quality TB screening, prevention, and treatment services.

Training and Education of Public and Private Health-Care Providers

Empowerment of at-risk groups in the community is a crucial element in TB control. This step begins with the public awareness campaigns described above because it is vitally important for members of at-risk populations to understand TB; its impact on the community; how it is diagnosed, treated, and prevented; and what services are available. These populations also should be able to influence the TB programs directed toward their communities.

1. Health departments should ensure that the sociodemographic composition of the communities being served is represented in the composition of the TB-control-program staff. The staff should be culturally and linguistically competent and sensitive to the populations being served.

2. All health department and other health-care staff who provide TB services should receive training to improve interpersonal skills needed to encourage open and effective communication with members of high-risk communities and groups. Continuous efforts must be made to establish and maintain the rapport needed to relate effectively to the communities being served and to the public and private health-care providers serving those communities.

3. Health-care providers serving at-risk areas should be given TB training on recommended procedures for examining, diagnosing, and treating TB cases, suspected cases, and contacts. The training should include information on procedures for rapidly reporting confirmed and suspected TB cases.

Coalition Building

Major progress toward elimination can be achieved by focusing TB screening and preventive therapy programs toward groups of persons at high risk of becoming infected or developing disease. Public and private health-care providers serving many at-risk clients in the community may not fully apply recommended prevention methods. Some at-risk population groups lack access to medical care, and special efforts are often required to provide them with needed services. Coalitions composed of representatives from groups and communities at increased risk of TB can assist in developing and implementing plans to improve access to health care.

1. Health departments should expand their efforts to reach community groups at high risk of TB and health-care providers serving these groups.
2. Decision makers, other key people, and agencies within at-risk communities should be identified and involved in TB elimination planning and implementation activities.
3. Coalitions should be established to advise health departments and health-care providers on how to design and carry out intensified community TB prevention and control efforts. These groups should be composed of representatives from affected communities, community-based organizations, health departments, private and public health-care providers, and the media serving high-risk populations and communities. These coalitions should be responsible for defining the problems and identifying obstacles related to excessive rates of TB in the at-risk communities; establishing short- and long-term goals; setting realistic and time-phased objectives; establishing priorities; and developing, implementing, and evaluating strategies. They should also analyze their communities to determine how strategies should be implemented and how to motivate and mobilize community members.
4. Coalitions should help identify and obtain resources needed by community programs and people serving the at-risk areas.
5. Credit for accomplishments should be given to members of the coalitions and the at-risk communities involved in these efforts.

Screening and Prevention

Screening at-risk populations for TB and tuberculous infection and providing appropriate treatment are crucial for achieving TB elimination. Screening is done to identify persons in need of preventive therapy (2). Responsibility for conducting screening will vary. For some groups, the local health department and health-care providers should assume responsibility for conducting the screening. For others, community-based organizations may conduct the screening with training and evaluation assistance from the health department.

1. Health departments should assess the prevalence, incidence, and sociodemographic characteristics of cases of TB and infected persons in their jurisdictions to identify high-risk areas in their communities. On the basis of this assessment, health departments should work with community-based organizations and health-care providers serving those communities to plan and initiate tuberculin screening and preventive therapy programs specifically adjusted to each community's at-risk groups.
2. Planning, developing, and implementing screening programs should be a joint effort coordinated among the local health department, public and pri-

vate community organizations, and health-care providers serving the affected community. Medicaid, Medicare, and private health-care funds should be sought to support screening and preventive treatment programs.

3. When possible, initiatives to systematically screen for TB should be established in specific high-risk settings such as correctional institutions, long-term-care facilities, nursing homes, drug treatment centers, in- and outpatient hospital facilities, and homeless shelters (2).

Case Reporting

Early reporting of TB is essential so that contacts can be examined for evidence of infection and disease and can be given appropriate therapy as quickly as possible.

1. Health departments should inform health-care providers serving at-risk groups and communities about the importance of early TB case reporting and about the services offered by the health departments. Health-care providers should become familiar with the TB case reporting system used in their particular areas.

2. Early TB case reporting can be encouraged by offering incentives, such as free laboratory services, to health-care providers and free antituberculosis drugs to their patients.

3. To facilitate TB case reporting for health-care providers, health departments should consider using facsimile machines or telephone-answering machines to receive reports. Large laboratories and health-care facilities should consider using computer-to-computer reporting systems.

4. All private physicians, public and private hospitals, clinics, medical/health centers, alcohol/drug treatment centers, nursing homes, laboratories, and correctional facilities should notify appropriate health departments about confirmed and suspected TB cases as quickly as possible. The development of a reporting system that includes all pharmacies that dispense antituberculosis drugs should also be considered.

Treatment and Adherence

The availability of TB health-care services and related transportation are frequently a problem in high-incidence and socioeconomically disadvantaged areas. Attracting competent health-care staff in some of these areas is sometimes a major obstacle. In addition, it is often difficult to establish and maintain rapport needed for effective diagnosis, treatment, and prophylaxis of patients with TB in at-risk areas and population groups. For many patients, a variety of health and socioeconomic-related problems (e.g., unemployment, low income, homelessness, lack of or limited access to health care, language barriers, and alcohol and drug abuse) may limit their ability to adhere to recommendations for treatment or to obtain other needed medical care. Much of their time and effort is understandably devoted to meeting day-to-day economic and survival needs, such as food, shelter, clothing, and safety. Nonadherence is a serious problem that can lead to treatment failure, drug resistance, continuing transmission of infection, increasing disability, and death (3). These are challenges that should be met with new and innovative strategies.

1. Quality TB treatment services and related transportation should be available at no cost to patients.
2. CDC should recruit, train, and assign a cadre of TB physicians, nurses, social workers, and public health advisors to work in high-incidence areas where TB is increasing and where it is extremely difficult to attract and retain qualified staff. The specific objective for these assignments should be to stabilize and begin to reduce the case rates within 3 years of assignment. As target rates are achieved in these areas, reassignment to other areas can be made.
3. Special treatment-housing centers should be established in cities with large numbers of persons at risk of TB who are homeless. These centers should provide continuous shelter, food, and treatment for homeless persons diagnosed with TB for the duration of their prescribed therapy regimen. The shelter and food act as incentives for patients to remain compliant with treatment. When patients complete their prescribed regimens or do not comply with therapy, they can be discharged from the centers and new patients admitted. The effectiveness of this concept has been demonstrated by existing programs in New York City and Denver. The resources necessary to establish similar centers might be shared through agreements between federal agencies (e.g., U.S. Department of Housing and Urban Development, Health Resources and Services Administration, or CDC), state/local agencies, or private organizations. Many identified at-risk areas contain properties that are federally owned and are suitable for conversion to treatment-housing centers.
4. Specific strategies for improving adherence to treatment regimens by individual patients or groups of patients should be established for each identified high-risk community and population group. These strategies should be broad-based and reflect an understanding of the difficulties associated with behavioral change and be sensitive and responsive to the patients' beliefs, cultures, and environments. This allows for the identification and removal of specific barriers to adherence.
5. Health-care providers of TB services should take the time to explain to patients, in simple language that is culturally and linguistically appropriate, the specific adherence behaviors expected. Patients must first know what is expected of them before they can comply.
6. Patient education and appointment reminders must be culturally sensitive and linguistically appropriate and should be used to effectively influence the cooperation of patients seeking TB services. Whenever possible, patients should be given reminders for pending appointments in person or by telephone. This removes any doubt about whether the patients received the messages. Patients also can be counseled over the telephone, thereby helping them overcome scheduling, transportation, or other problems that interfere with adherence.
7. Directly observed therapy should be considered for all TB patients.
8. Trained nurses or community outreach workers with the same cultural and linguistic background as the patients should help design treatment plans, administer directly observed therapy, and assist patients and health-care providers to identify and overcome obstacles to adherence.
9. Outreach workers should act as extensions of the clinician and nurse by locating patients, reminding them of appointments, resolving basic problems, encouraging adherence, delivering medication, observing its inges-

tion, and identifying, tracing, and examining contacts. They should also serve as a liaison between the clinic staff and the patient by helping to bridge cultural and linguistic gaps and by educating patients. Such employees can greatly enhance TB control efforts among at-risk populations.

10. Additional federal, state, local, and private resources will be required to increase the number of outreach workers. These outreach workers should be recruited and hired from the areas and communities being identified for service. They should have a knowledge of and be sensitive to the culture and language of the population to be served.

REFERENCES: AS NUMBERED IN ORIGINAL PUBLICATION

1. Advisory Committee for the Elimination of Tuberculosis. A strategic plan for the elimination of tuberculosis in the United States. MMWR 1989;38(Suppl. No. S-3):(inclusive page numbers).
2. Advisory Committee for the Elimination of Tuberculosis. Screening for tuberculosis and tuberculous infection in high-risk populations and the use of preventive therapy for tuberculous infection in the United States. MMWR 1990;39(No. RR-8):(inclusive page numbers).
3. Snider DE, Hutton MD. Improving patient compliance in tuberculosis treatment programs. Atlanta: CDC, revised February 1989.

Prevention and Control of Tuberculosis in Long-Term Care Facilities

Original Citation: Centers for Disease Control and Prevention. Prevention and control of tuberculosis in facilities providing long-term care to the elderly. Recommendations of the Advisory Committee for Elimination of Tuberculosis. MMWR 1990;39(RR-10):7–20.

Editor's Note: The information included here was based on an article which lists the Advisory Committee for Elimination of Tuberculosis (ACET) recommendations on tuberculosis control activities appropriate for nursing homes and other facilities providing long-term care for elderly persons.

GENERAL GUIDELINES

Each facility should assure that appropriate tuberculosis prevention and control measures are undertaken to protect residents and staff. In large facilities, an infection control committee will usually be responsible for operating the tuberculosis prevention and control program. In a system that has more than one facility providing long-term care to the elderly, a qualified person should oversee the control activities at all of the facilities. Responsibility for surveillance, containment, assessment, and education should be specified in this person's job description.

- Surveillance refers to identifying and reporting all cases of tuberculosis in the facility and identifying all infected residents and staff. When an infectious case is identified, additional cases and new infections (as indicated by skin-test conversion) should be identified with the help of the state or local health department, and appropriate therapy should be instituted.
- Containment refers to ensuring that transmission of tuberculous infection is stopped promptly. Persons for whom treatment of disease or preventive

treatment is indicated should complete the appropriate course of treatment under direct supervision (i.e., the actual ingestion of medication is observed by a staff member). In addition, appropriate ventilation control measures should be applied.

- Assessment refers to monitoring and evaluating the surveillance and containment activities throughout each facility.
- Education refers to providing information and imparting skills to patients, families, visitors, and employees so that they understand and cooperate with surveillance, containment, and assessment activities.

SURVEILLANCE

Diagnosis

The intracutaneous administration of 5 units of purified protein derivative tuberculin (PPD-T) (Mantoux test) should be used to identify persons infected with tubercle bacilli. Multiple-puncture devices are not recommended. False-negative reactions to the tuberculin test may occur for up to 30% of persons with tuberculosis but without acquired immunodeficiency syndrome (AIDS); in comparison, false-negative reactions may occur for up to 60% of persons with tuberculosis and AIDS (11; CDC, unpublished data). Therefore, a negative skin test does not exclude the diagnosis of tuberculosis. Chest radiography and bacteriologic examinations are indicated for all residents and staff with symptoms compatible with tuberculosis, regardless of the size of the skin-test reaction.

Skin tests should be administered to all new residents and employees as soon as their residency or employment begins unless they have documentation of a previous positive reaction. A two-step procedure is advisable for the initial testing of residents and employees in order to establish a reliable baseline (11–13). Appendix I explains this procedure and the rationale for using it. Each skin test should be administered and read by appropriately trained personnel and recorded (in mm induration) in the person's medical record. A record of all reactions of greater than or equal to 10 mm should be placed in a prominent location in order to facilitate the consideration of tuberculosis if the person develops signs or symptoms of tuberculosis, such as a cough of greater than 3 weeks' duration, unexplained weight loss, or unexplained fever. All persons with a reaction of greater than or equal to 10 mm should receive a chest radiograph to identify current or past disease.

Skin-test-negative employees and volunteers having contact (of greater than or equal to 10 hours per week) with elderly residents should periodically have repeat skin tests; the recommended frequency of repeat testing depends upon the risk of tuberculosis infection in that facility (13). Each tuberculin-positive resident should be evaluated annually, and a record should be kept that documents the presence or absence of symptoms of tuberculosis (e.g., weight loss, cough, fever). Repeat skin tests should be provided for tuberculin-negative residents and employees after any suspected exposure to a documented case of active tuberculosis. A skin-test conversion is defined as an increase of greater than or equal to 10 mm for a person less than 35 years of age or an increase of greater than or equal to 15 mm for a person greater than or equal to 35 years of age.*

Each skin-test converter should have a chest radiograph; if the radiograph is negative for tuberculosis, the individual should be treated preventively. If the source of infection is not known and/or if additional conversions occur, periodic retesting of residents and a careful search for the source case should be continued.

Persons with reactions greater than or equal to 10 mm and persons with symptoms suggesting tuberculosis (e.g., cough, anorexia, weight loss, fever), regardless of the size of the skin-test reaction, should have a chest radiograph within 72 hours. Persons with abnormal chest radiographs and/or symptoms compatible with tuberculosis should also have sputum smear and culture examinations. In addition, sputum should be submitted for smear and culture for acid-fast bacilli for persons with a chronic cough, pneumonia, or bronchitis who do not respond promptly and completely to antibiotic treatment. At least three sputum specimens should be submitted. In the absence of spontaneous production of sputum, suction of laryngeal or pharyngeal mucus is satisfactory if sterile water is used in clearing the catheter. Usually, the early detection of tuberculosis by such means either prevents or greatly diminishes the spread of infection.

Staff members who are considered to have infectious tuberculosis should be relieved of work responsibilities until the diagnosis is excluded or until they become noninfectious as a result of effective chemotherapy.

Case Reporting

Whenever tuberculosis is suspected or confirmed among residents or staff, this information should be recorded and kept on file (in the medical record, personnel record, or other appropriate place). A prototype tuberculosis record is shown in Appendix II. The local or state health department should also be notified, as required by state and local laws or regulations.

Tuberculosis and Human Immunodeficiency Virus Infection

Staff members and residents with tuberculosis or tuberculous infection should be assessed for human immunodeficiency virus (HIV) infection because the medical management of tuberculosis and tuberculous infection must be altered in the presence of HIV infection. Factors** that are associated with an increased

---

*The Committee chose a larger increase in reaction size to define a skin-test conversion among persons greater than or equal to 35 years of age because of the increased risk of isoniazid-associated hepatotoxicity in this age group. With the use of this criterion, the benefits of using isoniazid preventive therapy should clearly outweigh its risks.

**On the basis of seroprevalence studies, factors that place a person at risk for HIV infection include intravenous (IV)-drug use and homosexual/bisexual contact. Other factors that increase the risk for HIV infection among adults include having received blood or clotting-factor concentrate between 1978 and 1985 and having had sexual relations at any time since 1978 with (a) a person known to be infected with HIV or to have AIDS, (b) a man who has had homosexual/bisexual contact, (c) prostitutes, (d) IV-drug users, or (e) persons born in countries where most transmission of HIV is thought to occur through heterosexual sexual contact.

risk or prevalence of HIV infection should be routinely sought. If HIV infection is considered a possibility, counseling and HIV-antibody testing should be strongly encouraged. Previously published guidelines provide additional information about this topic (14).

CONTAINMENT

Isolation

Persons with suspected or confirmed tuberculosis can remain in their usual environment, provided (a) chemotherapy is promptly instituted at the time the diagnosis is suspected or confirmed, (b) recent and current contacts are evaluated and placed on appropriate therapy, and (c) new contacts can be prevented for a 1- to 2-week period. If these conditions cannot be met, the person with suspected or confirmed tuberculosis should be placed under appropriate isolation precautions to prevent the spread of infection (15). The local health department should be contacted regarding the need for isolation and the methods used for achieving it.

Treatment

ATS/CDC recommendations should be followed in treating and managing persons with confirmed or suspected tuberculosis (14, 16). For newly diagnosed, previously untreated patients, the treatment regimen should contain both isoniazid and rifampin. If the patient has been treated for tuberculosis in the past, other or additional drugs may be needed.

Antituberculosis medication should be given along with other medication administered by nursing home staff. Each dose of medication should be dispensed by a staff person who watches the patient swallow the pills and who is trained to monitor for evidence of drug toxicity. Persons with positive sputum smears or cultures at the beginning of therapy should be monitored by repeat sputum examinations for treatment response until smears become negative. Failure to achieve negative smears and cultures is usually due to the patient's noncompliance with therapy but may be due to the presence of drug-resistant organisms or other complications. Patients should also be monitored by trained personnel for signs and symptoms of adverse drug reactions during therapy (14, 16). Expert medical consultation should be sought when treating patients with complications (e.g., drug resistance, adverse reactions, nonpulmonary tuberculosis). Such consultation is usually available through the local or state health department.

Investigation for Contacts

Because tuberculosis is transmitted by the airborne route, persons who sleep, live, work, or who are otherwise in contact with an infectious person through a common ventilation system for a prolonged time are "close contacts" at risk of acquiring infection. These persons may include other residents, staff, and visitors. When a person with confirmed tuberculosis appears to be infectious (e.g., has pulmonary involvement as seen by chest radiograph and a cough and/or positive sputum smear), contacts who were previously tuberculin-negative should be retested (13). If the case occurs in a known tuberculin converter, a search for the person who has the source case (referred to hereafter as the "source patient") should be undertaken by performing chest radiographs for all persons known to be tuberculin reactors and by submitting sputum specimens for smear and culture for all patients with a cough.

General guidelines for conducting a contact investigation in a nursing home or other facility are given in Appendix III, but health department personnel should be consulted to help determine which contacts should be examined.

Preventive Therapy

Contacts who have documented skin-test conversions and whose chest radiographs do not reveal tuberculosis should be given at least 6 months' preventive therapy unless it is medically contraindicated. Other residents and staff with positive tuberculin reactions should be given preventive therapy and monitored according to previously published guidelines (17).

Preventive therapy for residents should be incorporated into the facility's routine for delivering medications (e.g., blister pack, cardex file) and should be dispensed by a staff person trained to monitor for signs and symptoms of drug toxicity (16). If such signs or symptoms appear, medication should be withheld pending evaluation by a physician.

If tuberculosis preventive therapy is recommended, but individuals refuse or are unable to complete the recommended course, they should be advised to seek prompt medical attention if they develop signs or symptoms compatible with tuberculosis (e.g., persistent cough, anorexia, weight loss, night sweats). Routine periodic chest radiographs are not useful for detecting disease in the absence of symptoms; however, chest radiographs should be obtained promptly for persons with a cough that persists for more than 3 weeks and/or with a prolonged and unexplained fever.

ASSESSMENT

A record-keeping system, such as that shown in Appendix II, is essential for tracking and assessing the status of persons with tuberculosis and tuberculous infection in nursing homes/facilities that provide long-term care for elderly persons. This system should also provide data needed to assess the overall effectiveness of tuberculosis control efforts. The following information should be reviewed annually with health department staff and should be compared with previous data and data from other facilities in the area:

- Percentage of residents and staff within each facility with positive skin tests
- Percentage of persons showing conversion of the tuberculin test if retesting is performed
- Description of therapy and supervision
- Percentage of persons recommended for therapy who complete the prescribed course (goal is greater than 95%)
- Number of persons experiencing drug toxicity or intolerance
- Number of persons discontinuing medication and reason for discontinuance

ROLE OF THE HEALTH DEPARTMENT

State and local health departments should assist in developing and updating policies, procedures, and record systems for tuberculosis control in nursing homes and other facilities that provide residential care for elderly persons. The health department should also provide access to expert tuberculosis medical consultation. A health department representative should be designated to provide epidemiologic and management assistance to such facilities, and this responsibility should be an element in that person's job performance plan. At a minimum, he or she should be required to complete an initial on-site consultation, to be available for telephone consultation, and to conduct an annual evaluation of individual facilities.

State health departments should assist local units in developing programs to train facility staff to administer, read, and record tuberculin skin tests; to identify signs and symptoms of tuberculosis; to initiate and observe therapy; to monitor for side effects; to collect diagnostic specimens; and to maintain record systems.

Health departments should also provide consultation for contact investigations within facilities, and they should assure appropriate examinations of nonresident contacts of persons with tuberculosis diagnosed in these facilities.

State health departments have a responsibility to maintain a tuberculosis registry with updated medical information on all persons who currently have tuberculosis within their jurisdiction, including persons in nursing homes and other facilities providing residential care for elderly persons. Records should be assessed annually, and necessary revisions in policies or procedures should be recommended. In addition, state health departments should periodically assess the impact of tuberculosis acquired in a residential facility and the impact of tuberculous infection on the community as a whole.

REFERENCES: AS NUMBERED IN ORIGINAL PUBLICATION

11. American Thoracic Society, CDC. Diagnostic standards and classification of tuberculosis. Am Rev Respir Dis 1989 (in press).
12. American Thoracic Society, CDC. The tuberculin skin test. Am Rev Respir Dis 1981;124:356–363.
13. American Thoracic Society, CDC. Control of tuberculosis. Am Rev Respir Dis 1983;128:336–342.
14. CDC. Tuberculosis and human immunodeficiency virus infection: recommendations of the Advisory Committee for Elimination of Tuberculosis. MMWR 1989;38:236–250.
15. CDC. Guidelines for prevention of TB transmission in hospitals. Atlanta: US Department of Health and Human Services, Public Health Service, 1982:DHHS publication no. (CDC)82–8371.
16. American Thoracic Society, CDC. Treatment of tuberculosis and tuberculosis infection in adults and children. Am Rev Respir Dis 1986;134:355–363.
17. CDC. Screening for tuberculosis and tuberculous infection in high-risk populations, and The use of preventive therapy for tuberculous infection in the United States: recommendations of the Advisory Committee for Elimination of Tuberculosis. MMWR 1990;39(no. RR-8):9–12.

APPENDIX I

Detection of Newly Infected Persons (Skin-Test Converters)

The tuberculin test can be especially valuable when it is repeated periodically in the surveillance of tuberculin-negative persons likely to be exposed to tuberculosis. However, special problems exist in identifying newly infected persons.

First, some errors may occur in even the most carefully performed tests. For this reason, small increases in reaction size are usually not meaningful. Only persons whose tuberculin reactions show marked increases in size (i.e., greater than or equal to 10 mm among persons less than 35 years of age and greater than or equal to 15 mm among those greater than or equal to 35 years) within a 2-year period should be considered newly infected.

A second problem in identifying newly infected persons is the "booster phenomenon." Repeated testing of uninfected persons does not sensitize them to tuberculin. However, delayed hypersensitivity to tuberculin, once it has been established by infection with any species of mycobacteria or by Bacillus of Calmette and Guerin (BCG) vaccination, may gradually wane over the years. When tested at this point, these persons may have negative reactions. The stimulus of this test may then boost or increase the size of the reaction to a subsequent test, sometimes causing an apparent conversion or development of sensitivity. Although the booster phenomenon may occur at any age, its importance increases with age.

When tuberculin skin testing of adults is to be repeated periodically, the use of two-step testing initially can reduce the likelihood that a boosted reaction will be interpreted as representing recent infection. If the reaction to the first test is negative, a second test should be given a week later. If the second test result remains below the cutting point for a positive test, the reaction is considered to be negative. If the reaction to the second test is positive, it probably represents a boosted reaction and not a new infection.

Multiple-puncture devices should not be used in tuberculin-testing surveillance programs designed to detect newly infected persons (such as in periodic testing programs for employees of hospitals and other institutions or in the evaluation of contacts).

APPENDIX II

Tuberculosis Summary Record

The Prototype Tuberculosis Summary Record is designed to update the tuberculosis status of each resident and employee in a facility. This record may be kept in a central location (e.g., in the infection control office) or may be kept in individual patient or staff medical records. The form should not replace the tuberculosis diagnostic and treatment information found in the medical records of persons with tuberculosis symptoms or of those persons receiving antituberculosis medications.

The form can also be used to prepare statistical reports and to track residents and employees requiring periodic skin testing. This information is important for assessing the overall effectiveness of tuberculosis control efforts in a facility. If kept current, the data on the forms can be summarized periodically and compared with previous data in order to determine:

- The number of staff and residents having positive tuberculin skin tests
- The number of persons whose tuberculin tests have shown conversions from negative to positive

- The number of persons in the home receiving tuberculosis therapy and supervision
- The number and percentage of persons recommended for therapy who complete the prescribed course (goal is greater than or equal to 95%)

When tuberculosis is diagnosed, the form contains the necessary information for reporting the case to the state or local health department. The form also reflects (a) if the case was reported, (b) if a contact investigation was completed, or (c) if HIV testing was performed. Summary information regarding the use of chemotherapy for infection or disease can also be recorded.

Many items on the form require only a check in the appropriate box. The format follows events in the order they are likely to occur in the diagnosis of tuberculosis infection and disease.

The first section can be completed at the time of admission or employment; it documents personal information, as well as baseline skin-testing results. Space is provided for recording the results of a second initial skin test when the two-step procedure is used.

If baseline skin testing is negative, the results of retesting can be recorded on the second section of the form.

The final section of the form can be used to document x-ray and bacteriologic results, diagnosis, chemotherapy, and other information. This part of the form is generally used only for those residents or employees who have tuberculous infection or disease, those who have tuberculosis symptoms, or those who require follow-up after exposure to tuberculosis.

APPENDIX III

Investigation for Contacts

Contacts of persons with newly diagnosed tuberculosis are at risk of infection and disease. The risk to contacts is related to various factors pertaining to the person who has the source case (the "source patient"), the contact, and the environment that they share. Many factors interact to influence the transmission of infectious particles (droplet nuclei) from the source patient to the contact.

As soon as the diagnosis is reasonably established on laboratory and/or clinical bases, investigation of contacts should begin. Health-care personnel should not wait for positive cultures if history, sputum smears, and chest radiographs are suggestive of tuberculosis.

DEVELOPMENT OF TRANSMISSION

Probability Data

When a source patient has been identified, the appropriate procedure in contact investigation entails the development of a data base and an evaluation of each of the factors noted below. These data are usually gathered by interviewing the source patient and by reviewing related historic and laboratory records. A visit to the source patient's home or place of employment will usually be necessary to assemble a satisfactory initial data base.

Source-Patient Characteristics

Any person who is generating aerosolized particles containing tubercle bacilli is a potential transmitter of infection. Factors that indicate the probability of spreading tuberculous infection are:

- If the source patient is not receiving adequate antituberculosis chemotherapy, the probability of his or her producing infectious particles is enhanced.
- The presence of acid-fast bacilli in the appropriately examined sputum smear is indicative of a greater potential for infection.
- The ability to culture Mycobacterium tuberculosis from secretions of the source patient is less important quantitatively as an indicator than is the positive sputum smear.
- The presence of tuberculous laryngitis increases infectiousness.
- The presence of cough increases the probability of aerosol generation.
- The volume and viscosity of respiratory secretions influence the production of infectious particles; high volume and watery sputum are regarded as risk factors.
- Forceful exhalation (e.g., singing or shouting) may increase the potential for producing infectious particles.
- Prolonged duration of respiratory symptoms may augment the likelihood that infection will be transmitted.

Environmental Air Factors

Air is the vehicle by which the infectious particle or droplet nucleus is transported from the source patient to susceptible persons. The greater the concentration of these droplet nuclei in air shared by the source patient and his or her associates, the greater the risk to these contacts. The following factors alter the concentration of infectious particles in the air:

- The volume of air common to the source patient and contact is critical. If low, the concentration of infectious particles is increased (e.g., as in sharing a small room).
- Ventilation with outside air dilutes the concentration of potentially infectious droplets.
- Recirculating air may result in the accumulation of high concentrations of infectious particles because droplet nuclei remain suspended in the air (e.g., ships, hospitals, and other structures with closed-circuit heating and air-conditioning systems).
- Filtering air by high-efficiency particulate air (HEPA) filters removes the droplet nuclei from recirculated air.
- Ultraviolet irradiation of the upper air within the shared space (when feasible) may reduce the spread of infection by killing the tubercle bacilli suspended in the droplet nuclei.

Contact Risk Factors

Persons who have recently shared air with the source patient may be considered potentially infected contacts. The following factors are known to modify the risk of infection for these persons:

- Prior infection with tuberculosis, as indicated by a significant skin-test reaction before exposure to the identified source patient, reduces risk.

- Increased time in association with the source patient influences the probability of infection.
- Physical closeness between the source patient and the contact may influence the likelihood of infection.

STRUCTURING A CONTACT INVESTIGATIONAL PROGRAM

Establishment of Investigational Priorities

The estimated probability of transmission, based on information obtained by following the steps described above, should influence the priority, rapidity, and thoroughness with which a contact investigation is conducted. By using this systematic approach, appropriate and productive public health programs can be implemented.

Classification of Contacts

For each source patient, the contact investigation should proceed in an orderly manner, starting with persons who are most likely to have been infected. Members of the immediate family or others who have shared accommodations with the source patient in the recent past usually are labeled household contacts. Contacts in working, leisure, or other settings are designated by other terms such as "close," "intimate," or "casual." The most important consideration in a contact investigation is the probability of infection among contacts; therefore, the first step is to allocate contacts into higher- and lower-risk contacts.

A higher-risk contact is defined as any person who shared the environment air with a source patient for a relatively longer time and who has other risk factors relatively higher than those of other known contacts. Nursing home/facility residents sharing the same wing or ventilation circuit should usually be considered close contacts.

ESTABLISHING LIMITS FOR CONTACT INVESTIGATIONS

By initially evaluating the higher-risk contacts for evidence of tuberculous infection and/or disease, the actual infectiousness of the source patient can be inferred. The following are guidelines for limiting the extent of a contact investigation:

- Initiate investigation with higher-risk contacts; if there is no evidence of recent transmission of infection in this group, extending the investigation is not appropriate.
- If data indicate recent infection in the higher-risk group, extend the limits of investigation to progressively lower-risk contacts until the levels of infection detected approximate the levels of infection in the local community.
- At each stage of the investigation, establish the number and identity of contacts to be examined. Establishing such a denominator helps to assure that no contact who should be examined is missed.

Screening for Tuberculosis and Tuberculosis Infection in High-Risk Populations

Original Citation: Centers for Disease Control and Prevention. Screening for tuberculosis and tuberculosis infection in high-risk populations. Recommendations of the Advisory Council for the Elimination of Tuberculosis. MMWR 1995;44(RR-11):18–34.

Original Author: Alan B. Bloch, MD, MPH

Editor's Note: The information included here was based on an updated MMWR Reports and Recommendations (Vol. 44;RR-11) which updates the Advisory Committee for Elimination of Tuberculosis (ACET) recommendations on screening high-risk populations for tuberculosis and tuberculous infection.

PRIORITY OF SCREENING AMONG TB PREVENTION AND CONTROL ACTIVITIES

Three basic strategies are critical to the prevention and control of TB. The first priority is identifying and completely treating all persons who have active TB (2, 3). The second priority is contact investigation (i.e., finding and evaluating persons who have had contact with TB patients, determining if they have TB infection or disease, and treating them appropriately) (4). Contact investigations are important for identifying persons who have active TB and infected persons at high risk for developing TB. The third priority is screening populations at high risk for TB to locate persons infected with TB and giving complete therapy to prevent the infection from progressing to active, contagious disease (3, 5). This screening also may identify cases of active disease.

Although screening high-risk populations for TB infection and providing preventive therapy are crucial to achieving the nation's goal of eliminating TB (6), completion of TB therapy and contact investigation should have priority over screening. Decisions to screen particular groups should be based on local epidemiologic data and made in consultation with local health jurisdictions to ensure appropriate follow-up, evaluation, and management of persons having TB infection or disease. Health-care agencies or other facilities should consult with the local health department before starting a skin-testing program to ensure that adequate provisions are made for the evaluation and treatment of persons whose tuberculin skin tests are positive. Tuberculin skin-testing programs that identify infected persons without current disease should be undertaken only if the diagnostic evaluation and a course of prescribed therapy can be initiated and completed.

Because most state and local TB control programs that report high TB morbidity have inadequate resources to screen all persons in high-risk groups and treat those persons who are infected, involvement of other health-care providers in screening and preventive treatment activities is important. These health-care providers can augment the limited resources of health departments by conducting appropriate screening efforts. This collaboration will necessitate additional efforts to train health-care workers in the administration, reading, and interpretation of the tuberculin skin test and in the appropriate use of preventive therapy. Priorities for screening activities should be determined by assessment of available resources and the probability of infection and disease among groups in the community.

Groups that have the highest priority in all areas of the country include contacts of persons who have suspected or confirmed TB and patients who have human immunodeficiency virus (HIV) infection or risk for HIV infection. In particular areas of the country, other groups at high risk may include persons who inject illicit drugs, persons who have certain medical risk factors, foreign-born persons recently arrived from countries with a high incidence or prevalence of TB, and residents of congregate settings where risk for transmitting M. tuberculosis is increased (e.g., correctional facilities, long-term care facilities, and homeless shelters). Screening persons in low-risk groups is not likely to be cost-effective and should be discontinued.

HIGH-RISK GROUPS

Based on published reports in the medical literature and CDC surveillance data, the Advisory Council for the Elimination of Tuberculosis (ACET) recommends that the following groups be screened for TB and TB infection:

- Close contacts (i.e., those sharing the same household or other enclosed environments) of persons known or suspected to have TB;
- Persons infected with HIV;
- Persons who inject illicit drugs or other locally identified high-risk substance users (e.g., crack cocaine users);
- Persons who have medical risk factors known to increase the risk for disease if infection occurs (see Persons Having Other Medical Risk Factors);
- Residents and employees of high-risk congregate settings (e.g., correctional institutions, nursing homes, mental institutions, other long-term residential facilities, and shelters for the homeless);
- Health-care workers who serve high-risk clients;
- Foreign-born persons, including children, recently arrived (within 5 years) from countries that have a high TB incidence or prevalence;
- Some medically underserved, low-income populations;
- High-risk racial or ethnic minority populations, as defined locally; and
- Infants, children, and adolescents exposed to adults in high-risk categories.

Flexibility is needed in defining high-priority groups for screening. The changing epidemiology of TB indicates that the risk for TB among groups currently considered high priority may decrease over time, and groups currently not identified as at risk subsequently may be considered as high priority. Local public health officials should identify community groups among whom TB and transmission of infection occur. Identification of these groups requires collecting and analyzing (a) data on newly reported cases available as part of TB surveillance (e.g., residence, occupation, race/ethnicity, country of origin, and status of HIV infection, injecting drug use, homelessness, and congregate settings), (b) data not routinely collected and/or analyzed (e.g., indicators of socioeconomic status), and (c) data from tuberculin screening programs (e.g., at correctional institutions and health-care facilities). These data will enable health departments and other local facilities to target screening and treatment programs to locally defined high-risk populations and areas.

Using surveillance information, local or state TB programs should take the lead in determining groups to be screened. Responsibility for conducting screening will vary, depending on local circumstances. For some groups, the local health department should conduct the screening. For others, the health department should discuss the need for screening with other appropriate persons (e.g., correctional facility staff, hospital infection control officers, and shelter operators) and offer assistance in training, evaluation, and, if necessary and possible, provision of supplies. In some areas, gaining the commitment of private health-care providers and community health centers to screen and provide follow-up for the high-risk patients they serve will be vital.

GENERAL COMMENTS ON SCREENING

Screening persons other than members of high-risk groups is not recommended because screening low-risk persons diverts resources from other priority activities and because many positive tests in low-risk persons do not represent TB infection. The goal of screening programs must be clearly defined: screening is usually conducted to identify infected persons who are at high risk for disease and who would benefit from preventive therapy or to find persons who have clinical disease and need treatment. Screening programs also can provide (a) epidemiologic data for assessing TB and its trends in a community, (b) data for assessing the value of continued screening, and (c) baseline data to help with assessment if subsequent exposure occurs (e.g., for nursing home residents and employees in some occupations). Screening programs should not be undertaken unless necessary facilities for patient evaluation and treatment are identified and made available and unless patients found to be positive are likely to complete preventive therapy.

To the extent possible, members of high-risk groups and their health-care providers should be involved in the design, implementation, and promotion of screening programs (6–8). Implementation may be enhanced by using health department or other staff (including trained volunteers) who have linguistic and cultural familiarity with the population at risk.

SCREENING METHODS

Tuberculin skin testing is the standard method for identifying persons infected with M. tuberculosis (1). The Mantoux test (i.e., the intracutaneous administration of five units of purified protein derivative [PPD] tuberculin) best detects infection. Because they are less specific than the Mantoux test, multiple puncture devices should not be used to screen high-risk populations (9).

Screening for disease rather than infection may be more appropriate in some circumstances (e.g., when the tuberculin skin-test results may be unreliable, when administering and reading the test or following up infected persons for preventive therapy may be impractical, when the risk for disease is high, or when the consequences of an undiagnosed case may be severe). Chest radiography is the preferred screening method when the objective is to identify persons who have current pulmonary TB and when preventive therapy for infected persons is not the primary goal (e.g., in high turnover jails or in some homeless shelters). In these screening programs, patients who have signs and/or symptoms suggesting pulmonary or pleural TB (e.g., cough of > 2 weeks' duration) should have a standard posterior-anterior chest radiograph, regardless of the tuberculin skin-test result. Although TB produces certain radiographic abnormalities more frequently than others, almost any form of pulmonary radiographic abnormality may result from TB, especially in immunosuppressed persons (1).

THE TUBERCULIN SKIN TEST

A detailed review of the tuberculin skin test has been published recently and is summarized here (10). Tuberculin skin-test results should be evaluated within the context of each patient's epidemiologic and environmental potential for infection (11).

SENSITIVITY, SPECIFICITY, AND POSITIVE PREDICTIVE VALUE OF THE TUBERCULIN SKIN TEST

Although the tuberculin skin test is now the only method for detecting M. tuberculosis infection, the test is neither 100% sensitive nor 100% specific. Sensitivity is a test's ability to identify correctly those persons who have a condition (e.g., those infected with M. tuberculosis). Specificity is a test's ability to identify correctly those persons who do not have a condition. In populations having a high prevalence of infection with nontuberculous mycobacteria or vaccination with Bacille Calmette-Guerin (BCG), the specificity of the tuberculin test will be low.

The positive predictive value of the tuberculin test is also variable. Positive predictive value reflects the ability of a positive test to identify those persons who have a condition (i.e., the probability that a condition is present when the test is positive). As the prevalence of TB infection in the population decreases, the positive predictive value of the tuberculin test also decreases. The prevalence of infection among the total adult population in the United States is an estimated 5%–10% (CDC, unpublished data). Among populations residing in areas where cross-reactions caused by nontuberculous mycobacteria are common, the positive predictive value of the tuberculin test is low if a cutoff of greater than or equal to 10 mm is used to define a positive test.

INTERPRETING TUBERCULIN SKIN-TEST RESULTS

The criteria endorsed by the American Thoracic Society and CDC for a positive tuberculin skin-test result are intended to increase the likelihood that persons at high risk for TB will be candidates for preventive therapy and that persons having tuberculin reactions not caused by M. tuberculosis will not receive unnecessary diagnostic evaluation or treatment (1, 3, 4).

For those persons who have had recent close contact with a person who has active TB and for those whose chest radiographic findings suggest TB, skin-test reactions are likely to represent infection with M. tuberculosis. Persons infected with HIV may have a limited ability to respond to tuberculin, even if they are infected with tubercle bacilli. These groups are at high risk for TB. Thus, to ensure that persons infected with TB are evaluated and appropriately treated, the sensitivity provided by a greater than or equal to 5-mm cutoff for a positive test is appropriate for these groups. Although persons having HIV infection have a decreased ability to respond to tuberculin, some severely immunosuppressed persons infected with tubercle bacilli may still manifest a positive reaction and benefit from tuberculin skin testing.

Other factors (e.g., certain medical conditions or injecting-drug use without simultaneous HIV infection) moderately increase the risk for active TB. A reaction of greater than or equal to 10 mm should be considered positive for these groups. This cutoff is also appropriate for other groups: persons born in countries with a high prevalence or incidence of TB; medically underserved, low-income populations; residents and employees of most correctional institutions and nursing homes; health-care workers in high-risk settings (as defined in CDC guidelines); and, because of the increased risk for severe disease, children < 4 years of age.

Routine screening is not recommended for populations at low risk for infection with M. tuberculosis. However, if these persons are tested, a higher cutoff of greater than or equal to 15 mm is recommended.

False-Positive Reactions

A small percentage of tuberculin reactions may be caused by errors in administering the test or in reading results. However, false-positive results are more commonly attributable to the presence in tuberculin of antigens shared with other mycobacteria. The potential sources of cross-reactions caused by these antigens are infection with nontuberculous mycobacteria and vaccination with BCG. Distinguishing clearly between reactions caused by infection with M. tuberculosis and those caused by other mycobacteria is difficult. However, the larger the induration, the greater is the likelihood that the reaction represents infection with M. tuberculosis. Similarly, clearly distinguishing between a tuberculin skin-test reaction caused by infection with M. tuberculosis and a reaction caused by BCG vaccination is difficult. The probability that a skin-test reaction results from infection with M. tuberculosis rather than from BCG vaccination increases (a) as the size of the reaction increases, (b) when the patient is a contact of a person who has TB (especially if that person has infected others), (c) when a family history of TB exists or when the patient's country of origin has a high incidence or prevalence of TB, and (d) as the interval between vaccination and tuberculin testing increases (because vaccination-induced reactivity wanes over time and is unlikely to persist for < 10 years) (12, 13). A history of BCG vaccination is not a contraindication to skin testing.

False-Negative Reactions

False-negative tuberculin skin-test reactions have many potential causes (1). Nonresponsiveness to delayed-type hypersensitivity-inducing antigens like tuberculin is common among persons having impaired immunity (e.g., HIV-infected persons). Delayed-type hypersensitivity can be assessed with skin-test antigens such as tetanus toxoid, mumps, and Candida. Most healthy persons in the population are sensitized to these antigens. However, the scientific basis for anergy testing is tenuous (14). Most skin-test antigens used for anergy testing have no standardization. Thus, anergy testing is usually not part of screening for TB infection.

All HIV-infected persons should be tuberculin tested (15, 16). Those who are tuberculin-positive (greater than or equal to 5 mm) should be evaluated for TB disease and placed on appropriate curative or preventive therapy. Preventive therapy should be administered to tuberculin-positive, HIV-infected persons, regardless of age. If they are at high risk for TB, persons failing to react to tuberculin may be evaluated for anergy (17), although the lack of standardization of anergy testing practices should be considered.

BOOSTER PHENOMENON AND TWO-STEP TUBERCULIN SKIN TESTING

Periodic use of the tuberculin skin test is valuable for the surveillance of tuberculin-negative persons at risk for exposure to M. tuberculosis. Repeated testing of uninfected persons does not sensitize them to tuberculin. However, delayed-type hypersensitivity resulting from mycobacterial infection or BCG vaccination may gradually wane with years. Although subsequent initial skin testing may be negative, the stimulus of a first test may boost or increase the size of the reaction to a second test administered 1 week to 1 year later and thus may suggest an apparent—but false—tuberculin conversion.

Although the booster phenomenon may occur at any age, its frequency increases with age and is highest among persons < 55 years of age and/or among those persons who have had prior BCG vaccination (18). When tuberculin skin testing of adults is repeated periodically, as in employee-health or institutional screening programs, an initial two-step approach can reduce the likelihood that a boosted reaction will be misinterpreted as a recent infection. If the first tuberculin test result is negative, a second 5-TU test should be administered 1 week to 3 weeks later. A positive second result probably indicates boosting from a past infection or prior BCG vaccination. Persons having a boosted reaction should be classified as reactors, not converters. If the second result is negative, the person is probably uninfected, and a positive reaction to subsequent tests indicates a true tuberculin skin-test conversion (see Definition of a Tuberculin Skin-Test Conversion).

Because of problems with continued cross-reactions with other mycobacteria, the specificity of the tuberculin test is less when serial skin testing is performed than when a single test is administered. Thus, serial skin-testing programs tend to overestimate the incidence of new TB infection in the tested population. Because of this potential for overestimation of incidence, serial skin-testing programs should be targeted to populations at high risk for continued exposure to infectious TB.

Definition of a Tuberculin Skin-Test Conversion

Recent tuberculin skin-test converters are considered at high risk. An increase in induration of greater than or equal to 10 mm within a 2-year period is classified as a conversion to a positive test among persons < 35 years of age. An increase in induration of greater than or equal to 15 mm within a 2-year period is classified as a conversion for persons greater than or equal to 35 years of age. Regardless of age, for employees in facilities where a person who has TB poses a hazard to many susceptible persons (e.g., health-care facilities, schools, and child-care facilities), an increase of greater than or equal to 10 mm induration should be considered positive.

TUBERCULIN TESTING DURING PREGNANCY

Studies in which the same patients were tested during and after pregnancy have demonstrated that pregnancy has no effect on cutaneous tuberculin hypersensitivity. Tuberculin skin testing is considered valid and safe throughout pregnancy. No teratogenic effects of testing during pregnancy have been documented (19).

RECOMMENDATIONS FOR SPECIFIC HIGH-RISK GROUPS

Contacts of Persons Who Have Infectious TB

Because the risk for infection and disease is particularly high among close contacts of persons having TB, these persons should be identified promptly (usually within 3 days) and examined soon (usually within 7 days) after identification of the potentially infectious patient (4, 6). State and local health departments should work with local health-care providers to ensure completion of these monitoring activities. Prompt notification of state and local agencies about suspected or newly diagnosed and potentially infectious cases is critical for contact investigation.

Persons Who Have HIV Infection

HIV infection is the strongest risk factor yet identified for the development of TB disease in persons having TB infection (20–23). All HIV-infected persons should receive a PPD-tuberculin skin test (5-TU, PPD by the Mantoux method) (15, 16).

Tuberculin testing for persons infected with HIV should be conducted in settings where HIV-infected persons or those at risk for HIV infection receive care. Administrators should ensure that the recommended screening is implemented and that prompt follow-up, evaluation, and treatment occurs. Because tuberculin skin-test results are less reliable as CD4 counts decline, screening should be completed as early as possible after HIV infection occurs. Those HIV-infected patients at high risk for continuing exposure to patients who have TB should be screened periodically for TB infection. If they have TB symptoms or if they are exposed to a patient who has pulmonary TB, HIV-infected persons should be evaluated promptly for TB. Because active disease can develop rapidly in HIV-infected persons, the highest priority for contact investigation should be given to persons potentially coinfected with HIV and TB.

Persons Who Inject Drugs

Because they are at high risk for TB and HIV infection, the priority for screening is high for persons who inject illicit drugs (16, 20–22, 24, 25). Drug treatment programs and other settings that provide care for persons who inject drugs should skin test injecting-drug users. If further evaluation and case management is necessary, adequate referral mechanisms should be in place. Coordination of these activities with local alcohol and other drug abuse treatment programs should be encouraged. Priority should be given to screening in facilities that are able to provide on-site, directly observed preventive therapy for 6–12 months to persons who have TB infection (e.g., clients of methadone maintenance treatment programs or residential treatment programs).

Persons Who Have Other Medical Risk Factors

Health-care providers should administer tuberculin tests to all patients who have medical risk factors that substantially increase the risk for TB (3, 22). These patients should be screened in settings where they receive primary or subspecialty care (e.g., infectious disease, immunology, endocrinology, hematology/oncology, nephrology, rheumatology, pulmonology, and gastroenterology) or on admission to a hospital. These medical risk factors include the following:

- HIV infection,
- Diabetes mellitus,
- Conditions requiring prolonged high-dose corticosteroid therapy and other immunosuppressive therapy (including bone marrow and organ transplantation),
- Chronic renal failure,
- Some hematologic disorders (e.g., leukemias and lymphomas),
- Other specific malignancies (e.g., carcinoma of the head or neck),
- Weight of greater than or equal to 10% below ideal body weight,
- Silicosis,
- Gastrectomy, and
- Jejunoileal bypass.

In addition, persons who have an abnormal chest radiograph showing fibrotic lesions consistent with old, healed TB should be skin tested. Regardless of age, persons who have a positive skin test and parenchymal lung scarring are at high risk for TB if they have not previously received TB treatment or preventive therapy.

Residents and Employees of High-Risk Congregate Settings

High-risk environments are settings where (a) persons who have infectious TB are more likely to live, (b) environmental characteristics (e.g., type of ventilation and size) are conducive to transmission, and (c) many susceptible persons at risk for prolonged exposure to potentially infectious patients may be located. These environments include prisons and jails (26, 27), nursing homes and other long-term facilities for the elderly (28), health-care facilities (29), homeless shelters (30), and residential settings for HIV-infected persons (31). Persons working in these settings should be educated about the risk for transmission, the signs and symptoms of TB, and proper procedures for minimizing the risk for transmitting TB infection. Clients and employees should be tuberculin tested on admission or initial employment.

Residents and Employees of Prisons and Jails

Recommendations for screening, treatment, and prevention in correctional facilities advise that on entry, all inmates should be screened for TB symptoms by a standardized interview process (26, 27). Persons who have symptoms suggesting pulmonary TB should be immediately isolated and evaluated for active TB. Initial screening of inmates may vary, depending on each inmate's length of stay and on an assessment of the risk for transmission of TB infection in the facility.

In long-term facilities, tuberculin skin-test screening of all inmates without a documented positive skin-test result should be mandatory. If boosting is common among the population served by the facility, two-step skin testing should be considered. Inmates who have HIV infection and those at risk for HIV infection but whose HIV status is unknown should have a chest radiograph as part of the initial screening, regardless of skin-test results.

In short-term facilities serving high-risk populations, tuberculin skin-test screening is generally not feasible, but is recommended for inmates who will remain in custody for greater than or equal to 14 days. Inmates who have HIV infection and those at risk for HIV infection but whose HIV status is unknown should have a chest radiograph as part of initial screening, regardless of skin-test status. In some large jails, officials should consider using on-site chest radiography to screen all inmates (short-term and long-term) for TB. In short-term facilities serving low-risk populations, screening inmates may be limited to screening for symptoms, provided that arrangements are made with a collaborating facility to receive inmates exhibiting symptoms.

Tuberculin skin-test screening also should be mandatory for all correctional staff in short-term or long-term facilities. Staff should be informed that if they are immunosuppressed, they should consult a health-care provider for appropriate follow-up and screening for TB.

Medical units within correctional facilities should conduct a thorough risk assessment and follow recommendations for prevention of transmission of TB infection in health-care facilities (29). Correctional authorities have primary responsibility for implementing these programs, but health departments should assist in program planning and training as well as regulating, advising, monitoring, and evaluating TB-control activities in correctional facilities.

Residents and Employees of Nursing Homes/Facilities for the Elderly

Because TB case rates increase with age among all racial and ethnic groups and both sexes, screening for TB in facilities providing long-term care to the elderly is recommended (28). The incidence of disease is two to seven times higher among nursing home residents in some areas than among demographically similar persons in other settings. Studies indicate that unsuspected transmission of M. tuberculosis in nursing homes/facilities presents a risk to residents and workers (32, 33). Residents should be screened for TB infection on admission by use of the two-step skin-testing method. Screening with chest radiographs alone is insufficient. Although few residents will be candidates for preventive therapy, baseline test results are essential to interpretation of subsequent tests if an acute exposure occurs. The two-step method also should be used for baseline screening of employees. Testing should be repeated in the event of exposure.

Residents and Workers at Homeless Shelters

Screening to find cases of active TB among the homeless consists of a chest radiograph (and possibly a sputum smear and culture) to determine current disease (30). Tuberculin skin-testing programs identifying infected persons who do not have current disease should be undertaken only if the diagnostic evaluation and course of preventive therapy can be initiated and completed. A special effort should be made to identify homeless persons coinfected with TB and HIV infection and to provide directly observed preventive therapy. Unless a shelter has its own health-care staff, the local government or a government-funded agency should assume responsibility for conducting screening programs for the homeless.

Health-Care Workers

Transmission of M. tuberculosis is a recognized risk in health-care facilities (29). Transmission is most likely to occur from patients who have unrecognized pulmonary or laryngeal TB, who are not on effective anti-TB therapy, and who have not been placed in TB isolation. Recent TB outbreaks in health-care facilities, including outbreaks of multidrug-resistant TB, have created heightened concern about nosocomial transmission. Increases of TB in some geographic areas are related to the high risk for TB among immunosuppressed persons infected with HIV. Transmission of M. tuberculosis to HIV-infected persons is of particular concern because, if infected with TB, these persons are at high risk for the rapid development of active TB. Thus, health-care facilities should be particularly alert to the need for preventing transmission of M. tuberculosis in settings where persons who have HIV infection receive care or work.

Health administrators and infection control departments in hospitals are responsible for ensuring the implementation of these recommendations. Implementing an effective TB control program requires risk assessment; early identification, isolation, and complete treatment of infectious TB patients; effective engineering controls; an appropriate respiratory protection program; and education, counseling, screening, and evaluation for health-care workers.

The Foreign-Born

TB is a problem among persons who arrive in the United States from countries having a high prevalence or incidence of TB (e.g., most countries in Africa, Asia, and Latin America) (34–37). Foreign-born persons at risk include immigrants (documented and undocumented), refugees, and some migrant workers and students. Because disease rates among the foreign-born are highest in the first few years after arrival in the United States, efforts should be made to screen new immigrants. Culturally and linguistically sensitive evaluation and treatment programs should be provided to help ensure a successful treatment outcome. Services should not be denied because of a real or perceived undocumented immigration status.

Other High-Incidence Population Groups

The incidence of TB is closely related to socioeconomic status; higher rates occur among persons in low-income groups (38). Special control strategies targeted toward these low-income groups are needed. In addition, community leaders from high-risk populations and service providers (e.g., health, welfare, and housing) for these groups should be involved in planning and implementing programs (8).

Implementation of TB prevention and control efforts among lower socioeconomic groups presents special problems because these groups usually have less access to care, are more likely to have coexisting diseases, lack adequate shelter and transportation, and encounter more obstacles to treatment and health-care delivery. However, screening programs have demonstrated success in reaching these groups (39, 40).

Screening for TB infection among certain occupational groups may occur at the worksite or other community sites. Screening migrant farm workers for TB infection is best conducted near home sites rather than at temporary work locations so that preventive therapy can be completed more easily for those who are infected (41). High-risk groups also may be screened whenever they have access to health care.

Persons Who Use Alcohol and Other Noninjecting Drugs

Because many persons who use alcohol and other noninjecting drugs are members of high-risk groups (e.g., HIV-infected persons, the homeless, residents of correctional facilities, and medically underserved, low-income persons), they should be included in screening activities if they also belong to a high-risk group. Because persons who use alcohol and other noninjecting drugs may be at risk for repeated exposure to others who have TB, a risk assessment and, if necessary, screening for TB infection should be administered on admission to a treatment program and on an annual basis, unless these persons are known to be tuberculin positive. Screening is not recommended for those persons who use alcohol and other noninjecting drugs but who are not members of high-risk groups because this screening diverts resources from higher priority activities.

RECOMMENDATIONS FOR SCREENING CHILDREN AND ADOLESCENTS

Although children in high-risk groups or those exposed to adults in high-risk groups may benefit from screening, most children are not members of high-risk groups. Mass or individual screening of children at low risk is not recommended because screening persons at low risk for TB infection diverts resources from higher priority activities and identifies few infected children (42, 43). In addition, the reactions in low-risk children are often false-positive.

School-based screening for TB infection among children was started in the 1950s when infection and disease rates were higher than at present. The major purpose of school testing is to identify infected children who can be treated before the infection progresses to infectious TB during adolescence or adulthood. Because broad-based school testing involves screening large numbers of low-risk children and because the majority of children who have pediatric TB are preschool age, generalized school screening as a public health measure is an ineffective method of detecting or preventing cases of childhood TB and should be discontinued (43).

Well-conducted contact tracing of infectious cases and refugee or immigration testing are more efficient methods than nonselective school-based testing for detecting children who have TB infection. However, targeted testing of high-risk children should be encouraged and may be conducted in the school setting (44). Before any testing program for children is implemented, arrangements for evaluation and treatment of children who test positive should be in place.

REPEAT SCREENING OF PERSONS AT CONTINUING RISK FOR EXPOSURE

The need for repeat skin testing should be determined by the likelihood of continued exposure to infectious TB. All tuberculin-negative persons should be retested if they are exposed to an infectious person. In some institutional and group-living environments (e.g., hospitals, prisons, nursing homes, and shelters for the homeless), the risk for exposure is enough to justify repeat testing at regular intervals. The frequency of repeat testing depends on the degree of risk for exposure, as determined by locally generated data. To assist in making these decisions, local facilities should compile and analyze their epidemiologic and programmatic data.

ROLE OF HEALTH DEPARTMENTS

In conjunction with local providers serving high-risk populations, health departments should assist in the development, implementation, and evaluation of TB screening programs appropriate for their communities by participating in specific activities:

ESTABLISHING PRIORITIES FOR PREVENTION AND CONTROL ACTIVITIES

Screening for TB infection should not be given preference over higher priority activities, especially complete treatment of patients having TB or TB/HIV infection as well as prompt, effective contact investigation.

DETERMINING PRIORITIES FOR SCREENING ACTIVITIES

This determination should be made by evaluating available resources, the probability of infection and disease among groups in the community, and the ability to ensure that those persons infected with TB will complete preventive therapy. Groups with the highest screening priorities include contacts of persons suspected or confirmed to have TB and patients having HIV infection.

REVIEWING EPIDEMIOLOGIC AND PROGRAMMATIC DATA TO IDENTIFY ADDITIONAL GROUPS FOR WHOM SCREENING PROGRAMS SHOULD BE DEVELOPED

This review includes (a) assessing the incidence, prevalence, and sociodemographic characteristics of persons having TB or TB infection; (b) identifying high-risk groups and settings to determine whether a need for screening is indicated; (c) designing tuberculin screening programs to reach the high-risk groups in communities; and (d) ensuring completion of preventive therapy.

IDENTIFYING AND ESTABLISHING WORKING RELATIONSHIPS WITH PERSONS, FACILITIES, AND AGENCIES PROVIDING HEALTH-CARE SERVICES TO HIGH-RISK POPULATIONS

These service providers should be assisted in the development, implementation, and evaluation of screening programs appropriate to the needs of the community. The decision to initiate a skin testing program for a high-risk group should be based primarily on the ability of the TB control program and health-care providers to provide adequate preventive therapy services (i.e., tuberculin skin testing, reading and interpreting the tests, evaluating persons who have positive results, initiating preventive therapy when appropriate, monitoring patients for adverse reactions, and ensuring that patients complete preventive therapy). To be effective, the plan for evaluation and treatment should be developed before testing begins.

ASSISTING HEALTH-CARE PROVIDERS WHO SERVE HIGH-RISK GROUPS

These providers should be assisted in providing screening services, evaluating data from screening programs to determine program effectiveness, and recommending appropriate future screening activities.

PROVIDING SUPPORT FOR STAFF TRAINING

Staff should be trained to perform, read, and record results of tuberculin skin tests; evaluate positive-tuberculin reactors for clinical TB and preventive therapy; provide preventive therapy and monitor for adherence and adverse drug reactions; and educate clients regarding the need for preventive therapy. The health department or facility may certify staff completing this training.

IDENTIFYING MEDICAL CONSULTANTS HAVING EXPERTISE IN TB PATIENT MANAGEMENT

These consultants should be able to assist with managing persons who have TB or are suspected to have TB, their contacts, and persons receiving preventive therapy.

ARRANGING REFERRALS AND MONITORING

Upon request, assistance should be provided in making arrangements for referring and monitoring persons who have clinical TB or adverse drug reactions while on preventive therapy.

REVIEWING SCREENING ACTIVITIES

Periodic assessments of screening activities are needed to examine the effectiveness of identifying infected persons and of ensuring that these persons complete preventive therapy.

EVALUATING SCREENING PROGRAMS

Regular assessments of screening programs are needed to determine their effectiveness. Recommendations for continuing or discontinuing screening programs should be made on the basis of their effectiveness.

REFERENCES: AS NUMBERED IN ORIGINAL PUBLICATION

1. American Thoracic Society/CDC. Diagnostic standards and classification of tuberculosis. Am Rev Respir Dis 1990;142:725–735.
2. CDC. Initial therapy for tuberculosis in the era of multidrug resistance: recommendations of the Advisory Council for the Elimination of Tuberculosis. MMWR 1993;42(No. RR-7).
3. American Thoracic Society/CDC. Treatment of tuberculosis and tuberculosis infection in adults and children. Am J Respir Crit Care Med 1994;149:1359–1374.
4. American Thoracic Society/CDC. Control of tuberculosis in the United States. Am Rev Respir Dis 1992;146:1623–1633.
5. CDC. The use of preventive therapy for tuberculous infection in the United States: recommendations of the Advisory Committee for Elimination of Tuberculosis. MMWR 1990;39(No. RR-8):9–12.
6. CDC. A strategic plan for the elimination of tuberculosis in the United States. MMWR 1989;38 (No. S-3).
7. CDC. Essential components of a tuberculosis program: recommendations of the Advisory Council for the Elimination of Tuberculosis. MMWR 1995;44(No. RR-11):1–16.
8. CDC. Prevention and control of tuberculosis in U.S. communities with at-risk minority populations: recommendations of the Advisory Council for the Elimination of Tuberculosis. MMWR 1992;41(No. RR-5):1–11.
9. Starke JR, Jacobs RF, Jereb J. Resurgence of tuberculosis in children. J Pediatr 1992;120:839–855.
10. Huebner RE, Schein MF, Bass JB Jr. The tuberculin skin test. Clin Infect Dis 1993;17:968–975.
11. Sbarbaro JA. Tuberculin test: a re-emphasis on clinical judgement [Editorial]. Am Rev Respir Dis 1985;132:177–178.
12. Snider DE Jr. Bacille Calmette-Guerin vaccinations and tuberculin skin tests. JAMA 1985;253:3438–3439.
13. CDC. Use of BCG vaccines in the control of tuberculosis: a joint statement by the ACIP and the Advisory Committee for Elimination of Tuberculosis. MMWR 1988;37:663–664, 669–675.
14. Caiaffa WT, Graham NMH, Galai N, Rizzo RT, Nelson KE, Vlahov D. Instability of delayed-type hypersensitivity skin test anergy in human immunodeficiency virus infection. Arch Intern Med (in press).
15. CDC. USPHS/IDSA guidelines for the prevention of opportunistic infections in persons infected with human immunodeficiency virus: a summary. MMWR 1995;44(No. RR-8).
16. CDC. Tuberculosis and human immunodeficiency virus infection: recommendations of the Advisory Committee for the Elimination of Tuberculosis (ACET). MMWR 1989;38:236–238, 243–250.
17. CDC. Purified protein derivative (PPD)-tuberculin anergy and HIV infection: guidelines for anergy testing and management of anergic persons at risk of tuberculosis. MMWR 1991;40(No. RR-5):27–33.
18. Sepulveda RL, Ferrer X, Latrach C, Sorensen RU. The influence of Calmette-Guerin Bacillus immunization on the booster effect of tuberculin testing in healthy young adults. Am Rev Respir Dis 1990;142:24–28.
19. Snider D. Pregnancy and tuberculosis. Chest 1984;86(Suppl):10S–13S.
20. Selwyn PA, Hartel D, Lewis VA, et al. A prospective study of the risk of tuberculosis among intravenous drug users with human immunodeficiency virus infection. N Engl J Med 1989;320:545–550.
21. Selwyn PA, Sckell BM, Alcabes P, Friedland GH, Klein RS, Schoenbaum EE. High risk of active tuberculosis in HIV-infected drug users with cutaneous anergy. JAMA 1992;268:504–509.
22. Rieder HL, Cauthen GM, Comstock GW, Snider DE Jr. Epidemiology of tuberculosis in the United States. Epidemiol Rev 1989;11:79–98.
23. Antonucci G, Girardi E, Raviglione MC, Ippolito G, Gruppo Italiano di Studio Tubercolosi e AIDS (GISTA). Risk factors for tuberculosis in HIV-infected persons: a prospective cohort study. JAMA 1995;274:143–148.
24. Reichman LB, Felton CP, Edsall JR. Drug dependence, a possible new risk factor for tuberculosis disease. Arch Intern Med 1979;139:337–339.
25. Braun MM, Byers RH, Heyward WL, et al. Acquired immunodeficiency syndrome and extrapulmonary tuberculosis in the United States. Arch Intern Med 1990;150:1913–1916.
26. CDC. Prevention and control of tuberculosis in correctional institutions: recommendations of the Advisory Committee for the Elimination of Tuberculosis. MMWR 1989;38:313–320, 325.
27. CDC. Prevention and control of tuberculosis in correctional facilities: recommendations of the Advisory Council for the Elimination of Tuberculosis. MMWR (in press).

28. CDC. Prevention and control of tuberculosis in facilities providing long-term care to the elderly: recommendations of the Advisory Committee for Elimination of Tuberculosis. MMWR 1990;39(No. RR-10):7–20.
29. CDC. Guidelines for preventing the transmission of Mycobacterium tuberculosis in health-care facilities, 1994. MMWR 1994;43(No. RR-13).
30. CDC. Prevention and control of tuberculosis among homeless persons: recommendations of the Advisory Council for the Elimination of Tuberculosis. MMWR 1992;41(No. RR-5):13–23.
31. Daley CL, Small PM, Schecter GF, et al. An outbreak of tuberculosis with accelerated progression among persons infected with the human immunodeficiency virus. N Engl J Med 1992;326:231–235.
32. Stead WW, Lofgren JP, Warren E, Thomas C. Tuberculosis as an endemic and nosocomial infection among the elderly in nursing homes. N Engl J Med 1985;312:1483–1487.
33. Hutton MD, Cauthen GM, Bloch AB. Results of a 29-state survey of tuberculosis in nursing homes and correctional facilities. Public Health Rep 1993;108:305–314.
34. Rieder HL, Cauthen GM, Kelly GD, Bloch AB, Snider DE Jr. Tuberculosis in the United States. JAMA 1989;262:385–389.
35. Cantwell MF, Snider DE Jr, Cauthen GM, Onorato IM. Epidemiology of tuberculosis in the United States, 1985 through 1992. JAMA 1994;272:535–539.
36. McKenna MT, McCray E, Onorato I. The epidemiology of tuberculosis among foreign-born persons in the United States, 1986 to 1993. N Engl J Med 1995;332:1071–1076.
37. CDC. Tuberculosis among foreign-born persons entering the United States: Recommendations of the Advisory Committee for Elimination of Tuberculosis. MMWR 1990;39(No. RR-18).
38. Hinman AR, Judd JM, Kolnik JP, Daitch PB. Changing risks in tuberculosis. Am J Epidemiol 1976;103:486–497.
39. Friedman LN, Sullivan GM, Bevilaqua RP, Loscos R. Tuberculosis screening in alcoholics and drug addicts. Am Rev Respir Dis 1987;136:1188–1192.
40. Grzybowski S, Allen EA, Black WA, et al. Inner-city survey for tuberculosis: evaluation of diagnostic methods. Am Rev Respir Dis 1987;135:1311–1315.
41. CDC. Prevention and control of tuberculosis in migrant farm workers: recommendations of the Advisory Council for the Elimination of Tuberculosis. MMWR 1992;41(No. RR-10).
42. American Academy of Pediatrics Committee on Infectious Diseases. Screening for tuberculosis in infants and children. Pediatrics 1994;93:131–134.
43. Starke JR. Universal screening for tuberculosis infection: school's out [Editorial]! JAMA 1995;274:652–653.
44. Mohle-Boetani JC, Miller B, Halpern M, et al. School-based screening for tuberculous infection: a cost-benefit analysis. JAMA 1995;274:613–619.

Essential Components of a Tuberculosis Prevention and Control Program

Original Citation: Centers for Disease Control and Prevention. Essential components of a tuberculosis prevention and control program: Recommendations of the Advisory Council for the Elimination of Tuberculosis. MMWR 1995;44(RR-11):1–16.

Original Author: Patricia M. Simone, MD.

Editor's Note: The information included here was based on a 1995 MMWR Reports and Recommendations issue (Vol. 44;RR-11) prepared by the Advisory Council for the Elimination of Tuberculosis (ACET) for the assessment of individual TB control programs by TB control program managers, policymakers, and other persons evaluating TB programs. The report defines essential components of a TB control program; the importance of prioritizing TB control activities and coordinating care, and using alternative approaches to TB control.

State and local health departments have primary responsibility for preventing and controlling TB. To meet this challenge successfully, TB control programs

should be able to administer activities that include the following core components:

- Conducting overall planning and development of policy,
- Identifying persons who have clinically active TB,
- Managing persons who have or who are suspected of having disease,
- Identifying and managing persons infected with M. tuberculosis,
- Providing laboratory and diagnostic services,
- Collecting and analyzing data, and
- Providing training and education.

In the United States, state and local health departments have legal responsibility for the prevention and control of TB in communities. Three strategies are
fundamental to the prevention and control of TB. The first priority is identifying and treating persons who have active TB; this priority entails identifying
persons who have TB, ensuring that they complete appropriate therapy, and,
in exceptional circumstances, using confinement measures. The second priority is finding and screening persons who have been in contact with TB patients
to determine whether they have TB infection or disease and providing them
with appropriate treatment. The third priority is screening high-risk populations to detect persons who are infected with M. tuberculosis and who could
benefit from therapy to prevent the infection from progressing to TB disease.

To implement these three strategies, public health TB control programs
should coordinate with health-care providers from several community organizations to ensure the provision of direct services for TB patients. Health departments are responsible for providing centralized, coordinated systems for
many activities extending beyond individual patient care (e.g., identifying TB
cases; ensuring that patients complete therapy; performing contact investigations; screening high-risk groups; and collecting, analyzing, and publishing epidemiologic and surveillance data).

PURPOSE

The Advisory Council for the Elimination of Tuberculosis (ACET) has prepared this report to
provide a national standard* for the assessment of individual TB control programs by TB control program managers, policymakers, and other persons evaluating TB programs. This report
also may be used to assist local programs in obtaining and maintaining adequate resources for
TB control activities. In addition to defining the essential components of a TB control program, these recommendations emphasize the importance of prioritizing TB control activities;
coordinating care with other health-care providers, facilities, and community organizations;
and using alternative approaches to TB control (e.g., the expanded use of directly observed
therapy, targeted screening and prevention programs to high-risk populations, and adoption
of current recommendations for the treatment of TB) (5–7). Although the size and structure
of TB control programs vary according to each community's specific needs, TB control program managers should attempt to incorporate each of these core components into program
activities.

---

*The word "standard" is being used to indicate a prototype established by authority, custom,
or general consent.

OVERALL PLANNING AND POLICY

To achieve effective TB control and progress toward TB elimination, TB control programs should develop an overall TB control strategy, including written policies and procedures, and should be able to provide guidance and oversight to local facilities and practitioners involved in TB control activities. TB control programs should ensure that appropriate laws and adequate staff and funding are available to support TB control activities. These programs also should form networks and coalitions with community groups to assist with implementing TB control activities.

AN OVERALL TB CONTROL STRATEGY AND WRITTEN POLICIES AND PROCEDURES

TB control programs should develop an overall TB control strategy in collaboration with local health-care providers, professional societies, and voluntary organizations. To determine specific needs, the program should use local TB morbidity data and standard indicators of program performance (e.g., the rate of completion of therapy). The plan should be developed by the state or local ACET in conjunction with community TB coalition representatives. The TB control strategy should outline program priorities and objectives reflecting the specific needs of the community and the roles of the various agencies, organizations, and providers. TB control programs should also have written policies and procedures that clearly define the standard of practice for TB treatment and prevention in the community (1, 5–18), and periodically revised as needed.

ADVISING LOCAL INSTITUTIONS AND PRACTITIONERS

TB control programs should provide consultation and oversight for the TB control activities of local facilities and practitioners (and local health departments where appropriate) to ensure that these efforts reflect current standards of care and public health practice. The consultation may be provided by either health department staff or local or regional medical experts who have agreed to act as consultants for the health department. Consultants should be available to advise local practitioners about patient management problems (e.g., monitoring treatment adherence); at least one consultant should be experienced in treating patients having drug-resistant TB. Information on the latest laboratory techniques and technology, guidance about appropriate laboratory methods for local facilities and laboratories, and assistance in conducting contact or outbreak investigations should be available from TB control programs or their consultants. TB programs should seek opportunities to inform persons or facilities about activities and technologies that can improve TB services.

APPROPRIATE LAWS AND REGULATIONS TO SUPPORT TB CONTROL ACTIVITIES

TB control programs periodically should review applicable laws, regulations, and policies to ensure their consistency with currently recommended medical and public health practices (8). States and municipalities should create laws, regulations, and policies that provide support and a legal basis for the following TB control activities:

- Ensuring the prompt, mandatory reporting of each confirmed and suspected case of TB;
- Observing state and local laws and regulations protecting patient confidentiality;
- Examining persons at high risk for TB infection and disease and prescribing and monitoring appropriate treatment for these persons;
- Ensuring that a treatment plan is devised for all hospitalized patients before their discharge;
- Ensuring rapid laboratory examination of specimens and reporting of results (including susceptibility-test results) to the appropriate health department and the requesting clinician;
- Ensuring that patients who have TB receive appropriate treatment until they are cured;
- Protecting the health of the public by isolating and treating persons who have infectious TB;

- Detaining persons who, though not infectious, are unwilling or unable to complete treatment and who are at risk for becoming infectious again and acquiring drug-resistant TB; and
- Treating patients without consideration of their ability to pay.

States also should require health-care facilities and congregate-living settings (e.g., correctional facilities) to apply recommended measures for infection control.

ADEQUATE AND APPROPRIATE STAFF TO CONDUCT TB CONTROL ACTIVITIES

TB control programs should have adequate and appropriate staff to ensure the fulfillment of TB control activities outlined in this report. The number and type of staff for these programs may vary, depending on the local TB morbidity and the specific needs of the community. Staff are necessary for program planning, program funding, record-keeping, education, and coordination of health department activities with other TB control activities in the community. All TB control programs should have a designated program manager. These programs should have access to, or have on staff, epidemiologists qualified to conduct data-based evaluation and surveillance activities.

Community outreach workers are needed to deliver directly observed TB therapy, thereby ensuring continuity and completion of treatment. Outreach workers may also be involved in other activities (e.g., educating patients, observing preventive therapy, conducting contact investigations, arranging or providing transportation, assisting patients with social services, serving as interpreters, and assisting clinicians with clinical services). These outreach workers may be nurses or lay persons specifically trained for these activities. The TB program should ensure that outreach workers have adequate clinical and administrative supervision.

Depending on clinic needs, clinic staff may be composed of various combinations of nurses, physicians, physician assistants, and other workers. In many areas, clinics have nurse managers responsible for providing most of the education, treatment, clinical monitoring, prevention services, and supervisory needs of the clinic. A physician who is qualified and trained in the diagnosis, management, and clinical monitoring of TB should be available on staff or employed on a contract basis. Clinic staff should have characteristics appropriate to the community's cultural and language needs.

ADEQUATE FUNDING TO CONDUCT TB CONTROL ACTIVITIES

TB control programs should seek funding for TB control activities from federal, state, local, and private sources. They should work with local organizations (e.g., state and local medical societies, lung associations, and TB coalition members) to educate policymakers about the local TB problem and local program priorities, needs, and objectives.

NETWORKS WITH COMMUNITY GROUPS

Optimal TB prevention and control activities require a multidisciplinary approach. Thus, TB control programs in communities having a high prevalence of TB should form networks and coalitions with local groups (e.g., cultural and ethnic organizations, community clinics, places of worship, professional societies, lung associations, and medical and nursing schools). In collaborating with these community groups, the TB control program should (a) ensure that community leaders, health-care providers, and policymakers are knowledgeable about TB; (b) help educate the public about TB; and (c) provide guidance and assistance for local screening and prevention services. Coalitions with community groups help TB control programs reach high-risk groups more effectively and provide culturally appropriate services. TB control programs should educate and advise community groups to ensure the quality and appropriateness of TB control activities in accordance with the community's needs. The National Coalition to Eliminate Tuberculosis exemplifies a national coalition involved in educating health-care providers and the public about TB.

MANAGING PERSONS WHO HAVE DISEASE OR WHO ARE SUSPECTED OF HAVING DISEASE

TB control programs should ensure that the services needed to evaluate, treat, and monitor TB patients are readily available in each community. In many areas, these services may be provided directly by the state TB control program. In other areas, local TB control programs or health-care professionals, with supervision and consultation from the state TB control program, provide treatment services to patients. Although some patients may undergo most of their evaluation and treatment in settings other than the health department, the major responsibility for monitoring and ensuring the quality of all TB-related activities in the community should be undertaken by the health department as part of its duties to protect the public health.

The public health goals of TB patient management are to initiate treatment promptly and ensure the completion of effective therapy to cure illness, reduce transmission, and prevent the development of drug-resistant TB.

CLINICAL SERVICES

Developing a Treatment Plan

A specific health department employee (case manager) should be assigned primary responsibility and held accountable for ensuring that each patient is educated about TB and its treatment, that therapy is continuous, and that contacts are examined. Some specific responsibilities also may be assigned to other persons (e.g., clinical supervisors [nurses, physicians, or physician assistants], outreach workers, health educators, and social workers).

As soon as TB is diagnosed or suspected, treatment should be started, and the TB case should be reported to the health department. Within 3 working days after the case is reported, a health department worker should visit the patient in the hospital or home to initiate patient education, identify contacts, make appropriate referrals for medical evaluation, and detect possible problems related to adherence to therapy. In cooperation with the other medical, nursing, and outreach staff providing care to the patient, the case manager should develop an initial treatment and monitoring plan based on the initial visit, the medical and nursing assessment, and other available information. The initial treatment plan should be developed within 1 week of diagnosis (i.e., within 1 week of initiation of therapy for a person suspected to have TB or within 1 week of identification of a person having a positive culture). This treatment plan should be reviewed regularly and modified as needed when additional relevant information becomes available (e.g., susceptibility-test results) or when the care of the patient is transferred from one provider to another.

The treatment plan should include the specifics of the medical regimen, a monitoring plan for toxicity and for clinical and bacteriologic response, and an assessment of the patient's social, behavioral, and additional medical needs that may affect continuity or completion of therapy (19). The health department employee responsible for monitoring treatment adherence should identify and implement methods that promote adherence and that are appropriate to the patient's needs and desires. A treatment plan should be designed for efficiency and economy of services and convenience to the patient.

When developing and implementing a treatment plan, TB control programs should work closely with health-care providers from local hospitals, drug-treatment centers, HIV clinics, correctional facilities, health maintenance organizations, private physicians' offices, and other facilities where TB patients receive medical care. TB control programs should fulfill their mandated responsibilities and also respect the relationship between patient and primary health-care provider.

Clinic Services

Clinic services provided by TB control programs should be accessible and acceptable to the members of the community served by the clinic. Clinic hours should be convenient and preferably should include some evening hours for persons who work or attend school during the day. The clinic should be easily accessible by public transportation, or transportation should be provided. Intervals between the time of referral and the time of appointment and waiting times in the clinic should be kept to a minimum. In busy TB clinics or multipurpose clinics, priority should be given to persons having TB or suspected of having TB and to persons receiving TB medications. Clinic services, including diagnostic evaluation, medications, and transportation, should be provided without consideration of the patient's ability to pay. The clinic should have staff members who speak the same language and have similar cultural and socioeconomic backgrounds as the community served by the clinic, or the clinic should employ persons trained to work in cross-cultural settings.

Promoting Adherence

Methods for promoting adherence to therapy should be tailored to the patient's needs, lifestyle, social support system, and beliefs about health. An assessment of these factors should be included in the development of a treatment plan (19, 20). Patients should be educated about the causes and effects of TB, the dosing and possible adverse reactions of their medication, and the importance of taking their medication according to the treatment plan. To facilitate adherence, the plan should use short-course treatment regimens and, for patients whose therapy is not directly observed, fixed-dose combination tablets. Providing transportation to the clinic also is important for promoting adherence. A welcoming and respectful atmosphere within the clinic setting is fundamental to maintaining adherence.

Consideration should be given to treating all patients with directly observed therapy (DOT) (6, 7). With DOT, a health-care provider or other responsible person observes the patient swallowing each dose of anti-TB medication. DOT may be administered with daily or intermittent regimens and may be given to patients in an office or clinic setting or by an outreach worker in the patient's home, place of employment, school, or other mutually agreed-upon place. In some instances, DOT may be administered by the staff of correctional facilities or drug-treatment programs, home health-care workers, staff of maternal and child health facilities, or a responsible community or family member.

Incentives and enablers should be available to enhance adherence to therapy. These incentives range from simple approaches (e.g., offering a cup of coffee or food discount coupons and talking with a patient while he or she is waiting in the clinic) to complex approaches (e.g., obtaining food and housing for a homeless patient).

Health-care professionals, including private practitioners, who become aware of a TB patient who has demonstrated an inability or unwillingness to adhere to a prescribed treatment regimen should consult the health department. The TB control program should assist in evaluating the patient for the causes of nonadherence to therapy and provide assistance (e.g., outreach-worker services) to enable the patient to complete the recommended therapy. If the patient still fails to adhere to treatment, the health department should take appropriate action based on local laws and regulations. This action could entail seeking court-ordered DOT or detention for those patients who are unwilling or unable to complete their treatment and who are infectious or who are at risk for becoming infectious or developing drug-resistant TB.

Additional services may be necessary to facilitate continuity and completion of therapy. Social workers, translators, and referral sources for drug-treatment services should be available in the clinic or easily accessible to the patients.

Referral System for Other Medical Problems

A system should be in place to facilitate referral of TB patients for evaluation and treatment of other medical problems, including those conditions (e.g., HIV infection, underlying malignancy, diabetes mellitus, and substance abuse) that may affect the course or outcome of TB treatment. Consultants should see referred patients in a timely fashion, and the assessment and recommendations of the consultant should be made available promptly to the referring health-care provider. If patients receive care in more than one setting, treatment should be coordinated with the other health-care providers to ensure continuity and completion of therapy, minimize drug interactions, and avoid duplication of efforts. The TB program should take primary responsibility for ensuring TB treatment and monitoring for adherence.

Clinical Consultative Services

Expert medical consultation should be available for management of all TB patients, including those who have drug-resistant TB. These consultative services should be available to the TB control program and health-care providers in the community. The consultation may be provided by a staff member of the TB control program or by a local or regional consultant collaborating with the health department.

INPATIENT CARE

Regardless of the patient's ability to pay, appropriate accommodations should be available for any TB patient requiring inpatient hospital care for TB or other conditions. The facility should have effective infection control measures in place to prevent transmission of TB infection in the hospital (12). Medical staff knowledgeable about the management of TB patients should be available to assist in the care of the patient while hospitalized. In addition, appropriate medications should be available in the facility so that the patient can continue therapy in the hospital. Appropriate diagnostic services (e.g., radiology and mycobacteriology) should be available to monitor the patient for adverse reactions, the progress of treatment, and other medical conditions. The local TB program and the facility should develop and implement protocols to ensure rapid reporting of known or suspected TB cases to the local health department.

CONFINEMENT CAPABILITY

To ensure that patients receive treatment until they are cured, TB control programs should have adequate legal authority and appropriate facilities available to isolate and treat patients who have infectious TB. When all less restrictive measures have failed, TB control programs also should have the authority to detain patients unwilling or unable to complete their treatment. This authority also should apply to nonadherent patients who are no longer infectious, but who are at risk for again becoming infectious or for the development of drug-resistant TB.

INFECTION CONTROL

TB control programs should serve the medical community as sources of information and consultation regarding appropriate infection control practices (12). During interactions with the medical community, TB control programs should emphasize the need to maintain a high level of suspicion for TB in evaluating patients who have TB symptoms and also the importance of early diagnosis and isolation and prompt initiation of therapy. The programs should give expert advice or provide referrals to experts for information about appropriate infection control measures for different settings (e.g., hospitals, clinics, nursing homes, correctional facilities, homeless shelters, and drug-treatment centers).

TB control programs should provide guidance to local facilities and the community to ensure the availability of an appropriate number of TB isolation rooms to meet community needs. Because local needs may change, the adequacy of the number of isolation rooms should be reassessed each year as part of the evaluation of the TB control program.

TB control programs should educate the staff of facilities providing care for TB patients about the need for routine periodic evaluation of infection control practices and may also assist in the evaluation process. Assistance may include providing current recommendations and regulations to the facility, providing names of experts in infection control, or providing access to personnel involved in programmatic evaluations.

COORDINATING CARE WITH OTHER HEALTH-CARE PROVIDERS AND FACILITIES

TB patients often receive care in multiple settings, including HIV clinics, drug-treatment centers, correctional facilities, hospitals, nursing homes, or primary care clinics. When patients move among these various settings, continuity and completion of therapy may be compromised unless a system for the coordination of care exists. Discharge planning for hospitalized patients should begin as soon as TB is diagnosed (i.e., at the time of initiation of therapy in a suspected case or identification of a positive culture in a confirmed case). A representative from the TB control program should visit the patient in the hospital to identify contacts, collect information for the initial treatment plan, and ensure that no obstacles to the patient's follow-up care exist (see Managing Persons Who Have Disease or Who Are Suspected of

Having Disease). To provide and coordinate continuous TB treatment and to facilitate transfers of care, TB control programs should communicate regularly with providers and facilities involved in TB patient care, including hospitals, infection-control practitioners, private practitioners, community clinics, correctional facilities, homeless shelters, and drug-treatment centers. TB control programs should consider using a computerized system for coordinating the care of TB patients.

IDENTIFYING PERSONS WHO HAVE CLINICALLY ACTIVE TB

DIAGNOSTIC METHODS

Clinics providing services for TB patients should have access to the basic methods necessary for the diagnosis of TB, including tuberculin skin testing, chest radiography, sputum induction, and mycobacteriology services for smears, cultures, and drug-susceptibility testing (see Laboratory and Diagnostic Services). TB control programs should provide guidance to facilities about appropriate diagnostic methods for different circumstances. Sputum smear examinations and cultures for mycobacteria should be performed on persons suspected of having active pulmonary or laryngeal TB. Tuberculin testing is the standard method for screening asymptomatic populations for infection with M. tuberculosis. However, screening initially for disease rather than infection may be more appropriate in some circumstances (e.g., when tuberculin skin-test results may be unreliable, when application and reading of the test may be impractical, or when the consequences of an undiagnosed case may be severe). For example, because elderly persons living in long-term care facilities are at high risk for the development of TB and may be anergic, all patients admitted to these facilities should have an initial screening chest radiograph. Chest radiography also may be the preferable screening method for persons incarcerated in jails or residing in other settings where TB is common and where diagnostic delays may result in large numbers of persons being exposed to TB.

CASE FINDING

Most persons who have TB are diagnosed when they seek medical care for symptoms caused by TB or other medical conditions. Therefore, for early identification of TB cases, health-care providers in the community must have an awareness of TB. Conducting contact investigations is another important way to find TB cases and may yield approximately 700 cases per 100,000 persons evaluated (CDC Program Management Reports 1990–1992, unpublished data). Health departments should seek cases of TB through active surveillance of mycobacteriology laboratories.

Routine screening with chest radiographs to identify persons who have disease is justifiable in certain situations, particularly when the prevalence of TB is extremely high (e.g., among homeless populations or certain immigrant or refugee populations from areas that have a high prevalence of TB) or when the consequences of an undiagnosed case of TB are severe (e.g., in residential facilities for HIV-infected persons, correctional facilities, homeless shelters [21, 22], or nursing homes). Using local epidemiologic data, TB programs should identify these high-risk groups and settings and determine whether screening is indicated.

CONTACT INVESTIGATION

Staff of TB control programs should begin a contact investigation as soon as they are notified of a suspected or confirmed case of TB. TB control programs should educate health-care providers in the community about the need for prompt reporting of suspected cases. Contact investigations are important for identifying persons who have TB infection and who are at high risk for the development of active disease. Contact investigations are also important for detecting cases of active TB (5).

The priority, speed, and extent of a contact investigation should be influenced by the likelihood of transmission (based on the characteristics of the source patient, environment, and contacts) and the possible consequences of infection (especially for HIV-infected contacts or contacts who are young children).

IDENTIFYING AND MANAGING PERSONS INFECTED WITH M. TUBERCULOSIS

TB SKIN TESTING OF HIGH-RISK GROUPS

TB control programs should assess the prevalence and incidence of TB and the sociodemographic characteristics of TB patients and infected persons in each community. On the basis of these data, TB control programs should design tuberculin screening programs to reach the community's high-risk groups (13, 16). Regular evaluation of the usefulness of these screening programs is extremely important because, in general, screening should not be given preference over higher priority activities (e.g., treatment of TB patients and contact investigation). The practice of screening low-risk groups should be discontinued.

TB control programs should identify and establish working relationships with persons, facilities, and agencies providing health-care services to high-risk populations and should assist them in developing and implementing screening programs appropriate for various situations. Decisions to initiate programs to skin test high-risk groups should be based on the ability of the TB control program and these community groups to provide adequate preventive therapy services. For appropriate implementation of screening programs, the TB control program and local facilities should be able to perform tuberculin skin tests, read and interpret the tests, evaluate those persons who have positive results, initiate preventive therapy when appropriate, monitor patients for adverse reactions, and ensure that patients complete preventive therapy. The plan for evaluation and treatment of patients should be developed before testing begins.

Health-care providers serving high-risk groups should receive assistance from TB control programs in planning and providing these services, including training staff and evaluating screening programs to determine their effectiveness. Members of high-risk groups should be educated about the problem of TB in their community and should be involved in the implementation of screening and prevention programs.

LABORATORY AND DIAGNOSTIC SERVICES

CHEST RADIOGRAPH AND INTERPRETATION

Outpatient and inpatient facilities offering TB treatment should have ready access to a sufficient quantity of radiology equipment and enough trained radiology technicians so that chest radiographs can be obtained each day during clinic hours for all patients needing them. Furthermore, the chest radiograph should be interpreted by a qualified person, and the report of the chest radiograph findings should be available within 24 hours.

MYCOBACTERIOLOGY LABORATORY

To ensure that results of acid-fast examinations of specimens are available promptly (ideally, within 24 hours of specimen collection), TB control programs should have access to adequate mycobacteriology laboratory services. Reports of isolation and identification of M. tuberculosis should be available within 10–14 days, and reports of drug-susceptibility tests should be available within 15–30 days of specimen collection. The TB control program should work closely with the laboratory to ensure rapid delivery of specimens to the laboratory and prompt laboratory reporting of acid-fast bacilli smears, culture results, and results of drug-susceptibility tests to the clinician and health department. The laboratory should use rapid laboratory methods, including fluorescent acid-fast staining procedures, inoculation of a liquid medium as primary culture, nucleic acid probes to identify M. tuberculosis, and, using radiometric (e.g., BACTEC®) or similar systems, testing of M. tuberculosis isolates for susceptibility to the first-line drugs (23). These mycobacteriology laboratory services also should be available to TB control programs for monitoring bacteriologic response to therapy.

DIAGNOSTIC SERVICES TO ASSESS DRUG TOXICITY

The outpatient and inpatient facilities where TB treatment is offered should provide, or have access to, diagnostic services for monitoring patients for potential adverse reactions to anti-TB medications. At least monthly during therapy, patients receiving anti-TB medications should be evaluated by a health-care professional (e.g., nurse, physician, or physician assistant) and questioned about possible adverse reactions. The facilities offering TB treatment should be able to perform visual acuity and color vision evaluations on site. Blood tests for liver enzymes, blood urea nitrogen, creatinine, uric acid, complete blood count, and platelets may be performed at an outside laboratory; however, phlebotomy services should be available on site. Audiometry should be available on site or at another accessible location. In geographic areas that have a high prevalence of drug-resistant TB, testing of serum levels for anti-TB medications, especially cycloserine, should be available through a reference laboratory.

HIV TESTING AND COUNSELING

All persons who have confirmed or suspected TB should be offered HIV counseling and antibody testing. If TB clinics are unable to perform on-site counseling and testing, they should coordinate with HIV-testing programs to make these services available. In geographic areas that have a high prevalence of HIV-infected persons, TB prevention and control staff should be trained and qualified to provide routine HIV counseling and antibody testing.

DATA COLLECTION AND ANALYSIS

CASE REPORTING

TB control programs should ensure and facilitate TB case reporting from various community sources (e.g., physicians, laboratories, hospitals, and pharmacies) and routinely monitor the completeness of reporting and the duration of time between diagnosis and reporting. TB control programs also should communicate regularly with infection-control practitioners in hospitals and other facilities that frequently diagnose TB. Case reporting is essential to the compilation of national, state, and local morbidity reports and to program planning and evaluation, and prompt reporting is necessary for effective contact tracing.

TB REGISTRY

To carry out mandatory community public health responsibilities, health department TB control programs should maintain a computerized record system (case registry) with up-to-date information on all current clinically active and suspected TB cases in the community. To ensure follow-up of all TB patients and those persons suspected of having TB, registry information (e.g., smear, culture, and susceptibility results; clinical status; chest radiograph results; and doses of medications being administered) should be obtained and updated on a continuing basis. A specific health department staff member should review detailed registry information for TB cases at least monthly to identify patients who have potential problems with adherence or response to therapy (e.g., patients who have persistently positive sputum or who are taking medications to which their TB organisms are resistant) and to ensure follow-up (e.g., initiating field follow-up visits or arranging medical consultation with providers). TB control programs also should maintain records on the examination and treatment status of the contacts of infectious TB patients and other groups of high-risk infected persons (e.g., persons coinfected with M. tuberculosis and HIV).

PROTECTION OF CONFIDENTIALITY

TB control programs should devise policies to ensure the data security and confidentiality of TB records. Strategies should be in place to protect all TB reports, records, and files containing patient names or other identifying information. Local policies regarding the security and confidentiality of such information, including HIV test results, must adhere to all laws applicable in state and local jurisdictions (8, 24). TB control programs should collaborate with HIV programs to develop and implement such policies.

DRUG RESISTANCE SURVEILLANCE

TB control programs should ensure that drug-susceptibility tests are performed on all initial isolates of M. tuberculosis and that the results are reported promptly to the primary care provider and the local health department. TB control programs should monitor local drug resistance rates to assess the effectiveness of local TB control efforts and to determine the appropriateness of the currently recommended initial TB treatment regimen for the area.

DATA ANALYSIS AND PROGRAM EVALUATION

To determine morbidity rates, trends, and demographic characteristics of the TB patient population in the area, TB control programs should analyze the data collected each year. Local health departments should rapidly report cases, including the necessary demographic information, to state health departments, and states should regularly forward the reports to CDC. Timely and complete reporting is essential for local, state, and national public health planning and assessment.

TB control programs should assess program performance by determining the rates for completion of therapy, contact identification, and initiation and completion of preventive therapy. At least annually, TB control program staff should assess progress toward achievement of program objectives. To facilitate the monitoring of TB morbidity and program performance, programs should implement computerized systems for data collection and analysis. Program evaluation reports should be shared with the appropriate public, private, and community groups.

TB control programs should periodically review screening activities to assess their effectiveness in identifying infected persons and in ensuring that these persons are completing courses of preventive therapy when appropriate. If reviews demonstrate that few or no new cases are being identified by particular screening activities, these activities should be discontinued.

Programs also should conduct periodic reviews of selected records systems (e.g., laboratory reports, pharmacy reports, AIDS registries, and death certificates) to validate the surveillance system and to detect any failure to report cases.

TB control programs should analyze each new TB case and each death caused by TB to determine whether the case or death could have been prevented. Based on such a review, new policies should be developed and implemented to reduce the number of preventable cases and deaths.

In collaboration with community-based organizations and professional societies, health departments should prepare annual reports based on these assessments. These reports should document the extent and nature of the TB problem in the area, assess the adequacy of prevention and control measures, and provide recommendations for program improvements. Some TB programs may determine that an outside review by experts from the state health department, CDC, local lung associations, or other TB experts may be helpful to determine methods for improving program performance and community TB control and for providing support for major changes (e.g., significant restructuring or acquisition of new resources).

TRAINING AND EDUCATION

STAFF TRAINING

TB control programs should provide appropriate training and evaluation for all program staff at time of employment and at regular intervals so that staff can maintain an accurate, up-to-date level of knowledge about TB, public health practice, management and evaluation skills, and other related topics.

FEALTH-CARE PROVIDERS AND MEMBERS OF THE COMMUNITY

TB control programs should provide leadership in TB education in the community. To determine needs for training and education, TB control programs should monitor the level of knowledge about TB among health-care providers, policymakers, and other community members who provide services to TB patients (e.g., the staff of social services departments, correctional services departments, mental health offices, and legal service offices). TB control programs should work closely with medical and nursing schools, schools of public health, community-based organizations, professional societies, minority advocacy groups, and others to meet the training and education needs of the community.

REFERENCES: AS NUMBERED IN ORIGINAL PUBLICATION

1. CDC. A strategic plan for the elimination of tuberculosis in the United States. MMWR 1989;38 (No. S-3).
5. American Thoracic Society/CDC. Control of tuberculosis in the United States. Am Rev Respir Dis 1992;146:1623–1633.
6. CDC. Initial therapy for tuberculosis in the era of multidrug resistance: recommendations of the Advisory Council for the Elimination of Tuberculosis. MMWR 1993;42(No. RR-7).
7. American Thoracic Society/CDC. Treatment of tuberculosis and tuberculosis infection in adults and children. Am J Respir Crit Care Med 1994;149:1359–1374.
8. CDC. Tuberculosis control laws—United States, 1993: recommendations of the Advisory Council for the Elimination of Tuberculosis (ACET). MMWR 1993;42(No. RR-15).
9. American Thoracic Society/CDC. Diagnostic standards and classification of tuberculosis. Am Rev Respir Dis 1990;142:725–735.
10. CDC. Tuberculosis and human immunodeficiency virus infection: recommendations of the Advisory Committee for the Elimination of Tuberculosis (ACET). MMWR 1989;38:236–238, 243–250.
11. CDC. Prevention and control of tuberculosis in correctional institutions: recommendations of the Advisory Committee for the Elimination of Tuberculosis. MMWR 1989;38:313–320, 325.
12. CDC. Guidelines for preventing the transmission of Mycobacterium tuberculosis in health-care facilities, 1994. MMWR 1994;43(No. RR-13).
13. CDC. Screening for tuberculosis and tuberculous infection in high-risk populations: recommendations of the Advisory Committee for Elimination of Tuberculosis. MMWR 1995;44(No. RR-11):19–34.
14. CDC. Prevention and control of tuberculosis in facilities providing long-term care to the elderly: recommendations of the Advisory Committee for Elimination of Tuberculosis. MMWR 1990;39(No. RR-10):7–20.
15. CDC. Tuberculosis among foreign-born persons entering the United States: recommendations of the Advisory Committee for Elimination of Tuberculosis. MMWR 1990;39(No. RR-18):1–21.
16. CDC. The use of preventive therapy for tuberculous infection in the United States: recommendations of the Advisory Committee for Elimination of Tuberculosis. MMWR 1990;39(No. RR-8):8–12.
17. CDC. Prevention and control of tuberculosis in migrant farm workers: recommendations of the Advisory Council for the Elimination of Tuberculosis. MMWR 1992;41(No. RR-10):1–15.
18. CDC. Prevention and control of tuberculosis among homeless persons: recommendations of the Advisory Council for the Elimination of Tuberculosis. MMWR 1992;41(No. RR-5):13–23.
19. CDC. Improving patient adherence to tuberculosis treatment. Atlanta: US Department of Health and Human Services, Public Health Service, CDC, 1994.
20. Sumartojo E. When tuberculosis treatment fails: a social behavioral account of patient adherence. Am Rev Respir Dis 1993;147:1311–1320.
21. McAdam J, Brickner PW, Glicksman R, Edwards D, Fallon B, Yanowitch P. Tuberculosis in the SRO/homeless population. In: Brickner PW, Scharer LK, Conanan B, Elvy A, Savarese M, eds. Health care of homeless people. New York: Springer, 1985:155–175.
22. Barry MA, Wall C, Shirley L, et al. Tuberculosis screening in Boston's homeless shelters. Public Health Rep 1986;101:487–498.
23. Tenover FC, Crawford JT, Huebner RE, Geiter LJ, Horsburgh CR, Good RC. The resurgence of tuberculosis: is your laboratory ready? J Clin Microbiol 1993;31:767–770.
24. Gostin LO. Controlling the resurgent tuberculosis epidemic: a 50-state survey of TB statutes and proposals for reform. JAMA 1993;269:255–261.

Guidelines for Preventing the Transmission of Mycobacterium Tuberculosis in Health-Care Facilities

Original Citation: Centers for Disease Control and Prevention. Guidelines for preventing the transmission of mycobacterium tuberculosis in health-care facilities, 1994. MMWR 1994;43(RR-13);1–132.

Editor's Note: The information included here was based on an MMWR Reports and Recommendations publication (Vol.43;RR-13). The April, 1992 National Action Plan to Combat Multidrug-Resistant Tuberculosis, published by the National MDR-TB Task Force, called for the update and revision of guidelines for preventing nosocomial transmission of Mycobacterium tuberculosis. The original document gives the background of these recommendations and the epidemiology, transmission, pathogenesis, and risk for nosocomial transmission of TB.

Supervisory responsibility for the TB infection-control program should be assigned to a designated person or group of persons who should be given the authority to implement and enforce TB infection-control policies. An effective TB infection-control program requires early identification, isolation, and treatment of persons who have active TB. The primary emphasis of TB infection-control plans in health-care facilities should be achieving these three goals by the application of a hierarchy of control measures, including (a) the use of administrative measures to reduce the risk for exposure to persons who have infectious TB, (b) the use of engineering controls to prevent the spread and reduce the concentration of infectious droplet nuclei, and (c) the use of personal respiratory protective equipment in areas where there is still a risk for exposure to M. tuberculosis (e.g., TB isolation rooms). Implementation of a TB infection-control program requires risk assessment and development of a TB infection-control plan; early identification, treatment, and isolation of infectious TB patients; effective engineering controls; an appropriate respiratory protection program; HCW TB training, education, counseling, and screening; and evaluation of the program's effectiveness.

Designated personnel at health-care facilities should conduct a risk assessment for the entire facility and for each area** and occupational group, determine the risk for nosocomial or occupational transmission of M. tuberculosis, and implement an appropriate TB infection-control program. The extent of the TB infection-control program may range from a simple program emphasizing administrative controls in settings where there is minimal risk for exposure to M. tuberculosis, to a comprehensive program that includes administrative controls, engineering controls, and respiratory protection in settings where the risk for exposure is high. In all settings, administrative measures should be used to minimize the number of HCWs exposed to M. tuberculosis while still providing optimal care for TB patients. HCWs providing care to patients who have TB should be informed about the level of risk for transmission of M. tuberculosis and the appropriate control measures to minimize that risk.

In this document, the term "HCWs" refers to all the paid and unpaid persons working in health-care settings who have the potential for exposure to M. tuberculosis. This may include, but is not limited to, physicians; nurses; aides; dental workers; technicians; workers in laboratories and morgues; emergency medical service (EMS) personnel; students; part-time personnel; temporary

---

**Area: a structural unit (e.g., a hospital ward or laboratory) or functional unit (e.g., an internal medicine service) in which HCWs provide services to and share air with a specific patient population or work with clinical specimens that may contain viable M. tuberculosis organisms. The risk for exposure to M. tuberculosis in a given area depends on the prevalence of TB in the population served and the characteristics of the environment.

staff not employed by the health-care facility; and persons not involved directly in patient care but who are potentially at risk for occupational exposure to M. tuberculosis (e.g., volunteer workers and dietary, housekeeping, maintenance, clerical, and janitorial staff).

Although the purpose of this document is to make recommendations for reducing the risk for transmission of M. tuberculosis in health-care facilities, the process of implementing these recommendations must safeguard, in accordance with applicable state and federal laws, the confidentiality and civil rights of persons who have TB.

D. Fundamentals of TB Infection Control

An effective TB infection-control program requires early identification, isolation, and effective treatment of persons who have active TB. The primary emphasis of the TB infection-control plan should be on achieving these three goals. In all health-care facilities, particularly those in which persons who are at high risk for TB work or receive care, policies and procedures for TB control should be developed, reviewed periodically, and evaluated for effectiveness to determine the actions necessary to minimize the risk for transmission of M. tuberculosis.

The TB infection-control program should be based on a hierarchy of control measures. The first level of the hierarchy, and that which affects the largest number of persons, is using administrative measures intended primarily to reduce the risk for exposing uninfected persons to persons who have infectious TB. These measures include (a) developing and implementing effective written policies and protocols to ensure the rapid identification, isolation, diagnostic evaluation, and treatment of persons likely to have TB; (b) implementing effective work practices among HCWs in the health-care facility (e.g., correctly wearing respiratory protection and keeping doors to isolation rooms closed); (c) educating, training, and counseling HCWs about TB; and (d) screening HCWs for TB infection and disease.

The second level of the hierarchy is the use of engineering controls to prevent the spread and reduce the concentration of infectious droplet nuclei. These controls include (a) direct source control using local exhaust ventilation, (b) controlling direction of airflow to prevent contamination of air in areas adjacent to the infectious source, (c) diluting and removing contaminated air via general ventilation, and (d) air cleaning via air filtration or ultraviolet germicidal irradiation (UVGI).

The first two levels of the hierarchy minimize the number of areas in the health-care facility where exposure to infectious TB may occur, and they reduce, but do not eliminate, the risk in those few areas where exposure to M. tuberculosis can still occur (e.g., rooms in which patients with known or suspected infectious TB are being isolated and treatment rooms in which cough-inducing or aerosol-generating procedures are performed on such patients). Because persons entering such rooms may be exposed to M. tuberculosis, the third level of the hierarchy is the use of personal respiratory protective equipment in these and certain other situations in which the risk for infection with M. tuberculosis may be relatively higher.

Specific measures to reduce the risk for transmission of M. tuberculosis include the following:

- Assigning to specific persons in the health-care facility the supervisory responsibility for designing, implementing, evaluating, and maintaining the TB infection-control program (Section II.A).
- Conducting a risk assessment to evaluate the risk for transmission of M. tuberculosis in all areas of the health-care facility, developing a written TB infection-control program based on the risk assessment, and periodically repeating the risk assessment to evaluate the effectiveness of the TB infection-control program (Section II.B).
- Developing, implementing, and enforcing policies and protocols to ensure early identification, diagnostic evaluation, and effective treatment of patients who may have infectious TB (Section II.C; Suppl. 2).
- Providing prompt triage for and appropriate management of patients in the outpatient setting who may have infectious TB (Section II.D).
- Promptly initiating and maintaining TB isolation for persons who may have infectious TB and who are admitted to the inpatient setting (Section II.E; Suppl. 1).
- Effectively planning arrangements for discharge (Section II.E).
- Developing, installing, maintaining, and evaluating ventilation and other engineering controls to reduce the potential for airborne exposure to M. tuberculosis (Section II.F; Suppl. 3).
- Developing, implementing, maintaining, and evaluating a respiratory protection program (Section II.G; Suppl. 4).
- Using precautions while performing cough-inducing procedures (Section II.H; Suppl. 3).
- Educating and training HCWs about TB, effective methods for preventing transmission of M. tuberculosis, and the benefits of medical screening programs (Section II.I).
- Developing and implementing a program for routine periodic counseling and screening of HCWs for active TB and latent TB infection (Section II.J; Suppl. 2).
- Promptly evaluating possible episodes of M. tuberculosis transmission in health-care facilities, including PPD skin-test conversions among HCWs, epidemiologically associated cases among HCWs or patients, and contacts of patients or HCWs who have TB and who were not promptly identified and isolated (Section II.K).
- Coordinating activities with the local public health department, emphasizing reporting, and ensuring adequate discharge follow-up and the continuation and completion of therapy (Section II.L).

II. RECOMMENDATIONS

A. Assignment of Responsibility

- Supervisory responsibility for the TB infection-control program should be assigned to a designated person or group of persons with expertise in infection control, occupational health, and engineering. These persons should be given the authority to implement and enforce TB infection-control policies.

- If supervisory responsibility is assigned to a committee, one person should be designated as the TB contact person. Questions and problems can then be addressed to this person.

B. Risk Assessment, Development of the TB Infection-Control Plan, and Periodic Reassessment

1. Risk Assessment

a. General

- TB infection-control measures for each health-care facility should be based on a careful assessment of the risk for transmission of M. tuberculosis in that particular setting. The first step in developing the TB infection-control program should be to conduct a baseline risk assessment to evaluate the risk for transmission of M. tuberculosis in each area and occupational group in the facility (Table 1; Figure 1). Appropriate infection-control interventions can then be developed on the basis of actual risk. Risk assessments should be performed for all inpatient and outpatient settings (e.g., medical and dental offices).
- Regardless of risk level, the management of patients with known or suspected infectious TB should not vary. However, the index of suspicion for infectious TB among patients, the frequency of HCW PPD skin testing, the number of TB isolation rooms, and other factors will depend on whether the risk for transmission of M. tuberculosis in the facility, area, or occupational group is high, intermediate, low, very low, or minimal.
- The risk assessment should be conducted by a qualified person or group of persons (e.g., hospital epidemiologists, infectious disease specialists, pulmonary disease specialists, infection-control practitioners, health-care administrators, occupational health personnel, engineers, HCWs, or local public health personnel).
- The risk assessment should be conducted for the entire facility and for specific areas within the facility (e.g., medical, TB, pulmonary, or HIV wards; HIV, infectious disease, or pulmonary clinics; and emergency departments or other areas where TB patients might receive care or where cough-inducing procedures are performed). This should include both inpatient and outpatient areas. In addition, risk assessments should be conducted for groups of HCWs who work throughout the facility rather than in a specific area (e.g., respiratory therapists; bronchoscopists; environmental services, dietary, and maintenance personnel; and students, interns, residents, and fellows).
- Classification of risk for a facility, for a specific area, and for a specific occupational group should be based on (a) the profile of TB in the community; (b) the number of infectious TB patients admitted to the area or ward, or the estimated number of infectious TB patients to whom HCWs in an occupational group may be exposed; and (c) the results of analysis of HCW PPD test conversions (where applicable) and possible person-to-person transmission of M. tuberculosis (Figure 1).
- All TB infection-control programs should include periodic reassessments of risk. The frequency of repeat risk assessments should be based on the results of the most recent risk assessment (Table 2; Figure 1).

Table 1. Elements of a Risk Assessment for Tuberculosis (TB) in Health-Care Facilities

1. Review the community TB profile (from public health department data).

2. Review the number of TB patients who were treated in each area of the facility (both inpatient and outpatient). (This information can be obtained by analyzing laboratory surveillance data and by reviewing discharge diagnoses or medical and infection-control records.)

3. Review the drug-susceptibility patterns of TB isolates of patients who were treated at the facility.

4. Analyze purified protein derivative (PPD)-tuberculin skin-test results of health-care workers (HCWs), by area or by occupational group for HCWs not assigned to a specific area (e.g., respiratory therapists).

5. To evaluate infection-control parameters, review medical records of a sample of TB patients seen at the facility.
   Calculate intervals from:
   —Admission until TB suspected;
   —Admission until TB evaluation performed;
   —Admission until acid-fast bacilli (AFB) specimens ordered;
   —AFB specimens ordered until AFB specimens collected;
   —AFB specimens collected until AFB smears performed and reported;
   —AFB specimens collected until cultures performed and reported;
   —AFB specimens collected until species identification conducted and reported;
   —AFB specimens collected until drug-susceptibility tests performed and reported;
   —Admission until TB isolation initiated;
   —Admission until TB treatment initiated; and
   —Duration of TB isolation.
   Obtain the following additional information:
   —Were appropriate criteria used for discontinuing isolation?
   —Did the patient have a history of prior admission to the facility?
   —Was the TB treatment regimen adequate?
   —Were follow-up sputum specimens collected properly?
   —Was appropriate discharge planning conducted?

6. Perform an observational review of TB infection control practices.

7. Review the most recent environmental evaluation and maintenance procedures.

- The "minimal-risk" category applies only to an entire facility. A "minimal-risk" facility does not admit TB patients to inpatient or outpatient areas and is not located in a community with TB (i.e., counties or communities in which TB cases have not been reported during the previous year). Thus, there is essentially no risk for exposure to TB patients in the facility. This category may also apply to many outpatient settings (e.g., many medical and dental offices).

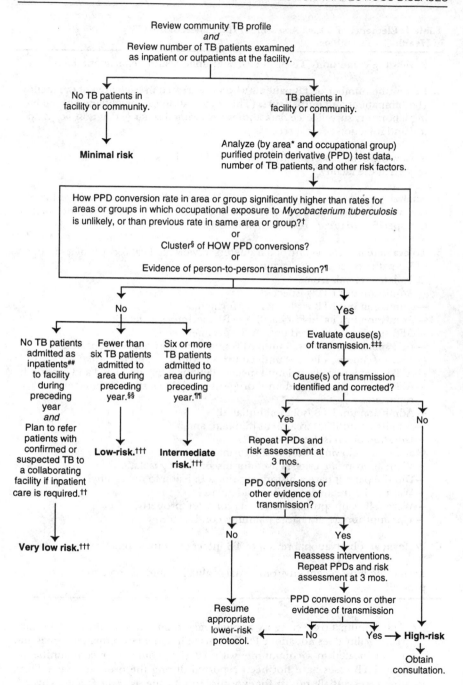

Figure 1. Protocol for conducting a tuberculosis (TB) risk assessment in a health-care facility.

*Area: a structural unit (e.g., a hospital ward or laboratory) or functional unit (e.g., an internal medicine service) in which HCWs provide services to share air with a specific patient population or work with clinical specimens that may contain viable *M. tuberculosis* organisms. The risk for exposure to *M. tuberculosis* in a given area depends on the prevalence of TB in the population served and the characteristics of the environment.

†With epidemiologic evaluation suggestive of occupational (nosocomial) transmission (see Problem Evaluation section in the text).

§Cluster: two or more PPD skin-test conversions occurring within a 3-month period among HCWs in a specific area or occupational group, and epidemiologic evidence suggests occupational (nosocomial) transmission.

¶For example, clusters of *M. tuberculosis* isolates with identical DNA fingerprint (RFLP) patterns or drug-resistance patterns, with epidemiologic evaluation suggestive of nosocomial transmission (see Problem Evaluation section in the text).

##Does not include patients identified in triage system and referred to a collaborating facility or patients being managed in outpatient areas.

††To prevent inappropriate management and potential loss to follow-up of patients identified in the triage system of a very low-risk facility as having suspected TB, an agreement should exist for referral between the referring and receiving facilities.

§§Or, for occupational groups, exposure to fewer than six TB patients for HCWs in the particular occupational group during the preceding year.

¶¶Or, for occupational groups, exposure to six or more TB patients for HCWs in the particular occupational group during the preceding year.

###See Problem Evaluation section in the text.

†††Occurrence of drug-resistant TB in the facility or community, or a relatively high prevalence of HIV infection among patients or HCWs in the area, may warrant a higher risk rating.

§§§For outpatient facilities, if TB cases have been documented in the community but no TB patients have been examined in the outpatient area during the preceding year, the area can be designated as very low risk.

Figure 1.—continued

- The "very low-risk" category generally applies only to an entire facility. A very low-risk facility is one in which (a) patients with active TB are not admitted to inpatient areas but may receive initial assessment and diagnostic evaluation or outpatient management in outpatient areas (e.g., ambulatory-care and emergency departments) and (b) patients who may have active TB and need inpatient care are promptly referred to a collaborating facility. In such facilities, the outpatient areas in which exposure to patients with active TB could occur should be assessed and assigned to the appropriate low-, intermediate-, or high-risk category. Categorical assignment will depend on the number of TB patients examined in the area during the preceding year and whether there is evidence of nosocomial transmission of M. tuberculosis in the area. If TB cases have been reported in the community, but no patients with active TB have been examined in the outpatient area during the preceding year, the area can be designated as very low risk (e.g., many medical offices).

  The referring and receiving facilities should establish a referral agreement to prevent inappropriate management and potential loss to follow-up of patients suspected of having TB during evaluation in the triage system of a very low-risk facility.

  In some facilities in which TB patients are admitted to inpatient areas, a very low-risk protocol may be appropriate for areas (e.g., administrative areas) or occupational groups that have only a very remote possibility of exposure to M. tuberculosis.

Table 2. Elements of a Tuberculosis (TB) Infection-Control Program

Element	Risk categories				
	Minimal	Very low	Low	Intermediate	High
Assigning responsibility (Section II.A)					
Designated TB control officer or committee	R	R	R	R	R
Conducting a risk assessment (Section II.B.1)					
Baseline risk assessment	R	R	R	R	R
Community TB profile: incidence, prevalence, and drug-susceptibility patterns	Y	Y	Y	Y	Y
Facility case surveillance (laboratory- and discharge-diagnosis-based)	C	C	C	C	C
Analysis of purified protein derivative (PPD) test results among health-care workers (HCWs)	N/A	V*	Y	every 6–12 mos	every 3 mos
Review of TB patient medical records	N/A	O+	Y	every 6–12 mos	every 3 mos
Observation of infection-control practices	N/A	N/A	Y	every 6–12 mos	every 3 mos
Evaluation of engineering control maintenance	O&	O&	Y	every 6–12 mos	every 3 mos
Developing a TB infection control plan (Section II.B.2)					
Written TB infection control plan	R	R	R	R	R
Periodically reassessing risk (Section II.B.3)					
Reassessment of risk	Y	Y	Y	every 6–12 mos	every 3 mos
Identifying, evaluating, and initiating treatment for patients who may have active TB (Section II.C)					
Protocol (clinical prediction rules)@ for identifying patients who may have active TB	R	R	R	R	R
Protocol for diagnostic evaluation of patients who may have active TB**	N/A	R	R	R	R

	Col 1	Col 2	Col 3	Col 4	Col 5
Protocol for reporting laboratory results to clinicians, infection-control practitioners, collaborating referral facilities, and appropriate health department(s)	N/A	R	R	R	R
Protocol for initiating treatment of patients who may have active TB**	N/A	R	R	R	R
Managing patients who may have TB in ambulatory-care settings and emergency departments (Section II.D)					
Triage system for identifying patients who have active TB in emergency departments and ambulatory-care settings	R	R	R	R	R
Protocol for managing patients who may have active TB in emergency departments and ambulatory-care settings	R	R	R	R	R
Protocol for referring patients who may have active TB to collaborating facility	R	R	N/A++	N/A++	N/A++
Managing hospitalized patients who may have TB (Section II.E)					
Appropriate number of TB isolation rooms&&	N/A	N/A	R	R	R
Protocol for initiating TB isolation	N/A	N/A	R	R	R
Protocol for TB isolation practices	N/A	N/A	R	R	R
Protocol for discontinuing TB isolation	N/A	N/A	R	R	R
Protocol for discharge planning	N/A	N/A	R	R	R
Engineering controls (Suppl. 3, Section II.F)					
Protocol(s) for maintenance of engineering controls	O&	O&	R	R	R
Respiratory protection (Suppl. 4, Section II.G)					
Respiratory protection program	N/A	V*	R	R	R

Table 2.—continued

Element	Minimal	Very low	Low	Intermediate	High
Cough-inducing and aerosol-generating procedures (Section II.H)					
Protocol(s) for performing cough-inducing or aerosol-generating procedures	O	O@@	R	R	R
Engineering controls for performing cough-inducing or aerosol-generating procedures	O&	O@@	R	R	R
Educating and Training HCWs (Section II.I)					
Educating and training HCWs regarding TB	R	R	R	R	R
Counseling and screening HCWs (Section II.J)					
Counseling HCWs regarding TB	R	R	R	R	R
Protocol for identifying and evaluating HCWs who have signs or symptoms of active TB	R	R	R	R	R
Baseline PPD testing of HCWs	O***	R	R	R	R
Routine periodic PPD screening of HCWs for latent TB infection	N/A	V*	Y	every 6–12 mos	every 3 mos
Protocol for evaluating and managing HCWs who have positive PPD tests	R	R	R	R	R
Protocol for managing HCWs who have active TB	R	R	R	R	R
Conducting a problem evaluation (Section II.K)					
Protocol for investigating possible PPD conversions and active TB in HCWs	R	R	R	R	R
Protocol for investigating possible patient-to-patient transmission of Mycobacterium tuberculosis	R	R	R	R	R

Protocol for investigating possible contacts of TB
  patients who were not diagnosed initially as having
  TB and were not placed in isolation   R   R   R

Coordination with the public health department
  (Section II.L)
Effective system for reporting patients who have
  suspected or confirmed TB to appropriate
  health department(s)   R   R   R

R = recommended; Y = yearly; C = continual; N/A = not applicable; O = optional; V = variable.

* Because very low-risk facilities do not admit patients who may have active TB to inpatient areas, most HCWs in such facilities do not need routine follow-up PPD screening after baseline PPD testing is done. However, those who are involved in the initial assessment and diagnostic evaluation of patients in the ambulatory-care, emergency, and admitting departments of such facilities or in the outpatient management of patients with active TB could be exposed potentially to a patient who has active TB. These HCWs may need to receive routine periodic PPD screening. Similarly, these HCWs may need to be included in a respiratory protection program.

+ Because very low-risk facilities do not admit patients suspected of having active TB, review of TB patient medical records is not applicable. However, follow-up of patients who were identified during triage as possibly having active TB and referred to another institution for further evaluation and management may be useful in evaluating the effectiveness of the triage system.

& Some minimal or very low-risk facilities may elect to use engineering controls (e.g., booths for cough-inducing procedures, portable high-efficiency particulate (HEPA) filtration units, ultraviolet germicidal irradiation units) in triage/waiting areas. In such situations, appropriate protocols for maintaining this equipment should be in place, and this maintenance should be evaluated periodically.

@ The criteria used in clinical prediction rules will probably vary from facility to facility depending on the prevalence of TB in the population served by the facility and on the clinical, radiographic, and laboratory characteristics of TB patients examined in the facility.

** The protocols should be consistent with CDC/American Thoracic Society recommendations (33).

++ Protocols for referring patients who require specialized treatment (e.g., patients with multidrug-resistant TB) may be appropriate.

&& Based on maximum daily number of patients requiring TB isolation for suspected or confirmed active TB. Isolation rooms should meet the performance criteria specified in these guidelines.

@@ If such procedures are used in the triage protocol(s) for identifying patients who may have active TB.

*** Minimal-risk facilities do not need to maintain an ongoing PPD skin-testing program. However, baseline PPD testing of HCWs may be advisable so that if an unexpected exposure does occur, conversions can be distinguished from positive PPD test results caused by previous exposures.

The very low-risk category may also be appropriate for outpatient facilities that do not provide initial assessment of persons who may have TB, but do screen patients for active TB as part of a limited medical screening before undertaking specialty care (e.g., dental settings).

- "Low-risk" areas or occupational groups are those in which (a) the PPD test conversion rate is not greater than that for areas or groups in which occupational exposure to M. tuberculosis is unlikely or than previous conversion rates for the same area or group, (b) no clusters*** of PPD test conversions have occurred, (c) person-to-person transmission of M. tuberculosis has not been detected, and (d) fewer than six TB patients are examined or treated per year.

- "Intermediate-risk" areas or occupational groups are those in which (a) the PPD test conversion rate is not greater than that for areas or groups in which occupational exposure to M. tuberculosis is unlikely or than previous conversion rates for the same area or group, (b) no clusters of PPD test conversions have occurred, (c) person-to-person transmission of M. tuberculosis has not been detected, and (d) six or more patients with active TB are examined or treated each year. Survey data suggest that facilities in which six or more TB patients are examined or treated each year may have an increased risk for transmission of M. tuberculosis (CDC, unpublished data); thus, areas in which six or more patients with active TB are examined or treated each year (or occupational groups in which HCWs are likely to be exposed to six or more TB patients per year) should be classified as "intermediate risk."

- "High-risk" areas or occupational groups are those in which (a) the PPD test conversion rate is significantly greater than for areas or groups in which occupational exposure to M. tuberculosis is unlikely or than previous conversion rates for the same area or group, and epidemiologic evaluation suggests nosocomial transmission; or (b) a cluster of PPD test conversions has occurred, and epidemiologic evaluation suggests nosocomial transmission of M. tuberculosis; or (c) possible person-to-person transmission of M. tuberculosis has been detected.

- If no data or insufficient data for adequate determination of risk have been collected, such data should be compiled, analyzed, and reviewed expeditiously.

b. Community TB Profile

- A profile of TB in the community that is served by the facility should be obtained from the public health department. This profile should include, at a minimum, the incidence (and prevalence, if available) of active TB in the community and the drug-susceptibility patterns of M. tuberculosis isolates (i.e., the antituberculous agents to which each isolate is susceptible and those to which it is resistant) from patients in the community.

c. Case Surveillance

- Data concerning the number of suspected and confirmed active TB cases among patients and HCWs in the facility should be systematically collected, re-

---

***Cluster: two or more PPD skin-test conversions occurring within a 3-month period among HCWs in a specific area or occupational group, and epidemiologic evidence suggests occupational (nosocomial) transmission.

viewed, and used to estimate the number of TB isolation rooms needed, to recognize possible clusters of nosocomial transmission, and to assess the level of potential occupational risk. The number of TB patients in specific areas of a facility can be obtained from laboratory surveillance data on specimens positive for AFB smears or M. tuberculosis cultures, from infection-control records, and from databases containing information about hospital discharge diagnoses.

- Drug-susceptibility patterns of M. tuberculosis isolates from TB patients treated in the facility should be reviewed to identify the frequency and patterns of drug resistance. This information may indicate a need to modify the initial treatment regimen or may suggest possible nosocomial transmission or increased occupational risk.

d. Analysis of HCW PPD Test Screening Data

- Results of HCW PPD testing should be recorded in the individual HCW's employee health record and in a retrievable aggregate database of all HCW PPD test results. Personal identifying information should be handled confidentially. PPD test conversion rates should be calculated at appropriate intervals to estimate the risk for PPD test conversions for each area of the facility and for each specific occupational group not assigned to a specific area (Table 2). To calculate PPD test conversion rates, the total number of previously PPD-negative HCWs tested in each area or group (i.e., the denominator) and the number of PPD test conversions among HCWs in each area or group (the numerator) must be obtained.
- PPD test conversion rates for each area or occupational group should be compared with rates for areas or groups in which occupational exposure to M. tuberculosis is unlikely and with previous conversion rates in the same area or group to identify areas or groups where the risk for occupational PPD test conversions may be increased. A low number of HCWs in a specific area may result in a greatly increased rate of conversion for that area, although the actual risk may not be significantly greater than that for other areas. Testing for statistical significance (e.g., Fisher's exact test or chi square test) may assist interpretation; however, lack of statistical significance may not rule out a problem (i.e., if the number of HCWs tested is low, there may not be adequate statistical power to detect a significant difference). Thus, interpretation of individual situations is necessary.
- An epidemiologic investigation to evaluate the likelihood of nosocomial transmission should be conducted if PPD test conversions are noted (Section II.K.1).
- The frequency and comprehensiveness of the HCW PPD testing program should be evaluated periodically to ensure that all HCWs who should be included in the program are being tested at appropriate intervals. For surveillance purposes, earlier detection of transmission may be enhanced if HCWs in a given area or occupational group are tested on different scheduled dates rather than all being tested on the same date (Section II.J.3).

e. Review of TB Patient Medical Records

- The medical records of a sample of TB patients examined at the facility can be reviewed periodically to evaluate infection-control parameters (Table 1). Parameters to examine may include the intervals from date of admission until (a) TB was suspected, (b) specimens for AFB smears were ordered, (c) these specimens were collected, (d) tests were performed, and (e) results were reported. Moreover, the adequacy of the TB treatment regimens that were used should be evaluated.

- Medical record reviews should note previous hospital admissions of TB patients before the onset of TB symptoms. Patient-to-patient transmission may be suspected if active TB occurs in a patient who had a prior hospitalization during which exposure to another TB patient occurred or if isolates from two or more TB patients have identical characteristic drug-susceptibility or DNA fingerprint patterns.
- Data from the case review should be used to determine if there is a need to modify (a) protocols for identifying and isolating patients who may have infectious TB, (b) laboratory procedures, (c) administrative policies and practices, or (d) protocols for patient management.

f. Observation of TB Infection-Control Practices

- Assessing adherence to the policies of the TB infection-control program should be part of the evaluation process. This assessment should be performed on a regular basis and whenever an increase occurs in the number of TB patients or HCW PPD test conversions. Areas at high risk for transmission of M. tuberculosis should be monitored more frequently than other areas. The review of patient medical records provides information on HCW adherence to some of the policies of the TB infection-control program. In addition, work practices related to TB isolation (e.g., keeping doors to isolation rooms closed) should be observed to determine if employers are enforcing, and HCWs are adhering to, these policies and if patient adherence is being enforced. If these policies are not being enforced or adhered to, appropriate education and other corrective action should be implemented.

g. Engineering Evaluation

- Results of engineering maintenance measures should be reviewed at regular intervals (Table 3). Data from the most recent evaluation and from maintenance procedures and logs should be reviewed carefully as part of the risk assessment.

2. Development of the TB Infection-Control Plan

- Based on the results of the risk assessment, a written TB infection-control plan should be developed and implemented for each area of the facility and for each occupational group of HCWs not assigned to a specific area of the facility (Table 2; Table 3).
- The occurrence of drug-resistant TB in the facility or the community, or a relatively high prevalence of HIV infection among patients or HCWs in the community, may increase the concern about transmission of M. tuberculosis and may influence the decision regarding which protocol to follow (i.e., a higher-risk classification may be selected).
- Health-care facilities are likely to have a combination of low-, intermediate-, and high-risk areas or occupational groups during the same time period. The appropriate protocol should be implemented for each area or group.
- Areas in which cough-inducing procedures are performed on patients who may have active TB should, at the minimum, implement the intermediate-risk protocol.

Table 3. Characteristics of an Effective Tuberculosis (TB) Infection-Control Program*

I. Assignment of responsibility
   A. Assign responsibility for the TB infection-control program to qualified person(s).
   B. Ensure that persons with expertise in infection control, occupational health, and engineering are identified and included.
II. Risk assessment, TB infection-control plan, and periodic reassessment
   A. Initial risk assessments
      1. Obtain information concerning TB in the community.
      2. Evaluate data concerning TB patients in the facility.
      3. Evaluate data concerning purified protein derivative (PPD)-tuberculin skin-test conversions among health-care workers (HCWs) in the facility.
      4. Rule out evidence of person-to-person transmission.
   B. Written TB infection-control program
      1. Select initial risk protocol(s).
      2. Develop written TB infection-control protocols.
   C. Repeat risk assessment at appropriate intervals.
      1. Review current community and facility surveillance data and PPD-tuberculin skin-test results.
      2. Review records of TB patients.
      3. Observe HCW infection-control practices.
      4. Evaluate maintenance of engineering controls.
III. Identification, evaluation, and treatment of patients who have TB
   A. Screen patients for signs and symptoms of active TB:
      1. On initial encounter in emergency department or ambulatory-care setting.
      2. Before or at the time of admission.
   B. Perform radiologic and bacteriologic evaluation of patients who have signs and symptoms suggestive of TB.
   C. Promptly initiate treatment.
IV. Managing outpatients who have possible infectious TB
   A. Promptly initiate TB precautions.
   B. Place patients in separate waiting areas or TB isolation rooms.
   C. Give patients a surgical mask, a box of tissues, and instructions regarding the use of these items.
V. Managing inpatients who have possible infectious TB
   A. Promptly isolate patients who have suspected or known infectious TB.
   B. Monitor the response to treatment.
   C. Follow appropriate criteria for discontinuing isolation.
VI. Engineering recommendations
   A. Design local exhaust and general ventilation in collaboration with persons who have expertise in ventilation engineering.
   B. Use a single-pass air system or air recirculation after high-efficiency particulate air (HEPA) filtration in areas where infectious TB patients receive care.
   C. Use additional measures, if needed, in areas where TB patients may receive care.
   D. Design TB isolation rooms in health-care facilities to achieve greater than or equal to 6 air changes per hour (ACH) for existing facilities and greater than or equal to 12 ACH for new or renovated facilities.

Table 3.—*continued*

      E. Regularly monitor and maintain engineering controls.

      F. TB isolation rooms that are being used should be monitored daily to ensure they maintain negative pressure relative to the hallway and all surrounding areas.

      G. Exhaust TB isolation room air to outside or, if absolutely unavoidable, recirculate after HEPA filtration.

  VII. Respiratory protection

      A. Respiratory protective devices should meet recommended performance criteria.

      B. Respiratory protection should be used by persons entering rooms in which patients with known or suspected infectious TB are being isolated, by HCWs when performing cough-inducing or aerosol-generating procedures on such patients, and by persons in other settings where administrative and engineering controls are not likely to protect them from inhaling infectious airborne droplet nuclei.

      C. A respiratory protection program is required at all facilities in which respiratory protection is used.

 VIII. Cough-inducing procedures

      A. Do not perform such procedures on TB patients unless absolutely necessary.

      B. perform such procedures in areas that have local exhaust ventilation devices (e.g., booths or special enclosures) or, if this is not feasible, in a room that meets the ventilation requirements for TB isolation.

      C. After completion of procedures, TB patients should remain in the booth or special enclosure until their coughing subsides.

  IX. HCW TB training and education

      A. All HCWs should receive periodic TB education appropriate for their work responsibilities and duties.

      B. Training should include the epidemiology of TB in the facility.

      C. TB education should emphasize concepts of the pathogenesis of and occupational risk for TB.

      D. Training should describe work practices that reduce the likelihood of transmitting M. tuberculosis.

   X. HCW counseling and screening

      A. Counsel all HCWs regarding TB and TB infection.

      B. Counsel all HCWs about the increased risk to immunocompromised persons for developing active TB.

      C. Perform PPD skin tests on HCWs at the beginning of their employment, and repeat PPD tests at periodic intervals.

      D. Evaluate symptomatic HCWs for active TB.

  XI. Evaluate HCW PPD test conversions and possible nosocomial transmission of M. tuberculosis.

  XII. Coordinate efforts with public health department(s).

---

*A program such as this is appropriate for health-care facilities in which there is a high risk for transmission of Mycobacterium tuberculosis.

3. Periodic Reassessment

- Follow-up risk assessment should be performed at the interval indicated by the most recent risk assessment (Figure 1; Table 2). Based on the results of the follow-up assessment, problem evaluation may need to be conducted or the protocol may need to be modified to a higher- or lower-risk level.
- After each risk assessment, the staff responsible for TB control, in conjunction with other appropriate HCWs, should review all TB control policies to ensure that they are effective and meet current needs.

4. Examples of Risk Assessment

Examples of six hypothetical situations and the means by which surveillance data are used to select a TB control protocol are described as follows:

HOSPITAL A

The overall HCW PPD test conversion rate in the facility is 1.6%. No areas or HCW occupational groups have a significantly greater PPD test conversion rate than areas or groups in which occupational exposure to M. tuberculosis is unlikely (or than previous rates for the same area or group). No clusters of PPD test conversions have occurred. Patient-to-patient transmission has not been detected. Patients who have TB are admitted to the facility, but no area admits six or more TB patients per year. The low-risk protocol will be followed in all areas.

HOSPITAL B

The overall HCW PPD test conversion rate in the facility is 1.8%. The PPD test conversion rate for the medical intensive-care unit rate is significantly higher than all other areas in the facility. The problem identification process is initiated (Section II.K). It is determined that all TB patients have been isolated appropriately. Other potential problems are then evaluated, and the cause for the higher rate is not identified. After consulting the public health department TB infection-control program, the high-risk protocol is followed in the unit until the PPD test conversion rate is similar to areas of the facility in which occupational exposure to TB patients is unlikely. If the rate remains significantly higher than other areas, further evaluation, including environmental and procedural studies, will be performed to identify possible reasons for the high conversion rate.

HOSPITAL C

The overall HCW PPD test conversion rate in the facility is 2.4%. Rates range from 0 to 2.6% for the individual areas and occupational groups. None of these rates is significantly higher than rates for areas in which occupational exposure to M. tuberculosis is unlikely. No particular HCW group has higher conversion rates than the other groups. No clusters of HCW PPD test conversions have occurred. In two of the areas, HCWs cared for more than six TB patients during the preceding year. These two areas will follow the intermediate-risk protocol, and all other areas will follow the low-risk protocol. This hospital is located in the southeastern United States, and these conversion rates may reflect cross-reactivity with nontuberculous mycobacteria.

HOSPITAL D

The overall HCW PPD test conversion rate in the facility is 1.2%. In no area did HCWs care for six or more TB patients during the preceding year. Three of the 20 respiratory therapists tested had PPD conversions, for a rate of 15%. The respiratory therapists who had PPD test conversions had spent all or part of their time in the pulmonary function laboratory, where induced sputum specimens were obtained. A low-risk protocol is maintained for all areas and occupational groups in the facility except for respiratory therapists. A problem evaluation is conducted in the pulmonary function laboratory (Section II.K). It is determined that the ventilation in this area is inadequate. Booths are installed for sputum induction. PPD testing and the risk assessment are repeated 3 months later. If the repeat testing at 3 months indicates that no more conversions have occurred, the respiratory therapists will return to the low-risk protocol.

HOSPITAL E

Hospital E is located in a community that has a relatively low incidence of TB. To optimize TB services in the community, the four hospitals in the community have developed an agreement that one of them (e.g., Hospital G) will provide all inpatient services to persons who have suspected or confirmed TB. The other hospitals have implemented protocols in their ambulatory-care clinics and emergency departments to identify patients who may have active TB. These patients are then transferred to Hospital G for inpatient care if such care is considered necessary. After discharge from Hospital G, they receive follow-up care in the public health department's TB clinic. During the preceding year, Hospital E has identified fewer than six TB patients in its ambulatory-care and emergency departments and has had no PPD test conversions or other evidence of M. tuberculosis transmission among HCWs or patients in these areas. These areas are classified as low risk, and all other areas are classified as very low risk.

HOSPITAL F

Hospital F is located in a county in which no TB cases have been reported during the preceding 2 years. A risk assessment conducted at the facility did not identify any patients who had suspected or confirmed TB during the preceding year. The facility is classified as minimal risk.

C. Identifying, Evaluating, and Initiating Treatment for Patients Who May Have Active TB

The most important factors in preventing transmission of M. tuberculosis are the early identification of patients who may have infectious TB, prompt implementation of TB precautions for such patients, and prompt initiation of effective treatment for those who are likely to have TB.

1. Identifying Patients Who May Have Active TB

- Health-care personnel who are assigned responsibility for TB infection control in ambulatory-care and inpatient settings should develop, implement, and enforce protocols for the early identification of patients who may have infectious TB.
- The criteria used in these protocols should be based on the prevalence and characteristics of TB in the population served by the specific facility. These protocols should be evaluated periodically and revised according to the results of the evaluation. Review of medical records of patients who were examined in the facility and diagnosed as having TB may serve as a guide for developing or revising these protocols.
- A diagnosis of TB may be considered for any patient who has a persistent cough (i.e., a cough lasting for greater than or equal to 3 weeks) or other signs or symptoms compatible with active TB (e.g., bloody sputum, night sweats, weight loss, anorexia, or fever). However, the index of suspicion for TB will vary in different geographic areas and will depend on the prevalence of TB and other characteristics of the population served by the facility. The index of suspicion for TB should be very high in geographic areas or among groups of patients in which the prevalence of TB is high (Section I.B). Appropriate diagnostic measures should be conducted and TB precautions implemented for patients in whom active TB is suspected.

2. Diagnostic Evaluation for Active TB

- Diagnostic measures for identifying TB should be conducted for patients in whom active TB is being considered. These measures include obtaining a medical history and performing a physical examination, PPD skin test, chest radiograph, and microscopic examination and culture of sputum or other appropriate specimens (6, 34, 35). Other diagnostic procedures (e.g., bronchoscopy or biopsy) may be indicated for some patients (36, 37).

- Prompt laboratory results are crucial to the proper treatment of the TB patient and to early initiation of infection control. To ensure timely results, laboratories performing mycobacteriologic tests should be proficient at both the laboratory and administrative aspects of specimen processing. Laboratories should use the most rapid methods available (e.g., fluorescent microscopy for AFB smears; radiometric culture methods for isolation of mycobacteria; r-nitro-a-acetylamino-b-hydroxy-proprophenone [NAP] test, nucleic acid probes, or high-pressure liquid chromatography [HPLC] for species identification; and radiometric methods for drug-susceptibility testing). As other more rapid or sensitive tests become available, practical, and affordable, such tests should be incorporated promptly into the mycobacteriology laboratory. Laboratories that rarely receive specimens for mycobacteriologic analysis should refer the specimens to a laboratory that more frequently performs these tests.

- Results of AFB sputum smears should be available within 24 hours of specimen collection (38).

- The probability of TB is greater among patients who have positive PPD test results or a history of positive PPD test results, who have previously had TB or have been exposed to M. tuberculosis, or who belong to a group at high risk for TB (Section I.B). Active TB is strongly suggested if the diagnostic evaluation reveals AFB in sputum, a chest radiograph suggestive of TB, or symptoms highly suggestive of TB. TB can occur simultaneously in immunosuppressed persons who have pulmonary infections caused by other organisms (e.g., Pneumocystis carinii or Mycobacterium avium complex) and should be considered in the diagnostic evaluation of all patients who have symptoms compatible with TB (Suppl. 1; Suppl. 2).

- TB may be more difficult to diagnose among persons who have HIV infection (or other conditions associated with severe suppression of cell-mediated immunity) because of a nonclassical clinical or radiographic presentation and/or the simultaneous occurrence of other pulmonary infections (e.g., P. carinii pneumonia and M. avium complex). The difficulty in diagnosing TB in HIV-infected persons may be further compounded by impaired responses to PPD skin tests (39, 40), the possibly lower sensitivity of sputum smears for detecting AFB (41), or the overgrowth of cultures with M. avium complex in specimens from patients infected with both M. avium complex and M. tuberculosis (42).

- Immunosuppressed patients who have pulmonary signs or symptoms that are ascribed initially to infections or conditions other than TB should be evaluated initially for coexisting TB. The evaluation for TB should be repeated if the patient does not respond to appropriate therapy for the presumed cause(s) of the pulmonary abnormalities (Suppl. 1; Suppl. 2).

- Patients with suspected or confirmed TB should be reported immediately to the appropriate public health department so that standard procedures for identifying and evaluating TB contacts can be initiated.

3. Initiation of Treatment for Suspected or Confirmed TB

- Patients who have confirmed active TB or who are considered highly likely to have active TB should be started promptly on appropriate treatment in accordance with current guidelines (Suppl. 2) (43). In geographic areas or facilities that have a high prevalence of MDR-TB, the initial regimen used may need to be enhanced while the results of drug-susceptibility tests are pending. The decision should be based on analysis of surveillance data.
- While the patient is in the health-care facility, anti-TB drugs should be administered by directly observed therapy (DOT), the process by which an HCW observes the patient swallowing the medications. Continuing DOT after the patient is discharged should be strongly considered. This decision and the arrangements for providing outpatient DOT should be made in collaboration with the public health department.

D. Management of Patients Who May Have Active TB in Ambulatory-Care Settings and Emergency Departments

- Triage of patients in ambulatory-care settings and emergency departments should include vigorous efforts to promptly identify patients who have active TB. HCWs who are the first points of contact in facilities that serve populations at risk for TB should be trained to ask questions that will facilitate identification of patients with signs and symptoms suggestive of TB.
- Patients with signs or symptoms suggestive of TB should be evaluated promptly to minimize the amount of time they are in ambulatory-care areas. TB precautions should be followed while the diagnostic evaluation is being conducted for these patients.
- TB precautions in the ambulatory-care setting should include (a) placing these patients in a separate area apart from other patients, and not in open waiting areas (ideally, in a room or enclosure meeting TB isolation requirements); (b) giving these patients surgical masks[+] to wear and instructing them to keep their masks on; and (c) giving these patients tissues and instructing them to cover their mouths and noses with the tissues when coughing or sneezing.
- TB precautions should be followed for patients who are known to have active TB and who have not completed therapy until a determination has been made that they are noninfectious (Suppl. 1).
- Patients with active TB who need to attend a health-care clinic should have appointments scheduled to avoid exposing HIV-infected or otherwise severely immunocompromised persons to M. tuberculosis. This recommenda-

---

[+]Surgical masks are designed to prevent the respiratory secretions of the person wearing the mask from entering the air. When not in a TB isolation room, patients suspected of having TB should wear surgical masks to reduce the expulsion of droplet nuclei into the air. These patients do not need to wear particulate respirators, which are designed to filter the air before it is inhaled by the person wearing the mask. Patients suspected of having or known to have TB should never wear a respirator that has an exhalation valve, because the device would provide no barrier to the expulsion of droplet nuclei into the air.

tion could be accomplished by designating certain times of the day for appointments for these patients or by treating them in areas where immunocompromised persons are not treated.

- Ventilation in ambulatory-care areas where patients at high risk for TB are treated should be designed and maintained to reduce the risk for transmission of M. tuberculosis. General-use areas (e.g., waiting rooms) and special areas (e.g., treatment or TB isolation rooms in ambulatory areas) should be ventilated in the same manner as described for similar inpatient areas (Sections II.E.3, II.F; Suppl. 3). Enhanced general ventilation or the use of air-disinfection techniques (e.g., UVGI or recirculation of air within the room through high-efficiency particulate air [HEPA] filters) may be useful in general-use areas of facilities where many infectious TB patients receive care (Section II.F; Suppl. 3).

- Ideally, ambulatory-care settings in which patients with TB are frequently examined or treated should have a TB isolation room(s) available. Such rooms are not necessary in ambulatory-care settings in which patients who have confirmed or suspected TB are seen infrequently. However, these facilities should have a written protocol for early identification of patients with TB symptoms and referral to an area or a collaborating facility where the patient can be evaluated and managed appropriately. These protocols should be reviewed on a regular basis and revised as necessary. The additional guidelines in Section II.H should be followed in ambulatory-care settings where cough-inducing procedures are performed on patients who may have active TB.

E. Management of Hospitalized Patients Who Have Confirmed or Suspected TB

1. Initiation of Isolation for TB

- In hospitals and other inpatient facilities, any patient suspected of having or known to have infectious TB should be placed in a TB isolation room that has currently recommended ventilation characteristics (Section II.E.3; Suppl. 3). Written policies for initiating isolation should specify (a) the indications for isolation, (b) the person(s) authorized to initiate and discontinue isolation, (c) the isolation practices to follow, (d) the monitoring of isolation, (e) the management of patients who do not adhere to isolation practices, and (f) the criteria for discontinuing isolation.

- In rare circumstances, placing more than one TB patient together in the same room may be acceptable. This practice is sometimes referred to as "cohorting." Because of the risk for patients becoming superinfected with drug-resistant organisms, patients with TB should be placed in the same room only if all patients involved (a) have culture-confirmed TB, (b) have drug-susceptibility test results available on a current specimen obtained during the present hospitalization, (c) have identical drug-susceptibility patterns on these specimens, and (d) are on effective therapy. Having isolates with identical DNA fingerprint patterns is not adequate evidence for placing two TB patients together in the same room, because isolates with the same DNA fingerprint pattern can have different drug-susceptibility patterns.

- Pediatric patients with suspected or confirmed TB should be evaluated for potential infectiousness according to the same criteria as are adults (i.e., on the basis of symptoms, sputum AFB smears, radiologic findings, and other criteria) (Suppl. 1). Children who may be infectious should be placed in isolation until they are determined to be noninfectious. Pediatric patients who may be infectious include those who have laryngeal or extensive pulmonary involvement, pronounced cough, positive sputum AFB smears, or cavitary TB or those for whom cough-inducing procedures are performed (44).

- The source of infection for a child with TB is often a member of the child's family (45). Therefore, parents and other visitors of all pediatric TB patients should be evaluated for TB as soon as possible. Until they have been evaluated, or the source case is identified, they should wear surgical masks when in areas of the facility outside of the child's room, and they should refrain from visiting common areas in the facility (e.g., the cafeteria or lounge areas).

- TB patients in intensive-care units should be treated the same as patients in noncritical-care settings. They should be placed in TB isolation and have respiratory secretions submitted for AFB smear and culture if they have undiagnosed pulmonary symptoms suggestive of TB.

- If readmitted to a health-care facility, patients who are known to have active TB and who have not completed therapy should have TB precautions applied until a determination has been made that they are noninfectious (Suppl. 1).

2. TB Isolation Practices

- Patients who are placed in TB isolation should be educated about the mechanisms of M. tuberculosis transmission and the reasons for their being placed in isolation. They should be taught to cover their mouths and noses with a tissue when coughing or sneezing, even while in the isolation room, to contain liquid drops and droplets before they are expelled into the air (46).

- Efforts should be made to facilitate patient adherence to isolation measures (e.g., staying in the TB isolation room). Such efforts might include the use of incentives (e.g., providing them with telephones, televisions, or radios in their rooms or allowing special dietary requests). Efforts should also be made to address other problems that could interfere with adherence to isolation (e.g., management of the patient's withdrawal from addictive substances [including tobacco]).

- Patients placed in isolation should remain in their isolation rooms with the door closed. If possible, diagnostic and treatment procedures should be performed in the isolation rooms to avoid transporting patients through other areas of the facility. If patients who may have infectious TB must be transported outside their isolation rooms for medically essential procedures that cannot be performed in the isolation rooms, they should wear surgical masks that cover their mouths and noses during transport. Persons transporting the patients do not need to wear respiratory protection outside the TB isolation rooms. Procedures for these patients should be scheduled at times when they can be performed rapidly and when waiting areas are less crowded.

- Treatment and procedure rooms in which patients who have infectious TB or who have an undiagnosed pulmonary disease and are at high risk for active TB receive care should meet the ventilation recommendations for isolation rooms (Section II.E.3; Suppl. 3). Ideally, facilities in which TB patients are frequently treated should have an area in the radiology department that is ventilated separately for TB patients. If this is not possible, TB patients should wear surgical masks and should stay in the radiology suite the minimum amount of time possible, then be returned promptly to their isolation rooms.

- The number of persons entering an isolation room should be minimal. All persons who enter an isolation room should wear respiratory protection (Section II.G; Suppl. 4). The patient's visitors should be given respirators to wear while in the isolation room, and they should be given general instructions on how to use their respirators.
- Disposable items contaminated with respiratory secretions are not associated with transmission of M. tuberculosis. However, for general infection-control purposes, these items should be handled and transported in a manner that reduces the risk for transmitting other microorganisms to patients, HCWs, and visitors and that decreases environmental contamination in the health-care facility. Such items should be disposed of in accordance with hospital policy and applicable regulations (Suppl. 5).

3. The TB Isolation Room

- TB isolation rooms should be single-patient rooms with special ventilation characteristics appropriate for the purposes of isolation (Suppl. 3). The primary purposes of TB isolation rooms are to (a) separate patients who are likely to have infectious TB from other persons; (b) provide an environment that will allow reduction of the concentration of droplet nuclei through various engineering methods; and (c) prevent the escape of droplet nuclei from the TB isolation room and treatment room, thus preventing entry of M. tuberculosis into the corridor and other areas of the facility.
- To prevent the escape of droplet nuclei, the TB isolation room should be maintained under negative pressure (Suppl. 3). Doors to isolation rooms should be kept closed, except when patients or personnel must enter or exit the room, so that negative pressure can be maintained.
- Negative pressure in the room should be monitored daily while the room is being used for TB isolation.
- The American Society of Heating, Refrigerating and Air-Conditioning Engineers, Inc. (ASHRAE) (47), the American Institute of Architects (AIA) (48), and the Health Resources and Services Administration (49) recommend a minimum of 6 air changes per hour (ACH) for TB isolation and treatment rooms. This ventilation rate is based on comfort and odor control considerations. The effectiveness of this level of airflow in reducing the concentration of droplet nuclei in the room, thus reducing the transmission of airborne pathogens, has not been evaluated directly or adequately.

    Ventilation rates of greater than 6 ACH are likely to produce an incrementally greater reduction in the concentration of bacteria in a room than are lower rates (50–52). However, accurate quantitation of decreases in risk that would result from specific increases in general ventilation levels has not been performed and may not be possible.

    For the purposes of reducing the concentration of droplet nuclei, TB isolation and treatment rooms in existing health-care facilities should have an airflow of greater than or equal to 6 ACH. Where feasible, this airflow rate should be increased to greater than or equal to 12 ACH by adjusting or modifying the ventilation system or by using auxiliary means (e.g., recirculation of air through fixed HEPA filtration systems or portable air cleaners) (Suppl. 3, Section II.B.5.a) (53). New construction or renovation of existing health-care facilities should be designed so that TB isolation rooms achieve an airflow of greater than or equal to 12 ACH.

- Air from TB isolation rooms and treatment rooms used to treat patients who have known or suspected infectious TB should be exhausted to the outside in accordance with applicable federal, state, and local regulations. The air should not be recirculated into the general ventilation. In some instances, recirculation of air into the general ventilation system from such rooms is unavoidable (i.e., in existing facilities in which the ventilation system or facility configuration makes venting the exhaust to the outside impossible). In such cases, HEPA filters should be installed in the exhaust duct leading from the room to the general ventilation system to remove infectious organisms and particulates the size of droplet nuclei from the air before it is returned to the general ventilation system (Section II.F; Suppl. 3). Air from TB isolation and treatment rooms in new or renovated facilities should not be recirculated into the general ventilation system.
- Although not required, an anteroom may increase the effectiveness of the isolation room by minimizing the potential escape of droplet nuclei into the corridor when the door is opened. To work effectively, the anteroom should have positive air pressure in relation to the isolation room. The pressure relationship between the anteroom and the corridor may vary according to ventilation design.
- Upper-room air UVGI may be used as an adjunct to general ventilation in the isolation room (Section II.F; Suppl. 3). Air in the isolation room may be recirculated within the room through HEPA filters or UVGI devices to increase the effective ACH and to increase thermal efficiency.
- Health-care facilities should have enough isolation rooms to appropriately isolate all patients who have suspected or confirmed active TB. This number should be estimated using the results of the risk assessment of the health-care facility. Except for minimal- and very low-risk health-care facilities, all acute-care inpatient facilities should have at least one TB isolation room (Section II.B).
- Grouping isolation rooms together in one area of the facility may reduce the possibility of transmitting M. tuberculosis to other patients and may facilitate care of TB patients and the installation and maintenance of optimal engineering (particularly ventilation) controls.

4. Discontinuation of TB Isolation

- TB isolation can be discontinued if the diagnosis of TB is ruled out. For some patients, TB can be ruled out when another diagnosis is confirmed. If a diagnosis of TB cannot be ruled out, the patient should remain in isolation until a determination has been made that the patient is noninfectious. However, patients can be discharged from the health-care facility while still potentially infectious if appropriate postdischarge arrangements can be ensured (Section II.E.5).
- The length of time required for a TB patient to become noninfectious after starting anti-TB therapy varies considerably (Suppl. 1). Isolation should be

discontinued only when the patient is on effective therapy, is improving clinically, and has had three consecutive negative sputum AFB smears collected on different days.

- Hospitalized patients who have active TB should be monitored for relapse by having sputum AFB smears examined regularly (e.g., every 2 weeks). Nonadherence to therapy (i.e., failure to take medications as prescribed) and the presence of drug-resistant organisms are the two most common reasons why patients remain infectious despite treatment. These reasons should be considered if a patient does not respond clinically to therapy within 2–3 weeks.
- Continued isolation throughout the hospitalization should be strongly considered for patients who have MDR-TB because of the tendency for treatment failure or relapse (i.e., difficulty in maintaining noninfectiousness) that has been observed in such cases.

5. Discharge Planning

- Before a TB patient is discharged from the health-care facility, the facility's staff and public health authorities should collaborate to ensure continuation of therapy. Discharge planning in the health-care facility should include, at a minimum, (a) a confirmed outpatient appointment with the provider who will manage the patient until the patient is cured, (b) sufficient medication to take until the outpatient appointment, and (c) placement into case management (e.g., DOT) or outreach programs of the public health department. These plans should be initiated and in place before the patient's discharge.
- Patients who may be infectious at the time of discharge should only be discharged to facilities that have isolation capability or to their homes. Plans for discharging a patient who will return home must consider whether all the household members were infected previously and whether any uninfected household members are at very high risk for active TB if infected (e.g., children less than 4 years of age or persons infected with HIV or otherwise severely immunocompromised). If the household does include such persons, arrangements should be made to prevent them from being exposed to the TB patient until a determination has been made that the patient is noninfectious.

F. Engineering Control Recommendations

1. General Ventilation

This section deals only with engineering controls for general-use areas of health-care facilities (e.g., waiting-room areas and emergency departments). Recommendations for engineering controls for specific areas of the facility (e.g., TB isolation rooms) are contained in the sections encompassing those areas. Details regarding ventilation design, evaluation, and supplemental approaches are described in Supplement 3.

- Health-care facilities should either (a) include as part of their staff an engineer or other professional with expertise in ventilation or (b) have this expertise available from a consultant who is an expert in ventilation engineering and who also has hospital experience. These persons should work closely with infection-control staff to assist in controlling airborne infections.

- Ventilation system designs in health-care facilities should meet any applicable federal, state, and local requirements.
- The direction of airflow in health-care facilities should be designed, constructed, and maintained so that air flows from clean areas to less-clean areas.
- Health-care facilities serving populations that have a high prevalence of TB may need to supplement the general ventilation or use additional engineering approaches (i.e., HEPA filtration or UVGI) in general-use areas where TB patients are likely to go (e.g., waiting-room areas, emergency departments, and radiology suites). A single-pass, nonrecirculating system that exhausts air to the outside, a recirculation system that passes air through HEPA filters before recirculating it to the general ventilation system, or upper air UVGI may be used in such areas.

2. Additional Engineering Control Approaches

a. HEPA Filtration

HEPA filters may be used in a number of ways to reduce or eliminate infectious droplet nuclei from room air or exhaust (Suppl. 3). These methods include placement of HEPA filters (a) in exhaust ducts discharging air from booths or enclosures into the surrounding room; (b) in ducts or in ceiling- or wall-mounted units, for recirculation of air within an individual room (fixed recirculation systems); (c) in portable air cleaners; (d) in exhaust ducts to remove droplet nuclei from air being discharged to the outside, either directly or through ventilation equipment; and (e) in ducts discharging air from the TB isolation room into the general ventilation system. In any application, HEPA filters should be installed carefully and maintained meticulously to ensure adequate functioning.

The manufacturers of in-room air cleaning equipment should provide documentation of the HEPA filter efficiency and the efficiency of the device in lowering room air contaminant levels.

b. UVGI

For general-use areas in which the risk for transmission of M. tuberculosis is relatively high, UVGI lamps may be used as an adjunct to ventilation for reducing the concentration of infectious droplet nuclei (Suppl. 3), although the effectiveness of such units has not been evaluated adequately. Ultra-violet (UV) units can be installed in a room or corridor to irradiate the air in the upper portion of the room (i.e., upper-room air irradiation), or they can be installed in ducts to irradiate air passing through the ducts. UV units installed in ducts should not be substituted for HEPA filters in ducts that discharge air from TB isolation rooms into the general ventilation system. However, UV units can be used in ducts that recirculate air back into the same room.

To function properly and decrease hazards to HCWs and others in the health-care facility, UV lamps should be installed properly and maintained adequately, which includes the monitoring of irradiance levels. UV tubes should be changed according to the manufacturer's instructions or when meter readings indicate tube failure. An employee trained in the use and handling of UV lamps should be responsible for these measures and for keeping maintenance records. Applicable safety guidelines should be followed. Caution should be exercised to protect HCWs, patients, visitors, and others from excessive exposure to UV radiation.

G. Respiratory Protection

- Personal respiratory protection should be used by (a) persons entering rooms in which patients with known or suspected infectious TB are being isolated, (b) persons present during cough-inducing or aerosol-generating procedures performed on such patients, and (c) persons in other settings where administrative and engineering controls are not likely to protect them from inhaling infectious airborne droplet nuclei (Suppl. 4). These other settings include transporting patients who may have infectious TB in emergency transport vehicles and providing urgent surgical or dental care to patients who may have infectious TB before a determination has been made that the patient is noninfectious (Suppl. 1).

- Respiratory protective devices used in health-care settings for protection against M. tuberculosis should meet the following standard performance criteria:

  a. The ability to filter particles 1 mm in size in the unloaded[++] state with a filter efficiency of greater than or equal to 95% (i.e., filter leakage of less than or equal to 5%), given flow rates of up to 50 L per minute.
  b. The ability to be qualitatively or quantitatively fit tested in a reliable way to obtain a face-seal leakage of less than or equal to 10% (54, 55).
  c. The ability to fit the different facial sizes and characteristics of HCWs, which can usually be met by making the respirators available in at least three sizes.
  d. The ability to be checked for facepiece fit, in accordance with standards established by the Occupational Safety and Health Administration (OSHA) and good industrial hygiene practice, by HCWs each time they put on their respirators (54, 55).

- The facility's risk assessment may identify a limited number of selected settings (e.g., bronchoscopy performed on patients suspected of having TB or autopsy performed on deceased persons suspected of having had active TB at the time of death) where the estimated risk for transmission of M. tuberculosis may be such that a level of respiratory protection exceeding the standard performance criteria is appropriate. In such circumstances, a level of respiratory protection exceeding the standard criteria and compatible with patient-care delivery (e.g., more protective negative-pressure respirators; powered air-purifying particulate respirators [PAPRs]; or positive-pressure air-line, half-mask respirators) should be provided by employers to HCWs who are exposed to M. tuberculosis. Information on these and other respirators is in the NIOSH Guide to Industrial Respiratory Protection (55) and in Supplement 4 of this document.

[++]Some filters become more efficient as they become loaded with dust. Health-care settings do not have enough dust in the air to load a filter on a respirator. Therefore, the filter efficiency for respirators used in health-care settings must be determined in the unloaded state.

- In some settings, HCWs may be at risk for two types of exposure: (a) inhalation of M. tuberculosis and (b) mucous membrane exposure to fluids that may contain bloodborne pathogens. In these settings, protection against both types of exposure should be used.
- When operative procedures (or other procedures requiring a sterile field) are performed on patients who may have infectious TB, respiratory protection worn by the HCW should serve two functions: (a) it should protect the surgical field from the respiratory secretions of the HCW, and (b) it should protect the HCW from infectious droplet nuclei that may be expelled by the patient or generated by the procedure. Respirators with exhalation valves and most positive-pressure respirators do not protect the sterile field.
- Health-care facilities in which respiratory protection is used to prevent inhalation of M. tuberculosis are required by OSHA to develop, implement, and maintain a respiratory protection program (Suppl. 4). All HCWs who use respiratory protection should be included in this program. Visitors to TB patients should be given respirators to wear while in isolation rooms, and they should be given general instructions on how to use their respirators.
- Facilities that do not have isolation rooms and do not perform cough-inducing procedures on patients who may have TB may not need to have a respiratory protection program for TB. However, such facilities should have written protocols for the early identification of patients who have signs or symptoms of TB and procedures for referring these patients to a facility where they can be evaluated and managed appropriately. These protocols should be evaluated regularly and revised as needed.
- Surgical masks are designed to prevent the respiratory secretions of the person wearing the mask from entering the air. To reduce the expulsion of droplet nuclei into the air, patients suspected of having TB should wear surgical masks when not in TB isolation rooms. These patients do not need to wear particulate respirators, which are designed to filter the air before it is inhaled by the person wearing the respirator. Patients suspected of having or known to have TB should never wear a respirator that has an exhalation valve, because this type of respirator does not prevent expulsion of droplet nuclei into the air.

H. Cough-Inducing and Aerosol-Generating Procedures

1. General Guidelines

Procedures that involve instrumentation of the lower respiratory tract or induce coughing can increase the likelihood of droplet nuclei being expelled into the air. These cough-inducing procedures include endotracheal intubation and suctioning, diagnostic sputum induction, aerosol treatments (e.g., pentamidine therapy), and bronchoscopy. Other procedures that can generate aerosols (e.g., irrigation of tuberculous abscesses, homogenizing or lyophilizing tissue, or other processing of tissue that may contain tubercle bacilli) are also covered by these recommendations.

- Cough-inducing procedures should not be performed on patients who may have infectious TB unless the procedures are absolutely necessary and can be performed with appropriate precautions.
- All cough-inducing procedures performed on patients who may have infectious TB should

be performed using local exhaust ventilation devices (e.g., booths or special enclosures) or, if this is not feasible, in a room that meets the ventilation requirements for TB isolation.

- HCWs should wear respiratory protection when present in rooms or enclosures in which cough-inducing procedures are being performed on patients who may have infectious TB.
- After completion of cough-inducing procedures, patients who may have infectious TB should remain in their isolation rooms or enclosures and not return to common waiting areas until coughing subsides. They should be given tissues and instructed to cover their mouths and noses with the tissues when coughing. If TB patients must recover from sedatives or anesthesia after a procedure (e.g, after a bronchoscopy), they should be placed in separate isolation rooms (and not in recovery rooms with other patients) while they are being monitored.
- Before the booth, enclosure, or room is used for another patient, enough time should be allowed to pass for at least 99% of airborne contaminants to be removed. This time will vary according to the efficiency of the ventilation or filtration used (Suppl. 3, Table S31).

2. Special Considerations for Bronchoscopy

- If performing bronchoscopy in positive-pressure rooms (e.g., operating rooms) is unavoidable, TB should be ruled out as a diagnosis before the procedure is performed. If the bronchoscopy is being performed for the purpose of diagnosing pulmonary disease and that diagnosis could include TB, the procedure should be performed in a room that meets TB isolation ventilation requirements.

3. Special Considerations for the Administration of Aerosolized Pentamidine

- Patients should be screened for active TB before prophylactic therapy with aerosolized pentamidine is initiated. Screening should include obtaining a medical history and performing skin testing and chest radiography.
- Before each subsequent treatment with aerosolized pentamidine, patients should be screened for symptoms suggestive of TB (e.g., development of a productive cough). If such symptoms are elicited, a diagnostic evaluation for TB should be initiated.
- Patients who have suspected or confirmed active TB should take, if clinically practical, oral prophylaxis for P. carinii pneumonia.

I. Education and Training of HCWs

All HCWs, including physicians, should receive education regarding TB that is relevant to persons in their particular occupational group. Ideally, training should be conducted before initial assignment, and the need for additional training should be reevaluated periodically (e.g., once a year). The level and detail of this education will vary according to the HCW's work responsibilities and the level of risk in the facility (or area of the facility) in which the HCW works. However, the program may include the following elements:

- The basic concepts of M. tuberculosis transmission, pathogenesis, and diagnosis, including information concerning the difference between latent TB infection and active TB disease, the signs and symptoms of TB, and the possibility of reinfection.
- The potential for occupational exposure to persons who have infectious TB in the health-care facility, including information concerning the prevalence of TB in the community and facility, the ability of the facility to properly isolate patients who have active TB, and situations with increased risk for exposure to M. tuberculosis.

- The principles and practices of infection control that reduce the risk for transmission of M. tuberculosis, including information concerning the hierarchy of TB infection-control measures and the written policies and procedures of the facility. Site-specific control measures should be provided to HCWs working in areas that require control measures in addition to those of the basic TB infection-control program.
- The purpose of PPD skin testing, the significance of a positive PPD test result, and the importance of participating in the skin-test program.
- The principles of preventive therapy for latent TB infection. These principles include the indications, use, effectiveness, and the potential adverse effects of the drugs (Suppl. 2).
- The HCW's responsibility to seek prompt medical evaluation if a PPD test conversion occurs or if symptoms develop that could be caused by TB. Medical evaluation will enable HCWs who have TB to receive appropriate therapy and will help to prevent transmission of M. tuberculosis to patients and other HCWs.
- The principles of drug therapy for active TB.
- The importance of notifying the facility if the HCW is diagnosed with active TB so that contact investigation procedures can be initiated.
- The responsibilities of the facility to maintain the confidentiality of the HCW while ensuring that the HCW who has TB receives appropriate therapy and is noninfectious before returning to duty.
- The higher risks associated with TB infection in persons who have HIV infection or other causes of severely impaired cell-mediated immunity, including (a) the more frequent and rapid development of clinical TB after infection with M. tuberculosis, (b) the differences in the clinical presentation of disease, and (c) the high mortality rate associated with MDR-TB in such persons.
- The potential development of cutaneous anergy as immune function (as measured by CD4+ T-lymphocyte counts) declines.
- Information regarding the efficacy and safety of BCG vaccination and the principles of PPD screening among BCG recipients.
- The facility's policy on voluntary work reassignment options for immunocompromised HCWs.

J. HCW Counseling, Screening, and Evaluation

A TB counseling, screening, and prevention program for HCWs should be established to protect both HCWs and patients. HCWs who have positive PPD test results, PPD test conversions, or symptoms suggestive of TB should be identified, evaluated to rule out a diagnosis of active TB, and started on therapy or preventive therapy if indicated (5). In addition, the results of the HCW PPD screening program will contribute to evaluation of the effectiveness of current infection-control practices.

1. Counseling HCWs Regarding TB

- Because of the increased risk for rapid progression from latent TB infection to active TB in HIV-infected or otherwise severely immunocompromised persons, all HCWs should know if they have a medical condition or are receiving a medical treatment that may lead to severely impaired cell-mediated immunity. HCWs who may be at risk for HIV infection should know their HIV status (i.e., they should be encouraged to voluntarily seek counseling and testing for HIV antibody status). Existing guidelines for counseling and testing should be followed routinely (56). Knowledge of these conditions allows the HCW to seek the appropriate preventive measures outlined in this document and to consider voluntary work reassignments. Of particular importance is that HCWs need to know their HIV status if they are at risk for HIV infection and they work in settings where patients who have drug-resistant TB may be encountered.

- All HCWs should be informed about the need to follow existing recommendations for infection control to minimize the risk for exposure to infectious agents; implementation of these recommendations will greatly reduce the risk for occupational infections among HCWs (57). All HCWs should also be informed about the potential risks to severely immunocompromised persons associated with caring for patients who have some infectious diseases, including TB. It should be emphasized that limiting exposure to TB patients is the most protective measure that severely immunosuppressed HCWs can take to avoid becoming infected with M. tuberculosis. HCWs who have severely impaired cell-mediated immunity and who may be exposed to M. tuberculosis may consider a change in job setting to avoid such exposure. HCWs should be advised of the option that severely immunocompromised HCWs can choose to transfer voluntarily to areas and work activities in which there is the lowest possible risk for exposure to M. tuberculosis. This choice should be a personal decision for HCWs after they have been informed of the risks to their health.

- Employers should make reasonable accommodations (e.g., alternative job assignments) for employees who have a health condition that compromises cell-mediated immunity and who work in settings where they may be exposed to M. tuberculosis. HCWs who are known to be immunocompromised should be referred to employee health professionals who can individually counsel the employees regarding their risk for TB. Upon the request of the immunocompromised HCW, employers should offer, but not compel, a work setting in which the HCW would have the lowest possible risk for occupational exposure to M. tuberculosis. Evaluation of these situations should also include consideration of the provisions of the Americans With Disabilities Act of 1990[+++] and other applicable federal, state, and local laws.

- All HCWs should be informed that immunosuppressed HCWs should have appropriate follow-up and screening for infectious diseases, including TB, provided by their medical practitioner. HCWs who are known to be HIV-infected or otherwise severely immunosuppressed should be tested for cutaneous anergy at the time of PPD testing (Suppl. 2). Consideration should be given to retesting, at least every 6 months, those immunocompromised HCWs who are potentially exposed to M. tuberculosis because of the high risk for rapid progression to active TB if they become infected.

- Information provided by HCWs regarding their immune status should be treated confidentially. If the HCW requests voluntary job reassignment, the confidentiality of the HCW should be maintained. Facilities should have written procedures on confidential handling of such information.

2. Screening HCWs for Active TB

- Any HCW who has a persistent cough (i.e., a cough lasting greater than or equal to 3 weeks), especially in the presence of other signs or symptoms com-

---

[+++]Americans With Disabilities Act of 1990. PL 101–336, 42 U.S.C. 12101 et seq.

patible with active TB (e.g., weight loss, night sweats, bloody sputum, anorexia, or fever), should be evaluated promptly for TB. The HCW should not return to the workplace until a diagnosis of TB has been excluded or until the HCW is on therapy and a determination has been made that the HCW is noninfectious.

3. Screening HCWs for Latent TB Infection

- The risk assessment should identify which HCWs have potential for exposure to M. tuberculosis and the frequency with which the exposure may occur. This information is used to determine which HCWs to include in the skin-testing program and the frequency with which they should be tested (Table 2).
- If HCWs are from risks groups with increased prevalence of TB, consideration may be given to including them in the skin-testing program, even if they do not have potential occupational exposure to M. tuberculosis, so that converters can be identified and preventive therapy offered.
- Administrators of health-care facilities should ensure that physicians and other personnel not paid by, but working in, the facility receive skin testing at appropriate intervals for their occupational group and work location.
- During the pre-employment physical or when applying for hospital privileges, HCWs who have potential for exposure to M. tuberculosis (Table 2), including those with a history of BCG vaccination, should have baseline PPD skin testing performed (Suppl. 2). For HCWs who have not had a documented negative PPD test result during the preceding 12 months, the baseline PPD testing should employ the two-step method; this will detect boosting phenomena that might be misinterpreted as a skin-test conversion. Decisions concerning the use of the two-step procedure for baseline testing in a particular facility should be based on the frequency of boosting in that facility.
- HCWs who have a documented history of a positive PPD test, adequate treatment for disease, or adequate preventive therapy for infection, should be exempt from further PPD screening unless they develop signs or symptoms suggestive of TB.
- PPD-negative HCWs should undergo repeat PPD testing at regular intervals as determined by the risk assessment (Section II.B). In addition, these HCWs should be tested whenever they have been exposed to a TB patient and appropriate precautions were not observed at the time of exposure (Section II.K.3). Performing PPD testing of HCWs who work in the same area or occupational group on different scheduled dates (e.g., test them on their birthdays or on their employment anniversary dates), rather than testing all HCWs in the area or group on the same day, may lead to earlier detection of M. tuberculosis transmission.
- All PPD tests should be administered, read, and interpreted in accordance with current guidelines by specified trained personnel (Suppl. 2). At the time their test results are read, HCWs should be informed about the interpretation of both positive and negative PPD test results. This information should indicate that the interpretation of an induration that is 5–9 mm in diameter depends on the HCW's immune status and history of exposure to persons who have infectious TB. Specifically, HCWs who have indurations of 5–9 mm in diameter should be advised that such results may be considered positive for HCWs who are contacts of persons with infectious TB or who

have HIV infection or other causes of severe immunosuppression (e.g., immunosuppressive therapy for organ transplantation).

- When an HCW who is not assigned regularly to a single work area has a PPD test conversion, appropriate personnel should identify the areas where the HCW worked during the time when infection was likely to have occurred. This information can then be considered in analyzing the risk for transmission in those areas.
- In any area of the facility where transmission of M. tuberculosis is known to have occurred, a problem evaluation should be conducted (Section II.K), and the frequency of skin testing should be determined according to the applicable risk category (Section II.B).
- PPD test results should be recorded confidentially in the individual HCW's employee health record and in an aggregate database of all HCW PPD test results. The database can be analyzed periodically to estimate the risk for acquiring new infection in specific areas or occupational groups in the facility.

4. Evaluation and Management of HCWs Who Have Positive PPD Test Results or Active TB

a. Evaluation

- All HCWs with newly recognized positive PPD test results or PPD test conversions should be evaluated promptly for active TB. This evaluation should include a clinical examination and a chest radiograph. If the history, clinical examination, or chest radiograph is compatible with active TB, additional tests should be performed (Section II.C.2). If symptoms compatible with TB are present, the HCW should be excluded from the workplace until either (a) a diagnosis of active TB is ruled out or (b) a diagnosis of active TB was established, the HCW is being treated, and a determination has been made that the HCW is noninfectious (Suppl. 2). HCWs who do not have active TB should be evaluated for preventive therapy according to published guidelines (Suppl. 2).
- If an HCW's PPD test result converts to positive, a history of confirmed or suspected TB exposure should be obtained in an attempt to determine the potential source. When the source of exposure is known, the drug-susceptibility pattern of the M. tuberculosis isolated from the source should be identified so that the correct curative or preventive therapy can be initiated for the HCW with the PPD test conversion. The drug-susceptibility pattern should be recorded in the HCW's medical record, where it will be available if the HCW subsequently develops active TB and needs therapy specific for the drug-susceptibility pattern.
- All HCWs, including those with histories of positive PPD test results, should be reminded periodically about the symptoms of TB and the need for prompt evaluation of any pulmonary symptoms suggestive of TB.

b. Routine and Follow-up Chest Radiographs

- Routine chest radiographs are not required for asymptomatic, PPD-negative HCWs. HCWs with positive PPD test results should have a chest radiograph as part of the initial evaluation of their PPD test; if negative, repeat chest radiographs are not needed unless symptoms develop that could be attributed to TB (58). However, more frequent monitoring for symptoms of TB may be considered for recent converters and other PPD-positive HCWs who are at increased risk for developing active TB (e.g., HIV-infected or otherwise severely immunocompromised HCWs).

c. Workplace Restrictions

1) Active TB
   - HCWs with pulmonary or laryngeal TB pose a risk to patients and other HCWs while they are infectious, and they should be excluded from the workplace until they are noninfectious. The same work restrictions apply to all HCWs regardless of their immune status.
   - Before the HCW who has TB can return to the work-place, the health-care facility should have documentation from the HCW's health-care provider that the HCW is receiving adequate therapy, the cough has resolved, and the HCW has had three consecutive negative sputum smears collected on different days. After work duties are resumed and while the HCW remains on anti-TB therapy, facility staff should receive periodic documentation from the HCW's health-care provider that the HCW is being maintained on effective drug therapy for the recommended time period and that the sputum AFB smears continue to be negative.
   - HCWs with active laryngeal or pulmonary TB who discontinue treatment before they are cured should be evaluated promptly for infectiousness. If the evaluation determines that they are still infectious, they should be excluded from the workplace until treatment has been resumed, an adequate response to therapy has been documented, and three more consecutive sputum AFB smears collected on different days have been negative.
   - HCWs who have TB at sites other than the lung or larynx usually do not need to be excluded from the workplace if a diagnosis of concurrent pulmonary TB has been ruled out.
2) Latent TB Infection
   - HCWs receiving preventive treatment for latent TB infection should not be restricted from their usual work activities.
   - HCWs with latent TB infection who cannot take or who do not accept or complete a full course of preventive therapy should not be excluded from the work-place. These HCWs should be counseled about the risk for developing active TB and instructed regularly to seek prompt evaluation if signs or symptoms develop that could be caused by TB.

K. Problem Evaluation

Epidemiologic investigations may be indicated for several situations. These include, but are not limited to, (a) the occurrence of PPD test conversions or active TB in HCWs; (b) the occurrence of possible person-to-person transmission of M. tuberculosis; and (c) situations in which patients or HCWs with active TB are not promptly identified and isolated, thus exposing other persons in the facility to M. tuberculosis. The general objectives of the epidemiologic investigations in these situations are as follows:

1. To determine the likelihood that transmission of and infection with M. tuberculosis has occurred in the facility;
2. To determine the extent to which M. tuberculosis has been transmitted;

3. To identify those persons who have been exposed and infected, enabling them to receive appropriate clinical management;

4. To identify factors that could have contributed to transmission and infection and to implement appropriate interventions; and

5. To evaluate the effectiveness of any interventions that are implemented and to ensure that exposure to and transmission of M. tuberculosis have been terminated.

The exact circumstances of these situations are likely to vary considerably, and the associated epidemiologic investigations should be tailored to the individual circumstances. The following sections provide general guidance for conducting these investigations.

1. Investigating PPD Test Conversions and Active TB in HCWs

a. Investigating PPD Test Conversions in HCWs

PPD test conversions may be detected in HCWs as a result of a contact investigation, in which case the probable source of exposure and transmission is already known (Section II.K.3.), or as a result of routine screening, in which case the probable source of exposure and infection is not already known and may not be immediately apparent.

If a skin-test conversion in an HCW is identified as part of routine screening, the following steps should be considered (Figure 2):

- The HCW should be evaluated promptly for active TB. The initial evaluation should include a thorough history, physical examination, and chest radiograph. On the basis of the initial evaluation, other diagnostic procedures (e.g., sputum examination) may be indicated.
- If appropriate, the HCW should be placed on preventive or curative therapy in accordance with current guidelines (Suppl. 2) (5).
- A history of possible exposure to M. tuberculosis should be obtained from the HCW to determine the most likely source of infection. When the source of infection is known, the drug-susceptibility pattern of the M. tuberculosis isolate from the source patient should be identified to determine appropriate preventive or curative therapy regimens.
- If the history suggests that the HCW was exposed to and infected with M. tuberculosis outside the facility, no further epidemiologic investigation to identify a source in the facility is necessary.
- If the history does not suggest that the HCW was exposed and infected outside the facility but does identify a probable source of exposure in the facility, contacts of the suspected source patient should be identified and evaluated. Possible reasons for the exposure and transmission should be evaluated (Table 4), interventions should be implemented to correct these causes, and PPD testing of PPD-negative HCWs should be performed immediately and repeated after 3 months.

    If no additional PPD test conversions are detected on follow-up testing, the investigation can be terminated.

    If additional PPD test conversions are detected on follow-up testing, the possible reasons for exposure and transmission should be reassessed, the appropriateness of and degree of adherence to the interventions implemented should be evaluated, and PPD testing of PPD-negative HCWs should be repeated after another 3 months.

    If no additional PPD test conversions are detected on the second round of follow-up testing, the investigation can be terminated. However, if additional PPD conversions are detected on the second round of follow-up testing, a high-risk protocol should be implemented in the affected area or occupational group, and the public health department or other persons with expertise in TB infection control should be consulted.

- If the history does not suggest that the HCW was exposed to and infected with M. tubercu-

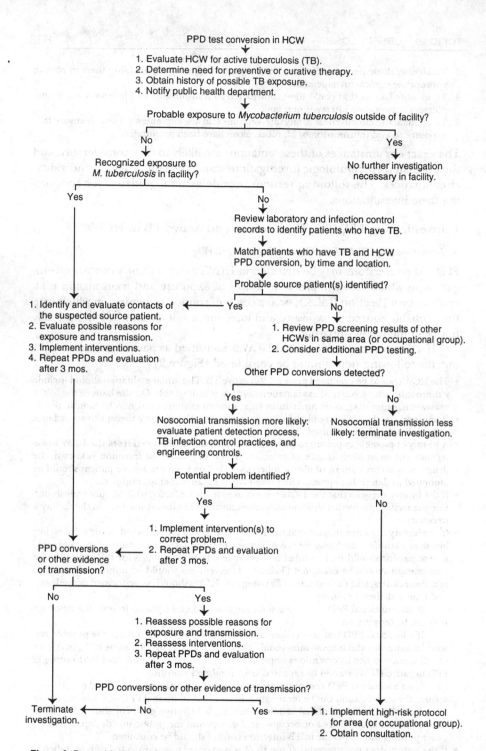

Figure 2. Protocol for investigating purified protein derivative (PPD)-tuberculin skin-test conversions in health-care workers (HCWs).

Table 4. Examples of Potential Problems that Can Occur When Identifying or Isolating Patients Who May Have Infectious Tuberculosis (TB)

Situation	Potential problem	Intervention
Patient identification during triage	Patient with signs or symptoms not identified. Patient had no symptoms listed in triage protocol.	Review triage procedures, facilities, and practices. Reevaluate triage protocol.
During review of laboratory results	Positive smear: results available >24 hours* after submitted	Change laboratory practices. Assess potential barriers. Explore alternatives.
	Positive smear: results available but action not taken promptly.	Educate appropriate personnel. Review protocol for management of positive smear results.
	Positive culture: results not available for >3 weeks.*	Change laboratory practices. Assess potential barriers. Explore alternatives.
	Positive culture: results available but action not taken promptly.	Educate appropriate personnel. Review protocol for management of positive culture results.
	Positive culture: susceptibility results not available for >6 weeks.*	Change laboratory practices. Assess potential barriers. Explore alternatives.
	Positive culture: susceptibility results available but action not taken promptly.	Educate appropriate personnel. Review protocol for management of positive culture susceptibility results.
At time of diagnosis and during isolation	Patient with signs/symptoms of TB: appropriate tests not ordered promptly.	Educate appropriate personnel. Evaluate protocols for TB detection.
	Isolation room unavailable.	Reassess need for number of isolation rooms.
	Isolation not ordered or discontinued too soon, or isolation policy not followed properly (e.g., patients going outside of room).	Educate patients and appropriate personnel. Evaluate institutional barriers to implementation of isolation policy.
	Personnel not properly using respiratory protection.	Educate appropriate personnel. Evaluate regularly scheduled re-education. Evaluate institutional barriers to use of respiratory protection.
	Isolation room or procedure room not at negative pressure relative to surrounding areas.	Make appropriate engineering modifications. Establish protocols for regularly monitoring and maintaining negative pressure.
	Inadequate air circulation.	Make appropriate engineering modifications.
	Door left open.	Educate appropriate personnel and patients. Evaluate self-closing doors, comfort levels in the room, and other measures to promote door closing.

*These time intervals are used as examples and should not be considered absolute standards.

losis outside the facility and does not identify a probable source of exposure in the facility, further investigation to identify the probable source patient in the facility is warranted.

The interval during which the HCW could have been infected should be estimated. Generally, this would be the interval from 10 weeks before the most recent negative PPD test through 2 weeks before the first positive PPD test (i.e., the conversion).

Laboratory and infection-control records should be reviewed to identify all patients or HCWs who have suspected or confirmed infectious TB and who could have transmitted M. tuberculosis to the HCW.

If this process does identify a likely source patient, contacts of the suspected source patient should be identified and evaluated, and possible reasons for the exposure and transmission should be evaluated (Table 4). Interventions should be implemented to correct these causes, and PPD testing of PPD-negative HCWs should be repeated after 3 months. However, if this process does not identify a probable source case, PPD screening results of other HCWs in the same area or occupational group should be reviewed for additional evidence of M. tuberculosis transmission. If sufficient additional PPD screening results are not available, appropriate personnel should consider conducting additional PPD screening of other HCWs in the same area or occupational group.

If this review and/or screening does not identify additional PPD conversions, nosocomial transmission is less likely, and the contact investigation can probably be terminated. Whether the HCW's PPD test conversion resulted from occupational exposure and infection is uncertain; however, the absence of other data implicating nosocomial transmission suggests that the conversion could have resulted from (a) unrecognized exposure to M. tuberculosis outside the facility; (b) cross-reactivity with another antigen (e.g., nontuberculous mycobacteria); c) errors in applying, reading, or interpreting the test; (d) false positivity caused by the normal variability of the test; or (e) false positivity caused by a defective PPD preparation.

If this review and/or screening does identify additional PPD test conversions, nosocomial transmission is more likely. In this situation, the patient identification (i.e., triage) process, TB infection-control policies and practices, and engineering controls should be evaluated to identify problems that could have led to exposure and transmission (Table 4).

If no such problems are identified, a high-risk protocol should be implemented in the affected area or occupational group, and the public health department or other persons with expertise in TB infection control should be consulted.

If such problems are identified, appropriate interventions should be implemented to correct the problem(s), and PPD skin testing of PPD-negative HCWs should be repeated after 3 months.

If no additional PPD conversions are detected on follow-up testing, the investigation can be terminated.

If additional PPD conversions are detected on follow-up testing, the possible reasons for exposure and transmission should be reassessed, the appropriateness of and adherence to the interventions implemented should be evaluated, and PPD skin testing of PPD-negative HCWs should be repeated after another 3 months.

If no additional PPD test conversions are detected on this second round of follow-up testing, the investigation can be terminated. However, if additional PPD test conversions are detected on the second round of follow-up testing, a high-risk protocol should be implemented in the affected area or occupational group, and the public health department or other persons with expertise in TB infection control should be consulted.

b. Investigating Cases of Active TB in HCWs

If an HCW develops active TB, the following steps should be taken:

- The case should be evaluated epidemiologically, in a manner similar to PPD test conversions in HCWs, to determine the likelihood that it resulted from occupational transmission and to identify possible causes and implement appropriate interventions if the evaluation suggests such transmission.

- Contacts of the HCW (e.g., other HCWs, patients, visitors, and others who have had intense exposure to the HCW) should be identified and evaluated for TB infection and disease (Section II.K.3; Suppl. 2). The public health department should be notified immediately for consultation and to allow for investigation of community contacts who were not exposed in the health-care facility.
- The public health department should notify facilities when HCWs with TB are reported by physicians so that an investigation of contacts can be conducted in the facility. The information provided by the health department to facilities should be in accordance with state or local laws to protect the confidentiality of the HCW.

2. Investigating Possible Patient-to-Patient Transmission of M. tuberculosis

Surveillance of active TB cases in patients should be conducted. If this surveillance suggests the possibility of patient-to-patient transmission of M. tuberculosis (e.g., a high proportion of TB patients had prior admissions during the year preceding onset of their TB, the number of patients with drug-resistant TB increased suddenly, or isolates obtained from multiple patients had identical and characteristic drug-susceptibility or DNA fingerprint patterns), the following steps should be taken:

- Review the HCW PPD test results and patient surveillance data for the suspected areas to detect additional patients or HCWs with PPD test conversions or active disease.
- Look for possible exposures that patients with newly diagnosed TB could have had to other TB patients during previous admissions. For example, were the patients admitted to the same room or area, or did they receive the same procedure or go to the same treatment area on the same day?

If the evaluation thus far suggests transmission has occurred, the following steps should be taken:

- Evaluate possible causes of the transmission (e.g., problem with patient detection, institutional barriers to implementing appropriate isolation practices, or inadequate engineering controls) (Table 4).
- Ascertain whether other patients or HCWs could have been exposed; if so, evaluate these persons for TB infection and disease (Section II.K.3; Suppl. 2).
- Notify the public health department so they can begin a community contact investigation if necessary.

3. Investigating Contacts of Patients and HCWs Who Have Infectious TB

If a patient who has active TB is examined in a health-care facility and the illness is not diagnosed correctly, resulting in failure to apply appropriate precautions, or if an HCW develops active TB and exposes other persons in the facility, the following steps should be taken when the illness is later diagnosed correctly:

- To identify other patients and HCWs who were exposed to the source patient before isolation procedures were begun, interview the source patient and all applicable personnel and review that patient's medical record. Determine the areas of the facility in which the source patient was hospitalized, visited, or worked before being placed in isolation (e.g., outpatient clinics, hospital rooms, treatment rooms, radiology and procedure areas, and patient lounges) and the HCWs who may have been exposed during that time (e.g., persons providing direct care, therapists, clerks, transportation personnel, housekeepers, and social workers).
- The contact investigation should first determine if M. tuberculosis transmission has occurred from the source patient to those persons with whom the source patient had the most intense contact.

- Administer PPD tests to the most intensely exposed HCWs and patients as soon as possible after the exposure has occurred. If transmission did occur to the most intensely exposed persons, then those persons with whom the patient had less contact should be evaluated. If the initial PPD test result is negative, a second test should be administered 12 weeks after the exposure was terminated.
- Those persons who were exposed to M. tuberculosis and who have either a PPD test conversion or symptoms suggestive of TB should receive prompt clinical evaluation and, if indicated, chest radiographs and bacteriologic studies should be performed (Suppl. 2). Those persons who have evidence of newly acquired infection or active disease should be evaluated for preventive or curative therapy (Suppl. 2). Persons who have previously had positive PPD test results and who have been exposed to an infectious TB patient do not require a repeat PPD test or a chest radiograph unless they have symptoms suggestive of TB.
- In addition to PPD testing those HCWs and patients who have been exposed to M. tuberculosis because a patient was not isolated promptly or an HCW with active TB was not identified promptly, the investigation should determine why the diagnosis of TB was delayed. If the correct diagnosis was made but the patient was not isolated promptly, the reasons for the delay need to be defined so that corrective actions can be taken.

L. Coordination with the Public Health Department

- As soon as a patient or HCW is known or suspected to have active TB, the patient or HCW should be reported to the public health department so that appropriate follow-up can be arranged and a community contact investigation can be performed. The health department should be notified well before patient discharge to facilitate follow-up and continuation of therapy. A discharge plan coordinated with the patient or HCW, the health department, and the inpatient facility should be implemented.
- The public health department should protect the confidentiality of the patient or HCW in accordance with state and local laws.
- Health-care facilities and health departments should coordinate their efforts to perform appropriate contact investigations on patients and HCWs who have active TB.
- In accordance with state and local laws and regulations, results of all AFB-positive sputum smears, cultures positive for M. tuberculosis, and drug-susceptibility results on M. tuberculosis isolates should be reported to the public health department as soon as these results are available.
- The public health department may be able to assist facilities with planning and implementing various aspects of a TB infection-control program (e.g., surveillance, screening activities, and outbreak investigations). In addition, the state health department may be able to provide names of experts to assist with the engineering aspects of TB infection control.

M. Additional Considerations for Selected Areas in Health-Care Facilities and Other Health-Care Settings

This section contains additional information for selected areas in health-care facilities and for other health-care settings.

1. Selected Areas in Health-Care Facilities

A. OPERATING ROOMS

- Elective operative procedures on patients who have TB should be delayed until the patient is no longer infectious.

- If operative procedures must be performed, they should be done, if possible, in operating rooms that have anterooms. For operating rooms without anterooms, the doors to the operating room should be closed, and traffic into and out of the room should be minimal to reduce the frequency of opening and closing the door. Attempts should be made to perform the procedure at a time when other patients are not present in the operative suite and when a minimum number of personnel are present (e.g., at the end of day).
- Placing a bacterial filter on the patient endotracheal tube (or at the expiratory side of the breathing circuit of a ventilator or anesthesia machine if these are used) when operating on a patient who has confirmed or suspected TB may help reduce the risk for contaminating anesthesia equipment or discharging tubercle bacilli into the ambient air.
- During postoperative recovery, the patient should be monitored and should be placed in a private room that meets recommended standards for ventilating TB isolation rooms.
- When operative procedures (or other procedures requiring a sterile field) are performed on patients who may have infectious TB, respiratory protection worn by the HCW must protect the field from the respiratory secretions of the HCW and protect the HCW from the infectious droplet nuclei generated by the patient. Valved or positive-pressure respirators do not protect the sterile field; therefore, a respirator that does not have a valve and that meets the criteria in Section II.G should be used.

B. AUTOPSY ROOMS

- Because infectious aerosols are likely to be present in autopsy rooms, such areas should be at negative pressure with respect to adjacent areas (Suppl. 3), and the room air should be exhausted directly to the outside of the building. ASHRAE recommends that autopsy rooms have ventilation that provides an airflow of 12 ACH (47), although the effectiveness of this ventilation level in reducing the risk for M. tuberculosis transmission has not been evaluated. Where possible, this level should be increased by means of ventilation system design or by auxiliary methods (e.g., recirculation of air within the room through HEPA filters) (Suppl. 3).
- Respiratory protection should be worn by personnel while performing autopsies on deceased persons who may have had TB at the time of death (Section II.G; Suppl. 4).
- Recirculation of HEPA-filtered air within the room or UVGI may be used as a supplement to the recommended ventilation (Suppl. 3).

C. LABORATORIES

- Laboratories in which specimens for mycobacteriologic studies (e.g., AFB smears and cultures) are processed should be designed to conform with criteria specified by CDC and the National Institutes of Health (59).

2. Other Health-Care Settings

TB precautions may be appropriate in a number of other types of health-care settings. The specific precautions that are applied will vary depending on the setting. At a minimum, a risk assessment should be performed yearly for these settings; a written TB infection-control plan should be developed, evaluated, and revised on a regular basis; protocols should be in place for identifying and managing patients who may have active TB; HCWs should receive appropriate training, education, and screening; protocols for problem evaluation should be in place; and coordination with the public health department should be arranged when necessary. Other recommendations specific to certain of these settings follow.

A. EMERGENCY MEDICAL SERVICES

- When EMS personnel or others must transport patients who have confirmed or suspected active TB, a surgical mask should be placed, if possible, over the patient's mouth and nose. Because administrative and engineering controls during emergency transport situations cannot be ensured, EMS personnel should wear respiratory protection when transporting such patients. If feasible, the windows of the vehicle should be kept open. The heating and air-conditioning system should be set on a nonrecirculating cycle.

- EMS personnel should be included in a comprehensive PPD screening program and should receive a baseline PPD test and follow-up testing as indicated by the risk assessment. They should also be included in the follow-up of contacts of a patient with infectious TB. [++++]

B. HOSPICES

- Hospice patients who have confirmed or suspected TB should be managed in the manner described in this document for management of TB patients in hospitals. General-use and specialized areas (e.g., treatment or TB isolation rooms) should be ventilated in the same manner as described for similar hospital areas.

C. LONG-TERM CARE FACILITIES

- Recommendations published previously for preventing and controlling TB in long-term care facilities should be followed (60).
- Long-term care facilities should also follow the recommendations outlined in this document.

D. CORRECTIONAL FACILITIES

- Recommendations published previously for preventing and controlling TB in correctional facilities should be followed (61).
- Prison medical facilities should also follow the recommendations outlined in this document.

E. DENTAL SETTINGS

In general, the symptoms for which patients seek treatment in a dental-care setting are not likely to be caused by infectious TB. Unless a patient requiring dental care coincidentally has TB, it is unlikely that infectious TB will be encountered in the dental setting. Furthermore, generation of droplet nuclei containing M. tuberculosis during dental procedures has not been demonstrated (62). Therefore, the risk for transmission of M. tuberculosis in most dental settings is probably quite low. Nevertheless, during dental procedures, patients and dental workers share the same air for varying periods of time. Coughing may be stimulated occasionally by oral manipulations, although no specific dental procedures have been classified as "cough-inducing." In some instances, the population served by a dental-care facility, or the HCWs in the facility, may be at relatively high risk for TB. Because the potential exists for transmission of M. tuberculosis in dental settings, the following recommendations should be followed:

- A risk assessment (Section II.B) should be done periodically, and TB infection-control policies for each dental setting should be based on the risk assessment. The policies should include provisions for detection and referral of patients who may have undiagnosed active TB; management of patients with active TB, relative to provision of urgent dental care; and employer-sponsored HCW education, counseling, and screening.
- While taking patients' initial medical histories and at periodic updates, dental HCWs should routinely ask all patients whether they have a history of TB disease and symptoms suggestive of TB.
- Patients with a medical history or symptoms suggestive of undiagnosed active TB should be referred promptly for medical evaluation of possible infectiousness. Such patients should not remain in the dental-care facility any longer than required to arrange a referral. While in the dental-care facility, they should wear surgical masks and should be instructed to cover their mouths and noses when coughing or sneezing.

[++++]The Ryan White Comprehensive AIDS Resource Emergency Act of 1990, P.L. 101–381, mandates notification of EMS personnel after they have been exposed to infectious pulmonary TB (42 U.S.C. 700ff; 82.54 Fed. Reg. 13417 [March 21, 1994]).

- Elective dental treatment should be deferred until a physician confirms that the patient does not have infectious TB. If the patient is diagnosed as having active TB, elective dental treatment should be deferred until the patient is no longer infectious.
- If urgent dental care must be provided for a patient who has, or is strongly suspected of having, infectious TB, such care should be provided in facilities that can provide TB isolation (Sections II.E and G). Dental HCWs should use respiratory protection while performing procedures on such patients.
- Any dental HCW who has a persistent cough (i.e., a cough lasting greater than or equal to 3 weeks), especially in the presence of other signs or symptoms compatible with active TB (e.g., weight loss, night sweats, bloody sputum, anorexia, and fever), should be evaluated promptly for TB. The HCW should not return to the work-place until a diagnosis of TB has been excluded or until the HCW is on therapy and a determination has been made that the HCW is noninfectious.
- In dental-care facilities that provide care to populations at high risk for active TB, it may be appropriate to use engineering controls similar to those used in general-use areas (e.g., waiting rooms) of medical facilities that have a similar risk profile.

F. HOME HEALTH-CARE SETTINGS

- HCWs who provide medical services in the homes of patients who have suspected or confirmed infectious TB should instruct such patients to cover their mouths and noses with a tissue when coughing or sneezing. Until such patients are no longer infectious, HCWs should wear respiratory protection when entering these patients' homes (Suppl. 4).
- Precautions in the home may be discontinued when the patient is no longer infectious (Suppl. 1).
- HCWs who provide health-care services in their patients' homes can assist in preventing transmission of M. tuberculosis by educating their patients regarding the importance of taking medications as prescribed and by administering DOT.
- Cough-inducing procedures performed on patients who have infectious TB should not be done in the patients' homes unless absolutely necessary. When medically necessary cough-inducing procedures (e.g., AFB sputum collection for evaluation of therapy) must be performed on patients who may have infectious TB, the procedures should be performed in a health-care facility in a room or booth that has the recommended ventilation for such procedures. If these procedures must be performed in a patient's home, they should be performed in a well-ventilated area away from other household members. If feasible, the HCW should consider opening a window to improve ventilation or collecting the specimen while outside the dwelling. The HCW collecting these specimens should wear respiratory protection during the procedure (Section II.G).
- HCWs who provide medical services in their patients' homes should be included in comprehensive employer-sponsored TB training, education, counseling, and screening programs. These programs should include provisions for identifying HCWs who have active TB, baseline PPD skin testing, and follow-up PPD testing at intervals appropriate to the degree of risk.
- Patients who are at risk for developing active TB and the HCWs who provide medical services in the homes of such patients should be reminded periodically of the importance of having pulmonary symptoms evaluated promptly to permit early detection of and treatment for TB.

G. MEDICAL OFFICES

In general, the symptoms of active TB are symptoms for which patients are likely to seek treatment in a medical office. Furthermore, the populations served by some medical offices, or the HCWs in the office, may be at relatively high risk for TB. Thus, it is likely that infectious TB will be encountered in a medical office. Because of the potential for M. tuberculosis transmission, the following recommendations should be observed:

- A risk assessment should be conducted periodically, and TB infection-control policies based on results of the risk assessment should be developed for the medical office. The policies should include provisions for identifying and managing patients who may have undiagnosed active TB; managing patients who have active TB; and educating, training, counseling, and screening HCWs.

- While taking patients' initial medical histories and at periodic updates, HCWs who work in medical offices should routinely ask all patients whether they have a history of TB disease or have had symptoms suggestive of TB.
- Patients with a medical history and symptoms suggestive of active TB should receive an appropriate diagnostic evaluation for TB and be evaluated promptly for possible infectiousness. Ideally, this evaluation should be done in a facility that has TB isolation capability. At a minimum, the patient should be provided with and asked to wear a surgical mask, instructed to cover the mouth and nose with a tissue when coughing or sneezing, and separated as much as possible from other patients.
- Medical offices that provide evaluation or treatment services for TB patients should follow the recommendations for managing patients in ambulatory-care settings (Section II.D).
- If cough-inducing procedures are to be administered in a medical office to patients who may have active TB, appropriate precautions should be followed (Section II.H).
- Any HCW who has a persistent cough (i.e., a cough lasting greater than or equal to 3 weeks), especially in the presence of other signs or symptoms compatible with active TB (e.g., weight loss, night sweats, bloody sputum, anorexia, or fever) should be evaluated promptly for TB. HCWs with such signs or symptoms should not return to the workplace until a diagnosis of TB has been excluded or until they are on therapy and a determination has been made that they are noninfectious.
- HCWs who work in medical offices in which there is a likelihood of exposure to patients who have infectious TB should be included in employer-sponsored education, training, counseling, and PPD testing programs appropriate to the level of risk in the office.
- In medical offices that provide care to populations at relatively high risk for active TB, use of engineering controls as described in this document for general-use areas (e.g., waiting rooms) may be appropriate (Section II.F; Suppl. 3).

Supplement 1: Determining the Infectiousness of a TB Patient

The infectiousness of patients with TB correlates with the number of organisms expelled into the air, which, in turn, correlates with the following factors: (a) disease in the lungs, airways, or larynx; (b) presence of cough or other forceful expiratory measures; (c) presence of acid-fast bacilli (AFB) in the sputum; (d) failure of the patient to cover the mouth and nose when coughing; (e) presence of cavitation on chest radiograph; (f) inappropriate or short duration of chemotherapy; and (g) administration of procedures that can induce coughing or cause aerosolization of M. tuberculosis (e.g., sputum induction).

The most infectious persons are most likely those who have not been treated for TB and who have either (a) pulmonary or laryngeal TB and a cough or are undergoing cough-inducing procedures, (b) a positive AFB sputum smear, or (c) cavitation on chest radiograph. Persons with extrapulmonary TB usually are not infectious unless they have (a) concomitant pulmonary disease; (b) nonpulmonary disease located in the respiratory tract or oral cavity; or (c) extrapulmonary disease that includes an open abscess or lesion in which the concentration of organisms is high, especially if drainage from the abscess or lesion is extensive (20, 22). Coinfection with HIV does not appear to affect the infectiousness of TB patients (63–65).

In general, children who have TB may be less likely than adults to be infectious; however, transmission from children can occur. Therefore, children with TB should be evaluated for infectiousness using the same parameters as for adults (i.e., pulmonary or laryngeal TB, presence of cough or cough-inducing procedures, positive sputum AFB smear, cavitation on chest radiograph, and adequacy and duration of therapy). Pediatric patients who may be infectious include those who (a) are not on therapy, (b) have just been started on therapy, or (c) are on inadequate therapy, and who (a) have laryngeal or extensive pulmonary involvement, (b) have pronounced cough or are undergoing cough-inducing procedures, (c) have positive sputum AFB smears, or (d) have cavitary TB. Children who have typical primary tuberculous lesions and do not have any of the indicators of infectiousness listed previously usually do not need to be placed in isolation. Because the source case for pediatric TB patients often occurs in a member of the infected child's family (45), parents and other visitors of all pediatric TB patients should be evaluated for TB as soon as possible.

Infection is most likely to result from exposure to persons who have unsuspected pulmonary TB and are not receiving anti-TB therapy or from persons who have diagnosed TB and are not receiving adequate therapy. Administration of effective anti-TB therapy has been associated with decreased infectiousness among persons who have active TB (66). Effective therapy reduces coughing, the amount of sputum produced, and the number of organisms in the sputum. However, the period of time a patient must take effective therapy before becoming noninfectious varies between patients (67). For example, some TB patients are never infectious, whereas those with unrecognized or inadequately treated drug-resistant TB may remain infectious for weeks or months (24). Thus, decisions about infectiousness should be made on an individual basis.

In general, patients who have suspected or confirmed active TB should be considered infectious if they (a) are coughing, (b) are undergoing cough-inducing procedures, or (c) have positive AFB sputum smears, and if they (a) are not on chemotherapy, (b) have just started chemotherapy, or (c) have a poor clinical or bacteriologic response to chemotherapy. A patient who has drug- susceptible TB and who is on adequate chemotherapy and has had a significant clinical and bacteriologic response to therapy (i.e., reduction in cough, resolution of fever, and progressively decreasing quantity of bacilli on smear) is probably no longer infectious. However, because drug-susceptibility results are not usually known when the decision to discontinue isolation is made, all TB patients should remain in isolation while hospitalized until they have had three consecutive negative sputum smears collected on different days and they demonstrate clinical improvement.

Supplement 2: Diagnosis and Treatment of Latent TB Infection and Active TB

I. DIAGNOSTIC PROCEDURES FOR TB INFECTION AND DISEASE

A diagnosis of TB may be considered for any patient who has a persistent cough (i.e., a cough lasting greater than or equal to 3 weeks) or other signs or symptoms compatible with TB (e.g., bloody sputum, night sweats, weight loss, anorexia, or fever). However, the index of suspicion for TB will vary in different geographic areas and will depend on the prevalence of TB and other characteristics of the population served by the facility. The index of suspicion for TB should be very high in areas or among groups of patients in which the prevalence of TB is high (Section I.B). Persons for whom a diagnosis of TB is being considered should receive appropriate diagnostic tests, which may include PPD skin testing, chest radiography, and bacteriologic studies (e.g., sputum microscopy and culture).

A. PPD SKIN TESTING AND ANERGY TESTING

1. Application and Reading of PPD Skin Tests

The PPD skin test is the only method available for demonstrating infection with M. tuberculosis. Although currently available PPD tests are less than 100% sensitive and specific for detection of infection with M. tuberculosis, no better diagnostic methods have yet been devised. Interpretation of PPD test results requires knowledge of the antigen used, the immunologic basis for the reaction to this antigen, the technique used to administer and read the test, and the results of epidemiologic and clinical experience with the test (2, 5, 6). The PPD test, like all medical tests, is subject to variability, but many of the variations in administering and reading PPD tests can be avoided by proper training and careful attention to details.

The intracutaneous (Mantoux) administration of a measured amount of PPD-tuberculin is currently the preferred method for doing the test. One-tenth milliliter of PPD (5 TU) is injected just beneath the surface of the skin on either the volar or dorsal surface of the forearm. A discrete, pale elevation of the skin (i.e., a wheal) that is 6–10 mm in diameter should be produced.

PPD test results should be read by designated, trained personnel between 48 and 72 hours after injection. Patient or HCW self-reading of PPD test results should not be accepted (68). The result of the test is based on the presence or absence of an induration at the injection site. Redness or erythema should not be measured. The transverse diameter of induration should be recorded in millimeters.

2. Interpretation of PPD Skin Tests

A. GENERAL

The interpretation of a PPD reaction should be influenced by the purpose for which the test was given (e.g., epidemiologic versus diagnostic purposes), by the prevalence of TB infection in the population being tested, and by the consequences of false classification. Errors in classification can be minimized by establishing an appropriate definition of a positive reaction (Table S21).

Table S21. Summary of Interpretation of Purified Protein Derivative (PPD)-Tuberculin Skin-Test Results

1. An induration of ≥5 mm is classified as positive in:
   —Persons who have human immunodeficiency virus (HIV) infection or risk factors for HIV infection but unknown HIV status;
   —Persons who have had recent close contact* with persons who have active tuberculosis (TB);
   —Persons who have fibrotic chest radiographs (consistent with healed TB).
2. An induration of ≥10 mm is classified as positive in all persons who do not meet any of the criteria above but who have other risk factors for TB, including:
   High-risk groups
   —Injecting-drug users known to be HIV seronegative;
   —Persons who have other medical conditions that reportedly increase the risk for progressing from latent TB infection to active TB (e.g., silicosis, gastrectomy or jejuno-ileal bypass; being ≥10% below ideal body weight; chronic renal failure with renal dialysis; diabetes mellitus; high-dose corticosteroid or other immunosuppressive therapy; some hematologic disorders, including malignancies such as leukemias and lymphomas; and other malignancies);
   —Children <4 years of age.
   High-prevalence groups
   —Persons born in countries in Asia, Africa, the Caribbean, and Latin America that have high prevalence of TB;
   —Persons from medically underserved, low-income populations;
   —Residents of long-term facilities (e.g., correctional institutions and nursing homes);
   —Persons from high-risk populations in their communities, as determined by local public health authorities.
3. An induration of ≥15 mm is classified as positive in persons who do not meet any of the above criteria.
4. Recent converters are defined on the basis of both size of induration and age of the person being tested:
   —≥10 mm increase within a 2-year period is classified as a recent conversion for persons <35 years of age;
   —≥15 mm increase within a 2-year period is classified as a recent conversion for persons ≥35 years of age.
5. PPD skin-test results in health-care workers (HCWs)
   —In general, the recommendations in sections 1, 2, and 3 of this table should be followed when interpreting skin-test results in HCWs.
   However, the prevalence of TB in the facility should be considered when choosing the appropriate cut-point for defining a positive PPD reaction. In facilities where there is essentially no risk for exposure to Mycobacterium tuberculosis (i.e., minimal- or very low-risk facilities Section II.B), an induration ≥15 mm may be a suitable cut-point for HCWs who have no other risk factors. In facilities where TB patients receive care, the cut-point for HCWs with no other risk factors may be ≥10 mm.
   —A recent conversion in an HCW should be defined generally as a ≥10 mm increase in size of induration within a 2-year period. For HCWs who work in facilities where exposure to TB is very unlikely (e.g., minimal-risk facilities), an increase of ≥15 mm within a 2-year period may be more appropriate for defining a recent conversion because of the lower positive-predictive value of the test in such groups.

*Recent close contact implies either household or social contact or unprotected occupational exposure similar in intensity and duration to household contact.

The positive-predictive value of PPD tests (i.e, the probability that a person with a positive PPD test is actually infected with M. tuberculosis) is dependent on the prevalence of TB infection in the population being tested and the specificity of the test (69, 70). In populations with a low prevalence of TB infection, the probability that a positive PPD test represents true infection with M. tuberculosis is very low if the cut-point is set too low (i.e., the test is not adequately specific). In populations with a high prevalence of TB infection, the probability that a positive PPD test using the same cut-point represents true infection with M. tuberculosis is much higher. To ensure that few persons infected with tubercle bacilli will be misclassified as having negative reactions and few persons not infected with tubercle bacilli will be misclassified as having positive reactions, different cut-points are used to separate positive reactions from negative reactions for different populations, depending on the risk for TB infection in that population.

A lower cut-point (i.e., 5 mm) is used for persons in the highest risk groups, which include HIV-infected persons, recent close contacts of persons with TB (e.g., in the household or in an unprotected occupational exposure similar in intensity and duration to household contact), and persons who have abnormal chest radiographs with fibrotic changes consistent with inactive TB. A higher cut-point (i.e., 10 mm) is used for persons who are not in the highest risk group but who have other risk factors (e.g., injecting-drug users known to be HIV seronegative; persons with certain medical conditions that increase the risk for progression from latent TB infection to active TB [Table S21]); medically underserved, low-income populations; persons born in foreign countries that have a high prevalence of TB; and residents of correctional institutions and nursing homes). An even higher cut-point (i.e., 15 mm) is used for all other persons who have none of the above risk factors.

Recent PPD converters are considered members of a high-risk group. A greater than or equal to 10 mm increase in the size of the induration within a 2-year period is classified as a conversion from a negative to a positive test result for persons less than 35 years of age. An increase of induration of greater than or equal to 15 mm within a 2-year period is classified as a conversion for persons greater than or equal to 35 years of age (5).

B. HCWS

In general, HCWs should have their skin-test results interpreted according to the recommendations in this supplement and in sections 1, 2, 3, and 5 of Table S21. However, the prevalence of TB in the facility should be considered when choosing the appropriate cut-point for defining a positive PPD reaction. In facilities where there is essentially no risk for exposure to TB patients (i.e., minimal- or very low-risk facilities [Section II.B]), an induration greater than or equal to 15 mm may be an appropriate cut-point for HCWs who have no other risk factors. In other facilities where TB patients receive care, the appropriate cut-point for HCWs who have no other risk factors may be greater than or equal to 10 mm.

A recent PPD test conversion in an HCW should be defined generally as an increase of greater than or equal to 10 mm in the size of induration within a 2-year period. For HCWs in facilities where exposure to TB is very unlikely (e.g., minimal-risk facilities), an increase of greater than or equal to 15 mm within a 2-year period may be more appropriate for defining a recent conversion because of the lower positive-predictive value of the test in such groups.

3. Anergy Testing

HIV-infected persons may have suppressed reactions to PPD skin tests because of anergy, particularly if their CD4+ T-lymphocyte counts decline (71). Persons with anergy will have a negative PPD test regardless of infection with M. tuberculosis. HIV-infected persons should be evaluated for anergy in conjunction with PPD testing (72). Two companion antigens (e.g., Candida antigen and tetanus toxoid) should be administered in addition to PPD. Persons with greater than or equal to 3 mm of induration to any of the skin tests (including tuberculin) are considered not anergic. Reactions of greater than or equal to 5 mm to PPD are considered to be evidence of TB infection in HIV-infected persons regardless of the reactions to the companion antigens. If there is no reaction (i.e., less than 3 mm induration) to any of the antigens, the person being tested is considered anergic. Determination of whether such persons are likely to be infected with M. tuberculosis must be based on other epidemiologic factors (e.g., the proportion of other persons with the same level of exposure who have positive PPD test results and the intensity or duration of exposure to infectious TB patients that the anergic person experienced).

4. Pregnancy and PPD Skin Testing

Although thousands (perhaps millions) of pregnant women have been PPD skin tested since the test was devised, thus far no documented episodes of fetal harm have resulted from use of the tuberculin test (73). Pregnancy should not exclude a female HCW from being skin tested as part of a contact investigation or as part of a regular skin-testing program.

5. BCG Vaccination and PPD Skin Testing

BCG vaccination may produce a PPD reaction that cannot be distinguished reliably from a reaction caused by infection with M. tuberculosis. For a person who was vaccinated with BCG, the probability that a PPD test reaction results from infection with M. tuberculosis increases (a) as the size of the reaction increases, (b) when the person is a contact of a person with TB, (c) when the person's country of origin has a high prevalence of TB, and (d) as the length of time between vaccination and PPD testing increases. For example, a PPD test reaction of greater than or equal to 10 mm probably can be attributed to M. tuberculosis infection in an adult who was vaccinated with BCG as a child and who is from a country with a high prevalence of TB (74, 75).

6. The Booster Phenomenon

The ability of persons who have TB infection to react to PPD may gradually wane. For example, if tested with PPD, adults who were infected during their childhood may have a negative reaction. However, the PPD could boost the hypersensitivity, and the size of the reaction could be larger on a subsequent test. This boosted reaction may be misinterpreted as a PPD test conversion from a newly acquired infection. Misinterpretation of a boosted reaction as a new infection could result in unnecessary investigations of laboratory and patient records in an attempt to identify the source case and in unnecessary prescription of preventive therapy for HCWs. Although boosting can occur among persons in any age group, the likelihood of the reaction increases with the age of the person being tested (6, 76).

When PPD testing of adults is to be repeated periodically (as in HCW skin-testing programs), two-step testing can be used to reduce the likelihood that a boosted reaction is misinterpreted as a new infection. Two-step testing should be performed on all newly employed HCWs who have an initial negative PPD test result at the time of employment and have not had a documented negative PPD test result during the 12 months preceding the initial test. A second test should be performed 1–3 weeks after the first test. If the second test result is positive, this is most likely a boosted reaction, and the HCW should be classified as previously infected. If the second test result remains negative, the HCW is classified as uninfected, and a positive reaction to a subsequent test is likely to represent a new infection with M. tuberculosis.

B. CHEST RADIOGRAPHY

Patients who have positive skin-test results or symptoms suggestive of TB should be evaluated with a chest radiograph regardless of PPD test results. Radiographic abnormalities that strongly suggest active TB include upper-lobe infiltration, particularly if cavitation is seen (77), and patchy or nodular infiltrates in the apical or subapical posterior upper lobes or the superior segment of the lower lobe. If abnormalities are noted, or if the patient has symptoms suggestive of extrapulmonary TB, additional diagnostic tests should be conducted.

The radiographic presentation of pulmonary TB in HIV-infected patients may be unusual (78). Typical apical cavitary disease is less common among such patients. They may have infiltrates in any lung zone, a finding that is often associated with mediastinal and/or hilar adenopathy, or they may have a normal chest radiograph, although this latter finding occurs rarely.

C. BACTERIOLOGY

Smear and culture examination of at least three sputum specimens collected on different days is the main diagnostic procedure for pulmonary TB (6). Sputum smears that fail to demonstrate AFB do not exclude the diagnosis of TB. In the United States, approximately 60% of patients with positive sputum cultures have positive AFB sputum smears. HIV-infected patients who have pulmonary TB may be less likely than immunocompetent patients to have AFB present on sputum smears, which is consistent with the lower frequency of cavitary pulmonary disease observed among HIV-infected persons (39, 41).

Specimens for smear and culture should contain an adequate amount of expectorated sputum but not much saliva. If a diagnosis of TB cannot be established from sputum, a bronchoscopy may be necessary (36, 37). In young children who cannot produce an adequate amount of sputum, gastric aspirates may provide an adequate specimen for diagnosis.

A culture of sputum or other clinical specimen that contains M. tuberculosis provides a definitive diagnosis of TB. Conventional laboratory methods may require 4–8 weeks for species identification; however, the use of radiometric culture techniques and nucleic acid probes facilitates more rapid detection and identification of mycobacteria (79, 80). Mixed mycobacterial infection, either simultaneous or sequential, can obscure the identification of M. tuberculosis during the clinical evaluation and the laboratory analysis (42). The use of nucleic acid probes for both M. avium complex and M. tuberculosis may be useful for identifying mixed mycobacterial infections in clinical specimens.

II. PREVENTIVE THERAPY FOR LATENT TB INFECTION AND TREATMENT OF ACTIVE TB

A. PREVENTIVE THERAPY FOR LATENT TB INFECTION

Determining whether a person with a positive PPD test reaction or conversion is a candidate for preventive therapy must be based on (a) the likelihood that the reaction represents true infection with M. tuberculosis (as determined by the cut-points), (b) the estimated risk for progression from latent infection to active TB, and (c) the risk for hepatitis associated with taking isoniazid (INH) preventive therapy (as determined by age and other factors).

HCWs with positive PPD test results should be evaluated for preventive therapy regardless of their ages if they (a) are recent converters, (b) are close contacts of persons who have active TB, (c) have a medical condition that increases the risk for TB, (d) have HIV infection, or (e) use injecting drugs (5). HCWs with positive PPD test results who do not have these risk factors should be evaluated for preventive therapy if they are less than 35 years of age.

Preventive therapy should be considered for anergic persons who are known contacts of infectious TB patients and for persons from populations in which the prevalence of TB infection is very high (e.g., a prevalence of greater than 10%).

Because the risk for INH-associated hepatitis may be increased during the peripartum period, the decision to use preventive therapy during pregnancy should be made on an individual basis and should depend on the patient's estimated risk for progression to active disease. In general, preventive therapy can be delayed until after delivery. However, for pregnant women who were probably infected recently or who have high-risk medical conditions, especially HIV infection, INH preventive therapy should begin when the infection is documented (81–84). No evidence suggests that INH poses a carcinogenic risk to humans (85–87).

The usual preventive therapy regimen is oral INH 300 mg daily for adults and 10 mg/kg/day for children (88). The recommended duration of therapy is 12 months for persons with HIV infection and 9 months for children. Other persons should receive INH therapy for 6–12 months. For persons who have silicosis or a chest radiograph demonstrating inactive fibrotic lesions and who have no evidence of active TB, acceptable regimens include (a) 4 months of INH plus rifampin or (b) 12 months of INH, providing that infection with INH-resistant organisms is unlikely (33). For persons likely to be infected with MDR-TB, alternative multidrug preventive therapy regimens should be considered (89).

All persons placed on preventive therapy should be educated regarding the possible adverse reactions associated with INH use, and they should be questioned carefully at monthly intervals by qualified personnel for signs or symptoms consistent with liver damage or other adverse effects (81–84, 88, 90, 91). Because INH-associated hepatitis occurs more frequently among persons greater than 35 years of age, a transaminase measurement should be obtained from persons in this age group before initiation of INH therapy and then obtained monthly until treatment has been completed. Other factors associated with an increased risk for hepatitis include daily alcohol use, chronic liver disease, and injecting-drug use. In addition, postpubertal black and Hispanic women may be at greater risk for hepatitis or drug interactions (92). More careful clinical monitoring of persons with these risk factors and possibly more frequent laboratory monitoring should be considered. If any of these tests exceeds three to five times the upper limit of normal, discontinuation of INH should be strongly considered. Liver function tests are not a substitute for monthly clinical evaluations or for the prompt assessment of signs or symptoms of adverse reactions that could occur between the regularly scheduled evaluations (33).

Persons who have latent TB infection should be advised that they can be reinfected with another strain of M. tuberculosis (93).

B. TREATMENT OF PATIENTS WHO HAVE ACTIVE TB

Drug-susceptibility testing should be performed on all initial isolates from patients with TB. However, test results may not be available for several weeks, making selection of an initial regimen difficult, especially in areas where drug-resistant TB has been documented. Current recommendations for therapy and dosage schedules for the treatment of drug-susceptible TB should be followed (Table S22; Table S23) (43). Streptomycin is contraindicated in the treatment of pregnant women because of the risk for ototoxicity to the fetus. In geographic areas or facilities in which drug-resistant TB is highly prevalent, the initial treatment regimen used while results of drug-susceptibility tests are pending may need to be expanded. This decision should be based on analysis of surveillance data.

When results from drug-susceptibility tests become available, the regimen should be adjusted appropriately (94–97). If drug resistance is present, clinicians unfamiliar with the management of patients with drug-resistant TB should seek expert consultation.

For any regimen to be effective, adherence to the regimen must be ensured. The most effective method of ensuring adherence is the use of DOT after the patient has been discharged from the hospital (43, 91). This practice should be coordinated with the public health department.

Supplement 3: Engineering Controls

I. INTRODUCTION

This supplement provides information regarding the use of ventilation (Section II) and UVGI (Section III) for preventing the transmission of M. tuberculosis in health-care facilities. The information provided is primarily conceptual and is intended to educate staff in the health-care facility concerning engineering controls and how these controls can be used as part of the TB infection-control program. This supplement should not be used in place of consultation with experts, who can assume responsibility for advising on ventilation system design and selection, installation, and maintenance of equipment.

The recommendations for engineering controls include (a) local exhaust ventilation (i.e., source control), (b) general ventilation, and (c) air cleaning. General ventilation considerations include (a) dilution and removal of contaminants, (b) airflow patterns within rooms, (c) airflow direction in facilities, (d) negative pressure in rooms, and (e) TB isolation rooms. Air cleaning or disinfection can be accomplished by filtration of air (e.g., through HEPA filters) or by UVGI.

II. VENTILATION

Ventilation systems for health-care facilities should be designed, and modified when necessary, by ventilation engineers in collaboration with infection-control and occupational health staff. Recommendations for designing and operating ventilation systems have been published by ASHRAE (47), AIA (48), and the American Conference of Governmental Industrial Hygienists, Inc. (98).

As part of the TB infection-control plan, health-care facility personnel should determine the number of TB isolation rooms, treatment rooms, and local exhaust devices (i.e., for

Table S22. Regimen Options for the Treatment of Tuberculosis (TB) in Children and Adults

Option	Indication	Total duration of therapy	Initial treatment phase		Continuation treatment phase		Comments
			Drugs*	Interval and duration	Drugs*	Interval and duration	
1	Pulmonary and extrapulmonary TB in adults and children	6 mos	INH RIF PZA EMB or SM	Daily for 8 wks	INH RIF	Daily or two or three times wkly+ for 16 wks	—EMB or SM should be continued until susceptibility to INH and RIF is demonstrated. —In areas where primary INH resistance is <4%, EMB or SM may not be necessary for patients with no individual risk factors for drug resistance.
2	Pulmonary and extrapulmonary TB in adults and children	6 mos	INH RIF PZA EMB or SM	Daily for 2 wks, then Two times wkly+ for 6 wks	INH RIF	Two times wkly+ for 16 wks^k	—Regimen should be directly observed. —After the initial phase, EMB or SM should be continued until susceptibility to INH and RIF is demonstrated, unless drug resistance is unlikely.
3	Pulmonary and extrapulmonary TB in adults and children	6 mos	INH RIF PZA EMB or SM	3 times wkly+ for 6 mos^k			—Regimen should be directly observed. —Continue all four drugs for 6 mos.@ —This regimen has been shown to be effective for INH-resistant TB.
4	Smear- and culture-negative pulmonary TB in adults	4 mos	INH RIF PZA EMB or SM	Follow option 1, 2, or 3 for 8 wks	INH RIF PZA EMB or SM	Daily or two or three times wkly+ for 8 wks	—Continue all four drugs for 4 mos. —If drug resistance is unlikely (primary INH resistance <4% and patient has no individual risk factors for drug resistance), EMB or SM may not be necessary and PZA may be discontinued after 2 mos.

Table S22. —*continued*

Option	Indication	Total duration of therapy	Initial treatment phase		Continuation treatment phase		Comments
			Drugs*	Interval and duration	Drugs*	Interval and duration	
5	Pulmonary and extrapulmonary TB in adults and children when PZA is contraindicated	9 mos	INH RIF EMG or SM**	Daily for 8 wks	INH RIF	Daily or two times wkly+ for 24 wks&	—EMB or SM should be continued until susceptibility to INH and RIF is demonstrated. —In areas where primary INH resistance is <4%, EMB or SM may not be necessary for patients with no individual risk factors for drug resistance.

*EMB = ethambutol; INH = isoniazid; PZA = pyrazinamide; RIF = rifampin; SM = streptomycin.

+All regimens administered intermittently should be directly observed.

&For infants and children with miliary TB, bone and joint TB, or TB meningitis, treatment should last at least 12 months. For adults with these forms of extrapulmonary TB, response to therapy should be monitored closely. If response is slow or suboptimal, treatment may be prolonged on a case-by-case basis.

@Some evidence suggests that SM may be discontinued after 4 months if the isolate is susceptible to all drugs.

**Avoid treating pregnant women with SM because of the risk for ototoxicity to the fetus.

Note: For all patients, if drug-susceptibility results show resistance to any of the first-line drugs, or if the patient remains symptomatic or smear- or culture-positive after 3 months, consult a TB medical expert.

Table S23. Dosage Recommendations for the Initial Treatment of Tuberculosis in Children* and Adults

| | Dosage schedule | | | | | |
| Drug | Daily dose (maximum dose) | | Two doses per week (maximum dose) | | Three doses per week (maximum dose) | |
	Children	Adults	Children	Adults	Children	Adults
Isoniazid	10–20 mg/kg (300 mg)	5 mg/kg (300 mg)	20–40 mg/kg (900 mg)	15 mg/kg (900 mg)	20–40 mg/kg (900 mg)	15 mg/kg (900 mg)
Rifampin	10–20 mg/kg (600 mg)	10 mg/kg (600 mg)	10–20 mg/kg (600 mg)	10 mg/kg (600 mg)	10–20 mg/kg (600 mg)	10 mg/kg (600 mg)
Pyrazinamide	15–30 mg/kg (2 gm)	15–30 mg/kg (2 gm)	50–70 mg/kg (4 gm)	50–70 mg/kg (4 gm)	50–70 mg/kg (3 gm)	50–70 mg/kg (3 gm)
Ethambutol	15–25 mg/kg (1 gm)	15–25 mg/kg	50 mg/kg	50 mg/kg	25–30 mg/kg	25–30 mg/kg
Streptomycin	20–40 mg/kg (1 gm)	15 mg/kg (1 gm)	20–40 mg/kg (1.5 gm)	20–40 mg/kg (1.5 gm)	20–40 mg/kg (1.5 gm)	20–40 mg/kg (1.5 gm)

*Persons ≤12 years of age.

cough-inducing or aerosol-generating procedures) that the facility needs. The locations of these rooms and devices will depend on where in the facility the ventilation conditions recommended in this document can be achieved. Grouping isolation rooms together in one area of the facility may facilitate the care of TB patients and the installation and maintenance of optimal engineering controls (particularly ventilation).

Periodic evaluations of the ventilation system should review the number of TB isolation rooms, treatment rooms, and local exhaust devices needed and the regular maintenance and monitoring of the local and general exhaust systems (including HEPA filtration systems if they are used).

The various types and conditions of ventilation systems in health-care facilities and the individual needs of these facilities preclude the ability to provide specific instructions regarding the implementation of these recommendations. Engineering control methods must be tailored to each facility on the basis of need and the feasibility of using the ventilation and air-cleaning concepts discussed in this supplement.

A. LOCAL EXHAUST VENTILATION

Purpose: To capture airborne contaminants at or near their source (i.e., the source control method) and remove these contaminants without exposing persons in the area to infectious agents (98).

Source control techniques can prevent or reduce the spread of infectious droplet nuclei into the general air circulation by entrapping infectious droplet nuclei as they are being emitted by the patient (i.e., the source). These techniques are especially important when performing procedures likely to generate aerosols containing infectious particles and when infectious TB patients are coughing or sneezing.

Local exhaust ventilation is a preferred source control technique, and it is often the most efficient way to contain airborne contaminants because it captures these contaminants near their source before they can disperse. Therefore, the technique should be used, if feasible, wherever aerosol-generating procedures are performed. Two basic types of local exhaust devices use hoods: (a) the enclosing type, in which the hood either partially or fully encloses the infectious source; and (b) the exterior type, in which the infectious source is near but outside the hood. Fully enclosed hoods, booths, or tents are always preferable to exterior types because of their superior ability to prevent contaminants from escaping into the HCW's breathing zone. Descriptions of both enclosing and exterior devices have been published previously (98).

1. Enclosing Devices

The enclosing type of local exhaust ventilation device includes laboratory hoods used for processing specimens that could contain viable infectious organisms, booths used for sputum induction or administration of acrosolized medications (e.g., aerosolized pentamidine) (Figure S31), and tents or hoods made of vinyl or other materials used to enclose and isolate a patient. These devices are available in various configurations. The most simple of these latter devices is a tent that is placed over the patient; the tent has an exhaust connection to the room discharge exhaust system. The most complex device is an enclosure that has a sophisticated self-contained airflow and recirculation system.

Both tents and booths should have sufficient airflow to remove at least 99% of airborne particles during the interval between the departure of one patient and the arrival of the next (99). The time required for removing a given percentage of airborne particles from an enclosed space depends on several factors. These factors include the number of ACH, which is determined by the number of cubic feet of air in the room or booth and the rate at which air is entering the room or booth at the intake source; the location of the ventilation inlet and outlet; and the physical configuration of the room or booth (Table S31).

2. Exterior Devices

The exterior type of local exhaust ventilation device is usually a hood very near, but not enclosing, the infectious patient. The airflow produced by these devices should be sufficient to

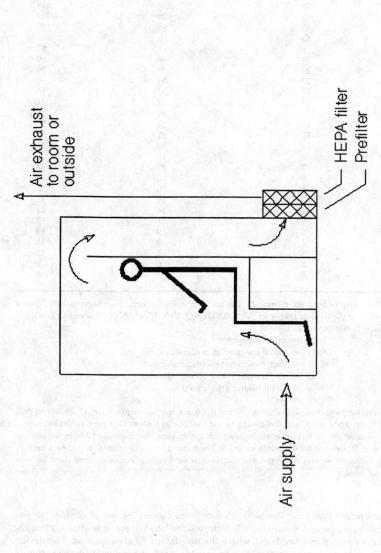

Air exhaust to room or outside

HEPA filter
Prefilter

Air supply

*Passage of air directly from the air supply to the exhaust (i.e., short-circuiting of air) is prevented by the structure on which patients sit and the wall on which patients rest their backs.

Figure S31. An enclosing booth designed to sweep air past a patient who has active tuberculosis and entrap the infectious droplet nuclei in a high-efficiency particulate air (HEPA) filter.

Table S31. Air Changes per Hour (ACH) and Time in Minutes Required for Removal Efficiencies of 90%, 99%, and 99.9% of Airborne Contaminants*

	Minutes required for a removal efficiency of:		
ACH	90%	99%	99.9%
1	138	276	414
2	69	138	207
3	46	92	138
4	35	69	104
5	28	55	83
6	23	46	69
7	20	39	59
8	17	35	52
9	15	31	46
10	14	28	41
11	13	25	38
12	12	23	35
13	11	21	32
14	10	20	30
15	9	18	28
16	9	17	26
17	8	16	24
18	8	15	23
19	7	15	22
20	7	14	21
25	6	11	17
30	5	9	14
35	4	8	12
40	3	7	10
45	3	6	9
50	3	6	8

*This table has been adapted from the formula for the rate of purging airborne contaminants (99). Values have been derived from the formula $t(1) = \ln(C(2)/C(1))/(Q/V) \times 60$, with $T(1) = 0$ and $C(2)/C(1) -$ (removal efficiency/100), and where:

$$
\begin{aligned}
t(1) &= \text{initial timepoint} \\
C(1) &= \text{initial concentration of contaminant} \\
C(2) &= \text{final concentration of contaminants} \\
Q &= \text{air flow rate (cubic feet per hour)} \\
V &= \text{room volume (cubic feet)} \\
Q/V &= \text{ACH}
\end{aligned}
$$

The times given assume perfect mixing of the air within the space (i.e., mixing factor = 1). However, perfect mixing usually does not occur, and the mixing factor could be as high as 10 if air distribution is very poor (98). The required time is derived by multiplying the appropriate time from the table by the mixing factor that has been determined for the booth or room. The factor and required time should be included in the operating instructions provided by the manufacturer of the booth or enclosure, and these instructions should be followed.

prevent cross-currents of air near the patient's face from causing escape of droplet nuclei. Whenever possible, the patient should face directly into the hood opening so that any coughing or sneezing is directed into the hood, where the droplet nuclei are captured. The device should maintain an air velocity of greater than or equal to 200 feet per minute at the patient's breathing zone to ensure capture of droplet nuclei.

3. Discharge Exhaust from Booths, Tents, and Hoods

Air from booths, tents, and hoods may be discharged into the room in which the device is located or it may be exhausted to the outside. If the air is discharged into the room, a HEPA filter should be incorporated at the discharge duct or vent of the device. The exhaust fan should be located on the discharge side of the HEPA filter to ensure that the air pressure in the filter housing and booth is negative with respect to adjacent areas. Uncontaminated air from the room will flow into the booth through all openings, thus preventing infectious droplet nuclei in the booth from escaping into the room. Most commercially available booths, tents, and hoods are fitted with HEPA filters, in which case additional HEPA filtration is not needed.

If the device does not incorporate a HEPA filter, the air from the device should be exhausted to the outside in accordance with recommendations for isolation room exhaust (Suppl. 3, Section II.B.5). (See Supplement 3, Section II.C, for information regarding recirculation of exhaust air.)

B. GENERAL VENTILATION

General ventilation can be used for several purposes, including diluting and removing contaminated air, controlling airflow patterns within rooms, and controlling the direction of airflow throughout a facility. Information on these topics is contained in the following sections.

1. Dilution and Removal

Purpose: To reduce the concentration of contaminants in the air.

General ventilation maintains air quality by two processes: dilution and removal of airborne contaminants. Uncontaminated supply (i.e., incoming) air mixes with the contaminated room air (i.e., dilution), which is subsequently removed from the room by the exhaust system (i.e., removal). These processes reduce the concentration of droplet nuclei in the room air.

A. TYPES OF GENERAL VENTILATION SYSTEMS

Two types of general ventilation systems can be used for dilution and removal of contaminated air: the single-pass system and the recirculating system. In a single-pass system, the supply air is either outside air that has been appropriately heated and cooled or air from a central system that supplies a number of areas. After air passes through the room (or area), 100% of that air is exhausted to the outside. The single-pass system is the preferred choice in areas where infectious airborne droplet nuclei are known to be present (e.g., TB isolation rooms or treatment rooms) because it prevents contaminated air from being recirculated to other areas of the facility.

In a recirculating system, a small portion of the exhaust air is discharged to the outside and is replaced with fresh outside air, which mixes with the portion of exhaust air that was not discharged to the outside. The resulting mixture, which can contain a large proportion of contaminated air, is then recirculated to the areas serviced by the system. This air mixture could be recirculated into the general ventilation, in which case contaminants may be carried from contaminated areas to uncontaminated areas. Alternatively, the air mixture could also be recirculated within a specific room or area, in which case other areas of the facility will not be affected (Suppl. 3, Section II.C.3).

B. VENTILATION RATES

Recommended general ventilation rates for health-care facilities are usually expressed in number of ACH. This number is the ratio of the volume of air entering the room per hour to the room volume and is equal to the exhaust airflow (Q [cubic feet per minute]) divided by the room volume (V [cubic feet]) multiplied by 60 (i.e., $ACH = Q / V \times 60$).

The feasibility of achieving specific ventilation rates depends on the construction and operational requirements of the ventilation system (e.g., the energy requirements to move and to heat or cool the air). The feasibility of achieving specific ventilation rates may also be different for retro-fitted facilities and newly constructed facilities. The expense and effort of achieving specific higher ventilation rates for new construction may be reasonable, whereas retro- fitting an existing facility to achieve similar ventilation rates may be more difficult. However, achieving higher ventilation rates by using auxiliary methods (e.g., room-air recirculation) in addition to exhaust ventilation may be feasible in existing facilities (Suppl. 3, Section II.C).

2. Airflow Patterns Within Rooms (Air Mixing)

Purpose: To provide optimum airflow patterns and prevent both stagnation and short-circuiting of air.

General ventilation systems should be designed to provide optimal patterns of airflow within rooms and prevent air stagnation or short-circuiting of air from the supply to the exhaust (i.e., passage of air directly from the air supply to the air exhaust). To provide optimal airflow patterns, the air supply and exhaust should be located such that clean air first flows to parts of the room where HCWs are likely to work, and then flows across the infectious source and into the exhaust. In this way, the HCW is not positioned between the infectious source and the exhaust location. Although this configuration may not always be possible, it should be used whenever feasible. One way to achieve this airflow pattern is to supply air at the side of the room opposite the patient and exhaust it from the side where the patient is located. Another method, which is most effective when the supply air is cooler than the room air, is to supply air near the ceiling and exhaust it near the floor (Figure S32). Airflow patterns are affected by large air temperature differentials, the precise location of the supply and exhausts, the location of furniture, the movement of HCWs and patients, and the physical configuration of the space. Smoke tubes can be used to visualize airflow patterns in a manner similar to that described for estimating room air mixing.

Adequate air mixing, which requires that an adequate number of ACH be provided to a room (Suppl. 3, Section II.B.1), must be ensured to prevent air stagnation within the room. However, the air will not usually be changed the calculated number of times per hour because the airflow patterns in the room may not permit complete mixing of the supply and room air in all parts of the room. This results in an "effective" airflow rate in which the supplied airflow may be less than required for proper ventilation. To account for this variation, a mixing factor (which

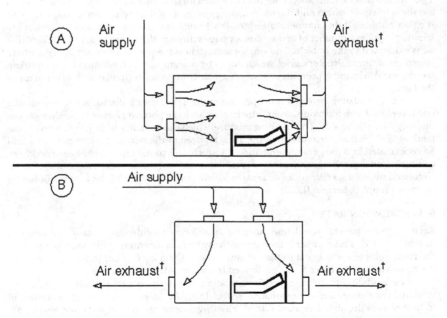

† Air should be exhausted to the outside (or through high-efficiency particulate air [HEPA] filters, if recirculated).

Figure S32. Room airflow patterns designed to provide mixing of air and prevent passage of air directly from the air supply to the exhaust.

ranges from 1 for perfect mixing to 10 for poor mixing) is applied as a multiplier to determine the actual supply airflow (i.e., the recommended ACH multiplied by the mixing factor equals the actual required ACH) (51, 98). The room air supply and exhaust system should be designed to achieve the lowest mixing factor possible. The mixing factor is determined most accurately by experimentally testing each space configuration, but this procedure is complex and time-consuming. A reasonably good qualitative measure of mixing can be estimated by an experienced ventilation engineer who releases smoke from smoke tubes at a number of locations in the room and observes the movement of the smoke. Smoke movement in all areas of the room indicates good mixing. Stagnation of air in some areas of the room indicates poor mixing, and movement of the supply and exhaust openings or redirection of the supply air is necessary.

3. Airflow Direction in the Facility

Purpose: To contain contaminated air in localized areas in a facility and prevent its spread to uncontaminated areas.

A. DIRECTIONAL AIRFLOW

The general ventilation system should be designed and balanced so that air flows from less contaminated (i.e., more clean) to more contaminated (less clean) areas (47, 48). For example, air should flow from corridors (cleaner areas) into TB isolation rooms (less clean areas) to prevent spread of contaminants to other areas. In some special treatment rooms in which operative and invasive procedures are performed, the direction of airflow is from the room to the hallway to provide cleaner air during these procedures. Cough-inducing or aerosol-generating procedures (e.g., bronchoscopy and irrigation of tuberculous abscesses) should not be performed in rooms with this type of airflow on patients who may have infectious TB.

B. NEGATIVE PRESSURE FOR ACHIEVING DIRECTIONAL AIRFLOW

The direction of airflow is controlled by creating a lower (negative) pressure in the area into which the flow of air is desired. For air to flow from one area to another, the air pressure in the two areas must be different. Air will flow from a higher pressure area to a lower pressure area. The lower pressure area is described as being at negative[&] pressure relative to the higher pressure area. Negative pressure is attained by exhausting air from an area at a higher rate than air is being supplied. The level of negative pressure necessary to achieve the desired airflow will depend on the physical configuration of the ventilation system and area, including the airflow path and flow openings, and should be determined on an individual basis by an experienced ventilation engineer.

4. Achieving Negative Pressure in a Room

Purpose: To control the direction of airflow between the room and adjacent areas, thereby preventing contaminated air from escaping from the room into other areas of the facility.

A. PRESSURE DIFFERENTIAL

The minimum pressure difference necessary to achieve and maintain negative pressure that will result in airflow into the room is very small (0.001 inch of water). Higher pressures (greater than or equal to 0.001 inch of water) are satisfactory; however, these higher pressures may be difficult to achieve. The actual level of negative pressure achieved will depend on the difference in the ventilation exhaust and supply flows and the physical configuration of the room, including the airflow path and flow openings. If the room is well sealed, negative pressures greater than the minimum of 0.001 inch of water may be readily achieved. However, if rooms are not well sealed, as may be the case in many facilities (especially older facilities), achieving higher negative pressures may require exhaust/supply flow differentials beyond the capability of the ventilation system.

[&]Negative is defined relative to the air pressure in the area from which air is to flow.

To establish negative pressure in a room that has a normally functioning ventilation system, the room supply and exhaust airflows are first balanced to achieve an exhaust flow of either 10% or 50 cubic feet per minute (cfm) greater than the supply (whichever is the greater). In most situations, this specification should achieve a negative pressure of at least 0.001 inch of water. If the minimum 0.001 inch of water is not achieved and cannot be achieved by increasing the flow differential (within the limits of the ventilation system), the room should be inspected for leakage (e.g., through doors, windows, plumbing, and equipment wall penetrations), and corrective action should be taken to seal the leaks.

Negative pressure in a room can be altered by changing the ventilation system operation or by the opening and closing of the room's doors, corridor doors, or windows. When an operating configuration has been established, it is essential that all doors and windows remain properly closed in the isolation room and other areas (e.g., doors in corridors that affect air pressure) except when persons need to enter or leave the room or area.

B. ALTERNATE METHODS FOR ACHIEVING NEGATIVE PRESSURE

Although an anteroom is not a substitute for negative pressure in a room, it may be used to reduce escape of droplet nuclei during opening and closing of the isolation room door. Some anterooms have their own air supply duct, but others do not. The TB isolation room should have negative pressure relative to the anteroom, but the air pressure in the anteroom relative to the corridor may vary depending on the building design. This should be determined, in accordance with applicable regulations, by a qualified ventilation engineer.

If the existing ventilation system is incapable of achieving the desired negative pressure because the room lacks a separate ventilation system or the room's system cannot provide the proper airflow, steps should be taken to provide a means to discharge air from the room. The amount of air to be exhausted will be the same as discussed previously (Suppl. 3, Section II.B.4.a).

Fixed room-air recirculation systems (i.e., systems that recirculate the air in an entire room) may be designed to achieve negative pressure by discharging air outside the room (Suppl. 3, Section II.C.3).

Some portable room-air recirculation units (Suppl. 3, Section II.C.3.b.) are designed to discharge air to the outside to achieve negative pressure. Air cleaners that can accomplish this must be designed specifically for this purpose.

A small centrifugal blower (i.e., exhaust fan) can be used to exhaust air to the outside through a window or outside wall. This approach may be used as an interim measure to achieve negative pressure, but it provides no fresh air and suboptimal dilution.

Another approach to achieving the required pressure difference is to pressurize the corridor. Using this method, the corridor's general ventilation system is balanced to create a higher air pressure in the corridor than in the isolation room; the type of balancing necessary depends on the configuration of the ventilation system. Ideally, the corridor air supply rate should be increased while the corridor exhaust rate is not increased. If this is not possible, the exhaust rate should be decreased by resetting appropriate exhaust dampers. Caution should be exercised, however, to ensure that the exhaust rate is not reduced below acceptable levels. This approach requires that all settings used to achieve the pressure balance, including doors, be maintained. This method may not be desirable if the corridor being pressurized has rooms in which negative pressure is not desired. In many situations, this system is difficult to achieve, and it should be considered only after careful review by ventilation personnel.

C. MONITORING NEGATIVE PRESSURE

The negative pressure in a room can be monitored by visually observing the direction of airflow (e.g., using smoke tubes) or by measuring the differential pressure between the room and its surrounding area.

Smoke from a smoke tube can be used to observe airflow between areas or airflow patterns within an area. To check the negative pressure in a room by using a smoke tube, hold the smoke tube near the bottom of the door and approximately 2 inches in front of the door, or at the face of a grille or other opening if the door has such a feature, and generate a small amount of smoke by gently squeezing the bulb (Figure S33). The smoke tube should be held parallel to the door,

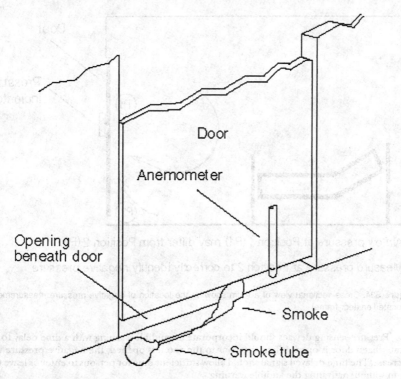

Figure S33. Smoke-tube testing and anemometer placement to determine the direction of airflow into and out of a room. Smoke flowing into the room indicates the room is at negative pressure relative to the corridor, and smoke flowing out of the room indicates the room is at positive pressure relative to the corridor. The anemometer, if used, is placed with the sensor in the airflow path at the bottom of the door.

and the smoke should be issued from the tube slowly to ensure the velocity of the smoke from the tube does not overpower the air velocity. The smoke will travel in the direction of airflow. If the room is at negative pressure, the smoke will travel under the door and into the room (e.g., from higher to lower pressure). If the room is not at negative pressure, the smoke will be blown outward or will stay stationary. This test must be performed while the door is closed. If room air cleaners are being used in the room, they should be running. The smoke is irritating if inhaled, and care should be taken not to inhale it directly from the smoke tube. However, the quantity of smoke issued from the tube is minimal and is not detectable at short distances from the tube.

Differential pressure-sensing devices also can be used to monitor negative pressure; they can provide either periodic (noncontinuous) pressure measurements or continuous pressure monitoring. The continuous monitoring component may simply be a visible and/or audible warning signal that air pressure is low. In addition, it may also provide a pressure readout signal, which can be recorded for later verification or used to automatically adjust the facility's ventilation control system.

Pressure-measuring devices should sense the room pressure just inside the airflow path into the room (e.g., at the bottom of the door). Unusual airflow patterns within the room can cause pressure variations; for example, the air can be at negative pressure at the middle of a door and at positive pressure at the bottom of the same door (Figure S34). If the pressure-sensing ports of the device cannot be located directly across the airflow path, it will be necessary to validate that the negative pressure at the sensing point is and remains the same as the negative pressure across the flow path.

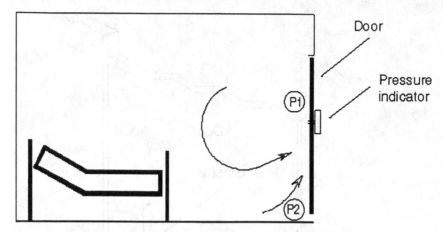

Airflow pressure at Position 1 (P1) may differ from Position 2 (P2).

Measure pressure at Position 2 to correctly identify negative pressure.

Figure S34. Cross-sectional view of a room showing the location of negative pressure measurement. (*Located on door frame)

Pressure-sensing devices should incorporate an audible warning with a time delay to indicate that a door is open. When the door to the room is opened, the negative pressure will decrease. The time-delayed signal should allow sufficient time for persons to enter or leave the room without activating the audible warning.

A potential problem with using pressure-sensing devices is that the pressure differentials used to achieve the low negative pressure necessitate the use of very sensitive mechanical devices, electronic devices, or pressure gauges to ensure accurate measurements. Use of devices that cannot measure these low pressures (i.e., pressures as low as 0.001 inch of water) will require setting higher negative pressures that may be difficult and, in some instances, impractical to achieve (Suppl. 3, Section II.B.4).

Periodic checks are required to ensure that the desired negative pressure is present and that the continuous monitoring devices, if used, are operating properly. If smoke tubes or other visual checks are used, TB isolation rooms and treatment rooms should be checked frequently for negative pressure. Rooms undergoing changes to the ventilation system should be checked daily. TB isolation rooms should be checked daily for negative pressure while being used for TB isolation. If these rooms are not being used for patients who have suspected or confirmed TB but potentially could be used for such patients, the negative pressure in the rooms should be checked monthly. If pressure-sensing devices are used, negative pressure should be verified at least once a month by using smoke tubes or taking pressure measurements.

C. HEPA FILTRATION

Purpose: To remove contaminants from the air.

HEPA filtration can be used as a method of air cleaning that supplements other recommended ventilation measures. For the purposes of these guidelines, HEPA filters are defined as air-cleaning devices that have a demonstrated and documented minimum removal efficiency of 99.97% of particles greater than or equal to 0.3 μm in diameter. HEPA filters have been shown to be effective in reducing the concentration of Aspergillus spores (which range in size from 1.5 μm to 6 μm) to below measurable levels (100–102). The ability of HEPA filters to remove tubercle bacilli from the air has not been studied, but M. tuberculosis droplet nuclei probably range from 1 μm to 5 μm in diameter (i.e., approximately the same size as

Aspergillus spores). Therefore, HEPA filters can be expected to remove infectious droplet nuclei from contaminated air. HEPA filters can be used to clean air before it is exhausted to the outside, recirculated to other areas of a facility, or recirculated within a room. If the device is not completely passive (e.g., it utilizes techniques such as electrostatics) and the failure of the electrostatic components permits loss of filtration efficiency to less than 99.97%, the device should not be used in systems that recirculate air back into the general facility ventilation system from TB isolation rooms and treatment rooms in which procedures are performed on patients who may have infectious TB (Suppl. 3, Section II.C.2).

HEPA filters can be used in a number of ways to reduce or eliminate infectious droplet nuclei from room air or exhaust. These methods include placement of HEPA filters (a) in exhaust ducts to remove droplet nuclei from air being discharged to the outside, either directly or through ventilation equipment; (b) in ducts discharging room air into the general ventilation system; and (c) in fixed or portable room-air cleaners. The effectiveness of portable HEPA room-air cleaning units has not been evaluated adequately, and there is probably considerable variation in their effectiveness. HEPA filters can also be used in exhaust ducts or vents that discharge air from booths or enclosures into the surrounding room (Suppl. 3, Section II.A.3). In any application, HEPA filters should be installed carefully and maintained meticulously to ensure adequate function.

Manufacturers of room-air cleaning equipment should provide documentation of the HEPA filter efficiency and the efficiency of the installed device in lowering room-air contaminant levels.

1. Use of HEPA Filtration When Exhausting Air to the Outside

HEPA filters can be used as an added safety measure to clean air from isolation rooms and local exhaust devices (i.e., booths, tents, or hoods used for cough-inducing procedures) before exhausting it directly to the outside, but such use is unnecessary if the exhaust air cannot reenter the ventilation system supply. The use of HEPA filters should be considered wherever exhaust air could possibly reenter the system.

In many instances, exhaust air is not discharged directly to the outside; rather, the air is directed through heat-recovery devices (e.g., heat wheels). Heat wheels are often used to reduce the costs of operating ventilation systems (103). If such units are used with the system, a HEPA filter should also be used. As the wheel rotates, energy is transferred into or removed from the supply inlet air stream. The HEPA filter should be placed upstream from the heat wheel because of the potential for leakage across the seals separating the inlet and exhaust chambers and the theoretical possibility that droplet nuclei could be impacted on the wheel by the exhaust air and subsequently stripped off into the supply air.

2. Recirculation of HEPA-filtered Air to Other Areas of a Facility

Air from TB isolation rooms and treatment rooms used to treat patients who have confirmed or suspected infectious TB should be exhausted to the outside in accordance with applicable federal, state, and local regulations. The air should not be recirculated into the general ventilation. In some instances, recirculation of air into the general ventilation system from such rooms is unavoidable (i.e., in existing facilities in which the ventilation system or facility configuration makes venting the exhaust to the outside impossible). In such cases, HEPA filters should be installed in the exhaust duct leading from the room to the general ventilation system to remove infectious organisms and particulates the size of droplet nuclei from the air before it is returned to the general ventilation system (Section II.F; Suppl. 3). Air from TB isolation rooms and treatment rooms in new or renovated facilities should not be recirculated into the general ventilation system.

3. Recirculation of HEPA-filtered Air Within a Room

Individual room-air recirculation can be used in areas where there is no general ventilation system, where an existing system is incapable of providing adequate airflow, or where an increase in ventilation is desired without affecting the fresh air supply or negative pressure system already in place. Recirculation of HEPA-filtered air within a room can be achieved in several ways: (a) by exhausting air from the room into a duct, filtering it through a HEPA filter

10% Exhaust to outside for negative
pressure if room has no ventilation

HEPA filter
and blower

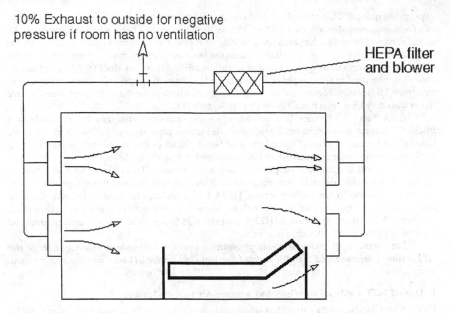

Figure S35. Fixed, ducted room-air recirculation system using a high-efficiency particulate air (HEPA) filter inside an air duct. Such a system can be used to increase the room ventilation rate.

installed in the duct, and returning it to the room (Figure S35); (b) by filtering air through HEPA recirculation systems mounted on the wall or ceiling of the room (Figure S36); or (c) by filtering air through portable HEPA recirculation systems. In this document, the first two of these approaches are referred to as fixed room-air recirculation systems, because the HEPA filter devices are fixed in place and are not easily movable.

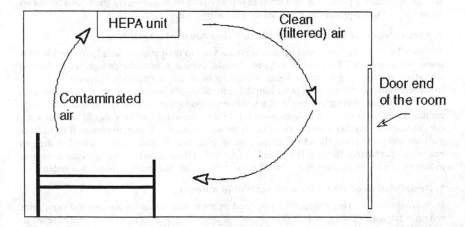

Figure S36. Fixed ceiling-mounted room-air recirculation system using a high-efficiency particulate air (HEPA) filter. Such a system can be used to increase the room ventilation rate. Position the HEPA unit one-third of the room's length from the patient's end of the room.

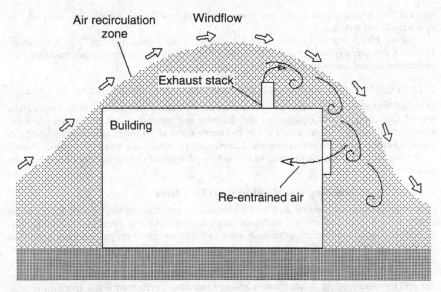

Figure S37. Air recirculation zone created by wind blowing over a building. Height of air recirculation zone may be variable. Air should be exhausted above the zone to prevent re-entrainment.

A. FIXED ROOM-AIR RECIRCULATION SYSTEMS

The preferred method of recirculating HEPA-filtered air within a room is a built-in system, in which air is exhausted from the room into a duct, filtered through a HEPA filter, and returned to the room (Figure S35). This technique may be used to add air changes in areas where there is a recommended minimum ACH that is difficult to meet with general ventilation alone. The air does not have to be conditioned, other than by the filtration, and this permits higher airflow rates than the general ventilation system can usually achieve. An alternative is the use of HEPA filtration units that are mounted on the wall or ceiling of the room (Figure S37). Fixed recirculation systems are preferred over portable (free-standing) units because they can be installed and maintained with a greater degree of reliability.

B. PORTABLE ROOM-AIR RECIRCULATION UNITS

Portable HEPA filtration units may be considered for recirculating air within rooms in which there is no general ventilation system, where the system is incapable of providing adequate airflow, or where increased effectiveness in room airflow is desired. Effectiveness depends on circulating as much of the air in the room as possible through the HEPA filter, which may be difficult to achieve and evaluate. The effectiveness of a particular unit can vary depending on the room's configuration, the furniture and persons in the room, and placement of the HEPA filtration unit and the supply and exhaust grilles. Therefore, the effectiveness of the portable unit may vary considerably in rooms with different configurations or in the same room if moved from one location to another in the room. If portable units are used, caution should be exercised to ensure they can recirculate all or nearly all of the room air through the HEPA filter. Some commercially available units may not be able to meet this requirement because of design limitations or insufficient airflow capacity. In addition, units should be designed and operated to ensure that persons in the room cannot interfere with or otherwise compromise the functioning of the unit. Portable HEPA filtration units have not been evaluated adequately to determine their role in TB infection-control programs.

Portable HEPA filtration units should be designed to achieve the equivalent of greater than or equal to 12 ACH. They should also be designed to ensure adequate air mixing in all areas of the hospital rooms in which they are used, and they should not interfere with the current ventilation system.

Some HEPA filtration units employ UVGI for disinfecting air after HEPA filtration. However, whether exposing the HEPA-filtered air to UV irradiation further decreases the concentration of contaminants is not known.

C. EVALUATION OF ROOM-AIR RECIRCULATION SYSTEMS AND UNITS

Detailed and accurate evaluations of room-air recirculation systems and units require the use of sophisticated test equipment and lengthy test procedures that are not practical. However, an estimate of the unit's ability to circulate the air in the room can be made by visualizing airflow patterns as was described previously for estimating room air mixing (Suppl. 3, Section II.B.1). If the air movement is good in all areas of the room, the unit should be effective.

4. Installing, Maintaining, and Monitoring HEPA Filters

Proper installation and testing and meticulous maintenance are critical if a HEPA filtration system is used (104), especially if the system used recirculates air to other parts of the facility. Improper design, installation, or maintenance could allow infectious particles to circumvent filtration and escape into the general ventilation system (47). HEPA filters should be installed to prevent leakage between filter segments and between the filter bed and its frame. A regularly scheduled maintenance program is required to monitor the HEPA filter for possible leakage and for filter loading. A quantitative leakage and filter performance test (e.g., the dioctal phthalate [DOP] penetration test [105]) should be performed at the initial installation and every time the filter is changed or moved. The test should be repeated every 6 months for filters in general-use areas and in areas with systems that exhaust air that is likely to be contaminated with M. tuberculosis (e.g, TB isolation rooms).

A manometer or other pressure-sensing device should be installed in the filter system to provide an accurate and objective means of determining the need for filter replacement. Pressure drop characteristics of the filter are supplied by the manufacturer of the filter. Installation of the filter should allow for maintenance that will not contaminate the delivery system or the area served. For general infection-control purposes, special care should be taken to not jar or drop the filter element during or after removal.

The scheduled maintenance program should include procedures for installation, removal, and disposal of filter elements. HEPA filter maintenance should be performed only by adequately trained personnel. Appropriate respiratory protection should be worn while performing maintenance and testing procedures. In addition, filter housing and ducts leading to the housing should be labelled clearly with the words "Contaminated Air" (or a similar warning).

When a HEPA filter is used, one or more lower efficiency disposable prefilters installed upstream will extend the useful life of the HEPA filter. A disposable filter can increase the life of a HEPA filter by 25%. If the disposable filter is followed by a 90% extended surface filter, the life of the HEPA filter can be extended almost 900% (98). These prefilters should be handled and disposed of in the same manner as the HEPA filter.

D. TB ISOLATION ROOMS AND TREATMENT ROOMS

Purpose: To separate patients who are likely to have infectious TB from other persons, to provide an environment that will allow reduction of the concentration of droplet nuclei through various engineering methods, and to prevent the escape of droplet nuclei from such rooms into the corridor and other areas of the facility using directional airflow.

A hierarchy of ventilation methods used to achieve a reduction in the concentration of droplet nuclei and to achieve directional airflow using negative pressure has been developed (Table S32). The methods are listed in order from the most desirable to the least desirable. The method selected will depend on the configuration of the isolation room and the ventilation system in the facility; the determination should be made in consultation with a ventilation engineer.

Table S32. Hierarchy of Ventilation Methods for Tuberculosis (TB) Isolation Rooms and Treatment Rooms

Reducing concentration of airborne tubercle bacilli*	Achieving directional airflow using negative pressure[+]
1. Facility heating, ventilation, and air-conditioning (HVAC) system.	1. Facility HVAC system.
2. Fixed room-air high-efficiency particulate air (HEPA) recirculation system.	2. Bleed air[&] from fixed room-air HEPA recirculation system.
3. Wall- or ceiling-mounted room-air HEPA recirculation system.	3. Bleed air from wall- or ceiling-mounted room-air HEPA recirculation system.
4. Portable room-air HEPA recirculation unit.	4. Bleed air from portable room-air HEPA recirculation unit.[@]
	5. Exhaust air from room through window-mounted fan.**

*Ventilation methods are used to reduce the concentration of airborne tubercle bacilli. If the facility HVAC system cannot achieve the recommended ventilation rate, auxiliary room-air recirculation methods may be used. These methods are listed in order from the most desirable to the least desirable. Ultraviolet germicidal irradiation may be used as a supplement to any of the ventilation methods for air cleaning.

[+]Directional airflow using negative pressure can be achieved with the facility HVAC system and/or the auxiliary air-recirculation—cleaning systems. These methods are listed in order from the most desirable to the least desirable.

[&]To remove the amount of return air necessary to achieve negative pressure.

[@]The effectiveness of portable room-air HEPA recirculation units can vary depending on the room's configuration, the furniture and persons in the room, the placement of the unit, the supply and exhaust grilles, and the achievable ventilation rates and air mixing. Units should be designed and operated to ensure that persons in the room cannot interfere with or otherwise compromise the function of the unit. Fixed recirculating systems are preferred over portable units in TB isolation rooms of facilities in which services are provided regularly to TB patients.

**This method simply achieves negative pressure and should be used only as a temporary measure.

1. Preventing the Escape of Droplet Nuclei from the Room

Rooms used for TB isolation should be single-patient rooms with negative pressure relative to the corridor or other areas connected to the room. Doors between the isolation room and other areas should remain closed except for entry into or exit from the room. The room's openings (e.g., windows and electrical and plumbing entries) should be sealed as much as possible. However, a small gap of ⅛ to ½ inch should be at the bottom of the door to provide a controlled airflow path. Proper use of negative pressure will prevent contaminated air from escaping the room.

2. Reducing the Concentration of Droplet Nuclei in the Room

ASHRAE (47), AIA (48), and the Health Resources and Services Administration (49) recommend a minimum of 6 ACH for TB isolation rooms and treatment rooms. This ventilation rate is based on comfort- and odor-control considerations. The effectiveness of this level of airflow in reducing the concentration of droplet nuclei in the room, thus reducing the transmission of airborne pathogens, has not been evaluated directly or adequately.

Ventilation rates greater than 6 ACH are likely to produce an incrementally greater reduction in the concentration of bacteria in a room than are lower rates (50–52). However, accurate quantitation of decreases in risk that would result from specific increases in general ventilation levels has not been performed and may not be possible.

To reduce the concentration of droplet nuclei, TB isolation rooms and treatment rooms in existing health-care facilities should have an airflow of greater than or equal to 6 ACH. Where feasible, this airflow rate should be increased to greater than or equal to 12 ACH by adjusting or modifying the ventilation system or by using auxiliary means (e.g., recirculation of air through fixed HEPA filtration units or portable air cleaners) (Suppl. 3, Section II.C) (53).

New construction or renovation of existing health-care facilities should be designed so that TB isolation rooms achieve an airflow of greater than or equal to 12 ACH.

3. Exhaust from TB Isolation Rooms and Treatment Rooms

Air from TB isolation rooms and treatment rooms in which patients with infectious TB may be examined should be exhausted directly to the outside of the building and away from air-intake vents, persons, and animals in accordance with federal, state, and local regulations concerning environmental discharges. (See Suppl. 3, Section II.C, for information regarding recirculation of exhaust air.) Exhaust ducts should not be located near areas that may be populated (e.g., near sidewalks or windows that could be opened). Ventilation system exhaust discharges and inlets should be designed to prevent reentry of exhausted air. Wind blowing over a building creates a highly turbulent recirculation zone, which can cause exhausted air to reenter the building (Figure S37). Exhaust flow should be discharged above this zone (Suppl. 3, Section II.C.1). Design guidelines for proper placement of exhaust ducts can be found in the 1989 ASHRAE Fundamentals Handbook (106). If recirculation of air from such rooms into the general ventilation system is unavoidable, the air should be passed through a HEPA filter before recirculation (Suppl. 3, Section II.C.2).

4. Alternatives to TB Isolation Rooms

Isolation can also be achieved by use of negative-pressure enclosures (e.g, tents or booths) (Suppl. 3, Section II.A.1). These can be used to provide patient isolation in areas such as emergency rooms and medical testing and treatment areas and to supplement isolation in designated isolation rooms.

III. UVGI

Purpose: To kill or inactivate airborne tubercle bacilli.

Research has demonstrated that UVGI is effective in killing or inactivating tubercle bacilli under experimental conditions (66, 107–110) and in reducing transmission of other infections in hospitals (111), military housing (112), and classrooms (113–115). Because of the results of numerous studies (116–120) and the experiences of TB clinicians and mycobacteriologists during the past several decades, the use of UVGI has been recommended as a supplement to other TB infection-control measures in settings where the need for killing or inactivating tubercle bacilli is important (2, 4, 121–125).

UV radiation is defined as that portion of the electromagnetic spectrum described by wavelengths from 100 to 400 nm. For convenience of classification, the UV spectrum has been separated into three different wave-length bands: UV-A (long wavelengths, range: 320–400 nm), UV-B (midrange wavelengths, range: 290–320 nm), and UV-C (short wavelengths, range: 100–290 nm) (126). Commercially available UV lamps used for germicidal purposes are low-pressure mercury vapor lamps (127) that emit radiant energy in the UV-C range, predominantly at a wavelength of 253.7 nm (128).

A. APPLICATIONS

UVGI can be used as a method of air disinfection to supplement other engineering controls. Two systems of UVGI can be used for this purpose: duct irradiation and upper-room air irradiation.

1. Duct Irradiation

Purpose: To inactivate tubercle bacilli without exposing persons to UVGI.

In duct irradiation systems, UV lamps are placed inside ducts that remove air from rooms to disinfect the air before it is recirculated. When UVGI duct systems are properly designed, installed, and maintained, high levels of UV radiation may be produced in the duct work. The only potential for human exposure to this radiation occurs during maintenance operations. Duct irradiation may be used:

- In a TB isolation room or treatment room to recirculate air from the room, through a duct containing UV lamps, and back into the room. This recirculation method can increase the overall room airflow but does not increase the supply of fresh outside air to the room.

- In other patients' rooms and in waiting rooms, emergency rooms, and other general-use areas of a facility where patients with undiagnosed TB could potentially contaminate the air, to recirculate air back into the general ventilation.
- Duct-irradiation systems are dependent on airflow patterns within a room that ensure that all or nearly all of the room air circulates through the duct.

2. Upper-Room Air Irradiation

Purpose: To inactivate tubercle bacilli in the upper part of the room, while minimizing radiation exposure to persons in the lower part of the room.

In upper-room air irradiation, UVGI lamps are suspended from the ceiling or mounted on the wall. The bottom of the lamp is shielded to direct the radiation upward but not downward. The system depends on air mixing to take irradiated air from the upper to the lower part of the room, and nonirradiated air from the lower to the upper part. The irradiated air space is much larger than that in a duct system.

UVGI has been effective in killing bacteria under conditions where air mixing was accomplished mainly by convection. For example, BCG was atomized in a room that did not have supplemental ventilation (120), and in another study a surrogate bacteria, Serratia marcescens, was aerosolized in a room with a ventilation rate of 6 ACH (129). These reports estimated the effect of UVGI to be equivalent to 10 and 39 ACH, respectively, for the organisms tested, which are less resistant to UVGI than M. tuberculosis (120). The addition of fans or some heating/air conditioning arrangements may double the effectiveness of UVGI lamps (130–132). Greater rates of ventilation, however, may decrease the length of time the air is irradiated, thus decreasing the killing of bacteria (117, 129). The optimal relationship between ventilation and UVGI is not known. Air irradiation lamps used in corridors have been effective in killing atomized S. marcescens (133). Use of UVGI lamps in an outpatient room has reduced culturable airborne bacteria by 14%–19%. However, the irradiation did not reduce the concentration of gram-positive, rod-shaped bacteria; although fast-growing mycobacteria were cultured, M. tuberculosis could not be recovered from the room's air samples because of fungal over-growth of media plates (134).

Upper-room air UVGI irradiation may be used:

- In isolation or treatment rooms as a supplemental method of air cleaning.
- In other patients' rooms and in waiting rooms, emergency rooms, corridors, and other central areas of a facility where patients with undiagnosed TB could potentially contaminate the air. Determinants of UVGI effectiveness include room configuration, UV lamp placement, and the adequacy of airflow patterns in bringing contaminated air into contact with the irradiated upper-room space. Air mixing may be facilitated by supplying cool air near the ceiling in rooms where warmer air (or a heating device) is present below. The ceiling should be high enough for a large volume of upper-room air to be irradiated without HCWs and patients being overexposed to UV radiation.

B. LIMITATIONS

Because the clinical effectiveness of UV systems varies, and because of the risk for transmission of M. tuberculosis if a system malfunctions or is maintained improperly, UVGI is not recommended for the following specific applications:

1. Duct systems using UVGI are not recommended as a substitute for HEPA filters if air from isolation rooms must be recirculated to other areas of a facility.
2. UVGI alone is not recommended as a substitute for HEPA filtration or local exhaust of air to the outside from booths, tents, or hoods used for cough-inducing procedures.
3. UVGI is not a substitute for negative pressure.

The use of UV lamps and HEPA filtration in a single unit would not be expected to have any infection-control benefits not provided by use of the HEPA filter alone.

The effectiveness of UVGI in killing airborne tubercle bacilli depends on the intensity of UVGI, the duration of contact the organism has with the irradiation, and the relative humidity (66, 108, 111). Humidity can have an adverse effect on UVGI effectiveness at levels greater than 70% relative humidity for S. marcescens (135). The interaction of these factors has not been fully defined, however, making precise recommendations for individual UVGI installations difficult to develop.

Old lamps or dust-covered UV lamps are less effective; therefore, regular maintenance of UVGI systems is crucial.

C. SAFETY ISSUES

Short-term overexposure to UV radiation can cause erythema and keratoconjunctivitis (136, 137). Broad-spectrum UV radiation has been associated with increased risk for squamous and basal cell carcinomas of the skin (138). UV-C was recently classified by the International Agency for Research on Cancer as "probably carcinogenic to humans (Group 2A)" (138). This classification is based on studies suggesting that UV-C radiation can induce skin cancers in animals; DNA damage, chromosomal aberrations and sister chromatid exchange and transformation in human cells in vitro; and DNA damage in mammalian skin cells in vivo. In the animal studies, a contribution of UV-B to the tumor effects could not be excluded, but the effects were greater than expected for UV-B alone (138). Although some more recent studies have demonstrated that UV radiation can activate HIV gene promoters (i.e., the genes in HIV that prompt replication of the virus) in laboratory samples of human cells (139–144), the implications of these in vitro findings for humans are unknown.

In 1972, the National Institute for Occupational Safety and Health (NIOSH) published a recommended exposure limit (REL) for occupational exposure to UV radiation (136). The REL is intended to protect workers from the acute effects of UV exposure (e.g., erythema and photokeratoconjunctivitis). However, photosensitive persons and those exposed concomitantly to photoactive chemicals may not be protected by the recommended standard.

If proper procedures are not followed, HCWs performing maintenance on such fixtures are at risk for exposure to UV radiation. Because UV fixtures used for upper-room air irradiation are present in rooms, rather than hidden in ducts, safety may be much more difficult to achieve and maintain. Fixtures must be designed and installed to ensure that UV exposure to persons in the room (including HCWs and inpatients) are below current safe exposure levels. Recent health hazard evaluations conducted by CDC have noted problems with over-exposure of HCWs to UVGI and with inadequate maintenance, training, labeling, and use of personal protective equipment (145–147).

The current number of persons who are properly trained in UVGI system design and installation is limited. CDC strongly recommends that a competent UVGI system designer be consulted to address safety considerations before such a system is procured and installed. Experts who might be consulted include industrial hygienists, engineers, and health physicists. Principles for the safe installation of UV lamp fixtures have been developed and can be used as guidelines (148, 149).

If UV lamps are being used in a facility, the general TB education of HCWs should include:

1. The basic principles of UVGI systems (i.e., how they work and what their limitations are).
2. The potential hazardous effects of UVGI if overexposure occurs.
3. The potential for photosensitivity associated with certain medical conditions or use of some medications.
4. The importance of general maintenance procedures for UVGI fixtures.

Exposure to UV intensities above the REL should be avoided. Light-weight clothing made of tightly woven fabric and UV-absorbing sunscreens with solar-protection factors (SPFs) greater than or equal to 15 may help protect photosensitive persons. HCWs should be advised that any eye or skin irritation that develops after UV exposure should be examined by occupational health staff.

D. EXPOSURE CRITERIA FOR UV RADIATION

The NIOSH REL for UV radiation is wavelength dependent because different wavelengths of UV radiation have different adverse effects on the skin and eyes (136). Relative spectral effectiveness (S sub l) is used to compare various UV sources with a source producing UV radiation at 270 nm, the wavelength of maximum ocular sensitivity. For example, the S sub l at 254 nm is 0.5; therefore, twice as much energy is required at 254 nm to produce an identical biologic effect at 270 nm (136). Thus, at 254 nm, the NIOSH REL is 0.006 joules per square centimeter (J/cm^2); and at 270 nm, it is 0.003 J/cm^2.

For germicidal lamps that emit radiant energy predominantly at a wavelength of 254 nm, proper use of the REL requires that the measured irradiance level (E) in microwatts per square centimeter ($\mu W/cm^2$) be multiplied by the relative spectral effectiveness at 254 nm (0.5) to obtain the effective irradiance (Eeff). The maximum permissible exposure time can then be determined for selected values of Eeff (Table S33), or it can be calculated (in seconds) by dividing 0.003 J/cm^2 (the NIOSH REL at 270 nm) by Eeff in $\mu W/cm^2$ (136, 150).

To protect HCWs who are exposed to germicidal UV radiation for 8 hours per workday, the measured irradiance (E) should be less than or equal to 0.2 $\mu W/cm^2$. This is calculated by obtaining Eeff (0.1 $\mu W/cm^2$) (Table S33) and then dividing this value by S sub 1 (0.5).

Table S33. Maximum Permissible Exposure Times* for Selected Values of Effective Irradiance

Permissible exposure time per day	Effective irradiance (Eeff)[+] ($\mu W/cm^2$)
8 hrs	0.1
4 hrs	0.2
2 hrs	0.4
1 hr	0.8
30 min	1.7
15 min	3.3
10 min	5.0
5 min	10.0
1 min	50.0
30 sec	100.0

*Permissible exposure times are designed to prevent acute effects of irradiation to skin and eyes (136). These recommended limits are wavelength dependent because different wave-lengths of ultraviolet (UV) radiation have different adverse effects on these organs.

[+]Relative spectral effectiveness (S sub 1) is used to compare various UV sources with a source producing UV radiation at 270 nm, the wavelength of maximum ocular sensitivity. For example, the relative spectral effectiveness at 254 nm is 0.5; therefore, twice as much energy is required at 254 nm to produce an identical biologic effect at 270 nm. At 254 nm, the NIOSH REL is 0.006 joules per square centimeter (J/cm^2); and at 270 nm, it is 0.003 J/cm^2. For germicidal lamps that emit radiant energy predominantly at a wavelength of 254 nm, proper use of the REL requires that the measured irradiance level (E) in microwatts per square centimeter ($\mu W/cm^2$) be multiplied by the relative spectral effectiveness at 254 nm (0.5) to obtain Eeff. The maximum permissible exposure time can be calculated (in seconds) by dividing 0.003 J/cm^2 (the NIOSH REL at 270 nm) by Eeff in $\mu W/cm^2$ (136,150). To protect health-care workers who are exposed to germicidal UV radiation for 8 hours per work day, the measured irradiance (E) should be ≤0.2 $\mu W/cm^2$, which is calculated by obtaining Eeff (0.1 $\mu W/cm^2$), then dividing this value by S sub 1 (0.5).

E. MAINTENANCE AND MONITORING

1. Labeling and Posting

Warning signs should be posted on UV lamps and wherever high- intensity (i.e., UV exposure greater than the REL) germicidal UV irradiation is present (e.g., upper-room air space and accesses to ducts [if duct irradiation is used]) to alert maintenance staff or other HCWs of the hazard. Some examples are shown below:

CAUTION

ULTRAVIOLET ENERGY:
TURN OFF LAMPS BEFORE
ENTERING UPPER ROOM

CAUTION

ULTRAVIOLET ENERGY:
PROTECT EYES & SKIN

2. Maintenance

Because the intensity of UV lamps fluctuates as they age, a schedule for replacing the lamps should be developed. The schedule can be determined from either a time/use log or a system based on cumulative time. The tube should be checked periodically for dust build-up, which lessens the output of UVGI. If the tube is dirty, it should be allowed to cool, then cleaned with a damp cloth. Tubes should be replaced if they stop glowing or if they flicker to an objectionable extent. Maintenance personnel must turn off all UV tubes before entering the upper part of the room or before accessing ducts for any purpose. Only a few seconds of direct exposure to the intense UV radiation in the upper-room air space or in ducts can cause burns. Protective equipment (e.g., gloves and goggles [and/or face shields]) should be worn if exposure greater than the recommended standard is anticipated.

Banks of UVGI tubes can be installed in ventilating ducts. Safety devices should be used on access doors to eliminate hazard to maintenance personnel. For duct irradiation systems, the access door for servicing the lamps should have an inspection window[&&] through which the lamps are checked periodically for dust build-up and malfunctioning. The access door should have a warning sign written in languages appropriate for maintenance personnel to alert them to the health hazard of looking directly at bare tubes. The lock for this door should have an automatic electric switch or other device that turns off the lamps when the door is opened.

Two types of fixtures are used in upper-room air irradiation: wall-mounted fixtures that have louvers to block downward radiation and ceiling-mounted fixtures that have baffles to block radiation below the horizontal plane of the UV tube. The actual UV tube in either type of fixture must not be visible from any normal position in the room. Light switches that can be locked should be used, if possible, to prevent injury to personnel who might unintentionally turn the lamps on during maintenance procedures.

In most applications, properly shielding the UV lamps to provide protection from most, if not all, of the direct UV radiation is not difficult. However, radiation reflected from glass, polished metal, and high-gloss ceramic paints can be harmful to persons in the room, particularly if more than one UV lamp is in use. Surfaces in irradiated rooms that can reflect UVGI into occupied areas of the room should be covered with non-UV reflecting material.

3. Monitoring

A regularly scheduled evaluation of the UV intensity to which HCWs, patients, and others are exposed should be conducted.

UV measurements should be made in various locations within a room using a detector designed to be most sensitive at 254 nm. Equipment used to measure germicidal UV radiation should be maintained and calibrated on a regular schedule.

A new UV installation must be carefully checked for hot spots (i.e., areas of the room where the REL is exceeded) by an industrial hygienist or other person knowledgeable in making UV measurements. UV radiation levels should not exceed those in the recommended guidelines.

Supplement 4: Respiratory Protection

I. CONSIDERATIONS FOR SELECTION OF RESPIRATORS

Personal respiratory protection should be used by (a) persons entering rooms where patients with known or suspected infectious TB are being isolated, (b) persons present during cough-inducing or aerosol-generating procedures performed on such patients, and (c) persons in other settings where administrative and engineering controls are not likely to protect them from inhaling infectious airborne droplet nuclei. These other settings should be identified on the basis of the facility's risk assessment.

Although data regarding the effectiveness of respiratory protection from many hazardous airborne materials have been collected, the precise level of effectiveness in protecting HCWs from M. tuberculosis transmission in health-care settings has not been determined. Information

---

[&&]Ordinary glass (not quartz) is sufficient to filter out UV radiation.

concerning the transmission of M. tuberculosis is incomplete. Neither the smallest infectious dose of M. tuberculosis nor the highest level of exposure to M. tuberculosis at which transmission will not occur has been defined conclusively (59, 151, 152). Furthermore, the size distribution of droplet nuclei and the number of particles containing viable M. tuberculosis that are expelled by infectious TB patients have not been defined adequately, and accurate methods of measuring the concentration of infectious droplet nuclei in a room have not been developed.

Nevertheless, in certain settings the administrative and engineering controls may not adequately protect HCWs from airborne droplet nuclei (e.g., in TB isolation rooms, treatment rooms in which cough-inducing or aerosol-generating procedures are performed, and ambulances during the transport of infectious TB patients). Respiratory protective devices used in these settings should have characteristics that are suitable for the organism they are protecting against and the settings in which they are used.

A. PERFORMANCE CRITERIA FOR PERSONAL RESPIRATORS FOR PROTECTION AGAINST TRANSMISSION OF M. TUBERCULOSIS

Respiratory protective devices used in health-care settings for protection against M. tuberculosis should meet the following standard criteria. These criteria are based on currently available information, including (a) data on the effectiveness of respiratory protection against noninfectious hazardous materials in workplaces other than health-care settings and on an interpretation of how these data can be applied to respiratory protection against M. tuberculosis; (b) data on the efficiency of respirator filters in filtering biological aerosols; (c) data on face-seal leakage; and (d) data on the characteristics of respirators that were used in conjunction with administrative and engineering controls in outbreak settings where transmission to HCWs and patients was terminated.

1. The ability to filter particles 1 mm in size in the unloaded state with a filter efficiency of greater than or equal to 95% (i.e., filter leakage of less than or equal to 5%), given flow rates of up to 50 L per minute.

   Available data suggest that infectious droplet nuclei range in size from 1 μm to 5 μm; therefore, respirators used in health-care settings should be able to efficiently filter the smallest particles in this range. Fifty liters per minute is a reasonable estimate of the highest airflow rate an HCW is likely to achieve during breathing, even while performing strenuous work activities.
2. The ability to be qualitatively or quantitatively fit tested in a reliable way to obtain a face-seal leakage of less than or equal to 10% (54, 55).
3. The ability to fit the different facial sizes and characteristics of HCWs, which can usually be met by making the respirators available in at least three sizes.
4. The ability to be checked for facepiece fit, in accordance with OSHA standards and good industrial hygiene practice, by HCWs each time they put on their respirators (54, 55).

In some settings, HCWs may be at risk for two types of exposure: (a) inhalation of M. tuberculosis and (b) mucous membrane exposure to fluids that may contain bloodborne pathogens. In these settings, protection against both types of exposure should be used.

When operative procedures (or other procedures requiring a sterile field) are performed on patients who may have infectious TB, respiratory protection worn by the HCW should serve two functions: (a) it should protect the surgical field from the respiratory secretions of the HCW and (b) it should protect the HCW from infectious droplet nuclei that may be expelled by the patient or generated by the procedure. Respirators with expiration valves and positive-pressure respirators do not protect the sterile field; therefore, a respirator that does not have a valve and that meets the criteria in Supplement 4, Section I.A, should be used.

B. SPECIFIC RESPIRATORS

The OSHA respiratory protection standard requires that all respiratory protective devices used in the workplace be certified by NIOSH.[&&&] NIOSH-approved HEPA respirators are the

---

[&&&]29 CFR Part 1910.134.

only currently available air-purifying respirators that meet or exceed the standard performance criteria stated above. However, the NIOSH certification procedures are currently being revised (153). Under the proposed revision, filter materials would be tested at a flow rate of 85 L/min for penetration by particles with a median aerodynamic diameter of 0.3 μm and, if certified, would be placed in one of the following categories: type A, which has greater than or equal to 99.97% efficiency (similar to current HEPA filter media); type B, greater than or equal to 99% efficiency; or type C, greater than or equal to 95% efficiency. According to this proposed scheme, type C filter material would meet or exceed the standard performance criteria specified in this document.

The facility's risk assessment may identify a limited number of selected settings (e.g., bronchoscopy performed on patients suspected of having TB or autopsy performed on deceased persons suspected of having had active TB at the time of death) where the estimated risk for transmission of M. tuberculosis may be such that a level of respiratory protection exceeding the standard criteria is appropriate. In such circumstances, a level of respiratory protection exceeding the standard criteria and compatible with patient-care delivery (e.g., negative-pressure respirators that are more protective; powered air-purifying particulate respirators [PAPRs]; or positive-pressure airline, half-mask respirators) should be provided by employers to HCWs who are exposed to M. tuberculosis. Information on these and other respirators may be found in the NIOSH Guide to Industrial Respiratory Protection (55).

C. THE EFFECTIVENESS OF RESPIRATORY PROTECTIVE DEVICES

The following information, which is based on experience with respiratory protection in the industrial setting, summarizes the available data about the effectiveness of respiratory protection against hazardous airborne materials. Data regarding protection against transmission of M. tuberculosis are not available.

The parameters used to determine the effectiveness of a respiratory protective device are face-seal efficacy and filter efficacy.

1. Face-seal leakage

Face-seal leakage compromises the ability of particulate respirators to protect HCWs from airborne materials (154–156). A proper seal between the respirator's sealing surface and the face of the person wearing the respirator is essential for effective and reliable performance of any negative-pressure respirator. This seal is less critical, but still important, for positive-pressure respirators. Face-seal leakage can result from various factors, including incorrect facepiece size or shape, incorrect or defective facepiece sealing-lip, beard growth, perspiration or facial oils that can cause facepiece slippage, failure to use all the head straps, incorrect positioning of the facepiece on the face, incorrect head strap tension or position, improper respirator maintenance, and respirator damage.

Every time a person wearing a negative-pressure particulate respirator inhales, a negative pressure (relative to the workplace air) is created inside the facepiece. Because of this negative pressure, air containing contaminants can take a path of least resistance into the respirator—through leaks at the face-seal interface—thus avoiding the higher-resistance filter material. Currently available, cup-shaped, disposable particulate respirators have from 0 to 20% face-seal leakage (55, 154). This face-seal leakage results from the variability of the human face and from limitations in the respirator's design, construction, and number of sizes available. The face-seal leakage is probably higher if the respirator is not fitted properly to the HCW's face, tested for an adequate fit by a qualified person, and then checked for fit by the HCW every time the respirator is put on. Face-seal leakage may be reduced to less than 10% with improvements in design, a greater variety in available sizes, and appropriate fit testing and fit checking.

In comparison with negative-pressure respirators, positive-pressure respirators produce a positive pressure inside the facepiece under most conditions of use. For example, in a PAPR, a blower forcibly draws ambient air through HEPA filters, then delivers the filtered air to the facepiece. This air is blown into the facepiece at flow rates that generally exceed the expected inhalation flow rates. The positive pressure inside the facepiece reduces face-seal leakage to low levels, particularly during the relatively low inhalation rates expected in health-care settings. PAPRs with a tight-fitting facepiece have less than 2% face-seal leakage under routine conditions (55). Powered-air respirators with loose-fitting facepieces, hoods, or helmets have less than 4% face-seal leakage under routine conditions (55). Thus, a PAPR may offer lower levels of face-seal leakage than nonpowered, half-mask respirators. Full facepiece, non-powered respirators have the same leakage (i.e., less than 2%) as PAPRs.

Another factor contributing to face-seal leakage of cup-shaped, disposable respirators is that some of these respirators are available in only one size. A single size may produce higher leakage for persons who have smaller or difficult-to-fit faces (157). The facepieces used for some reusable (including HEPA and replaceable filter, negative-pressure) and all positive-pressure particulate air-purifying respirators are available in as many as three different sizes.

2. Filter Leakage

Aerosol leakage through respirator filters depends on at least five independent variables: (a) the filtration characteristics for each type of filter, (b) the size distribution of the droplets in the aerosol, (c) the linear velocity through the filtering material, (d) the filter loading (i.e., the amount of contaminant deposited on the filter), and (e) any electrostatic charges on the filter and on the droplets in the aerosol (158).

When HEPA filters are used in particulate air-purifying respirators, filter efficiency is so high (i.e., effectively 100%) that filter leakage is not a consideration. Therefore, for all HEPA-filter respirators, virtually all inward leakage of droplet nuclei occurs at the respirator's face-seal.

3. Fit Testing

Fit testing is part of the respiratory protection program required by OSHA for all respiratory protective devices used in the workplace. A fit test determines whether a respiratory protective device adequately fits a particular HCW. The HCW may need to be fit tested with several devices to determine which device offers the best fit. However, fit tests can detect only the leakage that occurs at the time of the fit testing, and the tests cannot distinguish face-seal leakage from filter leakage.

Determination of facepiece fit can involve qualitative or quantitative tests (55). A qualitative test relies on the subjective response of the HCW being fit tested. A quantitative test uses detectors to measure inward leakage.

Disposable, negative-pressure particulate respirators can be qualitatively fit tested with aerosolized substances that can be tasted, although the results of this testing are limited because the tests depend on the subjective response of the HCW being tested. Quantitative fit testing of disposable negative-pressure particulate respirators can best be performed if the manufacturer provides a test respirator with a probe for this purpose.

Replaceable filter, negative-pressure particulate respirators and all positive-pressure particulate respirators can be fit tested reliably, both qualitatively and quantitatively, when fitted with HEPA filters.

4. Fit Checking

A fit check is a maneuver that an HCW performs before each use of the respiratory protective device to check the fit. The fit check can be performed according to the manufacturer's facepiece fitting instructions by using the applicable negative-pressure or positive-pressure test.

Some currently available cup-shaped, disposable negative-pressure particulate respirators cannot be fit checked reliably by persons wearing the devices because occluding the entire surface of the filter is difficult. Strategies for overcoming these limitations are being developed by respirator manufacturers.

5. Reuse of Respirators

Conscientious respirator maintenance should be an integral part of an overall respirator program. This maintenance applies both to respirators with replaceable filters and respirators that are classified as disposable but that are reused. Manufacturers' instructions for inspecting, cleaning, and maintaining respirators should be followed to ensure that the respirator continues to function properly (55).

When respirators are used for protection against noninfectious aerosols (e.g., wood dust), which may be present in the air in heavy concentrations, the filter material may become occluded with airborne material. This occlusion may result in an uncomfortable breathing resistance. In health-care settings where respirators are used for protection against biological aerosols, the concentration of infectious particles in the air is probably low; thus, the filter material in a respirator is very unlikely to become occluded with airborne material. In addition, there is no evidence that particles impacting on the filter material in a respirator are reaerosolized easily. For these reasons, the filter material used in respirators in the health-care setting should remain functional for weeks to months. Respirators with replaceable filters are reusable, and a respirator classified as disposable may be reused by the same HCW as long as it remains functional.

Before each use, the outside of the filter material should be inspected. If the filter material is physically damaged or soiled, the filter should be changed (in the case of respirators with replaceable filters) or the respirator discarded (in the case of disposable respirators). Infection-control personnel should develop standard operating procedures for storing, reusing, and disposing of respirators that have been designated as disposable and for disposing of replaceable filter elements.

II. IMPLEMENTING A PERSONAL RESPIRATORY PROTECTION PROGRAM

If personal respiratory protection is used in a health-care setting, OSHA requires that an effective personal respiratory protection program be developed, implemented, administered, and periodically reevaluated (54, 55).

All HCWs who need to use respirators for protection against infection with M. tuberculosis should be included in the respiratory protection program. Visitors to TB patients should be given respirators to wear while in isolation rooms, and they should be given general instructions on how to use their respirators.

The number of HCWs included in the respiratory protection program in each facility will vary depending on (a) the number of potentially infectious TB patients, (b) the number of rooms or areas to which patients with suspected or confirmed infectious TB are admitted, and (c) the number of HCWs needed in these rooms or areas. Where respiratory protection programs are required, they should include enough HCWs to provide adequate care for a patient with known or suspected TB should such a patient be admitted to the facility. However, administrative measures should be used to limit the number of HCWs who need to enter these rooms or areas, thus limiting the number of HCWs who need to be included in the respiratory protection program.

Information regarding the development and management of a respiratory protection program is available in technical training courses that cover the basics of personal respiratory protection. Such courses are offered by various organizations, such as NIOSH, OSHA, and the American Industrial Hygiene Association. Similar courses are available from private contractors and universities.

To be effective and reliable, respiratory protection programs must contain at least the following elements (55, 154):

1. Assignment of responsibility. Supervisory responsibility for the respiratory protection program should be assigned to designated persons who have expertise in issues relevant to the program, including infectious diseases and occupational health.
2. Standard operating procedures. Written standard operating procedures should contain information concerning all aspects of the respiratory protection program.
3. Medical screening. HCWs should not be assigned a task requiring use of respirators unless they are physically able to perform the task while wearing the respirator. HCWs should be screened for pertinent medical conditions at the time they are hired, then rescreened periodically (55). The screening could occur as infrequently as every 5 years. The screening process should begin with a general screening (e.g., a questionnaire) for pertinent

medical conditions, and the results of the screening should then be used to identify HCWs who need further evaluation. Routine physical examination or testing with chest radiographs or spirometry is not necessary or required.

Few medical conditions preclude the use of most negative-pressure particulate respirators. HCWs who have mild pulmonary or cardiac conditions may report discomfort with breathing when wearing negative-pressure particulate respirators, but these respirators are unlikely to have adverse health effects on the HCWs. Those HCWs who have more severe cardiac or pulmonary conditions may have more difficulty than HCWs with similar but milder conditions if performing duties while wearing negative-pressure respirators. Furthermore, these HCWs may be unable to use some PAPRs because of the added weight of these respirators.

4. Training. HCWs who wear respirators and the persons who supervise them should be informed about the necessity for wearing respirators and the potential risks associated with not doing so. This training should also include at a minimum:
   - The nature, extent, and specific hazards of M. tuberculosis transmission in their respective health-care facility.
   - A description of specific risks for TB infection among persons exposed to M. tuberculosis, of any subsequent treatment with INH or other chemoprophylactic agents, and of the possibility of active TB disease.
   - A description of engineering controls and work practices and the reasons why they do not eliminate the need for personal respiratory protection.
   - An explanation for selecting a particular type of respirator, how the respirator is properly maintained and stored, and the operation, capabilities, and limitations of the respirator provided.
   - Instruction in how the HCW wearing the respirator should inspect, put on, fit check, and correctly wear the provided respirator (i.e., achieve and maintain proper face-seal fit on the HCW's face).
   - An opportunity to handle the provided respirator and learn how to put it on, wear it properly, and check the important parts.
   - Instruction in how to recognize an inadequately functioning respirator.

5. Face-seal fit testing and fit checking. HCWs should undergo fit testing to identify a respirator that adequately fits each individual HCW. The HCW should receive fitting instructions that include demonstrations and practice in how the respirator should be worn, how it should be adjusted, and how to determine if it fits properly. The HCW should be taught to check the facepiece fit before each use.

6. Respirator inspection, cleaning, maintenance, and storage. Conscientious respirator maintenance should be an integral part of an overall respirator program. This maintenance applies both to respirators with replaceable filters and respirators that are classified as disposable but that are reused. Manufacturers' instructions for inspecting, cleaning, and maintaining respirators should be followed to ensure that the respirator continues to function properly (55).

7. Periodic evaluation of the personal respiratory protection program. The program should be evaluated completely at least once a year, and both the written operating procedures and program administration should be revised as necessary based on the results of the evaluation. Elements of the program that should be evaluated include work practices and employee acceptance of respirator use (i.e., subjective comments made by employees concerning comfort during use and interference with duties).

Supplement 5: Decontamination—Cleaning, Disinfecting, and Sterilizing of Patient-Care Equipment

Equipment used on patients who have TB is usually not involved in the transmission of M. tuberculosis, although transmission by contaminated bronchoscopes has been demonstrated (159, 160). Guidelines for cleaning, disinfecting, and sterilizing equipment have been published (161, 162). The rationale for cleaning, disinfecting, or sterilizing patient-care equipment can be understood more readily if medical devices, equipment, and surgical materials are divided into three general categories. These categories—critical, semicritical, and noncritical items—are defined by the potential risk for infection associated with their use (163, 164).

Critical items are instruments that are introduced directly into the bloodstream or into other normally sterile areas of the body (e.g., needles, surgical instruments, cardiac catheters, and implants). These items should be sterile at the time of use.

Semicritical items are those that may come in contact with mucous membranes but do not ordinarily penetrate body surfaces (e.g., noninvasive flexible and rigid fiberoptic endoscopes or bronchoscopes, endotracheal tubes, and anesthesia breathing circuits). Although sterilization is preferred for these instruments, high-level disinfection that destroys vegetative microorganisms, most fungal spores, tubercle bacilli, and small nonlipid viruses may be used. Meticulous physical cleaning of such items before sterilization or high-level disinfection is essential.

Noncritical items are those that either do not ordinarily touch the patient or touch only the patient's intact skin (e.g., crutches, bedboards, blood pressure cuffs, and various other medical accessories). These items are not associated with direct transmission of M. tuberculosis, and washing them with detergent is usually sufficient.

Health-care facility policies should specify whether cleaning, disinfecting, or sterilizing an item is necessary to decrease the risk for infection. Decisions about decontamination processes should be based on the intended use of the item, not on the diagnosis of the patient for whom the item was used. Selection of chemical disinfectants depends on the intended use, the level of disinfection required, and the structure and material of the item to be disinfected.

Although microorganisms are ordinarily found on walls, floors, and other environmental surfaces, these surfaces are rarely associated with transmission of infections to patients or HCWs. This is particularly true with organisms such as M. tuberculosis, which generally require inhalation by the host for infection to occur. Therefore, extraordinary attempts to disinfect or sterilize environmental surfaces are not indicated. If a detergent germicide is used for routine cleaning, a hospital-grade, EPA-approved germicide/disinfectant that is not tuberculocidal can be used. The same routine daily cleaning procedures used in other rooms in the facility should be used to clean TB isolation rooms, and personnel should follow isolation practices while cleaning these rooms. For final cleaning of the isolation room after a patient has been discharged, personal protective equipment is not necessary if the room has been ventilated for the appropriate amount of time (Table S31).

REFERENCES: AS NUMBERED IN ORIGINAL PUBLICATION

2. CDC. Guidelines for preventing the transmission of tuberculosis in health-care settings, with special focus on HIV-related issues. MMWR 1990;39(No. RR-17).
4. CDC. Guidelines for prevention of TB transmission in hospitals. Atlanta: US Department of Health and Human Services, Public Health Service, CDC, 1982:DHHS publication no. (CDC)82–8371.
5. CDC. Screening for tuberculosis and tuberculous infection in high-risk populations, and the use of preventive therapy for tuberculous infection in the United States: recommendations of the Advisory Committee for Elimination of Tuberculosis. MMWR 1990;39(No. RR-8).
6. American Thoracic Society/CDC. Diagnostic standards and classification of tuberculosis. Am Rev Respir Dis 1990;142:725–735.
20. Hutton MD, Stead WW, Cauthen GM, et al. Nosocomial transmission of tuberculosis associated with a draining tuberculous abscess. J Infect Dis 1990;161:286–295.
21. Kantor HS, Poblete R, Pusateri SL. Nosocomial transmission of tuberculosis from unsuspected disease. Am J Med 1988;84:833–838.
22. Lundgren R, Norrman E, Asberg I. Tuberculous infection transmitted at autopsy. Tubercle 1987;68: 147–150.
24. Beck-Sague C, Dooley SW, Hutton MD, et al. Outbreak of multidrug-resistant Mycobacterium tuberculosis infections in a hospital: transmission to patients with HIV infection and staff. JAMA 1992;268: 1280–1286.
33. American Thoracic Society. Treatment of tuberculosis and tuberculosis infection in adults and children. Am J Respir Crit Care Med 1994;149:1359–1374.
34. Strong BE, Kubica GP. Isolation and identification of Mycobacterium tuberculosis. Atlanta: US Department of Health and Human Services, Public Health Service, CDC, 1981:DHHS publication no. (CDC)81–8390.

35. CDC. Tuberculosis and human immunodeficiency virus infection: recommendations of the Advisory Committee for the Elimination of Tuberculosis (ACET). MMWR 1989;38:236–238, 243-2450.
36. Willcox PA, Benator SR, Potgieter PD. Use of flexible fiberoptic bronchoscope in diagnosis of sputum-negative pulmonary tuberculosis. Thorax 1982;37:598–601.
37. Willcox PA, Potgieter PD, Bateman ED, Benator SR. Rapid diagnosis of sputum-negative miliary tuberculosis using the flexible fiberoptic bronchoscope. Thorax 1986;41:681–684.
38. Tenover FC, Crawford JT, Huebner RE, Geiter LJ, Horsburgh CR Jr, Good RC. The resurgence of tuberculosis: is your laboratory ready? J Clin Microbiol 1993;31:767–770.
39. Pitchenik AE, Cole C, Russell BW, et al. Tuberculosis, atypical mycobacteriosis, and the acquired immunodeficiency syndrome among Haitian and non-Haitian patients in South Florida. Ann Intern Med 1984;101:641–645.
40. Maayan S, Wormscr GP, Hewlett D, et al. Acquired immunodeficiency syndrome (AIDS) in an economically disadvantaged population. Arch Intern Med 1985;145:1607–1612.
41. Klein NC, Duncanson FP, Lenox TH III, et al. Use of mycobacterial smears in the diagnosis of pulmonary tuberculosis in AIDS/ARC patients. Chest 1989;95:1190–1192.
42. Burnens AP, Vurma-Rapp U. Mixed mycobacterial cultures—occurrence in the clinical laboratory. Int J Med Microbiol 1989;27:85–90.
43. CDC. Initial therapy for tuberculosis in the era of multidrug resistance: recommendations of the Advisory Council for the Elimination of Tuberculosis. MMWR 1993;42(No. RR-7).
44. Rabalais G, Adams G, Stover B. PPD skin test conversion in health-care workers after exposure to Mycobacterium tuberculosis infection in infants [Letter]. Lancet 1991;338:826.
45. Wallgren A. On contagiousness of childhood tuberculosis. Acta Pediatr Scand 1937;22:229–234.
46. Riley RL. Airborne infection. Am J Med 1974;57:466–475.
47. American Society of Heating, Refrigerating and Air-Conditioning Engineers. Chapter 7: Health facilities. In: 1991 Application handbook. Atlanta: American Society of Heating, Refrigerating and Air-Conditioning Engineers, Inc., 1991.
48. American Institute of Architects, Committee on Architecture for Health. Chapter 7: General hospital. In: Guidelines for construction and equipment of hospital and medical facilities. Washington, DC: The American Institute of Architects Press, 1987.
49. Health Resources and Services Administration. Guidelines for construction and equipment of hospital and medical facilities. Rockville, MD: US Department of Health and Human Services, Public Health Service, 1984:PHS publication no. (HRSA)84–14500.
50. Riley RL, O'Grady F. Airborne infection: transmission and control. New York: McMillan, 1961.
51. Galson E, Goddard KR. Hospital air conditioning and sepsis control. ASHRAE Journal, 1968;(Jul): 33–41.
52. Kethley TW. Air: its importance and control. In: Proceedings of the National Conference on Institutionally Acquired Infections. Washington, DC: US Department of Health, Education, and Welfare, Public Health Service, Communicable Disease Center, Division of Hospital and Medical Facilities, 1963:35–46;PHS publication no. 1188.
53. Hermans RD, Streifel AJ. Ventilation design. In: Bierbaum PJ, Lippmann M, eds. Proceedings of the Workshop on Engineering Controls for Preventing Airborne Infections in Workers in Health Care and Related Facilities. Cincinnati: US Department of Health and Human Services, Public Health Service, CDC, 1994:DHHS publication no. (NIOSH)94–106.
54. American National Standards Institute. American national standard practices for respiratory protection. New York: American National Standards Institute, 1992.
55. NIOSH. Guide to industrial respiratory protection. Morgantown, WV: US Department of Health and Human Services, Public Health Service, CDC, 1987:DHHS publication no. (NIOSH)87–116.
56. CDC. Recommendations for HIV testing services for inpatients and outpatients in acute-care hospital settings; and Technical guidance on HIV counseling. MMWR 1993;42(No. RR-2).
57. Williams WW. Guidelines for infection control in hospital personnel. Infect Control 1983;4(Suppl): 326–349.
58. Barrett-Connor E. The periodic chest roentgenogram for the control of tuberculosis in health care personnel. Am Rev Respir Dis 1980;122:153–155.
59. CDC/National Institutes of Health. Agent: Mycobacterium tuberculosis, M. bovis. In: Biosafety in microbiological and biomedical laboratories. Atlanta: US Department of Health and Human Services, Public Health Service, 1993:95;DHHS publication no. (CDC)93–8395.
60. CDC. Prevention and control of tuberculosis in facilities providing long-term care to the elderly: recommendations of the Advisory Committee for Elimination of Tuberculosis. MMWR 1990;39(No. RR-10).
61. CDC. Prevention and control of tuberculosis in correctional institutions: recommendations of the Advisory Committee for the Elimination of Tuberculosis. MMWR 1989;38:313–320, 325.
62. Dueli RC, Madden RN. Droplet nuclei produced during dental treatment of tubercular patients. Oral Surg 1970;30:711–716.
63. Manoff SB, Cauthen GM, Stoneburner RL, Bloch AB, Schultz S, Snider DE Jr. TB patients with AIDS: are they more likely to spread TB [Abstract no. 4621]? Book 2. IV International Conference on AIDS. Stockholm, Sweden, June 12–16, 1988:216.

64. Cauthen GM, Dooley SW, Bigler W, Burr J, Ihle W. Tuberculosis (TB) transmission by HIV-associated TB cases [Abstract no. M.C.3326]. Vol 1. VII International Conference on AIDS. Florence, Italy, June 16–21, 1991.
65. Klausner JD, Ryder RW, Baende E, et al. Mycobacterium tuberculosis in household contacts of human immunodeficiency virus type 1-seropositive patients with active pulmonary tuberculosis in Kinshasa, Zaire. J Infect Dis 1993;168:106–111.
66. Riley RL, Mills CC, O'Grady F, Sultan LU, Wittstadt F, Shivpuri DN. Infectiousness of air from a tuberculosis ward. Am Rev Respir Dis 1962;85:511–525.
67. Noble RC. Infectiousness of pulmonary tuberculosis after starting chemotherapy: review of the available data on an unresolved question. Am J Infect Control 1981;9:6–10.
68. Howard TP, Solomon DA. Reading the tuberculin skin test: who, when, and how? Arch Intern Med 1988;148:2457–2459.
69. Snider DE Jr. The tuberculin skin test. Am Rev Respir Dis 1982;125:108–118.
70. Huebner RE, Schein MF, Bass JB Jr. The tuberculin skin test. Clin Infect Dis 1993;17:968–975.
71. Canessa PA, Fasano L, Lavecchia MA, Torraca A, Schiattone ML. Tuberculin skin test in asymptomatic HIV seropositive carriers [Letter]. Chest 1989;96:1215–1216.
72. CDC. Purified protein derivative (PPD)-tuberculin anergy and HIV infection: guidelines for anergy testing and management of anergic persons at risk of tuberculosis. MMWR 1991;40(No. RR-5).
73. Snider DE, Farer LS. Package inserts for antituberculosis drugs and tuberculins. Am Rev Respir Dis 1985;131:809–810.
74. Snider DE Jr. Bacille Calmette-Guerin vaccinations and tuberculin skin test. JAMA 1985;253:3438–3439.
75. CDC. Use of BCG vaccines in the control of TB: a joint statement by the ACIP and the Advisory Committee for the Elimination of Tuberculosis. MMWR 1988;37:663–664, 669–675.
76. Thompson NJ, Glassroth JL, Snider DE Jr, Farer LS. The booster phenomenon in serial tuberculin testing. Am Rev Respir Dis 1979;119:587–597.
77. Des Prez RM, Heim CR. Mycobacterium tuberculosis. In: Mandell GL, Douglas RG Jr, Bennett JE, eds. Principles and practice of infectious diseases. 3rd ed. New York: Churchill Livingstone, 1990:1877–1906.
78. Pitchenik AE, Rubinson HA. The radiographic appearance of tuberculosis in patients with the acquired immune deficiency syndrome (AIDS) and pre-AIDS. Am Rev Respir Dis 1985;131:393–396.
79. Kiehn TE, Cammarata R. Laboratory diagnosis of mycobacterial infection in patients with acquired immunodeficiency syndrome. J Clin Microbiol 1986;24:708–711.
80. Crawford JT, Eisenach KD, Bates JH. Diagnosis of tuberculosis: present and future. Semin Respir Infect 1989;4:171–181.
81. Moulding TS, Redeker AG, Kanel GC. Twenty isoniazid-associated deaths in one state. Am Rev Respir Dis 1989;140:700–705.
82. Snider DE Jr, Layde PM, Johnson MW, Lyle MA. Treatment of tuberculosis during pregnancy. Am Rev Respir Dis 1980;122:65–79.
83. Snider D. Pregnancy and tuberculosis. Chest 1984;86(Suppl):10S-13S.
84. Hamadeh MA, Glassroth J. Tuberculosis and pregnancy. Chest 1992;101:1114–1120.
85. Glassroth JL, White MC, Snider DE Jr. An assessment of the possible association of isoniazid with human cancer deaths. Am Rev Respir Dis 1977;116:1065–1074.
86. Glassroth JL, Snider DE Jr, Comstock GW. Urinary tract cancer and isoniazid. Am Rev Respir Dis 1977;116:331–333.
87. Costello HD, Snider DE Jr. The incidence of cancer among participants in a controlled, randomized isoniazid preventive therapy trial. Am J Epidemiol 1980;111:67–74.
88. CDC. The use of preventive therapy for tuberculous infection in the United States: recommendations of the Advisory Committee for Elimination of Tuberculosis. MMWR 1990;39(No. RR-8):9–12.
89. CDC. Management of persons exposed to multidrug-resistant tuberculosis. MMWR 1992;41(No. RR-11):59–71.
90. American Thoracic Society/CDC. Treatment of tuberculosis and tuberculosis infection in adults and children, 1986. Am Rev Respir Dis 1986;134:355–363.
91. American Thoracic Society/CDC. Control of tuberculosis in the United States. Am Rev Respir Dis 1992;146:1624–1635.
92. Snider DE Jr, Caras GJ. Isoniazid-associated hepatitis deaths: a review of available information. Am Rev Respir Dis 1992;145:494–497.
93. Small PM, Shafer RW, Hopewell PC, et al. Exogenous infection with multi-drug-resistant Mycobacterium tuberculosis in patients with advanced HIV infection. N Engl J Med 1993;328:1137–1144.
94. Iseman MD, Madsen LA. Drug-resistant tuberculosis. Clin Chest Med 1989;10:341–353.
95. Goble M. Drug-resistant tuberculosis. Semin Respir Infect 1986;1:220–229.
96. Goble M, Iseman MD, Madsen LA, Waite D, Ackerson L, Horsburgh CR Jr. Treatment of 171 patients with pulmonary tuberculosis resistant to isoniazid and rifampin. N Engl J Med 1993;328:527–532.
97. Simone PM, Iseman MD. Drug-resistant tuberculosis: a deadly—and growing—danger. J Respir Dis 1992;13:960–971.
98. American Conference of Governmental Industrial Hygienists. Industrial ventilation: a manual of recommended practice. Cincinnati: American Conference of Governmental Hygienists, Inc., 1992.

99. Mutchler JE. Principles of ventilation. In: NIOSH. The industrial environment—its evaluation and control. Washington, DC: US Department of Health, Education, and Welfare, Public Health Service, NIOSH, 1973.

100. Sherertz RJ, Belani A, Kramer BS, et al. Impact of air filtration on nosocomial Aspergillus infections. Am J Med 1987;83:709–718.

101. Rhame FS, Streifel AJ, Kersey JH, McGlave PB. Extrinsic risk factors for pneumonia in the patient at high risk of infection. Am J Med 1984;76:42–52.

102. Opal SM, Asp AA, Cannady PB, Morse PL, Burton LJ, Hammer PG. Efficacy of infection control measures during a nosocomial outbreak of disseminated Aspergillus associated with hospital construction. J Infect Dis 1986;153:63–67.

103. Woods JE. Cost avoidance and productivity in owning and operating buildings. Occup Med 1989;4:753–770.

104. Woods JE, Rask DR. Heating, ventilation, air-conditioning systems: the engineering approach to methods of control. In: Kundsin RB, ed. Architectural design and indoor microbial pollution. New York: Oxford University Press, 1988:123–153.

105. American Society of Heating, Refrigerating and Air-Conditioning Engineers. Chapter 25: Air cleaners for particulate contaminants. In: 1992 Systems and equipment fundamentals handbook. Atlanta: American Society of Heating, Refrigerating and Air-Conditioning Engineers, Inc., 1992:25.3–25.5.

106. American Society of Heating, Refrigerating and Air-Conditioning Engineers. Chapter 14: Air flow around buildings. In: 1989 Fundamentals handbook. Atlanta: American Society of Heating, Refrigerating and Air-Conditioning Engineers, Inc., 1989:14.1–14.13.

107. Riley RL, Wells WF, Mills CC, Nyka W, McLean RL. Air hygiene in tuberculosis: quantitative studies of infectivity and control in a pilot ward. Am Rev Tuberc 1957;75:420–431.

108. Riley RL, Nardell EA. Clearing the air: the theory and application of UV air disinfection. Am Rev Respir Dis 1989;139:1286–1294.

109. Riley RL. Ultraviolet air disinfection for control of respiratory contagion. In: Kundsin RB, ed. Architectural design and indoor microbial pollution. New York: Oxford University Press, 1988:175–197.

110. Stead WW. Clearing the air: the theory and application of ultraviolet air disinfection [Letter]. Am Rev Respir Dis 1989;140:1832.

111. McLean RL. General discussion: the mechanism of spread of Asian influenza. Am Rev Respir Dis 1961;83:36–38.

112. Willmon TL, Hollaender A, Langmuir AD. Studies of the control of acute respiratory diseases among naval recruits. I. A review of a four-year experience with ultraviolet irradiation and dust suppressive measures, 1943 to 1947. Am J Hyg 1948;48:227–232.

113. Wells WF, Wells MW, Wilder TS. The environmental control of epidemic contagion. I. An epidemiologic study of radiant disinfection of air in day schools. Am J Hyg 1942;35:97–121.

114. Wells WF, Holla WA. Ventilation in the flow of measles and chickenpox through a community: progress report, January 1, 1946 to June 15, 1949—Airborne Infection Study, Westchester County Department of Health. JAMA 1950;142:1337–1344.

115. Perkins JE, Bahlke AM, Silverman HF. Effect of ultra-violet irradiation of classrooms on spread of measles in large rural central schools. Am J Public Health Nations Health 1947;37:529–537.

116. Lurie MB. Resistance to tuberculosis: experimental studies in native and acquired defensive mechanisms. Cambridge, MA: Harvard University Press, 1964:160–164.

117. Collins FM. Relative susceptibility of acid-fast and non-acid-fast bacteria to ultraviolet light. Appl Microbiol 1971;21:411–413.

118. David HL, Jones WD Jr, Newman CM. Ultraviolet light inactivation and photoreactivation in the mycobacteria. Infect Immun 1971;4:318–319.

119. David HL. Response of mycobacteria to ultraviolet light radiation. Am Rev Respir Dis 1973;108:1175–1185.

120. Riley RL, Knight M, Middlebrook G. Ultraviolet susceptibility of BCG and virulent tubercle bacilli. Am Rev Respir Dis 1976;113:413–418.

121. American Thoracic Society/CDC. Control of tuberculosis. Am Rev Respir Dis 1983;128:336–342.

122. National Tuberculosis and Respiratory Disease Association. Guidelines for the general hospital in the admission and care of tuberculous patients. Am Rev Respir Dis 1969;99:631–633.

123. CDC. Notes on air hygiene: summary of Conference on Air Disinfection. Arch Environ Health 1971;22:473–474.

124. Schieffelbein CW Jr, Snider DE Jr. Tuberculosis control among homeless populations. Arch Intern Med 1988;148:1843–1846.

125. CDC. Prevention and control of tuberculosis in correctional institutions: recommendations of the Advisory Committee for the Elimination of Tuberculosis. MMWR 1989;38:313–320, 325.

126. International Commission on Illumination. International lighting vocabulary [French]. 4th ed. Geneva, Switzerland: Bureau Central de la Commission Electrotechnique Internationale, 1987:CIE publication no. 17.4.

127. Nagy R. Application and measurement of ultraviolet radiation. Am Ind Hyg Assoc J 1964;25:274–281.

128. Illuminating Engineering Society. IES lighting handbook. 4th ed. New York: Illuminating Engineering Society, 1966:25–27.
129. Kethley TW, Branch K. Ultraviolet lamps for room air disinfection: effect of sampling location and particle size of bacterial aerosol. Arch Environ Health 1972;25:205–214.
130. Riley RL, Permutt S, Kaufman JE. Convection, air mixing, and ultraviolet air disinfection in rooms. Arch Environ Health 1971;22:200–207.
131. Riley RL, Permutt S. Room air disinfection by ultraviolet irradiation of upper air. Arch Environ Health 1971;22:208–219.
132. Riley RL, Permutt S, Kaufman JE. Room air disinfection by ultraviolet irradiation of upper air: further analysis of convective air exchange. Arch Environ Health 1971;23:35–39.
133. Riley RL, Kaufman JE. Air disinfection in corridors by upper air irradiation with ultraviolet. Arch Environ Health 1971;22:551–553.
134. Macher JM, Alevantis LE, Chang Y-L, Liu K-S. Effect of ultraviolet germicidal lamps on airborne microorganisms in an outpatient waiting room. Applied Occupational and Environmental Hygiene 1992;7:505–513.
135. Riley RL, Kaufman JE. Effect of relative humidity on the inactivation of airborne Serratia marcescens by ultraviolet radiation. Appl Microbiol 1972;23:1113–1120.
136. NIOSH. Criteria for a recommended standard . . . occupational exposure to ultraviolet radiation. Washington, DC: US Department of Health, Education, and Welfare, Public Health Service, 1972:publication no. (HSM)73–110009.
137. Everett MA, Sayre RM, Olson RL. Physiologic response of human skin to ultraviolet light. In: Urbach F, ed. The biologic effects of ultraviolet radiation. Oxford: Pergamon Press, 1969.
138. International Agency for Research on Cancer. IARC monographs on the evaluation of carcinogenic risks to humans: solar and ultraviolet radiation. Vol 55. Lyon, France: World Health Organization, International Agency for Research on Cancer, 1992.
139. Valerie K, Delers A, Bruck C, et al. Activation of human immunodeficiency virus type 1 by DNA damage in human cells. Nature 1988;333:78–81.
140. Zmudzka BZ, Beer JZ. Activation of human immunodeficiency virus by ultraviolet radiation (yearly review). Photochem Photobiol 1990;52:1153–1162.
141. Wallace BM, Lasker JS. Awakenings—UV light and HIV gene activation. Science 1992;257:1211–1212.
142. Valerie K, Rosenberg M. Chromatin structure implicated in activation of HIV-1 gene expression by ultraviolet light. New Biol 1990;2:712–718.
143. Stein B, Rahmsdorf HJ, Steffen A, Litfin M, Herrlich P. UV-induced DNA damage is an intermediate step in UV-induced expression of human immunodeficiency virus type 1, collagenase, C-Fos, and metallathionein. Mol Cell Biol 1989;9:5169–5181.
144. Clerici M, Shearer GM. UV light exposure and HIV replication. Science 1992;258:1070–1071.
145. NIOSH. Hazard evaluation and technical assistance report: Onondaga County Medical Examiner's Office, Syracuse, New York. Cincinnati: US Department of Health and Human Services, Public Health Service, CDC, 1992:NIOSH report no. HETA 92–171-2255.
146. NIOSH. Hazard evaluation and technical assistance report: John C. Murphy Family Health Center, Berkeley, Missouri. Cincinnati: US Department of Health and Human Services, Public Health Service, CDC, 1992:NIOSH report no. HETA 91–148-2236.
147. NIOSH. Hazard evaluation and technical assistance report: San Francisco General Hospital and Medical Center, San Francisco, California. Cincinnati: US Department of Health and Human Services, Public Health Service, CDC, 1992:NIOSH report no. HETA 90–122-L2073.
148. Macher JM. Ultraviolet radiation and ventilation to help control tuberculosis transmission: guidelines prepared for California Indoor Air Quality Program. Berkeley, CA: Air and Industrial Hygiene Laboratory, 1989.
149. Riley RL. Principles of UV air disinfection. Baltimore, MD: Johns Hopkins University, School of Hygiene and Public Health, 1991.
150. American Conference of Governmental Industrial Hygienists. Threshold limit values and biological exposure indices for 1991–1992. Cincinnati: American Conference of Governmental Industrial Hygienists, Inc., 1991.
151. Bloom BR, Murray CJL. Tuberculosis: commentary on a reemergent killer. Science 1992;257:1055–1064.
152. Nardell EA. Dodging droplet nuclei: reducing the probability of nosocomial tuberculosis transmission in the AIDS era. Am Rev Respir Dis 1990;142:501–503.
153. US Department of Health and Human Services. 42 CFR Part 84: Respiratory protective devices; proposed rule. Federal Register 1994;59:26849-26889.
154. American National Standards Institute. ANSI Z88.2–1980: American national standard practices for respiratory protection. New York: American National Standards Institute, 1980.
155. Hyatt EC. Current problems and new developments in respiratory protection. Am Ind Hyg Assoc J 1963;24:295–304.
156. American National Standards Institute. ANSI Z88.2–1969: American national standard practices for respiratory protection. New York: American National Standards Institute, 1969.

157. Lowry PL, Hesch PR, Revoir WH. Performance of single-use respirators. Am Ind Hyg Assoc J 1977; 38:462–467.
158. Hyatt EC, et al. Respiratory studies for the National Institute for Occupational Safety and Health—July 1, 1972, through June 3, 1973. Los Alamos, NM: Los Alamos Scientific Laboratory; progress report no. LA-5620-PR.
159. Nelson KE, Larson PA, Schraufnagel DE, Jackson J. Transmission of tuberculosis by fiber broncho-scopes. Am Rev Respir Dis 1983;127:97–100.
160. Leers WD. Disinfecting endoscopes: how not to transmit Mycobacterium tuberculosis by bron-choscopy. Can Med Assoc J 1980;123:275–283.
161. Garner JS, Simmons BP. Guideline for isolation precautions in hospitals. Infect Control 1983; 4(Suppl):245–325.
162. Rutala WA. APIC guidelines for selection and use of disinfectants. Am J Infect Control 1990; 18:99–117.
163. Favero MS, Bond WW. Chemical disinfection of medical and surgical materials. In: Block SS, ed. Disinfection, sterilization, and preservation. 4th ed. Philadelphia: Lea & Febiger, 1991:617–641.
164. Garner JS, Favero MS. Guideline for handwashing and hospital environmental control. Atlanta: US Department of Health and Human Services, Public Health Service, CDC, 1985.

Glossary

This glossary contains many of the terms used in the guidelines, as well as others that are en-countered frequently by persons who implement TB infection-control programs. The defini-tions given are not dictionary definitions but are those most applicable to usage relating to TB.

ACID-FAST BACILLI (AFB)

Bacteria that retain certain dyes after being washed in an acid solution. Most acid-fast organ-isms are mycobacteria. When AFB are seen on a stained smear of sputum or other clinical specimen, a diagnosis of TB should be suspected; however, the diagnosis of TB is not con-firmed until a culture is grown and identified as M. tuberculosis.

ADHERENCE

Refers to the behavior of patients when they follow all aspects of the treatment regimen as pre-scribed by the medical provider, and also refers to the behavior of HCWs and employers when they follow all guidelines pertaining to infection control.

AEROSOL

The droplet nuclei that are expelled by an infectious person (e.g., by coughing or sneezing); these droplet nuclei can remain suspended in the air and can transmit M. tuberculosis to other persons.

AIA

The American Institute of Architects, a professional body that develops standards for building ventilation.

AIR CHANGES

The ratio of the volume of air flowing through a space in a certain period of time (i.e., the air-flow rate) to the volume of that space (i.e., the room volume); this ratio is usually expressed as the number of air changes per hour (ACH).

AIR MIXING

The degree to which air supplied to a room mixes with the air already in the room, usually ex-pressed as a mixing factor. This factor varies from 1 (for perfect mixing) to 10 (for poor mix-ing), and it is used as a multiplier to determine the actual airflow required (i.e., the recom-mended ACH multiplied by the mixing factor equals the actual ACH required).

ALVEOLI

The small air sacs in the lungs that lie at the end of the bronchial tree; the site where carbon diox-ide in the blood is replaced by oxygen from the lungs and where TB infection usually begins.

ANERGY

The inability of a person to react to skin-test antigens (even if the person is infected with the organisms tested) because of immunosuppression.

ANTEROOM

A small room leading from a corridor into an isolation room; this room can act as an airlock, preventing the escape of contaminants from the isolation room into the corridor.

AREA

A structural unit (e.g., a hospital ward or laboratory) or functional unit (e.g., an internal medicine service) in which HCWs provide services to and share air with a specific patient population or work with clinical specimens that may contain viable M. tuberculosis organisms. The risk for exposure to M. tuberculosis in a given area depends on the prevalence of TB in the population served and the characteristics of the environment.

ASHRAE

The American Society of Heating, Refrigerating and Air-Conditioning Engineers, Inc., a professional body that develops standards for building ventilation.

ASYMPTOMATIC

Without symptoms, or producing no symptoms.

BACILLUS OF CALMETTE AND GUERIN (BCG) VACCINE

A TB vaccine used in many parts of the world.

BACTEC®

One of the most often used radiometric methods for detecting the early growth of mycobacteria in culture. It provides rapid growth (in 7–14 days) and rapid drug-susceptibility testing (in 5–6 days). When BACTEC® is used with rapid species identification methods, M. tuberculosis can be identified within 10–14 days of specimen collection.

BOOSTER PHENOMENON

A phenomenon in which some persons (especially older adults) who are skin tested many years after infection with M. tuberculosis have a negative reaction to an initial skin test, followed by a positive reaction to a subsequent skin test. The second (i.e., positive) reaction is caused by a boosted immune response. Two-step testing is used to distinguish new infections from boosted reactions (see Two-Step Testing).

BRONCHOSCOPY

A procedure for examining the respiratory tract that requires inserting an instrument (a bronchoscope) through the mouth or nose and into the trachea. The procedure can be used to obtain diagnostic specimens.

CAPREOMYCIN

An injectable, second-line anti-TB drug used primarily for the treatment of drug-resistant TB.

CAVITY

A hole in the lung resulting from the destruction of pulmonary tissue by TB or other pulmonary infections or conditions. TB patients who have cavities in their lungs are referred to as having cavitary disease, and they are often more infectious than TB patients without cavitary disease.

CHEMOTHERAPY

Treatment of an infection or disease by means of oral or injectable drugs.

CLUSTER

Two or more PPD skin-test conversions occurring within a 3-month period among HCWs in a specific area or occupational group, and epidemiologic evidence suggests occupational (nosocomial) transmission.

CONTACT

A person who has shared the same air with a person who has infectious TB for a sufficient amount of time to allow possible transmission of M. tuberculosis.

CONVERSION, PPD

See PPD test conversion.

CULTURE

The process of growing bacteria in the laboratory so that organisms can be identified.

CYCLOSERINE

A second-line, oral anti-TB drug used primarily for treating drug-resistant TB.

DIRECTLY OBSERVED THERAPY (DOT)

An adherence-enhancing strategy in which an HCW or other designated person watches the patient swallow each dose of medication.

DNA PROBE

A technique that allows rapid and precise identification of mycobacteria (e.g., M. tuberculosis and M. bovis) that are grown in culture. The identification can often be completed in 2 hours.

DROPLET NUCLEI

Microscopic particles (i.e., 1–5 mm in diameter) produced when a person coughs, sneezes, shouts, or sings. The droplets produced by an infectious TB patient can carry tubercle bacilli and can remain suspended in the air for prolonged periods of time and be carried on normal air currents in the room.

DRUG RESISTANCE, ACQUIRED

A resistance to one or more anti-TB drugs that develops while a patient is receiving therapy and which usually results from the patient's nonadherence to therapy or the prescription of an inadequate regimen by a health-care provider.

DRUG RESISTANCE, PRIMARY

A resistance to one or more anti-TB drugs that exists before a patient is treated with the drug(s). Primary resistance occurs in persons exposed to and infected with a drug-resistant strain of M. tuberculosis.

DRUG-SUSCEPTIBILITY PATTERN

The anti-TB drugs to which the tubercle bacilli cultured from a TB patient are susceptible or resistant based on drug-susceptibility tests.

DRUG-SUSCEPTIBILITY TESTS

Laboratory tests that determine whether the tubercle bacilli cultured from a patient are susceptible or resistant to various anti-TB drugs.

ETHAMBUTOL

A first-line, oral anti-TB drug sometimes used concomitantly with INH, rifampin, and pyrazinamide.

ETHIONAMIDE

A second-line, oral anti-TB drug used primarily for treating drug-resistant TB.

EXPOSURE

The condition of being subjected to something (e.g., infectious agents) that could have a harmful effect. A person exposed to M. tuberculosis does not necessarily become infected (see Transmission).

FIRST-LINE DRUGS

The most often used anti-TB drugs (i.e., INH, rifampin, pyrazinamide, ethambutol, and streptomycin).

FIXED ROOM-AIR HEPA RECIRCULATION SYSTEMS

Nonmobile devices or systems that remove airborne contaminants by recirculating air through a HEPA filter. These may be built into the room and permanently ducted or may be mounted to the wall or ceiling within the room. In either situation, they are fixed in place and are not easily movable.

FLUOROCHROME STAIN

A technique for staining a clinical specimen with fluorescent dyes to perform a microscopic examination (smear) for mycobacteria. This technique is preferable to other staining techniques because the mycobacteria can be seen easily and the slides can be read quickly.

FOMITES

Linens, books, dishes, or other objects used or touched by a patient. These objects are not involved in the transmission of M. tuberculosis.

GASTRIC ASPIRATE

A procedure sometimes used to obtain a specimen for culture when a patient cannot cough up adequate sputum. A tube is inserted through the mouth or nose and into the stomach to recover sputum that was coughed into the throat and then swallowed. This procedure is particularly useful for diagnosis in children, who are often unable to cough up sputum.

HIGH-EFFICIENCY PARTICULATE AIR (HEPA) FILTER

A specialized filter that is capable of removing 99.97% of particles 30.3 mm in diameter and that may assist in controlling the transmission of M. tuberculosis. Filters may be used in ventilation systems to remove particles from the air or in personal respirators to filter air before it is inhaled by the person wearing the respirator. The use of HEPA filters in ventilation systems requires expertise in installation and maintenance.

HUMAN IMMUNODEFICIENCY VIRUS (HIV) INFECTION

Infection with the virus that causes acquired immunodeficiency syndrome (AIDS). HIV infection is the most important risk factor for the progression of latent TB infection to active TB.

IMMUNOSUPPRESSED

A condition in which the immune system is not functioning normally (e.g., severe cellular immunosuppression resulting from HIV infection or immunosuppressive therapy). Immunosuppressed persons are at greatly increased risk for developing active TB after they have been infected with M. tuberculosis. No data are available regarding whether these persons are also at increased risk for infection with M. tuberculosis after they have been exposed to the organism.

INDURATION

An area of swelling produced by an immune response to an antigen. In tuberculin skin testing or anergy testing, the diameter of the indurated area is measured 48–72 hours after the injection, and the result is recorded in millimeters.

INFECTION

The condition in which organisms capable of causing disease (e.g., M. tuberculosis) enter the body and elicit a response from the host' s immune defenses. TB infection may or may not lead to clinical disease.

INFECTIOUS

Capable of transmitting infection. When persons who have clinically active pulmonary or laryngeal TB disease cough or sneeze, they can expel droplets containing M. tuberculosis into the air. Persons whose sputum smears are positive for AFB are probably infectious.

INJECTABLE

A medication that is usually administered by injection into the muscle (intramuscular [IM]) or the bloodstream (intravenous [IV]).

INTERMITTENT THERAPY

Therapy administered either two or three times per week, rather than daily. Intermittent therapy should be administered only under the direct supervision of an HCW or other designated person (see Directly observed therapy [DOT]).

INTRADERMAL

Within the layers of the skin.

ISONIAZID (INH)

A first-line, oral drug used either alone as preventive therapy or in combination with several other drugs to treat TB disease.

KANAMYCIN

An injectable, second-line anti-TB drug used primarily for treatment of drug-resistant TB.

LATENT TB INFECTION

Infection with M. tuberculosis, usually detected by a positive PPD skin-test result, in a person who has no symptoms of active TB and who is not infectious.

MANTOUX TEST

A method of skin testing that is performed by injecting 0.1 mL of PPD-tuberculin containing 5 tuberculin units into the dermis (i.e., the second layer of skin) of the forearm with a needle and syringe. This test is the most reliable and standardized technique for tuberculin testing (see Tuberculin skin test and Purified protein derivative [PPD]-tuberculin test).

MULTIDRUG-RESISTANT TUBERCULOSIS (MDR-TB)

Active TB caused by M. tuberculosis organisms that are resistant to more than one anti-TB drug; in practice, often refers to organisms that are resistant to both INH and rifampin with or without resistance to other drugs (see Drug resistance, acquired and Drug resistance, primary).

M. TUBERCULOSIS COMPLEX

A group of closely related mycobacterial species that can cause active TB (e.g., M. tuberculosis, M. bovis, and M. africanum); most TB in the United States is caused by M. tuberculosis.

NEGATIVE PRESSURE

The relative air pressure difference between two areas in a health-care facility. A room that is at negative pressure has a lower pressure than adjacent areas, which keeps air from flowing out of the room and into adjacent rooms or areas.

NOSOCOMIAL

An occurrence, usually an infection, that is acquired in a hospital or as a result of medical care.

PARA-AMINOSALICYLIC ACID

A second-line, oral anti-TB drug used for treating drug-resistant TB.

PATHOGENESIS

The pathologic, physiologic, or biochemical process by which a disease develops.

PATHOGENICITY

The quality of producing or the ability to produce pathologic changes or disease. Some non-tuberculous mycobacteria are pathogenic (e.g., Mycobacterium kansasii), and others are not (e.g., Mycobacterium phlei).

PORTABLE ROOM-AIR HEPA RECIRCULATION UNITS

Free-standing portable devices that remove airborne contaminants by recirculating air through a HEPA filter.

POSITIVE PPD REACTION

A reaction to the purified protein derivative (PPD)-tuberculin skin test that suggests the person tested is infected with M. tuberculosis. The person interpreting the skin-test reaction determines whether it is positive on the basis of the size of the induration and the medical history and risk factors of the person being tested.

PREVENTIVE THERAPY

Treatment of latent TB infection used to prevent the progression of latent infection to clinically active disease.

PURIFIED PROTEIN DERIVATIVE (PPD)-TUBERCULIN

A purified tuberculin preparation that was developed in the 1930s and that was derived from old tuberculin. The standard Mantoux test uses 0.1 mL of PPD standardized to 5 tuberculin units.

PURIFIED PROTEIN DERIVATIVE (PPD)-TUBERCULIN TEST

A method used to evaluate the likelihood that a person is infected with M. tuberculosis. A small dose of tuberculin (PPD) is injected just beneath the surface of the skin, and the area is examined 48–72 hours after the injection. A reaction is measured according to the size of the induration. The classification of a reaction as positive or negative depends on the patient's medical history and various risk factors (see Mantoux test).

PURIFIED PROTEIN DERIVATIVE (PPD)-TUBERCULIN TEST CONVERSION

A change in PPD test results from negative to positive. A conversion within a 2-year period is usually interpreted as new M. tuberculosis infection, which carries an increased risk for progression to active disease. A booster reaction may be misinterpreted as a new infection (see Booster Phenomenon and Two-Step Testing).

PYRAZINAMIDE

A first-line, oral anti-TB drug used in treatment regimens.

RADIOGRAPHY

A method of viewing the respiratory system by using radiation to transmit an image of the respiratory system to film. A chest radiograph is taken to view the respiratory system of a person who is being evaluated for pulmonary TB. Abnormalities (e.g., lesions or cavities in the lungs and enlarged lymph nodes) may indicate the presence of TB.

RADIOMETRIC METHOD

A method for culturing a specimen that allows for rapid detection of bacterial growth by measuring production of CO_2 by viable organisms; also a method of rapidly performing susceptibility testing of M. tuberculosis.

RECIRCULATION

Ventilation in which all or most of the air that is exhausted from an area is returned to the same area or other areas of the facility.

REGIMEN

Any particular TB treatment plan that specifies which drugs are used, in what doses, according to what schedule, and for how long.

REGISTRY

A record-keeping method for collecting clinical, laboratory, and radiographic data concerning TB patients so that the data can be organized and made available for epidemiologic study.

RESISTANCE

The ability of some strains of bacteria, including M. tuberculosis, to grow and multiply in the presence of certain drugs that ordinarily kill them; such strains are referred to as drug-resistant strains.

RIFAMPIN

A first-line, oral anti-TB drug that, when used concomitantly with INH and pyrazinamide, provides the basis for short-course therapy.

ROOM-AIR HEPA RECIRCULATION SYSTEMS AND UNITS

Devices (either fixed or portable) that remove airborne contaminants by recirculating air through a HEPA filter.

SECOND-LINE DRUGS

Anti-TB drugs used when the first-line drugs cannot be used (e.g., for drug-resistant TB or because of adverse reactions to the first-line drugs). Examples are cycloserine, ethionamide, and capreomycin.

SINGLE-PASS VENTILATION

Ventilation in which 100% of the air supplied to an area is exhausted to the outside.

SMEAR (AFB SMEAR)

A laboratory technique for visualizing mycobacteria. The specimen is smeared onto a slide and stained, then examined using a microscope. Smear results should be available within 24 hours. In TB, a large number of mycobacteria seen on an AFB smear usually indicates infectiousness. However, a positive result is not diagnostic of TB because organisms other than M. tuberculosis may be seen on an AFB smear (e.g., nontuberculous mycobacteria).

SOURCE CASE

A case of TB in an infectious person who has transmitted M. tuberculosis to another person or persons.

SOURCE CONTROL

Controlling a contaminant at the source of its generation, which prevents the spread of the contaminant to the general work space.

SPECIMEN

Any body fluid, secretion, or tissue sent to a laboratory where smears and cultures for M. tuberculosis will be performed (e.g., sputum, urine, spinal fluid, and material obtained at biopsy).

SPUTUM

Phlegm coughed up from deep within the lungs. If a patient has pulmonary disease, an examination of the sputum by smear and culture can be helpful in evaluating the organism responsible for the infection. Sputum should not be confused with saliva or nasal secretions.

SPUTUM INDUCTION

A method used to obtain sputum from a patient who is unable to cough up a specimen spontaneously. The patient inhales a saline mist, which stimulates a cough from deep within the lungs.

SPUTUM SMEAR, POSITIVE

AFB are visible on the sputum smear when viewed under a microscope. Persons with a sputum smear positive for AFB are considered more infectious than those with smear-negative sputum.

STREPTOMYCIN

A first-line, injectable anti-TB drug.

SYMPTOMATIC

Having symptoms that may indicate the presence of TB or another disease (see Asymptomatic).

TB CASE

A particular episode of clinically active TB. This term should be used only to refer to the disease itself, not the patient with the disease. By law, cases of TB must be reported to the local health department.

TB INFECTION

A condition in which living tubercle bacilli are present in the body but the disease is not clinically active. Infected persons usually have positive tuberculin reactions, but they have no symptoms related to the infection and are not infectious. However, infected persons remain at lifelong risk for developing disease unless preventive therapy is given.

TRANSMISSION

The spread of an infectious agent from one person to another. The likelihood of transmission is directly related to the duration and intensity of exposure to M. tuberculosis (see Exposure).

TREATMENT FAILURES

TB disease in patients who do not respond to chemotherapy and in patients whose disease worsens after having improved initially.

TUBERCLE BACILLI

M. tuberculosis organisms.

TUBERCULIN SKIN TEST

A method used to evaluate the likelihood that a person is infected with M. tuberculosis. A small dose of PPD-tuberculin is injected just beneath the surface of the skin, and the area is examined 48–72 hours after the injection. A reaction is measured according to the size of the induration. The classification of a reaction as positive or negative depends on the patient's medical history and various risk factors (see Mantoux Test, PPD Test).

TUBERCULOSIS (TB)

A clinically active, symptomatic disease caused by an organism in the M. tuberculosis complex (usually M. tuberculosis or, rarely, M. bovis or M. africanum).

TWO-STEP TESTING

A procedure used for the baseline testing of persons who will periodically receive tuberculin skin tests (e.g., HCWs) to reduce the likelihood of mistaking a boosted reaction for a new infection.

If the initial tuberculin-test result is classified as negative, a second test is repeated 1–3 weeks later. If the reaction to the second test is positive, it probably represents a boosted reaction. If the second test result is also negative, the person is classified as not infected. A positive reaction to a subsequent test would indicate new infection (i.e., a skin-test conversion) in such a person.

ULTRAVIOLET GERMICIDAL IRRADIATION (UVGI)

The use of ultraviolet radiation to kill or inactivate microorganisms.

ULTRAVIOLET GERMICIDAL IRRADIATION (UVGI) LAMPS

Lamps that kill or inactivate microorganisms by emitting ultraviolet germicidal radiation, predominantly at a wavelength of 254 nm (intermediate light waves between visible light and X-rays). UVGI lamps can be used in ceiling or wall fixtures or within air ducts of ventilation systems.

VENTILATION, DILUTION

An engineering control technique to dilute and remove airborne contaminants by the flow of air into and out of an area. Air that contains droplet nuclei is removed and replaced by contaminant-free air. If the flow is sufficient, droplet nuclei become dispersed, and their concentration in the air is diminished.

VENTILATION, LOCAL EXHAUST

Ventilation used to capture and remove airborne contaminants by enclosing the contaminant source (i.e., the patient) or by placing an exhaust hood close to the contaminant source.

VIRULENCE

The degree of pathogenicity of a microorganism as indicated by the severity of the disease produced and its ability to invade the tissues of a host. M. tuberculosis is a virulent organism.

Tuberculosis Control Laws

Original Citation: Centers for Disease Control and Prevention. Tuberculosis Control Laws—United States, 1993. Recommendations of the Advisory Council for the Elimination of Tuberculosis (ACET). MMWR 1993;42(RR-15).

Editor's Note: The information included here was based on a 1993 MMWR Reports and Recommendations issue (Vol. 42;RR-15) which summarizes a survey of state TB control laws. The original text includes background history and methodology used in the survey.

SUMMARY

Because of its communicable nature, tuberculosis (TB) is treated differently than other airborne infectious diseases, as there are many state laws specific to the control of TB. Many of these laws predate the current public health recommendations for the prevention and control of TB. In 1989, CDC published A Strategic Plan for the Elimination of Tuberculosis in the United States that was developed by the Advisory Committee (now Council) for the Elimination of Tuberculosis (ACET) (1). The Plan called for the establishment of a national goal of TB elimination (i.e., achieving a case rate of less than 1 per million population) by the year 2010. One of the methods for improving disease containment in the Plan was for the use of quarantine measures for nonadherent patients. The Plan called for revision of state and local laws to "facilitate the cure of persons with infectious tuberculosis" (1). The issue of outdated state TB laws was also identified as a problem in the National Action Plan to Combat Multidrug-resistant Tuberculosis (2).

In response to this issue, CDC conducted a survey of state TB control laws and ACET developed recommendations to address discrepancies between previously published recommendations and guidelines for the control of TB and state TB control laws. In order to address these discrepancies, states updating TB control laws should incorporate current recommendations and guidelines from CDC, ACET, and the American Thoracic Society. State laws should permit policies and practices to be rapidly reviewed and amended as new data becomes available and new recommendations and guidelines are published.

The goal of state TB-control programs should be to prevent, control, and eventually eliminate TB. To protect the public from TB, these programs should ensure that persons with TB receive appropriate treatment. In addition, states should develop and encourage implementation of comprehensive programs that address the needs of persons who have TB, including the integration of TB services with drug and alcohol treatment programs and the expansion of public education, particularly for populations at increased risk for TB. States also should require the application of recommended infection control measures in health-care facilities and congregate-living settings (e.g., correctional facilities).

RESULTS AND RECOMMENDATIONS

Reporting Requirements

Persons Required to Report Cases of TB

All states require designated health-care professionals to report cases of TB to local or state health departments. Physicians are most frequently required to report cases of TB (42 states). Others required to report test results or cases are laboratory directors (33 states), hospitals and hospital administrators (31 states), other health-care workers (23 states), school authorities (22 states), nursing home administrators (15 states), and hospital infection control officers (six states). Eight states also require parents and guardians to report cases of TB among household members. Cases are reported by all states to CDC using the Report of Verified Case of Tuberculosis (CDC Form 72.9).

Recommendation

- States should require health-care providers and allied professionals who diagnose TB or treat or otherwise care for TB patients to report confirmed or suspected cases to the appropriate health agency. Among these providers and professionals are physicians, pharmacists, nurses, infection control officers, medical examiners, morticians, and the administrators of laboratories or other facilities where TB patients receive health-care services. Appropriate systems should be developed that maximize the reporting of new cases and minimize the reporting of duplicate cases and suspected cases and that protect the confidentiality of reports.

Time Frame for Reporting

State laws regarding the time allowed for reporting cases of TB vary from reporting at the time of diagnosis to within 1 week of diagnosis. Thirteen states require reporting at the time of diagnosis, 14 states within 24 hours of diagnosis, seven states within 48 hours, three states within 72 hours, and six states within 1 week. Six states do not specify a time frame for reporting. In nine states, the time frame for reporting cases of TB depends on the reporting source. For example, physicians may be required to report cases of TB within 7 days of diagnosis, whereas institutions in the same state are required to report cases within 48 hours. Reporting requirements for laboratory directors vary from reporting at the time of identification of Mycobacterium tuberculosis to reporting results once a week.

Recommendations

- Confirmed and suspected cases should be reported within 2 working days of identification of M. tuberculosis to the health agency with primary responsibility for TB control in that jurisdiction. Reporting should be based on a diagnosis or a presumptive diagnosis. Local health departments should report confirmed and suspected cases to the state TB-control agency within 1 working day of notification.
- When a case of TB is identified as being drug resistant, the case should be reported again within 2 working days in a manner consistent with the reporting of confirmed and suspected cases of TB. The report of drug-resistant TB also should include the results of susceptibility tests.
- All bacteriologic and pathologic laboratories that perform diagnostic services or perform related drug-susceptibility tests for M. tuberculosis should be required to report the results for any person whose sputa, gastric contents, or other specimens submitted for examination reveal the presence of tubercle bacilli. These results should be reported to the local health department within 1 working day of identification.
- Laboratories that perform diagnostic services on specimens from other states should be required to report the results to the state health department TB program from which the specimen was received. Reports should include the patient's name, address, and physician, and the person or agency referring the positive specimen for laboratory evaluation.

Failure to Report Cases of TB

Twenty-nine states have statutory authority to impose a penalty on persons who are required to report TB cases but fail to do so. Five states impose a penalty only when the failure to report a case is willful. Those persons found guilty of failing to report cases may be convicted of a misdemeanor and fined from $5 to $500.

Recommendation

- Because the rapid and accurate reporting of TB cases is critical to the management of TB patients, states should have the authority to impose a penalty for the willful failure to report confirmed and suspected cases of TB within the required time frame. In addition to imposing a penalty, states may refer reporting violations to professional licensing boards or, in the instance of a laboratory, to the licensing agency.

Duty to Report Nonadherent* Patients

Eleven states require health-care providers to report nonadherent patients. Two states also require the attending physician to notify the state health department when a patient has completed treatment for TB.

Recommendations

- TB patients who have demonstrated an inability or an unwillingness to adhere to a prescribed treatment regimen should be classified as nonadherent. Patients should be considered unable or unwilling to adhere to prescribed treatment if they do not report for directly observed therapy (DOT), refuse medication, or show other evidence of not taking medications as prescribed (e.g., incorrect pill counts or urine test showing no evidence of drug metabolites).
- Any health-care professional who is aware of a nonadherent TB patient should contact the appropriate health official for necessary interventions. The health official or a designated representative should meet with the patient to determine why the patient is nonadherent. The patient may be unwilling to continue treatment because the medication is causing side effects, because the patient may have difficulty obtaining additional medication, or because the patient believes the medication is no longer necessary. After determining why the patient is not adhering to the treatment regimen, the health official should take appropriate action, such as seeking court-ordered DOT.

Additional Reporting Recommendations

Reporting requirements should include any confirmed or suspected case of active disease caused by M. tuberculosis complex (i.e., M. tuberculosis, Mycobacterium bovis, and/or Mycobacterium africanum). State laws also should require drug susceptibility tests for all patients for whom a specimen is available. The results should be reported to local and/or state health departments. Reporting laws should require that all reports and records of clinical or laboratory examination for the presence of TB be kept in a confidential registry maintained by the state health agency.

When not prohibited by law, states also should require that information on the patient's HIV infection status, when known, be included in TB case reports. From a surveillance perspective, the inclusion of the patient's HIV status is important to determine the impact of the HIV epidemic on TB cases; this information also is important for case management and prioritizing contact investigations.

If HIV-related information is reported, states should ensure that this information is protected under their specific HIV and acquired immunodeficiency syndrome (AIDS) reporting laws and confidentiality laws. If a state does

---

*States use different terms to describe patients who do not follow a prescribed treatment regimen, including "noncompliant" and "noncooperative." Throughout this document, the term "nonadherent" is used to describe patients who do not follow a prescribed treatment regimen.

not have specific HIV or AIDS confidentiality laws, it should ensure that HIV-related information is protected by applicable confidentiality laws for infectious diseases, communicable diseases, or sexually transmitted diseases, or by other provisions for the protection of patient medical records.

Health agencies that maintain both an HIV or AIDS registry and a TB registry should permit the sharing of information between the registries to assist in case finding, particularly when the HIV or AIDS registry has information regarding persons infected with TB whose names have not been reported to the TB registry. Information about a person's HIV or AIDS status must be protected, even when it is reported to or shared with another division within a health department.

Federally assisted substance-abuse treatment programs must report HIV- and TB-related information for all patients in a manner consistent with federal regulations for completing Confidentiality of Alcohol and Drug Abuse Patient Records.** Once the information from such treatment programs is reported to states, the information should be protected in a manner consistent with the regulations.

MANAGEMENT OF TB CASES

Provision of Treatment

Sixteen states specify that state-supported outpatient treatment must be made available for persons with TB. Twenty-nine states recommend that TB patients voluntarily seek treatment before health officials seek state intervention.

Recommendations

- State laws should require that all TB patients receive immediate treatment according to the most recent ATS/CDC and ACET treatment guidelines. These guidelines include (a) the examination of persons exposed to TB and persons suspected of having active TB, (b) the treatment of persons who have latent infection or active TB, (c) the duration of treatment, and (d) the means for preventing TB patients from infecting other people. States also should require that health-care providers document patients' adherence to prescribed therapy.
- States should require that health-care workers providing care to patients with confirmed or suspected TB develop individualized, comprehensive treatment plans for all TB patients. The plans should be developed in cooperation with the patients and the appropriate health department and discussed with patients before they are discharged from treatment facilities. In addition, clinicians or other designated persons in all correctional facilities should develop individualized, comprehensive discharge plans for all TB-infected inmates who will be released from the facility before they complete the prescribed course of therapy.
- Patients who do not adhere to self-administered therapy should receive DOT. In addition, states should require the isolation of nonadherent, infec-

---

**42 CFR 2.32

tious patients while they are receiving treatment. Persons who have drug-resistant TB should be treated according to the most recent CDC treatment guidelines for drug-resistant TB.

Penalty for Nonadherent Patients

Three states have provisions for imposing a fine on TB patients who do not adhere to treatment. Four states specify certain behaviors that violate TB laws (e.g., breaking quarantine or willfully transmitting disease), and 29 states provide that anyone who violates the TB-control law may be quarantined. Two states have provisions for imposing an undefined penalty on nonadherent patients. In one state, violation of a treatment plan or disruptive behavior within an institution justifies transfer to a correctional facility where treatment will be provided.

Recommendation

- Penalties for nonadherent behavior should be levied only after the use of incentives, enablers, voluntary or ordered DOT, and commitment for inpatient management have failed to result in adherence to treatment.

Restrictions for Persons Infected with TB

Sixteen states require that persons infected or suspected of being infected with TB be restricted from various activities. Typically, state laws require that persons infected with TB be excluded from work until they are no longer infectious or until the absence of TB has been medically demonstrated.

Recommendation

- Restricting the activities of a person with TB should be based on whether the person has infectious TB and poses a risk to others. Restrictions should be terminated when the person is no longer infectious.

Quarantine of Persons with TB

Forty-three states provide for the quarantine of TB patients within their own homes. States define quarantine broadly and specifically. Statutes and regulations also provide guidelines for the movement of patients outside of the home. Thirty-five states specify that a quarantine should last until the person is no longer infectious. However, the health officer with jurisdiction over the patient frequently determines the exact length of quarantine.

Recommendation

- Quarantine, the traditional public health intervention of isolating persons who are exposed to an infectious disease but are not yet infected, is no longer an appropriate TB control measure. For patients with active TB who adhere to treatment, temporary restriction to their primary residence may adequately protect others from exposure. Such patients should be restricted to their residence until they are noninfectious. Appropriate residence facilities should be designated for the care of homeless persons infected with active TB.

Commitment of Persons with Infectious TB to Treatment Facilities

Forty-two states permit the commitment of TB patients to treatment facilities. However, the legal process for commitment and the duration of commitment vary in each state. Twenty-four states require that persons committed for TB treatment remain hospitalized until they no longer pose a health threat to others. Many state laws specify that this condition be met when a patient becomes noninfectious. Seven states recommend that a patient remain hospitalized until cured, and six states allow commitment of persons with infectious TB for an unspecified period of time.

Some states allow patients who have been committed to petition the court for a discharge and/or to appeal the decision. One state provides the patient the right to petition the court for discharge after 6 months, and nine states allow the patient to appeal the commitment.

Recommendations

- Before committing TB patients for inpatient treatment, states should adopt step-by-step interventions beginning with DOT and supplemented by incentives and enablers. If a patient does not voluntarily adhere to DOT, the next step may be DOT that is ordered by a public health official or a court. Only after the patient has demonstrated an inability or an unwillingness to adhere to treatment regimens should admission to a treatment facility be initiated. Commitment for inpatient management should be viewed as the last measure for treatment of persons infected with TB. However, when a person who has active, infectious TB refuses to be isolated, emergency detention to isolate the person is appropriate.
- State laws should permit the involuntary isolation and detention of noninfectious patients who, after being offered less restrictive alternatives, refuse to adhere to a treatment regimen or to complete treatment. These persons are at risk for drug-resistant TB, which can be transmitted to others.
- Commitment laws should specify (a) where patients will be treated, (b) the duration of commitment (e.g., until treatment is complete or until there is evidence that the patient will adhere to the remainder of the treatment regimen), and (c) the reimbursement mechanism for the treatment.
- States should authorize the examination of persons suspected of having TB and the emergency isolation and detention of persons who have infectious TB. Such laws will permit local health officers to examine the contacts of persons with infectious TB who are unwilling to seek evaluation and/or treatment. The laws would permit local health officers to isolate and detain persons who have infectious TB but who are unable or unwilling to receive treatment to prevent transmission. The court review of emergency detention should expeditiously follow the isolation of TB patients in a treatment facility. Voluntary treatment should be pursued; however, appropriate commitment procedures should be initiated immediately for patients who do not consent to isolation and treatment.
- As in commitment proceedings under state mental health laws, any law under which a person may be examined, isolated, detained, committed, and/or treated for TB must meet due process and equal protection requirements under state and federal statutes and constitutions. Also, all patients who are subject to these legal proceedings should be represented by legal counsel.

Commitment Orders

When determining whether the commitment of a person with TB is necessary to protect the health of the public, local health officers should determine whether that person presents a substantial risk for infecting others or developing drug-resistant disease. This determination should be based on an individualized assessment of the situation, including consideration of the following factors:

- Laboratory results or, in the absence of laboratory tests, clinical signs and symptoms of infectious TB;
- Previous treatment for TB but failure to complete therapy for reasons unrelated to access to treatment or medication;
- Adherence to prescribed therapy;
- Risk for infecting others depending on the patient's housing and employment situation;
- Laboratory tests or a history of nonadherence to anti-TB chemotherapy indicate possible infection with drug-resistant M. tuberculosis.

When local health officers determine that commitment is necessary to protect the health of the public, they should issue a commitment order in writing to local authorities. The order should specify the name of the infected person, the period of time during which the order is to remain effective, the facility to which the person will be committed, and other terms or conditions necessary to protect the health of the public. When an order is issued, a copy of the order should be given to the person named in the order.

The commitment order should require that the person infected with TB be isolated until he/she is determined to be noninfectious. This decision should be based on laboratory results demonstrating that the person is smear negative and asymptomatic or based on the local health officer's determination that the person has completed a course of therapy consistent with the most recent ATS/CDC treatment recommendations. The person also should be ordered to receive treatment in a hospital or other appropriate facility until cured, unless the person's voluntary completion of the ordered therapy can be ensured. If the person refuses to consent to the ordered treatment, the health officer should have the authority to extend the commitment order as necessary.

After receiving information that a commitment order has been violated, health officers should notify the appropriate official in the jurisdiction (e.g., a judge in the county where the person resides) that a violation of the order has occurred. This notification should be in writing and should explain the rationale for the hospitalization and the facts about the violation.

Treatment Facilities

State statutes and regulations provide for TB treatment at public hospitals, sanitoria, and private hospitals that have entered into agreements for such treatment with states. Thirty-three states provide or approve facilities for the treatment of TB patients. Twenty-one states have adopted detailed guidelines for the testing, monitoring, and care of the TB patient in treatment facilities.

Recommendations

- To more efficiently treat TB patients, states should permit cities, counties, or groups of counties to establish and maintain a variety of facilities for treating persons infected with TB. Such facilities include shelters for the homeless, halfway houses, and short- or long-term care facilities such as hospitals.
- State health departments should develop standards based on the current ATS/CDC recommendations and guidelines for local TB-control programs and facilities to use in treating TB and controlling its transmission.

Financing of Treatment

TB-control statutes in 46 states specify that the state will provide some reimbursement for patient care. Payment provisions vary among these states. For example, three states provide funding for the treatment of indigent patients only; three states offer sliding-scale payments according to the patient's financial status; and six states require that if a patient has third-party insurance, the third-party payor must be the first payor and the state the payor of last resort.

Recommendation

- States should specify how the treatment of TB patients will be paid. The patient's inability to pay for treatment should not be a barrier to receiving effective treatment. Assuring treatment for all patients, regardless of their ability to pay, is critical to preventing the transmission of TB in the community.

Investigation of TB Cases

Forty-nine states require the investigation of reported cases of TB. Forty-five states specify that an investigation can be conducted when a health official receives a report of a confirmed or suspected case of TB. Forty-one states authorize health departments to investigate under certain circumstances, such as when a health officer suspects or knows of a case of TB. Twenty-nine states specifically require contact investigations for reported cases of TB.

Recommendations

- States should require local health officers to conduct immediate contact investigations for all reported or suspected cases of pulmonary TB. During the investigations, each health officer should be authorized to examine and order the isolation of persons suspected of having or known to have infectious TB and to detain persons known to be nonadherent to prescribed therapy.
- Health officers should be authorized to order a physical examination of persons suspected of having TB. The examination order should be submitted in writing and should specify the name of the person to be examined, the time and the place where the examination is to be conducted, the medical basis for the examination order, and any other terms or conditions necessary to protect the health of the public. In addition, health officers should have the authority to review all patient records of both public and private institutions, clinics, and practices where TB patients are treated.

Screening for TB

Forty-four states require that certain populations be screened for TB. Screening is frequently required for school employees (20 states), employees of medical facilities (18 states), and day care employees (11 states). TB testing is typically required before the start of employment. Eleven states also require that schoolchildren be screened for TB.

Recommendation

- To eliminate TB, states must interrupt the transmission of tubercle bacilli by preventing, identifying, and treating TB-infected persons. TB screening may include screening for latent TB infection, active disease, or both. Screening requirements should be based on an analysis of epidemiologic data (including disease frequency and the demographic and geographic distribution of disease in the community) and morbidity trends, and ALA/ATS/CDC/ACET recommendations and guidelines for screening populations, institutions (including health-care and correctional facilities), and personnel.

TB-Control Officers

State laws and regulations generally do not designate a TB-control officer to supervise the state TB-control program. However, every state currently has a designated person responsible for their state TB-control program.

Recommendation

- Each state should designate a TB-control officer to supervise TB-control programs. These officers should have sufficient authority to address the current problems in TB control.

RESPONSIBILITIES

TB-control officers should be responsible for all statewide TB-control activities. They should cooperate with local health departments and other appropriate organizations to conduct or supervise clinics that diagnose, treat, and control TB throughout the state. The officers should maintain a registry of all cases, suspected cases, and contacts.

AUTHORITY

To conduct TB-control measures, TB-control officers must have the authority to examine all records, reports, and other data pertaining to confirmed and suspected TB patients. The records of the TB-control officer must be confidential and the identity of patients must not be disclosed, except where disclosure is necessary as part of official TB-control activities.

In addition, the officers should have the authority to examine or order the examination of any person known to have or suspected of having TB. The officers also should be authorized to perform or order any laboratory tests or radiographic examinations necessary to diagnose and treat any patient who has TB.

TB-control officers should have the authority to issue emergency examination, isolation, and detention orders for persons suspected of having active TB, and issue commitment orders for persons who have active TB or who are nonadherent to the prescribed therapy. Such decisions should be based on guidelines issued by the state health department. TB-control officers also should be directed to cooperate with state and federal agencies in the prevention and control of TB.

CONCLUSION

A survey of state TB-control laws and regulations indicates that states differ in their approach to the control of TB. This report provides recommendations from the ACET that can be used in revising state TB-control laws. The purpose of providing these recommendations is to increase uniformity among TB-control programs. These recommendations also are designed to encourage states to adopt flexible TB-control laws and regulations that will accommodate new TB-control recommendations and guidelines as they are published.

The goal of TB-control programs is to eliminate TB by appropriately treating persons infected with TB, to safeguard the confidentiality and civil liberties of persons who have TB, and to protect them from unlawful discrimination because of their disease (Table 1).

Table 1. Goals for State Tuberculosis Control Programs

States should have systems that incorporate the following guidelines:

Ensure the mandatory reporting of each confirmed and suspected case of TB, and observe local laws and regulations protecting patient confidentiality;

Table 1.—*continued*

Examine persons at high risk for TB infection and disease, prescribe the appropriate preventive or curative treatment for these persons, and monitor their treatment;

Monitor the treatment of patients, and require that a treatment plan be devised for all hospitalized patients before they are discharged;

Ensure the rapid laboratory examination of specimens and reporting of results to the appropriate health department and the requesting clinician;

Ensure that TB-infected patients receive treatment until they are cured;

Protect the health of the public by isolating and treating persons who have infectious TB and detaining persons who, although not infectious, are unwilling or unable to complete their treatment and are at risk for becoming infectious and for acquiring drug-resistant TB;

Finance the treatment of indigent patients.

REFERENCES: AS NUMBERED IN ORIGINAL PUBLICATION

1. CDC. A strategic plan for the elimination of tuberculosis in the United States. MMWR 1989;38(S-3).
2. CDC. National action plan to combat multidrug-resistant tuberculosis; meeting the challenge of multidrug-resistant tuberculosis: summary of a conference; management of persons exposed to multidrug-resistant tuberculosis. MMWR 1992;41(No. RR-11).

BIBLIOGRAPHY

American Thoracic Society/CDC. Control of tuberculosis in the United States. Am Rev Respir Dis 1992;146: 1623–1633.

CDC/American Thoracic Society. Core curriculum on tuberculosis. 2nd ed. Atlanta: US Department of Health and Human Services, Public Health Service, 1991.

American Thoracic Society/CDC. Diagnostic standards and classification of tuberculosis. Am Rev Respir Dis 1990;142:725–735.

CDC, Snider D, Hutton M. Improving patient compliance in tuberculosis treatment programs. 1989.

CDC. Prevention and control of tuberculosis among homeless persons: recommendations of the Advisory Council for the Elimination of Tuberculosis. MMWR 1992;41(No. RR-5):13–21.

CDC. Prevention and control of tuberculosis in U.S. communities with at-risk minority populations: recommendations of the Advisory Council for the Elimination of Tuberculosis. MMWR 1992;41(No. RR-5):1–11.

American Thoracic Society/CDC. Treatment of tuberculosis and tuberculosis infection in adults and children. Am Rev Respir Dis 1986;134:355–365.

CDC. The use of preventive therapy for tuberculosis infection in the United States: recommendations of the Advisory Committee for Elimination of Tuberculosis. MMWR 1990;39(No. RR-8):9–12.

CDC. Approaches to improving adherence to antituberculosis therapy—South Carolina and New York, 1986–1991. MMWR 1993;42:74–75, 81.

CDC. Screening for tuberculosis and tuberculous infection in high-risk populations: recommendations of the Advisory Committee for Elimination of Tuberculosis. MMWR 1990;39:(No. RR-8):9–12.

CDC. Prevention and control of tuberculosis in migrant farm workers: recommendations of the Advisory Council for the Elimination of Tuberculosis. MMWR 1992;41(No. RR-10).

CDC. Prevention and control of tuberculosis in facilities providing long-term care to the elderly: recommendations of the Advisory Council for the Elimination of Tuberculosis. MMWR 1990;39(No. RR-10).

CDC. Initial therapy for tuberculosis in the era of multidrug resistance: recommendations of the Advisory Council for the Elimination of Tuberculosis. MMWR 1992;42(No. RR-7).

CDC. Purified protein derivative (PPD)-tuberculin anergy and HIV infection: guidelines for anergy testing and management of anergic persons at risk of tuberculosis. MMWR 1991;40(No.RR-5):27–32.

CDC. Control of tuberculosis in correctional facilities: a guide for health-care workers. Atlanta: US Department of Health and Human Services, Public Health Service, 1992.

CDC. Prevention and control of tuberculosis in correctional institutions: recommendations of the Advisory Committee for the Elimination of Tuberculosis. MMWR 1989;38:313–332, 325.

CDC. Guidelines for preventing the transmission of tuberculosis in health-care settings, with special focus on HIV-related issues. MMWR 1990;39(No. RR-17).

APPENDIX

FREQUENTLY USED TERMS

The following are the recommended definitions for key terms in tuberculosis (TB) control laws:

Active TB. TB disease as demonstrated by clinical, bacteriologic, and/or radiographic evidence. Persons who have not completed a course of anti-TB treatment are considered to have active TB and may be infectious.

Adherent. Taking anti-TB medications as prescribed.

Case. An occurrence of active TB.

Commitment. The confinement of a person who has infectious TB or who is noninfectious, but who has not adhered to prescribed treatment. The purpose of commitment, which occurs under judicial or administrative order, is to prevent the transmission of tubercle bacilli to others, to prevent the development of drug-resistant organisms, or to ensure that persons receive a complete course of treatment.

Contact. A person exposed to a patient who has infectious TB. Contact investigation. Interviewing, counseling, educating, examining, and investigating activities directed at persons who have been in close contact with patients who have infectious TB.

Detention. The temporary confinement of a person who has or who is suspected of having TB.

Directly Observed Therapy (DOT). Treatment in which health-care providers or other designated persons observe patients ingesting anti-TB medications.

Enabler. Anything that helps the patient to more readily complete therapy (e.g., bus fare and gasoline).

Exposure. The sharing of air with a person who has infectious tuberculosis.

Incentive. Anything that motivates the patient to adhere to treatment (e.g., food, coupons, and personal items).

Infected. Having been exposed to someone with infectious tuberculosis, or having a positive response to a tuberculin skin test, but not having clinical or radiographic evidence of disease. Some patients who are anergic may not respond to a skin test but still be infected.

Infectious TB. TB disease in a communicable or infectious stage as determined by a chest radiograph, the bacteriologic examination of body tissues or secretions, or other diagnostic procedures.

Isolation. An infection control practice designed to prevent the transmission of tubercle bacilli.

Nonadherent. Not taking medications as prescribed or not following the recommendations of the attending physician or health officer for the management of TB.

Noninfectious. Not capable of transmitting tubercle bacilli. A determination of non-infectiousness can be made when a patient shows significant clinical improvement (e.g., the resolution of cough and/or fever) and has negative sputum smears on 3 consecutive days.

Quarantine. A limitation on the movement of persons exposed to, or infected with, TB to prevent the exposure of other persons.

Suspected Case. A person with signs or symptoms of TB for whom the results of diagnostic studies are still pending completion.

Tuberculosis (TB). Disease caused by Mycobacterium tuberculosis complex (i.e., M. tuberculosis, Mycobacterium bovis, or Mycobacterium africanum).

TB Control Officer. A person appointed by the state to be responsible for the administration of state TB programs.

Management of Persons Exposed to Multidrug-Resistant Tuberculosis

Original Citation: Centers for Disease Control and Prevention. Management of persons exposed to multidrug-resistant tuberculosis. MMWR 1992;41(RR-11):59–71.

Original Authors: Margarita E. Villarino, MD, MPH, Samuel W. Dooley, Jr., MD, Lawrence J. Geiter, MPH, Kenneth G. Castro, MD, Dixie E. Snider, Jr., MD, MPH.

Editor's Note: The information included here was based on a 1992 MMWR Reports and Recommendations issue (Vol. 41;RR-11). The original text gives a history of recent MDR-TB outbreaks and ends with a request to enroll patients for several studies related to MDR-TB.

PATHOGENESIS AND PREVENTION OF TUBERCULOSIS

Persons with recently acquired M. tuberculosis infection are at relatively high risk of developing active TB; in general, 5%–10% of persons develop active disease within 2 years of the primary infection (3–5). Coinfection with HIV increases this risk considerably; seven (41%) of 18 HIV-infected patients identified in a nosocomial TB outbreak investigation in Italy developed active disease within 60 days of their exposure to M. tuberculosis, and 11 (38%) of 29 persons in a residential facility for HIV-infected persons in San Francisco developed active disease within 4 months of exposure (6–8). To reduce the risk of active TB in persons newly infected with M. tuberculosis, the American Thoracic Society/CDC and the Advisory Council for the Elimination of Tuberculosis recommend INH preventive therapy (9–10). For HIV-infected persons, the higher disease attack rate and the shorter incubation period associated with newly acquired tuberculous infection and the high mortality rate associated with TB disease reinforce the rationale for the use of preventive therapy. In HIV-infected persons who become newly infected with M. tuberculosis, the use of drug therapy might be considered treatment of incubating or subclinical disease.

When the infecting strain of M. tuberculosis is susceptible to INH and patients adhere to the drug regimen, INH is highly effective for preventing active TB. In a wide variety of controlled studies, persons who were prescribed 12 months of INH preventive therapy had a 30%–93% reduction in the rate of active disease; the variation in effectiveness was almost entirely due to variation in patient adherence to the prescribed regimen (11, 12). In a more recent study, nursing-home residents in Arkansas who received 12 months of INH preventive therapy after a documented tuberculin skin-test conversion had a 98% reduction in the rate of active disease, compared with those who had a skin-test conversion but did not take preventive treatment (3). Most studies of preventive therapy have been conducted among immunocompetent subjects. However, early results of a recent study in Zambia indicated the efficacy of 6 months of INH preventive therapy in tuberculin-positive persons coinfected with HIV. This study showed a substantial reduction (87%) in the rate of active disease in the treated group when compared with a control group that received placebo (13).

RIF is recommended as an alternative to INH when the infecting strain of M. tuberculosis is resistant to INH but susceptible to RIF (9). When the infecting strain is multidrug resistant (i.e., resistant to both INH and RIF), treatment options are problematic because no studies have demonstrated the effectiveness of preventive therapy for persons infected with such strains of M. tuberculosis.

IDENTIFICATION AND EVALUATION OF PERSONS EXPOSED TO TUBERCULOSIS

Several factors should be considered in the management of persons exposed to TB (i.e., contacts): (a) the likelihood that the contact is newly infected with M. tuberculosis; (b) the likelihood that the infecting strain of M. tuberculosis is multidrug resistant; and (c) the estimated likelihood that the contact, if infected, will develop active TB.

Estimating the Likelihood of New Infection with M. tuberculosis and Preventive Therapy Decision-making

Because contacts of persons with infectious TB are at high risk for tuberculous infection, contacts should be rapidly identified and evaluated when a case of infectious TB (i.e., TB involving the respiratory tract or oral cavity) is identified (Figure 1) (14). Contacts who are not known or likely to be immunosuppressed and who have a documented prior positive tuberculin skin test (Mantoux test with 5 tuberculin units of purified protein derivative [PPD]) are probably not newly infected. These persons need no further evaluation for the current TB exposure unless they have symptoms suggestive of active TB; however, they should be evaluated for preventive therapy on the basis of the prior positive tuberculin skin-test result (10). Contacts who are not known or likely to be immunosuppressed and who have no history of a positive tuberculin skin-test reaction should receive a tuberculin skin test and, if indicated, chest radiograph and sputum examination. Those who have tuberculin skin-test reactions with greater than or equal to 5 mm induration should be considered probably newly infected with M. tuberculosis and should be evaluated for preventive therapy, after active TB is excluded (Figure 1) (15). Members of the immediate family, close social contacts, or others (e.g., hospital roommates, some health-care providers) who shared the same indoor environment with an infectious TB patient for substantial periods are considered high-risk contacts. High-risk contacts who have negative tuberculin skin-test reactions (< 5 mm induration) and who are not anergic should receive follow-up skin tests 12 weeks after their exposure to TB has ended. These initially tuberculin-negative, high-risk contacts should be considered possibly newly infected. They should receive a chest radiograph and be considered for preventive therapy until follow-up testing is complete if (a) there is evidence of TB contagion among other contacts with comparable exposure (i.e., tuberculin positivity or active TB), or (b) the contact is a child, HIV infected, or immunosuppressed for other reasons. Preventive therapy can be discontinued if follow-up tuberculin skin-test results are negative.

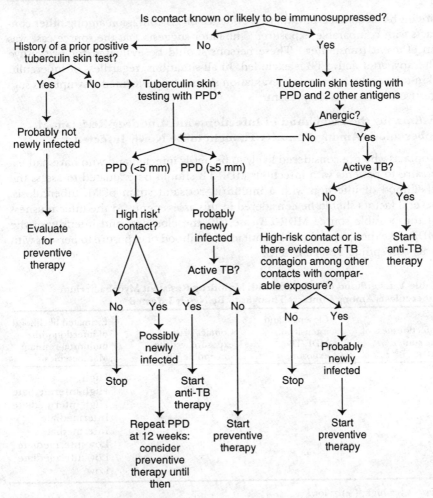

Is contact known or likely to be immunosuppressed?

History of a prior positive ◄——— No   Yes
tuberculin skin test?

Yes   No ——► Tuberculin skin   Tuberculin skin testing with
              testing with PPD*   PPD and 2 other antigens

Probably not   Anergic?
newly infected
                              ◄————————— No   Yes

                PPD (<5 mm)   PPD (≥5 mm)   Active TB?

Evaluate   No   Yes
for   High risk†   Probably
preventive   contact?   newly   High-risk contact or is   Start
therapy   infected   there evidence of TB   anti-TB
                                             contagion among other   therapy
                               Active TB?   contacts with compar-
                                             able exposure?

            No   Yes   Yes   No   No   Yes

                  Possibly
                  newly   Probably
                  infected   newly
                                                             infected
            Stop   Start
                        anti-TB   Stop
                        therapy

            Repeat PPD   Start   Start
            at 12 weeks: preventive   preventive
            consider   therapy   therapy
            preventive
            therapy until
            then

*PPD = purified protein derivative.
†Members of the immediate family, close social contacts, or others who shared the
 same indoor environment with an infectious TB patient for substantial periods.

Figure 1. Estimating the likelihood of infection with Mycobacterium tuberculosis and preventive therapy
decision-making for contacts of infectious tuberculosis (TB) cases.

Contacts who are known or likely to be HIV infected, or markedly immunosuppressed for other reasons, should be evaluated for anergy at the time
of tuberculin skin testing (Figure 1) (16). Immunosuppressed persons who
have a prior positive tuberculin skin test may be at risk for reinfection with M.
tuberculosis; these persons should also be evaluated with a tuberculin skin test
and a test for anergy. Those who are not anergic can be further evaluated in the
same way as contacts who are not known or likely to be immunosuppressed.
Those who are anergic should be considered probably newly infected if they

are high-risk contacts or if there is evidence of TB contagion among other contacts with comparable exposure. (The latter suggests that the source case was an efficient transmitter.) These persons should be evaluated for preventive therapy, after active TB is excluded. In all situations, regardless of tuberculin skin-test results, a diagnostic evaluation should be performed if symptoms suggestive of active TB are present.

Estimating the Likelihood of Infection with Multidrug-Resistant M. tuberculosis Among Contacts Thought to Be Newly Infected

Contacts who are considered likely to be newly infected and who have had exposure to patients with infectious MDR-TB should be evaluated to assess the likelihood of infection with a multidrug-resistant strain of M. tuberculosis. Several factors should be considered in this assessment: (a) the infectiousness of the possible source MDR-TB case, (b) the closeness and intensity of the MDR-TB exposure, and (c) the contact's likelihood of exposure to persons with drug-susceptible TB (Table 1).

Table 1. Likelihood of Infection with Multidrug-Resistant Mycobacterium tuberculosis Among Contacts Thought to Be Newly Infected*

Infectiousness of the source MDR-TB[@] case	Closeness and intensity of MDR-TB exposure	Contact's risk of exposure to drug-susceptible TB	Estimated likelihood of infection with multidrug-resistant M. tuberculosis[&]
+	+	−	High
+	−	−	High-intermediate
−	+	−	High-intermediate
−	−	−	Intermediate
+	+	+	Intermediate
+	−	+	Low-intermediate
−	+	+	Low-intermediate
−	−	+	Low

Key: (+) = high; (−) = low.

*Anergic contacts should be considered likely to be newly infected if there is evidence of contagion among contacts with comparable exposure.

[@]MDR-TB = multidrug-resistant tuberculosis.

[&]Multidrug preventive therapy should be considered for persons in high, high-intermediate, and intermediate categories.

Infectiousness of the Source Case

TB patients who cough and have acid-fast bacillus (AFB) smear-positive sputum are substantially more infectious than those who do not cough and have AFB smear-negative sputum. Evidence of tuberculin skin-test conversions among contacts of the TB case is another measure of infectivity.

Closeness and Intensity of the MDR-TB Exposure

Any person who shared the air space with an MDR-TB patient for a relatively prolonged time (e.g., household member, hospital roommate) is at higher risk for infection than those with a brief exposure to an MDR-TB patient, such as a one-time hospital visitor. Exposure of any length in a small, enclosed, poorly ventilated area is more likely to result in transmission than exposure in a large, well-ventilated space. Exposure during cough-inducing procedures (e.g., bronchoscopy, endotracheal intubation, sputum induction, administration of aerosol therapy), which may greatly enhance TB transmission, is also more likely to result in infection.

Contact History

Persons exposed to several sources of M. tuberculosis, including infectious TB patients with drug-susceptible M. tuberculosis, are less likely to have been infected with a multidrug-resistant strain than are those whose only known exposure to TB was to an infectious MDR-TB case.

Estimating the Likelihood that Infected Persons Will Develop Active Tuberculosis

The most potent factor that increases the probability that a person infected with M. tuberculosis will develop active TB is immunodeficiency, such as that caused by coinfection with HIV (Table 2) (17, 18); thus, health-care providers should routinely offer counseling and voluntary HIV antibody testing to all patients known or likely to be infected with M. tuberculosis. Other immunocompromising conditions, including treatment with immunosuppressive medications, renal failure, and diabetes mellitus, also increase the risk for progression to active disease, but to a considerably lesser extent than HIV infection (9, 18). Recentness of infection also contributes to the risk of developing active TB. In immunocompetent persons, the risk of developing active TB is highest within the first 2 years after infection, after which the risk declines markedly (18). This is probably different for HIV-infected persons, who have a progressive decline in cell-mediated immunity and may remain at high

Table 2. Risk Factors for the Development of Active Tuberculosis Among Persons Infected with Mycobacterium tuberculosis

Risk factor	Estimated increased risk for tuberculosis compared with persons with no known risk factor
Acquired immunodeficiency syndrome	170.0
Human immunodeficiency virus infection	113.0
Other immunocompromising conditions*	3.6–16.0
Recentness of infection (<2 years)	15.0
Age of contact (≤5 years and ≥ years)	2.2–5.0

*For example, diabetes mellitus type I, renal failure, carcinoma of head or neck, iatrogenic immunosuppression.

risk for an indefinite period or may even have an increasing risk as the immunosuppression progresses. Finally, the age of the contact needs to be considered. Children ages less than or equal to 5 years and persons greater than or equal to 60 years both have high TB disease attack rates and shorter incubation periods (3, 19).

PREVENTIVE THERAPY CONSIDERATIONS FOR PERSONS LIKELY TO BE INFECTED WITH A MULTIDRUG-RESISTANT STRAIN OF MYCOBACTERIUM TUBERCULOSIS

Before any preventive therapy regimen is initiated, the diagnosis of clinically active TB must be excluded (14, 20). Patients on preventive therapy should be monitored carefully for adverse reactions to the medications, evidence of active TB, and adherence to therapy. Patients on preventive therapy should be thoroughly educated about symptoms of TB and the need for immediate medical evaluation if symptoms do occur. As much as possible, alternative multidrug preventive therapy regimens should be selected, administered, and evaluated in a consistent and systematic way. All patients receiving one of these regimens should be on directly observed therapy. Clinicians who are not familiar with the management of patients with MDR-TB or those infected with multidrug-resistant organisms should seek expert consultation.

Considerations in Evaluating M. tuberculosis Isolates for Drug Susceptibility

Drug susceptibility test results of the M. tuberculosis isolate of the presumed source case should be considered in the selection of the drugs to be included in the preventive therapy regimen. The proportion method is commonly used for determining drug susceptibility of M. tuberculosis isolates (21). The results of this method of testing are reported to the clinician as the percentage of the total bacterial population resistant to a given drug, which is defined by the amount of growth on a drug-containing medium as compared with growth on a drug-free control medium. When greater than or equal to 1% of the bacillary population becomes resistant to the critical concentration of a drug, the M. tuberculosis isolate is considered resistant to that drug. The critical concentration of a drug is the concentration that inhibits the growth of most cells in wild strains of M. tuberculosis. One critical concentration is used for the susceptibility testing of most drugs; INH susceptibility testing is usually done by using two different drug concentrations (0.2 μg/mL and 1.0 μg/mL). Drug susceptibility testing of M. tuberculosis isolates is also possible through the use of radiometric techniques such as the BACTEC® system. Results of this method identify whether M. tuberculosis isolates are susceptible or resistant to the drugs tested. This method can reduce the time of identifying drug-resistant microorganisms from the 7 weeks needed for testing in solid media (proportion method) to 3 weeks. However, only five of the antituberculosis drugs (INH, RIF, PZA, EMB, and SM) are commercially available at this time for use in the BACTEC® system. Additional antibiotics may be tested with BACTEC® but require that dilutions be prepared by the laboratory.

General Approach to Selecting Drug Regimens for Preventive Therapy Candidates

Newly infected contacts who are thought to have a low to low-intermediate likelihood of infection with multidrug-resistant M. tuberculosis (Table 1) should be managed according to standard recommendations for infected contacts of non-MDR-TB patients (Figure 2) (10). Infected contacts who are thought to have an intermediate to high likelihood of being infected with a multidrug-resistant strain of M. tuberculosis need to be further categorized according to their risk of developing active TB. Those at high risk for disease include persons who are HIV infected, persons with risk factors for HIV infection who have unknown HIV status, and persons with other conditions known to cause severe immunosuppression. Preventive therapy regimens with at least two antituberculosis drugs should be strongly considered for persons likely to be infected with multidrug-resistant

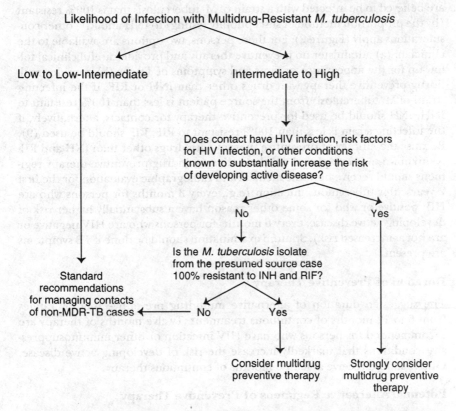

HIV = human immunodeficiency virus; INH = isoniazid; RIF = rifampin; MDR-TB = multidrug-resistant tuberculosis.

Figure 2. Approach to selecting drug regimens for preventive therapy candidates by likelihood of infection with multidrug-resistant Mycobacterium tuberculosis and by likelihood that persons will develop active tuberculosis.

M. tuberculosis who have a high risk of developing active disease (Figure 2). This suggestion is based on considerations of the extraordinarily high likelihood of progression to clinically active TB, especially in persons with advanced HIV disease; the severe consequences of clinically active MDR-TB in persons with HIV infection; and the possibility that MDR-TB may be more amenable to cure if treated when the bacterial burden is low rather than when the disease becomes clinically apparent and the bacterial burden is substantially higher. No clinical data exist on the risks and benefits of regimens that do not include INH or RIF; however, preventive therapy with more than one drug is recommended since efficacy of preventive monotherapy with alternative drugs has not been demonstrated.

For contacts who are not HIV infected, who do not have risk factors for HIV infection with unknown HIV status, who do not have another condition that substantially increases the likelihood of progression to active TB, and who are believed to be infected with a strain of M. tuberculosis that is 100% resistant (by the proportion method of susceptibility testing) to INH and RIF, other considerations apply (Figure 2). For these persons, two options are available to the clinician: (a) administer no preventive therapy and provide careful clinical follow-up for the appearance of signs and symptoms of TB, or (b) consider multidrug preventive therapy with drugs other than INH or RIF. If the infecting strain of M. tuberculosis from the source patient is less than 100% resistant to INH, INH should be used for preventive therapy for contacts; alternatively, if the infecting strain is less than 100% resistant to RIF, RIF should be used (9). Because the efficacy of preventive therapy with drugs other than INH and RIF is unknown, persons placed on alternative multidrug preventive therapy regimens should receive periodic medical and radiographic evaluation for the first 2 years after tuberculous infection (e.g., every 3 months for persons who are HIV positive or who for some other reason have a substantially higher risk of developing active disease; every 6 months for persons who are HIV negative or are not at increased risk). Sputum examination should be done if TB symptoms are present.

Duration of Preventive Therapy

The suggested duration of alternative multidrug preventive therapy ranges from 6 to 12 months of continuous treatment. Twelve months of therapy are recommended for persons who have HIV infection or other immunosuppressive conditions that markedly increase the risk of developing active disease. Others should receive at least 6 months of continuous therapy.

Potential Alternative Regimens of Preventive Therapy

The alternative regimens of preventive therapy suggested in this document do not represent approval from the Food and Drug Administration (FDA) or approved labeling for the particular products or indications in question. In the United States, the only drug approved by the FDA for TB preventive therapy is INH. Alternative drugs should be used for preventive therapy only when susceptibility to the drugs has been demonstrated by testing the M. tuberculosis isolate of the presumed source case.

One potential alternative preventive therapy regimen is a combination of PZA and EMB at the recommended dose for the therapy of TB (PZA, daily oral dose 25–30 mg/kg; EMB, daily oral dose 15–25 mg/kg) (9). Preventive therapy studies in a mouse model suggest that PZA may enhance the efficacy of a bactericidal drug, since a PZA-RIF combination was more effective than RIF alone (22). Both PZA and EMB have proved to be effective and well tolerated for the treatment of TB. EMB at the 15-mg/kg dose is considered bacteriostatic, and in vitro studies show that EMB may be bactericidal at the 25-mg/kg dose (23). If EMB is used at the higher dosage as part of a preventive therapy regimen, the potential for higher rates of toxicity must be recognized and carefully monitored. Because of the risk of retrobulbar neuritis, EMB should be used with caution in children who are too young for routine testing of visual acuity.

Another possible alternative preventive therapy regimen is PZA plus a fluoroquinolone with reported in vitro activity against M. tuberculosis. A recent report indicates that ofloxacin and ciprofloxacin have similar antimycobacterial potencies in vitro (24). Suggested doses for these agents include 400 mg twice a day of ofloxacin and 750 mg twice a day of ciprofloxacin. Sparfloxacin, another quinolone that has shown good in vitro activity against M. tuberculosis, is under investigation (25). However, to date, sparfloxacin is not licensed in the United States for any indication and would be available only under an investigational new drug (IND) agreement. For all quinolones, in vivo evidence of efficacy against M. tuberculosis is very limited. Short-term administration of quinolones is generally well tolerated, but therapy of 6–12 months' duration has not been studied. Arthropathy has been noted in experiments with immature animals (26); therefore, quinolones should be used in a preventive therapy regimen for children or pregnant females only if the potential benefits justify the potential side effects. Aminoglycosides—such as SM, KM, and amikacin—or the polypeptide antibiotic capreomycin might also be considered for inclusion in an alternative preventive therapy regimen. These drugs are at least partially bactericidal, but they have the disadvantage of requiring injection, creating problems both with logistics and with patient acceptability. The most common serious adverse effects of these drugs are ototoxicity and nephrotoxicity.

Para-aminosalicylic acid, ethionamide, and cycloserine are the other antituberculosis drugs sometimes used in the United States. None of these drugs is recommended for use as preventive therapy because of their high frequency of side effects and relatively low efficacy against M. tuberculosis.

REFERENCES: AS NUMBERED IN ORIGINAL PUBLICATION

3. Stead WW, To T, Harrison RW, Abraham JH. Benefit-risk considerations in preventive treatment for tuberculosis in elderly persons. Ann Intern Med 1987;107:843–845.
4. Styblo K. Epidemiology of tuberculosis. In: Broekmans JS, ed. Selected papers, vol. 24. The Hague, the Netherlands: Royal Netherlands Tuberculosis Association, 1991:1–136.
5. Zeidberg LD, Gass RS, Dillon A, et al. The Williamson County tuberculosis study. A twenty-four-year epidemiologic study. Am Rev Respir Dis 1963;87:1–88.
6. Di Perri G, Cruciani M, Danzi MC, et al. Nosocomial epidemic of active tuberculosis among HIV-infected patients. Lancet 1989;2:1502–1504.

7. CDC. Tuberculosis outbreak among persons in a residential facility for HIV-infected persons—San Francisco. MMWR 1991;40(38):649–652.
8. Daley CL, Small PM, Schecter GF, et al. An outbreak of tuberculosis with accelerated progression among persons infected with the human immunodeficiency virus. An analysis using restriction-fragment-length polymorphisms. N Engl J Med 1992;326:231–235.
9. American Thoracic Society/CDC. Treatment of tuberculosis and tuberculosis infection in adults and children. Am Rev Respir Dis 1986;134:355–363.
10. CDC. The use of preventive therapy for tuberculous infection in the United States: recommendations of the Advisory Committee for Elimination of Tuberculosis. MMWR 1990;39(RR-8):9–12.
11. International Union Against Tuberculosis Committee on Prophylaxis. Efficacy of various durations of isoniazid preventive therapy for tuberculosis: five years of follow-up in the IUAT trial. Bull WHO 1982;60:555–564.
12. Ferebee SH. Controlled chemoprophylaxis trials in tuberculosis. A general review. Adv Tuberc Res 1970;17:28–106.
13. Wadhawan D, Hira S, Mwansa N, Tembo G, Perine P. Preventive tuberculosis chemotherapy with isoniazid among persons infected with human immunodeficiency virus [Abstract W.B. 2261]. In: Proceedings of the Seventh International Conference on AIDS, Florence, Italy, June 16–21, 1991.
14. American Thoracic Society/CDC. Control of tuberculosis. Am Rev Respir Dis 1983;128:336–342.
15. American Thoracic Society/CDC. Diagnostic standards and classification of tuberculosis. Am Rev Respir Dis 1990;142:725–735.
16. CDC. Purified protein derivative (PPD)-tuberculin anergy and HIV infection: guidelines for anergy testing and management of anergic persons at risk of tuberculosis. MMWR 1991;40(RR-5):27–33.
17. Selwyn PA, Hartel D, Lewis VA, et al. A prospective study of the risk of tuberculosis among intravenous drug users with human immunodeficiency virus infection. N Engl J Med 1989;320:545–550.
18. Rieder HL, Cauthen GM, Comstock GW, Snider DE Jr. Epidemiology of tuberculosis in the United States. Epidemiol Rev 1989;11:79–98.
19. Comstock GW, Livesay VT, Woolpert SF. The prognosis of a positive tuberculin reaction in childhood and adolescence. Am J Epidemiol 1974;99:131–138.
20. CDC. Tuberculosis and human immunodeficiency virus infection: recommendations of the Advisory Committee for the Elimination of Tuberculosis. MMWR 1989;38(17):236–250.
21. Kent PT, Kubica GP. Public health mycobacteriology. A guide for the level III laboratory. Atlanta: CDC, 1985.
22. Lecoeur HF, Truffot-Pernot C, Grosset JH. Experimental short-course preventive therapy of tuberculosis with rifampin and pyrazinamide. Am Rev Respir Dis 1989;140:1189–1193.
23. Crowle AJ, Sbarbaro JA, Judson FN, May MH. The effect of ethambutol on tubercle bacilli within cultured human macrophages. Am Rev Respir Dis 1985;132:742–745.
24. Gorzynski EA, Gutman SI, Allen W. Comparative antimycobacterial activities of difloxacin, temafloxacin, enoxacin, pefloxacin, reference fluoroquinolones, and a new macrolide, clarithromycin. Antimicrob Agents Chemother 1989;33:591–592.
25. Rastogi N, Goh KS. In vitro activity of the new difluorinated quinolone sparfloxacin (AT-4140) against Mycobacterium tuberculosis compared with activities of ofloxacin and ciprofloxacin. Antimicrob Agents Chemother 1991;35:1933–1935.
26. Physicians' Desk Reference, 46th ed. Montvale, NJ: Medical Economics Data, 1992:1653–1654.

The Mantoux Tuberculin Skin Test

Original Citation: Centers for Disease Control and Prevention. Wall Poster.

- Give 0.1 cc of 5 Tuberculin Units PPD intradermally.
- All tests should be read between 48–72 hours. If more than 72 hours has elapsed and there is not an easily palpable positive reaction, repeat the test on the other arm and read at 48–72 hours.
- Measure induration—not erythema. Measure and report results in millimeters of induration.
- All persons with positive reactions should be evaluated for preventive therapy, once TB disease has been ruled out.

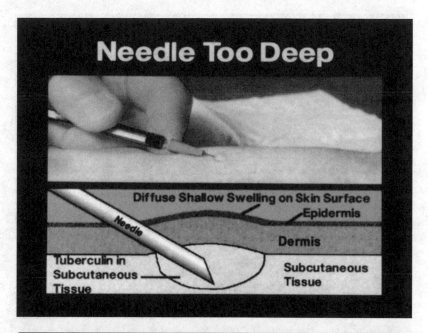

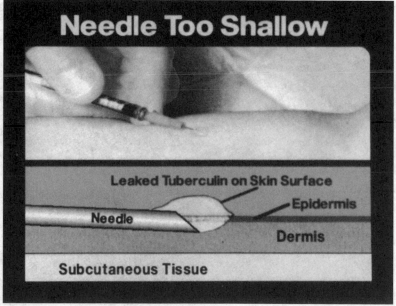

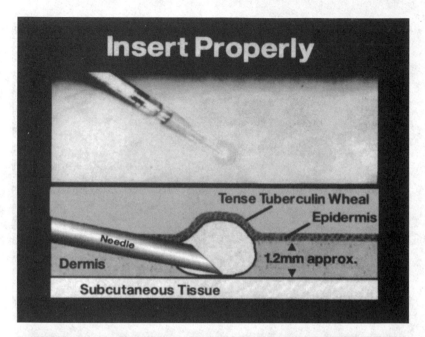

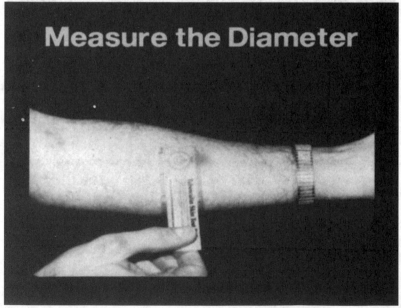

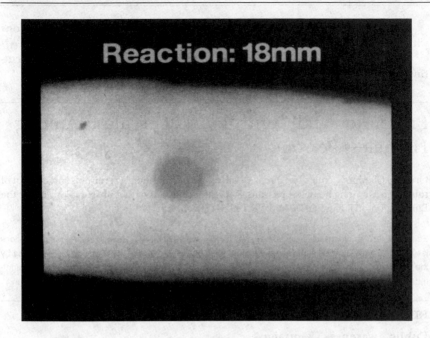

Five or more millimeters induration is considered positive for highest risk groups, such as:

- Persons with HIV infection;
- Persons who have had close contact with an infectious tuberculosis case;
- Persons who have chest radiographs consistent with old, healed tuberculosis;
- Intravenous drug users whose HIV status is unknown.

Ten or more millimeters induration is considered positive for other high risk groups, such as:

- Foreign-born persons from high prevalence areas (such as Asia, Africa, and Latin America);
- Intravenous drug users known to be HIV seronegative;
- Medically-underserved low income populations, including high-risk racial or ethnic minority populations (especially blacks, Hispanics, and Native Americans);
- Residents of long-term care facilities (such as correctional institutions, nursing homes, mental institutions);
- Persons with medical conditions which have been reported to increase the risk of tuberculosis such as silicosis, being ten percent or more below ideal body weight, chronic renal failure, diabetes mellitus, high dose corticosteroid and other immunosuppressive therapy, some hematologic disorders (such as leukemias and lymphomas), and other malignancies;
- Locally identified high risk populations;
- Children who are in one of the high risk groups listed above; and
- Health-care workers who provide services to any of the high risk groups.

Fifteen or more millimeters induration is considered positive for persons with no risk factors for tuberculosis.

Negative Reactions—For each of the categories, reactions below the cutting point are considered negative.

Prevention and Control of Tuberculosis Among Homeless Persons

Original Citation: Centers for Disease Control and Prevention. Prevention and control of tuberculosis among homeless persons. Recommendations of the Advisory Council for the Elimination of Tuberculosis. MMWR 1992;41(RR-5):1.

Editor's Note: The information included here was based on a 1992 MMWR Reports and Recommendations issue (Vol. 41;RR-5) which summarizes recommendations on prevention of TB among the homeless by the Advisory Council for the Elimination of Tuberculosis (ACET). The original text describes the magnitude and extent of tuberculosis in minority populations and the homeless.

RECOMMENDATIONS

Public Awareness Campaigns

Individuals in at-risk population groups, including local leaders, are often unaware of the extent of the TB problem in their communities and the potential for preventing infection. Public awareness campaigns can provide essential information.

1. A public awareness campaign should be initiated by national, state, and local organizations to alert communities at high risk for TB about the increasing TB threat and to the potential for eliminating the disease.
2. At the national level, this campaign should be designed and supported by CDC, the American Lung Association/American Thoracic Society (ALA/ATS), the American Public Health Association, and other national organizations that support or provide services to high-risk population groups.
3. At the state and local levels, health departments should collect and analyze epidemiologic data to identify local communities and population groups with high incidences so that TB prevention activities and public awareness campaigns can be appropriately directed. Local public awareness campaigns should be focused toward community members, health-care providers, and religious, social, economic, and other influential organizations. Awareness campaigns should be designed and supported by health departments and ALA/ATS affiliates working with recognized community leaders, organizations, and health-care providers.
4. The media (print, radio, and television) should be effectively utilized to disseminate information about TB prevention and related elimination efforts:
   a. Local community, minority, and ethnic media (newspapers, magazines, newsletters, radio, and television) should deliver the information to the general public, high-risk communities, and at-risk population groups.
   b. Messages should be disseminated through national and community-based organizations such as churches and forums focused on economic, medical, political, and social activities.
5. National and local TB awareness programs should be supported by the availability of convenient and high-quality TB screening, prevention, and treatment services.

Training and Education of Public and Private Health-Care Providers

Empowerment of at-risk groups in the community is a crucial element in TB control. This step begins with the public awareness campaigns described above because it is vitally important for members of at-risk populations to understand TB; its impact on the community; how it is diagnosed, treated, and prevented; and what services are available. These populations also should be able to influence the TB programs directed toward their communities.

1. Health departments should ensure that the sociodemographic composition of the communities being served is represented in the composition of the TB-control-program staff. The staff should be culturally and linguistically competent and sensitive to the populations being served.
2. All health department and other health-care staff who provide TB services should receive training to improve interpersonal skills needed to encourage open and effective communication with members of high-risk communities and groups. Continuous efforts must be made to establish and maintain the rapport needed to relate effectively to the communities being served and to the public and private health-care providers serving those communities.
3. Health-care providers serving at-risk areas should be given TB training on recommended procedures for examining, diagnosing, and treating TB cases, suspected cases, and contacts. The training should include information on procedures for rapidly reporting confirmed and suspected TB cases.

Coalition Building

Major progress toward elimination can be achieved by focusing TB screening and preventive therapy programs toward groups of persons at high risk of becoming infected or developing disease. Public and private health-care providers serving many at-risk clients in the community may not fully apply recommended prevention methods. Some at-risk population groups lack access to medical care, and special efforts are often required to provide them with needed services. Coalitions composed of representatives from groups and communities at increased risk of TB can assist in developing and implementing plans to improve access to health care.

1. Health departments should expand their efforts to reach community groups at high risk of TB and health-care providers serving these groups.
2. Decision makers, other key people, and agencies within at-risk communities should be identified and involved in TB elimination planning and implementation activities.
3. Coalitions should be established to advise health departments and health-care providers on how to design and carry out intensified community TB prevention and control efforts. These groups should be composed of representatives from affected communities, community-based organizations, health departments, private and public health-care providers, and the media serving high-risk populations and communities. These coalitions should be responsible for defining the problems and identifying obstacles related to excessive rates of TB in the at-risk communities; establishing short- and long-term goals; setting realistic and time-phased objectives; establishing priorities; and developing, implementing, and evaluating strategies. They should also analyze their communities to determine how strategies should be implemented and how to motivate and mobilize community members.
4. Coalitions should help identify and obtain resources needed by community programs and people serving the at-risk areas.
5. Credit for accomplishments should be given to members of the coalitions and the at-risk communities involved in these efforts.

Screening and Prevention

Screening at-risk populations for TB and tuberculous infection and providing appropriate treatment are crucial for achieving TB elimination. Screening is done to identify persons in need of preventive therapy (2). Responsibility for conducting screening will vary. For some groups, the local health department and health-care providers should assume responsibility for conducting the screening. For others, community-based organizations may conduct the screening with training and evaluation assistance from the health department.

1. Health departments should assess the prevalence, incidence, and sociodemographic characteristics of cases of TB and infected persons in their jurisdictions to identify high-risk areas in their communities. On the basis of this assessment, health departments should work with community-based organizations and health-care providers serving those communities to plan and initiate tuberculin screening and preventive therapy programs specifically adjusted to each community's at-risk groups.
2. Planning, developing, and implementing screening programs should be a joint effort coordinated among the local health department, public and private community organizations, and health-care providers serving the affected community. Medicaid, Medicare, and private health-care funds should be sought to support screening and preventive treatment programs.
3. When possible, initiatives to systematically screen for TB should be established in specific high-risk settings such as correctional institutions, long-term-care facilities, nursing homes, drug treatment centers, in- and outpatient hospital facilities, and homeless shelters (2).

Case Reporting

Early reporting of TB is essential so that contacts can be examined for evidence of infection and disease and can be given appropriate therapy as quickly as possible.

1. Health departments should inform health-care providers serving at-risk groups and communities about the importance of early TB case reporting and about the services offered by the health departments. Health-care providers should become familiar with the TB case reporting system used in their particular areas.
2. Early TB case reporting can be encouraged by offering incentives, such as free laboratory services, to health-care providers and free antituberculosis drugs to their patients.
3. To facilitate TB case reporting for health-care providers, health departments should consider using facsimile machines or telephone-answering machines to receive reports. Large laboratories and health-care facilities should consider using computer-to-computer reporting systems.
4. All private physicians, public and private hospitals, clinics, medical/health centers, alcohol/drug treatment centers, nursing homes, laboratories, and correctional facilities should notify appropriate health departments about confirmed and suspected TB cases as quickly as possible. The development of a reporting system that includes all pharmacies that dispense antituberculosis drugs should also be considered.

Treatment and Adherence

The availability of TB health-care services and related transportation are frequently a problem in high-incidence and socioeconomically disadvantaged areas. Attracting competent health-care staff in some of these areas is sometimes a major obstacle. In addition, it is often difficult to establish and maintain rapport needed for effective diagnosis, treatment, and prophylaxis of patients with TB in at-risk areas and population groups. For many patients, a variety of health and socioeconomic-related problems (e.g., unemployment, low income, homelessness, lack of or limited access to health care, language barriers, and alcohol and drug abuse) may limit their ability to adhere to recommendations for treatment or to obtain other needed medical care. Much of their time and effort is understandably devoted to meeting day-to-day economic and survival needs, such as food, shelter, clothing, and safety. Nonadherence is a serious problem that can lead to treatment failure, drug resistance, continuing transmission of infection, increasing disability, and death (3). These are challenges that should be met with new and innovative strategies.

1. Quality TB treatment services and related transportation should be available at no cost to patients.
2. CDC should recruit, train, and assign a cadre of TB physicians, nurses, social workers, and public health advisors to work in high-incidence areas where TB is increasing and where it is extremely difficult to attract and retain qualified staff. The specific objective for these assignments should be to stabilize and begin to reduce the case rates within 3 years of assignment. As target rates are achieved in these areas, reassignment to other areas can be made.
3. Special treatment-housing centers should be established in cities with large numbers of persons at risk of TB who are homeless. These centers should provide continuous shelter, food, and treatment for homeless persons diagnosed with TB for the duration of their prescribed therapy regimen. The shelter and food act as incentives for patients to remain compliant with treatment. When patients complete their prescribed regimens or do not comply with therapy, they can be discharged from the centers and new patients admitted. The effectiveness of this concept has been demonstrated by existing programs in New York City and Denver. The resources necessary to establish similar centers might be shared through agreements between federal agencies (e.g., U.S. Department of Housing and Urban Development, Health Resources and Services Administration, or CDC), state/local agencies, or private organizations. Many identified at-risk areas contain properties that are federally owned and are suitable for conversion to treatment-housing centers.
4. Specific strategies for improving adherence to treatment regimens by individual patients or groups of patients should be established for each identified high-risk community and population group. These strategies should be broad-based and reflect an understanding of the difficulties associated with behavioral change and be sensitive and responsive to the patients' beliefs, cultures, and environments. This allows for the identification and removal of specific barriers to adherence.
5. Health-care providers of TB services should take the time to explain to patients, in simple language that is culturally and linguistically appropriate, the specific adherence behaviors expected. Patients must first know what is expected of them before they can comply.
6. Patient education and appointment reminders must be culturally sensitive and linguistically appropriate and should be used to effectively influence the cooperation of patients seeking TB services. Whenever possible, patients should be given reminders for pending appointments in person or by telephone. This removes any doubt about whether the patients received the messages. Patients also can be counseled over the telephone, thereby helping them overcome scheduling, transportation, or other problems that interfere with adherence.
7. Directly observed therapy should be considered for all TB patients.
8. Trained nurses or community outreach workers with the same cultural and linguistic background as the patients should help design treatment plans, administer directly observed therapy, and assist patients and health-care providers to identify and overcome obstacles to adherence.
9. Outreach workers should act as extensions of the clinician and nurse by locating patients, reminding them of appointments, resolving basic problems, encouraging adherence, delivering medication, observing its ingestion, and identifying, tracing, and examining contacts. They should also serve as a liaison between the clinic staff and the patient by help-

ing to bridge cultural and linguistic gaps and by educating patients. Such employees can greatly enhance TB control efforts among at-risk populations.

10. Additional federal, state, local, and private resources will be required to increase the number of outreach workers. These outreach workers should be recruited and hired from the areas and communities being identified for service. They should have a knowledge of and be sensitive to the culture and language of the population to be served.

REFERENCES: AS NUMBERED IN ORIGINAL PUBLICATION

2. Advisory Committee for the Elimination of Tuberculosis. Screening for tuberculosis and tuberculous infection in high-risk populations and the use of preventive therapy for tuberculous infection in the United States. MMWR 1990;39(No. RR-8):(inclusive page numbers).

3. Snider DE, Hutton MD. Improving patient compliance in tuberculosis treatment programs. Atlanta: CDC, revised February 1989.

SUBTOPIC / TREATMENT

Treatment of Tuberculosis and Tuberculosis Infection in Adults and Children*

Original Citation: American Thoracic Society. Treatment of tuberculosis and tuberculosis infection in adults and children. Am J Resp Crit Care Med 1994;149:1359–1374.

Editor's Note: The information included here, based on a Joint Statement of CDC and the American Thoracic Society endorsed by the American Academy of Pediatrics printed in a 1994 issue of the American Journal of Respiratory and Critical Medicine, gives guidance on the treatment of tuberculosis and tuberculosis infection in adults and children. The original document includes extensive information on current drugs in use and potentially effective drugs that have not been widely used in the therapy of tuberculosis. Clinicians are urged to review this complete source of information thoroughly. In addition, the original document briefly describes the background for the development of these guidelines and the members of the Committee who prepared the statement. Clinicians who treat tuberculosis should have a copy of the Core Curriculum. Although the curriculum is not included in this book due to space limitations, it is available on the CD-ROM. The document includes the Epidemiology of Tuberculosis in the United States, transmission and pathogenesis, screening, preventive therapy, diagnosis and treatment of disease, infection control, community tuberculosis control, and BCG vaccination.

SUMMARY

Treatment of Tuberculosis

1. A 6-mo regimen consisting of isoniazid, rifampin, and pyrazinamide given for 2 mo followed by isoniazid and rifampin for 4 mo is the preferred treat-

---

*This Statement is one of a series of four Statements on diagnosis, treatment, and control of tuberculosis. For information on diagnostic methods, refer to (a) Diagnostic standards and classification of tuberculosis. Am Rev Respir Dis 1990;142:725–735; and (b) The tuberculin skin test. Am Rev Respir Dis 1981;124:356–363. For information on screening for tuberculosis, management of contacts, and organization of control programs, refer to (c) Control of tuberculosis. Am Rev Respir Dis 1992;146:1623–1633.

ment for patients with fully susceptible organisms who adhere to treatment. Ethambutol (or streptomycin in children too young to be monitored for visual acuity) should be included in the initial regimen until the results of drug susceptibility studies are available, unless there is little possibility of drug resistance (i.e., there is less than 4% primary resistance to isoniazid in the community, and the patient has had no previous treatment with antituberculosis medications, is not from a country with a high prevalence of drug resistance, and has no known exposure to a drug-resistant case). This four-drug, 6-mo regimen is effective even when the infecting organism is resistant to INH. This recommendation applies to both HIV-infected and uninfected persons. However, in the presence of HIV infection it is critically important to assess the clinical and bacteriologic response. If there is evidence of a slow or suboptimal response, therapy should be prolonged as judged on a case by case basis.

2. Alternatively, a 9-mo regimen of isoniazid and rifampin is acceptable for persons who cannot or should not take pyrazinamide. Ethambutol (or streptomycin in children too young to be monitored for visual acuity) should also be included until the results of drug susceptibility studies are available, unless there is little possibility of drug resistance (see Section 1 above). If INH resistance is demonstrated, rifampin and ethambutol should be continued for a minimum of 12 mo.

3. Consideration should be given to treating all patients with directly observed therapy (DOT).

4. Multiple-drug-resistant tuberculosis (i.e., resistance to at least isoniazid and rifampin) presents difficult treatment problems. Treatment must be individualized and based on susceptibility studies. In such cases, consultation with an expert in tuberculosis is recommended.

5. Children should be managed in essentially the same ways as adults using appropriately adjusted doses of the drugs. This document addresses specific important differences between the management of adults and children.

6. Extrapulmonary tuberculosis should be managed according to the principles and with the drug regimens outlined for pulmonary tuberculosis, except for children who have miliary tuberculosis, bone/joint tuberculosis, or tuberculous meningitis who should receive a minimum of 12 mo of therapy.

7. A 4-mo regimen of isoniazid and rifampin is acceptable therapy for adults who have active tuberculosis and who are sputum-smear and culture negative, if there is little possibility of drug resistance (see Section 1 above).

8. The major determinant of the outcome of treatment is patient adherence to the drug regimen. Careful attention should be paid to measures designed to foster adherence and to ensure that patients take the drugs as prescribed. The use of fixed drug combinations may enhance patient adherence and may reduce the risk of inappropriate monotherapy, and it may prevent the development of secondary drug resistance. For this reason, the use of such fixed drug combinations is strongly encouraged in adults. Virtually all the treatment regimens may be given intermittently if directly observed, thus assuring adherence.

Treatment of Tuberculosis Infection

1. Preventive therapy with isoniazid given for 6 to 12 mo is effective in decreasing the risk of future tuberculosis in adults and children with tuber-

culosis infection demonstrated by a positive tuberculin skin test reaction. The appropriate criterion for defining a positive skin test reaction depends on the population being tested. For adults and children with HIV infection, close contacts of infectious cases, and those with fibrotic lesions on chest radiograph, a reaction of greater than or equal to 5 mm is considered positive. For other at-risk adults and children, including infants and children younger than 4 yr of age, a reaction of greater than or equal to 10 mm is positive. Persons who are not likely to be infected with Mycobacterium tuberculosis should generally not be skin tested. If a skin test is performed on a person without a defined risk factor for tuberculosis infection, greater than or equal to 15 mm is positive.

2. Persons with a positive skin test and any of the following risk factors should be considered for preventive therapy regardless of age: persons with HIV infection; persons at risk for HIV infection with unknown HIV status; close contacts of sputum-positive persons with newly diagnosed infectious tuberculosis; newly infected persons (recent skin test converters); and persons with medical conditions reported to increase the risk of tuberculosis (i.e., diabetes mellitus, adrenocorticosteroid therapy and other immunosuppressive therapy, intravenous drug users, hematologic and reticuloendothelial malignancies, end-stage renal disease, and clinical conditions associated with rapid weight loss or chronic undernutrition). In some circumstances persons with negative skin tests should also be considered for preventive therapy. These include children who are close contacts of infectious cases and anergic HIV-infected adults at increased risk of tuberculosis. Tuberculin-positive adults with abnormal chest films that show fibrotic lesions likely representing old healed tuberculosis and adults with silicosis should usually receive 4-mo multidrug chemotherapy although 12 mo of isoniazid preventive therapy is an acceptable alternative. Persons who are known to be HIV-infected and who are contacts of patients with infectious tuberculosis should be carefully evaluated for evidence of tuberculosis. If there are no findings suggestive of current tuberculosis, preventive therapy with isoniazid should be given. Because HIV-infected contacts are not managed in the same way as those who are not HIV-infected, HIV testing is recommended if there are known or suspected risk factors for acquisition of HIV infection.

3. In the absence of any of the above risk factors, persons younger than 35 yr of age with a positive skin test in the following high incidence groups should also be considered for preventive therapy: foreign-born persons from high-prevalence countries; medically underserved low-income persons from high-prevalence populations (especially blacks, Hispanics, and Native Americans); and residents of facilities for long-term care (e.g., correctional institutions, nursing homes, and mental institutions).

4. Twelve months of preventive therapy is recommended for adults and children with HIV infection and other conditions associated with immunosuppression. Persons without HIV infection should receive at least 6 mo of preventive therapy. The American Academy of Pediatrics recommends that children receive 9 mo of therapy.

5. In patients who have positive tuberculin skin test and either silicosis or a chest radiograph demonstrating old fibrotic lesions, and who have no evidence of active tuberculosis, acceptable regimens include: (a) 4 mo of iso-

niazid plus rifampin, or (b) 12 mo of isoniazid, providing that infection with drug-resistant organisms is judged to be unlikely.

6. In persons younger than 35 yr of age, routine monitoring for adverse effects of isoniazid should consist of a monthly symptom review. For persons 35 yr of age and older, hepatic enzymes should be measured prior to starting isoniazid and monitored monthly throughout treatment, in addition to monthly symptom reviews. Other factors associated with an increased risk of hepatitis include daily use of alcohol, chronic liver disease, and injection drug use. There is also evidence to suggest that postpubertal black and Hispanic women are at greater risk for hepatitis. Certain medications taken concurrently with isoniazid may increase the risk of hepatitis or drug interactions. More careful monitoring should be considered in these groups, possibly including more frequent laboratory monitoring.

7. Persons who are presumed to be infected with isoniazid-resistant organisms should be treated with rifampin rather than with isoniazid.

8. As with treatment of tuberculosis, the key to success of preventive therapy is patient adherence to the prescribed regimen. Although not evaluated in clinical studies, directly observed, twice-weekly preventive therapy may be used for at-risk adults and children who cannot or will not reliably self-administer therapy.

TREATMENT OF TUBERCULOSIS

In the years since the advent of antituberculosis chemotherapy, controlled clinical trials have yielded three basic principles upon which recommendations for treatment are based: (a) regimens for treatment of disease must contain multiple drugs to which the organisms are susceptible, (b) the drugs must be taken regularly, and (c) drug therapy must continue for a sufficient period of time. The aim of treatment should be to provide the safest and most effective therapy in the shortest period of time (3). There are a large number of possible combinations of drugs and rhythms of administration. But the initial phase of treatment is crucial for preventing emerging drug resistance and determining the ultimate outcome of the regimen. Despite considerable price variation from time to time and place to place, short-course regimens rely heavily on generally expensive drugs; however, these regimens are probably more cost effective than cheaper regimens, and drug cost should not preclude access to effective and appropriate treatment. Utilization of resources and the potential for adverse reactions are also considerations in selecting a treatment regimen.

Any regimen is irrelevant if drugs do not enter the patient's body. Promoting and monitoring adherence to the drug regimen are essential for treatment to be successful. A variety of techniques have been developed to assist in identifying the nonadherent patient. All patients should be asked routinely about their adherence with medication taking, and sporadic urine tests and pill counts may be used to monitor drug ingestion. Record systems for clinic appointments and drug pickups are very important to identify persons who fail to return for follow-up visits. An effective communication system is also needed to ensure that failure to keep appointments comes to the attention of the responsible public health officials. To improve adherence a number of modifications in the organization of treatment have been tried with varying degrees of success. These include setting clinic hours and locations to suit the patients' needs and giving directly observed treatment in the clinic, home, workplace, or other location. The offering of incentives and enablers, such as food, carfare money, babysitting services, or small gifts, may improve adherence by facilitating the patients' medication-taking and appointment-keeping. Tuberculosis control depends on more than just the science of chemotherapy; chemotherapy can be successful only within the framework of the overall clinical and social management of patients and their contacts. The ultimate elimination of tuberculosis requires an organized and smoothly functioning network of primary and referral services based on cooperation between clinicians and public health officials, between health care facilities and community outreach programs, and between the private and public sectors of medical care.

Initial Treatment Regimens (see also Table 1)

A large number of studies performed during the past 45 yr have provided specific information concerning the use of combinations of antituberculosis agents. Several important generalizations can be made from these studies.

1. Isoniazid possesses the best combination of effectiveness, low frequency side effects, and cost of any of the antituberculosis agents and thus should be used for the duration of whatever regimen is used unless there are contraindications or the organisms are resistant to the drug.
2. Despite some scattered reports of good results with 4-mo regimens, in general, relapse rates with regimens of such short duration are unacceptably high. An exception is the adult who, after careful evaluation, is found to have sputum-culture-negative pulmonary tuberculosis. In such adults, 4-mo regimens have a high rate of success.
3. For regimens 6 mo in duration, rifampin and isoniazid are essential for the total duration of therapy.
4. Pyrazinamide, given in the initial phase, improves the efficacy of regimens of less than 9 mo duration.
5. In the doses usually given, substituting ethambutol or streptomycin for pyrazinamide in the initial phase decreases the effectiveness of a regimen.
6. There is good evidence that intermittent administration of appropriately adjusted doses of the drugs after an initial daily phase of treatment as short as 2 wk produces results equal to those of daily administration. Regimens of four drugs given three times weekly throughout the course of treatment give equally good results in adults. Although there are no data available for three times weekly regimens in children, experience with other intermittent regimens suggests that they would be equally efficacious in children.

The above treatment guidelines apply only when the disease is caused by organisms that are susceptible to the standard antituberculosis agents. Rates of initial resistance to antituberculosis drugs have remained low (< 4% to isoniazid) in some parts of the United States.

Outbreaks of disease caused by multiple drug-resistant organisms have been reported with increasing frequency (24–26). In these outbreaks the organisms isolated have been resistant at least to isoniazid and rifampin and fre-

Table 1. Regimen Options for the Preferred Initial Treatment of Children and Adults*

Option 1	Option 2	Option 3
Administer daily isoniazid, rifampin, and pyrazinamide for 8 wk followed by 16 wk of isoniazid and rifampin daily or 2–3 times/wk.[†] In areas where the isoniazid resistance rate is not documented to less than 4%, ethambutol or streptomycin should be added to the initial regimen until susceptibility to isoniazid and rifampin is demonstrated. Consult a TB medical expert if the patient is symptomatic or smear or culture positive after 3 mo.	Administer daily isoniazid, rifampin, pyrazinamide, and streptomycin or ethambutol for 2 wk followed by 2 times/wk[†] administration of the same drugs for 6 wk (by DOT), and subsequently, with 2 times/wk administration of isoniazid and rifampin for 16 wk (by DOT). Consult a TB medical expert if the patient is symptomatic or smear or culture positive after 3 mo.	Treat by DOT, 3 times/wk[†] with isoniazid, rifampin, pyrazinamide, and ethambutol or streptomycin for 6 mo.[‡] Consult a TB medical expert if the patient is symptomatic or smear or culture positive after 3 mo.

*Adapted from MMWR Vol. 42/no. RR-7.

[†]All regimens administered 2 times/wk or 3 times/wk should be monitored by directly observed therapy (DOT) for the duration of therapy.

[‡]The strongest evidence from clinical trials is the effectiveness of all four drugs administered for the full 6 mo. There is weaker evidence that streptomycin can be discontinued after 4 mo if the isolate is susceptible to all drugs. The evidence for stopping pyrazinamide before the end of 6 mo is equivocal for the 3 times/wk regimen, and there is no evidence on the effectiveness of this regimen with ethambutol for less than the full 6 mo.

quently to ethambutol and other agents as well. Not unexpectedly, tuberculosis caused by organisms resistant to isoniazid and rifampin has been notable for its poor response to treatment with standard initial regimens. In addition, because the outbreaks of multiple drug-resistant tuberculosis have occurred mainly, although not exclusively, among HIV-infected adults, there has been transmission of infection and rapid progression to disease among their contacts.

Because of the major impact of resistance to isoniazid and rifampin on the response to therapy and because of the public health issues involved, it is essential that physicians initiating therapy for tuberculosis be aware of the prevalence of drug resistance in their communities and of the epidemiologic features of persons most likely to be harboring these organisms. In addition, drug susceptibility testing should be performed on the organisms initially isolated from all patients with newly diagnosed tuberculosis. It is desirable to have access to a laboratory in which both identification of an organism and determination of its susceptibility pattern are done rapidly. At present radiometric or colorimetric detection techniques provide the earliest identification of growth. Even if there is no capability for performing full drug-susceptibility studies, testing for resistance to rifampin could identify strains likely to have multiple drug resistance.

The current minimal acceptable duration of treatment for all children and adults with culture-positive tuberculosis is 6 mo (27). The initial phase of a 6-mo regimen should consist of a 2-mo period of isoniazid, rifampin, and pyrazinamide. Ethambutol (or streptomycin in children too young to be monitored for visual acuity) should be included in the initial regimen until the results of drug susceptibility studies are available, unless there is little possibility of drug resistance (i.e., there is less than 4% primary resistance to isoniazid in the community, and the patient has had no previous treatment with antituberculosis medications, is not from a country with a high prevalence of drug resistance, and has no known exposure to a drug-resistant case). This recommendation is intended to prevent the development of multiple drug-resistant tuberculosis in areas where primary INH resistance is increased. The second phase of treatment should consist of isoniazid and rifampin given for 4 mo. In treating patients with HIV infection it is critically important to assess clinical and bacteriologic response. Treatment should be prolonged if the response is slow or otherwise suboptimal. There is probably a reduced margin of safety in treating patients with HIV infection; therefore, the effect of patient adherence on the outcome is much more crucial. For this reason, directly observed therapy is strongly recommended in this group.

Tuberculosis caused by multiple drug-resistant organisms should be suspected in patients who are not responding to initial therapy or when epidemiologic factors suggest the presence of multiple drug resistance. The principles of management in this setting are described below.

Because HIV-infected patients seem to have a greater frequency of adverse reactions to antituberculosis drugs compared with patients not infected with HIV, patient monitoring must take this into account.

Consideration should be given to treating all patients with directly observed therapy (DOT), which can be given on an intermittent schedule. DOT means observation of the patient by a health care provider or other responsible person as the patient ingests antituberculosis medications. DOT can be achieved with daily, twice-weekly, or thrice-weekly administration of medication. It may be administered to patients in the office or clinical setting, but it is frequently given by a health department worker in the "field;" i.e., the patient's home, place of employment, school, or other mutually agreed-upon place. In some cases, staff of correctional facilities or drug treatment programs, home health-care workers, maternal and child health staff, or responsible community or family members may administer DOT.

Several options exist for administering directly observed therapy. Intermittent (i.e., twice-weekly) therapy may be given during the second phase after daily therapy during the initial phase. For those for whom prolonged supervision of daily therapy during the initial phase is impractical, a regimen of daily isoniazid, rifampin, pyrazinamide, and streptomycin or ethambutol for 2 wk, followed by twice-weekly administration of the same drugs for 6 wk and subsequently twice-weekly isoniazid and rifampin for 18 wk has been shown to be highly effective in adults (28). Alternatively, three-times-weekly administration of isoniazid, rifampin, pyrazinamide, and either streptomycin or ethambutol for 6 mo yields equivalent results in adults (29).

These specific intermittent regimens have not been studied in children, but extrapolation from other intermittent regimens suggests that they would be effective. Nine-month regimens using isoniazid and rifampin are also effective when organisms are fully drug-susceptible (30). Ethambutol or streptomycin (or streptomycin in children too young to be monitored for visual acuity) should be included in the initial regimen until the results of drug-susceptibility studies are available, unless there is little possibility of drug resistance (i.e., there is less than 4% primary resistance to isoniazid in the community, and the patient has had no previous treatment with antituberculosis medications, is not from a country with a high prevalence of drug resistance, and has no known exposure to a drug-resistant case). Isoniazid and rifampin may be given twice weekly after an initial 1 or 2 mo of daily treatment (31).

Shorter treatment is possible in adults with sputum smear- and culture-negative active pulmonary tuberculosis. Four months of isoniazid and rifampin, preferably with pyrazinamide for the first 2 mo, yields results equivalent to those for patients with culture-positive disease treated with longer regimens (32, 33). This 4-mo regimen is also recommended for adult tuberculin reactors who have a chest film suggesting old healed tuberculosis and for adult reactors who have silicosis and are sputum smear- and culture-negative although 12 mo of isoniazid therapy is an acceptable alternative.

The frequency of adverse reactions to drugs in regimens of 6 to 9 mo in duration varies, depending in part on whether streptomycin is included in the regimen. With streptomycin-containing regimens, approximately 8% of patients have adverse reactions that require modification of the regimen. Without streptomycin, the frequency is approximately 3%. Because ethambutol can be used instead of streptomycin, and it appears to be equally effective, streptomycin toxicity should not be a major factor limiting the success of chemotherapy.

The use of fixed drug combinations may enhance patient adherence and may reduce the risk of inappropriate monotherapy and may prevent the development of secondary drug resistance. For this reason the use of such fixed-dose drug combinations is strongly encouraged in adults.

Monitoring for Adverse Reactions

Adults treated for tuberculosis with the regimens outlined above should have baseline measurements of hepatic enzymes, bilirubin, serum creatinine, a complete blood count, and a platelet count (or estimate). Serum uric acid should be measured if pyrazinamide is used, and a baseline examination of both visual acuity and red-green color perception should be obtained for patients to be treated with ethambutol. The purpose of these baseline tests is to detect any abnormality that would complicate the regimen or necessitate its modification. In addition, these baseline tests enable comparison with later measurements should a suspected adverse reaction occur. Baseline tests, except visual acuity, are unnecessary in children unless a complicating condition is known or clinically suspected.

All patients, adults and children, should be monitored clinically for adverse reactions during the period of chemotherapy. They should be instructed to look for symptoms associated with the most common adverse reactions to the medications they are receiving. Patients should be seen by medical personnel at least monthly during therapy and should be specifically questioned concerning such symptoms. All patients with abnormalities detected on baseline should have follow-up of these findings. Routine laboratory monitoring for toxicity in people with normal baseline is generally not necessary. However, if symptoms suggesting drug toxicity occur, then appropriate laboratory testing should be performed to confirm or exclude such toxicity.

EVALUATION OF RESPONSE TO TREATMENT

Patients with Positive Pretreatment Sputum

The response to antituberculosis chemotherapy in patients with positive bacteriology (M. tuberculosis identified in sputum) is best evaluated by repeated examinations of sputum. Sputum examinations at least at monthly intervals are desirable until sputum conversion is documented (weekly sputum smears with quantitation are encouraged). After 2 mo of treatment with regimens containing both isoniazid and rifampin, more than 85% of patients who had positive sputum cultures before treatment should have converted to negative.

Patients whose sputum cultures have not become negative after 2 mo of treatment should be carefully reevaluated. Drug susceptibility tests should be repeated, and treatment should be administered or continued under direct observation. Unless drug resistance is demonstrated, the treatment regimen should be continued with special attention to adherence. If organisms are found to be resistant, the treatment regimen should be modified to include at least two drugs to which the organisms are susceptible and administered under direct observation. Bacteriologic evaluations are valuable for detecting nonresponse to treatment and multidrug resistance, and they should be performed at least at monthly intervals thereafter until cultures become negative.

Patients whose sputum no longer contains M. tuberculosis after 2 mo of treatment should have at least one further sputum smear and culture performed at completion of therapy. Radiographic evaluations during treatment are of less importance than sputum examination. However, a chest film at completion of treatment provides a baseline for comparison with any future films.

Patients with susceptible organisms who have completed a standard period of treatment with an isoniazid-rifampin-containing regimen and who have had a prompt and satisfactory bacteriologic response do not need routine follow-up. In some circumstances, however, as when patients have been slow to respond, have significant residual radiographic findings on completion of treatment, or are immunosuppressed, reevaluation 6 mo after completion of treatment may be of value. Patients should be instructed to report promptly the development of any symptoms, particularly prolonged cough, fever, or weight loss. These statements apply to patients whose organisms were fully susceptible to the drugs being used. In patients with organisms resistant to isoniazid and/or rifampin, follow-up evaluations must be individualized.

Patients with Negative Pretreatment Sputum

In all adults with radiographic abnormalities consistent with tuberculosis, vigorous efforts should be made to establish a microbiologic diagnosis. These efforts should include induction of sputum by inhalation of hypertonic saline. Bronchoscopy with appropriate biopsies and bronchoalveolar lavage should be considered for patients unable to produce a satisfactory sputum specimen. If no other diagnosis can be established, presumptive treatment for tuberculosis may be indicated. In such adults, the major indicators of response to therapy are the chest radiograph and clinical evaluation. The intervals at which chest films should be repeated will depend on the clinical circumstances and the differential diagnosis being considered. Failure of the radiograph to improve after 3 mo of chemotherapy is strongly suggestive that the abnormality is the result of either previous (not current) tuberculosis or another process. If the tuberculin reaction is positive and other diagnoses have been excluded, isoniazid and rifampin can be continued for a total of 4 mo. In children with suspect tuberculosis, microbiologic data can be gained from early morning gastric aspirates or urine. In complicated cases or severely ill children, bronchoalveolar lavage should be considered. An aggressive diagnostic approach in children with HIV infection or pneumonia that is unresponsive to standard treatment should be taken. Specimens for smear, culture, and susceptibility tests should be collected from all children for whom culture and susceptibility information is not available in their adult contact whenever possible.

In patients with extrapulmonary tuberculosis, the nature of repeat evaluations should be determined by the site of involvement. In some instances, for example genitourinary tuberculosis, bacteriologic examinations may be quite feasible, whereas in disease involving lymph nodes or bones and joints, clinical evaluation is the most practical way of determining response. Evaluations should also be directed toward detecting and quantifying the effects of tuberculosis on the structure and function of the involved systems. For example, evidence of hemodynamic effects should be sought in patients with tuberculous pericarditis, and patients with genitourinary tuberculosis should be evaluated for the presence of ureteral strictures.

MANAGEMENT OF PATIENTS WHOSE TREATMENT HAS FAILED OR WHO HAVE RELAPSED

Patients whose sputum has not converted after 5 to 6 mo of treatment are treatment failures. Susceptibility tests should be obtained on a current sputum specimen. While results are pending, the original drug regimen may be continued or may be augmented by at least three drugs not given previously. The regimen should be adjusted in accordance with the results of the susceptibility tests. Therapy should be administered under direct observation.

In contrast to patients who are treatment failures, in patients who relapse after completing a regimen containing isoniazid and rifampin and whose organisms were susceptible to the drugs at the outset of treatment, the organisms usually remain susceptible (34). Thus, management of these patients generally consists of reinstitution of the regimen previously used. However, drug susceptibility testing should be performed and the regimen modified if resistance is detected. Directly observed therapy should be used.

Patients who relapse after receiving regimens that did not contain both isoniazid and rifampin should be assumed, until proved otherwise, to have organisms that are resistant to the agents that were used previously and managed accordingly.

MANAGEMENT OF PATIENTS WHO HAVE DRUG-RESISTANT DISEASE

Microbial resistance to antimycobacterial drugs may be either initial or secondary. Initial resistance occurs in patients who are not known to have had previous antimycobacterial treatment. Risk factors for initial resistance include exposure to a patient who has drug-resistant tuberculosis, being from a country with a high prevalence of drug resistance, and greater than 4% primary resistance to isoniazid in the community. Secondary resistance occurs in patients who have been treated in the past. The frequency of both types of resistance is to a large extent determined by the adequacy of tuberculosis treatment programs. Poor treatment programs enable resistant organisms to emerge, producing secondary resistance in inadequately treated patients. These organisms are then transmitted and, when disease occurs, the infected person has "primary" resistant disease. In the past, primary isoniazid resistance rates in most areas of the United States were < 4%; thus, two- and three-drug regimens for tuberculosis were considered adequate. Community rates of primary isoniazid resistance $< 4\%$ may be an indication that an initial regimen of fewer than four drugs is acceptable. However, continued surveillance of drug susceptibility patterns is necessary to ensure that low rates of primary drug resistance continue.

Recently, pockets of tuberculosis caused by organisms that are resistant to at least isoniazid and rifampin have been described. Resistance to both of these potent agents considerably complicates patient management, making a successful outcome much less likely than if susceptibility to one or the other of these two agents were maintained.

The basic principle of managing patients whose organisms are resistant to one or more drugs is administration of at least two agents to which there is demonstrated susceptibility. For patients with isolated isoniazid resistance the recommended 6-mo 4-drug regimen is effective (35). When isolated isoniazid resistance is documented, isoniazid should be discontinued and pyrazinamide should be continued for the entire 6-mo duration of therapy. When isoniazid resistance is documented in the 9-mo regimen without pyrazinamide, isoniazid should be discontinued. If ethambutol was included in the initial regimen, treatment with rifampin and ethambutol should be continued for a minimum of 12 mo (36). If ethambutol was not included initially, susceptibility tests should be repeated, isoniazid should be discontinued, and two new drugs (e.g., ethambutol and pyrazinamide) should be added. The regimen can be adjusted when the results of the susceptibility tests become available.

Unfortunately, good data are not available on the relative effectiveness of various regimens and the necessary duration of treatment for patients with organisms resistant to both isoniazid and rifampin. Moreover, many such patients will have resistance to other first-line drugs (e.g., ethambutol and streptomycin) when drug resistance is discovered. Because of the poor outcome in such cases, it is preferable to give at least three new drugs to which the organism is susceptible. This regimen should be continued at least until bacteriologic sputum conversion is documented, followed by at least 12 mo of two-drug therapy. Often, a total of 24 mo of therapy is given empirically. The role of new agents such as the quinolone derivatives and amikacin in the treatment of multidrug-resistant disease is not known, although these drugs are commonly being used in such cases. Finally, surgery appears to offer considerable benefit and significantly improved cure rate for those patients in whom the bulk of disease can be resected (37).

TUBERCULOSIS IN CHILDREN AND ADOLESCENTS

The basic principles of treatment of tuberculosis in children and adolescents are essentially the same as for adults (38). Nine-month regimens containing isoniazid and rifampin have been demonstrated to have a high rate of success in children and adolescents (39), and hilar adenopathy has been successfully treated with only 6 mo of this combination (40). More recent studies of 6-mo regimens containing pyrazinamide have also produced excellent results with minimal toxicity (41). There are no data related to the ultrashort 4-mo regimen in children and adolescents yet.

Therefore, the short-course regimens recommended for adults are also the regimens of choice for children with pulmonary tuberculosis. The usual doses for daily and twice-weekly treatment in children are shown in Table 2 and Table 3. Follow-up evaluations after successful completion of therapy should be the same as described for adults.

Beyond the basic approach to treatment of tuberculosis in children, there are several important management considerations.

1. Tuberculosis in infants and children younger than 4 yr of age is much more likely to disseminate; therefore, prompt and vigorous treatment should be started when the diagnosis is suspected.

2. Primary intrathoracic tuberculosis (parenchymal infiltration, hilar adenopathy, or both, in a child with a significant tuberculin skin test reaction) should be treated in the same manner as pulmonary tuberculosis. However, when drug resistance is unlikely, treatment with rifampin and isoniazid for 6 mo supplemented by pyrazinamide in the initial 2 mo is sufficient.

3. Because sputum specimens are less likely to be helpful in children, it may be necessary to rely on the results of cultures and susceptibility tests of specimens from the adult source case to "confirm" the diagnosis in the child and to guide the choice of drugs. In cases of suspect drug-resistant tuberculosis or where adult isolates are not available, the aggressive pursuit of early morning gastric aspirates, bronchoalveolar lavage, or tissue diagnosis may have to be entertained.

4. For the same reason, bacteriologic examinations are less useful in evaluating the response to treatment; thus, clinical and radiographic examinations are of relatively greater importance in children. However, hilar adenopathy frequently requires 2 to 3 yr of complete radiographic resolution; a normal chest radiograph is not a necessary criterion for discontinuing antituberculosis drugs.

5. Because it is difficult to monitor for ocular toxicity from ethambutol, this agent is less useful in young children. Streptomycin or pyrazinamide are alternatives.

6. In general, extrapulmonary tuberculosis, including cervical adenopathy, can be treated with the same regimens as pulmonary tuberculosis. Exceptions may be bone and joint disease, disseminated (miliary) disease, and meningitis for which there are inadequate data at present to support 6-mo therapy. In these situations, a minimum of 12 mo of therapy is recommended.

7. Directly observed therapy is preferable unless there is evidence that the patient or parent will comply with therapy.

8. Management of the newborn infant whose mother (or other household contact) has tuberculosis. Management of a newborn infant whose mother (or other household contact) is suspected of having tuberculosis is based on individual considerations. If possible, separation of the mother (or contact) and infant should be minimized. Differing circumstances and resulting recommendations are as follows: (a) Mother (or other household contact) who has a positive tuberculin skin test reaction and no evidence of current disease. Investigation of other members of the household or extended family to whom the infant may later be exposed is indicated. If no

Table 2. Dosage Recommendation for the Initial Treatment of Tuberculosis in Children* and Adults

	Dosage								
	Daily Dose		Twice-Weekly Dose		Thrice-Weekly Dose				
Drugs	Children	Adults	Children	Adults	Children	Adults			
Isoniazid, mg/kg	10–20 Max 300 mg	5 Max 300 mg	20–40 Max 900 mg	15 max Max 900 mg	20–40 Max 900 mg	15 max Max 900 mg			
Rifampin, mg/kg	10–20 Max 600 mg	10 Max 600 mg	10–20 Max 600 mg	10 Max 600 mg	10–20 Max 600 mg	10 Max 600 mg			
Pyrazinamide, mg/kg	15–30 Max 2 g	15–30 Max 2 g	50–70 Max 4 g	50–70 Max 4 g	50–70 Max 3 g	50–70 Max 3 g			
Ethambutol, mg/kg†	15–25	15–25	50	50	25–30	25–30			
Streptomycin, mg/kg	20–40 Max 1.0 g	15 Max 1.0 g	25–30 Max 1.5 g	25–30 Max 1.5 g	25–30 Max 1.5 g	25–30 Max 1.5 g			

*Children ≤12 yr of age.

†Ethambutol is generally not recommended for children whose visual acuity cannot be monitored (<8 yr of age). However, ethambutol should be considered for all children with organisms resistant to other drugs when susceptibility to ethambutol has been demonstrated or susceptibility is likely.

Table 3. Second-Line Antituberculosis Drugs*

Drug	Dosage Forms	Daily Dose in Children and Adults[†]	Maximal Daily Dose in Children and Adults	Major Adverse Reactions	Recommended Regular Monitoring
Capreomycin	Vials: 1 g	15 to 30 mg/kg, IM	1 g	Auditory, vestibular, and renal toxicity	Vestibular function audiometry, blood urea nitrogen, and creatinine
Kanamycin	Vials: 75 mg 500 mg 1 g	15 to 30 mg/kg, IM	1 g	Auditory and renal toxicity, rare vestibular toxicity	Vestibular function, audiometry, blood urea nitrogen, and creatinine
Ethionamide	Tablets: 250 mg	15 to 20 mg/kg, PO	1 g	Gastrointestinal disturbance, hepatotoxicity, hypersensitivity	
Para-aminosalicylic acid	Tablets: 500 mg, 1 g Bulk powder Delayed release granules	150 mg/kg, PO	12 g	Gastrointestinal disturbance, hypersensitivity hepatotoxicity, sodium load	Hepatic enzymes
Cycloserine	Capsules: 250 mg	15 to 20 mg/kg, PO	1 g	Psychosis, convulsions, rash	Assessment of mental status

*These drugs are more difficult to use than the drugs listed in Table 1. They should be used only when necessary, and they should be given and monitored by health providers experienced in their use.

[†]Doses based on weight should be adjusted as weight changes.

evidence of current disease is found in the mother or extended family, the infant should be tested with a Mantoux test (5 TU PPD) at 4 to 6 wk of age and at 3 to 4 mo of age. When the family cannot be promptly tested, consideration should be given to the administration of isoniazid (10 mg/kg/d) to the infant until skin testing of the family has excluded contact with a case of active tuberculosis. The infant does not need to be hospitalized during this time if adequate follow-up can be arranged. The mother should also be considered for isoniazid preventive therapy. (b) Mother who has current disease and is judged to be noncontagious at delivery. Careful investigation of household members and extended family is mandatory. A chest roentgenogram and Mantoux tuberculin test at 4 to 6 wk of age should be performed on the infant; if these are negative, the infant should be tested again at 3 to 4 mo and at 6 mo. Separation of the mother and infant is not necessary if adherence with treatment by the mother is ensured. The mother can breast feed. The infant should receive isoniazid even if the tuberculin skin test and chest roentgenogram do not suggest tuberculous disease since cell-mediated immunity of a degree sufficient to mount a significant reaction to tuberculin skin testing can only develop as late as 6 mo of age in an infant infected at birth. Isoniazid can be discontinued if the Mantoux skin test is negative at 6 mo of age and no active disease exists in family members. The infant should be examined carefully at monthly intervals. If nonadherence is documented, the mother has AFB-positive sputum (or smear), and supervision is impossible, bacillus Calmette-Guerin vaccine may be considered for the infant. However, the response to the vaccine in infants may be inadequate for prevention of tuberculosis. (c) Mother who has current disease and is suspected of being contagious at the time of delivery. The mother and the infant should be separated until the mother is judged to be noncontagious. Otherwise, management is the same as when the disease is judged to be noncontagious to the infant at delivery (see preceding paragraph). (d) Mother who has hematogenous spread of tuberculosis (e.g. meningitis, miliary disease, or bone involvement). If the mother has hematogenous spread of tuberculosis, congenital tuberculosis in the infant is possible. If the infant is suspected of having congenital tuberculosis, a PPD Mantoux skin test and chest roentgenogram should be performed promptly, and treatment of the infant should begin at once. If clinical or roentgenographic findings do not support the diagnosis of congenital tuberculosis, the infant should be separated from the mother until she is judged to be noninfectious. The infant should be given isoniazid until 6 mo of age at which time the skin test should be repeated. If the skin test is positive, isoniazid should be continued for a total of 9 mo (38).

SPECIAL CONSIDERATIONS IN TREATMENT

Extrapulmonary Tuberculosis

The basic principles that underlie the treatment of pulmonary tuberculosis also apply to extrapulmonary forms of the disease. Although there have not been the same kinds of carefully conducted controlled trials of treatment for extrapulmonary tuberculosis as for pulmonary disease, increasing clinical experience is indicating that 6- to 9-mo short-course regimens are effective (42). Because of insufficient data, miliary tuberculosis, bone/joint tuberculosis, and tuberculous meningitis in infants and children should receive 12 mo of therapy.

Bacteriologic evaluation of extrapulmonary tuberculosis may be limited by the relative inaccessibility of the sites of disease. Thus, response to treatment often must be judged on the basis of clinical and radiographic findings.

The use of adjunctive therapies such as surgery and corticosteroids is more commonly required in extrapulmonary tuberculosis than in pulmonary disease. Surgery may be necessary to obtain specimens for diagnosis and to treat such processes as constrictive pericarditis and spinal cord compression from Pott's Disease. Corticosteroids have been shown to be of benefit in preventing cardiac constriction from tuberculous pericarditis (43) and in decreasing the neurologic sequelae of all stages of tuberculous meningitis, especially when administered early in the course of disease (44).

Pregnancy and Lactation

Untreated tuberculosis represents a far greater hazard to a pregnant woman and her fetus than does treatment of the disease (45). However, tuberculosis during pregnancy is not an indication for therapeutic abortion. In a pregnant woman with tuberculosis it is essential that effective therapy be given. The initial treatment regimen should consist of isoniazid and rifampin. Ethambutol should be included unless primary isoniazid resistance is unlikely. Although the routine use of pyrazinamide in pregnancy is recommended by international tuberculosis organizations, recommendations for its general use in pregnancy in the United States cannot be made because of inadequate teratogenicity data.

Isoniazid, rifampin, and ethambutol all cross the placenta, but these drugs have not been demonstrated to have teratogenic effects. Pyridoxine is recommended for pregnant woman receiving isoniazid. Streptomycin, the only antituberculosis drug documented to have harmful effects on the fetus, interferes with development of the ear and may cause congenital deafness. This toxic potential is presumably shared by kanamycin and capreomycin; however, there is little specific information on the fetal effects of these two drugs. There is not enough information to determine the risk of cycloserine or ethionamide; they should be avoided if possible.

Because the small concentrations of antituberculosis drugs in breast milk do not produce toxicity in the nursing newborn, breast feeding should not be discouraged; conversely, drugs in breast milk should not be considered to serve as effective treatment for disease or as preventive treatment in a nursing infant (46).

Associated Disorders

Tuberculosis commonly occurs in association with other disease processes. An associated disorder may alter immune responsiveness, thereby predisposing a person to tuberculosis, or simply may be an illness that occurs frequently in the same social and cultural milieu as tuberculosis. Examples of the former class of disorders include HIV infection, hematologic or reticuloendothelial malignancies, immunosuppressive therapy, chronic renal failure, and malnutrition. Silicosis, by impairing pulmonary macrophage function, is a unique example of local immune dysfunction; treatment of culture-positive silicotuberculosis requires that the usual therapy be extended by at least 2 mo (47).

The latter group of disorders includes chronic alcoholism and its secondary effects. All of these conditions may influence the outcome of therapy. The response of the impaired host to treatment may not be as satisfactory as that of a person with normal host responsiveness. For this reason, therapeutic decisions for the impaired host must be individualized and steps taken when possible to try to correct the immune deficiency.

In patients with impairment of renal function, streptomycin, kanamycin, and capreomycin should be avoided if possible. If there is severe impairment of renal function, administration of drugs at more widely spaced intervals might be necessary, and measurement of blood concentrations might be helpful in adjusting dosage (48). Liver disease, particularly alcoholic hepatitis and cirrhosis, is commonly associated with tuberculosis. In one study, the complications of potentially hepatotoxic antituberculosis drugs were not found to be greater in patients with liver disease (49). However, detecting such adverse effects if they occur may be difficult because of the preexisting disorder of hepatic function. In such patients, routine monitoring of liver function should be performed. In patients with neuropsychiatric disorders, directly observed therapy is recommended.

TREATMENT OF TUBERCULOSIS INFECTION

Preventive therapy presumably acts by diminishing or eradicating the bacterial population in "healed" or radiographically invisible lesions. Follow-up studies have demonstrated that the beneficial effect of 12 mo of isoniazid preventive therapy given to persons with a positive tuberculin skin test reaction persists for as long as 20 yr (50). Presumably, in the absence of reinfection, this protection persists for life.

Sometimes isoniazid is given to persons who are exposed to tuberculosis but not yet infected in an attempt to prevent the establishment of tuberculosis infection (primary prophylaxis). In this situation isoniazid is protective only while the person is receiving the drug.

Although isoniazid is usually safe, it is occasionally associated with adverse reactions. The most significant of these is hepatitis. Elevation of serum aminotransferase (transaminase) activity, probably reflecting mild hepatic injury, occurs in 10 to 20% of persons receiving isoniazid (51). This type of abnormality usually occurs within the first 6 mo of treatment, but it can occur at any time during therapy. In most persons, enzyme levels return to normal despite continuation of medication. However, progressive liver damage and clinical hepatitis may occur. The frequency of progressive liver damage generally increases with age. Drinking alcohol, especially on a daily basis, may enhance the risk of isoniazid-associated hepatitis. Fatal hepatitis associated with isoniazid has been reported. A recent report suggests that this risk is greatest among women, particularly black and Hispanic women (52). The risk may also be increased during the postpartum period.

PERSONS FOR WHOM PREVENTIVE THERAPY IS RECOMMENDED

Priorities for preventive therapy take into consideration the risk of developing tuberculosis compared with the risk of isoniazid toxicity (53). Recommendations for the use of isoniazid are based on a comparison of the risk of hepatic injury during the period of treatment with the potential lifelong benefit of preventive therapy. Also of importance is the benefit to society derived from preventive therapy because prevention of tuberculosis precludes the spread of new infection.

The appropriate criterion for defining a positive skin test reaction depends on the likelihood of tuberculosis infection and the risk of tuberculosis if infection has occurred (54). For persons with HIV infection, close contacts of infectious cases, and those with fibrotic lesions on chest radiograph, a reaction of greater than or equal to 5 mm is considered positive. For other at-risk persons, including infants and children younger than 4 yr of age, a reaction of greater than or equal to 10 mm is positive. Persons who are not likely to be infected with M. tuberculosis should generally not be skin tested because the predicted value of a positive skin test in low risk populations is poor. If a skin test is performed on a person who is not in a high risk category or who is not exposed to a high risk environment, a cutoff point of greater than or equal to 15 mm is positive.

The following persons with positive tuberculin skin tests (as defined above) should be considered for isoniazid preventive therapy regardless of age.

1. Persons with HIV infection and persons with risk factors for HIV infection whose HIV infection status is unknown but who are suspected of having HIV infection. The risk of tuberculosis in a tuberculin-positive person with HIV infection may be as high as 8% per year (55). Thus, the identification of persons with dual infection and the administration of preventive therapy to these persons is of great importance. In addition, preventive therapy may be considered for HIV-infected persons who are tuberculin-negative but belong to groups in which the prevalence of tuberculosis infection is high (56).

2. Close contacts of persons with newly diagnosed infectious tuberculosis. Because persons in this group are likely to have been recently infected by the index case, their risk of developing tuberculosis will be relatively high, approximately 2 to 4% for the first year, with persons who have a positive tuberculin skin test having the greatest risk. The risk for very young children and adolescents may be as much as twice the adult risk. Furthermore, persons who do not develop disease in the period immediately following infection are at some risk of doing so for the remainder of their lives. In addition, tuberculin-negative (< 5 mm) children and adolescents who have been close contacts of infectious persons within the past 3 mo are candidates for preventive therapy until a repeat tuberculin skin test is done 12 wk after last contact with the infectious source. If the repeat skin test is positive (greater than or equal to 5 mm), therapy should be continued. If the reaction remains negative, therapy need not be continued unless there is continuing exposure to an infectious source case. If preventive therapy is not prescribed initially, the tuberculin skin test should be repeated in 3 mo and preventive therapy prescribed at that time if skin test conversion has occurred and the chest radiograph remains negative.

3. Recent tuberculin skin test converters (greater than or equal to 10 mm increase within a 2-yr period for those < 35 yr of age; greater than or equal to 15 mm increase for those greater than or equal to 35 yr of age). All infants and children younger than 4 yr of age with a greater than or equal to 10 mm skin test are included in this category. The excess risk of developing tuberculosis is concentrated in the first 1 to 2 yr after infection.

4. Persons with medical conditions that have been reported to increase the risk of tuberculosis. Persons in the following groups are generally considered at increased risk of developing tuberculosis, if infected (57). In most instances the risk is not well quantitated and probably varies from person to person.
   a. Diabetes mellitus. The risk for this group may be two to four times that of the general population. Particularly at risk are poorly controlled insulin-dependent diabetics.

b. Prolonged therapy with adrenocorticosteroids. The exact risk of tuberculosis associated with corticosteroid therapy is unknown. However, tuberculosis that develops during corticosteroid therapy is more likely to be disseminated or to present in an obscure fashion. Because > 15 mg of prednisone (or equivalent) given daily for 2 to 3 wk markedly reduces tuberculin reactivity, this is probably the lower limit of corticosteroid dose associated with an increased risk of tuberculosis. There are insufficient data at present to categorically recommend isoniazid preventive therapy for persons treated with < 15 mg prednisone daily (or its equivalent) or with alternate-day corticosteroids. However, because long-term corticosteroid requirements are unpredictable, and because the frequency of isoniazid-associated hepatitis increases with age, it may be prudent to consider some of these persons for preventive therapy.

c. Immunosuppressive therapy. Similar to those receiving corticosteroids, persons receiving other forms of immunosuppressive therapy are at increased risk of tuberculosis.

d. Some hematologic and reticuloendothelial diseases, such as leukemia or Hodgkin's disease. These conditions may be associated with suppressed cellular immunity and an increased risk of tuberculosis.

e. Injection drug users known to be HIV-seronegative. Through unknown mechanisms, persons injecting illicit drugs may be at increased risk of tuberculosis even if not infected with HIV.

f. End-stage renal disease. Persons with end-stage renal disease are at increased risk of developing tuberculosis and appear particularly predisposed to developing extrapulmonary and disseminated disease. Because many of these patients will be anergic, a documented history of a prior significant tuberculin skin test is an indication for preventive therapy unless the person has been treated previously.

g. Clinical situations associated with substantial rapid weight loss or chronic undernutrition. These situations include: intestinal bypass surgery for obesity, which appears to carry an increased risk particularly for extrapulmonary tuberculosis; the postgastrectomy state; chronic peptic ulcer disease; chronic malabsorption syndromes; chronic alcoholism; and carcinomas of the oropharynx and upper gastrointestinal tract that prevent adequate nutritional intake. The postgastrectomy state may increase the risk of developing tuberculosis even without weight loss.

In addition, even in the absence of any of the above risk factors persons < 35 yr of age in the following high-incidence groups are appropriate candidates for preventive therapy if their skin test is positive (greater than or equal to 10 mm).

1. Foreign-born persons from high-prevalence countries. These countries include those in Latin America, Asia, and Africa that have a high incidence of tuberculosis.

2. Medically underserved low-income populations, including high-risk racial or ethnic minority populations, especially blacks, Hispanics, and Native Americans.

3. Residents of facilities for long-term care (e.g., correctional institutions, nursing homes, and mental institutions).

The staff of facilities in which an individual with current tuberculosis would pose a risk to large numbers of susceptible persons (e.g., correctional institutions, nursing homes, mental institutions, other health-care facilities, schools, and child-care facilities) may also be considered for preventive therapy if their tuberculin reaction is greater than or equal to 10 mm induration.

Persons younger than 35 yr of age with none of the above risk factors who have a positive skin test (greater than or equal to 15 mm) may also be considered for preventive therapy based on individual assessment of risk and benefits.

SCREENING PROCEDURES

Before isoniazid preventive therapy is started for any of the above indications, it is important to undertake the following evaluations.

1. Exclude bacteriologically positive or radiographically progressive tuberculosis. Every person who has a significant tuberculin skin test reaction should have a chest radiograph. If there are findings consistent with pulmonary tuberculosis, further studies, including med-

ical evaluation, bacteriologic examinations, and comparison of the current and old radiographs, should be made to exclude progressive disease. Appropriate evaluation should be performed if extrapulmonary tuberculosis is suspected. Because of the risk of inducing isoniazid resistance when isoniazid is used alone in a person with current tuberculosis, the recommended regimens for treatment of disease should be used until the diagnosis is clarified. If the evaluation confirms previous (not current) tuberculosis, therapy of multidrug treatment may be stopped after 4 mo in adults and after 6 mo in children (32).

2. Question for a history of therapy or preventive therapy for tuberculosis to exclude those who have been adequately treated.

3. Question for a history of prior isoniazid preventive therapy to exclude those who have had an adequate course of the drug.

4. Check for contraindications to the administration of isoniazid for preventive therapy. These include:

   a. Previous isoniazid-associated hepatic injury.

   b. History of severe adverse reactions to isoniazid such as drug fever, rash, and arthritis.

   c. Acute or unstable liver disease of any etiology. Hepatitis B surface antigen positivity per se is not a contraindication.

5. Identify patients for whom special precautions are indicated. These include:

   a. Age greater than 35 yr.

   b. Concurrent use of any other medication on a long-term basis (in view of possible drug interactions).

   c. Daily use of alcohol, which may be associated with a higher incidence of isoniazid-associated hepatitis.

   d. History of previous discontinuation of isoniazid because of possible, but not definite, related side effects, e.g., headaches, dizziness, nausea.

   e. Current chronic liver disease.

   f. Existence of peripheral neuropathy or of a condition such as diabetes mellitus or alcoholism that might predispose to the development of neuropathy.

   g. Pregnancy. Although no harmful effects of isoniazid to the fetus have been observed, preventive therapy generally should be delayed until after delivery. There does not appear to be any substantial increase in tuberculosis risk for women as a result of pregnancy. However, for pregnant women likely to have been recently infected or with high-risk medical conditions, especially HIV infection, isoniazid preventive therapy should begin when the infection is documented.

   h. Injection drug use.

   i. A recent report suggests an increased risk of fatal hepatitis associated with isoniazid among women, particularly black and Hispanic women (52). The risk may also be increased during the postpartum period.

ADMINISTRATION OF ISONIAZID PREVENTIVE THERAPY

Isoniazid is used alone for preventive therapy. The drug is given in a single daily dose of 300 mg/d for adults and 10 to 15 mg/kg body weight/d, not to exceed 300 mg/d, for children. It is recommended to dispense isoniazid only in monthly allotments. In most clinical trials of isoniazid the drug has been given for 12 mo, but there is good evidence to suggest that 6 mo of preventive therapy confers a nearly comparable degree of protection (58, 59). Durations of less than 6 mo have been shown to be substantially less effective than 6 mo of therapy, and those of longer than 1 yr do not provide additional benefit. There are no data on the effectiveness of 9 mo of preventive therapy, but presumably it is intermediate between the effectiveness of 6 and 12-mo regimens. Every effort should be made to ensure adherence to preventive therapy for at least 6 mo. Persons with HIV infection should receive 12 mo of therapy. The American Academy of Pediatrics recommends that children receive 9 mo of preventive therapy (38).

For persons at especially high risk of tuberculosis whose adherence is questionable, directly observed preventive therapy may be indicated. When resources do not permit directly observed daily therapy, isoniazid may be given twice weekly at the dose of 15 mg/kg. Although there are limited data on intermittent isoniazid preventive therapy, results of chemotherapy studies in which isoniazid is given twice weekly in the sterilizing phase of treatment suggest that this would be an effective form of preventive therapy in both adults and children.

MONITORING PREVENTIVE THERAPY

The person receiving preventive therapy or a responsible adult in a household with children receiving preventive therapy should be questioned carefully at monthly intervals for symptoms or signs consistent with liver damage or other adverse effects. These include any of the following: unexplained anorexia, nausea, vomiting, dark urine, icterus, rash, persistent paresthesias of the hands and feet, persistent fatigue, weakness or fever of greater than 3 d duration, and/or abdominal tenderness (especially right upper quadrant discomfort).

If any of these or other signs or symptoms occur during preventive therapy, patients should be advised to report immediately to the clinic or health-care provider for evaluation, including biochemical tests for hepatitis. The use of a standardized form for interviewing will help ensure alertness to all signs and symptoms, expedite the interview process, and provide for standardized data collection.

As noted, 10 to 20% of those receiving isoniazid will develop some mild abnormality of liver function (an elevated aspartate aminotransferase). These abnormalities tend to resolve even if isoniazid is continued. Because there is a higher frequency of isoniazid-associated hepatitis among persons older than 35 yr of age, a transaminase measurement should be obtained prior to the starting and monthly during the course of preventive therapy in this age group. Other factors associated with an increased risk of hepatitis include daily use of alcohol, chronic liver disease, and injection drug use. There is also evidence to suggest that postpubertal black and Hispanic women are at greater risk for hepatitis or drug interactions. More careful monitoring should be considered in these groups, possibly including more frequent laboratory monitoring. If any of these tests exceeds three to five times the upper limit of normal, discontinuation of isoniazid should be strongly considered. Liver function tests are not a substitute for a clinical evaluation at monthly intervals or for the prompt assessment of signs or symptoms of adverse reactions occurring between regularly scheduled evaluations.

ALTERNATIVE FORMS OF TUBERCULOSIS PREVENTION

There are occasional situations in which alternative forms of preventive therapy might be desirable (60). Although other drugs might also be effective for preventive therapy, there are currently no data available documenting the clinical efficacy of any drug other than isoniazid.

MANAGEMENT OF CLOSE CONTACTS OF ISONIAZID-RESISTANT CASES

In the situation where there is confidence that the source case has isoniazid-resistant organisms, it appears reasonable to treat child contacts and those adult contacts who appear particularly susceptible to tuberculosis (e.g., immunocompromised hosts) with rifampin. Some clinicians would add a second drug such as ethambutol to which the organism is believed susceptible. The drug(s) should be given in standard therapeutic doses for 6 mo; a 9-mo treatment period for children is recommended. In situations in which there is less confidence that the infection is due to isoniazid-resistant organisms, isoniazid should be used.

MANAGEMENT OF PERSONS WITH A HIGH PROBABILITY OF INFECTION WITH MULTIDRUG-RESISTANT ORGANISMS

In persons likely to have been infected with bacilli resistant to both isoniazid and rifampin, observation without preventive therapy has usually been recommended because no other drugs have been evaluated for preventive therapy. However, in persons with an especially high risk of tuberculosis (e.g., persons with HIV infection), preventive therapy should be considered (61). If the organisms are thought to be susceptible, 6 mo of daily ethambutol and pyrazinamide at the usual therapeutic doses may be considered. If infection is due to organisms resistant to ethambutol as well, the combination of pyrazinamide plus a quinolone (ofloxacin or ciprofloxacin) for 6 mo is recommended. Careful assessment to exclude active tuberculosis prior to the initiation of preventive therapy is mandatory.

MANAGEMENT OF PERSONS INTOLERANT TO ISONIAZID

An approach similar to that taken for contacts of isoniazid-resistant cases can be used here with the exception that isoniazid is not one of the alternatives.

USE OF BCG

Bacille Calmette Guerin (BCG) was derived from a strain of M. bovis attenuated through years of serial passage in culture at the Pasteur Institute in Lille, France. There are many BCG vaccines available, most of which have not been recently studied. The protection obtained from studies of previous vaccines has varied from zero to 80% (62). The most recent large trial, conducted in South India, failed to show a protective effect despite the fact that the vaccines used were believed to be two of the most potent available (63). Subsequently, however, a large number of nonrandomized studies (case-control and cohort studies) have suggested that BCG vaccine does protect infants and young children from the more serious forms of tuberculosis, although the ability of BCG to prevent adult forms of tuberculosis remains questionable (64).

Even if vaccines of proved efficacy and safety were available, the potential benefit of BCG vaccination in a nation such as the United States would be small because most tuberculosis occurs in persons who have already been infected. Such persons will not benefit from BCG.

BCG rarely causes serious complications; osteomyelitis and death from disseminated BCG infection have occurred in only one case per million doses administered. The frequency of side effects, most commonly prolonged ulceration and local adenitis, occur in 1 to 10% of vaccines, varying with the vaccine used, the intensity with which adverse reactions are sought, and the population vaccinated. BCG vaccination may cause tuberculin skin test conversion, thus rendering the test less useful.

Because of these shortcomings, BCG is recommended only in the following situations (64).

1. BCG vaccine is strongly recommended for infants and children with negative tuberculin skin tests who: (a) are at high risk of intimate and prolonged exposure to persistently untreated or ineffectively treated patients with infectious pulmonary tuberculosis, cannot be removed from the source of exposure, and cannot be placed on long-term preventive therapy, or (b) are continuously exposed to persons with tuberculosis who have bacilli resistant to both isoniazid and rifampin.
2. BCG vaccination is also recommended for tuberculin-negative infants and children in groups in which the rate of new infections exceeds 1% per year and for whom the usual surveillance and treatment programs have been attempted but are not operationally feasible. These groups include persons without regular access to health care, those for whom usual health care is culturally or socially unacceptable, or groups who have demonstrated an inability to effectively use existing accessible care. In view of the recent outbreaks of multidrug-resistant tuberculosis, these recommendations are currently under review.

Vaccination should be administered only by the route indicated in the package labeling and only in the suggested dose. If a newborn is vaccinated, one-half the usual dose should be used. Depressed host immunity (from illness such as HIV infection or therapy with immunosuppressive drugs) is a contraindication to BCG administration.

REFERENCES: AS NUMBERED IN ORIGINAL PUBLICATION

3. Perez-Stable EJ, Hopewell PC. Chemotherapy of tuberculosis. Semin Respir Med 1988;9:459.
24. Centers for Disease Control. Nosocomial transmission of multidrug-resistant TB in health-care workers and HIV-infected patients in an urban hospital: Florida. MMWR 1990;39:718.
25. Centers for Disease Control. Nosocomial transmission of multidrug-resistant TB among HIV-infected persons: Florida and New York, 1988–1991. MMWR 1991;40:585.
26. Centers for Disease Control. Transmission of multidrug-resistant TB among immunocompromised persons in a correctional system: New York. MMWR 1991;41:507.
27. Combs DL, O'Brien RJ, Geiter LJ. USPHS tuberculosis short-course therapy trial 21: effectiveness, toxicity, and acceptability. The report of final results. Ann Intern Med 1990;112:397.
28. Cohn DL, Catlin BJ, Peterson KL, Judson FN, Sbarbaro JA. A 62-dose, 6-mo therapy for pulmonary and extrapulmonary tuberculosis. A twice-weekly, directly observed, and cost-effective regimen. Ann Intern Med 1990;112:407.

29. Hong Kong Chest Service/British Medical Research Council. Five-year follow-up of a controlled trial of five 6-month regimens of chemotherapy for pulmonary tuberculosis. Am Rev Respir Dis 1987;136:1339.
30. Slutkin G, Schecter GF, Hopewell PC. The results of 9-month isoniazid-rifampin therapy for pulmonary tuberculosis under program conditions in San Francisco. Am Rev Respir Dis 1988;138:1622.
31. Dutt AK, Moers D, Stead WW. Short-course chemotherapy for tuberculosis with mainly twice-weekly isoniazid and rifampin. Community physicians' seven-year experience with mainly outpatients. Am J Med 1984;77:233.
32. Hong Kong Chest Service/Tuberculosis Research Centre, Madras/British Medical Research Council. A controlled trial of 3-month, 4-month, and 6-month regimens of chemotherapy for sputum-smear negative pulmonary tuberculosis. Results at 5 years. Am Rev Respir Dis 1989;139:871.
33. Dutt AK, Moers D, Stead WW. Smear- and culture-negative pulmonary tuberculosis: four-month short course chemotherapy. Am Rev Respir Dis 1989;139:867.
34. Snider DE, Long MW, Cross FS, Farer LS. Six-months isoniazid-rifampin therapy for pulmonary tuberculosis. Am Rev Respir Dis 1984;129:573.
35. Singapore Tuberculosis Service/British Medical Research Council. Clinical trial of six-month and four-month regimens of chemotherapy in the treatment of pulmonary tuberculosis. Am Rev Respir Dis 1979;119:579-585.
36. Zierski M. Prospects of retreatment of chronic resistant pulmonary tuberculosis patients: a critical review. Lung 1977;154:91.
37. Iseman MD, Madsen L, Goble M, Pomerantz M. Surgical intervention in the treatment of pulmonary disease caused by drug-resistant Mycobacterium tuberculosis. Am Rev Respir Dis 1990;141:623.
38. American Academy of Pediatrics. Report of the Committee on Infectious Diseases. 22nd ed. Elk Grove, IL: American Academy of Pediatrics, 1991;487-508.
39. Abernathy AS, Dutt AK, Stead WW, Mowers DJ. Short-course chemotherapy for tuberculosis in children. Pediatrics 1983;72:801.
40. Jacobs RF, Abernathy RS. The treatment of tuberculosis in children. Pediatr Infect Dis J 1985;4:513.
41. Starke JR. Multidrug chemotherapy for tuberculosis in children. Pediatr Infect Dis J 1990;9:785-793.
42. Dutt AK, Stead WW. Treatment of extrapulmonary tuberculosis. Semin Respir Infect 1989;4:225.
43. Strang JIG, Kakaza HHS, Gibson DG, et al. Controlled trial of prednisolone as adjunct in treatment of tuberculous constrictive pericarditis in Transkei. Lancet 1987;2:1418.
44. Girgis NI, Farid Z, Kilpatrick ME, et al. Dexamethasone as an adjunct to treatment of tuberculous meningitis. Pediatr Infect Dis J 1991;10:179.
45. Snider DE, Layde RM, Johnson MW, Lyle MA. Treatment of tuberculosis during pregnancy. Am Rev Respir Dis 1980;122:65.
46. Snider DE, Powell KE. Should women taking antituberculosis drugs breast feed? Arch Intern Med 1984;144:589.
47. Hong Kong Chest Service/Tuberculosis Research Centre, Madras/British Medical Research Council. A controlled clinical comparison of 6 and 8 months of antituberculosis chemotherapy in the treatment of patients with silicotuberculosis in Hong Kong. Am Rev Respir Dis 1991;143:262-267.
48. Andrew OT, Schoenfeld PY, Hopewell PC, Humphrey MH. Tuberculosis in patients with end-stage renal disease. Am J Med 1980;68:59.
49. Cross FS, Long MW, Banner AS, Snider DE. Rifampin-isoniazid therapy of alcoholic and nonalcoholic tuberculosis patients in a U.S. Public Health Service cooperative therapy trial. Am Rev Respir Dis 1980;122:349.
50. Comstock GW, Baum C, Snider DF. Isoniazid prophylaxis among Alaskan Eskimos: a final report of the Bethel isoniazid studies. Am Rev Respir Dis 1979;119:827-830.
51. Mitchell JR, Zimmerman HJ, Ishak KG, et al. Isoniazid liver injury: clinical spectrum, pathology and probable pathogenesis. Ann Intern Med 1976;84:181.
52. Snider DE, Caras GJ. Isoniazid-associated hepatitis deaths: a review of available information. Am Rev Respir Dis 1992;145:484-497.
53. Advisory Committee for Elimination of Tuberculosis. The use of preventive therapy for tuberculous infection in the United States. MMWR 1990;39:9.
54. American Thoracic Society/Centers for Disease Control. Diagnostic standards and classification of tuberculosis. Am Rev Respir Dis 1990;142:725-735.
55. Selwyn PA, Hartel D, Lewis VA, et al. A prospective study of the risk of tuberculosis among intravenous drug users with human immunodeficiency virus infection. N Engl J Med 1989;320:545.
56. Centers for Disease Control. PPD-tuberculin anergy in persons with HIV infection. Guidelines for anergy testing and management of anergic persons at risk of tuberculous infection. MMWR 1991;40:27-33.
57. Rieder HL, Cauthen GM, Comstock GW, Snider DE. Epidemiology of tuberculosis in the United States. Epidemiol Rev 1989;11:79-98.
58. International Union against Tuberculosis. Efficacy of various durations of isoniazid preventive therapy for tuberculosis. Bull WHO 1982;60:555.
59. Snider DE, Caras GJ, Koplan JP. Preventive therapy with isoniazid. JAMA 1986;255:1579.
60. Koplan JP, Farer LS. Choice of preventive treatment for isoniazid resistant tuberculosis. JAMA 1980;244:2736.

61. Centers for Disease Control. Management of persons exposed to multidrug-resistant tuberculosis. MMWR 1992;41:59–71.
62. Luelmo F. BCG vaccination. Am Rev Respir Dis 1982;125:3(Part 2):70.
63. World Health Organization. Vaccination against tuberculosis. WHO/Technical Report Series 651, 1980.
64. Immunization Practices Advisory Committee and Advisory Committee for the Elimination of Tuberculosis. Use of BCG vaccines in the control of tuberculosis. MMWR 1988;37:663.

Initial Therapy for Tuberculosis in the Era of Multidrug Resistance

Original Citation: Centers for Disease Control and Prevention. Initial therapy for tuberculosis in the era of multidrug resistance—recommendations of the Advisory Council for the Elimination of Tuberculosis. MMWR 1993;42(RR-7):1.

Editor's Note: The information included here was based on an MMWR Reports and Recommendations document (Vol. 42;RR-7) which published the recommendations of the Advisory Council for the Elimination of Tuberculosis. The original publication gives an introduction which includes the epidemiology of MDR-TB and the rationale for multiple drug treatment.

TREATMENT

Because administration of a single drug often leads to the development of a bacterial population resistant to that drug, effective regimens for the treatment of TB must contain multiple drugs to which the organisms are susceptible. When two or more drugs are used simultaneously, each helps prevent the emergence of tubercle bacilli resistant to the others. However, when the in vitro susceptibility of a patient's isolate is not known—which is generally the case at the beginning of therapy—selecting two agents to which the patient's isolate is likely to be susceptible can be difficult. Improper selection of drugs for the treatment of drug-resistant TB (i.e., providing only one drug to which most organisms are susceptible) may subsequently result in the development of additional drug-resistant organisms.

A four-drug regimen with INH, RIF, pyrazinamide (PZA), and SM or EMB is preferred for the initial, empiric treatment of TB (Tables 1, 2). When adherence with the regimen is assured, such as with directly observed therapy (DOT), the four-drug regimen is highly effective even for INH-resistant organisms (7). Based on the prevalence and characteristics of drug-resistant organisms, at least 95% of patients will receive an adequate regimen (at least two drugs to which their organisms are susceptible) if this four-drug regimen is used at the beginning of therapy (CDC, unpublished data). Even with susceptible organisms, sputum conversion is accomplished more rapidly from positive to negative with a four-drug regimen than with a three-drug regimen of INH, RIF, and PZA (8). DOT is more easily managed with the four-drug regimen since it can be administered intermittently 3 times/week from the beginning of therapy (7). The four-drug regimen also can be administered 2 times/week following a 2-week induction phase of daily therapy (9). Finally, a patient who is

Table 1. Regimen Options for the Initial Treatment of TB Among Children and Adults—TB without HIV infection

Option 1	Option 2	Option 3	TB with HIV infection
Administer daily INH, or 3 can be RIF, and PZA for 8 weeks treatment followed by 16 weeks of should INH and RIF daily or 2–3 a total of 9 times/week* in areas least 6 where the INH resistance culture rate is not documented to be <4%. EMB or SM should be added to the initial regimen until susceptibility to INH and RIF is demonstrated. Continue treatment for at least 6 months and 3 months beyond culture conversion. Consult a TB medical expert if the patient is symptomatic or smear or culture positive after 3 months.	Administer daily INH, RIF, PZA, and SM or EMB for 2 weeks followed by 2 times/week* administration of the same drugs for 6 weeks (by DOT**), and subsequently, with 2 times/week administration of INH and RIF for 16 weeks (by DOT). Consult a TB medical expert if the patient is symptomatic or smear or culture positive after 3 months.	Treat by DOT, 3 times/week* with INH, RIF, PZA, and EMB or SM for 6 months[+] Consult a TB medical expert if the patient is symptomatic or smear or culture positive after 3 months.	Options 1, 2, used, but regimens continue for months and at months beyond conversion.

*All regimens administered 2 times/week or 3 times/week should be monitored by DOT for the duration of therapy.

[+]The strongest evidence from clinical trials is the effectiveness of all four drugs administered for the full 6 months. There is weaker evidence that SM can be discontinued after 4 months if the isolate is susceptible to all drugs. The evidence for stopping PZA before the end of 6 months is equivocal for the 3 times/week regimen, and there is no evidence on the effectiveness of this regimen with EMB for less than the full 6 months.

**DOT—Directly observed therapy.

Table 2. Dosage Recommendation for the Initial Treatment of TB Among Children* and Adults

| | Dosage | | | | | |
| | Daily | | 2 times/week | | 3 times/week | |
Drugs	Children	Adults	Children	Adults	Children	Adults
Isoniazid	10–20 mg/kg Max. 300 mg	5 mg/kg Max. 300 mg	20–40 mg/kg Max. 900 mg	15 mg/kg Max. 900 mg	20–40 mg/kg Max. 900 mg	15 mg/kg Max. 900 mg
Rifampin	10–20 mg/kg Max. 600 mg	10 mg/kg Max. 600 mg	10–20 mg/kg Max. 600 mg	10 mg/kg Max. 600 mg	10–20 mg/kg Max. 600 mg	10 mg/kg Max. 600 mg
Pyrazinamide	15–30 mg/kg Max. 2 gm	15–30 mg/kg Max 2 gm	50–70 mg/kg Max. 4 gm	50–70 mg/kg Max. 4 gm	50–70 mg/kg Max. 3 gm	50–70 mg/kg Max. 3 gm
Ethambutol+	15–25 mg/kg Max. 2.5 gm	5–25 mg/kg Max. 2.5 gm	50 mg/kg Max. 2.5 gm	50 mg/kg Max. 2.5 gm	25–30 mg/kg Max. 2.5 gm	25–30 mg/kg Max. 2.5 gm
Streptomycin	20–30 mg/kg Max. 1 gm	15 mg/kg Max. 1 gm	25–30 mg/kg Max. 1.5 gm	25–30 mg/kg Max. 1.5 gm	25–30 mg/kg Max. 1 gm	25–30 mg/kg Max. 1 gm

*Children ≤ 12 years of age.

+Ethambutol is generally not recommended for children whose visual acuity cannot be monitored (<6 years of age). However, ethambutol should be considered for all children with organisms resistant to other drugs, when susceptibility to ethambutol has been demonstrated, or susceptibility is likely.

treated with the four-drug regimen, but who defaults therapy is more likely to be cured and not relapse when compared with a patient treated for the same length of time with the three-drug regimen.

RECOMMENDATIONS

To avoid the emergence of drug-resistant organisms, the Advisory Council for the Elimination of Tuberculosis (ACET) recommends the following approach to beginning therapy for TB.

Susceptibility Testing

All persons with TB from whom M. tuberculosis is isolated should have drug susceptibility testing performed on their first isolate; these results should be reported promptly to the health-care provider and to the health department.

Such testing will provide the basis for clinical therapeutic decisions. In addition, surveillance of drug-susceptibility reports will help identify emerging drug resistance and help monitor control efforts in areas where resistance is already established. Drug-susceptibility testing also should be performed on additional isolates from patients whose cultures fail to convert to negative within 3 months of beginning therapy, or if there is clinical evidence of failure to respond to therapy. To monitor changes in drug susceptibility patterns in the United States, the "Report of Verified Cases of Tuberculosis" reporting form has been revised to include a section relating to drug susceptibility results from the initial isolate for all reported TB cases.

Initial Regimen

The initial treatment of TB should include four drugs. During the first 2 months, the drug regimen should include INH, RIF, PZA, and EMB or SM. When drug susceptibility results are available, the regimen should be altered as appropriate. This regimen should be administered to all patients unless the likelihood of INH or RIF resistance is low.

General Principles

Analysis of local rates of drug resistance provides the best basis for determining when the four-drug regimen might not be necessary. Local data may indicate that the population in general is at low risk for drug resistance or that specific and definable subgroups in the population can be defined that are at low risk for drug resistance. In the past, when national INH-resistance rates were about 4% and declining (10), two- and three-drug regimens were considered adequate. Community rates of INH resistance less than 4% may be an indication that an initial regimen with fewer than four drugs may be acceptable. However, continued surveillance of drug susceptibility patterns is necessary to ensure that low rates of drug resistance continue.

Institutions (e.g., health-care and correctional facilities) that are experiencing outbreaks of TB resistant to INH and RIF or that are resuming treatment for a patient with a prior history of anti-TB therapy may need to begin five-drug or six-drug regimens as initial therapy. These regimens should include the four-drug regimen and at least three drugs to which the suspected multidrug-resistant strain may be susceptible.

When the results of drug susceptibility tests become available, regimens should be specifically defined on the basis of those results. For example, patients whose TB organisms are susceptible to INH and RIF should receive a regimen of INH and RIF for a full 6 months, supplemented with PZA during the first 2 months. The treatment regimen of patients with drug-resistant organisms should be determined in consultation with physicians experienced in the treatment of drug-resistant TB.

When results of drug susceptibility tests are not available, either due to a failure to perform the tests or a failure of the test to yield definitive results, the decision to modify therapy should be based on the probability of drug resistance. Where the prevalence of drug resistance is sufficiently substantial to justify starting all patients on the four-drug regimen (i.e., a prevalence of INH resistance greater than or equal to 4%), PZA should be discontinued at 8 weeks, but EMB or SM should be continued (along with INH and RIF) for a total of 6 months.

Immunosuppressed Patients

HIV infection and other factors that compromise a patient's immune system are important considerations when clinicians select the most effective regimen for the treatment of TB. These factors are particularly important with drug-resistant TB because of the potential for rapid disease progression and death when patients receive inadequate treatment. Because data from controlled clinical trials are not available to determine if a 6-month regimen is adequate treatment for HIV-infected patients with TB, ACET recommends that such patients be treated for a total of 9 months and for at least 6 months after sputum conversion (11). No evidence suggests that intermittent therapy—2 times/week or 3 times/week—will not be as effective for the treatment of TB among HIV-infected persons when compared with TB treatment for persons who are not HIV positive.

If drug susceptibility results are not available, EMB or SM should be continued for the entire course of therapy because of the risk of rapid disease progression while the patient is on inadequate therapy.

Treatment of Extrapulmonary TB

Regimens that are adequate for treating adults and children with pulmonary TB also should be effective in treating extrapulmonary disease. However, some experts extend the duration of therapy to 9 months for patients with disseminated disease, miliary disease, disease involving the bones or joints, or tuberculous lymphadenitis. The use of adjunctive therapies, such as surgery and corticosteroids, may be beneficial (1).

Treatment of Infants and Children

Infants and children with TB should be treated with the same regimens recommended for adults; however, dosage may vary for some drugs (Table 2).

Further, EMB is generally not used for children whose visual acuity cannot be monitored (e.g., those less than 6 years of age); SM is an alternative. The inclusion of EMB in the treatment regimen should be considered, however, for all children with organisms resistant to other drugs when susceptibility to EMB has been demonstrated or when susceptibility is likely. Because the risk of dissemination of TB is greater among infants than adults, prompt and vigorous treatment should begin as soon as the diagnosis is suspected.

Treatment of TB During Pregnancy

Effective therapy for TB is essential for pregnant women with TB. However, the treatment regimen must be adjusted since SM may cause congenital deafness. SM is the only licensed anti-TB drug documented to have harmful effects on the fetus (1). Routine use of PZA also is not recommended during pregnancy because the risk of teratogenicity has not been determined. In addition, since the 6-month treatment regimen cannot be used and a minimum of 9 months of therapy is recommended, the preferred initial treatment regimen is INH, RIF, and EMB. If resistance to other drugs is likely and susceptibility to PZA also is likely, the use of PZA should be considered and the risks and benefits of the drug carefully weighed. Because the small concentrations of anti-TB drugs in breast milk do not produce toxicity in the nursing newborn, breast feeding should not be discouraged. Further, because these drug levels are so low in breast milk they cannot be relied upon for either prophylaxis or therapy for nursing infants.

Directly Observed Therapy (DOT)

A major cause of drug-resistant TB and treatment failure is patient nonadherence to prescribed treatment. Treatment failure and drug-resistant TB can be life-threatening and pose other serious public health risks because they can lead to prolonged infectiousness and increased transmission of TB in the community. DOT is one method of ensuring adherence; it requires that a healthcare provider or other designated person observe while the patient ingests anti-TB medications.

DOT should be considered for all patients because of the difficulty in predicting which patients will adhere to a prescribed treatment regimen. Decisions regarding the use of expanded or universal DOT should be based on a quantitative evaluation of local treatment completion rates. If the percentage of patients who complete therapy within 12 months is less than 90% or unknown, the use of DOT should be expanded. If greater than or equal to 90% of patients beginning therapy complete a recommended course of therapy within 12 months, the expanded use of DOT may not be necessary. However, even in these circumstances, consideration should be given to extending the use of DOT to increase the treatment completion rate. All patients with TB caused by organisms resistant to either INH or RIF and all patients receiving intermittent therapy should receive DOT.

DOT programs increase adherence in both rural and urban settings and provide effective treatment for TB (12, 13). A hospital in New York City reported that only 11% of patients under care for TB reported to an outpatient clinic for further treatment when discharged from the hospital (14). In contrast, a program in which DOT is routinely used for all patients had a completion rate of 98% (15).

Although expanding the use of DOT may require additional resources, intermittent, directly observed regimens are cost effective (16) (CDC unpublished data). DOT can be conducted with regimens given once a day, 2 times/week, or 3 times/week.

When TB is initially diagnosed, medical providers should explain to the patient about the disease, treatment, and the importance of completing the recommended course of therapy. Medical providers should also verify that the patient understands this information. When DOT is administered, the method must be specifically defined for each patient and be based on a thorough assessment of each patient's needs, living/employment conditions, and preferences. The patient and the provider should agree on a method that ensures the best possible DOT routine and maintains confidentiality. Patients who receive daily therapy can be successfully managed with self-administered therapy. Public health officials responsible for TB treatment should be notified when patients not receiving DOT miss appointments or demonstrate other nonadherent behaviors. These patients should be placed on DOT, and all regimens administered 2 times/week or 3 times/week should be administered as DOT for the duration of therapy.

Effective use of DOT sometimes requires an outreach worker to go into the community to locate a patient and administer each dose of medication. However, most patients can receive the daily, 2 times/week, or 3 times/week treatment at a location agreed on by both the provider and the patient. DOT can be arranged and administered in various settings, including TB clinics, community health centers, migrant clinics, homeless shelters, prisons or jails, nursing homes, schools, drug treatment centers, hospitals, HIV/AIDS clinics or hostels, or occupational health clinics.

In some situations, another responsible person other than a health-care worker may administer DOT. Persons administering DOT may include physicians, nurses, health care aides, nursing home staff, correctional facility personnel, staff of community-based organizations, school nurses or teachers, reliable volunteers, drug treatment center employees, social and welfare caseworkers, and clergy or other community leaders. These arrangements require careful supervision by the medical provider. The use of incentives or enablers (e.g., providing transportation or car/bus fare to the DOT site) may promote patient adherence to a DOT program. The use of combined preparations of INH and RIF (e.g., Rifamate Registered) or INH, RIF, and PZA (not available in the United States) may also improve patient adherence.

Poor patient adherence is a multifaceted problem; additional research is needed to clarify the role of operational, environmental, behavioral, and other factors in determining adherence. A research agenda is described in "Problem 38" of the National Action Plan to Combat Multidrug-Resistant Tuberculosis (17).

REFERENCES: AS NUMBERED IN ORIGINAL PUBLICATION

1. American Thoracic Society, CDC. Treatment of TB and TB infection in adults and children. Am Rev Respir Dis 1986;134:355–363.
7. Hong Kong Chest Service/British Medical Research Council. Controlled trial of 4 three-times-weekly regimens and a daily regimen given for 6 months for pulmonary TB. Second report: the results of final results up to 24-months. Tubercle 1982;63:89.
8. Combs DL, O'Brien RJ, Geiter LJ. USPHS TB short-course chemotherapy trial 21: effectiveness, toxicity, and acceptability. The report of final results. Ann Intern Med 1990;112:397.
9. Cohn DL, Catlin BJ, Peterson KL, Judson FN, Sbarbaro JA. A 62-dose 6-month therapy for pulmonary and extrapulmonary TB. A twice-weekly, directly observed, and cost effective regimen. Ann Int Med 1990;112(6):407.
10. CDC. Primary resistance to anti-TB drugs—United States. MMWR 1983;32(40):521.
11. CDC. TB and human immunodeficiency virus infection: recommendations of the advisory committee for the elimination of TB (ACET). MMWR 1989;38(17):236, 243.
12. Sbarbaro JA, Johnson S. TB chemotherapy for recalcitrant outpatients administered twice-weekly. Am Rev Respir Dis 1968;97:895.
13. Mcdonald RJ, Memon AM, Reichman LB. Successful supervised ambulatory management of TB treatment failures. Ann Intern Med 1982;96:297.
14. Brudney K, Dobkin J. Resurgent TB in New York City. Human immunodeficiency virus, homelessness and the decline of TB programs. Am Rev Respir Dis 1991;144:745.
15. CDC. Improving adherence to antituberculosis therapy—South Carolina and New York. MMWR 1993;42(4):74.
16. Iseman MD, Cohn DL, Sbarbaro JA. Directly observed treatment of tuberculosis—we can't afford not to try it. N Engl J Med 1993;328(8):576.
17. CDC. National action plan to combat multidrug-resistant tuberculosis; Meeting the challange of multidrug-resistant tuberculosis: summary of a conference; Management of persons exposed to multidrug-resistant tuberculosis. MMWR 1992;41(No. RR-11).

Tuberculosis Among Foreign-Born Persons Entering the United States

Original Citation: Centers for Disease Control and Prevention. Tuberculosis among foreign-born persons entering the United States—recommendations of the Advisory Committee for Elimination of Tuberculosis. MMWR 1990;39(RR-18):1–13, 18–21.

Editor's Note: The information included here was based on a 1990 MMWR Reports and Recommendations issue (Vol. 39;RR-18) written by the DHHS Advisory Committee for Elimination of Tuberculosis. The original text includes a summary of the document, an introductory paragraph, and background information on the epidemiology of tuberculosis in the foreign-born.

The ACET recommends that all foreign-born persons applying for permanent entry into the United States continue to be screened for disease. Deficiencies in the current screening methods should be corrected. The policy requiring that persons found to have infectious tuberculosis (known or suspected) be prevented from entering the country until treatment has rendered them noninfectious should be continued; however, persons with noninfectious tuberculosis should be permitted to enter the United States. Tuberculin skin testing and preventive therapy programs for foreign-born persons must be expanded both overseas and domestically if the goal of eliminating tuberculosis from the United States by the year 2010 is to be met.

DEFINITIONS OF TERMS

In these recommendations, use of the terms "alien" and "foreign-born" depends on whether the context is based on the Immigration and Nationality Act (alien) or on CDC's epidemiologic data base (foreign-born).

The following definitions were developed by CDC in consultation with INS. They have not been modified to conform to MMWR style.

ALIEN

Defined in the U.S. Immigration and Nationality Act as any person not a citizen or national of the United States.

UNDOCUMENTED ALIEN

Any alien who entered the United States without inspection, or someone in the United States in violation of the Immigration and Nationality Act or any other law of the United States.

IMMIGRANT

An alien who has been issued an immigrant visa by a consular officer outside the United States and has been lawfully accorded the privilege of residing permanently in the United States as an immigrant in accordance with the immigration laws.

NON-IMMIGRANT

An alien who has been issued a non-immigrant visa and has been admitted to the United States for such time and under such conditions as the Attorney General may by regulations prescribe.

ADJUSTMENT OF STATUS OF NON-IMMIGRANT TO THAT OF A PERSON ADMITTED FOR PERMANENT RESIDENCE

Under certain conditions, the status of an alien who was inspected and admitted or paroled into the United States may be adjusted by the Attorney General to that of an alien lawfully admitted for permanent residence. Also, under the Immigration Reform and Control Act of 1986, certain undocumented aliens already in the United States may apply for adjustment of status and undergo a medical examination similar to that for non-immigrants already in the country who apply for adjustment of status.

REFUGEE

Any person who is outside any country of such person's nationality or, in the case of a person having no nationality, is outside any country in which such person last habitually resided, and who is unable or unwilling to return to, and is unable or unwilling to avail himself or herself of, the protection of that country because of persecution or a well-founded fear of persecution on account of race, religion, nationality, membership in a particular social group, or political opinion; or any person who is within the country of such person's nationality or, in the case of a person having no nationality, within the country in which such person is habitually residing, and who is persecuted or who has a well-founded fear of persecution on account of race, religion, nationality, membership in a particular social group, or political opinion.

ENTRANT

An immigration designation given to a national of Cuba or Haiti who arrived in the United States between April 20, 1980, and October 11, 1981, and for whom a record was established by INS prior to January 1, 1982.

PAROLEE

An alien, appearing to be inadmissible to the inspecting officer, allowed to enter the United States under emergency (humanitarian) conditions or when that alien's entry is determined to be in the public interest. Parole does not constitute formal admission to the United States and confers temporary admission status only, requiring parolees to leave when the conditions supporting their parole cease to exist.

Definitions of Parolees Include

INDEFINITE PAROLEE

Parole is usually set for a specified period of time according to the conditions of parole. In some cases, as conditions warrant, the period of parole is specified as indefinite.

DEFERRED INSPECTION

Parole may be granted to an alien who appears not to be clearly admissible to the inspecting officer. An appointment will be made for the alien's appearance at another Service Office where more information is available and the inspection can be completed.

MEDICAL AND LEGAL PAROLEE

Parole may be granted to an alien who has a serious medical condition which would make detention or return inappropriate or who is to serve as a witness in legal proceedings or is subject to prosecution in the United States.

EXCLUDABLE MEDICAL CONDITION

Aliens shall be ineligible to receive a visa and shall be excluded from admission into the United States if found to have a condition described in Section 212(a)(1)-(6), Immigration and Nationality Act: "(1) Aliens who are mentally retarded; (2) Aliens who are insane; (3) Aliens who have had one or more attacks of insanity; (4) Aliens afflicted with psychopathic personality, or sexual deviation, or a mental defect; (5) Aliens who are narcotic drug addicts or chronic alcoholics; (6) Aliens who are afflicted with any dangerous contagious disease. (Public Health Service (PHS) Regulations define tuberculosis, active, as a 'dangerous contagious disease.')"

Waiver of Excludable Medical Condition

FOR IMMIGRANTS

Section 212(g), Immigration and Nationality Act, gives the Attorney General the authority to waive certain medical conditions, i.e., mental retardation, tuberculosis, and a past history of mental illness, for an alien who has been found to have one of these excludable medical conditions if the alien has certain relatives who are United States citizens or lawful permanent residents of the United States.

FOR REFUGEES

Section 207(c)(3), Immigration and Nationality Act, gives the Attorney General the authority to waive any of the health provisions listed in Section 212(a)(1)-(6) for humanitarian purposes, to assure family unity, or when it is otherwise in the public interest.

FOR NON-IMMIGRANTS

Section 212(d)(3), Immigration and Nationality Act, provides that an alien who has been found to have an excludable medical condition and is thus ineligible to receive a non-immigrant visa may, after approval by the Attorney General of a recommendation by the Secretary of State, be granted such a visa and may be admitted into the United States temporarily as a non-immigrant.

ABNORMAL CHEST RADIOGRAPH AS DEFINED BY THE ACET

All pulmonary parenchymal abnormalities suggestive of tuberculosis except when calcified granulomas are the sole abnormality.

CURRENT HEALTH SCREENING AND FOLLOW-UP REQUIREMENTS FOR ALIENS

PHS requirements and guidelines for the medical examination of aliens seeking entry into the United States are based on the Immigration and Nationality

Act and on INS and PHS regulations that exclude aliens with certain health conditions from entering the United States. (Note: New regulations for excludable medical conditions under the Immigration Act of 1990 are being developed and will be published in the Federal Register.)

Excludable Conditions

Currently, immigrants and refugees coming to the United States must have a physical and mental examination abroad. These examinations are performed by local "panel" physicians designated by Embassies and Consulates of the Department of State. The medical examinations are performed to identify, for the Department of State and the INS, those applicants for admission who have excludable mental and physical conditions, as specified in the Immigration and Nationality Act. Examining physicians follow a PHS medical examination manual. Required examinations done abroad include:

- A brief history of present and past illness.
- A chest X-ray examination for tuberculosis for persons greater than or equal to 15 years of age.
- A tuberculin skin test for persons less than 15 years of age if the person is ill or has a family member with suspected tuberculosis.

Any excludable or nonexcludable medical condition that is suspected or detected as a result of the screening examination may require a more comprehensive medical evaluation and may necessitate hospitalization or treatment before a visa is issued. Tuberculin skin testing has not been required as part of the medical examination for several reasons. First, it would be difficult to ensure quality control of testing materials and procedures. Second, there is a potential for fraudulent testing. Third, in most countries the medical examination is offered in one location and takes only 1 day. Requiring a return visit for reading a tuberculin test in 2–3 days would substantially increase the cost of the examination for the applicant (e.g., hotel stay and return travel).

Active Tuberculosis

The PHS medical examination manual specifies that the following criteria be used to diagnose "active tuberculosis": An abnormal chest radiograph or series of chest radiographs suggestive of current pulmonary tuberculosis, with or without compatible clinical symptoms, or a pathological condition suggestive of current extrapulmonary tuberculosis.

If the radiograph suggests current pulmonary tuberculosis, the panel physician is instructed to determine if a previous chest radiograph (at least 3 months old) is available for comparison. If no changes are evident from the previous film, the condition is classified as "Class B" or "Tuberculosis, not considered active," and the applicant may receive a visa and proceed to the United States. If changes are evident or if no previous film is available, the panel physician is instructed to perform two sputum smears. If both smears are negative for acid-fast bacilli (AFB), the condition is to be classified as "Class A" or "Tuberculosis, active, non-communicable for travel purposes," and the applicant is sent back to the United States Consular Officer for the determination of eligibility for a waiver of excludability. Travel is permitted for waiver cases only after negative sputum smears have been obtained on 2 consecutive days. In addition, a local health-care provider in the United States is identified in advance at the place of intended residence, and the provider's endorsement is obtained on the waiver application from the local health authority. When the immigrant or refugee with tuberculosis arrives in the United States, the quarantine officer at the port of entry notifies the local health department and instructs the immigrant or refugee to report for evaluation after reaching the final destination.

Because of limited diagnostic and therapeutic capabilities in many countries, PHS recommends that antituberculosis medications not be started abroad unless a positive smear is obtained, so that the immigrant can be evaluated in the United States by the local health-care provider and a decision made concerning the appropriate treatment regimen to be prescribed.

This procedure was designed to permit aliens with suspected tuberculosis to proceed to the United States with a minimum of delay and expense. The entire process—with its provisions for screening abroad, selected waivers of excludability, notification of arrival, and referral to the local health authority for evaluation upon reaching the destination in the United States—was designed to aid in the control of tuberculosis in the United States. However, some problems exist with the current process, as discussed in the following section.

PROBLEMS ASSOCIATED WITH CURRENT SCREENING AND FOLLOW-UP REQUIREMENTS

Aliens Enter with Active Tuberculosis That Was Missed During the Required Medical Examination

Misdiagnosis of tuberculosis may occur because of failure to correctly interpret the radiograph, poor quality of radiographs, improper performance of smear examinations, and other reasons related to equipment or technical competence. Administrative irregularities (e.g., clerical errors that occur during the visa medical examination process) may cause misclassification. Misclassification on the medical examination document may also occur as the result of intentional fraud. On occasion, there have been problems with X-ray or sputum substitutions when aliens with tuberculosis have sent someone else for the X-ray or have purchased a normal X-ray that they submitted to the panel physician instead of their own. In addition, applicants have sometimes been reluctant to produce a sputum specimen because they fear the implications of a positive result.

Finally, because a medical examination is valid for an entire year, a visa applicant who was free of tuberculosis at the time of examination may have developed tuberculosis in the interval before arriving in the United States.

Persons with Tuberculosis May Enter the United States under a Waiver but Fail to Comply with Waiver Provisions Calling for Further Examinations and/or Therapy

Active tuberculosis or suspected active tuberculosis is an excludable (Class A) condition. If an alien with tuberculosis is granted a waiver of excludability and is allowed to enter the United States, there is a requirement that medical care be sought immediately upon arrival in the United States. Local health departments are notified that an alien with tuberculosis will be arriving in the community so that appropriate evaluation can be undertaken. Despite these requirements, no federal mechanism exists for assuring that these aliens report for evaluation or comply with treatment recommendations. Although some health departments attempt to locate and refer such aliens, no federal action is taken if they do not comply.

The PHS currently notifies state or local tuberculosis control officials of the arrival of aliens with Class A or Class B tuberculosis and requests that necessary follow-up be provided within 30 days. The PHS asks for a report of the follow-up, indicating the diagnosis made by the local physician. In FY 1988, health departments returned confirmation follow-up reports for 67% of Class A arrivals and for 65% of Class B arrivals; however, the absence of a follow-up report on a tuberculosis notification does not necessarily mean that evaluations were not done.

Class A and Class B: The Classification System Does Not Accurately Distinguish Between Active and Inactive Disease

The problem is twofold. First, current procedures are not sensitive enough to identify all cases of active disease (i.e., some persons with active disease are not assigned Class A status). Second, current procedures are not specific enough to single out only those persons with active disease (i.e., some persons assigned Class A status do not have active disease).

Follow-up examinations completed in the United States reveal that 12% of the aliens assigned Class A status had active disease, and 1.2% of those assigned Class B status actually had active tuberculosis. Of the 1,161 Class A notifications in FY 1988 for which a report of follow-up was received and a diagnosis established, only 143 (12.3%) were in agreement with the overseas classification. The remaining notifications reported inactive tuberculosis (59.8%), extrapulmonary tuberculosis (0.4%), nontuberculous abnormality (13.9%), or normal (13.6%).

Of the 9,544 Class B notifications for which a report of follow-up was received and a diagnosis established, 5,603 (58.7%) were in agreement with the overseas classification. The remainder were found to be active tuberculosis (1.2%), extrapulmonary tuberculous abnormality (0.4%), nontuberculous abnormality (14.1%), or normal (25.6%).

Some Aliens Arrive in the United States with Inadequately Treated or Drug-Resistant Tuberculosis

Some applicants have had tuberculosis diagnosed before they applied for admission. Because resources for health care are severely limited in many countries where tuberculosis is highly prevalent, applicants from these countries with a history of past tuberculosis may have received delayed, inadequate, or inappropriate treatment and are at risk of relapsing with drug-resistant disease. In addition, applicants classified as having active or suspected active tuberculosis and who are not eligible for waivers must be treated abroad until rendered "not active" before a visa can be issued. Aliens who have positive sputum smears must be treated abroad until they convert to negative before a waiver can be issued. Although adequate treatment regimens are recommended in the PHS Guidelines, with the exception of certain persons with refugee status, no mechanism exists for ensuring that aliens with tuberculosis are treated in accordance with these guidelines, or that such treatment is available to them, or that they will comply. Inadequate treatment at this stage may also result in the development of drug-resistant disease or a high risk of relapse among aliens after they arrive in the United States.

Aliens in Certain Classifications May Enter the United States for Extended Periods Without Being Required to Have a Medical Evaluation for Tuberculosis

Although the Immigration and Nationality Act, Section 212(a)(1)–(6), provides for the exclusion of aliens with certain health conditions and subjects all aliens to these health exclusion provisions, PHS regulations (42 CFR, Part 34) and Department of State regulations (22 CFR, Part 41.108, and 22 CFR Part 42.66) establish which categories of aliens are routinely required to be medically examined as part of the visa application process. Currently, only aliens seeking permanent residence in the United States are required to be medically examined.

Others, such as students and exchange visitors, are examined at the discretion of a consular officer (generally when a consular officer believes an applicant may have an excludable medical condition).

Several such categories of aliens may enter the United States for protracted stays (greater than or equal to 1 year) without being required to undergo a medical examination before entry. In 1988, there were approximately 1 million such persons; they sometimes enter with active tuberculosis or develop tuberculosis while in the United States and then may infect others. College students pose a special problem because they often stay for greater than or equal to 4 years, and transmission may occur in dormitory settings.

Aliens with Tuberculosis Disease Come to the United States as Visitors Specifically to Obtain Treatment for Tuberculosis

Some aliens enter the United States as temporary visitors for the sole but undisclosed purpose of obtaining treatment for tuberculosis. Since non-immigrants are not routinely required to have a medical examination to obtain a visa, the number of such persons entering the United States is not known.

Aliens Enter the United States Infected with Tubercle Bacilli but Do Not Have Current Disease

Many tuberculosis cases in the United States occur among foreign-born persons who had asymptomatic infection but did not have current disease when they entered the United States. A large proportion of these persons are from countries where, according to available data, one-half or more of the adult population is infected and at risk of developing tuberculosis. Tuberculin skin testing is the only available method for identifying such persons.

Some Undocumented Aliens May Have Tuberculosis When They Enter the United States or May Develop it after Entry

Data are not available on the number of undocumented aliens who develop tuberculosis in the United States. The problems presented by undocumented aliens with tuberculous infection or clinical disease who illegally enter the country are much more difficult to address because (a) no mechanism exists for identifying them when they enter, and (b) they tend to avoid official public agencies because of fear of deportation.

Foreign-born Persons Who Enter the United States Often Have Language, Cultural, and Financial Adjustment Problems That Can Be Barriers to Obtaining Recommended Tuberculosis Treatment and Follow-up

Many local health departments do not have sufficient numbers of culturally sensitive outreach staff who speak foreign languages to effectively identify, follow up, and manage cases involving foreign-born patients (e.g., immigrants, refugees, and undocumented aliens).

RECOMMENDATIONS FOR IMPROVING PREVENTION AND CONTROL EFFORTS AMONG ALIENS SEEKING PERMANENT RESIDENCE IN THE UNITED STATES

The ACET supports continued tuberculosis screening for immigrants and refugees seeking entry into the United States.

IMMIGRANTS

1. Tuberculosis pre-entry screening for all immigrant visa applicants should continue to be required, including:
   a. A chest radiograph for all applicants greater than or equal to 15 years of age.
   b. A tuberculin skin test for applicants less than 15 years of age who are close contacts of

persons known to have or suspected of having tuberculosis, or if for any reason tuberculous infection is suspected.

2. All immigrant visa applicants with abnormal radiographs consistent with tuberculosis should be assigned Class A status. Although this approach will require a change in regulations, it will increase the sensitivity of the process to detect active disease (i.e., many active cases that erroneously would have been given Class B status will now be given Class A status). Follow-up work load for local health departments may increase substantially. However, the use of more standardized, rigorous, and restrictive criteria in the reading of chest radiographs as suggestive of active tuberculosis will focus the process on those persons at high risk of tuberculosis (see definition for abnormal chest radiograph). The degree to which local health departments can respond to an increased Class A work load will depend upon how well the upgraded classification procedures can reduce the number of false-positives and what priority can be given to this work load, considering available resources and other local needs.

   a. The requirement that all applicants for admission who have an abnormal chest radiograph and a positive smear for tuberculosis be started on a CDC/American Thoracic Society (CDC/ATS)-recommended antituberculosis regimen for persons at increased risk of drug-resistant disease (3) should be continued. Fully supervised therapy is strongly encouraged. After applicants have two consecutive negative sputum smears obtained on different days, the ACET recommends that they be granted a waiver of excludability and issued a visa for admission. This recommendation would require a change in law, since some of these persons are now ineligible for waivers.

   b. Other applicants who have an abnormal chest radiograph and who have had two consecutive negative sputum smears obtained on different days may be granted a waiver for conditional entry into the United States. The ACET recommends that antituberculosis medications not be started abroad unless a positive smear is obtained, so that the immigrant can be evaluated by a local health-care provider in the United States and a decision made concerning the appropriate regimen to prescribe. This recommendation would require a change in law, since some such persons are now ineligible for waivers.

   c. The recommendation to broaden the definition of Class A tuberculosis should not be implemented until legislative changes are made to broaden waiver authority. Otherwise, many persons who are now designated as having Class B tuberculosis would not be eligible for waivers.

3. Currently, immigrants with diagnosed tuberculosis or suspected tuberculosis entering the United States with a waiver of excludability (see Problems Associated With Current Screening and Follow-up Requirements: Aliens Enter With Active Tuberculosis That Was Missed During the Required Medical Examination, above) are required to make advance arrangements with a local U.S. physician provider and local health department official who agree to be responsible for necessary follow-up and treatment. Approval of this follow-up and treatment arrangement should be obtained from the official state or local health department at the site of intended residence. (Applicants known to have drug-resistant tuberculosis who are granted waivers should be identified to local health authorities and initiated on a regimen containing at least two antituberculosis drugs to which the organisms are likely to be susceptible.)

4. Quarantine officers at ports of entry should continue to notify local health departments of the arrival of immigrants who enter with a waiver, and the officers should instruct the immigrants to report to the agreed-upon health-care provider. Copies of the health department notification should be sent to the health-care provider.

5. Immigrants entering the United States with a waiver should be required to present themselves to the identified health-care provider for examination and evaluation for therapy within 10 days after arrival.

6. Providers not associated with a health department should notify local health departments within 1 week if an immigrant with an infectious case (smear-positive) undergoing treat-

ment fails to report for necessary examinations and follow-up or does not comply with therapy recommendations. For other immigrants referred for examination, providers should notify the health department within 30 days if the immigrant fails to report. The provider should also keep the health department informed on a timely basis as to the outcome of necessary examinations and the progress of treatment.

7. Immigrants who refuse to complete recommended tuberculosis treatment, after repeated attempts to encourage compliance through education, incentives, and directly supervised therapy, should be subject to the same quarantine provisions as U.S. citizens, according to state and local laws and regulations.

8. The Department of State should continue to designate physicians abroad to perform required initial medical examinations for visa applicants. The PHS should establish a written procedure for quality assurance and training concerning these examinations performed abroad and should conduct annual reviews of physician reports for accuracy and compliance with established guidelines. Written results of these reviews should be provided to the Department of State and to state and local health departments, as appropriate. Corrective action should be taken when necessary.

REFUGEES

1. The following tuberculosis screening procedures should be required for all aliens applying for refugee status:
   a. A chest radiograph for all refugees greater than or equal to 15 years of age.
   b. A chest radiograph for all Southeast Asian refugee children ages 2–14 years.
   c. A tuberculin skin test for all refugee children less than 15 years of age who are close contacts of persons known to have or suspected of having tuberculosis, or if for any reason tuberculous infection is suspected.

2. Refugees with abnormal radiographs consistent with tuberculosis should be assigned Class A status.

3. Refugees having an abnormal chest radiograph who are smear-positive and who have been approved for resettlement in the United States should be started on a CDC/ATS-recommended antituberculosis regimen for persons at increased risk of drug-resistant disease (3). Southeast Asian refugees who are required to receive English-language training and U.S. cultural orientation in overseas processing centers should continue to complete treatment, under supervision, before coming to the United States. Smear-positive refugees who receive care from designated examining physicians may be granted entry into the United States after they have been placed on a CDC/ATS-approved treatment regimen and have had two consecutive negative sputum smears obtained on consecutive days. Refugees with abnormal X-rays and negative sputum smears should be allowed to enter the United States and should be referred to the local health department for necessary evaluation, follow-up, and treatment. (Note: In many states, refugees are eligible for Medicaid assistance.)

4. Refugees less than 35 years of age from high-prevalence countries who are sent to overseas processing centers (for language training and cultural orientation) should be Mantoux-tuberculin tested, and those with positive reactions should be given a minimum of 6 months' preventive therapy for tuberculosis unless medically contraindicated. In addition, refugees greater than or equal to 35 years of age who have tuberculosis risk factors, including abnormal radiographs, should be tuberculin tested and considered for preventive therapy. The therapy regimen for tuberculin-positive refugees having abnormal chest radiographs should be initiated only after active disease has been ruled out. Refugees on preventive therapy should be monitored closely because of the possible existence of isoniazid-resistant disease in this group.

5. Refugees who enter the United States and who are known to have tuberculosis due to drug-resistant organisms should be identified to local health authorities and started on a regimen that contains at least two antituberculosis drugs to which the patient's organisms are likely to be susceptible.

6. Quarantine officers at the port of entry should continue to notify appropriate health de-

partments about all refugees who arrive in the United States, including those who have normal and abnormal chest radiographs (currently required by law).

7. Occasionally, refugees will enter the United States while on tuberculosis treatment or preventive therapy. In such instances, PHS should continue to forward this information to the appropriate health department at the site of current residence. The Department of State's Reception and Placement Cooperative Agreements specify that voluntary agencies are responsible for advising, encouraging, and assisting refugees in obtaining appropriate health screening and follow-up. Similarly, voluntary agencies should provide appropriate and timely information to state or local health departments regarding these examinations. Voluntary agency adherence to these recommendations should continue to be a part of the ongoing State Department review of initial resettlement service delivery.

8. Refugees who enter the United States and fail to comply with recommended treatment for tuberculosis should be subject to quarantine, as are U.S. citizens.

NON-IMMIGRANTS RESIDING IN THE UNITED STATES WHO REQUEST PERMANENT RESIDENCE

Section 245(a) of the Immigration and Nationality Act provides for adjustment of status in the United States to allow certain aliens who have been admitted or paroled into the United States to become permanent residents without the inconvenience and expense of having to go abroad to obtain immigrant visas. The aliens must be eligible to receive an immigrant visa and must be admissible to the United States for permanent residence, and an immigrant visa must be immediately available at the time the application is filed. Alien crewmen, aliens admitted in transit without a visa, and aliens who entered the United States without inspection are precluded by law from filing for this benefit.

The Immigration Reform and Control Act also permits certain undocumented aliens to apply for official status and permanent residency in the United States.

Applicants for adjustment of status and permanent residency in the United States should receive a Mantoux tuberculin skin test. Those with positive skin tests should receive a chest radiograph. In addition, persons with symptoms compatible with tuberculosis should receive a chest radiograph regardless of tuberculin test results. Those with active tuberculosis should be treated with a CDC/ATS-recommended antituberculosis regimen for persons at increased risk of drug-resistant disease (3). Persons less than 35 years of age with positive reactions should be given a minimum of 6 months' preventive therapy for tuberculosis unless medically contraindicated. In addition, those greater than or equal to 35 years of age who have tuberculosis risk factors, including abnormal radiographs, should be considered for preventive therapy.

Examinations should continue to be performed by physicians appointed by INS and designated as "civil surgeons." The ACET recommends that INS and CDC develop procedures for consulting with state or local health departments before designating a civil surgeon so that health department officials may help identify physicians who are willing to collaborate in tuberculosis follow-up and treatment.

RECOMMENDATIONS FOR THE SCREENING, PREVENTION, AND CONTROL OF TUBERCULOSIS AMONG FOREIGN-BORN PERSONS AFTER ARRIVAL IN THE UNITED STATES

Therapy for Infection and Disease

Immigrants and refugees less than 35 years of age who enter the United States and have a positive tuberculin test should be started on preventive therapy unless contraindicated. Those of any age having abnormal chest radiographs and who are infected but without disease should be started on preventive therapy within 30 days after their arrival unless they have a history of previous adequate therapy or unless there are medical contraindications. The preventive therapy regimen for tuberculin-positive refugees with abnormal chest radiographs should be for at least 12 months and should be initiated only after active disease has been ruled out. Preventive therapy should be monitored closely because of the possible development of drug-resistant organisms in this group. Persons with diagnosed active tuberculosis should be started on a CDC/ATS-recommended antituberculosis drug regimen for persons at risk of drug-resistant disease.

Health Departments

State and local health departments should ensure the provision of appropriate tuberculosis screening, prevention, and treatment when persons arrive in the United States from abroad. Immigrants, refugees, undocumented aliens, and other foreign-born persons who arrive in the United States often have linguistic, cultural, financial, or other barriers that impede their taking medication as prescribed or seeking necessary health care. Failure to seek appropriate examinations and treatment may lead to the spread of tuberculous infection in the United States. For this reason, these barriers to compliance must be addressed by health department officials when designing and providing tuberculosis services for the foreign-born. Many health departments have refugee health-care programs that can serve as models for providing tuberculosis-related services to all foreign-born persons, not just refugees. Such programs use outreach workers hired from the same cultural/ethnic/linguistic background as the patient populations they serve. These outreach staff members work closely with community, religious, and other organizations to set up appropriate screening and referral activities. They also work with individual patients to ensure necessary examinations and to provide directly observed therapy. Often, these outreach staff members work through government and community organizations to solve individual and family problems that hinder compliance (e.g., assist in providing housing, food stamps, transportation, and employment). All health departments that serve large numbers of foreign-born persons should have outreach workers for this purpose. Compliance should be further encouraged by health departments' use of incentives and enhancers for selected patients (e.g., cab fare, bus tokens, and child care). Effective health department record and follow-up systems must also be in place to ensure effective prevention and control procedures for new arrivals in the United States. To carry out these recommendations, health departments serving large numbers of refugees, immigrants, and other entrants will require additional outreach resources. In the United States, the Federal Government determines immigration policies; however, the impact of immigration is not felt equally by all states. A few states and many cities are heavily impacted by tuberculosis among the foreign-born. The ACET feels that the whole nation is responsible for helping heavily impacted areas deal with the problem and thus recommends that specific federal resources be made available for this purpose.

Local and state health departments, as part of routine tuberculosis-control activities, should analyze tuberculosis-morbidity patterns among foreign-born populations, including undocumented aliens. Screening and prevention activities should be carried out in identified high-risk groups. To facilitate this screening, the INS should set up a procedure to provide, when requested by state health departments, information on all new immigrants including the person's age, sex, family unit, and destination address, and the originating country. Health departments should work with community leaders and other organizations in planning programs to reach these groups. To encourage participation in such programs, health departments should provide free services and should not question the immigration status of participants. Since these recommended activities will substantially increase the work load for many health departments, resources should be identified to carry them out. Health departments should also work with other groups or individuals who provide health-care services to foreign-born persons and should encourage them—through training, consultation, and the provision of supplies—to carry out programs for tuberculosis screening and preventive therapy.

Health departments should make every effort to provide direct observation of tuberculosis therapy and preventive therapy prescribed for foreign-born persons after they arrive in the United States. Directly observed therapy should take place at a convenient location for the patient. The first choice should be the tuberculosis clinic or a satellite office of the health department, but if the patient is unable to come there, arrangements should be made for the therapy to be given elsewhere (e.g., the patient's residence or worksite). Culturally sensitive outreach workers who speak the same language as the new arrivals should be hired and trained to work with these persons. Responsibility for directly observing therapy should not be given to a family member or friend.

Schools and Colleges

Programs should be established by state and local governments or universities and colleges to make tuberculin-test screening mandatory for foreign-born students, their family members, and others who accompany foreign-born students entering the country. Requirements should state that the tuberculin test, reading, and initiation of appropriate follow-up and treatment should be completed within the first 6 weeks that a student starts school. Arrangements should be made for tuberculin-positive students to complete a full course of tuberculosis-preventive therapy unless medically contraindicated.

Programs should be established throughout the United States to require tuberculin-test screening at the preschool, elementary, and secondary levels for foreign-born students who enter the United States. Arrangements should be made for tuberculin-positive students to complete a full course of tuberculosis-preventive therapy unless medically contraindicated.

Medical-Care Providers

Medical-care providers, including those in community health centers and migrant and occupational health-care programs, should tuberculin test foreign-born persons under their care. Those with positive tuberculin reactions should receive preventive therapy unless it is contraindicated.

ORGANIZATIONAL GUIDELINES

Domestic

Regional staff of both INS and CDC should convene regional and subregional meetings among state and local health departments and INS staff at immigration entry points. These meetings should address operational issues relating to instructions given to Class A arrivals, the flow of information (e.g., implementing the recommendations listed above), information given to other foreign-born arrivals about tuberculosis, and other pertinent matters. CDC and INS should also promote the development of interagency cooperative programs at the local level that are tailored to local circumstances. The local staff should be instructed that time committed to such cooperative programs is a legitimate and priority use of staff resources.

International

The Office of the Assistant Secretary for Health, with input from appropriate components of the Department of Health and Human Services (e.g., the Office of International Health and CDC) should explore with the Department of State (including the Agency for International Development and the Peace Corps) and international health organizations (e.g., the World Health Organization, the Pan American Health Organization, and the International Union Against Tuberculosis) opportunities to upgrade the standards and levels of tuberculosis control programs. Particular attention—especially in the areas of quality assurance and training—should be given to the countries from which most immigrants may be expected over the next 10–20 years (e.g., Mexico, the Philippines, and selected Southeast Asian countries).

The ACET recommends that all foreign-born persons applying for permanent entry into the United States continue to be screened for disease. Deficiencies in the current screening methods should be corrected. The policy requiring that persons found to have infectious tuberculosis (known or suspected) be prevented from entering the country until treatment has rendered them noninfectious should be continued; however, persons with noninfectious tuberculosis should be permitted to enter the United States. Tuberculin skin testing and preventive therapy programs for foreign-born persons must be expanded both overseas and domestically if the goal of eliminating tuberculosis from the United States by the year 2010 is to be met.

REFERENCE: AS NUMBERED IN ORIGINAL PUBLICATION

3. American Thoracic Society/CDC. Treatment of tuberculosis and tuberculosis infection in adults and children. Am Rev Respir Dis 1986;134:355–363.

TOPIC 30 / **TYPHOID**

Typhoid Immunization

Original Citation: ACIP. Typhoid immunization recommendations of the Advisory Committee on Immunization Practices (ACIP). MMWR 1994;43(RR-14):1–7.

Original Authors: Paul R. Cieslak, MD, Robert V. Tauxe, MD, MPH, John C. Watson, MD, MPH.

SUMMARY

These revised recommendations of the Advisory Committee on Immunization Practices update previous recommendations (MMWR 1990;39[RR-10]:1–5). They include information on the Vi capsular polysaccharide (ViCPS) vaccine, which was not available when the previous recommendations were published.

INTRODUCTION

The incidence of typhoid fever declined steadily in the United States from 1900 to 1960 and has since remained low. From 1975 through 1984, the average number of cases reported annually was 464. During that period, 57% of reported cases occurred among persons greater than or equal to 20 years of age; 62% of reported cases occurred among persons who had traveled to other countries. From 1967 through 1976, only 33% of reported cases occurred among travelers to other countries (1).

TYPHOID VACCINES

Three typhoid vaccines are currently available for use in the United States: (a) an oral live-attenuated vaccine (Vivotif Berna-TM vaccine, manufactured from the Ty21a strain of Salmonella typhi (2) by the Swiss Serum and Vaccine Institute); (b) a parenteral heat-phenol-inactivated vaccine that has been widely used for many years (Typhoid Vaccine, manufactured by Wyeth- Ayerst); and (c) a newly licensed capsular polysaccharide vaccine for parenteral use (Typhim Vi, manufactured by Pasteur Merieux). A fourth vaccine, an acetone-inactivated parenteral vaccine, is currently available only to the armed forces.

Although no prospective, randomized trials comparing any of the three U.S.-licensed typhoid vaccines have been conducted, several field trials have demonstrated the efficacy of each vaccine. In controlled field trials conducted among schoolchildren in Chile, three doses of the Ty21a vaccine in enteric-coated capsules administered on alternate days reduced laboratory-confirmed infection by 66% over a period of 5 years (95% confidence interval [CI] = 50%–77%) (3, 4). In a subsequent trial in Chile, efficacy appeared to be lower: three doses resulted in only 33% (95% CI = 0%–57%) fewer cases of laboratory-confirmed infection over a period of 3 years. When the data were stratified by age in this trial, children greater than or equal to 10 years of age had a 53% reduction in incidence of culture-confirmed typhoid fever (95% CI = 7%–77%), whereas children 5–9 years of age had only a 17% reduction (95% CI = 0%–53%). This difference in age-related efficacy, however, is not statistically significant (5). In another trial in Chile, a significant decrease in the incidence of clinical typhoid fever occurred among persons receiving four doses of vaccine compared with persons receiving two (p less than 0.001) or three (p = 0.002) doses. Because no placebo group was included in this trial, absolute vaccine efficacy could not be calculated (6). Weekly and triweekly dosing regimens have been less effective than alternate-day dosing (3). A liquid formulation of Ty21a is more effective than enteric-coated capsules (5, 7, 8), but only enteric-coated capsules are available in the United States. The efficacy of vaccination with Ty21a has not been studied among persons from areas without endemic disease who travel to disease-endemic regions. The mechanism by which Ty21a vaccine confers protection is unknown; however, the vaccine does elicit both serum (2, 9) and intestinal (10) antibodies and cell-mediated immune responses (11). Vaccine organisms can be shed transiently in the stool of vaccine recipients (2, 9). However, secondary transmission of vaccine organisms has not been documented. In field trials involving a primary series of two doses of heat-phenol-inactivated typhoid vaccine (which is similar to the currently available parenteral inactivated vaccine), vaccine efficacy over the 2- to 3-year follow-up periods ranged from 51% to 77% (12–14). Efficacy for the acetone-inactivated parenteral vaccine, available only to the armed forces, ranges from 75% to 94% (12, 14, 15).

The newly licensed parenteral vaccine (Vi capsular polysaccharide [ViCPS]) is composed of purified Vi ("virulence") antigen, the capsular polysaccharide elaborated by S. typhi isolated from blood cultures (16). In recent studies, one 25-μg injection of purified ViCPS produced seroconversion (i.e., at least a four-fold rise in antibody titers) in 93% of healthy U.S. adults (17); similar results were observed in Europe (18). Two field trials in disease-endemic areas have demonstrated the efficacy of ViCPS in preventing typhoid fever. In a trial in Nepal, in which vaccine recipients were observed for 20 months, one dose of ViCPS among persons 5–44 years of age resulted in 74% (95% CI = 49%–87%) fewer cases of typhoid fever confirmed by blood culture than occurred with controls (19). In a trial involving schoolchildren in South Africa who were 5–15 years of age, one dose of ViCPS resulted in 55% (95% CI = 30%–71%) fewer cases of blood-culture-confirmed typhoid fever over a period of 3 years than occurred with controls. The reduction in the number of cases in years 1, 2, and 3, was 61%, 52%, and 50%, respectively (20, 21). The efficacy of vaccination with ViCPS has not been studied among persons from areas without endemic disease who travel to disease-endemic regions or among children less than 5 years of age. ViCPS has not been tested among children less than 1 year of age.

VACCINE USAGE

Routine typhoid vaccination is not recommended in the United States. However, vaccination is indicated for the following groups:

- Travelers to areas in which there is a recognized risk of exposure to S. typhi. Risk is greatest for travelers to developing countries (e.g., countries in Latin America, Asia, and Africa) who have prolonged exposure to potentially contaminated food and drink (22). Multidrug-resistant strains of S. typhi have become common in some areas of the world (e.g., the Indian subcontinent [23] and the Arabian peninsula [24, 25]), and cases of typhoid fever that are treated with ineffective drugs can be fatal. Travelers should be cautioned that typhoid vaccination is not a substitute for careful selection of food and drink. Typhoid vaccines are not 100% effective, and the vaccine's protection can be overwhelmed by large inocula of S. typhi.
- Persons with intimate exposure (e.g., household contact) to a documented S. typhi carrier.
- Microbiology laboratorians who work frequently with S. typhi (26).

Routine vaccination of sewage sanitation workers is not warranted in the United States and is indicated only for persons living in typhoid-endemic areas. Also, typhoid vaccine is not indicated for persons attending rural summer camps or living in areas in which natural disasters (e.g., floods) have occurred (27). No evidence has indicated that typhoid vaccine is useful in controlling common-source outbreaks.

CHOICE OF VACCINE

The parenteral inactivated vaccine causes substantially more adverse reactions but is no more effective than Ty21a or ViCPS. Thus, when not contraindicated, either oral Ty21a or parenteral ViCPS is preferable. Each of the three vaccines approved by the Food and Drug Administration has a different lower age limit for use among children (Table 1). In addition, the time required for primary vaccination differs for each vaccine. Primary vaccination with ViCPS can be ac-

Table 1. Dosage and schedules for typhoid fever vaccination

Vaccination	Age	Dose/mode of administration	Dosage Number of doses	Dosage Interval between doses	Boosting interval
Oral live-attenuated Ty21a vaccine					
Primary series	6 yrs	1 capsule*	4	2 days	—
Booster	≥6 yrs	1 capsule*	4	2 days	every 5 yrs
Vi capsular polysaccharide vaccine					
Primary series	≥2 yrs	0.50 mL$^+$	1	—	—
Booster	≥2 yrs	0.50 mL$^+$	1	—	every 2 yrs
Heat-phenol inactivated parenteral vaccine					
Primary series	6 mos–10 yrs	0.25 ml$^&$	2	≥4 wks	—
	≥10 yrs	0.50 mL$^&$	2	≥4 wks	—
Booster	6 mos–10 yrs	0.25 mL$^&$	1	—	every 3 yrs
	≥10 yrs	0.50 mL$^&$	1	—	every 3 yrs
	≥6 mos	0.10 mL$^@$	1	—	every 3 yrs

*Each orally administered capsule contains 2–6 × 10 (sup) 9 viable S. typhi Ty21a and 5–50 × 10 (sup) 9 nonviable S. typhi Ty21a.

$^+$Intramuscularly.

$^&$Subcutaneously.

$^@$Intradermally.

—Not applicable.

complished with a single injection, whereas 1 week is required for Ty21a, and 4 weeks are required to complete a primary series for parenteral inactivated vaccine (Table 1). Finally, the live-attenuated Ty21a vaccine should not be used for immunocompromised persons or persons taking antibiotics at the time of vaccination (see Precautions and Contraindications).

VACCINE ADMINISTRATION

Ty21a

Primary vaccination with live-attenuated Ty21a vaccine consists of one enteric-coated capsule taken on alternate days for a total of four capsules. The capsules must be kept refrigerated (not frozen), and all four doses must be taken to achieve maximum efficacy (6). Each capsule should be taken with cool liquid no warmer than 37°C (98.6°F), approximately 1 hour before a meal. Although adverse reactions to Ty21a are uncommon among children 1–5 years of age (28,29), data are unavailable regarding efficacy for this age group. This vaccine has not been studied among children less than 1 year of age. The vaccine manufacturer recommends that Ty21a not be administered to children less than 6 years of age.

ViCPS

Primary vaccination with ViCPS consists of one 0.5-mL (25-µg) dose administered intramuscularly. This vaccine has not been studied among children less than 1 year of age. The vaccine manufacturer does not recommend the vaccine for children less than 2 years of age.

Parenteral Inactivated Vaccine

Primary vaccination with parenteral inactivated vaccine consists of two 0.5-mL subcutaneous injections, each containing approximately 5×10^8 killed bacteria, separated by greater than or equal to 4 weeks. The vaccine manufacturer does not recommend the vaccine for use among children less than 6 months of age. If the two doses of parenteral inactivated vaccine cannot be separated by greater than or equal to 4 weeks because of time constraints, common practice has been to administer three doses of the vaccine at weekly intervals in the volumes listed above. Vaccines administered according to this schedule may be less effective, however.

Booster Doses

If continued or repeated exposure to S. typhi is expected, booster doses of vaccine are required to maintain immunity after vaccination with parenteral typhoid vaccines (Table 1). The ViCPS manufacturer recommends a booster dose every 2 years after the primary dose if continued or renewed exposure is expected. In a study in which efficacy was not examined, revaccination of U.S. adults at either 27 or 34 months after the primary vaccination increased mean antibody titers to the approximate levels achieved with the primary dose (17). The optimal booster schedule for persons administered Ty21a for primary vaccination has not been determined; however, the longest reported follow-up study of vaccine trial subjects indicated that efficacy continued for 5 years after vaccination (4). The manufacturer of Ty21a recommends revaccination with the entire four-dose series every 5 years if continued or renewed exposure to S. typhi is expected. This recommendation may change as more data become available about the period of protection produced by the Ty21a vaccine. If the parenteral inactivated vaccine is used initially, booster doses should be administered every 3 years if continued or renewed exposure is expected. A single booster dose of parenteral inactivated vaccine is sufficient, even if greater than 3 years have elapsed since the prior vaccination. When the heat-phenol-inactivated vaccine is used for booster vaccination, the intradermal route causes less reaction than the subcutaneous route (30). The acetone-inactivated vaccine should not be administered intradermally or by jet-injector gun because of the potential for severe local reactions (31).

No information has been reported concerning the use of one vaccine as a booster after primary vaccination with a different vaccine. However, using either the series of four doses of Ty21a or one dose of ViCPS for persons previously vaccinated with parenteral vaccine is a reasonable alternative to administration of a booster dose of parenteral inactivated vaccine.

ADVERSE REACTIONS

Ty21a produces fewer adverse reactions than either ViCPS or the parenteral inactivated vaccine. During volunteer studies and field trials with oral live-attenuated Ty21a vaccine, side effects were rare and consisted of abdominal discomfort, nausea, vomiting, fever, headache, and rash or urticaria (2, 7, 32) (Table 2). In placebo-controlled trials, monitored adverse reactions occurred with equal frequency among groups receiving vaccine and placebo.

In several trials, ViCPS produced fever (occurring in 0%–1% of vaccinees), headache (1.5%–3% of vaccinees), and erythema or induration greater than or equal to 1 cm (7% of vaccinees) (17, 20, 33) (Table 2). In the study conducted in Nepal, the ViCPS vaccine produced fewer local and systemic reactions than did the control (the 23-valent pneumococcal vaccine) (19). Among schoolchildren in South Africa, ViCPS produced less erythema and induration than did the control bivalent meningococcal vaccine (20). In a direct comparison, ViCPS produced reactions less than half as frequently as parenteral inactivated vaccine, probably because ViCPS contains negligible amounts of bacterial lipopolysaccharide (33).

Parenteral inactivated vaccines produce several systemic and local adverse reactions, including fever (occurring in 6.7%–24% of vaccinees), headache (9%–10% of vaccinees), and severe local pain and/or swelling (3%–35% of vaccinees) (Table 2); 21%–23% of vaccinees missed work or school because of adverse reactions (12, 13, 34). More severe reactions, including hypotension, chest pain, and shock, have been reported sporadically.

Table 2. Common adverse reactions of typhoid fever vaccines

| Vaccine | Reactions | | |
	Fever	Headache	Local reactions
Ty21a*	0%–5%	0%–5%	Not applicable
ViCPS	0%–1%	1.5%–3%	Erythema or induration ≥1 cm: 7%
Parenteral inactivated	6.7%–24%	9%–10%	Severe local pain or swelling: 3%–35%

*The side effects of Ty21a are rare and mainly consist of abdominal discomfort, nausea, vomiting, and rash or urticaria.

PRECAUTIONS AND CONTRAINDICATIONS

The theoretical possibility for decreased immunogenicity when Ty21a, a live bacterial vaccine, is administered concurrently with immunoglobulin, antimalarials, or viral vaccines has caused concern (35). However, because Ty21a is immunogenic even in persons with preexisting antibody titers (29), its immunogenicity should not be affected by simultaneous administration of immunoglobulin. Mefloquine can inhibit the growth of the live Ty21a strain in vitro; if this antimalarial is administered, vaccination with Ty21a should be delayed for 24 hours. The minimum inhibitory concentration of chloroquine for Ty21a is greater than 256 $\mu g/mL$; this antimalarial should not affect the immunogenicity of Ty21a (36, 37). The vaccine manufacturer advises that Ty21a should not be administered to persons receiving sulfonamides or other antimicrobial agents; Ty21a should be administered greater than or equal to 24 hours after an antimicrobial dose. No data exist on the immunogenicity of Ty21a when administered concurrently or within 30 days of viral vaccines (e.g., oral polio, measles/mumps/rubella, or yellow fever vaccines). In the absence of such data, if typhoid vaccination is warranted, it should not be delayed because of the administration of viral vaccines. No data have been reported on the use of any of the three typhoid vaccines among pregnant women. Live-attenuated Ty21a should not be used among immunocompromised persons, including those persons known to be infected with human immunodeficiency virus. The two available parenteral vaccines present theoretically safer alternatives for this group. The only contraindication to vaccination with either ViCPS or with parenteral inactivated vaccine is a history of severe local or systemic reactions following a previous dose.

REFERENCES

1. Ryan CA, Hargrett-Bean NT, Blake PA. Salmonella typhi infections in the United States, 1975–1984: increasing role of foreign travel. Rev Infect Dis 1989;11:1–8.
2. Gilman RH, Hornick RB, Woodward WE, et al. Evaluation of a UDP-glucose-4-epimeraseless mutant of Salmonella typhi as a live oral vaccine. J Infect Dis 1977;136:717–723.
3. Levine MM, Ferreccio C, Black RE, Germanier R, Chilean Typhoid Committee. Large-scale field trial of Ty21a live oral typhoid vaccine in enteric-coated capsule formulation. Lancet 1987;329:1049–1052.
4. Levine MM, Taylor DN, Ferreccio C. Typhoid vaccines come of age. Pediatr Infect Dis J 1989;8:374–381.
5. Levine MM, Ferreccio C, Cryz S, Ortiz E. Comparison of enteric-coated capsules and liquid formulation of Ty21a typhoid vaccine in randomised controlled field trial. Lancet 1990;336:891–894.
6. Ferreccio C, Levine MM, Rodriguez H, Contreras R, Chilean Typhoid Committee. Comparative efficacy of two, three, or four doses of TY21a live oral typhoid vaccine in enteric-coated capsules: a field trial in an endemic area. J Infect Dis 1989;159:766–769.
7. Simanjuntak CH, Paleologo FP, Punjabi NH, et al. Oral immunisation against typhoid fever in Indonesia with Ty21a vaccine. Lancet 1991;338:1055–1059.
8. Wahdan MH, Serie C, Cerisier Y, Sallam S, Germanier R. A controlled field trial of live Salmonella typhi strain Ty 21a oral vaccine against typhoid: three-year results. J Infect Dis 1982;145:292–295.
9. Hornick RB, Dupont HL, Levine MM, et al. Efficacy of a live oral typhoid vaccine in human volunteers. Dev Biol Stand 1976;33:89–92.
10. Cancellieri V, Fara GM. Demonstration of specific IgA in human feces after immunization with live Ty21a Salmonella typhi vaccine. J Infect Dis 1985;151:482–484.
11. Murphy JR, Baqar S, Munoz C, et al. Characteristics of humoral and cellular immunity to Salmonella typhi in residents of typhoid-endemic and typhoid-free regions. J Infect Dis 1987;156:1005–1009.
12. Yugoslav Typhoid Commission. A controlled field trial of the effectiveness of acetone-dried and inactivated and heat-phenol-inactivated typhoid vaccines in Yugoslavia. Bull WHO 1964;30:623–630.
13. Hejfec LB, Salmin LV, Lejtman MZ, et al. A controlled field trial and laboratory study of five typhoid vaccines in the USSR. Bull WHO 1966;34:321–329.
14. Ashcroft MT, Singh B, Nicholson CC, Ritchie JM, Sobryan E, Williams F. A seven-year field trial of two typhoid vaccines in Guyana. Lancet 1967;290:1056–1059.
15. Polish Typhoid Committee. Controlled field trials and laboratory studies on the effectiveness of typhoid vaccines in Poland, 1961–64. Bull WHO 1966;34:211–222.
16. Robbins JD, Robbins JB. Reexamination of the protective role of the capsular polysaccharide (Vi antigen) of Salmonella typhi. J Infect Dis 1984;150:436–449.
17. Keitel WA, Bond NL, Zahradnik JM, Cramton TA, Robbins JB. Clinical and serological responses following primary and booster immunization with Salmonella typhi Vi capsular polysaccharide vaccines. Vaccine 1994;12:195–199.
18. Ambrosch F, Fritzell B, Gregor J, et al. Combined vaccination against yellow fever and typhoid fever: a comparative trial. Vaccine 1994;12:625–628.
19. Acharya IL, Lowe CU, Thapa R, et al. Prevention of typhoid fever in Nepal with the Vi capsular polysaccharide of Salmonella typhi. N Engl J Med 1987;317:1101–1104.
20. Klugman KP, Gilbertson IT, Koornhof HJ, et al. Protective activity of Vi capsular polysaccharide vaccine against typhoid fever. Lancet 1987;330:1165–1169.

21. 21Klugman KP, Koornhof HJ, Robbins JB. Immunogenicity and protective efficacy of Vi vaccine against typhoid fever three years after immunization [Abstract]. Bangkok, Thailand: Second Asia-Pacific Symposium on Typhoid Fever and Other Salmonellosis, 1994.
22. Edelman R, Levine MM. Summary of an international workshop on typhoid fever. Rev Infect Dis 1986;8:329–349.
23. Rao PS, Rajashekar V, Varghese GK, Shivananda PG. Emergence of multidrug-resistant Salmonella typhi in rural southern India. Am J Trop Med Hyg 1993;48:108–111.
24. Wallace M, Yousif AA. Spread of multiresistant Salmonella typhi [Letter]. Lancet 1990;336:1065–1066.
25. Elshafie SS, Rafay AM. Chloramphenicol-resistant typhoid fever—an emerging problem in Oman. Scand J Infect Dis 1992;24:819–820.
26. Blaser MJ, Hickman FW, Farmer III JJ, Brenner DJ, Balows A, Feldman RA. Salmonella typhi: the laboratory as a reservoir of infection. J Infect Dis 1980;142:934–938.
27. Blake PA. Communicable disease control. In: Gregg MB, ed. The public health consequences of disasters. Atlanta: US Department of Health and Human Services, Public Health Service, CDC, 1989:7–12.
28. Murphy JR, Grez L, Schlesinger L, et al. Immunogenicity of Salmonella typhi Ty21a vaccine for young children. Infect Immun 1991;59:4291–4293.
29. Cryz SJ, Vanprapar N, Thisyakorn U, et al. Safety and immunogenicity of Salmonella-typhi Ty21a vaccine in young Thai children. Infect Immun 1993;61:1149–1151.
30. Iwarson S, Larsson P. Intradermal versus subcutaneous immunization with typhoid vaccine. J Hyg (Lond) 1978;84:11–16.
31. Edwards EA, Johnson DP, Pierce WE, Peckinpaugh RO. Reactions and serologic responses to monovalent acetone-inactivated typhoid vaccine and heat-killed TAB when given by jet-injection. Bull WHO 1974;51:501–505.
32. Cryz SJ Jr. Post-marketing experience with live oral Ty21a vaccine [Letter]. Lancet 1993;341:49–50.
33. Cumberland NS, Roberts JS, Arnold WSG, Patel RK, Bowker CH. Typhoid Vi: a less reactogenic vaccine. J Int Med Res 1992;20:247–253.
34. Ashcroft MT, Ritchie JM, Nicholson CC. Controlled field trial in British Guiana school children of heat-killed-phenolized and acetone-killed lyophilized typhoid vaccines. Amer J Hyg 1964;79:196–206.
35. Wolfe MS. Precautions with oral live typhoid (Ty 21a) vaccine [Letter]. Lancet 1990;336:631–632.
36. Brachman PS, Metchock B, Kozarsky PE. Effects of antimalarial chemoprophylactic agents on the viability of the Ty21a typhoid vaccine strain [Letter]. Clin Infect Dis 1992;15:1057–1058.
37. Horowitz H, Carbonaro CA. Inhibition of the Salmonella-typhi oral vaccine strain, Ty21a, by mefloquine and chloroquine [Letter]. J Infect Dis 1992;166:1462–1464.

TOPIC 31 / **VARICELLA**

Varicella

Original Citation: Varicella—U.S. Department of Health and Human Services, Public Health Services, Centers for Disease Control and Prevention, National Center for Prevention Services. Publication date: 12/01/1992.

HISTORY

Varicella (chickenpox) was not reliably distinguished from smallpox until the end of the 19th century. Herpes zoster (shingles) has been recognized since ancient times and was described in the early medical literature. Clinical observations of the relationship between varicella and herpes zoster were made in 1888 by Von Bokay, when susceptible children acquired varicella after contact with herpes zoster. Varicella virus (VZV) was isolated from vesicular fluid of both chickenpox and zoster lesions in cell culture by Weller in 1954. Subsequent laboratory studies of the virus have led to the development of a live attenuated varicella vaccine, Oka strain, in Japan in the 1970s. The vaccine has been shown to be safe and effective in healthy and immunocompromised children, and healthy adults. It will soon be licensed in the U.S., probably for use in healthy children.

VARICELLA ZOSTER VIRUS

VZV is a member of the herpes virus group, (alpha) herpes virus 3. It is a DNA virus. VZV has the capacity to persist as a latent infection in dorsal root or extra medullary cranial ganglia.

EPIDEMIOLOGY

Infectiousness

- Varicella is highly contagious (less so than measles, but more so than mumps and rubella), with secondary attack rates in susceptible household contacts of up to 90%.
- Virtually all persons in the U.S. acquire varicella by adulthood; thus, the number of cases occurring annually should approximate the U.S. birth cohort (3.5 to 4 million).

Epidemiologic Characteristics

- Varicella is endemic in the U.S. and has a seasonal fluctuation, with the highest incidence occurring in winter and early spring.
- Between 150,000 to 200,000 cases of varicella are reported annually to the Centers for Disease Control and Prevention (CDC), representing 4%–6% of all cases.
- Varicella is notifiable in approximately 33 reporting areas in the U.S.
- The majority of cases, approximately 90%, occur in children less than 15 years of age. The highest attack rates are in children 5 to 9 years of age, who represent 60% of all cases.
- By adulthood, 90%–95% of the U.S. population have antibodies to varicella.
- In the tropics, varicella occurs more often in adults; thus, immigrants from these areas are more likely to be susceptible than the remainder of the population at comparable ages.

Morbidity and Mortality

- Normal children usually have a relatively benign course.
- Complications are most likely to occur in the immunocompromised, newborns whose mothers develop rash close to the time of delivery, and adults.
- Approximately 40 to 90 deaths due to varicella are reported each year. The majority of these are in normal persons.

Herpes Zoster

- Reflects reactivation of latent VZV infection.
- Reactivation is associated with aging, immunosuppression, in utero exposure to varicella, and postnatal varicella occurring before 18 months of age.
- Approximately 300,000 cases are estimated to occur annually, and 5% are recurrences. No seasonal variation is known.
- Herpes zoster is not a notifiable condition.
- In the immunocompromised, zoster can disseminate, causing generalized skin lesions, and central nervous system (CNS), pulmonary, and hepatic involvement.

PATHOGENESIS AND SPREAD

Mode of Transmission

- Person to person—Via direct contact with vesicular fluid or via droplets from respiratory tract secretions.
- Airborne—Via aerosolized droplet nuclei.
- Indirect contact—For example, via articles containing fresh discharges of vesicular lesions.

Reservoir: Humans

Incubation Period

- The average length is 14 to 16 days from exposure, with a range of 10 to 21 days. This may be prolonged in immunocompromised patients and those who have received varicella zoster immune globulin (VZIG). The incubation period may be up to 28 days after VZIG.

Period of Communicability

- Extends from 1 to 2 days before the onset of rash through the first 5 to 6 days after rash onset. Immunocompromised patients with progressive varicella are probably contagious during the entire period new lesions are appearing. The virus has not been isolated from crusted lesions.

Mild and Inapparent Infections Occur Rarely (<5% of Infections)

Immunity Following Primary Infection Is Considered Long-lasting

- However, reexposure may lead to reinfection with boosts in antibody titers, usually without clinically apparent illness or detectable viremia.
- Path of entry of the virus into the susceptible host is assumed to be the upper respiratory tract

CLINICAL MANIFESTATIONS

- Prodrome—Adults may have 1 to 2 days of fever and malaise prior to rash onset, but in children the rash is often the first sign of disease.
- Rash—The rash is generalized, pruritic, and rapidly progresses from macules to papules to vesicular lesions before crusting. Lesions are usually 1 to 4 mm in diameter; the vesicles contain clear fluid on a erythematous base that may rupture or become purulent before they dry and crust. Successive crops appear over several days, with lesions present in several stages of maturity. The rash begins on the scalp, moves to the trunk, and then the extremities. Lesions also can occur on mucous membranes of the oropharynx, respiratory tract, vagina, conjunctiva, and the cornea.
- Other—The clinical course in normal children is typically benign, with mild malaise, pruritus, and fever up to 102°F for 2 to 3 days. Adults may have more marked systemic symptoms and they have a higher incidence of complications.
- Zoster—The vesicular eruption of zoster generally occurs unilaterally in the distribution of the dermatomes supplied by a dorsal root or extramedullary cranial nerve sensory ganglion. Most often, this involves the trunk or the area of cranial nerve V. Two to four days prior to the eruption there may be pain and paresthesia in the segment involved. There are few systemic symptoms. Post-herpetic neuralgia is a distressing complication of zoster, with no adequate therapy currently available. Ocular nerve and other organ involvement with zoster can occur, often with severe sequelae. Maternal varicella infection during pregnancy can lead to herpes zoster in the first year of life.

COMPLICATIONS

Varicella in Normal Children

- Low risk of complications.
- Accounts for >90% of cases, 75% of all varicella hospitalizations, 70% of cases of encephalitis, 40% to 60% of all deaths, and virtually 100% of Reye Syndrome cases.
- Most common complication is secondary bacterial infection of cutaneous lesions.
- CNS Complications: (a) Encephalitis (estimated rate = 1.7/100,000): Cerebellar ataxia is most common, and is associated with a good outcome; diffuse cerebral involvement is less common in children. (b) Reye Syndrome: Recent dramatic decrease in the incidence has occurred, presumably related to decreased use of aspirin in children. (c) Rare: Aseptic meningitis, transverse myelitis, and Guillain-Barré syndrome.
- Pneumonia: Viral or bacterial, more frequent in adults.
- Infrequent complications: Thrombocytopenia, hemorrhagic varicella, purpura fulminans, glomerulonephritis, myocarditis, arthritis, orchitis, uveitis, iritis, and clinical hepatitis.

Normal Adults

- Have a higher risk of complications than normal children.
- Less than 2% of reported cases are in persons > or equal to 20 years of age, but account for approximately 25% of mortality.
- Pneumonia: Case fatality rates of up to 30%.
- Diffuse cerebral encephalitis is more likely to affect adults than children, and has a case fatality rate of up to 37%.
- Hospitalization rate approximately 14–18/1,000 cases compared with 1–2/1,000 cases in normal children.

Immunocompromised Persons (i.e., Persons with Congenital or Acquired Immune Deficiencies, Malignancies, or on Immunosuppressive Therapy)

- Immunocompromised persons have a high risk of serious varicella infection.
- Immunocompromised persons have a high risk of disseminated disease (up to 36% in one report), resulting in multiple organ system involvement, often becoming fulminant and hemorrhagic.
- Most frequent complications include pneumonia and encephalitis.

- Increased risk of death; 7% in one report, however, this preceded the widespread use of VZIG and acyclovir and may not reflect current experience.

Congenital Infection

- Primary varicella infection in the first 16 weeks of gestation is rarely associated with a recognized constellation of abnormalities: low birth weight, hypoplasia of an extremity, cicatricial skin scarring, localized muscular atrophy, encephalitis, cortical atrophy, chorioretinitis, and microcephaly.
- Risk of congenital birth defects from primary maternal varicella infection during the first trimester is felt to be very low (1%–2%).
- Rare reports of congenital birth defects following maternal zoster exist; however, virologic confirmation of maternal lesions was lacking.
- Infection in utero with varicella, particularly after 20 weeks gestation, is associated with zoster in those infants at an earlier age; the exact risk is unknown.

Neonatal Infection Due to Maternal Chickenpox Close to Time of Delivery

- The onset of maternal varicella from 5 days before to 2 days after delivery may result in severe infection of the neonate (in an estimated 17% to 30%) and an estimated case fatality rate of 31% in the first 5 to 10 days of life.
- Fetal exposure to varicella virus without protection from sufficient maternal antibody results in severe disease.
- Infants born to mothers with onset of maternal varicella 5 days or more prior to delivery usually have a benign course, presumably due to passive transfer of sufficient maternal antibody.

Infants After Postnatal Exposure

- Normal full-term infants with normal birth weight are unlikely to develop serious complications.
- Premature infants may have medical conditions that put them at increased risk for serious varicella illness and those born before 28 weeks of gestation may not have received adequate maternal antibody.

Pregnancy

There is growing evidence that infection during pregnancy carries increased risk for serious varicella. Further study is needed.

Death

- Risk in normal children: approximately 1/100,000; in normal infants: approximately 6/100,000.
- Risk in normal adults: approximately 12/100,000.
- Risk in leukemics is higher than in normal children and has been reported at 7%.
- Risk for newborns (who do not receive VZIG) from maternal chickenpox close to time of delivery is estimated at 31%.
- Majority of deaths occur in normal individuals.

DIFFERENTIAL DIAGNOSIS

Chickenpox is associated with a very characteristic vesicular rash illness—"Your grandmother could diagnose it" (Fehrs, 1990). A history of chickenpox has been shown to be a reliable indicator of immunity; however, a lack of such history is not as reliable and does not always correlate with lack of immunity.

The differential diagnosis for chickenpox includes:

- Herpes simplex.
- Disseminated infection in the immunocompromised or neonate.
- Eczema herpeticum, vesicular lesions occur in the areas of eczematous involvement.
- Zoster-like lesions.

Enteroviral Infections

Papulovesicular lesions occur on palms and soles, with vesicular lesions on the buccal mucosa; usually self-limited.

Impetigo

Erythematous macules progress to vesiculopustular lesions that dry and crust. The infection can spread. Exposed areas such as the face, neck, and limbs are often involved. Skin breaks serve as the portal of entry. Group A Streptococcus is usually the etiologic agent, but superinfection by staphylococci often occurs.

Rickettsialpox

- Generalized erythematous papulovesicular lesions occur on the palms, soles, and mucous membranes after the bite of a house mouse mite, Liponyssoides sanguineus (the vector).
- A black scab occurs at the bite.
- Systemic disease consists of chills, fever, headache, myalgia, photophobia, and adenopathy. It is self-limited, nonfatal, and noncommunicable.

LABORATORY DIAGNOSIS

Not routinely required, but useful if confirmation of diagnosis or determination of susceptibility is necessary.

Viral Isolation

- Source—vesicular fluid; difficult to isolate from the respiratory tract.
- Tissue culture isolation.
- Vesicular scrapings (Tzanck smear) can identify multi-nucleated giant cells, consistent with VZV and herpes simplex virus (HSV) infection. In some instances, stains of vesicular scrapings may be tested using a fluorescent monoclonal antibody test which is very sensitive and specific.

Serologic Testing

- Antibody Tests
- Complement fixation (CF): Commercially available, but lacks sensitivity.
- Neutralization test (NT): Sensitive and specific; time consuming and difficult to perform; not readily available.
- Immunofluorescence assay for antibody to VZV-induced membrane antigen (FAMA): sensitive, time consuming, not readily available.
- Immune adherence hemagglutination (IAHA) sensitive; not readily available.
- Enzyme-linked immunosorbent assay (ELISA): Sensitive, simple, and commercially available; may be useful for routine testing.
- Cell Mediated Immunity
- Lymphocyte proliferative response to VZV antigen.
- Skin test antigen: Not commercially available.
- In normal individuals, the presence of detectable antibody can be considered evidence of immunity to VZV.
- Antibody levels in immunocompromised persons may be unreliable predictors of immunity, as they may reflect passively acquired antibody from blood products. Clinical varicella has developed in these persons. Laboratory tests must be interpreted cautiously in this population. History of prior chickenpox may be a more important indicator of immunity.

CURRENT METHODS OF CONTROL AND PREVENTION

VZIG

- Licensed in 1981.
- Prepared from plasma of normal blood donors with high antibody titers to VZV.
- Available from the American Red Cross.
- If administered within 96 hours of exposure, can modify or prevent clinical varicella and prevent complications or death, especially in susceptible immunocompromised individuals.

Indications for Use

Individuals with Significant Exposure

Continuous household contact; playmate contact of over an hour; hospital contact in the same 2- to 4-bed room, or prolonged direct contact; newborn of mother who had onset of varicella 5 days before to 2 days after delivery.

Individuals at Risk for Complications

- Immunocompromised children: Those with immune deficiencies, neoplastic disease, or on immunosuppressive therapy.
- Newborns of mothers with varicella onset 5 days before to 2 days after delivery.
- Premature infants with postnatal exposure:
- Those born > or equal to 28 weeks gestation and up to term, and > or equal to 1,000 grams; mother not immune.
- Those born <28 weeks or <1000 grams birth-weight, regardless of maternal history.
- Immunocompromised adults: If susceptible and have a history of significant exposure.
- Normal adults and pregnant females: Consider the type of exposure, susceptibility, risks for complications, and cost.
- No evidence that VZIG will prevent congenital varicella.

Dose

- 125 units/IO kg, up to a maximum of 625 units (five vials), IM. Volume 125 units per 1.25 ml (one vial). (Higher doses can be considered for immunosuppressed persons).
- Should be given within 96 hours of exposure, preferably as soon as possible.
- The administration of VZIG may prolong the incubation period of varicella to as long as 28 days post-exposure.

Special Varicella Zoster Exposure Situations

- Hospital personnel—If susceptible, with significant exposure, workers should be relieved from direct patient contact from day 10 to day 21 after exposure. If workers develop chickenpox, varicella lesions must be crusted before they should return to direct patient contact. Receipt of VZIG does not change this recommendation for reassignment. Since VZIG can prolong the incubation period, the period of removal from direct patient contact should be lengthened to 28 days after exposure.
- Newborn with maternal rash onset 5 days before to 2 days after delivery. Since about 50% of infants who receive VZIG will develop varicella, if these infants remain hospitalized beyond age 10 days, they should be kept in strict isolation until age 21 days.

Antiviral Therapy

- Acyclovir—The Advisory Committee on Immunization Practices (ACIP) has not set policy concerning acyclovir. The policy of the American Academy of Pediatrics (AAP) includes: Not routinely recommended for uncomplicated varicella in healthy children. Should be considered in individuals at high risk for severe varicella or complications.
- Healthy nonpregnant individuals 13 years of age or older.
- Children over 12 months of age with a chronic cutaneous or pulmonary disorder, or salicylate therapy.
- Children receiving short, intermittent or aerosolized courses of corticosteroids. If immunocompromised, intravenous administration is indicated.

Corticosteroids should be discontinued, if possible, after exposure. Dosage: Should be started within the first 24 hours of onset of rash, 20 mg/kg four times a day for 5 days, maximum 800 mg four times per day. Adequate fluid intake should be maintained. Intravenous acyclovir is recommended for primary varicella or recurrent zoster in immunocompromised children and for viral-mediated complications of varicella in normal individuals. Oral acyclovir is not recommended for pregnant women with uncomplicated varicella. Intravenous acyclovir should be considered in pregnant women with serious viral-mediated complications of varicella. Acyclovir should not be used prophylactically in normal children exposed to varicella to prevent infection or illness.

- Adenine Arabinoside (ara-A).
- Interferon—Currently under investigation.

VARICELLA VACCINE

Characteristics

- Oka strain.
- Vaccine virus isolated from vesicular fluid from a healthy child.
- Attenuated by passage 30 to 33 times in human diploid cells and guinea pig fibroblasts.
- Live attenuated vaccine developed in Japan in the early 1970s.
- Licensed for general use in Japan and Korea and in high-risk individuals in a number of European countries.
- Vaccine has been administered to over 15,000 people in Japan and the U.S., including healthy children, healthy adults, children with acute lymphocytic leukemia (ALL), and other immunocompromised patients.

See Table 1, Efficacy in Children.

Table 1. Efficacy In Children

	Normal Children	Children With ALL
1. Immunologic Response		
Humoral (seroconversion		One dose: 88%
rate)	94%–100%	Two doses: 98%
Cellular	>90%	Data difficult to interpret
2. Clinical Efficacy		
Pre-exposure	85%–95%	85% with 2 doses
3. Duration of Immunity		
Antibody	>90% (up to 3–10 years)	50%–80%
Cellular		Frequently lost
(Cell mediated)	90%	antibody
Cellular		
(Positive skin testing)	90%	90%
4. Breakthrough infections (about 2%/year in first few years post vaccination) are generally mild, with few skin lesions, and do not result in dissemination or serious illness.		

Normal Adults

- Seroconversion only 82% with one dose, 94% with two doses.
- Effective vaccination may require two doses.
- Efficacy of two doses only approximately 65%–70% after household exposure.
- Breakthrough infectious are mild, with few skin lesions, and do not result in dissemination of serious illness.

Adverse Events Following Varicella Vaccination

Normal Children/Adults.

- Rash.
  1. 4%–10%.
  2. Usually <50 lesions.
  3. Often maculopapular rather than vesicular.
- Injection site lesions, swelling, pain.
- System reactions rare.
- Reactivation (zoster)
  1. Adults: 1/302 at 3 years (wild-type virus isolated).
  2. Normal children:
     a. Six cases reported.
     b. 1.4/10,000 person-years (vs. 8/10,000 following natural disease).
     c. No virus isolated.

Children with acute lymphoblastic leukemia (ALL).

- Rash more frequent.
  1. Occurs in up to 40%.
  2. More frequent in patients:
     a. With recent steroid therapy.
     b. Receiving first dose.
     c. With no suspension of chemotherapy.
- Reactivation (zoster).
  1. May be less frequent than following natural disease (Hardy I, Gershon AA, Steinberg SP, LaRussa P, Varicella Vaccine Collaborative Study Group. The incidence of zoster after immunization with live attenuated varicella vaccine. A study in children with leukemia. N Engl J Med 1991;325[22]:1545–1550.)
  2. No severe illness or dissemination reported.
  3. More common in those with initial vaccine-related rash.
  4. Vaccine virus isolated.

Transmission of Varicella Vaccine Virus

- Transmission from normal recent vaccinees.
- No secondary clinical illnesses reported.
- <1% asymptomatic seroconversion documented in susceptible contacts (Weibel).
- Transmission from children with ALL.
- Only from recent vaccinees with rash.
- Transmission rate from those with post-vaccination rash is 9%–28%.
- Vaccine virus isolated from secondary cases.

- One case of tertiary transmission.
- Transmission has been documented from persons who initially seroconverted after vaccination but nevertheless developed mild breakthrough infection later.

Summary

- The vaccine appears to be safe and effective.
- Vaccination prevents illness in normal individuals.
- Vaccination prevents serious complications in the immunocompromised.
- Persistent immunity is produced in almost all normal vaccinees.
- Immunocompromised persons and adults may require two doses of vaccine.
- The risk for zoster appears to be less than the risk following natural varicella.
- Antibody levels following simultaneous administration of the vaccine with measles-mumps-rubella (MMR) at 15 months of age are similar to those detected when the vaccines are given alone.

COST/BENEFIT ANALYSIS

- Annual cost of caring for normal children estimated to be $400 million; 95% of costs are associated with wages lost when parents must provide home care of an ill child.
- Vaccine given with MMR at 15 months could reduce costs by 66%; benefit to cost ratio 6.9:1.

VARICELLA-ZOSTER IMMUNE GLOBULIN: REGIONAL DISTRIBUTION CENTERS

Service Area	Regional Center and 24-Hour Telephone
United States and territories	
Alabama	American Red Cross Blood Services
	Alabama Region (205) 322-5661
Alaska	(see Oregon)
Arizona	American Red Cross Blood Services
	Southern Arizona Region (602) 623-0541
Arkansas	(see Missouri)
California, northern	American Red Cross Blood Services
	L.A.-Orange Counties Region (213) 739-5200
Colorado	(see N. Mexico)
Connecticut	American Red Cross Blood Services
	Connecticut Region (203) 678-2730
Delaware	(see Pennsylvania)
Florida	South Florida Blood Service (305) 326-8888
	American Red Cross Blood Services
	Mid-Florida Region (904) 255-5444
Georgia	American Red Cross Blood Services
	Atlanta Region (404) 881-9800 (404) 881-6752 (night)
Hawaii	(see California, Southern)
Idaho	American Red Cross Blood Services
	Mid-America Region (312) 440-2222
Illinois, southern	(see Missouri)
Indiana	American Red Cross Blood Services
	Fort Wayne Region (219) 482-3781
Iowa	(see Wisconsin, S.E.)
Kansas	(see Missouri)
Kentucky	(see Missouri)
Louisiana	(see Texas [Gulf Coast])
Maine	American Red Cross Blood Services
	Northeast Region (207) 775-2367
Maryland	American Red Cross Blood Services
	(301) 764-4639 (also see Washington, DC)
Massachusetts	Massachusetts Public Health
	United States Biologics Laboratories (617) 522-3700
Michigan	American Red Cross Blood Services

	Southeastern Michigan Region (313) 494-2715
	American Red Cross Blood Services Wolverine Region
	(313) 232-1176
	American Red Cross Blood Services Great Lakes Region
	(517) 484-7461
Minnesota	American Red Cross Blood Services
	St. Paul Region (612) 291-6789 (612) 291-6767 (night)
Mississippi	(see Alabama)
Missouri	American Red Cross Blood Services
	(314) 658-2000 (314) 658-2136 (night)
Montana	(see Oregon)
Nebraska	American Red Cross Blood Services
	Midwest Region (402) 341-2723
Nevada	(see California, northern)
New Hampshire	(see Vermont)
New Jersey, northern	(see Greater New York Blood Program)
New Jersey, southern	(see Pennsylvania)
New Mexico	United Blood Services (505) 247-9831
New York	The Greater New York Blood Program
	(212) 468-2106 (212) 570-3068 (night)
	American Red Cross Blood Services
	Northeastern New York Region
	(518) 449-5020 or (518)462-7461 (518) 462-6964 (night)
	American Red Cross Blood Services Greater Buffalo Chapter
	(716) 886-6866
	American Red Cross Blood Services Rochester Region
	(716) 461-9800
	American Red Cross Blood Services Syracuse Region
	(315) 425-1647
North Carolina	American Red Cross Blood Services Carolinas Region
	(704) 376-1661
North Dakota	(see Wisconsin, S.E.)
Ohio	American Red Cross Blood Services
	Northern Ohio Region (216) 781-1800
	American Red Cross Blood Services Central Ohio Region
	(614) 253-7981
Oklahoma	(see Texas Gulf Coast)
Oregon	American Red Cross Blood Services Pacific Northwest Region
	(503) 243-5286
Puerto Rico	American Red Cross Servicio de Sangre Capitulo
	(809) 759-7979
Pennsylvania	American Red Cross Blood Services Penn-Jersey Region
	(215) 299-4126
Rhode Island	Rhode Island Blood Center (401) 863-8368
South Carolina	American Red Cross Blood Services South Carolina Region
	(803) 256-2301
South Dakota	(see Wisconsin, S.E.)
Tennessee	American Red Cross Nashville Region (6154) 327-1931,
	ext. 315
Texas	Gulf Coast Regional Blood Center (713) 791-6250
	American Red Cross Blood Services Central Texas Region
	(817) 776-8754
	American Red Cross Blood Services Red River Region
	(817) 322-8686
Utah	(see California, northern)
Vermont	American Red Cross Blood Services
	Vermont-New Hampshire Region (802) 658-6400, ext 217
Virginia	(also see Washington, DC)
	American Red Cross Blood Services Tidewater Region
	(804) 446-7709
	Richmond Metropolitan Blood Service (804) 359-5100
	ARC Blood Services Appalachian region (703) 985-3595
Washington	Puget Sound Blood Center (206) 292-6525
Washington, DC	American Red Cross Blood Services Washington Region
West Virginia	(see Washington, DC)

Wisconsin	The Blood Center of S.E. Wisconsin (414) 933-5000
	American Red Cross Blood Services Badger Region
	(608) 255-0021
Wyoming	(see California, northern)

Other countries

Canada	Canadian Red Cross Blood Transfusion Service National Office
	(416) 923-6692
Central and South America	South Florida Community Blood Center (305) 326-8888
All other countries	American Red Cross Blood Services Northeast Region
	(617) 449-0773
	American Red Cross Blood Services Blood Services
	(617) 731-2130

VARICELLA WORKSHOP

1. Which statement about varicella is not true?
    A. Varicella is highly contagious.
    B. Varicella is a notifiable disease in all states.
    C. Most adults are immune to varicella.
    D. Airborne transmission of varicella can occur.
2. Which statement about herpes zoster or shingles is not true?
    A. Zoster represents reactivation of latent varicella infection.
    B. About 5% of zoster episodes are recurrences of zoster.
    C. No seasonal variation in zoster is known.
    D. CDC receives reports of herpes zoster from states.
3. What is the incubation period for chickenpox?
4. If someone, such as a health care worker, is susceptible to varicella and is exposed to the disease, when should they be considered at risk for developing chickenpox and exposing others?
5. In the case in question 4, if the exposed person received VZIG, what effect would this treatment have on the incubation period? On recommendations for preventing exposure of high-risk persons to this person?
6. Which of the following is NOT true regarding varicella?
    A. The period of communicability (for normal persons) extends from 1 to 2 days before onset of the rash through the first 5 to 6 days after rash onset.
    B. Varicella zoster immune globulin (VZIG) is indicated for a healthy full-term infant who is exposed to chickenpox at home at age 2 weeks.
    C. Varicella vaccine is less immunogenic and effective in normal adults than in normal children, although it does prevent serious disease in this group.
    D. Herpes zoster is a reactivation of latent varicella infection.
    E. Normal adults have a higher risk of complications from the disease than do normal children.

Questions 7–16: Indicate whether the following persons should receive VZIG and why:

7. The normal newborn whose mother develops a varicella rash on the day of delivery.
    A. ____ Yes   B. ____ No   C. ____ VZIG should be considered
8. The normal newborn whose mother developed a rash 10 days before delivery.
    A. ____ Yes   B. ____ No   C. ____ VZIG should be considered
9. The 1500 g infant born at 30 weeks gestation who is exposed in the nursery to chickenpox.
    A. ____ Yes   B. ____ No   C. ____ VZIG should be considered
10. The infant born at 27 weeks gestation who is exposed to chickenpox in the nursery but whose mother is sure she had chickenpox several years ago, when she was in college.
    A. ____ Yes   B. ____ No   C. ____ VZIG should be considered
11. The pregnant woman who is exposed to a household member with chickenpox and whose doctor wants to protect her against the risk of complications of varicella in pregnancy.
    A. ____ Yes   B. ____ No   C. ____ VZIG should be considered
12. The pregnant woman who is exposed in the first trimester to a household member with varicella and who wants VZIG in order to protect her fetus against infection.
    A. ____ Yes   B. ____ No   C. ____ VZIG should be considered
13. The immunocompromised adult who is significantly exposed to varicella.
    A. ____ Yes   B. ____ No   C. ____ VZIG should be considered

14. The normal adult who is exposed to chickenpox and has no memory of ever having had chickenpox.
    A. ____ Yes B. ____ No C. ____ VZIG should be considered
15. The high-risk patient who was exposed to varicella 8 days ago.
    A. ____ Yes B. ____ No C. ____ VZIG should be considered
16. The susceptible high-risk patient who was exposed to varicella 3 days ago and whose doctor is unsuccessful in reaching CDC to obtain VZIG.
    A. ____ Yes B. ____ No C. ____ VZIG should be considered
17. What age group is currently most likely to develop chickenpox?
18. Name groups which have a higher risk for complications of varicella than do normal children.
19. For which persons is Merck Sharp & Dohme seeking FDA licensure of varicella vaccine?
20. Which of the following has not been observed following vaccination in trials of varicella vaccine in normal and immunocompromised children?
    A. Vaccine-associated rash associated with a low rate of transmission of vaccine virus
    B. Vaccine-associated fever
    C. Pain at injection site
    D. Zoster due to reactivation of vaccine virus
    E. Severe complications

Varicella Workshop Answers—

1. Which statement about varicella is not true?
   A. Varicella is highly contagious.
   B. Varicella is a notifiable disease in all states.
   C. Most adults are immune to varicella.
   D. Airborne transmission of varicella can occur.

Answer: B—Varicella is a notifiable disease in fewer states (less than 70%) than are measles, mumps, or rubella. This fact and the fact that many cases of varicella are mild and never come to medical attention contribute to the low rate of reporting of varicella to the CDC—only 4%–6% of the estimated annual total of U.S. cases.

2. Which statement about herpes zoster or shingles is not true?
   A. Zoster represents reactivation of latent varicella infection.
   B. About 5% of zoster episodes are recurrences of zoster.
   C. No seasonal variation in zoster is known.
   D. CDC receives reports of herpes zoster from states.

Answer: D—Unlike cases of primary varicella (or chickenpox), cases of herpes zoster are not tracked by the CDC through routine notifiable disease surveillance in States.

3. What is the incubation period for chickenpox?

Answer: An average of 14–16 days, with a range of 10–21 days.

4. If someone, such as a health care worker, is susceptible to varicella and is exposed to the disease, when should they be considered at risk for developing chickenpox and exposing others?

Answer: During the period of 10–21 days after exposure. This is the period during which they should not be in contact with susceptible persons at high risk for complications from varicella.

5. In the case in question 4, if the exposed person received VZIG, what effect would this treatment have on the incubation period? On recommendations for preventing exposure of high-risk persons to this person?

Answer: The incubation period could be lengthened to as long as 28 days. Therefore, the exposed person should not be in contact with susceptible persons at high risk for varicella complications during the period from 10 to 28 days post-exposure.

6. Which of the following is NOT true regarding varicella?
   A. The period of communicability (for normal persons) extends from 1 to 2 days before onset of the rash through the first 5 to 6 days after rash onset.
   B. Varicella zoster immune globulin (VZIG) is indicated for a healthy full-term infant who is exposed to chickenpox at home at age 2 weeks.

    C. Varicella vaccine is less immunogenic and effective in normal adults than in normal children, although it does prevent serious disease in this group.

    D. Herpes zoster is a reactivation of latent varicella infection. E. Normal adults have a higher risk of complications from the disease than do normal children.

Answer: B—Use of VZIG for infants and children is reserved primarily for susceptible, immunocompromised children after significant exposure. It is not indicated for healthy, normal-term infants, who are not known to be at any greater risk from complications of chickenpox than older children.

Questions 7–16: Indicate whether the following persons should receive VZIG and why:

    7. The normal newborn whose mother develops a varicella rash the day of delivery.

Answer: A—YES. This infant is likely to develop serious neonatal varicella because it was exposed in utero to varicella virus when the mother was viremic but was born before sufficient maternal antibody could be produced, transferred transplacentally, and moderate disease in the infant.

    8. The normal newborn whose mother developed a rash 10 days before delivery.

Answer: B—NO. This infant should have received maternal anti-body in utero and should have mild or no disease. Only infants whose mothers develop rash 5 days before to 2 days after delivery are at high-risk for serious varicella.

    9. The 1500 g infant born at 30 weeks gestation who is exposed in the nursery to chickenpox.

Answer: C—VZIG should be considered. Since this infant weighs > or equal to 1000 g and was born at > or equal to 28 weeks gestation, VZIG does not need to be given if there is a good maternal history of chickenpox, even though this infant is premature. If the mother does not have a history of chickenpox, VZIG should be given.

    10. The infant born at 27 weeks gestation who is exposed to chickenpox in the nursery but whose mother is sure she had chickenpox several years ago, when she was in college.

Answer: A—YES. Even though the mother should be immune to chickenpox, since the infant may have been born before maternal antibody was transferred transplacentally, the ACIP and AAP recommend that VZIG be given.

    11. The pregnant woman who is exposed to a household member with chickenpox and whose doctor wants to protect her against the risk of complications varicella in pregnancy.

Answer: C—VZIG should be considered. It is unclear if pregnant women have a higher risk for complications from varicella than do non- pregnant adults; however, adults do have a higher risk of complications than do children. Some obstetricians will administer VZIG to exposed pregnant women if adequate resources and time are available, especially if the exposure was high, as occurs within households.

    12. The pregnant woman who is exposed in the first trimester to a household member with varicella and who wants VZIG in order to protect her fetus against infection.

Answer: B—NO. There is no evidence that the administration of VZIG will prevent fetal infection. However, some obstetricians will give VZIG for a different reason (see above). The pregnant exposed women should be reassured that congenital varicella syndrome is rare and results from exposure during the first 16 weeks of pregnancy only.

    13. The immunocompromised adult who is significantly exposed to varicella.

Answer: C—VZIG should be considered. VZIG should be given if the adult does not have a carefully obtained history of varicella or has serologic evidence of lack of immunity.

    14. The normal adult who is exposed to chickenpox and has no memory of ever having had chickenpox.

Answer: C—VZIG should be considered. VZIG is expensive and not routinely recommended by the ACIP for such adults. However, since adults do have a higher rate of complications with varicella than do children, some physicians will offer adults the option of receiving VZIG.

    15. The high-risk patient who was exposed to varicella 8 days ago.

Answer: B—NO. VZIG should be administered within 96 hours of exposure. In this case, the patient would probably be treated with an anti-viral agent, such as acyclovir, at the first sign of illness.

16. The susceptible high-risk patient who was exposed to varicella 3 days ago and whose doctor is unsuccessful in reaching CDC to obtain VZIG.

Answer: A—YES. VZIG is obtained from the local American Red Cross, not from CDC.

17. What age group is currently most likely to develop chickenpox?

Answer: School-aged children, especially children 5–9 years of age.

18. Name groups which have a higher risk than do normal children for complications of varicella.

Answer:—Immunocompromised patients (including persons with AIDS).
   • Adults.
   • Newborns whose mothers develop a varicella rash 5 days before to 2 days after delivery.
   • Premature infants.
   • Normal infants under age 1 year (who have a lower risk than newborns with neonatal exposure but a higher risk than older children).
   • Pregnant women, possibly.

19. For which persons is Merck Sharp & Dohme seeking FDA licensure of varicella vaccine?

Answer: Children over 12 months of age and adults.

20. Which of the following have not been observed following vaccination in trials of varicella vaccine in normal and immunocompromised children?
   A. Vaccine-associated rash associated with a low rate of transmission of vaccine virus?
   B. Vaccine-associated fever.
   C. Pain at injection site.
   D. Zoster due to reactivation of vaccine virus.
   E. Severe complications.

Answer: E—Severe complications. While a few immunocompromised vaccines have developed extensive rashes similar to wild-type infection, no reports of serious complications or death due to vaccine infection exist.

TOPIC 32 / **VECTOR-BORNE DISEASES**

Vector-Borne Diseases (Lyme Disease, Japanese Encephalitis, Yellow Fever)

Original Citation: Vector-borne diseases (Lyme disease, Japanese encephalitis, Yellow Fever)—Centers for Disease Control and Prevention, Division of Vector-Borne Infectious Diseases, Fort Collins, CO, 1991.

GENERAL FACTS ABOUT LYME DISEASE AND ITS TRANSMISSION

Lyme disease is a bacterial infection caused by the bites of certain, very small, infected ticks.

Lyme disease can be diagnosed in the laboratory by isolating the bacteria or by detecting antibodies against the bacteria in blood. The first method, isolation of the bacteria, is difficult, and is frequently only done in research situations. Detecting antibodies in blood is the most common test performed. The detection of antibodies in blood is reliable in chronic cases of Lyme disease, but is frequently not positive in the early stages of illness. Research to remedy this problem is underway.

If you and your physician are concerned about the accuracy of your Lyme disease test results, your state health department laboratory can act as a reference laboratory to assist you.

Treatment of Lyme Disease

If your symptoms are diagnosed as due to Lyme disease, your physician will prescribe an antibiotic for treatment. The antibiotic he chooses for your treatment will usually be in one of four general groups; a penicillin, a cephalosporin, a tetracycline or a macrolide (erythromycin, azithromycin). The antibiotic chosen will depend on a number of factors such as allergic history, age, pregnancy, and stage of disease. Antibiotics may be given orally, intravenously or possibly intramuscularly as determined by your physician.

The response of patients to treatment for chronic Lyme disease is variable.

If a person has had untreated Lyme disease for many years, damage to the nervous system or joints may require a prolonged period for repair after the infection has been eradicated. In some instances, treatment seems to have little or no beneficial effect.

Prevention of Lyme Disease

The only certain way to prevent Lyme disease is to avoid all situations of exposure to infected ticks. For many people, this is not possible or is not acceptable. In these situations, there are a number of steps you can take which will greatly reduce your chances of acquiring Lyme disease.

1. Wear long pants. Tuck pants legs into long socks or seal pants legs with masking tape or rubber bands.
2. Spray a permethrin-containing tick repellent on clothes as directed by the manufacturer.
3. Use a repellent containing the compound DEET on your skin areas that are exposed except for the face area. Follow label directions carefully, and be especially cautious when using DEET on children.
4. Check your entire body carefully for ticks twice a day, including inspection of the neck and scalp. If you are alone, the use of a fine tooth comb will help locate adult ticks in your scalp.
5. Remove attached ticks from your skin immediately with tweezers by grasping the tick's mouth parts as close to your skin as possible. Do not attempt to get ticks out of your skin by burning them or coating them with anything such as nail polish remover or petroleum jelly. If you remove a tick before it has been attached for more than 24 hours, you greatly reduce your risk of infection.
6. There is presently no human vaccine commercially available for protection against Lyme disease.

Lyme Disease in Pregnancy and in Nursing Mothers

There is currently very limited information about Lyme disease infection during pregnancy. Presently there is no conclusive evidence that Lyme disease produces an increase in spontaneous abortions, stillbirths, or fetal abnormalities. Although not confirmed by cultural isolation, there have been several reports of the Lyme bacteria being found in stillborns, and in infants born with severe abnormalities. Therefore, pregnant women should be promptly treated if suspected of having been infected.

There is also no direct evidence to date that nursing mothers infected with Lyme disease transmit infection through their milk. If a nursing mother is suspected of being infected, she should be treated with an appropriate antibiotic other than a tetracycline. Nursing is not contraindicated during treatment.

JAPANESE ENCEPHALITIS VACCINE

The vaccine for Japanese encephalitis (JE) is commercially available in the United States and is distributed by Connaught Laboratories Inc. (JEVAX)

The ACIP does not recommend the vaccine for routine travel to Asia. The vaccine is recommended for expatriates and persons who will work or have extensive visits during the transmission season to rural areas of countries where JE is endemic. Risk of acquiring Japanese encephalitis is proportional to exposure to the mosquitos that breed chiefly in rural rice-growing and pig farming regions. Therefore, risk is low among persons whose itineraries are limited to cities or who will travel to the countryside for short periods (<30 days).

The vaccine is given in 3 doses on days, 0, 7 and 14 and protection can be expected 10 days following the last dose. No serious permanent side effects are known to be associated with the vaccine. Fever and local reactions such as redness, swelling and pain are reported in fewer than 10% of those vaccinated.

Because of the potential for other mosquito-borne diseases in Asia, all travelers, but particularly those who are unable to obtain Japanese encephalitis vaccine, are advised to use precautions to avoid mosquito bites. The mosquitoes which transmit Japanese encephalitis feed chiefly outdoors from dusk to dawn. Travelers are advised to minimize outdoor exposure at these times, to wear mosquito repellents containing DEET as an active ingredient, and to stay in air-conditioned or well-screened rooms. Travelers should bring a bed net, which can be obtained at army-navy surplus stores, and aerosol room insecticides to kill indoor mosquitoes. Repellents containing DEET should be used with care on children, because of the potential for neurological side effects.

Contraindications

There are some contraindications to the vaccine. The manufacturer recommends that the vaccine not be administered to the following persons:

- Those acutely ill or with active infections.
- Persons with heart, kidney, or liver disorders.
- Persons with generalized cancerous malignancies such as leukemia, lymphoma.
- Persons with a history of hypersensitivities.
- Pregnant women.

YELLOW FEVER VACCINE REQUIREMENTS

Yellow fever vaccine is the only vaccine that may be required for entry into certain countries in Africa and South America. After immunization an International

Certificate of Vaccination is issued and will meet entry requirements for all persons traveling to or arriving from countries where there is active or a potential for yellow fever transmission. The Certificate is good for 10 years. Most countries will accept a medical waiver for persons with a medical contraindication to vaccination (e.g., infants less than 4 months old, pregnant women, persons hypersensitive to eggs, or those with an immunosuppressed condition. CDC recommends obtaining written waivers from consular or embassy officials before departure.

The CDC maintains a 24-hour-a-day International Travelers Hotline where doctors or travelers can receive vaccine requirements based on their travel itineraries. Alternately, persons can contact state or local health departments for the most recent recommendations.

Vaccine is obtained from Yellow Fever Vaccine Centers designated by your state health department.

Yellow fever vaccine is a live attenuated viral vaccine. A single dose confers long-lived immunity lasting 10 years or more. Administration of immune globulin does not interfere with the antibody response to yellow fever vaccine. For some individuals, there are precautions and contraindications associated with this vaccine, and you are encouraged to listen to that section of these messages.

Contraindications

The vaccine generally is associated with few side effects: fewer than 5% of vaccinees develop mild headache, muscle pain, or other minor symptoms 5 to 10 days after vaccination.

However, three groups of individuals should not receive the vaccine, and a fourth group should be closely evaluated. The three groups contraindicated for the vaccine are:

1. Yellow fever vaccine should never be given to infants under 4 months of age due to a risk of developing viral encephalitis. In most cases, vaccination should be deferred until 9 to 12 months of age.
2. Pregnant women should not be vaccinated because of a theoretical risk that the developing fetus may become infected from the vaccine.
3. Persons hypersensitive to eggs should not receive the vaccine because it is prepared in embryonated eggs. If vaccination of a traveler with a questionable history of egg hypersensitivity is considered essential, an intradermal test dose may be administered under close medical supervision.

A fourth group should be closely evaluated before administering the vaccine:

1. Persons with an immunosuppressed condition associated with AIDS or HIV infection, or those with their immune system altered by either diseases such as leukemia and lymphoma or through drugs and radiation should not receive the vaccine. People with asymptomatic HIV infection may be vaccinated if exposure to yellow fever cannot be avoided.

In all cases, the decision to immunize an infant between 5 and 9 months of age, a pregnant woman, or an immunocompromised patient should be made on an individual basis. The physician should weigh the risks of exposure and contracting the disease, against the risks of immunization, and possibly consider alternative means of protection.

Most countries will accept a medical waiver for persons with a medical contraindication to vaccination. CDC recommends obtaining written waivers from consular or embassy officials before departure. Travelers should contact the embassy or consulate for specific advice. Typically, a physician's letter stating the contraindication for vaccination and written on letterhead stationery is required by the embassy or consulate.

ST. LOUIS ENCEPHALITIS

There are no drugs and no vaccines that can prevent or treat the disease. The best form of prevention is to avoid outdoor activity at night, especially at dusk and dawn when the mosquitoes are most active, and to repair screens on houses to prevent entry of mosquitoes indoors. While outdoors, wear clothing that completely covers the skin, and use mosquito repellents on clothing and any exposed skin. Repellents containing DEET are the most effective; however, they should always be used according to label directions. Use DEET sparingly on children, because in rare cases, DEET has caused seizures in children.

TOPIC 33 / YELLOW FEVER

Yellow Fever Vaccine

Original Citation: Yellow fever vaccine—recommendations of the Immunization Practices Advisory Committee (ACIP). MMWR 1990;39(No. RR-6).

These revised Immunization Practices Advisory Committee (ACIP) recommendations on yellow fever vaccine update previous recommendations (MMWR 1984;32:679–688). Changes have been made to clarify (a) the risks of acquiring yellow fever associated with travel to endemic areas, (b) the precautions necessary for vaccination of special groups (immunosuppressed individuals, infants, pregnant women), and (c) simultaneous administration of cholera vaccine and other vaccines.

INTRODUCTION

Yellow fever presently occurs only in Africa and South America. Two forms of yellow fever—urban and jungle—are epidemiologically distinguishable. Clinically and etiologically they are identical (1, 2).

Urban yellow fever is an epidemic viral disease of humans transmitted from infected to susceptible persons by Aedes aegypti mosquitoes, which breed in domestic and peridomestic containers (e.g., water jars, barrels, drums, tires, tin cans) and thus in close association with humans. In areas where Ae. aegypti has been eliminated or suppressed, urban yellow fever has disappeared. In the early 1900s, eradication of Ae. aegypti in a number of countries, notably Panama, Brazil, Ecuador, Peru, Bolivia, Paraguay, Uruguay, and Argentina, led to the disappearance of urban yellow fever. The last documented Ae. aegypti-borne yellow fever epidemic in the western hemisphere occurred in Trinidad in 1954. Ae. aegypti is suspected to have played a role in transmission in outbreaks occurring in Bolivia in 1989 and 1990, but that role was not proven. However, periodic reinfestations of some countries have occurred in recent years (Brazil, Bolivia, Ecuador, Panama). Other countries remain infested, including areas of Venezuela, Colombia, and the Guyanas, which include enzootic areas for jungle yellow fever. In West Africa, Ae. aegypti-transmitted epidemics continue to occur and involve human populations both in towns and in rural villages (3).

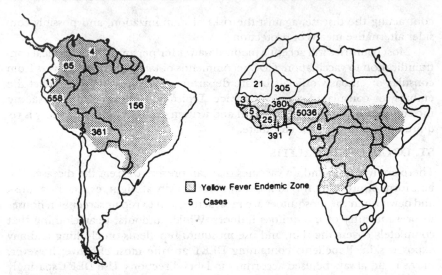

Figure 1. Yellow fever endemic zones in Americas and Africa; number of yellow fever cases reported to the World Health Organization,1980–1987.

Jungle yellow fever is an enzootic viral disease transmitted among nonhuman primate hosts by various mosquito vectors. It is currently observed only in forest-savannah zones of tropical Africa and in forested areas of South America but occasionally extends into parts of Central America and the island of Trinidad. In South America, approximately 100–300 cases are reported annually, mainly among men with occupational exposures in forested areas; however, the disease is believed to be greatly underreported. In Africa, epidemics involving tree-hole-breeding mosquito vectors affect tens of thousands of persons at intervals of a few years, but few cases are officially reported. Sometimes the disease is not detected in an area for years but then will reappear. Delineation of affected areas depends on surveillance of animal reservoirs and vectors, accurate diagnosis, and prompt reporting of all human cases. The jungle yellow fever cycle may be active but unrecognized in forested areas of countries within the yellow fever endemic zone (Figure 1). Urban yellow fever can be prevented by eradicating Ae. aegypti mosquitoes or by suppressing their numbers to the point that they no longer perpetuate infection. Jungle yellow fever can most effectively be prevented by vaccination of human populations at risk of exposure.

YELLOW FEVER VACCINE

Yellow fever vaccine is a live, attenuated virus preparation made from the 17D yellow fever virus strain (4). The 17D vaccine is safe and effective (5). The virus is grown in chick embryos inoculated with a seed virus of a fixed-passage level. The vaccine is a freeze-dried supernate of centrifuged embryo homogenate, packaged in 1-dose and 5-dose vials for domestic use.

Vaccine should be stored at temperatures between 5°C (41°F) and −30°C (−22°F)—preferably frozen, below 0°C (32°F)—until it is reconstituted by the addition of diluent sterile, physiologic saline supplied by the manufacturer. Multiple-dose vials of reconstituted vaccine should be held at 5°C–10°C (41°F–50°F); unused vaccine should be discarded within 1 hour after reconstitution.

Vaccine Usage

Persons Living or Traveling in Endemic Areas

1. Persons greater than or equal to 9 months of age traveling to or living in areas of South America and Africa where yellow fever infection is officially reported should be vaccinated. These areas are listed in the "Bi-Weekly Summary of Countries with Areas Infected with Quarantinable Diseases," available in state and local health departments. Information on known or

probably infected areas is also available from the World Health Organization (WHO) and Pan American Health Organization offices or the Division of Vector-Borne Infectious Diseases, Center for Infectious Diseases, CDC, Fort Collins, Colorado, telephone (303) 221-6400. Vaccination is also recommended for travel outside the urban areas of countries that do not officially report the disease but that lie in the yellow fever endemic zone (shaded area, (Figure 1). The actual areas of yellow fever virus activity far exceed the infected zones officially reported; in recent years, fatal cases of yellow fever have occurred among unvaccinated tourists visiting rural areas within the yellow fever endemic zone (6).

2. Infants less than 9 months of age and pregnant women should be considered for vaccination if traveling to areas experiencing ongoing epidemic yellow fever when travel cannot be postponed and a high level of prevention against mosquito exposure is not feasible. However, in no instance should infants less than 4 months of age receive yellow fever vaccine because of the risk of encephalitis (see Precautions and Contraindications).

3. Laboratory personnel who might be exposed to virulent yellow fever virus by direct or indirect contact or by aerosols should also be vaccinated.

Vaccination for International Travel

For purposes of international travel, yellow fever vaccines produced by different manufacturers worldwide must be approved by WHO and administered at an approved Yellow Fever Vaccination Center. State and territorial health departments have the authority to designate nonfederal vaccination centers; these can be identified by contacting state or local health departments. Vaccinees should receive an International Certificate of Vaccination completed, signed, and validated with the center's stamp where the vaccine is given. Vaccination for international travel may be required under circumstances other than those specified herein. Some countries in Africa require evidence of vaccination from all entering travelers. Some countries may waive the requirements for travelers coming from noninfected areas and staying less than 2 weeks. Because requirements may change, all travelers should seek current information from health departments. Travel agencies, international airlines, and/or shipping lines should also have up-to-date information. Some countries require an individual, even if only in transit, to have a valid International Certificate of Vaccination if s/he has been in countries either known or thought to harbor yellow fever virus. Such requirements may be strictly enforced, particularly for persons traveling from Africa or South America to Asia. Travelers should consult Health Information for International Travel 1989 (7) to determine requirements and regulations for vaccination.

Primary Vaccination

For persons of all ages, a single subcutaneous injection of 0.5 ml of reconstituted vaccine is used.

Booster Doses

The International Health Regulations require revaccination at intervals of 10 years. Revaccination boosts antibody titer; however, evidence from several studies (8–10) suggests that yellow fever vaccine immunity persists for at least 30–35 years and probably for life.

Reactions

Reactions to 17D yellow fever vaccine are generally mild. After vaccination, 2%–5% of vaccinees have mild headaches, myalgia, low-grade fevers, or other minor symptoms for 5–10 days. Fewer than 0.2% of the vaccinees curtail regular activities. Immediate hypersensitivity reactions, characterized by rash, urticaria, and/or asthma, are uncommon (incidence less than 1/1,000,000) and occur principally among persons with histories of egg allergy. Although greater than 34 million doses of vaccine have been distributed, only two cases of encephalitis temporally associated with vaccinations have been reported in the United States; in one fatal case, 17D virus was isolated from the brain.

Precautions and Contraindications

Age

Infants less than 4 months of age are more susceptible to serious adverse reactions (encephalitis) than older children. The risk of this complication appears to be age-related; whenever possible, vaccination should be delayed until age 9 months.

Pregnancy

Although specific information is not available concerning adverse effects of yellow fever vaccine on the developing fetus, pregnant women theoretically should not be vaccinated, and travel to areas where yellow fever is present should be postponed until after delivery. If international travel requirements constitute the only reason to vaccinate a pregnant woman, rather than an increased risk of infection, efforts should be made to obtain a waiver letter from the traveler's physician (see Hypersensitivity). Pregnant women who must travel to areas where the risk of yellow fever is high should be vaccinated. Under these circumstances, for both mother and fetus, the small theoretical risk from vaccination is far outweighed by the risk of yellow fever infection.

Altered Immune States

Infection with yellow fever vaccine virus poses a theoretical risk of encephalitis to patients with immunosuppression in association with acquired immunodeficiency syndrome (AIDS) or other manifestations of human immunodeficiency virus (HIV) infection, leukemia, lymphoma, generalized malignancy, or to those whose immunologic responses are suppressed by corticosteroids, alkylating drugs, antimetabolites, or radiation. Such patients should not be vaccinated. If travel to a yellow fever-infected zone is necessary, patients should be advised of the risk, instructed in methods for avoiding vector mosquitoes, and supplied with vaccination waiver letters by their physicians. Low-dose (10 mg prednisone or equivalent) or short-term (less than 2 weeks) corticosteroid therapy or intra-articular, bursal, or tendon injections with corticosteroids should not be immunosuppressive and constitute no increased hazard to recipients of yellow fever vaccine. Persons who have had previously diagnosed asymptomatic HIV infections and who cannot avoid potential exposure to yellow fever virus should be offered the choice of vaccination. Vaccinees should be monitored for possible adverse effects. Since the vaccination of such persons may be less effective than that for non-HIV-infected persons, their neutralizing antibody response to vaccination may be desired before travel. For such determinations, the appropriate state health department or CDC ((303) 221-6400) may be contacted. Family members of immunosuppressed persons, who themselves have no contraindications, may receive yellow fever vaccine.

Hypersensitivity

Live yellow fever vaccine is produced in chick embryos and should not be given to persons hypersensitive to eggs; generally, persons who are able to eat eggs or egg products may receive the vaccine. If international travel regulations are the only reason to vaccinate a patient hypersensitive to eggs, efforts should be made to obtain a waiver. A physician's letter stating the contraindication to vaccination has been acceptable to some governments. (Ideally, it should be written on letterhead stationary and bear the stamp used by health department and official immunization centers to validate the International Certificate of Vaccination.) Under these conditions, the traveler should also obtain specific and authoritative advice from the embassy or consulate of the country or countries s/he plans to visit. Waivers of requirements obtained from embassies or consulates should be documented by appropriate letters and retained for presentation with the International Health Certificate. If vaccination of an individual with a questionable history of egg hypersensitivity is considered essential because of a high risk of exposure, an intradermal test dose may be administered under close medical supervision. Specific directions for skin testing are found in the package insert.

Simultaneous Administration of Other Vaccines

Determination of whether to administer yellow fever vaccine and other immunobiologics simultaneously should be made on the basis of convenience to the traveler in completing the desired vaccinations before travel and on information regarding possible interference. The following will help guide these decisions.

Studies have shown that the serologic response to yellow fever vaccine is not inhibited by the administration of certain other vaccines concurrently or at various intervals of a few days to 1 month. Measles and yellow fever vaccines have been administered in combination with full efficacy of each of the components; Bacillus Calmette Guerin (BCG) and yellow fever vaccines have been administered simultaneously without interference. Additionally, severity of reactions to vaccination has not been amplified by the concurrent administration of yellow fever and other live virus vaccines (11). If live virus vaccines are not given concurrently, 4 weeks should elapse between sequential vaccinations.

Some data have indicated that persons given yellow fever and cholera vaccines simultaneously or 1–3 weeks apart had lower than normal antibody responses to both vaccines (12, 13). Unless there are time constraints, cholera and yellow fever vaccines should be administered at a minimal interval of 3 weeks. If the vaccines cannot be administered at least 3 weeks apart, the vaccines can be given simultaneously or at any time within the 3-week interval.

Hepatitis B and yellow fever vaccine may be given concurrently (14). No data exist on possible interference between yellow fever and typhoid, paratyphoid, typhus, plague, rabies, or Japanese encephalitis vaccines.

In a prospective study of persons given yellow fever vaccine and 5 cc of commercially available immune globulin, no alteration of the immunologic response to yellow fever vaccine was detected when compared with controls (15). Although chloroquine inhibits replication of yellow fever virus in vitro, it does not adversely affect antibody responses to yellow fever vaccine in humans receiving antimalaria prophylaxis (16).

REFERENCES

1. Strode GK, ed. Yellow fever. New York: McGraw Hill, 1951.
2. World Health Organization Expert Committee on Yellow Fever. Third report. WHO Tech Rep Ser No. 4791, 1971.
3. Nasidi A, Monath TP, DeCock K, et al. Urban yellow fever epidemic in western Nigeria, 1987. Trans R Soc Trop Med Hyg 1989;84:401–406.
4. Smithburn KC, Durieux C, Koerber R, et al. Yellow fever vaccination. WHO monograph series no. 30. Geneva, 1956.
5. Wisseman CL Jr, Sweet BH. Immunological studies with group B arthropod-borne viruses. III. Response of human subjects to revaccination with 17D strain yellow fever vaccine. Am J Trop Med Hyg 1962;11:570–575.
6. Rodhain F, Hannoun C, Jousset FX, Ravisse P. Isolement du virus de la fievre jaune a Paris a partir de deux cas humains importes. Bull Soc Pathol Exot 1979;72:411–415.
7. CDC. Health information for international travel 1989. Atlanta: CDC, 1989:HHS publication no. (CDC)89–8280.
8. Groot H, Ribeiro RB. Neutralizing and haemagglutination-inhibiting antibodies to yellow fever 17 years after vaccination with 17D vaccine. Bull WHO 1962;27:669–707.
9. Poland JD, Calisher CH, Monath TP, Downs WG, Murphy K. Persistence of neutralizing antibody 30–35 years after immunization with 17D yellow fever vaccine. Bull WHO 1981;59:895–900.
10. Rosenzweig EC, Babione RW, Wisseman CL Jr. Immunological studies with group B arthropod-borne viruses. IV. Persistence of yellow fever antibodies following vaccination with 17D strain yellow fever vaccine. Am J Trop Med Hyg 1963;12:230–235.
11. Tauraso NM, Myers MG, Nau EV, et al. Effect of interval between inoculation of live smallpox and yellow fever vaccines on antigenicity in man. J Infect Dis 1972;126:363–371.
12. Felsenfeld O, Wolf RH, Gyr K, et al. Simultaneous vaccination against cholera and yellow fever. Lancet 1973;1:457–458.
13. Gateff C. Influence de la vaccination anticholoerique sur l'immunisation antiamarile associee. Bull Soc Pathol Exot 1973;66:258–266.
14. Yvonnet B, Coursaget P, Deubel V, et al. Simultaneous administration of hepatitis B and yellow fever vaccines. J Med Virol 1986;19:307–311.
15. Kaplan JE, Nelson DB, Schonberger LB, et al. The effect of immune globulin on trivalent oral polio and yellow fever vaccinations. Bull WHO 1984;62:585–590.
16. Tsai TF, Bolin RA, Lazuick JS, et al. Chloroquine does not adversely affect the antibody response to yellow fever vaccine. J Infect Dis 1986;154:726.

section two

MATERNAL AND CHILD HEALTH/NUTRITION

CDC Criteria for Anemia in Children and Childbearing-Aged Women

Original Citation: Centers for Disease Control and Prevention. Current Trends: CDC criteria for anemia in children and childbearing-aged women. MMWR 1989;38(22):400–404.

Hemoglobin (Hb) and hematocrit (Hct) measurements are the laboratory tests used most commonly in clinical and public health settings for screening for anemia. Because most anemia in children and women of childbearing age is related to iron deficiency (1), the main purpose of anemia screening is to detect those persons at increased risk for iron deficiency. Proper anemia screening requires not only sound laboratory methods and procedures but also appropriate Hb and Hct cutoff values to define anemia. The "normal" ranges of Hb and Hct change throughout childhood and during pregnancy, and are higher for men than women (1, 2). Thus, criteria for anemia should be specific for age, sex, and stage of pregnancy. Current major reference criteria for anemia, however, are not based on representative samples and fail to take into account the normal hematologic changes occurring during pregnancy. To address these limitations, CDC has formulated new reference criteria for use in clinical practice for public health and nutrition programs and the CDC Pediatric and Pregnancy Nutrition Surveillance Systems. The new criteria may also be useful for defining anemia in clinical research and nutrition surveys.

The anemia reference values for children, nonpregnant women, and men are derived from the most current nationally representative sample—the Second National Health and Nutrition Examination Survey, 1976–1980 (NHANES II). Because representative data are not yet available for pregnant women, anemia reference values are based on the most current clinical studies available. Adjustment values of Hb and Hct cutoffs are provided for persons who reside at higher altitudes and for those who smoke cigarettes.

ANEMIA CUTOFFS FOR CHILDREN, NONPREGNANT WOMEN, AND MEN

Because hematologic values normally change as children grow older, it is necessary to use age-specific criteria for diagnosing anemia in children (1). The best hematologic reference data for the United States are available from the NHANES II. The Hb and Hct cutoffs recommended represent the age-specific fifth percentile values for "healthy" persons from NHANES II (Table 1) (3, 4). The healthy sample was defined by excluding persons who were likely to have iron deficiency based on ?multiple iron biochemical measures. The anemia cutoff values based on these NHANES II studies for younger children are in close agreement with the cutoff values recommended by the American Academy of Pediatrics, which were based on a sample of healthy white middle-class children (5). Even though no data are available from NHANES II to determine anemia cutoffs for infants less than 1 year of age, cutoff values for children 1–2 years can be extrapolated back to 6 months of age. In general, anemia screening to detect iron deficiency is not indicated for infants less than 6 months of age because younger infants usually have adequate iron nutritional status (6).

Table 1. Hemoglobin (Hb) and hematocrit (Hct) cutoffs for children, nonpregnant women, and men*

Age (yrs)/Sex	Hb (g/dL)	Hct (%)
Both sexes		
1–1.9	11.0	33.0
2–4.9	11.2	34.0
5–7.9	11.4	34.5
8–11.9	11.6	35.0
Female		
12–14.9	11.8	35.5
15–17.9	12.0	36.0
≥18	12.0	36.0
Male		
12–14.9	12.3	37.0
15–17.9	12.6	38.0
≥18	13.6	41.0

*Based on fifth percentile values from the Second National Health and Nutrition Examination Survey after excluding persons with a higher likelihood of iron deficiency (3, 4).

ANEMIA CUTOFFS DURING PREGNANCY

During a normal pregnancy, a woman's hematologic values change substantially (2). For women with adequate iron nutrition, Hb and Hct values start to decline during the early part of the first trimester, reach their nadir near the end of the second trimester, then gradually rise during the third trimester (2, 7–10). Because of the change of Hb and Hct during pregnancy, anemia must be characterized according to the specific stage of pregnancy. The normal range of Hb and Hct during pregnancy is based on data aggregated from four European studies of healthy iron-supplemented pregnant women (7–10). These studies provide similar findings at each specific month of pregnancy. The month-specific fifth percentile values for Hb of the pooled data have been adopted for use in the CDC Pregnancy Nutrition Surveillance System (Table 2). In addition, trimester-specific cutoffs also have been developed for use in the clinical setting (Table 2). These trimester-specific cutoffs are based on the mid-trimester values; cutoffs for the first trimester, the time at which most women are initially seen for prenatal care, are based on a late-trimester value. Adjustment of Hb and Hct Cutoffs for Altitude and Smoking Persons residing at higher altitudes (greater than 1000 meters (3300 feet)) have higher Hb and

Hct levels than those residing at sea level. This variation is due to the lower oxygen partial pressure at higher altitudes, a reduction in oxygen saturation of blood (11), and a compensatory increase in red cell production to ensure adequate oxygen supply to the tissues. Thus, higher altitude causes a generalized upward shift of the Hb and Hct distributions. This shift may be associated with the underdiagnosis of anemia for residents of higher altitudes when sea-level cutoffs are applied (CDC, unpublished data). Therefore, the proper diagnosis of anemia for those residing at higher altitudes requires an upward adjustment of Hb and Hct cutoffs. The values for altitude-specific adjustment of Hb and Hct are derived from data collected by the CDC Pediatric Nutrition Surveillance System on children residing at various altitudes in the mountain states (Table 3). Altitude affects Hb and Hct levels throughout pregnancy in a similar way (J.N. Chatfield, unpublished data).

Table 2. Pregnancy month-specific and trimester-specific hemoglobin (Hb) cutoffs*

Gestation (wks)	12	16	20	24	28	32	36	40
Trimester	1[†]	2	2[†]	2	3	3[†]	3	term
Mean Hb (g/dL)	12.2	11.8	11.6	11.6	11.8	12.1	12.5	12.9
5th percentile Hb values (g/dL)	11.0	10.6	10.5	10.5	10.7	11.0	11.4	11.9
Equivalent 5th percentile Hct[§] values (%)	33.0	32.0	32.0	32.0	32.0	33.0	34.0	36.0

*Based on pooled data from four European surveys of healthy women taking iron supplements (7–10).

[†]Hb values adopted for the trimester-specific cutoffs.

[§]Hematocrit.

Table 3. Altitude adjustments for hemoglobin (Hb) and hematocrit (Hct) cutoffs

Altitude (ft)	Hb (g/dL)	Hct (%)
<3000	0.0	0.0
3000–3999*	+0.2	+0.5
4000–4999*	+0.3	+1.0
5000–5999*	+0.5	+1.5
6000–6999*	+0.7	+2.0
7000–7999[†]	+1.0	+3.0
8000–8999[†]	+1.3	+4.0
9000–9999[†]	+1.6	+5.0
>10,000[†]	+2.0	+6.0

*Based on data from CDC Pediatric Nutrition Surveillance System and reference 11.

[†]Based on reference 11 only.

The influence of cigarette smoking is similar to that of altitude, in that smoking increases Hb and Hct levels substantially. The higher Hb and Hct of smokers is a consequence of an increased carboxyhemoglobin from inhaling carbon monoxide during smoking. Because carboxyhemoglobin has no oxygen carrying capacity, its presence causes a generalized upward shift of the Hb and Hct distribution curves (CDC, unpublished data). Therefore, a smoking-specific adjustment to the anemia cutoff is necessary for the proper diagnosis of anemia in smokers. The smoking-specific Hb and Hct adjustments are derived from the NHANES II data (Table 4).

The altitude and smoking adjustments are additive. For example, a woman living at 6000 feet and smoking two or more packs of cigarettes per day would have her cutoff for anemia adjusted upward by a total of 1.4 grams of Hb or 4% Hct.

Table 4. Smoking adjustments for hemoglobin (Hb) and hematocrit (Hct)

Characteristic	Hb (gm/dL)	Hct (%)
Nonsmoker	0.0	0.0
Smoker (all)	+0.3	+1.0
½–1 pack/day	+0.3	+1.0
1–2 packs/day	+0.5	+1.5
>2 packs/day	+0.7	+2.0

REFERENCES: AS NUMBERED IN ORIGINAL PUBLICATION

1. Dallman PR, Yip R, Johnson C. Prevalence and causes of anemia in the United States, 1976 to 1980. Am J Clin Nutr 1984;39:437–445.
2. Bothwell TH, Charlton RW. Iron deficiency in women: a report of the International Nutritional Anemia Consultative Group (INACG). New York: The Nutrition Foundation, 1981.
3. Pilch SM, Senti FR, eds. Assessment of the iron nutritional status of the U.S. population based on data collected in the Second National Health and Nutrition Examination Survey, 1976–1980. Bethesda, MD: Federation of American Societies for Experimental Biology, Life Sciences Research Office, 1984.
4. Yip R, Johnson C, Dallman PR. Age-related changes in laboratory values used in the diagnosis of anemia and iron deficiency. Am J Clin Nutr 1984;39:427–436.
5. American Academy of Pediatrics. Pediatric nutrition handbook. 2nd ed. Elk Grove Village, IL: American Academy of Pediatrics, Committee on Nutrition, 1985.
6. Smith NJ, Rosello S, Say MB, Yeya K. Iron storage in the first five years of life. Pediatrics 1955; 16:166–171.
7. Svanberg B, Arvidsson B, Norrby A, Rybo G, Solvell L. Absorption of supplemental iron during pregnancy: a longitudinal study with repeated bone-marrow studies and absorption measurements. Acta Obstet Gynecol Scand Suppl 1975;48:87–108.
8. Sjostedt JE, Manner P, Nummi S, Ekenved G. Oral iron prophylaxis during pregnancy: a comparative study on different dosage regimens. Acta Obstet Gynecol Scand Suppl 1977;60:3–9.
9. Puolakka J, Janne O, Pakarinen A, Jarvinen A, Vihko R. Serum ferritin as a measure of iron stores during and after normal pregnancy with and without iron supplements. Acta Obstet Gynecol Scand Suppl 1980;95:43–51.
10. Taylor DJ, Mallen C, McDougall N, Lind T. Effect of iron supplementation on serum ferritin levels during and after pregnancy. Br J Obstet Gynecol 1982;89:1011–1017.
11. Hurtado A, Merino C, Delgado E. Influence of anoxemia on the hemopoietic activity. Arch Intern Med 1945;75:284–323.

TOPIC 35 / **BIRTH DEFECTS**

Chorionic Villus Sampling and Amniocentesis: Recommendations for Prenatal Counseling

Original Citation: Centers for Disease Control and Prevention. Chorionic Villus Sampling and Amniocentesis: Recommendations for Prenatal Counseling. MMWR 1995;44(RR-9):1–12.

Original Authors: Richard S. Olney, MD, MPH, Cynthia A. Moore, MD, Muin J. Khoury, MD, PhD, Larry D. Edmunds, MSPH, Lorenzo D. Botto, MD, Hani K. Atrash, MD, MPH.

INTRODUCTION

Chorionic villus sampling (CVS) and amniocentesis are prenatal diagnostic procedures used to detect certain fetal genetic abnormalities. Both procedures increase the risk for miscarriage (1). In addition, concern has been increasing among health-care providers and public health officials about the potential occurrence of birth defects resulting from CVS (2).

USE OF CVS AND AMNIOCENTESIS

CVS utilizes either a catheter or needle to biopsy placental cells that are derived from the same fertilized egg as the fetus. During amniocentesis, a small sample of the fluid that surrounds the fetus is removed. This fluid contains cells that are shed primarily from the fetal skin, bladder, gastrointestinal tract, and amnion. Typically, CVS is done at 10–12 weeks' gestation, and amniocentesis is done at 15–18 weeks' gestation. In the United States, the current standard of care in obstetrical practice is to offer either CVS or amniocentesis to women who will be greater than or equal to 35 years of age when they give birth, because these women are at increased risk for giving birth to infants with Down syndrome and certain other types of aneuploidy. Karyotyping of cells obtained by either amniocentesis or CVS is the standard and definitive means of diagnosing aneuploidy in fetuses. The risk that a woman will give birth to an infant with Down syndrome increases with age. For example, for women 35 years of age, the risk is 1 per 385 births (0.3%), whereas for women 45 years of age, the risk is 1 per 30 births (3%) (1). The background risk for major birth defects (with or without chromosomal abnormalities) for women of all ages is approximately 3%.

Before widespread use of amniocentesis, several controlled studies were conducted to evaluate the safety of the procedure. The major finding from these studies was that amniocentesis increases the rate for miscarriage (i.e., spontaneous abortions) by approximately 0.5%. Subsequent to these studies, amniocentesis became an accepted standard of care in the 1970s. In 1990, more than 200,000 amniocentesis procedures were performed in the United States (4).

Although maternal age-related risk for fetal aneuploidy is the usual indication for CVS or amniocentesis, prospective mothers or fathers of any age might desire fetal testing when they are at risk for passing on certain Mendelian (single-gene) conditions. In a randomized trial conducted in the United States, 19% of women who underwent CVS were <35 years of age (10). DNA-based diagnoses of Mendelian conditions, such as cystic fibrosis, hemophilia, muscular dystrophy, and hemoglobinopathies, can be made by direct analysis of uncultured chorionic villus cells (a more efficient method than culturing amniocytes) (11). However, amniocentesis is particularly useful to prospective parents who have a family history of neural tube defects, because alpha-fetoprotein (AFP) testing can be done on amniotic fluid but cannot be done on CVS specimens.

When testing for chromosomal abnormalities resulting from advanced maternal age, CVS may be more acceptable than amniocentesis to some women because of the psychological and medical advantages provided by CVS through earlier diagnosis of abnormalities. Fetal movement is usually felt and uterine growth is visible at 17–19 weeks' gestation, the time when abnormalities are detected by amniocentesis; thus, deciding what action to take if an abnormality is detected at this time may be more difficult psychologically (12). Using CVS to diagnose chromosomal abnormalities during the first trimester allows a prospective parent to make this decision earlier than will amniocentesis.

Maternal morbidity and mortality associated with induced abortion increase significantly with increasing gestational age; thus, the timing of diagnosis of chromosomal abnormalities is important. Results of studies of abortion complications conducted by CDC from 1970 through 1978 indicated that the risk for major abortion complications (e.g., prolonged fever, hemorrhage necessitating blood transfusion, and injury to pelvic organs) increases with advancing gestational age. For example, from 1971 through 1974, the major complication rate was 0.8% at 11–12 weeks' gestation, compared with 2.2% at 17–20 weeks' gestation (13). However, the risk for developing major complications from abortion at any gestational age decreased during the 1970s. More contemporary national morbidity data based on current abortion practices are not yet available. CDC surveillance data also indicate an increase in the risk for maternal death with increasing gestation. From 1972 through 1987, the risk for abortion-related death was 1.1 deaths per 100,000 abortions performed at 11–12 weeks' gestation compared with 6.9 deaths per 100,000 abortions for procedures performed at 16–20 weeks' gestation (14). The lower risk associated with first-trimester abortions may be an important factor for prospective parents who are deciding between CVS and amniocentesis.

Amniocentesis is usually performed at 15–18 weeks' gestation, but more amniocentesis procedures are now being performed at 11–14 weeks' gestation. "Early" amniocentesis (defined as <15 weeks' gestation) remains investigational, because the safety of the procedure is currently being evaluated with controlled trials (15).

Risk estimates for miscarriage caused by either CVS or midtrimester amniocentesis have been adjusted to account for spontaneous fetal losses that occur early in pregnancy and are not procedure-related. Although one randomized trial indicated that the amniocentesis-related miscarriage rate may be as high as 1%, counselors usually cite risks for miscarriage from other amniocentesis studies ranging from 0.25%–0.50% (1/400–1/200) (1, 15). Rates of miscarriage after CVS vary widely by the center at which CVS was performed (16). Adjusting for confounding factors such as gestational age, the CVS-related miscarriage rate is approximately 0.5%–1.0% (1/200–1/100) (1).

Although uterine infection (i.e., chorioamnionitis) is one possible reason for miscarriage after either CVS or amniocentesis, infection has occurred rarely after either procedure. In one study, no episodes of septic shock were reported after 4,200 CVS procedures, although less severe infections may have been associated with 12 of the 89 observed fetal losses (5). Overall infection rates have been <0.1% after either CVS or amniocentesis (15).

Cytogenetically ambiguous results caused by factors such as maternal cell contamination or culture-related mosaicism are reported more often after CVS than after amniocentesis (2). In these instances, follow-up amniocentesis might be required to clarify results, increasing both the total cost of testing and the risk for miscarriage. However, ambiguous CVS results also may indicate a condition (e.g., confined placental mosaicism) that has been associated with adverse outcomes for the fetus (11). Thus, in these situations, CVS may be more informative than amniocentesis alone.

LIMB DEFICIENCIES AMONG INFANTS WHOSE MOTHERS UNDERWENT CVS

Certain congenital defects of the extremities, known as limb deficiencies or limb-reduction defects, have been reported among infants whose mothers underwent CVS. This section addresses (a) the expected frequency and classification of these birth defects, (b) the physical features of reported infants in relation to the timing of associated CVS procedures, and (c) cohort and case-control studies that have been done to systematically examine whether CVS increases the risk for limb deficiencies.

Population-Based Rates and Classification of Limb Deficiencies

Population-based studies indicate that the risk for all limb deficiencies is from 5–6 per 10,000 live births (17). Limb deficiencies usually are classified into distinct anatomic and pathogenetic categories. The most common subtypes are transverse terminal defects, which involve absence of distal structures with intact proximal segments, with the axis of deficiency perpendicular to the extremity. Approximately 50% of all limb deficiencies are transverse, and 50% of those defects are digital, involving the absence of parts of one or more fingers or toes. Transverse deficiencies occur as either isolated defects or with other major defects. The rare combination of transverse limb deficiencies with either absence or hypoplasia of the tongue and lower jaw—usually referred to as oromandibular-limb hypogenesis or hypoglossia/hypodactyly—occurs at a rate of approximately 1 per 200,000 births. Although the cause of many isolated limb deficiencies and multiple anomalies that include transverse deficiencies is unknown, researchers have hypothesized that these deficiencies are caused by vascular disruption either during the formation of embryonic limbs or in already-formed fetal limbs (17, 18).

Limb Deficiencies Reported in Infants Exposed to CVS

Reports of clusters of infants born with limb deficiencies after CVS were first published in 1991 (19). Three studies illustrate the spectrum of CVS-associated defects (19–21). Data from these studies suggest that the severity of the outcome is associated with the specific time of CVS exposure. Exposure at greater than or equal to 70 days' gestation has been associated with more limited defects, isolated to the distal extremities, whereas earlier exposures have been associated with more proximal limb deficiencies and orofacial defects. For example, in a study involving 14 infants exposed to CVS at 63–79 days' gestation and examined by a single pediatrician, 13 had isolated transverse digital deficiencies (20). In another study in Oxford of five infants exposed to CVS at 56–66 days' gestation, four had transverse deficiencies with oromandibular hypogenesis (19). In a review of published worldwide data, associated defects of the tongue or lower jaw were reported for 19 of 75 cases of CVS-associated limb deficiencies (21). Of those 19 infants with oromandibular-limb hypogenesis, 17 were exposed to CVS before 68 days' gestation. In this review, 74% of infants exposed to CVS at greater than or equal to 70 days' gestation had digital deficiencies without proximal involvement.

Cohorts of CVS-Exposed Pregnancies

Published CVS cohort studies of >1,000 CVS procedures include data from 65 CVS centers (Table 1). These rates include studies that describe affected limbs in sufficient detail to exclude nontransverse defects. Rates calculated for the smaller cohorts (i.e., centers performing <3,500 procedures) are less stable, but the overall rate of nonsyndromic transverse limb deficiency from these centers was 7.4 per 10,000 procedures.

Table 1. Rates of transverse terminal limb-deficiencies at 65 CVS centers*—selected geographical locations, 1984–1992

| Location[†] | CVS | | | |
	No. of Centers	No. of Cases	No. of Procedures	Rate
U.S. (NICHD[§]) (22, 23)	10	7	9,588	7.3
U.S. (24)	9	3	4,105	7.3
Netherlands—Rotterdam (25)	1	3	3,973	7.6
Italy—Sardinia (26)	1	3	3,082	9.7

Table 1.—*continued*

| Location[†] | No. of Centers | CVS | | Rate |
		No. of Cases	No. of Procedures	
U.S.—Beverly Hills, CA (27)	1	1	3,016	3.3
Germany—Münster (28)	1	2	2,836	7.1
Italy (GIDEF[1]) (29)	5	3	2,759	10.9
U.S.—Philadelphia, PA (30)	1	1	2,710	3.7
Denmark (31)	2	0	2,624	0.0
Australia—Victoria (32)	2	3	2,071	14.5
Europe (MRC**) (33)	31	2	1,609	12.4
U.S.—Evanston, IL (34)	1	1	1,048	9.5
Total	65	29	39,421	7.4

*Per 10,000 CVS procedures

[†]Excluded were centers (i.e., collaborating hospitals or other health-care facilities) reporting either ≤1,000 procedures or incomplete information about birth-defect outcomes.

[§]National Institute of Child Health and Human Development (combined data from two trials [5, 10]).

[1]Gruppo Italiano Diagnosi Embrio-Fetali.

**Medical Research Council, United Kingdom.

Case-Control Studies

Case-control approaches with a minimum of 100 cases and 100 control patients have greater statistical power than cohort studies of 10,000 or fewer births to detect a fourfold increase in risk for transverse deficiencies (the degree of relative risk suggested by data from the 65 CVS centers) (36). Investigators participating in multicenter birth-defect studies have used this case-control approach both to measure the strength of the association between CVS and limb deficiency and to determine if a dose-response (or gradient) effect of risk exists. The latter effect would be indicated by an increased relative risk for limb deficiency after earlier procedures, suggested in case reports of CVS-associated limb deficiencies by the high frequency of early exposures to CVS. Three case-control studies have used infants with limb deficiencies registered in surveillance systems and control infants with other birth defects to examine and compare exposure rates to CVS (36, 37, 39). The odds ratios for CVS exposure (an estimate of the relative risk for limb deficiency after CVS) are summarized in Table 3.

The U.S. Multistate Case-Control Study and the study of the Italian Multicentric Birth Defects Registry both indicated a significant association between CVS exposure and subtypes of transverse limb deficiencies (36, 37). The EUROCAT study did not analyze risk for transverse limb deficiencies (39); the risk for all limb deficiencies (odds ratio [OR] = 1.8, 95% confidence interval [CI] = 0.7–5.0) was similar to that measured in the U.S. Multistate Case-Control Study for all limb deficiencies (OR = 1.7, 95% CI = 0.4–6.3) (36).

Table 3. Risk for limb deficiencies and subtypes, by selected case-control studies of limb defects after chorionic villus sampling—by selected registries, 1984–1993

Registry	All limb deficiencies OR* (95% CI)[†]	Transverse limb deficiencies OR* (95% CI)[†]	Subsets of transverse deficiencies OR* (95% CI)[†]
U.S. Multistate Case-Control Study (36)	1.7 (0.4–6.3)	4.7 (0.8–28.4)	Digital: 6.4 (1.1.–38.6)
EUROCAT (European Registration of Congenital Anomalies and Twins) (39)	1.8 (0.7–5.0)	Not subclassified	Not subclassified
IMBDR (Italian Multicentric Birth Defects Registry)** (37)	Not included[§]	12.6 (6.2–23.9)	OMLH[¶]:223.8 (48.9–1006.8)

*Odds ratios.

[†]Confidence interval.

[§]Case definition included only transverse limb deficiencies.

[¶]Oromandibular-limb hypogenesis (hypoglossia/hypodactyly). (P. Mastroiacovo, personal communication).

**IPIMC (Indagine Policentrica Italiana sulle Malformazioni Congenite).

Analysis of subtypes in the U.S. study indicated a sixfold increase in risk for transverse digital deficiencies (36). In the U.S. study, no association between limb deficiencies and amniocentesis was observed. In the study of the Italian Multicentric Birth Defects Registry, the association between CVS exposure and transverse limb deficiencies was stronger (Table 3) (37).

GESTATIONAL AGE AT CVS

The lower risk observed in the United States may be related to the later mean gestational age of exposure. Increased risk was associated with decreased gestational age at the time of exposure (Table 4). The risk for transverse deficiencies was greatest at less than or equal to 9 weeks' gestation. An analysis of cohort studies regarding the timing of CVS indicated a similar gradient with a relative risk for transverse deficiencies of 6.2 at <10 weeks' and 2.4 at greater than or equal to 10 weeks' gestation (40). Because of reports of high rates of severe limb deficiencies after CVS at 6–7 weeks' gestation, a WHO-sponsored committee recommended that CVS be performed at 9–12 weeks after the last menstrual period (16).

ABSOLUTE RISK FOR LIMB DEFICIENCY

Subtypes of limb deficiencies rarely occur in the population of infants not exposed to CVS. Thus, even a sixfold increase in risk for such types as digital defects (the finding of the U.S. Multistate Case-Control Study) is comparable to a

Table 4. Risk for transverse limb deficiency after chorionic villus sampling (CVS), by gestational age—United States and Italy, 1988–1993

Gestational age (weeks)	United States*		Italy†	
	No. of CVS-exposed cases	OR§ (95% CI)¶	No. of CVS-exposed cases	OR§ (95% CI)¶
≤9	2	11.3 (1.0–131.6)	8	21.6 (9.0–47.7)
10	4	7.5 (1.5–36.7)	3	14.3 (3.2–47.2)
≥11	1	5.6 (0.3–94.7)	0	—**

*Includes transverse digital deficiencies only (36).

†Includes all types of transverse deficiencies (37).

§Odds ratio.

¶Confidence interval.

**No CVS-exposed cases.

small absolute risk (i.e., 3.46 cases per 10,000 CVS procedures [0.03%]) (36). The upper 95% confidence limit for this absolute risk estimate is approximately 0.1%. A range of absolute risk from 1 per 3,000 to 1 per 1,000 CVS procedures (0.03%–0.10%) for all transverse deficiencies is consistent with the overall increase in risk reported by the 65 centers (Table 1). In cohort studies that reported the timing of the CVS, the absolute risk for transverse limb deficiencies was 0.20% at less than or equal to 9 weeks, 0.10% at 10 weeks, and 0.05% at greater than or equal to 11 weeks (0.07% at greater than or equal to 10 weeks of gestation) (40).

The absolute risk for CVS-related birth defects is lower than the procedure-related risk for miscarriage that counselors usually quote to prospective parents (i.e., 0.5% to 1.0%) and also is lower than the risk for Down syndrome at age 35 (0.3%). Data from a decision analysis study supported the conclusion that, weighing a range of possible risks associated with prenatal testing, amniocentesis was preferred to CVS (43). This study was published in 1991 and did not consider risk for limb deficiency. Data indicate that publication of the initial case reports of limb deficiency decreased subsequent utilization of CVS (44, 45). However, one study demonstrated that prospective parents who were provided with formal genetic counseling, including information about limb deficiencies and other risks and benefits, chose CVS at a rate similar to a group of prospective parents who were counseled before published reports of CVS-associated limb deficiencies (44).

RECOMMENDATIONS

An analysis of all aspects of CVS and amniocentesis indicates that the occasional occurrence of CVS-related limb defects is only one of several factors that must be considered in counseling prospective parents about prenatal testing. Factors that can influence prospective parents' choices about prenatal testing include their risk for transmitting genetic abnormalities to the fetus and their perception of potential complications and benefits of both CVS and amniocentesis. Prospective parents who are considering the use of either procedure should be provided with current data for informed decision making. Individualized counseling should address the following:

Indications for Procedures and Limitations of Prenatal Testing

- Counselors should discuss the prospective parents' degree of risk for transmitting genetic abnormalities based on factors such as maternal age, race, and family history.
- Prospective parents should be made aware of both the limitations and usefulness of either CVS or amniocentesis in detecting abnormalities.

Potential Serious Complications from CVS and Amniocentesis

- Counselors should discuss the risk for miscarriage attributable to both procedures: the risk from amniocentesis at 15–18 weeks' gestation is approximately 0.25%- 0.50% (1/400–1/200), and the miscarriage risk from CVS is approximately 0.5%–1.0% (1/200–1/100).
- Current data indicate that the overall risk for transverse limb deficiency from CVS is 0.03%–0.10% (1/3,000–1/1,000). Current data indicate no increase in risk for limb deficiency after amniocentesis at 15–18 weeks' gestation.
- The risk and severity of limb deficiency appear to be associated with the timing of CVS: the risk at <10 weeks' gestation (0.20%) is higher than the risk from CVS done at greater than or equal to 10 weeks' gestation (0.07%). Most defects associated with CVS at greater than or equal to 10 weeks' gestation have been limited to the digits.

Timing of Procedures

- The timing of obtaining results from either CVS or amniocentesis is relevant because of the increased risks for maternal morbidity and mortality associated with terminating pregnancy during the second trimester compared with the first trimester (13, 14).
- Many amniocentesis procedures are now done at 11–14 weeks' gestation; however, further controlled studies are necessary to fully assess the safety of early amniocentesis.

REFERENCES: AS NUMBERED IN ORIGINAL PUBLICATION

1. Verp MS. Prenatal diagnosis of genetic disorders. In: Gleicher N., ed. Principles and practice of medical therapy in pregnancy. 2nd ed. Norwalk, CT: Appleton and Lange, 1992:159–170.
2. Lilford RJ. The rise and fall of chorionic villus sampling: midtrimester amniocentesis is usually preferable [Comment]. Br Med J 1991;303:936–937.
4. Meaney FJ, Riggle SM, Cunningham GC, Stern KS, Davis JG. Prenatal genetic services: toward a national data base. Clin Obstet Gynecol 1993;36:510–520.
5. Rhoads GG, Jackson LG, Schlesselman SE, et al. The safety and efficacy of chorionic villus sampling for early prenatal diagnosis of cytogenetic abnormalities. N Engl J Med 1989;320:609–617.
10. Jackson LG, Zachary JM, Fowler SE, et al. A randomized comparison of transcervical and transabdominal chorionic-villus sampling. N Engl J Med 1992;327:594–598.
11. Cohen MM, Rosenblum-Vos LS, Prabhakar G. Human cytogenetics: a current overview. Am J Dis Child 1993;147:1159–1166.
12. Burke BM, Kolker A. Clients undergoing chorionic villus sampling versus amniocentesis: contrasting attitudes toward pregnancy. Health Care Women Int 1993;14(2):193–200.

13. Cates W Jr, Grimes DA. Morbidity and mortality of abortion in the United States. In: Hodgson JE, ed. Abortion and sterilization: medical and social aspects. London: Academic Press Inc., 1981: 155–180.

14. Lawson HW, Frye A, Atrash HK, Smith JC, Shulman HB, Ramick M. Abortion mortality, United States, 1972 through 1987. Am J Obstet Gynecol 1994;171:1365–1372.

15. Schemmer G, Johnson A. Genetic amniocentesis and chorionic villus sampling. Obstet Gynecol Clin North Am 1993;20:497–521.

16. World Health Organization Regional Office for Europe (WHO/EURO). Risk evaluation of chorionic villus sampling (CVS): report on a meeting. Copenhagen: WHO/EURO, 1992.

17. Report of National Institute of Child Health and Human Development Workshop on Chorionic Villus Sampling and Limb and Other Defects, October 20, 1992. Am J Obstet Gynecol 1993;169:1–6.

18. Hoyme HE, Jones KL, Van Allen MI, Saunders BS, Benirschke K. Vascular pathogenesis of transverse limb reduction defects. J Pediatr 1982;101:839–843.

19. Firth HV, Boyd PA, Chamberlain P, MacKenzie IZ, Lindenbaum RH, Huson SM. Severe limb abnormalities after chorionic villus sampling at 56–66 days' gestation. Lancet 1991;337:762–763.

20. Burton BK, Schulz CJ, Burd LI. Spectrum of limb disruption defects associated with chorionic villus sampling [published erratum appears in Pediatrics 1993;92:722]. Pediatrics 1993;91:989–993.

21. Firth HV, Boyd PA, Chamberlain PF, MacKenzie IZ, Morriss-Kay GM, Huson SM. Analysis of limb reduction defects in babies exposed to chorionic villus sampling. Lancet 1994;343:1069–1071.

22. Mahoney MJ, for the USNICHD Collaborative CVS Study Group. Limb abnormalities and chorionic villus sampling [Letter]. Lancet 1991;337:1422–1423.

23. USNICHD Collaborative CVS Study Group. Limb defects, cavernous hemangiomas and other congenital anomalies in infants born to women in the United States Collaborative Trials of Chorionic Villus Sampling (CVS) [Abstract]. Teratology 1993;47:400.

24. Blakemore K, Filkins K, Luthy D, et al. Cook obstetrics and gynecology catheter multicenter chorionic villus sampling trial: comparison of birth defects with expected rates. Am J Obstet Gynecol 1993;169:1022–1026.

25. Jahoda MGJ, Brandenburg H, Cohen-Overbeek T, Los FJ, Sachs ES, Wladimiroff JW. Terminal transverse limb defects and early chorionic villus sampling: evaluation of 4,300 cases with completed follow-up. Am J Med Genet 1993;46:483–485.

26. Ibba RM, Monni G, Lai R, et al. Total fetal malformations following chorion villus sampling [Abstract]. Prenat Diag 1992;12(Suppl):S98.

27. Williams J III, Wang BBT, Rubin CH, Aiken-Hunting D. Chorionic villus sampling: experience with 3016 cases performed by a single operator. Obstet Gynecol 1992;80:1023–1029.

28. Schloo R, Miny P, Holzgreve W, Horst J, Lenz W. Distal limb deficiency following chorionic villus sampling? Am J Med Genet 1992;42:404–413.

29. GIDEF (Gruppo Italiano Diagnosi Embrio-Fetali). Transverse limb reduction defects after chorion villus sampling: a retrospective cohort study. Prenat Diagn 1993;13:1051–1056.

30. Godmilow L, Librizzi RJ, Donnenfeld AE. Congenital abnormalities following chorionic villus sampling [Abstract]. Am J Hum Genet 1992;51(Suppl 4):A409.

31. Smidt-Jensen S, Permin M, Philip J, et al. Randomised comparison of amniocentesis and transabdominal and transcervical chorionic villus sampling. Lancet 1992;340:1237–1244.

32. Halliday J, Lumley J, Sheffield LJ, Lancaster PAL. Limb deficiencies, chorion villus sampling, and advanced maternal age. Am J Med Genet 1993;47:1096–1098.

33. MRC Working Party on the Evaluation of Chorion Villus Sampling. Medical Research Council European Trial of chorion villus sampling. Lancet 1991;337:1491–1499.

34. Silver RK, Macgregor SN, Muhlbach LH, Knutel TA, Kambich MP. Congenital malformations subsequent to chorionic villus sampling: outcome analysis of 1048 consecutive procedures. Prenat Diagn 1994;14:421–427.

36. Olney RS, Khoury MJ, Alo CJ, et al. Increased risk for transverse digital deficiency after chorionic villus sampling: results of the United States Multistate Case-Control Study, 1988–1992. Teratology 1995;51: 20–29.

37. Mastroiacovo P, Botto LD. Chorionic villus sampling and transverse limb deficiencies: maternal age is not a confounder. Am J Med Genet 1994;53:182–186.

39. Dolk H, Bertrand F, Lechat MF, for the EUROCAT Working Group. Chorionic villus sampling and limb abnormalities [Letter]. Lancet 1992;339:876–877.

40. Olney RS, Khoury MJ, Botto LD, Mastroiacovo P. Limb defects and gestational age at chorionic villus sampling [Letter]. Lancet 1994;344:476.

43. Heckerling PS, Verp MS. Amniocentesis or chorionic villus sampling for prenatal genetic testing: a decision analysis. J Clin Epidemiol 1991;44:657–670.

44. Cutillo DM, Hammond EA, Reeser SL, et al. Chorionic villus sampling utilization following reports of a possible association with fetal limb defects. Prenat Diagn 1994;14:327–332.

45. James D, Bickley D, Davies T, McDermott A. Influence of The Lancet on chorionic villus sampling [Letter]. Lancet 1992;340:180–181.

Recommendations for the Use of Folic Acid to Reduce the Number of Cases of Spina Bifida and Other Neural Tube Defects

Original Citation: Centers for Disease Control and Prevention. Recommendations for the use of folic acid to reduce the number of cases of spina bifida and other neural tube defects. MMWR 1992;41(RR-14):1.

INTRODUCTION

Each year in the United States about 2,500 infants are born with the neural tube defects (NTDs) spina bifida and anencephaly. In addition, an unknown number of fetuses affected by these birth defects are aborted. All infants with anencephaly die shortly after birth, whereas the majority of babies born with spina bifida grow to adulthood with, in severe cases, paralysis and varying degrees of bowel and bladder incontinence. The evidence that consumption of folic acid, one of the B vitamins, before conception and during early pregnancy (the periconceptional period) can reduce the number of NTDs has been accumulating for several years. Published data are available from randomized controlled trials (1, 2), non-randomized intervention trials (3, 4), and observational studies (5–8) (Figure 1).

One of the most rigorously conducted studies was the randomized controlled trial sponsored by the British Medical Research Council (MRC) (2). The study showed that high-dose folic acid supplements (4.0 mg per day) used by women who had a prior NTD-affected pregnancy reduced the risk of having a subsequent NTD-affected pregnancy by 70%.

Preliminary results from the Hungarian randomized controlled trial of multivitamin/mineral supplementation (including 0.8 mg of folic acid) among women who had not had a prior NTD-affected pregnancy were reported in 1989 (9). This trial was stopped in May 1992 on the advice of an ad hoc scientific advisory committee because of evidence of an NTD-protective effect of the multivitamin/mineral preparation relative to the study placebo preparation (Czeizel AE, personal communication, May 1992).

Three of four published observational studies showed a lowered risk of NTDs for women who have not had a prior NTD-affected pregnancy and who consumed 0.4–0.8 mg (400–800 µg) of folic acid daily from multivitamin supplements (Figure 1).

Based on a synthesis of information from several studies, including those which used multivitamins containing folic acid at a daily dose level of greater than or equal to 0.4 mg, it was inferred that folic acid alone at levels of 0.4 mg per day will reduce the risk of NTDs.

RECOMMENDATIONS

The United States Public Health Service recommends that:

All women of childbearing age in the United States who are capable of becoming pregnant should consume 0.4 mg of folic acid per day for the purpose

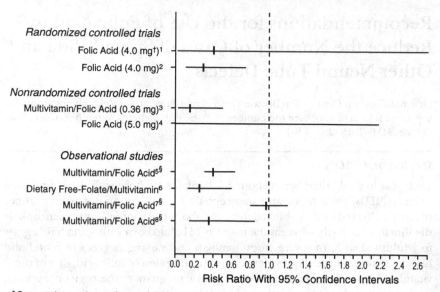

* Superscript numbers refer to references.
† Number in parentheses indicates daily dose of folic acid used in study.
§ Designated observational studies used low-dose folic acid (0.1–1.0 mg).

Figure 1. Risk ratios for multivitamin/folic acid use for preventing neural tube defects, by type of study, 1981–1990.

of reducing their risk of having a pregnancy affected with spina bifida or other NTDs. Because the effects of high intakes are not well known but include complicating the diagnosis of vitamin B_{12} deficiency, care should be taken to keep total folate consumption at less than 1 mg per day, except under the supervision of a physician. Women who have had a prior NTD-affected pregnancy are at high risk of having a subsequent affected pregnancy. When these women are planning to become pregnant, they should consult their physicians for advice.

COMMENT

There are three potential approaches for the delivery of folic acid to the general population in the dosage recommended: (a) improvement of dietary habits, (b) fortification of the U.S. food supply, and (c) use of dietary supplements. The Food and Drug Administration (FDA) will have to determine which approaches will best achieve the goal of increasing folic acid intake while ensuring that potential risks created by overfortification of food with folic acid, and thus overconsumption of this substance, are not reached. This process will require rulemaking and will include substantial efforts to involve the obstetrics community, other medical groups, the scientific community, consumers, industry, and other PHS agencies in a search for the best way to accomplish this goal. While this process is under way, and before the FDA issues final regulations on food fortification and permissible health claims on food labeling, further food fortification with folic acid would be inappropriate, and no health claims should be made. Folate intake greater than or equal to 0.4 mg per day can be obtained from the diet through careful selection of foods. Folate is a generic term for food compounds that have the biologic activity of folic acid; in general, folates obtained from foods are not as well absorbed as is folic acid. Although the average consumption of dietary folate by women in the United States has been estimated to be about 0.2 mg per day (10), women who select foods consistent with the U.S. Dietary Guidelines for Americans and the U.S. Dietary Pyramid are likely to consume diets containing greater than or equal to 0.4 mg of folate daily. Use of currently available fortified foods, such as some breakfast cereals, can also provide important sources of folic acid.

Folic acid supplement pills containing 0.4 mg of folic acid also are available, as are multivitamin preparations containing folic acid. About 20% of U.S. women now consume multivitamin preparations, which generally contain 0.4 mg of folic acid (11). Supplements for pregnant women generally contain up to 0.8 mg of folic acid.

Given these alternative routes for obtaining adequate amounts of folic acid, it is recommended that women be advised of the options available to them to obtain daily intakes of 0.4 mg of folic acid and be encouraged to meet this goal.

The research that serves as the basis for this recommendation generally focused on the use of supplements from at least 1 month before conception through early pregnancy, the periconceptional period. Development of the defect in the neural tube occurs within the first month after conception, before most women are aware of their pregnancy. Because greater than 50% of pregnancies in the United States are unplanned (12), it would be prudent for women to consume 0.4 mg of folic acid daily on a regular, continuous basis as long as they are capable of becoming pregnant.

Because supplements containing folic acid at the 0.4-mg level are widely available, this dosage has been the focus of the available observational research studies. It is possible that lower doses of folic acid may reduce the risk for NTDs, but further research would be needed to learn the minimum effective dose.

At this time, FDA allows food to be labeled according to the level of nutrients in the food relative to the U.S. Recommended Daily Allowances (USRDAs). Consumption of folic acid at USRDA-level doses (0.4 mg for nonpregnant women) is considered a safe and desirable practice. Over the years, RDAs have ranged from 0.18 to 0.4 mg of folic acid for women of childbearing age. RDAs for pregnant women have ranged from 0.4 to 0.8 mg per day. Folic acid is a water-soluble vitamin, and any excess consumed is rapidly excreted in the urine. The effects of higher doses are not well known, although they include complicating the diagnosis of vitamin B_{12} deficiency in certain people (13). Irreversible neurologic damage may occur if B_{12} deficiency is not diagnosed and treated. Therefore, women should be careful to keep their total daily folate consumption at less than 1 mg per day. Women may wish to consult their physicians or other health-care providers (nutritionists, dietitians) about how to best obtain the recommended amount of folic acid, while avoiding excessive consumption. Caution should also be taken to prevent excessive use of multivitamin supplements or fortified foods containing vitamin A, since excess vitamin A may cause birth defects. Further research will be needed to identify any unknown adverse effects.

The current recommendation is directed to all U.S. women, including women who have had a previous NTD-affected pregnancy. In August 1991, CDC issued a guideline (14) for women who have had a prior pregnancy affected by NTDs and who are planning to start a new pregnancy. The guideline called for the consumption of a 4.0-mg daily dose of folic acid, from at least 1 month before conception through the first 3 months of pregnancy. The guideline did not specifically address the issue of folic acid consumption among these women during the times when they are not planning to become pregnant. Women who have had an NTD-affected pregnancy should consume 0.4 mg of folic acid per day, unless they are planning a pregnancy. When these women are planning to become pregnant, they can follow the August 1991 guideline and consult their physicians about the desirability of using 4.0 mg of folic acid per day. Because 4.0 mg of folic acid per day is a very high dose, there may be risks associated with these levels. Although it appears that a lower dose, such as 0.4 mg, may have as great a beneficial effect as 4.0 mg, women who are at very high risk of having an NTD-affected pregnancy may choose to follow the August 1991 guideline (a) because it is based on data from the most rigorous study directly pertinent to their risk of NTDs, and (b) because their risk of having an NTD-affected pregnancy may outweigh any risk that may occur as the result of the use of 4.0 mg of folic acid.

REFERENCES: AS NUMBERED IN ORIGINAL PUBLICATION

1. Laurence KM, James N, Miller M, et al. Double blind randomized controlled trial of folate treatment before conception to prevent recurrence of neural-tube defects. Br Med J 1981;282:1509–1511.
2. MRC Vitamin Study Research Group. Prevention of neural tube defects: results of the Medical Research Council Vitamin Study. Lancet 1991;338:131–137.
3. Smithells RW, Nevin NC, Seller MJ, et al. Further experience of vitamin supplementation for the prevention of neural tube defect recurrences. Lancet 1983;1:1027–1031.
4. Vergel RG, Sanchez LR, Heredero BL, et al. Primary prevention of neural tube defects with folic acid supplementation: Cuban experience. Prenat Diagn 1990;10:149–152.
5. Mulinare J, Cordero JF, Erickson JD, Berry RJ. Periconceptional use of multivitamins and the occurrence of neural tube defects. JAMA 1988;260:3141–3145.
6. Bower C, Stanley FJ. Dietary folate as a risk factor for neural-tube defects: evidence from a case-control study in Western Australia. Med J Aust 1989;150:613–619.
7. Mills JL, Rhoads GG, Simpson JL, et al. The absence of a relation between the periconceptional use of vitamins and neural-tube defects. N Engl J Med 1989;321:430–435.
8. Milunsky A, Jick H, Jick SS, et al. Multivitamin/folic acid supplementation in early pregnancy reduces the prevalence of neural tube defects. JAMA 1989;262:2847–2852.
9. Czeizel AE, Fritz G. Letter to editor. JAMA 1989;262:1634.
10. National Academy of Sciences. Nutrition during pregnancy. Institute of Medicine, Food and Nutrition Board. Washington, DC: National Academy Press, 1990:365.
11. Moss AJ, Levy AS, Kim I, et al. Use of vitamin and mineral supplements in the United States: current users, types of products, and nutrients. Hyattsville, MD: National Center for Health Statistics, 1989 (Advance data, No. 174).
12. Grimes DA. Unplanned pregnancies in the U.S. Obstet Gynecol 1986;67:438–442.
13. Beck WS. Pernicious anemia. In: Wyngaarden JB, Smith LH, eds. Cecil textbook of medicine. 18th ed. Philadelphia: WB Saunders, 1988.
14. CDC. Use of folic acid for prevention of spina bifida and other neural tube defects—1983–1991. MMWR 1991;40:513–516.

Preventing Lead Poisoning in Young Children

Original Citation: Centers for Disease Control and Prevention. Preventing lead poisoning in young children, 1991.

Editor's Note: We have included the summary for pediatric health-care providers from this widely used document. Please refer to the full text for important chapters on sources of lead in the environment and abatement.

SUMMARY FOR THE PEDIATRIC HEALTH-CARE PROVIDER

Introduction and Background

Childhood lead poisoning is one of the most common pediatric health problems in the United States today, and it is entirely preventable. Enough is now known about the sources and pathways of lead exposure and about ways of preventing this exposure to begin the efforts to permanently eradicate this disease. The persistence of lead poisoning in the United States, in light of all that is known, presents a singular and direct challenge to public health authorities, clinicians, regulatory agencies, and society.

Previous lead statements issued by the Centers for Disease Control (CDC) have acknowledged the adverse effects of lead at lower and lower levels. In the most recent previous CDC lead statement, published in 1985, the threshold for action was set at a blood lead level of 25 µg/dL, although it was acknowledged that adverse effects occur below that level. In the past several years, however, the scientific evidence showing that some adverse effects occur at blood lead levels at least as low as 10 µg/dL in children has become so overwhelming and compelling that it must be a major force in determining how we approach childhood lead exposure.

Because 10 µg/dL is the lower level of the range at which effects are now identified, primary prevention activities—communitywide environmental interventions and nutritional and educational campaigns—should be directed at reducing children's blood lead levels at least to below 10 µg/dL. Blood lead levels between 10 and 14 µg/dL are in a border zone. While the overall goal is to reduce children's blood lead levels below 10 µg/dL, there are several reasons for not attempting to do interventions directed at individual children to lower blood lead levels of 10–14 µg/dL. First, laboratory measurements of blood lead levels may be variable, so a blood lead level in this range may, in fact, be below 10 µg/dL. Secondly, effective environmental and medical interventions for children with blood lead levels in this range have not yet been identified and evaluated. Finally, the sheer numbers of children in this range would preclude effective case management and would detract from the individualized followup required by children who have higher blood lead levels.

The Single, All-Purpose Definition of Childhood Lead Poisoning Has Been Replaced with a Multitier Approach

Community prevention activities should be triggered by blood lead levels > or = 10 μg/dL. Medical evaluation and environmental investigation and remediation should be done for all children with blood lead levels > or = 20 μg/dL. All children with blood lead levels > or = 15 μg/dL require individual followup, including nutritional and educational interventions. Furthermore, depending on the availability of resources environmental investigation and remediation should be done for children with blood lead levels of 15–19 μg/dL, if such levels persist. The highest priority should continue to be the children with the highest blood lead levels. Other differences between the 1985 and 1991 statements are as follows:

Screening Test of Choice

Because the erythrocyte protoporphyrin level is not sensitive enough to identify children with elevated blood lead levels below about 25 μg/dL, the screening test of choice is now blood lead measurement.

Universal Screening

Since virtually all children are at risk for lead poisoning, a phase in of universal screening is recommended, except in communities where large numbers or percentages of children have been screened and found not to have lead poisoning. The full implementation of this will require the ability to measure blood lead levels on capillary samples and the availability of cheaper and easier-to-use methods of blood lead measurement.

Primary Prevention

Efforts need to be increasingly focused on preventing lead poisoning before it occurs. This will require communitywide environmental interventions, as well as educational and nutritional campaigns.

Succimer

In January, 1991, the U.S. Food and Drug Administration approved succimer, an oral chelating agent, for chelation of children with blood lead levels over 45 μg/dL.

Sources and Pathways of Lead Exposure

A child's environment is full of lead. Children are exposed to lead from different sources (such as paint, gasoline, and solder) and through different pathways (such as air, food, water, dust, and soil). Although all U.S. children are exposed to some lead from food, air, dust, and soil, some children are exposed to high dose sources of lead. Lead-based paint is the most widespread and dangerous high-dose source of lead exposure for preschool children.

Lead-based paint (containing up to 50% lead) was in widespread use through the 1940s. Although the use and manufacture of interior lead-based paint declined during the 1950s and thereafter, exterior lead-based paint and lesser amounts of interior lead-based paint continued to be available until the mid-1970s. (Lead-based paint produced after the 1940s tended to have much lower lead concentrations than lead-based paint produced earlier.)

Pica, the repeated ingestion of nonfood substances, has been implicated in cases of lead poisoning; however, a child does not have to eat paint chips to become poisoned. More commonly, children ingest dust and soil contaminated with lead from paint which flaked or chalked as it aged or which has been disturbed during home maintenance and renovation. This lead-contaminated house dust, ingested via normal repetitive hand-to-mouth activity, is now recognized as a major contributor to the total body burden of lead in children. Because of the critical role of dust as an exposure pathway, children living in sub-standard housing and in homes undergoing renovation are at particular risk for lead poisoning.

Many cases of childhood lead poisoning that result from renovation or remodeling of homes have been reported. Before older homes undergo any renovation that may generate dust, they should be tested for the presence of lead-based paint. If such paint is found, contractors experienced in working with lead-based paint should do the renovations.

Other potentially important sources and pathways of lead exposure include soil and dust, water, "take home" exposures from parental occupations and hobbies, water, and food. Very high-dose exposure may occasionally result from sources other than lead-based paint in specific situations.

The Role of the Pediatric Health-Care Provider

Pediatric health-care providers, working as part of the public health team, must play a critical role in the prevention and management of childhood lead poisoning. Their roles include: (a) educating parents about key causes of childhood lead poisoning; (b) screening children and interpreting blood lead test results; (c) working with appropriate groups in the public and private sectors to make sure that poisoned children receive appropriate medical, environmental, and social service followup; and (d) coordinating with public health officials and others involved in lead-poisoning prevention activities.

Along with educating parents about nutrition and developmental stages, providers should discuss the potential hazards of lead. They should focus on the major likely preventable sources of high-dose lead poisoning in their communities. Parents should be told of the potential dangers of peeling lead-based paint, the potential hazards of renovating older homes, and the need for good work practices if their occupations or hobbies expose them to lead. In some communities parents should be warned about the potential for lead exposure from improperly fired ceramicware and imported pottery. In others, where water lead levels are a concern, parents could be advised to use only fully-flushed water (that is, water that has not been standing in pipes for a prolonged time) from the cold-water tap for drinking, cooking, or preparing infant formula. Pediatric health-care providers should provide information about simple ways parents can reduce exposure to lead. Some examples of these are discussed below.

Housekeeping Interventions

Particularly in older homes, which may have been painted with lead-based paint, interventions to reduce exposure to dust may help reduce blood lead levels. These include:

- Make sure your child does not have access to peeling paint. Pay special attention to windows and window sills and wells.
- If the house was built before about 1960 and has hard surface floors, wet mop them at least once a week with a high phosphate solution (for example, 6–8% phosphates). (The phosphate content of automatic dishwashing detergents and other cleaning substances is often listed on the label and may be high enough for this purpose. Otherwise, trisodium phosphate can be purchased in hardware stores.) Other hard surfaces (such as window sills and baseboards) should also be wiped with a similar solution. Do not vacuum hard surface floors or window sills or wells, since this will disperse dust. Vacuum cleaners with agitators remove dust from rugs more effectively than vacuum cleaners with suction only.
- Wash your child's hands and face before he/she eats.
- Wash toys and pacifiers frequently.

Other Interventions to Reduce Exposure to Lead

- If soil around the home is or is likely to be contaminated with lead (for example, if the home was built before 1960 or the house is near a major highway), plant grass or other ground cover. Since the highest concentrations of lead in a yard tend to be near surfaces that were once painted with lead paint, like exterior walls, if exterior lead paint was likely to be used, plant bushes around the outside of your house so your child cannot play there.
- In areas where the lead content of water exceeds the drinking water standard, use only fully-flushed water from the cold-water tap for drinking, cooking, and making formula. In communities where water conservation is a concern, use first-flush water for other purposes.
- Do not store food in open cans, particularly if the cans are imported.
- Do not use pottery or ceramicware that was improperly fired or is meant for decorative use for food storage or service.
- Make sure that take-home exposures are not occurring from parental occupations or hobbies (see Chapter 3 of original citation).

Not all aspects of a poisoned child's followup will be managed by the pediatric health-care provider, although the provider is an important part of the team. Through his or her interactions with the child and family and the responsible public health agency, the provider should make sure that any appropriate interventions are occurring. If the child needs a medical evaluation (for a blood lead level > or = 20 µg/dL) or pharmacologic treatment (see Chapter 7 of original citation), either the provider should do it or should refer the child to a place that treats large numbers of poisoned children. The provider should make sure that the child receives an appropriate environmental investigation and remediation with the help of the public health agencies. Particularly if the child is developmentally delayed, the provider should refer the child to an appropriate infant stimulation or child development program. In many cases, lead-poisoned children and their families will also benefit from social services followup.

THE ROLE OF STATE AND LOCAL PUBLIC AGENCIES

A variety of local, state and federal agencies play a role in preventing childhood lead poisoning. Pediatric health care providers and parents should know about what these agencies do so that they can use these resources effectively. In turn, these agencies must coordinate their activities to ensure that all aspects of childhood lead poisoning prevention—health, housing, and environment— are being addressed, and to provide the most comprehensive and cost-effective services to at-risk children, their parents, and their health-care providers.

SCREENING

Traditionally, the main purpose of a childhood lead poisoning screening program has been to identify asymptomatic lead-poisoned children and to intervene as quickly as possible to reduce their blood lead levels. An additional benefit of screening programs is that abatement of lead sources for poisoned children results in prevention of lead poisoning for children who would have been exposed to those sources in the future. As the focus in lead poisoning prevention turns more to primary prevention, an additional benefit of screening is that data generated can be used in targeting interventions to places with children at high risk for lead poisoning.

In 1984, the last year for which estimates are available, it is believed that between 3 and 4 million children younger than age 6 years (17% of all U.S. children in this age group) had blood lead levels above 15 µg/dL. Furthermore, about 74% of occupied, privately owned housing built before 1980 contains lead-based paint (defined as > or = 1 mg/square cm). BECAUSE ALMOST ALL U.S. CHILDREN ARE AT RISK FOR LEAD POISONING (ALTHOUGH SOME CHILDREN ARE AT HIGHER RISK THAN OTHERS), OUR GOAL IS THAT ALL CHILDREN SHOULD BE SCREENED, UNLESS IT CAN BE SHOWN THAT THE COMMUNITY IN WHICH THESE CHILDREN LIVE DOES NOT HAVE A CHILDHOOD LEAD POISONING PROBLEM. (Deciding that no problem exists requires that a large number or percentage of children be tested.) The full implementation of this will require the ability to measure blood lead levels on capillary samples and the availability of cheaper and easier-to-use methods of blood lead measurement. Children at highest risk for lead poisoning are the highest priority for screening. Table 6.1 provides guidance on the groups for which repeated screening is most strongly indicated.

Children ages 6 to 72 months who live in or are frequent visitors to deteriorated old buildings, including day care centers, make up the highest priority group. Because the highest concentrations of lead in paint were used in the early 1900s, homes built before about 1960 are of greatest concern. Children whose homes are being renovated are also at extremely high risk. Since sib-

Table 6.1. Priority groups for screening

Children, ages 6 to 72 months, who live in or are frequent visitors to deteriorated housing built before 1960.

Children, ages 6 to 72 months, who live in housing built before 1960 with recent, ongoing, or planned renovation or remodeling.

Children, ages 6 to 72 months, who are siblings, house mates, or playmates of children with known lead poisoning.

Children, ages 6 to 72 months, whose parents or other household members participate in a lead-related occupation or hobby.

Children, ages 6 to 72 months, who live near active lead smelters, battery recycling plant or other industries likely to result in atmospheric lead release.

lings, house mates, visitors, and playmates of children with confirmed lead poisoning may have similar exposures to lead, they also should be promptly screened. In communities with a high prevalence of lead poisoning, health departments should consider door-to-door screening, since many children with lead poisoning may be missed by fixed-site screening.

Children with parents whose work or hobbies involve lead may also risk lead exposure (see Chapter 3 of original citation). Also, children living near lead smelters or other industries where lead is processed may be at increased risk for lead poisoning.

In general, screening and assessment for lead poisoning should focus on children younger than 72 months of age, particularly on children younger than 36 months of age. Young children engage in the most hand-to-mouth activity (and therefore are at highest risk for lead exposure) and have the most rapidly developing nervous systems, making them more vulnerable to the effects of lead. Children with developmental delays, who may exhibit pica or have more extensive hand-to-mouth activity than other children, would be expected to be at increased risk for lead poisoning even if they are 72 months of age and older. These children may have to be screened more often during early infancy, and may require screening into their school years.

Children who have unexplained seizures, neurological symptoms, abdominal pain, or other symptoms that are consistent with lead poisoning should also have their blood lead levels measured. In addition, the possibility of lead poisoning should be considered in any child with growth failure, developmental delay, hyperactivity, behavior disorders, hearing loss, anemia, etc.

Screening Method

Since erythrocyte protoporphyrin (EP) is not sensitive enough to identify more than a small percentage of children with blood lead levels between 10 and 25 $\mu g/dL$ and misses many children with blood lead levels > or = 25 $\mu g/dL$, measurement of blood lead levels should replace the EP test as the primary screening method. Unless contamination of capillary blood samples can be prevented, lead levels should be measured on venous samples. Obtaining capillary specimens is more feasible at many screening sites. Contamination of capillary specimens obtained by finger prick can be minimized if trained personnel follow proper technique. Elevated blood lead results obtained on capillary specimens should be considered presumptive and must be confirmed using venous blood. At the present time, not all laboratories will measure lead levels on capillary specimens.

Anticipatory Guidance and Assessing Risk

Guidance on childhood lead poisoning prevention and assessment of the risk of lead poisoning should be part of routine pediatric care. Anticipatory guidance is discussed in detail in Chapter 4 of the original citation. The guidance and risk assessment should emphasize the sources and exposures that are of greatest concern in the child's community (see Chapter 3 of original citation). Because lead-based paint has been used in housing throughout the United States, in most communities it will be necessary to focus on this source.

Table 6.2 has sample questions for assessing a child's risk for high-dose lead exposure. Starting at 6 months of age and at each regular office visit thereafter, pediatric health-care providers should discuss childhood lead poisoning and assess the child's risk for high-dose exposure. The questions asked should be tailored to the likely sources of exposure in the community. THE QUESTIONS ARE NOT A SUBSTITUTE FOR A BLOOD LEAD TEST. On the basis of responses to questions such as those in (Table 6.2), children can be categorized as low or high risk for high-dose lead exposure. If the answers to all questions are negative, the child is at low risk for high-dose lead exposure and should be screened by a blood lead test at 12 months and again, if possible, at 24 months (since blood lead levels often peak at ages greater than 12 months). If the answer to any question is positive, the child is potentially at high risk for high-dose lead exposure, and a blood lead test should be obtained. FOR CHILDREN PREVIOUSLY AT LOW RISK, ANY HISTORY SUGGESTING THAT EXPOSURE TO LEAD HAS INCREASED SHOULD BE FOLLOWED UP WITH A BLOOD LEAD TEST.

Table 6.2. Assessing the risk of high-dose exposure to lead—sample questionnaire

Does your child
1. Live or regularly visit a house with peeling or chipping paint built before 1960? This could include a day care center, preschool, the home of a babysitter or relative, etc.
2. Live in or regularly visit a house built before 1960 with recent, ongoing, or planned renovation or remodeling?
3. Have a brother or sister, housemaid, or playmate being followed or treated for lead poisoning (that is, blood lead greater than or equal to 15 μg/dL)?
4. Live with an adult whose job or hobby involves exposure to lead?
5. Live near an active lead smelter, battery recycling plant, or other industry likely to release lead?

Screening Schedule

The following sections provide a minimum screening schedule for children aged 6 up to 36 and 36 to 72 months. The schedule is not rigid. Rather, it is a guide for pediatric health-care providers and screening programs to use in conjunction with other pertinent information in determining when an individual child should be tested. Programs and pediatric health-care providers may choose to screen more frequently than described below.

Children 6 up to 36 Months of Age

A questionnaire should be used at each routine office visit to assess the potential for high-dose lead exposure and, therefore, the appropriate frequency of screening.

Schedule If the Child Is at Low Risk for High Dose Lead Exposure by Questionnaire

A child at LOW RISK for exposure to high-dose lead sources by questionnaire should have an initial blood lead test at 12 months of age.

If the 12-month blood lead result is < 10 µg/dL, the child should be retested at 24 months if possible, since that is when blood lead levels peak.

If a blood lead test result is 10–14 µg/dL, the child should be retested every 3 to 4 months. After 2 consecutive measurements are < 10 µg/dL or three are < 15 µg/dL, the child should be retested in a year.

If any blood lead test result is > 15 µg/dL, the child needs individual case management and should be retested at least every 3 to 4 months.

Schedule If the Child Is at High Risk for High Dose Lead Exposure by Questionnaire

A child at HIGH RISK for exposure to high-dose lead sources by questionnaire should have an initial blood lead test at 6 months of age.

If the initial blood lead result is < 10 µg/dL, the child should be re-screened every 6 months. After 2 subsequent consecutive measurements are < 10 µg/dL or three are < 15 µg/dL, testing frequency can be decreased to once a year.

If a blood lead test result is 10–14 µg/dL, the child should be screened every 3 to 4 months. Once 2 subsequent consecutive measurements are < 10 µg/dL or three are < 15 µg/dL, testing frequency can be decreased to once a year.

If any blood lead test result is > OR = 15 µg/dL, the child needs individual case management and should be retested at least every 3 to 4 months.

Children > or = 36 Months and < 72 Months of Age

As for younger children, a questionnaire should be used at each routine office visit of children from 36 to 72 months of age. Any child at high risk by questionnaire who has not previously had a blood lead test should be tested. All children who have had venous blood lead tests > or = 15 μg/dL or who are at high risk by questionnaire should be screened at least once a year until their sixth birthday (age 72 months) or later, if indicated (for example, a retarded child with pica). Children should also be rescreened any time history suggests exposure has increased. Children with blood lead levels > or = 15 μg/dL should receive followup as described below.

Followup of Children with Blood Lead Levels > or = 15 μg/dL

Followup of children with blood lead levels > or = 15 μg/dL is discussed in more detail in later chapters of the original citation and is briefly summarized below. In general, such children should receive blood lead tests at least every 3 to 4 months.

IF THE BLOOD LEAD LEVEL IS 16–19 μg/dL, the child should be screened every 3–4 months, the family should be given education and nutritional counseling as described in Chapter 4 of the original citation, and a detailed environmental history should be taken to identify any obvious sources or pathways of lead exposure. When the venous blood lead level is in this range in two consecutive tests 3–4 months apart, environmental investigation and abatement should be conducted, if resources permit.

IF THE BLOOD LEAD LEVEL IS > OR = 20 μg/dL, the child should be given a repeat test for confirmation. If the venous blood lead level is confirmed to be > or = 20 μg/dL, the child should be referred for medical evaluation and followup as described in Chapter 7 of the original citation. Such children should continue to receive blood lead tests every 3–4 months or more often if indicated. Children with blood lead levels > or = 45 μg/dL must receive urgent medical and environmental followup, preferably at a clinic with a staff experienced in dealing with this disease. Symptomatic lead poisoning or a venous blood lead concentration > or = 70 μg/dL is a medical emergency, requiring immediate inpatient chelation therapy, as described in Chapter 7 of the original citation.

Classification on the Basis of Screening Test Results

On the basis of screening test results, children can be classified into categories according to their risk for adverse effects of lead. The urgency and type of followup are based on these risk classes. These classes are shown in (Table 6.3).

Measurement of Blood Lead Levels

Several factors can influence the quality of blood lead measurements. The ubiquity of lead in the environment makes contamination of specimens during collection a major source of error. Analytical variation in the laboratory can affect results. Accuracy and precision of blood lead measurements, particularly at low concentrations, can be assured by the use of appropriate analytical standards, maintenance of equipment, training of personnel, and participation in external proficiency testing programs.

Table 6.3. Class of child and recommended action according to blood lead measurement

Class	Blood Lead Concentration (μg/dL)	Action
I	≤9	Low risk for high-dose exposure: rescreen as described in text. High risk for high-dose exposure: rescreen as described in text.
IIA	10–14	Rescreen as described in text. If many children in the community have blood lead levels ≥10, community interventions (primary prevention activities) should be considered by appropriate agencies.
IIB	15–19	Rescreen as described in text. Take a history to assess possible high-dose sources of lead. Educate parents about diet, cleaning, etc. Test for iron deficiency. Consider environmental investigation and lead hazard abatement if levels persist.
III	20–44*	Conduct a complete medical evaluation. Identify and eliminate environmental lead sources.
IV	45–69*	Begin medical treatment and environmental assessment and remediation within 48 hours.
V	≥70*	Begin medical treatment and environmental assessment and remediation IMMEDIATELY.

*Based on confirmatory blood lead level.

Since blood collected by venipuncture has a low likelihood of contamination compared to blood collected by finger stick, venous blood is the preferred specimen for analysis and should be used for lead measurement whenever practicable. In addition, venous specimens provide a larger volume for analysis and are less prone to clotting and other problems that can be encountered with capillary specimens. At the present time, not all laboratories will accept capillary samples for lead analysis.

Finger stick specimens are acceptable for blood lead screening, provided that special collection procedures are followed to minimize the risk of contamination. Personnel must be thoroughly trained in collection procedures. A procedure for collecting finger stick specimens is described in Appendix I (in original publication).

Elevated blood lead results obtained on capillary specimens are presumptive and must be confirmed using venous blood. In general, children who have blood lead levels > or = 15 µg/dL on capillary samples should have these levels confirmed on venous samples, according to the timetable in (Table 6.4). A child with a blood lead level > or = 70 µg/dL or with symptoms of lead poisoning should be treated immediately while the results of an immediate confirmatory test are awaited.

Table 6.4. Suggested timetable for confirming capillary blood lead results with a venous blood measurement

Blood lead level (µg/dL)	Time within which blood lead level should be obtained
<10	Not applicable
10–14	Not applicable
15–19	Within 1 month
20–44	Within 1 week
45–69	Within 48 hours
≥70	Immediately

Blood Lead Levels—Additional Analytical Considerations

Blood lead levels can be determined by several analytic methods. The method used can affect the specimen volume required, the choice of anticoagulant (usually heparin or ethylenediaminetetraacetic acid (EDTA)), and other aspects related to specimen suitability. Specimen collection procedures and equipment must be checked for compatibility with laboratory requirements. Special lead-free evacuated tubes are available for blood collection, but standard tubes containing EDTA or heparin (lavender or green caps) can be acceptable after screening each lot to determine the lead content of the containers, needles, etc. Though reports of unsuitable levels of background lead in other collection materials are infrequent, all materials used should be determined to be lead-free before use.

Laboratories where blood is tested for lead levels should be successful participants in a blood lead proficiency testing program, such as the program conducted jointly by CDC, the Health Resources and Services Administration, and the University of Wisconsin. In interpreting laboratory results, it should be recognized that a "proficient" laboratory need only measure blood lead levels to within several µg/dL of the true value (for example, within 4 or 6 µg/dL of a target value). The blood lead level reported by a laboratory, therefore, may be several µg/dL higher or lower than the actual blood lead level.

Erythrocyte Protoporphyrin (EP)

EP is not a sensitive test to identify children with blood lead levels below about 25 µg/dL, and therefore it is no longer the screening test of choice. In some programs, however, it will continue to be used until the transition to blood lead measurements is complete.

Only fresh blood is suitable for analysis by hematofluorometer. Complete oxygenation of sample hemoglobin is necessary to prevent low results in some instruments. The hemoglobin concentration in the sample can also affect hematofluorometer EP readings. Results obtained by extraction methods are not affected by these factors and can be used to confirm hematofluorometer EP results.

In the past, an absorptivity of 241 L cm-1 mmol-1 has been used to determine EP levels. Recently, however, the correct absorptivity has been determined to be 297 L cm-1 mmol-1. Use of the correct absorptivity will result in EP values about 19% lower than those standardized using 241 L cm-1 mmol-1. Standardization of EP levels that are based on the correct absorptivity is expected to be widely adopted in 1992. Use of the correct standardization requires a change in calibration and is not simply a reduction of the screening cutoff value. Standardization criteria should also be considered when reviewing data in the literature.

An EP result of > or = 35 μg/dL standardized using 241 L cm-1 mmol-1 or > or = 28 μg/dL standardized using 297 L cm-1 mmol-1 is considered elevated. ALL ELEVATED EP RESULTS SHOULD BE FOLLOWED WITH A VENOUS BLOOD LEAD TEST TO DETERMINE IF LEAD POISONING IS RESPONSIBLE FOR THE ELEVATION. Elevated concentrations of EP also result from several health conditions other than lead intoxication, particularly iron deficiency. The iron status of children with elevated EP levels should always be determined, especially since iron deficiency and lead poisoning often coexist. In such cases, the EP may be disproportionately elevated in comparison to the blood lead level.

Some hematofluorometers report EP levels as μmol ZnPP/mol heme. For instruments that give results in these units, EP values > or = 70 μmol/mol should be considered elevated and should be promptly investigated.

DIAGNOSTIC EVALUATION AND MEDICAL MANAGEMENT OF CHILDREN WITH BLOOD LEAD LEVELS > OR = 20 MG/DL

Children with blood lead levels between 10 μg/dL and 19 μg/dL and their siblings need followup and repeat screening as described in previous sections. They do not, however, need medical evaluation as described in this chapter.

The cornerstones of clinical management are careful clinical and laboratory surveillance of the child, medical treatment when indicated, and eradication of controllable sources of environmental lead. THE MOST IMPORTANT FACTOR IN CASE MANAGEMENT IS TO DRASTICALLY REDUCE THE CHILD'S EXPOSURE TO LEAD.

All children with confirmed venous blood lead levels > or = 20 μg/dL require medical evaluation. The urgency of further medical evaluation depends on the blood lead level and whether symptoms are present.

The decision to institute medical management should virtually always be made on the basis of a venous blood lead measurement. No other screening test can be considered diagnostic. If the first evaluation was made on capillary blood, a confirmatory venous blood lead level must be done. Even if the first diagnostic measurement was on venous blood, it is preferable to retest before starting chelation therapy. For children with blood lead levels > or = 70 μg/dL or clinical symptoms of lead poisoning, chelation should not be postponed while awaiting results of the repeat test.

Symptoms of Lead Poisoning

SYMPTOMS OF LEAD POISONING IN A CHILD WITH AN ELEVATED BLOOD LEAD LEVEL CONSTITUTE A MEDICAL EMERGENCY, AND THE CHILD SHOULD BE HOSPITALIZED. Symptoms, which can mimic several other pediatric disorders, must be looked for so they are not missed.

Acute lead encephalopathy is characterized by some or all of these symptoms: coma, seizures, bizarre behavior, ataxia, apathy, incoordination, vomiting, alteration in the state of consciousness, and subtle loss of recently acquired skills. Any one or a mixture of these symptoms, associated with an elevated blood lead level, is an acute medical emergency. Lead encephalopathy is almost always associated with a blood lead level exceeding 100 μg/dL, although, occasionally, it has been reported at blood lead levels as low as 70 μg/dL. Even when identified and promptly treated, severe and permanent brain damage may result in 70%–80% of children with lead encephalopathy. Children with symptomatic lead poisoning with or without encephalopathy represent an acute medical emergency. THE POSSIBILITY OF LEAD ENCEPHALOPATHY SHOULD BE CONSIDERED IN THE DIFFERENTIAL DIAGNOSIS OF CHILDREN PRESENTING WITH COMA AND CONVULSIONS OF UNKNOWN ETIOLOGY.

Except for coma and seizures, symptomatic lead poisoning without encephalopathy is characterized by symptoms similar to those of lead encephalopathy. Symptomatic lead poisoning without encephalopathy is characterized by one or a combination of these symptoms: decrease in play activity, lethargy, anorexia, sporadic vomiting, intermittent abdominal pain, and constipation. These symptoms are usually associated with blood lead levels of at least 70 μg/dL, although occasionally cases have been associated with levels as low as 50 μg/dL. If the blood lead level is below 50 μg/dL, other causes of the symptoms should be sought. SINCE ACUTE LEAD ENCEPHALOPATHY MAY DEVELOP IN ANY SYMPTOMATIC CHILD, TREATMENT AND SUPPORTIVE MEASURES MUST BE STARTED IMMEDIATELY ON AN EMERGENCY BASIS.

Evaluation of the Child with a Blood Lead Level > or = 20 μg/dL

A child with a blood lead level > or = 20 μg/dL should have a pediatric evaluation, whether or not symptoms are present.

SPECIAL ATTENTION SHOULD BE GIVEN TO:

1. A detailed history, including the presence or absence of clinical symptoms, child's mouthing activities, the existence of pica, nutritional status (especially iron and calcium intake), dietary habits, family history of lead poi-

soning, potential sources of lead exposure (including exposure due to home renovation), and previous blood lead measurements.

2. Detailed environmental and occupational histories of adults in the household or other places the child spends a lot of time.

3. The physical examination, with particular attention to the neurologic examination and psychosocial and language development. A neurobehavioral assessment may be useful in children receiving chelation therapy both at the time of diagnosis and as the child approaches school age. Findings of language delay or other problems can prompt referral to appropriate programs.

4. Evaluation of iron status using measurement of iron and total iron binding capacity or of ferritin.

Tests

Tests for Iron Deficiency

BECAUSE IRON DEFICIENCY CAN ENHANCE LEAD ABSORPTION AND TOXICITY AND OFTEN COEXISTS WITH IT, ALL CHILDREN WITH BLOOD LEAD LEVELS > OR = 20 Mg/dL SHOULD BE TESTED FOR IRON DEFICIENCY. Measurements of hemoglobin, hematocrit, and reticulocyte are not adequately sensitive, and erythrocyte protoporphyrin (EP) is not specific enough to diagnose iron deficiency (although EP can be used to screen for iron deficiency).

SERUM IRON AND IRON BINDING CAPACITY (TRANSFERRIN SATURATION) AND FERRITIN are the most sensitive indicators of iron status. An abnormally low ratio of serum iron to iron binding capacity (transferrin saturation) of 0.2 is consistent with iron deficiency. The serum ferritin level, however, is the most definitive and accurate indication of overall iron status, although it is an acute phase reactant and may be falsely elevated in sick children; a value > or = 12 μg/dL indicates iron deficiency. Although all iron deficient children should receive treatment for this condition, the treatment should not be started until after chelation is completed in children receiving dimercaprol (BAL).

EP Level

An elevated EP level indicates impairment of the heme biosynthetic pathway. EP levels are sensitive screening tests for iron deficiency, and iron status should be assessed in any child with an elevated EP level (that is, > or = 35 μg/dL when standardized using 241 L cm-1 mmol-1, > or = 28 μg/dL when standardized using 297 L cm-1 mmol-1, or > or = 70 μmol/mol when measured in μmol/mol units).

Because EP levels take about 2 weeks to increase, EP levels may provide an indication of the duration of lead exposure. Similarly, monitoring the EP level after medical and environmental interventions for poisoned children may be useful. If exposure to lead has ceased, EP values elevated because of lead poisoning decline slowly over several weeks or months. A progressive decline in EP concentrations indicates that combined medical and environmental case management is proceeding efficaciously.

Edetate Disodium Calcium (CaNa2EDTA) Provocative Chelation Test

The mobilization test is used to determine whether a child with an initial confirmatory blood lead level of 25 to 44 μg/dL will respond to chelation therapy with a brisk lead diuresis. Because of the cost and staff time needed for quantitative urine collection, this test is used only in selected medical centers where large numbers of lead-poisoned children are treated. Children whose blood lead levels are > or = 45 μg/dL should not receive a provocative chelation test; they should be referred for appropriate chelation therapy immediately.

The outcome of the provocative chelation test is determined not by a decrease in the blood lead level but by the amount of lead excreted per dose of CaNa2EDTA given. This ratio correlates well with blood lead levels. In one study, almost all children with blood lead levels 45 μg/dL had positive provocative tests, 76% of the children with blood lead levels 35 to 44 μg/dL had positive test results, and 35% of the children with blood lead levels 25 to 34 μg/dL had positive test results. This test should not be done until the child is iron replete, since iron status may affect the outcome of the test. Details on how to conduct and interpret a provocative chelation test are in Chapter 7 of the original citation.

Radiologic Examination of the Abdomen

Radiologic examination of the abdomen (flat plate) may show radiopaque foreign material if the material has been ingested during the preceding 24 to 36 hours. Neither negative nor positive x-ray results are diagnostic or definitive. A flat plate of the abdomen may, however, provide information about the source of lead if paint chips or other lead objects are found.

Radiologic Examination of the Long Bones

X-rays of the long bones are unreliable for diagnosing acute lead poisoning, and they should not be obtained on a routine basis. They may provide some indication of whether lead poisoning has occurred in the past or has been ongoing for a length of time, and this may occasionally be important. Lines of increased density in the metaphyseal plate of the distal femur, proximal tibia, and fibula may be caused by lead which has disrupted the metabolism of bone matrix. Although these lines are sometimes called lead lines, they are areas of increased mineralization or calcification and not x-ray shadows of deposited lead.

The Following Tests Are Not Indicated for the Diagnosis or Clinical Management of Lead Poisoning

Microscopic examination of red cells for basophilic stippling. Since basophilic stippling is not always found in severe lead poisoning and is insensitive to lesser degrees of lead poisoning, it is not useful in diagnosis.

Tests of hair and fingernails for lead levels. The levels of lead in hair or fingernails do not correlate well with blood lead levels, except in extreme cases of symptomatic lead poisoning; therefore, these tests are not useful in diagnosis. Children should never receive chelating agents on the basis of analyses of lead levels in hair or fingernails.

Pharmacology of Chelating Agents

Several drugs are used in the treatment of lead poisoning. These drugs, capable of binding or chelating lead, deplete the soft and hard (skeletal) tissues of lead and thus reduce its acute toxicity. All drugs have potential side effects and must be used with caution. The basic pharmacologic characteristics of the various drugs are described below (Table 7.1).

Table 7.1. Chelating agents used in treating children with lead poisoning

Product Name	Generic Name	Chemical Name	Abbreviation
Calcium Disodium Versenate	Edetate disodium calcium	Calcium disodium ethylenediamine tetraacetate	CaNa2 EDTA
BAL in oil	Dimercaprol	2,3-dimercapto-1-propanol	BAL
Cuprimine	D-penicillamine	3-mercapto-D-valine	D-pencillamine
Chemet	Succimer	Meso 2,3-dimercaptosuccinic acid	DSMA

BAL

Mechanism of Action

Two molecules of dimercaprol (BAL) combine with one atom of heavy metal to form a stable complex. BAL enhances fecal and urinary excretion of lead and diffuses well into erythrocytes. Because it is predominantly excreted in bile, BAL can be administered in the presence of renal impairment.

Route of Administration and Dosage

BAL is available only in peanut oil for intramuscular administration. It is usually given every 4 hours, although it may be given every 8 hours; dosages are discussed below.

Precautions and Toxicity

For patients with glucose-6-phosphate dehydrogenase deficiency (G-6-PD), some clinicians recommend that BAL should be used only in life-threatening situations because it may induce hemolysis. Medicinal iron should never be administered during BAL therapy, because the combination of iron and BAL has been implicated in serious reactions. If iron deficiency coexists, it should not be treated until after BAL therapy has been completed. In cases of extreme anemia, blood transfusions are preferable.

Between 30% and 50% of patients who receive BAL will experience side effects. Mild febrile reactions and transient elevations of hepatic transaminases may be observed. Other minor adverse effects include, in order of frequency, nausea and occasional vomiting, headache, mild conjunctivitis, lacrimation, rhinorrhea, and salivation. Most side effects are transient and rapidly subside as the drug is metabolized and excreted. Intravenous hydration coupled with restricting oral intake can circumvent, in large part, gastrointestinal distress. BAL SHOULD NOT BE USED FOR CHILDREN WHO ARE ALLERGIC TO PEANUTS OR PEANUT PRODUCTS.

CaNa2EDTA

ONLY CaNa2EDTA CAN BE USED FOR TREATING CHILDREN WITH LEAD POISONING. Na2EDTA (DISODIUM EDETATE) SHOULD NEVER BE USED FOR TREATING CHILDREN WITH LEAD POISONING BECAUSE IT WILL INDUCE TETANY AND POSSIBLY FATAL HYPOCALCEMIA.

Mechanism of Action

CaNa2EDTA increases urinary lead excretion twentyfold to fiftyfold. CaNa2EDTA removes lead from the extracellular compartment only, because it does not enter cells.

Route of Administration and Dosage

The preferred route for administration of CaNa2EDTA is intravenous. CaNa2EDTA must be diluted to a concentration < 0.5% in dextrose and water or in 0.9% saline solution. It can be given as a continuous infusion or it can be given in two divided doses a day through a heparin lock over 30 to 60 minutes. CaNa2EDTA causes extreme pain when administered intramuscularly; therefore, when given by this route, it should be mixed with procaine so that the final concentration of procaine is 0.5%. CaNa2EDTA should never be given orally because it enhances absorption of lead from the gastrointestinal tract.

Dosages vary by situation and are detailed in Chapter 7 of the original citation. Individual courses should be limited to 5 days and repeated courses should be given at a minimum of 2- to 5-day intervals. Particularly when CaNa2EDTA is given on an outpatient basis, some clinicians use sequential 3-day courses of treatment.

Precautions and Toxicity

During chelation therapy with CaNa2EDTA, urine output, urine sediment, blood urea nitrogen (BUN), serum creatinine, and hepatocellular enzyme levels must be carefully monitored. The appearance of protein and formed elements in urinary sediment, and rising BUN and serum creatinine values reflect impending renal failure—the serious toxicity associated with inappropriately excessive or prolonged administration of CaNa2EDTA. Liver transaminases may increase by the fifth day of therapy, but return to pretreatment levels within a week after treatment has ended.

When CaNa2EDTA is used alone without concomitant BAL therapy, it may aggravate symptoms in patients with very high blood lead levels. Therefore, it should be used in conjunction with BAL when the blood lead level is > or = 70 µg/dL or overt clinical symptoms of lead poisoning are present. In such cases, the first dose of BAL should always precede the first dose of CaNa2EDTA by at least 4 hours.

The kidney is the principal site of potential toxicity. Renal toxicity is dose related, reversible, and rarely (if ever) occurs at doses < 1500 mg/square m when the patient is adequately hydrated. CaNa2EDTA must never be given in the absence of an adequate urine flow.

D-Penicillamine

The Food and Drug Administration (FDA) has approved d-penicillamine for the treatment of Wilson's disease, cystinuria, and severe, active rheumatoid arthritis. Although not approved for this use, it is used in some centers for treating lead poisoning. Until the recent approval of succimer, it was the only commercially available oral chelating agent. It can be given over a long period (weeks to months). D-Penicillamine has been used mainly for children with blood lead levels < 45 µg/dL.

Mechanism of Action

D-Penicillamine enhances urinary excretion of lead, although not as effectively as CaNa2EDTA. Its specific mechanism and site of action are not well understood.

Route of Administration and Dosage

D-Penicillamine is administered orally. It is available in capsules or tablets (125 mg and 250 mg). These capsules can be opened and suspended in liquid, if necessary. The usual dose is 25 to 35 mg/kg/day in divided doses. Side effects can be minimized, to an extent, by starting with a small dose and increasing it gradually, monitoring all the time for side effects. For example, 25% of the desired final dose could be given in week 1, 50% in week 2, and the full dose by week 3.

Precautions and Toxicity

Toxic side effects (albeit minor in most cases) occur in as many as 33% of patients given the drug. The main side effects of D-penicillamine are reactions resembling those of penicillin sensitivity, including rashes, leukopenia, thrombocytopenia, hematuria, proteinuria and hepatocellular enzyme elevations, and eosinophilia. Anorexia, nausea, and vomiting are infrequent. Of most concern, however, are isolated reports of nephrotoxicity, possibly from hypersensitivity reactions. For these reasons, patients should be carefully and frequently monitored for clinically obvious side effects, and frequent blood counts, urinalyses, and renal function tests should be performed. In particular, blood counts and urinalyses should be done on day 1, day 14, day 28, and monthly thereafter. If the absolute neutrophil count falls to < 1500/µL, the count should be rechecked immediately, and treatment should be stopped if it falls to < 1200/µL. D-Penicillamine should not be given on an outpatient basis if exposure to lead is continuing or the physician has doubts about compliance with the therapeutic regimen. D-PENICILLAMINE SHOULD NOT BE ADMINISTERED TO PATIENTS WITH KNOWN PENICILLIN ALLERGY.

Succimer

The FDA approved succimer in January, 1991 for treating children with blood lead levels > 45 µg/dL. Succimer appears to be an effective oral chelating agent.

Its selectivity for lead is high, whereas its ability to chelate essential trace metals is low. Although its use to date has been limited, succimer appears to have promising potential, and a broader range of clinical research studies in children are being undertaken.

Succimer is chemically similar to BAL but is more water soluble, has a high therapeutic index, and is absorbed from the gastrointestinal tract. It is effective when given orally and produces a lead diuresis comparable to that produced by CaNa2EDTA. This diuresis lowers blood lead levels and reverses the biochemical toxicity of lead, as indicated by normalization of circulating aminolevulinic acid dehydrase levels. Succimer is not indicated for prophylaxis of lead poisoning in a lead-containing environment. AS WITH ALL CHELATING AGENTS, SUCCIMER SHOULD ONLY BE GIVEN TO CHILDREN WHO RESIDE IN ENVIRONMENTS FREE OF LEAD DURING AND AFTER TREATMENT.

MECHANISM OF ACTION.

Succimer appears to be more specific for lead than the most commonly used chelating agent, CaNa2EDTA; the urinary loss of essential trace elements (for example, zinc) appears to be considerably less with succimer than with CaNa2EDTA. The site of lead chelation by succimer is not known.

Route of Administration and Dosage

Succimer is administered orally. It is available in 100 mg capsules. The recommended initial dose is 350 mg/square m (10 mg/kg) every 8 hours for 5 days, followed by 350 mg/square (10 mg/kg) every 12 hours for 14 days. A course of treatment, therefore, lasts 19 days. If more courses are needed, a minimum of 2 weeks between courses is preferred, unless blood lead levels indicate the need for immediate retreatment. These doses may be modified as more experience is gained in using succimer.

Patients who have received therapeutic courses of CaNa2EDTA with or without BAL may use succimer for subsequent treatment after an interval of 4 weeks. Data on the concomitant use of succimer and CaNa2EDTA with or without BAL are not available, and such use is not recommended.

If young children cannot swallow capsules, succimer can be administered by separating the capsule and sprinkling the medicated beads on a small amount of soft food or by putting them on a spoon and following with a fruit drink. Data are not available on how stable succimer is when it is suspended in soft foods for prolonged periods of time; succimer should be mixed with soft foods immediately before being given to the child.

Precautions and Toxicity

To date, toxicity due to succimer (transient elevations in hepatic enzyme activities) appears to be minimal. The most common adverse effects reported in clinical trials in children and adults were primarily gastrointestinal and included nausea, vomiting, diarrhea, and appetite loss. Rashes, some necessitating discontinuation of therapy, have been reported for about 4% of patients. THOUGH SUCCIMER HOLDS CONSIDERABLE PROMISE FOR THE OUTPATIENT MANAGEMENT OF LEAD POISONING, CLINICAL EXPERIENCE

WITH SUCCIMER IS LIMITED. Consequently, the full spectrum and incidence of adverse reactions, including the possibility of hypersensitivity or idiosyncratic reactions, have not been determined. Other precautions that need to
be taken with succimer are discussed in the full statement.

Treatment Guidelines for Children with Blood Lead Levels > or = 20 μg/dL

The single most important factor in managing of childhood lead poisoning is
the reducing the child's exposure to lead; some children, however, will benefit
from chelation therapy. Sample regimens for treating children with lead poisoning are described in Chapter 7 of the original publication.

Medical Management of Symptomatic Lead Poisoning (With or Without Encephalopathy)

Children with symptomatic lead poisoning (with or without encephalopathy)
must be treated only at a pediatric center that has an intensive care unit. They
should be managed by a multi disciplinary team that includes, as needed, critical care, toxicology, neurology, and neurosurgery. The child's neurological
status and fluid balance must be carefully monitored.

Medical Management of Asymptomatic Lead Poisoning

Blood Lead Level > or = 45 μg/dL

Children with blood lead levels > or = 45 μg/dL (with or without symptoms)
should undergo chelation therapy. A blood lead level > or = 70 μg/dL is a
medical emergency.

Blood Lead Level 25 to 44 μg/dL

For this blood lead range, the effectiveness of chelation therapy in decreasing
the adverse effects of lead on children's intelligence has not been shown.
Treatment regimens vary from clinic to clinic. Some practitioners treat children with lead levels in this range pharmacologically, some use D-penicillamine. The minimum medical management for children with these blood
lead levels is to decrease exposure to all sources of lead, to correct any iron deficiency and maintain an adequate calcium intake, and to test frequently to ensure that the child's blood lead levels are decreasing. Many experienced practitioners decide whether to use chelation therapy on the basis of the results of
carefully performed CaNa2EDTA mobilization tests.

Blood Lead Level 20 to 24 μg/dL

ONLY VERY MINIMAL DATA EXISTS ABOUT CHELATING CHILDREN
WITH BLOOD LEAD LEVELS BELOW 25 μg/dL, AND SUCH CHILDREN
SHOULD NOT BE CHELATED EXCEPT IN THE CONTEXT OF APPROVED
CLINICAL TRIALS. A child with a confirmed blood lead level of 20 to 24 μg/dL
will require individual case management by a pediatric health-care provider.
The child should have an evaluation with special attention to nutritional and

iron status. The parents should be taught about (a) the causes and effects of lead poisoning, (b) the need for more routine blood lead testing, (c) possible sources of lead intake and how to reduce them, (d) the importance of adequate nutrition and of foods high in iron and calcium, and (e) resources for further information. (This is described in more detail in Chapter 4 of the original publication.) Sequential measurements of blood lead levels along with review of the child's clinical status should be done at least every 3 months. Iron deficiency should be treated promptly. Children with blood lead levels in this range should be referred for environmental investigation and management. Identifying and eradicating all sources of excessive lead exposure is the most important intervention for decreasing blood lead levels (see Chapter 8 of original publication).

Post-Chelation Followup

At the end of each treatment cycle, the blood lead concentration usually declines to < 25 µg/dL. Within a few days, however, reequilibration among body lead compartments takes place and may result in a rebound; thus, THE BLOOD LEAD LEVEL MUST BE RECHECKED 7 TO 21 DAYS AFTER TREATMENT TO DETERMINE WHETHER RETREATMENT IS NECESSARY.

Children who undergo chelation treatment require long-term followup preferably from pediatric health-care providers, nutritionists, environmental specialists, and community out-reach workers. Community outreach workers provide a critical bridge between hospital-based or clinic-based (outpatient) medical care, health advocacy education, and environmental remediation outside the hospital. Children should NEVER be discharged from the hospital UNTIL THEY CAN GO TO A LEAD-FREE ENVIRONMENT. Lead-free safe housing (with friends, relatives, or in designated transitional housing), in which a treated child can live during the entire abatement process through the post-abatement clean-up, must be arranged. With appropriately carried-out public health measures, complete and safe abatement should be achieved during the treatment period.

Once a child is discharged to a safe environment, frequent followup is mandatory. In general, depending on the initial blood lead value, most children who require chelation therapy must be followed closely for at least one year or more. All children undergoing chelation treatment should be seen every other week for 6–8 weeks, then once a month for 4–6 months. A child treated with BAL and CaNa2EDTA should be followed more closely: weekly for 4 to 6 weeks, then monthly for 12 months.

MANAGEMENT OF LEAD HAZARDS IN THE ENVIRONMENT OF THE INDIVIDUAL CHILD

Eradicating childhood lead poisoning requires a long-term active program of primary lead-poisoning prevention, including abatement of lead-based paint hazards in homes, day-care centers, and other places where young children play and live. For the child who is lead poisoned, however, efficient and effective interventions are needed as quickly as possible. Abatement means making the source of lead inaccessible to the child.

Each situation in which a child gets poisoned is unique and must be evaluated by a person or team of persons skilled and knowledgeable about lead poisoning, hazard identification, and interventions to reduce lead exposure, including abatement of lead-based paint in housing. Childhood lead poisoning prevention programs need to work closely with other relevant agencies (for example, housing and environmental agencies) to ensure that the quickest and most effective approach is taken to remediating the environments of poisoned children.

Environmental case management includes a number of actions prescribed for a child with lead poisoning. Ideally, environmental case management should be conducted by a team of professionals in public health, environmental activities, medical management, and social management. A team approach to intervention will help ensure that followup is timely and effective. The management team may need to solve many related problems, such as whether to investigate supplemental addresses, where to find temporary alternative housing, and how to use community resources to assist the family in dealing with the lead-poisoned child.

MANAGEMENT OF LEAD HAZARDS IN THE COMMUNITY

In theory, primary prevention has always been the goal of childhood lead poisoning prevention programs. In practice, however, most programs focus exclusively on secondary prevention, dealing with children who have already been poisoned. As programs shift the emphasis to primary prevention, their efforts must be designed to systematically identify and remediate environmental sources of lead, including, most importantly, dwellings containing old lead paint.

The shift from case management to community-level intervention will require a fundamental shift in perspective. The focus must shift from the individual child to the population of children at risk and the environment in which they live. The purpose of community-level intervention is to identify and respond to sources, not cases, of lead poisoning. The responsibility for addressing lead poisoning will have to be expanded beyond health agencies to include a variety of housing, environmental and social service agencies at the local, county, state, and national level.

section three

CANCER

Mammography

Original Citation: Centers for Disease Control and Prevention. Public health focus: mammography. MMWR 1992;41(25):454–459.

EFFICACY

Results from large randomized clinical trials indicate that mammography screening has had favorable effects on breast-cancer mortality (Table 1). In these randomized trials that compared all women invited to screening (regardless of whether they participated) with an uninvited control group, mortality was reduced among women aged 50–69 years who were invited to screening. Among women who complied with the screening recommendations, calculations from the combined published data suggest a reduction in mortality of approximately 39% (4). These findings are consistent with studies with nonrandomized controls, comparisons to national rates, and several case-control studies on mammography screening. Although no studies have shown a statistically significant reduction in the risk for dying from breast cancer among women aged 40–49 years, more studies show a favorable trend for screening than studies showing no trend or harmful effects from screening for this age group (5).

EFFECTIVENESS

Data from the randomized trials have been used to estimate population mortality reductions that could be achieved through routine mammography programs (6–9). The estimated breast-cancer mortality reduction has ranged from 8% to 40%, reflecting different assumptions among the mathematical models about targeted age groups, screening intervals, sensitivity of the mammography, compliance with regular screening, and natural history of the disease. Among women who receive screening regularly, the mortality reduction should be substantially greater than these population estimates.

COST-EFFECTIVENESS

Estimates of the cost-effectiveness of mammography vary widely because of differences in methodologies, measures, assumptions, and the programs and policies evaluated. Factors affecting the estimates include the proportion of high-risk women screened, the sensitivity and specificity of the mammography technique, the interval between examinations, and the cost of each mammogram. In the Netherlands—where invitations were mailed to participants—the annual screening of women aged 50–69 years was estimated at a cost of $14,800 per life year gained (6). Simulated models based on the United Kingdom experience that assumed relatively low sensitivity and participation rates estimated costs ranging from $4500 to $5500 per life year saved (8). Estimates using data

Table 1. Summary of major controlled trials of breast cancer screening

Study location	Year of start	Age (yrs) at entry	No. women	Screening modality	Screening internal (months)	Follow-up (yrs)	Reduction in breast cancer deaths % (95% CI[a])
New York[b]	1963	40–64	62,000	Physical exam Mammography	12	10	29 (11–44)
Malmo Sweden[c]	1976	45–69	42,000	Mammography	18–24	9	4 (−35–32)
Two-county, Sweden[d]	1977	40–74	133,000	Mammography	21–33[e]	11	30 (15–42)
Edinburgh, Scotland[f]	1979	45–64	46,000	Physical exam Mammography	12–24[g]	7	17 (−18–42)
Stockholm, Sweden[h]	1981	40–64	60,000	Mammography	28	7	29 (−20–60)

[a]Confidence interval.

[b]Source: Shapiro S, Venet W, Strax P, et al. Ten-to-fourteen year effect of screening on breast cancer mortality. JNCI 1982;69:349–355.

[c]Source: Anderson I, Aspergren K, Janzon L, et al. Mammographic screening and mortality from breast cancer: the Malmo mammographic screening trial. Br Med J 1988;297:943–948.

[d]Source: Tabar L. Fagerberg G, Gad A, et al. Reduction in mortality from breast cancer after mass screening with mammography. Lancet 1985;1:829–832.

[e]Respective average for 40–49 year and 50–74 year age groups.

[f]Source: Roberts MM, Alexander FE, Anderson TJ, et al. Edinburgh trial of screening for breast cancer; mortality at seven years. Lancet 1990;335:241–246.

[g]Respective interval for physical examination and mammography.

[h]Source: Frisell J, Eklund G, Hellstrom L, Lidbrink E, Rutqvist LE, Somell A. Randomized study of mammography screening—preliminary report on mortality in the Stockholm trial. Breast Cancer Res Treat 1991;18:49–56.

from the U.S. Breast Cancer Detection Demonstration Project (BCDDP) (9) showed that annual screening of women aged 55–65 years with physical examination and mammography yielded a marginal cost of $22,000 per life year saved. Data from a 1960s trial that used less sensitive radiologic technology (the Health Insurance Plan of Greater New York (HIP)) indicated the estimated cost of saving one life year was less than or equal to $84,000. For women aged greater than 65 years, the estimated cost per life year saved ranged from $13,200 to $28,000. Estimates of the cost per life year saved among women aged 40–49 years ranged from $30,000 (BCDDP data) to $135,000 (HIP data) (10). However, screening programs with mortality reduction estimates as low as 8%–12% can be cost-effective (based on assumptions of lower sensitivity than shown in the most successful trials and participation rates of 50%–70%) (6, 8).

The estimated annual cost of illness for breast cancer is $3.8 billion, including $1.8 billion for medical-care costs (converted to 1987 dollars) (11). During the 1980s, in place of radical mastectomies, modified radical mastectomy and breast-preservation techniques were increasingly performed and contributed to a reduction in the average number of hospital days associated with the treatment for breast cancer (in 1982, an average of 10.0 days compared with 4.6 days during 1990) (Table 2).

Table 2. Breast cancer prevalence, mortality, and years of potential life lost before age 65 (YPLL), by race; and length of hospital stay—United States

Disease burden (year of most recent data)	Number	Rate[a]
Prevalence (1987)[b]		
White	1,160,807	977.3
Black	101,189	800.6
Other	15,572	431.3
Total	1,277,568	958.3
Mortality (1988)[c]		
White	37,324	31.0
Black	4,467	34.8
Other	378	11.6
Total	42,169	31.1
YPLL (1988)		
White	185,478	205.3
Black	37,887	278.4
Other	3.378	80.8
Total	226,743	207.5
Hospitalization (1990)[d]		
Discharged from short-stay hospitals	163,000	1.3
Average length of stay (days)	4.6	

[a]Per 100,000 women, age-adjusted to the 1990 U.S. population.

[b]Source: data from 1987 National Health Interview Survey, Cancer Supplement.

[c]Source: NCHS, underlying cause of death data. *International Classification of Diseases, Ninth Revision,* codes 174.0–174.9.

[d]Source: data from National Hospital Discharge Survey, annual summary 1990.

EDITORIAL NOTE

Widespread mammography screening may explain, in part, the increasing breast-cancer incidence in the United States; however, this increase also occurred among population groups not covered by screening and among industrialized countries before mammographic screening had been widely implemented. Screening with either mammography alone or in combination with physical breast examination can reduce the disease burden from breast cancer by reducing both morbidity and mortality. Breast-cancer screening studies illustrate that (a) high-quality mammography is needed to ensure breast tumors are diagnosed at a stage early enough to reduce mortality and (b) quantitative measures are available and can be used to evaluate and improve screening programs (12).

Differences in sensitivity of the screening tests might explain some of the differences in mortality reduction in different screening trials. Although data are not available on mortality reductions obtained from routine mammography screening that are not part of research programs, preliminary data from extensive screening programs are available from Australia, the Netherlands, and Scandinavia. Overall results indicate that acceptable levels of sensitivity and specificity of mammography can be achieved and suggest that these programs may result in a future reduction of breast-cancer mortality. However, early results from the carefully monitored national program in Finland (13) indicate that the sensitivity of mammography is 25%–50% lower than that measured in the major screening trials, highlighting the difficulty in maintaining high-quality imaging and interpretation.

Age is considered the only practical criterion on which to base screening guidelines. Targeting screening to only women who have one or more of the established breast-cancer risk factors would allow for 20%–50% of breast cancers to remain undetected by screening and, therefore, would undermine the cost-effectiveness of screening. Because of reduced sensitivity of screening and a lower incidence of breast cancer among younger women, the cost-effectiveness of screening younger women is less favorable than for older women. Mammography screening trials have not convincingly demonstrated mortality reduction among women less than 50 years of age. However, if more sensitive screening methods are developed, the cost-effectiveness of screening younger women might be improved. In addition, the value of screening women aged greater than or equal to 70 years has not been adequately addressed; whether cost-effective programs can be developed and successfully implemented for women aged greater than or equal to 70 years must be determined.

In addition, the optimum interval for mammography screening has not been firmly established; the best estimates are based on indirect calculations (14).

If routine screening programs are to have the favorable impact in reducing breast-cancer mortality as observed in randomized clinical trials, breast-cancer screening programs should have monitoring systems and require strict adherence to quality-assurance guidelines. Effective tracking and reminder systems must be an integral part of breast-cancer screening programs. In addition, if the benefits of early treatment are to be assured for women with a screening-detected cancer, physicians and health-care organizations must ensure timely referrals to diagnose and treat all women with abnormal screening results. Experiences from cervical cancer screening programs indicate that operational constraints on follow-up of abnormal screening exams can jeopardize the entire benefit of the program (15).

REFERENCES: AS NUMBERED IN ORIGINAL PUBLICATION

4. Day NE. Screening for breast cancer. Br Med Bull 1991;47:400–415.
5. Shapiro S. Periodic breast cancer screening in seven foreign countries. Cancer 1992;69(Suppl): 1919–1924.
6. Van der Maas PJ, de Koning HJ, van Ineveld BM, et al. The cost effectiveness of breast cancer screening. Int J Cancer 1989;43:1055–1060.
7. Prorok PC. Mathematical models of breast cancer screening. In: Day NE, Miller AB, eds. Screening for breast cancer. Toronto: Hans Huber Publishers, 1988:95–104 (International Union Against Cancer monograph).
8. Knox EG. Evaluation of a proposed breast cancer screening regimen. Br Med J 1988;297:650–654.
9. Eddy DM. Screening for breast cancer. Ann Intern Med 1989;111:389–399.
10. Eddy DM, Hasselblad V, McGivney W, Hendee W. The value of mammography screening in women under age 50 years. JAMA 1988;259:1512–1519.
11. Scitovsky AA, McCall N. Economic impact of breast cancer. Frontiers of Radiation Therapy and Oncology 1976;11:90–101.
12. Day NE, Williams DRR, Khaw KT. Breast cancer screening programmes: the development of a monitoring and evaluation system. Br J Cancer 1989;59:954–958.
13. Hakama M, Elovainio L, Kajantie R, Louhivuori K. Breast cancer screening as public health policy in Finland. Br J Cancer 1991;64:962–964.
14. Tabar L, Fagerberg G, Day NE, Holmberg L. What is the optimum interval between mammographic screening examinations?—An analysis based on the latest results of the Swedish Two-County Breast Cancer Screening Trial. Br J Cancer 1987;55:547–551.
15. Anonymous. Cancer of the cervix: death by incompetence [Editorial]. Lancet 1985;2:363–364.

section four

CHRONIC DISEASE

Physical Activity and Public Health

Original Citation: Pate RR, Pratt M, Blair SN, et al. Physical activity and public health—a recommendation from the Centers for Disease Control and Prevention and the American College of Sports Medicine. JAMA 1995;273:402–407.

Original Authors: Russell R. Pate, PhD, Michael Pratt, MD, MPH, Steven N. Blair, PED, William L. Haskell, PhD, Caroline A. Macera, PhD, Claude Bouchard, PhD, David Buchner, MD, MPH, Walter Ettinger, MD, Gregory W. Heath, DHSc, Abby C. King, PhD, Andrea Kriska, PhD, Arthur S. Leon, MD, Bess H. Marcus, PhD, Jeremy Morris, MD, Ralph S. Paffenbarger, Jr, MD, Kevin Patrick, MD, Michael L. Pollock, PhD, James M. Rippe, MD, James Sallis, PhD, Jack H. Wilmore, PhD.

INTRODUCTION

Regular physical activity has long been regarded as an important component of a healthy lifestyle. Recently, this impression has been reinforced by new scientific evidence linking regular physical activity to a wide array of physical and mental health benefits (1–7). Despite this evidence and the public's apparent acceptance of the importance of physical activity, millions of US adults remain essentially sedentary (8).

The focus of this article is on physical activity and the health benefits associated with regular, moderate-intensity physical activity. Physical activity has been defined as "any bodily movement produced by skeletal muscles that results in energy expenditure" (9). Moderate physical activity is activity performed at an intensity of 3 to 6 METs (work metabolic rate/resting metabolic rate)—the equivalent of brisk walking at 3 to 4 mph for most healthy adults. Physical activity is closely related to, but distinct from, exercise and physical fitness. Exercise is a subset of physical activity defined as "planned, structured, and repetitive bodily movement done to improve or maintain one or more components of physical fitness" (9). Physical fitness is "a set of attributes that people have or achieve that relates to the ability to perform physical activity" (9).

RELATIONSHIP BETWEEN PHYSICAL ACTIVITY AND HEALTH

Cross-sectional epidemiologic studies (15, 16) and controlled, experimental investigations (12) have demonstrated that physically active adults, as contrasted with their sedentary counterparts, tend to develop and maintain higher levels of physical fitness. Epidemiologic research has demonstrated protective effects of varying strength between physical activity and risk for several chronic diseases, including coronary heart disease (CHD) (1–3, 17, 18), hypertension (4, 19–21), non-insulin-dependent diabetes mellitus (22–24), osteoporosis (7, 25, 26), colon cancer (27), and anxiety and depression (5, 28).

Other epidemiologic studies have shown that low levels of habitual physical activity and low levels of physical fitness are associated with markedly increased all-cause mortality rates (1, 29). A midlife increase in physical activity is associated with a decreased risk of mortality (30). It has been estimated that as many as 250,000 deaths per year in the United States, approximately 12% of the total, are attributable to a lack of regular physical activity (31, 32).

The conclusions of these epidemiologic studies are supported by experimental studies showing that exercise training improves CHD risk factors and other health-related factors, including blood lipid profile (33), resting blood pressure in borderline hypertensives (4, 34–36), body composition (37–39), glucose tolerance and insulin sensitivity (40, 41), bone density (42), immune function (43, 44), and psychological function (45).

Epidemiologic criteria used to establish causal relationships can be applied to the association between physical activity and CHD (46). The following principles of causality appear to have been met:

Consistency

The association of physical inactivity and risk of CHD is observed in a number of settings and populations, with the better-designed studies showing the strongest associations.

Strength

The relative risk of CHD associated with physical inactivity ranges from 1.5 to 2.4, an increase in risk comparable with that observed for hypercholesterolemia, hypertension, and cigarette smoking (3, 47). Temporal sequencing: The observation of physical inactivity predates the diagnosis of CHD.

Dose Response

Most studies demonstrate that the risk of CHD increases as physical activity decreases.

Plausibility and Coherence

Physical activity reduces the risk of CHD through a number of physiological and metabolic mechanisms. These include the potential for increasing the level of high-density lipoprotein cholesterol; reducing serum triglyceride levels; reducing blood pressure; enhancing fibrinolysis and altering platelet function, thereby reducing the risk of acute thrombosis; enhancing glucose tolerance and insulin sensitivity; and reducing the sensitivity of the myocardium to the effects of catecholamines, thereby reducing the risk of ventricular arrhythmias (4, 33, 40, 48, 49).

PHYSICAL ACTIVITY RECOMMENDATION FOR ADULTS

The current low-participation rate may be due in part to the misperception of many people that to reap health benefits they must engage in vigorous, continuous exercise. The scientific evidence clearly demonstrates that regular, moderate-intensity physical activity provides substantial health benefits. After review of physiological, epidemiologic, and clinical evidence, an expert panel formulated the following recommendation:

Every US adult should accumulate 30 minutes or more of moderate-intensity physical activity on most, preferably all, days of the week.

This recommendation emphasizes the benefits of moderate-intensity physical activity and of physical activity that can be accumulated in relatively short bouts. Adults who engage in moderate-intensity physical activity—i.e., enough to expend approximately 200 calories per day—can expect many of the health benefits described herein. To expend these calories, about 30 minutes of moderate-intensity physical activity should be accumulated during the course of the day. One way to meet this standard is to walk 2 miles briskly. Table 2 provides examples of moderate-intensity physical activities.

Table 2. Examples of Common Physical Activities for Healthy US Adults by Intensity of Effort Required in MET Scores and Kilocalories per Minute*

Light (<3.0 METs or <4 kcal/min)	Moderate (3.0–6.0 METs or 4–7 kcal/min)	Hard/Vigorous (>6.0 METs or >7 kcal/min)
Walking, slowly (strolling) (1–2 mph)	Walking, briskly (3–4 mph)	Walking, briskly uphill or with a load
Cycling, stationary (<50 W)	Cycling for pleasure or transportation (≤10 mph)	Cycling, fast or racing (>10 mph)
Swimming, slow treading	Swimming, moderate effort	Swimming, fast treading or crawl
Conditioning exercise, light stretching	Conditioning exercise, general calisthenics	Conditioning exercise, stair ergometer, ski machine
—	Racket sports, table tennis	Racket sports, singles tennis, racketball)
Golf, power cart	Golf, pulling cart or carrying clubs	—
Bowling	—	—
Fishing, sitting	Fishing, standing/casting	Fishing in stream
Boating, power	Canoeing, leisurely (2.0–3.9 mph)	Canoeing, rapidly (≥4 mph)
Home care, carpet sweeping	Home care, general cleaning	Moving furniture
Mowing lawn, riding mower	Mowing lawn, power mower	Mowing lawn, hand mower
Home repair, carpentry	Home repair, painting	—

*Data from Ainsworth, et al. (69), Leon (70), and McCardle, et al. (71). The METS (work metabolic rate/resting metabolic rate) are multiples of the resting rate of oxygen consumption during physical activity. One MET represents the approximate rate of oxygen consumption of a seated adult at rest, or about 3.5 mL per min per kg. The equivalent energy cost of 1 MET in kilocalories per minute is about 1.2 for a 70-kg person, or approximately 1 kcal per kg per hour.

Intermittent activity also confers substantial benefits (1, 17, 72, 73). Therefore, the recommended 30 minutes of activity can be accumulated in short bouts of activity: walking up the stairs instead of taking the elevator, walking instead of driving short distances, doing calisthenics, or pedaling a stationary cycle while watching television. Gardening, housework, raking leaves, dancing, and playing actively with children can also contribute to the 30 minute-per-day total if performed at an intensity corresponding to brisk walking. Those who perform lower-intensity activities should do them more often, for longer periods of time, or both.

People who prefer more formal exercise may choose to walk or participate in more vigorous activities, such as jogging, swimming, or cycling for 30 minutes daily. Sports and recreational activities, such as tennis or golf (without riding a cart), can also be applied to the daily total.

Because most adults do not currently meet the standard described herein, almost all should strive to increase their participation in physical activity that is of at least moderate intensity. Those who do not engage in regular physical activity should begin by incorporating a few minutes of increased activity into their day, building up gradually to 30 minutes per day of physical activity. Those who are active on an irregular basis should strive to adopt a more consistent activity pattern.

The health benefits gained from increased physical activity depend on the initial activity level. Sedentary individuals are expected to benefit most from increasing their activity to the recommended level. People who are physically active at a level below the standard would also benefit from reaching the recommended level of physical activity. People who already meet the recommendation are also likely to derive some additional health and fitness benefits from becoming more physically active.

Most adults do not need to see their physician before starting a moderate-intensity physical activity program (74). However, men older than 40 years and women older than 50 years who plan a vigorous program (intensity $> 60\%$ individual maximum oxygen consumption) or who have either chronic disease or risk factors for chronic disease should consult their physician to design a safe, effective program (74).

PREVIOUS EXERCISE RECOMMENDATIONS

The recommendation presented in this article is intended to complement, not supersede, previous exercise recommendations. In the past, exercise recommendations (including those from the ACSM) were based on scientific studies that investigated dose-response improvements in performance capacity after exercise training, especially the effects of endurance exercise training on maximal aerobic power (maximum oxygen consumption). The recommendations usually involved 20 to 60 minutes of moderate- to high-intensity endurance exercise (60% to 90% of maximum heart rate or 50% to 85% of maximal aerobic power) performed three or more times per week.

Although the earlier exercise recommendations were based on documented improvements in fitness, they probably provide most of the disease prevention benefits associated with an increase in physical activity. However, it now appears that the majority of these health benefits can be gained by performing moderate-intensity physical activities outside of formal exercise programs.

UNIQUE ASPECTS OF THE NEW RECOMMENDATION

The new recommendation extends the traditional exercise-fitness model to a broader physical activity-health paradigm. The recommendation is distinct in two important ways. First, the health benefits of moderate-intensity physical activity are emphasized. Second, accumulation of physical activity in intermittent, short bouts is considered an appropriate approach to achieving the activity goal. These unique elements of the recommendation are based on mounting evidence indicating that the health benefits of physical activity are linked principally to the total amount of physical activity performed. This evidence suggests that amount of activity is more important than the specific manner in which the activity is performed (i.e., mode, intensity, or duration of the activity bouts).

The health benefits of physical activity appear to accrue in approximate proportion to the total amount of activity performed, measured as either caloric expenditure or minutes of physical activity (Figure 1). For example, observational studies have shown a significantly lower death rate from CHD in

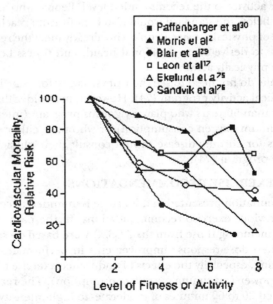

Figure 1. The relationship between level of physical activity (Paffenbanger, et al. (30), Morris, et al. (2), and Leon, et al. (17)) or exercise capatice (Blair, et al. (29), Ekelund, et al. (75), and Sandvik, et al. (76)) and coronary heart disease mortality. Values for more active or fit persons are expressed as the ratio of the event rate for more active or fit divided by the event rate for least active or fit.

people who perform an average of 47 minutes vs 15 minutes of activity per day (17), and in men who expend an estimated 2000 or more calories per week vs those who expend 500 or fewer calories per week (1). Five of the six studies shown in Figure 1 included men only; however, the relationship between physical fitness and cardiovascular disease mortality was identical for men and women in the one study that included both (29).

There is a clear association between total daily or weekly caloric expenditure and cardiovascular disease mortality. In most of the epidemiologic studies that have demonstrated this association, physical activity was assessed by questionnaires, and total activity was summed during periods ranging from 1 day to 1 year and then reported as average daily or weekly levels of physical activity. For example, among Harvard alumni the summed activity consisted of blocks walked, flights of stairs climbed, and moderate and vigorous sports play (1). In the Multiple Risk Factor Intervention Trial (17), the most frequently reported activities were lawn and garden work (80% of men), walking (65%), and home repairs (60%). It is not possible to ascertain with certainty whether the activity reported in these studies was performed in single, continuous daily bouts or was accumulated in multiple episodes. However, the nature of the most frequently reported activities suggests that it is unlikely that most of the activity was performed continuously. It is more likely that the daily or weekly caloric expenditures reflect accumulation of activity, most of which was performed intermittently. Also, the activities most commonly reported in these studies (e.g., walking, lawn work, and gardening) typically are performed at moderate intensity (Table 2).

Two published experimental studies have addressed the effects of continuous vs intermittent activity on fitness (72, 73). DeBusk, et al. (72), examined the effects of three 10-minute bouts of moderate to vigorous activity daily compared with a single 30-minute daily period of exercise of equal intensity in men. Ebisu (73) studied the effects of running on fitness and blood lipids in three groups of men. Subjects were divided into three exercise groups and one inactive control group. Each exercise group ran the same total distance, but in one, two, or three sessions daily. In both studies, fitness (measured as maximal oxygen uptake) increased significantly in all exercise groups, and the differences in fitness across the exercising groups were not significant. In the latter study, high-density lipoprotein cholesterol levels increased significantly only in the group that exercised three times per day (73).

Although more research is needed to better elucidate the health effects of moderate- vs high-intensity activity and intermittent vs continuous activity, clinicians and public health practitioners must rely on the most reasonable interpretation of existing data to guide their actions. We believe that the most reasonable interpretation of the currently available data is that (a) caloric expenditure and total time of physical activity are associated with reduced cardiovascular disease incidence and mortality; (b) there is a dose-response relationship for this association; (c) regular moderate physical activity provides substantial health benefits; and (d) intermittent bouts of physical activity, as short as 8 to 10 minutes, totaling 30 minutes or more on most days provide beneficial health and fitness effects.

MUSCULAR STRENGTH AND FLEXIBILITY

The preceding recommendation addresses the role of endurance exercise in preventing chronic diseases. However, two other components of fitness—flexibility and muscular strength—should not be overlooked. Clinical experience and limited studies suggest that people who maintain or improve their strength and flexibility may be better able to perform daily activities, may be less likely to develop back pain, and may be better able to avoid disability, especially as they advance into older age. Regular physical activity also may contribute to better balance, coordination, and agility, which in turn may help prevent falls in the elderly (77).

CONCLUSION

This statement and its recommendations are endorsed and supported by the Committee on Exercise and Cardiac Rehabilitation. Council on Clinical Cardiology, American Heart Association.

REFERENCES: AS NUMBERED IN ORIGINAL PUBLICATION

1. Paffenbarger RS, Hyde RT, Wing AL, Hsieh C-C. Physical activity, all-cause mortality, and longevity of college alumni. N Engl J Med 1986;314:605–613.
2. Morris JN, Clayton DG, Everitt MG, Semmence AM, Burgess EH. Exercise in leisure time: coronary attack and death rates. Br Heart J 1990;63:325–334.
3. Powell KE, Thompson PD, Caspersen CJ, Ford ES. Physical activity and the incidence of coronary heart disease. Annu Rev Public Health 1987;8:253–287.
4. Hagberg JM. Exercise, fitness, and hypertension. In: Bouchard C, Shephard RJ, Stephens T, Sutton JR, McPherson BD, eds. Exercise, fitness, and health. Champaign, IL: Human Kinetics Publishers, 1990: 455–566.
5. King AC, Taylor CB, Haskell WL, DeBusk RF. Influence of regular aerobic exercise on psychological health. Health Psychol 1989;8:305–324.
6. Dishman RK. Psychological effects of exercise for disease resistance and health promotion. In: Watson RR, Eisinher M, eds. Exercise and disease. Boca Raton, FL: CRC Press, 1992:179–207.
7. Marcus R, Drinkwater B, Dalsky G, et al. Osteoporosis and exercise in women. Med Sci Sports Exerc 1992;24(Suppl):S301–S307.
8. Centers for Disease Control and Prevention. Prevalence of sedentary lifestyle—behavioral risk factor surveillance system, United States, 1991. MMWR 1993;42:576–579.
9. Caspersen C J, Powell KE, Christenson GM. Physical activity, exercise, and physical fitness. Public Health Rep 1985;100:125–131.
12. American College of Sports Medicine. Position stand on the recommended quantity and quality of exercise for developing and maintaining cardiorespiratory and muscular fitness in healthy adults. Med Sci Sports Exert 1990;22:265–274.
15. Kohl HW, Blair SN, Paffenbarger RS, Macera CA, Kronenfeld JJ. A mall survey of physical activity habits as related to measured physical fitness. Am J Epidemiol 1988;127:1228–1239.
16. Taylor HL, Jacobs DR, Schucker B, Knudsen J, Leon AS, Debacker G. A questionnaire for the assessment of leisure time physical activities. J Chronic Dis 1978;31:741–755.
17. Leon AS, Connett J, Jacobs DR Jr, Rauramaa R. Leisure-time physical activity levels and risk of coronary heart disease and death: the Multiple Risk Factor Intervention trial. JAMA 1987;258:2388–2395.
18. Morris JN, Kagan A, Pattison DC, Chave SPW, Semmence AM. Incidence and prediction of ischemic heart disease in London busman. Lancet 1966;2:533–559.
19. Blair SN, Goodyear NN, Gibbons LW, Cooper KH. Physical fitness and incidence of hypertension in healthy normotensive men and women. JAMA 1984;252:487–490.
20. Paffenbarger RS. Wing AL, Hyde RT, Jung DL. Physical activity and incidence of hypertension in college alumni. Am J Epidemiol 1983;117:245–257.
21. American College of Sports Medicine. Position stand: physical activity, physical fitness, and hypertension. Med Sci Sports Exerc 1993;10:i–x.
22. Helmrich SP, Ragland DR, Leung RW, Paffenbarger RS. Physical activity and reduced occurrence of non-insulin-dependent diabetes mellitus. N Engl J Med 1991;325:147–152.

23. Manson JE, Nathan DM, Krolewski AS, Stampfer MJ, Willett WC, Hennekens CH. A prospective study of exercise and incidence of diabetes among US male physicians. JAMA 1992;268:63–67.
24. Manson JE, Rimm EB, Stampfer MJ, et al. Physical activity and incidence of non-insulin-dependent diabetes mellitus in women. Lancet 1991;338:774–778.
25. Cummings SR, Kelsey JL, Nevitt MD, O'Dowd KJ. Epidemiology of osteoporosis and osteoporotic fractures. Epidemiol Rev 1985;7:178–208.
26. Snow-Harter C, Marcus R. Exercise, bone mineral density, and osteoporosis. Exerc Sport Sci Rev 1991;19:351–388.
27. Lee I, Paffenbarger RS, Hsieh C. Physical activity and risk of developing colorectal cancer among college alumni. J Natl Cancer Inst 1991;83:1324–1329.
28. Taylor CB, Sallis JF, Needle R. The relationship of physical activity and exercise to mental health. Public Health Rep 1985;100:195–201.
29. Blair SN, Kohl HW, Paffenbarger RS, Clark DG, Cooper KH, Gibbons LW. Physical fitness and all-cause mortality. JAMA 1989;262:2395–2401.
30. Paffenbarger RS, Hyde RT, Wing AL, Lee I, Jung DL, Kampert JB. The association of changes in physical-activity level and other lifestyle characteristics with mortality among men. N Engl J Med 1993;328:538–545.
31. Hahn RA, Teutsch SM, Rothenberg RB, Marks JS. Excess deaths from nine chronic diseases in the United States. JAMA 1986;264:2654–2659.
32. McGinnis JM, Foege WH. Actual causes of death in the United States. JAMA 1993;270:2207–2212.
33. Haskell WL. The influence of exercise training on plasma lipids and lipoproteins in health and disease. Acta Med Scand 1986;711(Suppl):25–37.
34. Duncan JJ, Farr JE, Upton SJ, Hagan RD, Oglesby ME, Blair SN. The effects of aerobic exercise on plasma catecholamines and blood pressure in patients with mild essential hypertension. JAMA 1985; 254:2609–2613.
35. Hagberg JM, Montain S J, Martin WH, et al. Effect of exercise training on 60–69-year-old persons with essential hypertension. Am J Cardiol 1989;64:348–353.
36. Tipton CM. Exercise training and hypertension: an update. Exerc Sports Sci Rev 1991;19:447–505.
37. Bouchard C, Depres JP, Tremblay A. Exercise and obesity. Obesity Res 1993;1:133–147.
38. Pavlou K, Krey S, Steffee WP. Exercise as an adjunct to weight loss and maintenance in moderately obese subjects. Am J Clin Nutr 1989;49:1115–1123.
39. Wood PD, Stefanick ML, Williams PT, Haskell WL. The effects on plasma lipoproteins of prudent weight-reducing diet, with or without exercise, in overweight men and women. N Engl J Med 1991; 325:461–466.
40. Ivy JL. The insulin-like effect of muscle contraction. Exerc Sports Sci Rev 1987;15:29–51.
41. Koivisto VA, Yki-Jarvinen H, DeFronzo RA. Physical training and insulin sensitivity. Diabetes Metab Rev 1986;1:445–481.
42. Dalsky GP, Stoke KS, Ehsani AA, Slatopolsky E, Lee WC, Birge SJ. Weight-bearing exercise training and lumbar bone mineral content in postmenopausal women. Ann Intern Med 1988;108:824–828.
43. Nehlsen-Cannarella SL, Niemann DC, Balk-Lamberton AJ, et al. The effects of moderate exercise training on immune response. Med Sci Sports Exerc 1991;23:64–70.
44. Nieman DC. Physical activity, fitness, and infection. In: Bouchard C, Shephard RJ, Stephens T, eds. Physical activity, fitness, and health. Champaign, IL: Human Kinetics Publishers, 1994;796–813.
45. King AC, Taylor CB, Haskell WL. Effects of differing intensities and formats of 12 months of exercise training on psychological outcomes in older adults. Health Psychol 1993;12:292 300.
46. Hill AB. The environment and disease: association or causation? Proc R Soc Med 1965;58:295–300.
47. Centers for Disease Control and Prevention. Public health focus: physical activity and the prevention of coronary heart disease. MMWR 1993;42:669–672.
48. Rauramaa R, Salonen JT. Physical activity, fibrinolysis, and platelet aggregability. In: Bouchard C, Shephard RJ, Stephens T, eds. Physical activity, fitness, and health. Champaign, IL: Human Kinetics Publishers, 1994:471–479.
49. Moore S. Physical activity, fitness, and atherosclerosis. In: Bouchard C, Shephard RJ, Stephens T, eds. Physical activity, fitness, and health. Champaign, IL: Human Kinetics Publishers, 1994:570–578.
72. DeBusk RF, Stenestrand U, Sheehan M, Haskell WL. Training effects of long versus short bouts of exercise in healthy subjects. Am J Cardiol 1990;65:1010–1013.
73. Ebisu T. Splitting the distance of endurance running: on cardiovascular endurance and blood lipids. Jpn J Phys Educ 1985;30:37–43.
74. American College of Sports Medicine. Guidelines for exercise testing and prescription. 4th ed. Philadelphia, PA: Lea & Febiger, 1991.
75. Ekelund LG, Haskell WL, Johnson JL, Wholey FS, Criqui MH, Sheps DS. Physical fitness as a prevention of cardiovascular mortality in asymptomatic North American men. N Engl J Med 1988;319: 1379–1384.
76. Sandvik L, Erikssen J, Thaulow E, Erikssen G, Mundal R, Rodhal K. Physical fitness as a predictor of mortality among healthy, middle-aged Norweigan men. N Engl J Med 1993;328:533–537.

TOPIC 39 / **SMOKING/TOBACCO**

Guidelines for School Health Programs to Prevent Tobacco Use and Addiction

Original Citation: Centers for Disease Control and Prevention. Guidelines for school health programs to prevent tobacco use and addiction. MMWR 1994;43(RR-2):1–18.

BACKGROUND

School-based programs to prevent tobacco use can make a substantial contribution to the health of the next generation. In this report, the term "tobacco use" refers to the use of any nicotine-containing tobacco product, such as cigarettes, cigars, and smokeless tobacco.

Tobacco use is addictive and is responsible for more than one of every five deaths in the United States. However, many children and adolescents do not understand the nature of tobacco addiction and are unaware of, or underestimate, the important health consequences of tobacco use (1). On average, more than 3,000 young persons, most of them children and teenagers, begin smoking each day in the United States (21). Approximately 82% of adults ages 30–39 years who ever smoked daily tried their first cigarette before 18 years of age (8). National surveys indicate that 70% of high school students have tried cigarette smoking and that more than one-fourth (28%) reported having smoked cigarettes during the past 30 days (22).

THE NEED FOR SCHOOL HEALTH PROGRAMS TO PREVENT TOBACCO USE AND ADDICTION

The challenge to provide effective tobacco-use prevention programs to all young persons is an ethical imperative. Schools are ideal settings in which to provide such programs to all children and adolescents. School-based tobacco prevention education programs that focus on skills training approaches have proven effective in reducing the onset of smoking, according to numerous independent studies. A summary of findings from these studies demonstrates positive outcomes across programs that vary in format, scope, and delivery method (8).

To be most effective, school-based programs must target young persons before they initiate tobacco use or drop out of school. In 1992, 18% of surveyed U.S. high school seniors reported smoking their first cigarette in elementary school, and 30% started in grades seven to nine (23). Among persons age 17–18 years surveyed in 1989, substantially more high school dropouts (43%) than high school attendees or graduates (17%) had smoked cigarettes during the week preceding the survey (24).

Because considerable numbers of students begin using tobacco at or after age 15, tobacco-prevention education must be continued throughout high school. Among high school seniors surveyed in 1991 who had ever smoked a whole cigarette, 37% initiated smoking at age 15 or older (grades 10–12).

School-based programs offer an opportunity to prevent the initiation of tobacco use and therefore help persons avoid the difficulties of trying to stop after they are addicted to nicotine. The majority of current smokers (83%) wish they had never started smoking, and nearly one-third of all smokers quit for at least a day each year (25). Most smokers (93%) who try to quit resume regular smoking within 1 year (21, 26). Of those persons who successfully quit smoking for 1 year or longer, one-third eventually relapse (14).

By experimenting with tobacco, young persons place themselves at risk for nicotine addiction. Persons who start smoking early have more difficulty quitting, are more likely to become heavy smokers, and are more likely to develop a smoking-related disease (1, 27). Between 1975 and 1985, approximately 75% of persons who had smoked daily during high school were daily smokers 7–9 years later; however, only 5% of those persons had predicted as high school students that they would "definitely" smoke 5 years later (23). Smoking is addictive; three out of four teenagers who smoke have made at least one serious, yet unsuccessful, effort to quit (28). The 1994 Surgeon General's report on smoking and health concludes that the probability of becoming addicted to nicotine after any exposure is higher than that for other addictive substances (e.g., heroin, cocaine, or alcohol). Further, nicotine addiction in young people follows fundamentally the same process as in adults, resulting in withdrawal symptoms and failed attempts to quit (8). Thus, cessation programs are needed to help the young persons who already use tobacco (4).

School-based programs to prevent tobacco use should be provided for students of all ethnic/racial groups. In high school, more white (31%) and Hispanic (25%) students than black students (13%) are current smokers (29). Although ages and rates of initiation vary by race and ethnicity, tobacco use is a problem for all ethnic/racial groups. Given the diversity of cultures represented in many schools, it is important to tailor prevention programs for particular ethnic/racial subgroups of students. However, programs should be sensitive to, and representative of, a student population that is multicultural, multiethnic, and socioeconomically diverse.

Effective school-based programs to prevent tobacco use are equally important for both male and female students. From 1975 to 1987, daily smoking rates among 12th-grade females were as high or higher than males. Since 1988, smoking rates for males and females have been nearly identical (23). However, rates of smokeless tobacco use differ by sex: in 1991, 19% of male high school students and only 1% of females reported use during the past 30 days (22). Given the growing popularity of smokeless tobacco use, particularly among males (30), and given the prevalent misconception that smokeless tobacco is safe (23), school-based programs to prevent tobacco use must pointedly discourage the use of smokeless tobacco.

Despite gains made in the 1970s, progress in reducing smoking prevalence among adolescents slowed dramatically in the 1980s. For example, the percentage of seniors who report that they smoked on one or more days during the past month has remained unchanged since 1980—at approximately 29% (23). Further, despite negative publicity and restrictive legislation regarding tobacco use, the proportion of high school seniors who perceive that cigarette users are at great risk for physical or other harm from smoking a pack a day or more has increased only minimally—from 64% in 1980 to 69% in 1992 (23). Thus, efforts to prevent the initiation of tobacco use among children and adolescents must be intensified. School-based programs to prevent tobacco use also can contribute to preventing the use of illicit drugs, such as marijuana and cocaine, especially if such programs are also designed to prevent the use of these substances (31). Tobacco is one of the most commonly available and widely used drugs, and its use results in the most widespread drug dependency. Use of other drugs, such as marijuana and cocaine, is often preceded by the use of tobacco or alcohol. Although most young persons who use tobacco do not use illicit drugs, when further drug involvement does occur, it is typically sequential—from use of tobacco or alcohol to use of marijuana, and from marijuana to other illicit drugs or prescription psychoactive drugs (32). This sequence may reflect, in part, the widespread availability, acceptability, and use of tobacco and alcohol, as well as common underlying causes of drug use, such as risk-seeking patterns of behavior and deficits in communication and refusal skills. Recent reports on preventing drug abuse suggest that approaches effective in preventing tobacco use can also help prevent the use of alcohol and other drugs (33–35).

PURPOSES OF SCHOOL HEALTH PROGRAMS TO PREVENT TOBACCO USE AND ADDICTION

School-based health programs should enable and encourage children and adolescents who have not experimented with tobacco to continue to abstain from any use. For young persons who have experimented with tobacco use, or who are regular tobacco users, school health programs should enable and encourage them to immediately stop all use. For those young persons who are unable to stop using tobacco, school programs should help them seek additional assistance to successfully quit the use of tobacco.

RECOMMENDATIONS FOR SCHOOL HEALTH PROGRAMS TO PREVENT TOBACCO USE AND ADDICTION

Recommendation 1: Develop and Enforce a School Policy on Tobacco Use

A school policy on tobacco use must be consistent with state and local laws and should include the following elements (41):

- An explanation of the rationale for preventing tobacco use (i.e., tobacco is the leading cause of death, disease, and disability)
- Prohibitions against tobacco use by students, all school staff, parents, and visitors on school property, in school vehicles, and at school-sponsored functions away from school property
- Prohibitions against tobacco advertising in school buildings, at school functions, and in school publications

- A requirement that all students receive instruction on avoiding tobacco use
- Provisions for students and all school staff to have access to programs to help them quit using tobacco
- Procedures for communicating the policy to students, all school staff, parents or families, visitors, and the community
- Provisions for enforcing the policy

To ensure broad support for school policies on tobacco use, representatives of relevant groups, such as students, parents, school staff and their unions, and school board members, should participate in developing and implementing the policy. Examples of policies have been published (41), and additional samples can be obtained from state and local boards of education. Clearly articulated school policies, applied fairly and consistently, can help students decide not to use tobacco (42). Policies that prohibit tobacco use on school property, require prevention education, and provide access to cessation programs rather than solely instituting punitive measures are most effective in reducing tobacco use among students (43).

A tobacco-free school environment can provide health, social, and economic benefits for students, staff, the school, and the district (41). These benefits include decreased fires and discipline problems related to student smoking, improved compliance with local and state smoking ordinances, and easier upkeep and maintenance of school facilities and grounds.

Recommendation 2: Provide Instruction about the Short- and Long-term Negative Physiologic and Social Consequences of Tobacco Use, Social Influences on Tobacco Use, Peer Norms Regarding Tobacco Use, and Refusal Skills

Some tobacco-use prevention programs have been limited to providing only factual information about the harmful effects of tobacco use. Other programs have attempted to induce fear in young persons about the consequences of use (44). However, these strategies alone do not prevent tobacco use, may stimulate curiosity about tobacco use, and may prompt some students to believe that the health hazards of tobacco use are exaggerated (45–47).

Successful programs to prevent tobacco use address multiple psychosocial factors related to tobacco use among children and adolescents (48–51). These factors include:

- Immediate and long-term undesirable physiologic, cosmetic, and social consequences of tobacco use. Programs should help students understand that tobacco use can result in decreased stamina, stained teeth, foul-smelling breath and clothes, exacerbation of asthma, and ostracism by nonsmoking peers.
- Social norms regarding tobacco use. Programs should use a variety of educational techniques to decrease the social acceptability of tobacco use, highlight existing antitobacco norms, and help students understand that most adolescents do not smoke.
- Reasons that adolescents say they smoke. Programs should help students understand that some adolescents smoke because they believe it will

help them be accepted by peers, appear mature, or cope with stress. Programs should help students develop other more positive means to attain such goals.

- Social influences that promote tobacco use. Programs should help students develop skills in recognizing and refuting tobacco-promotion messages from the media, adults, and peers.
- Behavioral skills for resisting social influences that promote tobacco use. Programs should help students develop refusal skills through direct instruction, modeling, rehearsal, and reinforcement, and should coach them to help others develop these skills.
- General personal and social skills. Programs should help students develop necessary assertiveness, communication, goal-setting, and problem-solving skills that may enable them to avoid both tobacco use and other health risk behaviors.

School-based programs should systematically address these psychosocial factors at developmentally appropriate ages. Particular instructional concepts should be provided for students in early elementary school, later elementary school, junior high or middle school, and senior high school (Table 1). Local school districts and schools should review these concepts in accordance with student needs and educational policies to determine in which grades students should receive particular instruction.

Table 1. Instructional concepts (kindergarten through grade twelve)

Early Elementary School	Later Elementary School
KNOWLEDGE: Students will learn that	KNOWLEDGE: Students will learn that
A drug is a chemical that changes how the body works.	Stopping tobacco use has short- and long-term benefits.*
All forms of tobacco contain a drug called nicotine.	Environmental tobacco smoke is dangerous to health.*
Tobacco use includes cigarettes and smokeless tobacco.	Most young persons and adults do not use tobacco.*
Tobacco use is harmful to health.	Nicotine, contained in all forms of tobacco, is an addictive drug.
Stopping tobacco use has short-term and long-term benefits.	Tobacco use has short-term and long-term physiologic and cosmetic consequences.
Many persons who use tobacco have trouble stopping.	
Tobacco smoke in the air is dangerous to anyone who breathes it.	Personal feelings, family, peers, and the media influence decisions about tobacco use.
Many fires are caused by persons who smoke.	Tobacco advertising is often directed toward young persons.
Some advertisements try to persuade persons to use tobacco.	Young persons can resist pressure to use tobacco.
Most young persons and adults do not use tobacco.	Laws, rules, and policies regulate the sale and use of tobacco.
Persons who choose to use tobacco are not bad persons.	

Table 1.—*continued*

Early Elementary School	Later Elementary School

ATTITUDES: Students will demonstrate
  A personal commitment not to use
  tobacco.
  Pride about choosing not to use
  tobacco.
	ATTITUDES: Students will demonstrate
	  A personal commitment not to use
	  tobacco.*
	  Pride about choosing not to use
	  tobacco.*
	  Support for others' decisions not to
	  use tobacco.
	  Responsibility for personal health.

SKILLS: Students will be able to
  Communicate knowledge and per-
  sonal attitudes about tobacco use.
  Encourage other persons not to use
  tobacco.
	SKILLS: Students will be able to
	  Communicate knowledge and per-
	  sonal attitudes about tobacco use.*
	  Encourage other persons not to use
	  tobacco.*
	  Demonstrate skills to resist tobacco
	  use.
	  State the benefits of a smoke-free
	  environment.
	  Develop counterarguments to
	  tobacco advertisements and other
	  promotional materials.
	  Support persons who are trying to
	  stop using tobacco.

Middle School/Junior High School	Senior High School

KNOWLEDGE: Students will learn that
  Most young persons and adults do
  not smoke.*
  Laws, rules, and policies regulate the
  sale and use of tobacco.*
  Tobacco manufacturers use various
  strategies to direct advertisements
  toward young persons, and such as
  "image" advertising.*
  Tobacco use has short- and long-term
  physiologic, cosmetic, social, and
  economic consequences.*
  Cigarette smoking and smokeless
  tobacco use have direct health con-
  sequences.*
  Maintaining a tobacco-free environ-
  ment has health benefits.
  Tobacco use is an unhealthy way to
  manage stress or weight.
  Community organizations have infor-
  mation about tobacco use and can
  help persons stop using tobacco.
	KNOWLEDGE: Students will learn that
	  Most young persons and adults do
	  not smoke.*
	  Tobacco use has short- and long-term
	  physiologic, cosmetic, social, and
	  economic consequences.*
	  Cigarette smoking and smokeless
	  tobacco use have direct health
	  consequences.*
	  Community organizations have infor-
	  mation about tobacco use and can
	  help persons stop using tobacco.*
	  Smoking cessation programs can be
	  successful.*
	  Tobacco use is an unhealthy way to
	  manage stress or weight.*
	  Tobacco use during pregnancy has
	  harmful effects on the fetus.
	  Schools and community organiza-
	  tions can promote a smoke-free
	  environment.
	  Many persons find it hard to stop

Table 1.—*continued*

Middle School/Junior High School	Senior High School
Smoking cessation programs can be successful. Tobacco contains other harmful substances in addition to nicotine.	using tobacco, despite knowledge about the health hazards of tobacco use.
ATTITUDES: Students will demonstrate A personal commitment not to use tobacco.* Pride about choosing not to use tobacco.* Responsibility for personal health.* Support for others' decisions not to use tobacco.* Confidence in personal ability to resist tobacco use.	ATTITUDES: Students will demonstrate A personal commitment not to use tobacco.* Pride about choosing not to use tobacco.* Responsibility for personal health.* Support for others' decisions not to use tobacco.* Confidence in personal ability to resist tobacco use.* Willingness to use school and community resources for information about, and help with, resisting or quitting tobacco use.
SKILLS: Students will be able to Encourage other persons not to use tobacco.* Support persons who are trying to stop using tobacco.* Communicate knowledge end personal attitudes about tobacco use.* Demonstrate skills to resist tobacco use.* Identify and counter strategies used in tobacco advertisements and other promotional materials.* Develop methods for coping with tobacco use by parents and with other difficult personal situations, such as peer pressure to use tobacco. Request a smoke-free environment.	SKILLS: Students will be able to Encourage other persons not to use tobacco.* Support persons who are trying to stop using tobacco.* Communicate knowledge and personal attitudes about tobacco use.* Demonstrate skills to resist tobacco use.* Identify and counter strategies used in tobacco advertisements and other promotional materials.* Develop methods for coping with tobacco use by parents and with other difficult personal situations, such as peer pressure to use tobacco.* Use school and community resources for information about and help with, resisting or quitting tobacco use. Initiate school and community action to support a smoke-free environment.

*These concepts reinforce content introduced during earlier grades.

Recommendation 3: Provide Tobacco-Use Prevention Education in Kindergarten Through 12th Grade

This instruction should be especially intensive in junior high or middle school and should be reinforced in high school.

Education to prevent tobacco use should be provided to students in each grade, from kindergarten through 12th grade (4). Because tobacco use often begins in grades six through eight, more intensive instructional programs should be provided for these grade levels (4, 5). Particularly important is the year of entry into junior high or middle school when new students are exposed to older students who use tobacco at higher rates. Thereafter, annual prevention education should be provided. Without continued reinforcement throughout high school, successes in preventing tobacco use dissipate over time (52, 53). Studies indicate that increases in the intensity and duration of education to prevent tobacco use result in concomitant increases in effectiveness (54–56).

Most evidence demonstrating the effectiveness of school-based prevention of tobacco use is derived from studies of schools in which classroom curricula focused exclusively on tobacco use. Other evidence suggests that tobacco-use prevention also can be effective when appropriately embedded within broader curricula for preventing drug and alcohol use (57) or within comprehensive curricula for school health education (31). The effectiveness of school-based efforts to prevent tobacco use appears to be enhanced by the addition of targeted communitywide programs that address the role of families, community organizations, tobacco-related policies, antitobacco advertising, and other elements of adolescents' social environment (8).

Because tobacco use is one of several interrelated health risk behaviors addressed by schools, CDC recommends that tobacco-use-prevention programs be integrated as part of comprehensive school health education within the broader school health program (58).

Recommendation 4: Provide Program-Specific Training for Teachers

Adequate curriculum implementation and overall program effectiveness are enhanced when teachers are trained to deliver the program as planned (59, 60). Teachers should be trained to recognize the importance of carefully and completely implementing the selected program. Teachers also should become familiar with the underlying theory and conceptual framework of the program as well as with the content of these guidelines. The training should include a review of the program content and a modeling of program activities by skilled trainers. Teachers should be given opportunity to practice implementing program activities. Studies indicate that in-person training and review of curriculum-specific activities contribute to greater compliance with prescribed program components (4, 5, 61, 62).

Some programs may elect to include peer leaders as part of the instructional strategy. By modeling social skills (63) and leading role rehearsals (64), peer leaders can help counteract social pressures on youth to use tobacco.

These students must receive training to ensure accurate presentation of skills and information. Although peer-leader programs can offer an important adjunct to teacher-led instruction, such programs require additional time and effort to initiate and maintain.

Recommendation 5: Involve Parents or Families in Support of School-Based Programs to Prevent Tobacco Use

Parents or families can play an important role in providing social and environmental support for nonsmoking. Schools can capitalize on this influence by involving parents or families in program planning, in soliciting community support for programs, and in reinforcing educational messages at home. Homework assignments involving parents or families increase the likelihood that smoking is discussed at home and motivate adult smokers to consider cessation (65).

Recommendation 6: Support Cessation Efforts among Students and All School Staff Who Use Tobacco

Potential practices to help children and adolescents quit using tobacco include self-help, peer support, and community cessation programs. In practice, however, these alternatives are rarely available within a school system or community. Although the options are often limited, schools must support student efforts to quit using tobacco, especially when tobacco use is disallowed by school policy.

Effective cessation programs for adolescents focus on immediate consequences of tobacco use, have specific attainable goals, and use contracts that include rewards. These programs provide social support and teach avoidance, stress management, and refusal skills (66–69). Further, students need opportunities to practice skills and strategies that will help them remain nonusers (66, 67, 70).

Cessation programs with these characteristics may already be available in the community through the local health department or voluntary health agency (e.g., American Cancer Society, American Heart Association, American Lung Association). Schools should identify available resources in the community and provide referral and follow-up services to students. If cessation programs for youth are not available, such programs might be jointly sponsored by the school and the local health department, voluntary health agency, other community health providers, or interested organizations (e.g., churches).

More is known about successful cessation strategies for adults. School staff members are more likely than students to find existing cessation options in the community. Most adults who quit tobacco use do so without formal assistance. Nevertheless, cessation programs that include a combination of behavioral approaches (e.g., group support, individual counseling, skills training, family interventions, and interventions that can be supplemented with pharmacologic treatments) have demonstrated effectiveness (71). For all school staff, health promotion activities and employee assistance programs that include cessation programs might help reduce burnout, lower staff absenteeism, decrease health insurance premiums, and increase commitment to overall school health goals (41).

Recommendation 7: Assess the Tobacco-Use Prevention Program at Regular Intervals

Local school boards and administrators can use the following evaluation questions to assess whether their programs are consistent with CDC's Guidelines for School Health Programs to Prevent Tobacco Use and Addiction. Personnel in federal, state, and local education and health agencies also can use these questions to (a) assess whether schools in their jurisdiction are providing effective education to prevent tobacco use and (b) identify schools that would benefit from additional training, resources, or technical assistance. The following questions can serve as a guide for assessing program effectiveness:

1. Do schools have a comprehensive policy on tobacco use, and is it implemented and enforced as written?
2. Does the tobacco education program foster the necessary knowledge, attitudes, and skills to prevent tobacco use?
3. Is education to prevent tobacco use provided, as planned, in kindergarten through 12th grade, with special emphasis during junior high or middle school?
4. Is in-service training provided, as planned, for educators responsible for implementing tobacco-use prevention?
5. Are parents or families, teachers, students, school health personnel, school administrators, and appropriate community representatives involved in planning, implementing, and assessing programs and policies to prevent tobacco use?
6. Does the tobacco-use prevention program encourage and support cessation efforts by students and all school staff who use tobacco?

REFERENCES: AS NUMBERED IN ORIGINAL PUBLICATION

1. CDC. Reducing the health consequences of smoking: 25 years of progress—a report of the Surgeon General. Washington, DC: US Department of Health and Human Services, Public Health Service, CDC, 1989:DHHS publication no. (CDC)89–8411.
4. National Cancer Institute. School programs to prevent smoking: the National Cancer Institute guide to strategies that succeed. Rockville, MD: US Department of Health and Human Services, Public Health Service, National Institutes of Health, National Cancer Institute, 1990:DHHS publication no. (NIH)90–500.
5. Glynn T. Essential elements of school-based smoking prevention programs. J Sch Health 1989;59: 181–188.
8. CDC. Preventing tobacco use among young people: a report of the Surgeon General. Atlanta, GA: US Department of Health and Human Services, Public Health Service, CDC, 1994:DHHS publication no. S/N 017–001-00491–0.
14. CDC. The health benefits of smoking cessation: a report of the Surgeon General. US Department of Health and Human Services, Public Health Service, CDC, 1990:DHHS publication no. (CDC)90–8416.
21. Pierce JP, Fiore MC, Novotny TE, Hatziandreu EJ, Davis RM. Trends in cigarette smoking in the United States: projections to the Year 2000. JAMA 1989;261(1):61–65.
22. CDC. Tobacco, alcohol, and other drug use among high school students—United States, 1991. MMWR 1992;41:698–703.
23. National Institute on Drug Abuse. National survey results on drug use from Monitoring the Future Study, 1975–1992. Rockville, MD: US Department of Health and Human Services, Public Health Service, 1993:DHHS publication no. (NIH)93–3597.
24. CDC. Cigarette smoking among youth—United States, 1989. MMWR 1991;40:712–715.
25. Gallup G Jr., Newport F. Many Americans favor restrictions on smoking in public places. Gallup Poll Monthly 1990;298:19–27.

26. Hatziandreu EJ, Pierce JP, Lefkopoulou M, et al. Quitting smoking in the United States in 1986. J Natl Cancer Inst 1990;82;1402–1406.
27. Taioli E, Wynder E. Effect of the age at which smoking begins on frequency of smoking in adulthood. N Engl J Med 1991;325:968–969.
28. CDC. Recent trends in adolescent smoking, smoking-uptake correlates, and expectations about the future. Advance Data from vital and health statistics of the Centers for Disease Control and Prevention/National Center for Health Statistics, No. 221, Dec. 2, 1992.
29. Kann L, Warren W, Collins JL, Ross J, Collins B, Kolbe LJ. Results from the national school-based 1991 Youth Risk Behavior Survey and progress toward achieving related health objectives for the nation. Public Health Rep 1993;106(Suppl 1):47–55.
30. Office of the Inspector General. Spit tobacco and youth. Dallas, TX: US Department of Health and Human Services, 1992:DHHS publication no. (OEI)06–92-00500.
31. Errecart MT, Walberg HJ, Ross JG, Gold RS, Fiedler JL, Kolbe LJ. Effectiveness of teenage health teaching modules. J Sch Health 1991;61(Suppl 1):19–42.
32. Yamaguchi K, Kandel D. Patterns of drug use from adolescence to young adulthood. II. Sequences of progression. Am J Public Health 1984;74:668–672.
33. Tobler NS. Meta-analysis of 143 adolescent drug prevention programs: quantitative outcome results of program participants compared to a control or comparison group. J Drug Issues 1986;17:537–567.
34. Hansen WB. School-based substance abuse prevention: a review of the state of the art in curriculum. Health Educ Res 1992;7:3:403–430.
35. Botvin GJ, Botvin EM. School-based and community based prevention approaches. In: Lowinson J, Ruiz P, Millman R, eds. Comprehensive textbook of substance abuse. 2nd ed. Baltimore, MD: Williams & Wilkins, 1992:910–927.
41. National School Boards Association. No smoking: a board member's guide to nonsmoking policies for the schools. Alexandria, VA: National School Boards Association, 1987.
42. Grimes JD, Swisher JD. Educational factors influencing adolescent decision-making regarding use of alcohol and drugs. J Alcohol Drug Educ 1989;35:1–15.
43. Pentz MA, Brannon BR, Carlin VL, Barrett EJ, MacKinnon DP, Flay BR. The power of policy: the relationship of smoking policy to adolescent smoking. Am J Public Health 1989;79:857–862.
44. Office of Substance Abuse Prevention. Stopping alcohol and other drug use before it starts: the future of prevention. Rockville, MD: US Department of Health and Human Services, Public Health Service, 1989:DHHS publication no. (ADM)89–1645.
45. Swisher J, Crawford J, Goldstein R, Yura M. Drug education: pushing or preventing. Peabody J Educ 1971;49:68–75.
46. Flay B, Sobol J. The role of mass media in preventing adolescent substance abuse. In: Glenn T, Leukevald C, eds. Preventing adolescent drug abuse: intervention strategies. Washington, DC: National Institute on Drug Abuse, 1983:5–35.
47. Leventhal H, Cleary PD. The smoking problem: a review of research and theory in behavioral risk modification. Psychological Bull 1980;88:370–405.
48. Botvin G. Personal and social skills training: applications for substance abuse prevention. In: Proceedings of six regional workshops: strengthening health education for the 1990s. New York: Health and Safety Education Division, Medical Department, Metropolitan Life Insurance Company, 1991.
49. Flay B. Psychosocial approaches to smoking prevention: a review of findings. Health Psychol 1985;4:449–488.
50. Botvin GJ. Substance abuse prevention research: recent developments and future directions. J Sch Health 1986;56:369–374.
51. Best JA, Thomson SJ, Santi SM, Smith E, Brown KS. Preventing cigarette smoking among school children. Ann Rev Public Health 1988;9:161–201.
52. Murray DM, Pirie P, Luepker RV, Pallonen U. Five- and six-year follow-up results from four seventh-grade smoking prevention strategies. J Behav Med 1989;12:207–218.
53. Flay BR, Koepke D, Thomson SJ, Santi S, Best A. Six-year follow-up of the first Waterloo School Smoking Prevention Trial. Am J Public Health 1989;79:1371–1376.
54. Botvin GJ, Baker E, Dusenbury L, Tortu S, Botvin EM. Preventing adolescent drug abuse through a multimodal cognitive-behavioral approach: results of a three-year study. J Consul Clin Psychol 1990;58:437–446.
55. Botvin GJ, Renick NL, Baker E. The effects of scheduling format and booster sessions on a broad-spectrum psychosocial smoking prevention program. J Behav Med 1983;6:359–379.
56. Botvin GJ, Baker E, Dusenbury L, Botvin EM, Filazzola AD. Preventing adolescent drug abuse through a multi-modal cognitive-behavioral approach: results of a six-year study. Ithaca, NY: Cornell University Medical College, Institute for Prevention Research, 1993:Technical Report no. 93–10.
57. Hansen W, Graham J. Preventing alcohol, marijuana, and cigarette use among adolescents: peer pressure resistance training versus establishing conservative norms. Prev Med 1991;20:414–430.
58. The National Commission on the Role of the School and the Community in Improving Adolescent Health. Code blue: uniting for healthier youth. Alexandria, VA: National Association of State Boards of Education, 1990.

59. Connell DB, Turner RR, Mason EF. Summary of findings of the school health education evaluation: health promotion effectiveness, implementation, and costs. J Sch Health 1985;55:316–321.
60. Gold RS, Parcel GS, Walberg HJ, Luepker RV, Portnoy B, Stone EJ. Summary and conclusions of the THTM evaluation: the expert work group perspective. J Sch Health 1991;61:39–42.
61. Tortu S, Botvin GJ. School-based smoking prevention: the teacher training process. Prev Med 1989;18:280–290.
62. Perry CL, Murray DM, Griffin G. Evaluating the statewide dissemination of smoking prevention curricula: factors in teacher compliance. J Sch Health 1990;60:501–504.
63. Perry C, Telch M, Killen J, Burke A, Maccoby N. High school smoking prevention: the relative efficacy of varied treatments and instructors. Adolescence 1983;17:561–566.
64. Clarke J, MacPherson B, Holmes D, Jones R. Reducing adolescent smoking: a comparison of peer-led, teacher-led and expert interventions. J Sch Health 1986;56:102–106.
65. Perry CL, Pirie P, Holder W, Halper A, Dudovitz B. Parental involvement in cigarette smoking prevention: two pilot evaluations of the "unpuffables program." J Sch Health 1990;60:443–447.
66. Flay BR. Youth tobacco use: risks, patterns and control. In: Nicotine addiction: principles and management. New York: Oxford University Press, 1993.
67. Brink SG, Simons-Morton DG, Harvey CM, Parcel GS, Tiernan KM. Developing comprehensive smoking-control programs in schools. J Sch Health 1988;58:177–180.
68. St. Pierre RW, Shute RE, Jaycox S. Youth helping youth: a behavioral approach to the self-control of smoking. Health Educ 1983;14:28–31.
69. Weissman W, Glasgow R, Biglan A, Liechtenstein E. Development and preliminary evaluation of a cessation program for adolescent smokers. Psychol Addict Behav 1987;1:84–91.
70. Perry C, Killen J, Telch M, Slinkard LA, Danaher BG. Modifying smoking behavior of teenagers: a school-based intervention. Am J Public Health 1980;70:722–724.
71. CDC. The health consequences of smoking: nicotine addiction—a report of the Surgeon General. Rockville, MD: US Department of Health and Human Services, Public Health Service, CDC, 1988:DHHS publication no. (CDC)88–8406.

Preventing Tobacco Use Among Young People

Original Citation: Centers for Disease Control and Prevention. Preventing tobacco use among young people: a report of the surgeon general (executive summary). MMWR 1994;43(RR-4):1–10.

SUMMARY

Health Consequences of Tobacco Use Among Young People

Active smoking by young people is associated with significant health problems during childhood and adolescence and with increased risk factors for health problems in adulthood. Cigarette smoking during adolescence appears to reduce the rate of lung growth and the level of maximum lung function that can be achieved. Young smokers are likely to be less physically fit than young nonsmokers; fitness levels are inversely related to the duration and the intensity of smoking. Adolescent smokers report that they are significantly more likely than their nonsmoking peers to experience shortness of breath, coughing spells, phlegm production, wheezing, and overall diminished physical health. Cigarette smoking during childhood and adolescence poses a clear risk for respiratory symptoms and problems during adolescence; these health problems are risk factors for other chronic conditions in adulthood, including chronic obstructive pulmonary disease.

Cardiovascular disease is the leading cause of death among adults in the United States. Atherosclerosis, however, may begin in childhood and become clinically significant by young adulthood. Cigarette smoking has been shown to be a primary risk factor for coronary heart disease, arteriosclerotic peripheral vascular disease, and stroke. Smoking by children and adolescents is associated with an increased risk of early atherosclerotic lesions and increased risk factors for cardiovascular diseases. These risk factors include increased levels of low-density lipoprotein cholesterol, increased very-low-density lipoprotein cholesterol, increased triglycerides, and reduced levels of high-density lipoprotein cholesterol. If sustained into adulthood, these patterns significantly increase the risk for early development of cardiovascular disease.

Smokeless tobacco use is associated with health consequences that range from halitosis to severe health problems such as various forms of oral cancer. Use of smokeless tobacco by young people is associated with early indicators of adult health consequences, including periodontal degeneration, soft tissue lesions, and general systemic alterations. Previous reports have documented that smokeless tobacco use is as addictive for young people as it is for adults. Another concern is that smokeless tobacco users are more likely than nonusers to become cigarette smokers. Among addictive behaviors such as the use of alcohol and other drugs, cigarette smoking is most likely to become established during adolescence. Young people who begin to smoke at an earlier age are more likely than later starters to develop long-term nicotine addiction. Most young people who smoke regularly are already addicted to nicotine, and they experience this addiction in a manner and severity similar to what adult smokers experience. Most adolescent smokers report that they would like to quit smoking and that they have made numerous, usually unsuccessful attempts to quit. Many adolescents say that they intend to quit in the future and yet prove unable to do so. Those who try to quit smoking report withdrawal symptoms similar to those reported by adults. Adolescents are difficult to recruit for formal cessation programs, and when enrolled, are difficult to retain in the programs. Success rates in adolescent cessation programs tend to be quite low, both in absolute terms and relative to control conditions. Tobacco use is associated with a range of problem behaviors during adolescence. Smokeless tobacco or cigarettes are generally the first drug used by young people in a sequence that can include tobacco, alcohol, marijuana, and hard drugs. This pattern does not imply that tobacco use causes other drug use, but rather that other drug use rarely occurs before the use of tobacco. Still, there are a number of biological, behavioral, and social mechanisms by which the use of one drug may facilitate the use of other drugs, and adolescent tobacco users are substantially more likely to use alcohol and illegal drugs than are nonusers. Cigarette smokers are also more likely to get into fights, carry weapons, attempt suicide, and engage in high-risk sexual behaviors. These problem behaviors can be considered a syndrome, since involvement in one behavior increases the risk for involvement in others. Delaying or preventing the use of tobacco may have implications for delaying or preventing these other behaviors as well.

The Epidemiology of Tobacco Use Among Young People

Overall, about one-third of high-school-aged adolescents in the United States smoke or use smokeless tobacco. Smoking prevalence among U.S. adolescents declined sharply in the 1970s, but this decline slowed significantly in the 1980s, particularly among white males. Although female adolescents during the 1980s were more likely than male adolescents to smoke, female and male adolescents are now equally likely to smoke. Male adolescents are substantially more likely than females to use smokeless tobacco products; about 20 percent of high school males report current use, whereas only about 1 percent of females do. White adolescents are more likely to smoke and to use smokeless tobacco than are black and Hispanic adolescents.

Sociodemographic, environmental, behavioral, and personal factors can encourage the onset of tobacco use among adolescents. Young people from families with lower socioeconomic status, including those adolescents living in single-parent homes, are at increased risk of initiating smoking. Among environmental factors, peer influence seems to be particularly potent in the early stages of tobacco use; the first tries of cigarettes and smokeless tobacco occur most often with peers, and the peer group may subsequently provide expectations, reinforcement, and cues for experimentation. Parental tobacco use does not appear to be as compelling a risk factor as peer use; on the other hand, parents may exert a positive influence by disapproving of smoking, being involved in children's free time, discussing health matters with children, and encouraging children's academic achievement and school involvement. How adolescents perceive their social environment may be a stronger influence on behavior than the actual environment. For example, adolescents consistently overestimate the number of young people and adults who smoke. Those with the highest overestimates are more likely to become smokers than are those with more accurate perceptions. Similarly, those who perceive that cigarettes are easily accessible and generally available are more likely to begin smoking than are those who perceive more difficulty in obtaining cigarettes.

Behavioral factors figure heavily during adolescence, a period of multiple transitions to physical maturation, to a coherent sense of self, and to emotional independence. Adolescents are thus particularly vulnerable to a range of hazardous behaviors and activities, including tobacco use, that may seem to assist in these transitions. Young people who report that smoking serves positive functions or is potentially useful are at increased risk for smoking. These functions are associated with bonding with peers, being independent and mature, and having a positive social image. Since reports from adolescents who begin to smoke indicate that they have lower self-esteem and lower self-images than their nonsmoking peers, smoking can become a self-enhancement mechanism. Similarly, not having the confidence to be able to resist peer offers of tobacco seems to be an important risk factor for initiation. Intentions to use tobacco and actual experimentation also strongly predict subsequent regular use.

The positive functions that many young people attribute to smoking are the same functions advanced in most cigarette advertising. Young people are a strategically important market for the tobacco industry. Since most smokers try their first cigarette before age 18, young people are the chief source of new consumers for the tobacco industry, which each year must replace the many consumers who quit smoking and the many who die from smoking-related diseases. Despite restrictions on tobacco marketing, children and adolescents continue to be exposed to cigarette advertising and promotional activities, and young people report considerable familiarity with many cigarette advertisements. In the past, this exposure was accomplished by radio and television programs sponsored by the cigarette industry. Barred since 1971 from using broadcast media, the tobacco industry increasingly relies on promotional activities, including sponsorship of sports events and public entertainment, outdoor billboards, point-of-purchase displays, and the distribution of specialty items that appeal to the young. Cigarette advertisements in the print media persist; these messages have become increasingly less informational, replacing words with images to portray the attractiveness and function of smoking. Cigarette advertising frequently uses human models or human-like cartoon characters to display images of youthful activities, independence, healthfulness, and adventure-seeking. In presenting attractive images of smokers, cigarette advertisements appear to stimulate some adolescents who have relatively low self-images to adopt smoking as a way to improve their own self-image. Cigarette advertising also appears to affect adolescents' perceptions of the pervasiveness of smoking, images of smokers, and the function of smoking. Since these perceptions are psychosocial risk factors for the initiation of smoking, cigarette advertising appears to increase young people's risk of smoking.

Efforts to Prevent the Onset of Tobacco Use

Most of the U.S. public strongly favors policies that might prevent tobacco use among young people. These policies include mandated tobacco education in schools, a complete ban on smoking by anyone on school grounds, further restrictions on tobacco advertising and promotional activities, stronger prohibitions on the sale of tobacco products to minors, and increases in earmarked taxes on tobacco products. Interventions to prevent initiation among young people—even actions that involve restrictions on adult smoking or increased taxes—have received strong support among smoking and nonsmoking adults.

Numerous research studies over the past 15 years suggest that organized interventions can help prevent the onset of smoking and smokeless tobacco use. School-based smoking-prevention programs, based on a model of identifying social influences on smoking and providing skills to resist those influences, have demonstrated consistent and significant reductions in adolescent smoking prevalence; these program effects have lasted one to three years. Programs to prevent smokeless tobacco use have used a similar model to achieve modest reductions in initiation of use. The effectiveness of these school-based programs appears to be enhanced and sustained, at least until high school graduation, by adding coordinated communitywide programs that involve parents, youth-oriented mass media and counteradvertising, community organizations, or other elements of adolescents' social environments.

A crucial element of prevention is access: adolescents should not be able to purchase tobacco products in their communities. Active enforcement of age-at-sale policies by public officials and community members appears necessary to prevent minors' access to tobacco. Communities that have adopted tighter restrictions have achieved reductions in purchases by minors. At the state and national levels, price increases have significantly reduced cigarette smoking; the young have been at least as responsive as adults to these price changes. Maintaining higher real prices of cigarettes provides a barrier to adolescent tobacco use but depends on further tax increases to offset the effects of inflation. The results of this review thus suggest that a coordinated, multicomponent campaign involving policy changes, taxation, mass media, and behavioral education can effectively reduce the onset of tobacco use among adolescents.

Summary

Smoking and smokeless tobacco use are almost always initiated and established in adolescence. Besides its long-term effects on adults, tobacco use produces specific health problems for adolescents. Since nicotine addiction also occurs during adolescence, adolescent tobacco users are likely to become adult tobacco users. Smoking and smokeless tobacco use are associated with other problem behaviors and occur early in the sequence of these behaviors. The outcomes of adolescent smoking and smokeless tobacco use continue to be of great public health importance, since one out of three U.S. adolescents uses tobacco by age 18. The social environment of adolescents, including the functions, meanings, and images of smoking that are conveyed through cigarette advertising, sets the stage for adolescents to begin using tobacco. As tobacco products are available and as peers begin to try them, these factors become personalized and relevant, and tobacco use may begin. This process most affects adolescents who, compared with their peers, have lower self-esteem and self-images, are less involved with school and academic achievement, have fewer skills to resist the offers of peers, and come from homes with lower socioeconomic status. Tobacco-use prevention programs that target the larger social environment of adolescents are both efficacious and warranted.

CHAPTER CONCLUSIONS

Following are the specific conclusions for each chapter of this report (see chapters in original publication):

Chapter 2. The Health Consequences of Tobacco Use by Young People

1. Cigarette smoking during childhood and adolescence produces significant health problems among young people, including cough and phlegm production, an increased number and severity of respiratory illnesses, decreased physical fitness, an unfavorable lipid profile, and potential retardation in the rate of lung growth and the level of maximum lung function.

2. Among addictive behaviors, cigarette smoking is the one most likely to become established during adolescence. People who begin to smoke at an early age are more likely to develop severe levels of nicotine addiction than those who start at a later age.
3. Tobacco use is associated with alcohol and illicit drug use and is generally the first drug used by young people who enter a sequence of drug use that can include tobacco, alcohol, marijuana, and harder drugs.
4. Smokeless tobacco use by adolescents is associated with early indicators of periodontal degeneration and with lesions in the oral soft tissue. Adolescent smokeless tobacco users are more likely than nonusers to become cigarette smokers.

Chapter 3. Epidemiology of Tobacco Use Among Young People in the United States

1. Tobacco use primarily begins in early adolescence, typically by age 16; almost all first use occurs before the time of high school graduation.
2. Smoking prevalence among adolescents declined sharply in the 1970s, but the decline slowed significantly in the 1980s. At least 3.1 million adolescents and 25 percent of 17- and 18-year-olds are current smokers.
3. Although current smoking prevalence among female adolescents began exceeding that among males by the mid- to late-1970s, both sexes are now equally likely to smoke. Males are significantly more likely than females to use smokeless tobacco. Nationally, white adolescents are more likely to use all forms of tobacco than are blacks and Hispanics. The decline in the prevalence of cigarette smoking among black adolescents is noteworthy.
4. Many adolescent smokers are addicted to cigarettes; these young smokers report withdrawal symptoms similar to those reported by adults.
5. Tobacco use in adolescence is associated with a range of health-compromising behaviors, including being involved in fights, carrying weapons, engaging in higher-risk sexual behavior, and using alcohol and other drugs.

Chapter 4. Psychosocial Risk Factors for Initiating Tobacco Use

1. The initiation and development of tobacco use among children and adolescents progresses in five stages: from forming attitudes and beliefs about tobacco, to trying, experimenting with, and regularly using tobacco, to being addicted. This process generally takes about three years.
2. Sociodemographic factors associated with the onset of tobacco use include being an adolescent from a family with low socioeconomic status.
3. Environmental risk factors for tobacco use include accessibility and availability of tobacco products, perceptions by adolescents that tobacco use is normative, peers' and siblings' use and approval of tobacco use, and lack of parental support and involvement as adolescents face the challenges of growing up.
4. Behavioral risk factors for tobacco use include low levels of academic achievement and school involvement, lack of skills required to resist influences to use tobacco, and experimentation with any tobacco product.
5. Personal risk factors for tobacco use include a lower self-image and lower self-esteem than peers, the belief that tobacco use is functional, and lack of self-efficacy in the ability to refuse offers to use tobacco. For smokeless to-

bacco use, insufficient knowledge of the health con-sequences is also a factor.

Chapter 5. Tobacco Advertising and Promotional Activities

1. Young people continue to be a strategically important market for the tobacco industry.
2. Young people are currently exposed to cigarette messages through print media (including outdoor billboards) and through promotional activities, such as sponsorship of sporting events and public entertainment, point-of-sale displays, and distribution of specialty items.
3. Cigarette advertising uses images rather than information to portray the attractiveness and function of smoking. Human models and cartoon characters in cigarette advertising convey independence, healthfulness, adventure-seeking, and youthful activities—themes correlated with psychosocial factors that appeal to young people.
4. Cigarette advertisements capitalize on the disparity between an ideal and actual self-image and imply that smoking may close the gap.
5. Cigarette advertising appears to affect young people's perceptions of the pervasiveness, image, and function of smoking. Since misperceptions in these areas constitute psychosocial risk factors for the initiation of smoking, cigarette advertising appears to increase young people's risk of smoking.

Chapter 6. Efforts to Prevent Tobacco Use Among Young People

1. Most of the American public strongly favor policies that might prevent tobacco use among young people. These policies include tobacco education in the schools, restrictions on tobacco advertising and promotions, a complete ban on smoking by anyone on school grounds, prohibition of the sale of tobacco products to minors, and earmarked tax increases on tobacco products.
2. School-based smoking-prevention programs that identify social influences to smoke and teach skills to resist those influences have demonstrated consistent and significant reductions in adolescent smoking prevalence, and program effects have lasted one to three years. Programs to prevent smokeless tobacco use that are based on the same model have also demonstrated modest reductions in the initiation of smokeless tobacco use.
3. The effectiveness of school-based smoking-prevention programs appears to be enhanced and sustained by comprehensive school health education and by communitywide programs that involve parents, mass media, community organizations, or other elements of an adolescent's social environment.
4. Smoking-cessation programs tend to have low success rates. Recruiting and retaining adolescents in formal cessation programs are difficult.
5. Illegal sales of tobacco products are common. Active enforcement of age-at-sale policies by public officials and community members appears necessary to prevent minors' access to tobacco.
6. Econometric and other studies indicate that increases in the real price of cigarettes significantly reduce cigarette smoking; young people are at least as responsive as adults to such price changes. Maintaining higher real

prices of cigarettes depends on further tax increases to offset the effects of inflation.

REFERENCES

CDC. The health consequences of smoking: nicotine addiction—a report of the Surgeon General. Rockville, MD: US Department of Health and Human Services, Public Health Service, 1988:DHHS publication no. (CDC)88–8406.

CDC. Reducing the health consequences of smoking: 25 years of progress—a report of the Surgeon General. Rockville, MD: US Department of Health and Human Services, Public Health Service, 1989:DHHS publication no. (CDC)89–8411.

Public Health Service. The health consequences of using smokeless tobacco: a report of the advisory committee to the Surgeon General. Rockville, MD: US Department of Health and Human Services, Public Health Services, National Institutes of Health, 1986:DHHS publication no. (NIH)86–2874.

section five

ENVIRONMENTAL HEALTH

Managing Hazardous Materials Incidents Volume I, Emergency Medical Services

Original Citation: Managing hazardous materials incidents volume I, emergency medical services. U.S. Department of Human Services, Public Health Service, Agency for Toxic Substance and Disease Registry, 1992.

RESPONSE AND PATIENT MANAGEMENT

In the protocol for responding to potential hazardous materials incidents, the following primary considerations should be included: activities to undertake en route to the scene and upon arrival at the scene; guidelines for assessment, decontamination, and treatment of victims; and patient transport to the hospital.

En Route to a Hazardous Materials Scene

First responders need to be alert for hazardous materials when responding to every call. Hazardous materials can be obvious (i.e., noxious fumes, gasoline, or corrosive liquid spills) or they can be unnoticeable (odorless, but poisonous and/or flammable vapors and liquids, or radioactive). If a vehicle has a diamond-shaped placard or an orange-numbered panel on the side or rear, the cargo should be assumed to be hazardous. Unfortunately, not all hazardous materials carriers will be clearly marked. For example, delivery trucks regularly carry hazardous materials that can be released in a collision, yet rarely are marked. Therefore, first responders should use caution when attempting rescue at any incident scene. The hazard, or lack thereof, must be determined immediately—before first responders enter a chemically contaminated area.

The responder should pay attention to certain clues en route to an incident scene that could tip off the possibility of hazardous material involvement. Billowing smoke or clouds of vapor could give advanced warning that a dangerous substance may be involved. Senses are one of the best ways to detect chemicals, particularly the sense of smell. However, if you smell something you are too close and should remove yourself to a safe distance until you know more about the source of the odor. Failure to do so could cause injury. The nature of an incident should also be a key to identifying the possibility of a hazardous materials involvement. Tank trucks, train wrecks, and incidents at fixed facilities where chemicals are used could indicate hazardous materials involvement. The dispatcher may have clues that could indicate hazardous materials precautions are necessary. These could include the nature of an incident (e.g., leaking tank) and the nature of injuries (e.g., 25 workers with shortness of breath).

It is important that emergency responders pay attention to factors such as wind direction and topography when approaching a suspected hazardous materials incident. Responders should always approach upwind and upgrade from an incident, taking note that low lying areas such as stream beds and gulleys, or in urban areas, places such as courtyards or tall buildings, may contain vapor clouds that prevent dispersal by the wind.

Responders should also attempt to gather as much information as possible while en route to an incident. Using resources outlined in under Hazard Recognition, they can relay this information to a predesignated information center (e.g., regional poison control center, ATSDR) to obtain information about definitive care procedures including:

- Possible health effects
- Personal protective equipment (PPE) required
- Treatment/antidote therapy
- Decontamination procedures.

Information that will be needed to determine appropriate care will include:

- Knowledge of whether a chemical may be involved
- Chemical name of substance involved
- State of material (solid, liquid, gas)
- Quantities involved
- Number of victims
- Signs or symptoms
- Nature of exposure (inhalation, dermal, etc.)
- Length of exposure.

If a hazardous substance is involved and has been identified, responders should locate information concerning that substance using appropriate references, such as Material Safety Data Sheets (MSDS), the Department of Transportation (DOT) Emergency Response Guidebook, and CHEMTREC, as outlined under Hazard Recognition. This information can also help responders identify possible health hazards, including the nature of possible injuries; routes of exposure; proper level of PPE required; and the appropriate safe distance from the hazard to protect EMS personnel, the public, and property from exposure or other dangers, such as explosion or fire. This information may be available from a command post if one has been established. Emergency Medical Services Response to Hazardous Materials Incidents outlines these procedures for PPE, and Systems Approach to Planning describes guidelines for planning.

Communications with other agencies or services involved should also begin en route to an incident. If an Incident Command System (ICS) is implemented, interactions with an incident commander will identify the best route of approach, the possible dangers involved, and the estimated number of injuries. Communications between on-site response personnel and receiving facilities should be kept open to relay as much advance information as possible. Communications with other services should include the fire department, police, and hazardous materials response team (if one exists).

Arrival at the Scene

Many first responders (police, fire-rescue, and EMS personnel, including physicians and nurses) are accustomed to immediately attending an injured victim; often they disregard the possibility of danger to themselves. Consequently, a rescuer entering a contaminated area also risks exposure and the potential for becoming a victim. Even though rescue of any injured patient is important, it should only be attempted after it is certain that the responders, themselves, will not become injured. Responders must use judgement when assessing the dangers involved in a possible hazardous materials incident. Patient care should not be delayed unnecessarily when only minimal risk is involved, but many factors must be considered in determining the level of danger. Training and experience are essential for decision-making and those decisions, at best, are often a judgement call. As a rule, however, rescue should not be attempted by individuals who are not properly trained and equipped with appropriate PPE. Rescue should only be attempted by trained and equipped emergency personnel, fire department, or hazardous materials response team personnel. Figure 1 represents a typical decision tree that may be used in making decisions about risk and response.

Upon arrival at a scene, an initial assessment of the situation and the size of the incident should be conducted. Additional support should be requested, if necessary. Sources of on-scene assistance may include:

- Fire Departments
- Police Departments
- Health Departments
- Hazardous Materials Response Teams
- Local Industry Response Teams

Unless otherwise directed, responders should park upwind, upgrade, pointing away from, and a safe distance from any incident where hazardous materials are suspected. Safe distances for specific chemicals may be determined using the DOT Emergency Response Guidebook, by consulting CHEMTREC, or by using other response references. Responders should not drive or walk through any spilled or released materials (i.e., smoke and vapors as well as puddles). Also, a first-in responder should confirm that local authorities have been notified and are aware that hazardous materials might be involved.

Don't

- Don't drive or walk through any spilled materials.
- Don't allow unnecessary contamination of equipment.
- Don't attempt to recover shipping papers or manifests unless adequately protected.
- Don't become exposed while approaching a scene.
- Don't approach anyone coming from contaminated areas.
- Don't attempt rescue unless trained and equipped with appropriate PPE for the situation.

For first-in responders, the first priority is scene isolation. KEEP OTHERS AWAY! KEEP UNNECESSARY EQUIPMENT FROM BECOMING CONTAMINATED.

Sample EMS Decision Tree for Chemical Incidents

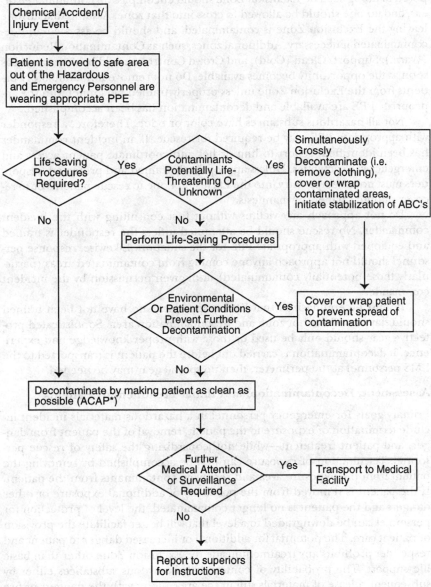

Figure 1. Sample EMS decision tree for chemical incidents.

Immediately establish an Exclusion (Hot) Zone, but do not become exposed in doing so. The Exclusion Zone should encompass all contaminated areas, and no one should be allowed to cross into that zone. Assume that anyone leaving the Exclusion Zone is contaminated, and should be assessed and decontaminated if necessary. Additional zones, such as Contamination Reduction (Warm), Support/Clean (Cold), and Crowd Control, should be determined as soon as the opportunity becomes available. Do not remove nonambulatory patients from the Exclusion Zone unless properly trained personnel with the appropriate PPE are available and decontamination has been accomplished.

Not all hazardous substances have color or odor. Therefore, a responder with appropriate PPE may be required for rescue. If an incident commander has been identified, report to him or her and coordinate patient access and emergency care activities. Unless appropriately trained and protected, responders must not attempt entry into the Exclusion Zone to rescue patients or to recover shipping papers or manifests.

Do not approach any victims without first consulting with the incident commander. No rescue should be attempted unless the responder is trained and equipped with appropriate PPE for the situation. Likewise, response personnel should not approach anyone coming from contaminated areas (particularly those potentially contaminated) until given permission by the incident commander.

It must be emphasized that EMS responders who have not been trained should stay out of the hot zone and decontamination area. Sophisticated protective gear should only be used by those with proper knowledge and experience. If decontamination is carried out before the patient is transported to the EMS personnel at the perimeter, then no special gear may be needed.

Assessment, Decontamination, and Initial Treatment of Patients

Primary goals for emergency personnel in a hazardous materials incident include termination of exposure to the patient, removal of the patient from danger, and patient treatment—while not jeopardizing the safety of rescue personnel. Termination of exposure can best be accomplished by removing the patient from the exposure area and removing contaminants from the patient. If the patient is removed from the possibility of additional exposure or other dangers and the patient is no longer contaminated, the level of protection for personnel can be downgraded to a level that will better facilitate the provision of patient care. The potential for additional or increased danger to patient and responder prohibits any treatment inside the Exclusion Zone other than basic life support. The probability of contact with hazardous substances either by subsequent release of materials still in the area, along with the dangers of fire or explosion, and the restriction of movement by necessary PPE outweighs the time saved by attempting patient care in a dangerous area. Gross management of Airway, Breathing, and Circulation (ABC) is all that should be undertaken while there is potential for further injury to patient or response personnel.

One of the most important steps in scene hazard assessment should be obtaining immediate assistance from a regional poison control center. The poison center can help determine the risk for secondary contamination, the need for special protective gear and decontamination procedures, and the toxic effects of the chemical.

Primary assessment can be undertaken while simultaneously performing decontamination in the Contamination Reduction Zone. Priority should be given to the ABC: Airway, Breathing, and Circulation. Once life-threatening matters have been addressed, rescue personnel can then direct attention to secondary patient assessment. It is important to remember that appropriate personal protective equipment and clothing must be worn until the threat of secondary exposure is no longer a danger. Therefore, the sooner the patient becomes decontaminated the sooner response personnel may reduce protective measures or downgrade the level of protection.

During initial patient stabilization, a gross decontamination should simultaneously be performed. This consists of cutting away or otherwise removing all suspected contaminated clothing, including jewelry and watches, and brushing or wiping off any obvious contamination. Care should be taken to protect any open wounds from contamination. Every effort should be made by personnel to avoid contact with any potentially hazardous substance.

Effective decontamination consists of making the patient As Clean As Possible (ACAP). This means that the contamination has been reduced to a level that is no longer a threat to the patient or the responder.

Decontamination

Directives for decontamination include the reduction of external contamination, containment of the contamination present, and prevention of the further spread of potentially dangerous substances. In other words, remove what you can and contain what you can't. With a few exceptions, intact skin is less absorptive than injured flesh, mucous membranes, or eyes. Therefore, decontamination should begin at the head of the patient and proceed downward with initial attention to contaminated eyes and open wounds. Once wounds have been cleaned, care should be exercised so as not to recontaminate them. This can be aided by covering the wounds with a waterproof dressing. For some chemicals, such as strong alkali, it may be necessary to flush exposed eyes with water or normal saline for several hours. Table 9 outlines the minimum equipment that is required for decontamination of patients by emergency response personnel. These lists are not detailed; they are only provided to guide departments in developing their own equipment lists based on their community needs and requirements. Many chemical substances, even though highly toxic, carry no intrinsic risk for contamination to others. Most toxic gases, such as carbon monoxide or arsine, are highly poisonous, but once the victim has been brought out of the exposure area and into the fresh air, the amount of leftover gas in and around the patient simply cannot poison others. Even many chemicals that have the potential for spreading contamination can be made less hazardous by simply diluting them with copious amounts of water.

Table 9. Suggested Decontamination Equipment

At a minimum, the protective equipment listed is necessary to participate in decontamination procedures. Protective equipment used for decontamination should be no less than one level below that used for entry into the hazardous environment. Positive-pressure self-contained breathing apparatus (SCBA) and fully encapsulated suits may be necessary in extreme cases.

Containment equipment	Sponges and soft brushes
Pool or tank	Large plastic bags for contaminated
Tarps	clothing
6-mil construction plastic	Small plastic bags for patients' valuables
Saw horses to support backboards	Tags and waterproof pens to mark bags
Fiberglass backboards	Disposable clothes and shoes for ambu-
Supports for ambulatory patients	latory patients
Water supply	Towels and blankets
Scissors for clothing removal	Clear, zip-front bags to minimize con-
Mild detergent (dishwashing liquid)	tamination to transport personnel and
Five-gallon buckets	ambulances
	Tape (duct, 4-inch)

External decontamination should be performed using the least aggressive methods. Limit mechanical or chemical irritation to the skin to prevent increased permeability. Wash contaminated areas gently under a gentle spray of water, and wash with a soft sponge using a mild soap such as dishwashing liquid. Use warm, never hot, water. The degree of decontamination should be completed based on the nature of the contaminant, the form of contaminant, the patient's condition, environmental conditions, and resources available. Care should be taken so that contaminants are not introduced into open wounds. Responders should try to contain all runoff from decontamination procedures for proper disposal. The patient should be isolated from the environment to prevent the spread of any remaining contaminants.

Ensure that all potentially contaminated patient clothing and belongings have been removed. Properly label bags that contain clothing or other potentially contaminated articles. Contaminated clothing and belongings should not be transported with the patient in the ambulance unless the incident commander approves, and the clothing and belongings have been adequately bagged.

Decontamination

- Decontaminate from the head down
- Take care not to introduce contaminants into open wounds
- Decontaminate exposed wounds and eyes before intact skin areas
- Cover wounds with a water-proof dressing after decontamination
- For external contamination, begin with the least aggressive methods
- Limit mechanical or chemical irritation of the skin
- Wash contaminated area gently under a stream of water, and scrub with a soft brush or surgical sponge

- Use warm, never hot, water
- Remove contaminants to the level that they are no longer a threat to patient or response personnel
- Isolate the patient from the environment to prevent the spread of any remaining contaminants
- If possible, contain all runoff from decontamination procedures for proper disposal
- Ensure that all potentially contaminated patient clothing and belongings have been removed
- properly label bags that contain clothing or other potentially contaminated articles

Considerations for Patient Treatment

Basically, a contaminated patient is like any other patient and may be treated as such except that responders must protect themselves and others from dangers due to contamination. Response personnel must first address life-threatening issues and then decontamination and supportive measures. Primary surveys will be accomplished simultaneously with decontamination; and secondary surveys should be completed as conditions allow. The chemical-specific information received from the hazardous materials response resources should be incorporated into the proper patient treatment procedures. In multiple patient situations, proper triage procedures should be implemented using local community emergency response plans (see Superfund Amendments and Reauthorization Act (SARA) Title 111). Treat presenting signs and symptoms as appropriate and when conditions allow. The sooner a patient has been decontaminated the sooner he or she can be treated like a "normal" patient. Administer orders of the designated poison control center when conditions allow. Unless required by life-threatening conditions prophylactic invasive procedures, such as intravenous injections (I.V.s) or intubation, should be performed only in fully decontaminated areas where conditions permit. These procedures may create a direct route for introducing the hazardous material into the patient. Oxygen should be given using a bag valve mask with reservoir device (rebreather) or manually triggered oxygen-powered breathing device. The contaminated atmosphere should not mix with the oxygen if possible. Reassess the patient frequently because many hazardous materials have latent physiological effects. While some cases may require treatment with antidotes, most cases will be handled with symptomatic care.

Patient Treatment

- Assign highest priorities to ABC and decontamination
- Complete primary and secondary surveys as conditions allow. Bear in mind the chemical specific information received from the designated poison control or information center
- In multiple patient situations, begin proper triage procedures
- Treat presenting signs and symptoms as appropriate and when conditions allow
- Administer orders of the designated poison control center when conditions allow

- Perform invasive procedures only in uncontaminated areas
- Reassess the patient frequently because many chemicals have latent physiological effects
- Delay prophylactic measures until the patient is decontaminated

Patient Transport to Hospital

When transporting a contaminated patient by ambulance, special care should be exercised in preventing contamination of the ambulance and subsequent patients. Exposed surfaces that the contaminated patient is likely to come into contact with should be covered with plastic sheeting.

Fiberglass backboards and disposable sheeting are recommended. If a wood backboard is used, it should be covered with disposable sheeting or it may have to be discarded afterwards. Equipment that comes in contact with the patient should be segregated for disposal or decontamination. EMS personnel should wear protective clothing appropriate for conditions (e.g., surgical gloves, CPC, etc.), and respirators, if indicated (see Section I of original publication, PPE). Table 10 outlines suggested equipment required for care and transport of contaminated patients. Like other listings provided, it is only for guidance, and items may be added or deleted with experience.

Table 10. Supplies

Enough 6-mil construction plastic* cut to size to:
    Cover floor of ambulance
    Cover squad seat
    Cover litter

Disposable sheets

One box of plastic trash bags to contain contaminated medical supply waste, gloves and the victim's clothes, and the like

Personal protection
    CVC disposable suits with built-in hoods and booty/boot covers
    Positive-pressure SCBA
    Full-face mask respirator with an orange- and purple-type cartridge (acid gas, organic vapor, highly toxic dust, mist and fumes, and radionuclides-rated cartridge)
    Poly-vinyl chloride (PVC) or duct type for taping closures
    Two-piece rainwear
    Rubber boots with steel toes
    Nitrite gloves with 14-inch cuffs
    Duct tape to seal suit seams if necessary

If the fire department's protective clothing is used, rainwear should be worn as an overgarment. Hydrocarbons and other chemicals may permeate the "bunker clothes."

NOTE: The protective equipment listed is to be used for patent care situations after initial decontamination. It is meant to be used when complete decontamination of the patients cannot be guaranteed or when assisting with decontamination procedures (in extreme cases positive-pressure SCBA and encapsulated suits may

Table 10.—*continued*

be required for decontamination procedures). It is not meant to be used in rescue operations of victims found in a hazardous area. Under no circumstances should this equipment be relied upon for entry into hazardous environments. Protective equipment for entry must be appropriate to and compatible with the products involved. This may include positive-pressure SCBA and fully encapsulated suits. Many factors must be taken into consideration when determining the appropriate level of protection. Consequently, selection of protective equipment must be done by a qualified individual.

*Wet plastic is slippery; stability is important.

The patient should be as clean as reasonably possible before transport, and further contact with contaminants should be avoided. Protective clothing should be worn by response personnel as appropriate. If decontamination cannot be performed adequately, responders should make every attempt to prevent the spread of contamination and at the very least remove patient clothing, wrap the patient in blankets, followed by body bags or plastic or rubber sheets to lessen the likelihood of contamination to equipment and others. Considerations should be made for chemicals that present the added danger of accelerated skin absorption due to heat. In these cases body bags and plastic or rubber sheets should not be used. Minimize contamination from shoes. The name of the involved chemicals, if identified, and any other data available, should be recorded before leaving the scene. Oxygen should be administered by rebreather mask for any victim with respiratory problems unless contraindicated (e.g., paraquat). Eyes that have been exposed should be irrigated with available saline or water, and such irrigation should be continued en route to the hospital. Personnel also should be alert for any respiratory distress.

In an ambulance during transport, personnel should use appropriate respiratory protection. Provide the maximum fresh air ventilation (e.g., open windows) that weather conditions permit to the patient and driver's compartment regardless of the presence or absence of odors.

Re-contact the receiving hospital and provide an update on treatment provided or required and any other information received from the designated poison control center. Instructions for the procedure to enter the hospital with a contaminated patient should also be requested. Facilities receiving a potential hazardous material patient will need as much information as possible.

A checklist should be developed and made available for all vehicles and telephone or radio communication centers. Information that will aid in initiating appropriate actions includes:

- Type and nature of incident
- Number of patients
- Signs/symptoms being experienced by the patients
- Nature of injuries
- Name of chemical(s) involved

- Information available at the site concerning the chemical(s)
- Extent of patient decontamination in the field
- Estimated time of arrival

The ambulance should park in an area away from the emergency room or go directly to a predesignated decontamination center or area, thereby limiting exposure to hospital facilities. In order to protect staff and other patients, the patient should not be brought into the emergency department before ambulance personnel receive permission from the hospital staff.

Upon the release of the patient to the hospital, any equipment that is believed to have become contaminated should be double-bagged. The use of disposable equipment is recommended whenever possible. Contaminated articles should be kept sealed until the Incident Commander or his designee gives further instructions. If possible, send any material safety data sheets concerning the involved hazardous materials with the patient.

The ambulance should not go back into service unless the vehicle is clean. This again emphasizes the importance of thorough patient decontamination; if the patient is clean, then the vehicle (interior) is clean. After the patient is unloaded from the ambulance, a check should be made with the hospital to determine where the ambulance can be safely decontaminated, and whether equipment is available for this purpose. When decontamination is required, the most appropriate method should be identified using information resources. In most cases soap and water are adequate for decontaminating of the vehicle.

Transport to Hospital

- Re-contact the receiving hospital
- Update the hospital on treatment provided and any other information received from the designated poison control center, and
- Obtain instructions on approaching and entering the hospital
- Avoid contact with contaminants; provide protection to the vehicle; wear protective clothing as appropriate
- Get patient as clean as possible prior to transport
- Administer oxygen by mask for any patient with respiratory problems (except as contraindicated)
- Before leaving the scene, write down the name of the involved chemicals, if identified, and any other data available
- Provide fresh air ventilation to patient and driver's compartment
- Continue to irrigate eyes that have been exposed with normal saline or water en route to the hospital and be alert for any respiratory distress
- Park the ambulance in an area away from the emergency department or go directly to a predesignated decontamination area
- Do not bring patients into the emergency department before ambulance personnel receive permission from the hospital staff
- After unloading the patient, check with the hospital to determine where the ambulance can be safely decontaminated, and the availability of equipment for this purpose
- Decontaminate exposed personnel

Air Transportation of Chemically Exposed Patients

There is a potential danger in transporting patients in a helicopter from a hazardous materials incident. Often decontamination is not complete, and the flight crew could experience difficulty breathing or seeing. Also the area of the incident needs to be clearly communicated with the flight crew to avoid traveling through an unsafe area. Furthermore, the downdraft from the helicopter could affect vapors or fumes on the scene. Considerations should be made for each specific incident and chemical.

Critique

As soon as possible after each incident, all participating units should send personnel involved to review the measures that were taken by each unit or agency. The purpose of this review is to examine which activities succeeded and which did not, and to evaluate the overall coordination effort.

Patient Management Under Mass Casualty Conditions Involving Hazardous Chemicals

Basic medical procedures in a large-scale hazardous materials incident are not substantially different from life-saving measures in other mass casualty disasters. Primary attention to the ABC (i.e., Airway, Breathing, and Circulation) continues to have first priority.

There are, however, several important differences in disasters involving hazardous materials. A chemical mass casualty incident may also require setting up mass screening and decontamination centers. It may also be necessary to establish casualty collection points to provide stabilizing care in the field prior to transport. A major chemical disaster may accompany other disasters such as an earthquake. Such an event would drastically increase the number of casualties and the complexity of the medical care that must be provided (crushing and broken bones vs. gas inhalation, for example). This would require increased numbers of personnel, perhaps more sophisticated medical equipment, and a better transport system for taking stabilized victims out of the area. Training in the appropriate procedures to be followed is essential for potential responders to a hazardous materials incident involving mass casualties. Triage may be complicated for chemical exposure by delayed onset of signs and symptoms. The patient, injured or not, must be decontaminated before being transported to the emergency department to protect EMS and emergency department staff.

SELECTED BIBLIOGRAPHY

Cashman JR. Hazardous materials emergencies, response and control. Revised. 2nd ed. Lancaster, PA: Technomic Publishing Co., 1988.

Currance PL, Bronstein AC. Emergency care for hazardous materials exposure. St. Louis, MO: C.V. Mosby, 1988.

Department of Transportation (DOT). Emergency response guidebook. Washington, DC: Department of Transportation, 1987:DOTP-5800.5

Federal Emergency Management Agency (FEMA). Disaster planning guidelines for fire chiefs. Prepared by International Association of Fire Chiefs, Inc. Washington, DC: FEMA, February 1981.

Federal Emergency Management Agency (FEMA). Guidance for developing state and local radiological emergency response plans and preparedness for transportation accidents. Washington, DC: FEMA, 1985.

Federal Emergency Management Agency (FEMA). Hazardous materials management system: a guide for local emergency managers. Prepared by the Multnomah County Office of Emergency Management. Washington, DC: FEMA, July 1981.

Federal Emergency Management Agency (FEMA). Hospital emergency department management of radiation accidents. Washington, DC: FEMA, 1984.

Goldfrank LR. Goldfrank's toxicological emergencies—a comprehensive handbook in problem solving. New York: Appleton Century Crofts, 1986.

Haddad LM, Winchester JF. Clinical management of poisoning and overdose. Philadelphia, PA: WB Saunders Co., 1983.

Leonard RB, Ricks R. Emergency department radiation accident protocol. Ann Emerg Med September, 1980.

Noji EK, Kelen GD. Manual of toxicologic emergencies. Chicago, IL: Year Book Medical Publishers, 1989.

Noll G, Hildebrand MS, Yvorra JG. Hazardous materials: managing the incident. Stillwater, OK: Fire Protection Publications, Oklahoma State University, 1988.

Ricks RC. Hospital emergency department management of radiation accidents. Oak Ridge, TN: Oak Ridge Associated Universities, 1984.

Stutz DR, Ricks R, Olsen M. Hazardous materials injuries: a handbook of prehospital care. Greenbelt, MD: Bradford Communications Corporation, 1982.

Managing Hazardous Materials Incidents
Volume II, Hospital Emergency Departments

Original Citation: Managing hazardous materials incidents volume II, hospital emergency departments. U.S. Department of Human Services, Public Health Service, Agency for Toxic Substance and Disease Registry, 1992.

PATIENT MANAGEMENT

Growing concern about the proper treatment of chemically contaminated patients has outpaced adequate guidance on the subject. However, definitive work has been done on cases that bear similar characteristics (e.g., radioactive exposure), and many of the same principles apply. Many of these principles can be found in the article "Emergency Department Radiation Accident Protocol" by R.B. Leonard, Ph.D., M.D., and R.C. Ricks, Ph.D., published in the September 1980 issue of Annals of Emergency Medicine. Further information on radiation response procedures is contained in Hospital Emergency Department Management of Radiation Accidents by Robert C. Ricks, Ph.D., prepared for the Federal Emergency Management Agency.

When a hospital receives a call that a patient exposed to hazardous materials is to be received, a planned course of action should be implemented. Steps in a protocol must be practiced before a hazardous materials emergency occurs. All staff members of an emergency department should know their responsibilities and how to perform them. All required equipment should be immediately available or readily accessed.

Individuals receiving a potential hazardous materials call should obtain as much information as possible. A checklist should be developed and made available for all telephone or radio communication centers. Information that will aid in initiating appropriate actions includes:

* Type and nature of incident
* Caller's telephone number

- Number of patients
- Signs/symptoms being experienced by the patients
- Nature of injuries
- Name of chemical(s) involved
- Extent of patient decontamination in the field
- Estimated time of arrival

After the above information is received, a predesignated resource center (e.g., regional poison control center, ATSDR) should be contacted for information regarding definitive care procedures, which should include decontamination methods that need to be performed. Communications should be kept open with on-site response personnel to obtain as much advance information as possible.

If incident notification comes from other than usual emergency communication channels, the call should be verified before a hazardous materials response plan is initiated. Ambulance personnel should be notified of any special approach or entrance to the emergency department and also advised not to bring the patient into the emergency department until the patient has been assessed and accepted by the emergency department.

Often patients contaminated by hazardous materials may be brought into the emergency department unannounced or not through regular EMS channels. This could be an ambulatory patient or a patient transported by private vehicle. The ideal response to this is to call a fire department which is properly trained and equipped or a hazmat team to come to the hospital and set up a decontamination area outside the ambulance entrance. In any event, these patients should be isolated from other patients and assessed and decontaminated as soon as possible.

Emergency Department Preparation

Every member of the emergency department should be familiar with the hospital's hazardous materials response plan and be required to participate in scheduled drills. Preparation for arrival of a contaminated patient should include: notification of all services involved, preparation of a Decontamination Area, and suiting up of the Decontamination Team.

Emergency Department Mobilization

The person receiving a call of incoming victims should notify the Nursing Supervisor who will in turn notify appropriate personnel according to the hospital's response plan. The hospital operator should be instructed to notify security and maintenance, and the nurse on duty should contact the predesignated resource center.

Decontamination Area Preparation

Any victim of a hazardous materials incident must be considered to be contaminated until demonstrated otherwise. Therefore, the route from the emergency entrance to the decontamination area may also become contaminated and all persons along that route should be removed by security personnel. Ideally, this area should be protected with plastic or paper sheeting. This barrier should be taped securely to the floor, and care should be taken while walking on it because plastic can be very slippery when wet.

Security personnel should be stationed at the main entrance of the emergency department close to the decontamination area to prevent unauthorized entry, to control the entrance of the contaminated patient into the department, and to direct the vehicle transporting the patient to the appropriate area. A reception area should be set up just outside the emergency department entrance, where arriving contaminated patients can be screened for adequate decontamination before entering the department.

A decontamination area should be large enough to facilitate decontamination of more than one patient and accommodate the many personnel involved in patient treatment and contamination reduction. The ventilation system should either be separate from the rest of the hospital or turned off in order to prevent spread of airborne contaminants throughout the facility. If the ventilation system is shut off during the handling of a contaminated victim in an enclosed area, the emergency department medical team could be endangered. Therefore, OSHA regulations (i.e., 29 CFR 1910.120(q)(3)(iv)) on monitoring the atmosphere should be adhered to, especially if APRs are used. The best place (weather permitting) to evaluate and initially treat contaminated patients is outside where ambient ventilation will keep cross-exposure low. Some hospitals have radiation decontamination facilities that can be used with minor changes. An outside or portable decontamination system is a viable substitute and would aid in preventing contamination of the emergency department and other patients. A practical alternative for facilities with limited resources is to have a warm shower nozzle, soap, a wading pool, and plastic garbage bags in a predesignated area outside the emergency department back door. The patient may be able to remove his or her own contaminated clothing, place it in a double bag, and do his or her own soap and water decontamination. A partial tent or curtain can provide privacy for the patients. In most circumstances, ordinary hospital gowns, plastic goggles, and plain latex gloves will adequately protect hospital staff in case they have to assist the patient in removing soaked clothing, wash exposed skin and hair, or perform eye irrigation. With large amounts of concentrated corrosives or very oily materials, such as pesticides, disposable CPC and unmilled nitrile gloves will offer additional protection. If it is anticipated that your facility is likely to receive heavily contaminated patients who have not received prior decontamination, then it may be appropriate to purchase appropriate protective gear and to fit and train emergency department staff in its use. However, no person should wear and use specialized PPE, especially respiratory protective gear, without prior training.

To prevent unnecessary contamination, all nonessential and nondisposable equipment should be removed from the decontamination area. All door knobs, cabinet handles, light switches, and other areas that have contact with hands should be taped, and the floors should be covered with plastic or paper sheeting to prevent contamination. The floor coverings should be securely taped to prevent slippage, and the entrance to the room marked with a wide strip of colored tape to indicate a contaminated area. Personnel should not enter the area unless properly protected, and no personnel or equipment should leave the area until properly decontaminated. A "clean" member of the staff should stand on the clean side of the entrance to hand in supplies and receive medical specimens. The essential requirements for any decontamination task are:

- A safe area to place a patient while undergoing decontamination
- A method for washing contaminants off a patient
- A means of containing the rinsate
- Adequate protection for personnel handling the patient
- Disposable or cleanable medical equipment to treat the patient

Decontamination Team Preparation

A decontamination team should be predesignated and trained in appropriate personal protection equipment and procedures. The team should consist of:

- Emergency physician
- Emergency department nurses and aides
- Support personnel
- Nursing Supervisor
- Occupational Health and Safety Officer
- Security
- Maintenance
- Recorder

The decontamination team should be equipped with personal protective clothing (as discussed in Section I of the original publication) for whatever level described as appropriate for the substance(s) involved. This may be determined by consulting reference guidebooks, database networks, or telephone hotlines.

Appropriate dress for the decontamination team should include:

- A scrub suit
- Plastic shoe covers
- Disposable CPC with hood and booties built in; tape hood at neck
- Poly Vinyl Chloride (PVC) gloves taped to sleeves
- Respiratory protection as appropriate
- Multiple layers of surgical gloves, neoprene or disposable nitrile gloves; change whenever torn; tape bottom layer
- Protective eyewear

A 2-inch-wide piece of masking tape with the team member's name placed on the back of the protective suits will often assist employee in communicating.

Patient Arrival

The emergency physician-in-charge or an emergency department nurse should meet the ambulance upon arrival and assess the condition of the patients as well as the degree of contamination. Personnel should keep in mind that the actual contamination may be (or become) a life-threatening condition. Triage

procedures should also be initiated at this point, if necessary. During initial patient survey and stabilization, contamination reduction should simultaneously
be performed. This consists of cutting away or otherwise removing all suspected
contaminated clothing, including jewelry and watches, and brushing or wiping
off any contamination. Care should be taken to protect any open wounds from
contamination. Emergency department personnel should make every effort to
avoid contact with any potentially hazardous substance.

Ideally, decontamination should be performed before patient transport;
however, field decontamination facilities are limited and emergency department personnel should consider that all hazardous materials patients need decontamination. If a patient's clothing was not removed at the incident site, it
should be removed outside the ambulance but before entry into the emergency
department. This will reduce further exposure to the patient and lessen the extent of contamination introduced to the emergency department. Contaminated
clothing should be double bagged in plastic bags, sealed, and labeled. The decontamination team should bring the prepared stretcher to the ambulance,
transfer the patient, and take him or her directly to the decontamination area
along the predesignated route.

Priority should be given to the ABC (Airway, Breathing, and Circulation)
and simultaneous contamination reduction. Once life-threatening matters have
been addressed, emergency department personnel can then direct attention to
thorough decontamination and secondary patient assessment. Identification of
hazardous materials involved can be simultaneously performed by other personnel. It is important to remember that appropriate personal protective clothing must be worn until personnel are no longer in danger. Therefore, the
sooner the patient becomes decontaminated the sooner personnel may reduce
protective measures.

Effective decontamination consists of making the patient As Clean As
Possible (ACAP). This means that the contamination has been reduced to a
level that is no longer a threat to the patient or the responder. The recorder
notes on a diagram of the body the areas found by the physician to be contaminated.

Decontamination of Patient

The basic purpose of decontamination is to reduce external contamination,
contain the contamination present, and prevent the further spread of potentially dangerous substances. In other words, remove what you can and contain
what you can't. With a few exceptions, intact skin is more resistant to hazardous
materials than injured flesh, mucous membranes, or eyes. Therefore, decontamination should begin at the head of the patient and proceed downward with
initial attention to contaminated eyes and open wounds. Once wounds have
been cleaned, care should be exercised so that the wounds are not recontami-
nated. This can be aided by covering the wounds with a waterproof dressing.
For some chemicals, such as strong alkali, it may be necessary to flush exposed
skin and eyes with water or normal saline for an extended period of time.

External decontamination should be performed using the least aggressive layer methods. Mechanical or chemical irritation to the skin should be limited to prevent damage to the epidermal layer, which would result in increased permeability. Contaminated areas should be gently washed under a spray of water, with a sponge and a mild soap. Warm, never hot, tap water should be used. Care should be taken so that contaminants are not introduced into open wounds. All run-off from decontamination procedures should be collected for proper disposal.

The first priority in the process of decontamination should be contaminated open wounds. These areas allow for rapid absorption of hazardous materials. Wounds should be irrigated with copious amounts of normal saline, and deep debridement and excision should be performed only when particles or pieces of material have been embedded in the tissues. Decontamination of eyes should also have high priority. Gentle irrigation of the eyes should be performed with the stream of normal saline diverted away from the medial canthus so that it does not force material into the lacrimal duct. Contaminated nares and ear canals should also be gently irrigated with frequent suction to prevent any material being forced deeper into those cavities. Washing with soap and tepid water is usually all that is needed to remove contamination. Hot water, stiff brushes, or vigorous scrubbing should never be used because they cause vasodilation and abrasion. This increases the chances for absorption of hazardous materials through the skin.

Considerations for Patient Treatment

Primary goals for emergency department personnel in handling a contaminated patient include termination of exposure to the patient, patient stabilization, and patient treatment—while not jeopardizing the safety of emergency department personnel. Termination of exposure can best be accomplished by removing the patient from the area of exposure and by removing contaminants from the patient. Basically, a contaminated patient is like any other and may be treated as such except that staff must protect themselves and others from dangers due to contamination.

Personnel must first address life-threatening issues and then decontamination and supportive measures. Priority should be given to the ABC with simultaneous contamination reduction. Once life-threatening matters have been addressed, emergency department personnel can then direct attention to thorough decontamination, secondary patient assessment, and identification of materials involved. It is important to remember that appropriate personal protective clothing must be worn until personnel are no longer in danger. Therefore, the sooner the patient becomes decontaminated the sooner personnel may reduce protective measures or downgrade the level of protection. Primary and secondary surveys should be completed as conditions allow. In treating patients, personnel should consider the chemical-specific information received from the hazardous materials response resources. In multiple patient situations, proper triage procedures should be implemented. Presenting signs and symptoms should be treated as appropriate and when conditions allow.

The sooner a patient has been decontaminated the sooner he or she can be treated like a "normal" patient. Orders of the designated poison control center and attending physician should be administered. Invasive procedures, such as IVs or intubation, should be performed only for life-threatening conditions, until decontamination is performed. These procedures may create a direct route for introducing the hazardous material into the patient. The patient should be frequently re-assessed because many hazardous materials have latent physiological effects.

Information on Materials Involved

Identification of materials involved should also be determined early in a hazardous material incident. Using resources outlined in this section, and in Section I under Hazard Recognition, personnel should identify and obtain detailed information involving treatment, decontamination procedures, and possible adverse health effects of the specific chemical(s) involved. Information that may be needed will include:

- Chemical name of substance involved
- Form of material (solid, liquid, gas)
- Length of exposure
- Routes of exposure
- Possible adverse health effects
- Treatment/antidote therapy
- Personal protection equipment (PPE) required
- Decontamination procedures

The importance of finding out as much as possible, as soon as possible, about an unknown substance cannot be emphasized enough; however, based on experience, NIOSH and EPA recommend that "Level B" protection is the minimum level to be worn when entering an area containing unknown substances. However, if the substance in question is suspected to involve the skin as a route of exposure or is otherwise noted to be dangerous by absorption, corrosion, and the like, "Level A" protection should be worn because it provides additional skin protection.

Removal of Patient from Decontamination Room

After the patient has been decontaminated, he or she should be discharged home or admitted to the hospital, depending on the patient's clinical condition. Place a clean piece of plastic on the floor for the patient and staff to use when exiting the clean area. If the patient is not ambulatory a clean stretcher or wheelchair should be brought to the doorway by an individual who has not been exposed. After the patient is transferred to the clean area, the physician can perform the physical examination and initiate routine patient management.

Note: The attending staff must remember that since exposure to some substances can result in serious delayed effects, sustained observation and monitoring are required.

Critique

As soon as possible after each incident, all participating units should send knowledgeable representatives to review the measures that were taken by each unit or agency. The purpose of this review is to examine which activities succeeded and which did not, and to evaluate the overall coordination effort.

Patient Management Under Mass Casualty Conditions Involving Hazardous Chemicals

Basic medical procedures in a large-scale hazardous materials incident are not substantially different from life-saving measures in other mass casualty disasters. Primary attention to the ABC continues to have first priority with decontamination performed at the same time. A chemical disaster may overwhelm any one hospital, particularly if it occurs along with another disaster such as an earthquake. Hospitals need to preplan what they will do if they are overwhelmed with hazmat patients.

There are, however, several important differences in disasters involving hazardous materials. Such differences include the need for the effective decontamination of exposed patients and response personnel, and the need for effective safety measures to protect response personnel. Training in the appropriate procedures to be followed is essential for potential responders to a hazardous materials incident involving mass casualties. Standard principles of triage apply in chemical disasters, except in exposures to very toxic substances. The patient, injured or not, must be decontaminated before being transported to the emergency department to protect EMS and emergency department staff.

SELECTED BIBLIOGRAPHY

Cashman JR. Hazardous materials emergencies, response and control. Revised. 2nd ed. Lancaster, PA: Technomic Publishing Co., 1988.

Currance PL, Bronstein AC. Emergency care for hazardous materials exposure. St. Louis, MO: C.V. Mosby, 1988.

Department of Transportation (DOT). Emergency response guidebook. Washington DC: Department of Transportation, 1987:DOTP-5800.5.

Federal Emergency Management Agency (FEMA). Disaster planning guidelines for fire chiefs. Prepared by International Association of Fire Chiefs, Inc. Washington DC: FEMA, February 1981.

Federal Emergency Management Agency (FEMA). Guidance for developing state and local radiological emergency response plans and preparedness for transportation accidents. Washington DC: FEMA, 1985.

Federal Emergency Management Agency (FEMA). Hazardous materials management system: a guide for local emergency managers. Prepared by the Multnomah County Office of Emergency Management. Washington DC: FEMA, July 1981.

Federal Emergency Management Agency (FEMA). Hospital emergency department management of radiation accidents. Washington DC: FEMA, 1984.

Goldfrank LR. Goldfrank's toxicological emergencies: a comprehensive handbook in problem solving. New York, Appleton Century Crofts, 1986.

Haddad LM, Winchester JF. Clinical management of poisoning and overdose. Philadelphia, PA: WB Saunders Co., 1983.

Leonard RB, Ricks R. Emergency department radiation accident protocol. Ann Emerg Med September, 1980.

Noji EK, Kelen GD. Manual of toxicologic emergencies. Chicago, IL: Year Book Medical Publishers, 1989.

Noll G, Hildebrand MS, Yvorra JG. Hazardous materials: managing the incident. Stillwater, OK: Fire Protection Publications, Oklahoma State University, 1988.

Ricks RC. Hospital emergency department management of radiation accidents. Oak Ridge, TN: Oak Ridge Associated Universities, 1984.

Stutz DR, Ricks R, Olsen M. Hazardous materials injuries: a handbook of prehospital care. Greenbelt, MD: Bradford Communications Corporation, 1982.

Impact of Lead-Contaminated Soil on Public Health

Original Citation: Impact of lead-contaminated soil on public health. U.S. Department of Health and Human Services, Public Health Service, Centers for Disease Control and Prevention, Agency for Toxic Substances and Disease Registry, 1992.

Original Author: Charles Xintaras, Sc.D.

FOREWORD

Lead in the environment and its effects on the health of people is a matter of great concern to the Agency for Toxic Substances and Disease Registry (ATSDR). The Agency was established by the Comprehensive Environmental Response, Compensation, and Liability Act of 1980 (CERCLA, also known as Superfund) to assess the public health impact of hazardous wastes in the general environment, to identify human populations at risk, and to effect actions to prevent adverse health effects from human contact with hazardous substances. The Agency's emphasis is on hazardous substances released from waste sites and substances released under emergency conditions (e.g., chemical spills). Lead left in the environment as hazardous waste is a matter of great public health concern to ATSDR.

ATSDR's concern about lead's toxicity derives from several factors. In a report to Congress, The Nature and Extent of Lead Poisoning in Children in the United States, published by ATSDR in July 1988, exposure to lead was identified as a serious public health problem, particularly for children. The report also identified six major environmental sources of lead, including leaded paint, gasoline, stationary sources, dust/soil, food, and water. For leaded paint, the number of potentially exposed children under 7 years of age in all housing with some lead paint at potentially toxic levels is about 12 million. An estimated 5.6 million children under 7 years old are potentially exposed to lead from gasoline at some level. The estimated number of children potentially exposed to U.S. stationary sources (e.g. smelters) is 230,000 children. The range of children potentially exposed to lead in dust and soil is estimated at 5.9 million to 11.7 million children. Some actual exposure to lead occurs for an estimated 3.8 million children whose drinking water lead level has been estimated at greater than 20 mcg/dl.

CERCLA requires ATSDR and the Environmental Protection Agency (EPA) to jointly rank, in order of priority, hazardous substances found at sites on EPA's National Priorities List (NPL). The current list of prioritized hazardous substances numbers 275. The three criteria for ranking were frequency of occurrence at NPL sites, toxicity, and potential for human exposure. Lead is ranked as the number one priority hazardous substance. In view of this, exposure to lead in populations close to hazardous waste sites continues to be a public health issue of concern. ATSDR, in reaction to this concern, recently established a Lead Initiative to systematically review Superfund sites for which the Agency's Public Health Assessments indicate the presence of site-related lead contamination. The goal of this ATSDR initiative is to prevent lead toxicity in persons, especially young children, exposed to lead released from Superfund sites and facilities. For all sites on the NPL, lead occurred at 853 (66%) of the 1300 sites. Thirteen sites have been selected for in-depth follow-up in fiscal year 1992 by ATSDR scientists.

This report provides background information on the complex and interactive factors that environmental health scientists need to consider when evaluating the impact of lead-contaminated soil on public health. A definitive analysis of the impact on public health of lead-contaminated soil is limited often by a lack of information on human exposure factors and soil conditions. Each waste site, therefore, poses a unique challenge to the health assessor and each site should be assessed in terms of its own characteristics.

The development of action levels for lead in soil lies outside the scope of the present report. However, the health assessor will find the information in this report useful in characterizing the significance of exposure pathways and the importance of the physical and chemical properties of the lead compounds that may impact on persons' uptake of lead.

The correlation between lead-contaminated soil and blood lead (PbB) level continues to challenge investigators. Correlations cited in the literature are influenced in specific studies by many factors, including access to soil, behavior patterns (especially of children), presence of ground cover, seasonal variation of exposure conditions, particle size and composition of the lead compounds found at various sites and the exposure pathway. These complex factors explain in some instances discrepant findings that are reported in the literature.

The reader is cautioned that much research is ongoing to clarify relationships between lead in soil and the amount absorbed by humans. Therefore, the associations and mathematical relationships between soil lead concentrations and blood-lead levels cited in this paper should be understood as being what has been published in the scientific literature, but subject to change as newer information becomes available.

Barry L. Johnson, PhD
Assistant Surgeon General
Assistant Administrator

INTRODUCTION

The Agency for Toxic Substances and Disease Registry (ATSDR) is mandated by the Comprehensive Environmental Response, Compensation, and Liability Act of 1980 (CERCLA or Superfund), as amended by the Superfund Amendments and Reauthorization Act of 1986 (SARA), to perform public health assessments for all sites on the National Priorities List (NPL). Data from health assessments for the first 951 sites show that metals and volatile organic compounds were the contaminants most often detected, and these commonly migrated from disposal areas to groundwater. Metallic substances occurred at 564 (59%) of the 951 sites, with lead, chromium, arsenic, and cadmium being cited most frequently (Susten, 1990).

The purpose of this analysis paper is to examine the relationship between exposure to lead-contaminated soil and the resulting impact on public health. The analysis will provide background information to ATSDR staff and other environmental health scientists responsible for preparing ATSDR documents, such as health assessments, health consultations, and emergency responses.

Emphasis in the analysis is given to the public health aspects of soil lead contamination at field sites. The analysis includes a review of the following areas: populations at high risk, sources of lead exposure, extent of lead poisoning in children, soil characterization, environmental fate of lead, bioavailability of lead, health effects of lead poisoning, correlations of soil lead and blood lead (PbB) in children, soil lead standards and recommendations, public health impact of exposure to lead-contaminated soil, general principles and limitations in field evaluations, and community prevention activities.

The Centers for Disease Control (CDC) Lead Statement for Preventing Lead Poisoning in Young Children is highlighted and provides guidelines on blood lead levels and childhood lead poisoning prevention (CDC, 1991). Examples in the use of the EPA Uptake/Biokinetic Model (Version 0.5) for estimating PbB levels from multiple exposure pathways are included.

Data gaps, such as usage patterns and soil condition, that limit a definitive analysis on the impact of soil on public health are discussed to the extent that information is available. Therefore, the development of action levels for lead in soil lies outside the scope of this document. Interactive and complex factors associated with multiple exposure pathways for lead require a site-specific approach in order to develop meaningful action levels for lead in soil. Identification and discussion of soil remediation protocols are also not within the scope of this analysis.

POPULATIONS AT RISK

Preschool-age children and fetuses are usually the most vulnerable segments of the population for exposures to lead (ATSDR, 1988). This increased vulnerability results from a combination of factors including: (a) the developing nervous system of the fetus or neonate has increased susceptibility to the neurotoxic effects of lead; (b) young children are more likely to play in dirt and to place their hands and other objects in their mouths, thereby increasing the opportunity for soil ingestion (pica—the eating of dirt and other non-food items—is more likely to occur in children); (c) the efficiency of lead absorption from the gastrointestinal tract is greater in children than in adults; and (d) nutritional deficiencies of iron or calcium, which are prevalent in children, may facilitate lead absorption and exacerbate the toxic effects of lead.

Among children, those in the 2–3 year-old age bracket may be most at risk for exposure to lead-contaminated soil. Mahaffey et al. (1982) reported that children in this age group had the highest PbB concentrations. This is also the age group in which pica tendencies are most prevalent (ATSDR, 1988).

SOURCES OF LEAD EXPOSURE

Several major sources of lead exposure have been identified (ATSDR, 1988). Leaded paint continues to cause most of the severe lead poisoning in children in the United States. It has the highest concentration of lead per unit of weight and is the most widespread of the various sources, being found in approximately 21 million pre-1940 homes. Dust and soil lead—derived from flaking, weathering, and chalking paint—plus airborne lead fallout and waste disposal over the years, are the major proximate sources of potential childhood lead exposure. Lead in drinking water is intermediate but highly significant as an exposure source for both children and the fetuses of pregnant women. Food lead also contributes to exposure of children and fetuses.

Individuals may be exposed to lead through several sources. When evaluating a site, a health assessor should be aware of multiple sources of lead exposure and the additive nature of the risks. An important source of lead exposure in older homes is contact with interior or exterior surfaces that have been painted with lead-based paints. Some individuals may be exposed to lead from occupational or hobby sources or from other less-common sources, such as the use of lead-glazed pottery, stained glass-working, and target practice in poorly ventilated indoor firing ranges.

EXTENT OF LEAD POISONING IN CHILDREN

The 1988 Agency for Toxic Substances and Disease Registry (ATSDR) report on the extent of lead poisoning in the United States estimated that in the 1984 standard metropolitan statistical areas 2.4 million white and black children aged 6 months through 5 years had PbB levels above 15 µg/dl and 200,000 children above 25 µg/dl. This would correspond to approximately 3 million and 250,000, respectively, for all children 6 months through 5 years in the total U.S. population.

The actual number of children exposed to lead in dust and soil at concentrations adequate to elevate PbB levels cannot be estimated with the data now available. However, the number of children potentially exposed to lead in dust and soil can be stated as a range of potential exposures to the primary sources of lead in dust and soil, namely, paint lead and atmospheric lead fallout. This range is estimated at 5.9 to 11.7 million children (ATSDR, 1988).

SOIL CHARACTERIZATION

Soil is contaminated by lead from various sources (American Academy of Pediatrics, 1987). Lead particles are deposited in the soil from flaking lead paint, from incinerators (and similar sources), and from motor vehicles that use leaded gasoline. Waste disposal is also a factor. Urban environments in general have received higher depositions of lead from vehicular emissions than have rural areas.

In many lead-mining districts, the predominant form of lead is galena or lead sulfide. However, the mineral deposits in Leadville, Colorado, are unusual (Colorado Department of Health, 1990). In Leadville, the mineral forms of lead are predominantly cerusite (lead carbonate), anglesite (lead sulfate), and massicot (lead oxide).

Wide variations in soil lead levels have been reported, ranging from less than 100 ppm to well over 11,000 ppm (National Research Council, 1980). Natural levels of lead in surface soils are usually below 50 ppm (Chaney et al., 1984; Reagan and Silbergeld, 1989). Soils adjacent to houses with exterior lead-based paints may have lead levels of $> 10,000$ $\mu g/g$ (EPA 1986).

PARTICLE SIZE AND LEAD CONTENT OF HOUSE DUST

Que Hee et al. (1985) measured the lead content in samples of house dust categorized into fractions by particle size collected in Cincinnati, Ohio (Table 1). The Que Hee et al. study shows that lead concentration is generally independent of particle size and that the bulk of the dust particles are concentrated in the smaller size ranges. Note that 77% of the lead was present in particles smaller than 149 μm. This distribution of lead in small particles would maximize intestinal absorption.

Table 1. Normal House Dust by Particle Size and Lead Content (Que Hee et al., 1985, adapted by Steele et al., 1990)

Size range (μm)	Weight % of fractionated dust	Lead content μg Pg/g of dust fraction	% Lead in unfractionated dust
<44	18	1440	21
44–149	58	1180	56
149–177	4.5	1330	4.9
177–246	2.7	1040	2.3
246–392	6.1	1110	5.6
392–833	11	1090	9.6
Unfractionated Dust	100	1214±13[a]	100

[a]Standard deviation

ENVIRONMENTAL FATE OF LEAD

AIR

Lead particles are emitted from automobiles to the atmosphere as lead halides (e.g., PbBrCl) and as the double salts with ammonium halides (e.g., $2PbBrCl \cdot NH_4Cl$); lead particles are emitted from mines and smelters primarily in the form of $PbSO_4$, $PbO \cdot PbSO_4$, and PbS (EPA, 1986). In the atmosphere, lead exists primarily in the form of $PbSO_4$ and $PbCO_3$ (EPA, 1986). How the chemical composition of lead changes in dispersion is not clear.

WATER

Lead has a tendency to form compounds of low solubility with the major anions found in natural water (Table 2). In the natural environment, the divalent form (Pb2+) is the stable ionic species of lead. Hydroxide, carbonate, sulfide, and, more rarely, sulfate may act as solubility controls in precipitating lead from water. A significant fraction of lead carried by river water is expected to be in an undissolved form. This can consist of colloidal particles or larger undissolved particles of lead carbonate, lead oxide, lead hydroxide, or other lead compounds incorporated in other components of surface particulate matter from runoff. The ratio of lead in suspended solids to lead in dissolved form has been found to vary from 4:1 in rural streams to 27:1 in urban streams (EPA, 1986).

Table 2. Solubility of Lead and Lead Compounds (ATSDR, 1992)

Element/Compound	Solubility	
	Water	Organic solvents
Lead	Insoluble	Insoluble
Lead acetate	221 g/100 mL at 50°C	Soluble in glycerol, very slight in alc.
Lead chloride	0.99 g/100 mL at 20°C	Insoluble in alcohol
Lead chromate	0.2 mg/L	Insoluble in acetic acid
Lead nitrate	37.65–56.5 g/100 mL at 0°C	1 g in 2,500 mL absolute alcohol 1 g in 75 mL absolute methanol
Lead oxide	0.001 g/100 cc at 20°C (Litharge)	Soluble in alkali chlorides
	0.0023 g/100 cc at 23°C (Massicot)	Soluble in alkali (Massicot)
Lead sulfate	42.5 mg/L at 25°C	Insoluble in alcohol

SOIL

Paint is a major contributor to soil lead contamination. Remediation of exterior lead-based paint hazards is critical if further contamination is to be avoided (Binder and Matte, 1992). The accumulation of lead in soil is primarily a function of the rate of deposition from the atmosphere. The fate of lead in soil is affected by the specific or exchange adsorption at mineral interfaces, the precipitation of sparingly soluble solid phases, and the formation of relatively stable organo-metal complexes or chelates with the organic matter in soil (EPA, 1986; NSF, 1977).

Evidence exists that atmospheric lead enters the soil as lead sulfate or is converted rapidly to lead sulfate at the soil surface. Lead sulfate is relatively soluble, and thus could leach through the soil if it were not transformed. In soils with pH of > or = 5 and with at least 5% organic matter, atmospheric lead is retained in the upper 2–5 cm of undisturbed soil (EPA, 1986).

Lead may mobilize from soil when lead-bearing soil particles run off to surface waters during heavy rains. Lead may also mobilize from soil to atmosphere by downwind transport of smaller lead-containing soil particles entrained in the prevailing wind (NSF, 1977). This latter process may be important in contributing to the atmospheric burden of lead around some lead-smelting and Superfund sites that contain elevated levels of lead in soil.

The downward movement of lead from soil by leaching is very slow under most natural conditions (NSF, 1977). The conditions that induce leaching are the presence of lead in soil at concentrations that either approach or exceed the sorption capacity of the soil, the presence in the soil of materials that are capable of forming soluble chelates with lead, and a decrease in the pH of the leaching solution (e.g., acid rain) (NSF, 1977). Partial favorable conditions for leaching may be present in some soils near lead-smelting and NPL sites that contain elevated levels of lead in soil.

BIOAVAILABILTY OF LEAD

Barltrop and Meek (1975) examined the absorption in rats of 12 different lead compounds following oral exposure, including solids and oily, viscous liquids, compared with lead acetate absorption. The kidney contents of lead were calculated as percentages of the relevant lead acetate values (Table 3). The absorption of metallic lead (particle size 180–250 μm) was lower than the absorption of lead salts (particle size < 50 μm). Lead carbonate had the highest absorption, which, the authors suggest, may reflect the greater solubility of this compound in gastric juice.

Table 3. Absorption by Rat Kidney of Lead Additives Compared with Lead Acetate (Barltrop and Meek, 1975)

Lead compound	Percent absorption compared with lead acetate
Control (no lead)	4
Metallic lead (particle size 180–250 μm)	14
Lead chromate	44
Lead octoate	62
Lead naphthenate	64
Lead sulfide	67
Lead tallate	121
Lead carbonate (basic)	164

A key factor in the solubility of lead is the pH of the fluid. Healy et al. (1982) measured the solubility of lead sulfide (particle size approximately 90 μm) in several fluids, including water, saliva, and gastric juice. The lead was relatively insoluble in water and saliva, but was 800 times more soluble in simulated gastric juice. Day et al. (1979) measured the solubility (extractability) in hydrochloric acid of lead from street dust collected in two industrial cities. The authors assumed that the lead compounds were primarily oxides and halides emitted from automobiles.

Under environmental conditions, these compounds can be converted to carbonates and sulfates. Less than 10% of the lead was extracted at pH 4 and higher; more than 80% was extracted at pH 1, the nominal pH of gastric juice. The significance of these findings is not clear because the temperature of extraction did not correspond to physiological conditions (37°C) and hydrochloric acid is a simplistic simulation of gastric juice. Other studies have supported the higher degree of solubilization at a pH about 1 of lead from street dust samples (Duggan and Williams, 1977; Harrison, 1979).

METABOLIC INTERACTIONS OF LEAD WITH NUTRIENTS

Mahaffey and co-workers (1976) reported that children with elevated PbB had lower dietary intakes of calcium and phosphorus than did a reference population. Heard and Chamberlain (1982) reported similar findings. Several studies have shown a strong inverse correlation between iron status and PbB (Chisolm, 1981; Yip et al., 1981; Watson et al., 1980). Zinc deficiency can also enhance lead absorption (Markowitz and Rosen, 1981).

The main conclusion to be drawn from studies of lead-nutrient interactions is that defects in nutrition will enhance lead absorption and retention and thus the toxicity risk. This problem is amplified when nutrient deficiencies are commonplace and lead exposure is highest, that is, in 2-to 4-year-old, underdeveloped children (ATSDR, 1988).

Improving the nutritional status of children who have a high risk of exposure and toxicity greatly increases the effectiveness of environmental lead abatement. However, nutritional supplement (calcium) only increases the lead level required for toxicity rather that eliminating lead uptake and its effects (Mahaffey, 1982).

The levels of phosphorus, which indicate Vitamin D levels, suggest that most poor children's intake of this vitamin is adequate (ATSDR, 1988). Vitamin D enhances lead uptake in the gut, but its intake is essential to health and cannot be reduced (ATSDR, 1988).

HEALTH EFFECTS OF LEAD EXPOSURE

Studies on the effects of lead in children have demonstrated a relationship between exposure to lead and a variety of adverse health effects. These effects include impaired mental and physical development, decreased heme biosynthesis, elevated hearing threshold, and decreased serum levels of vitamin D (Figure 1). The neurotoxicity of lead is of particular concern, because evidence from prospective longitudinal studies has shown that neurobehavioral effects, such as impaired academic performance and deficits in motor skills, may persist even after PbB levels have returned to normal (Needleman, 1990).

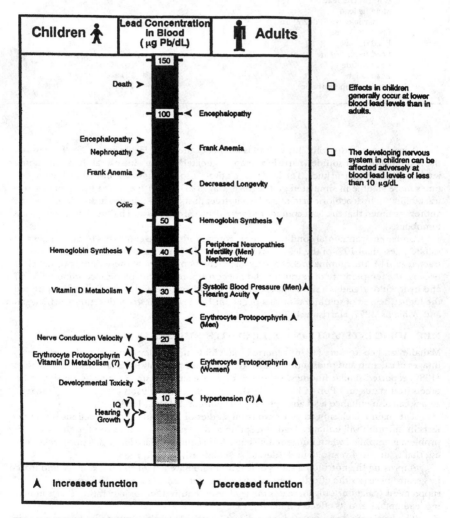

Figure 1. Effects of inorganic lead on children and adults—lowest observable adverse effects levels (adapted from case studies in Environmental medicine: lead toxicity, 1990, ATSDR).

Although no threshold level for these effects has been established, the available evidence suggests that lead toxicity may occur at PbB levels of 10–15 µg/dl or possibly less (ATSDR 1988).

Additional information on lead toxicity is contained in The Nature and Extent of Lead Poisoning in Children in the United States: A Report to Congress (ATSDR, 1988) and the ATSDR Toxicological Profile for Lead (ATSDR, 1992).

CORRELATIONS OF SOIL LEAD AND BLOOD LEAD IN CHILDREN

Every community and every study reflects a different range of soil lead concentrations and blood lead levels. Several comprehensive reviews have examined the quantitative relationship between exposure to lead-contaminated soil and PbB levels in children. This result is commonly expressed in the literature as a dose-response relationship and reflects a change in PbB levels with the change in soil lead concentrations (assuming a linear relationship between the two) scaled to a standard unit of soil lead concentration (either 1,000 µg/g or 100 µg/g) (Reagan and Silbergeld, 1989).

Duggan (1980), Duggin and Inskip (1985)

Duggan compiled data from published studies that reported a quantitative correlation between PbB concentrations and lead concentrations in soil or dust (Duggan, 1980; Duggin and Inskip, 1985). Duggan included data from sites with diverse sources of lead contamination (e.g., lead mining, smelting, lead paint, automobile exhaust emissions). The data indicated that the increase in PbB levels associated with exposures to lead in soil varied between 0.6 and 65 µg lead/dl blood per 1000 ppm lead in soil. As an average value, Duggan suggested that exposure to soil containing 1000 ppm of lead could increase the PbB level by 5 µg/dl. No value for an acceptable concentration of lead in soil was offered because such a value would depend on what constitutes an acceptable increase in the PbB concentration.

ATSDR (1988)

In the ATSDR document, The Nature and Extent of Lead Poisoning in Children in the United States: A Report to Congress, it was noted that several investigations have shown a highly significant correlation between PbB levels and lead concentrations in dust and soil. Several references were cited that describe quantitative relationships between PbB levels and soil or dust lead levels. The report concluded, "In general, lead in dust and soil at levels of 500 to 1,000 ppm begins to affect children's PbB levels."

Madhaven et al. (1989)

Madhaven et al. (1989) used the data compiled by Duggan (1980) to derive a "safe" or permissible level of lead in soil. The authors based their analysis on 8 of Duggan's 21 slope estimates for PbB vs. soil lead. Madhaven et al. selected those studies for which soil was believed to be the only source of lead and for which the susceptible population were children under 12 years of age. The geometric mean of the 8 studies was 3.41 μg lead/dl blood per 1000 ppm lead in soil, and the 95 percentile upper confidence interval was 8.59 μg/dl per 1000 ppm. The authors proposed permissible levels of lead in soil ranging from 250 to 1000 ppm depending on site conditions. The 250 ppm value applies to a worst-case scenario in which children below 5 years of age repeatedly used an area without grass cover and mouthed objects frequently. In this situation, a soil lead concentration of 250 ppm would add, at most, an estimated 2 μg/dl to the PbB level of children.

Reagan and Silbergeld (1989)

Recently Reagan and Silbergeld (1989) summarized the findings of several studies dealing with observed relationships between environmental lead concentrations and body lead burdens in young children (Table 4).

Table 4. Dose Response Relationships Between Soil Pb Concentrations and Blood Pb Levels (Reagan and Silbergeld, 1989)

	Dose response relationships[a]	
Study[b]	Change in blood Pb per 1000 μg/g soil lead	Change in blood Pb per 100 μg/g soil lead
Urban communities		
Angle and McIntire (1982)	15.5*	1.6
Brunekreef et al. (1983)	11.3*	1.1
Stark et al. (1982)	10.2*	1.0
Davies et al. (1987)	10.0	1.0
Haan (personal communication)	10.0	1.0
Madhaven et al. (1989)	9.0	.9
Reeves et al. (1982)	8.1*	0.8
Rabinowitz et al. (1985)	8.0	.8
Bornschein (1986)	6.2	0.6
Shellshear et al. (1975)	3.9	0.4
Lead industries communities		
Brunekreef et al. (1981)	12.6*	1.3
Landrigan et al. (1975)	11.7*	1.2
Neri et al. (1978)	11.2*	1.1
Yankel et al. (1977)	7.3*	0.7
Roberts et al. (1974)	5.3*	0.5
Galke et al. (1975)	4.9*	0.5
Mining communities		
Gallacher et al. (1974)	4.1	0.4
Barltrop et al. (1974)	0.6*	0.1
Review articles		
Brunekreef et al. (1986)	5–10	0.5–1.0
AAP (1987)	5–10	1.0–2.0[c]
Duggan (1980, 1983)	5	0.5
EPA (1986a)	2	0.2

[a]This table reflects unadjusted values (calculated by Brunekreef (1986) and noted by an * and values in other studies calculated by the authors of the study.

[b]See Reagan and Silbergeld (1989) for full citations for these references.

[c]Covering the range of 500–1,000 μg g^{-1} only.

Reagan and Silbergeld (1989) analyzed the review articles by Brunekreef (1986), American Academy of Pediatrics (AAP) (1987), Duggan (1980), Duggin and Inskip (1985), and EPA (1986) and reported several limitations in the articles. In the Brunekreef review, most studies reviewed "do not permit straightforward calculation of (a dose-response relationship) which are properly adjusted for relevant confounders." Nevertheless, Brunekreef concluded that the dose-response relationship was in the 5.0–10.0 ($\mu g/dl$ per 1,000 $\mu g/g$) range for lead in soil, house dust, street dust, and playground dust. After reviewing several studies Duggan also concluded that the dose-response relationship of PbB to soil lead concentration is 5 $\mu g/dl$ per 1000 $\mu g/g$ which is very close to his theoretical calculation of 7 $\mu g/dl$ per 1,000 $\mu g/g$. Brunekreef criticized Duggan's review because he relied heavily on studies in which one or more pathways were excluded and used adjusted instead of unadjusted values in some studies.

The review by the AAP notes that for each increase of 100 $\mu g/g$ in the lead content of surface soil above a level of 500 $\mu g/g$ a mean increase of 1 to 2 $\mu g/dl$ occurs in children's whole PbB (AAP 1987). No explanation was given in the AAP study for starting the slope at a soil lead value of 500 $\mu g/g$. Reagan and Silbergeld (1989) also criticized the EPA review for selecting only two studies (Stark et al., 1982; Angle and McIntire, 1982), which EPA believed provided good data for the slope estimates (2.2 $\mu g/dl$ and 6.8 $\mu g/dl$) and then selecting the lowest one as a "median estimate" without explaining why this selection technique is appropriate. Brunekreef also criticized the EPA conclusion because EPA mixed adjusted and unadjusted values and because use of an adjusted value in the Stark study was inappropriate.

The dose-response relationship differs between urban and industrial communities and lead-mining communities, with lead-mining communities having a shallower slope (Reagan and Silbergeld, 1989). This difference is probably due to a difference in the bioavailability of lead. Particle size and metal species are also thought to be major factors (Colorado Department of Health, 1990). However, differences in modulating factors (such as nutrition) may also have been important in these studies.

With regard to particle size, leaded gasoline, which is the predominant source of lead in urban communities, and industrial point sources emit small particles, whereas mines and tailing piles release relatively large particles, primarily as fugitive dusts (EPA, 1986). Smaller particles may be inhaled and ingested, increasing total exposure. Smaller particles are easily transferred to the hands and tend to remain on the hands longer, thereby increasing the potential for ingestion.

With respect to metal species, Steele et al. (1990) noted that the impact of lead in soil derived from mine waste (usually in the form of PbS) on blood lead is less than that for lead in soil derived from smelter, vehicle, or point sources. However, in an animal study, tailing material from Midvale, Utah, was found to be more available to young pigs than was reagent grade PbS when presented as a single large dose by intubation (LaVelle et al., 1991). This study does not lend support to the Steele finding.

Environmental Protection Agency (1990)

The U.S. Environmental Protection Agency (EPA) recently developed an Integrated Uptake/Biokinetic (IU/BK) model that examines the relationship between environmental exposure to lead and PbB levels. This model is not used to set clean-up standards per se. Rather, it allows the health assessor to make site-specific calculations for children 6 yrs of age and under for PbB levels resulting from exposures to lead in soil, dust, air, water, and the diet. Several assumptions and default exposure variables are built into the model for use when these parameters are not known. The model is still being validated by the EPA.

SOIL LEAD STANDARDS AND RECOMMENDATIONS

Many governments have promulgated soil lead standards or issued guidelines for lead in soil (Table 5).

Table 5. Soil Lead Standards for Residential Land Use (Adapted from Reagan and Silbergeld, 1989)

Location	Residential
U.S. (2–4)	500[a]
Minnesota (4, 5)	500[b]
OME, Canada (2, 6)	375[c]
	500[d]
Netherlands (9)	50[f]
	150[g]
	600[h]
England (8, 10)	500[i]
London (11)	500[j]

[a]600 μg g^{-1} repealed, changed to leachate standard, interim 500 μg g^{-1} guideline

[b]proposed emergency rule, interim 1,000 μg g^{-1} standard

[c]sandy soil

[d]non-sandy soil

[f]reference value

[g]further investigation

[h]clean up value

[i]redevelopment of industrial lands

[j]dust standard

Sources cited (see Reagan and Silbergeld, 1989, for full citations): (2) Rinne et al. (1986); (3) Office of Solid Waste and Emergency Response) (OSWER) (1989); (4) personal communication; (5) Minnesota Hazardous Waste Regulations; (6) Ontario Ministry of the Environment (OME) (1986); (8) Davies and Wixson (1986); (9) Assink and Vanderbrink (1986); (10) Department of the Environment (DOE, UK, 1987); (11) Wilson (1983).

Researchers have also calculated "acceptable" levels of lead in soil or dust (Table 6). Reagan and Silbergeld (1989) also noted an order of magnitude difference in the recommendations offered in the literature. The standards reflect four basic arguments to justify or advocate a specific lead limitation.

Table 6. Soil Lead Standard Recommendations (Adapted from Reagan and Silbergeld, 1989)

Author(s)	Standard (ppm)	Comments
Shellshear et al. (1975)	<100	Protect pica children
Mielke et al. (1989)	<150	Prevent lead toxicity (10 µg dl^{-1})
Chaney et al. (1986, 1989)	<150	Protect pica children
Duggan and Williams (1977)	300	Keep ADI <50 µg Pb Day^{-1} (street dust standard)
Boucier et al. (1985)	300	Keep blood lead below 25 µg dl^{-1}
Simms and Becket (1987)	500	Keep blood lead below 25 µg dl^{-1}
Madhaven et al. (1989)	600	Permit an increase in blood lead of 5 µg dl^{-1} above existing levels
	250	Protect children where there is no grass cover
Steenhout (1987)	900	Based upon an ADI of 200 µg Pb day^{-1}
Laxen et al. (1987)	1000	Allows dust to contribute 2.5–3.0 µg dl^{-1} (house dust)

1. To protect pica children, a lead soil standard should be below 100 µg/g (Shellshear et al. (1975)) or 150 µg/g, (Chaney et al. (1986, 1989)).
2. To keep PbB levels below 25 µg/dl a standard of 300 (Bourcier et al. (1985)) and 500 µg/g (Simms and Becket (1987)) is needed. Mielke et al. (1989) also argue that to keep PbB levels below 10 µg/dl the standard should be less than 150 µg/g.
3. Based on an Acceptable Daily Intake (ADI) of 50 and 200 µg Pb/day, respectively, soil levels of 300 (Duggan and Williams (1977)) and 900 µg/g (Steenhout (1987)) are recommended.
4. Laxen et al. (1987) and Madhaven et al. (1989) argue for a standard that would allow PbB levels to increase by 3–5 µg/dl over and above existing PbB levels. Madhaven et al. also argue that children exposed to lead at 250 µg/g in bare soils could have increased PbB levels of 2 µg/dl.

Reagan and Silbergeld (1989) have normalized the recommendations noted in the previous table (Table 7). They assumed a linear relationship and that all the lead comes from soil and dust. In recommending a soil lead standard, Reagan and Silbergeld argue that (a) no one should have a PbB level greater than 10 µg/dl; (b) pica children should be protected; (c) soil and dust lead exposure should not be allowed to increase PbB levels; and (d) (indirectly) the total allowable daily intake (ADI) of lead should not exceed 25 µg.

Reagan and Silbergeld (1989) caution that the "normalized" values reflect the assumption that all allowable lead came from soil or dust. A further downward revision should be made to allow for other sources that contribute to total body lead burden for all populations. The Laxen et al. value, Reagan and Silbergeld point out, was not adjusted for age (he examined 10–12-year-old children, instead of the high-risk, 2–4-year-old children).

Table 7. Normalized Soil Lead Standard Recommendations (Reagan and Silbergeld, 1989)

Author(s)	Recommended standard (ppm)	Normalized (ppm)
Shellshear et al. (1975)	<100	<100
Mielke et al. (1989)	<150	<150
Chaney et al. (1986, 1989)	<150	<150
Duggan and Williams (1977)	300	150
Bourcier et al. (1985)	300	120
Simms and Becket (1987)	500	200
Madhaven et al. (1989)	600	120
	250	50
Steenhout (1987)	900	112
Laxen et al. (1987)	1,000	333

Finally, Reagan and Silbergeld argue "that the literature as a whole supports a low soil lead standard of 100 µg/g or so."

In proposing this standard, Reagan and Silbergeld (1989) also proposed that the standard:

1. Be limited to residential areas;
2. Be a bare soil standard, if and only if, the community can guarantee adequate ground cover, essentially forever;
3. Be based on a soil survey;
4. Be applicable to property based on sample type;
5. Be enforceable;
6. Include a soil replacement standard;
7. Take into account soil type (i.e., the standard should be lower for sandy soil or soils having a low content of organic matter).

PUBLIC HEALTH IMPACT OF EXPOSURE TO LEAD-CONTAMINATED SOIL

A strong positive correlation is found between exposure to lead-contaminated soils and PbB levels. Generally, PbB levels rise 3–7 µg/dl for every 1000-ppm increase in soil or dust lead concentrations (CDC, 1991). This range reflects different sources of lead, different exposure conditions, and different exposed populations.

At all sites, ATSDR recommends that health assessors evaluate the need for any follow-up health activities. This effort should be coordinated with other health agencies, as appropriate, to ensure that all aspects of a site that impact the health of the community are evaluated. Environmental health scientists will find the recent statement by CDC, Preventing Lead Poisoning in Young Children, a very useful resource (CDC, 1991).

Ideally, to determine the public health impact of environmental lead contamination at a site, a biomarker of lead exposure in the exposed population should be available. The most commonly used biomarkers of lead exposure are the PbB concentration and the blood erythrocyte protoporphyrin (EP) concentration. Although blood EP levels are commonly used in lead screening programs, the EP test has poor sensitivity and specificity below a PbB level of 25 µg/dl (CDC, 1991). Therefore, PbB concentration is a more sensitive indicator of low-level lead exposures. CDC recommends PbB concentration as the screening test of choice (CDC, 1991).

To assess the potential for lead toxicity at a site, the health assessor should first examine the available PbB data. CDC has reported guidelines for interpreting PbB test results in children and recommendations for follow-up activities (Table 8). If PbB levels are elevated, exposure to lead-contaminated soil may not be the only source for the increased blood level. Other lead sources—such as lead from food, water, or air—could be partially or primarily responsible for the elevated PbB. These other potential exposure pathways should be thoroughly evaluated.

Table 8. Interpretation of Blood Lead Test Results and Follow-up Activities: Class of Child Based on Blood Lead Concentration

Class	Blood lead concentration (µg/dl)	Comment
I	≤9	A child in Class I is not considered to be lead-poisoned.
IIA	10–14	Many children (or a large proportion of children) with blood lead levels in this range should trigger community-wide childhood lead poisoning prevention activities. Children in this range need to be screened more frequently.
IIB	15–19	A child in Class IIB should receive nutritional and educational interventions and more frequent screening. If the blood lead levels persist in this range, environmental investigation and intervention should be done.
III	20–44	A child in Class III should receive environmental evaluation and remediation and a medical evaluation. Such a child may need pharmacologic treatment of lead poisoning.
IV	45–69	A child in Class IV will need both medical and environmental interventions, including chelation therapy.
V	≥70	A child with Class V lead poisoning is a **medical emergency.** Medical and environmental management must begin **immediately.**

(Adapted from CDC, *Preventing Lead Poisoning in Young Children.* A Statement by the Centers for Disease Control, October 1991. U.S. Department of Health and Human Services/Public Health Service.)

Even if PbB levels are not elevated, the site should not be dismissed as posing no potential public health hazard. Potential seasonal variation of exposure conditions; the half-life of lead in the blood stream; and limitations of any screening methods used, especially study design (power and representativeness of blood and soil samples), should be evaluated. If conditions at a site change dramatically, retesting exposed individuals may be necessary to determine the impact of altered conditions on PbB levels. Commonplace changes may also be significant in altering PbB levels.

The results of occupational studies indicate that increased exposures to lead are followed by elevations in PbB levels, which reach a new level in 60–120 days (Tola et al., 1973). Also, PbB levels may be higher in children during the summer months presumably as the result of increased opportunity for exposures through outdoor play.

The biologic fate of inorganic lead in the human body is well known. Inorganic lead is not metabolized but is directly absorbed, distributed, and excreted. Once in the blood, lead is distributed primarily among three compartments—blood, soft tissue (kidney, bone marrow, liver, and brain), and mineralizing tissue (bones and teeth). Mineralizing tissue contains about 95% of the total body burden of lead in adults (ATSDR, 1990).

In blood, 99% of the lead is associated with erythrocytes; the remaining 1% is in the plasma and is available for transport to the tissues. In single-exposure studies with adults, lead has a half-life in blood of approximately 25 days; in soft tissue, about 40 days; and in the non-labile portion of bone, more than 25 years. In bone there is both a labile component, which readily exchanges lead with the blood, and an inert pool. Lead in the inert pool poses a special risk because it is a potential endogenous source of lead. Because of these mobile lead stores, a person's PbB level can take several months or sometimes years to drop significantly, even after complete removal from the source of lead exposure (ATSDR, 1990).

In Leadville, Colorado, the Colorado Department of Health examined the impact of residential soil lead contamination on the PbB levels of children (Colorado Department of Health, 1990). Lead smelting operations in the area ended in 1961, and, at the time of the study in 1987, only one lead and zinc mine was still operating. An increase in soil lead concentration from 100 to 1100 ppm was associated with an estimated increase of 3.9 µg/dl in the PbB concentration.

The results of several studies have indicated that the increase in PbB concentration as a function of soil lead concentration is not linear. That is, at higher lead concentrations in soil, the rate of increase in PbB levels falls off. Using data from exposure studies conducted at Helena Valley in Montana and Silver Valley in Idaho, Schilling and Bain (1989) derived the following linear regression model for the correlation between PbB levels and soil lead levels:

$$ln(blood\ lead\ level) = 0.879 + 0.241\ ln(soil\ lead\ level)$$

Using this equation, an increase in soil lead from 100 ppm to 1100 ppm would increase the predicted PbB level from 7.3 µg/dl to 13.0 µg/dl, an increase of 5.7 µg/dl. A further increase in soil lead to 2100 ppm would increase the estimated PbB level to only 15.2 µg/dl.

The non-linearity of the dose-response curve for blood lead vs. soil lead is not unique to soil lead exposures. The rate of increase in PbB levels has also been observed to decrease upon exposure to high concentrations of lead in air or drinking water (Hammond, 1982).

Under the Superfund Amendments and Reauthorization Act of 1986, EPA (1991) initiated a "pilot program for the removal, decontamination, or other actions with respect to lead-contaminated soil in one to three metropolitan areas." One study, the Three City Urban Soil-Lead Demonstration Project, was designed to investigate whether the use of low-technology abatement methods to reduce environmental lead concentrations (soil, dust) would result in decreased PbB levels in children. Findings from this study are expected in the summer of 1992. It is possible that the impact of contaminated soil, like that of paint, is highly dependent on condition and usage patterns. This issue has not been adequately evaluated (Binder and Matte, 1992).

GENERAL PRINCIPLES AND LIMITATIONS IN FIELD EVALUATIONS

SCREENING TESTS

The erythrocyte protoporphyrin level is not sensitive enough to identify children with elevated PbB levels below about 25 µg/dl. The screening test of choice is now PbB measurement (CDC, 1991).

DOSE-RESPONSE CURVE

When assessing the public health impact of environmental lead contamination, the lower portion of the dose-response curve for PbB vs. soil lead should be used. This portion of the curve has the steepest slope, and it corresponds to conditions in which the impact on PbB is the greatest.

PbB levels generally rise 3–7 µg/dl for every 1,000-ppm increase in soil or dust lead concentrations (CDC, 1991). Access to soil, behavior patterns, presence of ground cover, seasonal variation of exposure conditions, and other factors may influence this relationship.

SAMPLE SIZE

Caution should be used in drawing conclusions when only one or a few soil samples from a site have been analyzed. Depending on the uniformity of lead distribution at a site, a single soil sample may significantly overestimate or underestimate the average lead concentration at a site.

SURFACE SOIL

Because lead is immobilized by the organic component of soil, lead deposited from the air is generally retained in the upper 2–5 centimeters of undisturbed soil (EPA, 1986). Urban soils and other soils that are disturbed or turned under may be contaminated down to far greater depths. Opportunity for exposure is much greater to surface soil than to subsurface soils.

Evidence for the non-uniformity of lead distribution in urban soils was demonstrated in a study that examined soil lead concentrations in urban Baltimore gardens (Chaney, 1984). Soil lead concentrations varied more than 10-fold within a single garden.

CHEMICAL FORM OF LEAD

The impact of exposure to lead-contaminated soil on PbB levels is also influenced by the chemical and physical form of the lead. Data from animal feeding studies suggest that the oral bioavailability of lead sulfide and lead chromate is significantly less than the bioavailability of other lead salts (oxide, acetate) (Barltrop and Meek, 1975).

PARTICLE SIZE

Increasing the particulate size also reduces the bioavailability of lead in the gastrointestinal tract. In animal feeding studies, decreasing the lead particulate size from 197 microns to 6 microns resulted in a 5-fold enhancement in absorption (Barltrop and Meek, 1979). The lead content of soil and dust has also been demonstrated to vary dramatically as a function of particle size (Duggan and Inskip, 1985). Several studies have reported that the lead content of soil, street dust, city dust, and house dust increases as the particle size decreases.

LEAD-MINING SITES

The results of studies at lead-mining sites have indicated that soil lead contamination from mine tailings may be less effective in increasing PbB levels than is lead contamination derived from urban lead pollution (paint, gasoline) or atmospheric lead fallout from lead smelting operations (Steele et al., 1990). However, an animal study by LaVelle et al. (1991) on the bioavailability of lead in mining wastes following oral intubation in young swine does not support these findings.

The reduced bioavailability of lead from mine tailings may be related to its chemical form (lead sulfide) and its larger particulate size. Evaluations of mining sites require analyses of these physical-chemical parameters.

COMMUNITY PREVENTION ACTIVITIES

Pathways of Exposure

Soil and dust act as pathways to children for lead deposited by primary lead sources such as lead paint, leaded gasoline, and industrial or occupational sources of lead (CDC, 1991).

Because lead does not dissipate, biodegrade, or decay, the lead deposited into dust and soil becomes a long-term source of lead exposure for children. For example, although lead emissions from gasoline have largely been eliminated, an estimated 4–5 million metric tons of lead previously used in gasoline remain in dust and soil, and children continue to be exposed to it (ATSDR 1988).

Prevention Activities

Community prevention activities should be triggered by PbB levels > or = 10 µg/dl, as recommended by the Centers for Disease Control (Table 8) (CDC, 1991). For community-level intervention to be successful at least five types of activities are necessary (CDC, 1991).

1. Screening and surveillance—determining populations at risk and the locations of the worst exposures;
2. Risk assessment and integrated prevention planning—analyzing all available data to assess sources of lead, exposure patterns, and high-risk populations; developing prevention plans;
3. Outreach and education—informing health-care providers, parents, property owners, and other key people about lead poisoning prevention;
4. Infrastructure development—finding the resources needed for a successful program of risk reduction;
5. Hazard reduction—reducing the hazards of lead-based paint and lead in dust and soil, particularly in high-risk buildings and neighborhoods.

Soil Lead Abatement

Soil lead abatement may consist of either establishing an effective barrier between children and the soil or the removal and replacement of at least the top few centimeters of soil.

SUMMARY

The health assessor should use caution in drawing conclusions when only one or a few soil samples from a site have been analyzed. Depending on the uniformity of lead distribution at a site, a single soil sample may significantly overestimate or underestimate the average lead concentration at a site. The impact of exposure to lead-contaminated soil on PbB levels is also influenced by the chemical and physical form of the lead.

At all sites, ATSDR recommends that health assessors evaluate the need for any follow-up health activities. This effort should be coordinated with other health agencies, as appropriate, to ensure that all aspects of a site that impact the health of the community are evaluated. The recent statement by the CDC, Preventing Lead Poisoning in Young Children, provides guidance and identifies community prevention activities that should be triggered by PbB levels > or = 10 µg/dl.

REFERENCES

American Academy of Pediatrics (AAP) (1987) (Committee on Environmental Hazards and Committee on Accident and Poison Prevention of the American Academy of Pediatrics). Statement on childhood lead poisoning. Pediatrics 1987;79:457–465.
Agency for Toxic Substances and Disease Registry (ATSDR) (1988). The nature and extent of lead poisoning in children in the United States: A report to Congress, July 1988.
Agency for Toxic Substances and disease Registry (ATSDR) (1990). Case studies in environmental medicine: Lead toxicity.
Agency for Toxic Substances and Disease Registry (ATSDR) (1992). Toxicological profile for lead. ATSDR/TP-88/17.
Barltrop D, Meek F. (1975). Absorption of different lead compounds. Postgrad Med J 1975;51:805–809.
Barltrop D, Meek F. (1979). Effect of particle size on lead absorption from the gut. Arch Environ Health 1979;34:280–285.
Binder S, Matte T. (1992). Personal Communication. Review of soil lead levels. May 8, 1992.
Centers for Disease Control (CDC), (1991). Preventing lead poisoning in young children, October 1991.

Chaney RL, et al. (1984). The potential for heavy metal exposure from urban gardens and soils, pages 37–84. In: Preer JR, ed. Proceedings of the symposium on heavy metals in urban gardens. Agricultural Experiment Station, University of the District of Columbia, Washington, DC.

Chisolm JJ Jr. (1981). Dose effect relationship for lead in young children; evidence in children for interactions among lead, zinc, and iron. (Cited in ATSDR 1988)

Colorado Department of Health, (1990). University of Colorado at Denver, Agency for Toxic Substances and Disease Registry, Leadville Metals Exposure Study, April 1990.

Day JP, et al. (1979). Solubility and potential toxicity of lead in urban street dust. Bull Environ Contam Toxicol 1979;23:497–502.

Duggan MJ, Williams S. (1977). Lead in dust in city streets. Sci Total Environ 1977;7:91–7.

Duggan MJ. (1980). Lead in urban dust: an assessment. Water, Air, Soil Pollution 1980;14:309–321.

Duggan MJ, Inskip MJ. (1985). Childhood exposure to lead in surface dust and soil: a community problem. Public Health Rev 1985;13:1–54.

EPA (Environmental Protection Agency) (1986). Air quality criteria for lead, June 1986 and Addendum, September 1986. Research Triangle Park, NC: EPA 600/8–83-018F.

EPA (Environmental Protection Agency) (1990). Uptake/biokinetic model for lead, Version 0.50 (December 1990).

EPA (Environmental Protection Agency) (1991). Three city urban soil-lead demonstration project, midterm project update.

Hammond PB. (1982). Inorganic lead in man's environment: sources and toxicological significance. J Appl Toxicol 1982;2(2):68–74.

Harrison RM. (1979). Toxic metals in street and household dusts. Sci Total Environ 1979;11:81–97.

Healy M, et al. (1982). Lead sulfide and traditional preparations: Routes for ingestion and solubility and reactions in gastric fluid. J Clin Hosp Pharm 1982;7:169–173.

Heard MJ, Chamberlain AC (1982). Effect of minerals and food on uptake of lead from the gastrointestinal track in humans. Hum Toxicol 1982;1:411–415.

LaVelle MJ, et al. (1991). Bioavailability of lead in mining wastes: an oral intubation study in young swine (submitted for publication).

Madhaven S, et al. (1989). Lead in soil: Recommended maximum permissible levels. Environ Res 1989; 49:136–142.

Mahaffey KR, et al. (1976). Difference in dietary intake of calcium, phosphorus, and iron of children having normal and elevated blood lead concentrations. J Nutr 1976;7:106. (Cited in ATSDR 1988.)

Mahaffey KR, et al. (1982). National estimates of blood lead levels: United States, 1976–1980. N Engl J Med 1982;307(10):573–579.

Markowitz ME, Rosen JF. (1981). Zinc (zn) and copper (Cu) metabolism in CaNa2 EDTA-treated children with plumbism. Pediatr Res 1981;15:635. (Cited in ATSDR 1988.)

National Research Council (1980). Lead in the human environment. Washington, DC: National Academy of Sciences.

Needleman HL, et al. (1990). The long-term effects of exposure to low doses of lead in childhood: an 11-year follow-up report. N Engl J Med 1990;322(2):83–88.

NSF (National Science Foundation) (1977). Lead in the environment. NSF/RA-770214. Bogess WR, ed. Washington, DC: NSF (cited in EPA 1986a).

Que Hee SS, et al. (1985). Evolution of efficient methods to sample lead sources, such as house dust and hand dust, in the homes of children. Environ Res 1985;38:77–95.

Reagan PL, Silbergeld EK. (1989). Establishing a health based standard for lead in residential soils. In: Hemphill and Cothern, eds. Trace substances in environmental health. Supplement to Volume 12 (1990) of Environmental Geochemistry and Health.

Schilling R, Bain RP. (1989). Prediction of children's blood lead levels on the basis of household-specific soil lead levels. Am J Epidemiol 1989;128(1):197–205.

Steele MJ, et al. (1990). Assessing the contribution from lead in mining wastes to blood lead. Regul Toxicol Pharmacol 1990;11:158–90.

Susten AS. (1990). The ATSDR health assessment: purpose, history, and findings. In: Andrews JS, et al., eds. Environmental issues: today's challenge for the future. Proceedings of Fourth National Environmental Health Conference, June 20–23, 1989, San Antonio, Texas. U.S. Department of Health and Human Services, Public Health Service.

Tola S, et al. (1973). Parameters indicative of absorption and biological effects in new lead exposure: a prospective study. Br J Ind Med 1973;30:134–41.

Watson WS, et al. (1980). Oral absorption of lead and iron. Lancet 1980;(8188):236–237.

Yip R, et al. (1981). Iron status of children with elevated blood lead concentrations. J Pediatr 1981;98: 922–925.

Famine-Affected, Refugee, and Displaced Populations

Original Citation: Centers for Disease Control and Prevention. Famine-affected, refugee, and displaced populations: recommendations for public health issues. MMWR 1992;41 (No. RR-13).

Original Authors: Mike J. Toole, MD, DTM&H, Rita M. Malkki, MPH

RECOMMENDATIONS

The technical recommendations in this report focus on the public health elements of an appropriate response program for refugees and displaced persons, however, the effectiveness of relief efforts will be enhanced if the affected communities and host countries have prepared for the emergency. Preparedness for sudden population displacement is critical and should be targeted at the most important public health problems identified in previous emergencies: malnutrition, measles, diarrheal diseases, malaria, ARI, and other communicable diseases (e.g., meningitis and hepatitis) that result in high death rates.

Preparedness requires that planning for emergencies be included as an integral part of routine health development programs in countries where sudden population displacements might occur. These programs include:

- Health Information Systems (HIS).
- Diarrheal Disease Control Programs.
- Expanded Programs on Immunization (EPI).
- Control Programs for Endemic Communicable Diseases.
- Nutrition Programs.
- Continuing Education Programs for Health Workers.

National public health programs should include detailed contingency planning for sudden population movements, both internally and from neighboring countries.

Response Preparedness

The critical components of a relief program responding to sudden population displacement comprise the provision of adequate food, clean water, sanitation, and shelter. In addition, the following elements of a health program should be established as soon as possible.

Health Information System

- Mortality surveillance.
- Nutrition surveillance.
- Surveillance for diseases of public health importance.

Diarrheal Disease Control

- ORT.
- Community hygiene education.
- Cholera preparedness.

Immunization

- Measles immunization immediately.
- Other EPI antigens later, when the emergency subsides.
- Identification of sources for meningitis vaccine.

Basic Curative Care

- Emphasis on maternal and child health (MCH).
- Establishment of a referral system.
- Development of an essential drugs list.
- Preparation of standard treatment guidelines (at least for Diarrhea, malaria, and ARI).
- Selection, training, and deployment of community health workers.

Endemic Disease Control and Epidemic Preparedness

- Establishment of surveillance, including standard case definitions.
- Development of standard case management protocols.
- Agreement on policies for prevention (including vaccination and prophylaxis).
- Identification of laboratory to confirm index cases of epidemic diseases.
- Identification of sources of relevant vaccines.
- Establishment of reserves of essential medical supplies (ORT, intravenous (IV) solutions).
- Identification of treatment sites, triage system, and training needs.
- Identification of expert assistance for epidemic investigation.
- Development of environmental management plans.
- Implementation of community education and prevention programs.

The detailed recommendations that follow are organized according to either disease group (e.g., diarrheal diseases or malnutrition) or technical methods (e.g., rapid assessment). Nevertheless, it is critical to keep in mind the demographic groups that are most at risk during emergencies, namely young children and women. It is important that health services in refugee settings be organized in a way that facilitates access by these groups. In general, MCH services should be given higher priority than general outpatient dispensaries and hospitals.

Maternal and Child Health Care

MCH clinics should be established (ideally one MCH clinic per 5,000 population) and staffed by trained personnel to provide routine screening and preventive, and curative services to pregnant and lactating women and to children less than 2 years of age. If resources are adequate, these services should be extended to children between 2 and 5 years of age. Services for children should include routine growth monitoring, immunization, nutritional rehabilitation, vitamin A supplementation, and curative care, as well as health education for their mothers.

Female health workers should be trained and employed to provide culturally appropriate health education both at MCH clinics and within the community, and to refer pregnant women to the clinic for antenatal care. At least some of these health workers should be recruited from among traditional birth attendants in the community. Antenatal care should include screening for high-risk pregnancies and providing iron and folic acid supplementation (as well as iodine supplementation in areas of endemic goiter), tetanus toxoid immunization, and health education. Postnatal care should include nutritional supplementation, counseling on family spacing, provision of contraceptives, and education about breast-feeding and infant care. In certain cultural situations, curative care may need to be provided to all women of child-bearing age in a setting physically segregated from male outpatient facilities.

Rapid Health Assessment

Rapid health assessment of an acute population displacement is conducted to:

- Assess the magnitude of the displacement.
- Determine the major health and nutrition needs of the displaced population.
- Initiate a health and nutrition surveillance system.
- Assess the local response capacity and immediate needs.

Preparations

The amount of time required to conduct an initial assessment of a refugee influx depends on the remoteness of the location, availability of transport, security situation in the area, availability of appropriate specialists, and willingness of the host country government to involve external agencies in refugee relief programs. In small countries with functioning communications facilities and secure borders, the assessment might be conducted in 4 days; in other countries, it might take 2 weeks.

Before the field visit, relevant information relating to the status of the incoming refugees, as well as the available resources of the host community, should be obtained from local ministries or organizations based in the capital city. Any maps of the area where the refugees are arriving and settling should likewise be obtained. Aerial photographs will also be of value, but may be considered sensitive by the military of the host country. International organizations like UNICEF, WHO, and the Red Cross/Red Crescent may also have demographic and health data concerning the refugee population.

In preparation for the field visit, establish whether food, medical supplies (including vaccines), or other relief supplies have been ordered or procured by any of the relief agencies involved. Additionally, the following conditions should be included in a field assessment.

Field Assessment

The following demographic information is required to determine the health status of the population.

- Total refugee or displaced population.
- Age-sex breakdown.
- Identification of at-risk groups; e.g., children less than 5 years of age, pregnant and lactating women, disabled and wounded persons, and unaccompanied minors.
- Average family or household size.

Why this Information Is Needed

The total population will be used as the denominator for all birth, death, injury, morbidity, and malnutrition rates to be estimated later. The total population is necessary for the calculation of quantities of relief supplies. The breakdown of the population by age and sex allows for the calculation of age- and sex-specific rates and enables interventions to be targeted effectively (e.g., immunization campaigns).

Sources of Information

Local government officials or camp authorities may be able to provide registration records. If no registration system is in effect, one should be established immediately. Information recorded should include the names of household heads, the number of family members by age and sex, former village and region of residence, and ethnic group, if applicable.

Refugee leaders may also have records, particularly if entire villages have fled together. In certain situations, political groups may have organized the exodus and may have detailed lists of refugee families.

A visual inspection of the settlement may provide a general impression of the demographic composition of the population. However, information obtained in this manner should be used judiciously as it is likely to provide a distorted view of the situation.

It may be necessary to conduct a limited survey on a convenience sample in order to obtain demographic information. Beginning at a randomly selected point, survey a sample (e.g., 50) of dwellings. Visit every fifth or 10th house until the predetermined number of houses have been surveyed. At each house, record the number of family members, the age and sex of each person, and the number of pregnant or lactating women. This process will establish an initial estimate of the demographic composition of the population. Estimate the number of persons in each house, as well as the total number of houses in the settlement, to gain a provisional estimate of the camp population. At the very least, this quick survey should give a rough estimate of the proportion of the total population made up of "vulnerable" groups; i.e., children less than 5 years of age and women of child bearing age. To determine the total population, a census may need to be conducted later.

Background Health Information

The information required includes:

- Main health problems in country of origin.
- Previous sources of health care (e.g., traditional healers).

- Important health beliefs and traditions (e.g., food taboos during pregnancy).
- Social structure (e.g., whether the refugees are grouped in their traditional villages and what type of social or political organization exists).
- Strength and coverage of public health programs in country of origin (e.g., immunization).

Why this Information Is Needed

Effective planning of health services will depend on this information. Planners need to be aware of traditional beliefs, taboos, and practices in order to avoid making costly mistakes and alienating the population.

Sources of Information

Obtain documents and reports from the host government, international organizations, and nongovernment organizations pertaining to endemic diseases and public health programs in the displaced population's region of origin.

Interview refugee leaders, heads of households, women leaders (e.g., traditional midwives), and health workers among the refugee population.

Seek information from development agencies, private companies, missionaries, or other groups having experience with the displaced population.

Nutritional Status

The information required includes:

- Prevalence of protein-energy undernutrition in the population less than 5 years of age.
- Nutritional status before arrival in host country.
- Prevalence of micronutrient deficiencies in the population less than 5 years of age.

Why this Information Is Needed

Evidence exists to support the fact that the nutritional status of displaced populations is closely linked with their chances of survival. Initial assessment of nutritional status serves to establish the degree of urgency in delivering food rations, the need for immediate supplementary feeding programs (SFPs), and the presence of micronutrient deficiencies that require urgent attention.

Sources of Nutritional Information

If refugees are still arriving at the site:

- Initiate nutritional screening of new arrivals immediately.
- Measure all children (or every third or fourth child, if insufficient trained personnel are available or the refugee influx is too great) for mid-upper arm circumference (MUAC) or, if time and personnel permit, WFH. Estimate the proportion of undernourished children using the methods described in the Rapid Nutrition Assessment Manual. (Available from IHPO, CDC, 1600 Clifton Road, MS F-03, Atlanta, GA 30333, 404-639-0308.)
- Look for clinical signs of severe anemia and vitamin A, B, and C deficiencies.
- If refugees are continuing to arrive, set up a permanent screening program

for new arrivals. A screening program also can be used to administer measles vaccination and vitamin A supplements to new arrivals.

If refugees are already located in a settlement:

- Walk through the settlement, select houses randomly, and observe the nutritional status of the children less than 5 years of age. Visual assessment should only be done by persons who are experienced in the assessment of malnutrition. The observer should enter the homes as malnourished children are likely to be bedridden.
- Combine the visual inspection with a rapid assessment of nutritional status, using either MUAC or WFH measurements. This can be done during the demographic survey described above. (See "Rapid Health Assessment")
- Review the records of local hospitals treating members of the displaced population. Note admissions or consultations for undernutrition and deaths related to undernutrition.
- Interview refugee leaders to establish food availability before displacement and the duration of the journey from place of origin to their present location.

In order to gather baseline data for evaluation of nutrition programs, plan to conduct a valid, cluster sample survey of the population as soon as possible (within 2 weeks). Appropriate technical expertise will be needed for the implementation and analysis of the survey.

Mortality Rates

The information required includes crude, age-, sex-, and cause-specific mortality rates.

Why this Information Is Needed

In the initial stages of a population displacement, mortality rates, expressed as deaths/10,000/day, are a critical indicator of improving or deteriorating health status.

In many African countries, the daily CMR (extrapolated from published annual rates) is approximately 0.5/10,000/day during non-emergency conditions. In general, health workers should be extremely concerned when CMRs in a displaced population exceed 1/10,000/day, or when less than 5 years of age mortality rates exceed 4/10,000/day.

Sources of Mortality Information

Check local hospital records and the records of local burial contractors. Interview community leaders.

Establish a mortality surveillance system. One approach is to designate a single burial site for the camp, which should be monitored by 24-hour grave watchers. Grave watchers should be trained to interview families, using a standard questionnaire, and then to record the data to determine gender, approximate age, and probable cause of death.

Other methods of collecting mortality data include registering deaths, issuing burial shrouds to families of the deceased to ensure compliance, or employing volunteer community informants who report deaths for a defined section of the population.

Demographic data are absolutely essential for calculating mortality rates. These provide the denominator for estimating death rates in the entire population and within specific vulnerable groups, such as children less than 5 years of age.

The population needs to be assured that death registration will have no adverse consequences (e.g., ration reductions).

Morbidity

The information required includes age- and sex-specific data regarding the incidence of common diseases of public health importance, i.e., measles, malaria, diarrheal diseases, and ARI, as well as diseases of epidemic potential such as hepatitis and meningitis. The data should be collected by all health facilities, including feeding centers.

Why this Information Is Needed

Data on diseases of public health importance may help plan an effective preventive and curative health program for refugees. These data will also facilitate the procurement of appropriate medical supplies and the recruitment and training of appropriate medical personnel, as well as focus environmental sanitation efforts (e.g., toward mosquito control in areas of high malaria prevalence).

Sources of Morbidity Information

Review the records of local clinics and hospitals to which refugees have access.

Where a clinic, hospital, or feeding center has already been established within the camp, examine patient records or registers and tally common causes of morbidity. Interview refugee leaders and health workers within the refugee population.

A simple morbidity surveillance system should be established as soon as curative services are established in the camp. Feeding centers should be included in the surveillance system. Community health workers should be trained as soon as possible to report diseases at the community level.

The initiation of certain public health actions should not be delayed until the disease appears. For example, measles immunization should be implemented immediately. Do not wait for the appearance of measles in the camp. Also, oral rehydration centers should be routinely established in all situations.

Environmental Conditions

The information required includes:

- Climatic conditions (average temperatures and rainfall patterns).
- Geographic features (soil, slope, and drainage).
- Water sources (local wells, reservoirs, rivers, tanks).

- Local disease epidemiology (endemic infectious diseases, e.g., malaria, schistosomiasis).
- Local disease vectors (mosquitoes, flies, ticks), including breeding sites.
- Availability of local materials for shelter and fuel.
- Existing shelters.
- Existing sanitation arrangements (latrines and open areas).

Why this Information Is Needed

Information on local environmental conditions affecting the health of displaced populations will help relief planners create priorities for public health programs. Sources of information. This assessment is made largely by visual inspection. In addition, interviews with local government and technical specialists will yield important information. In some cases, special surveys need to be conducted; e.g., entomologists may need to survey for local disease vectors, and water engineers may need to assess water sources.

Resources Available

Food Supplies

Efforts to evaluate food supplies should include:

- Attempting to assess the quantity and type of food currently available to the population.
- Calculating the average per capita caloric intake over the period of time for which records are available, if food is already being officially distributed.
- Inspecting any local markets for food availability and prices.
- Conducting a quick survey of dwellings and estimating the average food stores in each household. This should be done during the demographic survey (see "Rapid Health Assessment"). Look for obvious inequities between different families or different ethnic or regional groups.

Food Sources

Local, regional, and national markets need to be assessed. The cash and material resources of the displaced population should also be assessed in order to estimate its local purchasing power.

Food Logistics

Assess transport and fuel availability, storage facilities (size, security), and seasonal conditions of access roads.

Feeding Programs

Follow these guidelines to evaluate feeding programs:

- Look for any established feeding programs (mass, supplementary, and therapeutic feedings). These may have been set up by local officials, PVOs, church groups, or local villagers.
- Assess enrollment and discharge criteria, enrollment and attendance figures, quantity and quality of food being provided, availability of water, managerial competence, utensils, and storage.
- Determine whether measles vaccine is being administered.

Local Health Services

Follow these guidelines for assessing the capabilities of health services:

- Determine the ease of access by refugees (official attitudes, location, hours of operation).
- Evaluate the condition and size of facilities.
- Note the extent and appropriateness of medicines, equipment, and services.
- Determine the type and number of personnel.
- Review cold storage facilities, vaccine supplies, logistics, and communication systems.

Camp Health Services

Follow these guidelines for assessing camp health services:

- Note the type of facility (clinic, hospital, feeding center), as well as the size, capacity, and structure (tent, local materials).
- Determine the adequacy of health-facility water supply.
- Assess refrigeration facilities, fuel, and generator.
- Assess supplies of essential drugs (whether generic or brand-name) and medical supplies.
- Determine the need for essential vaccines and immunization equipment.
- Note the type of health personnel (doctors, nurses, nutritionists, sanitarians) and their relevant experience and skills.
- Review storage facilities.
- Assess adequacy of transport, fuel, and communications.
- Locate health workers in refugee population (traditional healers, birth attendants, "modern" practitioners).
- Determine whether there is a need for interpreters.

Taking Action

- An itemized summary of the findings should be prepared, following the sequence of activities outlined in this document.
- Estimate and quantify the need for outside assistance, based on preliminary findings.
- Prepare and convey assessment findings to appropriate emergency health officials at the local, national, and international levels.

Checklist For Rapid Health Assessment

Adapted from WHO Emergency Relief Operations. Emergency Preparedness and Response: Rapid Health Assessment in Sudden Population Displacements. WHO, in collaboration with CDC and other WHO Collaborating Centers for Emergency Preparedness and Response. Geneva: January 1990.

Preparation

- Obtain available information regarding refugees and resources from host country ministries and organizations.
- Obtain available maps or aerial photographs.
- Obtain demographic and health data from international organizations.

Field Assessment

- Determine total displaced population.
- Determine age and sex breakdown of population.
- Identify groups at increased risk.
- Determine average household size.

Health Information

- Identify primary health problems in country of origin.
- Identify previous sources of health care.
- Ascertain important health beliefs and traditions.
- Determine the existing social structure.
- Determine the strength and coverage of public health programs in country of origin.

Nutritional Status

- Determine prevalence of PEM in population less than 5 years of age.
- Ascertain prior nutritional status.
- Determine prevalence of micronutrient deficiencies in the population less than 5 years of age.

Mortality Rates

- Calculate crude, age-, sex-, and cause-specific mortality rates.

Morbidity

- Determine age- and sex-specific incidence rates of diseases that have public health importance.

Environmental Conditions

- Determine climatic conditions.
- Identify geographic features.
- Identify water sources.
- Ascertain local disease epidemiology.
- Identify local disease vectors.
- Assess availability of local materials for shelter and fuel.
- Assess existing shelters and sanitation arrangements.

Resources Available

- Assess food supplies and distribution systems.
- Identify and assess local, regional, and national food sources.
- Assess the logistics of food transport and storage.
- Assess feeding programs.
- Identify and assess local health services.
- Assess camp health services.

Health Information System

A health information system (HIS) provides continuous information on the health status of the refugee community and comprises both ongoing routine surveillance and intermittent population-based sample surveys. This information may be used to:

- Follow trends in the health status of the community and establish health-care priorities.
- Detect and respond to epidemics.
- Evaluate program effectiveness and service coverage.
- Ensure that resources are targeted to the areas of greatest need.
- Evaluate the quality of care delivered.

Data Collection

As soon as health services are established for a refugee population, a surveillance system should be instituted and should ideally be set up at the time of an initial, rapid assessment. Any agency or facility (including feeding centers) providing health services to the refugee population should be part of the reporting network. Any host community services to which the refugees might have access should also be part of the system.

Health information should be reported on a simple, standardized surveillance form. (A sample form, adapted from WHO Emergency Relief Operations, is located at the end of this section.) Each health facility should be held accountable for completing the reporting form at the appropriate interval and for returning it to the person or agency charged with compiling the reports, analyzing the information, and providing feedback. Each refugee settlement or camp should have a person responsible for coordinating the HIS. Forms should be translated into the appropriate local language(s) if community health workers are involved in information collection.

Health facilities should keep a daily record of patients; age, sex, clinical and laboratory diagnosis, and treatment should be specified. If personnel time is limited, a simple tally sheet should be used. In addition, the patient should be issued a health record card on which the date, diagnosis, and treatment are recorded. Each time a patient contacts the health-care system, whether for curative or preventive services, this should be noted on the health record card. Laboratory data should accompany diagnostic information whenever possible. Collecting Processing, Storing, and Shipping Diagnostic Specimens in Refugee Health-Care Environments (available from IHPO, CDC, 1600 Clifton Road, MS F-03, Atlanta, GA 30333, 404–639-0308) provides an overview of procedures for collecting and processing diagnostic specimens in the field.

Data collection should be limited to that information that can and will be acted upon. Information that is not immediately useful should not be collected during the emergency phase of a refugee relief operation. Overly detailed or complex reporting requirements will result in noncompliance.

The most valuable data are generally simple to collect and to analyze. Standard case definitions for the most common causes of morbidity and mortality should be developed and put in writing. The data collected will fall into one of the following categories: (a) demographic, (b) mortality, (c) morbidity, (d) nutritional status, and (e) health program activities.

Population

Camp registration records should provide most of the demographic information needed. If registration records are inadequate, a population census may be necessary. Conducting a census is often politically sensitive and may be delayed by the administrative authorities for a long period of time. Consequently, innovative methods may need to be devised. For example, organize a nutritional screening of all children less than 5 years of age. Count the children and estimate the percentage of the total population less than 5 years of age by doing a sample survey. From this information, estimate the total population size. For other methods to determine population size and structure see "Rapid Health Assessment".

It is important that population figures be updated on a regular basis, taking into account new arrivals, departures, births, and deaths. The total population is used as the denominator in the calculation of disease incidence, birth, and death rates. This total is also necessary to determine requirements for food and medical supplies and to estimate program coverage rates. Information about the population structure is needed to calculate age- and sex-specific morbidity and mortality rates, to estimate ration requirements, and to determine the target population for specific interventions, i.e., antenatal care and immunizations.

The rate of new arrivals and departures gives an indication of the stability of the population and will influence policy decisions about long-term interventions, such as TB therapy. This information is also used to predict future resource and program needs.

A birth registration system is usually simple, since the community expects an increase in the family food ration as a result of a new birth. Births might be reported in the community to volunteer health workers or traditional birth attendants. Alternatively, if good antenatal care services are established, follow-up of pregnant mothers will allow for a relatively complete registration of births. Examples of mortality surveillance systems are described in "Rapid Health Assessment". Deaths may be underreported if there is a fear of possible ration reduction; thus, an agreement might be negotiated with camp authorities not to decrease rations after a death occurs—at least during the emergency phase. Arrivals and departures should be monitored through the camp registration system.

Mortality

Each health facility should keep a log of all patient deaths (with cause of death and relevant demographic information) and report the deaths on a standardized form. Because many deaths occur outside of the health-care system, a community-based mortality surveillance system should be established. Such a system may include the employment of grave watchers, the routine issuance of burial shrouds, and the use of community informants (see "Rapid Health Assessment").

Death rates are the most specific indicators of a population's health status and are the category of data to which donors and relief agencies most readily respond. During the emergency phase of a relief operation, death rates should be expressed as deaths/10,000/day to allow for detection of sudden changes. In refugee camps, relief programs should aim at achieving a CMR of less than 1/10,000/day as soon as possible. This rate still represents approximately twice the "normal" CMR for non-displaced populations in most developing nations and should not signal a relaxation of efforts. After the emergency phase, death rates should be expressed as deaths/1,000/month to reflect the usual reporting frequency and to facilitate comparison with baseline, non-refugee death rates.

Age- and sex-specific mortality rates will indicate the need for interventions targeted at specific vulnerable groups. During the early stage of a relief operation, specific death rates for persons less than 5 years of age and greater than 5 years of age may suffice. Later, further disaggregation by age may be feasible— for example, less than 1 year, 1–4 years, 5–14 years, and greater than 15 years. Different male- and female-specific death rates may reflect inequitable access to resources or health services. Cause-specific mortality rates will reflect those health problems having the greatest impact on the refugee community and requiring the highest priority in public health program planning.

Morbidity

Health facilities and feeding centers should report morbidity information on the same form on which mortality is reported. Each disease reported in the system must have a written case definition that will guide health workers in their diagnosis and ensure the validity of data. Where practical, case definitions that rely on clinical signs and symptoms should be tested periodically for sensitivity and specificity as compared with a laboratory standard (e.g., malaria).

Knowledge of the major causes of illness and the groups in the affected population that are at greatest risk allows for the efficient planning of intervention strategies and the most effective use of resources. Morbidity rates are more useful than a simple tallying of cases, as trends can be followed over time, or rates compared with those from different populations. The monitoring of proportional morbidity (e.g., percentage of all morbidity caused by specific diseases) may be useful when specific control measures are being evaluated, although caution is needed in the interpretation of trends. A relative decrease in disease-specific proportional morbidity may merely reflect an absolute increase in the incidence of another disease.

Nutritional Status

Data regarding nutritional status can be obtained through a nutritional assessment survey or a mass screening exercise. Surveys should be repeated at regular intervals to determine changes in nutritional status; however, not so frequently as to obscure true differences between surveys. All children less than 5 years of age should undergo a nutritional screening upon arrival at the camp and should continue to be weighed and measured monthly at MCH clinics in the camp. Information collected during these screenings should be included in HIS reports. If the initial screening identifies high prevalence rates of undernutrition, cross-sectional surveys should be repeated at intervals of 6–8 weeks until the undernutrition prevalence rate is below 10%. Thereafter, surveys every 6–12 months will suffice, unless routine surveillance data indicate that nutritional status has deteriorated. Measurement of nutritional status is described in the Rapid Nutrition Assessment Manual (available from IHPO, CDC, 1600 Clifton Road, MS F-03, Atlanta, GA 30333, 404-639-0308).

The prevalence of acute malnutrition acts as an indicator of the adequacy of the relief ration. A high prevalence of malnutrition in the presence of an adequate average daily ration may indicate inequities in the food distribution system, or high incidence rates of communicable diseases (e.g., measles and diarrhea). The presence of nutritional deficiency disorders (i.e., pellagra, anemia, or xerophthalmia) indicates the need for ration supplementation.

Programs

Each health facility should keep a log of all activities. Immunizations should be recorded in a central record, as well as on the person's health record card. Records of health sector activities will be useful in determining whether certain groups in the population are underserved, and in planning measures to reach a broader population base. Although approximate immunization coverage may be estimated from the number of vaccine doses administered, the preferred method is by annual population surveys.

Analysis and Interpretation

Most data can be analyzed locally using a pen and paper. The use of computers and a data entry and analysis program, such as Epi Info, version 5, may be practical at the regional or national level. Trends in mortality, morbidity, and nutritional status should be monitored closely. Careful attention should be paid to changing denominators, and changes in proportional mortality or morbidity should be interpreted with particular caution. Where applicable, correlations between mortality, morbidity or nutritional status, and health sector activities should be examined. Likewise, the proportion of malnourished children identified in population surveys as enrolled in feeding programs can be used to estimate program coverage. All components of the HIS should be analyzed and interpreted in an integrated fashion. A single element examined alone will reveal only a small portion of the entire picture and may be easily misinterpreted. For example, an apparent decrease in malnutrition prevalence should be interpreted in the context of childhood mortality rates (1). The use of health information to guide program decision-making will be facilitated if targets and critical indicators are established at the beginning. For example, a measles incidence rate of 1/1,000/month might be an indicator that would initiate specific preventive actions. Similarly, during a cholera outbreak, a CFR of 3% in a given week might stimulate a critical review of case management procedures.

Control Measures

The information gathered through the HIS should be used to develop recommendations and to implement specific control measures. Objectives for disease control programs should be established and progress towards these objectives regularly assessed. The presentation of data to decision-makers should make use of simple, clear tables and graphs. Most importantly, there should be regular feedback to the data providers through newsletters, bulletins, and frequent supervisory visits.

Assessment

The HIS should be periodically assessed to determine its accuracy, completeness, simplicity, flexibility, and timeliness. The utilization of the data by program planners and key decision-makers should also be assessed. The HIS should evolve as the need for information changes.

REFERENCE: AS NUMBERED IN ORIGINAL PUBLICATION

1. Nieburg P, Berry A, Steketee R, Binkin N, Dondero T, Aziz N. Limitations of anthropometry during acute food shortages: high mortality can mask refugees' deteriorating nutritional status. Disasters 1988;12:253–258.

Nutrition

Rations

For populations totally dependent upon food aid, a general ration of at least 1,900 kcal/person/day is required. At least 10% of the calories in the general ration should be in the form of fats and at least 12% should be derived from proteins.

- Each of the rations above provides at least minimum quantities of energy, protein, and fat.
- Ration 2 provides additional quantities of various micronutrients through the inclusion of a fortified blended cereal. When provided in the general ration, fortified cereal blends should be used for the whole family.

The calculation of rations should account for calorie loss during transport and food preparation. Similarly, when the mean daily temperature falls below 20°C, the caloric requirement should be increased accordingly by 1% per degree of temperature below 20°C.

The standard requirement of 1,900 kcal is based on the following demographic structure of a population:

- Children less than 5 years of age (20%).
- Children 5–14 years of age (35%).
- Women 15–44 years of age (20%), of whom 40% are pregnant or lactating.
- Males 15–44 years of age (10%).
- Adults greater than 44 years of age (15%).

The calculation of ration requirements should be adjusted for deviations from the above population structure (age/gender breakdown), the underlying health and nutritional status of the population, and relative activity levels of the community.

Guidelines for Ration Distribution

- Food should be distributed in a community setting. Camps and mass feedings should be avoided if at all possible.

- Ration distribution should complement, not replace, any food that the refugees are able to provide for themselves.
- Distributed food should be familiar and culturally acceptable to the refugees.
- If food is distributed in uncooked form, adequate fuel and cooking utensils should be made available.
- Grains should be provided in ground form, or grinders must be made available.
- Distribution must be done on a regular basis, with no longer period than 10–14 days between distributions.
- If a specified food item in the ration cannot be supplied, the energy and nutrient content of the missing item should be provided by including additional quantities of another available commodity. This type of substitution is appropriate only as a short-term measure.
- Breast-feeding should be encouraged and supported.
- Lactating women should be provided with extra sources of calories and protein. Appropriate weaning foods should be included in the general ration (fats and oils).
- Bottle feeding should be discouraged. Infant bottles and formula should not be distributed.
- Dry skim milk (DSM) and other milk products should not be included in the ration as such, except where milk consumption is part of the traditional diet. Milk products should be mixed with milled grains to form a cereal. Any milk product that is included in the rations should be fortified with vitamin A.
- If fresh fruits and vegetables are not available, fortified blended foods (e.g., corn-soya milk (CSM)), CSB, or similar local products) should be provided to meet micronutrient requirements.
- Refugees should be encouraged to grow vegetables. Seeds, gardening implements, and suitable land should be made available for kitchen gardens. This is critical for the prevention of pellagra and scurvy.
- Refugees should be permitted access to local markets and be allowed to create markets. Trading or selling of ration commodities may be a necessary part of the camp economy. It enables refugees to supplement their diets with foods otherwise unavailable to them and to obtain essential nonfood items.
- It may be advisable to include certain culturally significant items i.e., tea, sugar, and spices in the food basket. Where such items are highly valued, refugees will sell or trade part of their ration to obtain them. This results in a reduction of caloric intake. Providing these items eliminates this overall reduction.

Supplementary Feeding Programs

SFPs are designed to help prevent severe malnutrition and to rehabilitate moderately malnourished persons. SFPs are not intended to be used as a method of targeting food during an emergency phase. Similarly, SFPs are inappropriate as a long-term supplement to an inadequate general ration.

Implementation of a SFP is necessary under the following circumstances:

- When the general ration is less than 1,500 kcal/person.
- Where nutritional assessment reveals that greater than 20% of children less than 5 years of age are acutely malnourished, as determined by a Z-score indicator of less than -2.

- When the acute malnutrition prevalence (as determined by a Z-score indicator of less than -2) falls between 10%–20% and the general ration is between 1,500–1,900 kcal.
- Where there is a high incidence of measles or diarrheal disease.

Inclusion and discharge criteria.   The following groups should be targeted for inclusion in a SFP:

- Acutely undernourished children less than 5 years of age (WFH Z-score less than -2 or less than 80% of reference median).
- Pregnant and lactating women.
- Elderly, chronically ill (e.g., TB patients), or disadvantaged groups.

Children should be discharged from the SFP after they have maintained greater than 85% of median WFH (or a Z-score greater than -1.5) for a period of 1 month.

Caloric requirements.   A SFP should provide at least 500 kcal and 15 g protein/day in one or two feedings.

High energy milk (HEM), a calorie-dense milk mixture, may be used in a SFP. One milliliter of HEM provides 1 kcal of energy. The formula below makes 5 L of HEM:

420 g dried skimmed milk, 250 g sugar, 320 g oil, and 4.4 L water.

If the general ration is inadequate (less than 1,900 kcal/person/day), the supplementary ration should provide 700–1,000 kcal/person/day in two to three feedings.

Types of SFPs.   SFPs fall into two categories, either on-site feeding or take-home rations. Listed below are some of the advantages and disadvantages of each type of SFP (1).

On-site feeding.   "Wet" rations are prepared by SFP staff and served to recipients in the feeding center. Listed below are the advantages of wet rations:

- The likelihood that the ration will be shared among family members is reduced.
- SFP staff maintain control over the preparation and consumption of the supplementary meals.
- Additional services can be incorporated into the feeding program.

These are the disadvantages of wet rations:

- Young children must be accompanied to the center. This may lead to poor attendance rates and create a hardship for many mothers who must also provide for other family members.
- Feeding centers must be located near the homes of the recipients.
- In order to increase motivation and attendance, other services may need to be offered.
- Feeding centers are a drain on health personnel resources.
- Feeding center meals may be substituted for meals at home, resulting in a net food intake deficit.
- On-site feedings are not appropriate for targeting entire families or community groups.

- Children less than 2 years of age are generally underserved by on-site feedings.
- On-site feedings remove the family's responsibility and control over providing for family members.
- The possibility of cross-contamination and infection is increased in mass feedings.

Take-home programs. "Dry" rations are provided on a regular basis to supplement the general ration normally received. These are the advantages of dry rations:

- Daily attendance of the enrollee or other family members is not required.
- Fewer centers are needed, and these may be located at a greater distance from homes.
- The supplementary ration increases the purchasing power of the family.
- The ration is intended to provide supplementation 365 days/year. (No missed days for holidays)
- Dry rations generally achieve higher coverage rates than wet rations.
- There is less disruption of family activities, as daily attendance is not required.
- The family is able to maintain control over feeding practices.

These are the disadvantages of dry rations:

- Dry rations are less effective at targeting person beneficiaries.
- Sharing of the ration among family members is increased.

Other elements of SFPs.

- Vitamin A should be administered upon admission to the SFP and every 3 months thereafter.
- If vitamin C is not included from the ration, vitamin C supplements should be administered weekly to all persons enrolled in SFPs.
- If iron deficiency anemia is highly prevalent, the provision of iron syrup to children enrolled in SFPs should be considered.
- All enrollees in the SFP should have their measles immunization status checked upon admission, and vaccine administered if needed.
- Mebendazole, an anthelminthic, should be administered along with the vitamin A, if it is available. Each child should be administered two 100 mg tablets to be chewed. Mebendazole should not be administered to infants less than 12 months of age or to pregnant women.
- On-site feeding centers require a regular supply of clean water and cooking fuel.

Therapeutic Feeding Programs

Therapeutic feeding programs (TFPs) are considered a medical intervention, the purpose of which is to save lives and restore the nutritional health of severely malnourished children. The recommendations listed below are adapted from the procedures for selective feeding (2).

Enrollment criteria. Children should be enrolled in a TFP if they meet one of the following criteria:

- Children less than 5 years of age (or less than 115 cm in height) with WFH Z-score of less than -3 (less than 70% median).
- Children with clinically evident edema.
- Children referred to TFP by medical personnel.

Caloric requirements.

- Children enrolled in a TFP should receive 150 kcal and 3 g of protein for each kg body weight/day.
- Feeding should be done in four to six meals/day. Feeding centers that provide meals on a 24-hour basis are likely to be most effective.
- HEM should be included in the TFP ration.
- All children enrolled in the TFP should receive a full course of vitamin A upon admission.
- Severely malnourished children typically have poor appetites and may require nasogastric feedings for short intervals. Trained and experienced personnel are needed for this procedure.

Discharge criteria. Discharge from a TFP to a SFP should occur when the following criteria are met:

- The child has maintained 80% WFH (or a Z-score of -2) for a period of 2 weeks.
- Weight gain has occurred without edema.
- The child is active and free from obvious illness.
- The child exhibits a good appetite.

Monitoring Requirements

- A register should be maintained with the details of each patient.
- Each patient should be given a personal ration card and an identification bracelet.
- Each patient should be weighed daily at first, and then twice weekly to monitor progress.
- TFPs should aim for a weight gain of 10 g/kg body weight/day.
- All absentees should be followed up at home and encouraged to resume attendance.
- Regular nutrition surveys should be conducted, and malnourished children who are not enrolled in a feeding program should be referred to either the SFP or the TFP. Feeding programs should aim for at least 80% enrollment and 80% daily attendance. In addition, health workers should be involved in active case-finding in the community.

Provision of Micronutrients

Ideally, the recommended daily allowances for all essential nutrients should be provided in the general rations. However, specific measures may be necessary to provide certain micronutrients.

Vitamin A.

Risk factors for vitamin A deficiency. Provide vitamin A supplements whenever any of the following conditions are present:

- The refugee population originates from a geographic area at high risk for vitamin A deficiency.

- There is evidence of severe vitamin A deficiency in the population.
- The general ration provides inadequate quantities of vitamin A (less than 2,000–2,500 IU/person/day).

Supplemental doses and schedule.

- Children 12 months 5 years of age should receive 200,000 IU every 3 months.
- Infants less than 12 months of age should receive 400,000 IU total dose in the first year of life, administered as follows:
- If a dose can be assured every 3 months: 100,000 IU to the infant every 3 months for 1 year.
- If 3-month dosing is impractical but 6-month dosing is anticipated: 200,000 IU to the infant every 6 months for 1 year.
- If any subsequent dosing is unlikely: 200,000 IU to the infant when examined.

In all cases, mothers should be administered 200,000 IU within 2 months of giving birth in order to provide adequate quantities of vitamin A in the breast milk. If it is not possible to provide supplements to the mother at or within 2 months of giving birth, then the mother should receive 100,000 IU during the third trimester of pregnancy.

- If xerophthalmia is observed in older children and adults, include the affected age groups in the standard 200,000 IU preventive vitamin A supplementation program administered to younger children.
- As a general practice, all doses of vitamin A should be documented on the child's growth record chart.

Full treatment schedule. A full treatment schedule of oral vitamin A should be administered to all persons suffering from severe malnutrition (WFH Z-score less than -3) or exhibiting eye symptoms of vitamin A deficiency (xerosis, Bitot's spots, keratomalacia, or corneal ulceration). The dose schedule is given below: 200,000 IU on day 1, 200,000 IU on day 2, and 200,000 IU 1 to 4 weeks later. Children less than 12 months of age receive half doses.

Anemia. The prevalence of anemia can be determined through a rapid anemia survey using a portable Hb photometer (HemoCue system).

The CDC has established the following criteria for defining anemia:

- Children 15 years of age: Hb less than 11.0 g/dL
- Pregnant women: Hb less than 11.0 g/dL
- Nonpregnant women: Hb less than 12 g/dL
- Men: Hb less than 13.5 g/dL

The risk of anemia is highest in pregnant and lactating women, and in children ages 9–36 months. If the general ration contains inadequate amounts of absorbable iron, folate, and vitamin C, anemia may be prevented through the daily administration of iron/folate tablets and vitamin C supplements. Supplementary feeding of high-risk groups with CSM will also help to reduce the likelihood of anemia (CSM contains 18 g iron/100 g).

Iron/folic acid. Routine iron/folate supplements should be provided to all pregnant and lactating women through antenatal and postnatal clinics. Female health workers should be employed to seek out pregnant and lactating women and encourage their participation in these programs.

Vitamin C. Fortification of foods with vitamin C is problematic because vitamin C is unstable. Further study is needed on the appropriate vehicle for fortification. The best solution is to provide a variety of fresh foods either by including them in the general ration or by promoting access to local markets. In addition, local cultivation of vitamin C-containing foods should be encouraged. Patients with clinical scurvy should be treated with 250 mg of oral vitamin C two times daily for 3 weeks.

Niacin. Maize-eating populations are at greatest risk for niacin deficiency, which causes pellagra. Recent studies of pellagra outbreaks among refugee populations found groundnut consumption, garden ownership, and home maize milling (as an indicator of higher socioeconomic status) to be protective factors. Niacin-fortified flour should be included in the general ration. The process of fortifying maize flour with niacin is simple and relatively inexpensive.

Clinical cases of pellagra can be treated with nicotinamide. The recommended treatment schedule is 100 mg three times daily for 3 weeks. The total daily dose of nicotinamide should not exceed 600 mg. Where the diet is deficient in niacin, vitamin B complex tablets can be used to prevent pellagra.

Iodine. If the general ration is naturally deficient of iodine, fortification of items such as salt or monosodium glutamate should be considered.

REFERENCES: AS NUMBERED IN ORIGINAL PUBLICATION

1. Peel S, Allegra DT, Knaub C, et al. Nutritional assessment and feeding programs in refugee centers: the Thailand experience. In: Allegra DT, Nieburg P, Grabe M, eds. Emergency refugee health care—a chronicle of the Khmer refugee-assistance operation 1979–1980. Atlanta: CDC, 1983:75–84.
2. Godfrey N. Supplementary feeding in refugee populations: comprehensive or selective feeding programmes? Health Policy Plan 1986;1:283–298.

SELECTED READING

Brown RE, Berry A. Prevention of malnutrition and supplementary feeding programs. In: Sandler RH, Jones TC, eds. Medical care of refugees. New York: Oxford University Press 1987:124.

CDC. Outbreak of pellagra among Mozambican refugees Malawi, 1990. MMWR 1991;40:209–213.

Desenclos JC, Berry AM, Padt R, Farah B, Segala C, Nabil AM. Epidemiological patterns of scurvy among Ethiopian refugees. Bull WHO 1989;67:309–316.

Nieburg P, Waldman RJ, Leavell R, Sommer A, DeMaeyer EM. Vitamin A supplementation for refugees and famine victims. Bull WHO 1988;66:689–697.

Peel S. Nutritional aspects of refugee assistance. In: Allegra DT, Nieburg P, Grabe M, eds. Emergency refugee health care—a chronicle of the Khmer refugee-assistance operation 1979–1980. Atlanta: CDC, 1983:121–127.

Peel S. Selective feeding procedures. Oxfam Working Paper no. 1. Oxford, 1979.

Seaman J, Rivers J. Strategies for the distribution of relief food. J R Statist Soc 1988;151:464–472.

United Nations Administrative Committee for Coordination, Subcommittee on Nutrition, and the International Nutrition Planners Forum. Nutrition in times of disaster. Presented as a report of an International Conference, September 27–30, 1988;Geneva, Switzerland.

UNHCR/WFP. Guidelines for calculation food rations for refugees. Geneva/Rome. August 1991.

Wallstam E, Nieburg P, Eie E, Lendorff A. Donated foods and their use in refugee-assistance operations. In: Allegra DT, Nieburg P, Grabe M, eds. Emergency refugee health care—a chronicle of the Khmer refugee-assistance operation 1979–1980. Atlanta: CDC, 1983:129–133.

Yip R, Gove S, Farah BH, Mursal HM. Rapid assessment of hematological status of refugees in Somalia: the potential value of hemoglobin distribution curves in assessing iron nutrition status. Presented at the APHA annual meeting, October 20, 1987.

Vaccine-Preventable Diseases

- Measles
- Diphtheria
- Pertussis
- Tetanus
- Polio
- Tuberculosis
- Meningitis

Overview

Only measles immunization should be part of the initial emergency relief effort; however, a complete EPI should be planned as an integral part of an ongoing long-term health program.

Diphtheria, tetanus toxoids (TT) and pertussis vaccine (DTP), oral polio vaccine (OPV), and bacille Calmette-Guerin (BCG) vaccinations are recommended. None should not be undertaken, however, unless the following criteria are met: the population is expected to remain stable for at least 3 months; the operational capacity to administer vaccine is adequate, and the program can be integrated into the national immunization program within a reasonable length of time.

It is essential that adequate immunization records be kept. At the very minimum, personal immunization cards (i.e., "Road to Health" cards) should be issued. In addition, a central register of all immunizations is desirable.

Measles

Priority

Measles vaccination campaigns should be assigned the highest priority early in emergency situations. Measles immunization programs should begin as soon as the necessary personnel, vaccine, cold chain equipment, and other supplies are available. Measles immunization should not be delayed until other vaccines become available or until cases of measles have been reported.

In refugee populations fleeing from countries with high immunization coverage rates, measles immunization should still be accorded high priority. Studies of urban populations (e.g., Kinshasa, Zaire) and densely populated refugee camps (e.g., camps in Malawi) have shown that large outbreaks of measles may still occur even if vaccine coverage rates exceed 80%. For example, in a camp of 50,000 refugees, approximately 10,000 would be children less than 5 years of age. If the vaccine coverage rate was 80% and vaccine efficacy was 90%, approximately 2,800 children in this camp would still be susceptible to measles. In addition, certain countries achieved high coverage in the 12 to 23 month age group, leaving large numbers of older children unprotected.

Program Management

Responsibilities for each aspect of the immunization program need to be explicitly assigned to agencies and persons by the coordination agency.

The national EPI should be involved from the outset of the emergency. National guidelines regarding immunization should be applied in refugee settings.

A pre-immunization count should be conducted to estimate the number of children eligible for vaccination. This should not be allowed, however, to delay the start of the vaccination program.

Choice of Vaccine

The standard Schwarz vaccine is recommended. The use of medium or high titer Edmonston-Zagreb (E-Z) vaccine is not yet recommended for refugee populations, since there are still concerns about its safety.

Target Population

During the emergency phase, defined as that time during which the CMR is higher than 1/10,000/day, all children ages 6 months-5 years should be vaccinated upon arrival at the camp.

In long-term refugee health programs, vaccination should be targeted at all children ages 9 months-5 years, except during outbreaks when the lower age limit should again be dropped to 6 months.

Any child who has been vaccinated between the ages of 6 and 9 months should be revaccinated as soon as possible after reaching 9 months of age, or 1 month later if the child was 8 months old at first vaccination.

If there is insufficient vaccine available to immunize all susceptible children, the immunization program should be targeted at the following high-risk groups, in order of priority:

- Undernourished or sick children ages 6 months-12 years who are enrolled in feeding centers or inpatient wards.
- All other children ages 6–23 months.
- All other children ages 24–59 months.

Older children, adolescents, and adults may also need to be immunized if surveillance data show that these groups are being affected during an outbreak.

Undernutrition is not a contraindication for measles vaccination! Undernutrition should be considered a strong indication for vaccination. Similarly, fever, respiratory tract infection, and diarrhea are not contraindications for measles vaccination. Unimmunized persons who are infected with HIV should receive the vaccine. Measles vaccine should also be administered in the presence of active TB (1).

Outbreak Control

Measles immunization programs should not be stopped or postponed because of the presence of measles in the camp or settlement. On the contrary, immunization efforts should be accelerated.

Among persons who have already been exposed to the measles virus, measles vaccine may provide some protection or modify the clinical severity of the disease, if administered within 3 days of exposure.

Isolation of patients with measles is not indicated in an emergency camp setting.

Case Management

All children who develop clinical measles in refugee camps should have their nutritional status monitored and be enrolled in a feeding program if indicated.

Children with measles complications should be administered standard treatment, e.g., ORT for diarrhea and antibiotics for acute lower respiratory infection (ALRI).

If they have not received vitamin A during the previous month, all children with clinical measles should receive 200,000 IU vitamin A orally. Children less than 12 months of age should receive 100,000 IU. This should be repeated every 3 months as part of the routine vitamin A supplementation schedule.

Children with complicated measles (pneumonia, otitis, croup, diarrhea with moderate or severe dehydration, or neurological problems) should receive a second dose of vitamin A on day 2.

If any eye symptoms of vitamin A deficiency are observed (xerosis, Bitot's spots, keratomalacia, or corneal ulceration), the following treatment schedule should be followed: 200,000 IU oral vitamin A on day 1; 200,000 IU oral vitamin A on day 2; 200,000 IU oral vitamin A 1–4 weeks later. Children less than 12 months of age receive half doses.

Diphtheria-Tetanus-Pertussis

Once a comprehensive EPI has been established, all children ages 6 weeks-5 years should receive three doses of DTP, 4–8 weeks apart.

Poliomyelitis

One dose of OPV should be administered at birth, followed by three doses 4–8 weeks apart to all children 6 weeks–5 years of age.

Tuberculosis

BCG vaccination should be offered as part of the comprehensive EPI, rather than as a separate TB program. One dose of BCG is administered subcutaneously at birth. Recommendations for TB control are presented in a separate section.

Neonatal Tetanus

All women between the ages of 15–44 years should receive a full schedule of TT vaccination. Vaccination should commence at a younger age if girls less than 15 years of age commonly bear children in the refugee community. TT vaccination should be included as part of a standard antenatal care program. Female health workers should be employed to educate women about the need for the TT vaccination and to refer pregnant women to the antenatal care clinic. Although WHO recommends a 5-dose schedule for TT vaccination (see "WHO Tetanus Toxoid Vaccination Schedule"), the number of doses of TT administered varies from country to country. The schedule in refugee camps should be consistent with host country national policies.

Meningococcal Meningitis

Surveillance

In areas where epidemics of meningococcal meningitis are known to occur, as in Africa's "meningitis belt," surveillance for meningitis should be a routine part of a HIS. Such surveillance requires a standard case definition, the identification (in advance) of laboratory facilities and a source of supplies (e.g., spinal needles, antiseptics, test tubes), and a clearly established reporting network.

Outbreak Identification and Control

If an outbreak of meningococcal meningitis is suspected, early priority should be given to the determination of etiology and serogroup. This may be accomplished through the use of latex agglutination tests. It is also important to determine antibiotic resistance patterns. Cerebral spinal fluid (CSF) or petechial washings should be placed in suitable transport media and kept at 37°C during transport to a local or regional laboratory with the capacity to perform the needed analysis. If transport media are unavailable, CSF specimens should be placed in a test tube and transported at body temperature as soon as possible.

After an outbreak has been confirmed, a presumptive diagnosis of meningococcal meningitis among persons with suggestive symptoms and signs can be made by visual inspection of CSF from lumbar punctures; CSF will appear cloudy in probable cases. Clinical characteristics include fever, severe headache, neck stiffness, vomiting, and photophobia.

Endemic rates of meningococcal disease vary by geographic area, season, and age; thus it is not possible to define a rate that can be applied universally to identify an epidemic disease. In one study, an average incidence rate of disease that exceeded 15 cases/100,000/week for a period of 2 consecutive weeks was predictive of an epidemic (defined as greater than 100 cases/100,000). Since this threshold may only be valid for populations greater than 100,000 and because the population in a refugee camp may be unknown, a doubling of the baseline number of cases from 1 week to the next over a period of 3 weeks may be used as a rough indicator of a meningitis outbreak.

Vaccination

Vaccination of refugees against meningococcal meningitis during non-epidemic periods is generally not considered to be an effective measure because of the short duration of protection in young children. If there are compelling reasons to believe that the refugee population is at high risk for an epidemic, preventive vaccination before the meningitis season may be warranted.

In the event of an outbreak, vaccination should be considered if the following criteria are met:

- The presence of meningococcal disease is laboratory confirmed.
- Serogrouping indicates the presence of group A or group C organisms.

* The disease is affecting children greater than 1 year of age (for group A) or greater than or equal to 2 years (for group C).

If it is logistically feasible, the household contacts of identified cases should be checked for vaccination status and immunized if necessary. It may be simpler to organize a mass immunization program.

Because cases of meningococcal meningitis are likely to cluster geographically within a refugee camp, it may be most efficient to focus the vaccination campaign on the affected area(s) first. Although the target group for immunization should be determined from the epidemiology of the specific outbreak, vaccination of children and young adults between the ages of 1–25 years will generally cover the at-risk population.

Chemoprophylaxis

Mass chemoprophylaxis is ineffective for control of epidemic meningococcal disease and is to be discouraged in a refugee setting.

If chemoprophylaxis is to be instituted, the following guidelines should be implemented:

* Chemoprophylaxis should be administered simultaneously to all members of a household where an infected person has been diagnosed to prevent reinfection. Recovering patients should receive chemoprophylaxis to eliminate carriage.
* Adults: 600 mg rifampicin twice a day for 2 days.
* Children greater than 1 month old: 10 mg/kg rifampicin twice a day for 2 days.
* Neonates: 5 mg/kg rifampicin twice a day for 2 days.

Rifampicin should not be administered to pregnant women. Patients should be warned that the drug will temporarily turn the urine and saliva orange.

Ceftriaxone and ciprofloxacin may be used as alternatives to rifampicin. These drugs, like rifampicin, are expensive and are generally not considered appropriate in a refugee setting. Because of widespread resistance, sulfonamides should not be used unless susceptibility tests show the organism to be sensitive. Widespread use of rifampicin may encourage drug resistance and could cause iatrogenic morbidity due to adverse drug reactions.

Treatment

IV-administered penicillin, which requires relatively intensive nursing care and medical equipment, is the treatment of choice for meningococcal disease in developed countries. However, in areas where such intensive care is not possible, a single intramuscular (IM) dose of long-acting chloramphenicol in oil suspension (Tifomycin) upon admission has been demonstrated to be effective. The dosage should be adjusted for age as follows:

* Greater than or equal to 15 years of age, 3.0 g (6 mL).
* 11–14 years of age, 2.5 g (5 mL).
* 7–10 years of age, 2.0 g (4 mL).

- 3–6 years of age, 1.5 g (3 mL).
- 1–2 years of age, 1.0 g (2 mL).
- less than 1 year old, 50 mg/kg.

In about 25% of cases, a second dose of chloramphenicol will be needed. Patients should be admitted as inpatients and monitored closely to determine whether the additional dose is required. The efficacy of this regimen of one or two doses of IM chloramphenicol has been proven in studies in both Europe and Africa.

Febrile seizures are common in small children, and acetaminophen (paracetamol) in either oral suspension or rectal suppositories should be administered to patients upon admission.

Typhoid and Cholera

Vaccination for typhoid or cholera is not recommended in refugee situations. The resources required for such a campaign are better spent on improving sanitation conditions (see "Diarrheal Diseases").

SELECTED READING

CDC monograph. Allegra DT, Nieburg P, Eriksen H, Thousig O, Grabe M. Measles Outbreak, Khao I-Dang Refugee Camp, Thailand. In: Allegra DT, Nieburg P, Brabe M, eds. Emergency refugee health-care—a chronicle of experience in the Khmer assistance operation 1979–1980. Atlanta, GA: CDC, 1983:49–55.
Moore PS, Toole MJ, Nieburg P, Waldman RJ, Broome CV. Surveillance and control of meningococcal meningitis epidemics in refugee populations. Bull WHO 1990;68:587–596.
CDC monograph. Preblud SR, Horan JM, Davis CE. Meningococcal disease among Khmer refugees in Thailand. In: Allegra DT, Nieburg P, Brabe M, eds. Emergency refugee health-care—a chronicle of experience in the Khmer assistance operation 1979–1980. Atlanta, GA: CDC, 1983:65–9.
CDC monograph. Preblud SR, Nieburg P, Allegra DT. Vaccination programs for refugees. In: Allegra DT, Nieburg P, Brabe M, eds. Emergency refugee health-care—a chronicle of experience in the Khmer assistance operation 1979–1980. Atlanta, GA: CDC, 1983:135–140.
CDC monograph. Toole MJ, Foster S. Famines. In: Gregg MB, ed. The public health consequences of disasters 1989. Atlanta, GA: CDC, 1989:85.
United Nations Children's Fund (UNICEF). Assisting in emergencies: a resource handbook for UNICEF field staff. New York: United Nations Children's Fund, 1986:269–277.

Diarrheal Diseases

The critical elements of a diarrheal disease control program in a refugee camp are: (a) prevention of morbidity, (b) prevention of mortality through appropriate case management, (c) surveillance for morbidity and mortality attributed to diarrheal diseases, and (d) preparedness for outbreaks of severe diarrheal diseases (e.g., cholera and dysentery). The objectives of a camp diarrheal diseases control program should include the following:

- Maintaining the incidence of diarrheal cases at less than 1% per month.
- Achieving a CFR of less than 1% for diarrheal cases, including cholera.

Prevention

Efforts aimed at reducing the incidence of diarrheal diseases and other enterically transmitted diseases should focus primarily on the provision of adequate quantities of clean water, improvements in camp sanitation, promotion of breast-feeding, and personal hygiene education.

The following recommendations relating to water and sanitation are largely based on the UNHCR Handbook for Emergencies (1) and Environmental Health Engineering in the Tropics (2).

Water

In general, the supply of adequate quantities of water to refugees in a camp setting has greater overall impact on health than a supply of small quantities of microbially pure water. The provision of adequate quantities of water is particularly effective in the prevention of bacillary dysentery. Nevertheless, whenever possible, sources of clean water should be sought or disinfection systems established. An additional health benefit derived from the provision of ample supplies of water, at a convenient distance from the camp, is the decrease in the daily workload of women, upon whom the burden of water collection usually falls.

Appropriate water sources should be identified before refugees arrive in an area. An adequate water supply is a crucial component of attempts to prevent disease and protect health and, as such, should be among the highest priorities for camp planners and administrators.

Standards. WHO has set standards for the microbiological quality of water supplies. These are as follows:

- For treated water supplies, the water entering the system should be free from coliforms. The water at the tap should be free of coliforms in 95% of samples taken over a 1-year period and should never have greater than 10 coliforms/100 mL. E. coli should never be present in the water.
- For untreated water supplies, less than 10 coliforms/100 mL and no evidence of E. coli.

The water quality should be tested before using a water source, at regular intervals thereafter, and during any outbreak of diarrheal disease in which the water source may be implicated. Sources. Whatever water source is chosen, it must be protected from contamination. Safety measures include:

- Springs protected by a spring box.
- Wells equipped with a well head, drainage apron, and a pulley, windlass, or pump.
- Surface water, such as lakes, dams, or rivers, provided there is a large mass of moving water. If surface water is to be used, water for drinking should be drawn upstream, away from obvious sources of contamination.
- Rainwater is not generally a practical source in a refugee setting.

Treatment. The selection of a water source should take into consideration the potential need for water treatment. Whether or not treatment is needed, the water should be tested routinely to ensure that it is of suitable quality.

When surface water is used as a communal source, covered storage will allow suspended particles to settle on the bottom, improving the quality of the water. Longer standing times and higher temperatures will yield a greater improvement in water quality.

Filtration and chlorination may require considerable effort and resources, but should be considered if the situation warrants.

Although boiling is an effective means of removing water pathogens, it is not generally a practical solution in refugee camps where fuel supplies are limited.

As a short-term measure during an emergency (e.g., a cholera outbreak, and when treatment of all water sources is not feasible), purification agents (such as chlorine) may be distributed to each household. In this way, water can be treated in household storage containers. However, a massive education effort is required and such measures usually cannot be maintained for longer than a few weeks.

Water storage containers with narrow necks or covers that prevent people from introducing their hands into the container are likely to reduce further contamination of water once it is stored in the home. The use of separate containers to store water for drinking and water for washing is preferable.

Supply. The chosen water supply should be adequate to meet the needs of the camp year-round. Seasonal variations in rainfall and in camp population should be taken into consideration when selecting a water source.

The UNHCR recommends that a minimum quantity of 20 L of water/person/day be provided. Health clinics, feeding centers, and hospitals require 40–60 L/patient/day.

Ideally, no individual dwelling should be located greater than 150 m from a water source. At any greater distance, the use of water for hygiene is greatly diminished.

Sanitation

Camp sanitation plans should be drawn up before refugees arrive. Because of the crucial role it plays in disease prevention, sanitation should be an early priority for camp planners.

Community attitudes and cultural practices regarding sanitation and disposal of excreta are vital to the success of a sanitation project and should be taken into careful consideration.

All efforts should be made to separate garbage and human waste from water and food supplies. Excreta should be contained within a specific area. Defecation fields may be used as a short-term measure until a more appropriate sanitation system can be implemented. This is particularly suitable in hot, dry climates.

The design and installation of latrines should also take into consideration the attitudes and practices of the refugee population. Latrines should be located so as to remove the possibility of contamination of the water source.

Latrines that are poorly maintained will not be used. For this reason, personal or family latrines are the best solution. However, limitations on building supplies, money, and space may make this impossible. If communal latrines are to be used, no more than 20 people should share one latrine and responsibility for maintaining cleanliness should be clearly assigned.

Breast-feeding

Breast-feeding is an effective measure for preventing diarrheal illness among infants. Exclusive breast-feeding for the first 4–6 months of a baby's life, and continued breast-feeding until the child is 2 years of age, should be encouraged through educational campaigns targeted at pregnant and lactating women. Distribution of milk products should be restricted, and feeding bottles should never be distributed within a camp (see "Nutrition").

Personal Hygiene

Community health education should reinforce the importance of handwashing with soap and of general domestic and personal hygiene, in particular safe food-handling practices. Soap should be made readily available by relief agencies.

Case Management

Assessment (see "Patient Assessment"). An adequate history should be taken from the patient or the patient's family. The duration of illness; quantity, frequency, and consistency of stool; presence or absence of blood in the stool; frequency of vomiting; and the presence of fever or convulsions should be assessed.

Assessment of dehydration and fluid deficit through careful physical examination should receive particular attention. Fever, rapid breathing, and hypovolemic shock may accompany severe dehydration.

Careful monitoring of the patient's weight and the signs of dehydration throughout the course of therapy will help assess the adequacy of rehydration. Adults with acute, dehydrating diarrhea should be carefully assessed by a physician to rule out cholera.

Management of Patients

In the camp setting, all patients with diarrhea should be encouraged to report to a clinic or health post for assessment, advice on feeding, fluid intake, and diarrhea prevention. The treatment of dehydration should always be initiated in the clinic. Ideally, a central clinic should be supplemented with several small ORT centers in the camp, staffed by trained community health workers.

Prevention of Dehydration

Case management should focus on the prevention of dehydration under two sets of circumstances: (a) when a patient with diarrhea shows no signs of dehydration, (b) when a patient has already been treated for dehydration in the ORT corner and is being released from medical care. Management of patients in these situations includes the following.

ORS. Mothers should be shown how to mix and give ORS and initially be given a 2-day supply. The amount to be given at home is as follows.

- Children less than 2 years old: 50–100 mL (¼ to ½ large cup) of ORS solution after each stool.

- Older children: 100–200 mL after each stool.
- Adults: As much as they want; however, dehydrated adults who fail to respond promptly to ORS should be reassessed to exclude cholera.

Increased fluids.   Patients should be instructed to increase their normal intake of fluids. Any locally available fluids known to prevent dehydration, especially those that can be prepared in the home (e.g., cereal-based gruels, soup, and rice water), should be encouraged. Soft drinks are not recommended because of their high osmolality.

Continued feeding.   Infants who are breast-fed should continue to receive breast milk. If an infant is receiving milk formula in a feeding center, the milk should be diluted with an equal volume of clean water until the diarrhea stops.
For children greater than 4–6 months of age:

- Give freshly prepared foods, including mixes of cereal and beans or cereal and meat, with a few drops of vegetable oil added.
- Offer food every 3–4 hours or more often for very young children.
- Encourage the child to eat as much as he or she wants.
- After the diarrhea stops, give one extra meal each day for a week.

Monitor condition.   The mother should be advised to return to the clinic with the child if he/she continues to pass many stools, is very thirsty, has sunken eyes, has a fever, or does not generally seem to be getting better.

Management of the Dehydrated Patient

Every health center in a refugee camp should have an area allocated for supervised oral rehydration (see "Guidelines for Rehydration Therapy"). Staff assigned to this activity need to be well-trained in the assessment and treatment of the dehydrated patient. Individual patients should be monitored to determine whether the recommended doses are adequate for their needs or whether rehydration proceeds faster than is expected.

For babies who are unable to drink but are not in shock, a nasogastric tube can be used to administer ORS solution at the rate of 15 mL/kg body weight/ hour. For infants in shock, a nasogastric tube should be used only if IV equipment and fluids are not available.

Reassessment

The patient's hydration status should be reassessed after 3–4 hours, and treatment continued according to the degree of dehydration at that time. Note: If the child is still dehydrated, rehydration should continue in the center. The mother should offer the child small amounts of food.

If the child is less than 12 months of age, the mother should be advised to continue breast-feeding. If the child is not being breast-fed, 100–200 mL of clean, plain water should be given before continuing the ORS. Older children and adults should consume plain water as often as they wish throughout the course of rehydration with ORS solution.

Nutritional Maintenance

Infants should resume feeding as outlined above. For children greater than 4–6 months old and adults, feeding should begin as soon as the appetite returns. Energy-rich, easily digestible foods will help maintain their nutritional status. There is no reason to delay feeding until the diarrhea stops and there is no justification for "resting" the bowel through fasting. Note: Children enrolled in SFPs or TFPs who develop diarrhea with dehydration should be fed HEM diluted with ORS in a ratio of 1:1, alternating with plain ORS. The overall volume of fluid should be calculated according to the child's weight and degree of dehydration.

Use of Chemotherapy

Antimicrobial drugs are contraindicated for the routine treatment of uncomplicated, watery diarrhea. Specific indications for their use include:

- Cholera.
- Shigella dysentery.
- Amoebic dysentery.
- Acute giardiasis.

For specific recommendations see "Cholera" and "Dysentery".

Anti-diarrheal agents are contraindicated for the treatment of diarrheal disease. Stimulants, steroids, and purgatives are not indicated for treatment of diarrheal disease and may produce adverse effects.

Surveillance for Diarrheal Diseases

All health facilities that serve the refugee population should maintain case records of diarrheal diseases as part of the routine HIS. Records should include the degree of dehydration at the time of presentation. Case definitions should be standardized. Dysentery cases should be recorded as a separate category.

Any increase in the number or severity of cases, change in the type of diarrhea, rise in diarrhea-specific mortality, or change in the demographic breakdown of the cases should be reported. A case definition for cholera should be established for the purpose of surveillance. Any suspected cholera cases should be reported immediately.

Sample case definitions for cholera and dysentery are provided below.

Cholera

Identification of the pathogen by laboratory culture is necessary to confirm the presence of cholera. Initially, rectal swabs of patients with suspected cholera should be transported to the laboratory in Cary-Blair transport medium (see Collecting, Processing, Storing and Shipping Diagnostic Specimens in Refugee Health-Care Environments, available from IHPO, CDC, 1600 Clifton Road, MS F-03, Atlanta, GA 30333, 404–639-0308.). The laboratory should determine the antibiotic sensitivity of the cultured strain. Once an outbreak is confirmed, it is not necessary to culture every case. Additionally, it is not necessary to wait until an outbreak has been confirmed to begin treatment and preventive measures.

Epidemics

In the event of an outbreak of cholera, early case-finding will allow for rapid initiation of treatment. Aggressive case-finding by trained community health workers should be coupled with community education to prevent panic and to promote good domestic hygiene.

Treatment centers should be easily accessible. Most patients can be treated with ORS alone in the local clinic and still achieve a CFR less than 1%. If the attack rate for cholera is high, it may be necessary to establish temporary cholera wards to handle the patient load. Health centers should be adequately stocked with ORS, IV fluids, and appropriate antibiotics. Health workers must be trained in the management of cholera.

Surveillance should be intensified and should change from passive to active case-finding. The number of new cholera cases and deaths should be reported daily, along with other relevant information (e.g., age, sex, location in camp, length of stay in camp).

Treatment

The goal of cholera treatment is to maintain the CFR at less than 1%.

Rehydration Therapy

Rehydration needs to be aggressive. However, careful supervision is necessary to prevent fluid overload, especially when children are rehydrated with IV fluids. Most cases of cholera can be treated through the administration of ORS solution (see "Patient Assessment" and "Guidelines for Rehydration Therapy"). Persons with severe disease may require IV fluid, which should be administered following the guidelines outlined in "Diarrheal Diseases".

Antibiotics

Antibiotics reduce the volume and duration of diarrhea in cholera patients. Antibiotics should be administered orally. Doxycycline should be used when available in a single dose of 300 mg for adults and 6 mg/kg/day for children less than 15 years of age. Tetracycline should be reserved for severely dehydrated persons, who are the most efficient transmitters because of their greater fecal losses. Tetracycline should be administered according to the following schedule.

- Adults: 500 mg every 6 hours for 72 hours
- Children: 50 mg/kg/day every 6 hours for 72 hours

Chloramphenicol can be used as an alternative to tetracycline; the dosage is the same. When tetracycline and chloramphenicol resistance is present, furazolidone, erythromycin, or trimethoprim-sulfamethoxazole (TMP-SMX) may be used.

Epidemiologic Investigation

Epidemiologic studies to determine the extent of the outbreak and the primary modes of transmission should be conducted so that specific control measures can be applied. The CFR should be monitored closely to evaluate the quality of treatment.

Case-control studies may be undertaken to identify risk factors for infection. Environmental sampling, examination of food, and the use of Moore swabs for sewage sampling may be useful to confirm the results of epidemiologic studies and define modes of transmission.

Control and Prevention

Health education. The community should be kept informed as to the extent and severity of the outbreak, as well as educated on the ease and effectiveness of treatment. Emphasis should be placed on the benefits of prompt reporting and early treatment. The community should be advised about suspected vehicles of transmission. The need for good sanitation, personal hygiene, and food safety should be stressed. Health workers involved in treating cholera patients need to observe strict personal hygiene, by washing their hands with soap after examining each patient. Smoking should be prohibited in cholera wards and clinics.

Water supply. Any water supplies implicated through epidemiologic studies should be tested. Any contaminated water sources should be identified and access to those sources cut off. Alternative sources of safe drinking water should be identified and developed as a matter of urgency.

Food safety. Community members should be informed of any food item that has been implicated as a possible vehicle of transmission. Health education messages regarding food preparation and storage should be disseminated.

During an outbreak, feeding centers should be extremely vigilant in the preparation of meals because of the potential for mass infection. Food workers should have easy access to soap and water for handwashing. Food workers should always wash their hands after defecating, and any food worker who is experiencing diarrhea should be prohibited from working.

Chemoprophylaxis. Mass chemoprophylaxis is not an effective cholera control measure and is not recommended. Although the WHO Guidelines for Cholera Control suggest that chemoprophylaxis may be justified for closed groups (such as refugee camps), CDC studies indicate that focusing on other preventive activities (i.e., providing an adequate water supply, improving camp sanitation, and providing adequate and prompt treatment) results in a more effective use of resources. If resources are adequate and transmission rates are high (greater than 15%), consideration should be given to providing a single dose of doxycycline to immediate family members of diagnosed patients.

Vaccines. Currently available vaccines are not recommended for the control of cholera among refugee populations. The efficacy of these vaccines is low and the duration of protection provided is short. Vaccination campaigns divert funds and personnel from more important cholera control activities and give refugee and surrounding populations a false sense of security.

Dysentery

When possible, patients presenting with signs and symptoms of dysentery should have stool specimens examined by microscopy to identify Entamoeba histolytica. Care should be taken to distinguish large white cells (a nonspecific indicator of dysentery) from trophozoites. Amebic dysentery tends to be misdiagnosed.

Shigellosis

If a microscope is unavailable for diagnosis, or if definite trophozoites are not seen, persons with bloody diarrhea should be treated initially for shigellosis. Appropriate treatment with antimicrobial drugs decreases the severity and duration of dysentery caused by Shigella and reduces the duration of pathogen excretion. The selection of an antimicrobial treatment regimen is often complicated by the presence of multiresistant strains of Shigella. The choice of a first-line drug should be based on knowledge of local susceptibility patterns. If no clinical response occurs within 2 days, the antibiotic should be changed to another recommended for that particular strain of shigellosis. If no improvement occurs after an additional 2 days of treatment, the patient should be referred to a hospital or laboratory for stool microscopy. At this stage, a diagnosis of resistant shigellosis is still more likely than amebiasis.

Drugs of Choice

Treatment guidelines for shigellosis are listed below.

- Ampicillin
- Children: 100 mg/kg/day in four divided doses for 5 days.
- Adults: 500 mg four times daily for 5 days
- TMP-SMX
- Children: 10 mg/kg/day TMP and 50 mg/kg/day SMX in two divided doses for 5 days.
- Adults: 160 mg TMP and 800 mg SMX twice daily for 5 days.

For strains resistant to these regimens, alternative treatment with nalidixic acid or tetracycline is indicated.

- Nalidixic acid
- 55 mg/kg/day in four divided doses for 5 days.
- Tetracycline
- 50 mg/kg/day in four divided doses for 5 days.

The fluoroquinolones (e.g., ciprofloxacin and ofloxacin) are highly effective for the treatment of shigellosis, but are expensive and have not yet been approved for treatment of children or pregnant or lactating women with shigellosis.

Because multiresistant strains of Shigella have become widespread and because Shigella strains can rapidly acquire resistance in epidemic settings, it is advisable that periodic antibiotic susceptibility testing be performed by a reference laboratory in the region. Note: WHO does not recommend mass prophylaxis or prophylaxis of family members as a control measure for shigellosis.

Amebiasis and Giardiasis

Treatment for amebiasis or giardiasis should not be considered unless microscopic examination of fresh feces shows amebic or Giardia trophozoites, or two different antibiotics given for shigellosis have not resulted in clinical improvement.

Treatment guidelines for amebiasis are as follows:

- Metronidazole
- Children: 30 mg/kg/day for 5–10 days.
- Adults: 750 mg/3 times/day for 5–10 days.

Treatment guidelines for giardiasis are as follows:

- Metronidazole
- Children: 15 mg/kg/day for 5 days.
- Adults: 250 mg/3 times/day for 5 days.

REFERENCES: AS NUMBERED IN ORIGINAL PUBLICATION

1.   United Nations High Commissioner for Refugees. Handbook for emergencies. Geneva, 1982.
2.   Cairncross S, Feachem RG. Environmental health engineering in the tropics: an introductory text. New York: John Wiley & Sons Ltd., 1983:28–33.

SELECTED READING

World Health Organization. A manual for the treatment of acute diarrhoea. 3rd ed. Geneva: Diarrhoeal Diseases Control Programme, 1990.
CDC. Shigella dysenteriae Type 1—Guatemala, 1991. MMWR 1991;40:421, 427–428.
Keusch GT, Bennish ML. Shigellosis: recent progress, persisting problems and research issues. Pediatr Infect Dis J 1989;8:713–719.
Smith M. Water and sanitation for disasters. Trop Doct 1991;21(Suppl 1):30–37.
World Health Organization. Guidelines for cholera control. 1991;80.4;Rev. 2.

Malaria

Knowledge of the epidemiology of transmission, including local vectors, is essential to a malaria control effort. Information regarding the local epidemiology may be available from the MOH, WHO, and regional health authorities. In certain instances, a vector survey may need to be done. The national malaria control program or WHO staff are often able to conduct such surveys.

Information on previous exposure can be obtained from the refugees themselves, or more detailed information on previous exposure to specific species can be obtained through international channels via WHO.

Within a camp, the proportion of fever illness attributable to malaria at a particular time can be determined by obtaining thick and thin blood smears from a sample of consecutive clinic patients with a history of recent fever (e.g., 50 children less than 5 years of age). The malaria infection prevalence rate among these patients can then be compared with a control group that is free of the signs and symptoms of malaria.

Laboratory examination will determine whether malaria illness is caused by Plasmodium falciparum or Plasmodium vivax.

Control of Transmission

Control of malaria transmission may be achieved through a combination of the following strategies.

Personal Protection

The use of protective clothing, insecticide-impregnated bed nets, and insect repellents will help limit human exposure to malaria-infected mosquitoes.

Residual Insecticides

Periodic spraying of the inside surfaces of permanent dwellings may reduce transmission. The use of residual insecticides, however, may be toxic to those involved in spraying and can also be detrimental to the environment. Spraying can be expensive and time consuming. Careful consideration should be given to the technical aspects of spraying, local vector behavior and susceptibility, personnel training, safety, and community motivation before undertaking such a program.

Source Reduction

The elimination of breeding sites by draining or filling may reduce the density of vectors in the area. Knowledge of the local vectors is essential to ensure that source reduction efforts are effectively targeted.

Ultra low-volume insecticide spraying. Adult mosquitoes may be killed through frequent fogging with nonresidual insecticides. Fogging is generally repeated on a daily basis.

Gametocidal drug use. Gametocidal drugs (e.g., primaquine) are not generally recommended for use in refugee camps.

Selection of control strategies will depend upon the local epidemiologic factors, availability of resources, and environmental and cultural factors.

Case Management

Case Definition

Malaria infection is defined as the presence of malaria parasites in the peripheral blood smear. Malaria illness is defined as the presence of "malaria signs and symptoms" in the presence of malaria infection. The signs and symptoms of malaria typically include fever, chills, body aches, and headache.

Diagnosis

If possible, a thick blood smear and Giemsa stain should be the basis for the diagnosis of malaria. These smears will also provide the basis for transmission surveillance in camps or geographic areas. If the patient load exceeds the capability of the laboratory to perform thick smears on all suspected cases, a system of microscopic diagnosis for a percentage of suspected cases should be established. When diagnoses are made by locally trained microscopists in small field laboratories, a randomly selected sample of both positive and negative slides should be sent to a reference laboratory for verification in order to maintain quality control.

When laboratory facilities are not available, clinical symptoms (paroxysmal fever, chills, sweats, and headache) and signs (measured fever) are the best predictors of malaria infection. In situations in which year-round high malaria endemicity has been established, all episodes of fever illness can be assumed to be caused by Plasmodium falciparum. However, health workers should bear in mind other causes of fever, including pneumonia, ALRI, or meningitis. In areas where transmission is highly seasonal, surveys should be conducted each year at the beginning of the high transmission season.

The presence of Plasmodium on blood smears does not prove that malaria is the cause of febrile illness, even in areas where malaria is highly prevalent. Other causes should be considered and ruled out.

Treatment with Chemotherapy

In areas without chloroquine resistance, the oral regimen of chloroquine usually employed in the treatment of uncomplicated attacks of malaria is as follows:

- Adults: A total dose of 1,500 mg chloroquine (approximately 25 mg/kg body weight) should be given during a 3-day period. This can be given as 600 mg, 600 mg, and 300 mg at 0, 24, and 48 hours, respectively.
- Pregnant women: Pregnant women with malaria should be treated aggressively using the regimen for adults. Chloroquine is safe during pregnancy. (Quinine is also safe although pregnant women receiving IV-administered quinine should be monitored carefully for hypoglycemia.)
- Children: A total dose of 25 mg/kg body weight chloroquine should be given during a 3-day period. This can be administered as 10 mg/kg, 10 mg/kg, and 5 mg/kg body weight at 0, 24 and 48 hours, respectively.

In areas where the likelihood of reinfection is low, consideration may be given to supplementation of chloroquine treatment with primaquine for persons infected with Plasmodium vivax.

- Adults: 15 mg daily for 14 days.
- Children: 0.3 mg/kg/day.

Among populations in which severe glucose-6-phosphate dehydrogenase (G-6-PD) deficiency is common (notably among Asians), however, primaquine should not be administered for greater than 5 days. Administration of primaquine for longer periods may result in life-threatening hemolysis. Whenever possible, persons needing primaquine should first have a blood test for G-6-PD deficiency.

When laboratory analysis is performed, the first dose of chloroquine should be administered when the blood smear is taken. The patient should be instructed to return the second day for the results of the smear. If the smear is positive, chemotherapy should be continued. If the smear is negative and the patient remains febrile, other causes of fever should be identified.

If supervised therapy during a 3-day period is not possible, the first dose of chloroquine should be given under supervision and the additional doses may be given to the patient with appropriate instructions.

Patients who remain symptomatic longer than 3 days into therapy should have a repeat thick smear examined. Alternative therapy should be instituted if the degree of parasitemia has not diminished markedly by this time.

In areas with chloroquine resistance, treatment of patients may be the same as in areas of chloroquine-sensitive malaria; or may include an alternative first-line drug. Additional care in the follow-up of patients is required.

- If the patient continues to have symptoms of malaria after 48–72 hours from the start of recommended chloroquine treatment, the patient should be treated with a second-line drug.
- The choice of an alternative drug depends on the availability of the drugs and the relative sensitivity of the parasites. Possible alternative drugs include sulfa drugs in combination with pyrimethamine (Fansidar, Maloprim), tetracycline, quinine, and newer drugs such as mefloquine. Use of alternative drugs should be consistent with national malaria control policies in the host country.

Fever Control

Antipyretics (i.e., acetaminophen, paracetamol) and anticonvulsives are often necessary for the care of the patient with malaria.

Children with high fevers should be frequently sponged with tepid water. Patients should increase their intake of fluids as the febrile illness will most likely be accompanied by mild dehydration. Patients with signs of moderate dehydration should be given ORS.

Chemoprophylaxis

During epidemics (seasons of high rates of transmission), malaria chemoprophylaxis should be considered for the following high-risk groups:

- Children less than 5 years of age, especially those suffering from malnutrition, anemia, or other debilitating diseases.
- Pregnant women.
- Other groups that are at increased risk for complications of malaria illness due to compromised health status.

The decision to provide chemoprophylaxis to high-risk persons should be based upon the capabilities of the health-care system to accomplish the following:

- At-risk persons can be readily identified and assembled.
- Follow-up can be assured.
- Sufficient personnel and medication are available to ensure regular administration of services.
- The parasite is known to be generally sensitive to the drug used.

Administration of chemoprophylaxis to high-risk groups can be logistically difficult and may be too great a strain on the capacities of the health-care system to be feasible.

Expatriates working in an endemic area should be on weekly chloroquine (300 mg chloroquine base) during the entire period of exposure and for an additional 6 weeks after leaving the area. In areas where chloroquine resistance is documented, prophylaxis with mefloquine is recommended (250 mg weekly dose).

Severe Malaria

Severe malaria is considered a medical emergency and demands prompt and specific medical care. Signs and symptoms of severe malaria include:

- Severe anemia.
- Hemoglobinuria, oliguria, or anuria.
- Hypotension and respiratory distress.
- Jaundice.
- Hemorrhagic diatheses.
- Cerebral malaria.

Signs of abnormal central nervous system (CNS) function, which may be present in cerebral malaria, include drowsiness, mental confusion, coma, and seizures.

Management of Severe Malaria

The following guidelines for the management of severe malaria are based upon those prepared by the MOH in Malawi.

Outpatient setting. If severe malaria is diagnosed in an outpatient setting, the patient should be referred for hospitalization. However, treatment should begin immediately and not be delayed until the patient has been transferred.

If the patient can swallow, sulfadoxine-pyrimethamine (SP) tablets (500 mg-25 mg) should be administered orally in the following doses according to the patient's age.

- Less than 3 years old: ¼ tablet
- 4–8 years old: 1 tablet
- 9–14 years old: 2 tablets
- Greater than 14 years old: 3 tablets

If the patient vomits within 30 minutes, the dose should be repeated.

If the patient cannot swallow or is vomiting repeatedly, an IM injection of quinine dihydrochloride (10 mg/kg) should be administered. This can be repeated every 4 hours for two additional doses, and every 8 hours thereafter if a long delay is anticipated for transport of the patient to a hospital.

The patient's fever should be reduced by sponging with lukewarm water or by using paracetamol or aspirin. Patients should be given ORS. In a patient who cannot drink, administer 20 mL/kg ORS with one teaspoon of glucose powder via naso-gastric tube every 4 hours.

If convulsions occur, administer 0.2 mL/kg paraldehyde by IM injection. If convulsions recur, repeat the treatment. If convulsions persist, give the patient a phenobarbitone 10-mg/kg IM injection.

In a child with altered consciousness or repeated convulsions, the physician should perform a lumbar puncture if possible. If the CSF is cloudy, treatment for meningococcal meningitis is indicated and anti-malarial treatment should be discontinued. If a lumbar puncture cannot be performed, treatment for meningitis should be administered while continuing treatment for malaria.

Inpatient Setting

The following tests should be performed immediately upon admission: thick blood film, hemoglobin, blood glucose, and lumbar puncture. If hemoglobin is below 4 g/dL, blood grouping and cross-matching should be done.

If the patient can swallow, give oral SP as described above. If the patient cannot swallow or has persistent vomiting, give IV-administered quinine as follows:

- An initial dose of 20 mg(salt)/kg body weight is injected into 10 mL/kg 5% dextrose (half-strength Darrow's solution) and infused during a 3-hour period. (If the patient has already received quinine before admission, the initial dose should be 10 mg/kg.)
- Subsequent doses of 10 mg/kg should be repeated as above every 12 hours. In between doses of quinine, the IV fluid (10 mL/kg during a 3-hour period) should be continued. Patients should be switched to oral medications as soon as their conditions allow.

In the presence of signs of volume depletion, fluid (which includes dextrose) should be administered to maintain cardiac output and renal perfusion.

- Care in the administration of fluid therapy is required, since fluid overload can precipitate pulmonary edema or adult respiratory distress syndrome (ARDS), which can worsen cerebral edema.
- The IV fluid of choice is 5% dextrose with ½ normal saline, since this mixture provides dextrose to prevent hypoglycemia and less salt to leak into pulmonary and cerebral tissues. Alternative IV fluids should be considered if this is unavailable.

Hypoglycemia is a complicating factor in patients with cerebral malaria and a risk factor for fatal outcome. When possible, blood glucose levels should be monitored. Hypoglycemia should be suspected whenever there is a deterioration in clinical status, especially in the presence of new neurologic findings. Hypoglycemia can be treated presumptively with 50 mL of 50% IV dextrose.

Blood transfusion is indicated when Hb less than 4 g/dL, or Hb less than 6 g/dL is detected and the patient has signs of heart failure (i.e., dyspnea, enlarging liver, gallop rhythm).

The administration of steroids has an adverse effect on outcome in cerebral malaria. Therefore, steroids are no longer recommended.

Anemia

Most anemias caused by malaria will reverse spontaneously after anti-malarial therapy. However, anemia may progress for several weeks after successful treatment of severe malaria and may require treatment.

For some patients (especially children), blood transfusion may be lifesaving. Recent studies indicate that blood transfusion should be given for Hb less than 4 g/dL or Hb less than 6 g/dL in the presence of symptoms of respiratory distress. Because of the potential for HIV or hepatitis B transmission, blood transfusion should be reserved for medical emergencies for which no alternative treatment exists. Facilities for screening blood for HIV antibodies are rare in refugee camps. Whenever feasible, patients requiring transfusion should be transferred to hospitals where such facilities exist.

The anemia of malaria is not associated with iron loss, and replacement is helpful only if a coexisting iron deficiency exists. Folic acid replacement may be helpful during the recovery period when rapid erythrocyte replacement occurs.

Renal Failure

Replacement of fluid losses (sweat, vomit, and diarrhea) is recommended to prevent renal failure. If renal failure is suspected, strict monitoring of fluid intake and output is necessary.

In the presence of oliguria, a fluid challenge followed by furosemide injection can help to differentiate acute renal failure from prerenal causes. If renal failure is demonstrated, fluid intake must be limited to daily replacement of insensible loss plus urine/vomitus volume in the previous 24 hours. Protein intake should be limited to less than 30 mg/day, and all drug doses should be adjusted for renal failure.

SELECTED READING

Ministry of Health. Malawi guidelines for the management of malaria. Malawi, October 1991.
CDC. Steketee RW, Campbell CC. Control of malaria among refugees and displaced persons. Atlanta, GA: CDC, 1988 (unpublished).

Tuberculosis

The TB control program should establish a policy covering areas of case definition, case-finding, treatment regimen, and the supervision of chemotherapy. This policy should be agreed upon and adhered to by all organizations and agencies providing health services to the refugees. During the emergency phase of a refugee relief operation, TB activities should be limited to the treatment of patients who present themselves to the health-care system and in whom tubercle bacilli have been demonstrated by sputum smear examination.

Control of Transmission

Target Population

Because of the limited resources available, efforts to control transmission of TB within a refugee settlement should focus on the primary sources of infection, i.e., those patients for whom microscopic analysis of sputum smears demonstrates the presence of acid-fast bacilli (AFB). (Specimens should be stained using the Ziehl-Neelsen method with the results graded quantitatively.)

Case Identification

Passive case-finding will be most efficient in the refugee setting. Patients with respiratory symptoms (chest pain, cough) of greater than 3 weeks' duration, hemoptysis of any duration, or significant weight loss should have a direct microscopic examination of their sputum for AFB. If the sputum smear is negative for AFB but pulmonary TB is still suspected, the patient should be given a 10-day course of antibiotics and then be re-examined after 2–4 weeks. Specific anti-TB chemotherapy should not begin unless the presence of AFB has been confirmed. Symptomatic family members of an identified patient should also have sputum specimens examined.

Children who show signs and symptoms compatible with TB and who are either: (a) a close contact of a patient with a confirmed case of TB, or (b) tuberculin skin-test positive (in the absence of a BCG vaccination scar) should undergo a full course of anti-TB treatment if they do not respond to an appropriate regimen of alternative antibiotics.

Case Management

The selection of a first-line chemotherapy regimen should generally be consistent with the national policy set forth by the host country MOH. However, it should be recognized that the crowded conditions of a refugee camp may foster an abnormally high rate of transmission. Additionally, uncertainty exists regarding the duration of stay in the country of asylum, and it may be more difficult to maintain adherence to an extended therapy regimen. Short-course therapy (6 months) should be considered for use in a refugee camp even when the national policy prescribes a longer course of treatment, provided the additional expense is not prohibitive.

Before enrolling refugees in a TB treatment program, consideration should be given to the stability of the populations and the capacity of the health-care program to supervise therapy and to follow-up patients who do not adhere to treatment. Administration of anti-TB drugs to persons in whom adherence is likely to be sporadic will foster increased drug resistance in that population.

The following drugs are used for the treatment of TB with chemotherapy: isoniazid, rifampin, pyrazinamide, streptomycin, ethambutol, and thiacetazone. The selection of a particular treatment regimen must take into consideration the organism susceptibility, cost, and duration of therapy. The decision regarding implementation of a specific therapeutic regimen will generally be made by the UNHCR in consultation with the MOH of the host government.

Case-holding

Whenever possible, chemotherapy should be observed by a health-care provider, especially during the first 2–3 months of treatment. Treatment efficacy should be assessed through a series of sputum smears. Patients participating in observed therapy who do not respond to treatment and whose sputum smears remain positive for AFB after 2 months should be reviewed by a physician and should begin a second-line treatment regimen.

Enrolling TB patients in a SFP may improve adherence to the treatment regimen and acts as a point of contact for follow-up.

The success of a TB control program depends on good management and close supervision. The responsibilities of staff assigned to the program need to be clearly defined, adequate records of patient progress should be maintained, and a system to follow-up patients who do not adhere to treatment should be established. The cooperation of the community is essential for success. A community education program should be established to help ensure adherence.

Prevention

Preventive chemotherapy for subclinical TB usually does not play a substantial role in TB control in a refugee camp. However, immediate family members of active TB patients should be examined for active TB and referred for treatment. This is particularly important for young children.

BCG vaccination should be administered as part of the comprehensive immunization schedule and not as a separate TB control activity. BCG vaccination is contraindicated for persons with symptomatic HIV infection, but can be administered to asymptomatic persons.

SELECTED READING

Rieder HL, Snider DE, Toole MJ, et al. Tuberculosis control in refugee settlements. Tubercle 1989;70:127–124.

Davis CE, Allegra DT, Buhrer M. Tuberculosis control programs, Sakaeo and Khao I-Dang. In: Allegra DT, Nieburg P, Grabe M, eds. Emergency refugee health care—a chronicle of the Khmer refugee-assistance operation 1979–1980. Atlanta, GA: CDC, 1983:61–64.

Epidemic Investigations

An epidemic is an unusually large or unexpected increase in the number of cases of a certain disease for a given place and time period. The general conditions of many refugee settlements (i.e., overcrowding, poor water and sanitation, inadequate rations) create an environment conducive to epidemics of infectious diseases. In the event of a suspected outbreak, an epidemiologic investigation should be conducted as quickly as possible.

Purpose

Epidemiologic investigations are conducted in order to:

- Confirm the threat or existence of an epidemic and identify the causative agent, its source and mode of transmission.
- Determine the geographic distribution and the public health impact of an epidemic, identifying those groups or persons who are at highest risk for disease.
- Assess local response capacity and identify the most effective control measures.

Preparations

Each camp should have an established HIS with standardized reporting practices. This will allow for prompt recognition of and rapid response to an epidemic.

An accurate assessment of available laboratory facilities is necessary in order to identify appropriate sites for microbiologic confirmation of an epidemic and to address deficiencies that may hamper an investigation.

Appropriate specimen containers and transport media should be procured. Arrangements should be made to meet the need for additional technical support.

A recognized administrative and reporting structure should be established, with a clear chain of command and delegation of responsibility. Lines of command should be well defined, and specific persons should be assigned responsibility for addressing the media and acting as liaisons to the camp leaders and the refugee population.

Current maps showing settlements, water sources, transport routes, and health facilities should be made available to investigators.

Conducting the Investigation

Determining the existence of an epidemic. An established HIS will allow for prompt recognition and confirmation of an epidemic. The need for routine health surveillance in a refugee camp cannot be overstated. Even if such a system is firmly in place and implemented, reports of an epidemic may be the result of artifactual causes, i.e., changes in reporting practices, an increased interest in a particular disease, a change in diagnostic methods, the arrival of new health staff, or an increase in the number of health facilities.

Confirming the Diagnosis

The diagnosis of an epidemic disease should be confirmed using standard clinical or laboratory techniques. However, once the presence of an epidemic is established, it is not necessary to confirm the diagnosis for each person before treatment. Ongoing laboratory confirmation of a sample of cases is generally sufficient.

Determining the Number of Cases

A workable case definition must be established in order to determine the scope of the outbreak. The sensitivity and specificity of the case definition depend upon:

- The usual apparent-to-inapparent case ratio.
- Whether pathognomonic signs and symptoms exist.
- The need for laboratory support for diagnosis.
- The accessibility of cases.
- The level of expertise of available health personnel.
- The amount of subjectivity involved in the diagnosis.

A case-finding mechanism should be established. The dynamics of this system will depend upon the disease being investigated and the specific attributes of the camp involved. Case-finding will be facilitated if a cadre of refugee community health workers has been identified and trained. The presence of an active camp health committee will also promote effective case-finding.

Time, Place, and Person

Certain information should be collected from each patient, or from their families, and recorded in a register. This should include:

- The date (and perhaps the time) of onset of symptoms.
- The length of time between arrival in camp and the onset of symptoms.
- Patient's age and gender.
- Place of residence.
- Ethnic group (if applicable).

Determining Who Is at Risk

The data collected from patients should be used in an ongoing analysis to determine who is at greatest risk and to target specific interventions most effectively.

Prepare a graph showing the number of cases per day. This "epidemic curve" will indicate the point at which the outbreak first occurred, the magnitude of the outbreak, the incubation period, and possible modes of transmission.

Using a current map of the camp, mark the residence or section of the camp of each case as it is reported. This will allow investigators to identify clusters of patients and may help to pinpoint a common source of infection.

A breakdown of cases by age, gender, length of stay in camp, vaccination status, if pertinent, and perhaps ethnic group will enable investigators to identify those groups or persons who are at highest risk for infection.

Testing a Hypothesis

As preliminary data are collected and analyzed, a hypothesis on the causative exposure should be developed and tested. A case-control study and analysis will help determine likely risk factors and sources of exposure. Laboratory analysis of environmental samples may be used to confirm a suspected source of infection.

Preparing a Report

Meetings should be held regularly with camp administrative officials, UNHCR and NGO representatives, local health officials, and refugee community leaders to discuss the evolution of the outbreak and to stress current control measures. In some cases, a written report may be necessary before any control and prevention efforts are undertaken. The report should include an estimate of the magnitude and health impact of the outbreak in numbers of projected cases and deaths. It should also include an estimation of the need for outside assistance and supplies. A written report will also provide a valuable record for use in future investigations. Moreover, the written report can serve as a useful teaching tool.

Control and Prevention

As the epidemiologic investigation progresses, it is important that decision-makers be informed as to the findings so that appropriate control measures may be instituted. Continued disease surveillance will determine the effectiveness of control measures.

SELECTED READING

CDC Monograph. Toole MJ, Foster S. Famines. In: Gregg MB, ed. The public health consequences of disasters 1989. Atlanta, GA: CDC, 1989.

Flood: A Prevention Guide to Promote Your Personal Health and Safety

Original Citation: Centers for Disease Control and Prevention. Flood: a prevention guide to promote your personal health and safety. Atlanta: US Department of Health and Human Services, Public Health Service, 1994.

INTRODUCTION

After a flood, the physical devastation to a community is obvious. But during the flood and its aftermath, there are some basic facts to remember that will help protect your personal health and safety. This pamphlet provides information that will help you and other flood victims prevent disease and injury and maintain good health in the days and weeks following a flood.

This information is provided by the Centers for Disease Control and Prevention (CDC) through state and local health departments. It includes general disease and injury prevention guidelines which may vary slightly from state to state. If in doubt, contact your local or state health departments, which will issue health advisories or recommendations particular to local conditions.

WATER QUALITY

Listen for public announcements on the safety of the municipal water supply. Flooded, private water wells will need to be tested and disinfected after floodwaters recede. Questions about testing should be directed to your local or state health departments.

Water for Drinking and Cooking

Safe drinking water includes bottled, boiled, or treated water. Your state of local health department can make specific recommendations for boiling or treating water in your area. Here are some general rules concerning water for drinking and cooking:

Remember:

- Do not use contaminated water to wash dishes, brush your teeth, wash and prepare food, or make ice.
- If you use bottled water, know where it came from. Otherwise, water should be boiled or treated before use. Drink only bottled, boiled, or treated water until your supply is tested and found safe.
- Boiling water kills harmful bacteria and parasites. Bringing water to a rolling boil for 1 minute will kill most organisms.
- Water may be treated with chlorine or iodine tablets, or by mixing six drops (⅛ teaspoon) of unscented, ordinary household chlorine bleach (5.25 percent sodium hypochlorite) per gallon of water. Mix the solution thoroughly, and let stand for about thirty minutes. However, this treatment will not kill parasitic organisms.

- Containers for water should be rinsed with a bleach solution before re-using them. Use water storage tanks and other types of containers with caution. For example, fire truck storage tanks, as well as previously used cans or bottles may be contaminated with microbes or chemicals. Do not rely on untested devices for decontaminating water.

Disinfecting Wells

If you suspect that your well may be contaminated, contact your local or state health department or agriculture extension agent for specific advice. Here are some general instructions for disinfecting wells. Source: Illinois Department of Public Health. Recommendations may vary from state to state.

To Disinfect Bored or Dug Wells
1. Use Table 1 to calculate how much bleach (liquid or granules) to use.
2. To determine the exact amount to use, multiply the amount of disinfectant needed (according to the diameter of the well) by the depth of the well. For example, a well 5 feet in diameter requires 4½ cups of bleach per foot of water. If the well is 30 feet deep, multiply 4½ by 30 to determine the total cups of bleach required (4½ x 30 = 135 cups). There are sixteen cups in each gallon of liquid bleach.
3. Add this total amount of disinfectant to about 10 gallons of water. Splash the mixture around the wall or lining of the well. Be certain the disinfectant solution contacts all parts of the well.
4. Seal the well top.
5. Open all faucets and pump water until a strong odor of bleach is noticeable at each faucet. Then stop the pump and allow the solution to remain in the well overnight.
6. The next day, operate the pump by turning on all faucets, continuing until the chlorine odor disappears. Adjust the flow of water faucets or fixtures that discharge to septic systems to a low flow to avoid overloading the disposal system.

To Disinfect Drilled Wells
1. Determine the amount of water in the well by multiplying the gallons per foot by the depth of the well in feet. For example, a well with a 6-inch diameter contains 1.5 gallons of water per foot. If the well is 120 feet deep, multiply 1.5 by 120 (1.5 x 120 = 180).

Table 1. Bleach for a Bored or Dug Well

Diameter of well (in feet)	Amount of 5.25% laundry bleach per foot of water	Amount of 70% OR chlorine granules per foot of water
3	1½ cups	1 ounce
4	3 cups	2 ounces
5	4½ cups	3 ounces
6	6 cups	4 ounces
7	9 cups	6 ounces
8	12 cups	8 ounces
10	18 cups	12 ounces

2. For each 100 gallons of water in the well, use the amount of chlorine (liquid or granules) indicated in Table 2. Mix the total amount of liquid or granules with about 10 gallons of water.
3. Pour the solution into the top of the well before the seal is installed.
4. Connect a hose from a faucet on the discharge side of the pressure tank to the well casing top. Start the pump. Spray the water back into the well and wash the sides of the casing for at least 15 minutes.
5. Open every faucet in the system and let the water run until the smell of chlorine can be detected. Then close all the faucets and seal the top of the well.
6. Let stand for several hours, preferably overnight.
7. After you have let the water stand, operate the pump by turning on all faucets, continuing until all odor of chlorine disappears. Adjust the flow of water from faucets of fixtures that discharge into septic tank systems to a low flow to avoid overloading the disposal system.

Table 2. Bleach for a Drilled Well

Diameter of Well (in inches)	Gallons per foot
3	0.37
4	0.65
5	1.0
6	1.5
8	2.6
10	4.1
12	6.0

Amount of Disinfectant Required for each 100 gallons of water: Laundry bleach (5.25% Chlorine) 3 cups* OR Hypochloride Granules (70% Chlorine) 2 ounces**

*1 cup = 8-ounce measuring cup
**1 ounce = 2 heaping tablespoons of granules

FOOD SAFETY

Do not eat any food that may have come into contact with flood water. Discard any food without a waterproof container if there is any chance that it has come into contact with flood water. Undamaged, commercially canned foods can be saved if you remove the can labels, thoroughly wash the cans, and then disinfect them with a solution consisting of one cup of bleach in 5 gallons of water. Re-label your cans, including expiration date, with a marker. Food containers with screw-caps, snap-lids, crimped caps (soda pop bottles), twist caps, flip tops, and home canned foods should be discarded if they have come into contact with flood water because they cannot be disinfected. For infants, use only pre-prepared canned baby formula that isn't condensed and doesn't require added water. Do not use powdered formulas prepared with treated water.

Frozen and Refrigerated Foods

If your refrigerator or freezer may be without power for a long period:

- Divide your frozen foods among friends' freezers if they have electricity;
- Seek freezer space in a store, church, school, or commercial freezer that has electrical service; or

- Use dry ice—25 pounds of dry ice will keep a 10-cubic-foot freezer below freezing for three to four days. (Exercise care when handling dry ice, because it freezes everything it touches. Wear dry, heavy gloves to avoid injury.)

Thawed food can usually be eaten or refrozen if it is still "refrigerator cold," or if it still contains ice crystals. To be safe, remember, "When in doubt, throw it out." Discard any food that has been at room temperature for two hours or more, and any food that has an unusual odor, color or texture. Your refrigerator will keep foods cool for about 4 hours without power. Add block or dry ice to your refrigerator if the electricity will be off longer than 4 hours.

SANITATION AND HYGIENE

One result of the flood may be a lapse in basic hygiene during the emergency period. It is critical for you to remember to practice basic hygiene. You must wash your hands with soap and water that has been boiled or disinfected:

- Before preparing or eating food;
- After toilet use;
- After participating in flood cleanup activities; and
- After handling articles contaminated with flood water or sewage.

Flood waters may contain fecal material from overflowing sewage systems, and agricultural and industrial byproducts. Although skin contact with flood water does not, by itself, pose a serious health risk, there is some risk of disease from eating or drinking anything contaminated with flood water. If you have any open cuts or sores that will be exposed to flood water, keep them as clean as possible by washing well with soap to control infection. If a wound develops redness, swelling, or drainage, seek immediate medical attention.

In addition, parents need to help children avoid water-borne illness. Do not allow children to play in flood water areas, wash children's hands frequently (especially before meals), and do not allow children to play with flood water contaminated toys that have not been disinfected. You can disinfect toys using a solution of one cup of bleach in 5 gallons of water.

PRECAUTIONS WHEN RETURNING TO YOUR HOME

Electrical power and natural gas or propane tanks should be shut off to avoid fire, electrocution, or explosions. Try to return to your home during the daytime so that you do not have to use any lights. Use battery-powered flashlights and lanterns, rather than candles, gas lanterns, or torches. If you smell gas or suspect a leak, turn off the main gas valve, open all windows, and leave the house immediately. Notify the gas company or the police or fire departments or State Fire Marshal's office, and do not turn on the lights or do anything that could cause a spark. Do not return to the house until you are told it is safe to do so.

Your electrical system may also be damaged. If you see frayed wiring or sparks, or if there is an odor of something burning but no visible fire, you should immediately shut off the electrical system at the circuit breaker.

Avoid any downed power lines, particularly those in water. Avoid wading in standing water, which also may contain glass or metal fragments.

You must consult your utility company about using electrical equipment, including power generators. Be aware that it is against the law and a violation of all electrical codes to connect generators to your home's electrical circuits without the approved, automatic-interrupt devices. If a generator is on line when electrical service is restored, it can become a major fire hazard. In addition, the improper connection of a generator to your home's electrical circuits may endanger line workers helping to restore power in your area. All electrical equipment and appliances must be completely dry before returning them to service. It is advisable to have a certified electrician check these items if there is any question. Also, remember not to operate any gas-powered equipment indoors.

CLEANUP

Walls, hard-surfaced floors, and many other household surfaces should be cleaned with soap and water and disinfected with a solution of 1 cup of bleach to five gallon of water. You need to be particularly careful to thoroughly disinfect surfaces that may come in contact with food, such as counter tops, pantry shelves, refrigerators, etc. Areas where small children play should also be carefully cleaned. Wash all linens and clothing in hot water, or dry clean them. For items that cannot be washed or dry cleaned, such as mattresses and upholstered furniture, air dry them in the sun and then spray them thoroughly with a disinfectant. Steam clean all carpeting.

If there has been a backflow of sewage into the house, wear rubber boots and waterproof gloves during cleanup. Remove and discard contaminated household materials that cannot be disinfected, such as wall coverings, cloth, rugs, and drywall.

IMMUNIZATIONS

Outbreaks of communicable diseases after floods are unusual. However, the rates of diseases that were present before a flood may increase because of decreased sanitation or overcrowding among displaced persons. Increases in infectious diseases that were not present in the community before the flood are not usually a problem. If you receive a puncture wound or a wound contaminated with feces, soil, or saliva, have a doctor or health department determine whether a tetanus booster is necessary based on individual records.

Specific recommendations for vaccinations should be made on a case by case basis, or as determined by local and state health departments.

MOSQUITOES

The large amount of pooled water remaining after the flood will lead to an increase in mosquito populations. The majority of these mosquitoes will be pests, but will not carry communicable diseases.

You should protect yourself from mosquitoes through the use of screens on dwellings, wearing long-sleeved and long-legged clothing, and using repellents containing DEET for personal protection. DEET is a common insect repellent chemical found in many repellent products. Products containing DEET are available from retail outlets and through local and state health departments.

Also after the flood, do not forget to drain all standing water left in containers around your home, an effective measure for controlling the mosquito population in the weeks ahead. Local, state, and federal public health authorities will be actively monitoring the situation in order to control the spread of any mosquito-borne diseases.

OTHER HAZARDS

Swiftly Flowing Water

If you enter swiftly flowing water, you risk drowning regardless of your ability to swim. Swiftly moving shallow water can be deadly, and even shallow standing water can be dangerous for small children. Cars or other vehicles do not provide adequate protection from flood waters. Cars can be swept away or may break down in moving water.

Animals

Many wild animals have been forced from their natural habitats by flooding, and many domestic animals are also without homes after the flood. Take care to avoid these animals, because some may carry rabies. Remember, most animals are disoriented and displaced, too. Do not corner an animal. If an animal must be removed, contact your local animal control authorities. Your local and state health department can provide information about the types of wild animals that carry rabies in your area.

Rats may be a problem during and after a flood. Take care to secure all food supplies, and remove any animal carcasses in the vicinity by contacting your local animal control authorities.

If you are bitten by any animal, seek immediate medical attention. If you are bitten by a snake, first try to accurately identify the type of snake so that, if poisonous, the correct anti-venom may be administered.

Chemical Hazards

Use extreme caution when returning to your area after a flood. Be aware of potential chemical hazards you may encounter during flood recovery. Flood waters may have buried or moved hazardous chemical containers of solvents or other industrial chemicals from their normal storage places.

If any propane tanks (whether 20-lb. tanks from a gas grill or household propane tanks) are discovered, do not attempt to move them yourself. These represent a very real danger of fire or explosion, and if any are found, police or fire departments or your State Fire Marshal's office should be contacted immediately.

Car batteries, even those in flood water, may still contain an electrical charge, and should be removed with extreme caution by using insulated gloves. Avoid coming in contact with any acid that may have spilled from a damaged car battery.

SUMMARY

The physical devastation that accompanies a flood is enormous. But as the flood waters recede, there may be more threats to your personal health and safety. By taking some basic precautions, you can help prevent many injuries as well as the possibility of some diseases.

In the midst of all this water, remember that it is summer, and heat will play a major role in your personal health. Drink plenty of fluids, avoid caffeine, and do not wait to get thirsty. When possible, take a break, being careful not to get any more exhausted than you already may be. Do not add weather-related health problems like heat stress or hypothermia to your other problems.

The weeks after a flood are going to be rough. In addition to your physical health, you need to take some time to consider your mental health as well. Remember that some sleeplessness, anxiety, anger, hyperactivity, mild depression, or lethargy are normal, and may go away with time. If you feel any of these symptoms acutely, seek some counseling. Your state and local health departments will help you find the local resources, including hospitals or health care providers, that you may need.

In addition to the information provided in this pamphlet, local and state health departments or emergency management agencies may issue health advisories particular to your location. For more information, contact your local or state health departments.

Hurricane: A Prevention Guide to Promote Your Personal Health and Safety

Original Citation: Centers for Disease Control and Prevention. Hurricane: a prevention guide to promote your personal health and safety. Atlanta: US Department of Health and Human Services, Public Health Service, 1994.

ABOUT HURRICANES

Hurricanes are powerful storms that form at sea with wind speeds of 74 mph or greater. Hurricanes are tracked by satellites from the moment they begin to form, so there is usually a warning 3–4 days before a storm strikes. A hurricane covers a circular area between 200 and 480 miles in diameter. In the storm, strong winds and rain surround a central, calm "eye," which is about 15 miles across. Winds in a hurricane can sometimes reach 200 miles per hour. However, the greatest damage to life and property is not from the wind, but from tidal surges and flash flooding.

Because of the destructive power of a hurricane, you should never ignore an evacuation order. Many victims of Hurricane Andrew who did ignore evacuation orders lost their lives or found that they could do nothing to protect their property against the storm.

PREPARING FOR THE HURRICANE

Hurricane Readiness

Hurricane readiness should begin long before the event occurs. If you live in a hurricane-prone area, you can prepare far in advance for the possible dangers to health and safety resulting from a hurricane by:

- Learning about your community's emergency plans, warning signals, evacuation routes, and locations of emergency shelters; and
- Taking a first aid and CPR course.

You should also prepare for a weather emergency by taking the following actions:

- Identify potential home hazards that could develop during a hurricane, such as those involving gas, electricity, chemicals, and structural damage;
- Install a smoke detector and check it monthly;
- Buy a fire extinguisher and make sure your family knows where to find it and how to use it;
- Conduct an evacuation drill for at least two ways out of your home;
- Provide escape ladders for multi-story structures;
- Establish an assembly point where the family meets in the event of fire or if a disaster occurs when the family is not together at home;
- Give your relatives and friends the name of a contact person who will know where you are and how you are doing;
- Know the location of your important papers, such as insurance policies, wills, licenses, stocks, etc.;
- Instruct family members about how to shut off the gas, water, and electric mains;
- Post emergency phone numbers at every phone;
- Inform local authorities about any special needs, i.e., elderly or bedridden people, or anyone with a disability; and
- Properly dispose of all chemicals, pesticides, and solvents not being used.

You should stock your home with supplies that may be needed during the emergency period. These supplies should include:

- Several clean containers for water, large enough for a 3–5 day supply of water (about five gallons for each person);
- A 3–5 day supply of nonperishable food;
- A first aid kit and manual;
- A battery-powered radio, flashlights, and extra batteries;
- Sleeping bags or extra blankets;
- A large supply of nonbreakable spoons, forks, knives, cups, plates, etc.;
- Water-purifying supplies, such as chlorine or iodine tablets or unscented, ordinary household chlorine bleach;
- Prescription medicines and special medical needs;
- Baby food and/or prepared formula, diapers, and other baby supplies;
- Disposable cleaning cloths, such as "baby wipes" for the whole family to use in case bathing facilities are not available;
- A portable toilet, and toilet paper;
- Personal hygiene supplies, such as soap, toothpaste, sanitary napkins, etc.;
- Alternate heat and cooking sources, such as a kerosene heater and a camp stove—use these only in well-ventilated areas;
- Shovels and hand tools;
- Candles and matches;
- A mop, bucket, and towels;
- One or more rolls of plastic sheeting, a staple gun with staples, and duct tape;
- Plastic trash bags and ties;
- An emergency kit for your car with food, flares, booster cables, maps, tools, a first aid kit, fire extinguisher, sleeping bags, etc.;
- A citizens band radio or a cellular phone, if possible;
- Games and favorite toys, etc.;

- Extra cash;
- Pet food;
- Insect repellent; and
- Rubber boots/rubber gloves.

Before the Storm

The National Weather Service will issue a hurricane watch when there is a threat to coastal areas of hurricane conditions within 24–36 hours. When a hurricane watch is issued, you should:

- BE PREPARED TO EVACUATE;
- Fill your automobile's gas tank;
- If no vehicle is available, make arrangements with friends or family for transportation;
- Fill your clean water containers;
- Review your emergency plans and supplies, checking to see if any items are missing;
- Tune in the radio or television for weather updates;
- Listen for disaster sirens and warning signals;
- If you must evacuate your home, pack only essential items, such as clothing, bedding, food, water, medicines, infant needs, vital family papers, and extra cash;
- Outside, secure any items which may damage property in a storm, such as bicycles, grills, propane tanks, etc.;
- Cover windows and doors with plywood or boards if possible. Otherwise, place large strips of masking tape or adhesive tape on the windows to reduce the risk of breakage and flying glass;
- Put livestock and family pets in a safe area if possible. Due to food and sanitation requirements, emergency shelters cannot accept animals;
- Place vehicles under cover, if at all possible;
- Fill sinks and bathtubs with water as an extra supply for washing; and
- Adjust the thermostat on refrigerators and freezers to the coolest possible temperature.

Evacuation

Expect the need to evacuate and prepare for it. Authorities will be most likely to direct you to leave if you are in a low-lying area, or within the greatest potential path of the storm. The National Weather Service will issue a hurricane warning when hurricane conditions are expected in a specified coastal area in 24 hours or less. If a hurricane warning is issued for your area or you are directed by authorities to evacuate the area:

- Take only essential items with you;
- Leave pets indoors in a safe, covered area with ample food and water;
- If you have time, turn off the gas, electricity, and water;
- Disconnect appliances to reduce the likelihood of electrical shock when power is restored;
- Make sure your automobile's emergency kit is ready;
- Follow the designated evacuation routes—others may be blocked—and expect heavy traffic; and
- Listen to the radio for emergency updates.

During the Storm

To get through the storm in the safest possible manner:

- Monitor the radio or television for weather conditions, if possible;
- Stay indoors until the authorities declare the storm is over;
- Do not go outside, even if the weather appears to have calmed the calm "eye" of the storm can pass quickly, leaving you outside when strong winds resume;
- Expect the loss of electricity, gas, and water;
- Stay away from all windows and exterior doors, seeking shelter in a bathroom or basement. Bathtubs can provide some shelter if you cover yourself with plywood or other materials;
- Prepare to evacuate to a shelter or to a neighbor's home if your home is damaged, or if you are instructed to do so by emergency personnel; and
- If you should lose electrical power, eat perishable food first.

HURRICANES AND YOUR HEALTH AND SAFETY

The great majority of injuries during a hurricane are cuts caused by flying glass or other debris. Other injuries include puncture wounds resulting from exposed nails, metal, or glass, and bone fractures.

State and local health departments may issue health advisories or recommendations particular to local conditions. If in doubt, contact your local or state health department.

WATER QUALITY

Hurricanes, especially if accompanied by a tidal surge or flooding, can contaminate the public water supply. Drinking contaminated water may cause illness. You cannot assume that the water in the hurricane-affected area is safe to drink.

In the area hit by a hurricane, water treatment plants may not be operating; even if they are, storm damage and flooding can contaminate water lines. Listen for public announcements about the safety of the municipal water supply. If your well has been flooded, it needs to be tested and disinfected after the storm passes and the flood waters recede. Questions about testing should be directed to your local or state health department. Information on disinfecting wells is available in later sections.

Water for Drinking and Cooking

Safe drinking water includes bottled, boiled, or treated water. Your state or local health department can make specific recommendations for boiling or treating drinking water in your area. Here are some general rules concerning water for drinking and cooking. Remember:

- Do not use contaminated water to wash dishes, brush your teeth, wash and prepare food, or make ice;
- If you use bottled water, know where it came from; otherwise, water should be boiled or treated before use. Drink only bottled, boiled, or treated water until your supply is tested and found safe.
- Boiling water kills harmful bacteria and parasites. Bringing water to a rolling boil for 1 minute will kill most organisms.
- Water may be treated with chlorine or iodine tablets, or by mixing six drops

(1/8 teaspoon) of unscented, ordinary household chlorine bleach (5.25 percent sodium hypochlorite) per gallon of water. Mix the solution thoroughly, and let stand for about 30 minutes. However, this treatment will not kill parasitic organisms.

Containers for water should be rinsed with a bleach solution before reusing them. Use water storage tanks and other types of containers with caution. For example, fire truck storage tanks, as well as previously used cans or bottles can be contaminated with microbes or chemicals. Do not rely on untested devices for decontaminating water.

Disinfecting Wells

If you suspect that your well may be contaminated, contact your local or state health department or agriculture extension agent for specific advice. Here are some general instructions for disinfecting wells. Source: Illinois Department of Public Health.

Recommendations may vary from state to state.

To Disinfect Bored or Dug Wells

1. Use Table 1 to calculate how much bleach (liquid or granules) to use.
2. To determine the exact amount to use, multiply the amount of disinfectant needed (according to the diameter of the well) by the depth of the well. For example, a well 5 feet in diameter requires 4½ cups of bleach per foot of water. If the well is 30 feet deep, multiply 4½ by 30 to determine the total cups of bleach required (4½ x 30 = 135 cups). There are sixteen cups in each gallon of liquid bleach.
3. Add this total amount of disinfectant to about 10 gallons of water. Splash the mixture around the wall or lining of the well. Be certain the disinfectant solution contacts all parts of the well.
4. Seal the well top.
5. Open all faucets and pump water until a strong odor of bleach is noticeable at each faucet. Then stop the pump and allow the solution to remain in the well overnight.
6. The next day, operate the pump by turning on all faucets, continuing until the chlorine odor disappears. Adjust the flow of water faucets or fixtures that discharge to septic systems to a low flow to avoid overloading the disposal system.

Table 1. Bleach for a Bored or Dug Well

Diameter of well (in feet)	Amount of 5.25% laundry bleach per foot of water	Amount of 70% OR chlorine granules per foot of water
3	1½ cups	1 ounce
4	3 cups	2 ounces
5	4½ cups	3 ounces
6	6 cups	4 ounces
7	9 cups	6 ounces
8	12 cups	8 ounces
10	18 cups	12 ounces

Table 2. Bleach for a Drilled Well

Diameter of Well (in inches)	Gallons per foot
3	0.37
4	0.65
5	1.0
6	1.5
8	2.6
10	4.1
12	6.0

Amount of Disinfectant Required for each 100 gallons of water: Laundry bleach (5.25% Chlorine) 3 cups* OR Hypochloride Granules (70% Chlorine) 2 ounces**

*1 cup = 8-ounce measuring cup

**1 ounce = 2 heaping tablespoons of granules

To Disinfect Drilled Wells

1. Determine the amount of water in the well by multiplying the gallons per foot by the depth of the well in feet. For example, a well with a 6-inch diameter contains 1.5 gallons of water per foot. If the well is 120 feet deep, multiply 1.5 by 120 (1.5 x 120 = 180).
2. For each 100 gallons of water in the well, use the amount of chlorine (liquid or granules) indicated in Table 2. Mix the total amount of liquid or granules with about 10 gallons of water.
3. Pour the solution into the top of the well before the seal is installed.
4. Connect a hose from a faucet on the discharge side of the pressure tank to the well casing top. Start the pump. Spray the water back into the well and wash the sides of the casing for at least 15 minutes.
5. Open every faucet in the system and let the water run until the smell of chlorine can be detected. Then close all the faucets and seal the top of the well.
6. Let stand for several hours, preferably overnight.
7. After you have let the water stand, operate the pump by turning on all faucets, continuing until all odor of chlorine disappears. Adjust the flow of water from faucets of fixtures that discharge into septic tank systems to a low flow to avoid overloading the disposal system.

FOOD SAFETY

Do not eat any food that may have come into contact with contaminated floodwater. Discard any food not in a waterproof container if there is any chance that it has come into contact with contaminated floodwater. Undamaged, commercially canned foods can be saved if you remove the can labels, thoroughly wash the cans, and then disinfect them with a solution consisting of one cup of bleach in five gallons of water. Re-label your cans, including expiration date, with a marker. Food containers with screw-caps, snap-lids, crimped caps (soda pop bottles), twist caps, flip tops, snap-open, and home canned foods should be discarded if they have come into contact with floodwater because they cannot be disinfected. For infants, use only pre-prepared canned baby formula that isn't condensed and doesn't require added water. Do not use powdered formulas prepared with treated water.

Frozen and Refrigerated Foods

If you will be without power for a long period:

- Ask friends to store your frozen foods in their freezers if they have electricity;
- See if freezer space is available in a store, church, school, or commercial freezer that has electrical service; or
- Use dry ice, if available. Twenty-five pounds of dry ice will keep a 10-cubic-foot freezer below freezing for 3–4 days. Use care when handling dry ice, and wear dry, heavy gloves to avoid injury.

Your refrigerator will keep foods cool for about four hours without power if it is unopened. Add block or dry ice to your refrigerator if the electricity will be off longer than four hours.

Thawed food can usually be eaten if it is still "refrigerator cold," or refrozen if it still contains ice crystals. To be safe, remember, "When in doubt, throw it out." Discard any food that has been at room temperature for two hours or more, and any food that has an unusual odor, color, or texture.

SANITATION AND HYGIENE

It is critical for you to remember to practice basic hygiene during the emergency period. Always wash your hands with soap and water that has been boiled or disinfected:

- Before preparing or eating food;
- After toilet use;
- After participating in cleanup activities; and
- After handling articles contaminated with floodwater or sewage.

If there is flooding along with a hurricane, the waters may contain fecal material from overflowing sewage systems and agricultural and industrial waste. Although skin contact with floodwater does not, by itself, pose a serious health risk, there is risk of disease from eating or drinking anything contaminated with floodwater. If you have any open cuts or sores that will be exposed to floodwater, keep them as clean as possible by washing them with soap and applying an antibiotic ointment to discourage infection. If a wound develops redness, swelling, or drainage, seek immediate medical attention.

Do not allow children to play in floodwater areas. Wash children's hands frequently(always before meals), and do not allow children to play with floodwater-contaminated toys that have not been disinfected. You can disinfect toys using a solution of one cup of bleach in five gallons of water.

IMMUNIZATIONS

Outbreaks of communicable diseases after hurricanes are unusual. However, the rates of diseases that were present before a hurricane may increase because of a lack of sanitation or overcrowding in shelters. Increases in infectious diseases that were not present before the hurricane are not a problem, so mass vaccination programs are unnecessary.

If you have wounds, you should be evaluated for a tetanus immunization, just as you would at any other time of injury. If you receive a puncture wound or a wound contaminated with feces, soil, or saliva, have a doctor or health department determine whether a tetanus booster is necessary based on individual records.

Specific recommendations for vaccinations should be made on a case-by-case basis, or as determined by local and state health departments.

MOSQUITOES

Rain and flooding in a hurricane area may lead to an increase in mosquitoes. Mosquitoes are most active at sunrise and sunset. In most cases, the mosquitoes will be pests but will not carry communicable diseases. It is unlikely that diseases which were not present in the area prior to the hurricane would be of concern. Local, state, and federal public health authorities will be actively working to control the spread of any mosquito-borne diseases.

To protect yourself from mosquitoes, use screens on dwellings, and wear clothes with long sleeves and long pants. Insect repellents that contain DEET are very effective. Be sure to read all instructions before using DEET. Care must be taken when using DEET on small children. Products containing DEET are available from stores and through local and state health departments.

To control mosquito populations, drain all standing water left in open containers outside your home.

MENTAL HEALTH

The days and weeks after a hurricane are going to be rough. In addition to your physical health, you need to take some time to consider your mental health as well. Remember that some sleeplessness, anxiety, anger, hyperactivity, mild depression, or lethargy are normal, and may go away with time. If you feel any of these symptoms acutely, seek counseling. Remember that children need extra care and attention before, during, and after the storm. Be sure to locate a favorite toy or game for your child before the storm arrives to help maintain his/her sense of security. Your state and local health departments will help you find the local resources, including hospitals or health care providers, that you may need.

SAFETY PRECAUTIONS WHEN RETURNING HOME

If your area is under a curfew, allow travel time to and from your home. Although unusual following a hurricane, crime can also increase. If your area is under martial law, obey all orders by authorities because they will be armed.

During a hurricane and in the cleanup, injuries occur. To avoid injury, use common sense and wear proper clothing, including clothes with long sleeves and long pants, and safety shoes or boots.

When returning to your home after a hurricane:

- Find out if the authorities have declared the area safe;
- Watch for debris on the road while driving;
- Return to your pre-determined assembly point and/or contact your pre-established out-of-area contact person. Make sure all family members have been accounted for and let others know of your status;
- Make sure the main electrical switch to your home is off before entering the structure;
- Be careful when entering a structure that has been damaged;
- If you suspect a gas leak, leave immediately and notify the gas company;

- If possible, listen to the radio or contact authorities to find out if sewage lines are intact before turning on the water or using the toilet;
- Report utility damage to the proper authorities;
- Continue to monitor your radio or television for up-to-date emergency information.

INSPECTING THE DAMAGE

Upon returning to dwellings evacuated before the hurricane's arrival, be aware of possible structural, electrical, or gas-leak hazards. Electrical power and natural gas or propane tanks should be shut off to avoid fire, electrocution, or explosions. Try to return to your home during the daytime so that you do not have to use any lights. Use battery-powered flashlights and lanterns, rather than candles, gas lanterns, or torches.

GAS LEAKS

If you smell gas or suspect a leak, turn off the main gas valve, open all windows, and leave the house immediately. Notify the gas company, the police, fire departments, or State Fire Marshal's office, and do not turn on the lights, light matches, smoke, or do anything that could cause a spark. Do not return to the house until you are told it is safe to do so.

ELECTRICAL DAMAGE

Your electrical system may have been damaged. If you see frayed wiring or sparks when you restore power, or if there is an odor of something burning but no visible fire, you should immediately shut off the electrical system at the main circuit breaker.

You should consult your utility company about using electrical equipment, including power generators. Be aware that it is against the law and a violation of electrical codes to connect generators to your home's electrical circuits without the approved, automatic-interrupt devices. If a generator is on line when electrical service is restored, it can become a major fire hazard. In addition, the improper connection of a generator to your home's electrical circuits may endanger line workers helping to restore power in your area.

All electrical equipment and appliances must be completely dry before returning them to service. It is advisable to have a certified electrician check these items if there is any question.

PLEASE NOTE: Several deaths following past hurricanes have occurred due to fires. In many cases, fires were caused by the careless use of candles to light homes without electrical power. Use battery-powered lanterns, if possible, rather than candles. If you use candles, make sure they are in safe holders away from curtains, paper, wood, or other flammable items. Never leave a candle burning when you are out of the room.

OTHER INJURY-PREVENTION MEASURES

To avoid other hurricane-related injuries, you should:

- Learn proper safety procedures and operating instructions before operating any gas-powered or electric chain saw;

- With an electric chain saw, use extreme caution to avoid electrical shock;
- When using any power equipment, always wear a safety face shield or eye-glasses, and gloves;
- Avoid all power lines, particularly those in water;
- Avoid wading in water. Broken glass, metal fragments, and other debris may be present in the water; and
- Be careful of nails and broken glass when removing boards covering the windows.

Contact your state or local health department or utility company if you need additional safety information.

CLEANUP

Once you have established that no structural, electrical, or gas-related hazards exist in your home, dry and disinfect all materials inside the house to prevent the growth of mold and mildew.

Walls, hard-surfaced floors, and many other household surfaces should be cleaned with soap and water and disinfected with a solution of one cup of bleach to five gallons of water. Be particularly careful to thoroughly disinfect surfaces that may come in contact with food, such as counter tops, pantry shelves, refrigerators, etc. Areas where small children play should also be carefully cleaned. Wash all linens and clothing in hot water, or dry clean them. For items that cannot be washed or dry cleaned, such as mattresses and upholstered furniture, air dry them in the sun and then spray them thoroughly with a disinfectant. Steam clean all carpeting. If there has been a backflow of sewage into the house, wear rubber boots and waterproof gloves during cleanup. Remove and discard contaminated household materials that cannot be disinfected such as wall coverings, cloth, rugs, and drywall.

OTHER HAZARDS

Downed Powerlines

If powerlines are lying on the ground or dangling near the ground, do not touch the lines. Notify your utility company as soon as possible that the lines have been damaged, or that the powerlines are down. Do not attempt to move or repair the powerlines.

Do not drive through standing water if downed powerlines are in the water. If a powerline falls across your car while you are driving, continue to drive away from the line. If the engine stalls, do not turn off the ignition. Stay in your car and wait for emergency personnel. Do not allow anyone other than emergency personnel to approach your vehicle.

Animals

Wild or stray domestic animals can pose a danger during or after the passage of a hurricane. Remember, most animals are disoriented and displaced, too. Do not corner an animal. If an animal must be removed, contact your local animal control authorities.

If you are bitten by any animal, seek immediate medical attention. If you are bitten by a snake, first try to accurately identify the type of snake so that, if poisonous, the correct anti-venom can be administered. Do not cut the wound or attempt to suck the venom out.

Certain animals may carry rabies. Although the virus is rare, care should be taken to avoid contact with stray animals and rodents. Health departments can provide information on the types of animals that carry rabies in your area.

Rats may also be a problem during and after a hurricane. Take care to secure all food supplies, and remove any animal carcasses in the vicinity by contacting your local animal control authorities.

Drowning

Although hurricane winds can cause an enormous amount of damage, wind is not the biggest killer in such a storm. Nine of every ten hurricane fatalities are drownings associated with swiftly moving waters. People who enter moving water with their cars, or who get on boats on lakes or bays when a hurricane strikes the area are at grave risk of drowning, regardless of their ability to swim. Even very shallow water that is moving swiftly can be deadly. Cars or other vehicles do not provide adequate protection. Cars can be swept away or may break down in moving water. Be alert and follow hazard warnings on roadways or those broadcast by the media. Police and public works departments should be contacted for up-to-date information regarding safe roadways.

Chemical Hazards

Be aware of potential chemical hazards you may encounter when returning to your home, especially if the hurricane is accompanied by flooding. Floodwaters and high winds may have moved or buried hazardous chemical containers of solvents or other industrial chemicals. Contact your local fire department about inspecting and removing hazardous chemical containers. Avoid inhaling chemical fumes.

If any propane tanks (whether 20-lb. tanks from a gas grill or household propane tanks) are discovered, do not attempt to move them yourself. These represent a very real danger of fire or explosion, and if any are found, the fire department, police, or your State Fire Marshal's office should be contacted immediately.

Car batteries, while flooded, may still contain an electrical charge and should be removed with extreme caution by using insulated gloves. Avoid coming in contact with any acid that may have spilled from a damaged car battery.

SUMMARY

Hurricanes are powerful storms formed at sea and consist of strong wind and rain. Because modern technology allows us to track a hurricane's progress, communities in the hurricane's path will usually be warned of the storm's strength. Evacuating the area may be necessary because of the strength of a particular storm. By taking some basic precautions, you will be prepared and able to help prevent many injuries, as well as the possibility of some diseases.

Before the hurricane, learn about the emergency procedures established by your community, and prepare a personal family action plan. Keep emergency supplies on hand such as extra food, water, and battery-operated radios and flashlights. If authorities issue an evacuation order, follow the route they suggest.

After the storm, listen for public announcements regarding the safety of your neighborhood and return only when the area is considered safe. Avoid downed powerlines and report any problems with your utilities to the appropriate companies. Be aware of possible structural, electrical, or gas-leak hazards.

If drinking water has been contaminated, treat the water before use. Discard any food that has come into contact with contaminated water. Remember the rule of thumb for food "when in doubt, throw it out."

The weeks after a hurricane will be physically and emotionally draining. To help manage stress, take frequent breaks during the cleanup, and get as much rest as possible. While some sleeplessness, anxiety, anger, hyperactivity, mild depression, or lethargy are normal, extreme or prolonged symptoms should be evaluated by a mental health professional.

Public Health Consequences of a Flood Disaster

Original Citation: Centers for Disease Control and Prevention. Public health consequences of a flood disaster—Iowa, 1993. MMWR 1993;42(34):653–656.

Flooding is the most common type of natural disaster worldwide, accounting for an estimated 40% of all natural disasters (1). In riverine flooding, water levels can rise to flood stage gradually or very rapidly (i.e., flash flood) from snow melt or heavy or repeated rains.

Flash flooding is the leading cause of weather-related mortality in the United States (accounting for approximately 200 deaths per year) (1). However, the public health impact of floods also includes damage or destruction to homes and displacement of the occupants that may, in turn, facilitate the spread of some infectious diseases because of crowded living conditions and compromised personal hygiene (i.e., hand washing). Stress-related mental health or substance-abuse problems may be associated with flood disasters (1, 2). As the findings in this report indicate, medical and public health services may be interrupted in affected communities. Finally, the occurrence of injuries may increase during the clean-up phase of a disaster (3).

The multiple environmental consequences of flooding can directly affect the public's health. For example, water sources can become contaminated with fecal material or toxic chemicals, water or sewer systems can be disrupted, dangerous substances can be released (e.g., propane from damaged storage tanks), and solid-waste collection and disposal can be disrupted. In addition, flooding can result in vector-associated problems, including increases in mosquito populations that, under certain circumstances, increase the risk for some mosquito-borne infectious diseases (e.g., viral encephalitis) (4, 5).

Floods and other natural disasters often are followed by rumors of epidemics (e.g., typhoid, cholera, or rabies) (6, 7) or unusual conditions such as increased snake or dog bites. Such unsubstantiated reports can gain public credibility when printed in newspapers or reported on television or radio as facts. The potential for such rumors underscores the need for valid and systematically collected data and the importance of basic public health surveillance in such settings. Elements to be considered in such surveillance efforts are described in the CDC publication Beyond the Flood: A Prevention Guide for Personal Health and Safety (8), which emphasizes the importance of (a) purification of drinking and cooking water; (b) disinfection of wells; (c) food safety (i.e., handling of food that may have come in contact with flood water or of refrigerated food after the interruption of electrical power); (d) sanitation and personal hygiene; (e) injury-prevention measures to be taken during the return to and cleaning up of flooded homes; (f) communicable diseases and vaccinations; (g) mosquito control; and (h) other hazards such as animals, chemicals, and swift-flowing water. Copies of the guide are available from state health departments.

REFERENCES: AS NUMBERED IN ORIGINAL PUBLICATION

1. French JG, Holt KW. Floods. In: Gregg MB, ed. The public health consequences of disasters. Atlanta: US Department of Health and Human Services, Public Health Service, CDC, 1989:69–78.
2. French JG, Ing R, Von Allmen S, Wood R. Mortality from flash floods: a review of National Weather Service reports, 1969–81. Public Health Rep 1983;98:584–588.
3. Lee LE, Fonseca V, Brett KM, et al. Active morbidity surveillance after Hurricane Andrew—Florida, 1992. JAMA 1993;270:591–594.
4. Cotton P. Health threat from mosquitoes rises as flood of the century finally recedes. JAMA 1993;270:685–686.
5. Nasci RS, Moore CG. Planning for emergency mosquito surveillance and control. Wing Beats 1993;4:4–7.
6. Seaman J, Leivesley S, Hogg C. Epidemiology of natural disasters. In: Klingberg MA, Papier C, eds. Contributions to epidemiology and biostatistics. Vol 5. Basel, New York: Karger, 1984:49–70.
7. Glass RI, Noji EK. Epidemiologic surveillance following disasters. In: Halperin WE, Baker EL, Monson RR, eds. Public health surveillance. New York: Van Nostrand Reinhold, 1992:195–205.
8. CDC. Beyond the flood: a prevention guide for personal health and safety. Atlanta: US Department of Health and Human Services, Public Health Service, 1993.

Extreme Heat

Original Citation: Centers for Disease Control. Extreme heat, June,1996.

DURING HOT WEATHER

To protect your health when temperatures are extremely high, remember to keep cool and use common sense. The following tips are important.

Drink Plenty of Fluid

Increase your fluid intake—regardless of your activity level. During heavy exercise in a hot environment, drink 2–4 glasses (16–32 ounces) of cool fluids each hour. **Caution:** If your doctor has prescribed a fluid-restricted diet or diuretics for you, ask your doctor how much you should drink.

During hot weather, you will need to drink more liquid than your thirst indicates. This is especially true for persons 65 years of age and older who often have a decreased ability to respond to external temperature changes. Drinking plenty of liquids during exercise is especially important. However, avoid very cold beverages because they can cause stomach cramps. In addition, avoid drinks containing alcohol because they will actually cause you to lose more fluid.

Replace Salt and Minerals

Heavy sweating removes salt and minerals from the body. These are necessary for your body and must be replaced. The easiest and safest way to replace salt and minerals is through your diet. Drink fruit juice or a sports beverage during exercise or any work in the heat. Do not take salt tablets unless directed by your doctor. If you are on a low-salt diet, ask your doctor before changing what you eat or drink—especially before drinking a sports beverage.

Wear Appropriate Clothing and Sunscreen

Wear as little clothing as possible when you are at home. Choose lightweight, light-colored, loose-fitting clothing. In the hot sun, a wide-brimmed hat will provide shade and keep the head cool.

Sunburn affects your body's ability to cool itself and causes a loss of body fluids. It also causes pain and damages the skin. A variety of sunscreens are available to reduce the risk of sunburn. The protection that they offer against sunburn varies. Check the sun protection factor (SPF) number on the label of the sunscreen container. Select SPF 15 or higher to protect yourself adequately. Apply sunscreen 30 minutes before going outdoors and reapply according to package directions.

Pace Yourself

If you are unaccustomed to working in a hot environment, start slowly. If you must work faster, pick up the pace gradually. If exertion in the heat makes your heart pound and leaves you gasping for breath, STOP all activity, get into a cool area, or at least in the shade, and rest, especially if you become lightheaded, confused, weak, or faint.

Stay Cool Indoors

The most efficient way to beat the heat is to stay in an air-conditioned area. If you do not have an air conditioner or evaporative cooling unit, consider a visit to a shopping mall or public library for a few hours. Contact your local health department to see if there are any heat-relief shelters in your area. Electric fans may be useful to increase comfort and to draw cool air into your home at night, but do not rely on a fan as your primary cooling device during a heat wave. When the temperature is in the high 90s or higher, a fan will not prevent heat-related illness. A cool shower or bath is a more effective way to cool off. Also, use your stove and oven less to maintain a cooler temperature in your home.

Schedule Outdoor Activities Carefully

If you must be out in the heat, try to plan your activities so that you are outdoors either before noon or in the evening. While outdoors, rest frequently in a shady area. Resting periodically will give your body's thermostat a chance to recover.

Use a Buddy System

When working in the heat, monitor the condition of your co-workers and have someone do the same for you. Heat-induced illness can cause a person to become confused or lose consciousness. If you are 65 years of age or older, have a friend or relative call to check on you twice a day during a heat wave. If you know anyone in this age group, check on them at least twice a day.

Monitor Those at High Risk

Those at greatest risk of heat-related illness include:

- Infants and children up to four years of age.
- People 65 years of age or older.
- People who are overweight.
- People who overexert during work or exercise.
- People who are ill or on certain medications.

Infants and children up to four years of age are sensitive to the effects of high temperatures and rely on others to regulate their environments and provide adequate liquids. People 65 years of age or older may not compensate for heat stress efficiently, and are less likely to sense and respond to changes in temperature. Overweight people may be prone to heat sickness because of their tendency to retain more body heat. Any health condition that causes dehydration makes the body more susceptible to heat sickness. If you or someone you know is at higher risk, it is important to drink plenty of fluids; avoid overexertion; and get your doctor or pharmacist's advice about medications taken for high blood pressure, depression, nervousness, mental illness, insomnia, or poor circulation.

Adjust to the Environment

Be aware that any sudden change in temperature, such as an early summer heat wave, will be stressful to your body. You will have a greater tolerance for the heat if you limit your physical activity, until you become accustomed to the heat. If traveling to a hotter climate, allow several days to become acclimated before attempting any vigorous exercise, and work up to it gradually.

Use Common Sense

Avoid hot foods and heavy meals—they add heat to your body. Do not leave infants or pets in a parked car. Dress infants in cool, loose clothing and monitor fluid intake. Give your pet plenty of fresh water, and leave the water in a shady area.

HOT WEATHER HEALTH EMERGENCIES

Even short periods of high temperatures can cause serious health problems. Two common problems are heat stroke and heat exhaustion.

Heat Stroke

Heat stroke occurs when the body becomes unable to control its temperature: the body's temperature rises rapidly, the sweating mechanism fails, and the body is unable to cool down. Body temperature may rise to 106°F or higher within 10–15 minutes. Heat stroke can cause death or permanent disability if emergency treatment is not given.

Recognizing Heat Stroke

Warning signs of heat stroke vary but may include:

- An extremely high body temperature (above 103°F, orally)
- Red, hot, and dry skin (no sweating)

- Rapid, strong pulse
- Throbbing headache
- Dizziness
- Nausea
- Confusion
- Unconsciousness

What to Do

If you see any of these signs, you may be dealing with a life threatening emergency. Have someone call for immediate medical assistance while you begin cooling the victim:

- Get the victim to a shady area.
- Cool the victim rapidly using whatever methods you can. For example, immerse the victim in a tub of cool water; place in a cool shower; spray with cool water from a garden hose; sponge with cool water: or if the humidity is low, wrap the victim in a cool, wet sheet and fan him or her vigorously.
- Monitor body temperature and continue cooling efforts until the body temperature drops to 101–102°F.
- If emergency medical personnel are delayed, call the hospital emergency room for further instructions.
- Do not give the victim alcohol to drink.
- Get medical assistance as soon as possible.

Sometimes a victim's muscles will begin to twitch uncontrollably as a result of heat stroke. If this happens, keep the victim from injuring himself, but do not place any object in the mouth and do not give fluids. If there is vomiting, make sure the airway remains open by turning the victim on his or her side.

Heat Exhaustion

Heat exhaustion is the body's response to an excessive loss of the water and salt contained in sweat. Those most prone to heat exhaustion are elderly people, people with high blood pressure, and people working or exercising in a hot environment.

Recognizing Heat Exhaustion

Warning signs of heat exhaustion include:

- Heavy sweating
- Paleness
- Muscle cramps
- Tiredness
- Weakness
- Dizziness
- Headache
- Nausea or vomiting
- Fainting

The skin may be cool and moist. The victim's pulse rate will be fast and weak, and breathing will be fast and shallow. If heat exhaustion is untreated it may progress to heat stroke. Seek medical attention immediately if:

- Symptoms are severe, or
- The victim has heart problems or high blood pressure.

Otherwise, help the victim to cool off, and seek medical attention if symptoms worsen or last longer than 1 hour.

What to Do

Cooling measures that may be effective include:

- Cool, non-alcoholic beverages, as directed by your physician.
- Rest.
- Cool shower, bath, or sponge bath.
- An air-conditioned environment.
- Lightweight clothing.

OTHER HEAT-RELATED HEALTH PROBLEMS

Heat Cramps

Heat cramps usually affect people who sweat a lot during strenuous activity. This sweating depletes the body's salt and moisture. The low salt level in the muscles causes painful cramps. Heat cramps may also be a symptom of heat exhaustion.

Recognizing Heat Cramps

Heat cramps are muscle pains or spasms—usually in the abdomen, arms, or legs—that may occur in association with strenuous activity. If you have heart problems or are on a low sodium diet, get medical attention for heat cramps.

What to Do

If medical attention is not necessary, take these steps:

- Stop all activity, and sit quietly in a cool place.
- Drink clear juice or a sports beverage.
- Do not return to strenuous activity for a few hours after the cramps subside because further exertion may lead to heat exhaustion or heat stroke.
- Seek medical attention for heat cramps if they do not subside in 1 hour.

Sunburn

Sunburn should be avoided because it is damaging to the skin. Although the discomfort is usually minor and healing often occurs in about a week, a more severe sunburn may require medical attention.

Recognizing Sunburn

Symptoms of sunburn are well known: skin becomes red, painful, and abnormally warm after sun exposure.

What to Do

Consult a doctor if the sunburn affects an infant under 1 year of age or if these symptoms are present:

- Fever.
- Fluid-filled blisters.
- Severe pain.

Also, remember these tips when treating sunburn:

- Avoid repeated sun exposure.
- Apply cold compresses or immerse the sunburned area in cool water.
- Apply moisturizing lotion to affected areas. Do not use salve, butter, or ointment.
- Do not break blisters.

Heat Rash

Heat rash is a skin irritation caused by excessive sweating during hot, humid weather. It can occur at any age but is most common in young children.

Recognizing Heat Rash

Heat rash looks like a red cluster of pimples or small blisters. It is more likely to occur on the neck and upper chest, in the groin, under the breasts, and in elbow creases.

What to Do

The best treatment for heat rash is to provide a cooler, less humid environment. Keep the affected area dry. Dusting powder may be used to increase comfort, but avoid using ointments or creams—keeping the skin warm and moist may make the condition worse.

Treating heat rash is simple and usually does not require medical assistance. Other heat-related problems can be much more severe.

Hypothermia-Related Deaths

Original Citation: Centers for Disease Control and Prevention. Hypothermia-related deaths—New Mexico, October 1993–March 1994. MMWR 1995;44(50):933–935.

Editor's Note: Hypothermia is an unintentional lowering of the body temperature to 95°F (35°C). From 1979 through 1992, 10,550 persons in the United States died from hypothermia, an average of 754 deaths per year (range: 557-1021). Although many deaths occur (as one would expect) in northern states, hypothermia can also strike those in southern states, where rapid drops in temperature occur, and in the west, due to high elevations and profound declines in temperatures at night.

EDITORIAL NOTE

From 1979 through 1992, the highest total number of deaths attributed to hypothermia occurred in Illinois (660), and the highest annual age-adjusted death rate (33 deaths per million persons) occurred in Alaska. However, the findings in this report underscore the risk for hypothermia-related deaths in states in other latitudes. Of the 10 states with the highest combined ranking for both number and rate of hypothermia deaths, only two (Illinois and Alaska) are characterized by severe winter weather; the winter climate is substantially milder in the other eight states (Alabama, Arizona, New Mexico, North Carolina, Oklahoma, South Carolina, Tennessee, and Virginia).

Factors associated with the increased risk for hypothermia in the very young and the elderly in mildly cool environments (65°F [18°C]) include an impaired shivering mechanism, lower levels of protective fat, limited mobility, lower metabolic rate, and chronic illness (2). Other risk factors associated with hypothermia for all groups include drinking alcoholic beverages, using neuroleptic medications, hypothyroidism, mental illness, starvation, dehydration, poverty, any immobilizing illnesses, and sustained contact with material that promotes conductive heat loss (e.g., water, solvents, and metals) (2).

The onset of hypothermia is insidious: early manifestations include shivering, numbness, fatigue, poor coordination, slurred speech, impaired mentation, blueness or puffiness of the skin, and irrationality (3). Early recognition and prompt treatment can prevent morbidity and death. Specific prevention measures during cold and inclement weather conditions include maintaining dry clothes and wearing layered, insulated clothing (particularly head gear, because 30% of heat loss occurs from the head) that does not retain moisture (e.g., wool or polypropylene). In addition, persons who are outdoors in such conditions for extended periods should increase their fluid and calorie intake, find adequate shelter, and avoid overexertion and sweating. Persons at increased risk for hypothermia during such periods should be monitored by family and neighbors.

High death rates in states with relatively mild winter climates reflect, in part, the need for increased efforts to inform the public and high-risk groups about the health risks of environmental cold and about measures for preventing hypothermia. During cold weather, health-care providers, public health agencies, community-services organizations, and others can reduce the occurrence of hypothermia-related morbidity and death by monitoring groups at elevated risk during cold weather and ensuring that adequate shelter is provided.

REFERENCES: AS NUMBERED IN ORIGINAL PUBLICATION

2. Merck Research Laboratories. The Merck manual of diagnosis and therapy. Rahway, NJ: Merck Research Laboratories, 1992.
3. CDC. Hypothermia—United States. MMWR 1983;32:46–48.

APPENDIX A
Telephone Information and Technical Support References

Resource	Contact	Services Provided
CHEMTRAC (Chemical Transportation Emergency Center)	1-800-424-9300	24-hour emergency number. Connection with manufacturers and/or shippers who will provide advice on handling rescue gear needed, decontamination considerations, etc. Also provides access to Chlorine Emergency Response Plan (CHLOREP)
ATSDR (Agency for Toxic Substances and Disease Registry)	1-404-639-0615	24-hour emergency number for health-related support in hazard materials emergencies, including on-site assistance, if necessary.
Bureau of Explosives	1-202-639-2222	24-hour emergency number for hazardous materials incidents involving railroads.
Emergency Planning and Community Right-to-Know Information Hotline	1-800-535-0202	8:30 A.M.-7:30 P.M. (EST) Provides information on SARA Title III. Provides list of extremely hazardous substances and planning guidelines.

APPENDIX A—*continued*

Telephone Information and Technical Support References

Resource	Contact	Services Provided
EPA (Environmental Protection Agency) Regional Offices	Region I 617-565-3698 CT, ME, MA, NH, RI, VT Region II 212-264-0504 NJ, NY, PR, VI Region III 215-597-0980 DE, DC, MD, PA, VA, WV Region IV 404-347-3454 AL, FL, GA, KY, MS, NC, SC, TN Region V 312-886-7579 IL, IN, MI, MN, OH, WI Region VI 214-655-6760 AR, LA, NM, OK, TX Region VII 913-236-2850 IA, KS, MO, NE Region VIII 303-293-1720 CO, MT, ND, SD, UT, WY Region IX 415-974-7460 AM, SAMOA, AZ, CA, GU, HI, NV, Trust Territory of the Pacific Isl., Marshall Isl., Palau, Ponape Region X 206-442-2782 AK, ID, OR, WA	Environmental response team available.
National Animal Poison Control Center	1-217-333-3611	24-hour consultation concerning animal poisonings or chemical contamination. Provides an emergency response team to investigate incidents and perform laboratory analysis.
National Response Center	1-800-424-8802	For reporting transportation incidents where hazardous materials are responsible for death, serious injury, property damage in excess of $50,000, or continuing danger to life and property.

APPENDIX B

Computerized Data Sources of Information and Technical Support

Data Systems	Contact	Description
ANSWER	ANSWER Specialized Information Svcs. National Library of Medicine Building 38A 8600 Rockville Pike Bethesda, Maryland 20894 (301) 496-6531	National Library of Medicine's Workstation of Emergency Response (ANSWER)—to advise emergency response health professionals on potential hazardous chemical emergencies.
CAMEO	CAMEO Database Manager National Oceanic and Atmospheric Administration (NOAA) Hazardous Materials Response Branch, N/OMA-34 7600 Sand Point Way, NE Seattle, Washington 98115 (206) 526-6317	Computer-Aided Management of Emergency Operations available to on-scene responder. Chemical identification database assists in: identifying substance involved, predicting downwind concentrations, providing response recommendations, and identifying potential hazards.

APPENDIX B—*continued*

Data Systems	Contact	Description
CHRIS	CIS, Inc. Fein Management Associates 7215 York Road Baltimore, Maryland 21212 (800) 247-8737	Chemical Hazard Response Information System, developed by the Coast Guard and comprised reviews on fire hazards, fire fighting recommendations, reactivities, physico chemical properties, health hazards, use of protective clothing, and shipping information for over chemicals.
HAZARDTEXT	Micromedex, Inc. 660 Bannock Street Denver, Colorado 80203-3527 (800) 525-9083	Assists responders dealing with incidents involving hazardous materials such as spills, leaks, and fires. Emergency medical treatment and recommendations for initial hazardous response are presented.
HMIS	David W. Donaldson Information Sys. Specialist Dept. of Trans/RSPA/OHMT 400 7th Street, S.W. Washington, D.C. 20590 (202) 366-5869	Hazardous Material Information Systems provides name and emergency phone number of manufacturer, chemical formula, NIOSH number, fire fighting, spill, and leak procedures.
HSDB	Toxicology Data Network (TOXNET) National Library of Medicine Toxicology Information Program 8600 Rockville Pike Bethesda, Maryland 20894 (301) 496-6531	Hazardous Substances Data Bank, compiled by the National Library of Medicine, provides reviews on the toxicity, hazards, and regulatory status of over 4,000 frequently used chemicals.
1st MEDICAL RESPONSE PROTOCOLS	Micromedex, Inc. 660 Bannock Street Denver, Colorado 80203-3527 (800) 525-9083	For use in developing training programs and establishing protocols for first aid or initial workplace response to a medical emergency.
MEDITEXT	Micromedex, Inc. 660 Bannock Street Denver, Colorado 80203-3527 (800) 525-9083	Provides recommendations regarding the evaluation and treatment of exposure to industrial chemicals.
OHMTADS	CIS, Inc. Fein Management Associates 7215 York Road Baltimore, Maryland 80203-3527 (800) 247-8737	Oil and Hazardous Materials Technical Assistance Data Systems provides effects of spilled chemical compounds and their hazardous characteristics and properties, assists in identifying unknown substances, and recommends procedures for handling and cleanup.
TOMES	Micromedex, Inc. 660 Bannock Street Denver, Colorado 80203-3527 (800) 525-9083	The Tomes Plus Information Systems is a series of comprehensive databases on a single CD-ROM disc. It provides information regarding hazardous properties of chemicals and medical effects from exposure. The Tomes Plus database contains Meditext, Hazardtext, HSDB CHRIS, OHMTADS, and 1st Medical Response Protocols.
TOXNET	Toxicology Data Network (TOXNET) National Library of Medicine Toxicology Information Prog. (301) 496-6531	Computerized system of three toxicologically oriented data banks operated by the National Library of Medicine—the Hazardous Substances Data Bank, the Registry of Toxic Effects of Chemical Substances, and the Chemical Carcinogenesis Research Information System. TOXNET provides information on the health effects of exposure to industrial and environmental substances.

section six

INJURIES

Injury-Control Recommendations: Bicycle Helmets

Original Citation: Centers for Disease Control and Prevention. Injury-control recommendations: bicycle helmets. MMWR 1995;44(RR-1):1–18.

Original Authors: Robert D. Brewer, MD, MSPH, Mary Ann Fenley, Pamela I. Protzel, MPH, Jeffrey J. Sacks, MD, MPH, Timothy N. Thornton, Nancy Dean Nowak, RN, MPH, Benjamin Moore, James Belloni, MA.

BACKGROUND

From 1984 through 1988, an annual average of 962 U.S. residents died from and 557,936 persons were treated in emergency departments for bicycle-related injuries (4). Approximately 6% of persons who are treated for bicycle-related injuries require hospitalization (5, 6). The annual societal cost of bicycle-related injuries and deaths is approximately $8 billion (7).

Head injury is the most common cause of death and serious disability in bicycle-related crashes (1). Head injury accounts for 62% of bicycle-related deaths (4). In addition, approximately 33% of all bicycle-related emergency department visits and 67% of all bicycle-related hospital admissions (5, 8) involve head injuries (1, 4, 5).

From 1984 through 1988, greater than 40% of all deaths from bicycle-related head injury were among persons less than 15 years of age (4). In all age groups, death rates were higher among males. Death rates from bicycle-related head injury were highest among males 10–14 years of age. During the same years, greater than 75% of persons treated in emergency departments for bicycle-related head injury were less than 15 years of age. Rates for bicycle-related head injury were also higher for males than females in all age groups; the rates were highest among males 5–15 years of age (4).

Nearly 90% of deaths from bicycle-related head injury result from collisions with motor vehicles (4). However, motor vehicle collisions cause less than 25% of the nonfatal bicycle-related head injuries that are treated in emergency departments (1, 11). Excluding collisions with motor vehicles, common causes of nonfatal bicycle-related head injuries include falls, striking fixed objects, and collisions with other bicycles (1, 11).

BICYCLE HELMETS AND THE PREVENTION OF HEAD INJURY

The implementation of effective bicycle helmet programs could have a substantial impact on rates for fatal and nonfatal bicycle-related head injury (4). For example, from 1984 through 1988, if a presumed helmet-use rate of 10%

had been increased to 100% (i.e., universal helmet use), an average of 500 fatal and 151,400 nonfatal bicycle-related head injuries could have been prevented each year (4).

The results of a case-control study in Seattle in 1989 indicated that the use of bicycle helmets reduced the risk for bicycle-related head injury by 74%–85% (1). The findings of other studies that have compared the proportions of helmeted and unhelmeted riders who sustained head injury in bicycle crashes (13–15) detected higher risks for head injury among unhelmeted riders (crude odds ratio = 4.2 [13], 19.6 [14], and 4.5 [15]). Although other strategies may be useful in preventing bicycle-related injuries (i.e., proper road design and maintenance; improvement in bicycle design, manufacturing, and repair; and bicycle safety training [5, 16, 17]), the use of these strategies does not eliminate the need for bicycle helmets.

Barriers to Helmet Use

Although bicycle helmets provide effective protection against bicycle-related head injury, only approximately 18% of bicyclists wear helmets all or most of the time (7). Rates of bicycle helmet use are lowest among those groups for whom rates for bicycle-related head injury are highest (i.e., school-age children). Approximately 15% of riders less than 15 years of age wear helmets (7), a prevalence substantially lower than the year 2000 objective—a helmet-use rate of at least 50% (32).

Barriers to helmet use include cost, the wearability of bicycle helmets, and a lack of knowledge regarding helmet effectiveness (33). In addition, some school-age children (i.e., children less than 15 years of age) believe that wearing a helmet will result in derision by their peers (34). Among older children and adults, rates for helmet use are influenced by some of the same demographic factors as rates for seat belt use (e.g., age, education, income, and marital status) (14, 33), and some of the reasons given for not wearing helmets are similar to those given for not wearing seat belts (e.g., rider was on a short trip, helmets are uncomfortable, and negligence) (14). Approaches to overcoming some of these barriers to helmet use include community-based programs (33) and bicycle helmet legislation, which may be particularly effective among school-age children (34–37).

INCREASING THE USE OF BICYCLE HELMETS

The goal of bicycle helmet programs is to increase the use of bicycle helmets, thereby reducing the number of head injuries and deaths caused by bicycle crashes. State and local health departments are in a unique position to undertake bicycle helmet campaigns because of their (a) knowledge of the specific problems affecting their states and communities; (b) ability to provide technical expertise and credibility in health matters that affect their states and communities; (c) ability to work with community groups that are involved with health issues; and (d) ability to place bicycle helmet programs within the framework of other injury and health activities.

State- or Local-Level Programs

State and local health departments may be responsible for the following tasks when conducting community campaigns:

- Collecting and analyzing data relevant to a bicycle helmet campaign or providing assistance to the local program in this task. These data include deaths and injuries attributable to bicycle-related head injury, age-group-specific rates for helmet use, and barriers to helmet use. In addition, state and local health departments can collect and provide information on programs or organizations responsible for similar or complementary activities.
- Overseeing the development of a coalition of individuals, agencies, and organizations that is interested in bicycle helmet programs; has the resources to support a bicycle helmet campaign; or has the influence necessary to establish credibility and support for the campaign in the community.
- Identifying resource needs and sources, including funding and training.
- Providing assistance to local programs in planning intervention activities and in developing educational and promotional materials.
- Developing a statewide process for program evaluation and collecting and analyzing data on the program to evaluate process, impact (i.e., the change in helmet- use rates), and outcome. This process should begin before the program is implemented.
- Conducting statewide educational campaigns to create an awareness of the need for and value of bicycle helmets.
- Developing legislation in conjunction with coalitions and local leaders that requires the use of bicycle helmets (Appendix A).

Community Programs

Educational and promotional campaigns for bicycle helmet use are usually most effective when conducted at the local (i.e., community) level. At this level, strategies that encourage persons to wear bicycle helmets can be adjusted to the needs of a specific community. Several organizations publish materials (e.g., program guides, videotapes, and training materials) that communities can use for developing a bicycle helmet program (Appendix B). Components of a community program include building a coalition and planning, implementing, and evaluating the program (Appendix C).

Legislation for Bicycle Helmet Use

Legislation that mandates the use of bicycle helmets effectively increases helmet use, particularly when combined with an educational campaign. Education often facilitates behavioral change; however, education alone is rarely effective. Laws mandating helmet use supplement and reinforce the message of an educational campaign, requiring people to act on their knowledge.

Several states and localities have enacted laws requiring bicycle helmet use (e.g., California; Connecticut; Georgia; Massachusetts; New Jersey; New York; Oregon; Pennsylvania; Tennessee; several counties in Maryland [Howard, Montgomery, and Allegheny]; and the city of Beechwood, Ohio). Other groups that require helmet use include the United States Cycling Federation—the governing body of amateur bicycle racing and Olympic training—and the Greater Arizona Bicyclist Association.

Once enacted, bicycle helmet laws should be enforced. However, enforcement of helmet laws should be carried out through education rather than punishment. For example, local police officers could tell persons who violate the bicycle helmet law about the benefits of helmet use and provide them with discount coupons for the purchase of a helmet. Fines for the first citation could be waived if the person shows that he or she has acquired a helmet.

Bicycle helmet laws contain stipulations concerning enforcement. For example, in the California and New York legislation, the first violation is dismissed if the person charged proves that a helmet meeting the standards has been purchased. Otherwise, the violation is punishable by a fine of not more than $20 and $50, respectively. Other areas have a fine for the first offense of $25-$50 and a fine of up to $100 for any subsequent offenses. The fines for noncompliance vary among jurisdictions.

Regardless of the specific penalties that are used to enforce the law, enforcement must be accompanied by the active involvement of the law enforcement community (e.g., participation in community education). This involvement should begin when the state or community is developing and advocating for a bicycle helmet law.

RECOMMENDATIONS

The following recommendations are based on current data regarding the occurrence of head injury among bicyclists and the ability of helmets to prevent or reduce these injuries. These recommendations are for state and local agencies and other organizations that are planning programs to increase the use of bicycle helmets.

Recommendation 1

Bicycle helmets should be worn by all persons (i.e., bicycle operators and passengers) at any age when bicycling. Although operators and passengers of all ages are at risk for bicycle-related head injuries, communities that must focus on a particular risk group should consider children less than 15 years of age as the primary target group for the following reasons:

- The majority of children ride bicycles.
- Rates for all bicycle-related head injuries are high among children.
- In most communities, helmet-use rates among children are lower than those among adults.
- Persons who begin using helmets as children are more likely to continue to use them as adults.

However, even in communities in which efforts or programs focus on children, adults also should be included in the bicycle helmet program because of their educational influence on children. As programs gain resources, they should expand to include older age groups because adults are also at risk for head injury.

Recommendation 2

Bicycle riders should wear helmets whenever and wherever they ride a bicycle.

Bicyclists are always at risk for falling and thus for head injury, regardless of where they are riding (e.g., a driveway, park, or sidewalk). Laws that encourage helmet use only in certain settings (e.g., riding to and from school) only partially address the problem and do not reinforce the need to wear helmets at all times.

Recommendation 3

Bicycle helmets should meet the standards of ANSI, the Snell Memorial Foundation, or ASTM.

Three organizations currently have voluntary standards for bicycle helmets; however, optimal helmet design (e.g., hard vs. soft shell helmets, differences in the needs of children less than 6 years of age, and how well different types of helmets protect in actual crash conditions) has not been established. Additional research is needed on the biomechanics of bicycle helmets before more definitive recommendations for biomechanical standards can be made. However, despite differences in helmet design, wearing an approved helmet is better than wearing no helmet at all. Furthermore, all standards emphasize that a helmet that has sustained an impact should be returned to the manufacturer for inspection or be destroyed and replaced.

Recommendation 4

To effectively increase helmet-use rates, states and communities must implement programs that include legislation, education and promotion, enforcement, and program evaluation.

Communities and states have used several strategies to increase helmet use, including laws that require helmet use among different age groups; community awareness campaigns; educational programs in schools and children's groups; and incentive campaigns that encourage use of helmets through giveaway programs, coupons, and rebates. Helmet-use laws should be implemented statewide; however, beginning this process with a demonstration program in one or several communities may be practical before expanding the program statewide. Laws are most effective when combined with educational programs.

REFERENCES: AS NUMBERED IN ORIGINAL PUBLICATION

1. Thompson RS, Rivara FP, Thompson DC. A case-control study of the effectiveness of bicycle safety helmets. N Engl J Med 1989;320:1361–1367.
4. Sacks JJ, Holmgreen P, Smith SM, Sosin DM. Bicycle-associated head injuries and deaths in the United States from 1984 through 1988:how many are preventable? JAMA 1991;266:3016–3018.
5. Friede AM, Azzara CV, Gallagher SS, Guyer B. The epidemiology of injuries to bicycle riders. Pediatr Clin North Am 1985;32:141–151.
6. Selbst SM, Alexander D, Ruddy R. Bicycle-related injuries. Am J Dis Child 1987;141:140–144.
7. Rodgers GB. Bicycle and bicycle helmet use patterns in the United States: a description and analysis of national survey data. Washington, DC: US Consumer Product Safety Commission, 1993.
8. Guichon MP, Myles ST. Bicycle injuries: one-year sample in Calgary. J Trauma 1975;15:504–506.
11. Belongia E, Weiss H, Bowman M, Rattanassiri P. Severity and types of head trauma among adult bicycle riders. Wis Med J 1988;87:11–14.

13. Dorsch MM, Woodward AJ, Somers RL. Do bicycle safety helmets reduce severity of head injury in real crashes? Accid Annal Prev 1987:19:183–190.
14. Wasserman RC, Waller JA, Monty MJ, et al. Bicyclists, helmets and head injuries: a rider-based study of helmet use and effectiveness. Am J Public Health 1988;78:1220–1221.
15. Wasserman RC, Buccini RV. Helmet protection from head injuries among recreational bicyclists. Am J Sports Med 1990;18:96–97.
16. CDC. Bicycle-related injuries: data from the National Electronic Injury Surveillance System. MMWR 1987;36:269–271.
17. Weiss BD. Childhood bicycle injuries: what can we do? Am J Dis Child 1987;141:135–136.
32. Public Health Service. Healthy people 2000: national health promotion and disease prevention objectives. Washington, DC: US Department of Health and Human Services 1990;DHHS publication no. (PHS)91–50213.
33. DiGuiseppi CG, Rivara FP, Koepsell TD, Polissar L. Bicycle helmet use by children: evaluation of community-wide helmet campaign. JAMA 1989;262:2256–2261.
34. Howland J, Sargent J, Weitzman M, et al. Barriers to bicycle helmet use among children. Am J Dis Child 1989;143:741–744.
35. Vulcan AP, Cameron MH, Heiman L. Evaluation of mandatory bicycle helmet use in Victoria, Australia. 36th Annual Proceedings. Portland, OR: Association for the Advancement of Automotive Medicine, 1992.
36. Cote T, Sacks JJ, Lambert-Huber DA, et al. Bicycle helmet use among Maryland children: effect of legislation and education. Pediatrics 1992;89:1216–1220.
37. Dannenberg AL, Gielen AC, Beilenson PL, Wilson MH, Joffe A. Bicycle helmet laws and educational campaigns: an evaluation of strategies to increase children's helmet use. Am J Public Health 1993; 83:667–674.

APPENDIX A

Bicycle Helmet Legislation

Legislation requiring bicycle helmet use can vary according to the needs of the state or county passing the law. Persons who draft laws requiring the use of bicycle helmets should consider the following components:

Ages Covered

Bicycle helmets should be worn by persons of all ages, including both bicycle operators and passengers, when they are on bicycles. Therefore, the most protective option is to include operators and passengers of all ages in the law. However, some states have been reluctant to pass laws that cover all ages because of difficulty with enforcement of the law. The alternative option is to include only children less than 15 years of age. (See Recommendation 1.)

Helmet Standards

Helmets worn by bicyclists should meet or exceed the current standards of either the American National Standards Institute, the Snell Memorial Foundation, or the American Society for Testing and Materials. (See Helmet Standards.)

Locations Where Riders Must Wear Helmets

The law should require helmet use in all places where bicyclists ride. A law that does not require helmet use in public parks, on trails, on boardwalks, or in other areas set aside for bicycle or pedestrian use does not provide adequate protection for the rider. (See Recommendation 2.)

Enforcement Provisions

Bicycle helmet laws can be enforced in several ways. In Howard County, Maryland, the law requires that children less than 16 years of age wear helmets and that a warning letter be given to a child's parent or guardian after the first and second offenses. On the third offense, a citation with a $50 fine is given. In New Jersey, the state law includes a $25 penalty for each incident in which a child less than 14 years of age fails to wear a bicycle helmet. Each subsequent fine is $100. In addition, all fines in New Jersey are deposited in a Bicycle Safety Fund to be used for bicycle safety education. Other methods of enforcement include confiscation of the bicycle. For example, in Beechwood, Ohio, the police can temporarily take possession of the child's bicycle until the child's parent or guardian has been notified. Several of the current laws waive the penalty if proof of helmet ownership or purchase is provided. Communities may decide to issue discount coupons along with a warning or citation to encourage the purchase of bicycle helmets. Existing laws also address the liability of the manufacturers and retailers of bicycle helmets and renters of bicycles.

APPENDIX B

Organizations that Provide Information on Bicycle Helmet Campaigns

Several organizations have guidelines or instructional manuals for conducting bicycle helmet campaigns. These materials outline strategies and activities that state and local organizations can use to develop campaigns that are consistent with the needs and resources of the communities they serve. Listed below are the names and addresses of several of these organizations as well as a listing of some of the materials that are available to the public:

- National SAFE KIDS Campaign, 111 Michigan Ave. NW, Washington, DC 20010 (202) 884-4993.

Materials include SAFE KIDS Cycle Smart, a guide for community bicycle safety programs and resource materials list; a kit for medical professionals regarding bicycle helmets and injury prevention; a teacher's guide on bicycle helmets; a brochure for parents; a bicycle helmet poster; a traffic safety magazine for children; public service announcements for television; and a chart of legislation mandating bicycle helmet use.

- American Trauma Society, 8903 Presidential Parkway Suite 512, Upper Marlboro, MD 20772-2656 (800) 556-7890.

Materials include a campaign kit and a resource catalog.

- National PTA, 330 North Wabash Avenue Suite 2100, Chicago, IL 60611-3690 (312) 670-6782.

Materials include a guide, Bike Injury/Bike Rodeos, which lists bicycle safety resources and provides guidelines to help local PTAs organize bicycle rodeos and promote bicycle safety.

- American Academy of Pediatrics, Publications Department, 141 Northwest Point Boulevard, Box 927, Elk Grove Village, IL 60009-0927 (800) 433-9016.

Materials include Physician's Resource Guide for Bicycle Safety Education; "Bicycle Safety Camp," which is a videotape for elementary school students concerning the importance of wearing helmets and other safety issues while riding bicycles; and bicycle safety sheets from The Injury Prevention Program. The safety sheets cover such topics as encouraging children to wear helmets, myths and facts about bicycle safety, choosing the right size bicycle for a child, and child passengers on adults' bicycles.

- Harborview Injury Prevention and Research Center, University of Washington, 325 Ninth Avenue, ZX-10, Seattle, WA 98104 (206) 521-1537.

Materials include Developing a Children's Bicycle Helmet Safety Program: A Guide for Local Communities.

- The Johns Hopkins Injury Prevention Center, The Johns Hopkins School of Hygiene and Public Health, 624 N. Broadway, 5th and 6th Floors, Baltimore, MD 21205-1996 (410) 955-7625.

Materials include Injuries to Bicyclists: A National Perspective. This monograph is available from the National Center for Injury Prevention and Control, CDC, mailstop F-36, 4770 Buford Highway, Atlanta, GA 30341-3724. A videotape produced by the Center, "ADVOKIDS: Kids Advocating Change," is available through AAA Foundation for Traffic Safety; telephone: (202) 638-5944.

APPENDIX C

Components of a Community-Based Bicycle Helmet Campaign

Bicycle helmet campaigns should include a number of specific components, regardless of the actual activities (e.g., bicycle rodeos, coupon programs, and helmet giveaways) that are included in the campaign.

A Coalition

A coalition of appropriate individuals, agencies, and organizations that represent all facets of the community should participate in all phases of the campaign, beginning with the development of a plan and the selection of target groups, through implementing the interventions and evaluating the effort. The following organizations should be considered for inclusion in campaigns: health departments; schools; parent-teacher-student organizations; police departments; churches; neighborhood and tenant associations; health care providers, including physicians, nurses, and emergency response personnel; community organizations (e.g., Kiwanis and Junior League); youth clubs (e.g., Girl Scouts of America, Boy Scouts of America, and 4-H); businesses, such as bicycle shop owners; and local government leaders and political organizations.

A Plan

A campaign to promote bicycle helmets should begin with a well-organized plan that includes the following components:

1. Goals and objectives that reflect what the community wants to achieve, what it determines is feasible, and the activities that are needed to achieve them. The goals and objectives should also reflect current rates of bicycle helmet use in the community.
2. A description of the primary target group for the campaign (e.g., children less than 15 years of age). Information on bicycle helmet use and rates of bicycle-related injury in the community should be used to select this target group.
3. A description of the intervention program(s) that will be used. The program should address barriers to helmet use in the target group (e.g., the cost of helmets) and include strategies for overcoming these barriers (e.g., discount coupons). In addition, the messages of the campaign should be designed so they are easily understood and accepted by the target group. Finally, programs should be offered in locations where the target group can be reached.

The following are educational and promotional strategies that have been used in some communities:

- Media campaigns often begin with a kick-off press conference and continue throughout the campaign to increase awareness and help create a community norm of wearing bicycle helmets. These campaigns can include public service announcements; newspaper articles; radio and television news programs and talk shows; and distribution of brochures, posters, fact sheets, and other printed materials.
- Educational campaigns may be offered through schools and youth organizations, churches, and civic and business organizations in the community. Speakers' bureaus are an effective way to conduct many of these activities.
- Events such as bicycle safety and skill rodeos combine fun and learning for both children and adults. These events demonstrate and promote helmet use along with other aspects of bicycle safety, provide good opportunities to distribute educational materials, and allow participants to interact with persons who have avoided injury by using bicycle helmets.
- Promotional activities, such as discount coupons for bicycle helmets and giveaway programs, provide incentives for acquiring bicycle helmets, particularly for persons who have difficulty affording one. Coupons can be obtained from helmet manufacturers or local bicycle shops. The program could also provide other incentives to obtain a helmet.

4. An evaluation component to determine if the program is reaching its goals. This evaluation should assess bicycle helmet use before and after the intervention(s) is conducted and at specific intervals thereafter.

5. A strategy for making bicycle helmet use a societal norm so that the public will maintain or increase levels of helmet use.

Deaths Resulting from Firearm- and Motor-Vehicle-Related Injuries

Original Citation: Centers for Disease Control and Prevention. Deaths resulting from firearm- and motor-vehicle-related injuries—United States, 1968–1991. MMWR 1994;43(3): 37–42.

Injury is the leading cause of death for persons aged 1–44 years in the United States. More than half (55%) of all injury-related deaths are caused by motor vehicles and firearms (1). Although the number of deaths from motor-vehicle crashes has exceeded those from firearms, since 1968, differences in the number of deaths have declined: from 1968 through 1991, motor-vehicle-related deaths decreased by 21% (from 54,862 to 43,536) while firearm-related deaths increased by 60% (from 23,875 to 38,317) (1). Based on these trends, by the year 2003, the number of firearm-related deaths will surpass the number of motor-vehicle crashes, and firearms will become the leading cause of injury-related death (Figure 1).

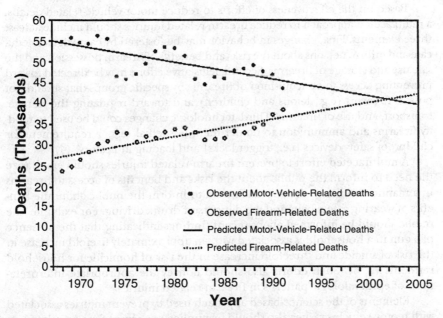

Figure 1. Observed and predicted firearm- and motor-vehicle-related injury deaths, by year—United States, 1968–2005 (the lines are predicted numbers of deaths based on linear regression).

These trends may reflect differences in the approaches to preventing motor-vehicle- and firearm-related injuries. In particular, reductions in the occurrence of motor-vehicle-related injuries have been associated with the development of a set of comprehensive and science-based interventions and policies (2); in contrast, there have been limited efforts to develop a systematic framework to reduce the incidence and impact of injuries associated with firearms.

Elements of the multifaceted, science-based approach to reduce mortality from motor-vehicle crashes have included public information programs, promotion of behavioral change, changes in legislation and regulations, and advances in engineering and technology. These strategies have resulted in safer vehicles (e.g., the addition of laminated windshields and interior padding), safer driving practices (e.g., reduced occurrence of alcohol-impaired driving and increased use of safety belts), safer travel environments (e.g., construction of safer highways and roads), and improved emergency medical services. Key elements of the science-based approach have included the establishment of a national data-collection system to routinely monitor motor-vehicle-related deaths, identification of modifiable risk factors, design and implementation of preventive measures, and evaluation of the effectiveness of these measures. Since 1966, when the federal government identified highway safety as a major goal and subsequently established the National Highway Traffic Safety Administration to help reduce death and injury on the highway, the annual number of motor-vehicle-related deaths in the United States has decreased, even though the annual number of vehicle-miles traveled has increased 114% (3).

Based on the effectiveness of efforts to reduce motor-vehicle-related deaths, a multifaceted approach to reduce firearm-related injuries should include at least three elements. First, changes in behavior may be fostered by campaigns to educate and inform persons about the risks and benefits of firearm possession and the safe use and storage of firearms. Second, legislative efforts may be directed toward preventing access to or acquisition of firearms by specific groups that should not possess firearms (e.g., felons and children) and toward regulating the storage, transport, and use of firearms. Third, technologic changes could be used to modify firearms and ammunition to render them less lethal (e.g., a requirement for childproof safety devices [i.e., trigger locks] and loading indicators) (4).

A multifaceted effort to prevent firearm-related injuries should emphasize the need to inform the public about the risks and benefits of access to firearms in a manner similar to the approach used to inform the public about the benefits of wearing safety belts and the dangers of drunk driving. For example, the public should be informed about recent findings indicating that the presence of a gun in a household is associated with an approximately fivefold increase in the risk of suicide and threefold increase in the risk of homicide for household residents (5, 6). Such efforts also should convey the appropriate interpretations of epidemiologic patterns in firearm-related injuries.

Elements of the science-based approach used to prevent injuries associated with motor-vehicle crashes also should be applied to prevent firearm-related injuries. These elements should include establishment of a national firearm injury surveillance system to enable systematic collection of data about fatal and nonfatal firearm-related injuries and about the patterns of firearm ownership and use, and continued efforts to define more precisely the risks and benefits of gun ownership and the modifiable factors that increase the risk of death and injury from firearms. In addition, despite the implementation of a variety of approaches to the prevention of firearm-related injuries and death, efforts to evaluate these approaches have been limited (8–10) and underscore the need for continued assessment of the effectiveness of such intervention strategies.

Because highway safety has been a national priority since 1966, an estimated 250,000 motor-vehicle-related deaths have been averted. Despite this progress, efforts to reduce the burden of motor-vehicle-related injuries and fatalities must be sustained. In addition, adoption of a similar multifaceted, science-based approach should assist in decreasing the public health impact and societal burden of injuries resulting from use of firearms.

REFERENCES: AS NUMBERED IN ORIGINAL PUBLICATION

1. Fingerhut LA, Jones C, Makuc D. Firearm and motor vehicle injury mortality—variation by state and race and ethnicity: United States, 1990–1991. Hyattsville, MD: US Department of Health and Human Services, Public Health Service, CDC, 1994 (Advance data from vital and health statistics; no. 242).
2. CDC/National Highway Traffic Safety Administration. Position papers from the Third National Injury Control Conference: setting the national agenda for injury control in the 1990s. Atlanta: US Department of Health and Human Services, Public Health Service, CDC, 1992.
3. National Highway Traffic Safety Administration. Fatal Accident Reporting System, 1991: a review of information on fatal traffic crashes in the United States. Washington, DC: US Department of Transportation, National Highway Traffic Safety Administration, 1993.
4. US General Accounting Office. Accidental shootings: many deaths and injuries caused by firearms could be prevented—report to the Chairman, Subcommittee on Antitrust, Monopolies, and Business Rights, Committee on the Judiciary, House of Representatives. Washington, DC: US General Accounting Office, 1991;report no. GAO/PEMD-91-9.
5. Kellermann AL, Rivara FP, Somes G, et al. Suicide in the home in relation to gun ownership. N Engl J Med 1992;327:467–472.
6. Kellermann AL, Rivara FP, Rushforth NB, et al. Gun ownership as a risk factor for homicide in the home. N Engl J Med 1993;329:1084–1091.
8. Rossman D, Paul F, Pierce GL, McDevitt J, Bowers W. Massachusetts' mandatory minimum sentence gun law: enforcement, prosecution, and defense impact. Crim Law Bull 1980;61:150–163.
9. McDowall D, Loftin C, Wiersema B. A comparative study of the preventive effects of mandatory sentencing laws for gun crimes. J Crim Law Criminol 1992;83:378–394.
10. Loftin C, McDowall D, Wiersema B, Cottey TJ. Effects of restrictive licensing of handguns on homicide and suicide in the District of Columbia. N Engl J Med 1991;325:1615–1620.

BB and Pellet Gun-Related Injuries

Original Citation: Centers for Disease Control and Prevention. BB and pellet gun-related injuries—United States, June 1992-May 1994. MMWR 1994;44(49):909–913.

Each year in the United States, approximately 30,000 persons with BB and pellet gun*-related injuries are treated in hospital emergency departments (EDs)

---

* In this report, the terms BB gun and pellet gun refer to nonpowder guns that use compressed air or gas to propel lead pellets or steel BBS.

(1). Most (95%) injuries are BB or pellet gunshot wounds (GSWs); 5% are other types of injuries (e.g., lacerations sustained inadvertently while cleaning or shooting a gun or contusions resulting from being struck with the butt of a gun) (1). Most (81%) persons treated for BB and pellet GSWs are children and teenagers (aged ≤19 years).

Despite the large number of BB and pellet gun-related injuries treated in hospital EDs each year (1), there are no nationally specified safety standards for nonpowder guns. Although voluntary industry standards were established in 1978 and revised in 1992 (7), the effectiveness of these standards for preventing injuries has not been determined. These voluntary standards specify two types of warning labels, including one on the gun itself ("WARNING: Before using read Owner's Manual available free from [company name]"), and one on the packaging ("WARNING: Not a toy. Adult supervision required. Misuse or careless use may cause serious injury or death. May be dangerous up to [specific distance]** yards ([specific distance] meters).") (7). The voluntary standards also specify that the owner's manual should provide instructions about handling and operating the gun safely, selecting safe and proper targets, caring for and maintaining the gun properly, storing of the gun in an unloaded state and in a safe and proper manner, and always confirming that the gun is unloaded when removed from storage or received from another person (7). However, these standards do not include specifications regarding other important injury-prevention measures pertinent to minors (e.g., limits on maximum velocity and impact force of BBS and pellets or design modifications to clearly indicate when a gun is loaded) (8).

In the United States, 14 states have enacted laws to regulate the sale or possession of nonpowder guns. Although most of these states restrict the purchase, possession, or use of these guns by minors aged <16 years or aged <18 years, such age restrictions on the purchase of these guns are void in most of these states when a minor has obtained permission from a parent or guardian.

Unintentional BB and pellet gun-related injuries that occur during unsupervised activities are preventable. Parents considering the purchase of a BB or pellet gun for their children should be aware of the potential hazards of these guns, and should help to ensure the safety of their children in the presence of a BB or pellet gun. Children and teenaged users should recognize that these guns are not toys but are designed and intended specifically for recreational and competitive sport use. Parents or other adults should provide direct supervision at all times for each child who is using or observing the use of these guns. Each user should be educated about the potential danger of these guns, the importance of gun-safety practices, and how to safely handle and fire the gun. The use of protective eyewear should be enforced during shooting activities. When not in use, all guns in the home should be kept locked up and unloaded. Subsequent efforts to reduce the severity and frequency of injuries associated with BB and pellet guns should include determination of the effectiveness of a variety of interventions (e.g., technological, regulatory, environmental, and behavioral).

** Distance is dependent on the type of gun and muzzle velocity.

REFERENCES: AS NUMBERED IN ORIGINAL PUBLICATION

1. McNeill AM, Annest JL. The ongoing hazard of BB and pellet gun-related injuries in the United States. Ann Emerg Med 1995;26:187–194.
7. Committee on Standards, American Society for Testing and Materials. Standard consumer safety specification for non-powder guns. Conshohocken, PA: American Society for Testing and Materials, 1992.
8. Greensher J, Aronow R, Bass JL, et al. Injuries related to "toy" firearms: Committee on Accident and Poison Prevention. Pediatrics 1987;79:473–474.

TOPIC 46 / **FIRES**

Deaths Resulting from Residential Fires

Original Citation: Centers for Disease Control and Prevention. Health objectives for the nation: deaths resulting from residential fires—United States, 1991. MMWR 1994;43 (49):901–904.

Data from the 1990 National Fire Incidence Reporting System (NFIRS) were used to estimate the numbers of fires and deaths associated with selected causes of residential fires during January, February, March, and December (2). During these months in 1990, residential electrical-distribution fires were associated with an estimated 40,000 fires and 266 deaths Table 1. Residential fires involving fireplaces and chimneys resulted in an estimated 26,200 fires, and portable kerosene and electrical heaters were involved in an estimated 1500 fires. Christmas tree fires caused approximately 600 residential fires and 29 deaths; the ratio of deaths to fires was 1:21. (Reported by Division of Unintentional Injury Prevention, National Center for Injury Prevention and Control, CDC.)

Table 1. Estimated number of residential fires, number of deaths, and ratio of deaths to fires, by selected causes—United States, 1990

Cause	No. deaths	Estimated no. fires	Ratio (deaths:fires)
Christmas trees	29	600	1:20
Portable heaters	56	1,500	1:27
Electrical distribution*	266	40,000	1:150
Fireplaces and chimneys	58	26,200	1:452

*Includes wiring, transformers, meter boxes, power switching gear, outlets, cords, plugs, and lighting fixtures as sources of heat.

Source: National Fire Incidence Reporting System, U.S. Fire Administration.

EDITORIAL NOTE

Despite the 37% decline in rates of residential-fire deaths from 1970 through 1991 (1), the overall rate in 1991 (1.5 per 100,000) exceeded the rate targeted by a national health objective for the year 2000 (reducing the rate of residential fire-related deaths to no more than 1.2 deaths per 100,000 persons [objective 9.6]). In particular, the rates for children aged less than 5 years (3.7 per

100,000 children) and for persons aged greater than or equal to 65 years (3.5 per 100,000)—the highest-risk groups—exceeded the age-group-specific target goal of 3.3 per 100,000 for each group (1, 3).

The increased occurrence of fire-related deaths during winter months (Figures 1 and 2) reflects the seasonal use of portable heaters, fireplaces and chimneys, and Christmas trees (2). Fires associated with electric portable heaters usually result from electrical shortages or device failure, rather than from ignition of nearby materials such as draperies. Electric cords for portable electric space heaters should be plugged directly into the wall and not linked through an extension cord, kept at least 3 feet from any combustible object, and unplugged when not in use. Fires attributed to the use of kerosene portable heaters usually result from using the wrong fuel, faulty switches and valves, and fuel leaks and spills that subsequently ignite. Kerosene heaters should be used only with K-1 kerosene, rather than gasoline or camp-stove fuel, and should be re-fueled outdoors after the heater has cooled. Chimney fires usually result from a build-up of creosote, a highly flammable by-product of wood fires. Chimneys should be cleaned or inspected annually to detect and prevent creosote build-up. A fire screen should be used in front of the fire-place; wood stoves and fireplaces should burn only seasoned wood—not green wood, trash, or wrapping paper.

Fires related to Christmas trees usually result from electrical problems (e.g., overloaded electrical circuits caused by using several extension cords in one outlet, or frayed wire and cords). In 1991, Christmas trees accounted for

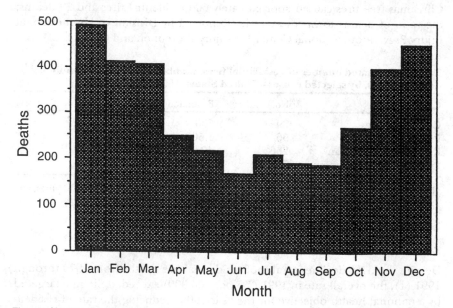

Figure 1. Number of deaths from residential fires (International Classification of Diseases, Ninth Revision, codes E890-E899) by month—United States, 1991. Source: National Center for Health Statistics, CDC.

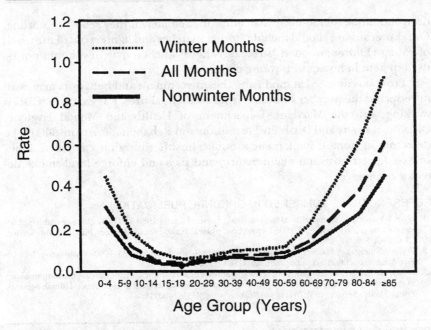

Figure 2. Rate (per 100,000 population) of deaths from residential fires (International Classification of Diseases, Ninth Revision, codes E890-E899) during winter months (January, February, March, and December) and nonwinter months (April through November), by age group of decedent—United States, 1991. Source: National Center for Health Statistics, CDC.

the lowest number of fires, but a substantially higher proportion of deaths than other types of residential fires described in this report Table 1. Persons in households with these holiday decorations should periodically examine the electric lights used and should not place trees near heating sources or fireplaces. In addition, live-cut trees should be sufficiently watered to reduce drying; dry trees ignite easily and burn rapidly.

To reduce the risk for death or injury resulting from fires, a smoke detector should be installed outside each sleeping area on every habitable level of a home and the battery changed at least annually. Occupants should develop escape plans that include the identification of two exits from every living area and should practice exit drills and meeting at a designated place at a safe location sufficiently distant from the home. In addition, every home should have a multipurpose fire extinguisher ready for use in extinguishing small fires. Residences should be evacuated for any fire that cannot be extinguished within 1 minute because of the rapid rate of accumulation of heat and smoke; once evacuated, residences should not be reentered. Persons who become trapped in a residence should crawl on the floor toward an exit to avoid inhalation of smoke that has risen.

Because children playing with fire-ignition sources were the leading cause of fires that resulted in the deaths of children aged less than 5 years, children should be taught not to play with matches or lighters. In addition, young children should be told to inform an adult immediately if they see a fire starting. Other precautions should include storing matches and lighters out of the reach of young children; wooden "strike anywhere" kitchen matches should not be used or kept in homes with young children.

Programs directed at modifying the environment and behaviors may assist in reducing the number of deaths from residential fires. For example, CDC is working with the Maryland Department of Health and Mental Hygiene, Division of Injury and Disability Prevention and Rehabilitation, to install smoke detectors in homes, implement a public health education campaign about smoke detector use and maintenance, and pass and enforce local smoke detector ordinances.

REFERENCES: AS NUMBERED IN ORIGINAL PUBLICATION

1. NCHS. Vital statistics mortality data, underlying cause of death, 1980–1991 [machine-readable public-use data tapes]. Hyattsville, MD: US Department of Health and Human Services, Public Health Service, CDC, NCHS, 1991.
2. Federal Emergency Management Agency. Fire in the United States, 1983–1990. Washington, DC: US Fire Administration, 1993:publication no. USFA/FA-140.
3. Public Health Service. Healthy people 2000: national health promotion and disease prevention objectives—full report, with commentary. Washington, DC: US Department of Health and Human Services, Public Health Service, 1991:DHHS publication no. (PHS)91–50212.

TOPIC 47 / **FIREWORKS**

Serious Eye Injuries Associated with Fireworks

Original Citation: Centers for Disease Control and Prevention. Serious eye injuries associated with fireworks—United States, 1990–1994. MMWR 1995;44(24):449–452.

Original Authors: S. Brown, MPH, C.D. Witherspoon, MD, R. Morris, MD, S.M. Hamilton, MD, F.I. Camesasca, MD, J.A. Kimble, MD.

Eye injuries caused by fireworks are often severe and can cause permanently reduced visual acuity or blindness. Findings from the National Electronic Injury Surveillance System database maintained by the U.S. Consumer Product Safety Commission (CPSC) indicate that approximately 12,000 persons are treated each year in U.S. emergency departments because of fireworks-related injuries; of these, an estimated 20% are eye injuries.

UNITED STATES EYE INJURY REGISTRY

United States Eye Injury Registry (USEIR), a nonprofit organization sponsored by the Helen Keller Eye Research Foundation, is a federation of state eye registries that uses a standardized form to obtain voluntarily reported data on eye injuries and to obtain 6-month follow-up information. Reports are made by ophthalmologists to the USEIR database in Birmingham, Alabama. The primary purpose of USEIR is to provide prospective, population-based, epidemiologic data to improve the prevention and control of eye injuries. The registry contains information only for patients who have sustained a serious eye injury, defined as "an injury resulting in permanent and significant, structural or functional ocular change." USEIR comprises 39 state registry affiliates (representing 89% of the U.S. population); 32 states registered injuries during 1990–1994, and 27 states reported fireworks-related injuries during this period.

From July 1990 through December 1994, a total of 4575 serious eye injuries from all causes were reported to USEIR; of the 274 (6%) fireworks-related injuries, 255 (93%) were unintentional injuries. Persons injured by fireworks were aged 4–63 years (median: 15 years); 211 (77%) were males. The largest proportion (123 [45%]) of injured persons were bystanders; 96 (35%) were fireworks operators, and for 55 (20%), status was unknown. Most (219 [80%]) injuries occurred during the Independence Day holiday period*; 44 (16%) occurred during the New Year's holiday period*, and 11 (4%) at other times. Most (67%) injuries occurred at home; injuries also occurred in recreational settings (14%), on a street or highway (5%), and in parking lots or occupational settings (1%). Location was unknown for 13%.

Most injuries were caused by bottle rockets (58%) (Figure 1). Bottle rockets accounted for 68% of the injuries to bystanders.

EDITORIAL NOTE

Irreversible consequences—including reduced visual acuity and blindness—can result from the use of consumer fireworks, especially bottle rockets. Analysis

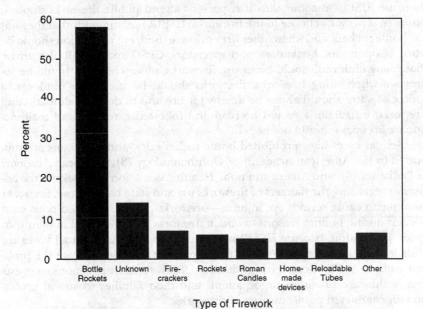

Figure 1. Percentage of fireworks-related serious eye injuries, by type of firework—United States Eye Injury Registry, 1990–1994.

---

* The number of days for the holiday period varied each year.

of the USEIR database indicated that a high proportion of fireworks-related injuries occurred among young males—a finding consistent with previous reports (1, 2). These findings are similar to the results of a study in Washington in which injuries were associated with improper use (both intentional and unintentional), product malfunctions (e.g., short fuses, erratic flight, or tip-over), and high temperature (2).

Consumer fireworks—including bottle rockets (classified as 1.4G [formally known as Class C] fireworks)—have been banned in 10 states (Arizona, Connecticut, Delaware, Georgia, Massachusetts, Minnesota, New Jersey, New York, Rhode Island, and Vermont). Six states (Illinois, Iowa, Maine, Maryland, Ohio, and Pennsylvania) permit the use only of sparklers and other novelties (e.g., poppers, wheels, and snaps). The District of Columbia and 32 states allow at least some 1.4G fireworks to be sold. Nevada and Hawaii have no laws regulating fireworks except for local ordinances. The CPSC has banned firecrackers with greater than 50 mg pyrotechnic composition (including cherry bombs, M-80s, and silver salutes) designed to detonate on or near the ground and reloadable shell devices with diameters exceeding 1.75 inches; bottle-rockets can contain up to 130 mg pyrotechnic composition.

Because of the risks for injury associated with bottle rockets and other fireworks, several organizations have made specific recommendations regarding their use. USEIR recommends that persons attend public fireworks displays; however, if persons choose to use fireworks, USEIR recommends that they not use bottle rockets, and when other fireworks are used, eye protection should be worn by operators, bystanders, and spectators. CPSC and USEIR also advise that young children should never use fireworks, older children should be supervised when using fireworks, fireworks should be used only outdoors, a source of water should always be nearby for fire and to douse malfunctioning fireworks, instructions should be read and followed carefully, and malfunctioning fireworks should not be relit.

Several states have prohibited bottle rocket sales, and such bans are supported by the American Academy of Ophthalmology (3), American Academy of Pediatrics (4), and American Public Health Association (5). Despite the advisories regarding the dangers of fireworks use and state bans on use, fireworks continue to cause serious eye injuries—fireworks purchasers often cross state borders during holiday seasons to obtain fireworks that are illegal in their own states. In addition, because USEIR is a voluntary registry and not all states are affiliated, the numbers presented in this report may underestimate the problem nationally. CDC, concurring with the USEIR recommendations, suggests that health-care providers urge patients and their families to attend professionally conducted public displays of fireworks.

REFERENCES: AS NUMBERED IN ORIGINAL PUBLICATION

1. CDC. Fireworks-related injuries—Marion County, Indiana, 1986–1991. MMWR 1992;41:451–454.
2. CDC. Fireworks-related injuries—Washington. MMWR 1983;32:285–286.
3. Eye Safety and Sports Ophthalmology Committee. Fireworks remain serious health hazard and cause of blindness. San Francisco: American Academy of Ophthalmology, May 1995.
4. Committee on Injury and Poison Prevention. Children and fireworks. Pediatr 1991;88:652–653.

5. American Public Health Association. Resolution 9111—banning bottle rockets: prevention of ocular injuries. In: American Public Health Association. Public policy statements of the American Public Health Association. Washington, DC: American Public Health Association, 1994:482–483.

TOPIC 48 / **MOTOR VEHICLES**

Air-Bag–Associated Fatal Injuries

Original Citation: Centers for Disease Control and Prevention. Air-bag-associated fatal injuries to infants and children riding in front passenger seats—United States. MMWR 1995;44(45):845–847.

Air bags, when used as a supplement to safety belts, effectively prevent deaths and serious injuries in frontal motor-vehicle crashes. Air bags are standard equipment in most new cars; federal safety standards require that all new passenger cars and light trucks be equipped with both driver- and passenger-side air bags by 1999. The safety of air bags is well documented, and air bags have saved an estimated 900 lives since the late 1980s (1); however, special precautions are needed to safely transport children in vehicles equipped with air bags. Reports of eight deaths of child passengers in crashes involving air-bag deployment are of special concern because they involved low-speed crashes that the children otherwise might have survived.

Although infants, children, and all other occupants always should be properly restrained in safety seats or safety belts, as many as 35% of young children ride unrestrained (3). Any child who rides unrestrained or incorrectly restrained in the front seat of a vehicle with a passenger-side air bag is at risk for serious injury or death if the air bag deploys. Precrash braking may propel an unrestrained child against the dashboard in immediate proximity to the point of air-bag deployment. The inflating air bag then can propel the child against structures inside the vehicle, causing serious injury or death.

Rear-facing child restraints also pose a hazard in vehicles with a passenger-side air bag and must never be placed in the front seat (4). To be properly protected, infants must ride in a rear-facing child restraint until they weigh 20 pounds or are approximately 1 year old (5). In a crash, a rear-facing child restraint placed in the front seat with its back close to the vehicle's instrument panel could be struck by the rapidly inflating air bag, and the child in the restraint could be seriously injured or killed.

Forward-facing safety seats are less likely to be affected by air bag interaction because of their greater distance from the point of air-bag deployment in the dashboard. However, because these seats usually place the child at least several inches closer to the dashboard than adults in the standard seating position, the safest practice is to place all child safety seats in the back seat of the vehicle. If a forward-facing safety seat must be placed in the front seat of a vehicle with a passenger-side air bag, the vehicle seat should be moved as far back as possible to maximize clearance with the dashboard.

As a result of an investigation of air-bag related fatalities and serious injuries to child passengers, the National Transportation Safety Board (NTSB) recently released safety recommendations regarding children and air bags (2). NTSB recommends collaboration between automobile and safety-seat manufacturers, the news media, health and medical organizations, and the National Highway Traffic Safety Administration (NHTSA) to inform motorists and parents of the correct procedures for transporting children in vehicles equipped with air bags. NHTSA has enacted several regulatory measures addressing the air bag/child passenger problem, including labeling requirements for vehicles and child safety seats and specifications for air-bag cutoff switches. CDC and NHTSA have developed recommendations to prevent air-bag associated injuries to infants and children (Table 1).

Table 1. Public Health Recommendations to Prevent Air-Bag-Associated Injuries to Infants and Children

- All infants and children should be properly restrained in child safety seats or lap and shoulder belts when riding in a motor vehicle.
- Infants riding in rear-facing child safety seats should never be placed in the front seat of a car or truck with a passenger-side air bag.
- Children should ride in a car's rear seat. If a vehicle does not have a rear seat, children riding in the front seat should be positioned as far back as possible from an air bag.

In addition to intensifying efforts to educate motorists, NHTSA has solicited public comment regarding further strategies to reduce adverse effects of air bags (published in the November 9, 1995, Federal Register (60 FR 56554)); written comments are due by December 26, 1995, to Docket Section, Room 5109, NHTSA, 400 Seventh St., SW, Washington, DC 20590 (refer to docket 74–14, notice #97).

Additional information is available from Child Safety Seats, c/o NHTSA, NTS-13, 400 Seventh St., SW, Washington, DC 20590; or from NHTSA's Auto Safety Hotline, telephone (800) 424-9393 or (202) 366-0123.

Air-bag-associated serious injuries and deaths to infants and children should be reported to Vernon Roberts, NTSB, telephone (202) 382-0660.

REFERENCES: AS NUMBERED IN ORIGINAL PUBLICATION

1. National Center for Statistics and Analysis, National Highway Traffic Safety Administration. Traffic safety facts 1994: occupant protection. Washington, DC: US Department of Transportation, National Highway Traffic Safety Administration, 1995.
2. National Transportation Safety Board. Safety recommendation, H-95–17. Washington, DC: National Transportation Safety Board, 1995.
3. National Center for Statistics and Analysis, National Highway Traffic Safety Administration. Research note. National occupant protection use survey: controlled intersection study. Washington, DC: US Department of Transportation, National Highway Traffic Safety Administration, May 1, 1995.
4. CDC. Warnings on interaction between air bags and rear-facing child restraints. MMWR 1993;42:280–282.
5. American Academy of Pediatrics. 1995 Family shopping guide to car seats: guidelines for parents. Elk Grove Village, Illinois: American Academy of Pediatrics, 1995.

Drivers With Repeat Convictions or Arrests for Driving While Impaired

Original Citation: Centers for Disease Control and Prevention. Current trends drivers with repeat convictions or arrests for driving while impaired—United States. MMWR 1994;43(41):759–761.

In 1992 (the latest year for which data are available), more than 1.6 million persons in the United States (approximately 1% of licensed drivers) were arrested for driving while impaired (DWI) (1). Persons arrested for DWI are at substantially greater risk for future death in a motor-vehicle crash involving alcohol than those who have not been arrested for DWI, and this risk increases directly in relation to the number of DWI arrests (2). In addition, drivers convicted of DWI are at greater risk of being involved in a fatal crash, regardless of whether they are killed (3).

EDITORIAL NOTE

Motor-vehicle crashes are the leading cause of death in the United States for persons in all age groups from ages 1 through 34 years (4). Approximately 44% of the 40,115 traffic fatalities in 1993 were alcohol-related (5). In 1990, alcohol-related crashes cost $46.1 billion, including $5.1 billion in medical expenses (6).

Although state laws have been effective in reducing drinking and driving and deaths associated with alcohol-related crashes (6), the findings in this report indicate that, in those states that provided data, approximately one third of drivers who were arrested or convicted for DWI had previous offenses for alcohol-impaired driving. Although this finding is consistent with previous unpublished reports of state data, it probably underestimates the prevalence of such drivers because convictions or arrests for DWI that occur out-of-state may not be included in a driver's record.

Because of the limited number of states with available data, the findings in this report may not be representative of all drivers with previous convictions or arrests for DWI. The need for such information underscores the importance for states and localities to develop systems to track DWI offenders (e.g., systems that combine criminal justice records with driver history data).

The risk for repeat arrests for DWI is higher among males and young persons (7); this risk is also higher among persons with histories of numerous traffic violations, a high alcohol concentration at arrest, and histories of alcohol problems (7). For example, of 461 drivers convicted of DWI in New York City during 1983–84, approximately 73% had histories of serious alcohol problems (8).

In addition to the influence of the risk factors, the percentage of drivers with previous convictions or arrests for DWI may reflect the aggressiveness with which states enforce laws against alcohol-impaired driving. Although the annual arrest rate for DWI nationally in 1992 was nine per 1000 licensed drivers (1), the rate varied by state and ranged from three to 22 per 1000 licensed drivers (1). In addition, most repeat arrests for DWI occur within 5 years of the previous arrest date (R. Peck, California Department of Motor Vehicles, unpublished data, 1994).

Effective strategies implemented by states and localities to prevent drinking and driving have included prompt license suspension for persons who drive while intoxicated; enactment of legislation lowering permissible blood alcohol content to 0.08 g/dL for adults and to 0.02 g/dL for drivers aged less than 21 years; and initiation of public education, community awareness, and media campaigns about the dangers of alcohol-impaired driving (6). Specific measures implemented to prevent repeat convictions and arrests for DWI include mandatory substance-abuse assessment and treatment, incarceration, and both; house arrest with electronic monitoring; ignition interlocks on vehicles; license plate tags that identify drivers with licenses suspended for DWI; vehicle impoundment or confiscation; fines; and increases in automobile insurance rates (9). The effectiveness of these specific measures must be evaluated further; however, the findings in this report suggest that, to prevent injuries and deaths in alcohol-related crashes, additional and stronger state legislation (e.g., mandatory substance-abuse assessment and treatment) should be directed toward persons arrested for or convicted of DWI.

REFERENCES: AS NUMBERED IN ORIGINAL PUBLICATION

1. Federal Bureau of Investigation, US Department of Justice. Uniform crime reports: crime in the United States, 1992. Washington, DC: US Department of Justice, Federal Bureau of Investigation, 1993.
2. Brewer RD, Morris PD, Cole T, Watkins S, Patetta MJ, Popkin C. The risk of dying in alcohol-related automobile crashes among habitual drunk drivers. N Engl J Med 1994;331:513–517.
3. Fell JC. Repeat DWI offenders: their involvement in fatal crashes. In: Utzelmann H-D, Berghaus G, Kroj G, eds. Proceedings of the 12th International Conference on Alcohol, Drugs, and Traffic Safety. Cologne, Germany: Verlag TUV Rheinland, 1993.
4. NCHS. Health, United States, 1993. Hyattsville, MD: US Department of Health and Human Services, Public Health Service, CDC, 1994:DHHS publication no. (PHS)94–1232.
5. National Highway Traffic Safety Administration, US Department of Transportation. Traffic safety facts, 1993: alcohol. Washington, DC: US Department of Transportation, National Highway Traffic Safety Administration, 1994.
6. CDC. Reduction in alcohol-related traffic fatalities—United States, 1990–1992. MMWR 1993;42:905–909.
7. Arstein-Kerslake GW, Peck RC. A typological analysis of California DUI offenders and DUI recidivism correlates. Sacramento, CA: California Department of Motor Vehicles, Research and Development Office, 1985.
8. Miller BA, Whitney R, Washousky R. Alcoholism diagnoses for convicted drinking drivers referred for alcoholism evaluation. Alcohol Clin Exp Res 1986;10:651–656.
9. Popkin CL, Wells-Parker E. A research agenda for the specific deterrence of DWI. J Traffic Med 1994;22:1–14.

Risky Driving Behaviors Among Teenagers

Original Citation: Centers for Disease Control and Prevention. Risky driving behaviors among teenagers—Gwinnett County, Georgia, 1993. MMWR 1994;43(22):405–409.

EDITORIAL NOTE

Young drivers account disproportionately for motor-vehicle crashes (MVCs) worldwide (4), reflecting, in part, the combination of immaturity and lack of driving experience (5). Adolescent drivers are more likely than adult drivers to report speeding, running red lights, making illegal turns, not wearing safety belts, riding with an intoxicated driver, and driving after using drugs or alcohol (6).

In the Gwinnett County study, most students—regardless of whether they were cases or controls—reported engaging in risky driving behaviors. Parents should recognize that driving is a complex task that can take several years to master and can assist in reducing the risk for MVCs among adolescent drivers by (a) providing young drivers a longer period of supervised driving in low-risk settings (e.g., with supervision, during daylight, and in safe environments) in addition to traditional driver's education courses, (b) serving as role models by practicing good driving behaviors and always obeying traffic laws, and (c) requiring all family members to be properly restrained each time they ride in a motor vehicle.

The findings in this report are subject to at least five limitations. First, because respondents were students who were licensed drivers enrolled in public schools, the study did not include students in private schools, youth not enrolled in school, and drivers with learners' permits. Second, because the study assessed only MVCs that occurred during January-March 1993, the effects of seasonal trends could not be analyzed. Third, the study did not include MVCs that resulted only in property damage or were not reported to the police. Fourth, other potential risk factors (e.g., alcohol use) were not analyzed in this report, although they were included in the study. Finally, the analysis of findings in this case-control study was influenced by the high prevalences of risky behaviors among members of both the case and control groups.

Graduated driver licensing is one strategy for promoting safe driving behaviors and reducing the incidence and severity of MVCs among young drivers. This method allows new drivers to accumulate driving experience in low-risk settings and gradually lifts restrictions until an unrestricted license is earned (7). In addition, because up to 24 months may be required to obtain an unrestricted license, drivers are older and more mature when they become fully licensed. Driving restrictions may include prohibiting unsupervised nighttime driving, requiring zero or near-zero blood alcohol concentration, requiring all occupants to be properly restrained, and limiting the number of passengers and the distances and types of roads traveled. The threshold for corrective action (e.g., a lengthened restriction period) may be lower for restricted drivers than for restricted drivers. Graduated licensing systems have been instituted in Australia, New Zealand, and Ontario, Canada. Although this system has not been implemented in the United States, the National Highway Traffic Safety Administration is providing funds to states to evaluate the impact of various elements of the graduated licensing system.

REFERENCES: AS NUMBERED IN ORIGINAL PUBLICATION

4. Evans L. Traffic Safety and the driver. New York: Van Nostrand Reinhold, 1991.
5. Mayhew DR, Simpson HM. New to the road: young drivers and novice drivers: similar problems and solutions? Ottawa: Traffic Injury Research Foundation of Canada, 1991.
6. Higson R, Howland J. Promoting safety in adolescents. In: Millstein SG, Petersen AC, Nightingdale EO, eds. Promoting the health of adolescents: new directions for the twenty-first century. New York: Oxford University Press, 1993.
7. Insurance Institute for Highway Safety. Slower graduation to full licensing means fewer teenage deaths. In: Status report. Arlington, VA: Insurance Institute for Highway Safety 1994;29(4):1-3.

Alcohol-Related Traffic Crashes

Original Citation: Centers for Disease Control and Prevention. Update: alcohol-related traffic crashes and fatalities among youth and young adults—United States, 1982–1994. MMWR 1995;44(47):869–874.

EDITORIAL NOTE

The findings in this report document that the overall decline in alcohol involvement among drivers in fatal crashes during 1982–1989 (5) continued through 1994. However, a substantial proportion of young drivers in fatal crashes had a BAC greater than or equal to 0.01 g/dL. The decline in alcohol involvement among drivers is consistent with the decline in the number and percentage of all ARTFs in the United States during 1982–1994. However, in 1994, 29% of crash-related deaths among persons aged 15–17 years and 44% of those among persons aged 18–20 years were alcohol-related. In addition, the prevalence of drinking and driving increases substantially among youth and young adults with the frequency of alcohol use and is strongly associated with binge drinking (1, 6). These findings highlight the need for additional prevention measures targeted specifically to young drivers.

Factors that may have contributed to the decline in both impaired driving and total ARTFs among young persons include prompt license suspension for persons who drive while intoxicated; increasing the minimum drinking age (since 1988, the minimum drinking age has been 21 years in all states); and the initiation of public education, community awareness, and media campaigns about the dangers of alcohol-involved driving (7). NHTSA efforts to prevent alcohol-involved driving among youth and young adults include supporting enforcement of minimum drinking age laws; providing grants to states to implement graduated licensing systems that both allow new drivers to accumulate driving experience in low-risk settings and gradually relax restrictions until an unrestricted license is earned (8); reducing legally permissible BACs to 0.08 g/dL for drivers aged greater than or equal to 21 years; promoting "zero-tolerance" laws, which lowers the legal BAC for drivers aged less than 21 years*; and developing workshops for judges and police officials to address the special problems associated with alcohol-related offenses among youth.

CDC is evaluating the effectiveness of mandatory substance-abuse assessment and treatment to reduce the risk for repeat arrests for driving while impaired among drivers of all ages and the effectiveness of intervention strategies to reduce both alcohol intake and future alcohol-related injuries among young adults hospitalized for motor-vehicle-crash-related injuries. Although addi-

---

* As of November 1995, 27 states and the District of Columbia had established a BAC of less than or equal to 0.02 g/dL as the legal limit for intoxication for drivers aged less than 21 years.

tional efforts are necessary to evaluate the effectiveness of interventions to prevent alcohol-impaired driving, the findings in this report indicate the need for intensified measures—including stronger state legislation (e.g., zero-tolerance laws)—to prevent ARTFs among youth and young adults.

REFERENCES: AS NUMBERED IN ORIGINAL PUBLICATION

1. Escobedo LG, Chorba TL, Waxweiler R. Patterns of alcohol use and the risk of drinking and driving among US high school students. Am J Public Health 1995;85:976–978.
5. CDC. Alcohol-related traffic fatalities among youth and young adults—United States, 1982–1989. MMWR 1991;40:178–179, 185–187.
6. Weschler H, Davenport A, Dowdall G, et al. Health and behavioral consequences of binge drinking in college. JAMA 1994;272:1672–1677.
7. CDC. Drivers with repeat convictions or arrests for driving while impaired—United States. MMWR 1994;43:759–761.
8. CDC. Risky driving behaviors among teenagers—Gwinnett County, Georgia, 1993. MMWR 1994;43:405–409.

TOPIC 49 / **SPORTS**

Injuries Associated with Soccer Goalposts

Original Citation: Centers for Disease Control and Prevention. Epidemiologic notes and reports injuries associated with soccer goalposts—United States, 1979–1993. MMWR 1994;43(9):153–155.

Injuries associated with sports can be related to a variety of factors, including participant's level of conditioning or training, failure to use safety equipment, contact, overexertion, difficulty in conducting the task required, mismatch in skill or size between players, and adverse environmental conditions. A rare but often fatal event is a blow caused by a falling soccer goalpost resulting from improper installation or use. From 1979 through 1993, 27 persons were injured or killed from falling soccer goalposts.

EDITORIAL NOTE

The findings in this report indicate the potential for serious injuries associated with improperly installed or used soccer goalposts. Regulation soccer goalposts can be manufactured from steel, aluminum, or metal pipe; measure approximately 8 feet by 24 feet; and weigh 250–800 pounds. Because the mouth of the goalpost is completely open to the playing field, only three sides are available for stabilizing the goalpost from forward falls. The reports to CPSC indicate that injuries typically result from climbing on goalposts, swinging or hanging from crossbars, or doing chin-ups on crossbars.

In the United States, soccer goalposts are manufactured by seven companies, and an undetermined number are produced by local machine shops without strict specifications. In 1990, CPSC issued a voluntary labeling standard for use of warning labels on the front and back of the crossbar and the front of the goalposts. Because of concerns about the inability of young children to read such warnings and the likelihood that older children would ignore these warnings, voluntary standards were adopted in 1992 by manufacturers; these standards specify the need to anchor or counterweight the goalposts using driving stakes, auger stakes, vertical pipe sleeves, or sandbags. If stakes are used, four are recommended—two on the rear and one on either side. Goalposts not in use should be chained to a fence or other permanent structure, placed goal-face down on the ground, or disassembled for storage. Additional information concerning these or other methods of anchoring is available from the Coalition to Promote Soccer Goal Safety, telephone (800) 527-7510 or (800) 531-4252.

In-Line Skating Injuries

Original Citation: Schieber RA, Branche-Dorsey CM. In-line skating injuries: epidemiology and recommendations for prevention. Sports Med 1995;19(6):427–432.

Original Authors: Richard A. Schieber, Christine M. Branche-Dorsey.

DISCUSSION AND RECOMMENDATIONS

The International In-line Skating Association recommends that skaters always wear full protective gear: helmet, wrist guards, and knee and elbow pads (6). Although use of wrist guards has been estimated at 46% in one affluent Michigan county (13), use in other geographical regions has been considerably lower (12) (Fig. 1. For all in-line skaters, roller-skaters and skateboarders, the wrist appears to be particularly vulnerable to injury, as might be expected in sports that commonly result in falling on outstretched arms with hyperextension of the wrist. By holding the wrist firmly against 1 or 2 stiff plastic or metal plates, wrist guards protect against such sudden hyperextension. They also provide a barrier to direct contact of the wrist with the hard skating surface. Until recently, the relative degree of effectiveness of wrist guards in preventing wrist injuries was not known. However, preliminary results of our case-control study of injured in-line skaters indicate that wrist guards are virtually completely protective against lacerations, sprains and strains, and that they reduce the overall odds of sustaining any wrist injury more than 6-fold (14). Because the wrist is at such high risk and because it is so readily protected, wrist guards should be worn by all in-line skaters (and probably by skateboarders and roller-skaters as well). Elbow- and knee-pad protectors might also help prevent local injuries, but their degree of effectiveness is unknown. Further evaluation of the effectiveness of wrist, knee and elbow pads in reducing or eliminating injuries is warranted.

The issue of protection against head injury is particularly important because of the potential for long term disability. Although the percentage of injured in-line skaters who sustain a head injury appears low (only about 5% in our study) (8), any such event has the potential to cause enormous and long-lasting medical, social and financial consequences. Approved cycle helmets and multipurpose helmets are effective in reducing the incidence of serious head injuries to

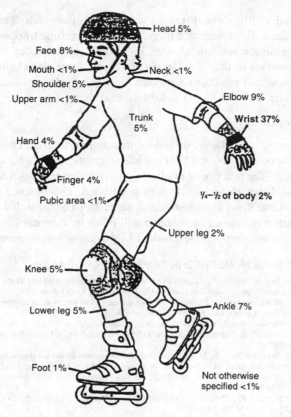

Head 5%
Face 8%
Mouth <1%
Shoulder 5%
Upper arm <1%
Neck <1%
Elbow 9%
Trunk 5%
Wrist 37%
Hand 4%
Finger 4%
Pubic area <1%
¼–½ of body 2%
Upper leg 2%
Knee 5%
Lower leg 5%
Ankle 7%
Foot 1%
Not otherwise specified <1%

Figure 1. Anatomical distribution of injuries sustained during in-line skating; expressed as a percentage of injured in-line skaters surveyed. From the National Electronic Injury Surveillance System, 1 July 1992 to 30 June 1993.

cyclists (15), and should offer similar protection to in-line skaters. Consequently, we recommend that in-line skaters also wear a helmet while skating.

Special Considerations for Novice Skaters

Novice skaters appear to be at particularly high risk of injury. Besides wearing protective gear, novices should avoid roadways with traffic, uneven surfaces, hills (even small ones) and obstacles. They should avoid roadways shared by cyclists and pedestrians until they are capable of steering away from them successfully. Skating instruction may reduce the likelihood of injury, and safe skating practices are likely to improve skills, especially in the early phases of learning.

Trails

Although more experienced skaters might be able to safely share the road with cyclists and pedestrians, separate trails are advisable where possible (6). Trail designs have been published, including recommendations for design speed, drainage, trail width, sight distances and surface materials. Trails should be kept free of sand, dirt, leaves and twigs, which can become trapped between the wheels and cause a sudden change in velocity with loss of balance. Good drainage is needed so that puddles do not form; water also changes the coefficient of friction and results in a sudden change in velocity. Trails should also flatten for at least 30 feet (9 m) before intersections.

General Measures

Equipment, especially wheels, should be maintained in good condition. Skaters should skate according to local bicycle traffic regulations and give way to pedestrians. "Skitching," the practice of holding onto a moving motor vehicle for propulsion while on skates, should be strongly prohibited. This practice potentially endangers the skater if the vehicle suddenly slows, stops or turns. If a skater fails for any reason, their enhanced momentum will result in a greater impact force with the roadway (or another vehicle), and is likely to cause a more severe injury.

REFERENCES: AS NUMBERED IN ORIGINAL PUBLICATION

6. International In-line Skating Association. Guidelines for establishing in-line skate trails in parks and recreational areas. Minneapolis: International In-line Skating Association, 1992.
8. Schieber RA, Branche-Dorsey CM, Ryan GW. Comparison of in-line skating injuries with rollerskating and skateboarding injuries. JAMA 1994:271:1856–1858.
12. Heller D. Rollerblading injuries. Hazard, Victoria, Australia 1993;10:11–16.
13. Jacques JB, Grzesiak E. Personal protective equipment used by in-line roller skaters. J Fam Prac 1994;38:486–488
14. Schieber RA, Branche-Dorsey CM. Effectiveness of wrist guards in preventing wrist injuries to in-line skaters [Abstract]. In: Abstract of the 122nd Annual Meeting and Exhibition, American Public Health Association; 1994 Oct 30-Nov 4, Washington, DC. Washington, DC: American Public Health Association, 1994:360.
15. Thompson RS, Rivara FP, Thompson DC. A case-control study of the effectiveness of bicycle safety helmets. N Engl J Med 1989;320:1361–1367.

TOPIC 50 / **SUICIDE**

Programs for the Prevention of Suicide Among Adolescents and Young Adults

Original Citation: Centers for Disease Control and Prevention. Programs for the prevention of suicide among adolescents and young adults—suicide contagion and the reporting of suicide: recommendations from a National Workshop. MMWR 1994;43(RR-6):1–7.

Original Authors: Patrick W. O'Carroll, MD, MPH, Lloyd B. Potter, PhD, MPH, James A. Mercy, PhD.

INTRODUCTION

The continued high rates of suicide among adolescents (i.e., persons aged 15–19 years) and young adults (persons aged 20–24 years) (Table 1) have heightened the need for allocation of prevention resources. To better focus these resources, CDC's National Center for Injury Prevention and Control recently published Youth Suicide Prevention Programs: A Resource Guide (1). The guide describes the rationale and evidence for the effectiveness of various suicide prevention strategies and identifies model programs that incorporate these strategies. It is intended as an aid for communities interested in developing or augmenting suicide prevention programs targeted toward adolescents and young adults. This report summarizes the eight prevention strategies described in the Resource Guide.

Table 1. Suicide rates* for persons 15–24 years of age, by age group and sex— United States, 1950, 1960, 1970, 1980, and 1990

Age group (yrs)/Sex	Year				
	1950	1960	1970	1980	1990
15–19					
Male	3.5	5.6	8.8	13.8	18.1
Female	1.8	1.6	2.9	3.0	3.7
Total	2.7	3.6	5.9	8.5	11.1
20–24					
Male	9.3	11.5	19.2	26.8	25.7
Female	3.3	2.9	5.6	5.5	4.1
Total	6.2	7.1	12.2	16.1	15.1
15–24					
Male	6.5	8.2	13.5	20.2	22.0
Female	2.6	2.2	4.2	4.3	3.9
Total	4.5	5.2	8.8	12.3	13.2

*Per 100,000 persons.

Source: National Center for Health Statistics, CDC.

METHODOLOGY

Suicide prevention programs were identified by contacting suicide prevention experts in the United States and Canada and asking them to name and describe suicide prevention programs for adolescents and young adults that, based on their experience and assessment, were likely to be effective in preventing suicide. After compiling an initial list, program representatives were contacted and asked to describe the number of persons exposed to the intervention, the number of years the program had been operating, the nature and intensity of the intervention, and the availability of data to facilitate evaluation. Program representatives were also asked to identify other programs that they considered exemplary. Representatives from these programs were contacted and asked to describe their programs. The list of programs was further supplemented by contacting program representatives who participated in the 1990 national meeting of the American Association of Suicidology and by soliciting program contacts through Newslink, the association's newsletter.

Suicide prevention programs on the list were then categorized according to the nature of the prevention strategy using a framework of eight suicide prevention strategies:

• School gatekeeper training. This type of program is designed to help school staff (e.g., teachers, counselors, and coaches) identify and refer students at risk for suicide. These programs also teach staff how to respond to suicide or other crises in the school.

- Community gatekeeper training. These programs train community members (e.g., clergy, police, merchants, and recreation staff) and clinical health-care providers who see adolescent and young adult patients (e.g., physicians and nurses) to identify and refer persons in this age group who are at risk for suicide.
- General suicide education. Students learn about suicide, its warning signs, and how to seek help for themselves or others. These programs often incorporate a variety of activities that develop self-esteem and social competency.
- Screening programs. A questionnaire or other screening instrument is used to identify high-risk adolescents and young adults and provide further assessment and treatment. Repeated assessment can be used to measure changes in attitudes or behaviors over time, to test the effectiveness of a prevention strategy, and to detect potential suicidal behavior.
- Peer support programs. These programs, which can be conducted in or outside of school, are designed to foster peer relationships and competency in social skills among high-risk adolescents and young adults.
- Crisis centers and hotlines. Trained volunteers and paid staff provide telephone counseling and other services for suicidal persons. Such programs also may offer a "drop-in" crisis center and referral to mental health services.
- Restriction of access to lethal means. Activities are designed to restrict access to handguns, drugs, and other common means of suicide.
- Intervention after a suicide. These programs focus on friends and relatives of persons who have committed suicide. They are partially designed to help prevent or contain suicide clusters and to help adolescents and young adults cope effectively with the feelings of loss that follow the sudden death or suicide of a peer. After categorizing suicide prevention efforts according to this framework, an expert group at CDC reviewed the list to identify recurrent themes across the different categories and to suggest directions for future research and intervention.

FINDINGS

The following conclusions were derived from information published in the Resource Guide:

- Strategies in suicide prevention programs for adolescents and young adults focus on two general themes. Although the eight strategies for suicide prevention programs for adolescents and young adults differ, they can be classified into two conceptual categories:
- Strategies to identify and refer suicidal adolescents and young adults for mental health care. This category includes active strategies (e.g., general screening programs and targeted screening in the event of a suicide) and passive strategies (e.g., training school and community gatekeepers, providing general education about suicide, and establishing crisis centers and hotlines). Some passive strategies are designed to lower barriers to self-referral, and others seek to increase referrals by persons who recognize suicidal tendencies in someone they know.
- Strategies to address known or suspected risk factors for suicide among adolescents and young adults. These interventions include promoting self-esteem and teaching stress management (e.g., general suicide education and peer support programs); developing support networks for high-risk adolescents and young adults (peer support programs); and providing crisis counseling (crisis centers, hotlines, and interventions to minimize contagion in the context of suicide clusters). Although restricting access to the means of committing suicide may be critically important in reducing risk, none of the programs reviewed placed major emphasis on this strategy.
- Suicide prevention efforts targeted for young adults are rare. With a few important exceptions, most programs have been targeted toward adolescents in high school, and these programs generally do not extend to include young adults. Although the reasons for this phenomenon are not clear, the focus of prevention efforts on adolescents may be because they are relatively easy to access in comparison with young adults, who may be working or in college. In addition, persons who design and implement such efforts may not realize that the suicide rate for young adults is substantially higher than the rate for adolescents (Table 1).
- Links between suicide prevention programs and existing community mental health resources are frequently inadequate. In many instances, suicide prevention programs directed

toward adolescents and young adults have not established close working ties with traditional community mental health resources. Inadequate communication with local mental health service agencies obviously reduces the potential effectiveness of programs that seek to identify and refer suicidal adolescents and young adults for mental health care.

- Some potentially successful strategies are applied infrequently, yet other strategies are applied commonly. Despite evidence that restricting access to lethal means of suicide (e.g., firearms and lethal dosages of drugs) can help to prevent suicide among adolescents and young adults, this strategy was not a major focus of any of the programs identified. Other promising strategies, such as peer support programs for those who have attempted suicide or others at high risk, are rarely incorporated into current programs. In contrast, school-based education on suicide is a common strategy. This approach is relatively simple to implement, and it is a cost-effective way to reach a large proportion of adolescents. However, evidence to indicate the effectiveness of school-based suicide education is sparse. Educational interventions often consist of a brief, one-time lecture on the warning signs of suicide—a method that is unlikely to have substantial or sustained impact and that may not reach high-risk students (e.g., those who have considered or attempted suicide). Further, students who have attempted suicide previously may react more negatively to such curricula than students who have not. The relative balance of the positive and the potentially negative effects of these general educational approaches is unclear.

- Many programs with potential for reducing suicide among adolescents and young adults are not considered or evaluated as suicide prevention programs. Programs designed to improve other psychosocial problem areas among adolescents and young adults (e.g., alcohol- and drug-abuse treatment programs or programs that provide help and services to runaways, pregnant teenagers, and/or high school dropouts) often address risk factors for suicide. However, such programs are rarely considered suicide prevention programs, and evaluations of such programs rarely consider their effect on suicidal behavior. A review of the suicide prevention programs discussed in the Resource Guide indicated that only a small number maintained working relationships with these other programs.

- The effectiveness of suicide prevention programs has not been demonstrated. The lack of evaluation research is the single greatest obstacle to improving current efforts to prevent suicide among adolescents and young adults. Without evidence to support the potential of a program for reducing suicidal behavior, recommending one approach over another for any given population is difficult.

RECOMMENDATIONS

Because current scientific information about the efficacy of suicide prevention strategies is insufficient, the Resource Guide does not recommend one strategy over another. However, the following general recommendations should be considered:

- Ensure that suicide prevention programs are linked as closely as possible with professional mental health resources in the community. Strategies designed to increase referrals of at-risk adolescents and young adults can be successful only to the extent that trained counselors are available and mechanisms for linking at-risk persons with resources are operational.
- Avoid reliance on one prevention strategy. Most of the programs reviewed already incorporate several of the eight strategies described. However, as noted, certain strategies tend to predominate despite insufficient evidence of their effectiveness. Given the limited knowledge regarding the effectiveness of any one program, a multi-faceted approach to suicide prevention is recommended.
- Incorporate promising, but underused, strategies into current programs where possible. Restricting access to lethal means of committing suicide may

be the most promising underused strategy. Parents should be taught to recognize the warning signs for suicide and encouraged to restrict their teenagers' access to lethal means. Peer support groups for adolescents and young adults who have exhibited suicidal behaviors or who have contemplated and/or attempted suicide also appear promising but should be implemented carefully. Establishment of working relationships with other prevention programs, such as alcohol- and drug-abuse treatment programs, may enhance suicide prevention efforts. Furthermore, when school-based education is used, program planners should consider broad curricula that address suicide prevention in conjunction with other adolescent health issues before considering curricula that address only suicide.

- Expand suicide prevention efforts for young adults. The suicide rate for persons in this age group is substantially higher than that for adolescents, yet programs targeted toward them are sparse. More prevention efforts should be targeted toward young adults at high risk for suicide.
- Incorporate evaluation efforts into suicide prevention programs. Planning, process, and outcome evaluation are important components of any public health effort. Efforts to conduct outcome evaluation are imperative given the lack of knowledge regarding the effectiveness of suicide prevention programs. Outcome evaluation should include measures such as incidence of suicidal behavior or measures closely associated with such incidence (e.g., measures of suicidal ideation, clinical depression, and alcohol abuse). Program directors should be aware that suicide prevention efforts, like most health interventions, may have unforeseen negative consequences. Evaluation measures should be designed to detect such consequences. For a copy of the full report, Youth Suicide Prevention Programs: A Resource Guide, write to Lloyd Potter, Ph.D., M.P.H., at the Centers for Disease Control and Prevention, National Center for Injury Prevention and Control, 4770 Buford Highway, Mailstop K-60, Atlanta, GA 30341-3724. Single copies are available free of charge.

REFERENCE: AS NUMBERED IN ORIGINAL PUBLICATION

1. CDC. Youth suicide prevention programs: a resource guide. Atlanta: US Department of Health and Human Services, Public Health Service, CDC, 1992.

Recommendations for a Community Plan for the Prevention and Containment of Suicide Clusters

Original Citation: Centers for Disease Control and Prevention. CDC recommendations for a community plan for the prevention and containment of suicide clusters. MMWR 1988;37(S-6):1–12.

Original Authors: Patrick W. O'Carroll, MD, MPH, James A. Mercy, PhD, John A. Steward, MPH.

INTRODUCTION

Recent suicide clusters among teenagers and young adults have received national attention, and public concern about this issue is growing. Unfortunately, our understanding of the causes and means of preventing suicide clusters is far from complete. A suicide cluster may be defined as a group of suicides or suicide attempts, or both, that occur closer together in time and space than would normally be expected in a given community. A statistical analysis of national mortality data indicates that clusters of completed suicide occur predominantly among adolescents and young adults, and that such clusters account for approximately 1%–5% of all suicides in this age group (1). Suicide clusters are thought by many to occur through a process of "contagion," but this hypothesis has not yet been formally tested (2, 3). Nevertheless, a great deal of anecdotal evidence suggests that, in any given suicide cluster, suicides occurring later in the cluster often appear to have been influenced by suicides occurring earlier in the cluster. Ecologic evidence also suggests that exposure of the general population to suicide through television may increase the risk of suicide for certain susceptible individuals (4, 5), although this effect has not been found in all studies (6, 7).

The Centers for Disease Control (CDC) has assisted several state and local health departments in investigating and responding to apparent clusters of suicide and suicide attempts. These clusters created a crisis atmosphere in the communities in which they occurred and engendered intense concern on the part of parents, students, school officials, and others. In the midst of these clusters of suicides or suicide attempts, community leaders were faced with the simultaneous tasks of trying to prevent the cluster from expanding and trying to manage the crisis that already existed. Potential opportunities for prevention were often missed during the early stages of response as community leaders searched for information on how best to respond to suicide clusters.

The recommendations contained in this report were developed to assist community leaders in public health, mental health, education, and other fields to develop a community response plan for suicide clusters or for situations that might develop into suicide clusters. A workshop for developing these recommendations was jointly sponsored by the New Jersey State Department of Health and CDC on November 16–17, 1987, in Newark, New Jersey. Participants in that workshop included persons who had played key roles in community responses to nine different suicide clusters. They were from a variety of different sectors including education, medicine, local government, community mental health, local crisis centers, and state public health and mental health. Also participating in this workshop were representatives from the National Institute of Mental Health (NIMH), the Indian Health Service (IHS), the American Association of Suicidology (AAS), and the Association of State and Territorial Health Officials (ASTHO).

These recommendations should not be considered explicit instructions to be followed by every community in the event of a suicide cluster. Rather, they are meant to provide community leaders with a conceptual framework for developing their own suicide-cluster-response plans, adapted to the particular needs, resources, and cultural characteristics of their communities. These recommendations will be revised periodically to reflect new knowledge in the field of suicide prevention and experience acquired in using this plan.

Certain elements of the proposed plan for the prevention and containment of suicide clusters are quite different from those of crisis-response plans for other community emergencies. These differences are primarily attributable to the potentially contagious nature of suicidal behavior and to the stigma and guilt often associated with suicide. Other elements of the proposed plan, however, are germane to crisis-response plans in general. Therefore, state and local health planners might consider whether the plan they develop from these recommendations should be integrated into existing guidelines for managing other emergencies or mental health crises.

I. A community should review these recommendations and develop its own response plan before the onset of a suicide cluster.

Comment. When a suicide cluster is occurring in a community—or when such a cluster seems about to occur—several steps in our recommended response plan should be taken right away. If such a timely reaction is to be possible, the response plan must necessarily already be developed, agreed upon, and understood by all the participants at the onset of the crisis. The recommended response requires a great deal of coordination among various sectors of the community. Such coordination is sometimes difficult to establish at the best of times and may be even more difficult to establish in the face of a crisis.

In the early days of an evolving suicide cluster there has typically been a great deal of confusion. There is often a sense of urgency in the community that something needs to be done to prevent additional suicides, but there has usually been little initial coordination of effort in this regard. Moreover, community members often disagree about precisely what should be done to prevent a cluster from expanding. In almost every case, communities ultimately develop some sort of plan for responding to the crisis in a coordinated manner, but opportunities for prevention are often missed in the crucial first hours of the response.

II. The response to the crisis should involve all concerned sectors of the community and should be coordinated as follows:

A. Individuals from concerned agencies—education, public health, mental health, local government, suicide crisis centers, and other appropriate agencies—should be designated to serve on a coordinating committee, which would be responsible for deciding when the response plan should be implemented and coordinating its implementation.

B. One agency should be designated as the "host" agency for the plan. The individual representing that agency would have the following responsibilities:

1. Call the initial meeting of the coordinating committee before any crisis occurs so that these recommendations can be incorporated into a plan that reflects the particular resources and needs of the community (see Section III, below).

2. Establish a notification mechanism by which the agency would be made aware of a potentially evolving suicide cluster (see Comment, below).

3. Convene the coordinating committee when it appears that a suicide cluster is occurring, or when it is suspected that a cluster may occur due to the influence of one or more recent suicides or other traumatic deaths (see Section IV, below). At this initial meeting, the members of the coordinating committee could decide whether to implement the community response plan and how extensive the response needs to be.

4. Maintain the suicide-cluster-response plan. The coordinating committee should meet periodically to assure that the plan remains operational.

5. Revise the community plan periodically to reflect new knowledge in the field of suicide prevention, the community's experiences in using the plan, and changes in the community itself.

Comment. Every effort should be made to promote and implement the proposed plan as a community endeavor. During past suicide clusters, a single agency has often found itself "in the hot seat," that is, as the focal point of demands that something be done to contain the suicide cluster. No single agency, however, has the resources or expertise to adequately respond to an evolving suicide cluster. Moreover, the emergence of one agency as the sole focus for responding to an apparent suicide cluster has several unfortunate consequences. The agency and its representatives run the danger of becoming scapegoats for a community's fear and anger over the apparent cluster. Such a focus can potentially blind a community to other valuable resources for responding to the crisis and to basic community problems that may have engendered the crisis.

The concept of a "host" agency was developed because—even though the response will involve a variety of different agencies and community groups—one person must necessarily take responsibility for establishing a notification mechanism, maintaining the response plan, and calling meetings of the coordinating committee as outlined above. Which agency should serve as the host agency should be decided by each community. In past clusters, for example, a school district, a municipal government, a mental health association, and even a private, nonprofit mental health center have taken the lead in organizing their community's response. State or local public health or mental health agencies might also serve as host agencies for the plan. The role of host agency might also be rotated among the various agencies represented on the coordinating committee.

The notification mechanism by which the host agency would be made aware of a potentially evolving suicide cluster would vary from community to community. In small communities, one death of a teenager by suicide might be unusual, and information about the death would be quickly transmitted to a county-level host agency. In some large communities, however, there are many suicides each year among young persons. Clearly, a more formal system would be needed in such a county to notify the host agency when an unusual number of suicides had occurred in a particular high school or municipality.

Determining whether to implement the response plan is not an all-or-nothing decision. Indeed, an important function of the coordinating committee is to decide to what extent the plan will be implemented. In situations in which it is feared that a cluster of suicides may be about to start, for example, the implementation of the plan might be quite subtle and limited, whereas in the event of a full-blown community crisis the implementation should be more extensive.

III.   The relevant community resources should be identified.

In addition to the agencies represented on the coordinating committee, the community should also seek to identify and enlist help from other community resources, including (but not limited to):

   (a) Hospitals and emergency departments;
   (b) Emergency medical services;
   (c) Local academic resources;
   (d) Clergy;
   (e) Parents groups (e.g., PTA);
   (f) Suicide crisis centers/hotlines;
   (g) Survivor groups;
   (h) Students;
   (i) Police;
   (j) Media;
   (k) Representatives of education, public health, mental health, and local government, if not already represented on the coordinating committee

Comment. The roles of each of the above groups should be defined as clearly as possible in the response plan before any crisis occurs. These roles should be agreed upon and reviewed by persons representing those groups. Most of those involved in the response will already know how to perform their particular duties. However, appropriate training for the staff of these groups should be provided as necessary (8). For example, if it is deemed desirable to conduct surveillance for suicide attempts through hospital emergency departments, officials at the state or local public health department might help design the system and train the emergency department staff. Other potential resources for training and counseling include state and local mental health agencies, mental health and other professional associations, and suicide crisis centers.

It is particularly important that representatives of the local media be included in developing the plan. In at least one community faced with a suicide cluster, the media collaborated in preparing voluntary guidelines for reporting suicide clusters. Although frequently perceived to be part of the problem, the media can be part of the solution. If representatives of the media are included in developing the plan, it is far more likely that their legitimate need for information can be satisfied without the sensationalism and confusion that has often been associated with suicide clusters.

The following example representing a composite of several actual suicide clusters illustrates the need for inclusion of and cooperation among many community organizations. Suppose that two high school students from the same school commit suicide in separate incidents on a weekend during the regular school year. The coordinating committee decides that these two deaths may increase the risk of suicide or attempted suicide among other students. The responsibilities of some of the relevant community resources might be as follows: School officials might be responsible for announcing the deaths to the students in an appropriate manner (discussed below, Section VI). School counselors and teachers might assist in identifying any students whom they think are at high risk; students in the school might also help in this regard. The local mental health agency might provide counselors to work with troubled students, as well as supply training and support for the teachers. Emergency departments of community hospitals might set up a suicide-attempt surveillance system that would increase the sensitivity with which suicide attempters were identified and would ensure proper referral of the attempters for counseling. Hotlines might help identify potential suicide attempters, and police might assist in locating such persons when appropriate. Police may also help by identifying and maintaining contact with such high-risk persons as high school dropouts and those with a history of delinquency. Local government or public health authorities might help coordinate these various efforts, if so designated by the coordinating committee.

IV. The response plan should be implemented under either of the following two conditions:

 A. When a suicide cluster occurs in the community; that is, when suicides or attempted suicides occur closer together in space and time than is considered by members of the coordinating committee to be usual for their community;

—OR—

 B. When one or more deaths from trauma occur in the community (especially among adolescents or young adults) which the members of the coordinating committee think may potentially influence others to attempt or complete suicide.

Comment. It is difficult to define a "suicide cluster" explicitly. Clearly, both the number and the degree of "closeness" of cases of suicide in time and space that would constitute a suicide cluster vary depending on the size of the community and on its background incidence of suicide. But when a community considers that it is facing a cluster of suicides, it is essentially irrelevant whether the incident cases of suicide meet some predefined statistical test of significance. With the suddenly heightened awareness of and concern about suicide in such a community, steps should be taken to prevent further suicides that may be caused in part by the atmosphere, or "contagion," of the crisis.

In several clusters of suicides or suicide attempts, the crisis situation was preceded by one or more traumatic deaths—intentional or unintentional—among the youth of the community. For example, in the 9 months preceding one cluster of four suicides and two suicide attempts among persons 15–24 years of age, there were four traumatic deaths among persons in the same age group and community—two from unintentional injuries, one from suicide, and one of undetermined intentionality. One of the unintentional-injury deaths was caused by a fall from a cliff. Two of the persons who later committed suicide in the cluster had been close friends of this fall victim; one of the two had witnessed the fall.

The hypothesis that a traumatic death can kindle a suicide cluster regardless of whether it is caused by intentional or unintentional injuries has not yet been tested. Nevertheless, the available anecdotal evidence suggests that some degree of implementation of the response plan be considered when a potentially influential traumatic death occurs in the community—especially if the person who dies is an adolescent or young adult.

We should emphasize that the fear of a contagious effect of suicide is not the only reason to implement this plan. For example, suppose that in the wake of some local economic downturn a community noted an excess of suicide deaths among persons who had been laid off from work. This would be a suicide cluster, and it would be entirely appropriate for the coordinating committee to implement the response plan. It is irrelevant that the suicides are not apparently related to contagion from previous suicides but to a "common-source" problem, since there is an identified population (laid-off workers) potentially at a suddenly increased risk of suicide.

Whether and when to implement the response plan should be determined by the coordinating committee. At this stage of our understanding of suicide clusters, we cannot specify that the response plan should be implemented only under a particular list of circumstances. Until further scientific investigation and experience with suicide clusters provides us with a more empirical basis for deciding when to implement the response plan, we must rely on prudent judgments by community leaders regarding the potential for further suicides in their communities.

V. If the response plan is to be implemented, the first step should be to contact and prepare the various groups identified above.

    A. Immediately notify those who will play key roles in the crisis response of the deaths that prompted the implementation of the response plan (if they are not already aware of them).

    B. Review the respective responsibilities and tasks with each of these key players.

    C. Consider and prepare for the problems and stresses that these persons may encounter—burnout, feelings of guilt if new suicides occur, and the like—as they carry out their assigned tasks.

Comment. Timely preparation of the groups involved is critical. In a past cluster that began with a scenario similar to that described in Section III above, the teachers and the students both heard about the suicide deaths at the same time over the school loudspeaker. The teachers were entirely unprepared to deal with the emotional response of the students and did not know what to say to them or where to refer those who were most upset. It would have been far preferable to have called a pre-school meeting with the teachers to outline the problem, discuss the appropriate roles of the teachers, and announce the various resources that were available (9). Support staff at the school—secretaries, bus drivers, janitors, nurses, and others—might also have been included at the meeting. Such preparation could have been of enormous help in several past suicide clusters.

VI. The crisis response should be conducted in a manner that avoids glorifying the suicide victims and minimizes sensationalism.

    A. Community spokespersons should present as accurate a picture as possible of the decedent(s) to students, parents, family, media, and others (see Section VIII, below).

    B. If there are suicides among persons of school age, the deaths should be announced (if necessary) in a manner that will provide maximal support for the students while minimizing the likelihood of hysteria.

Comment. Community spokespersons should avoid glorifying decedents or sensationalizing their deaths in any way (9). To do so might increase the likelihood that someone who identifies with the decedents or who is having suicidal thoughts will also attempt suicide, so as to be similarly glorified or to receive similar positive attention. One community that had had several suicides among high school students installed a "memorial bench" on the school grounds, with the names of the suicide victims engraved on the bench. Although this gesture was undoubtedly intended to demonstrate sincere compassion, such a practice is potentially very dangerous.

Spokespersons should also avoid vilifying the decedents in an effort to decrease the degree to which others might identify with them. In addition to being needlessly cruel to the families of the decedents, such an approach may only serve to make those who do identify with the decedents feel isolated and friendless. If the suicide victims are of school age, the deaths should be announced privately to those students who are most likely to be deeply affected by the tragedy—close friends, girl friends, boy friends, and the like. After the teachers are briefed (see Section V), the suicide deaths might be announced to the rest of the students either by individual teachers or over the school loudspeaker when all the students are in homeroom or some other similarly small, supervised groups. Funeral services should not be allowed to unnecessarily disrupt the regular school schedule.

VII. Persons who may be at high risk should be identified and have at least one screening interview with a trained counselor; these persons should be referred for further counseling or other services as needed.

    A. Active measures:

        1. Identify relatives (siblings, parents, children) of the decedents and provide an opportunity for them to express their feelings and to discuss their own thoughts about suicide with a trained counselor.

        2. Similarly, identify and provide counseling for boy friends/girl friends, close friends, and fellow employees who may be particularly affected by the deaths.

    a. Strategies to identify associates of the decedents or others who may be at increased risk of suicide might include: identifying the pall bearers at the funeral services of the decedent(s); checking with the funeral director regarding visitors who seemed particularly troubled at the services; keeping a list of hospital visitors of suicide attempters; and verifying the status of school absentees in the days following the suicide of a student.

3. In the case of suicides among school-age persons, enlist the aid of teachers and students in identifying any students whom they think may be at increased risk of suicide.

4. Identify and refer past and present suicide attempters for counseling if these persons were substantially exposed to suicide (see below), regardless of whether they were close friends of the decedents.

    a. "Substantially exposed" persons would include, for example, students in the same high school or workers at the same job location as the suicide victims. In past suicide clusters, such persons have committed or attempted suicide even though they did not personally know the victims who had committed suicide earlier in the cluster.

5. Identify and refer persons with a history of depression or other mental illness or with concurrent mental illness who were substantially exposed to suicide (see Section VII.A.4.a, above).

6. Identify and refer persons whose social support may be weakest and who have been substantially exposed to suicide. Examples of such persons include:

    a. Students who have recently moved into the school district;

    b. Students who come from a troubled family;

    c. Persons who have been recently widowed or divorced, or who have recently lost their jobs.

B. Passive measures:

1. Consider establishing hotlines or walk-in suicide crisis centers—even temporarily—if they do not already exist in the community; announce the availability of such hotlines/centers.

2. Provide counselors at a particular site (such as school, church, community center) and announce their availability for anyone troubled by the recent deaths.

    a. If suicides have occurred among school-age persons, provide counselors in the schools if possible; announce their availability to the students.

3. Enlist the local media to publish sources of help—hotlines, walk-in centers, community meetings, and other similar sources.

4. Make counseling services available to persons involved in responding to the crisis as well.

Comment. The recommendations for active measures to identify persons at high risk of suicide are based largely on scientific evidence that certain factors increase the risk of suicide. For example, mental illness (especially depressive illness) (10) and a history of past suicide attempts (11) are both strong risk factors for suicide. Certain sociologic factors such as unemployment (12), being widowed or divorced (13, 14), other bereavement (15, 16), and mobility (17), also appear to be important risk factors for suicide.

The role of imitation or "contagion" is, as we noted above, less well-established than the risk factors listed above. Nevertheless, the anecdotal evidence from suicide clusters is quite compelling, and several of the specific suggestions made above regarding who should be considered for screening are based on such evidence. For example, in one high school-based cluster, two persons who committed suicide late in the cluster had been pall bearers at the funerals of suicide victims who had died earlier in the cluster. It is likely that persons who are exposed to one or more of the aforementioned risk factors—depression or recent loss, for example—may be more susceptible to a contagious effect of suicide.

VIII. A timely flow of accurate, appropriate information should be provided to the media.
    A. Make certain that a single account of the situation is presented by appointing one person as information coordinator. This person's duties would include:
        1. meeting frequently with designated media spokespersons (see Section VIII.B, below) to share news and information, and to make certain that the spokespersons share a common understanding of the current situation
        2. "directing traffic"—referring requests for particular types of information to selected media spokespersons or to others (e.g., academic resources)
        3. maintaining a list of local and national resources for appropriate referral of media inquiries
        4. scheduling and holding press conferences.
    B. Appoint a single media spokesperson from each of the relevant community sectors—public health, education, mental health, local government, and the like.
        1. Each sector represented on the coordinating committee should have a spokesperson. This person is not necessarily the same representative who serves on the coordinating committee.
        2. Spokespersons from additional agencies or public groups may be designated as appropriate.
    C. These spokespersons should provide frequent, timely access to the media and present a complete and honest picture of the pertinent events. When appropriate, regularly scheduled press conferences should be held.
        1. Avoid "whitewashing"—that is, saying that everything is under control or giving other assurances that may later prove unwarranted. This practice would undermine the credibility of the community spokespersons.

2. Discuss the positive steps being taken, and try to get the media to help in the response by reporting where troubled persons can go for help.

D. The precise nature of the methods used by decedent(s) in committing suicide should not be disclosed. For example, it is accurate to state that an individual committed suicide by carbon monoxide poisoning. But it is not necessary—and is potentially very dangerous—to explain that the decedent acquired a hose from a hardware store, that s/he hooked it up to the tail pipe of a car, and then sat in a car with its engine running in a closed garage at a particular address. Such revelations can only make imitative suicides more likely and are unnecessary to a presentation of the manner of death.

E. Enlist the support of the community in referring all requests for information to these spokespersons.

Comment. If some suicide clusters spread through "contagion," the vehicle for such contagion is information, perhaps sensationalized information, about the suicides that have occurred. The role of the media in causing or exacerbating a suicide cluster is controversial, but some investigators will no longer even discuss an evolving suicide cluster with media representatives for fear that newspaper or television accounts will lead to further suicides. Although a definitive understanding of this issue must be left to future research, it is prudent in the meantime to try to prevent needlessly sensationalized or distorted accounts of evolving suicide clusters.

The media spokespersons should meet as a group and with the information coordinator regularly; under certain circumstances, they may need to check with each other several times a day. Gaining the cooperation of the community in referring requests to these spokespersons is a formidable task and will require early and ongoing efforts if it is to be accomplished. It may be helpful to assure community members that it is all right to say "no" to media phone calls or requests for interviews.

The cooperation of parents is especially essential in the context of a school-based suicide cluster. Interviews with students about the suicide of one or more of their peers can be very stressful. Parents who do not wish to have their children interviewed may be able to prevent such interviews by refusing to sign a release statement. A handout addressing how media requests should be handled might be prepared and distributed to parents, students, and other appropriate persons.

Gaining the cooperation of media representatives in this regard is also a formidable task. In the midst of a crisis, the frequent presentation of accurate and credible information is the best means of establishing such cooperation. It is preferable, however, to develop a working relationship with local media representatives before a crisis occurs.

IX. Elements in the environment that might increase the likelihood of further suicides or suicide attempts should be identified and changed.

Comment. If a particular method or site was used in previous suicides or suicide attempts, modification efforts should be addressed to these methods or sites first. For example, if the decedent(s) jumped off a particular building, bridge, or cliff, barriers might be erected to prevent other such attempts. If the decedent(s) committed suicide by carbon monoxide poisoning in a particular garage, access to that garage should be limited or monitored or both. If the decedent(s) committed suicide with a firearm or by taking an overdose of drugs, then restricting immediate access to firearms or to potentially lethal quantities of prescription drugs should be considered. In the case of suicides committed in jail, belts and other articles that may be used to commit suicide by hanging should be removed, and vigilance over the jail cells should be increased. Some of these modifications can be accomplished directly through the efforts of the coordinating committee, while others (limiting access to drugs or firearms) can only be suggested by the committee for others to consider.

Although immediate environmental modifications may be suggested by methods used in previous suicides, the modifications need not be limited only to those methods. If there is concern, for example, that the risk of suicide for particular adolescents may have been increased because of the influence of previous traumatic deaths, then common methods of suicide—firearm injury, carbon monoxide poisoning, overdose—should be made temporarily unavailable if possible. The coordinating committee should consider a variety of potentially relevant environmental factors in developing this element of the response strategy.

X. Long-term issues suggested by the nature of the suicide cluster should be addressed.

Comment. Common characteristics among the victims in a given suicide cluster may suggest that certain issues need to be addressed by the community. For example, if the decedent(s) in a particular suicide cluster tended to be adolescents or young adults who were outside the main stream of community life, efforts might be made to bring such persons back into the community. Or, if a large proportion of the suicide attempters or completers had not been suspected of having any problems, then a system should be developed (or the present system altered) so that troubled persons could receive help before they reached the stage of overt suicidal behavior.

Communities should consider establishing a surveillance system for suicide attempts as well as completed suicides. Suicide-attempt surveillance systems are almost nonexistent; yet the benefits of such systems are potentially great. In the context of a suicide cluster, such a system would allow persons who have attempted suicide in the past to be identified. Such persons are known to be at high risk of further suicide attempts. It would also allow for ongoing identification of high-risk persons during and after the current crisis. Communities should consider establishing suicide-attempt surveillance systems in their local emergency departments or wherever appropriate.

This plan should be modified according to the community's experience with its operation. Parts of the plan that have worked well in a given setting should be stressed in the updated plan, and parts that were inapplicable or that did not work should be excluded. Finally, the Centers for Disease Control requests that communities that use the plan notify us of their experiences with the plan to allow appropriate updating of this document. Please write to: Division of Violence Prevention, Mailstop K-60, Centers for Disease Control and Prevention, 1600 Clifton Road NE, Atlanta, GA 30333.

REFERENCES: AS NUMBERED IN ORIGINAL PUBLICATION

1. Gould MS, Wallenstein S, Kleinman M. A Study of time-space clustering of suicide. Final report. Atlanta: Centers for Disease Control, September 1987(contract no. RFP 200–85-0834).
2. Robbins D, Conroy C. A cluster of adolescent suicide attempts: is suicide contagious? J Adolesc Health Care 1983;3:253–255.
3. Davidson L, Gould MS. Contagion as a risk factor for youth suicide. In: Report of the Secretary's Task Force on Youth Suicide, vol. II: Risk factors for youth suicide. Washington, DC: US Government Printing Office (in press).
4. Phillips DP, Carstensen LL. Clustering of teenage suicides after television news stories about suicide. N Engl J Med 1986;315:685–689.
5. Gould MS, Shaffer D. The impact of suicide in television movies: evidence of imitation. N Engl J Med 1986;315:690–694.
6. Phillips DP, Paight DJ. The impact of televised movies about suicide: a replicative study. N Engl J Med 1987;317:809–811.
7. Berman AL. Fictional suicide and imitative effects. Am J Psychiatry 1988;(in press).
8. Dunne EJ, McIntosh JL, Dunne-Maxim K, eds. Suicide and its aftermath: understanding and counseling the survivors. New York: WW Norton & Company, 1987:151–182.
9. Lamb F, Dunne-Maxim K. Postvention in schools: policy and process. In: Dunne EJ, McIntosh JL, Dunne-Maxim K, eds. Suicide and its aftermath: understanding and counseling the survivors. New York: WW Norton & Company, 1987:245–260, and 248.
10. Hagnell O, Lanke J, Rorsman B. Suicide rates in the Lundby study: mental illness as a risk factor for suicide. Neuropsychobiology 1981;7:248–253.
11. Paerregaard G. Suicide among attempted suicides: a 10-year follow-up. Suicide 1975;5:140–144.
12. Platt S. Suicidal behavior and unemployment: a literature review. In: Wescott G, Svensson P-G, Zollner HFK, eds. Health policy implications of unemployment. Copenhagen: World Health Organization, 1985:87–132.
13. Monk M. Epidemiology of suicide. Epidemiol Rev 1987;9:51–69.
14. Smith JC, Mercy JA, Conn JM. Marital status and the risk of suicide. Am J Public Health 1988;78:78–80.
15. MacMahon B, Pugh TF. Suicide in the widowed. Am J Epidemiol 1965;81:23–31.
16. Bunch J, Barraclough B, Nelson B, et al. Suicide following bereavement of parents. Soc Psychiatry 1971;6:193–199.
17. South SJ. Metropolitan migration and social problems. Social Science Quarterly 1987;68:3–18.

Suicide Contagion and the Reporting of Suicide

Original Citation. Centers for Disease Control and Prevention. Suicide contagion and the reporting of suicide: recommendations from a National Workshop. MMWR 1994;43(RR-6):9–18.

Original Authors: Patrick W. O'Carroll, MD, MPH, Lloyd B. Potter, PhD, MPH.

INTRODUCTION

Suicide rates among adolescents and young adults have increased sharply in recent decades—from 1950 through 1990, the rate of suicide for persons 15–24 years of age increased from 4.5 to 13.5 per 100,000 (1, 2). In comparison with older persons, adolescents and young adults who commit suicide are less likely to be clinically depressed or to have certain other mental disorders (3) that are important risk factors for suicide among persons in all age groups (4). This has led to research directed at the identification of other preventable risk factors for suicide among young persons.

One risk factor that has emerged from this research is suicide "contagion," a process by which exposure to the suicide or suicidal behavior of one or more persons influences others to commit or attempt suicide (5). Evidence suggests that the effect of contagion is not confined to suicides occurring in discrete geographic areas. In particular, nonfictional newspaper and television coverage of suicide has been associated with a statistically significant excess of suicides (6). The effect of contagion appears to be strongest among adolescents (7, 8), and several well publicized "clusters" among young persons have occurred (9–11).

These findings have induced efforts on the part of many suicide-prevention specialists, public health practitioners, and researchers to curtail the reporting of suicide—especially youth suicide—in newspapers and on television. Such efforts were often counterproductive, and news articles about suicides were written without the valuable input of well-informed suicide-prevention specialists and others in the community. In November 1989, the Association of State and Territorial Health Officials and the New Jersey Department of Health convened a workshop* at which suicidologists, public health officials, researchers, psychiatrists, and psychologists worked directly with news media professionals from around the country to share their concerns and perspectives on this problem and explore ways in which suicide, especially suicide among persons 15–24 years of age, could be reported with minimal potential for suicide contagion and without compromising the independence or professional integrity of news media professionals.

A set of general concerns about and recommendations for reducing the possibility of media-related suicide contagion were developed at this workshop, and characteristics of news coverage that appear to foster suicide contagion were described. This report summarizes these concerns, recommendations, and characteristics.

GENERAL CONCERNS AND RECOMMENDATIONS

The following concerns and recommendations should be reviewed and understood by health professionals, suicidologists, public officials, and others who provide information for reporting of suicide:

- Suicide is often newsworthy, and it will probably be reported. The mission of a news organization is to report to the public information on events in the community. If a suicide is considered newsworthy, it will probably be reported. Health-care providers should realize that efforts to prevent news coverage may not be effective, and their goal should be to assist news professionals in their efforts toward responsible and accurate reporting.
- "No comment" is not a productive response to media representatives who are covering a suicide story. Refusing to speak with the media does not prevent

* CDC, which participated in developing the concepts for discussion and assisted in the operations of this workshop, supports these recommendations. Funding for the workshop was provided by the Maternal and Child Health Bureau, Health Resources and Services Administration, U.S. Department of Health and Human Services.

coverage of a suicide; rather, it precludes an opportunity to influence what will be contained in the report. Nevertheless, public officials should not feel obligated to provide an immediate answer to difficult questions. They should, however, be prepared to provide a reasonable timetable for giving such answers or be able to direct the media to someone who can provide the answers.

- All parties should understand that a scientific basis exists for concern that news coverage of suicide may contribute to the causation of suicide. Efforts by persons trying to minimize suicide contagion are easily misinterpreted. Health officials must take the time to explain the carefully established, scientific basis for their concern about suicide contagion and how the potential for contagion can be reduced by responsible reporting.

- Some characteristics of news coverage of suicide may contribute to contagion, and other characteristics may help prevent suicide. Clinicians and researchers acknowledge that it is not news coverage of suicide per se, but certain types of news coverage, that promote contagion. Persons concerned with preventing suicide contagion should be aware that certain characteristics of news coverage, rather than news coverage itself, should be avoided.

- Health professionals or other public officials should not try to tell reporters what to report or how to write the news regarding suicide. If the nature and apparent mechanisms of suicide contagion are understood, the news media are more likely to present the news in a manner that minimizes the likelihood of such contagion. Instead of dictating what should be reported, public officials should explain the potential for suicide contagion associated with certain types of reports and should suggest ways to minimize the risk for contagion (see Appendix in original publication).

- Public officials and the news media should carefully consider what is to be said and reported regarding suicide. Reporters generally present the information that they are given. Impromptu comments about a suicide by a public official can result in harmful news coverage. Given the potential risks, public officials and the media should seek to minimize these risks by carefully considering what is to be said and reported regarding suicide.

ASPECTS OF NEWS COVERAGE THAT CAN PROMOTE SUICIDE CONTAGION

Clinicians, researchers, and other health professionals at the workshop agreed that to minimize the likelihood of suicide contagion, reporting should be concise and factual. Although scientific research in this area is not complete, workshop participants believed that the likelihood of suicide contagion may be increased by the following actions:

- Presenting simplistic explanations for suicide. Suicide is never the result of a single factor or event, but rather results from a complex interaction of many factors and usually involves a history of psychosocial problems (12). Public officials and the media should carefully explain that the final precipitating event was not the only cause of a given suicide. Most persons who have committed suicide have had a history of problems that may not have been acknowledged during the acute aftermath of the suicide. Cataloguing the problems that could have played a causative role in a suicide is not necessary, but acknowledgment of these problems is recommended.

- Engaging in repetitive, ongoing, or excessive reporting of suicide in the news.

Repetitive and ongoing coverage, or prominent coverage, of a suicide tends to promote and maintain a preoccupation with suicide among at-risk persons, especially among persons 15–24 years of age. This preoccupation appears to be associated with suicide contagion. Information presented to the media should include the association between such coverage and the potential for suicide contagion. Public officials and media representatives should discuss alternative approaches for coverage of newsworthy suicide stories.

- Providing sensational coverage of suicide. By its nature, news coverage of a suicidal event tends to heighten the general public's preoccupation with suicide. This reaction is also believed to be associated with contagion and the development of suicide clusters. Public officials can help minimize sensationalism by limiting, as much as possible, morbid details in their public discussions of suicide. News media professionals should attempt to decrease the prominence of the news report and avoid the use of dramatic photographs related to the suicide (e.g., photographs of the funeral, the deceased person's bedroom, and the site of the suicide).

- Reporting "how-to" descriptions of suicide. Describing technical details about the method of suicide is undesirable. For example, reporting that a person died from carbon monoxide poisoning may not be harmful; however, providing details of the mechanism and procedures used to complete the suicide may facilitate imitation of the suicidal behavior by other at-risk persons.

- Presenting suicide as a tool for accomplishing certain ends. Suicide is usually a rare act of a troubled or depressed person. Presentation of suicide as a means of coping with personal problems (e.g., the break-up of a relationship or retaliation against parental discipline) may suggest suicide as a potential coping mechanism to at-risk persons. Although such factors often seem to trigger a suicidal act, other psychopathological problems are almost always involved. If suicide is presented as an effective means for accomplishing specific ends, it may be perceived by a potentially suicidal person as an attractive solution.

- Glorifying suicide or persons who commit suicide. News coverage is less likely to contribute to suicide contagion when reports of community expressions of grief (e.g., public eulogies, flying flags at half-mast, and erecting permanent public memorials) are minimized. Such actions may contribute to suicide contagion by suggesting to susceptible persons that society is honoring the suicidal behavior of the deceased person, rather than mourning the person's death.

- Focusing on the suicide completer's positive characteristics. Empathy for family and friends often leads to a focus on reporting the positive aspects of a suicide completer's life. For example, friends or teachers may be quoted as saying the deceased person "was a great kid" or "had a bright future," and they avoid mentioning the troubles and problems that the deceased person experienced. As a result, statements venerating the deceased person are often reported in the news. However, if the suicide completer's problems are not acknowledged in the presence of these laudatory statements, suicidal behavior may appear attractive to other at-risk persons—especially those who rarely receive positive reinforcement for desirable behaviors.

CONCLUSION

In addition to recognizing the types of news coverage that can promote suicide contagion, the workshop participants strongly agreed that reporting of suicide can have several direct benefits. Specifically, community efforts to address this problem can be strengthened by news coverage that describes the help and support available in a community, explains how to identify persons at high risk for suicide, or presents information about risk factors for suicide. An ongoing dialogue between news media professionals and health and other public officials is the key to facilitating the reporting of this information.

REFERENCES: AS NUMBERED IN ORIGINAL PUBLICATION

1. National Center for Health Statistics. Health, United States, 1991. Hyattsville, MD: US Department of Health and Human Services, Public Health Service, CDC, 1992.
2. National Center for Health Statistics. Mortality data tapes [machine-readable data tapes]. Hyattsville, MD: US Department of Health and Human Services, Public Health Service, CDC, 1993.
3. Shaffer D, Garland A, Gould M, Fisher P, Trautman P. Preventing teenage suicide: a critical review. J Am Acad Child Adolesc Psychiatry 1988;27:675–687.
4. O'Carroll PW. Suicide. In: Last JM, Wallace RB, eds. Maxcy-Rosenau-Last public health and preventive medicine. 13th ed. Norwalk, CT: Appleton & Lange, 1992:1054–1062.
5. Davidson LE, Gould MS. Contagion as a risk factor for youth suicide. In: Alcohol, drug abuse, and mental health administration. Report of the Secretary's Task Force on Youth Suicide. Vol 2. Risk factors for youth suicide. Washington, DC: US Department of Health and Human Services, Public Health Service, 1989:88–109;DHHS publication no. (ADM)89–1622.
6. Gould MS, Davidson L. Suicide contagion among adolescents. In: Stiffman AR, Felman RA, eds. Advances in adolescent mental health. Vol III. Depression and suicide. Greenwich, CT: JAI Press, 1988.
7. Gould MS, Wallenstein S, Kleinman MH, O'Carroll PW, Mercy JA. Suicide clusters: an examination of age-specific effects. Am J Public Health 1990;80:211–212.
8. Phillips DP, Carstensen LL. The effect of suicide stories on various demographic groups, 1968–1985. Suicide Life Threat Behav 1988;18:100–114.
9. CDC. Cluster of suicides and suicide attempts—New Jersey. MMWR 1988;37:213–216.
10. CDC. Adolescent suicide and suicide attempts—Santa Fe County, New Mexico, January 1985-May 1990. MMWR 1991;40:329–331.
11. Davidson LE, Rosenberg ML, Mercy JA, Franklin J, Simmons JT. An epidemiologic study of risk factors in two teenage suicide clusters. JAMA 1989;262:2687–2692.
12. O'Carroll PW. Suicide causation: pies, paths, and pointless polemics. Suicide Life Threat Behav 1993; 23:27–36.

section seven

OCCUPATIONAL HEALTH

Injuries Associated with Self-Unloading Forage Wagons

Original Citation: Centers for Disease Control and Prevention. Injuries Associated with Self-Unloading Forage Wagons—New York, 1991–1994. MMWR 1995;44(32):595–597, 603.

Editor's Note: Farming injuries kill and maim thousands of Americans every year, and children are at considerable risk. The injuries from forage equipment are very brutal. In the 1990s, the injuries have included amputation of the genitalia and deep tissue damage to the buttocks; multiple leg fractures with amputation of a foot; avulsion of the entire scrotal area; and bilateral above-the-knee amputations in a 9-year-old girl.

EDITORIAL NOTE

In the United States, farm machinery is a leading source of traumatic injuries to farmers, accounting for an estimated 34,000 lost-time work injuries to farmers nationally in 1993 (2). Mechanical devices are associated with approximately 30% of the work-related injuries on farms (2). Forage wagons are used most often on farms that raise large animals and grow their own feed grain. The fatal and severe nonfatal injuries described in this report were caused by a combination of factors. To unload feed grain, the forage wagon and silo blower must be in close proximity, which requires that the two tractors that power these machines also be in close proximity Figure 1. The speed-control lever for the wagon is often located on the discharge side near the silo blower (i.e., between the two pieces of equipment). Many older tractors are small enough that, when the forage wagon and blower are thus positioned for proper operation, sufficient space remains between the adjacent rear tires of the two tractors to allow the operator to dismount from either tractor seat and walk between the two tractors directly to the forage wagon speed control without crossing over a revolving power take-off (PTO) driveline. However, as both silos and self-unloading forage wagons have increased in capacity, both the size and horsepower of the associated tractors have increased concomitantly. When these larger tractors are used, their rear wheels abut, blocking access between the tractors and requiring the operator to cross over a revolving driveline to operate the forage wagon.

Since the 1930s, PTO drivelines have been manufactured with shields. However, shields are often damaged or removed during operation or maintenance of the farm equipment. Of the estimated 29,000 self-unloading wagons in use on New York farms, 3000–5000 are believed to lack shields to protect workers adequately from a revolving PTO driveline (J. Pollock, Cornell University, personal communication, 1995). Entanglement in PTO drivelines, including entanglement in those equipped with intact U-shaped shields that

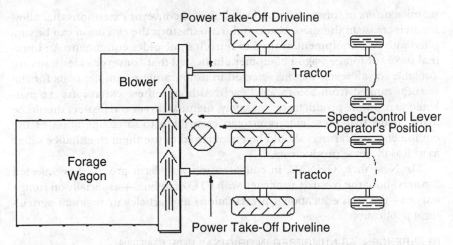

Figure 1. Typical arrangement of equipment used to transfer feed from a forage wagon (equipment used to transport and unload feed into a storage (e.g., silo or feed area) into a blower).

leave one side (generally the underside) unguarded, previously has been recognized as a hazard in the agricultural industry (3–6). Drivelines should be equipped with proper functioning guards in any work situation,*** especially when the worker must work between two operating PTO drivelines. Furthermore, workers must be trained in safe work practices, which include shutting off PTO drivelines whenever possible before dismounting tractors, maintaining warning decals, not wearing loose or bulky clothing around and avoiding close proximity to rotating PTO drivelines, and keeping bystanders—especially children—away from PTO-driven equipment (7). To assist in preventing injuries to children, farmers should recognize that farm equipment is designed for operation by adults; be aware of the physical, emotional, and mental characteristics and abilities of children; and select age-appropriate tasks for children (8). Because of the need for immediate response to serious injuries, workers should not work alone when using hazardous equipment; however, if persons do work alone, they should be monitored frequently to ensure immediate response in the event of injuries (7).

The National Institute for Farm Safety is reviewing approaches to reduce the risk for forage-wagon-related injuries. In addition to proper shielding of the drivelines, placement of the speed-control devices to enable operation of such devices from the tractor driver's seat or from another location on the wagon would eliminate the need for the operator to step over the driveline. Leading

---

*** 29 CFR section 1928.57. Occupational Safety and Health Administration (OSHA) Standard for Safety for Agricultural Equipment. Family-run farms with no other employees are exempt from compliance with federal OSHA standards, and those with less than or equal to 10 employees are generally not subject to OSHA inspection.

manufacturers of forage wagons have designed conveyor extensions that allow for an increase in the space between the two tractors; the extension can be supplied with new equipment or used to retrofit some older equipment. An informal survey of forage wagon equipment indicated that conveyor extensions are available for all seven wagons selected in a nonrandom sample; costs for the retrofits ranged from $35 to $600 each. Although these extensions are marketed to promote productivity, not safety, manufacturers and dealers should be made aware that these extensions can contribute to safer operation of the equipment, and farmers should be encouraged to use them to enhance safety as well as increase productivity.

In New York, OHNAC, in collaboration with farm groups, have alerted farmers about the hazards associated with PTO drivelines—especially on forage wagons—through educational presentations and articles in regional agricultural publications.

REFERENCES: AS NUMBERED IN ORIGINAL PUBLICATION

2. NIOSH. Traumatic injury surveillance of farmers: annual statistical abstract, 1993. Morgantown, WV: US Department of Health and Human Services, Public Health Service, CDC, NIOSH, 1995 (in press).
3. Cogbill TH, Steenlage ES, Landercasper J, Strutt PJ. Death and disability from agricultural injuries in Wisconsin: a 12-year experience with 739 patients. J Trauma 1991;31:1632–1637.
4. d. Heeg M, ten Duis HJ, Klasen HJ. Power take-off injuries. Br J Accident Surg 1986;17:28–30.
5. Roerig S. Scalping accidents with shielded PTO units: four case reports. Am Assoc Occup Health Nurs J 1993;41:437–439.
6. CDC. Scalping incidents involving hay balers—New York. MMWR 1992;41:489–491.
7. Demmin D, Hallman E. Cornell Cooperative Extension rural health and safety fact sheet: power take-off (PTO) safety. Ithaca, NY: Cornell University, 1995:publication no. 123FSF56.
8. Bean TL, Wojtowicz J. Farm safety for children: what job is right for my child? Columbus, OH: Ohio State University, 1992:publication no. AEX-991.1.

Agricultural Auger-Related Injuries and Fatalities

Original Citation: Centers for Disease Control and Prevention. Agricultural auger-related injuries and fatalities—Minnesota, 1992–1994. MMWR 1995;44(36):660–663.

Agriculture remains one of the most hazardous industries in the United States: in 1992, approximately 37 fatalities occurred per 100,000 agricultural workers and an estimated 140,000 disabling injuries to farmworkers (1). Recent surveillance for agricultural injuries and fatalities in Minnesota has helped characterize problems associated with the use of one type of implement—agricultural augers (large, corkscrew-like devices used to move dry materials [e.g., grains, animal feeds, and granular fertilizers]).

EDITORIAL NOTE

An agricultural auger consists of a continuous corkscrew blade attached to a long metal shaft and a round metal tube into which the blade is inserted. The metal tube contains the material as it is moved from the intake at one end of the auger to the discharge at the other end and protects the operator from contact with the rotating blade.*** Augers vary in size, generally ranging from 4 to 15 inches in diameter and from several feet to 100 feet or more in length (2). An auger can be independent and movable or it can be integrated with another piece of machinery or a grain storage system (e.g., as a fixed component of a combine, grain dryer, grain wagon, storage bin system, or silo unloader). In addition, augers can be self-powered (by an electric motor or a gasoline- or diesel-fueled engine) or driven by power transferred from a second piece of equipment through a power take-off shaft (PTO) or a series of gears, chains, belts, and/or pulleys. Auger-related injuries result from (a) contact with the exposed auger blade; (b) entanglement in a belt drive or PTO conveying power to the blade; (c) electrocution when an auger contacts overhead power lines (e.g., while it is being moved or positioned in an upright configuration); or (d) contact with a spinning crank, which is used to position the auger (3).

Although auger-related injuries are preventable, they remain a public health concern among farmers. On a per-hour-of-use basis, augers are one of the most dangerous types of farming equipment (4); severe injuries have resulted from entanglement and electrocution (2). The occupational injury surveillance and investigation data from Minnesota underscore the risks augers pose for both disabling and fatal injuries among farmers. In particular, the Minnesota data emphasize the risk for traumatic amputation resulting from entanglement of extremities.

NIOSH recommends the following precautions to substantially reduce the risks for hazards related to auger use:

1. Barriers (e.g., fences) should be used to prevent persons not involved in the operation of an auger from entering the area adjacent to the auger.
2. Children aged less than 18 years should not operate augers and should not enter the area near an auger.****
3. Before starting an auger, the operator should ensure that all protective shields, as supplied by the manufacturer, are in place and in good condition. The federal OSHA standard for safety of farm equipment requires placement of guards on augers consistent with their designed use (5).
4. Before service or repair, power should be shut off and the auger power source "locked-out" and "tagged." (Locking out prevents power from being restored while maintenance is in progress, and tagging the switch indicates that power is disabled and the reason).

*** An auger also may consist of only an exposed spiral corkscrew. A "sweep" auger, referred to in incident 1 (see original publication), is typically an exposed auger used to move material such as grain to a central discharge point inside a large storage structure. A sweep auger usually extends from the center of a round structure to its outside wall, is powered by a drive system that contacts the bin or silo wall, and slowly rotates (i.e., sweeps) around a pivot point at the center of the structure. The auger rests directly in the grain (or similar material), and the excess grain alongside the auger acts to confine the grain that is in contact with the auger.

**** Federal child labor laws prohibit employees aged less than 16 years from operating hazardous equipment (including agricultural augers). However, family members working on family farms are exempt from these provisions.

5. To prevent entanglement, persons wearing loose clothing or jewelry or persons with long, untied hair should not operate augers.
6. Workers should not step or jump on or over an auger while it is in operation.
7. Grain augers always should be lowered to a horizontal position before being moved from one location to another. Workers always should observe the presence and location of power lines before raising an auger into position.
8. Whenever possible, operators should ensure good footing while working around augers. Portable augers should be placed on dry, level ground or a gravel pad. Spilled grain should be removed between loads, after the equipment has been turned off.
9. Operators should never use their hands or feet to redirect the flow of grain or other materials into the auger.
10. All farm workers and auger operators should be educated about safe operating procedures and hazards associated with augers.
11. Augers should be clearly labeled as posing a hazard for entanglement and subsequent serious injury.

REFERENCES: AS NUMBERED IN ORIGINAL PUBLICATION

1. National Safety Council. Accident facts. Chicago: National Safety Council, 1993.
2. NIOSH. Preventing grain auger electrocutions. Cincinnati: US Department of Health and Human Services, Public Health Service, CDC, 1986:DHHS publication no. (NIOSH)86–119.
3. Linn R. Auger and elevator accident victim rescue. Bozeman, MT: Montana State University, Montguide Cooperative Extension Service, February 1987.
4. Aherin RA, Schultz L. Safe storage and handling of grain. St. Paul, MN: Minnesota Extension Service Bulletin, 1981:publication no. AG-FO-568.
5. Office of the Federal Register. Code of federal regulations: occupational safety and health standards. Subpart D: safety for agricultural equipment. Washington, DC: Office of the Federal Register, National Archives and Records Administration, 1994 (29 CFR section 1928.57[b]).

TOPIC 52 / **HOSPITALS AND OTHER HEALTH-CARE SETTINGS**

Editor's Note: "Guidelines on Intravascular Device-Related Infections Prevention" was recently revised and appeared in draft form with a solicitation for comment in the Federal Register (Vol. 60, No. 187, pp. 49978-50006) on September 27, 1995. A final version was not available as this book went to press.

Recommended Infection-Control Practices for Dentistry

Original Citation: Centers for Disease Control and Prevention. Recommended infection-control practices for dentistry, 1993. MMWR 1993;42(RR-8).

Editor's Note: The information included here was based on an MMWR Recommendations and Reports (Vol. 42, No. RR-8) and gives recommendations for infection-control practices for dental health care workers and their patients. The original text also contains information on transmission of HBV and HIV in dentistry.

VACCINES FOR DENTAL HEALTH-CARE WORKERS

Although HBV infection is uncommon among adults in the United States (1%–2%), serologic surveys have indicated that 10%–30% of health-care or dental workers show evidence of past or present HBV infection (6, 32). The OSHA bloodborne pathogens final rule requires that employers make hepatitis B vaccinations available without cost to their employees who may be exposed to blood or other infectious materials (4). In addition, CDC recommends that all workers, including dental health-care workers (DHCWs), who might be exposed to blood or blood-contaminated substances in an occupational setting be vaccinated for HBV (6–8). DHCWs also are at risk for exposure to and possible transmission of other vaccine-preventable diseases (33); accordingly, vaccination against influenza, measles, mumps, rubella, and tetanus may be appropriate for DHCWs.

PROTECTIVE ATTIRE AND BARRIER TECHNIQUES

For protection of personnel and patients in dental-care settings, medical gloves (latex or vinyl) always must be worn by DHCWs when there is potential for contacting blood, blood-contaminated saliva, or mucous membranes (1, 2, 4–6). Nonsterile gloves are appropriate for examinations and other nonsurgical procedures (5); sterile gloves should be used for surgical procedures. Before treatment of each patient, DHCWs should wash their hands and put on new gloves; after treatment of each patient or before leaving the dental operatory, DHCWs should remove and discard gloves, then wash their hands. DHCWs always should wash their hands and reglove between patients. Surgical or examination gloves should not be washed before use; nor should they be washed, disinfected, or sterilized for reuse. Washing of gloves may cause "wicking" (penetration of liquids through undetected holes in the gloves) and is not recommended (5). Deterioration of gloves may be caused by disinfecting agents, oils, certain oil-based lotions, and heat treatments, such as autoclaving.

Chin-length plastic face shields or surgical masks and protective eyewear should be worn when splashing or spattering of blood or other body fluids is likely, as is common in dentistry (2, 5, 6, 34, 35). When a mask is used, it should be changed between patients or during patient treatment if it becomes wet or moist. Face shields or protective eyewear should be washed with an appropriate cleaning agent and, when visibly soiled, disinfected between patients.

Protective clothing such as reusable or disposable gowns, laboratory coats, or uniforms should be worn when clothing is likely to be soiled with blood or other body fluids (2, 5, 6). Reusable protective clothing should be washed, using a normal laundry cycle, according to the instructions of detergent and machine manufacturers. Protective clothing should be changed at least daily or as soon as it becomes visibly soiled (9). Protective garments and devices (including gloves, masks, and eye and face protection) should be removed before personnel exit areas of the dental office used for laboratory or patient-care activities.

Impervious-backed paper, aluminum foil, or plastic covers should be used to protect items and surfaces (e.g., light handles or x-ray unit heads) that may become contaminated by blood or saliva during use and that are difficult or impossible to clean and disinfect. Between patients, the coverings should be removed (while DHCWs are gloved), discarded, and replaced (after ungloving and washing of hands) with clean material.

Appropriate use of rubber dams, high-velocity air evacuation, and proper patient positioning should minimize the formation of droplets, spatter, and aerosols during patient treatment. In addition, splash shields should be used in the dental laboratory.

HANDWASHING AND CARE OF HANDS

DHCWs should wash their hands before and after treating each patient (i.e., before glove placement and after glove removal) and after barehanded touching of inanimate objects likely to be contaminated by blood, saliva, or respiratory secretions (2, 5, 6, 9). Hands should be washed after removal of gloves because gloves may become perforated during use, and DHCWs' hands may become contaminated through contact with patient material. Soap and water will remove transient microorganisms acquired directly or indirectly from patient contact (9); therefore, for many routine dental procedures, such as examinations and nonsurgical techniques, handwashing with plain soap is adequate. For surgical procedures, an antimicrobial surgical handscrub should be used (10).

When gloves are torn, cut, or punctured, they should be removed as soon as patient safety permits. DHCWs then should wash their hands thoroughly and reglove to complete the dental procedure. DHCWs who have exudative lesions or weeping dermatitis, particularly on the hands, should refrain from all direct patient care and from handling dental patient-care equipment until the condition resolves (12). Guidelines addressing management of occupational exposures to blood and other fluids to which universal precautions apply have been published previously (6–8, 36).

USE AND CARE OF SHARP INSTRUMENTS AND NEEDLES

Sharp items (e.g., needles, scalpel blades, wires) contaminated with patient blood and saliva should be considered as potentially infective and handled with care to prevent injuries (2, 5, 6).

Used needles should never be recapped or otherwise manipulated utilizing both hands, or any other technique that involves directing the point of a needle toward any part of the body (2, 5, 6). Either a one-handed "scoop" technique or a mechanical device designed for holding the needle sheath should be employed. Used disposable syringes and needles, scalpel blades, and other sharp items should be placed in appropriate puncture-resistant containers located as close as is practical to the area in which the items were used (2, 5, 6). Bending or breaking of needles before disposal requires unnecessary manipulation and thus is not recommended.

Before attempting to remove needles from nondisposable aspirating syringes, DHCWs should recap them to prevent injuries. Either of the two acceptable techniques may be used. For procedures involving multiple injections with a single needle, the unsheathed needle should be placed in a location where it will not become contaminated or contribute to unintentional needlesticks between injections. If the decision is made to recap a needle between injections, a one-handed "scoop" technique or a mechanical device designed to hold the needle sheath is recommended.

STERILIZATION OR DISINFECTION OF INSTRUMENTS

Indications for Sterilization or Disinfection of Dental Instruments

As with other medical and surgical instruments, dental instruments are classified into three categories—critical, semicritical, or noncritical—depending on their risk of transmitting infection and the need to sterilize them between uses (9, 37–40). Each dental practice should classify all instruments as follows:

Critical

Surgical and other instruments used to penetrate soft tissue or bone are classified as critical and should be sterilized after each use. These devices include forceps, scalpels, bone chisels, scalers, and burs.

Semicritical

Instruments such as mirrors and amalgam condensers that do not penetrate soft tissues or bone but contact oral tissues are classified as semicritical. These devices should be sterilized after each use. If, however, sterilization is not feasible because the instrument will be damaged by heat, the instrument should receive, at a minimum, high-level disinfection.

Noncritical

Instruments or medical devices such as external components of x-ray heads that come into contact only with intact skin are classified as noncritical. Because these noncritical surfaces have a relatively low risk of transmitting infection, they may be reprocessed between patients with intermediate-level or low-level disinfection (see Cleaning and Disinfection of Dental Unit and Environmental Surfaces) or detergent and water washing, depending on the nature of the surface and the degree and nature of the contamination (9, 38).

Methods of Sterilization or Disinfection of Dental Instruments

Before sterilization or high-level disinfection, instruments should be cleaned thoroughly to remove debris. Persons involved in cleaning and reprocessing instruments should wear heavy-duty (reusable utility) gloves to lessen the risk of hand injuries. Placing instruments into a container of water or disinfectant/detergent as soon as possible after use will prevent drying of patient material and make cleaning easier and more efficient. Cleaning may be accomplished by thorough scrubbing with soap and water or a detergent solution, or with a mechanical device (e.g., an ultrasonic cleaner). The use of covered ultrasonic cleaners, when possible, is recommended to increase efficiency of cleaning and to reduce handling of sharp instruments.

All critical and semicritical dental instruments that are heat stable should be sterilized routinely between uses by steam under pressure (autoclaving), dry heat, or chemical vapor, following the instructions of the manufacturers of the instruments and the sterilizers. Critical and semicritical instruments that will not be used immediately should be packaged before sterilization.

Proper functioning of sterilization cycles should be verified by the periodic use (at least weekly) of biologic indicators (i.e., spore tests) (3, 9). Heat-sensitive chemical indicators (e.g., those that change color after exposure to heat) alone do not ensure adequacy of a sterilization cycle but may be used on the outside of each pack to identify packs that have been processed through the heating cycle. A simple and inexpensive method to confirm heat penetration to all instruments during each cycle is the use of a chemical indicator inside and in the center of either a load of unwrapped instruments or in each multiple instrument pack (41); this procedure is recommended for use in all dental practices. Instructions provided by the manufacturers of medical/dental instruments and sterilization devices should be followed closely.

In all dental and other health-care settings, indications for the use of liquid chemical germicides to sterilize instruments (i.e., "cold sterilization") are limited. For heat-sensitive instruments, this procedure may require up to 10 hours of exposure to a liquid chemical agent registered with the U.S. Environmental Protection Agency (EPA) as a "sterilant/disinfectant." This sterilization process should be followed by aseptic rinsing with sterile water, drying, and, if the instrument is not used immediately, placement in a sterile container.

EPA-registered "sterilant/disinfectant" chemicals are used to attain high-level disinfection of heat-sensitive semicritical medical and dental instruments. The product manufacturers' directions regarding appropriate concentration and exposure time should be followed closely. The EPA classification of the liquid chemical agent (i.e., "sterilant/disinfectant") will be shown on the chemical label. Liquid chemical agents that are less potent than the "sterilant/disinfectant" category are not appropriate for reprocessing critical or semicritical dental instruments.

CLEANING AND DISINFECTION OF DENTAL UNIT AND ENVIRONMENTAL SURFACES

After treatment of each patient and at the completion of daily work activities, countertops and dental unit surfaces that may have become contaminated with patient material should be cleaned with disposable toweling, using an appropriate cleaning agent and water as necessary. Surfaces then should be disinfected with a suitable chemical germicide.

A chemical germicide registered with the EPA as a "hospital disinfectant" and labeled for "tuberculocidal" (i.e., mycobactericidal) activity is recommended for disinfecting surfaces that have been soiled with patient material. These intermediate-level disinfectants include phenolics, iodophors, and chlorine-containing compounds. Because mycobacteria are among the most resistant groups of microorganisms, germicides effective against mycobacteria should be effective against many other bacterial and viral pathogens (9, 38–40, 42). A fresh solution of sodium hypochlorite (household bleach) prepared daily is an inexpensive and effective intermediate-level germicide. Concentrations ranging from 500 to 800 ppm of chlorine (a 1:100 dilution of bleach and tap water or ¨ cup of bleach to 1 gallon of water) are effective on environmental surfaces that have been cleaned of visible contamination. Caution should be exercised, since chlorine solutions are corrosive to metals, especially aluminum.

Low-level disinfectants—EPA-registered "hospital disinfectants" that are not labeled for "tuberculocidal" activity (e.g., quaternary ammonium compounds)—are appropriate for general housekeeping purposes such as cleaning floors, walls, and other housekeeping surfaces. Intermediate- and low-level disinfectants are not recommended for reprocessing critical or semicritical dental instruments.

DISINFECTION AND THE DENTAL LABORATORY

Laboratory materials and other items that have been used in the mouth (e.g., impressions, bite registrations, fixed and removable prostheses, orthodontic appliances) should be cleaned and disinfected before being manipulated in the laboratory, whether an on-site or remote location (43). These items also should be cleaned and disinfected after being manipulated in the dental laboratory and before placement in the patient's mouth (2). Because of the increasing variety of dental materials used intraorally, DHCWs are advised to consult with manufacturers regarding the stability of specific materials relative to disinfection procedures. A chemical germicide having at least an intermediate level of activity (i.e., "tuberculocidal hospital disinfectant") is appropriate for such disinfection. Communication between dental office and dental laboratory personnel regarding the handling and decontamination of supplies and materials is important.

USE AND CARE OF HANDPIECES, ANTIRETRACTION VALVES, AND OTHER INTRAORAL DENTAL DEVICES ATTACHED TO AIR AND WATER LINES OF DENTAL UNITS

Routine between-patient use of a heating process capable of sterilization (i.e., steam under pressure [autoclaving], dry heat, or heat/chemical vapor) is recommended for all high-speed dental handpieces, low-speed handpiece components used intraorally, and reusable prophylaxis angles. Manufacturers' instructions for cleaning, lubrication, and sterilization procedures should be followed closely to ensure both the effectiveness of the sterilization process and the longevity of these instruments. According to manufacturers, virtually all high-speed and low-speed handpieces in production today are heat tolerant, and most heat-sensitive models manufactured earlier can be retrofitted with heat-stable components.

Internal surfaces of high-speed handpieces, low-speed handpiece components, and prophylaxis angles may become contaminated with patient material during use. This retained patient material then may be expelled intraorally during subsequent uses (44–46). Restricted physical access—particularly to internal surfaces of these instruments—limits cleaning and disinfection or sterilization with liquid chemical germicides. Surface disinfection by wiping or soaking in liquid chemical germicides is not an acceptable method for reprocessing high-speed handpieces, low-speed handpiece components used intraorally, or reusable prophylaxis angles.

Because retraction valves in dental unit water lines may cause aspiration of patient material back into the handpiece and water lines, antiretraction valves (one-way flow check valves) should be installed to prevent fluid aspiration and to reduce the risk of transfer of potentially infective material (47). Routine maintenance of antiretraction valves is necessary to ensure effectiveness; the dental unit manufacturer should be consulted to establish an appropriate maintenance routine.

High-speed handpieces should be run to discharge water and air for a minimum of 20–30 seconds after use on each patient. This procedure is intended to aid in physically flushing out patient material that may have entered the turbine and air or water lines (46). Use of an enclosed container or high-velocity evacuation should be considered to minimize the spread of spray, spatter, and aerosols generated during discharge procedures. Additionally, there is evidence that overnight or weekend microbial accumulation in water lines can be reduced substantially by removing the handpiece and allowing water lines to run and to discharge water for several minutes at the beginning of each clinic day (48). Sterile saline or sterile water should be used as a coolant/irrigator when surgical procedures involving the cutting of bone are performed.

Other reusable intraoral instruments attached to, but removable from, the dental unit air or water lines—such as ultrasonic scaler tips and component parts and air/water syringe tips—should be cleaned and sterilized after treatment of each patient in the same manner as handpieces, which was described previously. Manufacturers' directions for reprocessing should be followed to ensure effectiveness of the process as well as longevity of the instruments.

Some dental instruments have components that are heat sensitive or are permanently attached to dental unit water lines. Some items may not enter the patient's oral cavity, but are likely to become contaminated with oral fluids during treatment procedures, including, for example, handles or dental unit attachments of saliva ejectors, high-speed air evacuators, and air/water syringes. These components should be covered with impervious barriers that are changed after each use or, if the surface permits, carefully cleaned and then treated with a chemical germicide having at least an intermediate level of activity. As with high-speed dental handpieces, water lines to all instruments should be flushed thoroughly after the treatment of each patient; flushing at the beginning of each clinic day also is recommended.

SINGLE-USE DISPOSABLE INSTRUMENTS

Single-use disposable instruments (e.g., prophylaxis angles; prophylaxis cups and brushes; tips for high-speed air evacuators, saliva ejectors, and air/water syringes) should be used for one patient only and discarded appropriately. These items are neither designed nor intended to be cleaned, disinfected, or sterilized for reuse.

HANDLING OF BIOPSY SPECIMENS

In general, each biopsy specimen should be put in a sturdy container with a secure lid to prevent leaking during transport. Care should be taken when collecting specimens to avoid contamination of the outside of the container. If the outside of the container is visibly contaminated, it should be cleaned and disinfected or placed in an impervious bag (49).

USE OF EXTRACTED TEETH IN DENTAL EDUCATIONAL SETTINGS

Extracted teeth used for the education of DHCWs should be considered infective and classified as clinical specimens because they contain blood. All persons who collect, transport, or manipulate extracted teeth should handle them with the same precautions as a specimen for biopsy (2). Universal precautions should be adhered to whenever extracted teeth are handled; because preclinical educational exercises simulate clinical experiences, students enrolled in dental educational programs should adhere to universal precautions in both preclinical and clinical settings. In addition, all persons who handle extracted teeth in dental educational settings should receive hepatitis B vaccine (6–8).

Before extracted teeth are manipulated in dental educational exercises, the teeth first should be cleaned of adherent patient material by scrubbing with detergent and water or by using an ultrasonic cleaner. Teeth should then be stored, immersed in a fresh solution of sodium hypochlorite (household bleach diluted 1:10 with tap water) or any liquid chemical germicide suitable for clinical specimen fixation (50).

Persons handling extracted teeth should wear gloves. Gloves should be disposed of properly and hands washed after completion of work activities. Additional personal protective equipment (e.g., face shield or surgical mask and protective eyewear) should be worn if mucous membrane contact with debris or spatter is anticipated when the specimen is handled, cleaned, or manipulated. Work surfaces and equipment should be cleaned and decontaminated with an appropriate liquid chemical germicide after completion of work activities (37, 38, 40, 51).

The handling of extracted teeth used in dental educational settings differs from giving patients their own extracted teeth. Several states allow patients to keep such teeth, because these teeth are not considered to be regulated (pathologic) waste (52) or because the removed body part (tooth) becomes the property of the patient and does not enter the waste system (53).

DISPOSAL OF WASTE MATERIALS

Blood, suctioned fluids, or other liquid waste may be poured carefully into a drain connected to a sanitary sewer system. Disposable needles, scalpels, or other sharp items should be placed intact into puncture-resistant containers before disposal. Solid waste contaminated with blood or other body fluids should be placed in sealed, sturdy impervious bags to prevent leakage of the contained items. All contained solid waste should then be disposed of according to requirements established by local, state, or federal environmental regulatory agencies and published recommendations (9, 49).

IMPLEMENTATION OF RECOMMENDED INFECTION-CONTROL PRACTICES FOR DENTISTS

Emphasis should be placed on consistent adherence to recommended infection-control strategies, including the use of protective barriers and appropriate methods of sterilizing or disinfecting instruments and environmental surfaces. Each dental facility should develop a written protocol for instrument reprocessing, operatory cleanup, and management of injuries (3). Training of all DHCWs in proper infection-control practices should begin in professional and vocational schools and be updated with continuing education.

ADDITIONAL NEEDS IN DENTISTRY

Additional information is needed for accurate assessment of factors that may increase the risk for transmission of bloodborne pathogens and other infectious agents in a dental setting. Studies should address the nature, frequency, and circumstances of occupational exposures. Such information may lead to the development and evaluation of improved designs for dental instruments, equipment, and personal protective devices. In addition, more efficient reprocessing techniques should be considered in the design of future dental instruments and equipment. Efforts to protect both patients and DHCWs should include improved surveillance, risk assessment, evaluation of measures to prevent exposure, and studies of postexposure prophylaxis. Such efforts may lead to development of safer and more effective medical devices, work practices, and personal protective equipment that are acceptable to DHCWs, are practical and economical, and do not adversely affect patient care (54, 55).

REFERENCES: AS NUMBERED IN ORIGINAL PUBLICATION

1. CDC. Recommended infection-control practices for dentistry. MMWR 1986;35:237–242.
2. CDC. Recommendations for prevention of HIV in health-care settings. MMWR 1987;36:(No. 2S).
3. US Department of Health and Human Services. Infection control file: practical infection control in the dental office. Atlanta, GA/Rockville, MD:CDC/FDA, 1989. (Available through the US Government Printing Office, Washington, DC, or the National Technical Information Services, Springfield, VA.)
4. Department of Labor, Occupational Safety and Health Administration. 29 CFR Part 1910.1030, occupational exposure to bloodborne pathogens; final rule. Federal Register 1991;56(235):64004-64182.
5. CDC. Update: universal precautions for prevention of transmission of human immunodeficiency virus, hepatitis B virus, and other bloodborne pathogens in health-care settings. MMWR 1988;37:377–382, 387–388.
6. CDC. Guidelines for prevention of transmission of human immunodeficiency virus and hepatitis B virus to health-care and public-safety workers. MMWR 1989;38(Suppl 6):1–37.
7. CDC. Protection against viral hepatitis: recommendations of the Immunization Practices Advisory Committee (ACIP). MMWR 1990;39(No. RR-2).
8. CDC. Hepatitis B virus: a comprehensive strategy for eliminating transmission in the United States through universal childhood vaccination. MMWR 1991;40(No. RR-13).
9. Garner JS, Favero MS. Guideline for handwashing and hospital environmental control, 1985. Atlanta: CDC, 1985:publication no. 99–1117.
10. Garner JS. Guideline for prevention of surgical wound infections, 1985. Atlanta: CDC, 1985:publication no. 99–2381.
12. CDC. Recommendations for preventing transmission of human immunodeficiency virus and hepatitis B virus during exposure-prone invasive procedures. MMWR 1991;40(No. RR-8).
32. Siew C, Gruninger SE, Mitchell EW, Burrell KH. Survey of hepatitis B exposure and vaccination in volunteer dentists. J Am Dent Assoc 1987;114:457–459.
33. CDC. Immunization recommendations for health-care-workers. Atlanta: CDC, Division of Immunization, Center for Prevention Services, 1989.
34. Petersen NJ, Bond WW, Favero MS. Air sampling for hepatitis B surface antigen in a dental operatory. J Am Dent Assoc 1979;99:465–467.
35. Bond WW, Petersen NJ, Favero MS, Ebert JW, Maynard JE. Transmission of type B viral hepatitis B via eye inoculation of a chimpanzee. J Clin Microbiol 1982;15:533–534.
36. CDC. Public Health Service statement on management of occupational exposure to human immunodeficiency virus, including considerations regarding zidovudine postexposure use. MMWR 1990;39(No. RR-1).
37. Miller CH, Palenik CJ. Sterilization, disinfection, and asepsis in dentistry. In: Block SS, ed. Disinfection, sterilization, and preservation. 4th ed. Philadelphia: Lea & Febiger, 1991:676–695.
38. Favero MS, Bond WW. Chemical disinfection of medical and surgical materials. In: Block SS, ed. Disinfection, sterilization, and preservation. 4th ed. Philadelphia: Lea & Febiger, 1991:617–641.

39. FDA, Office of Device Evaluation, Division of General and Restorative Devices, Infection Control Devices Branch. Guidance on the content and format of premarket notification [510 (k)] submissions for liquid chemical germicides. Rockville, MD: FDA, January 31, 1992:49.
40. Rutala WA. APIC guideline for selection and use of disinfectants. Am J Infect Control 1990;18:99–117.
41. Proposed American National Standard/American Dental Association Specification No. 59 for portable steam sterilizers for use in dentistry. Chicago: ADA, April 1991.
42. CDC. Recommendations for preventing transmission of infection with human T-lymphotropic virus type III/lymphadenopathy-associated virus in the workplace. MMWR 1985;34:682–686, 691–695.
43. Council on Dental Materials, Instruments, and Equipment, Dental Practice, and Dental Therapeutics, American Dental Association. Infection control recommendations for the dental office and the dental laboratory. J Am Dent Assoc 1988;1126:241–248.
44. Lewis DL, Boe RK. Cross infection risks associated with current procedures for using high-speed dental handpieces. J Clin Microbiol 1992;30:401–406.
45. Crawford JJ, Broderius RK. Control of cross infection risks in the dental operatory: prevention of water retraction by bur cooling spray systems. J Am Dent Assoc 1988;116:685–687.
46. Lewis DL, Arens M, Appleton SS, et al. Cross-contamination potential with dental equipment. Lancet 1992;340:1252–1254.
47. Bagga BSR, Murphy RA, Anderson AW, Punwani I. Contamination of dental unit cooling water with oral microorganisms and its prevention. J Am Dent Assoc 1984;109:712–716.
48. Scheid RC, Kim CK, Bright JS, Whitely MS, Rosen S. Reduction of microbes in handpieces by flushing before use. J Am Dent Assoc 1982;105:658–660.
49. Garner JS, Simmons BP. CDC guideline for isolation precautions in hospitals. Atlanta: CDC, 1983:HHS publication no. (CDC)83–8314.
50. Tate WH, White RR. Disinfection of human teeth for educational purposes. J Dent Educ 1991; 55:583–585.
51. Favero MS, Bond WW. Sterilization, disinfection, and antisepsis in the hospital. In: Balows A, Hausler WJ, Herrmann KL, Isenberg HD, Shadomy HJ, eds. Manual of clinical microbiology. 5th ed. Washington, DC: American Society for Microbiology, 1991:183–200.
52. The Michigan Medical Waste Regulatory Act of 1990, Act No. 368 of the Public Health Acts of 1978, Part 138, Medical Waste, Section 13807—Definitions.
53. Oregon Health Division. Infectious waste disposal; questions and answers pertaining to the Administrative Rules 333–18-040 through 333–18-070. Portland, OR: Oregon Health Division, 1989.
54. Bell DM. Human immunodeficiency virus transmission in health care settings: risk and risk reduction. Am J Med 1991;91(Suppl 3B):294–300.
55. Bell DM, Shapiro CN, Gooch BF. Preventing HIV transmission to patients during invasive procedures: the CDC perspective. J Public Health Dent (in press).

Recommendations for Preventing the Spread of Vancomycin Resistance

Original Citation: Centers for Disease Control and Prevention. Recommendations for preventing the spread of vancomycin resistance: recommendations of the Hospital Infection Control Practices Advisory Committee (HICPAC). MMWR 1995;44(RR-12):1–13.

SUMMARY

Since 1989, a rapid increase in the incidence of infection and colonization with vancomycin-resistant enterococci (VRE) has been reported by U.S. hospitals. This increase poses important problems, including (a) the lack of available antimicrobial therapy for VRE infections, because most VRE are also resistant to drugs previously used to treat such infections (e.g., aminoglycosides and ampicillin), and (b) the possibility that the vancomycin-resistant genes present in VRE can be transferred to other Gram-positive microorganisms (e.g., Staphylococcus aureus). An increased risk for VRE infection and colonization has been associated with previous vancomycin and/or multiantimicrobial therapy, severe underlying disease or immunosuppression, and intraabdominal surgery. Because enterococci can be found in the normal gastrointestinal and female genital tracts, most enterococcal infections have been attributed to endogenous sources within the individual patient. However, recent reports of outbreaks and endemic infections caused by enterococci, including VRE, have indicated that patient-to-patient transmission of the microorganisms can occur either through direct contact or through indirect contact via (a) the hands of personnel or (b) contaminated patient-care equipment or environmental surfaces.

This report presents recommendations of the Hospital Infection Control Practices Advisory Committee for preventing and controlling the spread of vancomycin resistance, with a special focus on VRE. Preventing and controlling the spread of vancomycin resistance will require coordinated, concerted efforts from all involved hospital departments and can be achieved only if each of the following elements is addressed: (a) prudent vancomycin use by clinicians, (b) education of hospital staff regarding the problem of vancomycin resistance, (c) early detection and prompt reporting of vancomycin resistance in enterococci and other Gram-positive microorganisms by the hospital microbiology laboratory, and (d) immediate implementation of appropriate infection-control measures to prevent person-to-person transmission of VRE.

INTRODUCTION

From 1989 through 1993, the percentage of nosocomial enterococcal infections reported to CDC's National Nosocomial Infections Surveillance (NNIS) system that were caused by vancomycin-resistant enterococci (VRE) increased from 0.3% to 7.9% (1). This overall increase primarily reflected the 34-fold increase in the percentage of VRE infections in patients in intensive-care units (ICUs) (i.e., from 0.4% to 13.6%), although a trend toward an increased percentage of VRE infections in non-ICU patients also was noted (1). The occurrence of VRE in NNIS hospitals was associated with larger hospital size (i.e., a hospital with greater than or equal to 200 beds) and university affiliation (1). Other hospitals also have reported increased endemic rates and clusters of VRE infection and colonization (2–8). The actual increase in the incidence of VRE in U.S. hospitals might be greater than reported because the fully automated methods used in many clinical laboratories cannot consistently detect vancomycin resistance, especially moderate vancomycin resistance (as manifested in the VanB phenotype) (9–11).

Vancomycin resistance in enterococci has coincided with the increasing incidence of high-level enterococcal resistance to penicillin and aminoglycosides, thus presenting a challenge for physicians who treat patients who have infections caused by these microorganisms (1, 4). Treatment options are often limited to combining antimicrobials or experimental compounds that have unproven efficacy (12–14). The epidemiology of VRE has not been clarified; however, certain patient populations are at increased risk for VRE infection or colonization. These populations include critically ill patients or those with severe underlying disease or immunosuppression (e.g., patients in ICUs or in oncology or transplant wards); persons who have had an intraabdominal or cardio-thoracic surgical procedure or an indwelling urinary or central venous catheter; and persons who have had a prolonged hospital stay or received multiantimicrobial and/or vancomycin therapy (2–8). Because enterococci are part of the normal flora of the gastrointestinal and female genital tracts, most infections with these microorganisms have been attributed to the patient's endogenous flora (15). However, recent studies have indicated that VRE and other enterococci can be transmitted directly by patient-to-patient contact or indirectly by transient carriage on the hands of personnel (16) or by contaminated environmental surfaces and patient-care equipment (3, 8, 17).

The potential emergence of vancomycin resistance in clinical isolates of Staphylococcus aureus and Staphylococcus epidermidis also is a public health concern. The vanA gene, which is frequently plasmid-borne and confers high-level resistance to vancomycin, can be transferred in vitro from enterococci to a variety of Gram-positive microorganisms (18, 19), including S. aureus (20). Although vancomycin resistance in clinical strains of S. epidermidis or S. aureus has not been reported, vancomycin-resistant strains of Staphylococcus haemolyticus have been isolated (21, 22).

In November 1993 and February 1994, the Subcommittee on the Prevention and Control of Antimicrobial-Resistant Microorganisms in Hospitals of CDC's Hospital Infection Control Practices Advisory Committee (HICPAC) responded to the increase in vancomycin resistance in enterococci by meeting with representatives from the American Hospital Association, the American Society for Microbiology, the Association for Professionals in Infection Control and Epidemiology, the Infectious Diseases Society of America, the Society for Healthcare Epidemiology of America, and the Surgical Infection Society. Meeting participants agreed with the need for prompt implementation of control measures; thus, recommendations to prevent the spread of VRE were developed. Public comments were solicited and incorporated into the draft recommendations. In November 1994, HICPAC ratified the following recommendations for preventing and controlling the spread of vancomycin resistance, with special focus on VRE. HICPAC recognizes that (a) data are limited and additional research will be required to clarify the epidemiology of VRE and determine cost-effective control strategies, and (b) many U.S. hospitals have concurrent problems with other antimicrobial-resistant organisms (e.g., methicillin-resistant S. aureus [MRSA] and beta-lactam and aminoglycoside-resistant Gram-negative bacilli) that might have different epidemiologic features and require different control measures.

RECOMMENDATIONS

Each hospital—through collaboration of its quality-improvement and infection-control programs; pharmacy and therapeutics committee; microbiology laboratory; clinical departments; and nursing, administrative, and housekeeping services—should develop a comprehensive, institution-specific, strategic plan to detect, prevent, and control infection and colonization with VRE. The following elements should be addressed in the plan.

Prudent Vancomycin Use

Vancomycin use has been reported consistently as a risk factor for infection and colonization with VRE (2, 4, 7, 8, 17) and may increase the possibility of the emergence of vancomycin-resistant S. aureus (VRSA) and/or vancomycin-resistant S. epidermidis (VRSE). Therefore, all hospitals and other health-care delivery services, even those at which VRE have never been detected, should (a) develop a comprehensive, antimicrobial-utilization plan to provide education for their medical staff (including medical students who rotate their training in different departments of the health-care facility), (b) oversee surgical prophylaxis, and (c) develop guidelines for the proper use of vancomycin (as applicable to the institution).

Guideline development should be part of the hospital's quality-improvement program and should involve participation from the hospital's pharmacy and therapeutics committee; hospital epidemiologist; and infection-control, infectious-disease, medical, and surgical staffs. The guidelines should include the following considerations:

° Situations in which the use of vancomycin is appropriate or acceptable:
  • For treatment of serious infections caused by beta-lactam-resistant Gram-positive microorganisms. Vancomycin may be less rapidly bactericidal than are beta-lactam agents for beta-lactam-susceptible staphylococci (23, 24).
  • For treatment of infections caused by Gram-positive microorganisms in patients who have serious allergies to beta-lactam antimicrobials.
  • When antibiotic-associated colitis fails to respond to metronidazole therapy or is severe and potentially life-threatening.

- Prophylaxis, as recommended by the American Heart Association, for endocarditis following certain procedures in patients at high risk for endocarditis (25).
- Prophylaxis for major surgical procedures involving implantation of prosthetic materials or devices (e.g., cardiac and vascular procedures [26] and total hip replacement) at institutions that have a high rate of infections caused by MRSA or methicillin-resistant S. epidermidis. A single dose of vancomycin administered immediately before surgery is sufficient unless the procedure lasts greater than 6 hours, in which case the dose should be repeated. Prophylaxis should be discontinued after a maximum of two doses (27–30).

° Situations in which the use of vancomycin should be discouraged:
- Routine surgical prophylaxis other than in a patient who has a life-threatening allergy to beta-lactam antibiotics (28).
- Empiric antimicrobial therapy for a febrile neutropenic patient, unless initial evidence indicates that the patient has an infection caused by Gram-positive microorganisms (e.g., at an inflamed exit site of Hickman catheter) and the prevalence of infections caused by MRSA in the hospital is substantial (31–37).
- Treatment in response to a single blood culture positive for coagulase-negative staphylococcus, if other blood cultures taken during the same time frame are negative (i.e., if contamination of the blood culture is likely). Because contamination of blood cultures with skin flora (e.g., S. epidermidis) could result in inappropriate administration of vancomycin, phlebotomists and other personnel who obtain blood cultures should be trained to minimize microbial contamination of specimens (38–40).
- Continued empiric use for presumed infections in patients whose cultures are negative for beta-lactam-resistant Gram-positive microorganisms (41).
- Systemic or local (e.g., antibiotic lock) prophylaxis for infection or colonization of indwelling central or peripheral intravascular catheters (42–48).
- Selective decontamination of the digestive tract.
- Eradication of MRSA colonization (49,50).
- Primary treatment of antibiotic-associated colitis (51).
- Routine prophylaxis for very low-birthweight infants (i.e., infants who weigh less than 1,500 g [3 lbs 4 oz]) (52).
- Routine prophylaxis for patients on continuous ambulatory peritoneal dialysis or hemodialysis (48, 53).
- Treatment (chosen for dosing convenience) of infections caused by beta-lactam-sensitive Gram-positive microorganisms in patients who have renal failure (54–57).

° Use of vancomycin solution for topical application or irrigation.
° Enhancing compliance with recommendations:
- Although several techniques may be useful, further study is required to determine the most effective methods for influencing the prescribing practices of physicians (58–61).
- Key parameters of vancomycin use can be monitored through the hospital's quality assurance/improvement process or as part of the drug-utilization review of the pharmacy and therapeutics committee and the medical staff.

Education Programs

Continuing education programs for hospital staff (including attending and consulting physicians, medical residents, and students; pharmacy, nursing, and laboratory personnel; and other direct patient-care providers) should include information concerning the epidemiology of VRE and the potential impact of this pathogen on the cost and outcome of patient care. Because detection and containment of VRE require an aggressive approach and high performance standards for hospital personnel, special awareness and educational sessions might be indicated.

Role of the Microbiology Laboratory in the Detection, Reporting, and Control of VRE

The microbiology laboratory is the first line of defense against the spread of VRE in the hospital. The laboratory's ability to promptly and accurately identify enterococci and detect vancomycin resistance is essential for recognizing VRE colonization and infection and avoiding complex, costly containment efforts that are required when recognition of the problem is delayed. In addition, cooperation and communication between the laboratory and the infection-control program will facilitate control efforts.

Identification of Enterococci

Presumptively identify colonies on primary isolation plates as enterococci by using colonial morphology, a Gram stain, and a pyrrolidonyl arylamidase (PYR) test. Although identifying enterococci to the species level can help predict certain resistance patterns (e.g., Enterococcus faecium is more resistant to penicillin than is Enterococcus faecalis) and may help determine the epidemiologic relatedness of enterococcal isolates, such identification is not routinely necessary if antimicrobial susceptibility testing is performed. However, under special circumstances or as laboratory resources permit, biochemical tests can be used to differentiate between various enterococcal species. Although most commercially available identification systems adequately differentiate E. faecalis from other species of enterococci, additional tests for motility and pigment production are required to distinguish Enterococcus gallinarum (motile and nonpigmented) and Enterococcus casseliflavus (motile and pigmented) from E. faecium (nonmotile and nonpigmented).

Tests for Antimicrobial Susceptibility

Determine vancomycin resistance and high-level resistance to penicillin (or ampicillin) and aminoglycosides (62) for enterococci isolated from blood, sterile body sites (with the possible exception of urine), and other sites as clinically indicated. Laboratories routinely may test wound and urine isolates for resistance to vancomycin and penicillin or ampicillin if resources permit (see Screening Procedures for Detecting VRE in Hospitals Where VRE Have Not Been Detected).

- Laboratories that use disk diffusion should incubate plates for 24 hours and read zones of inhibition by using transmitted light (62, 63).
- Minimum inhibitory concentrations can be determined by agar dilution, agar gradient dilution, broth macrodilution, or manual broth microdilution (62–64). These test systems should be incubated for 24 hours.

- The fully automated methods of testing enterococci for resistance to vancomycin currently are unreliable (9–11).

When VRE Are Isolated From a Clinical Specimen

Confirm vancomycin resistance by repeating antimicrobial susceptibility testing using any of the recommended methods (see Tests for Antimicrobial Susceptibility), particularly if VRE isolates are unusual in the hospital, OR streak 1 μL of standard inoculum (0.5 McFarland) from an isolated colony of enterococci onto brain heart infusion agar containing 6 μg/mL of vancomycin, incubate the inoculated plate for 24 hours at 35°C (95°F), and consider any growth indicative of vancomycin resistance (62, 63, 65). Immediately, while performing confirmatory susceptibility tests, notify the patient's primary caregiver, patient-care personnel, and infection-control personnel regarding the presumptive identification of VRE so that appropriate isolation precautions can be initiated promptly (see Preventing and Controlling VRE Transmission in All Hospitals). Follow this preliminary report with the (final) result of the confirmatory test. Additionally, highlight the report regarding the isolate to alert staff that isolation precautions are indicated.

Screening Procedures for Detecting VRE in Hospitals Where VRE Have Not Been Detected

In some hospital microbiology laboratories, antimicrobial susceptibility testing of enterococcal isolates from urine or nonsterile body sites (e.g., wounds) is not performed routinely; thus, identification of nosocomial VRE colonization and infection in hospitalized patients may be delayed. Therefore, in hospitals where VRE have not yet been detected, implementing special measures can promote earlier detection of VRE.

Antimicrobial Susceptibility Survey

Perform periodic susceptibility testing on an epidemiologic sample of enterococcal isolates recovered from all types of clinical specimens, especially from high-risk patients (e.g., those in an ICU or in an oncology or transplant ward). The optimal frequency of testing and number of isolates to be tested will vary among hospitals, depending on the patient population and number of cultures performed at the hospital. Hospitals that process large numbers of culture specimens need to test only a fraction (e.g., 10%) of enterococcal isolates every 1–2 months, whereas hospitals processing fewer specimens might need to test all enterococcal isolates during the survey period. The hospital epidemiologist can help design a suitable sampling strategy.

Culture Survey of Stools or Rectal Swabs

In tertiary medical centers and other hospitals that have many critically ill patients (e.g., ICU, oncology, and transplant patients) at high risk for VRE infection or colonization, periodic culture surveys of stools or rectal swabs of such patients can detect the presence of VRE. Because most patients colonized with VRE have intestinal colonization with this organism, fecal screening of patients is recommended even though VRE infections have not been identified clinically (2, 4, 16).

The frequency and intensity of surveillance should be based on the size of the population at risk and the specific hospital unit(s) involved. If VRE have been detected in other health-care facilities in a hospital's area and/or if a hospital's staff decides to determine whether VRE are present in the hospital despite the absence of recognized clinical cases, stool or rectal-swab culture surveys are useful. The cost of screening can be reduced by inoculating specimens onto selective media containing vancomycin (2, 17, 66) and restricting screening to those patients who have been in the hospital long enough to have a substantial risk for colonization (e.g., 5–7 days) or who have been admitted from a facility (e.g., a tertiary-care hospital or a chronic-care facility) where VRE have been identified.

After colonization with VRE has been detected, all the enterococcal isolates (including those from urine and wounds) from patients in the hospital should be screened routinely for vancomycin resistance, and efforts to contain the spread of VRE should be intensified (i.e., by strict adherence to handwashing and compliance with isolation precautions) (see Preventing and Controlling VRE Transmission in All Hospitals). Intensified fecal screening for VRE might facilitate earlier identification of colonized patients, leading to more efficient containment of the microorganism.

Preventing and Controlling Nosocomial Transmission of VRE

Eradicating VRE from hospitals is most likely to succeed when VRE infection or colonization is confined to a few patients on a single ward. After VRE have become endemic on a ward or have spread to multiple wards or to the community, eradication becomes difficult and costly. Aggressive infection-control measures and strict compliance by hospital personnel are required to limit nosocomial spread of VRE.

Control of VRE requires a collaborative, institution-wide, multidisciplinary effort. Therefore, the hospital's quality-assurance/improvement department should be involved at the outset to identify specific problems in hospital operations and patient-care systems and to design, implement, and evaluate appropriate changes in these systems.

Preventing and Controlling VRE Transmission in All Hospitals

The following measures should be implemented by all hospitals, including those in which VRE have been isolated infrequently or not at all, to prevent and control transmission of VRE.

- ° Notify appropriate hospital staff promptly when VRE are detected (see When VRE Are Isolated From a Clinical Specimen).
- ° Inform clinical staff of the hospital's policies regarding VRE-infected or colonized patients. Because the slightest delay can lead to further spread of VRE and complicate control efforts, implement the required procedures as soon as VRE are detected. Clinical staff are essential to limiting the spread of VRE in patient-care areas; thus, continuing education regarding the appropriate response to the detection of VRE is critical (see Education Programs).

° Establish system(s) for monitoring appropriate process and outcome measures (e.g., cumulative incidence or incidence density of VRE colonization, rate of compliance with VRE isolation precautions and handwashing, interval between VRE identification in the laboratory and implementation of isolation precautions on the wards, and the percentage of previously colonized patients admitted to the ward who are identified promptly and placed on isolation precautions). Relay these data to the clinical, administrative, laboratory, and support staff to reinforce ongoing education and control efforts (67).

° Initiate the following isolation precautions to prevent patient-to-patient transmission of VRE:

  • Place VRE-infected or colonized patients in private rooms or in the same room as other patients who have VRE (8).

  • Wear gloves (clean, nonsterile gloves are adequate) when entering the room of a VRE-infected or colonized patient because VRE can extensively contaminate such an environment (3, 8, 16, 17). When caring for a patient, a change of gloves might be necessary after contact with material that could contain high concentrations of VRE (e.g., stool).

  • Wear a gown (a clean, nonsterile gown is adequate) when entering the room of a VRE-infected or colonized patient (a) if substantial contact with the patient or with environmental surfaces in the patient's room is anticipated, (b) if the patient is incontinent, or (c) if the patient has had an ileostomy or colostomy, has diarrhea, or has a wound drainage not contained by a dressing (8).

  • Remove gloves and gown before leaving the patient's room and immediately wash hands with an antiseptic soap or a waterless antiseptic agent (68–71). Hands can be contaminated via glove leaks (72–76) or during glove removal, and bland soap does not always completely remove VRE from the hands (77).

  • Ensure that after glove and gown removal and handwashing, clothing and hands do not contact environmental surfaces in the patient's room that are potentially contaminated with VRE (e.g., a door knob or curtain) (3, 8).

° Dedicate the use of noncritical items (e.g., a stethoscope, sphygmomanometer, or rectal thermometer) to a single patient or cohort of patients infected or colonized with VRE (17). If such devices are to be used on other patients, adequately clean and disinfect these devices first (78).

° Obtain a stool culture or rectal swab from roommates of patients newly found to be infected or colonized with VRE to determine their colonization status, and apply isolation precautions as necessary. Perform additional screening of patients on the ward at the discretion of the infection-control staff.

° Adopt a policy for deciding when patients infected or colonized with VRE can be removed from isolation precautions. The optimal requirements remain unknown; however, because VRE colonization can persist indefinitely (4), stringent criteria might be appropriate, such as VRE-negative results on at least three consecutive occasions (greater than or equal to 1 week apart) for all cultures from multiple body sites (including stool or rectal swab, perineal area, axilla or umbilicus, and wound, Foley catheter, and/or colostomy sites, if present).

° Because patients with VRE can remain colonized for long periods after discharge from the hospital, establish a system for highlighting the records of infected or colonized patients so they can be promptly identified and placed on isolation precautions upon readmission to the hospital. This information should be computerized so that placement of colonized patients on isolation precautions will not be delayed because the patients' medical records are unavailable.

° Local and state health departments should be consulted when developing a plan regarding the discharge of VRE-infected or colonized patients to nursing homes, other hospitals, or home-health care. This plan should be part of a larger strategy for handling patients who have resolving infections and patients colonized with antimicrobial-resistant microorganisms.

Hospitals With Endemic VRE or Continued VRE Transmission

The following measures should be taken to prevent and control transmission of VRE in hospitals that have endemic VRE or continued VRE transmission despite implementation of measures described in the preceding section (see Preventing and Controlling VRE Transmission in All Hospitals).

° Focus control efforts initially on ICUs and other areas where the VRE transmission rate is highest (4). Such areas can serve as reservoirs for VRE, allowing VRE to spread to other wards when patients are well enough to be transferred.

° Where feasible, cohort the staff who provide regular, ongoing care to patients to minimize the movement/contact of health-care providers between VRE-positive and VRE-negative patients (4, 8).

° Hospital staff who are carriers of enterococci have been implicated rarely in the transmission of this organism (8). However, in conjunction with careful epidemiologic studies and upon the direction of the infection-control staff, examine personnel for chronic skin and nail problems and perform hand and rectal swab cultures of these workers. Remove from the care of VRE-negative patients those VRE-positive personnel linked epidemiologically to VRE transmission until their carrier state has been eradicated.

° Because the results of several enterococcal outbreak investigations suggest a potential role for the environment in the transmission of enterococci (3, 8, 16, 17, 79, 80), institutions experiencing ongoing VRE transmission should verify that the hospital has adequate procedures for the routine care, cleaning, and disinfection of environmental surfaces (e.g., bed rails, bedside commodes, carts, charts, doorknobs, and faucet handles) and that these procedures are being followed by housekeeping personnel. To verify the efficacy of hospital policies and procedures, some hospitals might elect to perform focused environmental cultures before and after cleaning rooms that house patients who have VRE. All environmental culturing should be approved and supervised by the infection-control program in collaboration with the clinical laboratory (3, 8, 16, 17, 79, 80).

° Consider sending representative VRE isolates to reference laboratories for strain typing by pulsed field gel electrophoresis or other suitable techniques to aid in defining reservoirs and patterns of transmission.

Detecting and Reporting VRSA and VRSE

The microbiology laboratory has the primary responsibility for detecting and reporting the occurrence of VRSA or VRSE in the hospital. All clinical isolates of S. aureus and S. epidermidis should be tested routinely, using standard methods, for susceptibility to vancomycin (62). If VRSA or VRSE is identified in a clinical specimen, confirm vancomycin resistance by repeating antimicrobial susceptibility testing using standard methods (62). Restreak the colony to ensure that the culture is pure. The most common causes of false-positive VRSA reports are susceptibility testing on mixed cultures and misidentifying VRE, Leuconostoc, S. haemolyticus, or Pediococcus as VRSA (81, 82).

Immediately (i.e., while performing confirmatory testing) notify the hospital's infection-control personnel, the patient's primary caregiver, and patient-care personnel on the ward on which the patient is hospitalized so that the patient can be placed promptly on isolation precautions (depending on the site[s] of infection or colonization) adapted from previous CDC guidelines (83) and those recommended for VRE infection or colonization in this report (see Preventing and Controlling Nosocomial Transmission of VRE). Furthermore, immediately notify the state health department and CDC, and send the isolate through the state health department to CDC (telephone [404] 639-6413) for confirmation of vancomycin resistance.

REFERENCES: AS NUMBERED IN ORIGINAL PUBLICATION

1. CDC. Nosocomial enterococci resistant to vancomycin—United States, 1989–1993. MMWR 1993;42:597–599.
2. Rubin LG, Tucci V, Cercenado E, Eliopoulos G, Isenberg HD. Vancomycin-resistant Enterococcus faecium in hospitalized children. Infect Control Hosp Epidemiol 1992;13:700–705.
3. Karanfil LV, Murphy M, Josephson A, et al. A cluster of vancomycin-resistant Enterococcus faecium in an intensive care unit. Infect Control Hosp Epidemiol 1992;13:195–200.
4. Handwerger S, Raucher B, Altarac D, et al. Nosocomial outbreak due to Enterococcus faecium highly resistant to vancomycin, penicillin, and gentamicin. Clin Infect Dis 1993;16:750–755.
5. Frieden TR, Munsiff SS, Low DE, et al. Emergence of vancomycin-resistant enterococci in New York City. Lancet 1993;342:76–79.
6. Boyle JF, Soumakis SA, Rendo A, et al. Epidemiologic analysis and genotypic characterization of a nosocomial outbreak of vancomycin-resistant enterococci. J Clin Microbiol 1993;31:1280–1285.
7. Montecalvo MA, Horowitz H, Gedris C, et al. Outbreak of vancomycin-, ampicillin-, and aminoglycoside-resistant Enterococcus faecium bacteremia in an adult oncology unit. Antimicrob Agents Chemother 1994;38:1363–1367.
8. Boyce JM, Opal SM, Chow JW, et al. Outbreak of multi-drug resistant Enterococcus faecium with transferable vanB class vancomycin resistance. J Clin Microbiol 1994;32:1148–1153.
9. Tenover FC, Tokars J, Swenson J, Paul S, Spitalny K, Jarvis W. Ability of clinical laboratories to detect antimicrobial agent-resistant enterococci. J Clin Microbiol 1993;31:1695–1699.
10. Sahm DF, Olsen L. In vitro detection of enterococcal vancomycin resistance. Antimicrob Agents Chemother 1990;34:1846–1848.
11. Zabransky RJ, Dinuzzo AR, Huber MB, Woods GL. Detection of vancomycin resistance in enterococci by the Vitek AMS System. Diagn Microbiol Infect Dis 1994;20:113–116.
12. Moellering RC Jr. The Garrod lecture: the enterococcus—a classic example of the impact of antimicrobial resistance on therapeutic options. J Antimicrob Chemother 1991;28:1–12.
13. Hayden MK, Koenig GI, Trenholme GM. Bactericidal activities of antibiotics against vancomycin-resistant Enterococcus faecium blood isolates and synergistic activities of combinations. Antimicrob Agents Chemother 1994;38:1225–1229.
14. Mobarakai N, Landman D, Quale JM. In-vitro activity of trospectomycin, a new aminocyclitol antibiotic against multidrug-resistant Enterococcus faecium. J Antimicrob Chemother 1994;33:319–321.
15. Murray BE. The life and times of the enterococcus. Clin Microbiol Rev 1990;3:46–65.
16. Rhinehart E, Smith N, Wennersten C, et al. Rapid dissemination of beta-lactamase-producing aminoglycoside-resistant Enterococcus faecalis among patients and staff on an infant and toddler surgical ward. N Engl J Med 1990;323:1814–1818.
17. Livornese LL Jr, Dias S, Samel C, et al. Hospital-acquired infection with vancomycin-resistant Enterococcus faecium transmitted by electronic thermometers. Ann Intern Med 1992;117:112–116.
18. Uttley AH, George RC, Naidoo J, et al. High-level vancomycin-resistant enterococci causing hospital infections. Epidemiol Infect 1989;103:173–181.

19. Leclercq R, Derlot E, Weber M, Duval J, Courvalin P. Transferable vancomycin and teicoplanin resistance in Enterococcus faecium. Antimicrob Agents Chemother 1989;33:10–15.
20. Noble WC, Virani Z, Cree R. Co-transfer of vancomycin and other resistance genes from Enterococcus faecalis NCTC12201 to Staphylococcus aureus. FEMS Microbiol Lett 1992;72:195–198.
21. Veach LA, Pfaller MA, Barrett M, Koontz FP, Wenzel RP. Vancomycin resistance in Staphylococcus haemolyticus causing colonization and bloodstream infection. J Clin Microbiol 1990;28:2064–2068.
22. Degener JE, Heck MEOC, Vanleeuwen WJ, et al. Nosocomial infection by Staphylococcus haemolyticus and typing methods for epidemiological study. J Clin Microbiol 1994;32:2260–2265.
23. Small PM, Chambers HF. Vancomycin for Staphylococcus aureus endocarditis in intravenous drug users. Antimicrob Agents Chemother 1990;34:1227–1231.
24. Cantoni L, Glauser MP, Bille J. Comparative efficacy of daptomycin, vancomycin, and cloxacillin for the treatment of Staphylococcus aureus endocarditis in rats and role of test conditions in this determination. Antimicrob Agents Chemother 1990;34:2348–2353.
25. American Heart Association Committee on Rheumatic Fever and Infective Endocarditis. Prevention of bacterial endocarditis. Circulation 1984;70:1123–1124.
26. Maki DG, Bohn MJ, Stolz SM, Kroncke GM, Acher CW, Myerowitz PD. Comparative study of cefazolin, cefamandole, and vancomycin for surgical prophylaxis in cardiac and vascular operations: a double-blind randomized trial. J Thorac Cardiovasc Surg 1992;104:1423–1434.
27. Classen DC, Evans RS, Pestotnik SL, Horn SD, Menlove RL, Burke JP. The timing of prophylactic administration of antibiotics and the risk of surgical-wound infection. N Engl J Med 1992;326:281–286.
28. Conte JE Jr, Cohen SN, Roe BB, Elashoff RM. Antibiotic prophylaxis and cardiac surgery: a prospective double-blind comparison of single-dose versus multiple-dose regimens. Ann Intern Med 1972;76:943–949.
29. DiPiro JT, Cheung RP, Bowden TA Jr, Mansberger JA. Single-dose systemic antibiotic prophylaxis of surgical wound infections. Am J Surg 1986;152:552–559.
30. Heydemann JS, Nelson CL. Short-term preventive antibiotics. Clin Orthop 1986;205:184–187.
31. Rubin M, Hathorn JW, Marshall D, Gress J, Steinberg SM, Pizzo PA. Gram-positive infections and the use of vancomycin in 550 episodes of fever and neutropenia. Ann Intern Med 1988;108:30–35.
32. Shenep JL, Hughes WT, Roberson PK, et al. Vancomycin, ticarcillin, and amikacin compared with ticarcillin-clavulanate and amikacin in the empirical treatment of febrile neutropenic children with cancer. N Engl J Med 1988;319:1053–1058.
33. Pizzo PA, Hathorn JW, Hiemenz J, et al. A randomized trial comparing ceftazidime alone with combination antibiotic therapy in cancer patients with fever and neutropenia. N Engl J Med 1986;315:552–558.
34. Karp JE, Dick JD, Angelopulos C, et al. Empiric use of vancomycin during prolonged treatment-induced granulocytopenia: randomized, double-blind, placebo-controlled clinical trial in patients with acute leukemia. Am J Med 1986;81:237–242.
35. European Organization for Research and Treatment of Cancer (EORTC) International Antimicrobial Therapy Cooperative Group, National Cancer Institute of Canada Clinical Trials Group. Vancomycin added to empirical combination antibiotic therapy for fever in granulocytopenic cancer patients. J Infect Dis 1991;163:951–958.
36. Riikonen P. Imipenem compared with ceftazidime plus vancomycin as initial therapy for fever in neutropenic children with cancer. Pediatr Infect Dis 1991;10:918–923.
37. Lamy T, Michelet C, Dauriac C, Grulois I, Donio PY, Le Prise PY. Benefit of prophylaxis by intravenous systemic vancomycin in granulocytopenic patients: a prospective, randomized trial among 59 patients. Acta Haematol 1993;90:109–113.
38. Isaacman DJ, Karasic RB. Lack of effect of changing needles on contamination of blood cultures. Pediatr Infect Dis J 1990;9:274–278.
39. Krumholz HM, Cummings S, York M. Blood culture phlebotomy: switching needles does not prevent contamination. Ann Intern Med 1990;113:290–292.
40. Strand CL, Wajsbort RR, Sturmann K. Effect of iodophor vs iodine tincture skin preparation on blood culture contamination rate. JAMA 1993;269:1004–1006.
41. Maki DG, Schuna AA. A study of antimicrobial misuse in a university hospital. Am J Med Sci 1978;275:271–282.
42. Ranson MR, Oppenheim BA, Jackson A, Kamthan AG, Scarffe JH. Double-blind placebo controlled study of vancomycin prophylaxis for central venous catheter insertion in cancer patients. J Hosp Infect 1990;15:95–102.
43. Henrickson KJ, Powell KR, Schwartz CL. A dilute solution of vancomycin and heparin retains antibacterial and anticoagulant activities. J Infect Dis 1988;157:600–601.
44. Schwartz C, Henrickson KJ, Roghmann K, Powell K. Prevention of bacteremia attributed to luminal colonization of tunneled central venous catheters with vancomycin-susceptible organism. J Clin Oncol 1990;8:1591–1597.
45. Henrickson KJ, Dunne WM Jr. Modification of central venous catheter flush solution improves in vitro antimicrobial activity. J Infect Dis 1992;166:944–946.
46. Gaillard JL, Merlino R, Pajot N, et al. Conventional and nonconventional modes of vancomycin ad-

ministration to decontaminate the internal surface of catheters colonized with coagulase-negative staphylococci. J Paren Enter Nutr 1990;14:593–597.

47. Spafford PS, Sinkin RA, Cox C, Reubens L, Powell KR. Prevention of central venous catheter-related co-agulase-negative staphylococcal sepsis in neonates. J Pediatr 1994;125:259–263.

48. Kaplan AH, Gilligan PH, Facklam RR. Recovery of resistant enterococci during vancomycin prophylaxis. J Clin Microbiol 1988;26:1216–1218.

49. Gradon JD, Wu EH, Lutwick LI. Aerosolized vancomycin therapy facilitating nursing home placement. Ann Pharmacother 1992;26:209–210.

50. Weathers L, Riggs D, Santeiro M, Weibley RE. Aerosolized vancomycin for treatment of airway colonization by methicillin-resistant Staphylococcus aureus. Pediatr Infect Dis 1990;9:220–221.

51. Johnson S, Homann SR, Bettin KM, et al. Treatment of asymptomatic Clostridium difficile carriers (fecal excretors) with vancomycin or metronidazole. Ann Intern Med 1992;117:297–302.

52. Kacica MS, Horgan MJ, Ochoa L, Sandler R, Lepow ML, Venezia RA. Prevention of gram-positive sepsis in neonates weighing less than 1500 grams. J Pediatr 1994;125:253–258.

53. Lam TY, Vas SI, Oreopoulos DG. Long-term intraperitoneal vancomycin in the prevention of recurrent peritonitis during CAPD: preliminary results. Perit Dial Int 1991;11:281–282.

54. Bastani B, Freer K, Read D, et al. Treatment of gram-positive peritonitis with two intraperitoneal doses of vancomycin in continuous ambulatory peritoneal dialysis patients. Nephron 1987;45:283–285.

55. Newman LN, Tessman M, Hanslik T, Schulak J, Mayes J, Friedlander M. A retrospective view of factors that affect catheter healing: four years of experience. Adv Perit Dial 1993;9:217–222.

56. Capdevila JA, Segarra A, Planes AM, et al. Successful treatment of haemodialysis catheter-related sepsis without catheter removal. Nephrol Dial Transplant 1993;8:231–234.

57. Edell LS, Westby GR, Gould SR. An improved method of vancomycin administration to dialysis patients. Clin Nephrol 1988;29:86–87.

58. Soumerai SB, McLaughlin TJ, Avorn J. Quality assurance for drug prescribing. Qual Assur Health Care 1990;2:37–58.

59. Everitt DE, Soumerai SB, Avorn J, Klapholz H, Wessels M. Changing surgical antimicrobial prophylaxis practices through education targeted at senior department leaders. Infect Control Hosp Epidemiol 1990;11:578–583.

60. Soumerai SB, Avorn J, Taylor WC, Wessels M, Maher D, Hawley SL. Improving choice of prescribed antibiotics through concurrent reminders in an educational order form. Med Care 1993;31:552–558.

61. Soumerai SB, McLaughlin TJ, Avorn J. Improving drug prescribing in primary care: a critical analysis of the experimental literature. Milbank Q 1989;67:268–317.

62. National Committee for Clinical Laboratory Standards. Methods for dilution antimicrobial susceptibility tests for bacteria that grow aerobically. 3rd ed. Villanova, PA: National Committee for Clinical Laboratory Standards, 1993:publication M7-A3.

63. Swenson JM, Ferraro MJ, Sahm DF, Charache P, Tenover FC, National Committee for Clinical Laboratory Standards Working Group on Enterococci. New vancomycin disk diffusion breakpoints for enterococci. J Clin Microbiol 1992;30:2525–2528.

64. CDC. Recommendations for prevention of HIV transmission in health-care settings. MMWR 1987;36(No. 2S).

65. Swenson JM, Clark NC, Ferraro MJ, et al. Development of a standardized screening method for detection of vancomycin-resistant Enterococci. J Clin Microbiol 1994;32:1700–1704.

66. Edberg SC, Hardalo CJ, Kontnick C, Campbell S. Rapid detection of vancomycin-resistant enterococci. J Clin Microbiol 1994;32:2182–2184.

67. Nettleman MD, Trilla A, Fredrickson M, Pfaller M. Assigning responsibility: using feedback to achieve sustained control of methicillin-resistant Staphylococcus aureus. Am J Med 1991;91(Suppl 3B):228S-232S.

68. Doebbeling BN, Stanley GL, Sheetz CT, et al. Comparative efficacy of alternative hand-washing agents in reducing nosocomial infections in intensive care units. N Engl J Med 1992;327:88–93.

69. Jones MV, Rowe GB, Jackson B, Pritchard NJ. The use of alcohol paper wipes for routine hand cleansing: results of trials in two hospitals. J Hosp Infect 1986;8:268–274.

70. Nicoletti G, Boghossian V, Borland R. Hygienic hand disinfection: a comparative study with chlorhexidine detergents and soap. J Hosp Infect 1990;15:323–337.

71. Butz AM, Laughon BE, Gullette DL, Larson EL. Alcohol-impregnated wipes as an alternative in hand hygiene. Am J Infect Control 1990;18:70–76.

72. Korniewicz DM, Laughon BE, Butz A, Larson E. Integrity of vinyl and latex procedure gloves. Nurs Res 1989;38:144–146.

73. Korniewicz DM, Kirwin M, Cresci K, Markut C, Larson E. In-use comparison of latex gloves in two high-risk units: surgical intensive care and acquired immunodeficiency syndrome. Heart Lung 1992;21:81–84.

74. DeGroot-Kosolcharoen J, Jones JM. Permeability of latex and vinyl gloves to water and blood. Am J Infect Control 1989;17:196–201.

75. Paulssen J, Eidem T, Kristiansen R. Perforations in surgeons' gloves. J Hosp Infect 1988;11:82–85.

76. Korniewicz DM, Laughon BE, Cyr WH, Lytle CD, Larson E. Leakage of virus through used vinyl and latex examination gloves. J Clin Microbiol 1990;28:787–788.

77. Wade JJ, Desai N, Casewell MW. Hygienic hand disinfection for the removal of epidemic vancomycin-resistant Enterococcus faecium and gentamicin-resistant Enterobacter cloacae. J Hosp Infect 1991;18:211–218.
78. Favero MS, Bond WW. Sterilization, disinfection, and antisepsis in the hospital. In: Balows A, Hausler WJ Jr, Herrman KL, Isenberg HD, Shadomy HJ, eds. Manual of clinical microbiology. 5th ed. Ch. 24. Washington, DC: American Society for Microbiology, 1991:183–200.
79. Zervos MJ, Kauffman CA, Therasse PM, Bregman AG, Mikesell TS, Schaberg DR. Nosocomial infection by gentamicin-resistant Streptococcus faecalis: an epidemiologic study. Ann Intern Med 1987;106:687–691.
80. Wells VD, Wong ES, Murray BE, Coudron PE, Williams DS, Markowitz SM. Infections due to beta-lactamase-producing, high-level gentamicin-resistant Enterococcus faecalis. Ann Intern Med 1992;116:285–292.
81. Orberg PK, Sandine WE. Common occurrence of plasmid DNA and vancomycin resistance in Leuconostoc spp. Appl Environ Microbiol 1984;48:1129–1133.
82. Schwalbe RS, Ritz WJ, Verma PR, Barranco EA, Gilligan PH. Selection for vancomycin resistance in clinical isolates of Staphylococcus haemolyticus. J Infect Dis 1990;161:45–51.
83. Garner JS, Simmons BP. Guideline for isolation precautions in hospitals. Infect Control 1983;4(Suppl): 245–325.

Guideline for Handwashing and Hospital Environmental Control

Original Citation: Centers for Disease Control and Prevention. Guideline for handwashing and hospital environmental control, 1985 (supersedes guideline for hospital environmental control published in 1981). MMWR 1988;37(No. 24).

Original Authors: Revised by Julia S. Garner, RN, MN, Martin S. Favero, PhD.

RANKING SCHEME FOR RECOMMENDATIONS

Category I

Measures in Category I are strongly supported by well-designed and controlled clinical studies that show their effectiveness in reducing the risk of nosocomial infections, or are viewed as effective by a majority of expert reviewers. Measures in this category are viewed as applicable for most hospitals- regardless of size, patient population, or endemic nosocomial infection rates.

Category II

Measures in Category II are supported by highly suggestive clinical studies in general hospitals or by definitive studies in specialty hospitals that might not be representative of general hospitals. Measures that have not been adequately studied but have a logical or strong theoretical rationale indicating probable effectiveness are included in this category. Category II recommendations are viewed as practical to implement in most hospitals.

Category III

Measures in Category III have been proposed by some investigators, authorities, or organizations, but, to date, lack supporting data, a strong theoretical rationale, or an indication that the benefits expected from them are cost effective. Thus, they are considered important issues to be studied. They might be considered by some hospitals for implementation, especially if the hospitals have specific nosocomial infection problems, but they are not generally recommended for widespread adoption.

SECTION 1: HANDWASHING
Introduction

Handwashing is the single most important procedure for preventing nosocomial infections. Handwashing is defined as a vigorous, brief rubbing together of all surfaces of lathered hands, followed by rinsing under a stream of water. Although various products are available, handwashing can be classified simply by whether plain soap or detergents or antimicrobial-containing products are used (1). Handwashing with plain soaps or detergents (in bar, granule, leaflet, or liquid form) suspends microorganisms and allows them to be rinsed off; this process is often referred to as mechanical removal of microorganisms. In addition, handwashing with antimicrobial-containing products kills or inhibits the growth of microorganisms; this process is often referred to as chemical removal of microorganisms. Routine handwashing is discussed in this Guideline; the surgical hand scrub is discussed in the Guideline for Prevention of Surgical Wound Infections.

EPIDEMIOLOGY

The microbial flora of the skin consists of resident and transient microorganisms; the resident microorganisms survive and multiply on the skin and can be repeatedly cultured, while the transient microbial flora represent recent contaminants that can survive only a limited period of time. Most resident microorganisms are found in superficial skin layers, but about 10%–20% can inhabit deep epidermal layers (2, 3). Hand washing with plain soaps and detergents is effective in removing many transient microbial flora (4–6). Resident microorganisms in the deep layers may not be removed by handwashing with plain soaps and detergents, but usually can be killed or inhibited by handwashing with products that contain antimicrobial ingredients.

Many resident skin microorganisms are not highly virulent and are not implicated in infections other than skin infections. However, some of these microorganisms can cause infections in patients when surgery or other invasive procedures allow them to enter deep tissues or when a patient is severely immunocompromised or has an implanted device, such as a heart valve. In contrast, the transient microorganisms often found on the hands of hospital personnel can be pathogens acquired from colonized or infected patients and may cause nosocomial infections. Several recent studies have shown that transient and resident hand carriage of aerobic gram-negative microorganisms by hospital personnel may be more frequent than previously thought (7–10). More study on the bacteriology of hands is needed to fully understand the factors that contribute to persistent hand carnage of such microorganisms (11).

CONTROL MEASURES

The absolute indications for and the ideal frequency of handwashing are generally not known because of the lack of well-controlled studies. Listing all circumstances that may require handwashing would be a lengthy and arbitrary task. The indications for handwashing probably depend on the type, intensity, duration, and sequence of activity. Generally, superficial contact with a source not suspected of being contaminated, such as touching an object not visibly soiled or taking a blood pressure, does not require handwashing. In contrast, prolonged and intense contact with any patient should probably be followed by handwashing. In addition, handwashing is indicated before performing invasive procedures, before taking care of particularly susceptible patients, such as those who are severely immunocompromised or newborn infants, and before and after touching wounds. Moreover, handwashing is indicated, even when gloves are used, after situations during which microbial contamination of the hands is likely to occur, especially those involving contact with mucous membranes, blood and body fluids, and secretions or excretions, and after touching inanimate sources that are likely to be contaminated, such as urine-measuring devices. In addition, handwashing is an important component of the personal hygiene of all hospital personnel, and hand washing should be encouraged when personnel are in doubt about the necessity for doing so.

The circumstances that require handwashing are frequently found in high-risk units, because patients in these units are often infected or colonized with virulent or multiply-resistant microorganisms, and are highly susceptible to infection because of wounds, invasive procedures, or diminished immune function. Handwashing in these units is indicated between direct contact with different patients and often is indicated more than once in the care of one patient, for example, after touching excretions or secretions, before going on to another care activity for the same patient.

The recommended handwashing technique depends on the purpose of the handwashing. The ideal duration of handwashing is not known, but washing times of 15 seconds (6) or less (5) have been reported as effective in removing most transient conrruminants from the skin. Therefore, for most activities, a vigorous, brief (at least 10 seconds) rubbing together of all surfaces of lathered hands followed by rinsing under a stream of water is recommended. If hands are visibly soiled, more time may be required for handwashing.

The absolute indications for handwashing with plain soaps and detergents versus handwashing with antimicrobial-containing products are not known because of the lack of well-controlled studies comparing infection rates when such products are used. For most routine activities, handwashing with plain soap appears to be sufficient, since soap will allow most transient microorganisms to be washed off (4–6).

Handwashing products for use in hospitals are available in several forms. It is important, however, that the product selected for use be acceptable to the personnel who will use it (6). When plain soap is selected for handwashing, the bar, liquid, granule, or soap-impregnated tissue form may be used. It is preferable that bar soaps be placed on racks that allow water to drain. Since liquid-soap containers can become contaminated and might serve as reservoirs of microorganisms, reusable liquid containers need to be cleaned when empty and refilled with fresh soap. Completely disposable containers obviate the need to empty and clean dispensers but may be more expensive. Most antimicrobial-containing handwashing products are available as liquids. Antimicrobial-containing foams and rinses are also available for use in areas without easy access to sinks.

In addition to handwashing, personnel may often wear gloves as an extra margin of safety. As with handwashing, the absolute indications for wearing gloves are not known. There is general agreement that wearing sterile gloves is indicated when certain invasive procedures are performed or when open wounds are touched. Nonsterile gloves can be worn when hands are likely to become contaminated with potentially infective material such as blood, body fluids, or secretions, since it is often not known which patients' blood, body fluids, or secretions contain hepatitis B virus or other pathogens. Further, gloves can be worn to prevent gross microbial contamination of hands, such as when objects soiled with feces are handled. When gloves are worn, handwashing is also recommended because gloves may become perforated during use and because bacteria can multiply rapidly on gloved hands.

The convenient placement of sinks, handwashing products. and paper towels is often suggested as a means of encouraging frequent and appropriate handwashing. Sinks with faucets that can be turned off by means other than the hands (e.g., foot pedals) and sinks that minimize splash can help personnel avoid immediate recontamination of washed hands.

Although handwashing is considered the most important single procedure for preventing nosocomial infections, two reports showed poor compliance with handwashing protocols by personnel in medical intensive care units, especially by physicians (12) and personnel taking care of patients on isolation precautions (13). Failure to wash hands is a complex problem that may be caused by lack of motivation or lack of knowledge about the importance of handwashing. It may also be caused by obstacles such as under staffing, inconveniently located

sinks, absence of paper towels, an unacceptable handwashing product, or the presence of dermatitis caused by previous handwashing. More study is needed to identify which of these factors, alone or in combination, contribute significantly to the problem of poor compliance with
handwashing recommendations.

Recommendations

    1. Handwashing Indications

      a. In the absence of a true emergency, personnel should always wash
their hands

        i.   Before performing invasive procedures; Category I.

        ii. Before taking care of particularly susceptible patients, such as
those who are severely immunocompromised and newborns;
Category I.

        iii. Before and after touching wounds, whether surgical, traumatic,
or associated with an invasive device; Category I.

        iv. After situations during which microbial contamination of hands is
likely to occur, especially those involving contact with mucous
membranes. blood or body fluids, secretions, or excretions;
Category I.

        v.   After touching inanimate sources that are likely to be contami-
nated with virulent or epidemiologically important microorganisms; these sources include urine-measuring devices or secretion
collection apparatuses; Category I.

        vi. After taking care of an infected patient or one who is likely to be col-
onized with microorganisms of special clinical or epidemiologic significance. For example, multiply-resistant bacteria; Category I.

        vii. Between contacts with different patients in high-risk units.
Category I.

      b. Most routine, brief patient-care activities involving direct patient con-
tact other than that discussed in 1.a. above, e.g., taking a blood pressure, do not require handwashing; Category II.

      c. Most routine hospital activities involving indirect patient contact, e.g.,
handing a patient medications, food, or other objects, do not require
handwashing; Category I.

    2. Handwashing Technique

      For routine handwashing, a vigorous rubbing together of all surfaces of
lathered hands for at least 10 seconds. followed by thorough rinsing under a stream of water is recommended; Category I.

    3. Handwashing with Plain Soap

      a. Plain soap should be used for handwashing unless otherwise indi-
cated; Category II.

      b. If bar soap is used, it should be kept on racks that allow drainage of
water; Category II.

      c. If liquid soap is used, the dispenser should be replaced or cleaned and
filled with fresh product when empty; liquids should not be added to
a partially full dispenser; Category II.

4. Handwashing with Antimicrobial-Containing Products (Health-Care Personnel Handwashes)
    a. Antimicrobial handwashing products should be used for handwashing before personnel care for newborns and when otherwise indicated during their care, between patients in high-risk units, and before personnel take care of severely immunocompromised patients; Category III. (Hospitals may choose from products in the product category defined by the FDA as health-care personnel handwashes. Persons responsible for selecting commercially marketed antimicrobial health-care personnel handwashes can obtain information about categorization of products from the Center for Drugs and Biologics, Division of OTC Drug Evaluation, FDA. 5600 Fishers Lane, Rockville, MD 20857. In addition, information published in the scientific literature, presented at scientific meetings, documented by manufacturers, and obtained from other sources deemed important may be considered.)
    b. Antimicrobial-containing products that do not require water for use, such as foams or rinses, can be used in areas where no sinks are available; Category II.
5. Handwashing Facilities
    a. Handwashing facilities should be conveniently located throughout the hospital; Category I.
    b. A sink should be located in or just outside every patient room. More than one sink per room may be necessary if a large room is used for several patients; Category II.
    c. Handwashing facilities should be located in or adjacent to rooms where diagnostic or invasive procedures that require handwashing are performed (e.g., cardiac catheterization, bronchoscopy, sigmoidoscopy, etc.); Category I.

REFERENCES: AS NUMBERED IN ORIGINAL PUBLICATION

1. The tentative final monograph for OTC topical antimicrobial products. Federal Register Jan 6, 1978;43 FR 1210:1211–1249 T.
2. Price PB. New studies in surgical bacteriology and surgical technique. JAMA 1938;111:1993–1996.
3. Ulrich JA. Techniques of skin sampling for microbial contaminants. Hosp Topics 1965;43:121–123.
4. Lowbury EJL, Lilly HA, Bull JP. Disinfection of hands: removal of transient organisms. Br Med J 1964;2:230–233.
5. Sprunt K, Redman W, Leidy G. Antibacterial effectiveness of routine handwashing. Pediatrics 1973; 52:264–271.
6. Ojajarvi J. The importance of soap selection for routine hygiene in hospital. J Hyg (Camb) 1981; 8:275–283.
7. Knittle MA, Eitzman DV, Bear H. Role of hand contamination of personnel in the epidemiology of gram-negative nosocomial infections. J Pediatr 1975;86:433–437.
8. Larson EL. Persistent carriage of gram-negative bacteria on hands. Am J Infect Control 1981;9:112–119.
9. Adams BG, Marrie TJ. Hand carriage of aerobic gram-negative rods may not be transient. J Hyg (Camb) 1982;89:33–46.
10. Adams BG, Marrie TJ. Hand carriage of aerobic gram-negative rods by health care personnel. J Hyg (Camb) 1982;89:23–31.
11. Larson E. Current handwashing issues. Infect Control 1984;5:15–17.
12. Albert RK, Condie F. Handwashing patterns in medical intensive-care units. N Engl J Med 1981; 304:1465–1466.
13. Larson E. Compliance with isolation techniques. Am J Infect Control 1983;11:221–225.

SECTION 2: CLEANING, DISINFECTING, AND STERILIZING PATIENT-CARE EQUIPMENT

INTRODUCTION

Cleaning, the physical removal of organic material or soil from objects, is usually done by using water with or without detergents. Generally, cleaning is designed to remove rather than to kill microorganisms. Sterilization, on the other hand, is the destruction of all forms of microbial life; it is carried out in the hospital with steam under pressure, liquid or gaseous chemicals, or dry heat. Disinfection, defined as the intermediate measures between physical cleaning and sterilization, is carried out with pasteurization or chemical germicides.

Chemical germicides can be classified by several systems. We have used the system originally proposed by Spaulding (1) in which three levels of disinfection are defined: high, intermediate, and low (Table 1). In contrast, EPA uses a system that classifies chemical germicides as sporicides, general disinfectants, hospital disinfectants, sanitizers, and others. Formulations registered by the EPA as sporicides are considered sterilants if the contact time is long enough to destroy all forms of microbial life, or high-level disinfectants if contact times are shorter. Chemical germicides registered by the EPA as sanitizers probably fall into the category of low-level disinfectants. Numerous formulations of chemical germicides can be classified as either low- or intermediate-level disinfectants. depending on the specific label claims. For example, some chemical germicide formulations are claimed to be efficacious against Mycobacterium tuberculosis; by Spaulding's system, these formulations would be classified at least as intermediate-level disinfectants. However, chemical germicide formulations with specific label claims for effectiveness against Salmonella choleraesuis. Staphylococcus aureus, and Pseudomonas aeruginosa (the challenge microorganisms required for EPA classification as a "hospital disinfectant") could fall into intermediate- or low-level disinfectant categories.

Table 1. Levels of disinfection according to type of microorganism

		Bacteria			Viruses	
Levels	Vegetative	Tubercle Bacillus	Spores	Fungi[1]	Lipid & Medium size	Nonlipid & Small
High	+[2]	+	+[3]	+	+	+
Intermediate	+	+	±[4]	+	+	±[5]
Low	+	−	−	±	+	−

[1]Includes asexual spores but not necessarily chlamydospores or sexual spores.

[2]Plus sign indicates that a killing effect can be expected when the normal use-concentrations of chemical disinfectants or pasteurization are properly employed; a negative sign indicates little or no killing effect.

[3]Only with extended exposure times are high-level disinfectant chemicals capable of actual sterilization.

[4]Some intermediate-level disinfectants can be expected to exhibit some sporicidal action.

[5]Some intermediate-level disinfectants may have limited virucidal activity.

The rationale for cleaning, disinfecting, or sterilizing patient-care equipment can be understood more readily if medical devices, equipment, and surgical materials are divided into three general categories (critical items, semicritical items, and noncritical items) based on the potential risk of infection involved in their use. This categorization of medical devices also is based on the original suggestions by Spaulding (1).

Critical items are instruments or objects that are introduced directly into the bloodstream or into other normally sterile areas of the body. Examples of critical items are surgical instruments. cardiac catheters, implants, pertinent components of the heart-lung oxygenator, and the blood compartment of a hemodialyzer. Sterility at the time of use is required for these items; consequently, one of several accepted sterilization procedures is generally recommended.

Items in the second category are classified as semicritical in terms of the degree of risk of infection. Examples are noninvasive flexible and rigid fiber optic endoscopes, endotracheal tubes, anesthesia breathing circuits, and cystoscopes. Although these items come in contact with intact mucous membranes, they do not ordinally penetrate body surfaces. If steam sterilization can be used, it is often cheaper to sterilize many of these items, but sterilization is not absolutely essential; at a minimum, a high-level disinfection procedure that can be expected to destroy vegetative microorganisms, most fungal spores, tubercle bacilli, and small nonlipid viruses is recommended. In most cases, meticulous physical cleaning followed by an appropriate high-level disinfection treatment gives the user a reasonable degree of assurance that the items are free of pathogens.

Noncritical items are those that either do not ordinarily touch the patient or touch only intact skin. Such items include crutches, bed boards, blood pressure cuffs, and a variety of other medical accessories. These items rarely, if ever, transmit disease. Consequently, depending on the particular piece of equipment or item, washing with a detergent may be sufficient.

The level of disinfection achieved depends on several factors, principally contact time, temperature, type and concentration of the active ingredients of the chemical germicide, and the nature of the microbial contamination. Some disinfection procedures are capable of producing sterility if the contact times used are sufficiently long; when these procedures are continued long enough to kill all but resistant bacterial spores, the result is high-level disinfection. Other disinfection procedures that can kill many types of viruses and most vegetative microorganisms (but cannot be relied upon to kill resistant microorganisms such as tubercle bacilli, bacterial spores, or certain viruses) are considered to be intermediate- or low-level disinfection (Table 1).

The tubercle bacillus, lipid and nonlipid viruses, and other groups of microorganisms in Table 1 are used in the context of indicator microorganisms that have varying degrees of resistance to chemical germicides and not necessarily because of their importance in causing nosocomial infections. For example, cells of M. tuberculosis or M. bovis, which are used in routine efficacy tests, are among the most resistant vegetative microorganisms known and. after bacterial endospore, constitute the most severe challenge to a chemical germicide. Thus, a tuberculocidal chemical germicide may be used as a high or intermediate-level disinfectant targeted to many types of nosocomial pathogens but not specifically to control respiratory tuberculosis.

CONTROL MEASURES

Since it is neither necessary nor possible to sterilize all patient-care items, hospital policies can identify whether cleaning, disinfecting, or sterilizing of an item is indicated to decrease the risk of infection. The process indicated for an item will depend on its intended use. Any microorganism, including bacterial spores, that come in contact with normally sterile tissue can cause infection. Thus, it is important that all items that will touch normally sterile tissues be sterilized. It is less important that objects touching mucous membranes be sterile. Intact mucous membranes are generally resistant to infection by common bacterial spores but are not resistant to many other microorganisms, such as viruses and tubercle bacilli; therefore, items that touch mucous membranes require a disinfection process that kills all but resistant bacterial spores. In general, intact skin acts as an effective barrier to most microorganisms; thus, items that touch only intact skin need only be clean.

Items must be thoroughly cleaned before processing, because organic material (e.g., blood and proteins) may contain high concentrations of microorganisms. Also, such organic material may inactivate chemical germicides and protect microorganisms from the disinfection or sterilization process. For many noncritical items, such as blood pressure cuffs or crutches, cleaning can consist only of (a) washing with a detergent or a disinfectant-detergent, (b) rinsing, and (c) thorough drying.

Steam sterilization is the most inexpensive and effective method for sterilization. Steam sterilization is unsuitable, however, for processing plastics with low melting points, powders, or anhydrous oils. Items that are to be sterilized but not used immediately need to be wrapped for storage. Sterility can be maintained in storage for various lengths of time, depending on the type of wrapping material, the conditions of storage, and the integrity of the package.

Several methods have been developed to monitor steam sterilization processes. One method is to check the highest temperature that is reached during sterilization and the length of time that this temperature is maintained. In addition, heat- and steam-sensitive chemical indicators can be used on the outside of each pack. These indicators do not reliably document sterility, but they do show that an item has not accidentally bypassed a sterilization process. As an additional precaution, a large pack might have a chemical indicator both on the outside and the inside to verify that steam has penetrated the pack.

Microbiological monitoring of steam sterilizers is recommended at least once a week with commercial preparations or spores of Bacillus stearorhermophilus (a microorganism having spores that are particularly resistant to moist heat, thus assuring a wide margin of safety). If a sterilizer is working properly and used appropriately, the spores are usually killed. One positive spore test (spores not killed) does not necessarily indicate that items processed in the sterilizer are not sterile, but it does suggest that the sterilizer should be rechecked for proper temperature, length of cycle, loading, and use and that the test be repeated. Spore testing of steam sterilization is just one of several methods for assuring adequate processing of patient-care items (Table 2).

Implantable items, such as orthopedic devices, require special handling before and during sterilization thus, packs containing implantable objects need to be clearly labeled so they will be appropriately processed. To guarantee a wide margin of safety, it is recommended that each load of such items be tested with a spore test and that the sterilized item not be released

Table 2. Methods of assuring adequate processing and Safe use of medical devices

Object and Classification	Example	Method	Comment
Patient-care objects Critical			
Sterilized in the hospital	Surgical instruments and devices; trays and sets	1. Thoroughly clean objects and wrap or package for sterilization. 2. Follow manufacturer's instructions for use of each sterilizer or use recommended protocol. 3. Monitor time-temperature charts. 4. Use commercial spore preparations to monitor sterilizers. 5. Inspect package for integrity and for exposure of sterility indicator before use. 6. Use before maximum safe storage time has expired if applicable.	Sterilization processes are designed to have a wide margin of safety. If spores are not killed, the sterilizer should be checked for proper use and function; if spore tests remain positive, discontinue use of the sterilizer until properly serviced. Maximum safe storage time of items processed in the hospital varies according to type of package or wrapping material(s) used; follow manufacturer's instructions for use and storage times.
Purchased as sterile	Intravenous fluids; irrigation fluids; normal saline; trays and sets	1. Store in safe, clean area. 2. Inspect package for integrity before use. 3. Use before expiration date if one is given. 4. Culture only if clinical circumstances suggest infection related to use of the item.	Notify the Food and Drug Administration, local and state health departments, and CDC if intrinsic contamination is suspected.

Table 2.—*continued*

Object and Classification	Example	Method	Comment
Semicritical Should be free of vegetative bacteria. May be subjected to high-level disinfection rather than sterilization process	Respiratory therapy equipment and instruments that will touch mucous membranes	1. Sterilize or follow a protocol for high-level disinfection. 2. Bag and store in safe, clean area. 3. Conduct quality control monitoring after any important changes in the disinfection process.	Bacterial spores may survive after high-level disinfection, but these usually are not pathogenic. Microbiologic sampling can verify that a high-level disinfection process has resulted in destruction of vegetative bacteria; however, this sampling is not routinely recommended.
Non critical Usually contaminated with some bacteria	Bedpans; crutches; rails; EKG leads	1. Follow a protocol for cleaning or, if necessary a low-level disinfection process.	
Water-produced or treated	Water used for hemodialysis fluids	1. Assay water and dialysis fluids monthly. 2. Water should not have more than 200 bacteria/ml and dialysis fluids not more than 2000 bacteria/ml.	Gram-negative water bacteria can grow rapidly in water and dialysis fluids and can place dialysis patients at risk of pyrogenic reactions or septicemia. These water sources and pathways should be disinfected routinely.

for use until the spore test is negative at 48 hours. If it is not possible to process an implantable object with a confirmed 48-hour spore test before use, it is recommended that the unwrapped object receive the equivalent of full-cycle steam sterilization and not flash sterilization. Flash sterilization [270°F (132°C) for 3 minutes in a gravity displacement steam sterilizer] is not recommended for implantable items because spore tests cannot be used reliably and the margin of safety is lower.

Because ethylene oxide gas sterilization is a more complex and expensive process than steam sterilization, it is usually restricted to objects that might be damaged by heat or excessive moisture. Before sterilization, objects also need to be cleaned thoroughly and wrapped in a material that allows the gas to penetrate. Chemical indicators need to be used with each package to show that it has been exposed to the gas sterilization process. Moreover, it is recommended that gas sterilizers be checked at least once a week with commercial preparations of spores, usually Bacillus subtilis var. niger. Because ethylene oxide gas is toxic, precautions (e.g., local exhaust ventilation) should be taken to protect personnel (2). All objects processed by gas sterilization also need special aeration according to manufacturer's recommendations before use to remove toxic residues of ethylene oxide.

Powders and anhydrous oils can be sterilized by dry heat. Microbiological monitoring of dry heat sterilizers and following manufacturers' recommendations for their use and maintenance usually provides a wide margin of safety for dry heat sterilization.

Liquid chemicals can be used for sterilization and disinfection when steam, gas, or dry heat sterilization is not indicated or available. With some formulations, high-level disinfection can be accomplished in 10–30 minutes, and sterilization can be achieved if exposure is for significantly longer times. Nevertheless, not all formulations are equally applicable to all items that need to be sterilized or disinfected. No formulation can be considered as an "all purpose" chemical germicide. In each case, more detailed information can be obtained from the EPA, descriptive brochures from the manufacturers, peer-review journal articles, and books. The most appropriate chemical germicide for a particular situation can be selected by responsible personnel in each hospital based on the object to be disinfected, the level of disinfection needed, and the scope of services, physical facilities, and personnel available in the hospital. It is also important that the manufacturer's instructions for use be consulted.

Gloves may be indicated to prevent skin reactions when some chemical disinfectants are used. Items subjected to high-level disinfection with liquid chemicals need to be rinsed in sterile water to remove toxic or irritating residues and then thoroughly dried. Subsequently, the objects need to be handled aseptically with sterile gloves and towels and stored in protective wrappers to prevent recontamination.

Hot-water disinfection (pasteurization) is a high-level, nontoxic disinfection process that can be used for certain items, e.g., respiratory therapy breathing circuits.

In recent years, some hospitals have considered reusing medical devices labeled disposable or single use only. In general, the primary, if not the sole, motivation for such reuse is to save money. For example, the disposable hollow-fiber hemodialyzer has been reprocessed and reused on the same patient in hemodialysis centers since the early 1970s. By 1984, 51% of the 1,200 U.S. dialysis centers were using dialyzer reprocessing programs. It has been estimated that this practice saves more than 100 million dollars per year (3). When standard protocols for cleaning and disinfecting hemodialyzers are used, there does not appear to be any significant infection risk to dialysis patients (4). Moreover, the safety and efficacy of dialyzer reuse programs are supported by several major studies (5–7). Few, if any, other medical devices that might be considered candidates for reprocessing have been evaluated in this manner.

Arguments for and against reprocessing and reusing single-use items in the 1980s have been summarized (4). Since there is lack of evidence indicating increased risk of nosocomial infections associated with reusing all single-use items, a categorical recommendation against all types of reuse is not considered justifiable. Rather than recommending for or against reprocessing and reuse of all single-use items, it appears more prudent to recommend that hospitals consider the safety and efficacy of the reprocessing procedure of each item or device separately and the likelihood that the device will function as intended after reprocessing. In many instances it may be difficult if not impossible to document that the device can be reprocessed without residual toxicity and still function safely and effectively. Few, if any, manufacturers of disposable or single-use medical devices provide reprocessing information on the product label.

Hydrotherapy pools and immersion tanks present unique disinfection problems in hospitals. It is generally not economically feasible to drain large hydrotherapy pools that contain thousands of gallons of water after each patient use. Typically, these pools are used by a large number of patients and are drained and cleaned every one to two weeks. The water temperature is typically maintained near 37°C. Between cleanings, water can be contaminated by organic material from patients, and high levels of microbial contamination are possible. One method to maintain safe pool water is to install a water filter of sufficient size to filter all the water at least three times per day and to chlorinate the water so that a free chlorine residual of approximately 0.5 mg/L is maintained at a 7.2 to 7.6. Local public health authorities can provide consultation regarding chlorination, alternate halogen disinfectants, and hydrotherapy pool sanitation.

Hubbard and immersion tanks present entirely different problems than large pools, since they are drained after each patient use. All inside surfaces need to be cleaned with a disinfectant-detergent, then rinsed with tap water. After the last patient each day, an additional disinfection step is performed. One general procedure is to circulate a chlorine solution (200–300 mg/L) through the agitator of the tank for 15 minutes and then rinse it out. It is also recommended that the tank be thoroughly cleaned with a disinfectant-detergent, rinsed, wiped dry with clean cloths, and not filled until ready for use.

An alternative approach to control of contamination in hydrotherapy tanks is to use plastic liners and create the "whirlpool effect" without agitators. Such liners make it possible to minimize contact of contaminated water with the interior surface of the tank and also obviate the need for agitators that may be very difficult to clean and decontaminate.

Recommendations

1. Cleaning
   All objects to be disinfected or sterilized should first be thoroughly cleaned to remove all organic matter (blood and tissue) and other residue; Category I.
2. Indications for Sterilization and High-Level Disinfection
   a. Critical medical devices or patient-care equipment that enter normally sterile tissue or the vascular system or through which blood flows should be subjected to a sterilization procedure before each use; Category I.
   b. Laparoscopes, arthroscopes, and other scopes that enter normally sterile tissue should be subjected to a sterilization procedure before each use; if this is not feasible, they should receive at least high-level disinfection; Category I.
   c. Equipment that touches mucous membranes, e.g., endoscopes, endotracheal tubes, anesthesia breathing circuits, and respiratory therapy equipment, should receive high-level disinfection; Category I.
3. Methods of Sterilization
   a. Whenever sterilization is indicated, a steam sterilizer should be used unless the object to be sterilized will be damaged by heat, pressure, or moisture or is otherwise inappropriate for steam sterilization. In this case, another acceptable method of sterilization should be used; Category II.
   b. Flash sterilization [270°F (132°C) for 3 minutes in a gravity displacement steam sterilizer] is not recommended for implantable items; Category II.
4. Biological Monitoring of Sterilizers
   a. All sterilizers should be monitored at least once a week with commercial preparations of spores intended specifically for that type of sterilizer (i.e., Bacillus stearothermophilus for steam sterilizers and Bacillus subtilis for ethylene oxide and dry heat sterilizers); Category II.
   b. Every load that contains implantable objects should be monitored. These implantable objects should not be used until the spore test is found to be negative at 48 hours; Category II.
   c. If spores are not killed in routine spore tests, the sterilizer should immediately be checked for proper use and function and the spore test repeated. Objects, other than implantable objects, do not need to be recalled because of a single positive spore test unless the sterilizer or the sterilization procedure is defective; Category II.
   d. If spore tests remain positive, use of the sterilizer should be discontinued until it is serviced; Category I.
5. Use and Preventive Maintenance
   Manufacturers' instructions should be followed for use and maintenance of sterilizers; Category II.

6. Chemical Indicators

Chemical indicators that will show a package has been through a sterilization cycle should be visible on the outside of each package sterilized; Category II.

7. Use of Sterile Items

An item should not be used if its sterility is questionable, e.g., its package is punctured, torn, or wet; Category I.

8. Reprocessing Single-Use or Disposable Items

a. Items or devices that cannot be cleaned and sterilized or disinfected without altering their physical integrity and function should not be reprocessed; Category I.

b. Reprocessing procedures that result in residual toxicity or compromise the overall safety or effectiveness of the items or devices should be avoided; Category I.

REFERENCES: AS NUMBERED IN ORIGINAL PUBLICATION

1. Favero MS. Chemical disinfection of medical and surgical materials. In: Block SS, ed. Disinfection, sterilization and preservation. 3rd ed. Philadelphia: Lea and Febiger, 1983;469–492.
2. Fed Reg June 22, 1984; 29 CFR 1910 (Occupational Exposure to Ethylene Oxide).
3. Romeo AA. The economics of reuse. In: Reuse of disposable medical devices in the 1980's. Proceedings of International Conference on the Reuse of Disposable Medical Devices in the 1980's, The Institute for Health Policy Analysis. Georgetown University Medical Center. March 29–30, 1984. Washington, DC: Institute for Health Policy Analysis, 1984:43–49.
4. Institute for Health Policy Analysis. Georgetown University Medical Center. Proceedings of International Conference on the Reuse of Disposable Medical Devices in the 1980's. March 29–30, 1984. Washington, DC.
5. Jacobs C, Brunner FP, Chantler C, et al. Combined report on regular dialysis and transplantation in Europe VII. 1976. Proc Eur Dial Transplant Assoc 1977;14:3–69.
6. Levin N. Dialyzer re-use in a hospital. Dial and Transplant 1980;9(1):40–46.
7. Wing AJ, Brunner FP, Brynger H, et al. Mortality and morbidity of reusing dialyzers. Br Med J 1978;2:853–855.

SECTION 3: MICROBIOLOGIC SAMPLING

INTRODUCTION

Before 1970, regularly scheduled culturing of the air and environmental surfaces such as floors, walls, and table tops was widely practiced in U.S. hospitals. By 1970, CDC and the American Hospital Association were advocating that hospitals discontinue routine environmental culturing, since rates of nosocomial infection had not been related to levels of general microbial contamination of air or environmental surfaces, and meaningful standards for permissible levels of microbial contamination of environmental surfaces did not exist (1, 2). Between 1970 and 1975, 25% of U.S. hospitals reduced the extent of such routine environmental culturing (3), and this trend has continued.

In the last several years, there has also been a trend toward reducing routine microbiologic sampling for quality control purposes. In 1982, CDC recommended that the disinfection process for respiratory therapy equipment should not be monitored by routine microbiologic sampling (4). Moreover, the recommendation for microbiologic sampling of infant formulas prepared in the hospital has been removed from this Guideline, since there is no epidemiologic evidence to show that such quality control testing influences the infection rate in hospitals.

CONTROL MEASURES

The only routine or periodic microbiologic sampling that is recommended is of the water and dialysis fluids used with artificial kidney machines in hospital-based or free standing chronic hemodialysis centers. Microbiologic sampling of dialysis fluids and water used to prepare dialysis fluids is recommended because gram-negative bacteria are able to grow rapidly in water and other fluids associated with the hemodialysis system; high levels of these microorganisms place dialysis patients at risk of pyrogenic reactions, bacteremia, or both (5). It is suggested that the water that is used to prepare dialysis fluid also be sampled periodically, because high levels of bacteria in water often become amplified downstream in a hemodialysis system and are sometimes predictive of bacterial contamination in dialysis fluids. Although it is difficult to determine the exact frequency of such a sampling program in the absence of pyrogenic reactions and bacteremia, sampling water and dialysis fluid monthly appears to be reasonable.

Routine microbiologic sampling of patient-care items purchased as sterile is not recommended because of the difficulty and expense of performing adequate sterility testing with low-frequency contamination.

Microbiologic sampling is indicated during investigation of infection problems if environmental reservoirs are implicated epidemiologically in disease transmission. It is important, however, that such culturing be based on epidemiologic data and follow a written plan that specifies the objects to be sampled and the actions to be taken based on culture results.

Recommendations

1. Routine Environmental Culturing of Air and Environmental Surfaces
   Routine microbiologic sampling of the air and environmental surfaces should not be done; Category I.
2. Microbiologic Sampling of Dialysis Fluids
   Water used to prepare dialysis fluid should be sampled once a month; it should not contain a total viable microbial count greater than 200 colony-forming units (CFU)/ml. The dialysis fluid should be sampled once a month at the end of a dialysis treatment and should contain less than 2,000 CFU/ml; Category II.
3. Microbiologic Sampling for Specific Problems Microbiologic sampling, when indicated, should be an integral part of an epidemiologic investigation; Category I.
4. Sampling for Manufacturer-Associated Contamination
   a. Routine microbiologic sampling of patient-care objects purchased as sterile is not recommended; Category I.
   b. If contamination of a commercial product sold as sterile is suspected, infection control personnel should be notified, suspect lot numbers should be recorded, and items from suspected lots should be segregated and quarantined. Appropriate microbiologic assays may be considered; however, the nearest district office of the FDA, local and state health departments, and CDC should be notified promptly; Category I.

REFERENCES: AS NUMBERED IN ORIGINAL PUBLICATION

1. Eickhoff TC. Microbiologic sampling. Hospitals 1970;44:86–87.
2. American Hospital Association Committee on Infections Within Hospitals. Statement on microbiologic sampling in the hospital. Hospitals 1974;48:125–126.
3. Haley RW, Shachtrnan RS. The emergence of infection surveillance and control programs in U.S. hospitals: an assessment, 1976. Am J Epidemiol 1980;111:574–591.
4. Simmons BP, Wong ES. Guideline for prevention of nosocomial pneumonia. Infect Control 1982;3:327–333.
5. Favero MS, Petersen NJ. Microbiologic guidelines for hemodialysis systems. Dialys Transpl 1977;6:34–36.

SECTION 4: INFECTIVE WASTE

INTRODUCTION

There is no epidemiologic evidence to suggest that most hospital waste is any more infective than residential. Moreover, there is no epidemiologic evidence that hospital waste disposal practices have caused disease in the community. Therefore, identifying wastes for which special precautions are indicated is largely a matter of judgment about the relative risk of disease transmission. Aesthetic and emotional considerations may override the actual risk of disease transmission, particularly for pathology wastes.

Since a precise definition of infective waste that is based on the quantity and type of etiologic agents present is virtually impossible, the most practical approach to infective waste management is to identify those wastes that represent a sufficient potential risk of causing infection during handling and disposal and for which some special precautions appear prudent. Hospital wastes for which special precautions appear prudent include microbiology laboratory waste, pathology waste, and blood specimens or blood products. Moreover, the risk of either injury or infection from certain sharp items (e.g., needles and scalpel blades) contaminated with blood also needs to be considered when such items are disposed of. While any item that has had contact with blood, exudates, or secretions may be potentially infective, it is not normally considered practical or necessary to treat all such waste as infective. CDC has published general recommendations for handling infective waste from patients on isolation precautions (1). Additional special precautions may be necessary for certain rare diseases or conditions such as Lassa fever (2). The EPA has published a draft manual (Environmental Protection Agency, Office of Solid Waste and Emergency Response: Draft Manual for Infectious Waste Management, SW-957, 1982. Washington, DC: 1982) that identifies and categorizes other specific types of waste that may be generated in some research-oriented hospitals. In addition to the above guidelines, local and state environmental regulations may also exist.

CONTROL MEASURES

Solid waste from the microbiology laboratory can be placed in steam-sterilizable bags or pans and steam sterilized in the laboratory. Alternatively, it can be transported in sealed, impervious plastic bags to be burned in a hospital incinerator. A single bag is probably adequate if the bag is sturdy (not easily penetrated) and if the waste can be put in the bag without contaminating the outside of the bag; otherwise, double-bagging is indicated. All slides or tubes with small amounts of blood can be packed in sealed, impervious containers and sent for incineration or steam sterilization in the hospital. Exposure for up to 90 minutes at 250°F (121°C) in a steam sterilizer, depending on the size of the load and type container, may be necessary to assure an adequate sterilization cycle (3, 4). After steam sterilization, the residue can be safely handled and discarded with all other nonhazardous hospital solid waste. All containers with more than a few milliliters of blood remaining after laboratory procedures and/or bulk blood may be steam sterilized, or the contents may be carefully poured down a utility sink drain or toilet.

Waste from the pathology laboratory is customarily incinerated at the hospital. Although no national data are available, in one state 96% of the hospitals surveyed reported that they incinerate pathology waste (5). Any hospital incinerator should be capable of burning, within applicable air pollution regulations, the actual waste materials to be destroyed. Improper incineration of waste with high moisture and low energy content, such as pathology waste, can lead to emission problems.

Disposables that can cause injury, such as scalpel blades and syringes with needles, should be placed in puncture-resistant containers. Ideally, such containers are located where these items are used. Syringes and needles can be placed intact directly into the rigid containers for safe storage until terminal treatment. To prevent needle-stick injuries, needles should not be recapped, purposely bent, or broken by hand. When some needle cutting devices are used, blood may be aerosolized or spattered onto environmental surfaces; however, currently no data are available from controlled studies examining the effect, if any, of the use of these devices on the incidence of needle-transmissible infections.

It is often necessary to transport or store infective waste within the hospital prior to terminal treatment. This can be done safely if proper and common-sense procedures are used. The EPA draft manual mentioned above contains guidelines for the storage and transport, both on-site and off-site, of infective waste. For unique and specialized problems, this manual can be consulted.

Recommendations

1. Identification of Infective Waste
   a. Microbiology laboratory wastes, blood and blood products, pathology waste, and sharp items (especially needles) should be considered as potentially infective and handled and disposed of with special precautions; Category II.
   b. Infective waste from patients on isolation precautions should be handled and disposed of according to the current edition of the Guideline for Isolation Precautions in Hospitals. (This recommendation is not categorized since the recommendations for isolation precautions are not categorized.)

2. Handling, Transport, and Storage of Infective Waste
   a. Personnel involved in the handling and disposal of infective waste should be informed of the potential health and safety hazards and trained in the appropriate handling and disposal methods; Category II.
   b. If processing and/or disposal facilities are not available at the site of infective waste generation (i.e., laboratory, etc.) the waste may be safely transported in sealed impervious containers to another hospital area for appropriate treatment; Category II.
   c. To minimize the potential risk for accidental transmission of disease or injury, infective waste awaiting terminal processing should be stored in an area accessible only to personnel involved in the disposal process; Category III.

3. Processing and Disposal of Infective Waste
   a. Infective waste, in general, should either be incinerated or should be autoclaved prior to disposal in a sanitary landfill; Category III.
   b. Disposable syringes with needles, scalpel blades, and other sharp items capable of causing injury should be placed intact into puncture-resistant containers located as close to the area in which they were used as is practical. To prevent needle-stick injuries, needles should not be recapped, purposely bent, broken, or otherwise manipulated by hand; Category I.
   c. Bulk blood, suctioned fluids, excretions, and secretions may be carefully poured down a drain connected ro a sanitary sewer. Sanitary sewers may also be used for the disposal of other infectious wastes capable of being ground and flushed into the sewer; Category II (special precautions may be necessary for certain rare diseases or conditions such as Lassa fever (2)).

REFERENCES: AS NUMBERED IN ORIGINAL PUBLICATION

1. Garner JS, Simmons BP. Guideline for isolation precautions in hospitals. Infect Control 1983;4: 245–325.
2. Centers for Disease Control. Viral hemorrhagic fever: initial management of suspected and confirmed cases. MMWR 1983;32(Suppl):275–405.

3. Rutala WA, Stiegel MM, Sarubbi FA. Decontamination of laboratory microbiological waste by steam sterilization. Appl Environ Microbiol 1982;43:1311–1316.
4. Lauer JL, Battles DR, Vesley D. Decontaminating infectious laboratory waste by autoclaving. Appl Environ Microbiol 1982;44:690–694.
5. Rutala WA, Sarubbi FA. Management of infectious waste from hospitals. Infect Control 1983;4:198–203.

SECTION 5: HOUSEKEEPING

INTRODUCTION

Although microorganisms are a normal contaminant of walls, floors, and other surfaces, these environmental surfaces rarely are associated with transmission of infections to patients or personnel. Therefore, extraordinary attempts to disinfect or sterilize these environmental surfaces are rarely indicated. However, routine cleaning and removal of soil are recommended. Recommendations for cleaning in the rooms of patients on isolation precautions have been published (1).

CONTROL MEASURES

Cleaning schedules and methods vary according to the area of the hospital, type of surface to be cleaned, and the amount and type of soil present. Horizontal surfaces (for example, beside tables and hard-surfaced flooring) in patient-care areas are usually cleaned on a regular basis, when soiling or spills occur, and when a patient is discharged. Cleaning of walls, blinds, and curtains is recommended only if they are visibly soiled. Disinfectant fogging is an unsatisfactory method of decontaminating air and surfaces and is not recommended.

Recommendations against use of carpets in patient-care areas have been removed from this Guideline, since there is no epidemiologic evidence to show that carpets influence the nosocomial infection rate in hospitals (2). Carpets, however, may contain much higher levels of microbial contamination than hard-surfaced flooring and can be difficult to keep clean in areas of heavy soiling or spillage; therefore, appropriate cleaning and maintenance procedures are indicated.

Disinfectant-detergent formulations registered by the EPA can be used for environmental surface cleaning, but the actual physical removal of microorganisms by scrubbing is probably as important, if not more so, than any antimicrobial effect of the cleaning agent used. Therefore, cost, safety, and acceptability by housekeepers can be the main criteria for selecting any such registered agent. The manufacturers' instructions for appropriate use should be followed.

Special precautions for cleaning incubators, mattresses, and other nursery surfaces with which neonates have contact have been recommended (3), since inadequately diluted solutions of phenolics used for such cleaning and poor ventilation have been associated with hyperbilirubinemia in newborns (4).

Recommendations

1. Choice of Cleaning Agent for Environmental Surfaces in Patient-Care Areas
   Any hospital-grade disinfectant-detergent registered by the EPA may be used for cleaning environmental surfaces. Manufacturers' instructions for use of such products should be followed; Category II.
2. Cleaning of Horizontal Surfaces in Patient-Care Areas
   a. Uncarpeted floors and other horizontal surfaces, e.g., bedside tables, should be cleaned regularly and if spills occur; Category II.
   b. Carpeting should be vacuumed regularly with units designed to efficiently filter discharged air, cleaned if spills occur, and shampooed whenever a thorough cleaning is indicated. Category II
3. Cleaning Walls, Blinds, and Curtains
   Terminal cleaning of walls, blinds, and curtains is not recommended unless they are visibly soiled; Category II.

4. Disinfectant Fogging
Disinfectant fogging should not be done; Category I.

REFERENCES: AS NUMBERED IN ORIGINAL PUBLICATION

1. Garner JS, Simmons BP. Guideline for isolation precautions in hospitals. Infect Control 1983;4: 245–325.
2. Anderson RL, Mackel DC, Stoler BS, Mallison GF. Carpeting in hospitals: An epidemiological evaluation. J Clin Microbiol 1982;15:408–415.
3. American Academy of Pediatrics, American College of Obstetricians and Gynecologists. Guidelines for perinatal care. Evanston, IL/Washington, DC: AAP, ACOG, 1983.
4. Wysowski DK, Flynt JW, Goldfield M, et al. Epidemic neonatal hyperbilirubinemia and use of a phenolic disinfectant detergent. Pediatrics 1978;61:165–170.

SECTION 6: LAUNDRY

INTRODUCTION

Although soiled linen has been identified as a source of large numbers of pathogenic microorganisms, the risk of actual disease transmission appears negligible. Rather than rigid rules and regulations, hygienic and common sense storage and processing of clean and soiled linen are recommended. Guidelines for laundry construction and operation for health care facilities have been published (1, 2).

CONTROL MEASURES

Soiled linen can be transported in the hospital by cart or chute. Bagging linen is indicated if chutes are used, since improperly designed chutes can be a means of spreading microorganisms throughout the hospital (3). Recommendations for handling soiled linen from patients on isolation precautions have been published (4).

Soiled linen may or may not be sorted in the laundry before being loaded into washer/extractor units. Sorting before washing protects both machinery and linen from the effects of objects in the linen and reduces the potential for recontamination of clean linen that sorting after washing requires. Sorting after washing minimizes the direct exposure of laundry personnel to infective material in the soiled linen and reduces airborne microbial contamination in the laundry (5). Protective apparel and appropriate ventilation (2) can minimize these exposures.

The microbicidal action of the normal laundering process is affected by several physical and chemical factors (5). Although dilution is not a microbicidal mechanism, it is responsible for the removal of significant quantities of microorganisms. Soaps or detergents loosen soil and also have some microbicidal properties. Hot water provides an effective means of destroying microorganisms, and a temperature of at least 71°C (160°F) for a minimum of 25 minutes is commonly recommended for hot-water washing. Chlorine bleach provides an extra margin of safety. A total available chlorine residual of 50–150 ppm is usually achieved during the bleach cycle. The last action performed during the washing process is the addition of a mild acid to neutralize any alkalinity in the water supply, soap, or detergent. The rapid shift in pH from approximately 12 to 5 also may tend to inactivate some microorganisms.

Recent studies have shown that a satisfactory reduction of microbial contamination can be achieved at lower water temperatures of 22–50°C when the cycling of the washer, the wash formula, and the amount of chlorine bleach are carefully monitored and controlled (6, 7). Instead of the microbicidal action of hot water, low temperature laundry cycles rely heavily on the presence of bleach to reduce levels of microbial contamination. Regardless of whether hot or cold water is used for washing, the temperatures reached in drying and especially during ironing provide additional significant microbicidal action.

Recommendations

1. Routine Handling of Soiled Linen
  a. Soiled linen should be handled as little as possible and with minimum

agitation to prevent gross microbial contamination of the air and of persons handling the linen; Category II.

    b. i. All soiled linen should be bagged or put into carts at the location where it was used; it should not be sorted or prerinsed in patient-care areas; Category II.

      ii. Linen soiled with blood or body fluids should be deposited and transported in bags that prevent leakage; Category II.

    c. If laundry chutes are used, linen should be bagged, and chutes should be properly designed; Category II.

2. Hot-Water Washing

If hot water is used, linen should be washed with a detergent in water at least 71°C (160°F) for 25 minutes; Category II.

3. Low-Temperature Water Washing

If low temperature (<70°C) laundry cycles are used, chemicals suitable for low-temperature washing at proper use concentration should be used; Category II.

4. Transportation of Clean Linen

Clean linen should be transported and stored by methods that will ensure its cleanliness; Category II.

REFERENCES: AS NUMBERED IN ORIGINAL PUBLICATION

1. U.S. Department of Health and Human Services. Guidelines for construction and equipment of hospital and medical facilities. Washington, DC: Government Printing Office, July 1984:DHHS publication No. (HRS-M-HF) 84–1.
2. Joint Committee on Health Care Laundry Guidelines. Guidelines for health care linen service. Mallandale, FL: Textile Rental Services Association of America, 1983:TILSA publication no. 71482.
3. Hughes HG. Chutes in hospitals. J Can Hosp Assoc 1964;41:56–57.
4. Garner JS, Simmons BP. Guideline for isolation precautions in hospitals. Infect Control 1983; 4:245–325.
5. Waiter WG, Schillinger JE. Bacterial survival in laundered fabrics. Appl Microbiol 1975;29:368–373.
6. Christian RR, Manchester JT, Melior MT. Bacteriological quality of fabrics washed at lower-than-standard temperatures in a hospital laundry facility. Appl Env Microbiol 1983;45:591–597.
7. Blaser MJ, Smith PF, Cody HJ, Wang WL, LaForce FM. Killing of fabric-associated bacteria in hospital laundry by low temperature washing. J Infect Dis 1984;149:48–57.

Guideline for Prevention of Catheter-Associated Urinary Tract Infections

Original Citation: Centers for Disease Control and Prevention. Guideline for prevention of catheter-associated urinary tract infections, 1981.

Original Authors: Edward S. Wong, MD, in consultation with Thomas M. Hooton, MD.

INTRODUCTION

The urinary tract is the most common site of nosocomial infection, accounting for more than 40% of the total number reported by acute-care hospitals and affecting an estimated 600,000 patients per year (1).

Most of these infections—66% to 86%—follow instrumentation of the urinary tract, mainly urinary catheterization (2). Although not all catheter associated urinary tract infections can be prevented, it is believed that a large number could be avoided by the proper management of the indwelling catheter. The following recommendations were developed for the care of patients with temporary indwelling urethral catheters. Patients who require chronic indwelling catheters or individuals who can be managed with intermittent catheterization may have different needs. Determination of the optimal catheter care for these and other patients with different drainage systems requires separate evaluation.

EPIDEMIOLOGY

The risk of acquiring a urinary tract infection depends on the method and duration of catheterization, the quality of catheter care, and host susceptibility. Reported infection rates vary widely, ranging from 1%–5%, after a single brief catheterization (3) to virtually 100% for patients with indwelling urethral catheters draining into an open system for longer than 4 days (4). Adoption of the closed method of urinary drainage has markedly reduced the risk of acquiring a catheter-associated infection, but the risk is still substantial. As recent studies have shown, over 20% of patients catheterized and maintained on closed drainage on busy hospital wards may be expected to become infected (5, 6). In these studies, errors in maintaining sterile closed drainage were common and predisposed patients to infection. Host factors which appear to increase the risk of acquiring catheter-associated urinary tract infections include advanced age, debilitation, and the postpartum state (7, 8).

Catheter-associated urinary tract infections are generally assumed to be benign. Such infection in otherwise healthy patients is often asymptomatic and is likely to resolve spontaneously with the removal of the catheter. Occasionally, infection persists and leads to such complications as prostatitis, epididymitis, cystitis, pyelonephritis, and gram-negative bacteremia, particularly in high-risk patients (8). The last complication is serious since it is associated with a significant mortality, but fortunately occurs in fewer than 1% of catheterized patients (9, 10). The natural history of catheter associated urinary tract infections has been largely unstudied. Catheter-associated urinary tract infections are caused by a variety of pathogens, including Escherichia coli, Klebsiella, Proteus, enterococcus, Pseudomonas, Enterobacter, Serratia, and Candida. Many of these microorganisms are part of the patient's endogenous bowel flora, but they can also be acquired by cross-contamination from other patients or hospital personnel or by exposure to contaminated solutions or non-sterile equipment (11, 12). Urinary tract pathogens such as Serratia marcescens and Pseudomonas cepacia have special epidemiologic significance. Since these microorganisms do not commonly reside in the gastrointestinal tract, their isolation from catheterized patients suggests acquisition from an exogenous source (13, 14).

Whether from endogenous or exogenous sources, infecting microorganisms gain access to the urinary tract by several routes. Microorganisms that inhabit the meatus or distal urethra can be introduced directly into the bladder when the catheter is inserted. Generally, however, low rates of infection have been reported after single brief catheterization (4), suggesting that microorganisms introduced by this method are usually removed from healthy individuals by voiding or by antibacterial mechanisms of the bladder mucosa (15). With indwelling catheters, infecting microorganisms can migrate 10 the bladder along the outside of the catheter in the periurethral mucous sheath (16, 17) or along the internal lumen of the catheter after the collection bag or catheter-drainage tube junction has been contaminated (5, 6). The importance of intraluminal ascension is suggested by the substantial reduction in infections that has been achieved through the use of the closed urinary drainage system. However, if sterile closed drainage can be maintained, extraluminai migration of microorganisms in the periurethral space becomes a relatively more important pathway of entry into the bladder (17).

CONTROL MEASURES

An estimated 4 million patients are subjected yearly to urinary catheterization and, therefore, are at risk for catheter-associated infection and its related sequelae. One of the most important infection control measures is to limit the use of urinary catheters to carefully selected patients, thereby reducing the size of the population at risk. Generally, urinary catheterization is indicated (a) to relieve urinary tract obstruction, (b) to permit urinary drainage in patients with neurogenic bladder dysfunction and urinary retention, (c) to aid in urologic surgery or other surgery on contiguous structures, and (d) to obtain accurate measurements of urinary output in critically ill patients. Specifically, urinary catheterization should be discouraged as a means of obtaining urine for culture or certain diagnostic tests such as urinary electrolytes when the patient can voluntarily void or as a substitute for nursing care in the incontinent patient.

In selected populations, other methods of urinary drainage exist as possible alternatives to the use of the indwelling urethral catheter. Condom catheter drainage may be useful for incontinent male patients without outlet obstruction and with an intact voiding reflex. Its use, however, requires meticulous nursing care if local complications such as skin maceration or phimosis are to be avoided. In addition, frequent manipulation of the condom catheter drainage system (e.g., by agitated patients) has been associated with an increased risk of urinary tract infection (18). Another alternative, suprapubic catheter drainage, is most frequently used in patients on urologic or gynecologic services. Although preliminary data on the risk of infection are encouraging (19, 20), the benefit of the suprapubic catheter with regard to infection control has not been proven by controlled clinical studies. For certain types of patients with bladder-emptying dysfunction, such as those with spinal cord injuries or children with meningomyelocele, a third alternative, intermittent catheterization, is commonly employed. The "no-touch" method of intermittent catheterization advocated by Guttmann (21) is generally reserved for patients hospitalized during the acute phase of their spinal cord injury, while the clean, nonsterile method of Lapides (22) is frequently used by ambulatory patients for whom the practice of aseptic catheter insertion is difficult to maintain. As with suprapubic catheterization, however, well-designed clinical trials comparing the efficacy of intermittent catheterization by either method to indwelling catheterization in minimizing the risk of infection are lacking.

For patients who require indwelling urethral catheterization, adherence to the sterile continuously closed system of urinary drainage is the cornerstone of infection control. For short-term catheterization, this measure alone can reduce the rate of infection from an inevitable 100% when open drainage is employed to less than 25% (5). All other interventions can be viewed as adjunctive measures since none have proven to be as effective in reducing the frequency of catheter-associated urinary tract infections.

Efforts have been made to improve the design of the closed urinary drainage system by modifying or adding to the basic unit introduced and widely adopted in the 1960s. Two modifications, the addition of a urine sampling port in the drainage tubing and the preconnected catheter/collecting tube system seem to have been logical advances since they discourage or prevent opening the closed system which has been well-documented to predispose patients to infection (6). Other alterations have included the insertion of air vents, drip chambers, and one-way valves that were designed to prevent the reflux of contaminated urine. Although these modifications have some theoretical basis, none have been shown to be effective in reducing the frequency of catheter-associated infections. Additionally, overly complex drainage systems can affect the ease of operation or more easily real function (5). These latter factors can influence the acceptance of different systems by hospital personnel and ultimately affect infection control.

Other efforts to reduce the incidence of catheter associated infections have been directed toward (a) preventing microorganisms at the meatus from entering the bladder and (b) eradicating microorganisms that gain entry into the urinary tract before they can proliferate (23). Measures directed toward the first objective include aseptic catheter insertion. daily meatal cleansing, and daily application of antimicrobial ointments or solutions. On the basis of recent studies that have shown that catheterized patients colonized at the meatus with gram-negative bacilli or enterococci are at increased risk for subsequent infection (17, 24), these measures have some theoretical value and can be expected to delay or prevent the onset of infection. Generally, clinical trials that have attempted to demonstrate their efficacy have not been well designed or did not include the use of the closed system of urinary drainage. However, 2 recent prospective, controlled studies conducted by the same research group have shown that meatal care as it is currently commonly practiced (either twice-a-day cleansing with povidone-iodine solution followed by povidone iodine ointment or daily cleansing with soap and water) was ineffective in reducing the frequency of catheter-associated infections in patients on closed urinary drainage (25, 26). The value of different regimens (e.g., more frequent application, other concentrations, or other antimicrobial agents) is not known and requires further evaluation.

Infection control measures for purposes of eradicating microorganisms in the urinary tract before they can proliferate and cause infection include irrigation of the bladder and the use of prophylactic systemic antibiotics. In one controlled study, continuous irrigation of the bladder with nonabsorbable antibiotics was associated with frequent interruption of the closed drainage system and did not bring about a reduction in the frequency of catheter associated infections (27). It is not known, however, whether such irrigation would be effective if the integrity of the closed drainage system could be maintained. Several recent studies have shown that prophylactic systemic antibiotics delay the emergence of catheter-related infection (6, 28), but this protective effect was transient and was associated with the selection of antibiotic-resistant microorganisms. Thus, controversy regarding the value of prophylactic systemic antibiotics remains.

When cross-infection is likely to be responsible for the spread of catheter-associated infections, additional measures have been proposed (29). In several outbreaks of nosocomial urinary tract infections, catheterized patients with asymptomatic infections served as unrecognized reservoirs of infecting organisms, and the mechanism of transmission appeared to be carriage on the hands of patient-care personnel (13, 14). In these outbreaks, the implementation of control measures to prevent cross infection, including renewed emphasis on hand washing and spatial separation of catheterized patients, particularly infected from uninfected ones, effectively ended the outbreak. In the absence of epidemic spread or frequent cross-infection, spatial separation of catheterized patients is probably less effective in controlling catheter-associated infections.

Regular bacteriologic monitoring of catheterized patients has been advocated to ensure early diagnosis and treatment of urinary tract infections (8). Its possible value as an infection measure lies in its potential usefulness in detecting and initiating treatment of clinically inapparent infections, which may serve as reservoirs of hospital pathogens, and thus, reducing the likelihood of cross-infection. However, the potential benefit of bacteriologic monitoring for such a purpose has not been adequately investigated.

RECOMMENDATIONS

1. Personnel
   a. Only persons (e.g., hospital personnel, family members, or patients themselves) who know the correct technique of aseptic insertion and maintenance of the catheter should handle catheters (5, 6, 8); Category I.
   b. Hospital personnel and others who take care of catheters should be given periodic in service training stressing the correct techniques and potential complications of urinary catheterization; Category 11.
2. Catheter Use
   a. Urinary catheters should be inserted only when necessary and left in place only for as long as necessary. They should not be used solely for the convenience of patient-care personnel; Category I.
   b. For selected patients, other methods of urinary drainage such as condom catheter drainage, suprapubic catheterization. and intermittent urethral catheterization can be useful alternatives to indwelling urethral catheterization (8, 9, 21, 22); Category III.
3. Handwashing: Handwashing should be done immediately before and after any manipulation of the catheter site or apparatus (14, 30); Category I.

4. Catheter Insertion
   a. Catheters should be inserted using aseptic technique and sterile equipment (8, 16, 31); Category I.
   b. Gloves, drape, sponges, an appropriate antiseptic solution for periurethral cleaning, and a single-use packet of lubricant jelly should be used for insertion; Category II.
   c. As small a catheter as possible, consistent with good drainage, should be used to minimize urethral trauma (8); Category II.
   d. Indwelling catheters should be properly secured after insertion to prevent movement and urethral traction (31); Category I.
5. Closed Sterile Drainage
   a. A sterile, continuously closed drainage system should be maintained (5, 6, 27); Category I.
   b. The catheter and drainage tube should not be disconnected unless the catheter must be irrigated (see Irrigation Recommendation 6); Category I.
   c. If breaks in aseptic technique, disconnection, or leakage occur, the collecting system should be replaced using aseptic technique after disinfecting the catheter-tubing junction; Category III.
6. Irrigation
   a. Irrigation should be avoided unless obstruction is anticipated (e.g., as might occur with bleeding after prostatic or bladder surgery); closed continuous irrigation may be used to prevent obstruction. To relieve obstruction due to clots, mucus, or other causes, an intermittent method of irrigation may be used. Continuous irrigation of the bladder with antimicrobial has not proven to be useful (28) and should not be performed as a routine infection prevention measure; Category II.
   b. The catheter-tubing junction should be disinfected before disconnection; Category II.
   c. A large-volume sterile syringe and sterile irrigant should be used and then discarded. The person performing irrigation should use aseptic technique; Category I.
   d. If the catheter becomes obstructed and can be kept open only by frequent irrigation, the catheter should be changed if it is likely that the catheter itself is contributing to the obstruction (e.g., formation of concretions); Category II.
7. Specimen Collection
   a. If small volumes of fresh urine are needed for examination, the distal end of the catheter, or preferably the sampling port if present, should be cleansed with a disinfectant, and urine then aspirated with a sterile needle and syringe (5, 8); Category I.
   b. Larger volumes of urine for special analyses should be obtained aseptically from the drainage bag; Category. I.
8. Urinary Flow
   a. Unobstructed flow should be maintained (6, 8); Category I. (Occasionally, it is necessary to temporarily obstruct the catheter for specimen collection or other medical purposes.)
   b. To achieve free flow of urine (a) the catheter and collecting tube should be kept from kicking; (b) the collecting bag should be emptied regularly using a separate collecting container for each patient (the draining spigot and nonsterile collecting container should never come in contact) (33); (c) poorly functioning or obstructed catheters should be irrigated (see Irrigation Recommendation 6) or if necessary, replaced; and (d) collecting bags should always be kept below the level of the bladder; Category I.
9. Meatal Care: Twice daily cleansing with povidone-iodine solution and daily cleansing with soap and water have been shown in 2 recent studies not to reduce catheter-associated urinary tract infection (25, 26). Thus, at this time, daily meatal care with either of these 2 regimens cannot be endorsed; Category II.
10. Catheter Change Interval: Indwelling catheters should not be changed at arbitrary fixed intervals (34); Category II.
11. Spatial Separation of Catheterized Patients: To minimize the chances of cross-infection,

infected and uninfected patients with indwelling catheters should not share the same room or adjacent beds (29); Category III.

12. Bacteriologic Monitoring: The value of regular bacteriologic monitoring of catheterized patients as an infection control measure has not been established and is not recommended (35); Category III.

SUMMARY OF MAJOR RECOMMENDATIONS

Category I. Strongly Recommended for Adoption*

Educate personnel in correct techniques of catheter insertion and care.

Catheterize only when necessary.

Emphasize handwashing.

Insert catheter using aseptic technique and sterile equipment.

Secure catheter properly.

Maintain closed sterile drainage.

Obtain urine samples aseptically.

Maintain unobstructed urine flow.

Category II. Moderately Recommended for Adoption

Periodically re-educate personnel in catheter care.

Use smallest suitable bore catheter.

Avoid irrigation unless needed to prevent or relieve obstruction.

Refrain from daily meatal care with either of the regimens discussed in text.

Do not change catheters at arbitrary fixed intervals.

Category III. Weakly Recommended for Adoption

Consider alternative techniques of urinary drainage before using an indwelling urethral catheter.

Replace the collecting system when sterile closed drainage has been violated.

Spatially separate infected and uninfected patients with indwelling catheters.

Avoid routine bacteriologic monitoring.

REFERENCES: AS NUMBERED IN ORIGINAL PUBLICATION

1. Centers for Disease Control. National Nosocomial Infections Study Report. Atlanta: Centers for Disease Control, November 1979:2–14.
2. Martin CM, Bookrajian EN. Bacteriuria prevention after indwelling urinary catheterization. Arch Intern Med 1962;110:703–711.
3. Turck M, Goffe B. Petersdoff RG. The urethral catheters and urinary tract infection. J Urol 1962; 88:834–837.
4. Kass EH. Asymptomatic infections of the urinary tract. Trans Assoc Am Physicians 1956:69:56–63.
5. Kunin CM, McCormack RC. Prevention of catheter induced urinary tract infections bysterile closed drainage. N Engl J Med 1966;274:1155–1162.

---

*Refer to Introduction of manual for full explanation of the ranking scheme for recommendations.

 6. Garibaldi RA, Burke JP, Dickman ML, Smith CB. Factors predisposing to bacteriuria during indwelling urethral catheterization. N Engl J Med 1974;291:215–218.
 7. Bruinrite W, Davies BL, Rosser E. The urethral catheter as a cause of urinary tract infection in pregnancy and puerperium. Lancet 1961;2:1059–1061.
 8. Kunin CM. Detection, prevention, and management of urinary tract infections. 3rd ed. Philadelphia: Lea & Febiger, 1979.
 9. Seeere AC, Starnrn WE, Martin SM, Bennett JV. Gram-negative rod bacteremia. In: Bennett IV, Brachman PS, eds. Hospital infections. Boston: Little, Brown and Company, 1979:507–518.
10. Kreger BE, Craven DE, McCabe WR. Gram-negative bacterernia IV. Re-evaluation of clinical features and treatment in 612 patients. Am J Med 1980;68;344–355.
11. Selden R, Lee S, Wang WLL, et al Nosocomial KIebsieiia infections: intestinal colonization as a reservoir. Ann Intern Med 1971;74:2657–2664.
12. McLeod J. The hospital urine bottle and bedpan as reservoirs of infection by Pseudomonas. Lancet 1958:1:394–395.
13. Maki DG, Hennekens CH, Bennett JV, et al. Nosocomial urinary tract infection with Serratia marcesceus: an epidemiologic study. J Infect Dis 1973;128:579–587.
14. Kaslov RA, Lindsey JO, Bisno AL, Price A. Nosocomial infection with highly resistant Proleus rettgeri. Report of an epidemic. Am J Epidemiol 1976;104:278–286.
15. Norden CW, Green GM, Kass EH. Antibacterial mechanisms of the urinary bladder. J Clin Invest 1968;47:2689–2700.
16. Kass EH, Schneiderman LJ. Entry of bacteria into the urinary tract of patients with inlying catheters. N Engl J Med 1957;256:556–557.
17. Garibaldi RA, Burke JP, Britt MR, Miller WA, Smith CB. Meatal colonization and catheter-associated bacteriuria. N Engl J Med 1980;303;316–318.
18. Hirsh DD, Fainstein V, Musher DM. Do condom catheter collecting systems cause urinary tract infection? JAMA 1979;242:2340–2341.
19. Hodgkinson CP, Hodart AA. Trocar suprapubic cystostomy for postoperative bladder drainage in the female. J Obstet Gynecol 1966;96;773–783.
20. Marcus RT. Narrow-bore suprapubic bladder drainage in Uganda. Lancet 1967:1:748–750.
21. Guttman L, Frankel H. The value of intermittent catheterization in the early management of traumatic paraplegia and tetraplegia. Paraplegia 1966;4:63–83.
22. Lapides J, Diokno AC, Gould FR, Lowe BS. Further observations on self-catheterization. J Urol 1976;116:169–171.
23. Sanford JP. Hospital-acquired urinary tract infections. Ann Intern Med 1964;60:903–914.
24. Garibaldi RA, Britt MR, Miller WA, Steinmuller P, Burke JP. Evaluation of periurethral colonization as a risk factor for catheter-associated bacteriuria. In: Proceedings of the 16th Interscience Conference on Antimicrobial Agents and Chemotherapy, 1976:142.
25. Britt MR, Burke JP, Miller VA, Steinmiller P, Garibaldi RA. The non-effectiveness of daily meatal care in the prevention of catheter-associated bacteriuria. In: Proceedings of the 16th Interscience Conference on Antimicrobial Agents and Chemotherapy, 1976:141.
26. Burke JP, Garibaldi RA, Britt MR, Jacobson JA, Conti M, Alling DW. Prevention of catheter-associated urinary tract infections. Efficacy of daily meatal care regimens. In: Proceedings of the 2nd International Conference on Nosocomial Infections, Atlanta, August 4–8, 1980. Am J Med 1981:70:655–658.
27. Warren J, Platt R, Thomas KI, Rosner B, Kass EH. Antibiotic irrigation and catheter-associated urinary tract infections. N Engl J Med 1978;299:570–573.
28. Britt MR, Garibaldi RA, Miller WA, Hebertson RM, Burke JP. Antimicrobial prophylaxis for catheter-associated bacteriuria. Antimicrob Agents Chemother 1977;11:240–243.
29. Maki DG, Hennekens CH, Bennett JV. Prevention of catheter-associated urinary tract infection: an additional measure. JAMA 1972;221:1270–1271.
30. Steere AC, Mallison GF. Handwashing practices for the prevention of nosocomial infections. Ann Intern Med 1975;83:683–690.
31. Desautels RF, Walter CW, Graves RC, et al. Technical advances in the prevention of urinary tract infection. J Urol 1962;87:487–490.
32. Viant AC, Linton KB, Gillespie WA. Improved method for preventing movement of indwelling catheters in female patients. Lancet 1971;1:736–737.
33. Marfie TJ, Major H, Gurwith M, et al. Prolonged outbreak of nosocomial urinary tractinfection with a single strain of Pseudomonas aeruginosa. Can Med J 1978;119:593–596.
34. Stature WE. Guidelines for the prevention of catheter associated urinary tract infections. Ann Intern Med 1975;82;386–390.
35. Mooney BS, Garibaldi RA, Britt MR. Natural history of catheter-associated bacteriuria (colonization, infection, bacteremia): implication for protection. In: Proceedings of the 11th International Congress of Chemotherapy and the 19th Interscience Conference on Antimicrobial Agents and Chemotherapy, Boston, October 8–12, 1979. Washington, DC: American Society of Microbiology, 1980:1083–1085.

Guideline for Prevention of Nosocomial Pneumonia

Original Citation: Centers for Disease Control and Prevention. Guideline for prevention of nosocomial pneumonia: Part 1. Issues on prevention of nosocomial pneumonia, 1994. Respir Care 1994;39(12):1191–1236.

Original Authors: Ofelia C. Tablan, MD, Larry J. Anderson, MD, Nancy H. Arden, MN, Robert F. Breiman, MD, Jay C. Butler, MD, Michael M. McNeil, MD, and the Hospital Infection Control Practices Advisory Committee.

INTRODUCTION

This 2-part document updates and replaces the previously published Centers for Disease Control and Prevention Guideline for Prevention of Nosocomial Pneumonia (Infection Control 1982;3:327–333, Respir Care 1983;28:221–232, and Am J Infect Control 1983;11:230–244). The revised guideline is designed to reduce the incidence of nosocomial pneumonia and intended for use by personnel who are responsible for surveillance and control of infections in acute-care hospitals. The guideline may not be applicable in long-term care facilities because of the unique characteristics of these settings.

The revised guideline addresses common problems encountered by infection control practitioners regarding the prevention and control of nosocomial pneumonia in U.S. hospitals. Sections on the prevention of bacterial pneumonia in mechanically ventilated and/or critically ill patients, care of respiratory-therapy devices, prevention of cross-contamination, and prevention of viral lower respiratory tract infections, such as respiratory syncytial virus (RSV) and influenza infections, have been expanded and updated. New sections on Legionnaires' disease and pneumonia due to Aspergillus spp. have been added. Lower respiratory tract infection due to Mycobacterium tuberculosis is not addressed in this document; it is covered in separate guidelines (1).

A working draft of the guideline has been reviewed by experts in infection control, pulmonology, respiratory therapy, anesthesiology, internal medicine, and pediatrics. However, all recommendations in the guideline may not reflect the opinions of all reviewers.

Part I, "Issues on Prevention of Nosocomial Pneumonia—1994," provides the background for the consensus recommendations of the Hospital Infection Control Practices Advisory Committee (HICPAC) in Part II, "Recommendations for Prevention of Nosocomial Pneumonia." HICPAC was established in 1991 to provide advice and guidance to the Secretary and Assistant Secretary for Health, Department of Health and Human Services; the Director, CDC; and the Director, NCID, CDC, regarding the practice of hospital infection control and strategies for surveillance, prevention, and control of nosocomial infections in U.S. hospitals. The committee also advises the CDC on periodic updating of guidelines and other policy statements regarding prevention of nosocomial infections. The Guideline for Prevention of Nosocomial Pneumonia is the first of a series of CDC guidelines being revised by HICPAC and NCID, CDC.

Part I can be an important resource for educating health-care workers regarding prevention and control of nosocomial respiratory tract infections. Because education of health-care workers is the cornerstone of an effective infection control program, hospitals should give high priority to continuing infection control educational programs for these staff members.

Summary

Pneumonia is the second most common nosocomial infection in the United States and is associated with substantial morbidity and mortality. Most patients with nosocomial pneumonia are those with extremes of age, severe underlying disease, immunosuppression, depressed sensorium, and cardiopulmonary disease, and those who have had thoraco-abdominal surgery. Although patients with mechanically assisted ventilation do not comprise a major proportion of patients with nosocomial pneumonia, they have the highest risk of developing the infection.

Most bacterial nosocomial pneumonias occur by aspiration of bacteria colonizing the oropharynx or upper gastrointestinal tract of the patient. Intubation and mechanical ventilation greatly increase the risk of nosocomial bacterial pneumonia because they alter first-line patient defenses. Pneumonias due to Legionella spp., Aspergillus spp., and influenza virus are often caused by inhalation of contaminated aerosols. Respiratory syncytial virus (RSV) infection usually follows viral inoculation of the conjunctivae or nasal mucosa by contaminated hands.

Traditional preventive measures for nosocomial pneumonia include decreasing aspiration by the patient, preventing cross-contamination or colonization via hands of personnel, appropriate disinfection or sterilization of respiratory-therapy devices, use of available vaccines to protect against particular infections, and education of hospital staff and patients. New measures under investigation involve reducing oropharyngeal and gastric colonization by pathogenic microorganisms.

BACTERIAL PNEUMONIA

ETIOLOGIC AGENTS

The reported distribution of etiologic agents causing nosocomial pneumonia varies between hospitals because of differences in patient populations and diagnostic methods employed (2–10). In general, however, bacteria have been the most frequently isolated pathogens (2–6, 9, 11–13). Schaberg et al reported that in 1986–1989, aerobic bacteria comprised at least 73%, and fungi 4%, of isolates from sputum and tracheal aspirates from pneumonia patients at the University of Michigan Hospitals and hospitals participating in the National Nosocomial Infection Surveillance System (NNIS); very few anaerobic bacteria and no viruses were reported, probably because anaerobic and viral cultures were not performed routinely in the reporting hospitals (Table 1) (3). Similarly, cultures of bronchoscopic specimens from mechanically ventilated patients with pneumonia have rarely yielded anaerobes (5–7, 9, 11, 14, 15). Only the report by Bartlett, which was based mainly on cultures of transtracheal aspirates from patients not receiving mechanically assisted ventilation, showed a predominance of anaerobes (4).

Table 1. Microorganisms isolated from respiratory tract specimens obtained by various representative methods from adult patients with a diagnosis of nosocomial pneumonia

	Schaberg (3)	Bartlett (4)	Fagon (5)	Torres (6)
Hospital Type	NNIS & UMH*	Veterans	General	General
Patients Studied:				
Ventilated or nonventilated	Mixed	Mixed	Ventilated	Ventilated
Number	N/A[†]	159	49	78
Number of Episodes of Pneumonia	N/A	159	52	78
Specimen(s) Cultured	Sputum, tracheal aspirate	Transtracheal aspirate, pleural fluid, blood	Protected specimen brushing	Protected specimen brushing, lung aspirate, pleural fluid, blood
Culture Results:				
No organism isolated	N/A	0	0	54%[‡]
Polymicrobial	N/A	54%[‡]	40%[‡]	13%[‡]
Number of isolates	15,499	314	111	N/A
Aerobic Bacteria				
Gram-Negative Bacilli	50%**	46%[††]	75%[††]	16%[‡‡]
Pseudomonas aeruginosa	17%**	9%[††]	31%[††]	5%[‡‡]
Enterobacter sp.	11	4	2	0
Klebsiella sp.	7	23	4	0
Escherichia coli	6	14	8	0
Serratia sp.	5	0	0	1
Proteus sp.	3	11	15	1
Citrobacter sp.	1	0	2	0
Acinetobacter calcoaceticus	N/A	0	12	9
Others	N/A	0	10	0
Haemophilus influenzae	6%**	17%[††]	10%[††]	0%[‡‡]
Legionella sp.	N/A	N/A	2%[††]	2%[‡‡]
Gram-Positive Cocci	17%**	56%[††]	52%[††]	4%[‡‡]
Staphylococcus aureus	16%**	25%[††]	33%[††]	2%[‡‡]
Streptococcus sp.	1	31	21	2
Others	0	0	8	0
Anaerobes	N/A	35%[††]	2%[††]	0
Peptostreptococcus	N/A	14%[††]	N/A	0
Fusobacterium sp.	N/A	10	N/A	0
Peptococcus sp.	N/A	11	N/A	0
Bacteroides melaninogenicus	N/A	9	N/A	0
Bacteroides fragilis	N/A	8	N/A	0
Fungi	4%**	N/A	0	1%[‡‡]
Aspergillus sp.	N/A	N/A	0	1%[‡‡]
Candida sp.	4%**	N/A	0	0
Viruses	N/A	N/A	N/A	N/A

*NNIS & UMH = National Nosocomial Infections Surveillance System and University of Michigan Hospitals.

[†]N/A = Not applicable: not tested or not reported.

[‡]Percent episodes.

**Percent isolates.

[††]Percent episodes (percentages not additive due to polymicrobial etiology in some episodes).

[‡‡]Percent patients with pure culture.

References appear at the end of the document.

Nosocomial bacterial pneumonias are frequently polymicrobial (4, 7, 9, 11, 12, 15–19), and gram-negative bacilli are the usual predominant organisms (Table 1) (2–6, 9, 11–13). However, Staphylococcus aureus (especially methicillin-resistant S. aureus) (5, 7, 10, 15, 20, 21) and other gram-positive cocci, including Streptococcus pneumoniae (5, 7), have recently emerged as significant isolates (14). In addition, Haemophilus influenza has been isolated from mechanically ventilated patients with pneumonia that occurs within 48–96 hours after intubation (3–5, 12, 15, 22). In NNIS hospitals, Pseudomonas aeruginosa, Enterobacter sp., Klebsiella pneumoniae, Escherichia coli, Serratia marcescens, and Proteus spp. comprised 50% of the isolates from cultures of respiratory tract specimens from patients for whom nosocomial pneumonia was diagnosed by using clinical criteria; S. aureus accounted for 16%, and H. influenzae, for 6% (Table 1) (3). Fagon and co-workers reported that gram-negative bacilli were present in 75% of quantitative cultures of protected-specimen brushings (PSB) from patients who had received mechanically assisted ventilation and acquired nosocomial pneumonia; 40% of the cultures were polymicrobial (5). In the report by Torres, et al., 20% of pathogens recovered from cultures of PSB, blood, pleural fluid, or percutaneous lung aspirate were gram-negative bacilli in pure culture, and 17% were polymicrobial; however, 54% of specimens did not yield any microorganism, probably because of receipt of antibiotics by patients (6).

DIAGNOSIS

Nosocomial bacterial pneumonia has been difficult to diagnose (7, 8, 16, 23–32). Frequently, the criteria for diagnosis have been fever, cough, and development of purulent sputum, in combination with radiologic evidence of a new or progressive pulmonary infiltrate, a suggestive Gram's stain, and cultures of sputum, tracheal aspirate, pleural fluid, or blood (3, 4, 23, 25, 33–36). Although clinical criteria together with cultures of sputum or tracheal specimens may be sensitive for bacterial pathogens, they are highly nonspecific, especially in patients with mechanically assisted ventilation (8, 9, 12–15, 18, 24–26, 29, 31, 37–42); on the other hand, cultures of blood or pleural fluid have very low sensitivity (8, 18, 19, 43).

Because of these problems, a group of investigators recently formulated consensus recommendations for standardization of methods to diagnose pneumonia in clinical research studies of ventilator-associated pneumonia (44–46). These methods involve bronchoscopic techniques, e.g., quantitative culture of PSB (5, 7–9, 13, 15, 27, 31, 38, 41, 47, 48), bronchoalveolar lavage (BAL) (7, 12, 41, 47, 49–54), and protected BAL (pBAL) (14). The reported sensitivities and specificities of these methods have ranged between 70% to 100% and 60% to 100%, respectively, depending on the tests or diagnostic criteria they were compared with. Because these techniques are invasive, they may cause complications such as hypoxemia, bleeding, or arrhythmia (8, 13, 42, 44, 52, 55, 56). In addition, the sensitivity of the PSB procedure may decrease for patients receiving antibiotic therapy (9, 13, 27). Nonbronchoscopic (NB) procedures, e.g., NB-pBAL(12, 27, 57, 58) or NB-PSB (13), which utilize blind catheterization of the distal airways, and quantitative culture of endotracheal aspirate (59, 60), have been developed recently. Of these, endotracheal aspirate culture appears to be the most practical. The use of these bronchoscopic and nonbronchoscopic diagnostic tests can be a major step in better defining the epidemiology of nosocomial pneumonia, especially in patients with mechanically assisted ventilation; however, further studies are needed to determine each test's applicability in daily clinical practice.

EPIDEMIOLOGY

NNIS reports that pneumonias (diagnosed on the basis of the CDC surveillance definition of nosocomial pneumonia) account for approximately 15% of all hospital-associated infections and are the second most common nosocomial infections after those of the urinary tract (2, 61). In 1984, the overall incidence of lower respiratory tract infection was 6 per 1,000 discharged patients (2). The incidence per 1,000 discharged patients ranged from 4.2 in nonteaching to 7.7 in university-affiliated hospitals, probably reflecting institutional differences in the level of patients' risk for acquiring nosocomial pneumonia.

Nosocomial bacterial pneumonia often has been identified as a postoperative infection (62, 63). In the Study of the Efficacy of Nosocomial Infection Control in the 1970s, 75% of reported cases of nosocomial bacterial pneumonia occurred in patients who had had a surgical operation; the risk was 38 times greater for thoracoabdominal procedures than for those involving other body sites (63). More recent epidemiologic studies, including NNIS studies, have identified other subsets of patients at high risk of developing nosocomial bacterial pneumonia: patients with endotracheal intubation and/or mechanically assisted ventilation, depressed level of consciousness (particularly those with closed-head injury), prior episode of a large-volume aspiration, or underlying chronic lung disease, and patients >70 years of age. Other risk factors include 24-hour ventilator-circuit changes, fall-winter season, stress-bleeding prophylaxis with cimetidine with or without antacid, administration of antimicrobials, presence of a nasogastric tube, severe trauma, and recent bronchoscopy (6, 34, 35, 64–74).

Recently, NNIS stratified the incidence density of nosocomial pneumonia by patients' use of mechanical ventilator and type of intensive care unit (ICU). From 1986 to 1990, the median rate of ventilator-associated pneumonia per 1,000 ventilator-days ranged from 4.7 in pediatric ICUs to 34.4 in burn ICUs (66). In contrast, the median rate of nonventilator-associated pneumonia per 1,000 ICU-days ranged from 0 in pediatric and respiratory ICUs to 3.2 in trauma ICUs.

Nosocomial pneumonia has been associated with high fatality rates. Crude mortality rates of 20%–50% and attributable mortality rates of 30%–33% have been reported; in one study, pneumonia comprised 60% of all deaths due to nosocomial infections (17, 35, 74–80). Patients receiving mechanically assisted ventilation have higher mortality rates than do patients not receiving ventilation support; however, other factors, such as a patient's underlying disease(s) and organ failure, are stronger predictors of death in patients with pneumonia (34, 74).

Analyses of pneumonia-associated morbidity have shown that pneumonia could prolong hospitalization by 4–9 days (79–83). A conservative estimate of the direct cost of excess hospital stay due to pneumonia is $1.2 billion a year for the nation (83). Because of its reported frequency, associated high fatality rate, and attendant costs, nosocomial pneumonia is a major infection control problem.

PATHOGENESIS

Bacteria may invade the lower respiratory tract by aspiration of oropharyngeal organisms, inhalation of aerosols containing bacteria, or, less frequently, by hematogenous spread from a distant body site (Figure 1). In addition, bacterial translocation from the gastrointestinal tract has been recently hypothesized as a mechanism for infection. Of these routes, aspiration is believed to be the most important for both nosocomial and community-acquired pneumonia.

In radioisotope-tracer studies, 45% of healthy adults were found to aspirate during sleep (84). Persons with abnormal swallowing, such as those who have depressed consciousness, respiratory tract instrumentation and/or mechanically assisted ventilation, or gastrointestinal tract instrumentation or diseases, or who have just undergone surgery, are particularly likely to aspirate (6, 34, 35, 63, 85–87).

The high incidence of gram-negative bacillary pneumonia in hospitalized patients appears to be the result of factors that promote colonization of the pharynx by gram-negative bacilli and the subsequent entry of these organisms into the lower respiratory tract (33, 88–91). Whereas aerobic gram-negative bacilli are recovered infrequently or are found in small numbers in pharyngeal cultures of healthy persons (88, 92), colonization dramatically increases in patients with coma, hypotension, acidosis, azotemia, alcoholism, diabetes mellitus, leukocytosis, leukopenia, pulmonary disease, or nasogastric or endotracheal tubes in place, and in patients given antimicrobial agents (33, 91, 93, 94).

Oropharyngeal or tracheobronchial colonization by gram-negative bacilli begins with the adherence of the microorganisms to the host's epithelial cells (90, 95–97). Adherence may be affected by multiple factors related to the bacteria (presence of pili, cilia, capsule, or production of elastase or mucinase), host cell (surface proteins and polysaccharides), and environment (pH and presence of mucin in respiratory secretions) (89, 90, 95, 98–107). The exact interactions among these factors have not been fully elucidated, but studies indicate that certain substances, such as fibronectin, can inhibit the adherence of gram-negative bacilli to host cells (98, 100, 108). Conversely, certain conditions, such as malnutrition, severe illness, or post-operative state, can increase adherence of gram-negative bacteria (89, 98, 102, 107, 109).

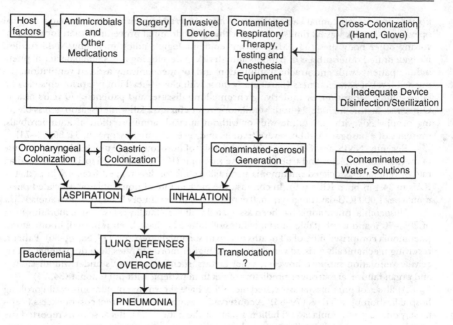

Figure 1. Pathogenesis of nosocomial bacterial pneumonia.

Besides the oropharynx, the stomach has been postulated to be an important reservoir of organisms that cause nosocomial pneumonia (34, 110–114). The stomach's role may vary depending on the patient's underlying conditions and on prophylactic or therapeutic interventions (22, 111, 115–118). In healthy persons, few bacteria entering the stomach survive in the presence of hydrochloric acid at pH <2 (119, 120). However, when gastric pH increases from the normal levels to >4, microorganisms are able to multiply to high concentrations in the stomach (117, 119, 121–123). This can occur in patients with advanced age (121), achlorhydria (119), ileus, or upper gastrointestinal disease, and in patients receiving enteral feeding, antacids, or histamine-2 [H-2] antagonists (111, 117, 118, 123–125). The contribution of other factors, such as duodeno-gastric reflux and the presence of bile, to gastric colonization in patients with impaired intestinal motility has been suggested and needs further investigation (116).

Bacteria can also gain entry into the lower respiratory tract of hospitalized patients through inhalation of aerosols generated primarily by contaminated respiratory-therapy or anesthesia-breathing equipment (126–129). Outbreaks related to the use of respiratory-therapy equipment have been associated with contaminated nebulizers, which are humidification devices that produce large amounts of aerosol droplets <4 μm via ultrasound, spinning disk, or the Venturi mechanism (126, 129, 130). When the fluid in the reservoir of a nebulizer becomes contaminated with bacteria, the aerosol produced may contain high concentrations of bacteria that can be deposited deep in the patient's lower respiratory tract (126, 130, 131). Because endotracheal and tracheal tubes provide direct access to the lower respiratory tract, contaminated aerosol inhalation is particularly hazardous for intubated patients. In contrast to nebulizers, bubble-through or wick humidifiers mainly increase the water-vapor (or molecular-water) content of inspired gases. Although heated bubble-through humidifiers generate aerosol droplets, they do so in quantities that may not be clinically significant (127, 132); wick humidifiers do not generate aerosols.

Rarely, bacterial pneumonia can result from hematogenous spread of infection to the lung from another infection site, e.g., pneumonia resulting from purulent phlebitis or right-sided endocarditis. Another mechanism, translocation of bacteria via the passage of viable bacteria from the lumen of the gastrointestinal tract through epithelial mucosa to the mesenteric lymph nodes and to the lung, has been shown in animal models (133). Translocation is postulated to occur in patients with immunosuppression, cancer, or burns (133); however data are lacking regarding this mechanism in humans (134).

RISK FACTORS AND CONTROL MEASURES

Several large studies have examined potential risk factors for nosocomial bacterial pneumonia (Table 2) (6, 34, 35, 135, 136). Although specific risk factors may differ between study populations, they can be grouped into the following general categories: (a) host factors such as extremes of age and severe underlying conditions, including immunosuppression; (b) factors, such as administration of antimicrobials, admission to the ICU, underlying chronic lung disease, or coma, that enhance colonization of the oropharynx and/or stomach by microorganisms; (c) conditions favoring aspiration or reflux, including endotracheal intubation, insertion of nasogastric tube, or supine position; (d) conditions requiring prolonged use of mechanical ventilatory support with potential exposure to contaminated respiratory equipment and/or contact with contaminated or colonized hands of health-care workers; and (e) factors that impede adequate pulmonary toilet, such as surgical procedures involving the head, neck, thorax, or upper abdomen, and immobilization due to trauma or illness (6, 33–35, 62, 73, 74, 135).

Table 2. Risk factors and suggested infection control measures for prevention of nosocomial pneumonia

Risk Factors	Infection Control Measures Suggested to Prevent Nosocomial Pneumonia
Bacterial Pneumonia	
Host-related; age >65 years	
Underlying illness:	
Chronic obstructive pulmonary disease (COPD)	Perform incentive spirometry; positive end expiratory pressure or continuous positive airway pressure by face mask.
Immunosuppression	Avoid exposure to potential nosocomial pathogens; decrease duration of immunosuppression, such as by administration of granulocyte macrophage colony stimulating factor (GMCSF).
Depressed consciousness	Administer central nervous system depressants cautiously.
Surgery (thoracic/abdominal)	Properly position patients; promote early ambulation; appropriately control pain.
Device-related	Properly clean, sterilize or disinfect, and handle devices; remove devices as soon as the indication for their use ceases.
Endotracheal intubation and mechanical ventilation	Gently suction secretions; place patient in semirecumbent position, i.e., 30° to 45° head-elevation; use nonalkalinizing gastric cytoprotective agent on patients at risk for stress bleeding; do not routinely change ventilator circuits more often than every 48 hours; drain and discard inspiratory-tubing condensate, or use heat-moisture exchanger if indicated.
Nasogastric tube (NGT) placement and enteral feeding	Routinely verify appropriate tube placement; promptly remove NGT when no longer needed. Drain residual; place patient in semirecumbent position as described above.
Personnel- or procedure-related	
Cross-contamination by hands	Educate and train personnel; wash hands adequately and wear gloves appropriately; conduct surveillance for cases of pneumonia, and give feedback to personnel.
Antibiotic administration	Use antibiotics prudently, especially on high-risk intensive-care unit (ICU) patients.

Table 2.—*continued*

Risk Factors	Infection Control Measures Suggested to Prevent Nosocomial Pneumonia
Legionnaires' Disease	
Host-related	
Immunosuppression	Decrease duration of immunosuppression.
Device-related	
Contaminated aerosol from devices	Sterilize/disinfect aerosol-producing devices before use; use only sterile water for respiratory humidifying devices; do not use cool-mist room-air "humidifiers" without adequate sterilization or disinfection.
Environment-related	
Aerosols from contaminated water supply	Hyperchlorinate or superheat hospital water system; routinely maintain water-supply system; consider use of sterile water for drinking by immunosuppressed patients.
Cooling-tower draft	Properly design, place, and maintain cooling towers.
Aspergillosis	
Host-related	
Severe granulocytopenia	Decrease duration of immunosuppression, such as by administration of GMCSF; place patients with severe and prolonged granulocytopenia in protected environment.
Environment-related	
Construction activity	Remove granulocytopenic patients from vicinity of construction; if not already done, place severely granulocytopenic patients in protected environment; make severely granulocytopenic patients wear a mask when they leave their protected environment.
Other environmental sources of aspergilli	Routinely maintain hospital air-handling system and rooms of immunosuppressed patients.
Respiratory Syncytial Virus Infection	
Host-related	
Age (<2 Years; congenital pulmonary/cardiac disease, immunosuppression	Consider routine preadmission screening of patients at high-risk for severe RSV infection, followed by cohorting of patients and nursing personnel during hospital outbreaks of RSV infection.
Personnel- or procedure-related	
Cross-contamination by hands	Educate personnel; wash hands; wear gloves; wear a gown; during outbreaks, use private rooms or cohort patients and nursing personnel, and limit visitors.
	Place infected patients in private rooms or cohort them.
Influenza	
Host-related	
Age >65 years; immunosuppression	Vaccinate high-risk patients before the influenza season each year; use amantadine or rimantadine for chemoprophylaxis during an outbreak
Personnel-related	
Infected personnel	Before the influenza season each year, vaccinate personnel caring for high-risk patients; use amantadine or rimantadine for prophylaxis during an outbreak.

Oropharyngeal, Tracheal, and Gastric Colonization

The association between colonization of the oropharynx (88, 137), trachea (138), or stomach (110, 111, 117, 123) and predisposition to gram-negative bacillary pneumonia prompted attempts to prevent infection either by prophylactic local application of antimicrobial agent(s) (139, 140) or by utilizing the phenomenon of local bacterial interference (141, 142). Although early work suggested that the former method, use of aerosolized antimicrobials, could eradicate common gram-negative pathogens from the upper respiratory tract (138), superinfection occurred in some patients receiving this therapy (139–141, 143, 144). The latter method, bacterial interference (with alpha-hemolytic streptococci), has been successfully used by some investigators to prevent oropharyngeal colonization by aerobic gram-negative bacilli (141). However, the efficacy of this method for use in general has not been evaluated.

The administration of antacids and H-2 blockers for prevention of stress bleeding in critically ill, postoperative, and/or mechanically ventilated patients has been associated with gastric bacterial overgrowth in many studies (34, 112, 113, 118, 122, 123, 145–147). Sucralfate, a cytoprotective agent that has little effect on gastric pH and may have bactericidal properties of its own, has been suggested as a potential substitute for antacids and H-2 blockers (148–150). The results of clinical trials comparing the risk of pneumonia in patients receiving sucralfate to that in patients given antacids and/or H-2 blockers have been variable (112, 118, 147, 148, 151–153). In most randomized trials, ICU patients receiving mechanically assisted ventilation and antacids with or without H-2 blockers had increased gastric pH, high bacterial counts in the gastric fluid, and increased risk of pneumonia compared with patients given sucralfate (112, 118, 147, 148, 151). In one report with a large number of study patients, the incidence of early-onset pneumonia (occurring <4 days after intubation) did not differ between patient groups, but late-onset pneumonia occurred in 5% of 76 patients who received sucralfate, 16% of 69 given antacids, and 21% of 68 who received an H-2 blocker (147). On the other hand, a meta-analysis of data from eight earlier studies (154) and a later study comparing sucralfate with ranitidine (153) did not show a strong association between nosocomial pneumonia and drugs that raise gastric pH. Further comparative studies are underway in which bronchoscopy with PSB or BAL is utilized for the diagnosis of pneumonia.

Selective decontamination of the digestive tract (SDD) is another strategy designed to prevent bacterial colonization and lower respiratory tract infection in mechanically ventilated patients (155–179). SDD is aimed at preventing oropharyngeal and gastric colonization with aerobic gram-negative bacilli and Candida spp., without altering the anaerobic flora (Table 3). A variety of SDD regimens use a combination of locally administered nonabsorbable antibiotic agents such as polymyxin and an aminoglycoside (tobramycin, gentamicin, or, rarely, neomycin), or a quinolone (norfloxacin or ciprofloxacin), coupled with either amphotericin B or nystatin. The local antimicrobial preparation is applied as a paste to the oropharynx and given orally or via the nasogastric tube four times a day. In addition, in many studies, a systemic (intravenous) antimicrobial such as cefotaxime or trimethoprim is administered to the patient.

While most clinical trials (155–158, 160–167, 169, 170, 175–177), including two meta-analyses (171, 178), of SDD have demonstrated a decrease in the rates of nosocomial respiratory infections, these trials have been difficult to assess because they have differed in study design and population, and many have had short follow-up periods (Table 3). In most of these studies, the diagnosis of pneumonia was based on clinical criteria; bronchoscopy with BAL or PSB was used in only a few studies (159, 162, 173, 175–177, 179).

Two recently published large double-blind, placebo-controlled trials demonstrated no benefit from SDD (173, 174). In one, a large French multicenter study by Gastinne et al, a significant decrease in incidence of gram-negative bacillary pneumonia was not accompanied by a decrease in pneumonia from all causes (173). In the other study, by Hammond, et al., no differences were noted between patients randomized to SDD or to placebo; however, both patient groups received intravenous cefotaxime (174).

Although an earlier meta-analysis suggested a trend toward decreased mortality in patients given SDD (171), a more recent and more extensive analysis highlights the equivocal effect of SDD on patient mortality, as well as the high cost of using SDD to prevent pneumonia

Table 3. Controlled studies on nosocomial lower respiratory tract infections and other associated outcomes of selective decontamination of the digestive tract in adult patients with mechanically assisted ventilation

Author	Study Patients	Lower Respiratory Tract Infection			Colonization or Infection with Resistant Microorganisms[B]		Overall Mortality In Hospital		Mean Total Number of Days in ICU[C]	
		Diagnostic Method	Infection Rate							
			SDD[D] (%)	Controls (%)	SDD[D] (%)	Controls (%)	SDD[D] (%)	Controls (%)	SDD[D]	Controls
Stoutenbeek (155) (1984)	Trauma; SDD = 63; controls = 59	Clinical & radiologic;[E] TS culture[F]	8	59	"No increase"		3	8	Not reported	
Unertl (156) (1987)	General ICU; SDD = 19; controls = 20	Clinical & radiologic[E]	21	70	21[G]	20[G]	26	30	18[H]	23[H]
Kerver (157) (1988)	Surgical ICU; SDD = 49; controls = 47	Clinical & radiologic[E]	12	85	"Not recorded"		29; IR[I] = 4	32; IR[I] = 17	17	20
Ledingham (158) (1988)	General ICU; SDD = 163; controls = 161	Clinical & radiologic[E]	2	11	"No increase"		24	24	Not reported	
Brun-Buisson (159) (1989)	Medical ICU; SDD = 36; controls = 50	Clinical & radiologic,[E] TS & PSB culture[F]	20	22	3[G]	16[G]	22; IR[I] = 9	24; IR[I] = 10	14	15
Ulrich (160) (1989)	General ICU; SDD = 48; controls = 52	Clinical & radiologic;[E] TS culture[F]	15	50	GP = 78[I] GN = 3[I]	GP = 44[I] GN = 2[I]	31; IR[I] = 0	54; IR[I] = 15	15	17
Flaherty (161) (1990)	Cardiac surgery ICU; SDD = 51; controls = 56	Clinical & radiologic[E]	2	9	GN = 22[G]	GN = 21[G]	0	2	Not reported	
Godard (162) (1990)	General ICU; SDD = 97; controls = 84	Clinical & radiologic,[E] TS & PSB culture[F]	2	15	GN = 15[I]	GN = 15[I]	12	18	11	16
McClelland (163) (1990)	Renal & respiratory failure; SDD = 15; controls = 12	TS culture[F]	7	50	Not reported		60; IR[I] = 27	58; IR[I] = 8	Not reported	
Rodriquez-Roldan (164) (1990)	General ICU: SDD = 13; controls = 15	Clinical & radiologic;[E] TS culture[F]	Pn = 0[K] TB = 23[K]	Pn = 73[K] TB = 20[K]	"None noticed"		30; IR[I] = 0	33; IR[I] = 13	Not reported	

Source (Year)	Patients	Diagnosis	Infection, SDD	Infection, Control	Resistance, SDD	Resistance, Control	Mortality¹, SDD	Mortality¹, Control	Mortality², SDD	Mortality², Control
Tetteroo (165) (1990)	Esophageal resection; SDD = 56; controls = 56	Clinical & radiologic[3] culture of bronchial aspirate	2	14	2[G]	4[G]	5; IR[I] = 4	IR[I] = 0	6	5
Aerdts (166) (1991)	General ICU; SDD = 17; controls-A = 18[L]; controls-B = 21[L]	Clinical & radiologic[3] TS culture[F]	6	A = 78; B = 62	"Not Observed"		12; IR[I] = 6	A = 22; IR[I] = 11; B = 10; IR[I] = 0	19; 23	A = 30; B = 25
Blair (167) (1991)	General ICU; SDD = 126; controls = 130	Clinical & radiologic[E]	10	35	"No evidence of increased resistance"		14	19	8	8
Fox (168) (1991)	Cardiac bypass; SDD = 12; controls = 12	TS culture[F]	66	50	Not reported		17	66	12	12
Hartenauer (169) (1991)	Surgical ICU ICU-1; SDD = 50; controls = 61	Clinical & radiologic[E] TS culture[F]	10	46	S = 34[G]; GN = 0[G]	S = 37[G]; GN = 0[G]	38 IR[I] = 8	35; IR[I] = 21	12	13
	ICU-2; SDD = 49; controls = 40		10	45	S = 33[G]; GN = 0[G]	S = 37[G]; GN = 0[G]	31; IR[I] = 6	43; IR[I] = 25	13	17
Pugin (170) (1991)	Surgical ICU; SDD = 25; controls = 27	Clinical & radiologic[E] TS culture[F]	16	78	"No new antibiotic resistance"		28	26	13	15
Vandenbroucke-Grauls (171) (1991)	ICUs (pooled data),[M] SDD-A = 488; controls-A (historical) = 540; SDD-B = 225; controls-B (random) = 266	Clinical & radiologic[E] TS culture[F]	A = 7; B = 8	A = 28; B = 45	"No increase in resistant microorganisms in 10 of 11 studies"		A = 25; B = 21	A = 26; B = 26	Not reported	
Cockerill (172) (1992)	Surgical and medical ICUs; SDD = 75; controls = 75	Clinical & radiologic[E] TS culture[F]	Pn = 5[K]; TB = 4[K]	Pn = 16[K]; TB = 5[K]	16[J]	11[J]	15	21	10	12
Gastinne (173) (1992)	Medical ICU; SDD = 220; controls = 225	Clinical & radiologic[E] TS ± PSB culture[F]	12	15	Not reported		40, 34[N]	36, 34[N]	18	19
Hammond (174) (1992)	General ICU; SDD = 114; controls = 125	Clinical & radiologic[E] TS culture[F]	Pn = 15[K]; Br = 6[K]	Pn = 15[K]; Br = 6[K]	Not reported[O]		18; IR[I] = 6	17; IR[I] = 6	16	17
Rocha (175) (1992)	General ICU; SDD = 47; controls = 54	Clinical & radiologic[E]	26	63	GP = 62[J]; GN = 43[J]	GN = 38[J]; GN = 30[J]	21; IR[I] = 2	44; IR[I] = 20	19	18

Table 3.—continued

| Author | Study Patients | Lower Respiratory Tract Infection | | | Colonization or Infection with Resistant Microorganisms[B] | | Overall Mortality In Hospital | | Mean Total Number of Days in ICU[C] | |
| | | Diagnostic Method | Infection Rate | | | | | | | |
			SDD[D] (%)	Controls (%)	SDD[D] (%)	Controls (%)	SDD[D] (%)	Controls (%)	SDD[D]	Controls
Winter (176) (1992)	General ICU; SDD = 91; control-A = 84; control-B = 92	Clinical & radiologic;[E] BAL culture[F]	3	A = 11; B = 23	1-8[J]	A = 1-7;[J] B = 1-17[J]	36	A = 43; B = 43	6	A = 7; B = 8
Korinek (177) (1993)	Neurosurgical ICU; SDD = 63; controls = 60	Clinical & Radiologic;[E] TS & PSB culture[F]	24	42	"No evidence of increased resistance"		8	7	24	29
SDD Trialists (178) (1993)	ICU's (pooled data);[M] SDD = 2047; controls = 2095	Variable	Odds ratio = 0.37;[P] CI$_{95}$,[Q] 0.31-0.43		Not analyzed		27 Odds ratio = 0.90; CI$_{95}$,[Q] 0.79-1.04	29	Not analyzed	
Ferrer (179) (1994)	Respiratory ICU; SDD = 39; controls = 41	Clinical & radiologic;[E] TS + PSB or BAL culture[F] ± autopsy histology	18	24	Not reported[R]		31	27	Not reported	

[A] Resistant to at least one antimicrobial in the SDD regimen

[B] During the study period

[C] ICU = intensive care unit

DSDD = selective digestive tract decontamination

EClinical criteria included temperature >38°C, purulent bronchorrhea, WBC >(12,000–15,000/mm³). Radiologic criterion was evidence of new and progressive infiltrate(s)

FTS = tracheal secretions; PSB = protected-specimen brushing; EAL = broncho-alveolar lavage

GPercentage of patients infected or colonized with gram-positive (GP) and/or gram-negative bacillary (GN) organisms at any body site; GP = percentage of patients infected or colonized with gram-positive organisms at any body site; GN = percentage of patients infected or colonized with gram-negative bacillary organisms at any body site; S = Percentage of patients with coagulase-negative staphylococcal infection or colonization

HMedian

IIR = Infection-related

JPercentage of isolates; GP = percentage of gram-positive isolates GN = percentage of gram-negative bacillary isolates

KPn = pneumonia; TB = tracheo-bronchial infection; Br = bronchial infection

LControl-A = patients given penicillin (ampicillin, piperacillin, or flucloxacillin) for clinical infection(s); Control-B = patients given cephalosporin (cephadrine, cefuroxime, or cefotaxime) for clinical infection(s)

MMeta-analysis

NIn ICU

OHowever, at 4 weeks, 13% and 5%, respectively, of oropharyngeal cultures of SDD and control patients had MRSA, and 41% of SDD and control patients were colonized with enterococci.

PComputed using data from 3,836 patients and 526 events, 260 in SDD- and 366 in control-patients

QCI₉₅ = 95% confidence interval

RHowever, MRSA bronchial colonization occurred in 45% of SDE patients and 21% of controls or death (i.e., in order to prevent one case of nosocomial pneumonia, or one death due to nosocomial pneumonia, 6 [range: 5–9] or 23 [range: 13–39] patients, respectively, would have to be given SDD) (178). Furthermore, there are concerns over the development of antimicrobial resistance and superinfection with gram-positive bacteria and other antibiotic-resistant nosocomial pathogens (156, 158, 159, 161, 175, 180). Thus, currently available data do not justify the routine use of SDD for prevention of nosocomial pneumonia in ICU patients. SDD may be ultimately useful for specific subsets of ICU patients, such as those with trauma or severe immunosuppression, e.g., bone-marrow transplant recipients.

A new approach advocated to prevent oropharyngeal colonization in patients receiving enteral nutrition is to reduce bacterial colonization of the stomach by acidifying the enteral feed (181). Although the absence of bacteria from the stomach has been confirmed in patients given acidified enteral feeding, the effect on the incidence of nosocomial pneumonia has not been evaluated (181).

Aspiration of Oropharyngeal and Gastric Flora

Clinically significant aspiration usually occurs in patients who have one or more of the following conditions: a depressed level of consciousness, dysphagia due to neurologic or esophageal disorders, an endotracheal (naso- or oro-tracheal), tracheostomy, or enteral (naso- or oro-gastric tube) in place, and receipt of enteral feeding (35, 84, 85, 182–186). Placement of an enteral tube may increase nasopharyngeal colonization, cause reflux of gastric contents, or allow bacterial migration via the tube from the stomach to the upper airway (183, 186–188). When enteral feedings are administered, gross contamination of the enteral solution during preparation (189–191) and elevated gastric pH (70, 192, 193) may lead to gastric colonization with gram-negative bacilli. In addition, gastric reflux and aspiration may occur because of increased intragastric volume and pressure (70, 117, 183).

Prevention of pneumonia in such patients may be difficult, but methods that make regurgitation less likely (for example, placing the patient in a semirecumbent position by elevating the head of the bed and withholding enteral feeding when the residual volume in the stomach is large or if bowel sounds are not heard upon auscultation of the abdomen) may be beneficial (185, 194–197). On the other hand, administering enteral nutrition intermittently in small boluses rather than continuously (70, 193), using flexible, small-bore enteral tubes (186, 198), or placing the enteral tube below the stomach (e.g., in the jejunum) (199, 200) have yielded equivocal results.

Mechanically Assisted Ventilation and Endotracheal Intubation

Patients receiving continuous, mechanically assisted ventilation have 6–21 times the risk of developing nosocomial pneumonia compared with patients not receiving ventilatory support (34, 63, 65, 75). Data from the study by Fagon and co-workers indicate that the risk of developing ventilator-associated pneumonia increases by 1% per day (5). This increased risk is partly due to carriage of oropharyngeal organisms upon passage of the endotracheal tube into the trachea during intubation, as well as to depressed host defenses secondary to the patient's severe underlying illness (6, 34, 35, 201). In addition, bacteria can aggregate on the surface of the tube over time and form a glycocalyx (biofilm) that protects the bacteria from the action of antimicrobial agents or host defenses (202). Some investigators believe that these bacterial aggregates may become dislodged by ventilation flow, tube manipulation, or suctioning and subsequently embolize into the lower respiratory tract and cause focal pneumonia (203, 204). Removing tracheal secretions by gentle suctioning and using aseptic technique to reduce cross-contamination to patients from contaminated respiratory therapy equipment or contaminated or colonized hands of personnel have been utilized traditionally to help prevent pneumonia in patients receiving mechanically assisted ventilation.

The risk of pneumonia is also increased by the direct access of bacteria to the lower respiratory tract, often because of leakage around the endotracheal cuff (86, 205), which allows pooled secretions above the cuff to enter the trachea (206). In one recent study, the occurrence of nosocomial pneumonia was delayed and decreased in intubated patients whose endotracheal tubes had a separate dorsal lumen that allowed drainage (by suctioning) of secretions in the space above the endotracheal tube cuff and below the glottis (206). However, further studies are needed to determine the cost-benefit ratio of using this device.

Cross-Colonization Via Hands of Personnel

Pathogens causing nosocomial pneumonia, such as gram-negative bacilli and Staphylococcus aureus, are ubiquitous in the hospital, especially in intensive or critical care areas (207, 208). Transmission of these microorganisms to patients frequently occurs via health-care workers' hands that become contaminated or transiently colonized with the microorganisms (209–215). Procedures such as tracheal suctioning and manipulation of ventilator circuit or endotracheal tubes increase the opportunity for cross-contamination (215, 216). The risk of cross-contamination can be reduced by using aseptic technique and sterile or disinfected equipment when appropriate (65) and eliminating pathogens from the hands of personnel (65, 215, 217–219).

In theory, adequate handwashing is an effective way of removing transient bacteria from the hands (218, 219), but personnel compliance with handwashing has been generally poor (220–223). For this reason, the routine use of gloves has been advocated to help prevent cross-contamination (224, 225). Routine gloving (in addition to gowning) was associated with a decrease in the incidence of nosocomial respiratory syncytial virus (RSV) (226) and other ICU infections (227). However, nosocomial pathogens can colonize gloves (228), and outbreaks have been traced to health-care workers who did not change gloves after contact with one patient and before providing care to another (229, 230). In addition, gloved hands may get contaminated via leaks in the gloves (231).

Contamination of Devices Used on the Respiratory Tract

Devices used on the respiratory tract for respiratory therapy (e.g., nebulizer), diagnostic examination (e.g., bronchoscope or spirometer), or administration of anesthesia are potential reservoirs or vehicles for infectious microorganisms (65, 232–236). Routes of transmission may be from device to patient (127, 129, 234–244), from one patient to another (245, 246), or from one body site to the lower respiratory tract of the same patient via hand or device (233, 246–248). Contaminated reservoirs of aerosol-producing devices, e.g., nebulizers, can allow the growth of hydrophilic bacteria that may be subsequently aerosolized during device use (126, 129, 130, 242). Gram-negative bacilli such as Pseudomonas spp., Xanthomonas spp., Flavobacterium spp., Legionella spp., and nontuberculous mycobacteria can multiply to substantial concentrations in nebulizer fluid (241, 249–251) and increase the device-user's risk of acquiring pneumonia (127–130, 241, 242, 252, 253).

Proper cleaning and sterilization or disinfection of reusable equipment are important components of a program to reduce infections associated with respiratory therapy and anesthesia equipment (234, 235, 237–240, 242, 254–259). Many devices or parts of devices used on the respiratory tract have been categorized as semicritical in the Spaulding classification system for appropriate sterilization or disinfection of medical devices because they come into direct or indirect contact with mucous membranes but do not ordinarily penetrate body surfaces (see Appendix A), and the associated infection risk following the use of these devices in patients is less than that associated with devices that penetrate normally sterile tissues (260). Thus, if it is not possible or cost-effective to sterilize these devices by steam autoclave or ethylene oxide (261), they can be subjected to high-level disinfection by pasteurization at 75°C for 30 min (262–265), or by using liquid chemical disinfectants approved by the Environmental Protection Agency (EPA) as sterilants/disinfectants and cleared for marketing for use on medical instruments by the Food and Drug Administration (225, 266–268).

When rinsing is needed (to remove residual liquid chemical sterilant/disinfectant) after a respiratory device has been chemically disinfected, sterile water has been preferred because tap or locally prepared distilled water may harbor microorganisms that can cause pneumonia (249, 250, 269–272). In some hospitals, a tap-water rinse followed by air-drying with or without an alcohol rinse (to hasten drying) is used (273). In theory, if complete drying is achieved following a tap-water rinse, the risk of nosocomial pneumonia associated with the use of the device is probably low. Drying has been shown to lower the level of microbial contamination of gastrointestinal endoscopes and washed hands (274–276). However, many semicritical items used on the respiratory tract (e.g., corrugated tubing, jet or ultrasonic nebulizers, bronchoscopes) are difficult to dry and the degree of dryness of a device is difficult to assess (265). Data are lacking regarding the safety of routinely using tap water for rinsing (followed by drying) reusable semicritical respiratory devices after their disinfection or between their uses on the same patient (242, 258, 273, 277).

MECHANICAL VENTILATORS, BREATHING CIRCUITS, HUMIDIFIERS, HEAT-MOISTURE EXCHANGERS AND IN-LINE NEBULIZERS

Mechanical ventilators

The internal machinery of mechanical ventilators used for respiratory therapy is not considered an important source of bacterial contamination of inhaled gas (278). Thus, routine sterilization or high-level disinfection of the internal machinery is considered unnecessary. Using high-efficiency bacterial filters at various positions in the ventilator breathing circuit had been advocated previously (279, 280). Filters interposed between the machinery and the main breathing circuit can eliminate contaminants from the driving gas and prevent retrograde contamination of the machine by the patient but may also alter the functional specifications of the breathing device by impeding high gas flows (279–281). Placement of a filter or condensate trap at the expiratory-phase tubing of the mechanical-ventilator circuit may help prevent cross-contamination of the ventilated patient's immediate environment (247, 282), but the importance of such filters in preventing nosocomial pneumonia needs further evaluation.

Breathing circuits, humidifiers, and heat-moisture exchangers

Most U.S. hospitals currently use ventilators with either bubble-through or wick humidifiers that produce either insignificant (132, 283) or no aerosols, respectively, for humidification. Thus, they do not seem to pose an important risk for pneumonia in patients. In addition, bubble-through humidifiers are usually heated to temperatures that reduce or eliminate bacterial pathogens (283, 284). Sterile water, however, is still generally used to fill these humidifiers (285) because tap or distilled water may harbor microorganisms, such as Legionella spp., that are more heat-resistant than other bacteria (252, 271).

The potential risk for pneumonia in patients using mechanical ventilators with heated bubble-through humidifiers stems primarily from the condensate that forms in the inspiratory-phase tubing of the ventilator circuit as a result of the difference in the temperatures of the inspiratory-phase gas and ambient air; condensate formation increases if the tubing is unheated (286). The tubing and condensate can rapidly become contaminated, usually with bacteria that originate from the patient's oropharynx (286). In the study by Craven, et al., 33% of inspiratory circuits were colonized with bacteria from patients' oropharynx within 2 hours and 80% within 24 hours of use (286). Spillage of the contaminated condensate into the patient's tracheobronchial tree, as can occur during procedures in which the tubing may be moved (e.g., suctioning, adjusting the ventilator setting, or feeding or caring for the patient), may increase the risk of pneumonia in the patient (286). Thus, in many hospitals, health-care workers are trained to prevent such spillage and to drain the fluid periodically. Microorganisms contaminating ventilator-circuit condensate can be transmitted to others patient via hands of the health-care worker handling the fluid, especially if the health-care worker fails to wash his or her hands after handling the condensate.

The role of ventilator-tubing changes in preventing pneumonia in patients using mechanical ventilators with bubble-through humidifiers has been investigated. Initial studies of in-use contamination of mechanical ventilator circuits with humidifiers have shown that neither the rate of bacterial contamination of inspiratory-phase gas nor the incidence of pneumonia was significantly increased when tubing was changed every 24 hours rather than every 8 or 16 hours (287). Craven, et al., later showed that changing the ventilator circuit every 48 hours rather than 24 hours did not result in an increase in contamination of the inspiratory-phase gas or tubing of the ventilator circuits (288). In addition, the incidence of nosocomial pneumonia was not significantly higher when circuits were changed every 48 hours than when changes were done every 24 hours (288). More recent reports suggest that the risk of pneumonia may not increase when the interval for circuit change is prolonged beyond 48 hours. Dreyfuss and others showed that the risk of pneumonia (8 [29%] of 28) was not significantly higher when the circuits were never changed for the duration of use by the patient, than (11 [31%] of 35) when the circuits were changed every 48 hours (289).

These findings indicate that the recommended daily change in ventilator circuits may be extended to >48 hours. This change in recommendation is expected to result in large savings in device use and personnel time for U.S. hospitals (285, 288). The maximum time, however, that a circuit can be safely left unchanged on a patient has yet to be determined.

Condensate formation in the inspiratory-phase tubing of a ventilator breathing circuit can be decreased by elevating the temperature of the inspiratory-phase gas with a heated wire in the inspiratory-phase tubing. However, in one report, three cases of endotracheal- or tracheostomy-tube blockage by dried-up patient secretions were attributed to the decrease in the relative humidity of inspired gas that results from the elevation of the gas temperature (290). Until further data are available about the frequency of the occurrence of such cases, users of heated ventilator tubing should be aware of the advantages and potential complications of using heated tubing.

Condensate formation can be eliminated by using a heat-moisture exchanger (HME) or a hygroscopic condenser humidifier ("artificial nose") (291–296). An HME recycles heat and moisture exhaled by the patient, and eliminates the need for a humidifier. In the absence of a humidifier, no condensate forms in the inspiratory-phase tubing of the ventilator circuit. Thus, bacterial colonization of the tubing is prevented, and the need to routinely change the tubing periodically is obviated (216). Some models of HMEs are equipped with bacterial filters, but the advantage of these filters remains unknown. HMEs can increase the dead space and resistance to breathing, may leak around the endotracheal tube, and may result in drying of sputum and blockage of the tracheo-bronchial tree (297). Although recently developed HMEs with humidifiers increase airway humidity without increasing colonization with bacteria (293, 298), more studies are needed to determine whether the incidence of pneumonia is decreased (299–302).

Small-volume ("in-line") medication nebulizers

Small-volume medication nebulizers that are inserted in the inspiratory circuit of mechanical ventilators can produce bacterial aerosols (242). If they become contaminated by condensate in the inspiratory tubing of the breathing circuit, they can increase the patient's risk of pneumonia because the nebulizer aerosol is directed through the endotracheal tube and bypasses many of the normal host defenses against infection (286).

LARGE-VOLUME NEBULIZERS

Nebulizers with large volume (>500 cc) reservoirs, including those used in intermittent positive-pressure breathing (IPPB) machines and ultrasonic or spinning-disk room-air "humidifiers," pose the greatest risk of pneumonia to patients, probably because of the total amount of aerosol they generate (237–241, 252, 303). These reservoirs can become contaminated by hands of personnel, unsterile humidification fluid, or inadequate sterilization or disinfection between uses (126). Once introduced into the reservoir, various bacteria, including Legionella spp., can multiply to sufficiently large numbers within 24 hours to pose a risk of infection in patients who receive inhalation therapy (128, 129, 241, 253, 303). Sterilization or high-level disinfection of these nebulizers can eliminate vegetative bacteria from their reservoirs and make them safe for patient use (260). Unlike nebulizers attached to IPPB machines, however, room-air "humidifiers" have a high cost-benefit ratio: evidence of clinical benefits from their use in hospitals is lacking, and the potential cost of daily sterilization or disinfection of, and use of sterile water to fill, such devices is substantial.

HAND-HELD SMALL-VOLUME MEDICATION NEBULIZERS

Small-volume medication nebulizers for administration of bronchodilators, including those that are hand-held, can produce bacterial aerosols. Hand-held nebulizers have been associated with nosocomial pneumonia, including Legionnaires' disease, resulting from contamination with medications from multidose vials (304) or Legionella-contaminated tap water used for rinsing and filling the reservoir (258).

SUCTION CATHETERS, RESUSCITATION BAGS, OXYGEN ANALYZERS, AND VENTILATOR SPIROMETERS.

Tracheal suction catheters can introduce microorganisms into a patient's lower respiratory tract. Currently, there are two types of suction-catheter systems used in U.S. hospitals, the open single-use catheter system and the closed multi-use catheter system. Studies comparing the two systems have involved small numbers of patients; results suggest that the risk of catheter contamination or pneumonia is not different between patients on whom the single-use suction method is used and those on whom the closed multi-use catheter system is used (305–307). While advantages of cost and decreased environmental contamination have been attributed to the use of the closed-suction system (308, 309), larger studies are needed to weigh the advantages and disadvantages of one system over the other (310).

Reusable resuscitation bags are particularly difficult to clean and dry between uses; microorganisms in secretions or fluid left in the bag may be aerosolized and/or sprayed into the lower respiratory tract of the patient on whom the bag is used; in addition, contaminating microorganisms may be transmitted from one patient to another via hands of staff members (311–313). Oxygen analyzers and ventilator spirometers have been associated with outbreaks of gram-negative respiratory tract colonization and pneumonia resulting from patient-to-patient transmission of organisms via hands of personnel (233, 245). These devices require sterilization or high-level disinfection between uses on different patients. Education of physicians, respiratory therapists, and nursing staff regarding the associated risks and appropriate care of these devices is essential.

ANESTHESIA EQUIPMENT

The contributory role of anesthesia equipment in outbreaks of nosocomial pneumonia were reported before hospitals implemented routine after-use cleaning and disinfection/sterilization of reusable anesthesia-equipment components that may become contaminated with pathogens during use (314, 315).

Anesthesia machine

The internal components of anesthesia machines, which include the gas sources and outlets, gas valves, pressure regulators, flowmeters, and vaporizers, are not considered an important source of bacterial contamination of inhaled gases (316). Thus, routine sterilization or high-level disinfection of the internal machinery is considered unnecessary.

Breathing system or patient circuit

The breathing system or patient circuit, through which inhaled and/or exhaled gases flow to and from a patient (and may include the tracheal tube or face mask, inspiratory and expiratory tubing, y-piece, CO_2 absorber and its chamber, the anesthesia ventilator bellows and tubing, humidifier, adjustable pressure-limiting valve, and other devices and accessories), can become contaminated with microorganisms that may originate from the patient's oropharynx or trachea. Recommendations for in-use care, maintenance, and reprocessing (i.e., cleaning and disinfection or sterilization) of the components of the breathing system have been published (317, 318). In general, reusable components of the breathing system that directly touch the patient's mucous membranes (e.g., face mask or tracheal tube) or become readily contaminated with the patient's respiratory secretions (e.g., y-piece, inspiratory and expiratory tubing and attached sensors) are cleaned and subjected to high-level disinfection or sterilization between patients. The other parts of the breathing system (e.g., carbon dioxide absorber and its chamber), for which an appropriate and cost-effective schedule of reprocessing has not been firmly determined (319), are changed, cleaned, and sterilized or subjected to high-level disinfection periodically, according to published guidelines (317, 318) and/or their manufacturers' instructions.

Using high-efficiency bacterial filters at various positions in the patient circuit, e.g., at the y-piece or on the inspiratory and expiratory sides of the patient circuit, has been advocated (317, 320, 321) and shown to decrease contamination of the circuit (321–323). However, the use of bacterial filters to prevent nosocomial pulmonary infections has not been shown effective and needs further study (324–326).

PULMONARY FUNCTION TESTING APPARATUS

Internal parts of pulmonary function testing apparatus

In general, the internal parts of pulmonary function testing apparatus are not considered an important source of bacterial contamination of inhaled gas (327). However, because of concern about possible carry-over of bacterial aerosols from an infectious patient-user of the apparatus to the next patient (246, 328), placement of bacterial filters (that remove exhaled bacteria) between the patient and the testing equipment has been recently advocated (246, 329). More studies are needed to evaluate the need for and efficacy of these filters in preventing nosocomial pneumonia (330).

Tubing, rebreathing valves, and mouthpieces

Tubing, connectors, rebreathing valves, and mouthpieces may become contaminated with patient secretions during use of the pulmonary function testing apparatus. Thus, they are cleaned and subjected to high-level disinfection or sterilization between uses on different patients.

Thoracoabdominal Surgical Procedures

Certain patients are at high risk of developing postoperative pulmonary complications, including pneumonia. These persons include those who are more than 70 years of age, are obese, or have chronic obstructive pulmonary disease (331–334). Abnormal pulmonary function tests (especially decreased maximum expiration flow rate), a history of smoking, the presence of tracheostomy or prolonged intubation, or protein depletion that can cause respiratory-muscle weakness are also risk factors (62, 68, 136). Patients who undergo surgery of the head, neck, thorax, or abdomen may suffer from impairment of normal swallowing and respiratory clearance mechanisms as a result of instrumentation of the respiratory tract, anesthesia, or increased use of narcotics and sedatives (332, 335, 336); patients who undergo upper abdominal surgery usually suffer from diaphragmatic dysfunction that results in decreased functional residual capacity of the lungs, closure of airways, and atelectasis (337, 338). Interventions aimed at reducing the postoperative patient's risk of pneumonia have been developed (339). These include deep breathing exercises, chest physiotherapy, use of incentive spirometry, IPPB, and continuous positive airway pressure (CPAP) by face mask (339–349). Studies evaluating the relative efficacy of these modalities have shown variable results, and have been difficult to compare because of differences in outcome variables assessed, patient populations studied, and study design (339, 341, 342, 348–350). Nevertheless, many studies have found deep breathing exercises, use of incentive spirometry, and IPPB as advantageous maneuvers, especially in patients with preoperative pulmonary dysfunction (342, 343, 345, 346, 348–350). In addition, control of pain that interferes with cough and deep breathing during the immediate postoperative period has been shown to decrease the incidence of pulmonary complications after surgery; several methods of controlling pain have been used; these include intramuscular or intravenous (including patient-controlled) administration, or regional (e.g., epidural) analgesia (351–358).

Other Prophylactic Measures

VACCINATION OF PATIENTS

Although pneumococci are not a major cause of nosocomial pneumonia, they have been identified as etiologic agents of serious nosocomial pulmonary infection and bacteremia (359–361). The following factors render patients at high risk of complications from pneumococcal infections: >65 years of age, chronic cardiovascular or pulmonary disease, diabetes mellitus, alcoholism, cirrhosis, cerebrospinal fluid leaks, immunosuppression, functional or anatomic asplenia, or HIV infection. Pneumococcal vaccine is effective in preventing pneu-

mococcal disease (362, 363). Because two-thirds or more of patients with serious pneumococcal disease have been hospitalized at least once within 5 years before their pneumococcal
illness, offering pneumococcal vaccine in hospitals, e.g., at the time of patient discharge,
should contribute substantially to preventing the disease (362, 364).

PROPHYLAXIS WITH SYSTEMIC ANTIMICROBIAL AGENTS

Systemic antimicrobial administration has been a prevalent practice in the prevention of nosocomial infections (365), including pneumonia (366), especially in patients who are weaned
off mechanical ventilators, postoperative, and/or critically ill (367). However, the efficacy of
such practice is questionable and the potential for superinfection, which may result from any
antimicrobial therapy, is a problem (74, 91, 366–371).

USE OF "KINETIC BEDS" OR CONTINUOUS LATERAL ROTATIONAL THERAPY (CLRT) FOR THE IMMOBILIZED STATE

Use of kinetic beds or CLRT is a maneuver for prevention of pulmonary and other complications from prolonged immobilization or bed rest, such as in patients with acute stroke, critical illness, head injury or traction, blunt chest trauma, and/or mechanically assisted ventilation (372–377). This involves the use of a bed that turns continuously and slowly (from <40°
for CRLT to >40° for kinetic therapy) along its longitudinal axis. Among the hypothesized
benefits are improved drainage of secretions within the lungs and lower airways, increased
tidal volume, and reduction of venous thrombosis with resultant pulmonary embolization
(378–381). However, the efficacy in preventing pneumonia needs further evaluation because
studies have yielded variable results (372–376). In addition, the studies either involved small
numbers of patients (373), lacked adequate randomization (372), had no clear definition of
pneumonia (372), did not distinguish between community-acquired and nosocomial pneumonia (373, 377), or did not adjust for possible confounding factors such as mechanical ventilation, endotracheal intubation, nasogastric intubation, and enteral feeding (372).

LEGIONNAIRES' DISEASE

Legionnaires' disease is a multisystem illness, with pneumonia, caused by Legionella spp. In
contrast, Pontiac fever is a self-limited influenza-like illness, without pneumonia, that is associated with Legionella spp (382).

EPIDEMIOLOGY

Since identification of the etiologic agent, numerous outbreaks of nosocomial Legionnaires'
disease have been reported and have provided the opportunity to study the epidemiology of
epidemic legionellosis. In contrast, the epidemiology of sporadic (i.e., nonoutbreak-related)
nosocomial Legionnaires' disease has not been well elucidated. However, data suggest that
when one case is recognized, the presence of additional cases should be suspected. Of 196
cases of nosocomial Legionnaires' disease reported in England and Wales during 1980 to
1992, 69% occurred during 22 nosocomial outbreaks (defined as two or more cases occurring
at an institution during a 6-month period) (383). Nine per cent of cases occurred >6 months
before or after a hospital outbreak. Another 13% were in hospitals where other sporadic cases
(but no outbreaks) were identified. Only 9% occurred at institutions where no outbreaks or
additional sporadic cases were identified.

The overall proportion of nosocomial pneumonias due to Legionella spp. in the North
America has not been determined, although individual hospitals have reported ranges of
0%–14% (384–386). Because diagnostic tests for Legionella spp. infection are not routinely
performed on all patients with hospital-acquired pneumonia in most U.S. hospitals, these
ranges probably underestimate the incidence of Legionnaires' disease.

Legionella spp. are commonly found in a variety of natural and man-made aquatic environments (387, 388) and may enter hospital water systems in low or undetectable numbers
(389, 390). Cooling towers, evaporative condensers, heated potable-water-distribution systems
within hospitals, and locally produced distilled water can provide a suitable environment for
legionellae to multiply. Factors known to enhance colonization and amplification of le-

gionellae in man-made water environments include temperatures of 25–42°C (392–396), stagnation (397), scale and sediment (393), and the presence of certain free-living aquatic amoebae that are capable of supporting intracellular growth of legionellae (398, 399).

A person's risk of acquiring legionellosis following exposure to contaminated water depends on a number of factors, including the type and intensity of exposure and the exposed person's health status (400–402). Persons with severe immunosuppression or chronic underlying illnesses, such as hematologic malignancy or end-stage renal disease, are at markedly increased risk for legionellosis (402–405). Persons in the later stages of acquired immunodeficiency syndrome are also probably at increased risk of legionellosis, but data are limited because of infrequent testing of patients (402). Persons with diabetes mellitus, chronic lung disease, or non-hematologic malignancy, those who smoke cigarettes, and the elderly are at moderately increased risk (382). Nosocomial Legionnaires' disease has also been reported among patients at children's hospitals (406, 407).

Underlying disease and advanced age are not only risk factors for acquiring Legionnaires' disease but also for dying from the illness. In a multivariate analysis of 3,524 cases reported to CDC from 1980 through 1989, immunosuppression, advanced age, end-stage renal disease, cancer, and nosocomial acquisition of disease were each independently associated with a fatal outcome (402). The mortality rate among 803 persons with nosocomially acquired cases was 40% compared with 20% among 2,721 persons with community-acquired cases (402), probably reflecting increased severity of underlying disease in hospitalized patients.

DIAGNOSIS

The clinical spectrum of disease due to Legionella spp. is broad and ranges from asymptomatic infection to rapidly progressive pneumonia. Legionnaires' disease cannot be distinguished clinically or radiographically from pneumonia caused by other agents (408, 409), and evidence of infection with other respiratory pathogens does not rule out the possibility of concomitant Legionella spp. infection (410–412).

The diagnosis of legionellosis may be confirmed by any one of the following: culture isolation of Legionella from respiratory secretions or tissues, or microscopic visualization of the bacterium in respiratory secretions or tissue by immunofluorescent microscopy; and, for legionellosis due to L. pneumophila serogroup 1, detection of L. pneumophila serogroup-1 antigens in urine by radioimmunoassay, or observation of a four-fold rise in L. pneumophila serogroup-1 antibody titer to >1:128 in paired acute and convalescent serum specimens by use of an indirect immunofluorescent antibody test (IFA) (413, 419). A single elevated antibody titer does not confirm a case of Legionnaires' disease because IFA titers ≥1:256 are found in 1%–16% of healthy adults (411, 414–417).

Because the above tests complement each other, performing each test when Legionnaires' disease is suspected increases the probability of confirming the diagnosis (418). However, because none of the laboratory tests is 100% sensitive, the diagnosis of legionellosis is not ruled out even if one or more of the tests are negative (418, 419). Of the available tests, the most specific is culture isolation of Legionella spp. from any respiratory tract specimen (420, 421).

MODES OF TRANSMISSION

Inhalation of aerosols of water contaminated with Legionella spp. is believed to be the primary mechanism of entry of these organisms into a patient's respiratory tract (382). In several hospital outbreaks, patients were considered to be infected through exposure to contaminated aerosols generated by cooling towers, showers, faucets, respiratory therapy equipment, and room-air humidifiers (11, 241, 258, 422–428). In other studies, aspiration of contaminated potable water or pharyngeal colonizers has been proposed as the mode of transmission to certain patients (426, 429–431). Person-to-person transmission, however, has not been observed.

DEFINITION OF NOSOCOMIAL LEGIONNAIRES' DISEASE

The incubation period for Legionnaires' disease is generally 2–10 days (432); thus, for epidemiologic purposes, in this document and in the accompanying recommendations by the HICPAC, laboratory-confirmed legionellosis that occurs in a patient who has spent >10 days continuously in the hospital prior to onset of illness is considered **definite** nosocomial Legionnaires' disease, and laboratory-confirmed infection that occurs 2–9 days after hospitalization is **possible** nosocomial infection.

PREVENTION AND CONTROL MEASURES

Prevention of Legionnaires' Disease in Hospitals with No Identified Cases (Primary Prevention)

Prevention strategies in healthcare facilities with no cases of nosocomial legionellosis have varied by institution, depending on the immunologic status of the patients, the design and construction of the facility, resources available for implementation of prevention strategies, and state and local regulations.

There are at least two schools of thought regarding the most appropriate and cost-effective approach to prevent nosocomial legionellosis, especially in hospitals where no cases or only sporadic cases of the illness are detected. However, a study comparing the cost-benefit ratios of these strategies has not been done.

The first approach is based on periodic, routine culturing of water samples from the hospital's potable water system, for Legionella spp (433, 434). When >30% of the samples obtained are culture-positive for Legionella spp., the hospital's potable water system is decontaminated (434) and diagnostic laboratory tests for legionellosis are made available to clinicians in the hospital's microbiology department so that active surveillance for cases can be instituted (434, 435). This approach is based on the premise that no cases of nosocomial legionellosis can occur in the absence of Legionella spp. from the potable water system, and, conversely, once Legionella spp. are cultured from the water, cases of nosocomial legionellosis may occur (429, 436). Proponents of this strategy indicate that when physicians are informed that the potable water system of the hospital is culture-positive for Legionella spp., they are more inclined to conduct the necessary tests for legionellosis (435). A potential advantage of this approach is the lower cost of culturing a limited number of water samples, if the testing is done infrequently, compared with the cost of routine laboratory diagnostic testing for legionellosis in all patients with nosocomial pneumonia in hospitals that have had no cases of nosocomial legionellosis.

The main argument against this approach is that in the absence of cases, the relationship between the results of water cultures and the risk of legionellosis remains undefined. The bacterium has been frequently present in hospital water systems (437), often without being associated with known cases of disease (271, 385, 438, 439). In a study of 84 hospitals in Quebec, 68% were found to be colonized with Legionella spp., and 26% were colonized at >30% of sites sampled; however, cases of Legionnaires' disease were rarely reported from these hospitals (271). Similarly, at one hospital where active surveillance for legionellosis and environmental culturing for Legionella spp. were done, no cases of legionellosis occurred in a urology ward during a 3.5-month period when 70% of water samples from the ward were culture-positive for L. pneumophila serogroup 1 (385). Interpretation of the results of routine culturing of water may be confounded by variable culture results among sites sampled within a single water system and by fluctuations in the concentration of Legionella spp. in the same site (440, 441). In addition, the risk of illness following exposure to a given source may be influenced by a number of factors other than the presence or concentration of organisms; these include the degree to which contaminated water is aerosolized into respirable droplets, the proximity of the infectious aerosol to potential host, the susceptibility of the host, and the virulence properties of the contaminating strain (442–444). Thus, data are insufficient to assign a level of risk of disease even on the basis of the number of colony-forming units detected in samples from the hospital environment. By routinely culturing water samples, many hospitals will have to be committed to water-decontamination programs to eradicate Legionella spp. Because of this problem, routine monitoring of water from the hospital's potable water system and from aerosol-producing devices is not widely recommended (445).

The second approach to prevent and control nosocomial legionellosis is by (a) maintaining a high index of suspicion for legionellosis and appropriately using diagnostic tests for legionellosis in patients with nosocomial pneumonia who are at high risk of developing the disease and dying from the infection (385, 446), (b) initiating an investigation for a hospital source of Legionella spp. upon identification of one case of definite or two cases of possible nosocomial Legionnaires' disease, and (c) routinely maintaining cooling towers and using only sterile water for filling and terminal rinsing of nebulization devices.

Measures aimed at creating an environment that is not conducive to survival or multiplication of Legionella spp. have been advocated and utilized in hospitals where cases of nosocomial legionellosis have been identified; these include routine maintenance of potable water at >50°C or <20°C at the tap or chlorination of heated water to achieve 1–2 mg/L free residual chlorine at the tap, especially in areas where immunosuppressed and other high-risk patients are located (385, 429, 440, 447–450). However, the cost-benefit ratio of such measures in hospitals with no identified cases of legionellosis needs further study.

Prevention of Legionnaires' Disease in Hospitals with Identified Cases (Secondary Prevention)

The indications for a full-scale environmental investigation to search for and subsequently decontaminate identified sources of Legionella spp. in hospital environments remain to be elucidated, and probably vary from hospital to hospital. In institutions where as few as 1–3 nosocomial cases are identified over a period of up to several months, intensified surveillance for Legionnaires' disease has frequently detected numerous additional cases (404, 423, 426, 448). This suggests the need for a low threshold for initiating an investigation following the identification of nosocomial, laboratory-confirmed cases of legionellosis. However, when developing a strategy to respond to such an identification, infection-control personnel should consider the level of risk of nosocomial acquisition of, and mortality from, Legionella spp. infection at their particular hospital.

An epidemiologic investigation of the source of Legionella spp. involves several important steps, including retrospective review of microbiologic and medical records; active surveillance to identify all recent or ongoing cases of legionellosis; identification of potential risk factors (including environmental exposures for infection, such as showering or use of respiratory-therapy equipment) by line listing of cases, analysis by time, place, and person, and comparison with appropriate controls; collection of water samples from environmental sources implicated by the epidemiologic investigation and from other potential sources of aerosolized water; and subtype-matching between legionellae isolated from patients and environmental samples (428, 452–454). The latter step can be crucial in supporting epidemiologic evidence of a link between human illness and a specific source (455).

In hospitals where the heated-water system has been identified as the source of the organism, the system has been decontaminated by pulse (one-time) thermal disinfection or superheating (i.e., flushing for at least 5 minutes each distal outlet of the hot-water system with water at ≥65°C) and hyperchlorination (flushing all outlets of the hot-water system with water containing >10 mg/L free residual chlorine) (450, 456–458). Following either of these procedures, most hospitals maintain heated water at >50°C or <20°C at the tap or chlorinate heated water to achieve 1–2 mg/L free residual chlorine at the tap (385, 429, 440, 447–450). Additional measures, such as physical cleaning or replacement of hot-water storage tanks, water-heaters, faucets, and showerheads, may be required because scale and sediment that provide organisms protection from the biocidal effects of heat and chlorine, may accumulate in them (393, 450). Alternative methods for control and eradication of legionellae in water systems, such as treatment of water with ozone, ultraviolet light, or heavy metal ions, have limited the growth of legionellae under laboratory and/or operating conditions (391, 459–463). However, further data are needed regarding the efficacy of these methods before they can be considered standard. In hospitals where the cooling towers are contaminated, measures for decontamination have been previously published (464).

For highly immunocompromised patients, other preventive measures have been used. At one hospital, immunosuppressed patients were restricted from taking showers, and, for these patients, only sterile water was used for drinking or flushing nasogastric tubes (430). In another hospital, a combined approach, consisting of continuous heating, particulate filtration, ultraviolet treatment, and monthly pulse hyperchlorination of the water supply of the bone-marrow transplant unit, was used to decrease the incidence of Legionnaires' disease (459).

In view of the high cost of an environmental investigation and of instituting control measures to eradicate Legionella spp. from sources in the hospital (465, 466) and the differential risk, based on host factors, for acquiring nosocomial legionellosis and of having severe and fatal infection with the microorganism, the decision to search for and the choice of procedures to eradicate hospital environmental sources of Legionella spp. should take into account the type of patient population served by the hospital.

ASPERGILLOSIS

EPIDEMIOLOGY

Aspergillus spp. are ubiquitous fungi, commonly occurring in soil, water, and decaying vegetation. Aspergillus spp. have been cultured from unfiltered air, ventilation systems, contaminated dust dislodged during hospital renovation and construction, horizontal surfaces, food, and ornamental plants (467).

A. fumigatus and A. flavus are the most frequently isolated Aspergillus spp. in patients with proven aspergillosis (468). Nosocomial aspergillosis has been recognized increasingly as a cause of severe illness and mortality in highly immunocompromised patients, e.g., patients undergoing chemotherapy and/or organ transplantation, including bone-marrow transplantation for hematologic and other malignant neoplasms (469–473).

The most important nosocomial infection due to Aspergillus spp. is pneumonia (474, 495). Hospital outbreaks of pulmonary aspergillosis have occurred mainly in granulocytopenic patients, especially in bone-marrow transplant units (474–480). Although invasive aspergillosis has been reported in recipients of solid-organ transplants (e.g., heart or kidney) (481–485), the incidence of Aspergillus spp. infections in these patients has been lower than in recipients of bone-marrow transplants, probably because granulocytopenia is less severe in solid-organ transplant recipients and the use of corticosteroids has decreased with the introduction of cyclosporine (483, 486). In solid-organ transplant recipients, the efficacy of infection control measures, such as provision of protected environments and prophylaxis with antifungal agents, in preventing aspergillosis has not been well evaluated (483, 484, 486, 489). In one study of heart-transplant recipients, protective isolation of patients alone failed to prevent fungal infections (490).

The reported attributable mortality from invasive pulmonary aspergillosis has varied, depending on the patient population studied. Rates have been as high as 95% in recipients of allogeneic bone-marrow transplants and patients with aplastic anemia, compared with rates of 13%–80% in leukemic patients (491–493).

PATHOGENESIS

In contrast to most bacterial pneumonias, the primary route of acquiring Aspergillus spp. infection is by inhalation of the fungal spores. In severely immunocompromised patients, primary Aspergillus spp. pneumonia results from local lung tissue invasion (468, 494, 495). Subsequently, the fungus may disseminate via the bloodstream to involve multiple other deep organs (468, 495, 496). A role for nasopharyngeal colonization with Aspergillus spp., as an intermediate step before invasive pulmonary disease, has been proposed, but remains to be elucidated (488, 497, 498). On the other hand, colonization of the lower respiratory tract by Aspergillus spp., especially in patients with preexisting lung disease such as chronic obstructive lung disease, cystic fibrosis, or inactive tuberculosis, has predisposed patients to invasive pulmonary and/or disseminated infection (468, 495, 499).

DIAGNOSIS

Diagnosing pneumonia due to Aspergillus spp. is often difficult without performing invasive procedures. Bronchoalveolar lavage has been a useful screening test (500–502), but lung biopsy is still considered the most reliable technique (503). Histopathologic demonstration of tissue invasion by fungal hyphae has been required in addition to isolation of Aspergillus spp. from respiratory tract secretions because the latter, by itself, may indicate colonization (504). However, when Aspergillus spp. is grown from the sputum of a febrile, granulocytopenic patient with a new pulmonary infiltrate, it is highly likely that the patient has pulmonary aspergillosis (497, 505). Routine blood cultures are remarkably insensitive for detecting Aspergillus spp. (506), and systemic antibody responses in immunocompromised patients are likely to be unreliable indicators of infection (507–509). Antigen-based serologic assays are now being developed in an attempt to allow for the rapid and specific diagnosis of Aspergillus spp. infections; however, their clinical usefulness is presently undefined (510, 511).

RISK FACTORS AND CONTROL MEASURES

The major risk factor for invasive aspergillosis is severe and prolonged granulocytopenia, both disease- and therapy-induced (512). Since bone-marrow transplant recipients experience the most severe degree of granulocytopenia, they probably constitute the population at highest risk of developing invasive aspergillosis (492, 513). The tendency of bone-marrow transplant recipients to develop severe granulocytopenia (<1,000 polymorphonuclears/µL) is associated with the type of graft they receive. While both autologous and allogeneic bone-marrow transplant recipients are severely granulocytopenic for up to 4 weeks after the transplant procedure, allogeneic-transplant recipients may, in addition, develop acute or chronic graft-versus-host disease. The latter may occur up to several months after the procedure, and the disease and/or its therapy (often with high doses of corticosteroids, cyclosporine, and other immunosuppressive agents) may result in severe granulocytopenia. Consequently, in developing strategies to prevent invasive Aspergillus spp. infection in bone-marrow-transplant patients, infection control personnel should consider exposures of the patient to the fungus not only during the patient's immediate posttransplantation period, but also other exposures (e.g., at home or in an ambulatory-care setting) subsequent to the immediate posttransplant period, when the patient (especially allogeneic-transplant recipients) may again manifest severe granulocytopenia. To help address this problem, various studies are now in progress to evaluate newer methods of enhancing host resistance to invasive fungal (and other) infections, and of eliminating or suppressing respiratory fungal colonization of the upper respiratory tract. These methods include, respectively, the use of granulocyte-colony-stimulating factors and intranasal application of amphotericin B, or oral or systemic antifungal drug prophylaxis (467, 514–517). For solid-organ transplant recipients, risk factors for invasive aspergillosis have not been as extensively studied. In one study of liver-transplant recipients, risk factors for invasive infection with Aspergillus spp. identified by univariate analysis included preoperative and postoperative receipt of steroids and antimicrobial agents, and prolonged duration of transplant surgery (518).

The presence of aspergilli in the hospital environment is the major extrinsic risk factor for the occurrence of opportunistic invasive Aspergillus spp. infection (487, 519). Environmental disturbances due to construction and/or renovation activities in and around hospitals markedly raise the airborne Aspergillus spp. spore counts in such hospitals and have been associated with nosocomial aspergillosis (476, 478, 479, 520–523). In addition, aspergillosis in high-risk immunosuppressed patients has been associated with other hospital environmental reservoirs, including bird droppings in air ducts supplying high-risk patient areas (524), and contaminated fireproofing material or damp wood (478, 525).

A single case of nosocomial Aspergillus spp. pneumonia is often difficult to link to a specific environmental exposure. However, additional cases may remain undetected without an active search that includes an intensive retrospective review of microbiologic, histopathologic, and postmortem records; notification of clinicians caring for high-risk patients; and establishment of a system for prospective surveillance for additional cases. When additional cases are detected, the likelihood is increased that a hospital environmental source of Aspergillus spp. can be identified (476, 478, 520–525). Previous investigations have shown the importance of construction activities and/or fungal "contamination" of hospital air-handling systems as major sources for outbreaks (474, 476, 478, 520–524). New molecular typing techniques, namely karyotyping (526) and DNA endonuclease profiling (now available for A. fumigatus) (527), may significantly aid in identifying the source of an outbreak.

Outbreaks of invasive aspergillosis reinforce the importance of maintaining an environment as free of Aspergillus spp. spores as possible for patients with severe granulocytopenia. To achieve this goal, specialized services in many large hospitals, in particular bone-marrow transplant services, have installed "protected environments" for the care of their high-risk, severely granulocytopenic patients, and increased their vigilance during hospital construction and routine maintenance of hospital air-filtration and ventilation systems, to prevent exposing high-risk patients to bursts of fungal spores (476, 478, 520–524, 528–533).

While the exact configuration and specifications of the protected environments may vary between hospitals, these patient-care areas are built to minimize fungal spore counts in air by maintaining (a) high-efficiency filtration of incoming air by using central or point-of-use HEPA filters that are 99.97% efficient in filtering 0.3-μm-sized particles, (b) directed room airflow—from intake on one side of the room, across the patient, and out through the exhaust on the opposite side of the room, (c) positive room-air pressure relative to the corridor, (d) well-sealed rooms, and (e) high rates of room-air changes (range: 15 to >400 per hour) although air-change rates at the higher levels may pose problems of patient comfort (474, 529–531, 533–535). The oldest and most studied protected environment is a room with laminar airflow, consisting of a bank of HEPA filters along an entire wall through which air is pumped by blowers into the room at a uniform velocity (90 + 20 feet/minute), forcing the air to move in a laminar, or at least unidirectional, pattern (536). The air usually exits at the opposite end of the room, and ultra-high air-change rates (100–400 per hour) are achieved (474, 528). The net effects are essentially sterile air in the room, minimal air turbulence, minimal opportunity for microorganism build-up, and a consistently clean environment (474).

The efficacy of a laminar-airflow system in decreasing or eliminating the risk of nosocomial aspergillosis in high-risk patients has been demonstrated (474, 529, 534, 535). However, such a system is costly to install and maintain. Less expensive alternative systems with lower air-change rates (10–15 per hour) have been utilized in some centers (530, 531, 537). However, studies comparing the efficacy of these alternative systems with laminar-airflow rooms in eliminating Aspergillus spp. spores and preventing nosocomial aspergillosis are limited. One institution employing cross-flow ventilation, point-of-use high-efficiency filters, and 15 air changes per hour reported that cases of nosocomial aspergillosis in patients housed in these rooms have occurred, albeit at a low rate (3.4%) (531, 537). The infections, however, were due to A. flavus—a species that was never cultured from the room air, suggesting that the patients were probably exposed to fungal spores when they were allowed outside their rooms (531).

Copper-8-quinolinolate has been used on environmental surfaces contaminated with Aspergillus spp. to control a reported outbreak (538), and incorporated in fireproofing material of a newly constructed hospital (531) to help decrease the environmental spore burden, but its general applicability is yet to be established.

VIRAL PNEUMONIAS

Viruses can be an important and often unappreciated cause of nosocomial pneumonia (539–541). In one prospective study of endemic nosocomial infections, approximately 20% of patients with pneumonia had viral infections (540). Although early diagnosis and treatment of viral infections have become possible in recent years (542–545), many hospitalized patients remain at high risk for developing severe and sometimes fatal viral infections (539, 546–553). Based on these data and on well-documented outbreaks with nosocomial viral transmission (554–557), measures to prevent viral transmission should be instituted.

Nosocomial respiratory viral infections (a) usually follow community outbreaks that occur during a particular period every year (556, 558–561), (b) confer only short-term immunity (562), (c) affect healthy and ill persons (548, 549, 555, 563–565), and (d) have exogenous sources. A number of viruses, including adenoviruses, influenza virus, measles virus, parainfluenza viruses, respiratory syncytial virus (RSV), rhinoviruses, and varicella-zoster virus can cause nosocomial pneumonia (549, 556, 557, 566–572, 574); however, adenoviruses, influenza viruses, parainfluenza viruses, and RSV have been reported to account for most (70%) of nosocomial pneumonias due to viruses (573).

Because influenza and RSV infections substantially contribute to patient morbidity and mortality associated with viral pneumonia and have been well studied epidemiologically, this section focuses on the principles and approaches to control these infections. Prevention of nosocomial infections due to other viral pathogens are addressed in another document (224).

RSV INFECTION

EPIDEMIOLOGY

RSV infection is most common during infancy and early childhood, but may also occur in adults (563, 566, 575, 576). Infection usually causes mild or moderately severe upper respiratory illness. However, life-threatening pneumonia or bronchiolitis has been reported in children with chronic cardiac and pulmonary disease, immunocompromised patients, and the elderly (548, 550, 565, 566, 577, 578).

Recent surveillance of 10 U.S. hospital laboratories performing cultures for RSV suggests that community outbreaks occur yearly between December and March, last from 3–5 months, and are associated with increased hospitalization and deaths among infants and young children (579). During community outbreaks of RSV, children admitted to the hospital with respiratory symptoms often serve as reservoirs for RSV (554, 556).

DIAGNOSIS

The clinical characteristics of RSV infection, especially in neonates, are often indistinguishable from those of other viral respiratory tract infections (566, 567). Culture of RSV from respiratory secretions remains the "gold standard" for diagnosis. Although rapid antigen-detection kits utilizing direct immunofluorescence or enzyme-linked immunosorbent assay are available and can provide results within hours, the benefit of using these tests to identify infected patients depends on the sensitivity and specificity of the test. The reported sensitivity and specificity of RSV enzyme immunoassays vary between 80% and 95%, and may even be lower in actual practice (580–583). In general, once laboratory-confirmed cases of RSV infection are identified in a hospital, a presumptive diagnosis of RSV infection in subsequent cases with manifestations suggestive of RSV infection may be acceptable for infection control purposes.

MODES OF TRANSMISSION

RSV is present in large numbers in the respiratory secretions of symptomatic persons infected with the virus and can be transmitted directly via large droplets during close contact with such persons, or indirectly via RSV-contaminated hands or fomites (554, 584, 585). The portal of entry is usually the conjunctiva or the nasal mucosa (586). Inoculation by RSV-contaminated hands is the usual way of depositing the virus onto the eyes or nose (554, 584–586). Hands can become contaminated through handling of infected persons' respiratory secretions or contaminated fomites (584, 585).

In nosocomial RSV outbreaks in which the viral isolates were typed, more than one strain of RSV has often been identified (555, 564, 587), suggesting multiple sources of the virus. Potential sources include patients, hospital staff, and visitors. Because infected infants shed large amounts of virus in their respiratory secretions and easily contaminate their immediate surroundings, they are a major reservoir for RSV (588). Hospital staff may become infected after exposure in the community (589) or in the hospital, and in turn, infect patients, other health-care workers, or hospital visitors (567, 590).

CONTROL MEASURES

Various combinations of control measures ranging from the simple to the complex have been effective, to some degree or other, in preventing and controlling nosocomial RSV infection (226, 590–597). Successful programs have had two elements in common: implementation of contact-isolation precautions, and compliance with these precautions by healthcare personnel. In theory, strict handwashing should prevent most nosocomial RSV infections. However, health-care workers' handwashing practices have always been poor (221, 222). Thus, other preventive measures are usually relied upon to prevent RSV infection.

The basic precautions that have been associated with decreased incidence of nosocomial RSV infections are gloving and gowning (226). Gloving has helped decrease transmission probably because gloves remind patient-care personnel to comply with handwashing and other precautions, and deter persons from touching their eyes or noses. The benefits from gloving, however, are offset if gloves are not changed between patients or after contact with contaminated fomites, and if hands are not adequately washed after glove removal (229). Gowning, in combination with gloving, during contact with RSV-infected infants or their immediate environment has been used successfully to prevent infection (226). In addition, the use of eye-nose goggles rather than masks has protected health-care workers from infection; however, eye-nose goggles are not widely available and are inconvenient to wear (594, 598).

Additional measures may be indicated to control ongoing nosocomial transmission of RSV or to prevent transmission to patients at high risk for serious complications of infections, such as those with compromised cardiac, pulmonary, or immune systems. The following additional control measures have been used in various combinations: (a) use of private rooms for infected patients OR cohorting of infected patients, with or without pre-admission screening by rapid laboratory diagnostic tests; (b) cohorting of personnel; (c) exclusion of health-care workers who have symptoms of upper respiratory tract infection from the care of uninfected patients at high risk of severe or fatal RSV infection, e.g., infants; (d) limiting visitors; and (e) postponing admission of patients at high risk of complications from RSV infection (224, 591, 593, 595, 597). Although the exact role of each of these measures has not been fully elucidated, their use for control of outbreaks seems prudent.

INFLUENZA

EPIDEMIOLOGY

Pneumonia in patients with influenza may be due to the influenza virus itself, secondary bacterial infection, or a combination of both (599–601). Influenza-associated pneumonia can occur in any person, but is more common in the very young or old and in persons in any age group with immunosuppression or certain chronic medical conditions such as severe underlying heart or lung disease (576, 602–604).

Influenza typically occurs annually in the winter between December and April; peak activity in a community usually lasts from 6 to 8 weeks during this period (605, 606). During influenza epidemics in the community, nosocomial outbreaks can occur and are often characterized by abrupt onset and rapid transmission (607–609). Most reported institutional outbreaks of influenza have occurred in nursing homes; however, hospital outbreaks have been reported on pediatric and chronic-care wards, as well as on medical and neonatal intensive care units (557, 610–613).

Influenza is believed to be spread from person to person by direct deposition of virus-laden large droplets onto the mucosal surfaces of the upper respiratory tract of an individual during close contact with an infected person, as well as by droplet nuclei or small-particle aerosols (614–617). The extent to which transmission may occur by virus-contaminated hands or fomites is unknown; however, it is not the primary mode of spread (618).

The most important reservoirs of influenza virus are infected persons, and the period of greatest communicability is during the first 3 days of illness; however, the virus can be shed before onset of symptoms, and up to 7 or more days after illness onset (451, 557, 605).

DIAGNOSIS

Influenza is clinically indistinguishable from other febrile respiratory illnesses, but during outbreaks with laboratory-confirmed cases, a presumptive diagnosis of the infection can be made in cases with similar manifestations (619). In the past, diagnosis of influenza was made by virus isolation from nasopharyngeal secretions or by serologic conversion, but recently developed rapid diagnostic tests that are similar to culture in sensitivity and specificity allow early diagnosis and treatment of cases and provide a basis for prompt initiation of antiviral prophylaxis as part of outbreak control (620–625).

PREVENTION AND CONTROL OF INFLUENZA

Vaccination of persons at high risk for complications of influenza is currently the most effective measure for reducing the impact of influenza, and should be done before the influenza season each year. High-risk persons include those >65 years of age; those in long-term-care units; those with chronic disorders of the pulmonary or cardiovascular systems, those with diabetes mellitus, renal dysfunction, hemoglobinopathies, or immunosuppression; and children 6 months–18 years of age who are receiving long-term aspirin therapy (612, 626–628). Patients with musculo-skeletal disorders that impede adequate respiration may also be at high risk of developing complications of influenza. When high vaccination rates are achieved in closed or semi-closed settings, the risk of outbreaks is reduced because of induction of herd immunity (629, 630).

When an institutional outbreak is caused by influenza type A, antiviral agents may be used both for treatment of ill persons and as prophylaxis for others (642). Two related antiviral agents, amantadine hydrochloride and rimantadine hydrochloride, are effective against influenza type A, but not influenza type B, virus (544, 632–634). These agents can be used to prevent influenza type A (a) as short-term prophylaxis after late vaccination of high-risk persons; (b) as prophylaxis for persons for whom vaccination is contraindicated; (c) as prophylaxis for immunocompromised persons who may not produce protective levels of antibody in response to vaccination; (d) as prophylaxis for unvaccinated health-care workers who provide care to high-risk patients, either for the duration of influenza activity in the community or until immunity develops after vaccination; and (e) when vaccine strains do not closely match the epidemic virus strain (642).

Amantadine has been available in the United States for many years; rimantadine has been approved for use since 1993. Both drugs protect against all naturally-occurring strains of type A influenza virus; thus, antigenic changes in the virus that may reduce vaccine efficacy do not alter the effectiveness of amantadine or rimantadine. Both drugs are 70%–90% effective in preventing illness if taken before exposure to influenza A virus (632, 635). In addition, they can reduce the severity and duration of illness due to influenza type A when administered within 24–48 hours after onset of symptoms (636, 637). These drugs can limit nosocomial spread of influenza type A if they are administered to all or most patients when influenza type A illnesses begin in a facility (610, 638, 639).

Compared to rimantadine, amantadine has been associated with a higher incidence of adverse central nervous system (CNS) reactions such as mild and transitory nervousness, insomnia, impaired concentration, mood changes, and light-headedness. These symptoms have been reported in 5%–10% of healthy young adults receiving 200 mg of amantadine per day (544, 632). In the elderly, CNS side effects may be more severe; in addition, dizziness and ataxia are more common in this age group (640, 641). Dose reductions of both amantadine and rimantadine are recommended for certain patient groups, such as persons >65 years of age and/or those who have renal insufficiency. The drug package insert for amantadine or rimantadine contains important information regarding administration of either drug. Guidelines for the use of these drugs and considerations for the selection of amantadine or rimantadine have been developed by the Advisory Committee for Immunization Practices (642).

Emergence of amantadine- and rimantadine-resistant strains of influenza A virus has been observed in persons who have received these drugs for treatment of the infection (643, 644). Because of the potential risk of transmission of resistant viral strains to contacts of persons receiving amantadine or rimantadine for treatment (644, 645), to the extent possible, infected persons taking either drug should avoid contact with others during treatment and for 2 days after discontinuing treatment (645, 646). This is particularly important if the contacts are uninfected high-risk persons (645, 647).

Vaccination of high-risk patients and of hospital personnel before the influenza season is the primary focus of efforts to prevent and control nosocomial influenza (628, 631, 648). The decision to use amantadine or rimantadine as an adjunct to vaccination in the prevention and control of nosocomial influenza is based in part on results of virologic and epidemiologic surveillance in the hospital and the community. When outbreaks of influenza type A occur in a hospital, and antiviral prophylaxis of high-risk persons and/or treatment of cases is undertaken, administration of amantadine or rimantadine is begun as early in the outbreak as possible to reduce transmission (610, 642, 638, 647).

Measures other than vaccination and chemoprophylaxis have been recommended for control of nosocomial influenza outbreaks. Because influenza can be transmitted during contact with an infected person, contact-isolation precautions, placing a patient symptomatic with influenza in a private room, cohorting of patients with influenza-like illness, and masking upon entering a room with persons with suspected or proven influenza have been recommended (224). Handwashing, gloving, and gowning by health-care workers during the patient's symptomatic period have also been recommended, but the exact role of these measures in preventing influenza transmission remains to be elucidated (224, 609, 649). Although influenza can be transmitted via the airborne route, the efficacy of placing infected persons in rooms with negative pressure in relation to their immediate environment has not been assessed. In addition, this measure may be impractical during institutional outbreaks that occur in the midst of a community epidemic of influenza because many newly admitted patients and health-care workers may be infected with the virus; thus, the hospital would face the logistical problem of accommodating all ill persons in rooms with special ventilation. Although controlled studies are not available to measure their effectiveness, the following additional measures have been recommended for consideration, particularly during severe outbreaks: (a) curtailment or elimination of elective admissions, both medical and surgical; (b) restriction of cardiovascular and pulmonary surgery; (c) restriction of hospital visitors, especially those with acute respiratory illnesses; and (d) work restriction for health-care workers with acute respiratory illness (649).

PART II. RECOMMENDATIONS FOR PREVENTION OF NOSOCOMIAL PNEUMONIA

THE HOSPITAL INFECTION CONTROL PRACTICES ADVISORY COMMITTEE

INTRODUCTION

The recommendations are presented according to the etiology of the infection, in the following order: bacterial pneumonia, including Legionnaires' disease; fungal pneumonia (aspergillosis); and virus-associated pneumonia (respiratory syncytial virus [RSV] and influenza infections). Each topic is subdivided according to the following general approaches for nosocomial infection control, as applicable to the infection:

1. Staff education and infection surveillance;
2. Interruption of transmission of microorganisms by eradicating infecting microorganisms from their epidemiologically important reservoirs, and/or preventing person-to-person transmission; and
3. Modifying host risk for infection.

As in previous CDC guidelines, each recommendation is categorized on the basis of existing scientific evidence, theoretical rationale, applicability, and economic impact (224, 225, 650–654). However, the previous CDC system of categorizing recommendations has been modified as follows:

CATEGORY IA   Strongly recommended for all hospitals and strongly supported by well-designed experimental or epidemiologic studies.

CATEGORY IB   Strongly recommended for all hospitals and viewed as effective by experts in the field and a consensus of HICPAC based on strong rationale and suggestive evidence, even though definitive scientific studies may not have been done.

CATEGORY II   Suggested for implementation in many hospitals. Recommendations may be supported by suggestive clinical or epidemiologic studies, a strong theoretical rationale, or definitive studies applicable to some but not all hospitals.

NO RECOMMENDATION; UNRESOLVED ISSUE. Practices for which insufficient evidence or consensus regarding efficacy exists.

BACTERIAL PNEUMONIA

I. Staff Education and Infection Surveillance

   A. Staff Education

     Educate health-care workers regarding nosocomial bacterial pneumonias and infection control procedures to prevent their occurrence (655–661).

     CATEGORY IA

   B. Surveillance

     1. Conduct surveillance for bacterial pneumonia in ICU patients at high risk for nosocomial bacterial pneumonia (e.g., patients with mechanically assisted ventilation, selected postoperative patients) to determine trends and identify potential problems (6, 34, 35, 62, 63, 662–664). Include data regarding the causative microorganisms and their antimicrobial susceptibility patterns (2, 3). Express data as rates (e.g., number of infected patients or infections per 100 ICU days or per 1,000 ventilator-days) to facilitate intra-hospital comparisons and determining trends (66, 665–667).

     CATEGORY IA

     2. Do not **routinely** perform surveillance cultures of patients or of equipment or devices used for respiratory therapy, pulmonary-function testing, or delivery of inhalation anesthesia (65, 668, 669).

     CATEGORY IA

II. Interruption of Transmission of Microorganisms

   A. Sterilization or Disinfection, and Maintenance of Equipment and Devices

     1. General Measures

       a. Thoroughly clean all equipment and devices to be sterilized or disinfected (266, 267, 670).

       CATEGORY IA

       b. Sterilize or use high-level disinfection for semicritical equipment or devices, i.e., items that come into direct or indirect contact with mucous membranes of the lower respiratory tract (see examples, Appendix A). High-level disinfection can be achieved either by wet heat pasteurization at 76°C for 30 minutes or by using liquid chemical disinfectants approved as sterilants/disinfectants by the Environmental Protection Agency and cleared for marketing for use on medical instruments by the Office of Device Evaluation, Center for Devices and Radiologic Health, Food and Drug Administration (260, 262, 264, 267, 671). Follow disinfection with appropriate rinsing, drying, and packaging, taking care not to contaminate the items in the process.

       CATEGORY IB

       c. (i) Use sterile (not distilled, nonsterile) water for rinsing reusable semicritical equipment and devices used on the respiratory

tract after they have been chemically disinfected (241, 249, 250, 258, 269).
CATEGORY IB

(ii) No Recommendation for using tap water (as an alternative to sterile water) to rinse reusable semicritical equipment and devices used on the respiratory tract, after they have been subjected to high-level disinfection, whether or not rinsing is followed by drying with or without the use of alcohol (241, 249, 250, 258, 269, 273, 277).
UNRESOLVED ISSUE

d. Do not reprocess an equipment or device that is manufactured for single use only, unless data show that reprocessing the equipment or device poses no threat to the patient, is cost-effective, and does not change the structural integrity or function of the equipment or device (672, 673).
CATEGORY IB

2. Mechanical Ventilators, Breathing Circuits, Humidifiers and Nebulizers
   a. Mechanical Ventilators
      Do not routinely sterilize or disinfect the internal machinery of mechanical ventilators. (126, 128, 674)
      CATEGORY IA
   b. Ventilator Circuits with Humidifiers
      (i) Do not routinely change more frequently than every 48 hours the breathing circuit, including tubing and exhalation valve, and the attached bubbling or wick humidifier of a ventilator that is in use on an individual patient (34, 283, 288).
      CATEGORY IA

      (ii) No Recommendation for the maximum length of time after which the breathing circuit and the attached bubbling or wick humidifier of a ventilator in use on a patient should be changed (289).
      UNRESOLVED ISSUE

      (iii) Sterilize reusable breathing circuits and bubbling or wick humidifiers, or subject them to high-level disinfection between their uses on different patients (259, 260, 262, 264, 267).
      CATEGORY IB

      (iv) Periodically drain and discard any condensate that collects in the tubing of a mechanical ventilator, taking precautions not to allow condensate to drain toward the patient. Wash hands after performing the procedure or handling the fluid. (215, 282, 286)
      CATEGORY IB

      (v) No Recommendation for placing a filter or trap at the distal end of the expiratory-phase tubing of the breathing circuit to collect condensate (247, 282).
      UNRESOLVED ISSUE

(vi) Do not place bacterial filters between the humidifier reservoir and the inspiratory-phase tubing of the breathing circuit of a mechanical ventilator.
CATEGORY IB

(vii) Humidifier fluids

(a) Use sterile water to fill bubbling humidifiers (132, 241, 249, 250, 286).
CATEGORY II

(b) Use sterile, distilled, or tap water to fill wick humidifiers (249, 250, 286).
CATEGORY II

(c) No Recommendation for preferential use of a closed, continuous-feed humidification system.
UNRESOLVED ISSUE

c. Ventilator Breathing Circuits with Hygroscopic Condenser-Humidifiers or Heat-Moisture Exchangers

(i) No Recommendation for preferential use of hygroscopic condenser-humidifier or heat-moisture exchanger rather than a heated humidifier to prevent nosocomial pneumonia (298–302).
UNRESOLVED ISSUE

(ii) Change the hygroscopic condenser-humidifier or heat-moisture exchanger according to manufacturer's recommendation and/or when evidence of gross contamination or mechanical dysfunction of the device is present (298).
CATEGORY IB

(iii) Do not routinely change the breathing circuit attached to a hygroscopic condenser-humidifier or heat-moisture exchanger while it is in use on a patient (298, 301).
CATEGORY IB

3. Wall humidifiers

a. Follow manufacturers' instructions for use and maintenance of wall oxygen humidifiers unless data show that the modification in their use or maintenance poses no threat to the patient and is cost-effective (675–679).
CATEGORY IB

b. Between patients, change the tubing, including any nasal prongs or mask, used to deliver oxygen from a wall outlet.
CATEGORY IB

4. Small-Volume Medication Nebulizers: "In-Line" and Hand-Held Nebulizers

a. (i) Between treatments on the same patient, disinfect, rinse with sterile water, or air-dry small-volume medication nebulizers (242, 258).
CATEGORY IB

(ii) No Recommendation for using tap water as an alternative to

sterile water to rinse reusable small-volume medication nebulizers between treatments on the same patient (242, 258, 273).
UNRESOLVED ISSUE

b. Between patients, replace nebulizers with those that have undergone sterilization or high-level disinfection (126, 128, 129, 269, 680).
CATEGORY IB

c. Use only sterile fluids for nebulization, and dispense these fluids aseptically (238, 241, 249, 250, 258, 269, 304).
CATEGORY IA

d. If multidose medication vials are used, handle, dispense, and store them according to manufacturers' instructions (238, 304, 680–682).
CATEGORY IB

5. Large-volume nebulizers and Mist Tents

a. Do not use large-volume room-air humidifiers that create aerosols (e.g., by venturi principle, ultrasound, or spinning disk) and thus are really nebulizers, unless they can be sterilized or subjected to high-level disinfection at least daily and filled only with sterile water. (239–241, 252, 303, 683)
CATEGORY IA

b. Sterilize large-volume nebulizers that are used for inhalation therapy, e.g., for tracheostomized patients, or subject them to high-level disinfection between patients and after every 24 hours of use on the same patient (126, 128, 129).
CATEGORY IB

c. (i) Use mist-tent nebulizers and reservoirs that have undergone sterilization or high-level disinfection and replace them between patients (684).
CATEGORY IB

(ii) No Recommendation regarding the frequency of changing mist-tent nebulizers and reservoirs while in use on one patient.
UNRESOLVED ISSUE

6. Other Devices Used in Association with Respiratory Therapy

a. Between patients, sterilize or subject to high-level disinfection portable respirometers, oxygen sensors, and other respiratory devices used on multiple patients (233, 245).
CATEGORY IB

b. (i) Between patients, sterilize or subject to high-level disinfection reusable hand-powered resuscitation bags (for example, Ambu bags) (255, 311–313).
CATEGORY IA

(ii) No Recommendation regarding the frequency of changing hydrophobic filters placed on the connection port of resuscitation bags.
UNRESOLVED ISSUE

7. Anesthesia Machines and Breathing Systems or Patient Circuits

a. Do not routinely sterilize or disinfect the internal machinery of anesthesia equipment (316).
CATEGORY IA

b. Clean and then sterilize or subject to high-level liquid chemical disinfection or pasteurization reusable components of the breathing system or patient circuit (e.g., tracheal tube or face mask; inspiratory and expiratory breathing tubing; y-piece; reservoir bag; humidifier and tubing) between uses on different patients, by following the device manufacturer's instructions for their reprocessing (260, 264, 267, 317, 685).
CATEGORY IB

c. No Recommendation for the frequency of routinely cleaning and disinfecting unidirectional valves and carbon dioxide absorber chambers (317–319).
UNRESOLVED ISSUE

d. Follow published guidelines and/or manufacturers' instructions regarding in-use maintenance, cleaning, and disinfection or sterilization of other components or attachments of the breathing system or patient circuit of anesthesia equipment (317, 318).
CATEGORY IB

e. Periodically drain and discard any condensate that collects in the tubing of a breathing circuit, taking precautions not to allow condensate to drain toward the patient. After performing the procedure or handling the fluid, wash hands with soap and water or with a waterless handwashing preparation (218, 219, 686, 687).
CATEGORY IB

f. No Recommendation for placing a bacterial filter in the breathing system or patient circuit of anesthesia equipment (1, 317, 318, 321–326, 688).
UNRESOLVED ISSUE

8. Pulmonary-Function Testing Equipment

a. Do not routinely sterilize or disinfect the internal machinery of pulmonary-function testing machines between uses on different patients (327, 328).
CATEGORY II

b. Sterilize or subject to high-level liquid chemical disinfection or pasteurization reusable mouthpieces and tubing or connectors between uses on different patients, OR follow device manufacturer's instructions for their reprocessing (260, 261, 263–267).
CATEGORY IB

B. Interruption of Person-to-Person Transmission of Bacteria

1. Handwashing
Wash hands after contact with mucous membranes, respiratory secretions, or objects contaminated with respiratory secretions,

whether or not gloves are worn. Wash hands before and after contact with a patient who has an endotracheal or tracheostomy tube in place, and before and after contact with any respiratory device that is used on the patient, whether or not gloves are worn (210, 212, 218, 219, 231, 689, 690).
CATEGORY IA

2. Barrier Precautions
  a. Wear gloves for handling respiratory secretions or objects contaminated with respiratory secretions of any patient (226, 227).
     CATEGORY IA
  b. Change gloves and wash hands between patients; after handling respiratory secretions or objects contaminated with secretions from one patient and before contact with another patient, object, or environmental surface; and between contacts with a contaminated body site and respiratory tract of, or respiratory device on, the same patient (226, 228–230).
     CATEGORY IA
  c. Wear a gown when soiling with respiratory secretions from a patient is anticipated, and change the gown after such contact and before providing care to another patient (226).
     CATEGORY IB

3. Care of Patients with Tracheostomy
  a. Perform tracheostomy under sterile conditions.
     CATEGORY IB
  b. When changing a tracheostomy tube, use aseptic technique and replace the tube with one that has undergone sterilization or high-level disinfection.
     CATEGORY IB

4. Suctioning of Respiratory Tract Secretions
  a. No Recommendation for wearing sterile rather than clean gloves when suctioning a patient's respiratory secretions.
     UNRESOLVED ISSUE
  b. If the open suction system is employed, use a sterile single-use catheter.
     CATEGORY II
  c. Use only sterile fluid to remove secretions from the suction catheter if the catheter is to be used for re-entry into the patient's lower respiratory tract (691).
     CATEGORY IB
  d. No Recommendation for preferential use of the multi-use closed-system suction catheter or the single-use open-system catheter for prevention of pneumonia (305–308, 310).
     UNRESOLVED ISSUE
  e. Change suction collection tubing (up to the canister) between patients.
     CATEGORY IB

    f. Change suction collection canisters between uses on different patients except when used in short-term care units.
CATEGORY IB

III. Modifying Host Risk for Infection
  A. Precautions for Prevention of Endogenous Pneumonia
Discontinue enteral-tube feeding and remove devices such as endotracheal, tracheostomy, and/or enteral (i.e., oro- or naso-gastric, or jejunal) tubes from patients as soon as the clinical indications for these are resolved (6, 34, 35, 85–87, 117, 183, 185, 186, 202, 692).
CATEGORY IB

    1. Prevention of Aspiration Associated with Enteral Feeding
      a. If there is no contraindication to the maneuver, elevate at an angle of 30–45° the head of the bed of a patient at high risk of aspiration pneumonia, e.g., a person receiving mechanically assisted ventilation and/or has an enteral tube in place (74, 185).
CATEGORY IB

      b. Routinely verify appropriate placement of the feeding tube (693–695).
CATEGORY IB

      c. Routinely assess the patient's intestinal motility (e.g., by auscultating for bowel sounds and measuring residual gastric volume or abdominal girth) and adjust the rate and volume of enteral feeding to avoid regurgitation (692).
CATEGORY IB

      d. No Recommendation for the preferential use of small-bore tubes for enteral feeding (694).
UNRESOLVED ISSUE

      e. No Recommendation for administering enteral feeding continuously or intermittently (70, 193, 198).
UNRESOLVED ISSUE

      f. No Recommendation for preferentially placing the feeding tubes, e.g., jejunal tubes, distal to the pylorus (199, 200).
UNRESOLVED ISSUE

    2. Prevention of Aspiration Associated with Endotracheal Intubation
      a. No Recommendation for using orotracheal rather than nasotracheal tube to prevent nosocomial pneumonia (699).
UNRESOLVED ISSUE

      b. No Recommendation for routinely using an endotracheal tube with a dorsal lumen above the endotracheal cuff to allow drainage (by suctioning) of tracheal secretions that accumulate in the patient's subglottic area (206).
UNRESOLVED ISSUE

      c. Before deflating the cuff of an endotracheal tube in preparation for tube removal, or before moving the tube, ensure that secretions are cleared from above the tube cuff.
CATEGORY IB

3. Prevention of Gastric Colonization

   a. If stress-bleeding prophylaxis is needed for a patient with mechanically assisted ventilation, use an agent that does not raise the patient's gastric pH (22, 34, 112, 118, 122, 147–154).
   CATEGORY II

   b. No Recommendation for selective decontamination of a critically ill, mechanically ventilated, or ICU patient's digestive tract with oral and/or intravenous antimicrobials to prevent gram-negative bacillary (or Candida spp.) pneumonia (155–180).
   UNRESOLVED ISSUE

   c. No Recommendation for routine acidification of gastric feedings to prevent nosocomial pneumonia (181).
   UNRESOLVED ISSUE

B. Prevention of Postoperative Pneumonia

   1. Instruct preoperative patients, especially those at high risk of developing pneumonia, regarding frequent coughing, taking deep breaths, and ambulating as soon as medically indicated in the postoperative period (346, 348). High-risk patients include those who will receive anesthesia, especially those who will have an abdominal, thoracic, head, or neck operation, or who have substantial pulmonary dysfunction, such as patients with chronic obstructive lung disease, a musculoskeletal abnormality of the chest, or abnormal pulmonary function tests (331–334, 337, 338).
   CATEGORY IB

   2. Encourage postoperative patients to cough frequently, take deep breaths, move about the bed, and ambulate unless it is medically contraindicated (345, 346, 348).
   CATEGORY IB

   3. Control pain that interferes with coughing and deep breathing during the immediate postoperative period by using systemic analgesia (352, 701), including patient-controlled analgesia (353–355), with as little cough-suppressant effect as possible; appropriate support for abdominal wounds, such as tightly placing a pillow across the abdomen; or regional (e.g., epidural) analgesia (356–358).
   CATEGORY IB

   4. Use an incentive spirometer or intermittent positive pressure breathing on patients at high risk of developing postoperative pneumonia (339, 342, 343, 346, 348, 349). (See III.B.1 above for definition of high-risk patients.)
   CATEGORY II

C. Other Prophylactic Procedures for Pneumonia

   1. Vaccination of Patients
   Vaccinate patients at high risk for complications of pneumococcal infections with pneumococcal polysaccharide vaccine. High-risk patients include persons >65 years old; adults with chronic car-

diovascular or pulmonary disease, diabetes mellitus, alcoholism, cirrhosis, or cerebrospinal fluid leaks; and children and adults with immunosuppression, functional or anatomic asplenia, or HIV infection (362–364).
CATEGORY IA

2. Antimicrobial Prophylaxis
Do not routinely administer systemic antimicrobial agents to prevent nosocomial pneumonia (74, 91, 201, 366–370, 702).
CATEGORY IA

3. Use of Rotating "Kinetic" Beds or Continuous Lateral Rotational Therapy
No Recommendation for the routine use of "kinetic" beds or continuous lateral rotational therapy (i.e., placing patients on beds that turn on their longitudinal axes intermittently or continuously) for prevention of nosocomial pneumonia in patients in the ICU, critically ill patients, or patients immobilized by illness and/or trauma (372–377, 703).
UNRESOLVED ISSUE

PREVENTION AND CONTROL OF LEGIONNAIRES' DISEASE

I. Staff Education and Infection Surveillance
A. Staff Education
Educate (a) physicians to heighten their suspicion for cases of nosocomial Legionnaires' disease and to use appropriate methods for its diagnosis, and (b) patient-care, infection-control, and engineering personnel about measures to control nosocomial legionellosis (659–661).
CATEGORY IA

B. Surveillance
1. Establish mechanism(s) to provide clinicians with appropriate laboratory tests for the diagnosis of Legionnaires' disease (386, 414, 415, 419, 704).
CATEGORY IA

2. Maintain a high index of suspicion for the diagnosis of nosocomial Legionnaires' disease, especially in patients who are at high-risk of acquiring the disease (patients who are immunosuppressed, including organ-transplant patients, patients with AIDS, and patients receiving systemic steroids; are >65 years of age; or have chronic underlying disease such as diabetes mellitus, congestive heart failure, and chronic obstructive lung disease) (385, 386, 400, 402–406, 412). Refer to the accompanying background document for definition of nosocomial legionellosis.
CATEGORY II

3. No Recommendation for routinely culturing water systems for Legionella spp. (271, 385, 429, 433, 435, 436, 438–440, 456, 705).
UNRESOLVED ISSUE

II. Interruption of Transmission of Legionella Spp.

A. Primary Prevention (Preventing Nosocomial Legionnaires' Disease When No Cases Have Been Documented)

1. Nebulization and other devices

a. (i) Use sterile (not distilled, nonsterile) water for rinsing nebulization devices and other semicritical respiratory-care equipment after they have been cleaned and/or disinfected (258, 271, 706). CATEGORY IB

(ii) No Recommendation for using tap water as an alternative to sterile water to rinse reusable semicritical equipment and devices used on the respiratory tract, after they have been subjected to high-level disinfection, whether or not rinsing is followed by drying with or without the use of alcohol. UNRESOLVED ISSUE

b. Use only sterile (not distilled, nonsterile) water to fill reservoirs of devices used for nebulization (241, 252, 258, 271, 706). CATEGORY IA

c. Do not use large-volume room-air humidifiers that create aerosols (e.g., by venturi principle, ultrasound, or spinning disk) and thus are really nebulizers, unless they can be sterilized or subjected to high-level disinfection daily and filled only with sterile water (252, 706). CATEGORY IA

2. Cooling towers

a. When a new hospital building is constructed, place cooling tower(s) in such a way that the tower drift is directed away from the hospital's air-intake system, and design the cooling towers such that the volume of aerosol drift is minimized (422, 707). CATEGORY IB

b. For operational cooling towers, install drift eliminators, regularly use an effective biocide, maintain the tower according to manufacturers' recommendations, and keep adequate maintenance records. (See Appendix D.) (422, 464, 708) CATEGORY IB

3. Water-Distribution System

a. No Recommendation for routinely maintaining potable water at the outlet at $\geq 50°C$ or $<20°C$, or chlorinating heated water to achieve 1–2 mg/L free residual chlorine at the tap (385, 429, 440, 447–450). UNRESOLVED ISSUE

b. No Recommendation for treatment of water with ozone, ultraviolet light, or heavy-metal ions (391, 460–463, 466). UNRESOLVED ISSUE

B. Secondary Prevention (Response to Identification of Laboratory-Confirmed Nosocomial Legionellosis)

When a single case of laboratory-confirmed, definite nosocomial Legionnaires' disease is identified, OR if two or more cases of laboratory-confirmed, possible nosocomial Legionnaires' disease occur within 6 months of each other (refer to background document for definition of definite and possible nosocomial Legionnaires' disease.):

1. Contact the local or state health department or the CDC if the disease is reportable in the state or if assistance is needed.
CATEGORY IB

2. If a case is identified in a severely immunocompromised patient such as an organ-transplant recipient, OR if the hospital houses severely immunocompromised patients, conduct a combined epidemiologic and environmental investigation (as outlined from II.B.3.b(i) through II.B.5, below) to determine the source(s) of Legionella spp.
CATEGORY IB

3. If the hospital does not house severely immunocompromised patients, conduct an epidemiologic investigation via a retrospective review of microbiologic, serologic, and postmortem data to identify previous cases, and begin an intensive prospective surveillance for additional cases of nosocomial Legionnaires' disease.
CATEGORY IB

   a. If there is no evidence of continued nosocomial transmission, continue the intensive prospective surveillance (as in II.B.3, above) for at least 2 months after surveillance was begun.
   CATEGORY II

   b. If there is evidence of continued transmission:

      (i) Conduct an environmental investigation to determine the source(s) of Legionella spp. by collecting water samples from potential sources of aerosolized water, following the methods described in Appendix C and saving and subtyping isolates of Legionella spp. obtained from patients and environment (241, 258, 422–428, 452, 454).
      CATEGORY IB

      (ii) If a source is not identified, continue surveillance for new cases for at least 2 months, and, depending on the scope of the outbreak, decide on either deferring decontamination pending identification of the source(s) of Legionella spp., or proceeding with decontamination of the hospital's water distribution system, with special attention to the specific hospital areas involved in the outbreak.
      CATEGORY II

      (iii) If a source of infection is identified by epidemiologic and environmental investigation, promptly decontaminate it (466).
      CATEGORY IB

         (a) If the heated-water system is implicated:
            i. Decontaminate the heated-water system either by superheating (flushing for at least 5 minutes each distal outlet of the system with water at $\geq 65°C$), OR by hyperchlorination (flushing for at least 5 minutes all

outlets of the system with water containing >10 mg/L free residual chlorine) (450, 452, 456, 457). Post warning signs at each outlet being flushed to prevent scald injury to patients, staff, or visitors.
CATEGORY IB

ii. Depending on local and state regulations regarding potable water temperature in public buildings (458), maintain potable water at the outlet at ≥50°C or <20°C, or chlorinate heated water to achieve 1–2 mg/L free residual chlorine at the tap in hospitals housing patients who are at high risk of acquiring nosocomial legionellosis (e.g., immunocompromised patients) (385, 429, 440, 447–450). (See Appendix B.)
CATEGORY II

iii. No Recommendation for treatment of water with ozone, ultraviolet light, or heavy-metal ions (391, 460, 461, 463).
UNRESOLVED ISSUE

iv. Clean hot-water storage tanks and waterheaters to remove accumulated scale and sediment (393).
CATEGORY IB

v. Restrict immunocompromised patients from taking showers, and use only sterile water for their oral consumption until Legionella spp. becomes undetectable by culture in the hospital water (430).
CATEGORY II

(b) If cooling towers or evaporative condensers are implicated, decontaminate the cooling-tower system using the protocol outlined in Appendix D (464).
CATEGORY IB

(iv) Assess the efficacy of implemented measures in reducing or eliminating Legionella spp. by collecting specimens for culture at 2-week intervals for 3 months.
CATEGORY II

(a) If Legionella spp. are not detected in cultures during 3 months of monitoring, collect cultures monthly for another 3 months.
CATEGORY II

(b) If Legionella spp. are detected in one or more cultures, reassess the implemented control measures, modify them accordingly, and repeat decontamination procedures. Options for repeat decontamination include the intensive use of the same technique utilized for initial decontamination, or a combination of superheating and hyperchlorination.
CATEGORY II

(v) Keep adequate records of all infection control measures, including maintenance procedures, and of environmental test results for cooling towers and potable-water systems.
CATEGORY II

PREVENTION AND CONTROL OF NOSOCOMIAL PULMONARY ASPERGILLOSIS

I. Staff Education and Infection Surveillance
A. Staff Education
Educate health-care workers regarding nosocomial pulmonary aspergillosis especially in immunocompromised patients, and about infection control procedures to decrease its occurrence. (659–661)
CATEGORY IA
B. Surveillance
1. Maintain a high index of suspicion for the diagnosis of nosocomial pulmonary aspergillosis in high-risk patients, i.e., patients with prolonged, severe granulocytopenia (<1,000 polymorphonuclear cells/mm^3 for 2 weeks or <100 polymorphonuclear cells/mm^3 for 1 week), most notably bone-marrow transplant recipients (512, 513, 709). Consider solid-organ transplant recipients and patients with hematologic malignancies who are receiving chemotherapy also to be at high risk of developing the infection when they are severely granulocytopenic as defined above (473, 485, 512, 710).
CATEGORY IB
2. Maintain surveillance for cases of nosocomial pulmonary aspergillosis by periodically reviewing the hospital's microbiologic, histopathologic, and postmortem data.
CATEGORY IB
3. No Recommendation for performing routine, periodic cultures of the nasopharynx of high-risk patients, or devices, air samples, dust, ventilation ducts, and filters in rooms occupied by high-risk patients (467, 478, 487, 488, 521–523).
UNRESOLVED ISSUE
II. Interruption of Transmission of Aspergillus Spp. Spores
A. Planning New Specialized-Care Units for High-Risk Patients
1. When constructing new specialized-care units for high-risk patients, ensure that patient rooms have adequate capacity to minimize fungal spore counts via maintenance of (a) high-efficiency air filtration (b), directed room airflow (c), positive air pressure in patient's room in relation to the corridor (d), properly sealed room, and (e) high rates of room-air changes (474, 529–531, 534, 538, 711, 712).
CATEGORY IB
a. Air filtration. Install high efficiency particulate air (HEPA) filters that are 99.97% efficient in filtering 0.3 μm-sized particles, either centrally or at the point of use, i.e., at the room-air intake site (474, 529–531, 534, 538, 711, 712).
CATEGORY IB

b. Directed room airflow. Place air-intake and exhaust ports such that room air comes in from one side of the room, flows across the patient's bed, and exits on the opposite side of the room (530, 531).
CATEGORY IB

c. Well-sealed room. Construct windows, doors, and intake and exhaust ports to achieve complete sealing of the room against air leaks (530, 531).
CATEGORY IB

d. Room-air pressure. Ensure that room-air pressure can be maintained continuously above that of corridor, e.g., as can be demonstrated by performance of the smoke-tube test, unless there are clinical-care or infection-control contraindications to do so (530, 531).
CATEGORY IB

(i) To maintain positive room-air pressure in relation to the corridor, supply room air at a rate that is 10–20% more than the rate of exhausting air from the room (530, 531).
CATEGORY IB

(ii) For placement of patients at high risk of aspergillosis who also have an infection (e.g., varicella or infectious tuberculosis) requiring negative room-air pressure in relation to the corridor, provide optimal conditions to prevent the spread of the airborne infection from and acquisition of aspergillosis by the patient, e.g., by providing anterooms with an independent exhaust (530).
CATEGORY II

e. Room-air changes. Maintain room-air changes at >12 per hour (1, 530, 536, 537).
CATEGORY II

2. No Recommendation for the preferential installation of a particular system, such as one with ultra-high air change rates (100–400 per hour), e.g., laminar airflow, over other systems that meet the conditions in II.A.1.a through II.A.1.e above (474, 529–531, 534, 538, 711, 712).
UNRESOLVED ISSUE

3. Formulate hospital policies to minimize exposures of high-risk patients to potential sources of Aspergillus spp., such as hospital construction and renovation, cleaning activities, carpets, food, potted plants, and flower arrangements (467, 487, 523, 528, 713–715).
CATEGORY IB

4. No Recommendation for prophylactic use of copper-8-quinolinolate biocide in fireproofing material (467, 477, 531, 538).
UNRESOLVED ISSUE

B. In Existing Facilities with No Cases of Nosocomial Aspergillosis

1. Place high-risk patients in protected environment that meets the con-

ditions outlined in Section II.A.1.a through II.A.1.e above (474, 487, 529, 538, 711, 712, 716).
CATEGORY IB

2. Routinely inspect air-handling systems in high-risk patient-care areas, maintain adequate air exchanges and pressure differentials, and eliminate air leakages. Coordinate repairs of the system with relocation of high-risk patients to other areas with optimal air-handling capabilities (467, 478, 487).
CATEGORY IB

3. Minimize the time high-risk patients spend outside their rooms for diagnostic procedures and other activities; and when high-risk patients leave their rooms, require them to wear well-fitting masks capable of filtering Aspergillus spp. spores.
CATEGORY IB

4. Prevent dust accumulation by daily damp-dusting horizontal surfaces, regularly cleaning ceiling tiles and air-duct grates when the rooms are not occupied by patients, and maintaining adequate seals on windows to prevent room infiltration by outside air, especially in areas occupied by patients at high-risk for developing aspergillosis (487).
CATEGORY IB

5. Systematically review and coordinate infection-control strategies with personnel in charge of hospital engineering, maintenance, central supply and distribution, and catering (467, 523).
CATEGORY IB

6. When planning hospital construction and renovation activities, assess whether patients at high-risk for aspergillosis are likely to be exposed to high ambient-air spore counts of Aspergillus spp. from construction and renovation sites, and develop a plan to prevent such exposures (467, 523).
CATEGORY IB

7. During construction or renovation activities:
   a. Construct barriers between patient-care and construction areas to prevent dust from entering patient-care areas; these barriers (e.g., plastic or drywall), should be impermeable to Aspergillus spp (467, 478, 522, 523).
   CATEGORY IB
   b. In construction/renovation areas inside the hospital, create and maintain negative pressure relative to that in adjacent patient-care areas if there are no contraindications for such pressure differential, e.g., there are patients with infectious tuberculosis in the adjacent patient-care areas (467, 478, 522, 523, 538).
   CATEGORY II
   c. Direct pedestrian traffic from construction areas away from patient-care areas to limit opening and closing of doors (or other

barriers) that may cause dust dispersion, entry of contaminated air, or tracking of dust into patient areas (467, 478, 522, 523).
CATEGORY IB

   d. Clean newly constructed areas before allowing patients to enter the areas (467, 523).
   CATEGORY IB

8. Eliminate exposures of patients at high-risk for aspergillosis to activities, such as floor or carpet vacuuming, that may cause spores of Aspergillus spp. and other fungi to be aerosolized (467, 487, 523).
CATEGORY IB

9. Eliminate exposures of patients at high-risk for aspergillosis to potential environmental sources of Aspergillus spp., such as Aspergillus-contaminated food, potted plants, or flower arrangements (467, 487, 523, 713–715).
CATEGORY II

10. Prevent birds from gaining access to hospital air-intake ducts (524).
CATEGORY IB

C. When A Case of Nosocomial Aspergillosis Occurs

   1. Begin a prospective search for additional cases in hospitalized patients and an intensified retrospective review of the hospital's microbiologic, histopathologic, and postmortem records.
   CATEGORY IB

   2. If there is no evidence of continuing transmission, continue routine maintenance procedures to prevent nosocomial aspergillosis, as in Section II.B.1 through II.B.10 above.
   CATEGORY IB

   3. If evidence of continuing Aspergillus spp. infection exists, conduct an environmental investigation to determine and eliminate the source. If assistance is needed, contact the local or state health department (474, 477, 478, 522, 534, 538).
   CATEGORY IB

      a. Collect environmental samples from potential sources of Aspergillus spp., especially those sources implicated in the epidemiologic investigation, by using appropriate methods (474, 477, 478, 522, 534, 538, 717), e.g., use of a high-volume air sampler rather than settle plates (474).
      CATEGORY IB

      b. Perform molecular subtyping of Aspergillus spp. obtained from patients and the environment to establish strain identity, depending on test availability (526, 527).
      CATEGORY IB

      c. If air-handling systems supplying high-risk patient-care areas are not optimal, consider temporary deployment of portable HEPA filters until rooms with optimal air-handling systems are available for all patients at high risk of invasive aspergillosis.
      CATEGORY II

　　　　d. If an environmental source is identified, perform corrective mea-
　　　　　sures as needed to eliminate the source from the high-risk pa-
　　　　　tients' environment.
　　　　　CATEGORY IB
　　　　e. If an environmental source is not identified, review existing in-
　　　　　fection-control measures, including engineering aspects, to iden-
　　　　　tify potential areas that can be corrected or improved.
　　　　　CATEGORY IB
　　III. Modifying Host Risk for Infection
　　A. Administer cytokines, including granulocyte colony-stimulating factor
　　　　and granulocyte-macrophage stimulating factor, to increase host resis-
　　　　tance to aspergillosis by decreasing the duration and severity of
　　　　chemotherapy-induced granulocytopenia (514, 515).
　　　　CATEGORY II
　　B. No Recommendation for administration of intranasal amphotericin B or
　　　　oral antifungal agents (including amphotericin B and triazole compounds)
　　　　in high-risk patients for prophylaxis against aspergillosis (516, 517, 718).
　　　　UNRESOLVED ISSUE

PREVENTION AND CONTROL OF RESPIRATORY SYNCYTIAL VIRUS INFECTION

　　I. Staff Education and Infection Surveillance
　　A. Staff Education
　　　　Educate personnel about the epidemiology, modes of transmission
　　　　and means of preventing spread of respiratory syncytial virus (RSV)
　　　　(226, 659–661).
　　　　CATEGORY IA
　　B. Surveillance
　　　1. Establish mechanism(s) by which the appropriate hospital personnel are
　　　　promptly alerted to any increase in RSV activity in the local community.
　　　　CATEGORY IB
　　　2. During periods of increased prevalence of RSV in the community
　　　　(and during December-March), attempt prompt diagnosis of RSV in-
　　　　fection by using rapid diagnostic techniques as clinically indicated in
　　　　pediatric patients, especially infants, and in immunocompromised
　　　　adults admitted to the hospital with respiratory illness (593, 597).
　　　　CATEGORY IB
　　II. Interruption of Transmission of RSV
　　A. Prevention of Person-to-Person Transmission
　　　1. Primary measures for contact isolation
　　　　a. Handwashing
　　　　　Wash hands after contact with a patient, or after touching respi-
　　　　　ratory secretions or fomites potentially contaminated with respi-
　　　　　ratory secretions, whether or not gloves are worn (218, 231, 554,
　　　　　584–586, 595).
　　　　　CATEGORY IA

b. Gloving
  (i) Wear gloves for handling patients or respiratory secretions of patients with proven or suspected RSV infection, or fomites potentially contaminated with patient secretions (226, 554, 584, 585, 591, 597).
       CATEGORY IA
  (ii) Change gloves between patients, or after handling respiratory secretions or fomites contaminated with secretions from one patient before contact with another patient (226, 228). Wash hands after removing gloves. (See II.A.1.a, above.)
       CATEGORY IA

c. Gowning
   Wear a gown when soiling with respiratory secretions from a patient is anticipated, e.g., when handling infants with RSV infection or other viral respiratory illness, and change the gown after such contact and before caring for another patient (226, 590, 592, 597).
   CATEGORY IB

d. Staffing
   Restrict health-care workers in the acute stages of an upper respiratory illness, i.e., those who are sneezing and/or coughing) from taking care of infants and other patients at high risk for complications from RSV infection (e.g., children with severe underlying cardio-pulmonary conditions, children receiving chemotherapy for malignancy, premature infants, and patients who are otherwise immunocompromised) (595, 597).
   CATEGORY IB

e. Limiting visitors
   Do not allow persons with symptoms of respiratory infection to visit uninfected pediatric, immunosuppressed, and cardiac patients (591).
   CATEGORY II

2. Control of RSV outbreaks
  a. Use of private room, cohorting, and patient-screening
     To control ongoing RSV transmission in the hospital, admit young children with symptoms of viral respiratory illness to single rooms when possible, OR perform RSV-screening diagnostic tests on young children upon admission and cohort them according to their RSV-infection status. (591, 593, 595, 597)
     CATEGORY II

  b. Personnel cohorting
     During an outbreak of nosocomial RSV, cohort personnel as much as practical, i.e., restrict personnel who give care to infected patients from giving care to uninfected patients, and vice-versa (591, 595, 597).
     CATEGORY II

    c. Postponing patient admission

    During outbreaks of nosocomial RSV, postpone elective admission of uninfected patients at high risk of complications from RSV infection.

    CATEGORY II

    d. Wearing eye-nose goggles

    No Recommendation for wearing eye-nose goggles for close contact with an RSV-infected patient (594, 598).

    UNRESOLVED ISSUE

PREVENTION AND CONTROL OF INFLUENZA

I. Staff Education and Infection Surveillance

  A. Staff Education

    Educate personnel about the epidemiology, modes of transmission, and means of preventing the spread of influenza (659–661, 719, 720).

    CATEGORY IA

  B. Surveillance

    1. Establish mechanism(s) by which the appropriate hospital personnel are promptly alerted of any increase in influenza activity in the local community.

    CATEGORY IB

    2. Arrange for laboratory tests to be available to clinicians, for use when clinically indicated, to promptly confirm the diagnosis of influenza and other acute viral respiratory illnesses, especially during November–April (620–625).

    CATEGORY IB

II. Modifying Host Risk to Infection

  A. Vaccination

    1. Patients

    Offer vaccine to outpatients and inpatients at high risk of complications from influenza, beginning in September and continuing until influenza activity has begun to decline (628, 631, 648, 721–723). Patients at high risk of complications from influenza include those >65 years of age; in long-term-care units; with chronic disorders of the pulmonary or cardiovascular systems, diabetes mellitus, renal dysfunction, hemoglobinopathies, or immunosuppression; and children 6 months–18 years of age who are receiving long-term aspirin therapy (628). In addition, consider patients with musculo-skeletal disorders that impede adequate respiration to be at risk of complications from influenza.

    CATEGORY IA

    2. Personnel

    Vaccinate health-care workers before the influenza season each year, preferably between mid-October and mid-November. Until influenza activity declines, continue to make vaccine available to newly hired personnel and to those who initially refuse vaccination. If vaccine supply is limited, give highest priority to staff caring for patients at great-

est risk of severe complications from influenza infection, as listed in Section II.A.1 above (628).
CATEGORY IB

B. Use of Antiviral Agents (See Section IV below, Control of Influenza Outbreaks)

III. Interruption of (Person-to-Person) Transmission

A. Keep a patient for whom influenza is suspected or diagnosed in a private room, or in a room with other patients with proven influenza, unless there are medical contraindications to doing so.
CATEGORY IB

B. As much as feasible, maintain negative air pressure in rooms of patients for whom influenza is suspected or diagnosed, or place together persons with influenza-like illness in a hospital area with an independent air-supply and exhaust system (614, 615, 617, 724).
CATEGORY II

C. Institute masking of individuals (except those immune to the infecting strain) who enter the room of a patient with influenza (614, 615, 724).
CATEGORY IB

D. As much as possible during periods of influenza activity in the community, have the hospital's employee health service evaluate patient-care staff who have symptoms of febrile upper respiratory tract infection suggestive of influenza for possible removal from duties that involve direct patient contact. Use more stringent guidelines for staff working in certain patient-care areas, e.g., ICUs, nurseries, and units with severely immunosuppressed patients (649, 725).
CATEGORY II

E. When community and/or nosocomial outbreaks occur, especially if they are characterized by high attack rates and severe illness:

   1. Restrict hospital visitors who have a febrile respiratory illness.
   CATEGORY IB

   2. Curtail or eliminate elective medical and surgical admissions as necessary.
   CATEGORY IB

   3. Restrict cardiovascular and pulmonary surgery to only emergency cases.
   CATEGORY IB

IV. Control of Influenza Outbreaks

A. Determining the Outbreak Strain
Early in the outbreak, obtain nasopharyngeal-swab or nasal-wash specimens from patients with recent-onset symptoms suggestive of influenza for influenza virus culture or antigen detection.
CATEGORY IB

B. Vaccination of Patients and Personnel
Administer current influenza vaccine to unvaccinated patients and staff, especially if the outbreak occurs early in the influenza season (610, 628).
CATEGORY IB

C. Amantadine or Rimantadine Administration
1. When a nosocomial outbreak of influenza A is suspected or recognized:
   a. Administer amantadine or rimantadine for prophylaxis to all uninfected patients in the involved unit for whom it is not contraindicated. Do not delay administration of amantadine or rimantadine unless the results of diagnostic tests to identify the infecting strain(s) can be obtained within 12 to 24 hours after specimen collection (634, 642).
   CATEGORY IB
   b. Administer amantadine or rimantadine for prophylaxis to unvaccinated staff members for whom it is not medically contraindicated, and who are in the involved unit or taking care of high-risk patients (642).
   CATEGORY II
2. Discontinue amantadine or rimantadine if laboratory tests confirm or strongly suggest that influenza type A is not the cause of the outbreak (632).
   CATEGORY IA
3. If the cause of the outbreak is confirmed or believed to be influenza type A AND vaccine has been administered only recently to susceptible patients and personnel, continue amantadine or rimantadine prophylaxis until 2 weeks after the vaccination (726).
   CATEGORY IB
4. To the extent possible, do not allow contact between those at high risk of complications from influenza and patients or staff who are taking amantadine or rimantadine for treatment of acute respiratory illness; prevent contact during and for two days after the latter discontinue treatment (633, 643–647).
   CATEGORY IB
D. Interruption of (Person-to-Person) Transmission of Microorganisms (See Section III, A-E above.)

REFERENCES: AS NUMBERED IN ORIGINAL PUBLICATION

1. Centers for Disease Control and Prevention. Guidelines for preventing the transmission of tuberculosis in health-care facilities, 1994. MMWR 1994;43:1–132.
2. Horan TC, White JW, Jarvis WR, et al. Nosocomial infection surveillance, 1984. MMWR 1986;35:17SS–29SS.
3. Schaberg DR, Culver DH, Gaynes RP. Major trends in the microbial etiology of nosocomial infection. Am J Med 1991;91(Suppl 3B):72S-75S.
4. Bartlett JG, O'Keefe P, Tally FP, et al. Bacteriology of hospital-acquired pneumonia. Arch Intern Med 1986;146:868–871.
5. Fagon JY, Chastre J, Domart Y, et al. Nosocomial pneumonia in patients receiving continuous mechanical ventilation: Prospective analysis of 52 episodes with use of a protected specimen brush and quantitative culture techniques. Am Rev Respir Dis 1989;139:877–884.
6. Torres A, Aznar R, Gatell JM, et al. Incidence, risk, and prognosis factors of nosocomial pneumonia in mechanically ventilated patients. Am Rev Respir Dis 1990;142:523–528.
7. Chastre J, Fagon JY, Soler P, et al. Diagnosis of nosocomial bacterial pneumonia in intubated patients undergoing ventilation: comparison of the usefulness of bronchoalveolar lavage and the protected specimen brush. Am J Med 1988;85:499–506.
8. Fagon J, Chastre J, Hance AJ, et al. Detection of nosocomial lung infection in ventilated patients: Use

of a protected specimen brush and quantitative culture technique in 147 patients. Am Rev Respir Dis 1988;138:110–116.

9. Chastre J, Viau F, Brun P, et al. Prospective evaluation of the protected specimen brush for the diagnosis of pulmonary infections in ventilated patients. Am Rev Respir Dis 1984;130:924–929.

10. Rello J, Quintana E, Ausina V, et al. Incidence, etiology, and outcome of nosocomial pneumonia in mechanically ventilated patients. Chest 1991;100:439–444.

11. Jimenez P, Torres A, Rodriguez-Riosin R, et al. Incidence and etiology of pneumonia acquired during mechanical ventilation. Crit Care Med 1989;17:882–885.

12. Pugin J, Auckenthaler R, Mili N, Janssens JP, Lew PD, Suter PM. Diagnosis of ventilator-associated pneumonia by bacteriologic analysis of bronchoscopic and nonbronchoscopic blind bronchoalveolar lavage fluid. Am Rev Respir Dis 1991;143:1121–1129.

13. Torres A, De La Bellacasa JP, Rodriguez-Riosin R, De Anta MT, Agusti-Vidal A. Diagnostic value of telescoping plugged catheters in mechanically ventilated patients with bacterial pneumonia using the metras catheter. Am Rev Respir Dis 1988;138:117–120.

14. Meduri GU, Beals DH, Meijub AG, Baselski V. Protected bronchoalveolar lavage: a new bronchoscopic technique to retrieve uncontaminated distal airway secretions. Am Rev Respir Dis 1991;143:855–864.

15. De Castro FR, Violan JS, Capuz BL, Luna JC, Rodriguez BG, Alonso JLM. Reliability of bronchoscopic protected catheter brush in the diagnosis of pneumonia in mechanically ventilated patients. Crit Care Med 1991;19:171–175.

16. Davidson M, Tempest B, Palmer DL. Bacteriologic diagnosis of acute pneumonia. JAMA 1976;235: 158–163.

17. Fagon JY, Chastre J, Hance AJ, Montravers P, Novara A, Gilbert C. Nosocomial pneumonia in ventilated patients: a cohort study evaluating attributable mortality and hospital stay. Am J Med 1993;94:281–288.

18. Higuchi JH, Coalson JJ, Johanson WG Jr. Bacteriologic diagnosis of nosocomial pneumonia in primates: usefulness of the protected specimen brush. Am Rev Respir Dis 1982;125:53–57.

19. Bryan CS, Reynolds KL. Bacteremic nosocomial pneumonia: analysis of 172 episodes from a single metropolitan area. Am Rev Respir Dis 1984;129:668–671.

20. Espersen F, Gabrielsen J. Pneumonia due to Staphylococcus aureus during mechanical ventilation. J Infect Dis 1981;144:19–23.

21. Inglis TJJ, Sproat LJ, Hawkey PM, Gibson JS. Staphylococcal pneumonia in ventilated patients: a twelve month review of cases in an intensive care unit. J Hosp Infect 1993;25:207–210.

22. Reusser P, Zimmerli W, Scheidegger D, Marbet GA, Buser M, Gyr K. Role of gastric colonization in nosocomial infections and endotoxemia: a prospective study in neurosurgical patients on mechanical ventilation. J Infect Dis 1989;160:414–421.

23. Johanson WG Jr, Pierce AK, Sanford JP, et al. Nosocomial respiratory infections with gram-negative bacilli: the significance of colonization of the respiratory tract. Ann Intern Med 1972;77:701–706.

24. Berger R, Arango L. Etiologic diagnosis of bacterial nosocomial pneumonia in seriously ill patients. Crit Care Med 1985;13:833–836.

25. Andrews CP, Coalson JJ, Smith JD, et al. Diagnosis of nosocomial bacterial pneumonia in acute, diffuse lung injury. Chest 1981;80:254–258.

26. Salata RA, Lederman MM, Shlaes DM, et al. Diagnosis of nosocomial pneumonia in intubated, intensive care unit patients. Am Rev Respir Dis 1987;136:426–432.

27. Pham LH, Brun-Buisson C, Legrand P, et al. Diagnosis of nosocomial pneumonia in mechanically ventilated patients: comparison of a plugged telescoping catheter with the protected specimen brush. Am Rev Respir Dis 1991;143:1055–1061.

28. Meduri GU. Ventilator-associated pneumonia in patients with respiratory failure. Chest 1990;97: 1208–1219.

29. Bell RC, Coalson JJ, Smith JD, Johanson WG Jr. Multiple organ system failure and infection in adult respiratory distress syndrome. Ann Intern Med 1983;99:293–298.

30. Tobin MJ, Grenvik A. Nosocomial lung infection and its diagnosis. Crit Care Med 1984;12:191–200.

31. Villers D, Deriennic M, Raffi R, et al. Reliability of the bronchoscopic protected catheter brush in intubated and ventilated patients. Chest 1985;88:527–530.

32. Guckian JC, Christensen WD. Quantitative culture and gram stain of sputum in pneumonia. Am Rev Respir Dis 1978;118:997–1005.

33. Lowry FD, Carlisle PS, Adams A, Feiner C. The incidence of nosocomial pneumonia following urgent endotracheal intubation. Infect Control 1987;8:245–248.

34. Craven DE, Kunches LM, Kilinsky V, Lichtenberg DA, Make BJ, McCabe WR. Risk factors for pneumonia and fatality in patients receiving continuous mechanical ventilation. Am Rev Respir Dis 1986;133:792–796.

35. Celis R, Torres A, Gatell JM, et al. Nosocomial pneumonia—a multivariate analysis of risk and prognosis. Chest 1988;93:318–324.

36. Garner JS, Jarvis WR, Emori TG, Horan TC, Hughes JM. CDC definitions for nosocomial infections, 1988. Am J Infect Control 1988;16:128–140.

37. Fagon JY, Chastre J, Hance AJ, Domart Y, Trouillet JL, Gibert C. Evaluation of clinical judgment in the identification and treatment of nosocomial pneumonia in ventilated patients. Chest 1993;103:547–553.

38. Baughman RP, Thorpe JE, Staneck J, et al. Use of the protected specimen brush in patients with endotracheal or tracheostomy tubes. Chest 1987;91:233–235.
39. Meduri GU, Wunderink RG, Leeper KV, Beals DH. Management of bacterial pneumonia in ventilated patients. The role of protected bronchoalveolar lavage. Chest 1992;101:500–508.
40. Bryant LR, Trinkle JK, Mobin-Uddin K, Baker J, Griffin WO. Bacterial colonization profile with tracheal intubation and mechanical ventilation. Arch Surg 1972;104:647–651.
41. Torres A, De La Bellacasa JP, Xaubet A, et al. Diagnostic value of quantitative cultures of bronchoalveolar lavage and telescoping plugged catheter in mechanically ventilated patients with bacterial pneumonia. Am Rev Respir Dis 1989;140:306–310.
42. Lambert RS, Vereen LE, George RB. Comparison of tracheal aspirates and protected brush catheter specimens for identifying pathogenic bacteria in mechanically ventilated patients. Am J Med Sci 1989;297:377–382.
43. Seidenfeld JJ, Pohl DF, Bell RC, et al. Incidence, site and outcome of infections in patients with the adult respiratory distress syndrome. Am Rev Respir Dis 1986;134:12–16.
44. Meduri GU, Chastre J. The standardization of bronchoscopic techniques for ventilator-associated pneumonia. Chest 1992;102(Suppl 1):557S-563S.
45. Baselski V, El-Torky M, Coalson SS, Griffin J. The standardization of criteria for processing and interpreting laboratory specimens. Chest 1992;102:571S-579S.
46. Wunderink RG, Mayhall G, Gibert C. Methodology for clinical investigation of ventilator-associated pneumonia: epidemiology and therapeutic intervention. Chest 1992;102(Suppl 1):580S-588S.
47. Martos JA, Ferrer M, Torres A, et al. Specificity of quantitative cultures of protected specimen brush and bronchoalveolar lavage in mechanically ventilated patients [Abstract]. Am Rev Respir Dis 1990;141:A276.
48. Marquette CH, Ramon P, Courcol R, et al. Bronchoscopic protected catheter brush for the diagnosis of pulmonary infections. Chest 1988;93:746–755.
49. Kahn FW, Jones JM. Diagnosing bacterial respiratory infection by bronchoalveolar lavage. J Infect Dis 1987;155:862–869.
50. Thorpe JE, Baughman RP, Frame PT, Wesseler TA, Staneck JL. Bronchoalveolar lavage for diagnosing acute bacterial pneumonia. J Infect Dis 1987;155:855–861.
51. Johanson WG Jr, Seidenfeld JJ, Gomez P, De los Santos R, Coalson JJ. Bacteriologic diagnosis of nosocomial pneumonia following prolonged mechanical ventilation. Am Rev Respir Dis 1988;137:259–264.
52. Guerra LF, Baughman PP. Use of bronchoalveolar lavage to diagnose bacterial pneumonia in mechanically ventilated patients. Crit Care Med 1990;18:169–173.
53. Chastre J, Fagon JY, Soler P, et al. Quantification of BAL cells containing intracellular bacteria rapidly identifies ventilated patients with nosocomial pneumonia. Chest 1989;95:190S–192S.
54. Rouby JJ, Rossignon MD, Nicolas MH, et al. A prospective study of protected bronchoalveolar lavage in the diagnosis of nosocomial pneumonia. Anesthesiology 1989;71:679–685.
55. Trouillet JL, Guiget M, Gibert C, et al. Fiberoptic bronchoscopy in ventilated patients. Evaluation of cardiopulmonary risk under midazolam sedation. Chest 1990;97:927–933.
56. Lindholm CE, Ollman B, Snyder JV, et al. Cardiorespiratory effects of flexible fiberoptic bronchoscopy in critically ill patients. Chest 1978;74:362–368.
57. Rouby JJ, De lasalle EM, Poete P, et al. Nosocomial bronchopneumonia in the critically ill. Am Rev Respir Dis 1992;146:1059–1066.
58. Piperno D, Gaussorgues P, Bachmann P, Jaboulay M, Robert D. Diagnostic value of nonbronchoscopic bronchoalveolar lavage during mechanical ventilation [Letter]. Chest 1988;93:223.
59. El-ebiary M, Torres A, Gonzalez J, et al. Quantitative cultures of endotracheal aspirates for the diagnosis of ventilator-associated pneumonia. Am Rev Respir Dis 1993;148:1552–1557.
60. Marquette CH, Georges H, Wallet F, et al. Diagnostic efficiency of endotracheal aspirates with quantitative bacterial cultures in intubated patients with suspected pneumonia. Am Rev Respir Dis 1993;148:138–144.
61. Emori TG, Gaynes RP. An overview of nosocomial infections, including the role of the microbiology laboratory. Clin Microbiol Rev 1993;6:428–442.
62. Garibaldi RA, Britt MR, Coleman ML, Reading JC, Pace NL. Risk factors for postoperative pneumonia. Am J Med 1981;70:677–680.
63. Haley RW, Hooton TM, Culver DH, et al. Nosocomial infections in U.S. hospitals, 1975–1976; estimated frequency by selected characteristics of patients. Am J Med 1981;70:947–959.
64. Emori TG, Banerjee SN, Culver DH, et al. Nosocomial infections in elderly patients in the United States, 1986–1990. Am J Med 1991;91(Suppl 3B):289S-293S.
65. Cross AS, Roup B. Role of respiratory assistance device in endemic nosocomial pneumonia. Am J Med 1981;70:681–685.
66. Jarvis WR, Edwards JR, Culver DH, et al. Nosocomial infection rates in adult and pediatric intensive care units in the United States. Am J Med 1991;91(Suppl 3B):185S-191S.
67. Rello J, Quintana E, Ausina V, et al. Risk factors for Staphylococcus aureus pneumonia in critically ill patients. Am Rev Respir Dis 1990;142:1320–1324.
68. Gaynes R, Bizek B, Mowry-Hanley J, et al. Risk factors for nosocomial pneumonia after coronary artery bypass graft operations. Ann Thorac Surg 1991;51:215–218.

69. Joshi N, Localio AR, Hamory BH. A predictive risk index for nosocomial pneumonia in the intensive care unit. Am J Med 1992;93:135–142.
70. Jacobs S, Chang RWS, Lee B, Bartlett FW. Continuous enteral feeding: a major cause of pneumonia among ventilated intensive care unit patients. J Parent Enter Nutr 1990;14:353–356.
71. Ashbaugh DC, Petty TL. Sepsis complicating the acute respiratory distress syndrome. Surg Gynecol Obstet 1972;135:865–868.
72. Chevret S, Hemmer M, Carlet J, Langer M, et al. Incidence and risk factors of pneumonia acquired in intensive care units. Intensive Care Med 1993;19:256–264.
73. Hanson LC, Wever DJ, Rutala WA. Risk factors for nosocomial pneumonia in the elderly. Am J Med 1992;92:161–166.
74. Kollef MH. Ventilator-associated pneumonia. JAMA 1993;270:1965–1970.
75. Craven DE, Kunches LM, Lichtenberg DA, et al. Nosocomial infection and fatality in medical and surgical intensive care unit patients. Arch Intern Med 1988;148:1161–1168.
76. Graybill JR, Marshall LW, Charache P, Wallace CK, Melvin VB. Nosocomial pneumonia—a continuing major problem. Am Rev Respir Dis 1973;108:1130–1140.
77. Gross PA, Van Antwerpen C. Nosocomial infections and hospital deaths. Am J Med 1983;75:658–662.
78. Stevens RM, Teres D, Skillman JJ, Feingold DS. Pneumonia in an intensive care unit. A 30-month experience. Arch Intern Med 1974;134:106–111.
79. Craig CP, Connelly S. Effect of intensive care unit nosocomial pneumonia on duration of stay and mortality. Am J Infect Control 1984;4:233–238.
80. Leu HS, Kaiser DL, Mori M, Woolson RF, Wenzel RP. Hospital-acquired pneumonia: attributable mortality and morbidity. Am J Epidemiol 1989;129:1258–1267.
81. Haley RW, Schaberg DR, Crowley KH, Von Allmen SD, McGowan JE Jr. Extra charges and prolongation of stay attributable to nosocomial infections: a prospective interhospital comparison. Am J Med 1981;70:51–58.
82. Freeman J, Rosner BA, McGowan JE. Adverse effects of nosocomial infection. J Infect Dis 1979;140:732–740.
83. Martone WJ, Jarvis WR, Culver DH, Haley RW. Incidence and nature of endemic and epidemic nosocomial infections. In: Bennett JV, Brachman PS, eds. Hospital Infections. 3rd ed. Boston: Little, Brown and Co., 1993:577–596.
84. Huxley EJ, Viroslav J, Gray WR, Pierce AK. Pharyngeal aspiration in normal adults and patients with depressed consciousness. Am J Med 1973;64:564–568.
85. Olivares L, Segovia A, Revuelta R. Tube feeding and lethal aspiration in neurologic patients: A review of 720 autopsy cases. Stroke 1974;5:654–657.
86. Spray SB, Zuidema GD, Cameron HL. Aspiration pneumonia: incidence of aspiration with endotracheal tubes. Am J Surg 1976;131:701–703.
87. Cameron JL, Reynolds J, Zuidema GD. Aspiration in patients with tracheostomies. Surg Gynecol Obstet 1973;136:68–70.
88. Johanson WG Jr, Pierce AK, Sanford JP. Changing pharyngeal bacterial flora of hospitalized patients. N Engl J Med 1969;281:1137–1140.
89. Niederman MS, Merrill WW, Ferranti RD. Nutritional status and bacterial binding in the lower respiratory tract in patients with chronic tracheostomy. Ann Intern Med 1984;100:795–800.
90. Reynolds HY. Bacterial adherence to respiratory tract mucosa: A dynamic interaction leading to colonization. Semin Respir Infect 1987;2:8–19.
91. Louria DB, Kanimski T. The effects of four antimicrobial drug regimens on sputum superinfection in hospitalized patients. Am Rev Respir Dis 1962;85:649–665.
92. Rosenthal S, Tager IB. Prevalence of gram-negative rods in the normal pharyngeal flora. Ann Intern Med 1975;83:355–357.
93. Mackowiak PA, Martin RM, Jones SR. Pharyngeal colonization by gram-negative bacilli in aspiration-prone persons. Arch Intern Med 1978;138:1224–1227.
94. Valenti WM, Trudell RG, Bentley DW. Factors predisposing to oropharyngeal colonization with gram-negative bacilli in the aged. N Engl J Med 1978;298:1108–1111.
95. Woods DE, Straus DC, Johanson WG, Berry VK, Bass JA. Role of pili in adherence of Pseudomonas aeruginosa to mammalian buccal epithelial cells. Infect Immun 1980;29:1146–1151.
96. Niederman MS. Bacterial adherence as a mechanism of airway colonization. Eur J Clin Microbiol Infect Dis 1989;8:15–20.
97. Johanson WG Jr, Higuchi JH, Chaudhuri TR. Bacterial adherence to epithelial cells in bacillary colonization of the respiratory tract. Am Rev Respir Dis 1980;121:55–63.
98. Abraham SN, Beachey EH, Simpson WA, et al. Adherence of Streptococcus pyogenes, Escherichia coli, and Pseudomonas aeruginosa to fibronectin-coated and uncoated epithelial cells. Infect Immun 1983;41:1261–1268.
99. Beachey EH. Bacterial adherence: adhesin-receptor interactions mediating the attachment of bacteria to mucosal surfaces. J Infect Dis 1981;143:325–345.
100. Woods DE, Straus DC, Johanson WG, Bass JA. Role of fibronectin in the prevention of adherence of Pseudomonas aeruginosa to buccal cells. J Infect Dis 1981;143:784–790.

101. Woods DE, Straus DC, Johanson WG, Bass JA. Role of salivary protease activity in adherence of gram-negative bacilli to mammalian buccal epithelial cells in vitro. J Clin Invest 1981;68:1435–1440.
102. Ramphal R, Small PM, Shands JW Jr, et al. Adherence of Pseudomonas aeruginosa to tracheal cells injured by influenza infection or by endotracheal intubation. Infect Immun 1980;27:614–619.
103. Niederman MS, Merrill WW, Polomski LM, Reynolds HY, Gee JBL. Influence of sputum IgA and elastase on tracheal cell bacterial adherence. Am Rev Respir Dis 1986;133:255–260.
104. Niederman MS, Raferty TD, Sasaki CT, et al. Comparison of bacterial adherence to ciliated and squamous epithelial cells obtained from the human respiratory tract. Am Rev Respir Dis 1983;127:85–90.
105. Franklin AL, Todd T, Gurman G, et al. Adherence of Pseudomonas aeruginosa to cilia of human tracheal epithelial cells. Infect Immun 1987;55:1523–1525.
106. Palmer LB, Merrill WW, Niederman MS, et al. Bacterial adherence to respiratory tract cells: relationships between in vivo and in vitro pH and bacterial attachments. Am Rev Respir Dis 1986:133:784–788.
107. Dal Nogare AR, Toews GB, Pierce AK. Increased salivary elastase precedes gram-negative bacillary colonization in postoperative patients. Am Rev Respir Dis 1987;135:671–675.
108. Proctor RA. Fibronectin: a brief overview of its structure, function, and physiology. Rev Infect Dis 1987;9:S317–S321.
109. Niederman MS, Mantovani R, Schoch P, et al. Patterns and routes of tracheobronchial colonization in mechanically ventilated patients: The role of nutritional status in colonization of the lower airway by Pseudomonas species. Chest 1989;95:155–161.
110. Atherton ST, White DJ. Stomach as source of bacteria colonising respiratory tract during artificial ventilation. Lancet 1978;2:968–969.
111. Du Moulin GC, Paterson DG, White JH, Lisbon A. Aspiration of gastric bacteria in antacid-treated patients: a frequent cause of postoperative colonisation of the airway. Lancet 1982;2:242–245.
112. Kappstein I, Friedrich T, Hellinger P. Incidence of pneumonia in mechanically ventilated patients treated with sucralfate or cimetidine as prophylaxis for stress bleeding: bacterial colonization of the stomach. Am J Med 1991;91(Suppl 2A):125S–131S.
113. Daschner F, Kappstein I, Reuschenbach K, Pfisterer J, Krieg N, Vogel W. Stress ulcer prophylaxis and ventilation pneumonia: prevention by antibacterial cytoprotective agents? Infect Control 1988; 9:59–65.
114. Torres A, El-ebiary M, Gonzalez J, et al. Gastric and pharyngeal flora in nosocomial pneumonia acquired during mechanical ventilation. Am Rev Respir Dis 1993;148:352–357.
115. Martin LF, Booth FVM, Karlstadt RG, et al. Continuous intravenous cimetidine decreases stress-related upper gastrointestinal hemorrhage without promoting pneumonia. Crit Care Med 1993;21:19–29.
116. Inglis TJJ, Sherratt MJ, Sproat LJ, Gibson JS, Hawkey PM. Gastroduodenal dysfunction and bacterial colonisation of the ventilated lung. Lancet 1993;341:911–913.
117. Pingleton SK, Hinthron DR, Liu C. Enteral nutrition in patients receiving mechanical ventilation: Multiple sources of tracheal colonization include the stomach. Am J Med 1986;80:827–832.
118. Driks MR, Craven DE, Celli BR, et al. Nosocomial pneumonia in intubated patients given sucralfate as compared with antacids or histamine type 2 blockers. N Engl J Med 1987;317:1376–1382.
119. Drasar BS, Shiner M, McLeod GM. Studies of the intestinal flora. I. The bacterial flora of the gastrointestinal tract in healthy and achlorhydric persons. Gastroenterology 1969;56:71–79.
120. Garrod LP. A study of the bactericidal power of hydrochloric acid and of gastric juice. St Barth Hosp Rep 1939;72:145–167.
121. Arnold I. The bacterial flora within the stomach and small intestine: the effect of experimental alterations of acid-base balance and the age of the subject. Am J Med Sci 1933;186:471–481.
122. Ruddell WSJ, Axon ATR, Findlay JM. Effect of cimetidine on the gastric bacterial flora. Lancet 1980;1:672–674.
123. Donowitz LG, Page MC, Mileur BL, Guenthner SH. Alteration of normal gastric flora in critical patients receiving antacid and cimetidine therapy. Infect Control 1986;7:23–26.
124. Priebe HJ, Skillman JJ, Bushnell LS, Long PC, Silen W. Antacid versus cimetidine in preventing acute gastrointestinal bleeding. N Engl J Med 1992;302:426–430.
125. Zinner MJ, Zuidema GD, Smith PL, Mignosa M. The prevention of upper gastrointestinal tract bleeding in patients in an intensive care unit. Surg Gynecol Obstet 1981;153:214–220.
126. Reinarz JA, Pierce AK, Mays BB, Sanford JP. The potential role of inhalation therapy equipment in nosocomial pulmonary infection. J Clin Invest 1965;44:831–839.
127. Schulze T, Edmondson EB, Pierce AK, Sanford JP. Studies on a new humidifying device as a potential source of bacterial aerosol. Am Rev Respir Dis 1967;96:517–519.
128. Pierce AK, Sanford JP, Thomas GD, Leonard JS. Long-term evaluation of decontamination of inhalation-therapy equipment and the occurrence of necrotizing pneumonia. N Engl J Med 1970; 292:528–531.
129. Edmondson EB, Reinarz JA, Pierce AK, Sanford JP. Nebulization equipment: a potential source of infection in gram-negative pneumonias. Am J Dis Child 1966;111:357–360.
130. Pierce AK, Sanford JP. Bacterial contamination of aerosols. Arch Intern Med 1973;131:156–159.
131. Brain JD, Valberg PA. Deposition of aerosol in the respiratory tract. Am Rev Respir Dis 1979;120:1325–1373.

132. Rhame FS, Streifel A, McComb C, Boyle M. Bubbling humidifiers produce microaerosols which can carry bacteria. Infect Control 1986;7:403–407.
133. Deitch EA, Berg R. Bacterial translocation from the gut: a mechanism of infection. J Burn Care Rehab 1987;8:475–482.
134. Fiddian-Green RG, Baaker S. Nosocomial pneumonia in the critically ill: product of aspiration or translocation? Crit Care Med 1991;19:763–769.
135. Harkness GA, Bentley DW, Roghmann KJ. Risk factors for nosocomial pneumonia in the elderly. Am J Med 1990;89:457–463.
136. Windsor JA, Hill GL. Risk factors for postoperative pneumonia. Ann Surg 1988;208:209–214.
137. Penn RG, Sanders WE, Sanders CC. Colonization of the oropharynx with gram-negative bacilli: a major antecedent to nosocomial pneumonia. Am J Infect Control 1981;9:25–34.
138. Lepper MH, Kofman S, Blatt N, et al. Effect of eight antibiotics used singly and in combination on the tracheal flora following tracheostomy in poliomyelitis. Antibiot Chemother 1954;4:829–833.
139. Klick JM, Du Moulin GC, Hedley-Whyte J, Teres D, Bushnell LS, Feingold DS. Prevention of gram-negative bacillary pneumonia using polymyxin aerosol as prophylaxis. J Clin Invest 1975;55:514–519.
140. Feeley TW, Du Moulin GC, Hedley-Whyte J, Bushnell LS, Gilbert JP, Feingold DS. Aerosol polymyxin and pneumonia in seriously ill patients. N Engl J Med 1975;293:471–475.
141. Sprunt K, Redman W. Evidence suggesting importance of role of interbacterial inhibition in maintaining balance of normal flora. Ann Intern Med 1968;68:579–590.
142. Sprunt K, Leidy G, Redman W. Abnormal colonization of neonates in an ICU: conversion to normal colonization by pharyngeal implantation of alpha hemolytic streptococcus strain 215. Petiatr Res 1980;14:308–313.
143. Klastersky J, Huysmans E, Werts D, Hensgens C, Daneau D. Endotracheally administered gentamicin for the prevention of infections of the respiratory tract in patients with tracheostomy: a double-blind study. Chest 1974;65:650–654.
144. Greenfield S, Teres D, Bushnell LS, Hedley-Whyte J, Feingold DS. Prevention of gram-negative bacillary pneumonia using aerosol polymyxin as prophylaxis. J Clin Invest 1973;52:2935–2940.
145. Daschner F. Stress ulcer prophylaxis and the risk of nosocomial pneumonia in artificially ventilated patients. Eur J Clin Microbiol 1987;6:129–131.
146. Goularte TA, Lichtenberg DA, Craven DE. Gastric colonization in patients receiving antacids and mechanical ventilation: a mechanism for pharyngeal colonization [Abstract]. Am J Infect Control 1986;14:88.
147. Prod'hom G, Leuenberger PH, Koerfer J, et al. Nosocomial pneumonia in mechanically ventilated patients receiving antacid, ranitidine, or sucralfate as prophylaxis for stress ulcer. Ann Intern Med 1994;120:653–662.
148. Tryba M. Risk of acute stress bleeding and nosocomial pneumonia in ventilated intensive care unit patients: sucralfate versus antacids. Am J Med 1987;83(Suppl 3B):117–124.
149. Tryba M, Mantey-Stiers F. Antibacterial activity of sucralfate in human gastric juice. Am J Med 1987;83(Suppl 3B):125–127.
150. Lacroix J, Infante-Rivard C, Jenicek M, Gauthier M. Prophylaxis of upper gastrointestinal bleeding in intensive care units: a meta-analysis. Crit Care Med 1991;19:942–949.
151. Laggner AN, Lenz K, Base W, Druml WC, Schneeweiss B, Grimm G. Prevention of upper gastrointestinal bleeding in long-term ventilated patients. Sucralfate versus ranitidine. Am J Med 1989;86(Suppl 6A):81–84.
152. Ryan P, Dawson J, Teres D, Navab F. Continuous infusion of cimetidine versus sucralfate: Incidence of pneumonia and bleeding compared [Abstract]. Crit Care Med 1990;18(Suppl):253.
153. Pickworth KK, Falcone RE, Hoogeboom JE, Santanello SA. Occurrence of nosocomial pneumonia in mechanically ventilated trauma patients: a comparison of sucralfate and ranitidine. Crit Care Med 1993;21:1856–1862.
154. Cook DJ, Laine LA, Guyatt GH, Raffin TA. Nosocomial pneumonia and the role of gastric pH. A meta-analysis. Chest 1991;100:7–13.
155. Stoutenbeek CP, Van Saene HKF, Miranda DR, Zandstra DF. The effect of selective decontamination of the digestive tract on colonisation and infection rate in multiple trauma patients. Intensive Care Med 1984;10:185–192.
156. Unertl K, Ruckdeschel G, Selbmann K, et al. Prevention of colonization and respiratory infections in long-term ventilated patients by local antimicrobial prophylaxis. Intensive Care Med 1987;13:106–113.
157. Kerver JH, Rommes JH, Mevissen-Verhage EAE, et al. Prevention of colonization and infection in critically ill patients: a prospective study. Crit Care Med 1988;16:1087–1093.
158. Ledingham IM, Alcock SR, Eastaway AT, McDonald JG, Mckay I, Ramsay G. Triple regimen of selective decontamination of the digestive tract, systemic cefotaxime, and microbiological surveillance for prevention of acquired infection in intensive care. Lancet 1988;i:785–790.
159. Brun-Buisson C, Legrand P, Rauss A, et al. Intestinal decontamination for control of nosocomial multiresistant gram-negative bacilli: study of an outbreak in an intensive care unit. Ann Intern Med 1989;110:873–881.
160. Ulrich C, Harinck-de Weerd JE, Bakker NC, Jacz K, Doornbos L, de Ridder VA. Selective decontami-

nation of the digestive tract with norfloxacin in the prevention of ICU-acquired infections: a prospective randomized study. Intensive Care Med 1989;15:424–431.

161. Flaherty J, Nathan C, Kabins SA, Weinstein RA. Pilot trial of selective decontamination for prevention of bacterial infection in an intensive care unit. J Infect Dis 1990;162:1393–1397.

162. Godard J, Guillaume C, Reverdy ME, et al. Intestinal decontamination in a polyvalent ICU. Intensive Care Med 1990;16:307–311.

163. McClelland P, Murray AE, Williams PS, et al. Reducing sepsis in severe combined acute renal and respiratory failure by selective decontamination of the digestive tract. Crit Care Med 1990;18:935–939.

164. Rodriguez-Roldan JM, Altuna-Cuesta A, Lopez A, et al. Prevention of nosocomial lung infection in ventilated patients: use of an antimicrobial pharyngeal nonabsorbable paste. Crit Care Med 1990;180:1239–1242.

165. Tetteroo GWM, Wagenvoort JHT, Casterlein A, Tilanus HW, Ince C, Buining HA. Selective decontamination to reduce gram-negative colonisation and infections after oesophageal resection. Lancet 1990;335:704–707.

166. Aerdts SJA, van Daelen R, Clasener HAL, Festen J, Van Lier HJJ, Vollaard EJ. Antibiotic prophylaxis of respiratory tract infection in mechanically ventilated patients: a prospective, blinded, randomized trial of the effect of a novel regimen. Chest 1991;100:783–791.

167. Blair P, Rowlands BJ, Lowry K, Webb H, Armstrong P, Smilie J. Selective decontamination of the digestive tract: a stratified, randomized, prospective study in a mixed intensive care unit. Surgery 1991;110:303–310.

168. Fox MA, Peterson S, Fabri BM, Van Saene HKF, Williets T. Selective decontamination of the digestive tract in cardiac surgical patients. Crit Care Med 1991;19:1486–1490.

169. Hartenauer U, Thulig B, Diemer W, et al. Effect of selective flora suppression on colonization, infection, and mortality in critically ill patients: a one-year, prospective consecutive study. Crit Care Med 1991;19:463–473.

170. Pugin J, Auckenthaler R, Lew DP, Suter PM. Oropharyngeal decontamination decreases incidence of ventilator-associated pneumonia: a randomized, placebo-controlled, double-blind clinical trial. JAMA 1991;265:2704–2710.

171. Vandenbroucke-Grauls CMJE, Vandenbroucke JP. Effect of selective decontamination of the digestive tract on respiratory tract infections and mortality in the intensive care unit. Lancet 1991;338:859–862.

172. Cockerill FR, Muller SM, Anhalt JP, et al. Prevention of infection on critically ill patients by selective decontamination of the digestive tract. Ann Intern Med 1992;117:545–553.

173. Gastinne H, Wolff M, Destour F, Faurisson F, Chevret S. A controlled trial in intensive care units of selective decontamination of the digestive tract with nonabsorbable antibiotics. N Engl J Med 1992;326:594–599.

174. Hammond JMJ, Potgieter PD, Saunders GL, Forder AA. A double blind study of selective decontamination in intensive care. Lancet 1992;340:5–9.

175. Rocha LA, Martin MJ, Pita S, et al. Prevention of nosocomial infection in critically ill patients by selective decontamination of the digestive tract. Intensive Care Med 1992;18:398–404.

176. Winter R, Humphreys H, Pick A, MacGowan P, Wilatts SM, Speller DCE. A controlled trial of selective decontamination of the digestive tract in intensive care and its effect on nosocomial infection. J Antimicrob Chemother 1992;30:73–87.

177. Korinek AM, Laisne MJ, Nicolas MH, Raskine S, Deroin V, Sanson-Lepors MJ. Selective decontamination of the digestive tract in neurosurgical intensive care unit patients: a double-blind, randomized, placebo-controlled study. Crit Care Med 1993;21:1466–1473.

178. Selective Decontamination of the Digestive Tract Trialists' Collaborative Group. Meta-analysis of randomised controlled trials of selective decontamination of the digestive tract. Br Med J 1993;307:525–532.

179. Ferrer M, Torres A, Gonzalez J, et al. Utility of selective decontamination in mechanically ventilated patients. Ann Intern Med 1994;120:389–395.

180. Nau R, Ruchel R, Mergerian H, Wegener U, Winkelmann T, Prange HW. Emergence of antibiotic-resistant bacteria during selective decontamination of the digestive tract. J Antimicrob Chemother 1990;25:881–883.

181. Heyland D, Bradley C, Mandell LA. Effect of acidified enteral feedings on gastric colonization in the critically ill patient. Crit Care Med 1992;20:1388–1394.

182. Bartlett JG, Gorbach SL. The triple threat of aspiration pneumonia. Chest 1975;68:560–566.

183. Winterbauer RH, Durning RB, Barron E, McFadden MC. Aspirated nasogastric feeding solution detected by glucose strips. Ann Intern Med 1981;95:67–68.

184. Nair P, Jani K, Sanderson PJ. Transfer of oropharyngeal bacteria into the trachea during endotracheal intubation. J Hosp Infect 1986;8:96–103.

185. Treolar DM, Stechmiller J. Pulmonary aspiration of tube-fed patients with artificial airways. Heart Lung 1984;13:667–671.

186. Metheny NA, Eisenberg P, Spies M. Aspiration pneumonia in patients fed through nasoenteral tubes. Heart Lung 1986;15:256–261.

187. Cheadle WG, Vitale GC, Mackie CR, Cuschiere A. Prophylactic postoperative nasogastric decompression. Ann Surg 1985;202:361–366.

188. Ibanez J, Penafiel A, Raurich J. Gastroesophageal reflux and aspiration of gastric contents during nasogastric feeding; the effect of posture [Abstract]. Intensive Care Med 1988;14(Suppl 2):296.
189. Anderson KR, Norris DJ, Godfrey LB, et al. Bacterial contamination of the tube-feeding formulas. J Parent Enter Nutr 1984;8:673–678.
190. Schroeder P, Fisher D, Volz M. Microbial contamination of enteral feeding solutions in a community hospital. J Parent Enter Nutr 1983;7:459–461.
191. Thurn J, Crossley K, Gerdts A, et al. Enteral hyperalimentation as a source of nosocomial infection. J Hosp Infect 1990;15:203–217.
192. Civil ID, Schwab CW. The effect of enteral feeding on gastric pH. Am Surg 1987;12:688–690.
193. Lee B, Chang RWS, Jacobs S. Intermittent nasogastric feeding: a simple and effective method to reduce pneumonia among ventilated ICU patients. Clin Intensive Care 1990;1:100–102.
194. Torres A, Serra-Battles J, Ros E, et al. Pulmonary aspiration of gastric contents in patients receiving mechanical ventilation: the effect of body position. Ann Intern Med 1992;116:540–542.
195. Wynne JW, Modell JH. Respiratory aspiration of stomach contents. Ann Intern Med 1977;87:466–474.
196. Betcher E, Seltzer M, Slocum M, et al. Complications occurring during enteral nutritional support: a prospective study. J Parent Enter Nutr 1983;7:546–552.
197. Bernard M, Forlaw L. Complications and their prevention. In: Rombeau J, Caldwell M, eds. Clinical nutrition. Vol. I: Enteral and tube feeding. Philadelphia: W.B. Saunders, Co., 1984:534.
198. Dohbie RP, Hoffmeister JA. Continuous pump-tube enteric hyperalimentation. Surg Gynecol Obstet 1976;143:273–276.
199. Strong RM, Condon SC, Solinger MR, et al. Equal aspiration rates from postpylorus and intragastric-placed feeding tubes: a randomized, prospective study. J Parent Enter Nutr 1992;16:59–63.
200. Montecalvo M, Steger KA, Farber HW, et al. Nutritional outcome and pneumonia in critical care patients randomized to gastric versus jejunal tube feedings. Crit Care Med 1992;20:1377–1387.
201. Sanderson PJ. Colonisation of the trachea in ventilated patients. What is the bacterial pathway? J Hosp Infect 1983;4:15–18.
202. Sottile FD, Marrie TJ, Prough DS, et al. Nosocomial pulmonary infection: possible etiologic significance of bacterial adhesion to endotracheal tubes. Crit Care Med 1986;14:265–270.
203. Inglis TJJ, Jones JG, Newman SP. Gas-liquid interaction with tracheal tube biofilm: a means of bacterial colonisation of the lung. Br J Hosp Med 1989;42:141–142.
204. Inglis TJJ, Millar MR, Jones JG, Robinson DA. Tracheal tube biofilm as a source of bacterial colonisation of the lung. J Clin Microbiol 1989;27:2014–2018.
205. McCrae W, Wallace P. Aspiration around high volume, low pressure endotracheal cuff. Br Med J 1981;2:1220–1221.
206. Mahul Ph, Auboyer C, Jospe R, et al. Prevention of nosocomial pneumonia in intubated patients: respective role of mechanical subglottic drainage and stress ulcer prophylaxis. Intensive Care Med 1992;18:20–25.
207. Weinstein RA, Nathan C, Gruensfelder R. Endemic aminoglycoside resistance in gram-negative bacilli: epidemiology and mechanisms. J Infect Dis 1980;141:338–345.
208. Maki DG. Control of colonization and transmission of pathogenic bacteria in the hospital. Ann Intern Med 1979;89:777–780.
209. Larson E. Persistent carriage of gram-negative bacteria on hands. Am J Infect Control 1981;9:112–119.
210. Adams BG, Marrie TJ. Hand carriage of gram-negative rods may not be transient. J Hyg 1982;89:33–46.
211. Daschner FD. The transmission of infections in hospitals by staff carriers, methods of prevention and control. Infect Control 1985;6:97–98.
212. Adams BG, Marrie TJ. Hand carriage of aerobic gram-negative rods by health care personnel. J Hyg 1982;89:23–31.
213. Marples RR, Towers AG. A laboratory model for the investigation of contact transfer of micro-organisms. J Hyg 1979;82:237–248.
214. Casewell M, Phillips I. Hands as a route of transmission of Klebsiella species. Br Med J 1977;2:1315–1317.
215. Gorman LJ, Sanai L, Notman AW, Grant IS, Masterton RG. Cross infection in an intensive care unit by Klebsiella pneumoniae from ventilator condensate. J Hosp Infect 1993;23:27–34.
216. Cadwallader HL, Bradley CR, Ayliffe GAJ. Bacterial contamination and frequency of changing ventilator circuitry. J Hosp Infect 1990;15:65–72.
217. Mortimer EA, Lipsitz PJ, Wolinsky E, et al. Transmission of staphylococci between newborns. Am J Dis Child 1962;104:289–295.
218. Lowbury EJL, Lilly HA, Bull JP. Disinfection of hands: removal of transient organisms. Br Med J 1964;2:230–233.
219. Sprunt K, Redman W, Leidy G. Antibacterial effectiveness of routine handwashing. Pediatrics 1973;52:264–271.
220. Steere AC, Mallison GF. Handwashing practices for the prevention of nosocomial infections. Ann Intern Med 1975;83:683–690.
221. Albert RK, Condie F. Hand-washing patterns in medical intensive care units. N Engl J Med 1981;304:146–147.

222. Doebbeling BN, Stanley GL, Sheetz CT, et al. Comparative efficacy of alternative hand-washing agents in reducing nosocomial infections in intensive care units. N Engl J Med 1992;327:88–93.
223. Simmons B, Bryant J, Neiman K, Spencer L, Arheart K. The role of handwashing in prevention of endemic intensive care unit infections. Infect Control Hosp Epidemiol 1990;11:589–594.
224. Garner JS, HICPAC. Draft guideline for isolation precautions in hospitals. Federal Register 1994;59(Part V):55552–55570.
225. Garner JS, Simmons BP. Guideline for handwashing and environmental control. Infect Control 1986;7:231–242.
226. LeClair JM, Freeman J, Sullivan BF, Crowley CM, Goldmann DA. Prevention of nosocomial respiratory syncytial virus infections through compliance with glove and gown isolation precautions. N Engl J Med 1987;317:329–333.
227. Klein BS, Perloff WH, Maki DG, et al. Reduction of nosocomial infection during pediatric intensive care by protective isolation. N Engl J Med 1989;320:1714–1721.
228. Doebbeling BN, Pfaller MA, Houston AK, Wenzel RP. Removal of nosocomial pathogens from the contaminated glove. Ann Intern Med 1988;109:394–398.
229. Maki DG, McCormick RD, Zilz MA, et al. An MRSA outbreak in a SICU during universal precautions: new epidemiology for nosocomial MRSA; downside for universal precautions (UPs) [Abstract]. Abstracts of the 30th Interscience Conference on Antimicrobial Agents and Chemotherapy 1990;165.
230. Patterson JE, Vecchio J, Pantelick EL, et al. Association of contaminated gloves with transmission of Acinetobacter calcoaceticus var. anitratus in an intensive care unit. Am J Med 1991;91:479–483.
231. Korniewicz DM, Laughon BE, Cyr WH, Lytle CD, Larson E. Leakage of virus through used vinyl and latex examination gloves. J Clin Microbiol 1990;28:787–788.
232. Pandit SK, Mehta S, Agarwal SC. Risk of cross-infection from inhalation anesthetic equipment. Br J Anaesth 1967;39:838–844.
233. Cunha BA, Klimek JJ, Gracewski J, McLaughlin JC, Quintiliani R. A common source outbreak of Acinetobacter pulmonary infection traced to Wright respirometers. Postgrad Med J 1980;56:169–172.
234. Phillips J. Pseudomonas aeruginosa respiratory tract infections in patients receiving mechanical ventilation. J Hyg 1967;65:229–235.
235. Wheeler PW, Lancaster D, Kaiser AB. Bronchopulmonary cross-colonization and infection related to mycobacterial contamination of suction valves of bronchoscopes. J Infect Dis 1989;159:954–958.
236. Fraser VJ, Jones M, Murray PR, Medoff F, Zhang Y, Wallace RJ. Contamination of flexible fiberoptic bronchoscopes with Mycobacterium chelonae linked to an automated bronchoscope disinfection machine. Am Rev Respir Dis 1992;145:853–855.
237. Grieble HG, Colton FR, Thomas MS, et al. Fine particle humidifiers: source of Pseudomonas aeruginosa infections in a respiratory-disease unit. N Engl J Med 1970;282:531–533.
238. Mertz JJ, Scharer L, McClement JH. A hospital outbreak of Klebsiella pneumonia from inhalation therapy with contaminated aerosols. Am Rev Respir Dis 1967;95:454–460.
239. Ringrose RE, McKown B, Felton FG, Barclay BO, Muchmore HG, Rhoades ER. A hospital outbreak of Serratia marcescens associated with ultrasonic nebulizers. Ann Intern Med 1968;69:719–729.
240. Rhoades ER, Ringrose R, Mohr JA, Brooks L, McKown BA, Felton F. Contamination of ultrasonic neb ulization equipment with gram negative bacteria. Arch Intern Med 1971;127:228–232.
241. Arnow PM, Chou T, Weil D, Shapiro EN, Kretzschmar C. Nosocomial Legionnaires' disease caused by aerosolized tap water from respiratory devices. J Infect Dis 1982;146:460–467.
242. Craven DE, Lichtenberg DA, Goularte TA, Make BJ, McCabe WR. Contaminated medication nebulizers in mechanical ventilator circuits. Am J Med 1984;77:834–838.
243. Babington PCB, Baker AB, Johnson HH. Retrograde spread of organisms from ventilator to patient via the expiratory limb. Lancet 1971;1:61–63.
244. Smith JR, Howland WS. Endotracheal tube as a source of infection. JAMA 1959;169:343–345.
245. Irwin RS, Demers RR, Pratter MR. An outbreak of Acinetobacter infection associated with the use of a ventilator spirometer. Respir Care 1980;25:232–237.
246. Gough J, Kraak WAG, Anderson EC, Nichols WW, Slack MPE, McGhie D. Cross-infection by non-encapsulated Haemophilus influenzae. Lancet 1990;336:159–160.
247. Dyer ED, Peterson DE. How far do bacteria travel from the exhalation valve of IPPB equipment? Anesth Analg 1972;51:516–519.
248. Hovig B. Lower respiratory tract infections associated with respiratory therapy and anesthesia equipment. J Hosp Infect 1981;2:301–315.
249. Carson LA, Favero MS, Bond WW, Petersen NJ. Morphological, biochemical, and growth characteristics of Pseudomonas cepacia from distilled water. Appl Microbiol 1973;25:476–483.
250. Favero MS, et al. Pseudomonas aeruginosa: growth in distilled water from hospitals. Science 1971;173:836–838.
251. Carson LA, Petersen NJ, Favero MS, Aguero SM. Growth characteristics of atypical mycobacteria in water and their comparative resistance to disinfectants. Appl Environ Microbiol 1978;36:839–846.
252. Zuravleff JJ, Yu VL, Shonnard JW, Best M. Legionella pneumophila contamination of a hospital humidifier: demonstration of aerosol transmission and subsequent subclinical infection in exposed guinea pigs. Am Rev Respir Dis 1983;128:657–661.

253. Gorman GW, Yu VL, Brown A. Isolation of Pittsburgh pneumonia agent from nebulizers used in respiratory therapy. Ann Intern Med 1980;93:572–573.
254. Habeeb AFSA, Hiramoto R. Reaction of proteins with glutaraldehyde. Arch Biochem 1968;126:16.
255. Fierer J, Taylor PM, Gezon HM. Pseudomonas aeruginosa epidemic traced to delivery-room resuscitators. N Engl J Med 1967;276:991–996.
256. Berthelot P, Grattard F, Mahul P, et al. Ventilator temperature sensors: an unusual source of Pseudomonas cepacia in nosocomial infection. J Hosp Infect 1993;25:33–43.
257. Weems JJ. Nosocomial outbreak of Pseudomonas cepacia associated with contamination of reusable electronic ventilator temperature probes. Infect Control Hosp Epidemiol 1993;14:583–586.
258. Mastro TD, Fields BS, Breiman RF, Campbell J, Plikaytis BD, Spika JS. Nosocomial Legionnaires' disease and use of medication nebulizers. J Infect Dis 1991;163:667–670.
259. Cefai C, Richards J, Gould FK, McPeake P. An outbreak of Acinetobacter respiratory tract infection resulting from incomplete disinfection of ventilatory equipment. J Hosp Infect 1990;15:177–182.
260. Spaulding EH. Chemical sterilization of surgical instruments. Surg Gynecol Obstet 1939;69:738–744.
261. Snow JC, Mangiaracine AB, Anderson ML. Sterilization of anesthesia equipment with ethylene oxide. N Engl J Med 1962;266:443–445.
262. Roberts FJ, Cockcroft WH, Johnson HE. A hot water disinfection method for inhalation therapy equipment. Can Med Assoc J 1969;101:30–32.
263. Nelson EJ, Ryan KJ. A new use for pasteurization: disinfection of inhalation therapy equipment. Respir Care 1971;16:97–103.
264. Craig DB, Cowan SA, Forsyth W, Parker SE. Disinfection of anesthesia equipment by a mechanical pasteurization method. Can Anaesth Soc J 1975;22:219–223.
265. Smith MD, Box T, Pocklington ML, Kelsey MC. An evaluation of the Hamo LS-76 washing, drying and disinfecting machine for anaesthetic equipment. J Hosp Infect 1992;22:149–157.
266. Favero MS. Principles of sterilization and disinfection. Anesth Clin N Am 1989;7:941–949.
267. Favero MS, Bond WW. Clinical disinfection of medical and surgical materials. In: Block S, ed. Disinfection, sterilization, and preservation. 4th ed. Philadelphia: Lea and Febiger, 1991:617–641.
268. Haselhuhn DH, Brason FW, Borick PM. "In-use study" of buffered glutaraldehyde for cold sterilization of anesthesia equipment. Anesth Analg 1967;46:468–474.
269. Moffet HL, Williams T. Bacteria recovered from distilled water and inhalation therapy equipment. Am J Dis Child 1967;114:7–12.
270. Highsmith AK, Emori TG, Aguero SM, Favero MS, Hughes JM. Heterotrophic bacteria isolated from hospital water system. International Symposium on Water-Related Health Issues 1986;181–187.
271. Alary MA, Joly JR. Factors contributing to the contamination of hospital water distribution systems by Legionellae. J Infect Dis 1992;165:565–569.
272. Olson BH, Nagy LA. Microbiology of potable water. In: Laskin AI, ed. Advances in applied microbiology. Orlando, FL: Academic Press, Inc., 1984:73–132.
273. Rutala WA, Clontz EP, Weber DJ, Hoffman KK. Disinfection practices for endoscopes and other semicritical items. Infect Control Hosp Epidemiol 1991;12:282–288.
274. Gerding DN, Peterson LR, Vennes JA. Cleaning and disinfection of fiberoptic endoscopes: Evaluation of glutaraldehyde exposure time and forced-air drying. Gastroenterology 1982;83:613–618.
275. Alfa MJ, Sitter DL. In-hospital evaluation of contamination of duodenoscopes: a quantitative assessment of the effect of drying. J Hosp Infect 1991;19:89–98.
276. Ansari SA, Springhope VS, Sattar SA, Tostowaryk W, Wells GA. Comparison of cloth, paper, and warm air drying in eliminating viruses and bacteria from washed hands. Am J Infect Control 1991;19:243–249.
277. Martin MA, Reichelderfer M, APIC 1991, 1992, and 1993 APIC Guidelines Committee. APIC guideline for infection prevention and control in flexible endoscopy. Am J Infect Control 1994;22:19–38.
278. Holdcroft A, Lumley J, Gaya H, et al. Why disinfect ventilators? Lancet 1973;1:240–242.
279. Bishop C, Roper WAG, Williams SR. The use of an absolute filter to sterilize the inspiratory air during intermittent positive pressure respiration. Br J Anaesth 1963;35:32–34.
280. Hellewell J. The Williams bacterial filter, use in the intensive care unit. Anaesthesia 1967;22:497–503.
281. Buckley PM. Increase in resistance of in-line breathing filters in humidified air. Br J Anaesth 1984;56:637–643.
282. Christopher KL, Saravolatz LD, Bush TL. Cross-infection: a study using a canine model for pneumonia. Am Rev Respir Dis 1983;128:271–275.
283. Goularte TA, Manning M, Craven DE. Bacterial colonization in humidifying cascade reservoirs after 24 and 48 hours of continuous mechanical ventilation. Infect Control 1987;8:200–203.
284. Vesley D, Anderson J, Halbert MM, Wyman L. Bacterial output from three respiratory therapy humidifying devices. Respir Care 1979;24:228–234.
285. Boyce JM, White RL, Spruill EY, Wall M. Cost-effective application of the Centers for Disease Control guideline for prevention of nosocomial pneumonia. Am J Infect Control 1985;13:228–232.
286. Craven DE, Goularte TA, Make BA. Contaminated condensate in mechanical ventilator circuits—risk factor for nosocomial pneumonia? Am Rev Respir Dis 1984;129:625–628.
287. Lareau SC, Ryan KJ, Diener CF. The relationship between frequency of ventilator circuit changes and infectious hazard. Am Rev Respir Dis 1978;118:493–496.

288. Craven DE, Connolly MG, Lichtenberg DA, Primeau PJ, McCabe WR. Contamination of mechanical ventilators with tubing changes every 24 or 48 hours. N Engl J Med 1982;306:1505–1509.
289. Dreyfuss D, Djedaini K, Weber P, et al. Prospective study of nosocomial pneumonia and of patient and circuit colonization during mechanical ventilation with circuit changes every 48 hours vs no change. Am Rev Respir Dis 1991;143:738–743.
290. Miyao H, Hirokawa T, Miyasaka K, Kawazoe T. Relative humidity, not absolute humidity, is of great importance when using a humidifier with a heating wire. Crit Care Med 1992;20:674–679.
291. MacIntyre NR, Anderson HR, Silver RM. Pulmonary function in mechanically-ventilated patients using 24-hour use of a hygroscopic condenser humidifier. Chest 1983;84:560–564.
292. Make BJ, Craven DE, O'Donnell C. Clinical and bacteriologic comparison of hygroscopic and cascade humidifiers in ventilated patients [Abstract]. Am Rev Respir Dis 1987;135:A212.
293. Suzukawa M, Usuda Y, Numata K. The effects on sputum characteristics of combining an unheated humidifier with a heat-moisture exchanging filter. Respir Care 1989;34:976–984.
294. Hay R, Millar WC. Efficacy of a new hygroscopic condenser humidifier. Crit Care Med 1982;10:49–51.
295. Mebius C. A comparative study of disposable humidifiers. Acta Anaesth Scand 1983;27:403–409.
296. Shelly MP, Bethune DW, Latimer RD. A comparison of five heat and moisture exchangers. Anaesthesia 1986;41:527–532.
297. Branson RD, Hurst JM. Laboratory evaluation of moisture output of seven airway heat and moisture exchangers. Respir Care 1987;32:741–747.
298. Branson RD, Campbell RS, Davis KJ, Johnson DJ, Porombka D. Humidification in the intensive care unit. Prospective study of a new protocol utilizing heated humidification and a hygroscopic condenser humidifier. Chest 1993;104:1800–1805.
299. Roustan JP, Kienlen J, Aubas P, Aubas S, du Cailar J. Comparison of hydrophobic heat and moisture exchanger with heated humidifier during prolonged mechanical ventilation. Intensive Care Med 1992;18:97–100.
300. Misset B, Escudier B, Rivara D, Leclercq B, Nitenberg G. Heat and moisture exchanger vs heated humidifier during long-term mechanical ventilation: a prospective randomized study. Chest 1991;100:160–163.
301. Gallagher J, Strangeways JE, Allt-Graham J. Contamination control in long term ventilation: a clinical study using heat and moisture exchanging filter. Anaesthesia 1987;42:476–481.
302. Martin C, Perrin G, Gevaudan MJ, Saux P, Gouin F. Heat and moisture exchangers and vaporizing humidifiers in the intensive care unit. Chest 1990;97:144–149.
303. Kaan JA, Simoons-Smit AM, MacLaren DM. Another source of aerosol causing nosocomial Legionnaire's disease. J Infect 1985;11:145–148.
304. Sanders CV, Luby JP, Johanson WG, Barnett JA, Sanford JP. Serratia marcescens infections from inhalation therapy medications: nosocomial outbreak. Ann Intern Med 1970;73:15–21.
305. Decker MD, Lancaster AD, Latham RH, Bunce CP, Becker NR, Burns K. Influence of closed suctioning system on ventilator-associated pneumonias [Abstract]. Third Annual Meeting of the Society for Hospital Epidemiology of America 1993;A6.
306. Deppe SA, Kelly JW, Thoi LL, et al. Incidence of colonization, nosocomial pneumonia, and mortality in critically ill patients using Trach Care closed-suction system versus open-suction system: prospective, randomized study. Crit Care Med 1990;18:1389–1393.
307. Ritz R, Scott LR, Coyle MB, Pierson DJ. Contamination of a multiple-use suction catheter in a closed-circuit system compared to contamination of a disposable, single-use suction catheter. Respir Care 1986;31:1087–1091.
308. Johnson KL, Kearney PA, Johnson SB, Niblett JB, Mcmillan NL, McClain RE. Closed versus open endotracheal suctioning: costs and physiologic consequences. Crit Care Med 1994;22:658–666.
309. Cobley M, Atkins M, Jones FL. Environmental contamination during tracheal suction. A comparison of disposable conventional catheters with a multiple-use closed system device. Anaesthesia 1991;46:957–961.
310. Mayhall CCG. The Trach Care closed tracheal suction system: a new medical device to permit tracheal suctioning without interruption of ventilatory assistance. Infect Control Hosp Epidemiol 1988;9:125–126.
311. Stone JW, Das BC. Investigation of an outbreak of infection with Acinetobacter calcoaceticus in a special care baby unit. J Hosp Infect 1986;7:42–48.
312. Thompson AC, Wilder BJ, Powner DJ. Bedside resuscitation bags: a source of bacterial contamination. Infect Control 1985;6:231–232.
313. Weber DJ, Wilson MB, Rutala WA, Thomann CA. Manual ventilation bags as a source for bacterial colonization of intubated patients. Am Rev Respir Dis 1990;142:892–894.
314. Olds JW, Kisch AL, Eberle BS, Wilson JN. Pseudomonas aeruginosa respiratory tract infection acquired from a contaminated anesthesia machine. Am Rev Respir Dis 1972;105:628–632.
315. Albrecht WH, Dryden GE. Five-year experience with development of an individually clean anesthesia system. Anesth Analg 1974;52:24–28.
316. Du Moulin GC, Sauberman AJ. The anesthesia machine and circle system are not likely to be sources of bacterial contamination. Anesthesiology 1977;47:353–358.

317. American Association of Nurse Anesthetists. Infection control guide. 2nd ed. Illinois: American Association of Nurse Anesthetists, 1993:12–28.
318. American Society for Anesthesiologists . Prevention of nosocomial infections in patients. In: Recommendations for infection control for the practice of anesthesiology. Park Ridge, IL: American Society of Anesthesiologists, 1991:1–9.
319. Bengtson JP, Brandberg A, Brinkhoff B, Sonander H, Stenqvist O. Low-flow anesthesia does not increase the risk of microbial contamination through the circle absorber system. Acta Anaesth Scand 1989;33:89–92.
320. Centers for Disease Control. Draft guidelines for preventing the transmission of tuberculosis in health-care facilities. Federal Register 1993;58:52810–52854.
321. Parmley JB, Tahir AH, Dascomb HE, Adriani J. Disposable versus reusable rebreathing circuits: advantages, disadvantages, hazards and bacteriologic studies. Anesth Analg 1972;51:888–894.
322. Shiotani GM, Nicholes P, Ballinger CM, et al. Prevention of contamination of the circle system and ventilators with a new disposable filter. Anesth Analg 1971;50:844–855.
323. Luttropp HH, Berntman L. Bacterial filters protect anaesthetic equipment in a low-flow system. Anaesthesia 1993;48:520–523.
324. Garibaldi RA, Britt MR, Webster C, Pace NL. Failure of bacterial filters to reduce the incidence of pneumonia after inhalation anesthesia. Anesthesiology 1981;54:364–368.
325. Feeley TW, Hamilton WK, Xavier B, Moyers J. Sterile anesthesia breathing circuits do not prevent postoperative pulmonary infection. Anesthesiology 1981;54:369–372.
326. Berry AJ, Nolte FS. An alternative strategy for infection control of anesthesia breathing circuits: A laboratory assessment of the Pall HME filter. Anesth Analg 1991;72:651–655.
327. Rutala DR, Rutala WA, Weber DJ, Thomann CA. Infection risks associated with spirometry. Infect Control Hosp Epidemiol 1991;12:89–92.
328. Hazaleus RE, Cole J, Berdischewsky M. Tuberculin skin test conversion from exposure to contaminated pulmonary function testing apparatus. Respir Care 1980;26:53–55.
329. Kirk YL, Kendall K, Ashworth HA, Hunter PR. Laboratory evaluation of a filter for the control of cross-infection during pulmonary function testing. J Hosp Infect 1992;20:193–198.
330. Leeming JP, Kendrick AH, Pryce-Roberts D, Smith DR, Smith EC. Use of filters for the control of cross-infection during pulmonary function testing [Letter]. J Hosp Infect 1992;20:245–246.
331. Djokovic JL, Hedley-White J. Prediction of outcome of surgery and anesthesia in patients over 80. JAMA 1979;242:2301–2306.
332. Tisi GM. Preoperative evaluation of pulmonary function: validity, indications and benefits. Am Rev Respir Dis 1979;119:293–310.
333. Gould AB. Effect of obesity in respiratory complications following general anesthesia. Anesth Analg 1962;41:448–452.
334. Cain HD, Stevens PM. Preoperative pulmonary function and complications after cardiovascular surgery. Chest 1979;76:130–135.
335. Wightman JAK. A prospective study of the incidence of postoperative pulmonary complications. Br J Surg 1968;55:85–91.
336. Culver GA, Makel HP, Beecher HK. Frequency of aspiration of gastric contents by lungs during anesthesia and surgery. Ann Surg 1961;133:289–292.
337. Rigg JDA. Pulmonary atelectasis after anaesthesia: Pathophysiology and management. Can Anaesth Soc J 1981;28:306–311.
338. Simonneau G, Vivien A, Sartene R, et al. Diaphragm dysfunction induced by upper abdominal surgery. Am Rev Respir Dis 1983;128:899–903.
339. Bartlett RH, Gazzaniga AB, Geraghty TR. Respiratory maneuvers to prevent postoperative pulmonary complications. JAMA 1973;234:1017–1021.
340. Ali J, Serette C, Wood LDM, et al. Effect of postoperative intermittent positive pressure breathing on lung function. Chest 1984;85:192–196.
341. Pontoppidan H. Mechanical aids to lung expansion in non-intubated surgical patients. Am Rev Respir Dis 1980;122(Suppl):109–119.
342. Morran CG, Finlay IG, Mithieson M, McKay AJ, Wilson N, McArdle CS. Randomized controlled trial of physiotherapy for postoperative pulmonary complications. Br J Anaesth 1983;55:1113–1116.
343. Castillo R, Haas A. Chest physical therapy: comparative efficacy of preoperative and postoperative in the elderly. Arch Phys Med Rehabil 1985;66:376–379.
344. Cordier P, Squifflet JP, Carlier M, Alexandre GPJ. Postoperative continuous positive airway pressure helps to prevent pulmonary infection after human renal transplantation. Transplant Proc 1984;16:1337–1339.
345. Vraciu JK. Effectiveness of breathing exercises in preventing pulmonary complications following open heart surgery. Phys Ther 1977;57:1367–1371.
346. Celli BR, Rodriguez KS, Snider GL. A controlled trial of intermittent positive pressure breathing, incentive spirometry, and deep breathing exercises in preventing pulmonary complications after abdominal surgery. Am Rev Respir Dis 1984;1304:12–15.
347. Schwieger I, Gamulin ZB, Forster A, Meyer P, Gemperle MB, Suter PM. Absence of benefit of incen-

tive spirometry in low-risk patients undergoing elective cholecystectomy: a controlled randomized study. Chest 1986;89:652–656.

348. Roukema JA, Carol EJ, Prins JG. The prevention of pulmonary complications after upper abdominal surgery in patients with noncompromised pulmonary status. Arch Surg 1988;123:30–34.

349. Stock MC, Downs JB, Gauer PK, Alster JM, Imrey PB. Prevention of postoperative pulmonary complications with CPAP, incentive spirometry, and conservative therapy. Chest 1985;87:151–157.

350. Stein M, Cassara EL. Preoperative pulmonary evaluation and therapy for surgery patients. JAMA 1970;211:787–790.

351. Yeager MP, Glass DD, Neff RK, Brinck-Johnson T. Epidural anesthesia and analgesia in high-risk surgical patients. Anesthesiology 1987;66:729–736.

352. Rutter PC, Murphy D, Dudley HAF. Morphine: controlled trial of different methods of administration for postoperative pain. Br Med J 1980;280:12–13.

353. Wasylak TJC, Abbott FV, English MJM, Jeans ME. Reduction of postoperative morbidity following patient-controlled morphine. Can J Anaesth 1990;37:726–731.

354. Egbert AM, Leland HP, Short LM, Burnett ML. Randomized trial of postoperative patient-controlled analgesia vs. intramuscular narcotics in frail elderly men. Arch Intern Med 1990;150:1897–1903.

355. Lange MP, Dahn MS, Jacobs LA. Patient-controlled analgesia versus intermittent analgesia dosing. Heart Lung 1988;17:495–498.

356. Addison NV, Brear FA, Budd K, Whitaker M. Epidural analgesia following cholecystectomy. Br J Surg 1974;61:850–852.

357. Rawal N, Shostrand U, Christofferson E, Dahlstrom B, Arvill A, Rydman H. Comparison of intramuscular and epidural morphine for postoperative analgesia in the grossly obese: influence on postoperative ambulation and pulmonary function. Anesth Analg 1984;63:583–592.

358. Cushieri RJ, Morran CG, Howie JC, McArtle CS. Postoperative pain and pulmonary complications: comparison of three analgesic regimens. Br J Surg 1985;72:495–498.

359. Gould FK, Magee JG, Ingham HR. A hospital outbreak of antibiotic-resistant Streptococcus pneumoniae. J Infect 1987;15:77–79.

360. Moore EP, Williams EW. Hospital transmission of multiply antibiotic resistant Streptococcus pneumoniae. J Infect 1988;16:199–208.

361. Alvarez S, Shell CG, Wooley TW, et al. Nosocomial infections in long-term care facilities. J Gerontol 1992;43:M9-M12.

362. Advisory Committee on Immunization Practices. Pneumococcal polysaccharide vaccine. MMWR 1989; 38:64–76.

363. Shapiro ED, Clemens JD. A controlled evaluation of the protective efficacy of pneumococcal vaccine for patients at high risk of serious pneumococcal infections. Ann Intern Med 1984;101:325–330.

364. Williams WW, Hickson MA, Kane MA, Kendal AP, Spika JS, Hinman AR. Immunization policies and vaccine coverage among adults: the risk for missed opportunities. Ann Intern Med 1988;108:616–625.

365. Langer M, Cigada M, Mandelli M, et al. Early onset pneumonia: a multicenter study in intensive care units. Intensive Care Med 1987;13:342–346.

366. Mandelli M, Mosconi P, Langer M, Cigada M. Prevention of pneumonia in an intensive care unit: a randomized multicenter clinical trial. Crit Care Med 1989;17:501–505.

367. Petersdorf RG, Curtin JA, Hoeprich PD, Peeler RN, Bennet LL. A study of antibiotic prophylaxis in unconscious patients. N Engl J Med 1957;257:1001–1009.

368. Tillotson JR, Finland M. Bacterial colonization and clinical superinfection of the respiratory tract complicating antibiotic treatment of pneumonia. J Infect Dis 1969;119:597–624.

369. Sen P, Kapila P, Chmel H, Armstrong DA, Louria DB. Superinfection: another look. Am J Med 1982;73:706–718.

370. Nord CE, Kager L, Hemdahl A. Impact of antimicrobial agents on the gastrointestinal microflora and the risk of infections. Am J Med 1984;80:99–106.

371. Goodpasture HC, Romig DA, Voth DW. A prospective study of tracheobronchial bacterial flora in acute brain-injured patients with and without antibiotic prophylaxis. J Neurosurg 1977;47:228–235.

372. Kelley RE, Vibulsresth S, Bell L, Duncan RC. Evaluation of kinetic therapy in the prevention of complications of prolonged bed rest secondary to stroke. Stroke 1987;18:638–642.

373. Gentilello L, Thompson DA, Tonnesen AS, et al. Effect of a rotating bed on the incidence of pulmonary complications in critically ill patients. Crit Care Med 1988;16:783–786.

374. Summer WR, Curry P, Haponik EF, Nelson S, Elston R. Continuous mechanical turning of intensive care unit patients shortens length of stay in some diagnostic-related groups. J Crit Care 1989;4:45–53.

375. Fink MP, Helsmoortel CM, Stein KL, Lee PC, Cohn SM. The efficacy of an oscillating bed in the prevention of lower respiratory tract infection in critically ill victims of blunt trauma: a prospective study. Chest 1990;97:132–137.

376. Nelson LD, Choi SC. Kinetic therapy in critically ill trauma patients. Clin Intensive Care 1992;37: 248–252.

377. deBoisblanc BP, Castro M, Everret B, Grender J, Walker CD, Summer WB. Effect of air-supported, continuous, postural oscillation on the risk of early ICU pneumonia in nontraumatic critical illness. Chest 1993;103:1543–1547.

378. Zack MB, Pontoppidan H, Kazemi H. The effect of lateral positions on gas exchange in pulmonary disease: a prospective evaluation. Am Rev Respir Dis 1974;110:49–54.
379. Wong JW, Keens TG, Wannamaker EM, Crozier DN, Levison H, Aspin N. The effects of gravity on tracheal mucous transport rates in normal subjects and patients with cystic fibrosis. Pediatrics 1977;60:146–152.
380. Blake JR. On the movement of mucous in the lung. J Biochem 1975;8:175–190.
381. Becker DM, Gonzalez M, Gentili A, Eismont F, Green BA. Prevention of deep venous thrombosis in patients with acute spinal cord injuries: use of rotating treatment tables. Neurosurgery 1987;20:675–677.
382. Hoge CW, Breiman RF. Advances in the epidemiology and control of Legionella infections. Epidemiol Rev 1991;13:329–340.
383. Joseph CA, Watson JM, Harrison TG, Bartlett CLR. Nosocomial Legionnaires' disease in England and Wales, 1980–92. Epidemiol Infect 1994;112:329–345.
384. Brennen C, Vickers JP, Yu VL, Puntereri A, Yee YC. Discovery of occult Legionella pneumonia in a long-stay hospital: results of prospective serologic survey. Br Med J 1987;295:306–307.
385. Marrie TJ, MacDonald S, Clarke K, Haldane D. Nosocomial Legionnaires' disease: lessons from a four-year prospective study. Am J Infect Control 1991;19:79–85.
386. Muder RR, Yu VL, McClure JK, Kroboth FJ, Kominos SD, Lumish RN. Nosocomial Legionnaires' disease uncovered in a prospective pneumonia study: implications for underdiagnosis. JAMA 1983;249:3184–3188.
387. Fliermans CD, Cherry WB, Orrison LH, Smith SJ, Tison DL, Pope DH. Ecologic distribution of Legionella pneumophila. Appl Environ Microbiol 1981;41:9–16.
388. Morris GK, Patton CM, Feeley JC, et al. Isolation of the Legionnaires' disease bacterium from environmental samples. Ann Intern Med 1979;90:664–666.
389. Hsu SC, Martin R, Wentworth BB. Isolation of Legionella species from drinking water. Appl Environ Microbiol 1984;48:830–832.
390. Tison DL, Seidler RJ. Legionella incidence and density in potable drinking water. Appl Environ Microbiol 1983;45:337–339.
391. Muraca P, Stout JE, Yu VL. Comparative assessment of chlorine, heat, ozone, and UV light for killing Legionella pneumophila within a model plumbing system. Appl Environ Microbiol 1987;53:447–453.
392. Farrell ID, Barker JE, Miles EP, Hutchinson JCP. A field study of the survival of Legionella pneumophila in a hospital hot-water system. Epidemiol Infect 1990;104:381–387.
393. Stout JE, Yu VL, Best MG. Ecology of Legionella pneumophila within water distribution systems. Appl Environ Microbiol 1985;49:221–228.
394. Sanden GN, Fields BS, Barbaree JM, et al. Viability of Legionella pneumophila in chlorine-free water at elevated temperatures. Curr Microbiol 1989;18:61–65.
395. Schulze-Robbecke R, Rodder M, Exner M. Multiplication and killing temperatures of naturally occurring legionellae. Zbl Bakt Hyg B 1987;184:495–500.
396. Habicht W, Muller HE. Occurrence and parameters of frequency of Legionella in warm water systems of hospitals and hotels in Lower Saxony. Zbl Bakt Hyg B 1988;186:79–88.
397. Ciesielski CA, Blaser MJ, Wang WL. Role of stagnation and obstruction of water flow in isolation of Legionella pneumophila from hospital plumbing. Appl Environ Microbiol 1984;48:984–987.
398. Rowbotham TJ. Preliminary report on the pathogenicity of Legionella pneumophila for freshwater and soil amoebae. J Clin Path 1980;33:1179–1183.
399. Fields BS, Sanden GN, Barbaree JM, et al. Intracellular multiplication of Legionella pneumophila in amoebae isolated from hospital hot water tanks. Curr Microbiol 1989;18:131–137.
400. Le Saux NM, Sekla L, McLeod J, et al. Epidemic of nosocomial Legionnaires' disease in renal transplant recipients: a case-control and environmental study. Can Med Assoc J 1989;140:1047–1053.
401. Berendt RF, Young HW, Allen RG, Knutsen GL. Dose-response of guinea pigs experimentally infected with aerosols of Legionella pneumophila. J Infect Dis 1980;141:186–192.
402. Marston BJ, Lipman HB, Breiman RF. Surveillance for Legionnaires' disease in the eighties: risk factors for morbidity and mortality related to infection with Legionella. Arch Intern Med 1994;(in press).
403. Kirby BD, Snyder KM, Meyer RD, et al. Legionnaires' disease. Report of 65 nosocomially acquired cases and review of the literature. Medicine 1980;59:188–205.
404. Haley CE, Cohen ML, Halter J, Meyer RD. Nosocomial Legionnaires' disease: a continuing common-source epidemic at Wadsworth Medical Center. Medicine 1979;90:583–586.
405. Bock BV, Kirby BD, Edelstein PH, et al. Legionnaires' disease in renal transplant recipients. Lancet 1978;1:410–413.
406. Brady MT. Nosocomial Legionnaires' disease in a children's hospital. J Pediatr 1989;115:46–50.
407. Horie H, Kawakami H, Minoshima K, et al. Neonatal Legionnaires' disease: histologic findings in an autopsied neonate. Acta Pathol Jpn 1992;42:427–431.
408. Helms CM, Viner JP, Sturm RH, et al. Comparative features of pneumococcal, mycoplasma, and Legionnaires' disease pneumonias. Ann Intern Med 1979;90:543–547.
409. Yu V, Kroboth FJ, Shonnard J, Brown A, McDearman S, Magnussen M. Legionnaires' disease: new clinical perspectives from a prospective pneumonia study. Am J Med 1982;73:357–361.

410. Marston B, Plouffe J, File T, et al. Evidence of mixed infection in patients with antibody to Chlamydia pneumoniae [Abstract]. Abstracts of the 32nd Interscience Conference on Antimicrobial Agents and Chemotherapy 1992;808.
411. Ussery XT, Butler JC, Breiman R, et al. Outbreak of Legionnaires' disease associated with Mycoplasma infection [Abstract]. Abstracts of the 32nd Interscience Conference on Antimicrobial Agents and Chemotherapy 1992;815.
412. Jimenez ML, Aspa J, Padilla B, et al. Fiberoptic bronchoscopic diagnosis of pulmonary disease in 151 HIV-infected patients with pneumonitis. Eur J Clin Microbiol Infect Dis 1991;10:491–497.
413. Centers for Disease Control. Case definitions for public health surveillance. MMWR 1990;39(RR-13):18.
414. Helms CM, Renner ED, Viner JP, Hierholzer WJ, Wintermeyer LA, Johnson W. Indirect immunofluorescence antibodies to Legionella pneumophila: frequency in a rural community. J Clin Microbiol 1980;12:326–328.
415. Wilkerson HW, Reingold AL, Brake BJ, McGiboney DL, Gorman GW, Broome CV. Reactivity of serum from patients with suspected legionellosis against 29 antigens of Legionellaceae and Legionella-like organisms by indirect immunofluorescence assay. J Infect Dis 1983;147:23–31.
416. Nichol KL, Parenti CM, Johnson JE. High prevalence of positive antibodies to Legionella pneumophila among outpatients. Chest 1991;100:663–666.
417. Storch G, Hayes PS, Hill DL, Baine W. Prevalence of antibody to Legionella pneumophila in middle-aged and elderly Americans. J Infect Dis 1979;140:784–788.
418. Plouffe J, Marston B, Straus W, Breiman R, Hackman B, Moyenuddin M. Utility of diagnostic studies in Legionnaires' disease: Franklin County [Abstract]. Abstracts of the 32nd Interscience Conference on Antimicrobial Agents and Chemotherapy 1992;817.
419. Edelstein PH. The laboratory diagnosis of Legionnaires' disease. Semin Respir Infect 1987;2:235–241.
420. Bridge JA, Edelstein PH. Oropharyngeal colonization with Legionella pneumophila. J Clin Microbiol 1983;18:1108–1112.
421. Fukunaga H, Akagi K, Yabuchi E. Asymptomatic infection of Legionella pneumophila in four cases with pulmonary disease in Japanese. Nippon Saikingaku Zasshi 1990;45:833–840.
422. Dondero TJ, Rendtorff RC, Mallison GF, et al. An outbreak of Legionnaires' disease associated with a contaminated air-conditioning cooling tower. N Engl J Med 1980;302:365–370.
423. Garbe PL, Davis BJ, Weisfield JS, et al. Nosocomial Legionnaires' disease: epidemiologic demonstration of cooling towers as a source. JAMA 1985;254:521–524.
424. O'Mahony MC, Stanwell-Smith RE, Tillett HE, et al. The Stafford outbreak of Legionnaires' disease. Epidemiol Infect 1990;104:361–380.
425. Breiman RF, Fields BS, Sanden G, Volmer L, Meier A, Spika J. An outbreak of Legionnaires' disease associated with shower use: possible role of amoebae. JAMA 1990;263:2924–2926.
426. Hanrahan JP, Morse DL, Scharf VB, et al. A community hospital outbreak of Legionellosis: Transmission by potable hot water. Am J Epidemiol 1987;125:639–649.
427. Breiman RF, VanLoock FL, Sion JP, et al. Association of "sink bathing" and Legionnaires' disease [Abstract]. Abstracts of the 91st Meeting of the American Society for Microbiology 1991;L18.
428. Struelens MJ, Maes N, Rost F, et al. Genotypic and phenotypic methods for the investigation of a nosocomial Legionella pneumophila outbreak and efficacy of control measures. J Infect Dis 1992;166:22–30.
429. Johnson JT, Yu VL, Best MG, et al. Nosocomial legionellosis in surgical patients with head and neck cancer: Implications for epidemiological reservoir and mode of transmission. Lancet 1985;2:298–300.
430. Marrie TJ, Haldane D, MacDonald S, et al. Control of endemic nosocomial Legionnaires' disease by using sterile potable water for high risk patients. Epidemiol Infect 1991;107:591–605.
431. Blatt SP, Parkinson MD, Pace E, et al. Nosocomial Legionnaires' disease: aspiration as a primary mode of disease acquisition. Am J Med 1993;95:16–22.
432. Fraser DW, Tsai TR, Orenstein W, et al. Legionnaires' disease: description of an epidemic of pneumonia. N Engl J Med 1977;297:1189–1197.
433. Yu VL. Routine culturing for Legionella in the hospital environment may be a good idea: a three-hospital prospective study. Am J Med 1987;294:97–99.
434. Allegheny County Health Department. Approaches to prevention and control of Legionella infection in Allegheny County health care facilities. Pittsburgh: Allegheny County Health Department, 1993:1–13.
435. Goetz A, Yu VL. Screening for nosocomial legionellosis by culture of the water supply and targeting of high-risk patients for specialized laboratory testing. Am J Infect Control 1991;19:63–66.
436. Yu VL. Nosocomial legionellosis: current epidemiologic issues. In: Remington JS, Swartz MN, eds. Current clinical topics in infectious diseases. New York: McGraw-Hill, 1986:239–253.
437. Vickers RM, Yu VL, Hanna SS. Determinants of Legionella pneumophila contamination of water distribution systems: 15-hospital prospective study. Infect Control 1987;8:357–363.
438. Tobin JO, Swann RA, Bartlett CLR. Isolation of Legionella pneumophila from water systems: methods and preliminary results. Br Med J 1981;282:515–517.
439. Dennis PJ, Fitzgeorge RB, Taylor JA, et al. Legionella pneumophila in water plumbing systems. Lancet 1982;1:949–951.

440. Marrie TJ, Haldane D, Bezanson G, Peppard R. Each water outlet is a unique ecologic niche for Legionella pneumophila. Epidemiol Infect 1992;108:261–270.
441. Marrie TJ, Bezanson G, Fox J, Kuehn R, Haldane D, Birbridge S. Dynamics of Legionella pneumophila in the potable water of one floor of a hospital. In: Barbaree JM, Breiman RF, Dufow AP, eds. Legionella: current status and emerging perspectives. Washington, DC: ASM, 1993:238–240.
442. Plouffe JF, Para MF, Maher WE, Hackman B, Webster L. Subtypes of Legionella pneumophila serogroup 1 associated with different attack rates. Lancet 1983;2:649–650.
443. Fraser DW. Sources of legionellosis. In: Thornsberry C, Balows A, Feeley JC, Jakubowski W, eds. Legionella: proceedings of the 2nd International Symposium. Washington, DC: American Society for Microbiology, 1984:277–280.
444. Dourmon E, Bibb WF, Rajagopalan P, Desplaces N, McKinney RM. Monoclonal antibody reactivity as a virulence marker for Legionella pneumophila serogroup 1 strain. J Infect Dis 1992;165:569–573.
445. Brundrett GW. Guides on avoiding Legionnaires' disease. In: Legionella and building services. Oxford: Butterworth Heineman, 1992:346–373.
446. Kugler JW, Armitage JO, Helms CM, et al. Nosocomial Legionnaires' disease. Occurrence in recipients of bone marrow transplants. Am J Med 1983;74:281–288.
447. Department of Health. The control of legionella in health care premises: a code of practice. London: HMSO, 1991:
448. Helms CM, Massanari RM, Wenzel RP, et al. Legionnaires' disease associated with a hospital water system: a five-year progress report on continuous hyperchlorination. JAMA 1988;259:2423–2427.
449. Snyder MB, Siwicki M, Wireman J, et al. Reduction of Legionella pneumophila through heat flushing followed by continuous supplemental chlorination of hospital hot water. J Infect Dis 1990;162:127–132.
450. Ezzeddine H, Van Ossel C, Delmee M, Wauters G. Legionella spp. in a hospital hot water system: effect of control measures. J Hosp Infect 1989;13:121–131.
451. Kilbourne ED. Influenza. New York: Plenum Publishing, 1987.
452. Johnston JM, Latham RH, Meier FA, et al. Nosocomial outbreak of Legionnaires' disease: molecular epidemiology and disease control measures. Infect Control 1987;8:53–58.
453. Joly JR, McKinney RM, Tobin JO, Bibb WF, Watkins ID, Ramsay D. Development of a standardized subgrouping scheme for Legionella pneumophila serogroup 1 using monoclonal antibodies. J Clin Microbiol 1986;23:768–771.
454. Schoonmaker D, Helmberger T, Birkhead G. Comparison of ribotyping and restriction enzyme analysis using pulsed-field gel electrophoresis for distinguishing Legionella pneumophila isolates obtained during a nosocomial outbreak. J Clin Microbiol 1992;30:1491–1498.
455. Barbaree JM. Selecting a subtyping technique for use in investigations of legionellosis epidemics. In: Barbaree JM, Breiman RF, Dufow AP, eds. Legionella: current status and emerging perspectives. Washington, DC: ASM, 1993.
456. Best M, Yu VL, Stout J, Goetz A, Muder RR, Taylor F. Legionellaceae in the hospital water supply: epidemiologic link with disease and evaluation of a method for control of nosocomial Legionnaires' disease and Pittsburgh pneumonia. Lancet 1983;2:307–310.
457. Meenhorst PL, Reingold AL, Groothuis DG, et al. Water-related nosocomial pneumonia caused by Legionella pneumophila serogroups 1 and 10. J Infect Dis 1985;152:356–364.
458. Mandel AS, Sprauer MA, Sniadack DH, Ostroff SM. State regulation in hospital water temperature. Infect Control Hosp Epidemiol 1993;14:642–645.
459. Matulonis U, Rosenfeld CS, Shadduck RK. Prevention of Legionella infections in a bone marrow transplant unit: multifaceted approach to decontamination of a water system. Infect Control Hosp Epidemiol 1993;14:571–583.
460. Domingue EL, Tyndall RL, Mayberry WR, Pancorbo OC. Effects of three oxidizing biocides of Legionella pneumophila serogroup 1. Appl Environ Microbiol 1988;54:741–747.
461. Landeen LK, Yahya MT, Gerba CP. Efficacy of copper and silver ions and reduced levels of free chlorine in inactivation of Legionella pneumophila. Appl Environ Microbiol 1989;55:3045–3050.
462. Liu Z, Stout JE, Tedesco L, et al. Controlled evaluation of copper-silver ionization in eradicating Legionella pneumophila from a hospital water distribution system. J Infect Dis 1994;169:919–922.
463. Edelstein PH, Whittaker RE, Kreiling RL, Howell CL. Efficacy of ozone in eradication of Legionella pneumophila from hospital water fixtures. Appl Environ Microbiol 1982;44:1330–1334.
464. Wisconsin Department of Health and Social Services. Control of Legionella in cooling towers: summary guidelines. Madison, WI: Wisconsin Division of Health, 1987.
465. Best MG, Goetz A, Yu VL. Heat eradication measures for control of nosocomial Legionnaire's disease: implementation, education, and cost analysis. Infect Control 1984;12:26–30.
466. Muraca PW, Yu VL, Goetz A. Disinfection of water distribution systems for Legionella: a review of application procedures and methodologies. Infect Control Hosp Epidemiol 1990;11:79–88.
467. Walsh TJ, Dixon DM. Nosocomial aspergillosis: environmental microbiology, hospital epidemiology, diagnosis and treatment. Eur J Epidemiol 1989;5:131–142.
468. Bodey GP, Vartivarian S. Aspergillosis. Eur J Clin Microbiol Infect Dis 1989;8:413–437.
469. Fraser DW, Ward JL, Ajello L, Plikaytis BD. Aspergillosis and other systemic mycoses: the growing problem. JAMA 1979;242:1631–1635.

470. Iwen PC, Reed EC, Armitage JO, et al. Nosocomial invasive aspergillosis in lymphoma patients treated with bone marrow or peripheral stem cell transplants. Infect Control Hosp Epidemiol 1993;14:131–139.
471. Cordonnier C, Bernaudin JF, Bierling P, Huet Y, Vernant JP. Pulmonary complications occurring after allogeneic bone marrow transplantation: a study of 130 consecutive transplanted patients. Cancer 1986;58:1047–1054.
472. Klimowski LL, Rotstein C, Cummings KM. Incidence of nosocomial aspergillosis in patients with leukemia over a twenty-year period. Infect Control Hosp Epidemiol 1989;10:299–305.
473. Walmsley S, Devi S, King S, Schneider R, Richardson S, Ford-Jones L. Invasive Aspergillus infections in a pediatric hospital: a ten-year review. Pediatr Infect Dis 1993;12:673–682.
474. Sherertz RJ, Belani A, Kramer BS, et al. Impact of air filtration on nosocomial aspergillus infections. Unique risk of bone marrow transplant recipients. Am J Med 1987;83:709–718.
475. Rhame FS. Lessons from the Roswell Park bone marrow transplant aspergillosis outbreak. Infect Control 1985;6:345–346.
476. Rotstein C, Cummings KM, Tiddings J, et al. An outbreak of invasive aspergillosis among bone marrow transplants: a case-control study. Infect Control 1985;6:347–355.
477. Aisner J, Schimpff SC, Bennett JE, et al. Aspergillus infections in cancer patients. Association with fireproofing materials in a new hospital. JAMA 1976;235:411–412.
478. Arnow PM, Anderson RI, Mainous PD, Smith EJ. Pulmonary aspergillosis during hospital renovation. Am Rev Respir Dis 1978;118:49–53.
479. Streifel AJ, Laner JL, Vesley D, et al. Aspergillus fumigatus and other thermotolerant fungi generated by hospital building demolition. Appl Environ Microbiol 1983;46:375–378.
480. Hopkins CC, Weber DJ, Rubin RH. Invasive aspergillosis infection: possible non-ward common source within the hospital environment. J Hosp Infect 1989;13:19–25.
481. Gurwith MJ, Stinson EB, Remington JS. Aspergillus infection complicating cardiac transplantation: report of five cases. Arch Intern Med 1971;128:541–545.
482. Weiland D, Ferguson RM, Peterson PK, Snover DC, Simmons RL, Najarian JS. Aspergillosis in 25 renal transplant patients. Ann Surg 1983;198:622–629.
483. Hofflin JM, Potasman I, Baldwin JC, Oyster PE, Stinson EB, Remington JS. Infectious complications in heart transplant recipients receiving cyclosporine and corticosteroids. Ann Intern Med 1987;106:209–216.
484. Schulman LL, Smith CR, Drusin R, Rose EA, Enson Y, Reemtsma K. Respiratory complications of cardiac transplantation. Am J Med Sci 1988;296:1–10.
485. Gustafson TL, Schaffner W, Lavely GB, Stratton CW, Johnson HK, Hutcheson RH. Invasive aspergillosis in renal transplant recipients: correlation with corticosteroid therapy. J Infect Dis 1983; 148:230–238.
486. Ho M, Dummer JS. Risk factors and approaches to infections in transplant recipients. In: Mandell GL, Douglas RG Jr, Bennett JE, eds. Principles and practice of infectious diseases. 3rd ed. New York: Churchill Livingstone, Inc., 1990:2284–2291.
487. Rhame FS, Streifel AJ, Kersey JHJ. Extrinsic risk factors for pneumonia in the patient at high risk for infection. Am J Med 1984;76:42–52.
488. Aisner J, Murillo J, Schimpff SC, Steere AC. Invasive aspergillosis in acute leukemia: correlation with nose cultures and antibiotic use. Ann Intern Med 1979;90:4–9.
489. Ho M, Dummer JS, Peterson PK, Simmons RL. Infections in solid organ transplant recipients. In: Mandell GL, Douglas RG Jr, Bennett JE, eds. Principles and practice of infectious diseases. 3rd ed. New York: Churchill Livingstone, 1990:2294–2303.
490. Walsh TR, Guttendorf J, Dummer S, et al. The value of protective isolation procedures in cardiac transplant recipients. Ann Thorac Surg 1989;47:539–545.
491. Denning DW, Stevens DA. Antifungal and surgical treatment of invasive aspergillosis: review of 2121 published cases. Rev Infect Dis 1990;12:1147–1201.
492. Pannuti CS, Pfaller MA, Wenzel RP. Nosocomial pneumonia in adult patients undergoing bone marrow transplantation: a 9-year study. J Clin Oncol 1991;9:77–84.
493. Weinberger M, Elattaar I, Marshall D, et al. Patterns of infection in patients with aplastic anaemia and the emergence of aspergillus as a major cause of death. Medicine 1992;71:24–43.
494. Orr DP, Myerowitz RL, Jenkins R, et al. Patho-radiologic correlation of invasive pulmonary aspergillosis in the compromised host. Case report and review of literature. Cancer 1978;41:2028–2039.
495. Young RC, Bennett JE, Vogel CL, Carbone PP, DeVita VT. Aspergillosis: the spectrum of the disease in 98 patients. Medicine 1970;49:147–173.
496. Meyer RD, Young LS, Armstrong D, et al. Aspergillosis complicating neoplastic disease. Am J Med 1973;54:6–15.
497. Yu VL, Muder RR, Poorsattar A. Significance of isolation of Aspergillus from the respiratory tract in diagnosis of invasive pulmonary aspergillosis. Results of a three-year prospective study. Am J Med 1986;81:249–254.
498. Martino P, Raccah R, Gentile G, Venditti M, Girmenea C, Mandelli F. Aspergillus colonization of the nose and pulmonary aspergillosis in neutropenic patients: a retrospective study. Hematologica 1989;74:263–265.

499. Richet HM, McNeil MM, Davis BJ, et al. Aspergillus fumigatus sternal wound infections in patients undergoing open heart surgery. Am J Epidemiol 1992;135:48–58.
500. Albelda SM, Talbot GH, Gerson SL, Miller WT, Cassileth PA. Role of fiberoptic bronchoscopy in the diagnosis of invasive pulmonary aspergillosis in patients with acute leukemia. Am J Med 1984;76:1027–1034.
501. Kahn FW, Jones JM, England DM. The role of bronchoalveolar lavage in the diagnosis of invasive pulmonary aspergillosis. Am J Clin Pathol 1986;86:518–523.
502. Saito H, Anaissie EJ, Morice RC, Dekmezian R, Bodey GP. Bronchoalveolar lavage in the diagnosis of pulmonary infiltrates in patients with acute leukemia. Am J Med 1984;76:1027–1034.
503. Cohen J. Clinical manifestations and management of aspergillosis in the compromised patient. In: Warnock DW, Richardson MD, eds. Fungal infections in the compromised patient. London: John Wiley & Sons Ltd., 1991:117–152.
504. Pepys J, Riddell RW, Citron KM, Clayton YM, Short EI. Clinical and immunologic significance of Aspergillus fumigatus in the sputum. Am Rev Respir Dis 1959;80:167–180.
505. Karam GH, Griffin JR. Invasive pulmonary aspergillosis in nonimmunocompromised, non-neutropenic hosts. Rev Infect Dis 1986;8:357–363.
506. Kammer RB, Utz JP. Aspergillus species endocarditis: the new face of a not so rare disease. Am J Med 1974;56:506–521.
507. Holmberg K, Berdischewsky M, Young LS. Serologic immunodiagnosis of invasive aspergillosis. J Infect Dis 1980;141:656–664.
508. Matthews R, Burnie JP, Fox A, Tabaqchali S. Immunoblot analysis of serological responses in invasive aspergillosis. J Clin Path 1985;38:1300–1303.
509. Burnie JP, Matthews RC, Clark I, Milne LJ. Immunoblot fingerprinting of Aspergillus fumigatus. J Immunol Methods 1989;118:179–186.
510. Talbot GH, Weiner MH, Person SL, Provencher M, Hurwitz S. Serodiagnosis of invasive aspergillosis in patients with hematologic malignancy: validation of the Aspergillus fumigatus antigen radioimmunoassay. J Infect Dis 1987;155:12–27.
511. Dupont B, Huber M, Kim SJ, Bennett JE. Galactomannan antigenemia and antigenuria in aspergillosis: studies in patients and experimentally infected rabbits. J Infect Dis 1987;155:1–11.
512. Gerson SL, Talbot GH, Hurwitz S, Strom B, Lusk EJ. Prolonged granulocytopenia: the major risk factor for invasive pulmonary aspergillosis in patients with leukemia. Ann Intern Med 1984;100:345–351.
513. Wingard JR, Beals SU, Santos GW, Mertz WG, Saral R. Aspergillus infections in bone marrow transplant recipients. Bone Marrow Transplant 1987;2:175–181.
514. Peters WP. Use of cytokines during prolonged neutropenia associated with autologous bone marrow transplantation. Rev Infect Dis 1991;13:993–996.
515. Lieschke GJ, Burgess AW. Granulocyte colony-stimulating factor and granulocyte-macrophage colony-stimulating factor. N Engl J Med 1992;327:28–35.
516. Karp JE, Burch PA, Merz WG, et al. An approach to intensive antileukemia therapy in patients with previous invasive aspergillosis. Am J Med 1988;85:203–206.
517. Meunier-Carpentier F, Snoeck R, Gerain J, et al. Chemoprophylaxis of fungal infections. Am J Med 1984;76:652–656.
518. Wajszczuk CP, Dummer JS, Ho M, et al. Fungal infections in liver transplant recipients. Transplantation 1985;40:347–353.
519. Rhame FS, Streifel A, Stevens P, et al. Endemic Aspergillus airborne spore levels are a major risk factor for aspergillosis in bone marrow transplant patients [Abstract]. Abstracts of the 25th Interscience Conference on Antimicrobial Agents and Chemotherapy 1985;A147.
520. Lentino JR, Rosenkranz MA, Michaels JA, et al. Nosocomial aspergillosis: a retrospective review of airborne disease secondary to road construction and contaminated air conditioners. Am J Epidemiol 1982;116:430–437.
521. Sarubbi FA, Kopf HB, Brejetta Wilson M, et al. Increased recovery of Aspergillus flavus from respiratory specimens during hospital construction. Am Rev Respir Dis 1982;125:33–38.
522. Krasinski K, Holzman RS, Hanna B, et al. Nosocomial fungal infection during hospital renovation. Infect Control 1985;6:278–282.
523. Weems JJ, Davis BJ, Tablan OC, Kaufman L, Martone WJ. Construction activity: an independent risk factor for invasive aspergillosis and zygomycosis in patients with hematologic malignancy. Infect Control 1987;8:71–75.
524. Cage AA, Dean DC, Schimert G, Minsley N. Aspergillus infection after cardiac surgery. Arch Surg 1970;101:384–387.
525. Streifel AJ, Stevens PP, Rhame FS. In-hospital source of airborne Penicillium spores. J Clin Microbiol 1987;25:1–4.
526. Keller NP, Cleveland TE, Bhatnagar D. Variable electrophoretic karyotypes of members of Aspergillus flavi. Curr Genet 1992;21:371–375.
527. Denning DW, Clemons KV, Hanson LH, Stevens DA. Restriction endonuclease analysis of total cellular DNA of Aspergillus fumigatus isolates of geographically and epidemiologically diverse origin. J Infect Dis 1990;162:1151–1158.

528. Rhame FS. Prevention of nosocomial aspergillosis. J Hosp Infect 1991;18:466–472.
529. Buckner CD, Clift RA, Sanders AJ, et al. Protective environment for marrow transplant recipients. Ann Intern Med 1978;89:893–901.
530. Murray WA, Streifel AJ, O'Dea TJ, Rhame FS. Ventilation for protection of immune compromised patients. ASHRAE Transactions 1988;94:1185–1191.
531. Streifel AJ, Vesley D, Rhame FS, Murray B. Control of airborne fungal spores in a university hospital. Environment International 1989;12:441–444.
532. Streifel AJ, Rhame FS. Hospital air filamentous fungal spore and particle counts in a specially designed hospital. Proc Indoor Air 1993;4:161–163.
533. Perry S, Penland WZ. The portable laminar flow isolator: new unit for patient protection in a germ-free environment. In: Recent results in cancer research. New York: Springer-Verlag, 1970.
534. Barnes RA, Rogers TR. Control of an outbreak of nosocomial aspergillosis by laminar air-flow isolation. J Hosp Infect 1989;14:89–94.
535. Levine AS, Siegel SE, Schrelber AD, et al. Protected environments and prophylactic antibiotics. N Engl J Med 1973;288:477–483.
536. ASHRAE. Handbook, heating ventilation air conditioning applications. Atlanta: ASHRAE, 1991: 7.1–7.12.
537. Rhame FS. Nosocomial aspergillosis: how much protection for which patients? Infect Control Hosp Epidemiol 1989;10:296–298.
538. Opal SM, Asp AA, Cannady PB, Morse PL, Burton LJ, Hammer PG. Efficacy of infection control measures during a nosocomial outbreak of disseminated aspergillosis associated with hospital construction. J Infect Dis 1986;153:634–637.
539. Welliver RC, McLaughlin S. Unique epidemiology of nosocomial infections in a children's hospital. Am J Dis Child 1984;138:131–135.
540. Valenti WM, Hall CB, Douglas RG, Jr., Menegus MA, Pincus PH. Nosocomial viral infections: I. Epidemiology and significance. Infect Control 1980;1:33–37.
541. Goldwater PN, Martin AJ, Ryan B, et al. A survey of nosocomial respiratory viral infections in a children's hospital: occult respiratory infection in patients admitted during an epidemic season. Infect Control Hosp Epidemiol 1991;12:231–238.
542. Mintz L, Ballard RA, Sniderman SH, et al. Nosocomial respiratory syncytial virus infections in an intensive care nursery: rapid diagnosis by direct immunofluorescence. Pediatrics 1979;64:149–153.
543. Hall CB, McBride JT, Walsh EE, et al. Aerosolized ribavirin treatment in infants with respiratory syncytial virus infection. N Engl J Med 1983;308:1443–1447.
544. Betts RF. Amantadine and rimantadine for the prevention of influenza A. Semin Respir Infect 1989;4:304–310.
545. Rodriguez WJ, Parrott RH. Ribavirin aerosol treatment of serious respiratory syncytial virus infection in infants. Infect Dis Clin N Am 1987;2:425.
546. Krasinski K. Severe respiratory syncytial virus infection: clinical features, nosocomial acquisition and outcome. Pediatr Infect Dis 1985;4:250–256.
547. Meissner HC, Murray SA, Kiernan MA, et al. A simultaneous outbreak of respiratory syncytial virus and parainfluenza virus type 3 in a newborn nursery. J Pediatr 1984;104:680–684.
548. Hall CB, Powell KR, MacDonald NE, et al. Respiratory syncytial virus infection in children with compromised immune function. N Engl J Med 1986;315:77–81.
549. Mathur U, Bentley DW, Hall CB. Concurrent respiratory syncytial virus and influenza A infections in the institutionalized elderly and chronically ill. Ann Intern Med 1980;93:49–52.
550. MacDonald NE, Hall CB, Suffin SC, Alexon C, Harris PJ, Manning JA. Respiratory syncytial viral infection in infants with congenital heart disease. N Engl J Med 1982;307:397–400.
551. Drescher J, Zink P, Verhagen W, et al. Recent influenza virus A infections in forensic cases of sudden unexplained death. Virology 1987;92:63–76.
552. Hertz MI, Englund JA, Snover D, Bitterman PB, McGlave PB. Respiratory syncytial virus-induced acute lung injury in adult patients with bone marrow transplants: a clinical approach and review of the literature. Medicine 1989;68:269–281.
553. Baron RC, Dicker RC, Bussell KE, Herndon JL. Assessing trends in mortality in 121 U.S. cities, 1970–1979, from all causes and from pneumonia and influenza. Public Health Rep 1988;103:120–128.
554. Hall CB. The nosocomial spread of respiratory syncytial viral infections. Ann Rev Med 1983;34: 311–319.
555. Finger F, Anderson LJ, Dicker RC, et al. Epidemic infections caused by respiratory syncytial virus in institutionalized young adults. J Infect Dis 1987;155:1335–1339.
556. Hall CB. Nosocomial viral infections: perennial weeds on pediatric wards. Am J Med 1981;70:670–676.
557. Hall CB, Douglas RG Jr. Nosocomial influenza infection as a cause of intercurrent fevers in infants. Pediatrics 1975;55:673–677.
558. Glezen WP. Viral pneumonia as a cause and result of hospitalization. J Infect Dis 1983;147:765–770.
559. Wenzel RP, Deal EC, Hendley JO. Hospital-acquired viral respiratory illness on a pediatric ward. Pediatrics 1977;60:367–371.
560. Hall CB. Hospital-acquired pneumonia in children. Semin Respir Infect 1987;2:48–56.

561. Glezen WP, Loda FA, Clyde WA, Jr., et al. Epidemiologic patterns of acute lower respiratory diseases in pediatric group practice. J Pediatr 1971;78:397–406.

562. Henderson FW, Collier AM, Clyde WA, Jr., et al. Respiratory-syncytial-virus infections, reinfections and immunity: a prospective, longitudinal study in young children. N Engl J Med 1979;300:530–534.

563. Hall WJ, Hall CB, Speers DM. Respiratory syncytial virus infection in adults: clinical, virologic, and serial pulmonary function studies. Ann Intern Med 1978;88:203–205.

564. Englund JA, Anderson LJ, Rhame FS. Nosocomial transmission of respiratory syncytial virus in immunocompromised adults. J Clin Microbiol 1991;29:115–119.

565. Falsey AR, Walsh EE, Betts RF. Serologic evidence of respiratory syncytial virus infection in nursing home patients. J Infect Dis 1990;162:568–569.

566. Hall CB, Kopelman AE, Douglas G, Jr., Griman JM, Meagher MP. Neonatal respiratory syncytial virus infection. N Engl J Med 1979;300:393–396.

567. Hall CB, Douglas RG, Jr., Geiman JM, et al. Nosocomial respiratory syncytial virus infections. N Engl J Med 1975;203:1343–1346.

568. Centers for Disease Control. Parainfluenza outbreaks in extended-care facilities. MMWR 1978;27:475–476.

569. De Fabritus AM, Riggio RR, David DS, et al. Parainfluenza type 3 in a transplant unit. JAMA 1979;241:384–385.

570. Mufson MA, Mocega HE, Krause HE. Acquisition of parainfluenza 3 virus infection by hospitalized children. I. Frequencies, rates, and temporal data. J Infect Dis 1973;128:141–147.

571. McNamara MJ, Phillips IA, Williams OB. Viral and Mycoplasma pneumoniae infections in exacerbations of chronic lung disease. Am Rev Respir Dis 1969;100:19–24.

572. Meyers JD, MacQuarrie MB, Merigan TC, Jennison MH. Nosocomial varicella—Part I. Outbreak in oncology patients at a children's hospital. West J Med 1979;130:196–199.

573. Graman PS, Hall CB. Epidemiology and control of nosocomial viral infections. Infect Dis Clin N Am 1989;3:815–841.

574. Atkinson WL, Markowitz LE, Adams NC, Seastrom GR. Transmission of measles in medical settings: United States, 1985–1989. Am J Med 1991;91(Suppl 3B):252S–255S.

575. Brandt CD, Kim HW, Arrobio JO, et al. Epidemiology of respiratory syncytial virus in Washington, DC. III. Composite analysis of 11 consecutive yearly epidemics. Am J Epidemiol 1973;98:355–364.

576. Glezen WP, Denny FW. Epidemiology of acute lower respiratory disease in children. N Engl J Med 1973;288:498–505.

577. Englund JA, Sullivan CJ, Jordan C, Dehner LP, Vercellotti GM, Balfour HH. Respiratory syncytial virus infection in immunocompromised adults. Ann Intern Med 1988;109:203–208.

578. Sorvillo FJ, Huie SF, Strassburg MA, Butsumyo A, Shandera WX, Fannin SL. An outbreak of respiratory syncytial virus pneumonia in a nursing home for the elderly. J Infect 1984;9:252–256.

579. Anderson LJ, Parker RA, Strikas RL. Association between respiratory syncytial virus outbreaks and lower respiratory tract deaths in infants and young children. J Infect Dis 1990;161:640–646.

580. Waner JL, Whitehurst NJ, Todd SJ, et al. Comparison of Directigen RSV with viral isolation and direct immunofluorescence for identification of respiratory syncytial virus. J Clin Microbiol 1990;28:480–483.

581. Ray CG, Minnich LL. Efficacy of immunofluorescence for rapid diagnosis of common respiratory viruses. J Clin Microbiol 1987;25:355–357.

582. Popow-Kraupp T, Kern G, Binder C, et al. Detection of RSV in nasopharyngeal secretions by enzyme-linked immunosorbent assay, indirect immunofluorescence and virus isolation. J Med Virol 1986;19:123–134.

583. Kellogg JA. Culture vs direct antigen assays for detection of microbial pathogens from lower respiratory tract specimens suspected of containing the respiratory syncytial virus. Arch Pathol Lab Med 1991;115:451–458.

584. Hall CB, Douglas RG Jr. Modes of transmission of respiratory syncytial virus. J Pediatr 1981;99:100–103.

585. Hall CB, Douglas RG Jr, Geiman JM. Possible transmission by fomites of respiratory syncytial virus. J Infect Dis 1980;141:98–102.

586. Hall CB, Douglas RG Jr, Schnabel KC, Geiman JM. Infectivity of respiratory syncytial virus by various routes of inoculation. Infect Immun 1981;33:779–783.

587. Storch GA, Park CS, Dohner DE. RNA fingerprinting of respiratory syncytial virus using ribonuclease protection: application to molecular epidemiology. J Clin Invest 1989;83:1894–1902.

588. Hall CB, Douglas RG Jr, Geiman J. Respiratory syncytial virus infections in infants: quantitation and duration of shedding. J Pediatr 1976;89:11–15.

589. Berglund M. Respiratory syncytial virus infections in families: a study of family members of children hospitalized for acute respiratory disease. Acta Pediatr Scand 1967;56:395–404.

590. Hall CB, Douglas RG Jr. Nosocomial respiratory syncytial viral infections. Should gowns and masks be used? Am J Dis Child 1981;135:512–515.

591. Snydman DR, Greer C, Meissner HC, McIntosh K. Prevention of nosocomial transmission of respiratory syncytial virus in a newborn nursery. Infect Control Hosp Epidemiol 1988;9:105–108.

592. Murphy D, Todd JK, Chao RK, et al. The use of gowns and masks to control respiratory illness in pediatric hospital personnel. J Pediatr 1981;99:746–750.
593. Krasinski K, LaCouture R, Holzman RS, Waithe E, Bank S, Hanna B. Screening for respiratory syncytial virus and assignment to a cohort at admission to reduce nosocomial transmission. J Pediatr 1990;116:894–898.
594. Agah R, Cherry JD, Garakian AJ, et al. Respiratory syncytial virus (RSV) infection rate in personnel caring for children with RSV infections: routine isolation procedure vs routine procedure supplemented by use of masks and goggles. Am J Dis Child 1987;141:695–697.
595. Hall CB, Geiman JM, Douglas RG Jr. Control of nosocomial respiratory syncytial viral infections. Pediatrics 1978;62:728–732.
596. Itano A, Sorvillo F. Infection control practices for respiratory syncytial virus (RSV) among acute care hospitals in Los Angeles County [Abstract]. Am J Infect Control 1991;19:107.
597. Madge P, Paton JY, McColl JH, Mackie PLK. Prospective controlled study of four infection control procedures to prevent nosocomial infection with respiratory syncytial virus. Lancet 1992;340:1079–1083.
598. Gala CL, Hall CB, Schnabel MA, et al. The use of eye-nose goggles to control nosocomial respiratory syncytial virus infection. JAMA 1986;256:2706–2708.
599. Louria DB, Blumenfeld HL, Ellis JT, Kilbourne ED, Rogers DE. Studies on influenza in the pandemic of 1957–58. II. Pulmonary complications of influenza. J Clin Invest 1959;38:213–265.
600. Lindsay MI Jr, Herrman EC Jr, Morrow GW Jr, et al. Hong Kong influenza: clinical, microbiologic, and pathologic features of 127 cases. JAMA 1970;214:1825–1832.
601. Schwarzmann SW, Adler JL, Sullivan RJ, et al. Bacterial pneumonia during the Hong Kong influenza epidemic of 1968–1969. Arch Intern Med 1971;127:1037–1041.
602. Barker WH, Mullooly JP. Pneumonia and influenza deaths during epidemics. Arch Intern Med 1982;142:85–89.
603. Mullooly JP, Barker WH. Impact of type A influenza on children: a retrospective study. Am J Public Health 1982;72:1008–1016.
604. Eickhoff TC, Sherman IL, Serfling RE. Observations on excess mortality associated with epidemic influenza. JAMA 1961;176:104–110.
605. Noble GR. Epidemiological and clinical aspects of influenza. In: Beare AS, ed. Basic and applied influenza research. Boca Raton, FL: CRC Press, 1982:11–49.
606. Monto AS, Kioumehr F. The Tecumseh study of respiratory illness. IX. Occurrence of influenza in the community, 1966–1971. Am J Epidemiol 1975;102:553–563.
607. Blumenfeld HL, Kilbourne ED, Louria DB, et al. Studies on influenza in the pandemic of 1957–1958. I. An epidemiologic, clinical, and serologic investigation of an intra-hospital epidemic, with a note on vaccine efficacy. J Clin Invest 1959;38:199–212.
608. Bean B, Rhame FS, Hughes RS, et al. Influenza B: hospital activity during a community epidemic. Diag Microbiol Infect Dis 1983;1:177–183.
609. Hoffman PC, Dixon RE. Control of influenza in the hospital. Ann Intern Med 1977;87:725–728.
610. Arden NH, Patriarca PA, Fasano MB, et al. The roles of vaccination and amantadine prophylaxis in controlling an outbreak of influenza A (H3N2) in a nursing home. Arch Intern Med 1988;148:865–868.
611. Arroyo JC, Postic B, Brown A, et al. Influenza A/Philippines/2/82 outbreak in a nursing home: limitations of influenza vaccination in the elderly. Am J Infect Control 1984;12:329–334.
612. Patriarca PA, Weber JA, Parker RA, et al. Efficacy of influenza vaccine in nursing homes: reduction in illness and complications during influenza A (H3N2) epidemic. JAMA 1985;253:1136–1139.
613. Saah AJ, Neufeld R, Rodstein M, et al. Influenza vaccine and pneumonia mortality in a nursing home population. Arch Intern Med 1986;146:2353–2357.
614. Alford RH, Kasel JA, Gerone PJ, Knight V. Human influenza resulting from aerosol inhalation. Proc Soc Exp Biol Med 1966;122:800–804.
615. Moser MR, Bender TR, Margolis HS, Noble GR, Kendal AP, Ritter DG. An outbreak of influenza aboard a commercial airliner. Am J Epidemiol 1979;110:1–6.
616. Knight V. Airborne transmission and pulmonary deposition of respiratory viruses. In: Mulder J, Hers JFP, eds. Influenza. Groningen, Netherlands: Wolters-Noordhoff, 1972:1–9.
617. Loosli CG, Lemon HM, Robertson OH, et al. Experimental air-borne influenza infection. I. Influence of humidity on survival of virus in air. Proc Soc Exp Biol Med 1943;53:205–206.
618. Bean B, Moore BM, Sterner B, et al. Survival of influenza viruses on environmental surfaces. J Infect Dis 1982;146:47–52.
619. Glezen WP, Decker M, Joseph SW, Mercready RG Jr. Acute respiratory disease associated with influenza epidemics in Houston, 1981–1983. J Infect Dis 1987;155:1119–1126.
620. McQuillin J, Madeley CR, Kendal AP. Monoclonal antibodies for the rapid diagnosis of influenza A and B virus infections by immunofluorescence. Lancet 1985;2:911–914.
621. Berg RA, Yolken RH, Rennard SI, et al. New enzyme immunoassay for measurement of influenza A/Victoria/3/75 virus in nasal washes. Lancet 1980;1:851–853.
622. Espy MJ, Smith TF, Harmon MW, et al. Rapid detection of influenza virus by shell vial assay with monoclonal antibodies. J Clin Microbiol 1986;24:677–679.

623. Chomel JJ, Pardon D, Thouvenot D, Allard JP, Aynard M. Comparison between three rapid methods for direct diagnosis of influenza and the conventional isolation procedure. Biologicals 1991;19:287–292.
624. Bucher DJ, Mikhail A, Popple S, et al. Rapid detection of type A influenza viruses with monoclonal antibodies to the M protein (M1) by enzyme-linked immunosorbent assay and time-resolved fluoroimmunoassay. J Clin Microbiol 1991;29:2484–2488.
625. Spada B, Biehler K, Chegas P, Kaye J, Riepenhoff-Talty M. Comparison of rapid immunofluorescence assay to cell culture isolation for the detection of influenza A and B viruses in nasopharyngeal secretions from infants and children. J Virol Methods 1991;33:305–310.
626. Barker WH, Mullooly JP. Influenza vaccination of elderly persons: reduction in pneumonia and influenza hospitalizations and deaths. JAMA 1980;244:2547–2549.
627. Foster DA, Tolsma AN, Newson AF, et al. Influenza vaccine effectiveness in preventing hospitalizations for pneumonia in the elderly. Am J Epidemiol 1992;136:286–307.
628. Advisory Committee on Immunization Practices. Prevention and control of influenza: Part I, vaccines. Recommendations of the Advisory Committee on Immunization Practices (ACIP). MMWR 1993; 42(RR-6):1–14.
629. Patriarca PA, Weber JA, Parker RA, et al. Risk factors for outbreaks of influenza in nursing homes: a case control study. Am J Epidemiol 1986;124:114–119.
630. Fox JP, Elveback L, Scott W, Gatewood L, Ackerman E. Herd immunity: basic concept and relevance to public health immunization practices. Am J Epidemiol 1971;94:171–189.
631. Advisory Committee on Immunization Practices. Prevention and control of influenza: Part I, vaccines. MMWR 1994;43:(No. RR-9).
632. Tominack RL, Hayden FG. Rimantadine hydrochloride and amantadine hydrochloride use in influenza A virus infections. Infect Dis Clin N Am 1987;1:459–478.
633. Hall CB, Dolin R, Gala CL, et al. Children with influenza A infection: treatment with rimantadine. Pediatrics 1987;80:275–282.
634. Dolin R, Reichman RC, Madore HP, et al. A controlled trial of amantadine and rimantadine prophylaxis of influenza infection. N Engl J Med 1982;307:580–584.
635. Douglas RG. Drug therapy: prophylaxis and treatment of influenza. N Engl J Med 1990;322:443–450.
636. Younkin SW, Betts RF, Roth FK, et al. Reduction in fever and symptoms in young adults with influenza A/Brazil/78 H1N1 infection after treatment. Antimicrob Agents Chemother 1983;23:577–582.
637. Van Voris LP, Betts RF, Hayden FG. Successful treatment of naturally occurring influenza A/USSR/77/H1N1. JAMA 1981;245:1128–1131.
638. Atkinson WL, Arden NH, Patriarca PA, et al. Amantadine prophylaxis during an institutional outbreak of type A(H1N1) influenza. Arch Intern Med 1986;146:1751–1756.
639. O'Donoghue JM, Ray CG, Terry DW Jr, Beaty HN. Prevention of nosocomial influenza infection with amantadine. Am J Epidemiol 1973;97:276–282.
640. Leeming JK. Amantadine hydrochloride and the elderly. Lancet 1969;1:313–314.
641. Postma JU, Tilburg WV. Visual hallucinations and delirium during treatment with amantadine (Symmetrel). J Am Geriatr Soc 1975;23:212–215.
642. Advisory Committee on Immunization Practices. Prevention and control of influenza; Part II, antiviral agents. MMWR 1994;43:1–10.
643. Hayden FG, Sperber SJ, Belshe RB, Clover RD, Hay AJ, Pyke S. Recovery of drug-resistant influenza A virus during therapeutic use of rimantadine. Antimicrob Agents Chemother 1991;35:1741–1747.
644. Mast EE, Harmon MW, Gravenstein S, et al. Emergence and possible transmission of amantadine-resistant viruses during nursing home outbreaks of influenza A(H3N2). Am J Epidemiol 1991;13:988–997.
645. Hayden PG, Blake RB, Clover RD, Hey AJ, Oakes MG, Soo W. Emergence and apparent transmission of rimantadine-resistant influenza A virus in families. N Engl J Med 1989;321:1696–1702.
646. Hayden FG, Couch RB. Clinical and epidemiological importance of influenza A viruses resistant to amantadine and rimantadine. Rev Med Virol 1992;2:89–96.
647. Monto AS, Arden NH. Implications of viral resistance to amantadine in control of influenza A. Clin Infect Dis 1992;15:362–367.
648. Fedson DS. Immunizations for health care workers and patients in hospitals. In: Wenzel RP, ed. Prevention and control of nosocomial infection. Baltimore: Williams and Wilkins, 1987:116–174.
649. Valenti WM, Betts RF, Hall CB, Hruska JF, Douglas RG Jr. Nosocomial viral infections: II. Guidelines for prevention and control of respiratory viruses, herpesviruses, and hepatitis viruses. Infect Control 1981;1:165–178.
650. Williams WW. Guideline for infection control in hospital personnel. Infect Control 1983;4:326–349.
651. Wong ES, Hooton TM. Guideline for prevention of catheter-associated urinary tract infections. Am J Infect Control 1983;11:28–33.
652. Simmons BP, Hooton TM, Wong ES, Allen JR. Guideline for prevention of intravascular infections. Infect Control 1982;3:61–72.
653. Simmons BP, Wong ES. Guideline for prevention of nosocomial pneumonia. Infect Control 1982;3:327–333.
654. Garner JS. Guideline for prevention of surgical wound infections. Infect Control 1986;7:193–200.

655. Britt MR, Schleupner CJ, Matsumiya S. Severity of underlying disease as a predictor of nosocomial infection. JAMA 1978;239:1047–1051.
656. Conly JM, Hill S, Ross J, Lertzman J, Louie TJ. Handwashing practices in an intensive care unit: the effects of an educational program and its relationship to infection rates. Am J Infect Control 1989;17:330–339.
657. Seto WH, Ching TY, Yuen KY, Chu YB, Seto WL. The enhancement of infection control in-service education by ward opinion leaders. Am J Infect Control 1991;19:86–91.
658. Haiduven DJ, DeMaiao TM, Stevens DA. A five-year study of needlestick injuries: significant reduction associated with communication, education, and convenient placement of sharps containers. Infect Control Hosp Epidemiol 1992;13:265–271.
659. Johnson MW, Mitch WE, Heller AH, Spector R. The impact of an educational program on gentamicin use in a teaching hospital. Am J Med 1982;73:9–14.
660. Soumerai SB, Salem-Schatz S, Avorn J, Casteris CS, Ross-Degnan D, Popovsky MA. A controlled trial of educational outreach to improve blood transfusion practice. JAMA 1993;270:961–966.
661. Eisenberg JM. An education program to modify laboratory use by house staff. J Med Educ 1977;52:578–581.
662. Haley RW, Culver DH, White JW, et al. The efficacy of infection surveillance and control programs in preventing nosocomial infections in US hospitals. Am J Epidemiol 1985;121:182–205.
663. Gross AS, Roup B. Role of respiratory assistance devices in endemic nosocomial pneumonia. Am J Med 1981;70:681–685.
664. Hall JC, Tarala RA, Hall JL, Mander J. A multivariate analysis of the risk of pulmonary complications after laparotomy. Chest 1991;99:923–927.
665. Josephson A, Karanfil L, Alonso H, Watson A, Blight J. Risk-specific nosocomial infection rates. Am J Med 1991;91(Suppl 3B):131S–137S.
666. Freeman J, McGowan JE. Methodologic issues in hospital epidemiology. I. Rates, case finding and interpretation. Rev Infect Dis 1981;3:658–667.
667. Madison R, Afifi AA. Definition and comparability of nosocomial infection rates. Am J Infect Control 1982;10:49–52.
668. American Hospital Association Committee on Infection within Hospitals. Statement on microbiologic sampling. Hospitals 1974;48:125–126.
669. Eickhoff TC. Microbiologic sampling. Hospitals 1970;44:86–87.
670. Bond WW, Ott BJ, Franke KA, McCracken JE. Effective use of liquid chemical germicides on medical devices: instrument design problems. In: Block SS, ed. Disinfection, sterilization, and preservation. 4th ed. Philadelphia: Lea and Febiger, 1991:1097–1106.
671. McDonald WL, Welch HJ, Keet JE. Antisepsis of endotracheal tubes and face masks. Anesthesiology 1955;16:206.
672. Institute for Health Policy Analysis. Proceedings of International Conference on the Reuse of Disposable Medical Devices in the 1980's. Washington, DC: Georgetown University Medical Center, 1984.
673. Bosomworth PP, Hamelberg W. Effect of sterilization on safety and durability of endotracheal tubes and cuffs. Anesth Analg 1965;44:576–586.
674. Comhaire A, Lamy RM. Contamination rate of sterilized ventilators in an ICU. Crit Care Med 1981;9:546–548.
675. Seto WH, Ching TY, Yuen KY, Lam WK. Evaluating the sterility of disposable wall oxygen humidifiers, during and between use on patients. Infect Control 1990;11:604–605.
676. Stoler BS. Sterility of a disposable oxygen humidification system. Respir Care 1972;17:572–573.
677. Meehan TP. Sterility in oxygen humidifiers. Respir Tech 1977;14:15–22.
678. Golar SD, Sutherland LLA, Ford GT. Multipatient use of prefilled disposable oxygen humidifiers for up to 30 days: patient safety and cost analysis. Respir Care 1993;38:343–347.
679. Henderson E, Ledgerwood D, Hope KM, et al. Prolonged and multipatient use of prefilled disposable oxygen humidifier bottles: safety and cost. Infect Control Hosp Epidemiol 1993;14:463–468.
680. Cabrera HA. An outbreak of Serratia marcescens, and its control. Arch Intern Med 1969;123:650–655.
681. Longfield R, Longfield J, Smith LP, Hyams K, Strohmer ME. Multidose medication vial sterility: an in-use study and a review of the literature. Infect Control 1984;5:165–169.
682. Sheth NK, Post GT, Wisniewski TR, Uttech BV. Multi-dose vials versus single-dose vials: a study in sterility and cost-effectiveness. J Clin Microbiol 1983;17:377–379.
683. Smith PW, Massanari RM. Room humidifiers as the source of Acinetobacter infections. JAMA 1977;237:795–797.
684. Moffet HL, Allan D. Survival and dissemination of bacteria in nebulizers and incubators. Am J Dis Child 1967;114:13–20.
685. Berry AJ. Infection control in anesthesia. Anesth Clin N Am 1989;7:967.
686. Larson EL, Eke PI, Laughon BE. Efficacy of alcohol-based hand rinses under frequent-use conditions. Antimicrob Agents Chemother 1986;30:542–544.
687. Jones MV, Rowe GB, Jackson B, Pritchard NJ. The use of alcohol paper wipes for routine hand cleansing: results of trials in two hospitals. J Hosp Infect 1986;8:268–274.

688. Ping FC, Oulton JL, Smith JA, Skidmore AG, Jenkins LC. Bacterial filters—are they necessary on anesthetic machines? Can Anaesth Soc J 1979;26:415–419.
689. Knittle MA, Eitzman DV, Baer H. Role of hand contamination of personnel in the epidemiology of gram-negative nosocomial infections. J Pediatr 1975;86:433–437.
690. Reybrouck G. Role of the hands in the spread of nosocomial infections. J Hosp Infect 1983;41: 103–110.
691. Sutter VL, Hurst V, Grossman M, Calonje R. Source and significance of Pseudomonas aeruginosa in sputum. JAMA 1966;197:854–856.
692. Bernard M, Braunstein N, Stevens R, et al. Incidence of aspiration pneumonia in enteral hyperalimentation [Abstract]. J Parent Enter Nutr 1982;6:588.
693. Harvey P, Bell P, Harris O. Accidental intrapulmonary clinifeed. Anesth Analg 1981;36:518–522.
694. Hand R, Kempster M, Levy J, Rogol R, Spirin P. Inadvertent transbronchial insertion of narrow-bore feeding tubes into the pleural space. JAMA 1984;251:2396–2397.
695. Dorsey J, Cogordan J. Nasotracheal intubation and pulmonary parenchymal perforation: an unusual complication of nasoenteral feeding with small-diameter feeding tubes. Chest 1985;87:131–132.
696. Heymsfield SB, Bethel RA, Ansley JD, Nixon DW, Rudman D. Enteral hyperalimentation: an alternative to central venous hyperalimentation. Ann Intern Med 1979;90:63–71.
697. Bury KD, Jambanathan G. Effects of elemental diets on gastric emptying and gastric secretion in man. Am J Surg 1974;127:59–64.
698. Douglas RG, Jr. Influenza in man. In: Kilbourne ED, ed. The influenza viruses and influenza. New York: New York Academy Press, 1975.
699. Holzapfel L, Chevret S, Madinier G, et al. Influence of long-term oro- or nasotracheal intubation on nosocomial maxillary sinusitis and pneumonia: results of a prospective, randomized clinical trial. Crit Care Med 1993;21:1132–1138.
700. Cerra FB, Maddaus MA, Dunn DL, et al. Selective gut decontamination reduces nosocomial infections and length of stay but not mortality or organ failure in surgical intensive care unit patients. Arch Surg 1992;127:163–169.
701. Nayman J. Measurement and control of postoperative pain. Ann R Coll Surg Engl 1979;61:419–426.
702. Roberts NJ, Douglas RG, Jr. Gentamicin use and Pseudomonas and Serratia resistance: effect of a surgical prophylaxis regimen. Antimicrob Agents Chemother 1978;13:214–220.
703. Gentinello L, Thompson DA, Tonnesen AS, et al. Effect of a rotating bed on the incidence of pulmonary complications in critically ill patients. Crit Care Med 1988;16:783–786.
704. Ruf B, Schurmann D, Horbach I, et al. Prevalence and diagnosis of Legionella pneumonia: a 3-year prospective study with emphasis on application of urinary antigen detection. J Infect Dis 1990;162: 1341–1348.
705. Redd SC, Cohen ML. Legionella in water: what should be done? JAMA 1987;257:1221–1222.
706. Woo AH, Yu VL, Goetz A. Potential in-hospital modes of transmission of Legionella pneumophila: demonstration experiments for dissemination by showers, humidifiers, and rinsing of ventilation bag apparatus. Am J Med 1986;80:567–573.
707. World Health Organization. Environmental aspects of the control of Legionellosis. 14th ed. Copenhagen: World Health Organization, 1986:118–120.
708. Bhopal RS, Barr G. Maintenance of cooling towers following two outbreaks of Legionnaires' disease in a city. Epidemiol Infect 1990;104:29–38.
709. Pannuti C, Gingrich R, Pfaller MA, Kao C, Wenzel RP. Nosocomial pneumonia in patients having bone marrow transplant: attributable mortality and risk factors. Cancer 1992;69:2653–2662.
710. Mahoney DH, Steuber CP, Starling KA, Barrett FF, Goldberg J, Fernbach DJ. An outbreak of aspergillosis in children with acute leukemia. J Pediatr 1979;95:70–72.
711. Rogers TR. Infections in hematologic malignancy. Infect Control 1986;7S:124–125.
712. McWhinney PHM, Kibbler CC, Hamon MD, et al. Progress in the diagnosis and management of aspergillosis in bone marrow transplantation: 13 years. J Infect Dis 1993;17:397–404.
713. Staib F. Ecological and epidemiological aspects of aspergilli pathogenic for man and animal in Berlin (West). Zbl Bakt Hyg A 1984;257:240–245.
714. Staib F, Folkens U, Tompak B, Abel T, Thiel D. A comparative study of antigens of Aspergillus fumigatus isolates from patients and soil of ornamental plants in the immunodiffusion test. Zbl Bakt Hyg I Abt Orig A 1978;242:93–99.
715. Lie TS, Hofer M, Hohnke C, et al. Aspergillose nach lebertransplantation als hospitalismusinfekion. Dtsch Med Wschr 1987;112:297–301.
716. Bodey GP. Current status of prophylaxis of infection with protected environments. Am J Med 1984;76: 678–684.
717. Grossman ME, Fithian EC, Behrens C, Bissinger J, Fracaro M, Neu HC. Primary cutaneous aspergillosis in six leukemic children. J Am Acad Dermatol 1985;12:313–318.
718. Walsh TJ, Van Cutsem J, Polak AM, Graybill JR. Immunomodulation and antifungal treatment of experimental invasive candidosis, histoplasmosis, and aspergillosis. Recent advances and concepts. J Med Vet Mycol 1992;30(Suppl 1):225–240.
719. Nichol KL. Preventing influenza: The physician's role. Semin Respir Infect 1992;7:71–77.

720. Pachucki CT, Lentino JR, Jackson CG. Attitudes and behavior of health care personnel regarding the use and efficacy of influenza vaccine. J Infect Dis 1985;151:1170–1171.
721. Fedson DS, Kessler HA. A hospital-based influenza immunization program, 1977–78. Am J Public Health 1983;73:442–445.
722. Williams WW, Hickson MA, Kane MA, et al. Immunization policies and vaccine coverage among adults. Ann Intern Med 1988;108:616–625.
723. Arden N, Patriarca PA, Kendal AP. Experiences in the use and efficacy of inactivated vaccines in nursing homes. In: Kendal AP, Patriarca PA, eds. Options for the control of influenza. New York: Alan Liss, 1985:155–168.
724. Ksiazek TG, Olson JG, Irving GS, Settle CS, White R, Petrusso R. An influenza outbreak due to A/USSR/77-like (H1N1) virus aboard a US navy ship. Am J Epidemiol 1980;112:487–494.
725. Berlinberg CD, Weingarten SR, Bolton LB, Waterman SH. Occupational exposure to influenza—introduction of an index case to a hospital. Infect Control Hosp Epidemiol 1989;10:70–73.
726. Askonas BA, McMichael AJ, Webster RG. The immune response to influenza viruses and the problem of protection against infection. In: Beare AS, ed. Basic and applied influenza research. Boca Raton, FL: CRC Press, 1982:159–182.
727. Schulze-Robbecke R, Jung KD, Pullman H, Hundgeburth J. Control of Legionella pneumophila in a hospital hot water system. Zbl Hyg 1990;190:84–100.
728. Groothis DG, Veenendaal HR, Dijkstra HL. Influence of temperature on the number of Legionella pneumophila in hot water systems. J Appl Bacteriol 1985;59:529–536.
729. Colbourne JS, Pratt DJ, Smith MG, Fisher-Hoch SP, Harper D. Water fittings as sources of Legionella pneumophila in a hospital plumbing system. Lancet 1984;1:210–213.
730. Environmental Protection Agency. National interim primary drinking water regulations: control of trihalothanes in drinking water: final rules. Federal Register 1979;44:68624-68705.
731. Environmental Protection Agency. National interim primary drinking water regulations: trihalothanes. Federal Register 1983;48:8406–8414.
732. Centers for Disease Control and Prevention. Procedures for the recovery of Legionella from the environment. Atlanta: Public Health Service, 1992:1–13.
733. Alary MA, Joly JR. Comparison of culture methods and an immunofluorescence assay for the detection of Legionella pneumophila in domestic hot water devices. Curr Microbiol 1992;25:19–25.
734. Vickers RM, Stout JE, Yu VL. Failure of a diagnostic monoclonal immunofluorescent reagent to detect Legionella pneumophila in environmental samples. Appl Environ Microbiol 1990;56:2912–2914.
735. Fluornoy DJ, Belobraydic KA, Silberg SL, Lawrence CH, Guthrie PJ. False-positive Legionella pneumophila direct immunofluorescent monoclonal antibody test caused by Bacillus cereus spores. Diag Microbiol Infect Dis 1988;9:123–125.
736. Bej AK, Mahbubani MH, Atlas RM. Detection of viable Legionella pneumophila in water by polymerase chain reaction and gene probe methods. Appl Environ Microbiol 1991;57:597–600.
737. Barbaree JM, Gorman GW, Martin WT, Fields BS, Morrill WE. Protocol for sampling environmental sites for Legionellae. Appl Environ Microbiol 1987;53:1454–1458.

APPENDIX A

Examples of Semicritical Items* Used on the Respiratory Tract

Anesthesia device or equipment including:
Face mask or tracheal tube
Inspiratory and expiratory tubing
Y-piece
Reservoir bag
Humidifier
Breathing circuits of mechanical ventilators
Bronchoscopes and their accessories, except for biopsy forceps and specimen brush, which are considered critical items and are sterilized before reuse.
Endotracheal and endobronchial tubes
Laryngoscope blades
Mouthpieces and tubing of pulmonary-function testing equipment
Nebulizers and their reservoirs
Oral and nasal airways

---

* Items that directly or indirectly contact mucous membranes of the respiratory tract. They are sterilized or subjected to high-level disinfection before reuse.

Probes of CO_2 analyzers, air-pressure monitors
Resuscitation bags
Stylets
Suction catheters
Temperature sensors

APPENDIX B

Maintenance Procedures to Decrease Survival and Multiplication of Legionella spp. in Potable-Water Distribution Systems

Providing Water at ≥50°C at All Points in the Heated Water System, Including the Taps

This requires that water in calorifiers (water heaters) be maintained at ≥60°C. In the United Kingdom, where maintenance of water temperatures at ≥50°C in hospitals has been mandated, installation of blending or mixing valves at or near taps to reduce the water temperature to ≤43°C has been recommended in certain settings to reduce the risk of scald injury to patients, visitors, and health-care workers (447). However, Legionella spp. can multiply even in short segments of pipe containing water at this temperature. Increasing the flow rate from the hot-water-circulation system may help lessen the likelihood of water stagnation and cooling (450, 727). Insulation of plumbing to ensure delivery of cold (<20°C) water to water heaters (and to cold-water outlets) may diminish the opportunity for bacterial multiplication (392). "Dead legs" or capped spurs within the plumbing system provide areas of stagnation and cooling to <50°C regardless of the circulating-water temperature; these segments may need to be removed to prevent colonization (728). Rubber fittings within plumbing systems have been associated with persistent colonization, and replacement of these fittings may be required for Legionella spp. eradication (729).

Continuous Chlorination to Maintain Concentrations of Free Residual Chlorine at 1–2 mg/L at the Tap

This requires the placement of flow-adjusted, continuous injectors of chlorine throughout the water distribution system. Adverse effects of continuous chlorination include accelerated corrosion of plumbing resulting in system leaks and production of potentially carcinogenic trihalomethanes. However, when levels of free residual chlorine are below 3 mg/L, trihalomethane levels are kept below the maximum "safety level" recommended by the Environmental Protection Agency (448, 730, 731).

APPENDIX C

Culturing Environmental Specimens for Legionella spp.

I. Recommended Procedure for Collecting and Processing Environmental Specimens for Legionella spp (732).

    A. Collect water (if possible, one-liter samples) in sterile, screw-top bottles, preferably containing sodium thiosulfate at a concentration of 0.5 cc of 0.1 N solution of sample water. (Sodium thiosulfate inactivates any residual halogen biocide).

    B. Collect culture-swabs of the internal surfaces of faucets, aerators, and showerheads; in a sterile, screw-top container, such as a 50-cc plastic centrifuge tube, submerge each swab in 5–10 cc of sample water taken from the same device from which the sample was obtained.

    C. As soon as possible after collection, water samples and swabs should be transported to and processed in a laboratory proficient at culturing water specimens for Legionella spp. Samples may be transported at room temperature but must be protected from temperature extremes.

    D. Test samples for the presence of Legionella spp. by using semi-selective culture media. Use standard laboratory procedures. (Detection of Legionella spp. antigen by the direct fluorescent antibody technique is not suitable for environmental samples (733–735). In addition, the use of polymerase chain reaction (PCR) for identification of Legionella spp. is not recommended until more data on the sensitivity and specificity of this procedure are available (736).)

II. Possible Samples and Sampling Sites for Legionella Spp. in the Hospital (737)

Water Samples
Potable Water System
    Incoming water main
    Water softener
    Holding tanks/cisterns
    Water heater tanks (inflow and outflow sites)
    Potable water outlets (faucets or taps, showers) especially outlets located in or near case-patients' rooms
    Cooling Tower/Evaporative Condenser
Make-up water (water added to system to replace water lost by evaporation, drift, and leakage)
    Basin (area under tower for collection of cooled water)
    Sump (section of basin from which cooled water returns to heat source)
    Heat source (e.g., chillers)
Other Sources
Humidifiers (Nebulizers)
    Bubblers for oxygen
    Water used for respiratory therapy equipment
    Decorative fountains
    Irrigation equipment
    Fire sprinkler system (if recently used)
Whirlpools/spas
    Swabs
Potable Water System
    Faucets (proximal to aerators)
    Faucet aerators
    Shower heads
Cooling Towers
    Internal components (e.g., splash bars and other fill surfaces)
    Areas with visible biofilm accumulation

APPENDIX D

Procedure for Cleaning Cooling Towers and Related Equipment

(Adapted from the Emergency Protocol in Control of Legionella spp. in Cooling Towers: Summary Guidelines (464).)

I. Preparatory to Chemical Disinfection and Mechanical Cleaning

    A. Provide protective equipment to workers who would perform the disinfection, to prevent their exposure to (a) chemicals used for disinfection and (b) aerosolized water containing Legionella spp. Protective equipment may include full-length protective clothing, boots, gloves, goggles, and a full- or half-face mask that combines high efficiency particulate air filter and chemical cartridges to protect against airborne chlorine levels of up to 10 mg/L.

    B. Shut off cooling-tower.
        1. If possible, shut off heat source.
        2. Shut off fans, if present, on the cooling tower/evaporative condenser (CT/EC).
        3. Shut off the system blowdown (purge) valve. Shut off automated blowdown controller, if present, and set system controller to manual.
        4. Keep make-up water valves open.
        5. Close building air-intake vents within at least 30 meters of the CT/EC until after the cleaning procedure is complete.
        6. Continue operating pumps for water circulation through the CT/EC.

II. Chemical Disinfection

    A. Add fast-release, chlorine-containing disinfectant in pellet, granular, or liquid form, and follow safety instructions on the product label. Examples of disinfectants include sodium hypochlorite (NaOCl) or calcium hypochlorite (Ca[OCl]$_2$), calculated to achieve initial free residual chlorine (FRC) of 50 mg/L, i.e., 3.0 lbs (1.4 kg) industrial grade NaOCl (12–15% available Cl) per 1,000 gallons of CT/EC water; 10.5 lbs (4.8 kg) domestic grade NaOCl (3–5% available Cl) per 1,000 gallons of CT/EC water; or 0.6 lb (0.3 kg) Ca(OCl)$_2$ per 1,000 gallons of CT/EC water. If significant biodeposits are present, additional chlorine may be required. If the volume of water in CT/EC is not known, it can be estimated (in gallons) by multiplying the recirculation rate in gallons/minute by 10, or the refrigeration capacity in tons by 30. Other appropriate compounds may be suggested by a water-treatment specialist.

    B. Record the type and quality of all chemicals used for disinfection, exact time the chemicals are added to the system, and time and results of measurements of (FRC) and pH.

    C. Add dispersant simultaneously with or within 15 minutes of adding disinfectant. The dispersant is best added by first dissolving it in water and adding the solution to a turbulent zone in the water system. Examples of low or non-foaming, silicate-based dispersants are: automatic-dishwasher compounds, such as Cascade** or Calgonite** or an equivalent product. Dispersants are added at 10–25 lbs. (4.5–11.25 kg) per 1,000 gallons of CT/EC water.

    D. After adding disinfectant and dispersant, continue circulating the water through the system. Monitor FRC by using an FRC-measuring device, such as a swimming pool test kit, and measure the pH with a pH meter every 15 minutes for 2 hours. Add chlorine as needed to maintain FRC at >10 mg/L. Since the biocidal effect of chlorine is reduced at higher pH, adjust pH to 7.5–8.0. The pH may be lowered by using any acid (e.g., muriatic acid or sulfuric acid used for maintenance of swimming pools) that is compatible with the treatment chemicals.

    E. Two hours after adding disinfectant and dispersant or after FRC level is stable at ≥10 mg/L, monitor at 2-hour intervals and maintain FRC at ≥10 mg/L for 24 hours.

    F. After FRC level has been maintained at ≥10 mg/L for 24 hours, drain the system. CT/EC water may be safely drained to the sanitary sewer. Municipal water and sewerage authorities should be contacted regarding local regulations. If a sanitary sewer is not available, consult local or state authorities (e.g., Department of Natural Resources) regarding disposal of water. If necessary, the drain-off may be dechlorinated by dissipation or chemical neutralization with sodium bisulfite.

    G. Refill system with water and repeat procedure outlined in steps 2–6 in I.B above.

III. Mechanical Cleaning

    A. After water from the second chemical disinfection has been drained, shut down the CT/EC.

    B. Inspect all water contact areas for sediment, sludge, and scale. Using brushes and/or a low-pressure water hose, thoroughly clean all CT/EC water contact areas including basin, sump, fill, spray nozzles, and fittings. Replace components as needed.

    C. If possible, clean CT/EC water contact areas within the chillers.

IV. After Mechanical Cleaning

    A. Fill the system with water, and add chlorine to achieve FRC level of 10 mg/L.

    B. Circulate water for one hour, then open blowdown valve and flush the entire system until the water is free of turbidity.

    C. Drain the system.

    D. Open any air intake vents that were closed prior to cleaning.

    E. Fill the system with water. CT/EC may be put back into service using an effective water-treatment program.

** Use of product names is for identification only and does not imply endorsement by the Public Health Service or the U.S. Department of Health and Human Services.

Guideline for Infection Control in Hospital Personnel

Original Citation: Centers for Disease Control and Prevention. Guideline for infection control in hospital personnel. U.S. Department of Health and Human Services, Public Health Service, Center for Disease Control. Infect Control 1983;4(Suppl):326–349.

Original Author: Walter W. Williams, MD, MPH

CDC GUIDELINES ON INFECTION CONTROL

The Guideline for Infection Control in Hospital Personnel is part of the Guidelines for Prevention and Control of Nosocomial Infections. The CDC guidelines were developed to provide a central reference for professionals involved in infection control that contains CDC recommendations and is easily accessible to the infection control personnel in hospitals. It should be emphasized that these guidelines represent the advice of CDC on questions commonly asked of the Hospital Infections Program, but are not intended to have the force of law or regulation. These guidelines can be expected to change in response to the acquisition of new knowledge.

Each guideline begins with a preamble that describes the approaches that have been used or advocated to deal with infection control issues and evaluate, where data exist, their efficacy. The preamble is followed by a group of succinct recommendations. The guidelines are assembled in a loose-leaf notebook to allow for the addition of new guidelines as they are developed and revisions as necessary.

Optimally, recommendations should be based on rigorously controlled scientific studies because recommendations of this type have the highest probability of value. There are some recommended practices that have not been adequately evaluated by controlled scientific trials, but are based on such inherent logic and broad experience that experts generally agree that they are useful. At the other extreme are recommendations that are of uncertain benefit and may be quite controversial. To address these last 2 types of practices, realizing that hospitals must make decisions in the absence of definitive data, we have sought the advice of working groups composed of non-CDC experts with broad experience in infection control. CDC has endorsed such recommendations if members of the working group have determined that the recommended practices are likely to be effective.

To assist infection control staff in critically assessing the value of these recommendations, we developed a ranking scheme that takes into account considerations of scientific validity, applicability, and practicality (Table 1). The last 2 considerations are clearly important since scientifically valid infection control practices that are applicable in one setting (e.g., debilitated patients in tertiary referral centers) might not necessarily be applicable or practical in another (e.g., acutely ill patients in community hospitals). Cost effectiveness, another important consideration, is taken into account in the ranking process when possible, although adequate data are generally lacking. We have ranked each recommendation according to the degree to which it has been substantiated by scientific data or the strength of the working group's opinion on the effectiveness and practical value of the particular practice. The rankings thus provide additional useful information for hospital officials who must decide on the recommendations (e.g., those in Category II and, especially, Category III) that best suit their hospital's needs and resources.

Finally, the adoption of these recommendations by hospitals does not guarantee that hospital personnel will adhere to them. The reduction of nosocomial infection risks depends largely on the actual performance of correct patient-care practices. Personnel may be motivated to follow those practices if they are given adequate training, followed by periodic in-service education. Continuous or periodic evaluation of patient-care practices, preferably under the supervision of the infection control staff, might assure continued performance of correct practices.

Table 1. Ranking scheme for recommendations*

Category I. Strongly Recommended for Adoption:
  Measures in Category I are strongly supported by well-designed and controlled clinical studies that
  show effectiveness in reducing the risk of nosocomial infections or are viewed as useful by the majority
  of experts in the field. Measures in this category are judged to be applicable to the majority of hospitals—regardless of size, patient population, or endemic nosocomial infection rate—and are considered
  practical to implement.
Category II. Moderately Recommended for Adoption:
  Measures in Category II are supported by highly suggestive clinical studies or by definitive studies in institutions that might not be representative of other hospitals. Measures that have not been adequately
  studied, but have a strong theoretical rationale indicating that they might be very effective are included
  in this category. Category II measures are judged to be practical to implement. They are *not* to be considered a standard of practice for every hospital.
Category III. Weakly Recommended for Adoption:
  Measures in Category III have been proposed by some investigators, authorities, or organizations, but,
  to date, they lack both supporting data and a strong theoretical rationale. Thus, they might be considered as important issues that require further evaluation; they might be considered by some hospitals
  for implementation, especially if such hospitals have specific nosocomial infection problems or sufficient resources.

Recommendations that advise against the adoption of certain measures can be found in the guidelines.
These negative recommendations are also ranked into 1 of the 3 categories depending on the strength of
the scientific backing or opinions of the members of the working group. A negative recommendation in
Category I means that scientific data or prevailing opinion strongly indicate that the measure not be adopted.
A negative recommendation in Category III means that, given the available information, the measure under
consideration should probably not be adopted; such a measure, however, requires further evaluation.

GUIDELINE FOR INFECTION CONTROL IN
HOSPITAL PERSONNEL

Introduction

In the United States, about 5 million persons work in more than 7,000 hospitals. These personnel may become infected through exposure to infected patients if proper precautions are not used, or acquire infection outside the hospital. They may then transmit the infection to susceptible patients or other
hospital personnel, members of their households, or other community contacts. In this guideline, we focus on diseases that are of particular concern to
hospital personnel because of the possibility of transmission. In some instances
we focus our discussion on transmission of infectious disease from patient-care
personnel to patients. In other instances we focus on transmission of disease
from patients to patient-care personnel. Recommendations for prevention and
control are limited to these areas. We frequently refer to the Guideline for
Isolation Precautions in Hospitals, where suggestions can be found on precautions that personnel may use when taking care of patients to prevent the spread
of infection to themselves, other personnel or patients, and visitors.

   Personnel who have direct contact with patients include nursing personnel,
medical house staff, clinical faculty, attending physicians, paramedical staff, and
nursing and medical students. Since other hospital personnel may have exposure to patients that is comparable in quality, intensity, and duration to that of
patient-care personnel, hospitals may also consider them in applying these recommendations. Risk to patients from personnel with whom patients have only
brief casual contact, or risk to these personnel, is generally felt to be low.

In the glossary key words or phrases used in this guideline are defined. Issues related to management of outbreaks, exposure to agents in microbiologic and biomedical laboratories, and risks from exposure to noninfectious hazards are not discussed in this guideline.

Objectives of a Personnel Health Service for Infection Control

The infection control objectives of a personnel health service should be part of the hospital's general programs for infection control. The objectives can include (a) stressing maintenance of sound habits in personal hygiene and individual responsibility in infection control; (b) monitoring and investigating infectious diseases, potentially harmful infectious exposures, and outbreaks of infections among personnel; (c) providing care to personnel for work-related illnesses or exposures; (d) identifying infection risks related to employment and instituting appropriate preventive measures; and (e) containing costs by eliminating unnecessary procedures and by preventing infectious disease that results in absenteeism and disability. For these objectives to be met, the support of the administration, medical staff, and other hospital staff is essential.

Whether programs or services other than those for infection control are offered will depend on whether the hospital's personnel health service is devoted mainly to controlling infectious diseases or to providing a comprehensive health program for personnel.

Elements of a Personnel Health Service for Infection Control

The organization of a health service for hospital personnel will depend on many factors, for example, the size of the institution, the number of personnel, and the services offered. These factors will determine the size, location, and staffing of the service. Regardless of how the service is provided, certain elements will assist in effectively attaining infection control goals. These elements are as follows:

1. Placement evaluations.
2. Personnel health and safety education.
3. Immunization programs.
4. Protocols for surveillance and management of job-related illnesses and exposures to infectious diseases.
5. Counseling services for personnel regarding infection risks related to employment or special conditions.
6. Guidelines for work restriction because of infectious disease.
7. Maintenance of health records.

Placement Evaluations

When personnel are initially appointed or are reassigned to different jobs or areas, a placement evaluation can be used to ensure that persons are not placed in jobs that would pose undue risk of infection to them, other personnel, patients, or visitors. A health inventory is an important part of this evaluation. This inventory can include determining a health worker's immunization status and obtaining a history of any conditions that may predispose the health worker to acquiring or transmitting infectious diseases; for example, a history of such childhood diseases as chickenpox and measles, history of exposure to or treatment for tuberculosis, history of hepatitis, dermatologic conditions, chronic draining infections or open wounds, and immunodeficient conditions. Physical examinations may be useful to detect conditions that may increase the likelihood of transmitting disease to patients, or unusual susceptibility to infection, and to serve as a baseline for determining whether any future problems are work-related. There are no data, however, to suggest that routine complete physical examinations are needed for infection control purposes. Neither are there data to suggest that routine laboratory testing (such as complete blood counts, serologic tests for syphilis, urinalysis, chest roentgenograms) or pre-employment screening for enteric or other pathogens are cost-beneficial. The health inventory can be used to determine whether physical examinations or laboratory tests are needed. In some areas, however, local public health ordinances may still mandate that certain screening procedures be used.

It is important that initial placement evaluations be done when personnel are hired or as soon alter as possible. After the placement evaluation, later appraisals may be done as needed to ongoing programs or evaluation of work-related problems.

Personnel Health and Safety Education

Personnel are more likely to comply with an infection control program if they understand its rationale. Thus, staff education should be a central focus of the infection control program. Clearly written policies, guidelines, and procedures are needed in many instances for uniformity, efficiency, and effective coordination of activities. Since job categories vary, not all personnel need the same degree of instruction in infection control. Educational programs should be matched to the needs of each group.

Immunization Programs

Since hospital personnel are at risk of exposure to and possible transmission of vaccine-preventable diseases because of their contact with patients or material from patients with infections, maintenance of immunity is an essential part of a hospital's personnel health and infection control program. Optimal use of immunizing agents will not only safeguard the health of personnel but also protect patients from becoming infected by personnel. Following a consistent program of immunizations could eliminate the problem of susceptible personnel and avoid unnecessary work restrictions.

Immunization recommendations are made by the U.S. Public Health Service Immunization Practices Advisory Committee (ACIP) and are published periodically in the Morbidity and Mortality Weekly Report (MMWR). Indications for use of licensed vaccines are generally the same for hospital personnel as for the general population; however, immunity to some diseases, such as rubella, may be more important for persons who work in hospitals. Decisions about which vaccines to include in immunization programs can be made by considering (a) the risk of exposure to an agent in a given area, (b) the nature of employment, and (c) the size and kind of institution. The suggestions included in this guideline summarize ACIP recommendations as they apply to hospital personnel. The categories reflect the views of the Working Group for this guideline. The ACIP guidelines should be consulted for a detailed discussion of the rationale for active or passive immunization of hospital personnel and the general population. The ACIP guidelines can be requested from Public Inquiries, Building 1, Room B63, Centers for Disease Control, Atlanta, Georgia 30333.

Screening for Susceptibility to Hepatitis B or Rubella

The decision to screen potential vaccine recipients for susceptibility to hepatitis B virus (HBV) is an economic one, because vaccinating HBV carriers or persons already immune does not appear to present a hazard (1, 2). In the United States the prevalence of previous infection in any targeted group, the cost of screening, and the cost of immunizing personnel determine whether screening would be cost-effective (3, 4).

Routinely performing serologic tests to determine susceptibility to rubella to be sure vaccine is given only to proven susceptibles may be very expensive. The ACIP believes that rubella immunization of men and women not known to be pregnant is justifiable without serologic testing (5).

Vaccine Administration

The most efficient use of vaccines with high-risk groups is to immunize personnel before they enter high-risk situations. It is crucial that persons administering immunizing agents be well-informed about indications, storage, dosage, preparation, and contraindications for each of the vaccines, toxoids, and immune globulins they may use. Product information should be available at all times, and pertinent health history should be obtained from each health worker before an agent is given.

How immunizations are provided to personnel and who pays for vaccines are topics not addressed in this guideline.

Work Restrictions and Management of Job-related Illnesses and Exposures

Major functions of the personnel health service include arranging for prompt diagnosis and management of job-related illnesses and providing prophylaxis for certain preventable diseases to which personnel may be exposed. If susceptible personnel contract a serious infection that is potentially transmissible or are exposed to an illness that leads to a period during which infection may be spread, the hospital's responsibility to prevent the spread of infection to patients and other personnel may sometimes require that these persons be excluded from direct patient contact. For any exclusion policy to be enforceable and effective, all personnel—especially department heads, area supervisors, and head nurses—must know when an illness must be reported. Any policy for work restriction should be designed to encourage personnel to report their illnesses or exposures and not penalize them with loss of wages, benefits, or job status.

Health Counseling

Access to health counseling about illnesses they may acquire from or transmit to patients is especially important for all hospital personnel, but particularly for women of childbearing age and persons with special clinical conditions. All personnel should know about infection risks related to employment. Female personnel who may be pregnant or who might become pregnant should know about potential risks to the lotus due to work assignments and preventive measures that will reduce those risks. Among the diseases with potential for risk to a lotus if contracted by the mother are cytomegalovirus infection, hepatitis B, and rubella.

Coordinated Planning With Other Departments

For infection control objectives to be achieved, the activities of the personnel health service must be coordinated with the infection control program and with various hospital departments. This coordination will help assure adequate surveillance of infections in personnel and maintenance of effective infection control programs. During case investigations, outbreaks, and other epidemiologic studies that involve hospital personnel, coordinating activities will help to assure that investigations can be conducted efficiently and control measures implemented promptly.

EPIDEMIOLOGY AND CONTROL OF SELECTED INFECTIONS TRANSMITTED AMONG HOSPITAL PERSONNEL AND PATIENTS

Almost any transmissible infection may occur in the community at large or within the hospital and can affect both personnel and patients. However, only those infectious diseases that occur frequently in the hospital setting or are most important to personnel are discussed below. These diseases have been divided into 2 groups, according to what we know about the epidemiology and whether the primary concern is (a) preventing transmission of infection both to and from personnel and patients or (b) preventing transmission of infection primarily from infected patients to personnel. Within each section, diseases are listed alphabetically. Relevant epidemiology, microbiology, and preventive measures are reviewed for each disease. Infections that are unusual or are not major nosocomial problems in this country receive only a brief comment or none at all.

In all patient-care activities, personnel can decrease the risk of acquiring or transmitting infection by careful handwashing and by taking care of patients with potentially transmissible infections according to the CDC Guideline for Isolation Precautions in Hospitals.

GROUP I INFECTIONS: TRANSMISSION TO AND FROM PERSONNEL

ACQUIRED IMMUNODEFICIENCY SYNDROME (AIDS)

Personnel have been exposed to patients with AIDS and to their clinical specimens; however, there is currently no evidence of AIDS transmission to hospital personnel or from hospital personnel to patients. The etiology of the underlying immune deficiencies of patients with AIDS is unknown. One current hypothesis is that a transmissible agent is involved. If so, the agent appears to be transmitted most commonly through intimate, direct contact with mucosal surfaces or through parenteral spread. Airborne spread and interpersonal spread through casual contact do not seem likely. These patterns resemble the distribution of disease and modes of spread of hepatitis B virus.

With our present knowledge, it appears prudent for hospital personnel to use similar precautions when taking care of patients with AIDS as those used for patients with hepatitis B virus infection (6) (see Guideline for Isolation Precautions in Hospitals). It also appears prudent for hospital personnel who have AIDS to use similar precautions as those suggested for known carriers of HBsAg to minimize their infectious risk to others (see hepatitis discussion below). Precautions have been advised for persons and specimens from persons in certain patient categories considered to be part of the AIDS spectrum. These categories include persons with the following illnesses: opportunistic infections that are not associated with underlying immunosuppressive disease or therapy; Kaposi's sarcoma (patients under 60 years of age); chronic generalized lymphadenopathy, unexplained weight loss, and/or prolonged unexplained fever in persons who belong to groups with apparently increased risk of AIDS (homosexual men, intravenous-drug abusers, Haitian immigrants, hemophiliacs) (6). However, since AIDS has been diagnosed in persons not in identified high-risk groups, personnel may also use precautions when taking care of patients whose clinical condition and epidemiologic history suggest a risk for developing AIDS. Any new information on the cause and transmission of AIDS should be considered when precautions are designed or changed.

Extraordinary care must be taken to avoid accidental wounds from sharp instruments contaminated with potentially infective material and to avoid contact of mucous membranes and open skin lesions with materials from AIDS patients. Because of the lack of pertinent information, no particular course of action can be recommended in the event of accidental percutaneous or mucosal exposure to potentially infective material from patients with AIDS. Since these patients are often in high-risk groups for hepatitis B, following the suggestions for handling exposures to blood at high risk of being positive for hepatitis B surface antigen (HBsAg) may be considered (Table 2). Currently, no information is available on the potential benefits or problems associated with administering passive or active immunizing agents or therapy in this situation.

Table 2. Summary of postexposure prophylaxis for acute percutaneous (needlestick) exposures to HBV*

Status of the patient's blood the health worker was exposed to	HBsAg testing recommended	Recommended prophylaxis
HBsAg-positive		HBIG (0.06 ml/kg) immediately and 1 month after needle-stick
HBsAg status unknown Source known:		
Blood is at *High Risk* (β) of being HBsAg-positive	Yes§	IG (0.06 ml/kg) immediately and if *test positive* HBIG (0.06 ml/kg) immediately and 1 month after needle-stick or if *test negative* nothing
Blood is at *Low Risk* (¶) of being HBsAg-positive	No	Nothing or IG (0.06 ml/kg)
HBsAg status unknown Source unknown	No	Nothing or IG (0.06 ml/kg)

*Consult current ACIP recommendation for important details.

(β) *High risk that the source is HBsAG-positive*—such as patients with acute, unconfirmed viral hepatitis; patients institutionalized with Down's syndrome; patients on hemodialysis; persons of Asian origin; homosexual men; users of illicit, intravenous drugs.

§If results can be known within 7 days after exposure. Although prophylaxis may be given up to 7 days after exposure, it is most effective when given as soon after exposure as possible, preferably within 24–48 hours. Screening of exposed personnel to determine susceptibility may also be considered, but the decision to screen should not delay the administration of globulin.

(¶) *Low risk that the source is HBsAG-positive*—such as the average hospital patient.

HBIG = Hepatitis B immune globulin

IG = Immune globulin (formerly called "immune serum globulin," ISG, or "gamma globulin")

ACUTE DIARRHEA

Various agents may cause diarrhea in patients and hospital personnel. Salmonella, Shigella, and Campylobacter species are among the common bacterial enteric pathogens. Infection with these agents may produce mild symptoms but is often accompanied by other symptoms, such as abdominal cramps, fever, or bloody diarrhea. Diarrheal illness accompanied by such symptoms suggests a bacterial cause. Rotavirus and the 27-nanometer (Norwalk and Norwalk-like) agents are among the chief causes of sporadic and epidemic viral gastroenteritis. Giardia lamblia and other protozoa are also frequent causes of diarrhea. Any of these agents may be nosocomially transmitted via the hands of personnel who are infected.

If personnel contract an acute diarrheal illness accompanied by fever, cramps, or bloody stools, they are likely to be excreting potentially infective organisms in high titer in their feces. The specific cause of acute diarrhea, however, cannot be determined solely on the basis of clinical symptoms; thus, appropriate laboratory tests are important. Not allowing these persons to take care of patients pending evaluation will prevent transmission. Evaluation of personnel may usually be limited to an initial culture for bacterial pathogens and stool examination for intestinal protozoa; repeat studies may be indicated if the results of the first tests are negative and the illness persists.

Carriage of Enteric Pathogens by Personnel

Carnage of enteric pathogens may persist after resolution of the acute illness. Once the person has clinically recovered and is having formed stools, however, there should be little hazard to patients, provided normal hygienic practices are observed. Existing data suggest that appropriate antibiotic therapy may eradicate fecal excretion of Shigella or Campylobacter. If persons take antibiotics, any follow-up cultures are best taken 48 hours after the last dose. Carriage of Salmonella, however, calls for special concern, because carnage may be prolonged and because the clinical sequelae of acute salmonellosis are often severe in high-risk patients, such as newborns, the elderly, immunocompromised patients, and the severely ill, such as those in intensive care units. Antibiotic therapy may prolong Salmonella excretion or lead to emergence of resistant strains and is not generally indicated. Thus, special precautions regarding contact with high-risk patients may be needed for personnel who are convalescent carriers of Salmonella.

Generally, personal hygiene, particularly handwashing by personnel before and after all patient contacts, will minimize the risk of transmitting enteric pathogens to patients. Maintaining good hygiene when away from the work setting will minimize the risk of transmission to family contacts.

Food-service personnel are not discussed in this guideline. Precautions for personnel taking care of patients who have gastroenteritis are discussed in the Guideline for Isolation Precautions in Hospitals.

HEPATITIS

Viral hepatitis has long been recognized as a nosocomial hazard. The agents that most commonly cause vital hepatitis are hepatitis A virus (HAV), hepatitis B virus (HBV), and 1 or more viruses currently designated non-A, non-B (NANB).

Hepatitis A

Nosocomial hepatitis A occurs infrequently and is associated with 2 unusual circumstances: (a) the source of infection is a patient hospitalized for other reasons whose hepatitis is not apparent, and (b) the patient is fecally incontinent. These circumstances may occur in adult and pediatric patients.

Hepatitis A is transmitted primarily by the fecal-oral route. It has not been reported to occur after inadvertent needle sticks or other contact with blood. Personnel who have frequent contact with blood, such as those who work in dialysis units, do not have evidence of increased infections with HAV (7). Hepatitis A has, however, been reported to be transmitted by blood transfusion (8).

Fecal excretion of HAV is greatest during the incubation period of disease before the onset of jaundice. Once disease is clinically obvious, the risk of transmitting infection is decreased. However, some patients admitted to the hospital with hepatitis A may still be shedding virus (9, 10) and are potentially infective. Fecal shedding of HAV can continue for up to 2 to 3 weeks after onset of dark urine; however, in most persons, viral shedding is complete about 7 days after dark urine appears (9). Anicteric infection may also occur, especially in young children. There is no evidence supporting the existence of a chronic HAV carrier state.

Personnel can help protect themselves and others from infection with HAV by always maintaining good personal hygiene, practicing thorough handwashing at all times, and taking care of patients known to be infected with HAV according to published recommendations (see Guideline for Isolation Precautions in Hospitals). If personnel become infected with HAV, the risk of transmitting infection is very low or negligible after about 7 days after onset of jaundice. Foodborne transmission of hepatitis A is not discussed in this guideline.

Hepatitis B

Most nosocomial cases of hepatitis B unrelated to the transfusion of blood or blood products occur in hospital personnel rather than patients. Transmission occurs by parenteral or mucosal exposure to HBsAg-positive blood from persons who are carriers or have acute HBV infection. Often carriers of HBsAg and persons with acute infections are unrecognized and are therefore not known to be infective. The infectivity of blood is best correlated with the presence of hepatitis B "e" antigen (HBeAg); however, any blood that is HBsAg-positive is potentially infective. Presence of HBeAg correlates strongly with the number of infective HBV in the serum.

The principal modes of HBV transmission are given below in order of decreasing efficiency:

1. Overt Parenteral Transmission

   Direct percutaneous inoculation by needle or instrument contaminated with serum or plasma (for example, accidental needle-sticks, transfusion of contaminated blood or blood products, and acupuncture).

2. Inapparent Parenteral Transmission
   a. Percutaneous inoculation with infective serum or plasma without overt needle puncture (for example, contamination of fresh cutaneous scratches, abrasions, burns, or other lesions).
   b. Contamination of mucosal surfaces with infective serum or plasma (for example, mouth pipetting accidents, accidental eye splash, and other direct contact with mucous membranes of the eyes or mouth, such as hand to mouth or eye when contaminated with infective blood or serum).
   c. Transfer of infective material to skin lesions or mucous membranes via inanimate environmental surfaces (for example, surfaces of various types of hospital equipment, devices, and rubber gloves).
   d. Contamination of mucosal surfaces with infective secretions other than serum or plasma (for example, contact involving saliva or semen).

   Fecal-oral transmission of HBV does not appear to occur; however, transmission among homosexual men has been described, possibly via contamination from asymptomatic rectal mucosal lesions at sites of sexual contact (11). Airborne spread of HBV by droplet nuclei does not appear to be epidemiologically important (12, 13). Transmission of HBV in dental operatories, however, by large droplets that may strike mucous membranes or contaminate environmental surfaces has not been ruled out (13).

   Within the hospital setting certain work locations and occupational categories have been identified as showing increased risk for hepatitis B infection (7, 14, 20). Generally, the highest risk of HBV infection is associated with locations and occupations in which contact with blood from infected patients is frequent. The locations and occupations are as follows (adapted from Maynard JE. Nosocomial viral hepatitis. Am J Med 1981;70:440):

Work locations	Occupational categories
Blood banks	Dentists and dental surgeons
Dental clinics	Dialysis technicians
Clinical laboratories	Laboratory technicians
Dialysis wards	Nurses
Emergency rooms	Physicians (especially surgeons and pathologists)
Hematology/oncology wards	
Operating and recovery rooms	
Pathology laboratories	

Hospital personnel who do not have physical exposure to blood are at no greater risk than the general population. Patient contact without physical exposure to blood has not been documented to be a risk factor.

To prevent transmission of hepatitis B, hospital staff must be aware of the modes of transmission and the appropriate precautions in taking care of infected patients or handling their clinical specimens (see Guideline for Isolation Precautions in Hospitals). In general, the major emphasis is on applying blood precautions, practicing proper handwashing, having minimal contact with blood or blood-contaminated excretions, and handling the blood of all patients as potentially infective material (21).

Since droplets from the patient's mouth reach the face of the dentist during certain procedures, dentists might consider protecting their eyes, nose, and mouth from such exposure by using masks and protective eyewear. They can prevent direct contact with infective material in the mouth by routinely wearing gloves during dental procedures.

ACUTE HBV INFECTION IN PERSONNEL AND HBsAG CARRIERS

A career is defined as a person who is HBsAg-positive on at least 2 occasions at least 6 months apart. After acute infection with HBV, the likelihood of developing the carrier state lessens as the person gets older and depends on the host's immune responsiveness. Carriers and persons with acute cases have the highest concentrations of HBV in the blood and serous fluids. The risk of transmission of HBV by HBsAg-positive health professionals has been examined in recent reports (22–28). Transmission has been documented in a few instances from oral surgeons, gynecologists performing complex pelvic surgery, and a general practitioner. HBsAg-positive personnel with exudative dermatitis on body areas that may contact patients may also pose a risk to patients (28).

Among dental practitioners who do not routinely wear gloves, a greater risk of transmitting infection appears to be associated with highly traumatic dental work, such as tooth extractions and surgery, than with less traumatic work such as examinations and restorations. Transmission by surgeons has been related to type of surgery, in particular, major operative procedures, such as laparotomy, hysterectomy, and major repairs, during which the chance of accidental puncture wounds is presumably greater. In 1 instance, transmission by a hospital worker with a severe exudative dermatitis on both hands appeared to be related to contamination of indwelling arterial catheters (28).

The asymptomatic carrier of HBsAg and the person with an acute case do not appear to endanger susceptible persons except through direct inoculation of his or her blood or contaminated secretions. Thus, these persons need not be restricted from patient-care responsibilities, unless there is epidemiologic evidence that the worker is transmitting infection.

Personnel who are HBsAg-positive may be able to reduce or eliminate their risk of infecting patients by wearing gloves during high-risk procedures in which their blood or body fluids may contact patients (22, 23). Double-gloving during complex surgery might also help interrupt transmission (26). Furthermore, it is crucial to counsel known carriers of HBsAg about practicing good personal hygiene, preventing their blood and potentially infective body fluids from contacting other persons, and not donating blood.

HEMODIALYSIS CENTERS

Infection with HBV has represented a great hazard to both patients and personnel in hemodialysis centers. If adequate infection control strategies are not practiced, hepatitis B infection, once introduced, can become endemic, with patients and environmental surfaces acting as reservoirs. Isolating or segregating patients who are HBV carriers, combined with assigning seropositive personnel to take care of these patients, has greatly decreased transmission of HBV in this environment. A complete discussion of the modes of transmission and control measures for hepatitis B in dialysis centers has been published (29).

PREGNANT PERSONNEL

Pregnant personnel are at no greater risk of contracting hepatitis than other personnel; however, if a woman develops hepatitis B during pregnancy and is HBsAg-positive at the time of delivery, the infant is at high risk of developing neonatal hepatitis and becoming an HBsAg carrier (30, 31). Because of this risk, it is important that pregnant personnel know the dangers of working in high-risk departments and be familiar with precautions that should be used (29). Female personnel of childbearing age may also consider immunization with hepatitis B virus vaccine (see below).

HEPATITIS B VIRUS (HBV) VACCINE

An inactivated vaccine of high immunogenicity and efficacy is commercially available. The application of the vaccine in acute-care hospitals will depend on the risk of HBV infection for hospital personnel and the cost of vaccine.

Present estimates of risk have been based primarily on studies of the prevalence of hepatitis serum markers in selected groups (14–17, 19, 20). Incidence studies of HBV infection among hospital personnel have been few (18, 32, 33) and have not included all groups of hospital personnel and appropriate community controls. Thus, data that can be used to analyze the cost-effectiveness of administering vaccine to hospital personnel are not complete.

Because the risk that hospital personnel will acquire hepatitis B varies among hospitals and among different occupational groups within hospitals, each hospital should formulate its own specific immunization strategy. In developing specific immunization strategies, hospitals may use available published data (14–20, 32, 33) about the risk of infection. Some institutions may instead choose to serologically screen personnel in various occupational categories or work locations to determine the prevalence of seropositivity in these groups.

The decision to screen potential vaccine recipients for susceptibility to hepatitis B is an economic decision; immunizing HBV carriers and persons already immune does not appear to present a hazard (1, 2). In the United States, the prevalence of previous infection in any targeted group, the cost of screening, and the cost of immunizing personnel determine whether screening would be cost-effective (3, 4).

HBV vaccine is reported to be safe (34–38). The Immunization Practices Advisory Committee (ACIP) has published a discussion of this vaccine and its use (3).

Non-A, Non-B Hepatitis

The epidemiology of NANB hepatitis in the United States more closely resembles that of hepatitis B than that of hepatitis A. Important aspects of NANB infections are as follows: (a) the NANB agent(s) circulates in the blood in acute cases, (b) there appears to be a chronic blood carrier state during which blood may remain infective, and (c) transmission of NANB infection is usually associated with percutaneous needle exposure or other exposure to blood, or with inapparent parenteral transmission. Since blood containing HBsAg is not used for transfusion, most post-transfusion hepatitis in the United States is NANB. Thus, emphasis on blood precautions, as with hepatitis B, seems the most reasonable current approach to preventing transmission from patients to personnel. For personnel who contract this illness, precautions suggested for hepatitis B should be adequate to prevent transmission to patients. Techniques are not yet available to detect specific antigens and antibodies or to determine the period of infectivity after acute infection.

NEEDLESTICK INJURIES

Needlestick injuries account for a large number of the work-related accidents reported in hospitals (39). Most injuries happen on patient-care units when personnel are (a) disposing of used needles, (b) administering parenteral injections or infusion therapy (especially to uncooperative patients), (c) drawing blood, (d) recapping needles after use, (e) handling linens or trash containing uncapped needles, or (f) cleaning up after patient-care procedures in which needles are used. Although other infections have been reported to be transmitted by accidental needle sticks, hepatitis B and probably NANB pose the greatest risks to hospital personnel. In the absence of immunoprophylaxis, the risk of acquiring overt hepatitis B through an accidental puncture wound from a needle used on an HBsAg-positive patient is about 6% (40).

The risk of needlestick injuries can be reduced by discarding used needles in punctureresistant disposal units without first recapping them or purposely bending or breaking them by hand. Risk of injury may also be reduced if personnel obtain assistance when administering injections or infusion therapy to uncooperative patients and if personnel use caution when cleaning up after procedures that include the use of needles. Additionally, the incidence of needlestick injuries may be reduced by providing needle-disposal units throughout the hospital in locations that facilitate their immediate use, for example, in nursing stations, patient rooms, laboratories, and utility rooms (41). When some needle-cutting devices are used, blood may spatter onto environmental surfaces. Currently, no data are available from controlled studies examining the effect, if any, of needle-cutting devices on the incidence of needle-stick injuries.

After some needlestick injuries, immunoprophylaxis for hepatitis B or NANB may be advisable (42). Immune globulins for protection against vital hepatitis are most effective when given soon after exposure.

HERPES SIMPLEX VIRUSES

Herpes simplex viruses (HSV) can be transmitted among personnel and patients through either primary or recurrent lesions or through secretions (such as saliva, vaginal secretions, infected amniotic fluid) that can contain the virus when no lesions are obvious. Although many sites can become infected, exposed areas of skin are most likely to be involved, particularly when minor cuts, abrasions, or other skin lesions are present. Direct contact with lesions or infected secretions is the principal mode of spread.

Transmission of HSV From Patients to Personnel

Personnel may develop an infection of the fingers (herpetic whitlow or paronychia) from exposure to contaminated oral secretions. Such exposure is a distinct hazard for nurses, anesthesiologists, dentists, respiratory care personnel, and other personnel who may have direct (usually hand) contact with either oral lesions or respiratory secretions from patients. Less frequently, personnel may develop infection of the fingers from exposure to contaminated genital secretions or lesions on skin or mucous membranes. Personnel can protect themselves from such infections by (a) avoiding direct contact with lesions, (b) wearing gloves on both hands or using "no-touch" technique for all contact with oral or vaginal secretions, and (c) thorough handwashing after patient contact (see Guideline for Isolation Precautions in Hospitals).

Transmission of HSV From Personnel to Patients

Currently, there is no evidence that personnel with genital infections pose a high risk to patients if personnel follow good patient-care practices. The risk posed by personnel with orofacial herpes to patients is unknown. Personnel with oral infections, however, can reduce the risk of infecting patients by (a) wearing an appropriate barrier—such as a mask or gauze dressing—to prevent hand contact with the lesion, (b) washing hands well before all patient care, and (c) whenever possible, not taking care of patients at high risk of severe infection such as neonates, patients with severe malnutrition, severely burned patients, and patients in immunodeficient states. The potential risk of infecting high-risk patients must be weighed against the possibility of compromising patient care by excluding personnel with orofacial herpes.

Personnel with herpetic whitlow may be more likely to transmit infection by contact. Personnel can prevent transmission of HSV to patients by not working when they have active infections of the hands. Although some have suggested that personnel with herpetic whitlow may have patient contact if they wear gloves (43, 44), the adequacy of this method of preventing transmission of infection is unknown.

STAPHYLOCOCCUS AUREUS AND STREPTOCOCCUS, GROUP A AND GROUP B

Carnage of potential pathogens by hospital personnel has been a traditional concern of infection control practitioners. Management of personnel who are infected with Staphylococcus aureus or camera of Staphylococcus aureus or group A or group B Streptococcus is discussed here. Carnage of enteric pathogens and meningococci by hospital personnel are covered elsewhere; carnage of other organisms, such as gram-negative bacteria, has rarely been implicated as a source of nosocomial infection and is not discussed.

Staphylococcus aureus Infection and Carriage

Staphylococcal carnage or infection occurs frequently in humans. In nosocomial transmission, there are 2 sources: a person with a lesion or an asymptomatic carrier. Persons with skin lesions due to S. aureus are most likely to disseminate these organisms. Direct contact is the major route of transmission. Even a single boil in an occult body site (for example, the axilla) caused by S. aureus may increase the likelihood of dissemination. One way to decrease the possibility of dissemination is to not allow patient-care personnel to work until skin infection caused by this organism is resolved.

The anterior nares is one of the most commonly colonized sites, but carnage of S. aureus may occur at other sites, such as the axilla or perineum. The epidemiology of methicillin-resistant staphylococci does not appear to be different, except that nasal carriage may be less frequent, and outbreaks tend to occur more frequently in intensive care and burn units.

Culture surveys of personnel can detect carriers of S. aureus but do not indicate whether carriers are likely to disseminate their organisms. Thus, such data are difficult to interpret. A more reasonable approach is to emphasize effective surveillance that permits prompt recognition of staphylococcal infections in both personnel and patients. If certain personnel are linked epidemiologically to an increased number of infections, these persons can be cultured and, if positive, removed from patient contact until carnage is eradicated. Treatment regimens, followup of implicated personnel, and management of outbreaks are not discussed in this guideline.

Group A Streptococcus Carriage

For nosocomial transmission, the main reservoirs for group A Streptococcus appear to be the pharynx, the skin, the rectum, and the female genital tract. Direct contact and large droplets are the major modes of transmitting this organism; however, airborne spread has been suggested (45, 46).

Although pharyngeal and skin infections are the most common group A streptococcal infections, outbreaks of surgical wound infections caused by this organism have been more important in the hospital. Since group A streptococcal surgical wound infections occur infrequently, the occurrence of cases should prompt a search for a carrier. If personnel are linked epidemiologically to the occurrence of disease, they should be cultured, and if positive, removed from patient contact until carnage is eradicated. Treatment regimens, followup of implicated personnel, and management of outbreaks are not discussed here.

Group B Streptococcus Carriage

Carnage of group B Streptococcus by personnel does not appear to be important in nosocomial transmission. The epidemiology of group B streptococcal infections in neonates suggests that maternal colonization with group B Streptococcus, followed by the infant's acquisition during passage through the birth canal, accounts for most infections that have onset soon after birth. Spread of the organism from colonized to uncolonized infants via the hands of personnel, however, may play a role in late onset neonatal infections. Careful handwashing by personnel will minimize the risk of spread from colonized to uncolonized infants.

TUBERCULOSIS

Even though the risk of nosocomial infection with Mycobacterium tuberculosis is low, tuberculosis (TB) continues to pose a problem for health-care personnel. In the hospital, infection is most likely to occur when a patient has unsuspected pulmonary or laryngeal TB, has bacilli-laden sputum or respiratory secretions, and is coughing or sneezing into air that remains in circulation. The best ways to protect others from a patient with TB are to maintain a high index of suspicion for TB and to institute appropriate precautions (see Guideline for Isolation Precautions in Hospitals). A complete discussion of the transmission of tuberculosis in hospitals has been published elsewhere (47).

Screening Programs

A tuberculosis screening and prevention program for personnel is important in protecting personnel and patients (48, 49). It is important that all institutions have a screening program; however, the program should be based on local epidemiologic dam, because risk of transmission varies broadly among different segments of the population and in different localities. It is important to identify hospital personnel with tuberculous infection without evidence of current (active) disease, because preventive treatment with isoniazid may be indicated (50). Persons with tuberculous infection are those with a significant skin-test reaction, usually defined as 10 mm or more of induration to 5 Tuberculin Units (TU) of Purified Protein Derivative-Standard (PPD-S) administered via the Mantoux technique.

The tuberculin skin test is the method of choice for TB screening. The Mantoux technique (intracutaneous injection of 0.1 ml of PPD-tuberculin containing 5 TU) is preferred for screening persons for TB infection (51), because it is the most accurate test available. A 2-step procedure (52) can be used to minimize the likelihood of misinterpreting a boosted reaction as a true conversion due to recent infection (52, 53). In the 2-step procedure, an initial tuberculin skin test (Mantoux, 5 TU PPD) is given. If this test result is 0–9 mm of induration, a second test is given at least 1 week and no more than 3 weeks after the first. The results of the second test should be used as the baseline test in determining treatment and follow-up of these personnel. A skin test result of 10 mm of induration or more is considered to be significant.

The 2-step procedure, however, may not always be necessary. Personnel in the second or third decade of life may be less likely to have had remote infection with M. tuberculosis. Thus, the age of personnel in an institution and the epidemiology of nontuberculous mycobacterial infection in the geographic location may determine the frequency of the booster phenomenon (54). Depending on these factors, the 2-step method may not detect any more reactors than a single test. A pilot study may be useful to assess the frequency of the booster phenomenon in a given hospital and, thus, the need for the 2-step test (54).

Multipuncture skin-test methods deliver an unknown quantity of antigen and may produce both false-positive and false-negative results. When repeated tuberculin testing is required or in postexposure testing, multipuncture methods do not allow precise interpretation of test results and proper counseling.

After the initial TB screening test, policies for repeat testing can be established by considering factors that contribute to the risk that a person will acquire new infection (49). These factors include the location and prevalence of untreated TB in the community, in the institution, and among personnel (49). For personnel considered to be at significant risk, repeat skin tests may be necessary on a routine basis (for example, every 3–6 months or yearly). If the risk of exposure to TB is small, it is not necessary to repeat skin tests routinely.

During TB screening, it is important to obtain an initial chest roentgenogram on those persons with significant skin test reactions, those who convert their skin tests, or those who have pulmonary symptoms that may be due to TB. There is no need to obtain routine chest films of asymptomatic, tuberculin-negative personnel.

After initial chest films of persons with significant reactions, repeated chest X-ray examinations have not been found to be of sufficient clinical value or to be cost-effective in monitoring persons for development of disease (55). Thus, personnel known to have a significant reaction and significant reactors who have completed adequate preventive treatment do not need repeat chest films unless they have pulmonary symptoms that may be due to TB (55, 56).

Management of Personnel After Exposure

If personnel are exposed to an infective patient with TB and do not use proper precautions, it is important to skin test these personnel 10 weeks after the exposure. Ten weeks is the upper limit of the time required for an infected person to develop hypersensitivity to tuberculin. Unless a recent skin test was given, for example, during the 3 months before the exposure, a baseline test may be needed as soon as possible after the exposure, to help in deciding whether a significant reaction at 10 weeks represents a recent conversion related to the exposure.

Because the size of the skin-test reaction can be so important, the Mantoux technique is preferred for postexposure evaluations. Those already known to have significant reactions need not be skin-tested. Those who have significant reactions upon testing need chest roentgenograms to exclude the possibility of tuberculous pulmonary disease. If chest films are normal, these persons can be advised to receive preventive treatment, unless such treatment is contraindicated. If the chest film has abnormalities compatible with pulmonary TB, these personnel need evaluation to rule out the possibility of current disease.

BCG Vaccination

Many Bacille Calmette-Guerin (BCG) vaccines are available today, and they vary in immunogenicity, efficacy, and reactogenicity. Controlled trials of previous vaccines conducted before 1955 showed protection ranging from 0 to 80%; however, the efficacy of vaccines currently available in the United States has not been demonstrated directly and can only be inferred. Thus, the skin-test reaction after BCG vaccination may be quite variable, and it cannot be distinguished from that due to virulent tuberculous infection. Caution is necessary in attributing a significant skin test to prior BCG vaccination, especially if the vaccinee has recently been exposed to infective tuberculosis. A history of BCG vaccination, then, should not preclude an initial screening test, and it is important to manage a significant reaction in BCG-vaccinated persons as a possible tuberculous infection.

Skin testing after BCG vaccination or natural infection with mycobacteria may be associated with adverse reactions, including severe or prolonged ulceration at the test site. Initial use of 1 TU PPD or a partial dose of 5 TU PPD may be useful in avoiding untoward reactions in persons who might be expected to have a severe reaction, such as those with an undocumented history of a large reaction in the past. A full 5 TU dose may be used safely if the initial skin test is negative. The efficacy of this method, however, has not been examined in controlled trials.

Generally in the United States, adequate surveillance and control measures rather than BCG vaccination are all that is necessary to protect hospital personnel and patients.

Preventive Treatment and Work Restrictions

Preventive treatment of persons with significant tuberculin reactions may decrease the risk that their subclinical infections will progress to clinical disease. In determining priorities for preventive therapy the decision-maker must weigh the risk of the person's developing current tuberculosis against the risk of isoniazid toxicity, the ease of identifying and supervising those to whom preventive therapy is offered, and the likelihood of their infecting others. About 5% of persons who are recent converters will develop current disease in the first 1–2 years after infection; the risk of developing current disease gradually declines thereafter. Persons for whom preventive treatment is recommended include newly infected persons, significant reactors with abnormal chest roentgenograms and negative bacteriologic findings, persons with special clinical conditions, significant reactors less than 35 years old, even in the absence of additional risk factors, and household members of persons with newly discovered TB (50). Contraindications to treatment include (a) previous isoniazid-associated hepatic injury or other severe adverse reactions (for example, drug fever, chills, and arthritis), and (b) acute liver disease of any etiology. Persons of age 35 years or more may need preventive treatment, if the potential exists for transmitting disease if it develops (50). Since the risk of developing current disease is low, work restrictions may not be necessary for otherwise healthy persons who do not accept preventive therapy. However, it is essential that they be instructed to seek evaluation promptly if symptoms develop that may be caused by TB, especially if they have contact with high-risk patients.

Personnel with current pulmonary or laryngeal TB pose a risk to patients and other personnel while they are infective. Stringent requirements regarding work restrictions for hospital personnel are necessary because of this special situation. Objective measures of lack of infectivity are negative cultures and sputum smears that are free of bacilli. Criteria for removing from or returning to work should always be tailored to the individual. Multiple factors should be considered, including those that influence the expulsion of infective particles in the work air space, mainly coughing, and the characteristics of potential contacts in the work environment and possible consequences, if they become infected (57).

VARICELLA ZOSTER

Varicella-zoster virus (VZV) is the etiologic agent of varicella (chickenpox) and zoster (shingles). Nosocomial transmission of varicella-zoster infection among personnel and patients is well recognized. Appropriate isolation of hospitalized patients with known or suspected varicella or zoster can reduce the risk of transmission to personnel (see Guideline for Isolation Precautions in Hospitals). It is advisable to allow only personnel who have had varicella or those with serologic evidence of immunity to take care of these patients.

Varicella

Varicella is transmitted primarily via airborne spread by small particle aerosols (droplet nuclei) and by large particles (droplets). The virus may also be spread by direct contact but is not likely to be spread by inanimate objects because the virus is extremely labile. The incubation period for varicella in the normal host ranges from 10 to 21 clays.

Even though personnel who are susceptible to varicella may be few, it is useful to identify such persons at the time of the placement evaluation. Most persons with a clearly positive history of previous varicella are probably immune. Many with negative or unknown histories may be immune, but some may also be susceptible (58). When available, serologic screening may be used to define susceptibility more precisely. In institutions where varicella is prevalent or where there are many high-risk patients, it may be useful to screen those personnel who have a negative or equivocal history of varicella for the presence of serum antibodies to VZV to document susceptibility or immunity. This knowledge will help in assigning personnel to areas where VZV infection is present, avoiding unnecessary work restrictions and disruption of patient service if exposure occurs, and reducing the chance of nosocomial transmission (59). Sensitive screening techniques exist, for example, fluorescent antibody to membrane antigen (FAMA), immune adherence hemagglutination (IAH), or enzyme-linked immunosorbent assay (ELISA), but they may not be readily available. The complement fixation (CF) test is not considered to be reliable because of the false-negative results obtained by this method.

If susceptible personnel are exposed to persons with varicella, these personnel are potentially infective during the incubation period (10 to 21 days after exposure). If varicella occurs, transmission is possible until all lesions are dry and crusted.

Zoster

Zoster appears to occur as a result of activation of latent VZV. There is scant evidence to support the view that zoster can be contracted by exposure to persons with varicella or zoster. However, varicella-zoster virus can be transmitted by direct contact with a person with zoster. If susceptible personnel are exposed to zoster, varicella may occur; thus, these persons may transmit VZV during the incubation period of varicella.

Because of the possibility of transmission and development of severe illness in high-risk patients, it may be advisable to exclude personnel with zoster from taking care of high-risk patients until all lesions are crusted. Personnel with zoster may not pose a special risk to other patients if the lesions can be covered.

VIRAL RESPIRATORY INFECTIONS

Viral respiratory infections are common problems for infection control programs. The role of viruses in nosocomial infections has been recently discussed (60–62) (also, see Guideline for Prevention of Nosocomial Pneumonia). Hospital personnel, visitors, and patients are important sources of viruses.

The 3 chief mechanisms of transmission of respiratory viruses are (a) small-particle aerosols (droplet nuclei), (b) large particles (droplets), and (c) inoculation of viruses after direct contact with infective areas or materials. Different respiratory viruses may vary in the way in which they are transmitted.

Small-particle aerosols are produced by talking, sneezing, or coughing and may transmit infection over a considerable distance (more than 3 feet). Large particles (droplets) are produced by sneezing and coughing and require close person-to-person contact for transmission. Person-to-person transmission can also occur by contaminating the hands by direct contact with infective areas or materials, then transferral of infective virus to mucous membranes of a susceptible person. Self-inoculation can also occur in this way. The nose and eyes, rather than the mouth, appear to be important portals of entry.

Pediatric patients appear to be at particular risk for complications from nosocomial respiratory tract infections. Infection in the elderly, patients with chronic underlying illness, and immunocompromised patients may also be associated with significant morbidity. Thus, it may be prudent to exclude personnel with viral respiratory infections from the care of these high-risk patients. Because large numbers of personnel may have viral respiratory illnesses during the winter, it may not be possible to restrict all such personnel from taking care of patients not in high-risk groups. In all instances, careful handwashing before patient contact is essential in preventing transmission. If handwashing is done appropriately, gloves and routine use of gowns may have no additional benefit in preventing transmission to patients (63, 64). Masks might be beneficial in preventing transmission by large droplets from personnel to patients upon close contact. However, masks probably will not completely protect personnel from patients with respiratory illnesses because large particles and aerosols may still reach the eyes, and self-inoculation from contaminated hands can still occur by touching the eyes.

Influenza epidemics may require other measures. Because influenza epidemics are unpredictable, hospitals may want to determine their policy on influenza immunization each year, taking note of the recommendations from the Immunization Practices Advisory Committee (ACIP), which are revised annually. Nosocomial spread of influenza might be reduced by immunizing personnel and high-risk patients several weeks or longer before the influenza season. An antiviral drug, amantadine, may be useful to limit spread to and from patients and unimmunized personnel during an epidemic of influenza A.

GROUP 11 INFECTIONS: TRANSMISSION FROM PATIENTS TO PERSONNEL

CYTOMEGALOVIRUS

Personnel may be exposed to patients with cytomegalovirus (CMV) infection, but the risk of acquiring CMV infection from patients appears to be small. There are 2 principal reservoirs of CMV in the hospital: (a) infants infected with CMV and (b) immunocompromised patients, such as oncology patients and those undergoing kidney or bone marrow transplant. Available data have shown no evidence of an excess risk of transmission of CMV to personnel working in dialysis units (65), oncology wards (66), or pediatric areas, when compared with personnel with no patient contact (67, 68). However, evidence is accumulating to suggest sexual contact as a significant mode of transmission of CMV outside the hospital environment (69–70). Large, well-controlled studies are needed to document the validity of these observations.

The precise mechanism of transmission is unknown; however, infection appears to be acquired only through intimate, direct contact with an excreter of CMV or contact with contaminated secretions. Virus can be shed in the urine, saliva, respiratory secretions, tears, feces, breast milk, semen, and cervical secretions.

Screening Programs for CMV Infection

Because infection with CMV during pregnancy may damage the fetus, protecting women of childbearing age from persons who are excreting the virus is of primary concern. Most infants who are infected with CMV are asymptomatic. Screening programs to detect such patients, however, are not practical, because the tests are time-consuming and costly and would entail screening all newborns. Mass screening of personnel is not likely to provide useful information because the available complement fixation (CF) tests are not reliable indicators of immunity, since these tests lack sensitivity and since the antigen most commonly used for serologic testing (the AD 169 strain) may not cross-react with all other known CMV strains. Furthermore, identifying seropositive women would not necessarily provide a group who, if they become pregnant, are at no risk of transmitting infection to the lotus, because congenital infection may result from reactivation of latent infection (72), and, theoretically, from exogenous reinfection. In addition, since there are no studies to indicate clearly that personnel may be protected by transfer to areas with less contact with infants and children (67, 68), identifying seronegative women in order to institute such measures may not reduce the number of primary infections.

Preventing Transmission of CMV

When hygienic precautions (appropriate handwashing, not kissing infants, etc.) are satisfactory, the risk of acquiring infection through patient contact is low (68). Therefore, a practical approach to reducing the risk of infection with CMV is to stress careful handwashing after all patient contacts and avoiding contact with areas or materials that are potentially infective (see Guideline for Isolation Precautions in Hospitals). Patients known to be infected with CMV can be identified, and this information can be used in counseling pregnant personnel and determining their work assignments.

Personnel who contract illnesses thought to be due to CMV need not be restricted from work. They can reduce the risk of transmission to patients or other personnel by careful handwashing and exercising care to prevent their body fluids from contacting other persons.

MENINGOCOCCAL DISEASE

Nosocomial transmission of Neisseria meningitidis to hospital personnel taking care of patients with meningococcemia, meningococcal meningitis, or lower respiratory infections is uncommon. In rare instances transmission to personnel from patients with meningococcemia or meningococcal meningitis has occurred through intensive direct contact with the infected person and direct contact with respiratory secretions without use of proper precautions. The most likely mode of spread from a person with infections at these sites is by large droplet secretions. Risk to personnel from casual contact (for example, as usually occurs with housekeepers and with laboratory contact with clinical specimens) appears to be negligible.

Meningococcal lower respiratory infections, however, may present a greater risk of transmission than meningococcemia or meningitis alone (73, 74), especially if the patient has an active, productive cough (73). Possible airborne transmission to other persons who did not have close contact with the infected patient has been suggested (73); however, droplet spread could not be excluded.

When taking care of patients with suspected N. meningitidis infection at any site, personnel can decrease the risk of infection by using proper precautions (see Guideline for Isolation Precautions in Hospitals).

Prophylaxis After Unprotected Exposure

Antimicrobial prophylaxis can eradicate carriage of N. meningitidis and prevent infections in personnel who have unprotected exposure to patients with meningococcal infections. Prophylaxis is indicated for persons who have intensive direct contact with infected patients and who do not use proper precautions. Personnel who have close contact with patients who have unrecognized meningococcal lower respiratory infection and therefore do not use proper precautions might also need prophylaxis (73). Further studies will be important to define the need for prophylaxis in this situation.

When prophylaxis is deemed necessary, it is important to begin treatment immediately. Often prophylaxis must be started before results of antimicrobial testing are available. Rifampin is now the drug of choice for prophylaxis. Because sulfonamide-resistant meningococci are prevalent, sulfonamides should be used only if the organism has been found to be sulfonamide sensitive.

Carriage of N. meningitidis by Personnel

Carriage of N. meningitidis in the nasopharynx of healthy persons has been recognized for many years, but the prevalence is quite variable. Carriage may be transient, intermittent, or chronic. Surveillance of hospital personnel to determine carriage is useful only during special epidemiologic studies. Generally, in non-outbreak situations, asymptomatic carriers among personnel need not be identified, treated, or removed from patient-care activities. Management of comers identified during special studies is not within the scope of this guideline.

PERTUSSIS

Pertussis, caused by Bordetella pertussis, is highly communicable. The secondary attack rate is determined primarily by the immune status of those exposed; age may also be a factor. Unless infected persons are treated with an effective antibiotic, the period of communicability extends from the beginning of the catarrhal stage to approximately 3 weeks after onset of paroxysms.

Nosocomial transmission of pertussis has been reported infrequently. Although infection occurs less commonly in adults and may be limited to mild respiratory illness, personnel with pediatric patient contact may be involved in transmission of pertussis to patients (75, 76). However, the risk of pertussis infection and dissemination is probably not serious enough to warrant routine immunization of hospital personnel with current vaccines. Immunizing persons over age 6 is not recommended, because of the increased frequency of adverse reactions. In addition, current vaccines do not confer complete immunity, and protection against pertussis may decrease as the interval between immunization and reexposure increases. Natural immunity appears to be long-lasting, although infection in persons who reportedly had pertussis in the past has been reported (76).

During an outbreak, removal of personnel with cough or upper respiratory tract symptoms from the care of patients may be important in preventing further spread (75). Erythromycin prophylaxis of exposed susceptibles who are infected may abort or attenuate illness if administered in the early pre-paroxysmal cough stage of the illness. Prophylaxis for less than 14 days is frequently followed by bacteriologic relapse. Infected contacts may be identified rapidly by the fluorescent antibody (FA) technique; however, culture techniques identify infection more reliably than FA examination, because of both false-positive and false-negative results with the FA method. "Carriers" of pertussis are very unusual, because persons with positive cultures generally develop symptoms.

SCABIES

Scabies is a disease caused by infestation with the mite Sarcoptes scabiei. It is transmitted in hospitals primarily through intimate direct contact with an infested person, even when high levels of personal hygiene are maintained (77–79). Transmission to personnel has occurred during activities such as sponge-bathing patients or applying body lotions. Transmission between patients may also be possible when patients are ambulatory. Transmission by casual contact, such as holding hands, has been infrequently reported (80). Transmission via inanimate objects, such as infested bedding, clothes, or other fomites has not been implicated as a major mode of transferring mites (77, 81).

Treatment is recommended for persons with active infestation. A single, correct application (77, 81) of agents used to treat scabies is curative in most cases and appears to eliminate the risk of transmission immediately after the first treatment (77, 78, 81). Treatment destroys both eggs and the active forms of the mites; however, ovicidal activity has not been fully substantiated for all available agents. Repeating the treatment 7–10 days after the initial therapy will kill any newly hatched mites. Between treatments the risk of transmission is felt to be negligible.

Using appropriate precautions when taking care of infested patients will decrease the risk of transmission to personnel (see Guideline for Isolation Precautions in Hospitals). If personnel are infested with the mite, transmission can be prevented by excluding them from work until they are treated.

GLOSSARY

EXPOSURE

An important exposure is one in which a person is subjected to an infectious agent in a way considered likely to lead to acquisition of disease. Whether an exposure to an infectious agent is important depends on various factors, including (a) the mechanism of transmission of the agent involved and the person's infective potential; for example, a non-coughing patient with pulmonary tuberculosis poses little threat; (b) the type and duration of contact; (c) host susceptibility; and (d) whether or not suggested precautions are used. The persons in each hospital who have been given the responsibility, in consultation with others who may be involved, will have to determine whether an important exposure has occurred and if some intervention after the exposure is needed.

TRANSMISSION

Microorganisms are transmitted by various routes, and the same microorganism may be transmitted by more than 1 route. For example, varicella-zoster virus can spread either by the airborne route (droplet nuclei) or by direct contact. The differences in infectivity and in the mode of transmission of the various agents form the basis for the differences in precautions that are recommended in this guideline.

There are 4 main routes of transmission—contact, vehicle, airborne, and vectorborne.

A. Contact transmission, the most important and frequent means of transmission of nosocomial infections, can be divided into 3 subgroups: direct contact, indirect contact, and droplet contact.

1. Direct contact—This involves direct physical transfer between a susceptible host and an infected or colonized person, such as occurs between patient and hospital personnel when personnel are turning patients, giving baths, changing dressings, or performing other procedures requiring direct personal contact. Taking care of patients generally involves some direct contact. Direct contact can also occur between 2 patients, 1 serving as the source of infection and the other as a susceptible host.

2. Indirect contact—This involves personal contact of the susceptible host with a contaminated intermediate object, usually inanimate, such as instruments, dressings, or other infective material. If proper care is not taken, personnel can contaminate objects when assembling or handling critical equipment (such as respiratory therapy equipment, pressure-monitoring devices, cardiac bypass pumps) or during other procedures that involve inanimate objects.

3. Droplet contact—Infectious agents may come in contact with the conjunctivae, nose, or mouth of a susceptible person as a result of coughing, sneezing, or talking by an infected person. This occurrence is considered "contact" transmission rather than airborne since droplets usually travel no more than about 3 feet. "Close contact" is used to mean within 3 feet of an infected person.

B. The vehicle route applies in diseases transmitted through contaminated items, such as transmission of hepatitis non-A, non-B by contaminated blood.

C. Airborne transmission occurs by dissemination of either droplet nuclei (residue of evaporated droplets that may remain suspended in the air for long periods of time) or dust particles in the air containing the infectious agent. Organisms carried in this manner are then inhaled by or deposited on the susceptible host.

D. Vectorborne transmission is of greater concern in developing countries, for example, mosquito-transmitted malaria.

Since agent and host factors are more difficult to control, interruption of the chain of infection in the hospital is directed primarily at transmission. The precautions recommended in this guideline are based on this concept.

RECOMMENDATIONS*

1. Elements of a Personnel Health Service for Infection Control
   a. Placement Evaluation
      (i) A health inventory should be obtained from personnel who will have patient contact. Category I

---

* The recommendations in this guideline are limited to prevention and control of infectious disease transmission among patient-care personnel and patients (see Introduction). These suggestions, however, can include other personnel. This guideline and other guidelines in the manual include all of the current recommendations of the Hospital Infections Program, CDC, on personnel health. Hospitals may choose to establish additional policies for personnel.

(ii) For infection control, complete physical and laboratory examinations should not be routinely required for all personnel but should be done when indicated; for example, the need for an examination or laboratory test may be determined from results of the health inventory. Category I

(iii) Health assessments of personnel other than placement evaluations should be done depending only on need; for example, as required to evaluate work-related illness or exposures to infectious diseases. Category I

(iv) Routine culturing of personnel, such as taking cultures of the nose, throat, or stool, should not be done as part of the placement evaluation or thereafter. Category I (See Guideline for Hospital Environmental Control: Microbiologic Surveillance of the Environment and of Personnel in the Hospital)

b. Personnel Health and Safety Education

(i) Initial job orientation and ongoing in-service education should include the infection control aspects of personnel health and the proper use of the personnel health service. Category I

(ii) Specific written policies and procedures for control of infections in hospital personnel should be readily available. Category I

c. Job-Related Illnesses and Exposures

(i) A record should be maintained on hospital personnel that includes information obtained during the placement evaluation, immunization records, results of tests obtained in any screening or control programs, and reports of work-related illnesses or exposures. Category I

(ii) A readily available mechanism should be established for personnel to obtain advice about illnesses they may acquire from or transmit to patients. Category I

(iii) Evaluation of job-related illnesses or important exposures and postexposure prophylaxis, when indicated, should be provided. Category I

(iv) Written protocols should be established for handling job-related infectious diseases or important exposures. These occurrences should be recorded in the person's record and, when applicable, the appropriate member of the infection control committee and personnel health service should be notified. Category I

d. Coordinated Planning and Administration

(i) Each hospital should have ways to coordinate policy-making and planning among the administration, personnel health service, infection control program, and various departments. Category I

(ii) A system should be established for notifying the infection control program of (a) infections in personnel that require work restrictions or exclusion from work, (b) clearance for work after an infectious illness that required work restrictions or exclusion, (c) other work-related infections and exposures, and (d) when appropriate, results of epidemiologic investigations. Category I

(iii) A representative of the personnel health program should be on the infection control committee. Category I

2. Immunization of Hospital Personnel**
  a. Hospitals should formulate a written comprehensive policy on immunizing hospital personnel. Category I
  b. The following recommendations should be considered by the hospital in formulating its policies:
    (i) Rubella
      (a) All personnel (male or female) who are considered to be at increased risk of contact with patients with rubella or who are likely to have direct contact with pregnant patients should be immune to rubella.*** Category I
      (b) Before immunizing, serologic screening for rubella need not be done unless the hospital considers it cost-effective or the potential vaccinee requests it. Category I (Persons can be considered susceptible unless they have laboratory evidence of immunity or documented immunization with live virus vaccine on or after their first birthday. Consideration should be given to giving rubella vaccine in combination with measles and mumps vaccines [measles-mumps-rubella (MMR) trivalent vaccine].)
    (ii) Hepatitis B
      (a) Persons at substantial risk of HBV infection who are demonstrated or judged likely to be susceptible should be actively immunized (see text). Category II
      (b) Before immunizing, serologic screening for hepatitis B need not be done unless the hospital considers it cost-effective or the potential vaccinee requests it. Category I
      (c) Prophylaxis with an immune globulin (passive immunization) should be used when indicated, such as following needlestick exposure to blood that is at high-risk of being HbsAg-positive. Category I
      (d) Immune globulins should not be used as a substitute for active immunization. Category I
    (iii) Measles
      All persons susceptible by history or serology who are considered to be at increased risk of contact with patients infected with measles should be protected.*** Category I (Most persons born before 1957 have probably been infected naturally and generally need not be considered susceptible. Younger persons can be considered immune only if they have documentation of (a) physician-diagnosed measles, (b) laboratory evidence of measles immunity, or (c) adequate immunization with live measles vaccine on or after the first birthday. Consideration should be

---

** Consult current ACIP recommendations for a detailed discussion of the rationale for each recommendation. See earlier for information on obtaining the full ACIP guidelines.

*** Pregnancy is a contraindication. Vaccine should not be given to pregnant women or those who may become pregnant within 3 months.

given to administering measles vaccine in combination with rubella and mumps vaccines [measles-mumps-rubella (MMR) trivalent vaccine].)

(iv) Poliomyelitis

(a) Routine primary immunization for adults in the United States is not recommended. Personnel who may have direct contact with patients who may be excreting polioviruses should complete a primary series. Primary immunization with inactivated polio vaccine (IPV) instead of oral polio vaccine (OPV) is recommended for these persons whenever feasible. Category I (IPV is preferred because the risk of vaccine-associated paralysis following OPV is slightly higher in adults than in children and because personnel may shed virus after OPV and inadvertently expose susceptible or immunocompromised patients to live virus.)

(b) In an outbreak, OPV should be provided to anyone who has not been completely immunized or whose immunization status is unknown.**** Category I

(v) Influenza

To avoid problems with staffing during the influenza season and to prevent spread of influenza from personnel to patients, efforts should be made to immunize hospital personnel against influenza in the fall of each year. Category II

c. Hospital personnel are not at substantially higher risk than the general adult population of acquiring diphtheria, pneumococcal disease, mumps, or tetanus. Therefore, hospital personnel should seek these immunizations from their primary care provider, according to the recommendations of ACIP. Category I

d. Hospitals should not assume responsibility for routine immunization of hospital personnel against pertussis, tuberculosis, cholera, meningococcal disease, plague, rabies, typhoid, typhus, or yellow fever. Category I (Smallpox vaccine is no longer recommended for general use.**)

3. Protection of Personnel and Other Patients from Patients with Infections

a. Patients with potentially transmissible infections should be placed on isolation precautions using recommendations in the current Guideline for Isolation Precautions in Hospitals. (This recommendation is not categorized. The working group for the Guideline for Isolation Precautions in Hospitals did not rank the isolation recommendations into categories. Although the isolation recommendations are based on well-documented modes of transmission identified in epidemiologic studies or on a reasonable theoretical rationale, there have been few studies to test the efficacy of isolation recommendations.)

** Consult current ACIP recommendations for a detailed discussion of the rationale for each recommendation. See earlier for information on obtaining the full ACIP guidelines.

**** Exceptions to this recommendation are discussed in the current ACIP recommendations under the heading Precautions and Contraindications: Immunodeficiency.

4. Prevention of Needlestick Injuries

  a. Training or instruction of personnel should include discussions of methods to prevent needlestick injuries. Category I

  b. Used needles should be placed in a prominently labeled, puncture-resistant container designated specifically for their disposal. Category I

  c. Used needles should not be recapped, purposely bent, or broken by hand. Category II

5. Prophylaxis After Exposure

  a. When prophylactic treatment with drugs, vaccines, or immune globulins is deemed necessary and is offered, personnel should be informed of alternative means of prophylaxis, the risk (if this is known) of infection if treatment is not accepted, the degree of protection provided by the therapy, and the potential side effects. Category I

  b. Hepatitis A

  (i) Personnel who have had direct fecal-oral exposure to excretions from a patient found to have been incubating hepatitis A should be given immune globulin (IG) (0.02 ml/kg). Category I

  (ii) Prophylaxis with immune globulin (IG) for all personnel who take care of patients with hepatitis A (other than as suggested in recommendation 5.b.i above) should not be given. Category I

  c. Hepatitis B

  For prophylaxis against hepatitis B after percutaneous (needle-stick) or mucous membrane exposure to blood that might be infective, the recommendations in Table 1 should be followed. Category I

  d. Hepatitis Non-A, Non-B

  If needlestick exposures occur involving patients known to have hepatitis non-A, non-B, IG (0.06 ml/kg) should be given. Category II

  e. Meningococcal disease

  Antimicrobial prophylaxis against meningococcal disease should be offered immediately to personnel who have had intensive direct contact with an infected patient without using proper precautions. If prophylaxis is deemed necessary, treatment should not await results of antimicrobial sensitivity testing. Category I

  f. Pertussis

  Antimicrobial prophylaxis against pertussis should be offered immediately to personnel who have had intensive contact with an infected patient without using proper precautions. Category II

  g. Rabies

  Hospital personnel who either have been bitten by a human with rabies or have scratches, abrasions, open wounds, or mucous membranes contaminated with saliva or other potentially infective material from a human with rabies should receive a full course of anti-rabies treatment. Category I

6. Personnel Restriction Because of Illnesses or Special Conditions

  a. (i) Hospitals should have well-defined policies concerning contact of personnel with patients when personnel have potentially transmissible conditions. Policies should govern personnel responsibility in using the health service and reporting illness, removal of personnel from direct contact with patients, and clearance for work after an infectious disease that required work restriction. Category I

(ii) Hospitals should identify those with authority to relieve personnel of duties. Category I

(iii) Policies for exclusion from work should be designed to encourage personnel to report their illnesses or exposures and not penalize them with loss of wages, benefits, or job status. Category I

b. Personnel who have responsibilities for patient care and have signs and symptoms of a transmissible infectious disease should report promptly to their supervisor. Category I

c. Acute Diarrhea

(i) Personnel with an acute diarrheal illness that is severe, is accompanied by other symptoms (such as fever, abdominal cramps, or bloody stools) or lasts longer than 24 hours should be excluded from direct patient contact pending evaluation. Category II

(ii) Whenever appropriate, specific treatment for documented infection with enteric pathogens should be made available to infected personnel. Category I

(iii) Personnel with non-typhoidal Salmonella enteric infections should be excluded from the direct care of high-risk patients until stool cultures are Salmonella-free on 2 consecutive specimens collected not less than 24 hours apart. Category II

(iv) (a) Personnel infected by enteric pathogens other than Salmonella may return to work after symptoms resolve. Category II

(b) These persons should be individually counseled before they return to work about the importance of handwashing. Category I

(v) Follow-up cultures or examinations of stool for pathogens other than Salmonella may be done to determine when the stool is free of the infecting organism. Category III

d. Herpes Simplex Infections

(i) Personnel with primary or recurrent orofacial herpes simplex infections should not take care of high-risk patients, for example, newborns, patients with burns, or severely immunocompromised patients, until the lesions are healed. Category II

(ii) Personnel with herpes simplex infections of the fingers or hands (herpetic whitlow) should not have direct contact with patients until lesions are healed. Category I

e. Respiratory Infections

(i) Personnel with respiratory infections should not be assigned to the direct care of high-risk patients, for example, neonates, young infants, patients with chronic obstructive lung disease, or immunocompromised patients. Category I

(ii) If an influenza epidemic is anticipated, a prevention program should be started for all patient-care personnel and high-risk patients. This program could include use of influenza vaccine and antiviral chemo-prophylaxis. Category II

f. Streptococcal Disease

If group A streptococcal disease is suspected, appropriate cultures should be taken, and the health worker should be excluded from work until she or he has received adequate therapy for 24 hours or until streptococcal infection has been ruled out. Category I

g. Management of Personnel Who Are Linked to Outbreaks

Personnel who are linked epidemiologically to an increase in bacterial infections caused by a pathogen associated with a carrier state should be cultured and, if positive, excluded from patient contact until carriage is eradicated or the risk of disease transmission is eliminated. Category I

7. Detection and Control of Tuberculosis

a. Skin Tests

(i) During the placement evaluation a tuberculin skin test should be given to all personnel, unless a previously significant reaction (10 mm or more of induration by Mantoux or vesiculation by a multiple puncture test) can be documented. The results should be used as the baseline test in determining treatment and follow-up of these personnel. Category I

(ii) The Mantoux technique using 5 TU PPD should be used. Category II

(iii) The 2-step test should be used to minimize the likelihood of interpreting a boosted reaction as a true conversion due to recent infection. Category II (Evaluation of the efficacy of the 2-step method in a given area may be necessary.)

(iv) If there is a likelihood of a severe reaction to skin testing, an initial test using a 2-step method with 1 TU PPD or a partial dose of 5 TU PPD should be considered. Category II

(v) After the initial skin test, the need for repeat testing should be determined in each hospital by the risk of acquiring new infection; for example, personnel need not have repeat testing if the incidence of tuberculosis in the community and in personnel is very low and personnel have not been exposed to an infective case. Category II

(vi) All personnel with significant reactions should be informed about risks of developing disease, risks they may pose to their contacts, and preventive treatment (see also recommendation 7.c.). Category I

b. Skin Tests After BCG Vaccination

(i) Persons who have had prior BCG vaccination should be skin-tested using the Mantoux method, unless a previously significant reaction can be documented. Category I

(ii) The results of skin tests in persons who have had prior BCG vaccination should be interpreted and acted on in the same manner as those in personnel who have not been vaccinated with BCG (see Preventive Treatment and Work Restrictions below). Category I

c. Chest Roentgenograms

 (i) Chest roentgenograms should be taken on those persons with signifi-
     cant tuberculin skin test results (a) who have never been evaluated,
     (b) who have had recent conversions, (c) who have never received ad-
     equate treatment for tuberculosis, or (d) who have pulmonary symp-
     toms that may be due to tuberculosis. If the chest film suggests pul-
     monary TB, these persons should be evaluated to rule out the
     possibility of current disease. Category I

 (ii) Routine follow-up roentgenograms should not be taken. Category I

d. Preventive Treatment and Work Restrictions

 (i) Personnel with current pulmonary or laryngeal tuberculosis whose
     sputum smear shows bacilli should be excluded from work until ade-
     quate treatment has begun and the sputum is free of bacilli on 3 con-
     secutive smears obtained on separate days or until sputum cultures
     show no growth. Category I

 (ii) Personnel who have current TB at a site other than the lung or larynx
      should be allowed to continue their usual activities. Category I

 (iii) Personnel who discontinue medications for current pulmonary or la-
       ryngeal disease before the recommended course of therapy has been
       completed should not be allowed to work. Category I

 (iv) (a) All personnel with significant skin-test reactions who do not have
          current tuberculosis and who have not had previous adequate
          therapy should be advised to receive preventive treatment, unless
          such therapy is specifically contraindicated. Category I

      (b) These personnel, if otherwise healthy and receiving preventive treat-
          ment, should be allowed to continue usual activities. Category I

 (v) (a) Personnel who cannot take or do not accept or complete preven-
         tive treatment should have their work situations evaluated and may
         require reassignment. A change in assignment should be consid-
         ered, if these persons work with high-risk patients. Category III

     (b) These persons should be counseled about the risk of developing
         disease and risks they may pose to their contacts and should be in-
         structed to seek evaluation of any signs or symptoms that may be
         due to TB. Category I

 (vi) All persons with a history of TB and all personnel with significant re-
      actions are at risk for developing current disease. These persons
      should be instructed to report promptly for evaluation if symptoms
      that may be due to TB develop. Category I

 (vii) Personnel who have completed preventive treatment or adequate
       therapy for current disease should be exempt from further screening
       unless symptomatic. Category I

e. Postexposure Prophylaxis

 (i) After exposure to an infective case of tuberculosis during which
     proper precautions were not used, all personnel, except those already
     known to have significant skin-test reactions, should be skin-tested 10

weeks after the exposure. Personnel whose skin test converts should have a chest roentgenogram taken and, unless specifically contraindicated, be advised to receive preventive treatment, provided current disease has been ruled out. If the chest film suggests pulmonary TB, these persons should be evaluated to rule out current disease. Category I

(ii) Unless a skin test was given during the 3 months before exposure, a baseline skin test should be done as soon as possible after the exposure to assist in interpreting the 10-week postexposure skin test. Category II

(iii) Personnel already known to have significant reactions should not have a chest roentgenogram taken unless they have pulmonary symptoms that may be due to tuberculosis. Category I

8. Personnel Exposed to Varicella or Zoster

a. After exposure to varicella (chickenpox) or zoster (shingles) personnel not known to be immune to varicella (by history or serology) should be excluded from work beginning on the tenth day after exposure and remain away from work for the maximum incubation period of varicella (21 days). Category I

b. Personnel who have onset of varicella should be excluded from work at least until all lesions have dried and crusted. Category I

9. Control of Hepatitis Infections

a. Personnel who are suspected of being infected with hepatitis A virus (HAV) should not take care of patients until 7 days after the onset of jaundice. Category III

b. Screening for evidence of prior infection with hepatitis B virus (HBV) in personnel who work in dialysis centers or other high-risk areas should be done only when needed to institute appropriate control measures. Category I

c. Personnel who are known careers of HBsAg should be counseled about precautions to minimize their risk of infecting others. Category I

d. (i) Personnel who have no exudative lesions on the hands and who are acutely infected with HBV, are known to be careers of HBsAg, or have hepatitis non A/non B (NANB) should not be restricted from patient-care responsibilities, unless there is evidence of disease transmission. Category I

(ii) Personnel who have no exudative lesions on the hands and who are acutely infected with HBV, are known to be careers of HBsAg, or have hepatitis NANB should wear gloves for procedures that involve trauma to tissues or direct contact with mucous membranes or non-intact skin. Category II

e. Personnel with exudative lesions on the hands who are HBsAg-positive should either wear gloves for all direct patient contact and when handling equipment that will touch mucous membranes or non-intact skin or abstain from all direct patient care. Category I

Table 3. Summary of important recommendations and work restriction for personnel with other infectious diseases

Disease/Problem	Relieve from direct patient contact	Partial work restriction	Duration	Category
Conjunctivitis, infectious	Yes		Until discharge ceases	II
Cytomegalovirus infections	No			II
Diarrhea (see 6.c.)				
Acute stage (diarrhea with other symptoms)	Yes		Until symptoms resolve and infection with Salmonella is ruled out	II
Convalescent stage				
Salmonella (non-typhoidal)	No	Personnel should not take care of high-risk patients	Until stool is free of the infecting organism on 2 consecutive cultures not less than 24 hours apart	II
Other enteric pathogens	No	(See text & recommendation 6.c.)		II
Enteroviral infections	No	Personnel should not take care of infants and newborns	Until symptoms resolve	II
Group A streptococcal disease	Yes		Until 24 hours after adequate treatment is started	I
Hepatitis, viral				
Hepatitis A	Yes		Until 7 days after onset of jaundice	III
Hepatitis B				
Acute	No	Personnel should wear gloves for procedures that involve trauma to tissues or contact with mucous membranes or non-intact skin	Until antigenemia resolves	II
Chronic antigenemia	No	Same as acute illness	Until antigenemia resolves	II
Hepatitis NANB	No	Same as acute hepatitis B	Period of infectivity has not been determined	II

Table 3.—continued

Disease/Problem	Relieve from direct patient contact	Partial work restriction	Duration	Category
Herpes simplex				
Genital	No			II
Hands (herpetic whitlow)	Yes	(Note: It is not known whether gloves prevent transmission)	Until lesions heal	I
Orofacial	No	Personnel should not take care of high-risk patients	Until lesions heal	II
Measles				
Active	Yes		Until 7 days after the rash appears	I
Postexposure (Susceptible personnel)	Yes		From the 5th through the 21st day after exposure and/or 7 days after the rash appears	II
Mumps				
Active	Yes		Until 9 days after onset of parotitis	I
Postexposure	Yes*		From the 12th through the 26th day after exposure or until 9 days after onset of parotitis	III
Pertussis				
Active	Yes		From the beginning of the catarrhal stage through the 3rd week after onset of paroxysms or until 7 days after start of effective therapy	I
Postexposure (asymptomatic personnel)	No			II

Postexposure (symptomatic personnel)	Yes	Same as active pertussis	I
Rubella			
Active	Yes	Until 5 days after the rash appears	I
Postexposure (susceptible personnel)	Yes	From the 7th through the 21st day after exposure and/or 5 days after rash appears	II
Scabies	Yes	Until treated	I
Staphylococcus aureus (skin lesions)	Yes	Until lesions have resolved	II
Upper respiratory infections (high-risk patients)	Yes	Personnel with upper respiratory infections should not take care of high-risk patients (See 6.e.)	II
Zoster (Shingles)			
Active	No	Appropriate barrier desirable; personnel should not take care of high-risk patients	II
Postexposure (susceptible personnel)	Yes	From the 10th through the 21st day after exposure or if varicella occurs until all lesions dry and crust	I
Varicella (Chickenpox)			
Active	Yes	Until all lesions dry and crust	I
Postexposure	Yes	From the 10th through the 21st day after exposure or if varicella occurs until all lesions dry and crust	I

*Mumps vaccine may be offered to susceptible personnel. When given after exposure to susceptible personnel. When given after exposure, mumps vaccine may not provide protection. However, if exposure did not result in infection, immunizing exposed personnel should protect against subsequent infection. Neither mumps immune globulin nor immune serum globulin (ISG) is of established value in postexposure prophylaxis. Transmission of mumps among personnel and patients has not been a major problem in hospitals in the United States, probably due to multiple factors, including high levels of natural and vaccine-induced immunity.

f. Dental personnel should consider routine use of gloves, masks, and protective eyewear when performing dental procedures. Category III

10. Precautions for AIDS*****

a. Personnel considered to have any of the clinical features described in the AIDS spectrum should be counseled about precautions to minimize their risk of infecting others (see discussion of AIDS and HbsAg careers in text). Category I

b. Personnel considered to have any of the clinical features described in the AIDS spectrum who have no exudative lesions on the hands should wear gloves for procedures that involve trauma to tissues or direct contact with mucous membranes or non-intact skin. Category II

c. Personnel considered to have any of the clinical features described in the AIDS spectrum and who have exudative lesions on the hands should either wear gloves for all direct patient contact and when handling equipment that will touch mucous membranes or non-intact skin or abstain from all direct patient care. Category II

d. Dental personnel taking care of patients considered to have any of the clinical features in the AIDS spectrum should consider routine use of gloves, masks, and protective eyewear when performing dental procedures. Category II

11. Personnel with Other Infectious Diseases

Table 3 is a summary of the important recommendations above and work restrictions for personnel with other infectious diseases not mentioned previously.

REFERENCES: AS NUMBERED IN ORIGINAL PUBLICATION

1. Dienstag JL, Stevens CE, Bhan AK, Szmuness W. Hepatitis B vaccine administered to chronic carders of hepatitis B surface antigen. Ann Intern Med 1982;96:575–579.
2. Szmuness W, Stevens CE, Oleszko WR, Goodman A. Passive-active immunization against hepatitis B: immunogenicity studies in adult Americans. Lancet 1981;1:575–577.
3. Immunization Practices Advisory Committee. Recommendation on inactivated hepatitis B virus vaccine. MMWR 1982;31:317–328.
4. Mulley AG, Silverstein MD, Dienstag JL. Indications for use of hepatitis B vaccine based on cost effectiveness analysis. N Engl J Med 1982;307:644–652.
5. Immunization Practices Advisory Committee. Recommendation on rubella prevention. MMWR 1981;30:37–47.
6. Centers for Disease Control. Acquired immune deficiency syndrome (AIDS): precautions for clinical and laboratory staffs. MMWR 1982;31:557–580.
7. Maynard JE. Viral hepatitis as an occupational hazard in the health care profession. In: Vyas GN, Cohen SN, Schmid R, eds. Viral hepatitis: a contemporary assessment of epidemiology, pathogenesis and prevention. Philadelphia: Franklin Institute Press, 1978;321–331.
8. Seeberg S, Bandberg A, Hermodsson S, et al. Hospital outbreak of hepatitis A secondary to blood exchange in a baby [Letter]. Lancet 1981;1:1155–1156.
9. Coulepis AG, Locamini SA, Lehmann NI, Gust ID. Detection of hepatitis A virus in the feces of patients with naturally acquired infections. J Infect Dis 1980;141:151–156.
10. Carl M, Kantor RJ, Webster HM, et al. Excretion of hepatitis A virus in the stools of hospitalized patients. J Med Virol 1982;9:125–129.
11. Reiner NE, Judson FN, Bond WW, et al. Asymptomatic rectal mucosai lesions and hepatitis B surface antigen at sites of sexual contact in homosexual men with persistent hepatitis B virus infection: evidence for de facto parenteral transmission. Ann Intern Med 1982;96:170–173.

***** These suggestions are not meant to restrict hospitals from using additional precautions.

12. Petersen NJ, Bond WW, Marshall JH, et al. An air sampling technique for hepatitis B surface antigen. Health Lab Sci 1976;13:233–237.
13. Petersen NJ, Bond WW, Favero MS. Air sampling for hepatitis B surface antigen in a dental operatory. JADA 1979;99:465–467.
14. Pattison CP, Maynard JE, Berquist KR, et al. Epidemiology of hepatitis B in hospital personnel. Am J Epidemiol 1975;101:59–64.
15. Dienstag JL, Ryan DM. Occupational exposure to hepatitis B virus in hospital personnel: infection or immunization? Am J Epidemiol 1982;115:26–39.
16. Janzen J, Tripatzis I, Wagner U, et al. Epidemiology of hepatitis B surface antigen (HBsAg) and antibody to HBsAg in hospital personnel. J Infect Dis 1978;137:261–265.
17. Levy BS, Hams JC, Smith JL, et al. Hepatitis B in ward and clinical laboratory employees of a general hospital. Am J Epidemiol 1977;106:330–335.
18. Hirschowitz BA, Dasher CA, Whitt FJ, Cole GW. Hepatitis B antigen and antibody and tests of liver function—a prospective study of 310 hospital laboratory workers. Am J Clin Pathol 1980;73:63–68.
19. Leers WD, Kouroupis GM. Prevalence of hepatitis B antibodies in hospital personnel. Can Med Assoc J 1975;113:844–847.
20. Tabor E, Gerety RJ, Mott M, Wilbur J. Prevalence of hepatitis B in a high risk setting: a serologic study of patients and staff in a pediatric oncology unit. Pediatrics 1978;61:711–715.
21. Favero MS. Maynard JE, Leger RT, Graham DR, Dixon RE. Guidelines for care of patients hospitalized with viral hepatitis. Ann Intern Med 1979;91:872–876.
22. Hadler SC, Sorlev DL, Acree KH, et al. An outbreak of hepatitis B in a dental practice. Ann Intern Med 1981;95:133–138.
23. Rimland D, Parkin WE. Miller GB, Schrack WD. Hepatitis B outbreak traced to an oral surgeon. N Engl J Med 1977;296:953–958.
24. Communicable Disease Surveillance Centre and the Epidemiological Research Laboratory of the Public Health Laboratory Service, London. Acute hepatitis B associated with gynecological surgery. Lancet 1980;1:1–6.
25. Reingold AL, Kane MA, Murphy BL, et al. Transmission of hepatitis B by an oral surgeon. J Infect Dis 1982:145:262–268.
26. Carl M, Francis DP, Blakey DL, Maynard JE. Interruption of hepatitis B transmission by modification of a gynecologist's surgical technique. Lancet 1982;1:731–733.
27. Alter HJ, Chalmers TC, Freeman BM, et al. Health-care workers positive for hepatitis B surface antigen: are their contacts at risk? N Engl J Med 1975;292:454–457.
28. Snydman DR, Hindman SH, Wineland MD, et al. Nosocomial viral hepatitis B: a cluster among staff with subsequent transmission to patients. Ann Intern Med 1976;85:573–577.
29. Center for Disease Control. Control measures for hepatitis B in dialysis centers. Atlanta: Department of Health, Education and Welfare, Public Health Service, Viral Hepatitis Investigations and Control Series, November 1977 (HEW publication no. [CDC]78–8358).
30. Tong MJ, Thursby M, Rakela J, et al. Studies on the maternal-infant transmission of the viruses which cause acute hepatitis. Gastroenterology 1981;80:999–1004.
31. Schweitzer IL, Dunn AE, Peters RL, Spears RL. Viral hepatitis B in neonares and infants. Am J Med 1973;55:762–771.
32. Craig CP, Gribble C, Suarez K. Risk of hepatitis B among phlebotomists. Am J Infect Control 1981;9:11–14.
33. Centers for Disease Control. Hepatitis surveillance report no. 47 (December), 1981:3.
34. Szmuness W, Stevens CE, Harley EJ, et al. Hepatitis B vaccine: demonstration of efficacy in a controlled clinical trial in a high-risk population in the United States. N Engl J Med 1980;303:833–841.
35. Francis DP, Hadlet SC, Thompson SE, et al. The prevention of hepatitis B with vaccine: report of the CDC multi-center efficacy trial among homosexual men. Ann Intern Med 1982;97:362–366.
36. Szmuness W, Stevens CE, Zang EA, et al. A controlled clinical trial of the efficacy of the hepatitis B vaccine (Heptavax-B): a final report. Hepatology 1981;1:377–385.
37. Centers for Disease Control. Hepatitis B virus vaccine safety: report of an interagency group. MMWR 1982;31:465–468.
38. Centers for Disease Control. The safety of hepatitis B virus vaccine. MMWR 1983;32:134–136.
39. McConnick RD, Maki DG. Epidemiology of needle-stick injuries in hospital personnel. Am J Med 1981;70:928–932.
40. Seeff LB, Wright EC, Zimmerman HJ, et al. Type B hepatitis after needle-stick exposure: prevention with hepatitis B immune globulin: final report of the Veterans Administration Cooperative Study. Ann Intern Med 1978;88:285–293.
41. Osterman CA. Relationship of new disposal unit to risk of needle puncture injuries. Hosp Top 1975;53:12–13.
42. Immunization Practices Advisory Committee. Recommendation on immune globulins for protection against vital hepatitis. MMWR 1981;30:423–428, 433–435.
43. American Academy of Pediatfics Committee on Fetus and Newborn. Perinatal herpes simplex viral infections. Pediatrics 1980;66:147–149.

44. Greaves WL, Kaiser AB, Afford RH, Schaffner W. The problem of herpetic whitlow among hospital personnel. Intect Control 1980;1:381–385.
45. Stamm WE, Feeley JC, Facklam RR. Wound infections due to group A Streptococcus traced to a vaginal carrier. J Infect Dis 1978;38:287–292.
46. Berkelman RL, Martin D, Graham DR, et al. Streptococcal wound infections caused by a vaginal carrier. JAMA 1982:247:2680–2682.
47. Centers for Disease Control. Guidelines for prevention of TB transmission in hospitals. Atlanta: U.S. Department of Health and Human Services (HHS publication no. [CDC]82–8371), 1982.
48. Craven RB, Wenzel RP, Atuk NO. Minimizing tuberculosis risk to hospital personnel and students exposed to unsuspected disease. Ann Intern Med 1975;82:628–632.
49. American Thoracic Society, Ad Hoc Committee of the Scientific Assembly on Tuberculosis. Screening for pulmonary tuberculosis in institutions. Am Rev Respir Dis 1977;115:901–906.
50. American Thoracic Society, American Lung Association, and Centers for Disease Control. Preventive therapy of tuberculous infection. Am Rev Respir Dis 1974;110:371–374.
51. American Thoracic Society Executive Committee. The tuberculin skin test. Am Rev Respir Dis 1981;124:356–363.
52. Thompson NJ, Glassroth JL, Snider DE, Farer ES. The booster phenomenon in serial tuberculin testing. Am Rev Respir Dis 1979;119:587–597.
53. American Thoracic Society Executive Comtmttee. Diagnostic standards and classification of tuberculosis and other mycobacterial diseases. 14th ed. Am Rev Respir Dis 1981;123:343–358.
54. Valenti WM, Andrews BA, Presley BA, Reifler CB. Absence of the booster phenomenon in serial tuberculin skin testing. Am Rev Respir Dis 1982;125:323–325.
55. Barrett-Connor E. The periodic chest roentgenogram for the control of tuberculosis in health care personnel. Am Rev Respir Dis 1980;122:153–155.
56. American Thoracic Society, Ad Hoe Committee of the Scientific Assembly on Tuberculosis. Discharge of tuberculosis patients from medical surveillance. Am Rev Respir Dis 1976;113:709–710.
57. American Thoracic Society. Guidelines for work for patients with tuberculosis. Am Rev Respir Dis 1973;108:160–161.
58. Ross AH. Modification of chickenpox in family contacts by administration of gamma globulin. N Engl J Med 1962;267:369–376.
59. Hayden GF, Meyers JD, Dixon RE. Nosocomial vancella: II. Suggested guidelines for management. West J Med 1979:130:300–303.
60. Valenti WM, Hall CB, Douglas RG Jr, et al. Nosocomial viral infections: I. Epidemiology and significance. Infect Control 1980;1:33–37.
61. Valenti WM, Betts RF, Hall CB, et al. Nosocomial viral infections: II. Guidelines for prevention and control of respiratory viruses, herpes viruses, and hepatitis viruses. Infect Control 1981:1:165–178.
62. Valenti WM, Hruska JF, Menegus MA, Freeburn MJ. Nosocomial viral infections: III. Guidelines for prevention and control of exanthematous viruses, gastroenteritis viruses, picornaviruses, and uncommonly seen viruses. Infect Control 1981;2:38–49.
63. Hall CD, Douglass RG Jr. Nosocomial respiratory, syncytial viral infections: should gowns and masks be used? Am J Dis Child 1981;135:512–515.
64. Hail CB, Douglass RG Jr. Modes of transmission of respiratory syncytial virus. J Pediatr 1981;99:100–103.
65. Tolkoff-Rubin NE, Rubin RH, Keller EE, et al. Cytomegalovirus intection in dialysis patients and personnel. Ann Intern Med 1978;89:625–628.
66. Duvall CP, Casazza AR, Grimley PM, et al. Recovery of cytomegalovirus from adults with neoplastic disease. Ann Intern Med 1966;65:531–539.
67. Yeager AS. Longitudinal serological study of cytomegalovirus infections in nurses and in personnel without patient contact. J Clin Microbiol 1975;2:448–452.
68. Ahlfors K, Ivarsson S-A, Johnsson T, Renmarker K. Risk of cytomegalovirus infection in nurses and congenital infection in their offspring. Acta Paediatr Scand 1981;70:819–823.
69. Jordan MC, Rousseau WE, Noble GR, et al. Association of cervical cytomegalovirus with venereal disease. N Engl J Med 1973;288:932–934.
70. Davis LE, Steward JA, Garvin S. Cytomegalovirus infection: a seroepidemiologic comparison of nuns and women from a venereal disease clinic. Am J Epidemiol 1975;102:327–330.
71. Stagno S, Reynolds DW, Huang E-S, et al. Congenital cytomegalovirus infection: occurrence in an immune population. N Engl J Med 1977;296:1254–1258.
72. Ahlfors K, Ivarsson S-A, Johnsson T, Svanberg L. Primary and secondary maternal cytomegalovirus infections and their relation to congenital infection. Acta Paediatr Scand 1982;71:109–113.
73. Cohen MS, Steere AC, Baltimore R, et al. Possible nosocomial transmission of group Y Neisseria meningitidis among oncology patients. Ann Intern Med 1979;91:7–12.
74. Rose HD, Lenz IE, Sheth NK. Meningococcal pneumonia: a source of nosocomial infection. Arch Intern Med 1981;141:575–577.
75. Limemann CC Jr, Ramundo N, Peristein PH, Minton SD. Use of pertussis vaccine in an epidemic involving hospital staff. Lancet 1975;2:540–543.
76. Kurt TL, Yeager AS, Guenette S, Dunlop S. Spread of pertussis by hospital staff. JAMA 1972;221:264–267.

77. Gooch JJ, Strasius SR, Beamer B, et al. Nosocomial outbreak of scabies. Arch Dermatol 1978;114:897–898.
78. Belle EA, D'Souza TJ, Zarzour JY, et al. Hospital epidemic of scabies: diagnosis and control. Can J Pub Health 1979;70:133–135.
79. Bernstein B, Mihan R. Hospital epidemic of scabies. J Pediatr 1973;83:1086–1087.
80. Haydon JR Jr, Caplan RM. Epidemic scabies. Arch Dermatol 1971;103:168–173.
81. Estes SA. Diagnosis and management of scabies. Med Clin N Am 1982;66:955–963.

FURTHER READING

1. National Institute for Occupational Safety and Health (NIOSH). Hospital occupational health services study, NIOSH I-VII. Cincinnati: U.S. Department of Health, Education and Welfare, Public Health Service, Center for Disease Control. July 1974 to April 1976 (HEW publication Nos. [NIOSH] 75–101, 75–137, 76–107, 76–115, 76–116, 77–140).
2. Haley RW, Emori TG. The employee health service and infection control in U.S. hospitals. 1976–1977: I. Screening procedures. JAMA 1981;246:844–847.
3. Haley RW, Emori TG. The employee health service and infection control in U.S. hospitals, 1976–1977: II. Managing employee illness. JAMA 1981;246:962–966.
4. Werdegar D. Guidelines tbr infection control aspects of employee health. J Assoc Pract Intect Cont 1977;5(Sept):17–22.
5. Werdegar D. Guidelines for infection control aspects of employee health. J Assoc Pract Infect Cont 1977;5(Dec):15–22.
6. Werdegar D. Employee health. Nurs Clin N Am 1980;15:769–787.
7. Gardner P, Oxman MN, Breton S. Hospital management of patients and personnel exposed to communicable diseases. Pediatrics 1975;56:700–709.
8. Klein JO. Management of infections in hospital employees. Am J Med 1981;70:919–923.

Guideline for Prevention of Surgical Wound Infections

Original Citation: Centers for Disease Control and Prevention. Guideline for prevention of surgical wound infections, 1985 (supersedes Guideline for Prevention of Surgical Wound Infections published in 1982).

Original Author: Revised by Julia S. Garner, RN, MN.

RANKING SCHEME FOR RECOMMENDATIONS

Category I

Measures in Category I are strongly supported by well-designed and controlled clinical studies that show their effectiveness in reducing the risk of nosocomial infections or are viewed as effective by a majority of expert reviewers. Measures in this category are viewed as applicable for most hospitals—regardless of size, patient population, or endemic nosocomial infection rates.

Category II

Measures in Category II are supported by highly suggestive clinical studies in general hospitals or by definitive studies in specialty hospitals that might not be representative of general hospitals. Measures that have not been adequately studied but have a logical or strong theoretical rationale indicating probable effectiveness are included in this category. Category II recommendations are viewed as practical to implement in most hospitals.

Category III

Measures in Category III have been proposed by some investigators, authorities, or organizations, but, to date, lack supporting data, a strong theoretical rationale, or an indication that the benefits expected from them are cost effective. Thus, they are considered important issues to be studied. They might be considered by some hospitals for implementation, especially if the hospitals have specific nosocomial infection problems, but they are not generally recommended for widespread adoption.

INTRODUCTION

Surgical wound infections are the second most frequent nosocomial infection in most hospitals and are an important cause of morbidity, mortality, and excess hospital costs (1–4). They are divided into infections (a) confined to the incisional wound and (b) involving structures adjacent to the wound that were entered or exposed during an operation (sometimes called "deep infections"). Some 60%–80% of infections are incisional, and the rest are at adjacent sites, for example, intraabdominal/retroperitoneal and deep soft tissue (5, 6). This Guideline deals primarily with incisional infections, although many, recommendations in it will also help prevent infections at adjacent sites. Burn wounds are not discussed.

EPIDEMIOLOGY

In general, a wound can be considered infected if purulent material drains from it, even without the confirmation of a positive culture (7). This clinical definition has advantages compared with those based on culture results, because (a) a positive culture does not necessarily indicate infection, since many wounds, infected or not, are colonized by bacteria, and (b) infected wounds may not yield pathogens by culture because some pathogens are fastidious, culture techniques are inadequate, or the patient has received antimicrobial therapy. On the other hand, infections, for example, those in the granulocytopenic patient, may not always produce purulent material. It is therefore also useful to consider a wound infected if the attending surgeon believes it to be. Unless the incision is involved, stitch abscesses should not be counted as surgical wound infections; they can be counted as skin or cutaneous infections.

Wounds can be classified according to the likelihood and degree of wound contamination at the time of operation. A widely accepted classification scheme (7–9) is listed below:

CLEAN WOUNDS

These are uninfected operative wounds in which no inflammation is encountered and the respiratory, alimentary, genital, or uninfected urinary tracts are not entered. In addition, clean wounds are primarily closed, and if necessary, drained with closed drainage. Operative incisional wounds that follow nonpenetrating (blunt) trauma should be included in this category if they meet the criteria.

Clean-Contaminated Wounds

These are operative wounds in which the respiratory, alimentary, genital, or urinary tract is entered under controlled conditions and without unusual contamination. Specifically, operations involving the biliary tract, appendix, vagina, and oropharynx are included in this category, provided no evidence of infection or major break in technique is encountered.

Contaminated Wounds

These include open, fresh, accidental wounds, operations with major breaks in sterile technique or gross spillage from the gastrointestinal tract, and incisions in which acute, nonpurulent inflammation is encountered.

Dirty or Infected Wounds

These include old traumatic wounds with retained devitalized tissue and those that involve existing clinical infection or perforated viscera. This definition suggests that the organisms causing postoperative infection were present in the operative field before the operation.

This classification scheme has been shown in numerous studies to predict the relative probability that a wound will become infected. Clean wounds have a 1%–5% risk of infection; clean-contaminated, 3%–11%; contaminated, 10%–17%; and dirty, over 27% (2, 3, 7). These infection rates were affected by many appropriate prevention measures taken during the studies, such as use of prophylactic antimicrobials, and would have been higher if no prevention measures had been taken. In addition to the scheme's application to predicting the probability of infection, this classification has other uses. For a given operation, the clean-wound infection rate, in particular, can be used by surgeons to compare their own infection rates, and by inference, their operating techniques, with those of other surgeons (2, 10). The classification also can alert personnel to wounds at high risk of infection and thus enable personnel to take appropriate perioperative preventive measures (3, 11).

Although the degree or operative contamination of wounds is important in determining the risk of infection, so are host and local wound factors. The host factors leading to increased risk may include very young or old age, presence of a perioperative infection, and possibly diabetes and severe malnutrition (7). Local wound factors associated with high risk include presence of devitalized tissue or foreign bodies and poor blood supply to the wound.

A multivariate index combining patient susceptibility and wound contamination was developed and tested during the CDC Study on the Efficacy of Nosocomial Infection Control (SENIC) (12). This index, which involved 4 risk factors, predicted the surgical wound infection risk about twice as well as the traditional wound classification system. The 4 risk factors were: having an abdominal operation, having an operation that lasted longer than 2 hours, having a contaminated, dirty, or infected operation by the traditional classification system, and having 3 or more discharge diagnoses. Since this index includes discharge diagnoses, some modification and a prospective evaluation of the index are needed before it can be recommended for adoption.

Surgical wound infections are most often localized to the wound and with appropriate treatment usually do not result in major complications. Local complications include destruction of tissue, wound dehiscence, incisional and deep hernias, septic thrombophlebitis, recurrent pain, and disfiguring and disabling scars. The numerous potential systemic complications include fever, increased metabolic demands that sometimes result in malnutrition, toxemia, bacteremia, shock, metastatic infection, failure of vital organs remote from the infection, and death. The severity of each complication depends in large part on the infecting pathogen and on the site of infection. For example, viridans group streptococci are unlikely to cause a severe infection unless they invade the vascular system, but a group A streptococcal infection is likely to be severe regardless of the site. Further, any infection involving an implanted foreign body or substantial necrotic tissue is likely to have serious sequelae, regardless of the pathogen involved.

As determined by reports to the National Nosocomial Infection Study, gram-negative aerobic bacteria make up approximately 40% of pathogens isolated from surgical wounds. However, Staphylococcus aureus remains the single most frequently isolated species (13). Pathogens other than bacteria, for example, fungi and viruses, are uncommonly reported.

Pathogens that infect surgical wounds can be acquired from the patient, the hospital environment, or personnel. The patient's own flora appears to be responsible for most infections, especially if clean-wound infections are excluded (8). Sources of contamination include the gastrointestinal, respiratory, genital, and urinary tracts and the skin and anterior nares.

Exogenous contamination appears responsible for a substantial proportion of infections of clean wounds. During epidemic periods, exogenous contamination may be responsible for many more infections (14, 15). Exogenous contamination may come from any personnel or environmental source, although direct contact with the wound by the surgical team is probably the final pathway for spread of most such contamination. Epidemics of infections due to group A streptococci and some outbreaks of S. aureus wound infections indicate that personnel carriers can be a source. Epidemics due to gram-negative microorganisms may be spread from environmental sources, especially those containing water (for example, irrigating solutions). Most infections, endogenous or exogenous, appear to result from contamination acquired in the operating room. Few infections are acquired after the operation if wounds are closed primarily, that is, before leaving the operating room, and if drains are not used, probably because the normal healing process seals most wounds within 24 hours after closure.

CONTROL MEASURES

The risk of developing a surgical wound infection is largely determined by 3 factors: (a) the amount and type of microbial contamination of the wound, (b) the condition of the wound at the end of the operation (largely determined by surgical technique and disease processes encountered during the operation), and (c) host susceptibility, that is, the patient's intrinsic ability to deal with microbial contamination. These factors interact in a complex manner. For example, a wound in healthy tissue is surprisingly resistant to infection even when contaminated with many microorganisms, but a wound containing foreign or necrotic material is highly susceptible to infection even if few microorganisms are present. Measures intended to prevent surgical wound infections are directed at all 3 factors just mentioned. Since most infections are acquired in the operating room and good surgical practices are crucial to their prevention, most prevention measures should be directed at influencing the practices of the surgical team.

Measures aimed at preventing microbial contamination of the wound begin before the operation. One important preoperative and postoperative measure is the treatment of active infections. A patient who has an active bacterial infection, even if it is at a site remote from the surgical wound, has a greater risk of wound infection than does an uninfected patient (7). Treating a "remote" infection that is present before or after an operation is believed to reduce the risk of wound infection.

Other preoperative measures involving the patient are keeping the preoperative hospital stay short, avoiding hair removal or, if necessary, removing hair with clippers or depilatories rather than a razor, and preparing the operative site with an antiseptic. A short preoperative stay has been associated with low wound infection rates (2, 5, 7, 16). Bathing by the patient with antimicrobial-containing products has been suggested as an effective preoperative prevention measure, because it reduces colonization with typical wound pathogens such as S. aureus (16). Although such bathing is relatively easy, safe, and inexpensive, it has not been proven to reduce colonization with S. aureus in the host's natural reservoir—the anterior nares—or to reduce infection rates.

Hair adjacent to the operative site is often removed to prevent the wound from becoming contaminated with hair during the operation. However, several studies (2, 17, 18) have suggested that shaving with a razor can injure the skin and increase the risk of infection. Clipping hair, using a depilatory, or no shaving at all has been suggested in place of shaving. Results of 2 studies (2, 17) suggest that if shaving is necessary, it be performed immediately before the operation.

The skin at the operative site is thoroughly cleaned to remove superficial flora, soil, and debris before the operation to reduce the risk of contaminating the wound with a patient's skin flora. Immediately before the operation, a preoperative skin preparation is applied to the patient's skin to kill or inhibit more adherent, deep, resident flora. A patient preoperative skin preparation is defined as "a safe, fast-acting, broad-spectrum antimicrobial-containing preparation which significantly reduces the number of microorganisms on intact skin" (19).

The surgical team must also take perioperative measures to prevent microbial contamination of the wound. Contamination from the surgical team may result from direct contact, usually with hands or from shedding from skin or mucous membranes. Transfer of microorganisms from hands to the wound is reduced by scrubbing the hands and wearing sterile gloves. The surgical scrub is designed to kill or remove as many bacteria as possible, including resident bacteria. A surgical scrub preparation is defined as: "a nonirritating antimicrobial-containing preparation that significantly reduces the number of microorganisms on the intact skin. A surgical hand scrub should be broad-spectrum, fast-acting, and persistent." (19) The ideal duration of the surgical scrub is not known, but times as short as 5 minutes appear safe (20, 21). Once hands are scrubbed, sterile gloves act as an additional barrier to transfer of microorganisms to the wound. However, bacteria can multiply rapidly under gloves and can contaminate the wound through punctures in gloves, which occur frequently (22); use of surgical hand scrubs before putting on gloves should retard bacterial growth.

Air is also a potential source of microorganisms that can contaminate surgical wounds; its role in wound infections has been demonstrated in certain clean operations (7), such as operations in which a foreign body is implanted. Operating room (OR) air is often contaminated with microorganisms that are usually attached to other airborne particles such as dust, lint, skin squames, or respiratory droplets. Many of these microorganisms are potential pathogens. The number of viable airborne microorganisms for a given amount of OR ventilation is largely proportional to human activity. Greater numbers of airborne microorganisms can be expected with increased numbers of persons, especially if OR doors are being opened and the persons are moving, talking, or have uncovered skin areas. Airborne contamination decreases with (a) decreased numbers and activity of personnel, (b) increased ventilation that dilutes contaminated air with relatively clean filtered or outdoor air, (c) ultraviolet light, which kills microorganisms, and (d) proper use of occlusive clothing, masks, and gloves, which reduce shedding into air. Movement or activity in the OR can be decreased by closing the OR door and by limiting the number of personnel in the OR and adjacent corridors. In addition to limiting unnecessary activity, closing the door will decrease mixing of the OR air with corridor air, which may contain higher counts of bacteria. Limiting personnel movement in the OR and adjacent corridors takes planning. The goal of such planning, often called "traffic control," is to make the OR self-sufficient, or nearly so, once an operation has begun.

To reduce airborne contamination, a ventilation system producing a minimum of 20 changes of highly filtered air per hour is recommended for modern ORs (23). Some hospitals have installed "laminar flow" ventilation units for use in ORs (24), especially for rooms used for orthopedic procedures, because these ventilation units can provide nearly sterile air with minimal air turbulence. Investigators from a British multicenter study recently reported that several factors, including ultraclean air in ORs, systemic prophylactic antimicrobials for patients, and exhaust-ventilated suits for personnel reduced the incidence of deep wound infection after total joint replacement operations (25). An editorial about the study suggested that prophylactic antimicrobials are at least as effective as ultraclean air and exhaust ventilated suits in reducing deep sepsis and that cheaper alternatives such as prophylactic antimicrobials "should be exhausted" before any of the substantially more expensive provisions, such as ultraclean air and exhaust ventilated suits, are considered (26). A follow-up report from the multicenter study that examined the cost implications for the British National Health Service of ultraclean air and other infection control measures for total joint replacement suggested that antimicrobial prophylaxis was more cost effective than an ultraclean air system (27). In addition to the above findings, lower baseline rates of deep wound sepsis have been reported following total hip arthroplasty performed in conventional ORs in U.S. hospitals (28–31) than in hospitals in the British multicenter study.

Ultraviolet (UV) irradiation may decrease airborne microorganisms to low levels. Although UV-irradiation of ORs has been shown to result in a small but statistically significant decrease in infections of clean surgical wounds, infections of all surgical wounds combined were not reduced (7). Further, use of UV irradiation in ORs has several distinct disadvantages. UV light requires routine use of a visor or goggles and skin protection to prevent burns. UV lights also require frequent, routine maintenance to monitor the intensity of the light and can be costly to install or replace.

Microorganisms are constantly being shed from posed skin and mucous membranes, so masks, drapes, hoods, and gowns are used as barriers to decrease shedding into the air and prevent wound contamination. These barriers, even when wet, are most effective when their pore size prevents passage of bacteria. Several woven fabrics and nonwoven materials are virtually impermeable to bacteria (32). When drapes and gowns made from such nonwoven disposable material were used in a recent study, a reduction in wound infections occurred (33). Reusable gowns made of tightly woven cotton treated with a water repellent prevent passage of bacteria, provided they have not been laundered and sterilized more than 75 times (34). Some gowns are made entirely of impermeable materials, and others have these materials in critical areas, such as in the front and on the sleeves. Surgical team members may get uncomfortably hot in gowns made only of impermeable materials unless the room temperature is lowered or ventilation is increased.

Wearing shoe covers or regularly cleaned shoes has been recommended as a means of preventing transmission of bacteria from shoes (9). However, in one study, no significant differences in floor contamination were seen when ordinary shoes, clean shoes, or shoe covers were worn (35), There have been no controlled clinical studies to evaluate the role of shoe covers in preventing or reducing surgical wound infections. Furthermore, there is no strong theoretical rationale for their use or indication that the benefits expected from them are cost effective.

In the modern, well-managed OR, the risk of infection related to the inanimate environment appears low. This is due, in great part, to adequate sterilization of surgical devices, ventilation systems that provide clean air, and adequate cleaning of the OR. Environmental culturing and special cleaning after "dirty" cases are not recommended. There is no evidence that special cleaning procedures, e.g., "dirty case routines," are necessary. Some architectural designs incorporated into ORs may be useful in maintaining a clean environment (36). Others, however, such as floor plans including a central clean area and a peripheral traffic corridor, have not been proven to be especially useful. In addition, tacky or antiseptic mats placed at the entrance to OR suites to reduce carriage of microorganisms on shoes or stretcher wheels have not been shown to reduce the risk of infection.

The most important measure to prevent wound infections is operative technique. Poor technique can result in inadvertent contamination of the wound (for example, an accidental perforation of the bowel during an abdominal operation), may prolong the operation, and may result in a wound that cannot adequately resist infection because it contains devitalized tissues or foreign bodies. Since the risk of wound infection increases with the length of the operation, an expeditious operation is important (2, 5, 7, 12). However, the surgeon must balance the need to operate quickly with the need to handle tissues gently, reduce bleeding and hematoma formation, eradicate dead space, and minimize devitalized tissue and foreign materials in the wound. Other prevention techniques are not as well established as those just mentioned but appear prudent to use when possible. These are use of fine and monofilament rather than thick or braided suture and minimal use of suture and cautery. Technique applies not only to a surgeon's skill in handling the wound, but also to skill in supervising the surgical team and maintaining professional decorum that facilitates expeditious and successful operations. Poor discipline in the OR can result in mistakes and sloppy aseptic technique.

Once a surgeon has finished training, surgical habits might not be easy to change, but improvement may be stimulated by calculating and informing surgeons of their rates of wound infections. Traditionally, such efforts have been primarily focused on measuring the surgical wound infection rates following clean operations and reporting these rates to practicing surgeons (2, 10). Two recent reports, however, demonstrate the effectiveness of not limiting surgical wound surveillance and reporting programs exclusively to clean operations (3, 11). The first report, from the CDC SENIC Project, showed that establishing an infection surveillance and control program which included reporting surgeon-specific rates led to a reduction in hospitals' overall surgical wound infection rates of approximately 35% (11). Moreover, the report indicated that programs reporting such surgical wound infection rates, were just as effective in reducing infection rates in contaminated or dirty cases as in clean or clean-contaminated cases. The other report, a 5-year prospective study in a large Veterans Administration Medical Center that involved surveillance and reporting of clean, clean-contaminated, and contaminated surgical wound infection rates, demonstrated a 55% reduction in the incidence of surgical wound infections and a savings of nearly $750,000 in hospital costs over the study period (3). Overall wound infection rates and clean-contaminated wound infection rates were significantly lower than baseline rates in each year of the study.

The postoperative period usually does not contribute greatly to the risk of surgical wound infections. Nevertheless, wounds can become contaminated and later become infected if they are touched by contaminated hands or objects after the operation, especially if the wound is left open or if a drain is used. Until wound edges are sealed and the wound is healing (about 24 hours after the operation for most wounds), wounds are covered with sterile dressings to reduce the risk of such contamination. A transparent, semipermeable membrane dressing has been developed for use on wounds because the dressing does not need to be removed for the wound to be observed; the effect of use of this dressing on wound infection rates is unknown. Most dressings are occasionally removed to observe the wound; the frequency of removal depends on such factors as the type of wound and the presence of infection, drainage, moisture, pain, or fever. Personnel taking care of wounds can reduce the risk of contamination by washing their hands and using instruments to handle dressings and tissues (the no-touch technique) or, if touching the wound is necessary, wearing sterile gloves.

In the postoperative period, the risk of wound infection can be reduced by adequate wound drainage. If not allotted to drain freely, blood, body fluids, pus, and necrotic material collect in a wound and provide a growth medium for microorganisms. However, if a wound is drained, the skin cannot be completely closed, and microorganisms can enter the wound or deeper structures and cause infection. Thus, surgeons routinely drain only wounds expected to produce significant amounts of blood or other drainage and use closed drainage in preference to open drainage (37, 38). If a drain is used, having it enter through an adjacent, separate stab wound rather than the primary surgical wound will reduce the risk of infection. For dirty wounds, delaying wound closure is preferable to inserting a drain which increases the risk of infection (39); delayed wound closure is also useful for many contaminated wounds.

A patient's intrinsic susceptibility to infection is also important in determining the risk of infection. Unlike many other risk factors, host susceptibility is often not easily altered. If the operation can be delayed, some host factors can be altered: (a) Some diabetics can have their blood glucose better controlled, (b) some patients on adrenal glucocorticoids may be able to discontinue them or have the dosage reduced, and (c) severely malnourished patients can receive oral or parenteral hyperalimentation. However, there is no definitive evidence that these interventions will reduce the risk of infection. In each example, and in others in which host susceptibility can be altered, the physician must weigh the potential benefits of the alteration against the risks of a delayed operation and potential complications of the intervention.

For some operations, prophylactic antimicrobials are a means of reducing the risk of wound infections. Reviews of antimicrobial prophylaxis for surgery that deal with selection of agents and duration of therapy are available (9, 40–42). Prophylaxis is most useful for operations associated with a moderate level of contamination (clean-contaminated operations). Prophylaxis is not generally indicated for clean operations unless the consequences of infection are severe or life-threatening, for example, prosthetic (implant) orthopedic and cardiovascular surgery.

RECOMMENDATIONS

1. Preparation of the Patient Before Operation
   a. If the operation is elective, all bacterial infections that are identified, excluding ones for which the operation is performed, should be treated and controlled before the operation. Category I
   b. If the operation is elective, the hospital stay before the operation should be as short as possible. Category II
   c. If the operation is not urgent and the patient is malnourished, the patient should receive enteral or parenteral nutrition before the operation. Category II
   d. If the operation is elective, the patient should bathe (or be bathed) the night before with an antimicrobial soap. Category II
   e. (i) Unless hair near the operative site is so thick that it will interfere with the surgical procedure, it should not be removed. Category II

    (ii) If hair removal is necessary, it should be done either by clipping or using a depilatory rather than shaving. Category II

f. The area around and including the operative site should be washed and an antimicrobial preoperative skin preparation applied from the center to the periphery. This area should be large enough to include the entire incision and an adjacent area large enough for the surgeon to work during the operation, without contacting unprepared skin. Category II (Persons responsible for selecting commercially marketed antimicrobial preoperative skin preparations can obtain information about categorization of products from the Center for Drugs and Biologics, Division of OTC Drug Evaluation, FDA. In addition, information published in the scientific literature, presented at scientific meetings, documented by manufacturers and obtained from other sources deemed important may be considered.)

g. For major operations involving an incision and requiring use of the operating room (OR), the patient should be covered with sterile drapes in such a manner that no part of the patient is uncovered except the operative field and those parts necessary for anesthesia to be administered and maintained. Category II

2. Preparation of the Surgical Team

a. Everyone who enters the OR during an operation should at all times wear a high-efficiency mask to fully cover the mouth and nose and a cap or hood to fully cover hair on the head and face. Category I

b. Everyone who enters the OR should wear shoe covers. Category III

c. (i) The surgical team, that is, those who will touch the sterile surgical field, sterile instruments, or an incisional wound, should scrub their hands and arms to the elbows with an antimicrobial surgical hand scrub preparation before each operation. Scrubbing should be done before every procedure and take at least 5 minutes before the first procedure of the day. Category I (Persons responsible for selecting commercially marketed surgical hand scrubs can obtain information about categorization of products from the Center for Drugs and Biologics, Division of OTC Drug Evaluation, FDA. In addition, information published in the scientific literature, presented at scientific meetings, documented by manufacturers, and obtained from other sources deemed important may be considered.)

   (ii) Between consecutive operations, scrubbing times of 2 to 5 minutes may be acceptable. Category II

d. (i) After the hands are scrubbed and dried with sterile towels, the surgical team should don sterile gowns. Category I

   (ii) Gowns used in the OR should be made of reusable or disposable fabrics that have been shown to be effective barriers to bacteria, even when wet. Category II

e. (i) The surgical team should wear sterile gloves. If a glove is punctured during the operation, it should be changed as promptly as safety permits. Category I

(ii) For open bone operations and orthopedic implant operations, 2 pairs of sterile gloves should be worn. Category II

3. Preparation and Maintenance of Operating Room Environment

a. OR ventilation should include a minimum of 20 air changes per hour, of which at least 4 should be fresh air. All inlets should be located as high above the floor as possible and remote from exhaust outlets of all types. All air, recirculated or fresh, should be filtered (at least 90% efficiency) before it enters the OR. The surgical suite should be under positive pressure relative to the surrounding area. Category II

b. All OR doors should be kept closed except as needed for passage of equipment, personnel, and the patient—the number of personnel allowed to enter the OR, especially after an operation has started, should be kept to a minimum. Category II

c. The OR should be cleaned between surgical operations. Category II

d. Routine microbiologic sampling of the air or environmental surfaces should not be done. Category I

e. Use of tacky or antiseptic mats at the entrance to the OR is not recommended for purposes of infection control. Category I

f. Surgical instruments and supplies should be sterilized as outlined in the current edition of the CDC Guideline for Handwashing and Hospital Environmental Control. (This recommendation is not categorized since it refers to multiple recommendations that have been categorized elsewhere.)

4. Operative Technique

a. The surgical team should work as efficiently as possible in order to handle tissues gently, prevent bleeding, eradicate dead space, minimize devitalized tissue and foreign material in the wound, and reduce the length of the operation. Category I

b. Incisional wounds that are classified as "dirty and infected" should not ordinarily have skin closed over them at the end of an operation; that is, they should not ordinarily be closed primarily. Category II

c. If drainage is necessary for an uninfected wound, a closed suction drainage system should be used and placed in an adjacent stab wound rather than the main incisional wound. Category II

5. Wound Care

a. Personnel should wash their hands before and after taking care of a surgical wound. Category I

b. Personnel should not touch an open or fresh wound directly unless they are wearing sterile gloves or use no-touch technique. When the wound has sealed dressings may be changed without gloves. Category I

c. Dressings over closed wounds should be removed or changed if they are wet or if the patient has signs or symptoms suggestive of infection; for example, fever or unusual wound pain. When the dressing is removed, the wound should be evaluated for signs of infection. Any drainage from a wound that is suspected of being infected should be cultured and smeared for Gram stain. Category I

6. Prophylactic Antimicrobials
   a. Parenteral antimicrobial prophylaxis is recommended for operations that (a) are associated with a high risk of infection or (b) are not frequently associated with infection but, if infection occurs, are associated with severe or life-threatening consequences; for example, cardiovascular and orthopedic operations involving implantable devices. Category I
   b. Antimicrobials selected for use for prophylaxis should have been shown to be safe and effective for prophylaxis of operative wound infections in well-designed, controlled trials whose results have been published. Category I
   c. Parenteral antimicrobial prophylaxis should be started shortly before the operation and should be promptly discontinued after the operation. Category I (For cesarean sections, prophylaxis is usually given intraoperatively after the umbilical cord is clamped.)
7. Protection of Patients from Other Infected Patients or Personnel
   a. Patients with potentially transmissible wound or skin infections should be placed on isolation precautions according to the current edition of the CDC Guideline for Isolation Precautions in Hospitals. (This recommendation is not categorized, since the recommendations for isolation precautions are not categorized.)
   b. Personnel with potentially transmissible conditions, for example, Herpes simplex infections of fingers and hands, group A streptococcal disease, or S. aureus skin lesions, should be managed according to the current edition of the CDC Guideline for Infection Control in Hospital Personnel. (This recommendation is not categorized since it refers to several recommendations that have been categorized elsewhere.)
   c. Routine culturing of personnel should not be done. Category I
8. Surveillance and Classification
   a. At the time of operation or shortly after, all operations should be classified and recorded as clean, clean-contaminated, contaminated, or dirty and infected (see text for definitions). Category II
   b. The person in charge of surveillance of surgical patients should gather the information necessary to compute the classification-specific wound infection for all operations in the hospital. These rates should be computed periodically and made available to the infection control committee and the department of surgery. Category II
   c. Procedure-specific wound infection rates should be computed periodically for the hospital and all active surgeons so that they can compare their own rates with those of others; the rates can be coded so that names do not appear. Category II
   d. Increases in wound infection rates should be evaluated. If an outbreak is confirmed, appropriate epidemiologic studies should be initiated. Category I
   e. An effort should be made to contact discharged patients to determine the infection rate for the 30 days after operation. Category III

REFERENCES: AS NUMBERED IN ORIGINAL PUBLICATION

1. Brachman PS, Dan BB, Haley RW, Hooton TM, Garner IS, Allen JR. Nosocomial surgical infections: incidence and cost. Surg Clin North Am 1980;60:15–25.
2. Cruse PJE, Foord R. The epidemiology of wound infection. A ten-year prospective study of 62,939 wounds. Surg Clin North Am 1980;60:27–40.
3. Olson M, O'Connor MO, Schwartz ML. A 5-year prospective study of 20,193 wounds at the Minneapolis VA Medical Center. Ann Surg 1984:199:253–259.
4. Green JW, Wenzel RP. Postoperative wound infection: a controlled study of increased duration of hospital stay and direct cost of hospitalization. Ann Surg 1977;285:264–268.
5. Haley RW, Hooton TM, Culver DH, et al. Nosocomial infections in U.S. hospitals. 1975–1976: estimated frequency by selected characteristics of patients. Am J Med 1981;70:947–959.
6. Allen JR, Hightower AW, Martin SM, Dixon RE. Secular trends in nosocomial infections: 1970–1979. Am J Med 1981:70:389–392.
7. Howard JM, Barker WE, Culbertson WR, et al. Postoperative wound infections: the influence of ultraviolet irradiation of the operating room and various other factors. Ann Surg 1964;160(Suppl):l-192.
8. Alterneier WA. Surgical infections: incisional wounds. In: Bennett JV, Brachman PS, eds. Hospital infections. Boston: Little, Brown and Co., 1979:287–306.
9. American College of Surgeons Committee on Control of Surgical Infections. Manual on control of infection in surgical patients. 2nd ed. Philadelphia: JB Lippincott, 1984.
10. Condon RE, Schulte WJ, Malangoni MA, Anderson-Teschendorf MJ. Effectiveness of a surgical wound surveillance program. Arch Surg 1983;118:303–307.
11. Haley RW, Culver DH, White JW, et al. The efficacy of infection surveillance and control programs in preventing nosocornial infections in U.S. hospitals. Am J Epidemiol 1985;121:182–205.
12. Haley RW, Culver DH, Morgan WM, Emori TG, Munn VP, Hooten TM. Identifying patients at high risk of surgical wound infection: a simple multivariate index of patient susceptibility and wound contamination. Am J Epiderniol 1985;121:206–215.
13. Centers for Disease Control. Nosocomial infection surveillance, 1983. In: CDC Surveillance Summaries 1984;33(No. 2SS):9SS-21SS.
14. Garner JS, Dixon RE, Aber RC. Epidemic infections in surgical patients. AORN J 1981;34:700–724.
15. Aber RC, Garner JS. Postoperative wound infections. In: Wenzel RP, ed. Handbook of hospital acquired infections. Boca Raton, FL: CRC Press, Inc. 1981;303–316.
16. Bruun J. Postoperative wound infection: predisposing factors and the effect of a reduction in the dissemination of staphylococci. Acta Med Scand 1970;514(Suppl):1–89.
17. Seroplan R, Reynolds BM. Wound infections after preoperatire depilatory versus razor preparation. Ann J Surg 1971;121:251–254.
18. Alexander JW, Fischer JE, Boyajian M, Palmquist J, Morris MJ. The influence of hair-removal methods on wound infections. Arch Surg 1983;118:347–352.
19. The tentative final monograph for OTC topical antimicrobial products. Federal Register 1978 Jan 6; 43 FR 1210:1211–1249.
20. Dineen P. An evaluation of the duration of the surgical scrub. Surg Gynecol Obstet 1969;129: 1181–1184.
21. Galle PC, Homesley HD, Rhyne AL. Reassessment of the surgical scrub. Surg Gynecol Obstet 1978; 147:215–218.
22. Walter CW, Kundsin RB. The bacteriologic study of surgical gloves from 250 operations. Surg Gynecol Obstet 1969;129:949–952.
23. U.S. Department of Health and Human Services. Guideline for construction and equipment of hospital and medical facilities. Washington, DC: Government Printing Office, July 1984:(DHHS publication no. (HR5-M-HF) 84–1).
24. Garner JS, Emori TG, Haley RW. Operating room practices for the control of infection in U.S. hospitals, October 1976-July 1977. Surg Gynecol Obstet 1982;155:873–880.
25. Lidwell OM, Lowbury EJL, Whyte W, Blowers R, Stanley SJ, Lowe D. Effect of ultraclean air in operating rooms on deep sepsis in the joint after total hip or knee replacement: a randomized study. Br Med J 1982;285:10–14.
26. Meers PD. Ventilation in operating rooms. Br Med J 1983;286:244–245.
27. Lidwell OM. The cost implications of clean air systems and antibiotic prophylaxis in operations for total joint replacement. Infect Control 1984;5:36–37.
28. Fitzgerald RH, Nolan DR, Ilstrup DM, VanScoy RE, Washington JA, Coventry MB. Deep wound sepsis following total hip arthroplasty. J Bone Joint Surg 1977;59A:847–855.
29. Fitzgerald RH, Bechtol CO, Eftekhar N, Nelson JP. Reduction of deep sepsis after total hip arthroplasty. Arch Surg 1979;114:803–804.
30. Fitzgerald RH. Microbiologic environment, of the conventional operating room. Arch Surg 1979;114:772–775.
31. Coilis DK, Steinhaus K. Total hip replacement without deep infection in a standard operating room. J Bone Joint Surg 1976;58A:446–450.

32. Schwartz JT, Saunders DE. Microbial penetration of surgical gown materials. Surg Gynecol Obstet 1980;150:507–512.
33. Moylan JA, Kennedy BV. The importance of gown and drape barriers in the prevention of wound infection. Surg Gynecol Obstet 1980;151:465–470.
34. Laufman H, Eudy WW, Vandernoot AM, Liu D, Harris CA. Strike-through of moist contamination by woven and nonwoven surgical materials. Ann Surg 1975;181:857–862.
35. Hambraeus A, Maimborg AS. The influence of different footwear on floor contamination. Scand J Infect Dis 1979;11:243–246.
36. Laufman H. Surgical hazard control: effect of architecture and engineering. Arch Surg 1973;107:552–559.
37. Mcllrath DC, Van Heerden J, Edis AJ. Closure of abdominal incisions with subcutaneous catheters. Surgery 1976;4:4112–4116.
38. van der Linden W, Gedda S, Edlund G. Randomized trial of drainage after cholecystectomy: suction versus static drainage through a main wound versus a stab incision. Am J Surg 1981;141:289–294.
39. Verrier ED, Bossart KJ, Heer FW. Reduction of infection rates in abdominal incisions by delayed wound closure techniques. Am J Surg 1979;138:22–28.
40. Antimicrobial prophylaxis for surgery. Med Lett Drugs Ther 1983;25:113–116.
41. Conte JE, Jacob LS, Polk HC. Antibiotic prophylaxis in surgery. Philadelphia: JB Lippincott, 1984:296.
42. Gorbach SL, Bartlett JG, Nichols RL. Manual of surgical infections. Boston: Little, Brown and Co., 1984:405.

Guideline for Isolation Precautions in Hospitals

Original Citation: Centers for Disease Control and Prevention. Guideline for isolation precautions hospitals, 1994.

Original Author: Julia S. Garner, RN, MN.

PART I: EVOLUTION OF ISOLATION PRACTICES

INTRODUCTION

To assist hospitals in maintaining up-to-date isolation practices, the Centers for Disease Control and Prevention (CDC) and the Hospital Infection Control Practices Advisory Committee (HIC-PAC) have revised the "CDC Guideline for Isolation Precautions in Hospitals." HICPAC was established in 1991 to provide advice and guidance to the Secretary, Department of Health and Human Services (DHHS); the Assistant Secretary for Health, DHHS; the Director, CDC; and the Director, National Center for Infectious Diseases regarding the practice of hospital infection control and strategies for surveillance, prevention, and control of nosocomial infections in US hospitals. HICPAC also advises the CDC on periodic updating of guidelines and other policy statements regarding prevention of nosocomial infections.

The revised guideline contains two parts. Part I, "Evolution of Isolation Practices," reviews the evolution of isolation practices in US hospitals, including their advantages, disadvantages, and controversial aspects, and provides the background for the HICPAC-consensus recommendations contained in Part II, "Recommendations for Isolation Precautions in Hospitals." The guideline supersedes previous CDC recommendations for isolation precautions in hospitals (24).

The guideline recommendations are based on the latest epidemiologic information on transmission of infection in hospitals. The recommendations are intended primarily for use in the care of patients in acute-care hospitals, although some of the recommendations may be applicable for some patients receiving care in subacute care or extended care facilities. The recommendations are not intended/or use in day care, well care, or domiciliary care programs. Because there have been few studies to test the efficacy of isolation precautions and gaps still exist in the knowledge of the epidemiology and modes of transmission of some diseases, disagreement with some of the recommendations is expected. A working draft of the guideline was reviewed by experts in infection control and published in the Federal Register for public comment. However, all recommendations in the guideline may not reflect the opinions of all reviewers.

HICPAC recognizes that the goal of preventing transmission of infections in hospitals can be accomplished by multiple means and that hospitals will modify the recommendations according to their needs and circumstances and as directed by federal, state, or local regulations. Modification of the recommendations is encouraged if (a) the principles of epidemiology and disease transmission are maintained, and (b) precautions are included to interrupt spread of infection by all routes that are likely to be encountered in the hospital.

Summary

The "Guideline for Isolation Precautions in Hospitals" was revised to meet the following objectives: (a) to be epidemiologically sound; (b) to recognize the importance of all body fluids, secretions, and excretions in the transmission of nosocomial pathogens; (c) to contain adequate precautions for infections transmitted by the airborne, droplet, and contact routes of transmission; (d) to be as simple and user friendly as possible; and, (e) to use new terms to avoid confusion with existing infection control and isolation systems.

The revised guideline contains two tiers of precautions. In the first, and most important, tier are those precautions designed for the care of all patients in hospitals regardless of their diagnosis or presumed infection status. Implementation of these "Standard Precautions" is the primary strategy for successful nosocomial infection control. In the second tier are precautions designed only for the care of specified patients. These additional "Transmission-Based Precautions" are used for patients known or suspected to be infected or colonized with epidemiologically important pathogens that can be transmitted by airborne or droplet transmission or by contact with dry skin or contaminated surfaces.

Standard Precautions synthesize the major features of Universal (Blood and Body Fluid) Precautions (designed to reduce the risk of transmission of blood borne pathogens) and Body Substance Isolation (designed to reduce the risk of transmission of pathogens from moist body substances). Standard Precautions apply to (a) blood; (b) all body fluids, secretions, and excretions except sweat, regardless of whether or not they contain visible blood; (c) nonintact skin; and (d) mucous membranes. Standard Precautions are designed to reduce the risk of transmission of microorganisms from both recognized and unrecognized sources of infection in hospitals.

Transmission-Based Precautions are designed for patients documented or suspected to be infected or colonized with highly transmissible or epidemiologically important pathogens for which additional precautions beyond Standard Precautions are needed to interrupt transmission in hospitals. There are three types of Transmission-Based Precautions: Airborne Precautions, Droplet Precautions, and Contact Precautions. They may be combined for diseases that have multiple routes of transmission. When used either singularly or in combination, they are to be used in addition to Standard Precautions.

The revised guideline also lists specific clinical syndromes or conditions in both adult and pediatric patients that are highly suspicious for infection and identifies appropriate Transmission-Based Precautions to use on an empiric, temporary basis until a diagnosis can be made; these empiric, temporary precautions are also to be used in addition to Standard Precautions.

EARLY ISOLATION PRACTICES

The first published recommendations for isolation precautions in the United States appeared as early as 1877, when a hospital handbook recommended placing patients with infectious diseases in separate facilities (5) which ultimately became known as infectious disease hospitals. Although this practice segregated infected patients from noninfected patients, nosocomial transmission continued to occur because infected patients were not separated from each other according to their disease, and few, if any, aseptic procedures were practiced. Personnel in infectious disease hospitals began to combat problems of nosocomial transmission by setting aside a floor or ward for patients with similar diseases and by practicing aseptic procedures recommended in nursing textbooks published from 1890 to 1900 (5).

In 1910, isolation practices in US hospitals were altered by the introduction of the cubicle system of isolation, which placed patients in multiple-bed wards (6). With the cubicle system, hospital personnel used separate gowns, washed their hands with antiseptic solutions after patient contact, and disinfected objects contaminated by the patient These nursing procedures, designed to prevent transmission of pathogenic organisms to other patients and personnel, became known as "barrier nursing." Use of the cubicle system of isolation and barrier nursing procedures provided general hospitals with an alternative to placing some patients in infectious disease hospitals.

During the 1950s, US infectious disease hospitals, except those designated exclusively for tuberculosis, began to close. In the mid-1960s, tuberculosis hospitals also began to close, partly because general hospital or outpatient treatment became preferred for patients with tuberculosis. Thus, by the late 1960s, patients with infectious diseases were housed in wards in general hospitals, either in specially designed, single-patient isolation rooms or in regular single or multiple-patient rooms.

CDC ISOLATION SYSTEMS

CDC Isolation Manual

In 1970, CDC published a detailed manual entitled "Isolation Techniques for Use in Hospitals" to assist general hospitals with isolation precautions (2). A revised edition appeared in 1975. The manual could be applied in small community hospitals with limited resources, as well as in large, metropolitan, university associated medical centers.

The manual introduced the category system of isolation precautions. It recommended that hospitals use one of seven isolation categories (Strict Isolation, Respiratory Isolation, Protective Isolation, Enteric Precautions, Wound and Skin Precautions, Discharge Precautions, and Blood Precautions). The precautions recommended for each category were determined almost entirely by the epidemiologic feature's of the diseases grouped in the category, primarily their routes of transmission. Certain isolation techniques, believed to be the minimum necessary to prevent transmission of all diseases in the category, were indicated for each isolation category. Because all diseases in a category did not have the same epidemiology (i.e., were not spread by exactly the same combination of modes of transmission), with some requiring fewer precautions than others, more precautions were suggested for some diseases than were necessary. This disadvantage of "over isolation" for some diseases was offset by the convenience of having a small number of categories. More importantly, the simple system required personnel to learn only a few established routines for applying isolation precautions. To make the system even more user friendly, instructions for each category were printed on color-coded cards and placed on the door, beds, or charts of patients on isolation precautions.

By the mid-1970s, 93% of US hospitals had adopted the isolation system recommended in the manual. However, neither the efficacy of the category approach in preventing spread of infections nor the costs of using the system were evaluated by empirical studies.

By 1980, hospitals were experiencing new endemic and epidemic nosocomial infection problems, some caused by multidrug-resistant microorganisms and others caused by newly recognized pathogens, which required different isolation precautions from those specified by any existing isolation category. There was increasing need for isolation precautions to be directed more specifically at nosocomial transmission in special-care units, rather than the intra-hospital spread of infectious diseases acquired in the community (8). Infection control professionals and nursing directors in hospitals with particularly sophisticated nursing staffs increasingly were tiling for new isolation systems that would tailor precautions to the modes of transmission for each and avoid the over-isolation inherent in category-specific approach. Further, new facts the epidemiology and modes of transmission of some diseases made it necessary for CDC to revise isolation manual. Toward that end, during 1981 CDC Hospital

Infections Program personnel consulted with infectious disease specialists in medicine, pediatrics, and surgery; hospital epidemiologists; and infection control practitioners about the manual.

CDC Isolation Guideline

In 1983, the CDC Guideline for Isolation Precautions in Hospitals (4) (hereafter referred to as the isolation guideline) was published to take the place of the 1975 isolation manual; it contained many important changes. One of the most important was the increased emphasis on decision making on the part of users. Unlike the 1975 manual, which encouraged few decisions on the part of users, the isolation guideline encouraged decision making at several levels (9, 10). First, hospital infection control committees were given a choice of selecting between category-specific or disease-specific isolation precautions or using the guideline to develop a unique isolation system appropriate to their hospitals' circumstances and environments. Second, personnel who placed a patient on isolation precautions were encouraged to make decisions about the individual precautions to be taken (e.g. whether the patient's age, mental status, or condition indicated that a private room was needed to prevent sharing of contaminated articles). Third, personnel taking care of patients on isolation precautions were encouraged to decide whether they needed to wear a mask, gown, or gloves based on the likelihood of exposure to infective material. Such decisions were deemed necessary to isolate the infection, but not the patient, and to reduce the costs associated with unnecessary isolation precautions.

In the category-specific section of the guideline, existing categories were modified, new categories were added, and many infections were reassigned to different categories. The old category of Blood Precautions, primarily directed toward patients with chronic carriage of hepatitis B virus (HBV), was renamed Blood and Body Fluid Precautions and was expanded to include patients with AIDS and body fluids other than blood. The old category of Protective Isolation was deleted because of studies demonstrating its lack of efficacy in general clinical practice in preventing the acquisition of infection by the immunocompromised patient for whom it had been described originally (11, 12). The 1983 guideline contained the following categories of isolation: Strict Isolation, Contact Isolation, Respiratory Isolation, Tuberculosis (acid-fast bacilli [AFB]) Isolation, Enteric Precautions, Drainage/Secretion Precautions, and Blood and Body Fluid Precautions. As with the category approach in the former CDC isolation manuals, these categories tended to over-isolate some patients.

In the disease-specific section of the guideline, the epidemiology of each infectious disease was considered individually by advocating only those precautions (e.g., private room, mask, gown, and gloves) needed to interrupt transmission of the infection. In place of the categories and signs of the category specific approach, a chart listed all diseases posing the threat of in-hospital transmission, with checks in columns indicating which precautions were required for each. Because precautions were individualized for each disease, hospitals using the system were encouraged to provide more initial training and inservice education and to encourage a much higher level of attention from patient-care personnel. Although disease-specific isolation precautions eliminated over-isolation, personnel might be prone to mistakes in applying the precautions, particularly if the disease was not seen regularly in the hospital (9, 10), if there was a delay in diagnosis, or if there was a misdiagnosis. Placing disease-specific isolation precautions in a hospital computerized information system resulted in more accurate use of the system (13).

Because gaps existed in the knowledge of the epidemiology of some diseases, disagreement was expected, and occurred, regarding the placement of individual diseases within given categories, especially diseases with a respiratory component of transmission (14). Placing measles in Respiratory Isolation (designed to prevent transmission of large-particle droplets) rather than in a category that had provisions for preventing transmission by airborne droplet nuclei and placing rubella and respiratory syncytial virus (RSV) infection in Contact Isolation were controversial (15). There also was disagreement about the lack of a recommendation for adult patients with influenza, the need for private rooms for pediatric patients with RSV infections. and the length of time that precautions should be maintained (15). The lack of empiric studies on the efficacy and costs of implementing the recommendations contributed to the disagreements.

As new epidemiologic data became available, several subsequent CDC reports (16, 18) updated portions of the isolation guideline. Updated recommendations for management of patients with suspected hemorrhagic fever were published in 1988 (16). The recommendation for Respiratory Isolation for acute erythema infectiosum was superseded by a 1989 report that recommended Respiratory Isolation for human parvovirus B19 (the causative agent for erythema infectiosum) only when infected patients were in transient aplastic crisis or had immunodeficiency and chronic human parvovirus B19 infection (17).

Recommendations for Tuberculosis (AFB) Isolation were updated in 1990 (18) because of heightened concern about nosocomial transmission of multidrug-resistant tuberculosis (19, 20) particularly in settings where persons with human immunodeficiency virus (HIV) infection were receiving care. The 1990 tuberculosis guidelines emphasized (a) placing a hospital patient with confirmed or suspected tuberculosis in a private room that has lower, or negative, air pressure compared with surrounding areas; (b) reducing mycobacterial contamination of air by dilution and removal of airborne contaminants; and (c) wearing particulate respirators, rather than standard surgical masks, when hospital personnel shared air space with an infectious tuberculosis patient Subsequent recommendations reemphasized the importance of early diagnosis and treatment of tuberculosis (21). In 1993, a second edition of the guidelines for preventing the transmission of tuberculosis in health care facilities was published in draft for public comment (22). After review of written comments, the guidelines were modified and published (23).

UNIVERSAL PRECAUTIONS

In 1985, largely because of the HIV epidemic, isolation practices in the United States were altered dramatically by the introduction of a new strategy for isolation precautions, which became known as Universal Precautions (UP). Following the initial reports of hospital personnel becoming infected with HIV through needle sticks and skin contamination with patients' blood, a widespread outcry created the urgent need for new isolation strategies to protect hospital personnel from blood borne infections. The subsequent modification of isolation precautions in some hospitals produced several major strategic changes and sacrificed some measures of protection against patient-to-patient transmission in the process of adding protection against patient-to-personnel transmission. In acknowledgment of the fact that many patients with blood borne infections are not recognized, the new UP approach for the first time placed emphasis on applying Blood and Body Fluid Precautions universally to all persons regardless of their presumed infection status (24). Until this time, most patients placed on isolation precautions were those for whom a diagnosis of an infectious disease had been made or was suspected. This provision led to the new name of Universal Precautions.

In addition to emphasizing prevention of needle stick injuries and the use of traditional barriers such as gloves and gowns, UP expanded Blood and Body Fluid Precautions to include use of masks and eye coverings to prevent mucous membrane exposures during certain procedures and the use of individual ventilation devices when the need for resuscitation was predictable. This approach, and particularly the techniques for preventing mucous membrane exposures, was reemphasized in subsequent CDC reports that contained recommendations for prevention of HIV transmission in health care settings (25–28).

In 1987, one of these reports (27) stated that implementation of UP for all patients eliminated the need for the isolation category of Blood and Body Precautions for patients known or suspected to be infected with blood borne pathogens; however, the report stated that other category- or disease-specific isolation precautions recommended in the CDC isolation guideline (4) should be used as necessary if infections other than blood borne infections were or suspected.

The 1987 report was updated by a 1988 report that emphasized two important points: (a) blood was the single most important source of HIV, HBV, and other blood borne pathogens in the occupational setting, and (b) infection control efforts for preventing transmission of blood borne pathogens in health care settings must focus on preventing exposures blood, as well as on delivery of HBV immunization. The report stated that UP applied to blood, to body fluids that had been implicated in the transmission of blood borne infections (semen and vaginal secretion, to body fluids from which the risk of transmission of unknown (amniotic, cerebrospinal, pericardial toneal, pleural, and synovial fluids), and to any other body fluid visibly contaminated with blood, but not to feces, nasal secretions, sputum, sweat, tears, urine, or vomitus unless they contained visible blood. Although HIV and HBV surface antigen (HBsAg had been found in some of the fluids, secretions, and excretions to which UP did not apply, epidemiologic studies in the health care and community settings had not implicated these substances in the transmission of HIV and HBV infections. However, the report noted that some of the fluids, secretions, and excretions not covered under UP represented a potential source for nosocomial and community-acquired infections with other pathogens and referred reader to the CDC isolation guideline.

BODY SUBSTANCE ISOLATION

In 1987, a new system of isolation, called Body Substance Isolation (BSI), was proposed after 3 years of study by infection control personnel at the Harborview Medical Center in Seattle, Washington. and the University of California at San Diego, California, as an alternative to diagnosis-driven isolation systems (29). BSI focused on the isolation of all moist and potentially infectious body substances (blood, feces, urine, sputum, saliva, wound drainage, and other body fluids) from all patients, regardless of their presumed infection status, primarily through the use of gloves. Personnel were instructed to put on clean gloves just before contact with mucous membranes and nonintact skin, and to wear gloves for anticipated contact with moist body substances in addition, a "Stop Sign Alert" was used to instruct persons wishing to enter the room of some patients with infections transmitted exclusively, or in part, by the airborne route to check with the floor nurse, who would determine whether a mask should be worn. Personnel were to be immune to or immunized against selected infectious diseases transmitted by airborne or droplet routes (measles, mumps, rubella, varicella), or they were not to enter the rooms housing patients with these diseases. Other issues related to implementing BSI in a university teaching hospital were described (30).

Among the advantages cited for BSI were that it was a simple, easy to learn and administer system, that it avoided the assumption that individuals with our known or suspected diagnoses of transmissible infectious diseases were free of risk to patients and personnel, and that only certain body fluids were associated with transmission of infections. The disadvantages of BSI included the added cost of increased use of barrier equipment, particularly gloves (31); the difficulty in maintaining routine application of the protocol for all patients; the uncertainty about the precautions to be taken when entering a room with a "Stop Sign Alert"; and the potential for misapplication of the protocol to overprotect personnel at the expense of the patient (32).

In a prospective study (33) a combination use of gown and glove protocols similar to BSI led to lower infection rates in a pediatric intensive care unit (ICU), and, in other studies, similar combinations of barriers were associated with lower rates of nosocomial RSV infection in a pediatric ICU (34) and of resistant gram-negative organisms in an acute-care hospital (35). However, in none of these studies, initiated before publication of BSI, were the authors attempting to evaluate BSI, nor were they able to separate the effect of gloves from that of gowns or from gloves and gowns used in combination.

Controversial aspects of BSI have been summarized (35, 36). BSI appeared to replace some, but not all, of the isolation precautions necessary to prevent transmission of infection. BSI did not contain adequate provisions to prevent (a) droplet transmission of serious in pediatric populations (e.g., invasive Hemophilus influenza, Neisseria meningitides meningitis and pneumonia and pertussis); (b) direct or indirect contact transmission of epidemiologically important microorganisms from dry skin or environmental sources (e.g.. Clostridium difficile and vancomycin-resistant enterococci); or (c) true airborne transmission of infections transmitted over long distances by floating droplet nuclei. Although BSI emphasized that a private room was indicated for some patients with some diseases transmitted exclusively, or in part by the true airborne route, it did not emphasize the need for special ventilation for patients known or suspected of having pulmonary tuberculosis or other diseases transmitted by airborne droplet nuclei. The lack of emphasis on special ventilation was of particular concern to CDC in the early 1990s because of multidrug-resistant tuberculosis (18, 19).

BSI and UP shared many similar features designed to prevent the transmission of blood borne pathogens in hospitals. However, there was an important difference in the recommendation for glove use and handwashing. Under UP, gloves were recommended for anticipated contact with blood and specified body fluids, and hands were to be washed immediately after gloves were removed (27, 28). Under BSI, gloves were recommended for anticipated contact with any moist body substance, but hand washing after glove removal was not required unless the hands visibly were soiled (29). The lack of emphasis on hand washing after glove removal was cited as one of the theoretical disadvantages of BSI (15, 37, 38). Using gloves as a protective substitute for hand washing may have provided a false sense of security, resulted in less hand washing, increased the risk of nosocomial transmission of pathogens, because hands can become contaminated even when gloves are used (39) and are contaminated easily in the process of removing gloves, and contributed to skin problems and allergies associated with the use of gloves (40, 41). On the other hand, proponents of BSI have noted that studies of hand washing have indicated that there is relatively low compliance by hospital personnel (42, 43), that glove use may have been easier to manage than hand washing, and that frequent hand washing may have led to eczema, skin cracking, or, in some persons, clinical damage to the skin of the hands (44). Although use of gloves may have been better than no hand washing, the efficacy of using gloves as a substitute for hand washing has not been demonstrated.

OSHA BLOOD BORNE PATHOGENS REGULATIONS

In 1989, the Occupational Safety and Health Administration (OSHA) published a proposed rule regarding occupational exposure to blood borne pathogens in hospitals and other health care settings (45). The proposed rule, based on the concept of UP, raised concerns in the infection control community. Among them were concerns about the use of "visibly bloody" as a marker for the infectious risk of certain body fluids and substances, the imbalance toward precautions to protect personnel and away from protection for patients, the lack of proven efficacy of UP and the costs for implementing the proposed regulations (46–50). After a series of OSHA public hearings and the review of written comments, the proposed rule was modified, and the final rule on occupational exposure to blood borne pathogens was published in 1991 (51). Although the final rule was expected to improve occupational safety in the care of patients infected with blood borne pathogens, its impact on the cost of patient care and on nosocomial infection control has remained undefined. Information on complying with the OSHA final rule has been made available by the American Hospital Association (52) and others (53).

THE NEED FOR A NEW ISOLATION GUIDELINE

By the early 1990s, isolation had become an infection control conundrum (54). Although many hospitals had incorporated all or portions of UP into their category- or disease-specific isolation system and others had adopted all or portions of BSI (55, 56), there was much local variation in the interpretation and use of UP and BSI, and a variety of combinations was common. Further, there was considerable confusion about which body fluids or substances required precautions under UP and BSI. Many hospitals espousing UP really were using BSI and vice versa. Moreover, there was continued lack of agreement about the importance of hand washing when gloves were used (14, 15, 27–29, 37, 38, 57, 58) and the need for additional precautions beyond BSI to prevent airborne, droplet, and contact transmission (14, 15, 27–29, 31, 36, 59, 60). Some hospitals had not implemented appropriate guidelines for preventing transmission of tuberculosis, including multidrug-resistant tuberculosis (61). As other multidrug-resistant microorganisms (62, 63) were emerging, some hospitals failed to recognize them as new problems and to add appropriate precautions that would contain them.

In view of these problems and concerns, no simple adjustment to any of the existing approaches—UP, BSI, the CDC isolation guideline, or other isolation systems—appeared likely to solve the conundrum. Clearly what was needed was a new synthesis of the various systems that would provide a guideline with logistically feasible recommendations for preventing the many infections that occur in hospitals through diverse modes of transmission. To achieve this, the new guideline would (a) have to be epidemiologically sound; (b) have to recognize the importance of all body fluids, secretions, and excretions in the transmission of nosocomial pathogens; (c) have to contain adequate precautions for infections transmitted by the airborne, droplet, and contact routes of transmission; (d) have to be as simple and user friendly as possible; and (e) have to use new terms to avoid confusion with existing systems.

Based on these considerations, this guideline subsequently was developed. It contains three important changes from previous recommendations. First, it synthesizes the major features of UP (27, 28) and BSI (29, 30) into a single set of precautions to be used for the care of all patients in hospitals regardless of their presumed infection status. These precautions, called Standard Precautions, are designed to reduce the risk of transmission of blood borne and other pathogens in hospitals. As a result of this synthesis, a large number of patients with diseases or conditions that previously required category- or disease-specific precautions in the 1983 CDC isolation guideline (4) now are covered under Standard Precautions and do not require additional precautions. Second, it collapses the old categories of isolation precautions (Strict Isolation, Contact Isolation, Respiratory Isolation, Tuberculosis Isolation, Enteric Precautions, and Drainage/Secretion Precautions) and the old disease specific precautions into three sets of precautions based on routes of transmission for a smaller number of specified patients known or suspected to be infected or colonized with highly transmissible or epidemiologically important pathogens. These Transmission-Based Precautions, designed to reduce the risk of airborne, droplet, and contact transmission in hospitals, are to be used in addition to Standard Precautions. Third, it lists specific syndromes in both adult and pediatric patients that are highly suspicious for infection and identifies appropriate Transmission-Based Precautions to use on an empiric, temporary basis until a diagnosis can be made. These empiric, temporary precautions also are designed to be used in addition to Standard Precautions. The details of the guideline recommendations are presented in Part II, "Recommendations for Isolation Precautions in Hospitals."

In summary, this new guideline is another step in the evolution of isolation practices in US hospitals. It now is recommended for review and use by hospitals with the following provision. No guideline can address all of the needs of the more than 6,000 US hospitals, which range in size from five beds to more than 1,500 beds and serve very different patient populations. Hospitals are encouraged to review the recommendations and to modify them according to what is possible, practical, and prudent.

PART II: RECOMMENDATIONS FOR ISOLATION PRECAUTIONS IN HOSPITALS

RATIONALE FOR ISOLATION PRECAUTIONS IN HOSPITALS

Transmission of infection within a hospital requires three elements: a source of infecting microorganisms, a susceptible host, and a means of transmission for the microorganism.

Source

Human sources of the infecting microorganisms in hospitals may be patients, personnel, or, on occasion, visitors, and may include persons with acute disease, persons in the incubation period of a disease, persons who are colonized by an infectious agent but have no apparent disease, or persons who are chronic carriers of an infectious agent. Other sources of infecting microorganisms can be the patients own endogenous flora, which may be difficult to control, and inanimate environmental objects that have become contaminated, including equipment and medications.

Host

Resistance among persons to pathogenic microorganisms varies greatly. Some persons may be immune to infection or may be able to resist colonization by an infectious agent; others exposed to the same agent may establish a commensal relationship with the infecting microorganism and become asymptomatic carriers; still others may develop clinical disease. Host factors such as age; underlying diseases; certain treatments with antimicrobials, corticosteroids, or other immunosuppressive agents; irradiation; and breaks in the first line of defense mechanisms caused by such factors as surgical operations, anesthesia, and indwelling catheters may render patients more susceptible to infection.

Transmission

Microorganisms are transmitted in hospitals by several routes, and the same microorganism may be transmitted by more than one route. There are five main routes of transmission—contact, droplet, airborne, common vehicle, and vector borne. For the purpose of this guideline, common vehicle and vector borne transmission will be discussed only briefly, because neither play a significant role in typical nosocomial infections.

1. Contact transmission, the most important and frequent mode of transmission of nosocomial infections, is divided into two subgroups: direct-contact transmission and indirect-contact transmission.
   a. Direct-contact transmission involves a direct body surface-to-body surface contact and physical transfer of microorganisms between a susceptible host and an infected or colonized person, such as occurs when a person turns a patient, gives a patient a bath, or performs other patient-care activities that require direct personal contact. Direct-contact transmission also can occur between two patients, with one serving as the source of the infectious microorganisms and the other as a susceptible host.
   b. Indirect-contact transmission involves contact of a susceptible host with a contaminated intermediate object, usually inanimate, such as contaminated instruments, needles, or dressings, or contaminated hands that are not washed and gloves that are not changed between patients.
2. Droplet transmission, theoretically, is a form of contact transmission. However, the mechanism of transfer of the pathogen to the host is quite distinct from either direct- or indirect-contact transmission. Therefore, droplet transmission will be considered a separate route of transmission in this guideline. Droplets are generated from the source person primarily during coughing, sneezing, and talking, and during the performance of certain procedures such as suctioning and bronchoscopy. Transmission occurs when droplets containing microorganisms generated from the infected person are propelled a short distance through the air and deposited on the host's conjunctivae, nasal mucosa, or mouth. Because droplets do not remain suspended in the air, special air handling and ventilation are not required to prevent droplet transmission; that is, droplet transmission must not be confused with airborne transmission.
3. Airborne Transmission occurs by dissemination of either airborne droplet nuclei (small-particle residue [5 μm or smaller in size] of evaporated droplets containing microorganisms that remain suspended in the air for long periods of time) or dust particles containing the infectious agent. Microorganisms carried in this manner can be dispersed widely by air currents and may become inhaled by a susceptible host within the same room or over a longer distance from the source patient, depending on environmental factors; therefore, special air handling and ventilation are required to prevent airborne transmission. Microorganisms transmitted by airborne transmission include Mycobacterium tuberculosis and the rubeola and varicella viruses.
4. Common Vehicle Transmission applies to microorganisms transmitted by contaminated items such as food, water, medications, devices, and equipment.
5. Vector Borne Transmission occurs when vectors such as mosquitoes, flies, rats, and other vermin transmit microorganisms; this route of transmission is of less significance in hospitals in the United States than in other regions of the world.

Isolation precautions are designed to prevent transmission of microorganisms by these routes in hospitals. Because agent and host factors are more difficult to control, interruption of transfer of microorganisms is directed primarily at transmission. The recommendations presented in this guideline are based on this concept.

Placing a patient on isolation precautions, however, often presents certain disadvantages to the hospital, patients, personnel, and visitors. Isolation precautions may require specialized equipment and environmental modifications that add to the cost of hospitalization. Isolation precautions may make frequent visits by nurses, physicians, and other personnel inconvenient, and they may make it more difficult for personnel to give the prompt and frequent care that sometimes is required. The use of a multi-patient room for one patient uses valuable space that otherwise might accommodate several patients. Moreover, forced solitude deprives the patient of normal social relationships and may be psychologically harmful, especially to children. These disadvantages, however, must be weighed against the hospital's mission to prevent the spread of serious and epidemiologically important microorganisms in the hospital.

FUNDAMENTALS OF ISOLATION PRECAUTIONS

A variety of infection control measures are used for decreasing the risk of transmission of microorganisms in hospitals. These measures make up the fundamentals of isolation precautions.

Hand Washing and Gloving

Hand washing frequently is called the single most important measure to reduce the risks of transmitting microorganisms from one person to another or from one site to another on the same patient. The scientific rationale, indications, methods, and products for hand washing have been delineated in other publications (64–72).

Washing hands as promptly and thoroughly as possible between patient contacts and after contact with blood, body fluids, secretions, excretions, and equipment or articles contaminated by them is an important component of infection control and isolation precautions. In addition to hand washing, gloves play an important role in reducing the risks of transmission of microorganisms.

Gloves are worn for three important reasons in hospitals. First, gloves are worn to provide a protective barrier and to prevent gross contamination of the hands when touching blood, body fluids, secretions, excretions, mucous membranes, and nonintact skin (27–29); the wearing of gloves in specified circumstances to reduce the risk of exposures to blood borne pathogens is mandated by the OSHA Blood Borne Pathogens final rule (51). Second, gloves are worn to reduce the likelihood that microorganisms present on the hands of personnel will be transmitted to patients during invasive or other patient-care procedures that involve touching a patient's mucous membranes and nonintact skin. Third, gloves are worn to reduce the likelihood that hands of personnel contaminated with microorganisms from a patient or a fomite can transmit these microorganisms to another patient. In this situation, gloves must be changed between patient contacts and hands should be washed after gloves are removed.

Wearing gloves does not replace the need for hand washing, because gloves may have small, apparent defects or may be torn during use, and hands can become contaminated during removal of gloves (14, 15, 39, 72–76). Failure to change gloves between patient contacts is an infection control hazard (32).

Patient Placement

Appropriate patient placement is a significant component of isolation precautions. A private room is important to prevent direct- or indirect-contact transmission when the source patient has poor hygienic habits, contaminates the environment, or cannot be expected to assist in maintaining infection control precautions to limit transmission of microorganisms (i.e., infants, children, and patients with altered mental status). When possible, a patient with highly transmissible or epidemiologically important microorganisms is placed in a private room with hand washing and toilet facilities, to reduce opportunities for transmission of microorganisms.

When a private room is not available, an infected patient is placed with an appropriate roommate. Patients infected by the same microorganism usually can share a room, provided they are not infected with other potentially transmissible microorganisms and the likelihood of reinfection with the same organism is minimal. Such sharing of rooms, also referred to as cohorting patients, is useful especially during outbreaks or when there is a shortage of private rooms. When a private room is not available and cohorting is not achievable or recommended (23), it is very important to consider the epidemiology and mode of transmission of the infecting pathogen and the patient population being served in determining patient placement. Under these circumstances, consultation with infection control professionals is advised before patient placement. Moreover, when an infected patient shares a room with a noninfected patient, it also is important that patients, personnel, and visitors take precautions to prevent the spread of infection and that roommates are selected carefully.

Guidelines for construction, equipment, air handling, and ventilation for isolation rooms have been delineated in other publications (77–79). A private room with appropriate air handling and ventilation is particularly important for reducing the risk of transmission of microorganisms from a source patient to susceptible patients and other persons in hospitals when the microorganism is spread by airborne transmission. Some hospitals use an isolation room with an anteroom as an extra measure of precaution to prevent airborne transmission. Adequate data regarding the need for an anteroom, however, is not available. Ventilation recommendations for isolation rooms housing patients with pulmonary tuberculosis have been delineated in other CDC guidelines (23).

Transport of Infected Patients

Limiting the movement and transport of patients infected with virulent or epidemiologically important microorganisms and ensuring that such patients leave their rooms only for essential purposes reduces opportunities for transmission of microorganisms in hospitals. When patient transport is necessary, it is important that (a) appropriate barriers (e.g., masks, impervious dressings) are worn or used by the patient to reduce the opportunity for transmission of pertinent microorganisms to other patients, personnel, and visitors and to reduce contamination of the environment; (b) personnel in the area to which the patient is to be taken are notified of the impending arrival of the patient and of the precautions to be used to reduce the risk of transmission of infectious microorganisms; and (c) patients are informed of ways by which they can assist in preventing the transmission of their infectious microorganisms to others.

Masks, Respiratory Protection, Eye Protection, Face Shields

Various types of masks, goggles, and face shields are worn alone or in combination to provide barrier protection. A mask that covers both the nose and the mouth, and goggles or a face shield are worn by hospital personnel during procedures and patient care activities that are likely to generate splashes or sprays of blood, body fluids, secretions, or excretions to provide protection of the mucous membranes of the eyes, nose, and mouth from contact transmission of pathogens. The wearing of masks, eye protection, and face shields in specified circumstances to reduce the risk of exposures to blood borne pathogens is mandated by the OSHA Blood Borne Pathogens final rule (51). A surgical mask generally is worn by hospital personnel to provide protection against spread of infectious large-particle droplets that are transmitted by close contact and generally travel only short distances (up to 3 ft) from infected patients who are coughing or sneezing.

An area of major concern and controversy over the last several years has been the role and selection of respiratory protection equipment and the implications of a respiratory protection program for prevention of transmission of tuberculosis in hospitals. Traditionally, although the efficacy was not proven, a surgical mask was worn for isolation precautions in hospitals when patients were known or suspected to be infected with pathogens spread by the airborne route of transmission. In 1990, however, the CDC tuberculosis guidelines (18) stated that surgical masks may not be effective in preventing the inhalation of droplet nuclei and recommended the use of disposable particulate respirators, despite the fact that the efficacy of particulate respirators in protecting persons from the inhalation of M tuberculosis had not been demonstrated. By definition, particulate respirators included dust-mist (DM), dust-fume-mist (DFM), or high-efficiency particulate air (HEPA) filter respirators certified by the CDC National Institute for Occupational Safety and Health (NIOSH); because the generic term "particulate respirator" was used in the 1990 guidelines, the implication was that any of these respirators provided sufficient protection (80).

In 1993, a draft revision of the CDC tuberculosis guidelines (22) outlined performance criteria for respirators and stated that some DM or DFM respirators might not meet these criteria. After review of public comments, the guidelines were finalized in October 1994 (23), with the draft respirator criteria unchanged. At that time, the only class of respirators that were known to consistently meet or exceed the performance criteria outlined in the 1994 tuberculosis guidelines and that were certified by NIOSH (as required by OSHA) were HEPA filter respirators. Subsequently, NIOSH revised the testing and certification requirements for all types of air-purifying respirators, including those used for tuberculosis control (81). The new rule, effective in July 1995, provides a broader range of certified respirators that meet the performance criteria recommended by CDC in the 1994 tuberculosis guidelines. NIOSH has indicated that the N95 (N category at 95% efficiency) meets the CDC performance criteria for a tuberculosis respirator. The new respirators are likely to be available in late 1995. Additional information on the evolution of respirator recommendations, regulations to protect hospital personnel, and the role of various federal agencies in respiratory protection for hospital personnel has been published (80).

Gowns and Protective Apparel

Various types of gowns and protective apparel are worn to provide barrier protection and to reduce opportunities for transmission of microorganisms in hospitals. Gowns are worn to prevent contamination of clothing and to protect the skin of personnel from blood and body fluid exposures. Gowns especially treated to make them impermeable to liquids, leg coverings, boots, or shoe covers provide greater protection to the skin when splashes or large quantities of infective material are present or anticipated. The wearing of gowns and protective apparel under specified circumstances to reduce the risk of exposures to blood borne pathogens, is mandated by the OSHA Blood Borne Pathogens final rule (51).

Gowns also are worn by personnel during the care of patients infected with epidemiologically important microorganisms to reduce the opportunity for transmission of pathogens from patients or items in their environment to other patients' environments; when gowns are worn for this purpose, they are removed before leaving the patient's environment, and hands are washed. Adequate data regarding the efficacy of gowns for this purpose, however, is not available.

Patient-Care Equipment and Articles

Many factors determine whether special handling and disposal of used patient-care equipment and articles are prudent or required, including the likelihood of contamination with infective material; the ability to cut, stick, or otherwise cause injury (needles, scalpels, and other sharp instruments [sharps]); the severity of the associated disease; and the environmental stability of the pathogens involved (27, 51, 82–84). Some used articles are enclosed in containers or bags to prevent inadvertent exposures to patients, personnel, and visitors and to prevent contamination of the environment. Used sharps are placed in puncture-resistant containers; other articles are placed in a bag. One bag is adequate if the bag is sturdy and the article can be placed in the bag without contaminating the outside of the bag (85); otherwise, two bags are used.

The scientific rationale, indications, methods, products, and equipment for reprocessing patient-care equipment have been delineated in other publications (68, 84–86, 91). Contaminated, reusable critical medical devices or patient-care equipment (i.e., equipment that enters normally sterile tissue or through which blood flows) or semicritical medical devices or patient-care equipment (i.e., equipment that touches mucous membranes) are sterilized or disinfected (reprocessed) after use to reduce the risk of transmission of microorganisms to other patients; the type of reprocessing is determined by the article and its intended use, the manufacturer's recommendations, hospital policy, and any applicable guidelines and regulations.

Noncritical equipment (i.e., equipment that touches intact skin) contaminated with blood, body fluids, secretions, or excretions is cleaned and disinfected after use, according to hospital policy. Contaminated disposable (single-use) patient-care equipment is handled and transported in a manner that reduces the risk of transmission of microorganisms and decreases environmental contamination in the hospital; the equipment is disposed of according to hospital policy and applicable regulations.

Linen and Laundry

Although soiled linen may be contaminated with pathogenic microorganisms, the risk of disease transmission is negligible if it is handled, transported, and laundered in a manner that avoids transfer of microorganisms to patients, personnel, and environments. Rather than rigid rules and regulations, hygienic and common sense storage and processing of clean and soiled linen are recommended (27, 83, 92, 93). The methods for handling, transporting, and laundering of soiled linen are determined by hospital policy and any applicable regulations.

Dishes, Glasses, Cups, and Eating Utensils

No special precautions are needed for dishes, glasses, cups, or eating utensils. Either disposable or reusable dishes and utensils can be used for patients on isolation precautions. The combination of hot water and detergents used in hospital dishwashers is sufficient to decontaminate dishes, glasses, cups, and eating utensils.

Routine and Terminal Cleaning

The room, or cubicle, and bedside equipment of patients on Transmission-Based Precautions are cleaned using the same procedures used for patients on Standard Precautions, unless the infecting microorganism(s) and the amount of environmental contamination indicate special cleaning. In addition to thorough cleaning, adequate disinfection of bedside equipment and environmental surfaces (e.g., bed rails, bedside tables, carts, commodes, doorknobs, faucet handles) is indicated for certain pathogens, especially enterococci, which can survive in the inanimate environment for prolonged periods of time (94). Patients admitted to hospital rooms that previously were occupied by patients infected or colonized with such pathogens are at increased risk of infection from contaminated environmental surfaces and bedside equipment if they have not been cleaned and disinfected adequately. The methods, thoroughness, and frequency of cleaning and the products used are determined by hospital policy.

HICPAC ISOLATION PRECAUTIONS

There are two fibers of HICPAC isolation precautions. In the first, and most important, tier are those precautions designed for the care of all patients in hospitals, regardless of their diagnosis or presumed infection status. Implementation of these "Standard Precautions" is the primary strategy for successful nosocomial infection control. In the second tier, are precautions designed only for the care of specified patients. These additional "Transmission-Based Precautions" are for patients known or suspected to be infected by epidemiologically important pathogens spread by airborne or droplet transmission or by contact with dry skin or contaminated surfaces.

STANDARD PRECAUTIONS

Standard Precautions synthesize the major features of UP (Blood and Body Fluid Precautions) (27, 28) (designed to reduce the risk of transmission of blood borne pathogens) and BSI (29, 30) (designed to reduce the risk of transmission of pathogens from moist body substances) and applies them to all patients receiving care in hospitals, regardless of their diagnosis or presumed infection status. Standard Precautions apply to (a) blood; (b) all body fluids, secretions, and excretions except sweat, regardless of whether or not they contain visible blood; (c) nonintact skin; and, (d) mucous membranes. Standard Precautions are designed to reduce the risk of transmission of microorganisms from both recognized and unrecognized sources of infection in hospitals.

Transmission-Based Precautions

Transmission-Based Precautions are designed for patients documented or suspected to be infected with highly transmissible or epidemiologically important pathogens for which additional precautions beyond Standard Precautions are needed to interrupt transmission in hospitals. There are three types of Transmission-Based Precautions: Airborne Precautions, Droplet Precautions, and Contact Precautions. They may be combined for diseases that have multiple routes of transmission. When used either singularly or in combination, they are to be used in addition to Standard Precautions.

Airborne Precautions are designed to reduce the risk of airborne transmission of infectious agents. Airborne transmission occurs by dissemination of either airborne droplet nuclei (small-particle residue [5 µm or smaller in size] of evaporated droplets that may remain suspended in the air for long periods of time) or dust particles containing the infectious agent. Microorganisms carried in this manner can be dispersed widely by air currents and may become inhaled by or deposited on a susceptible host within the same room or over a longer distance from the source patient, depending on environmental factors; therefore, special air handling and ventilation are required to prevent airborne transmission. Airborne Precautions apply to patients known or suspected to be infected with epidemiologically important pathogens that can be transmitted by the airborne route.

Droplet Precautions are designed to reduce the risk of droplet transmission of infectious agents. Droplet transmission involves contact of the conjunctivae or the mucous membranes of the nose or mouth of a susceptible person with large-particle droplets (larger than 5 μm in size) containing microorganisms generated from a person who has a clinical disease or who is a carrier of the microorganism. Droplets are generated from the source person primarily during coughing, sneezing, or talking and during the performance of certain procedures such as suctioning and bronchoscopy. Transmission via large-particle droplets requires close contact between source and recipient persons, because droplets do not remain suspended in the air and generally travel only short distances, usually 3 ft or less, through the air. Because droplets do not remain suspended in the air, special air handling and ventilation are not required to prevent droplet transmission. Droplet Precautions apply to any patient known or suspected to be infected with epidemiologically important pathogens that can be transmitted by infectious droplets.

Contact Precautions are designed to reduce the risk of transmission of epidemiologically important microorganisms by direct or indirect contact. Direct-contact transmission involves skin-to-skin contact and physical transfer of microorganisms to a susceptible host from an infected or colonized person, such as occurs when personnel turn patients, bathe patients, or perform other patient-care activities that require physical contact. Direct-contact transmission also can occur between two patients (e.g., by hand contact), with one serving as the source of infectious microorganisms and the other as a susceptible host. Indirect-contact transmission involves contact of a susceptible host with a contaminated intermediate object, usually inanimate, in the patient's environment. Contact Precautions apply to specified patients known or suspected to be infected or colonized (presence of microorganism in or on patient but without clinical signs and symptoms of infection) with epidemiologically important microorganisms that can be transmitted by direct or indirect contact.

A synopsis of the types of precautions and the patients requiring the precautions is listed in Table 1.

Table 1. Synopsis of types of precautions and patients requiring the precautions*

Standard Precautions
  Use Standard Precautions for the care of all patients
Airborne Precautions
  In addition to Standard Precautions, use Airborne Precautions for patients known or suspected to have serious illness transmitted by airborne droplet nuclei. Examples of such illnesses include:
    Measles
    Varicella (including disseminated zoster) [+]
    Tuberculosis [++]
Droplet Precautions
  In addition to Standard Precautions, use Droplet Precautions for patients known or suspected to have serious illnesses transmitted by large particle droplets. Examples of such illnesses include:
    Invasive Haemophilus influenzae type b disease, including meningitis, pneumonia, epiglottitis, and sepsis
    Invasive Neisseria meningitidis disease, including meningitis, pneumonia, and sepsis
    Other serious bacterial respiratory infections spread by droplet transmission, including:
      Diphtheria (pharyngeal)
      Mycoplasma pneumonia
      Pertussis
      Pneumonic plague
      Streptococcal pharyngitis, pneumonia, or scarlet fever in infants and young children
    Serious viral infections spread by droplet transmission, including:
      Adenovirus [+]
      Influenza
      Mumps
      Parvovirus B19
      Rubella

Table 1.—continued

Contact Precautions

In addition to Standard Precautions, use Contact Precautions for patients known or suspected to have serious illnesses easily transmitted by direct patient contact or by contact with items in the patient's environment. Examples of such illnesses include:

Gastrointestinal, respiratory, skin, or wound infections or colonization with multidrug-resistant bacteria judged by the infection control program, based on current state, regional, or national recommendations, to be of special clinical and epidemiologic significance

Enteric infections with a low infectious dose or prolonged environmental survival, including:

Clostridium difficile

For diapered or incontinent patients: enterohemorrhagic Escherichia coil O157:H7, Shigella, hepatitis A, or rotavirus

Respiratory syncyfial virus, parainfluenza virus, or enteroviral infections in infants and young children

Skin infections that are highly contagious or that may occur on dry skin, including:

Diphtheria (cutaneous)

Herpes simples virus (neonatal or mucocutaneous)

Impetigo

Major (noncontained) abscesses, cellulitis, or decubiti

Pediculosis

Scabies

Staphylococcal furunculosis in infants and young children

Zoster (disseminated or in the immunocompromised host) [+]

Viral/hemorrhagic conjunctiivitis

Viral hemorrhagic infections (Ebola, Lassa, or Marburg) [*]

---

*See Appendix A for a complete listing of infections requiring precautions, including appropriate footnotes.

[+]Certain infections require more than one type of precaution.

[++]See CDC "Guidelines for Preventing the Transmission of Tuberculosis in Health-Care Facilities" (23).

EMPIRIC USE OF AIRBORNE, DROPLET, OR CONTACT PRECAUTIONS

In many instances, the risk of nosocomial transmission of infection may. be highest before a definitive diagnosis can be made and before precautions based on that diagnosis can be implemented. The routine use of Standard Precautions for all patients should reduce greatly this risk for conditions other than those requiring Airborne, Droplet, or Contact Precautions. While it is not possible to prospectively identify all patients needing these enhanced precautions, certain clinical syndromes and conditions carry a sufficiently high risk to warrant the empiric addition of enhanced precautions while a more definitive diagnosis is pursued. A listing of such conditions and the recommended precautions beyond Standard Precautions is presented in Table 2.

Table 2. Clinical syndromes or conditions warranting additional empiric precautions to prevent transmission of epidemiologically important pathogens pending confirmation of diagnosis*

Clinical Syndrome or Condition*	Potential Pathogens[++]	Empiric Precautions
Diarrhea		
Acute diarrhea with a likely infectious cause in an incontinent or diapered patient	Enteric Pathogens[&]	Contact
Diarrhea in an adult with a history of recent antibiotic use	Clotridium difficile	Contact
Meningitis	Neisseria meningitidis	Droplet
Rash or exanthems, generalized, etiology unknown		
Petechial/ecchymotic with fever	Neisseria meningitidis	Droplet
Vesicular	Varicella	Airborne/Contact
Maculopapular with coryza and fever	Rubeola (measles)	Airborne
Respiratory infections		
Cough/fever/upper lobe pulmonary infiltrate in an HIV-negative patient or a patient at low risk for HIV infection	Mycobacterium tuberculosis	Airborne

Table 2.—continued

Clinical Syndrome or Condition*	Potential Pathogens[++]	Empiric Precautions
Cough/fever/pulmonary infiltrate in any lung location in an HIV-infected patient or a patient at high risk for HIV infection (23)	Mycobacterium tuberculosis	Airborne
Paroxysmal or severe persistent cough during periods of pertussis activity	Bordetella pertussis	Droplet
Respiratory infections, particularly bronchiolitis and croup, in infants and young children	Respiratory syncytial or parainfluenza virus	Contact
Risk of multidrug-resistant microorganisms		
History of infection or colonization with multidrug-resistant organisms	Resistant bacteria	Contact
Skin, wound, or urinary tract infection in a patient with a recent hospital or nursing home stay in a facility where multidrug-resistant organisms are prevalent	Resistant bacteria	Contact
Skin or Wound Infection		
Abscess or draining wound that cannot be covered	Staphylococcus aureus, Group A streptococcus	Contact

*Infection control professionals are encouraged to modify or adapt this table according to local conditions. To ensure that appropriate empiric precautions are implemented always, hospitals must have systems in place to evaluate patients routinely according to these criteria as part of their preadmission care.

[+]Patients with the syndromes or conditions listed below may present with atypical signs or symptoms (e.g., pertussis in neonates and adults may not have paroxysmal or severe cough). The clinician's index of suspicion should be guided by the prevalence of specific conditions in the community, as well as clinical judgment.

[++]The organisms listed under the column "Potential Pathogens" are not intended to represent the complete, or even most likely, diagnoses, but rather possible etiologic agents that require additional precautions beyond Standard Precautions until they can be ruled out.

&These pathogens include enterohemorrhagic Escherichia coli O157:H7, Shigella, hepatitis A, and rotavirus.

Resistant bacteria judged by the infection control program, based on current state, regional or national recommendations, to be of special clinical of epidemiological significance.

The organisms listed under the column "Potential Pathogens" are not intended to represent the complete or even most likely diagnoses, but rather possible etiologic agents that require additional precautions beyond Standard Precautions until they can be ruled out. Infection control professionals are encouraged to modify or adapt this Table according to local conditions. To ensure that appropriate empiric precautions are implemented always, hospitals must have systems in place to evaluate patients routinely according to these criteria as part of their preadmission and admission care.

IMMUNOCOMPROMISED PATIENTS

Immunocompromised patients vary in their susceptibility to nosocomial infections, depending on the severity and duration of immunosuppression. They generally are at increased risk for bacterial, fungal. parasitic, and viral infections from both endogenous and exogenous sources. The use of Standard Precautions for all patients and Transmission-Based Precautions for specified patients, as recommended in this guideline, should reduce the acquisition by these patients of institutionally acquired bacteria from other patients and environments.

It is beyond the scope of this guideline to address the various measures that may be used for immunocompromised patients to delay or prevent acquisition of potential pathogens during temporary periods of neutropenia. Rather, the primary objective of this guideline is to prevent transmission of pathogens from infected or colonized patients in hospitals. Users of this guideline, however, are referred to the "Guideline for Prevention of Nosocomial Pneumonia"

(95, 96) for the HICPAC recommendations for prevention of nosocomial aspergillosis and Legionnaires disease in immunocompromised patients.

RECOMMENDATIONS

The recommendations presented below are categorized as follows:

Category IA: Strongly recommended for all hospitals and strongly supported by well-designed experimental or epidemiologic studies.

Category IB: Strongly recommended for all hospitals and reviewed as effective by experts in the field and a consensus of HICPAC based on strong rationale and suggestive evidence, even though definitive scientific studies have not been done.

Category II: Suggested for implementation in many hospitals. Recommendations may be supported by suggestive clinical or epidemiologic studies, a strong theoretical rationale, or definitive studies applicable to some, but not all, hospitals.

No Recommendation; Unresolved Issue: Practices for which insufficient evidence or consensus regarding efficacy exists.

The recommendations are limited to the topic of isolation precautions. Therefore, they must be supplemented by hospital policies and procedures for other aspects of infection and environmental control, occupational health, administrative and legal issues, and other issues beyond the scope of this guideline.

I. Administrative Controls
   A. Education
      Develop a system to ensure that hospital patients, personnel, and visitors are educated about use of precautions and their responsibility for adherence to them. Category IB
   B. Adherence to Precautions
      Periodically evaluate adherence to precautions, and use findings to direct improvements. Category IB
II. Standard Precautions
   Use Standard Precautions, or the equivalent, for the care of all patients. Category IB
   A. Hand washing
      1. Wash hands after touching blood, body fluids, secretions, excretions, and contaminated items, whether or not gloves are worn. Wash hands immediately after gloves are removed, between patient contacts, and when otherwise indicated to avoid transfer of microorganisms to other patients or environments. It may be necessary to wash hands between tasks and procedures on the same patient to prevent cross-contamination of different body sites. Category IB
      2. Use a plain (nonantimicrobial) soap for routine hand washing. Category IB
      3. Use an antimicrobial agent or a waterless antiseptic agent for specific circumstances (e.g., control of outbreaks or hyperendemic infections), as defined by the infection control program. Category IB

(See Contact Precautions for additional recommendations on using antimicrobial and antiseptic agents.)

B. Gloves

Wear gloves (clean, nonsterile gloves are adequate) when touching blood, body fluids, secretions. excretions, and contaminated items. Put on clean gloves just before touching mucous membranes and nonintact skin. Change gloves between tasks and procedures on the same patient after contact with material that may contain a high concentration of microorganisms. Remove gloves promptly after use, before touching noncontaminated items and environmental surfaces, and before going to another patient, and wash hands immediately to avoid transfer of microorganisms to other patients or environments. Category IB

C. Mask, Eye Protection, Face Shield

Wear a mask and eye protection or a face shield to protect mucous membranes of the eyes, nose, and mouth during procedures and patient-care activities that are likely to generate splashes or sprays of blood, body fluids, secretions, and excretions. Category IB

D. Gown

Wear a gown (a clean, nonsterile gown is adequate) to protect skin and to prevent soiling of clothing during procedures and patient-care activities that are likely to generate splashes or sprays of blood, body fluids, secretions, or excretions. Select a gown that is appropriate for the activity and amount of fluid likely to be encountered. Remove a soiled gown as promptly as possible, and wash hands to avoid transfer of microorganisms to other patients or environments. Category IB

E. Patient-Care Equipment

Handle used patient-care equipment soiled with blood, body fluids, secretions, and excretions in a manner that prevents skin and mucous membrane exposures, contamination of clothing, and transfer of microorganisms to other patients and environments. Ensure that reusable equipment is not used for the care of another patient until it has been cleaned and reprocessed appropriately. Ensure that single-use items are discarded properly. Category IB

F. Environmental Control

Ensure that the hospital has adequate procedures for the routine care, cleaning, and disinfection of environmental surfaces, beds, bed rails, bedside equipment, and other frequently touched surfaces and ensure that these procedures are being followed. Category IB

G. Linen

Handle, transport, and process used linen soiled with blood, body fluids, secretions, and excretions in a manner that prevents skin and mucous membrane exposures and contamination of clothing, and that avoids transfer of microorganisms to other patients and environments. Category IB

H. Occupational Health and Blood Borne Pathogens

    1. Take care to prevent injuries when using needles, scalpels, and other sharp instruments or devices; when handling sharp instruments after procedures; when cleaning used instruments; and when disposing of used needles. Never recap used needles, or otherwise manipulate them using both hands, or use any other technique that involves directing the point of a needle toward any part of the body; rather, use either a one-handed "scoop" technique or a mechanical device designed for holding the needle sheath. Do not remove used needles from disposable syringes by hand, and do not bend, break, or otherwise manipulate used needles by hand. Place used disposable syringes and needles, scalpel blades, and other sharp items in appropriate puncture-resistant containers, which are located as close as practical to the area in which the items were used, and place reusable syringes and needles in a puncture-resistant container for transport to the reprocessing area. Category IB

    2. Use mouthpieces, resuscitation bags, or other ventilation devices as an alternative to mouth-to-mouth resuscitation methods in areas where the need for resuscitation is predictable. Category IB

I. Patient Placement

Place a patient who contaminates the environment or who does not (or cannot be expected to) assist in maintaining appropriate hygiene or environmental control in a private room. If a private room is not available. consult with infection control professionals regarding patient placement or other alternatives. Category IB

III. Airborne Precautions

In addition to Standard Precautions, use Airborne Precautions, or the equivalent, for patients known or suspected to be infected with microorganisms transmitted by airborne droplet nuclei (small-particle residue [5 μm or smaller in size] of evaporated droplets containing microorganisms that remain suspended in the air and that can be dispersed widely by air currents within a room or over a long. distance). Category IB

A. Patient Placement

Place the patient in a private room that has (a) monitored negative air pressure in relation to the surrounding area, (b) 6 to 12 changes per hour, and (c) appropriate discharge of air outdoors or monitored high-efficiency filtration of room air is circulated to other areas in the hospital (23). Keep the room door closed and the patient in the room. When a private room is not available, place the patient in a room with a patient who has active infection with the same microorganism, unless otherwise recommended (23), but with no other infection. When a private room is not available and cohorting is not desirable, consultation with infection control professionals is advised before patient placement. Category IB

B. Respiratory Protection

Wear respiratory protection when entering the room of a patient with known or suspected infectious pulmonary tuberculosis (23, 81). Susceptible persons should not enter the room of patients known or suspected to have measles or (rubeola) or varicella (chickenpox) if other immune care givers are available. If susceptible persons must enter the room of a patient known or suspected to have measles (rubeola) or varicella, they should wear respiratory protection (81). Persons immune to measles (rubeola) or varicella need not wear respiratory protection. Category IB

C. Patient Transport

Limit the movement and transport of the patient from the room to essential purposes only. If transport or movement is necessary, minimize patient dispersal of droplet nuclei by placing a surgical mask on the patient, if possible. Category IB

D. Additional Precautions for Preventing Transmission of Tuberculosis

Consult CDC "Guidelines for Preventing the Transmission of Tuberculosis in Health-Care Transmission of Facilities" (23) for additional prevention strategies.

IV. Droplet Precautions

In addition to Standard Precautions, use Droplet Precautions, or the equivalent for a patient known or suspected to be infected with microorganisms transmitted by droplets (large-particle droplets [larger than 5 μm in size] that can be generated by the patient during coughing, sneezing, talking, or the performance of procedures). Category IB

A. Patient Placement

Place the patient in a private room. When a private room is not available, place the patient in a room with a patient(s) who has active infection with the same microorganism but with no other infection (cohorting). When a private room is not available and cohorting is not achievable, maintain spatial separation of at least 3 ft between the infected patient and other patients and visitors. Special air handling and ventilation are not necessary, and the door may remain open. Category IB

B. Mask

In addition to standard precautions, wear a mask when working within 3 ft of the patient, (Logistically, some hospitals may want to implement the wearing of a mask to enter the room.) Category IB

C. Patient Transport

Limit the movement and transport of the patient from the room to essential purposes only. If transport or movement is necessary, minimize patient dispersal of droplets by masking the patient, if possible. Category IB

V. Contact Precautions

In addition to Standard Precautions, use Contact Precautions, or the equivalent, for specified patients known or suspected to be infected or colonized with epidemiologically important microorganisms that can be transmitted by direct contact with the patient (hand or skin-to-skin contact that occurs when performing patients are activities that require touching the patients dry skin) or indirect contact (touching) with environmental surfaces or patient-care items in the patient's environment, Category IB

A. Patient Placement

Place the patient in a private room. When a private room is not available, place the patient in a room with a patient(s) who has active infection with the same microorganism but with no other infection (cohorting). When a private room is not available and cohorting is not achievable, consider the epidemiology of the microorganism and the patient population when determining patient placement. Consultation with infection control professionals is advised before patient placement. Category IB

B. Gloves and Hand Washing

In addition to wearing gloves as outlined under Standard Precautions, wear gloves (clean, nonsterile gloves are adequate) when entering the room. During the course of providing care for a patient, change gloves after having contact with infective material that may contain high concentrations of microorganisms (fecal material and wound drainage). Remove gloves before leaving the patient's environment and wash hands immediately with an antimicrobial agent or a waterless antiseptic agent (72, 94). After glove removal and hand washing, ensure that hands do not touch potentially contaminated environmental surfaces or items in the patients room to avoid transfer of microorganisms to other patients or environments. Category IB

C. Gown

In addition to wearing a gown as outlined under Standard Precautions, wear a gown (a clean, nonsterile gown is adequate) when entering the room if you anticipate that your clothing will have substantial contact with the patient, environmental surfaces, or items in the patient's room, or if the patient is incontinent or has diarrhea, an ileostomy, a colostomy, or wound drainage not contained by a dressing. Remove the gown before leaving the patient's environment. After gown removal, ensure that clothing does not contact potentially contaminated environmental surfaces to avoid transfer of microorganisms to other patients or environments. Category IB

D. Patient Transport

Limit the movement and transport of the patient from the room to essential purposes only. If the patient is transported out of the room, ensure that precautions are maintained to minimize the risk of transmission of microorganisms to other patients and contamination of environmental surfaces or equipment. Category IB

E. Patient-Care Equipment

When possible, dedicate the use of noncritical patient-care equipment to a single patient (or cohort of patients infected or colonized with the pathogen requiting precautions) to avoid sharing between patients. If use of common equipment or items is unavoidable, then adequately clean and disinfect them before use for another patient Category IB

F. Additional Precautions for Preventing the Spread of Vancomycin Resistance

Consult the HICPAC report on preventing the spread of vancomycin resistance for additional prevention strategies (94).

REFERENCES: AS NUMBERED IN ORIGINAL PUBLICATION

1. Garner JS. The CDC Hospital Infection Control Practices Advisory Committee. Am J Infect Control 1993;21:160–162.
2. National Communicable Disease Center. Isolation techniques for use in hospitals. 1st ed. Washington, DC: US Government Printing Office, 1970:PHS publication no. 2054.
3. Centers for Disease Control. Isolation techniques for use in hospitals. 2nd ed. Washington, DC: US Government Printing Office, 1975:HHS publication no. (CDC) 83–8314.
4. Garner JS, Simmons BE. CDC guideline for isolation precautions in hospitals. Atlanta: US Department of Health and Human Services, Public Health Service, Centers for Disease Control, HHS publication no. (CDC) 83–8314;Infect Control 1983;4:245–325; and Am J Infect Control 1984;12:103–163.
5. Lynch T. Communicable disease nursing. St. Louis: Mosby, 1949.
6. Gage ND, Landon JF, Sider MT, Communicable diseases. Philadelphia: FA Davis, 1959.
7. Haley RW, Shachtman RH. The emergence of infection surveillance and control programs in US hospitals; an assessment; 1976. Am J Epidemiol 1980;111:574–591.
8. Schaffner W. Infection control; old myths and new realities. Infect Control 1980;1:330–334.
9. Garner JS. Comments on CDC guideline for isolation precautions in hospitals, 1984. Am J Infect Control 1984;12:163–164.
10. Haley RW, Garner JS, Simmons BP. A new approach to the isolation of patients with infectious diseases: alternative systems. J Hosp Infect 1985;6:128–139.
11. Nausef WM, Make DG. A study of the value of simple protective isolation in patients with granulocytopenia. N Engl J Med 1981;304:448–453.
12. Pizzo PA. The value of protective isolation in preventing nosocomial infections in high risk patients. Am J Med 1981;70:631–637.
13. Jacobson JT, Johnson DS, Ross CA, Conti MT, Evans RS, Burke JP. Adapting disease-specific isolation guidelines to a hospital information system. Infect Control 1986;7:411–418.
14. Goldmann DA. The role of barrier precautions in infection control. J Hosp Infect 1991;18:515–523.
15. Goldmann DA, Platt R, Hopkins C. Control of hospital-acquired infections. In: Gorbach SL, Bartlett JG, Blacklow NR, eds. Infectious diseases. Philadelphia: WB Saunders, 1992:378–390.
16. Centers for Disease Control. Management of patients with suspected hemorrhagic fever. MMWR 1988;37(3S):1–16.
17. Centers for Disease Control. Risks associated with human parvovirus B19 infection. MMWR 1989;38: 81–88, 93–97.
18. Centers for Disease Control. Guidelines for preventing the transmission of tuberculosis in health-care settings, with special focus on HIV-related issures. MMWR 1990;39(RR-17):1–29.
19. Centers for Disease Control. Nosocomial transmission of multidrug-resistant tuberculosis to health-care workers and HIV-infected patients in an urban hospital-Florida. MMWR 1990;39:718–722.
20. Centers for Disease Control. Nosocomial transmission of multidrug-resistant tuberculosis among HIV-infected persons—Florida and New York, 1988–91. MMWR 1991;39(RR-17):1–29.
21. Centers for Disease Control and Prevention. Initial therapy for tuberculosis in the era of multidrug resistance: recommendations of the advisory Council for the Elimination of Tuberculosis. MMWR 1993;39:718–722.
22. Centers for Disease Control and Prevention. Draft guidelines for preventing the transmission of tuberculosis in health-care facilities, second edition. Federal Register 1993;58(195):52810-52850.
23. Centers for Disease Control and Prevention. Guidelines for preventing the transmission of tuberculosis in health-care facilities, 1994. MMWR 1993;43(RR-13):1–132, and Federal Register 1994;59(208): 54242-54303.
24. Centers for Disease Control. Recommendations for preventing transmission of infection with human

T-lymphotrophic virus type III/lymphadenopathy-associated virus in the workplace. MMWR 1985;34:681–686, 691–695.

25. Centers for Disease Control. Recommendations for preventing transmission of infection with human T-lymphotropic virus type III/lymphadenopathy-associated virus during invasive procedures. MMWR 1986;35:221–223.

26. Centers for Disease Control. Update: human immunodeficiency virus infections in health-care workers exposed to blood of infected patients. MMWR 1987;36:285–289.

27. Centers for Disease Control. Recommendations for prevention of HIV transmission in health-care settings. MMWR 1987;36:(2S):1S-18S.

28. Centers for Disease Control. Update: universal precautions for prevention of transmission of human immunodeficiency virus, hepatitis B, and other bloodborne pathogens in health-care setting. MMWR 1988;37:377–382, 387–388.

29. Lynch E, Jackson MM, Cummings MJ, Stamm WE. Rethinking the role of isolation practices in the prevention of nosocomial infections. Ann Intern Med 1987;107:245–246.

30. Lynch E, Cummings MJ, Roberts PL, Herriott MJ, Yates B, Stamm WE. Implementing and evaluating a system of generic infection precautions: body substance isolation. Am J Infect Control 1990;18:1–12.

31. McPherson DC, Jackson MM, Rogers JC. Evaluating the cost of the body substance isolation system. J Healthcare Material Mgmt 1988;6:20–28.

32. Patterson JE, Vecchio J, Pantelick EL, et al. Association of contaminated gloves with transmission of Aciutabader calcoaceticus var. anitratus in an intensive care unit. Am J Med 1991;91:479–483.

33. Klein BS, Perioff WH, Maid DG. Reduction of nosocomial infection during pediatric intensive care by protective isolation. N Engl J Med 1989;320:1714–1721.

34. Leclair JM, Freeman J, Sullivan BF, Crowley CM, Goldmann DA. Prevention of nosocomial respiratory syncytial virus infections through compliance with gown and glove isolation precautions. N Engl J Med 1987;317:329–334.

35. Weinstein RK, Kabins SK. Strategies for prevention and control of multiple drug-resistant nosocomial infection. Am J Med 1981;70:449–454.

36. Garner JS, Hierholzer WJ. Controversies in isolation policies and practices. In: Wenzel RP, ed. Prevention and control nosocomial infections. 2nd ed. Baltimore: Williams & Wilkins, 1993:70–81.

37. Garner JS, Hughes JM. Options for isolation precautions. Ann Intern Med 1987;107:248–250.

38. Weinstein RA, Kabins SA. Isolation practices in hospitals [Letter]. Ann Intern Med 1987;107:781–782.

39. Doebbeling BN, Pfaller MA, Houston AK, Wenzel RE. Removal of nosocomial pathogens from the contaminated glove: implications for glove reuse and handwashing. Ann Intern Med 1988;109:394–398.

40. Sussman GL, Tario S, Dolovich J. The spectrum of IgE-mediated response to latex. JAMA 1991;255:2844–2847.

41. Bubak ME, Reed CE, Fransway AF, et al. Allergic reactions to latex among health-care workers. Mayo Clin Proc 1992;67:1075–1079.

42. Albert RK, Condie E. Hand-washing patterns in medical intensive care units. N Engl J Med 1981;304:1465–1466.

43. Preston GA, Larson EL, Stamm WE. The effect of private isolation rooms on patient care practices, colonization, and infection in an intensive care unit Am J Med 1981;70:641–645.

44. Larson E, Leyden JJ, McGinley KI, Grove GL, Talbot GH. Physiologic and microbiologic changes in skin related to frequent handwashing. Infect Control 1986;7:59–63.

45. Department of Labor, Occupational Safety and Health Administration. Occupational exposure to bloodborne pathogens; proposed rule and notice of hearings. Federal Register 1989;54(102):23042-23139.

46. Doebbelling BN, Wenzel RE. The direct costs of universal precautions in a teaching hospital. JAMA 1990;264:2083–2087.

47. Eickhoff TC. The cost of prevention. Infect Dis News 1991;4:6.

48. Fahey BJ, Koziol DE, Banks SM, Henderson DK. Frequency of nonparenteral occupational exposures to blood and body fluids before and after universal precautions training. Am J Med 1991;90:145–153.

49. Klein RS. Universal precautions for preventing occupational exposures to human immunodeficiency virus type 1. Am J Med 1991;90:141–153.

50. Wong ES, Stotka JL, Chinchiili VM, Williams DS, Stuart CG, Markowitz SM. Are universal precautions effective in reducing the number of occupational exposures among health care workers? JAMA 1991;265:1123–1128.

51. Department of Labor, Occupational Safety and Health Administration. Occupational exposure to blood borne pathogens; final rule. Federal Register 1991;56(235):64175-64182.

52. American Hospital Association. OSHA's final bloodborne pathogens standard. A special briefing. 1992:item no. 155904.

53. Bruning LM. The bloodborne pathogens final rule. AORN J 1993;57:439–461.

54. Jackson MM, Lynch E. An attempt to make an issue less murky: a comparison of four systems for infection precautions. Infect Control Hosp Epidemiol 1991;12:448–450.

55. Pugliese G, Lynch E, Jackson MM. Univesal precautions: policies, procedures, and resources. Chicago: American Hospital Association, 1991:7–87.

56. Birnbaum D, Schulzer M, Mathjag RG, Kelly M, Chow AW. Adoption of guidelines for universal precautions and body substance isolation in Camulian acute-care hospitals. 1990;11:465–472.
57. Lynch E, Cummings MI, Stamm WE, Jacka OA. Handwashing versus gloving [Letter]. Infect Control Hosp Epidemiol 1991;12:139.
58. Birnbaum D, Schulzer M, Mathias RG, Kelly M, Chow AW. Handwashing versus gloving [Letter]. Infect Control Hosp Epidemiol 1991;12:140.
59. Gurevich I. Body substance isolation [Letter]. Infect Control Hosp Epidemiol 1992;13:191.
60. Jackson MM, Lynch E. Body substance isolation [Letter]. Infect Control Hosp Epidemiol 1992;13: 191–192.
61. Rudnick JR, Kroc K, Manangan L, Banerjee S, Pugliese G, Jarvis W. Are US hospitals prepared to control nosocomial transmission of tuberculosis [Abstract]? Epidemic Intelligence Service Annual Conference, 1993;60.
62. Institute of Medicine. Emerging infections: microbial threats to health in the United States. 1st ed. Washington, DC: National Academy Press, 1992.
63. Centers for Disease Control and Prevention. Nosocomial enterococci resistant to vancomycin—United States, 1989–1983. MMWR 1993;42:597–599.
64. Lowbury FJL, Lilly HA, Bull JE. Disinfection of hands: removal of transient organisms. Br Med J 1964;2:230–233.
65. Sprunt K, Redmon W, Leidy G. Antibacterial effectiveness of routine handwashing. Pediatrics 1973;52: 264–271.
66. Steere AC, Manison GE. Handwashing practices for the prevention of nosocomial infections. Ann Intern Med 1975;83:6834–6890.
67. Food and Drug Administration. The tentative final monograph for over-the-counter topical antimicrobial products. Federal Register 1978;43:12104-12249.
68. Garner JS, Favero MS. Guidelines for handwashing and hospital environmental control. Atlanta: US Department of Health and Human Services, Public Health Service, Centers for Disease Control, 1985.
69. Larson E. APIC guideline for use of topical antimicrobial products. Am J Infect Control 1988;16:253–266.
70. Ehrenkranz NJ. Bland soap handwash or hand antisepsis? The pressing need for clarity. Infect Control Hosp Epidemiol 1992;13:299–301.
71. Larson E. Skin cleansing. In: Wenzel RE, ed. Prevention and control of nosocomial infections. 2nd ed. Baltimore: Williams & Wilkins, 1993:450–459.
72. Larson EL, 1992, 1993, and 1994 Association for Professionals in Infection Control and Epidemiology Guidelines Committee. APIC guideline for handwashing and hand antisepsis in health care settings. Am J Infect Control 1995;23:251–269.
73. Paulssen J, Eidem T, Kristiansen R. Perforations in surgeons gloves. J Hosp Infect 1988;11:82–85.
74. DeGroot-Kosolcharoen J, Jones JM. Permeability of latex and vinyl gloves to water and blood. Am J Infect Control 1989;17:196–201.
75. Kotilainen HR, Brinker JP, Avato JL, Gantz NM. Latex and vinyl examination gloves quality control procedures and implications for health care workers. Arch Intern Med 1989;149;2749–2753.
76. Olsen RJ, Lynch P, Coyle MB, Cuntmings MJ, Bokete T, Stature WE. Examination gloves as barriers to hand contamination and clinical practice. JAMA 1993;270:350–353.
77. Health Resources and Services Administration. Guidelines for construction and equipment of hospital and medical facilities. Rockville, MD: US Department of Health and Human Services, Public Health Service, 1984: PHS publication no. (HRSA)84–14500.
78. American Institute of Architects, Committee on Architecture for Health. General hospital. In: Guidelines for construction and equipment of hospital and medical facilities. Washington, DC: The American Institute of Architects Press; 1993.
79. American Society of Heating, Refrigerating, and Air Conditioning Engineers. Health facilities. In: 1991 Application handbook. Atlanta: American Society of Heating, Refrigerating, and Air Conditioning Engineers, Inc., 1991.
80. Jarvis WR, Bolyard FA, Boza CJ, et al Respirators, recommendations, and regulations: the controversy surrounding protection of health care workers from tuberculosis. Ann Intern Med 1995;122:142–146.
81. Department of Health and Human Services, Department of Labor. Respiratory protective devices: final rules and notice. Federal Register 1995;60(110):30336-30402.
82. Rutula WK, Mayhall CG. The Society for Hospital Epidemiology of America position paper: medical waste. Infect Control Hosp Epidemiol 1992;13:38–48.
83. Rhame FS. The inanimate environment. In: Bennett JV, Brachman PS, eds. Hospital infections. 3rd ed. Boston: Little, Brown and Co., 1992:299–333.
84. Rumla WA. Disinfection, sterilization, and waste disposal. In: Wenzel RE, ed. Prevention and control of nosocomial infections. 2nd ed. Baltimore: Williams & Wilkins, 1993:460–495.
85. Maid DG, Alvarado C, Hassemer C. Double-bagging of items from isolation rooms is unnecessary as an infection control measure: a comparative study of surface contamination with single and double bagging. Infect Control 1986;7:535–537.
86. American Society for Healthcare Central Services. Recommended practices for central service: sterilization. Chicago: American Hospital Association, 1988.

87. American Society for Healthcare Central Services. Recommended practices for central service: decontamination. Chicago: American Hospital Association, 1990.
88. Rumla WA. APIC guideline for selection and use of disinfectants. Am J Infect Control 1990;18:90–117.
89. Bond WW, Ott BJ, Franke KA, McCracken JE. Effective use of liquid chemical germicides on medical devices: instrument design problems. In: Block SS, ed. Disinfection, sterilization, and preservation. 4th ed. Philadelphia: Lea and Febiger, 1991:1097–1106.
90. Favero MS, Bond WW. Sterilization, disinfection, and antisepsis. In: Ballows A, Hausler WJ, Herrmann KL, Isenberg HO, Shadomy HJ, eds. Manual of clinical microbiology. 5th ed. Washington, DC: American Society for Microbiology, 1991:183–200.
91. Favero MS, Bond WW. Chemical disinfection of medical and surgical materials. In: Block SS, ed. Disinfection, sterilization, and preservation. 4th ed. Philadelphia: Lea and Febiger, 1991:617–641.
92. Pugliese G, Hunstiger CA. Central services, linens, and laundry. In: Bennett JV, Brachman PS, eds. Hospital infections. 3rd ed. Boston: Little, Brown and Co., 1992:335–344.
93. Joint Committee on Healthcare Laundry Guidelines. Guidelines for healthcare linen service—1994. Hallmadale, FL: Textile Rental Services Association of America, 1994.
94. Hospital Infection Control Practices Advisory Committee. Recommendations for preventing the spread of vancomycin resistance. Am J Infect Control 1995;23:87–94; Infect Control Hosp Epidemiol 1995; 16:105–113;. and MMWR 1995;44(No. RR-12):1–13.
95. Tablan OC, Anderson LJ, Arden NH, Breiman RF, Butler JC, McNeil MM, Hospital Infection Control Practices Advisory Committee. Guideline for prevention of nosocomial pneumonia, Part I: issues on prevention of nosocomial pneumonia-1994. Am J Infect Control 1994;22:247–266; Infect Control Hosp Epidemiol 1994;15:587–604; and American Association of Respiratory Care 1994;12:1191–1209.
96. Hospital Infection Control Practices Advisory Committee. Guideline for prevention of nosocomial pneumonia, Part II: recommendations for prevention of nosocomial pneumonia. Am J Infect Control 1994;22:266–292; Infect Control Hosp Epidemiol 1994;15:604–627; and American Association of Respiratory Care 1994;12:1209–1236.
97. Centers for Disease Control and Prevention. Update: management of patients with suspected viral hemorrhagic fever—United States. MWWR 1995;44:475–479.

APPENDIX A
Type and Duration of Precautions Needed for Selected Infections and Conditions

Infection/Conditions	Precautions Type*	Duration
Abscess		
Draining, major[1]	C	DI
Draining, minor or limited[2]	S	
Acquired immunodeficiency syndrome[3]	S	
Actinomycosis	S	
Adenovirus infection, infants and young children	D,C	DI
Amebiasis	S	
Anthrax		
Cutaneous	S	
Pulmonary	S	
Antibiotic-associated colitis (see Clostridium difficile)		
Arthropodborne viral encephalitides (eastern, western, Venezuelan equine encephalomyelitis; St. Louis, California encephalitis	S[4]	
Arthropodborne viral fevers (dengue, yellow fever, Colorado tick fever)	S[4]	
Ascariasis	S	
Aspergillosis	S	
Babesiosis	S	
Blastomycosis, North American, cutaneous or pulmonary	S	
Botulism	S	
Bronchiolitis (see respiratory infections in infants and young children)		
Brucellosis (undulant, Malta, Mediterranean fever)	S	
Campylobacter gastroenteritis (see gastroenteritis)		
Candidiasis, all forms including mucocutaneous	S	
Cat-scratch fever (benign inoculation lymphoreticulosis)	S	
Cellulitis, uncontrolled drainage	C	DI
Chancroid (soft chancre)	S	
Chickenpox (varicella; see F[5] for varicella exposure)	A,C	F[5]

APPENDIX A—*continued*

Infection/Conditions	Precautions	
	Type*	Duration
Chlamydia trachomatis		
Conjunctivitis	S	
Genital	S	
Respiratory	S	
Cholera (see gastroenteritis)		
Closed-cavity infection		
Draining, limited or minor	S	
Not draining	S	
Clostridium		
C botulinum	S	
C difficile	C	DI
C perfringens		
Food poisoning	S	
Gas gangrene	S	
Coccidioidomycosis (valley fever)		
Draining lesions	S	
Pneumonia	S	
Colorado tick fever	S	
Congenital rubella	C	F[6]
Conjunctivitis		
Acute bacterial	S	
Chlamydia	S	
Gonococcal	S	
Acute viral (acute hemorrhagic)	C	DI
Coxsackie virus disease (see enteroviral infection)		
Creutzfeldt-Jakob disease	S[7]	
Croup (see respiratory infections in infants and young children)		
Cryptococcosis	S	
Cryptosporidiosis (see gastroenteritis)		
Cysticerosis	S	
Cytomegalovirus infection, neonatal or inununosuppressed	S	
Decubitus ulcer, infected		
Major[1]	C	DI
Minor or limited[2]	S	
Dengue	S[4]	
Diarrhea, acute—infective etiology suspected (see gastroenteritis)		
Diphtheria		
Cutaneous	C	CN[8]
Pharyngeal	D	CN[8]
Ebola vital hemorrhagic fever	C[9]	DI
Echinococcosis (hydatidosis)	S	
Echovirus (see enteroviral infection)		
Encephalitis or encephalomyelitis (see specific etiologic agents)		
Endometritis	S	
Enterobiasis (pinworm disease, oxyuriasis)		
Enterococcus species (see multidrug-resistant organisms or epidemiologically	S	
significant or vancomycin resistant)		
Enterocolitis, Clostridium difficile	C	DI
Enteroviral infections		
Adults	S	
Infants and young children	C	DI
Epiglottitis, due to Haemophilus influenzae	D	U24 hrs
Epstein-Barr virus infection, including infectious mononucleosis	S	
Erythema infectiosum (also see Parvovirus B19)	S	
Escherichia coli gastroenteritis (see gastroenteritis)		
Food poisoning		
Botulism	S	
Clostridium perfringens or welchii	S	
Staphylococcal	S	

APPENDIX A—*continued*

Infection/Conditions	Precautions	
	Type*	Duration
Furunculosis—staphylococcal		
Infants and young children	C	DI
Gangrene (gas gangrene)	S	
Gastroenteritis		
Campylobacter species	S[10]	
Cholera	S[10]	
Clostridium difficile	C	DI
Cyptosporidium species	S[10]	
Escherichia coli		
Enterohemorrhagic O157:H7	S[10]	
Diapered or incontinent	C	DI
Other species	S[10]	
Giardia lamblia	S[10]	
Rotavirus	S[10]	
Diapered or incontinent	C	DI
Salmonella species including S typhi)	S[10]	
Shigella species	S[10]	
Diapered or incontinent	C	DI
Vibrio parahaemolvticus	S[10]	
Viral (if not covered elsewhere)	S[10]	
Yersinia enterocolitica	S[10]	
German measles (rubella)	D	F[22]
Giardiasis (see gastroenteritis)		
Gonococcal ophthalmia neonatorum (gonorrheal opthalmia acute conjunctivitis of newborn)	S	
Gonorrhea	S	
Granuloma inguinale (donovanosis, granuloma venereum)	S	
Guillain-Barré syndrome	S	
Hand, foot, and mouth disease (see enteroviral infection)		
Hantavirus pulmonary syndrome	S	
Helicobacter pylori	S	
Hemorrhagic fevers (for example, Lassa and Ebola)	C[9]	DI
Hepatitis, viral		
Type A	S	
Diapered or incontinent patients	C	F[11]
Type B—HBsAg positive	S	
Type C and other unspecified non-A, non-B	S	
Type E	S	
Herpangina (see enteroviral infection)		
Herpes simplex (Herpesvirus hominis)		
Encephalitis	S	
Neonatal[12] (see F for neonatal exposure)	C	DI
Mucocutaneous, disseminated or primary, severe	C	DI
Mucocutaneous, recurrent (skin, oral, genital)	S	
Herpes zoster (varicella-zoster)		
Localized in immunocompromised patient, or disseminated	A,C	DI[13]
Localized in normal patient Histoplasmosis	S[13]	
HIV (see human immunodefidency virus)	S	
Hookworm disease (ancylostomiasis, uncinansis)	S	
Human immunodeficiency virus (HIV) infection[3]	S	
Impetigo	C	U24 hrs
Infectious mononucleosis	S	
Influenza	D	DI
Kawasaki syndrome	S	
Lassa fever	C[19]	DI
Legionnaire's disease	S	
Leprosy	S	
Leptospirosis	S	
Lice (pediculosis)	C	U24

APPENDIX A—*continued*

Infection/Conditions	Precautions	
	Type*	Duration
Listeriosis	S	
Lyme disease	S	
Lymphocytic choriomeningitis	S	
Lymphogranuloma venereum	S	
Malaria	S[4]	
Marburg virus disease	C[9]	DI
Measles (rubeola), all presentations	A	DI
Melioidosis, all forms	S	
Meningitis	S	
Aseptic (nonbacterial or viral meningitis gram-negative bacterial)	S	
Burkholderia cepacia in cystic fibrosis (CF) patients, including respiratory tract colonization	S[20]	
Chlamydia	S	
Fungal	S	
Haemophilus influenzae		
Adults	S	
Infants and children (any age)	D	U24 hrs
Legionella	S	
Meningococcal	D	U24 hrs
Multidrug-resistant bacterial (see multidrug-resistant organisms)		
Mycoplasma (primary atypical pneumonia)	D	DI
Multidrug-resistant (see multidrug-resistant organisms)		
Pneumocystis carinii	S[21]	
Pseudomonas cepacia (see Burkholderia cepacia)	S[20]	
Staphylococcus aureus	S	
Streptococcus, Group A		
Adults	S	
Infants and young children	D	U24 hrs
Viral		
Adults	S	
Infants and young children (see respiratory infectious disease, acute)		
Poliomyetilis	S	
Psittacosis (ornithosis)	S	
Q fever	S	
Rabies	S	
Rat-bite fever (Streptobacillus moniliformis disease, Spirillum minus disease)	S	
Relapsing fever	S	
Resistant bacterial infection or colonization (see multidrug-resistant organisms)		
Respiratory infectious disease, acute (if not covered elsewhere)		
Adults	S	
Infants and young children[3]	C	DI
Respiratory syncyfial virus infection, in infants and young children, and immunocompromised adults	C	DI
Reye's syndrome	S	
Rheumatic fever	S	
Rickettsial fevers, tickborne (Rocky Mountain [also see enteroviral infections])		
Bacterial, gram-negative enteric, in neonates	S	
Fungal	S	
Haemophilas influenzae, known or suspected	D	U24 hrs
Listeria monocytogenes	S	
Neisseria meningitidis (meningococcal) known or suspected	D	U24 hrs
Pneumococcal	S	
Tuberculosis[15]	S	
Other diagnosed bacterial	S	
Meningococcal pneumonia	D	U24 hrs
Meningococcemia (meningococcal sepsis)	D	U24 hrs
Molluscum contagiosum	S	
Mucormycosis	S	

APPENDIX A—_continued_

Infection/Conditions	Precautions Type*	Duration
Multidrug-resistant organisms, infection or colonization[16]		
Gastrointestinal	C	CN
Respiratory	C	CN
Pneumococcal	S	
Skin, wound, or burn	C	CN
Mumps (infectious parotitis)	D	F[17]
Mycobacteria nontuberculosis (atypical)		
Pulmonary	S	
Wound	S	
Mycoplasma pneumonia	D	
Necrotizing enterocolitis	S	
Nocardiosis, draining lesions or other presentations	S	
Norwalk agent gastroenteritis (see viral gastroenteritis)		
Orf	S	
Parainfluenza virus infection, respiratory in infants and young children	C	DI
Parovirus B19	D	F[18]
Pediculosis (lice)	C	U24 hrs
Pertussis (whooping cough)	D	F[19]
Pinworm infection	S	
Plague		
Bubonic	S	
Pneumonic	D	U72 hrs
Pleurodynia (see enteroviral infection)		
Pneumonia		
Adenovirus	D,C	DI
Bacterial not listed elsewhere (including spotted fever, tickborne typhus fever)	S	
Rickettsialpox (vesicular rickettsiosis)	S	
Ringworm (dermatophytosis, dermatomycosis, tinea)	S	
Ritter's disease (staphylococcal scalded skin syndrome)	S	
Rocky Mountain spotted fever	S	
Roseola infanmm (exanthem subitum)	S	
Rotavirus infection (see gastroenteritis)		
Rubella (German measles; also see congenital rubella)	D	F[22]
Salmonellosis (see gastroenteritis)		
Scabies	C	U24 hrs
Scalded skin syndrome, staphylococcal (Ritter's disease)	S	
Schistosorniasis (bilharziasis)	S	
Shigellosis (see gastroenteritis)		
Sporotrichosis	S	
Spirillum minas disease (rat-bite fever)	S	
Staphylococcal disease (S aureas)	S	
Skin, wound, or burn		
Major[1]	C	DI
Minor or limited[2]	S	
Enterocolitis	S[10]	
Multidrug resistant (see multidrug-resistant organisms)		
Pneumonia	S	
Scalded skin syndrome	S	
Toxic shock syndrome	S	
Streptobacillus monilformis disease (rat-bite fever)	S	
Streptococcal disease (group A streptococcus)		
Skin, wound, or burn		
Major[1]	C	U24 hrs
Minor or limited[2]	S	
Endometritis (puerperal sepsis)	S	
Pharyngitis in infants and young children	D	U24 hrs
Pneumonia in infants and young children	D	U24 hrs
Scarlet fever in infants and young children	D	U24 hrs
Streptococcal disease (group B streptococcus), neonatal	S	

APPENDIX A—*continued*

Infection/Conditions	Precautions	
	Type*	Duration
Streptococcal disease (not group A or B) unless covered elsewhere	S	
Multidrug-resistant (see multidrug-resistant organisms)		
Strongyloidiasis	S	
Syphilis		
Skin and mucous membrane, including congenital, primary, secondary	S	
Latent (tertiary) and seropositivity without lesions	S	
Tapeworm disease		
Hymenolepis nana	S	
Taenia solium (pork)	S	
Other	S	
Tetanus	S	
Tinea (fungus infection dermatophytosis, dermatomycosis, ringworm)	S	
Toxoplasmosis	S	
Toxic shock syndrome (staphylococcal disease)	S	
Trachoma, acute	S	
Trench mouth (Vincent's angina)	S	
Trichinosis	S	
Trichomoniasis	S	
Trichuriasis (whipworm disease)	S	
Tuberculosis		
Extrapulmonary, draining lesion (including scrofula)	S	
Extrapulmonary, meningitis[15]	S	
Pulmonary, confirmed or suspected or laryngeal disease	A	F[23]
Skin-test positive with no evidence of current pulmonary disease	S	
Tularemia		
Draining lesion	S	
Pulmonary	S	
Typhoid (Salmonella typhi) fever (see gastroenteritis)		
Typhus, endemic and epidemic	S	
Urinary tract infection (including pyelonephritis), with or without urinary	S	
catheter		
Varicella (chickenpox)	A,C	F[5]
Vibrio parahaemolyticus (see gastroenteritis)		
Vincent's angina (trench mouth)	S	
Viral diseases		
Respiratory (if not covered elsewhere)		
Adults	S	
Infants and young children (see respiratory infectious disease, acute)		
Whooping cough (pertussis)	D	F[19]
Wound infections		
Major[1]	C	DI
Minor or limited[12]	S	
Yersinia enaterocolitica gastroenteritis (see gastroenteritis)		
Localized in immunocompromised patient, disseminated	A,C	DI[13]
Localized in normal patient	S[13]	
Zygomycosis (phycomycosis, mucormycosis)	S	
Zoster (varicella-zoster)		

Abbreviations: type of precautions: A, Airborne; C, Contact; D, Droptet; S, Standard; when A, C, and D are specified, also use S.

⁺Duration of precautions: CN, until off antibiotics and culture-negative; DH, duration of hospitalization; DI duration of illness (with wound lesions, DI means until they stop draining); U, until time specified in hours (hr.) after initiation of effective therapy; F, see footnote number.

[1]No dressing or dressing does not contain drainage adequately.

[2]Dressing covers and contains drainage adequately.

[3]Also see syndromes of conditions listed in Table 2.

APPENDIX A—*continued*

[4]Install screens in windows and doors in endemic areas.

[5]Maintain precautions until all lesions are crusted. The average incubation period for varicella is 10 to 21 days. After exposure, use varicella zoster immune globin (VZIG) when appropriate, and discharge susceptible patients if possible. Placed exposed susceptible patients on Airborne Precautions beginning 10 days after exposure and continuing until 21 after the last exposure (up to 28 days if VZIG has been given). Susceptible persons should not enter the room of patients on precautions if other immune caregivers are available.

[6]Place infant on precautions during any admission until 1 year of age, unless nasapharyngeal and urine cultures are negative for virus after age 3 months.

[7]Additional special precautions are necessary for handling and decontamination of blood, body fluids and tissues, and contaminated items from patients with confirmed or suspected disease. See latest College of American Pathologists (Northfield, Illinois) guidelines or other references.

[8]Until two cultures taken at least 24 hours apart are negative.

[9]Call state health department and CDC for specific advice about management of a suspected case. During the 1995 Ebola outbleak in Zaire, interim recommendations were published (97). Pending a comprehensive review of the epidemiologic data from the outbreak and evaluation of the interim recommendations, the 1988 guidelines for management of patients with suspected vital hemorrhagic infections (16) will be reviewed and updated if indicated.

[10]Use Contact Precautions for diapered or incontinent children <6 years of age for duration of illness.

[11]Maintain precautions in infants and children <3 years of age for duration of hospitalization; in children 3 to 14 yeas of age, until 2 weeks after onset of symptoms; and in others, until 1 week after onset of symptoms.

[12]For infants delivered vaginally or by C-section and if mother has active infection and membranes have been ruptured for more than 4 to 6 hours.

[13]Persons susceptible to varicella are also at risk for developing varicella when exposed to patients with herpes zoster lesions; therefore, susceptibles should not enter the room if other immune caregivers are available.

[14]The "Guideline for Prevention of Nosocomial Pneunmonia" (95,96) recommends surveillance, vaccination, antiviral agents, and use of private rooms with negative air pressure as much as feasible for patients for whom influenza is suspected or diagnosed. Many hospitals encounter logistic difficulties and physical plant limitations when admitting multiple patients with suspected influenza during community outbreaks. If sufficient private rooms are unavailable, consider cohorting patients or, at the very least, avoid room sharing with high-risk patients. See "Guideline for Prevention of Nosocomial Pneumonia" (95,96) for additional prevention and control strategies.

[15]Patient should be examined for evidence of current (active) pulmonary tuberculosis. If evidence exists, additional precautions are necessary (see tuberculosis).

[16]Resistant bacteria judged by the infection control program based on current state, regional, or national recommendations, to be of special clinical and epidemiologic significance.

[17]For 9 days after onset of swelling.

[18]Maintain precautions for duration of hospitalization when chronic disease occurs in an immunodeficient patient. For patients with transient aplastic crisis or red-cell crisis, maintain precautions for 7 days.

[19]Maintain precautions until 5 days after patient is placed on effective therapy.

[20]Avoid cohorting or placement in the same room with a CF patient who is not infected or colonized with B cepacia. Persons with CF who visit or provide care and are not infected or colonized with B cepacia may elect to wear a mask when within 3 ft of a colonized or infected patient.

[21]Avoid placement in the same room with an immunocompromised patient.

[22]Until 7 days after onset of rash.

[23]Discontinue precautions only when TB patient is on effective therapy, is improving clinically, and has three consecutive negative sputum smears collected on different days, or TB is ruled out. Also see CDC "Guidelines for preventing the Transmission of Tuberculosis in Health-Care Facilities" (23).

TOPIC 53 / **CHEMICAL AND INFECTIOUS AGENTS**

Effectiveness in Disease and Injury Prevention Control of Excessive Lead Exposure in Radiator Repair Workers

Original Citation: Centers for Disease Control and Prevention. Effectiveness in disease and injury prevention control of excessive lead exposure in radiator repair workers. MMWR 1991;40(8):139–141.

Editor's Note: Among automotive repair workers for whom a job category is specified, radiator repair work is often the principal source of lead exposure. The major sources of exposure are lead fumes generated during soldering and lead dust produced during radiator cleaning. This report describes three control technologies that are effective in reducing lead exposures in radiator repair shops.

Airborne lead levels as high as 500 $\mu g/m^3$ (10 times greater than the Occupational Safety and Health Administration (OSHA) permissible exposure limit (PEL) of 50 $\mu g/m^3$) have been reported in small radiator repair shops (3). Engineering controls in such facilities typically consist of wall- or roof-mounted propeller fans, which provide general area ventilation, or electrostatic precipitators suspended from the ceiling, which remove airborne particulates (2). However, neither method reduces worker lead exposures to levels below the OSHA PEL. In 1989, to meet the need for effective engineering controls in radiator repair shops, NIOSH researchers studied three exhaust-ventilation control systems for radiator shops. Each of the three local control systems effectively reduced radiator repair workers' lead exposures to levels substantially below the OSHA PEL. The performance of each control system was documented by collecting personal breathing-zone samples for lead and by measuring local exhaust-ventilation system airflow capacities.

VENTILATED ENCLOSURE

An enclosure resembling a laboratory hood surrounds the workstation (4). The enclosure's walls are curtains of silicone-coated fibrous glass cloth, which have a temperature rating of 1000°F (538°C), cannot be set on fire by a mechanic's torches, and will not corrode. The curtains are suspended from the building's ceiling and extend to the top outer edges of a water bath (used to leak-test radiators). The ceiling forms the top of the enclosure; the back wall of the building, which has a propeller exhaust fan, forms the rear wall. A 3-foot by 3-foot opening in the front of the enclosure permits the mechanic access to repair the radiator, which remains within the enclosure. The fan exhausts air at a rate of 2000 cubic feet per minute (cfm), producing an air flow of 200 feet per minute (fpm) through the enclosure opening.

The approximate cost of the enclosure was $1000 (1990 dollars), which included structural materials, installation, and a wall-mounted axial fan with motor. During the study of this system, lead exposures for the radiator repair worker using the ventilated enclosure averaged 9.9 $\mu g/m^3$. Comparison personal breathing-zone samples obtained from a radiator repair mechanic in the same shop who worked at an identical workstation without ventilation control averaged 453 $\mu g/m^3$.

MOVABLE EXHAUST HOOD

A canopy-shaped exhaust hood with a 24-inch by 36-inch opening is connected to an 8-inch diameter flexible duct that permits the hood to be moved directly to the work that generates lead fumes. The face velocity at the hood opening is approximately 100 fpm. The cost of the hood and duct work for each workstation was $1000 (1990 dollars). Lead exposures for the busiest mechanic averaged 12 $\mu g/m^3$. In comparison, personal sampling data collected at this shop by the Virginia Occupational Safety and Health Department before the exhaust hood installation found time-weighted average lead exposures for workers at levels as high as 193 $\mu g/m^3$ (R.D. Mitchell, Virginia Occupational Safety and Health Department, personal communication, December 20, 1988).

VENTILATED BOOTH

A shop owner, using design information provided by NIOSH, relocated the shop's two existing radiator repair benches against an outside wall and enclosed them in a booth. Cement-block walls form the sides, a welding curtain encloses the top of the booth, and a strip of plastic across the bottom 3 feet of the front of the booth creates a front opening 11.5 feet wide by 4 feet high. An axial, belt-driven fan (exhaust capacity 14,000 cfm) was installed in the outside wall at the rear of the booth, which produced a 250 fpm face velocity airflow through the front opening. The cost of the control system, including materials and labor, for two workstations was approximately $2200 (1990 dollars); this included a set of high-intensity lights costing $250. The average lead exposure for radiator repair workers using this system was 9 $\mu g/m^3$, a reduction of 91% compared with an average lead exposure of 98 $\mu g/m^3$ (range: 30–220 $\mu g/m^3$) measured during a NIOSH health hazard evaluation conducted before installation of the control (5).

Reported by: A. Miller, MD, Occupational Health and Safety Center, Univ. of Illinois at Chicago; Div. of Physical Sciences and Engineering, Div. of Surveillance, Hazard Evaluations, and Field Studies, National Institute for Occupational Safety and Health, CDC.

EDITORIAL NOTE

In general, environmental monitoring and medical surveillance for lead exposure in radiator repair workers is inadequate. For example, in California in 1986, only 1.4% of these workers were employed in positions where environmental monitoring was ever done; only 7.9% of the surveyed radiator repair shops performed any routine biologic monitoring (11). Inadequate medical surveillance of these workers can result in substantial underestimation of the number of workers at risk for lead toxicity and further underscores the need for both improved monitoring and effective engineering controls to protect the health of these workers. The three economic and effective ventilation control systems described in this report have potential for widespread application in relatively small radiator shops that lack resources for purchase of elaborate ventilation systems.***

REFERENCES: AS NUMBERED IN ORIGINAL PUBLICATION

2. Goldman RH, Baker EL, Hannan M, et al. Lead poisoning in automobile radiator mechanics. N Engl J Med 1987;317:214–218.
3. Gunter BJ, Pryor RD, NIOSH. Health hazard evaluation report no. HETA 80–89-723. Cincinnati: US Department of Health and Human Services, Public Health Service, CDC, 1980.
4. Goldfield J, Sheehy JW, Gunter BJ, Daniels WJ. Cost-effective radiator repair ventilation control. Appl Occup Environ Hyg (in press).
5. Gunter BJ, Hales T, NIOSH. Health hazard evaluation report no. HETA 89–232-2015. Cincinnati: US Department of Health and Human Services, Public Health Service, CDC, 1990.
11. Rudolph L, Sharp DS, Samuels S, Perkins C, Rosenberg J. Environmental and biological monitoring for lead exposure in California workplaces. Am J Public Health 1990;80:921–925.

Carbon Monoxide Poisoning from Use of Gasoline-Fueled Power Washers in an Underground Parking Garage

Original Citation: Carbon monoxide poisoning from use of gasoline-fueled power washers in an underground parking garage—District of Columbia, 1994. MMWR 1995; 44(18):356–357, 363–364.

Editor's Note: In 1992, CO exposure in the United States accounted for 867 nonfatal work-related poisonings that resulted in days away from work and 32 fatal work-related poisonings. The occurrence of nonfatal work-related CO poisonings probably is underestimated because workers with mild symptoms may not seek treatment, medical providers may not recognize nonspecific symptoms as manifestations of CO poisoning, and some correctly diagnosed cases may not be reported as work-related.

EDITORIAL NOTE

CO is a potentially lethal gas with nonspecific warning properties. Levels of CO uptake vary among persons and are a function of air concentration, level of exertion and ventilatory rate, and duration of exposure. For example, among workers engaged in light work and who were exposed to a CO con-

---

*** To obtain the latest reports on engineering controls for radiator repair shops, contact John W. Sheehy, NIOSH, CDC, Mailstop R-5, 4676 Columbia Parkway, Cincinnati, OH 45226; telephone (513) 841-4221.

centration of 700 ppm, COHb levels were 20% after 35 minutes and 40% after approximately 1 hour (4). In general, COHb levels greater than 20% are associated with symptoms; dizziness and unsteady gait may result from levels greater than 30% (5).

Since November 1990, Division of Occupational and Environmental Medicine (DOEM) has identified four other cases of CO poisoning among construction workers; all required emergency medical treatment (1). Two cases involved use of gasoline-powered forklifts in an enclosed warehouse, and two involved use of gasoline-fueled saws. Similar incidents have been reported among workers in other industries, including farmers using gasoline-fueled pressure washers to clean structures housing animals (6; NIOSH, unpublished data, 1993) and workers using liquid propane-powered floor burnishers to clean floors in a retail establishment (7). During January 1985–February 1995, the Colorado Department of Public Health and Environment (CDPHE) received reports of 147 cases of occupational CO poisoning related to the use of gasoline-powered equipment; of these, 13 (9%) were associated with use of pressure washers (CDPHE, unpublished data, 1995).

The investigation described in this report and other incidents indicate that many workers may not be aware of the risks of CO poisoning associated with gasoline-fueled engines and may not be able to assess accurately whether ventilation is adequate for their safe use. For example, in 1993, to characterize risk awareness and behavior related to the indoor use of small engines, NIOSH surveyed 416 persons involved in flood-cleanup activities in Missouri. Of those who had ever used a gasoline-powered pressure washer, 38% reported bringing the engine component of the washer inside a building (NIOSH, unpublished data, 1993).

The risk for CO exposure to workers can be reduced through improved ventilation. In addition, however, risk-reduction efforts must include air monitoring for CO levels. Reliable air monitoring includes the requirement for persons who have been trained to perform the monitoring and for equipment that has been properly calibrated and maintained. Training and warning labels can increase awareness among contractors and workers about the risks associated with use of gasoline-fueled equipment in enclosed spaces.

REFERENCES: AS NUMBERED IN ORIGINAL PUBLICATION

1. Hunting KL, Nessel-Stephens L, Sandford SM, Shesser R, Welch LS. Surveillance of construction worker injuries through an urban emergency department. J Occup Med 1994;36:356–364.
4. Forbes WH, Sargent F, Foughton FJW. The rate of CO uptake by normal man. Am J Physiol 1945;143: 594–608.
5. Seger DL, Welch L. Carbon monoxide. In: Sullivan JB, Krieger GR, eds. Hazardous materials toxicology: clinical principles of environmental health. Baltimore: Williams and Wilkins, 1992: 1160–1164.
6. CDC. Unintentional carbon monoxide poisoning from indoor use of pressure washers—Iowa, January 1992–January 1993. MMWR 1993;42:777–779, 785.
7. CDC. Carbon monoxide poisoning associated with a propane-powered floor burnisher—Vermont, 1992. MMWR 1993;42:726–728.

Workplace Hazards: Falls Through Skylights and Roof Openings, Deaths of Farm Workers in Manure Pits, and Exposure to Dimethylformamide

Original Citation: Centers for Disease Control and Prevention. Notices to readers NIOSH alerts on workplace hazards: falls through skylights and roof openings, deaths of farm workers in manure pits, and exposure to dimethylformamide. MMWR 1991;40(8):142–143.

CDC's National Institute for Occupational Safety and Health (NIOSH) periodically issues alerts on workplace hazards that have caused injury, illness, or death to workers. Three alerts are now available about the serious hazards posed by skylights and roof openings, manure pits, and the organic solvent dimethylformamide (DMF).* Each alert is summarized briefly below.

NIOSH ALERT: REQUEST FOR ASSISTANCE IN PREVENTING WORKER DEATHS AND INJURIES FROM FALLS THROUGH SKYLIGHTS AND ROOF OPENINGS (1)

Fatal falls frequently result from inadequate guarding and fall protection for work around skylights, skylight openings, and other roof openings. More frequent use of skylights in new construction has increased the risk to workers for such falls. This alert describes eight incidents in which workers died from falls through skylights or roof openings. NIOSH recommends four steps to prevent fatal falls through skylights and roof openings: (a) strict adherence to applicable Occupational Safety and Health Administration (OSHA) regulations, (b) adequate worker training to recognize fall hazards, (c) placement of decals on skylights to warn workers against sitting or stepping on them, and (d) design of skylights to support the weight of a worker who steps, sits, or falls on one.

NIOSH ALERT: REQUEST FOR ASSISTANCE IN PREVENTING DEATHS OF FARM WORKERS IN MANURE PITS (2)

Farm workers who enter manure pits risk death from exposure to oxygen-deficient, toxic, or explosive atmospheres resulting from fermentation of the animal wastes in these confined spaces. Gases commonly encountered in manure pits include methane, hydrogen sulfide, carbon dioxide, and ammonia. The hazards

---

* Single copies are available without charge from the Publications Dissemination Section, Division of Standards Development and Technology Transfer, NIOSH, CDC, 4676 Columbia Parkway, Cincinnati, OH 45226; telephone (513) 533-8287.

of manure pits have been known for several years, but recent NIOSH investigations suggest that many farm workers are unaware of the danger, and deaths continue to occur after entry into these pits. This alert describes two incidents (3) that resulted in seven deaths from asphyxiation in manure pits. Victims in both incidents included rescuers who were members of the same family. Deaths in manure pits occur most frequently from April through September, when warm weather may result in increased gas accumulation. Manure pits should be treated as confined spaces, with proper ventilation, testing of the atmosphere before entry, presence of a standby person outside the manure pit, and use of a safety belt or harness with a lifeline attached to mechanical lifting equipment. A positive-pressure, self-contained breathing apparatus should be used if an oxygen-deficient or toxic atmosphere is detected. No one should enter a manure pit unless it is absolutely necessary and proper precautions have been taken.

NIOSH ALERT: REQUEST FOR ASSISTANCE IN PREVENTING ADVERSE HEALTH EFFECTS FROM EXPOSURE TO DIMETHYLFORMAMIDE (DMF) (4)

NIOSH estimates that greater than 100,000 U.S. workers may be exposed to DMF, an organic solvent that is readily absorbed through the skin. This chemical is toxic to the liver and can cause skin problems and alcohol intolerance. Some reports also suggest an increase in cancer among workers exposed to DMF, but the evidence is not conclusive. DMF is used in acrylic fiber spinning, chemical manufacturing, and pharmaceutical production; it is also present in textile dyes and pigments, paint stripping solvents, and coating, printing, and adhesive formulations. Workers exposed to DMF should be informed about its adverse health effects and trained to avoid skin contact and to use appropriate protective equipment and work practices. Employers should institute engineering controls to ensure that DMF exposures do not exceed the NIOSH recommended exposure limit/OSHA permissible exposure limit of 10 ppm as an 8-hour time-weighted average (5). Environmental and biological monitoring should be instituted if skin contact with liquid DMF is possible, and medical screening should be performed under certain circumstances, as outlined in the alert.

REFERENCES: AS NUMBERED IN ORIGINAL PUBLICATION

1. NIOSH. NIOSH alert: request for assistance in preventing worker deaths and injuries from falls through skylights and roof openings. Cincinnati: US Department of Health and Human Services, Public Health Service, CDC, 1990:DHHS publication no. (NIOSH)90–100.
2. NIOSH. NIOSH alert: request for assistance in preventing deaths of farm workers in manure pits. Cincinnati: US Department of Health and Human Services, Public Health Service, CDC, 1990:DHHS publication no. (NIOSH)90–103.
3. CDC. Fatalities attributed to methane asphyxia in manure waste pits—Ohio, Michigan, 1989. MMWR 1989;38:583–586.
4. NIOSH. NIOSH alert: request for assistance in preventing adverse health effects from exposure to dimethylformamide (DMF). Cincinnati: US Department of Health and Human Services, Public Health Service, CDC, 1990:DHHS publication no. (NIOSH)90–105.
5. Office of the Federal Register. Code of federal regulations: occupational safety and health standards. Subpart Z: air contaminants—permissible exposure limits. Table Z-1-A. Washington, DC: Office of the Federal Register, National Archives and Records Administration, 1989 (29 CFR 1910.1000).

Back Belts—Do They Prevent Injury?

Original Citation: Workplace use of back belts: review and recommendations. NIOSH, Back Belt Working Group, 1994.

Editor's Note: Back injuries account for nearly 20% of all injuries and illnesses in the workplace and cost the nation an estimated 20 to 50 billion dollars per year.

In the Autumn of 1992, the Director of the National Institute for Occupational Safety and Health (NIOSH) formed a Working Group to review the scientific literature related to back belts. The Group's objective was to evaluate the adequacy of the data supporting the use of back belts to reduce work-related back injuries in healthy, previously uninjured workers. The NIOSH Back Belt Working Group has reviewed the most recent, published scientific information contained in refereed or peer-reviewed literature. Research excluded from this review related to the use of back belts prescribed by medical care providers for the treatment and rehabilitation of injured persons.

Back belts are also known as weight lifting devices, supports, or aids, and abdominal belts, which are primarily designed for use in the general population. The term "back belt" is also applied to therapeutic devices such as spinal braces, supports, corsets, and orthoses.

The term back injury is used throughout the text to refer to all back disorders, injuries, or pain. These disorders can be precipitated by a single traumatic event such as twisting, slipping, or lifting, or by the cumulative effect of repetitive trauma.

OVERALL CONCLUSIONS AND RECOMMENDATIONS

On the basis of the review of pertinent literature, the Working Group has formulated the following conclusions and recommendations.

Conclusions

The Working Group concludes that the effectiveness of using back belts to lessen the risk of back injury among uninjured workers remains unproven.

The Working Group does not recommend the use of back belts to prevent injuries among uninjured workers, and does not consider back belts to be personal protective equipment.

The Working Group further emphasizes that back belts do not mitigate the hazards to workers posed by repeated lifting, pushing, pulling, twisting, or bending.

The Working Group also concludes that:

- There are insufficient data indicating that typical industrial back belts significantly reduce the biomechanical loading of the trunk during manual lifting.

- There is insufficient scientific evidence to conclude that wearing back belts reduces risk of injury to the back based on changes in intra-abdominal pressure (GAP) and trunk muscle electromyography (EMG).
- The use of back belts may produce temporary strain on the cardiovascular system.
- There are insufficient data to demonstrate a relationship between the prevalence of back injury in healthy workers and the discontinuation of back belt use.

Recommendations

The Working Group recommends that the most effective means of minimizing the likelihood of back injury is to develop and implement a comprehensive ergonomics program. The program should include ergonomic assessments of jobs and workstations to ensure that work activity can be accomplished without exceeding the physical capabilities and capacities of the workers (Waters, et al., 1993); on-going, comprehensive training for all workers on lifting mechanics and techniques; a surveillance program to identify potential work-related musculoskeletal problems; and a medical management program.

The Working Group also recommends:

- Caution in interpreting the results of studies that evaluated the effects of belt use on predictions of biomechanical loading of the spine.
- Caution in interpreting the results of epidemiological studies; the experience with these studies should be used to develop better designed epidemiological research.
- Future research should be designed to evaluate the efficacy of wearing back belts to prevent work-related back injury.

EPIDEMIOLOGICAL STUDIES

In a retrospective study of 1,316 workers who routinely perform manual lifting activities, Mitchell, et al. [1994], investigated the effectiveness of back belts in reducing back injuries and the associated costs. The study consisted of a self-administered questionnaire to determine exposure information on lift frequency, weight of lifts and proportion of the workday spent lifting, belt use, history of back problems, and treatment for the period from 1985–1991. For the period from 1985–1986, leather belts were used, and after 1986, a standard Velcro back support with suspenders was used. Univariate analyses of factors related to initial injury revealed that previous lifting training ($P < 0.01$), previous back problems ($P < 0.001$), and amount of weight lifted per day ($P < 0.001$) were significantly correlated with initial injury, but belt use at time of injury was not ($P = 0.438$). Subsequent logistic regression analyses revealed that a history of previous back problems (Odds Ratio [OR] = 5.56, 95% Confidence Interval [CI] = 3.35, 9.26) and the amount of weight lifted per day (OR = 1.01, CI = 1.01, 1.02) were positively related to first occurrences of back injury, and that previous training (OR = 0.65, CI = 0.45, 0.93) and back belt use (OR = 0.60, CI = 0.36, 1.00) were negatively related to first back injury. It should be pointed out that the protective effects of back belts are only weakly supported. This study was limited in that back belt usage was not controlled during the course of the study and recall bias may have been introduced because the self-reported exposure and injury data covered the 6 years prior to the study and were not validated by objective data. Although the data indicate that back belts appear to be minimally effective in preventing low back injuries, the Working Group concluded that this study did not provide conclusive evidence that back belts significantly reduce risk of injury. The results do suggest, however, that certain work-related factors, namely a history of previous back problems and the daily amount of weight lifted, significantly increase the risk of back injuries.

The purpose of the prospective study by Reddell, et al. [1992], was to evaluate the efficacy of a commercially available, fabric, weight-lifting belt to lower the lumbar injury incident rate and severity of injuries over an 8-month period. At the beginning of the study, 896 airline baggage handlers who performed manual materials-handling tasks were selected and randomly placed into one of four test groups: belt only, belt and training, training only, and control group. At the end of the study, only 642 of the 896 workers were located and interviewed about back injuries and comfort of the belt. Of the 272 participants in the belt groups, 6.3% never used the belt and 52% used it less than 50% of the time (noncompliant group). A total of 28 (4.4%) job-related injuries were self-reported but were not validated: 3 (1.2%) in controls, 1 (0.8%) in training only, 3 (5.2%) in belt only and 3 (5.2%) in belt and training. The remaining 17 (10.7%) injuries occurred among the noncompliant group. Although the data are not shown, the authors report no differences among the groups for incidence rates of total injuries, restricted workday case injuries, and for severity. Yet, severity of injury based on lost workday case incidence rates indicated a significant difference among the groups. The authors concluded that 'neither the belt nor the training group had a significant effect on injury reduction' and that discontinuing belt use may increase the risk of back injury, although no data are reported to support this statement.

The Working Group concluded that these results must be tempered by the severe limitations of the data, including low participation (72%) and compliance rates (42%), potential recall biases related to self-reported injury rates, and the inclusion of previously injured workers in the study. The low, overall incidence rate of self-reported back injuries suggest that the study period was too short and the realized sample size was too small. Because of these limitations, this study could not evaluate the effectiveness of back belts on incident back injuries.

In a 2-month prospective study of construction workers, Holmstrom and Mortiz [1992] investigated the effects of two types of belts on maximal isometric trunk muscle strength and endurance. Twelve healthy male construction workers with negligible or no low back symptoms wore soft Neoprene heat-retaining belts (Group SB). Twenty-four male construction workers who had current low back pain or experienced low back pain of more than 8 days duration during the preceding year wore leather weight-lifting belts (Group WB). These previously injured workers were not considered in the Working Group's review.

The subjects wore the assigned belts during their working days, recorded daily use, and rated the intensity of pain at its occurrence. The following strength and endurance tests were measured at the start of the study and after 1 and 2 months: maximum voluntary isometric contraction of the trunk flexors and extensors, and maximum voluntary isometric endurance of trunk extensors. The differences in the mean of trunk extensor strength (start = 1.264 N, 1 month = 1.258 N, 2 months = 1.311 N) and endurance measurements (start = 182.6s, 1 month = 179.3 s, 2 months = 198.3 s) from before using the belt and after two months of belt use were not statistically significant. The 13% increase in trunk flexor strength was significant (P <0.01). The authors concluded that 2 months of daily use of a soft heat-retaining belt did not influence the trunk extensor strength or endurance, but was associated with a significant increase in trunk flexor strength.

The Working Group noted that the study is limited by a number of factors, including: the short duration of the study; the absence of an unbelted control group and assessment of the type of tasks each subject did on the job; the measurement of flexion and extension in the sagittal plane, only when the activities of construction work require various postures and motions including twisting. The Working Group also concluded that given the short duration of the observation period, the study was unable to determine the relationship between increased trunk flexor strength and worker back injury.

Walsh and Schwartz [1990] studied three groups of 81 male warehouse workers in a 6-month intervention trial. Three equal sized groups (n = 27), were separated into a control group and two intervention groups. The controls (group 1) received no training or low-back orthoses. One intervention group (group 2) received a 1-hour training session on lifting mechanics and back pain prevention, and no orthoses. The other intervention group (group 3) received 1 training session and a custom-fitted lumbosacral orthoses. This device differs from many commonly used back belts and included a heat-molded hard insert customized to the individual. No group was assigned belts without training. The trial evaluated the effect of intervention on abdominal flexion strength, injury rate, productivity, and lost work time. The authors report controls and group 2 (training only group) showed no changes in abdominal flexion strength, injury rate, productivity, or lost time. Group 3 (orthoses and training) also showed no changes in abdominal flexion strength, injury rate, or productivity. Group 3 however, lost less work time, post-training. The authors concluded that the use of intermittent prophylactic bracing had no adverse effects on abdominal flexor strength and may contribute to a decrease in lost work time from work injuries.

The selection of workers and assignment to the three groups was random and excluded individuals "currently being treated for back pain or back injury." However, exclusion from the study on the basis of prior injury was not required if treatment was not ongoing at the time of entry into the study. As a result, both control and treatment groups included previously injured workers. In fact the authors subdivided the groups into high-risk (those patients with previous injury) and low-risk (those without a history of previous injury) during the 6 months before the study.

Pretraining workdays lost were higher in the two treatment groups than in controls, suggesting a selection bias for workers with previous injuries to wear back belts. The apparent effect of decreased lost time from work injury in group 3 (training and orthoses) was only seen in those workers with previous low back injury. No difference in lost workdays was observed for any of the treatment groups composed of workers without a prior history of injury. The findings from this study may more accurately define the therapeutic benefit of back belts in previously injured workers rather than clarifying the preventive role of these belts in previously healthy workers.

Early physiological and biomechanical studies suggested that discontinuing the use of back belts after a period of prolonged use may place a worker at greater risk of back injury. This hypothesis, proposed by Harman in 1989 in relation to IAP changes, received support by Reddell, et al. [1992], who reported that workers who discontinued the use of belts had injury rates higher than the control group and the group that did not discontinue. However, the Reddell results are open to different interpretations because of severe limitations of the data. In addition, a recent study by Holmstrom and Moritz [1992], found that after 2 months of soft belt wearing, trunk extensor strength and endurance were unchanged, and trunk flexor strength increased, casting doubt on the muscle detraining-injury hypothesis. Finally, McGill, et al. [1990], found the contraction level of abdominal muscles was so slight during experimental lifting with or without a belt, that a detraining effect from belt wearing is highly unlikely. The Working Group concluded that because of critical methodological limitations of published epidemiologic studies, there is insufficient data to demonstrate a relationship between the prevalence of back injury in healthy workers and the discontinuation of back belt use. However, this theory should be evaluated in future epidemiologic investigations of long-term back belt users.

SUMMARY CONCLUSIONS AND RECOMMENDATIONS FOR REVIEWED STUDIES

Biomechanical Studies

The Working Group concludes that there are insufficient data to indicate that typical industrial-type back belts (i.e., those designed for use in the workplace, as compared to medical or therapeutic orthoses) significantly reduce the biomechanical loading of the trunk during manual lifting. No studies provided conclusive evidence that actual trunk muscle forces, predicted spinal compression, or shear forces were significantly reduced by wearing a back belt.

This conclusion is based on our review of studies that evaluated the effects of belt usage on predictions of biomechanical loading of the spine. These reductions were determined from various physiological and biomechanical parameters that were measured during lifting, such as IAP, EMG activity, IDP, anthropometry, body kinematics, and ground reaction forces.

The results of studies reviewed by the Working Group were inconclusive regarding the effects of back belts on spinal loading. Some suggested that back belts reduce spinal loading under certain conditions, while others were less conclusive. The Working Group recommends caution in interpreting these results, however, for the following reasons. First, the results are based on numerous assumptions about the relationship between spinal loading and measurable physiological and biomechanical parameters, which may not be valid when a belt is worn. For example, the addition of a belt may impose other unknown mechanical effects that alter the relationship between IAP and spinal compression. A more basic question, which has not been sufficiently addressed, is the validity of the core assumption that IAP reduces intra-abdominal pressure and spinal compression. Second, it is not possible to verify the accuracy of the predictions of changes in spinal loading. Because of ethical considerations, measurement of IDP, which may be the best measure of spinal compression to date, has been limited to a few studies. Third, if lifting belts' appreciably affect the magnitude of spinal loading, then the resulting spinal loading from wearing a belt would be significantly affected by the mechanical characteristics of the various belt designs and the way they are worn. In the studies reviewed, however, these factors were not controlled.

A few studies suggest that back belts may reduce the range of spinal motion for a person wearing a belt during a lifting activity. Theoretically, this reduction in range of motion could diminish the necessary torque around the lower spine by reducing the muscle force required to support the body. This in turn would reduce the compression force on the spine. The limited studies available, however, do not indicate that typical industrial-type belts sufficiently reduce range of motion about the spine to significantly reduce loading on the spinal structures. Moreover, it is possible that the resistance provided by a belt may increase loading on the spine, especially during asymmetric lifting, because of the necessity to increase muscle forces to overcome the resistance of the belt. Therefore, the Working Group concludes that there is insufficient evidence to recommend the use of back belts on the basis of reduction in range of motion.

Based on an analysis of available literature, the Working Group recommends that intervention strategies other than back belts be used to reduce biomechanical loading on the spine during manual material handling.

Physiological Studies

A number of studies have evaluated various physiologic parameters during back belt use, including IAP, EMG, heart rate and blood pressure. Other studies have suggested that abdominal and back extensor muscle strength changes with prolonged back belt use.

Some authors have extrapolated beyond their results to argue that a hypothesized protective effect of increased IAP exists. These extrapolations are based on assumptions about the role of IAP in reducing spinal forces; such assumptions have yet to be validated. IAP fairly conclusively increases when belt is worn in the ranges of lifted weights reported, and at least some other indicators (mainly psychophysical) have also been in the "good" direction during increased IAP. Therefore, it is implied that belt-wearing and its increased IAP is good or "protective." While belt-wearing may increase IAP during lifting activities, the studies that have simultaneously assessed muscle EMG have been inconclusive; the lack of consistency is caused by a variety of technical problems, methodological deficiencies, and incomplete analyses. At present, no scientific evidence exists for concluding that belt-wearing is protective to an industrial population on the basis of changes in IAP and trunk muscle EMG.

The nature of the exact physiological and biomechanical mechanism that could result in the hypothesized protection remains to be determined. Presently, an adequate model of increased-IAP effects has yet to be developed. Restriction of motion coincident with the increased IAP is possibly more important than muscle EMG readings in "protection"; in that case, even the absence of an inverse relationship between IAP and EMG may be irrelevant.

Consideration of the effects of prolonged back-belt use on back and abdominal muscle tone and cardiovascular health is also necessary. The results of a single, well-conducted study found significant increases in heart rate during aerobic activity and systolic blood pressure during both aerobic and isometric exercises. The Working Group concluded that the use of back belts can put a strain on the cardiovascular system and that individuals with a compromised cardiovascular system may be at greater risk when exercising or working with back supports.

Biomechanical studies have suggested that long-term use of back supports may decrease abdominal muscle tone, thereby increasing the likelihood of back injury if the user discontinued use of the back belt. The Working Group concluded that because of critical methodological limitations of published epidemiologic studies, there is insufficient data to demonstrate a relationship between the prevalence of back injury in healthy workers and the discontinuation of back belt use. However, this theory should be evaluated in future epidemiologic investigations of long-term back-belt users.

Psychophysical Studies

Only a limited number of studies use psychophysical techniques to assess the subject's perception of acceptable lifting loads or back pain and discomfort while lifting either with and without back belts. No study has evaluated the relationship between the subject or worker is perception of maximum acceptable workload and low back injury. The available data suggest that subjects lifted significantly heavier loads with the belt than without and report less discomfort lifting with a back belt than without. This perception of protection while wearing a back belt may not reflect the individual's ability to lift a heavier load or lack of discomfort, but may reflect the effect of using a treatment, also known as the "Hawthorne Effect." No study that used psychophysical techniques suggested that its results may have been biased by the prestudy assumptions of the subjects relative to back belt use. Additional studies are necessary to delineate these possible effects.

As a result, the Working Group has concerns about how wearing a belt may alter a worker's perception of capacity to lift heavy workloads when wearing a belt (i.e., belt wearing may foster an increased sense of security, which may not be warranted or substantiated).

Epidemiologic Studies

The use of epidemiologic methods to evaluate the effectiveness of back belts in reducing and preventing low back injury in uninjured workers is relatively recent. Three of the four studies in this review suffer at least some of the pitfalls of intervention studies that, by design, attempt to change long-standing attitudes, personal behaviors and work practices. Unfortunately, methodological limitations of most, if not all of the studies, also restrict the ability to interpret the results concerning the assessment of back belts' efficacy in reducing work-related back injuries. A few of the critical problems include, but are not limited to, low participation rates, inadequate observation periods, small sample sizes, relatively low back-injury rates, inclusion of individuals with previous back injuries, and recall and reporting biases of current and previous injuries and exposures.

The Working Group recommends that the results of the epidemiologic studies be interpreted with caution and that the experience of these studies be used to develop better designed epidemiologic research. The Working Group also recommends that future research designed to evaluate the efficacy of back belts in reducing and preventing work-related back injury include only previously uninjured female and male workers representative of the age range of the U.S. working population. The group further recommends that the belts be the types that are typically used in the workplace rather than for medical orthoses, that the jobs of workers wearing belts be analyzed as part of the study, that self-reports of back injury be validated using medical records, and that the term "back injury" be defined using codes from the International Classification of Diseases (ICD) or some other standard terminology.

REFERENCES

Bourne ND, Reilly T. Effect of a weight lifting belt on spinal shrinkage. Br J Sports Med 1991;25(4):209–212.

Grew ND, Deane G. The physical effects of lumbar spine supports. Prosthet Orthot Int 1982;6:79–87.

Harman EA, Rosenstein RM, Frykman PN, Nigro GA. Effects of a belt on intra-abdominal pressure during weight lifting. Med Sci Sports Exerc 1989;21(2):186–190.

Hilgen TH, Smith LA. The minimum abdominal belt-aided lifting weight. In: Karwoski W, Yates JW, eds. Advances in industrial ergonomics and safety HI. New York: Taylor & Francis, 1991:217–224.

Holmstrom E, Moritz U. Effect of lumbar belts on trunk muscle strength and endurance: a follow-up study of construction workers. J Spinal Disord 1992;5(3):260–266.

Hunter GR, McGuirk J, Mitrano N, Pearman P, Thomas B, Arrington R. The effects of a weight training belt on blood pressure during exercise. J Appl Sport Sci Res 1989;3:13–18.

Kumar S, Godfrey CM. Spinal braces and abdominal support. In: Karwoski W, ed. Trends in ergonomics/human factors III. New York: Elsevier Science Publishers, 1986:717–725.

Lander JE, Simonton RL, Giacobbe JKF. The effectiveness of weight-belts during the squat exercise. Med Sci Sports Exerc 1990;22:117–126.

Lander JE, Hundley JR, Simonton RL. The effectiveness of weight-belts during multiple repetitions of the
    squat exercise. Med Sci Sports Exerc 1992;24:603–609.
Lantz SA, Schultz AB. Lumbar spine orthosis wearing: I. Restrictions of gross body motions. Spine 1986a;
    11:834–837.
Lantz SA, Schultz AB. Lumbar spine orthosis wearing: II. Effect on trunk muscle myoelectric activity. Spine
    1986b;11:838–842.
McCoy MA, Congleton JJ, Johnson WL. The role of lifting belts in manual lifting. Int J Ind Ergon 1988;
    2:259–266.
McGill SM, Norman RW, Sharratt MT. The effect of an abdominal belt on trunk muscle activity and intra-
    abdominal pressure during squat lifts. Ergonomics 1990;323:147–160.
McGill S, Seguin J, Bennett G. Passive stiffness of the upper torso in flexion, extension, lateral bending, and
    axial rotation: effect of belt wearing and breath holding. Spine 1994;19(6):696–704.
Mitchell LV, Lawler FH, Bowen D, Mote W, Asundi P, Purswell J. Effectiveness and cost-effectiveness of em-
    ployer-issued back belts in areas of high risk for back injury. J Occup Med 1994;36(1):90–94.
Nachemson A, Schultz A, Andersson G. Mechanical effectiveness studies of lumbar spine orthoses. Scand J
    Rehabil Med 1983;9:139–149.
Reddell CR, Congleton JJ, Huchingson RD, Montgomery JF. An evaluation of a weightlifting belt and back
    injury prevention training class for airline baggage handlers. Appl Ergon 1992;223:319–329.
Walsh NE, Schwartz RK. The influence of prophylactic orthoses on abdominal strength and low back injury
    in the workplace. Am J Phys Med Rehabil 1990;69:245–250.
Waters RL, Morris JM. Effect of spinal supports on the electrical activity of muscles of the trunk. J Bone Joint
    Surg 1970;52A(1):51–60.
Waters TR, Anderson VP, Garg A, Fine LJ. Revised NIOSH equation for the design and evaluation of man-
    ual lifting tasks. Ergonomics 1993;366:749–776.
Woodhouse ML, Heinen JR, Shall L, Bragg K. Selected isokinetic lifting parameters of adult male athletes
    utilizing lumbar/sacral supports. JOSPT 1990;11:467–473.

Applications Manual for the Revised NIOSH Lifting Equation

Original Citation: Centers for Disease Control and Prevention. Applications manual for
the revised NIOSH lifting equation, January 1994.

Original Authors: Thomas R. Waters, PhD, Vern Putz-Anderson, PhD, Arun Garg, PhD.

Editor's Note: We have included only a precis of this long and technical manual, which is a must for anyone working to reduce back injuries associated with lifting. The detailed equations and tables are brought
to life with 15 very clearly worked-out and illustrated real-life examples.

FOREWORD

This Manual was developed to provide users of the revised NIOSH lifting equation (1991 version) with methods for accurately applying the lifting equation to
a variety of lifting tasks. All necessary terms, definitions, and data requirements
for the revised equation are provided in Section 1. Procedures for analyzing sin-
gle-task and multi-task lifting jobs are described in Section 2. A series of ten lifting tasks is included in Section 3 to illustrate application of the procedure. For
each task, a brief **job description** is provided, followed by a **job analysis,** and a
hazard assessment, including a completed worksheet. Suggestions for redesign
of the task are also provided.

The rationale and supporting criteria for the development of the revised
NIOSH lifting equation are described in a journal article, Revised NIOSH
Equation for the Design and Evaluation of Manual Lifting Tasks, by T. Waters,

V. Putz-Anderson, A. Garg, and L. Fine, Ergonomics 1993. The revised equation reflects research findings published subsequent to the publication of the original NIOSH equation (1981) and includes consideration of additional components of lifting tasks such as asymmetrical lifting and quality of hand-container couplings as well as a larger range of work durations and lifting frequencies than did the 1981 equation. It must be noted that application of this equation is limited to those conditions for which it was designed. It does not, for example, address such task factors as one-handed lifting, lifting extremely hot or cold objects, or factors that may increase the risk of a slip or fall and other non-lifting components of job tasks.

Although the revised lifting equation has not been fully validated, the recommended weight limits derived from the revised equation are consistent with, or lower than, those generally reported in the literature (Waters, et al., 1993, Tables 2, 4, and 5). Moreover, the proper application of the revised equation is more likely to protect healthy workers for a wider variety of lifting tasks than methods that rely only a single task factor or single criterion.

Finally, it should be stressed that the NIOSH lifting equation is only one tool in a comprehensive effort to prevent work-related low back pain and disability. [Other approaches to prevention are described elsewhere (ASPH/NIOSH, 1986)]. Moreover, lifting is only one of the causes of work-related low back pain and disability. Other causes which have been hypothesized or established as risk factors include whole body vibration, static postures, prolonged sitting, and direct trauma to the back. Psychosocial factors, appropriate medical treatment, and job demands (past and present) also may be particularly important in influencing the transition of acute low back pain to chronic disabling pain.

REFERENCES

ASPH/NIOSH. Proposed national strategies for the prevention of leading work-related diseases and injuries, Part I. Washington, DC: Association of Schools of Public Health under a cooperative agreement with the National Institute for Occupational Safety and Health, 1986.

Ayoub MM, Mital A. Manual materials handling. London: Taylor & Francis, 1989.

Chaffin DB, Andersson GBJ. Occupational biomechanics. New York: John Wiley and Sons, 1984.

DOL(BLS). Back injuries associated with lifting. Bulletin No. 2144. Washington, DC: U.S. Department of Labor, Bureau of Labor Statistics, 1982.

Eastman Kodak Company, Ergonomics Group. Ergonomic design for people at work. Vol. 2. New York: Van Nostrand Reinhold, 1986.

Gallagher S, Marras WS, Bobick TG. Lifting in stooped and kneeling postures: effects on lifting capacity, metabolic costs, and electromyography of eight trunk muscles Intern J Indus Ergonomics 1988;3:65–76.

Gallagher S, Unger RL. Lifting in four restricted lifting conditions: psychophysical, physiological and biomechanical effects of lifting in stooped and kneeling postures. App Ergonomics 1990;21:237–245.

Gallagher S. Acceptable weights and physiological costs of performing combined manual handling tasks in restricted postures. Ergonomics 1991;34(7):939–952.

Garg A. Epidemiological basis for manual lifting guidelines. 1991:NIOSH project report (available from the National Technical Information Service, NTIS number 91–227-348).

Garg A, Chaffin DC, Herrin GD. Prediction of metabolic rates for manual materials handling jobs. Am Indus Hyg Assoc J 1978;39(8):661–764.

National Safety Council. Accident facts. Chicago: National Safety Council, 1990.

NIOSH. Work practices guide for manual lifting. NIOSH technical report no. 81–122. Cincinnati: U.S. Department of Health and Human Services, National Institute for Occupational Safety and Health, 1981.

Waters TR. Strategies for assessing multi-task manual lifting jobs. Proceedings of the Human Factors Society 35th Annual Meeting—1991. San Francisco, CA: 1991.

Waters TR, Putz-Anderson V, Garg A, Fine LJ. Revised NIOSH equation for the design and evaluation of manual lifting tasks. Ergonomics 1993;36(7):749–776.

Preventing Deaths and Injuries of Adolescent Workers

Original Citation: NIOSH. Preventing deaths and injuries of adolescent workers. DHHS (NIOSH) Publication No. 95–125.

RISK OF WORK-RELATED INJURIES AMONG ADOLESCENTS

Deaths

The U.S. Bureau of Labor Statistics identified 136 work-related deaths of adolescents under age 18 in 1992 and 1993 (68 deaths each year) [Derstine 1994; Toscano and Windau 1994]. Agricultural businesses and retail trade accounted for the most deaths (Table 1). Many of the deaths of adolescents under age 16 occurred in family-owned businesses.

Table 1. Fatal work-related injury deaths of U.S. adolescents by industry and age, 1992–93

Age of worker and industry	Number of deaths
Workers under age 14:	
Agriculture, forestry and fishing	21 (16 in family businesses)
Other	6
Total	27
Workers aged 14 and 15:	
Agriculture, forestry and fishing	12 (7 in family businesses)
Retail trade	6
Services	3
Other	8
Total	29
Workers aged 16 and 17:	
Retail trade	25 (3 in family businesses)
Agriculture, forestry and fishing	20 (5 in family businesses)
Construction	11
Services	10
Wholesale trade	5
Manufacturing	4
Other	5
Total	80

Source: Derstine [1994].

Adolescent and adult workers have similar risks of fatal occupational injuries. NIOSH has determined that in 1980–89, the risk of injury death for workers aged 16 and 17 was 5.1 per 100,000 full-time equivalent workers compared with 6.0 for adult workers aged 18 and older [Castillo et al. 1994]. This similarity in risk is cause for concern because adolescents are employed less frequently in especially hazardous jobs. The rate of fatal injuries among adolescents should therefore be much lower than for adults.

NONFATAL INJURIES

NIOSH estimates that 64,000 adolescents required treatment in hospital emergency rooms for work-related injuries in 1992 [Layne et al. 1994]. However, research indicates that only one-third of work-related injuries are seen in emergency rooms [CDC 1983]. NIOSH therefore estimates that nearly 200,000 adolescents suffer work-related injuries each year. A substantial number of injured adolescents require hospitalization. From July through December 1992, an estimated 950 adolescents were hospitalized for their injuries [Layne et al. 1994].

Compared with adult workers, adolescents have a high risk of work-related injuries requiring treatment in hospital emergency rooms. Nearly 6 of every 100 full-time equivalent adolescent workers obtain treatment in hospital emergency rooms each year [Layne et al. 1994]. Data from a 1982 study that collected data for workers of all ages suggest that workers under age 18 have higher injury rates than adult workers [CDC 1983].

Sixty-eight percent of occupationally injured 14- to 16-year-olds experienced limitations in their normal activities (including work, school, and play) for at least 1 day, and 25% experienced limitation in their normal activities for more than a week [Knight et al. 1995]. More than half of these adolescents reported that they had not received any training in how to prevent the injury they sustained. A supervisor was present at the time of the injury in only about 20% of the cases.

WORK ASSOCIATED WITH LARGE NUMBERS OF DEATHS AND SERIOUS INJURIES

Federal child labor laws prohibit some work associated with large numbers of deaths and serious injuries—such as driving a motor vehicle and operating a forklift. Other hazardous activities, such as working alone in retail businesses and cooking, are typically permitted.

WORKING IN OR AROUND MOTOR VEHICLES

Motor-vehicle-related deaths accounted for nearly one-fourth of the work-related injury deaths of 16- and 17-year-olds during the period 1980–89 [Castillo et al. 1994]. These deaths include those of workers who were drivers and passengers in motor vehicles, pedestrians, and bicyclists involved in crashes with motor vehicles.

The following jobs are examples of work that may be associated with motor-vehicle-related deaths and injuries:

- Delivery of passengers or goods (such as furniture, appliances, parcels, messages, newspapers, pizzas, groceries, and pharmaceuticals).
- Services that require routine travel to provide home-based service such as cable television installation and repair, appliance repair, and landscaping services.
- Residential trash pickup.
- Road maintenance (such as operation of sweepers).
- Work at road construction sites (including flagpersons).
- Work at gas stations, truck stops and auto repair shops.

OPERATING TRACTORS AND OTHER HEAVY EQUIPMENT

Machine-related deaths were the second leading cause of work-related injury death for 16- and 17-year-olds for the years 1980–89 [Castillo et al. 1994]. Tractors alone accounted for 44% of the machine-related deaths.

The following lists examples of heavy equipment associated with deaths:

- Tractors used in farm settings and nonfarm settings such as construction
- Forklifts.
- Excavating machinery such as backhoes, bulldozers, steam and power shovels, and trenchers.
- Loaders such as bucket loaders, end loaders, and front-end loaders.
- Road grading and surfacing machinery such as asphalt and mortar spreaders, graders, levelers, planers, scrapers, road linemarking machinery, steam rollers, and road pavers.

WORKING NEAR ELECTRICAL HAZARDS

Electrocution was the third leading cause of work-related injury death among 16-and 17-year-olds for the years 1980–89 [Castillo et al. 1994]. Electrocution accounted for a greater proportion of work-related injury deaths in adolescents than in adults (12% versus 7%). Contact with an energized power line caused more than 50% of the electrocutions.

The following types of work pose an increased risk for electrocution:

- Using poles, pipes, and ladders near overhead power lines during construction work, painting, and pool cleaning.
- Working on roofs to perform jobs such as roofing, roof maintenance, cleaning of rain gutters, installation and repair of heating and cooling equipment, installation and repair of television antennas, and cleaning of chimneys and smoke stacks.
- Operating or contacting boomed vehicles, such as bucket trucks, telescopic forklifts, and telescopic cranes.
- Using grain augers and moving grain elevators and irrigation pipes near power lines.
- Tree trimming.
- Wiring of electrical circuits and other work involving exposure to electrical circuitry, including work performed by electricians' helpers.

WORKING AT JOBS WITH A HIGH RISK FOR HOMICIDE

In 1993, assaults and violent acts accounted for about one-fourth of all work-related injury deaths of adolescents [Toscano and Windau 1994]. Most work-related homicides are associated with robbery (75% in 1993).

The following types of jobs involve increased risk for work-related homicide:

- Working alone or in small numbers in businesses where money is exchanged with the public and the risk for robbery-related homicide is high—for example, in convenience stores, gas stations, restaurants, hotels, and motels.
- Working alone in contact with large numbers of people where there may be opportunities for uninterrupted assaults—for example, working in motel housekeeping, delivery of passengers or goods, and door-to-door sales.

WORKING WITH FALL HAZARDS

Falls were the fifth leading cause of work-related injury death for 16- and 17-year-olds during the years 1980–89 [Castillo et al. 1994]; they accounted for 8% of these deaths in 1993 [Toscano and Windau 1994]. Forty percent of fatal falls were from or out of a building or other structure [Castillo et al. 1994]. Fatal falls were documented for distances ranging from 10 feet to 14 floors.

The following types of jobs are associated with work-related falls:

- Using ladders and scaffolds to work at heights—such as, in building construction, building maintenance (brick cleaning and window washing), painting, and harvesting fruit from trees.
- Working on structures or near openings in building construction.
- Working on roofs.
- Tree trimming.

COOKING AND WORKING AROUND COOKING APPLIANCES

Severe burns are a risk for adolescents involved in cooking. An estimated 5,200 adolescents sought emergency-room treatment for work-related burns associated with cooking or working in a place where food was prepared during the 18-month period from July 1992 through December 1993 [NIOSH 1994].

The following types of work involve burn hazards associated with cooking:

- Cooking in restaurants and other commercial settings.
- Servicing cooking equipment—adding, filtering, and removing hot grease from fryers, and cleaning grills and fryers and their associated vents.
- Working near cooking appliances where workers may slip into or against equipment.

HAZARDOUS MANUAL LIFTING

From July 1992 through December 1993, overexertion accounted for approximately 4,500 work-related injuries of adolescents treated in hospital emergency rooms; about 2,500 of these injuries were attributed to lifting [NIOSH 1994]. These estimates are conservative, since sprains and strains that result from repeated stress on the body (as opposed to a single injurious event) are often not treated in emergency rooms but by private physicians or clinics. Sprains and strains associated with lifting are frequently severe [Parker et al. 1994]. Although an individual's ability to safely lift objects varies, work for adolescents should not generally require them to lift objects weighing greater than 15 pounds more than once per minute or to lift objects weighing greater than 30 pounds; tasks involving continuous lifting should never last more than 2 hours [NIOSH 1994].

The following types of work may involve hazardous manual lifting:

- Working in warehouses.
- Delivering furniture and appliances.
- Retrieving, carrying, or stocking shelves with relatively heavy items.
- Working in health care settings where patients are lifted and moved.
- Installing or removing carpet or tile.
- Baling hay.

OTHER HAZARDOUS WORK

Many particularly hazardous jobs are prohibited by Federal child labor laws. These are summarized in the Appendix [DOL 1990a,b]. Other particularly hazardous work that is not typically prohibited by Federal child labor laws includes work in petroleum and gas extraction, commercial fishing, many jobs that require use of respirators, work in sewage treatment plants or sewers, work on industrial conveyors, many uses of compressed air or pneumatic tools such as nail guns, farm work using all-terrain vehicles, and work around many types of machines with power take-offs or similarly rotating drivelines [NIOSH 1994].

ADDITIONAL HEALTH CONCERNS FOR ADOLESCENT WORKERS

In addition to injuries, hazardous materials and working conditions are also a concern for adolescent workers. Less is known about them than the effects of injuries (which have an immediate impact and can be counted and classified as to cause). Exposures of adolescent workers to hazardous materials and working conditions may result in an immediate illness; however, illness might not be detected for months or years after exposure. Adolescent workers may be exposed to pesticides in farm work and lawn care, benzene at gasoline stations, lead in auto body repair, asbestos and silica in construction and maintenance work, and high levels of noise in manufacturing, construction, and agriculture [Committee on Environmental Health 1995; Pollack et al. 1990; NIOSH 1994]. Concerns have also been raised that fatigue from balancing work and school may contribute to injuries among adolescent workers [Miller 1995].

EXISTING REGULATIONS

Occupational safety and health regulations apply to adolescent and adult workers. Federal and State child labor laws provide additional protection for workers under age 18. When Federal and State regulations differ on the same issue, the more protective law applies.

OSHA

The Occupational Safety and Health Administration (OSHA) within the Department of Labor is the Federal agency with primary responsibility for setting and enforcing standards to promote safe and healthful working conditions for all workers. OSHA standards may require specific conditions in the workplace or the use of specific practices, methods, or processes to promote safe work. Employers are responsible for becoming familiar with standards applicable to their establishments and for ensuring a safe working environment.

Violations of occupational safety and health regulations have been associated with deaths of adolescents. Of the 104 deaths of adolescents under age 18 investigated by OSHA between

1984 and 1987, citations for safety violations were issued in 70% of the deaths [Suruda and Halperin 1991].

FEDERAL CHILD LABOR LAWS

The primary law governing the employment of workers under age 18 is the Fair Labor Standards Act, which is enforced by the Wage and Hour Division of the Employment Standards Administration within the Department of Labor. Child labor provisions of this act are designed to protect the educational opportunities of minors and prohibit their employment in jobs and under conditions that could harm their health or well-being.

Federal child labor laws restrict hours and types of work for 14- and 15-year-olds and set minimum ages for work declared hazardous under the law. Hazardous farm work (see Appendix A) is prohibited for adolescents under age 16 [DOL 1990a], but children working on family farms are exempt from Federal child labor laws. Hazardous work in nonfarm businesses including family businesses (see Appendix A) is prohibited for adolescents under age 18 [DOL 1990b].

Violations of Federal child labor laws are common and have been associated with serious injury and death. An estimated 1,475 youths incurred serious injuries as a result of illegal employment between 1983 and 1990 [GAO 1991]. Research on work-related deaths of adolescents has found that 38% to 86% of the deaths are associated with prohibited activities [Castillo et al. 1994; Dunn and Runyan 1993; Suruda and Halperin 1991; GAO 1990].

STATE CHILD LABOR LAWS

States also have child labor laws. They may be stricter than Federal child labor laws.

RECOMMENDATIONS

EMPLOYERS

NIOSH recommends that employers take the following steps to protect adolescent workers:

- Know and comply with child labor laws and occupational safety and health regulations that apply to your business. Post these regulations for workers to read.
- Assess and eliminate the potential for injury or illness associated with tasks required of adolescents.
- Provide training to ensure that adolescents recognize hazards and are competent in safe work practices.
- Routinely verify that the adolescents continue to recognize hazards and employ safe work practices.
- Evaluate equipment that adolescents are required to operate to ensure that it is both legal and safe for use by adolescents.
- Ensure that adolescents are appropriately supervised to prevent injuries and hazardous exposures.
- Involve supervisors and experienced workers in developing an injury and illness prevention program and in identifying and solving safety and health problems.

PARENTS

Parents should take the following steps to protect adolescent workers:

- Take an active role in the employment decisions of your children.
- Discuss the types of work involved and the training and supervision provided by the employer.

EDUCATORS

Educators should take the following steps to protect adolescent workers:

- If you are responsible for signing work permits, know the State and Federal child labor laws.
- Talk to students about safety and health hazards in the workplace and students' rights and responsibilities as workers.

- Ensure that school-based work experience programs (such as vocational education programs and School-to-Work programs) provide students with work experience in safe and healthful environments free of recognized hazards.
- Ensure that school-based work experience programs incorporate information about workers' legal rights and responsibilities and training in hazard recognition and safe work practices.
- Consider incorporating information about workers' rights and responsibilities and occupational safety and health into high school and junior high curricula to prepare students for the world of work.

ADOLESCENTS

Adolescent workers should take the following steps to protect themselves:

- Be aware that you have the right to work in a safe and healthful work environment free of recognized hazards and that you have the right to refuse unsafe work tasks and conditions.
- Know that you have the right to file complaints with the U.S. Department of Labor when you feel your rights have been violated or your safety has been jeopardized.
- Remember that adolescent workers are entitled to workers' compensation in the event of work injury or illness.
- Obtain information about your rights and responsibilities as workers from school counselors and State labor departments.
- Participate in any training programs offered by your employer, or request training if none is offered.
- Recognize the potential for injury at work and seek information about safe work practices from employers and State labor departments.
- Follow safe work practices.

REFERENCES

Castillo DN, Landen DD, Layne LA. Occupational injury deaths of 16- and 17-year-olds in the United States. Am J Public Health 1994;84(4):646–649.

CDC (Centers for Disease Control and Prevention). Surveillance of occupational injuries treated in hospital emergency departments. MMWR 1983;32(2SS):31SS-37SS.

Committee on Environmental Health. The hazards of child labor. Pediatrics 1995;95(2):311–313.

DOL. Child labor requirements in agriculture under the Fair Labor Standards Act. Washington, DC: U.S. Department of Labor, Employment Standards Administration, Wage and Hour Division, Child Labor Bulletin No. 102, 1990a.

DOL. Child labor requirements in nonagricultural occupations under the Fair Labor Standards Act. Washington, DC: U.S. Department of Labor, Employment Standards Administration, Wage and Hour Division, WH 1330, 1990b.

Derstine B. Youth worker at risk of fatal injuries. Paper presented at the 122nd Annual Meeting of the American Public Health Association, October 30, 1994. Washington, DC: 1994.

Dunn KA, Runyan CW. Deaths at work among children and adolescents. Am J Dis Child 1993;147: 1044–1047.

GAO. Child labor: characteristics of working children. Washington, DC: U.S. General Accounting Office, 1991:GAO/HRD-91-83BR.

GAO. Child labor: increases in detected child labor violations throughout the United States. Washington, DC: U.S. General Accounting Office, 1990:GAO/HRD-90-116.

Knight EB, Castillo DN, Layne LA. A detailed analysis of work-related injury among youth treated in emergency departments. Am J Ind Med 1995;27:793–805.

Layne LA, Castillo DN, Stout N, Cutlip P. Adolescent occupational injuries requiring hospital emergency department treatment: a nationally representative sample. Am J Public Health 1994;84(4): 657–660.

Miller M. Occupational injuries among adolescents in Washington State, 1988–1991: a review of workers' compensation data. Olympia, WA: Washington State Department of Labor and Industries, 1995:Technical Report No. 35-1-1995.

NIOSH. Comments of the National Institute for Occupational Safety and Health on the Department of Labor/Wage and Hour Division advance notice of proposed rulemaking on child labor regulations, orders and statements of interpretation. Cincinnati: U.S. Department of Health and Human Services, Public Health Service, Centers for Disease Control and Prevention, National Institute for Occupational Safety and Health, Division of Standards Development and Technology Transfer, 1994.

Parker DL, Carl WR, French LR, Martin FB. Characteristics of adolescent work injuries reported to the Minnesota Department of Labor and Industry. Am J Public Health 1994;84(4):606–611.

Pollack SH, Landrigan PJ, Mallino DL. Child labor in 1990: prevalence and health hazards. Ann Rev Public Health 1990;11:359–375.

Suruda A, Halperin W. Work-related deaths in children. Am J Ind Med 1991;19(6):739–745.

Toscano G, Windau J. The changing character of fatal work injuries. Monthly Labor Review 1994; 118:17–28.

APPENDIX A

Extremely Hazardous Jobs Prohibited by Federal Child Labor Laws

Farm work declared hazardous under Federal child labor laws [DOL 1990a]:

- Operating a tractor of more than 20 power-take-off horsepower, or connecting or disconnecting an implement or any of its parts to or from such a tractor
- Operating or helping to operate any of the following machines:
  - Corn picker
  - Cotton picker
  - Grain combine
  - Hay mower
  - Forage harvester
  - Hay baler
  - Potato digger
  - Mobile pea viner
  - Feed grinder
  - Crop dryer
  - Forage blower
  - Auger conveyor
  - Unloading mechanism of a nongravity-type, self-unloading wagon or trailer
  - Power post-hole digger
  - Power post driver
  - Nonwalking-type rotary tiller
  - Trencher or earthmoving equipment
  - Forklift
  - Potato combine
  - Power-driven circular, band, or chain saw
- Working on a farm in a yard, pen, or stall occupied by one or more of the following:
  - Bull, boar, or stud horse maintained for breeding purposes
  - Sow with suckling pigs
  - Cow with newborn calf (with umbilical cord present)
- Felling, bucking, skidding, loading, or unloading timber with a butt diameter of more than 6 inches
- Working from a ladder or scaffold (painting, repairing, or building structures, pruning trees, picking fruit, etc.) at a height greater than 20 feet
- Driving a bus, truck, or automobile when transporting passengers, or riding on a tractor as a passenger or helper
- Working inside one of the following:
  - A fruit, forage, or grain storage area designed to retain an oxygen-deficient or toxic atmosphere
  - An upright silo within 2 weeks of adding silage or with a top unloading device in operating position
  - A manure pit

- A horizontal silo while operating a tractor for packing purposes
- Handling or applying agricultural chemicals identified by the word "Danger," "Poison" with skull and crossbones, or "Warning" on the label
- Handling or using a blasting agent—including (but not limited to) dynamite, black powder, sensitized ammonium nitrate, blasting caps, and primer cord
- Transporting, transferring, or applying anhydrous ammonia

Nonfarm work declared hazardous under Federal child labor laws [DOL 1990b]:

- Manufacturing and storing explosives
- Motor vehicle driving and working as outside helper
- Coal mining
- Logging and sawmilling
- Operating power-driven woodworking machines
- Work involving exposure to radioactive substances
- Operating power-driven hoisting apparatus
- Operating power-driven metal-forming, punching, and shearing machines
- Mining, other than coal mining
- Power-driven bakery machines
- Slaughtering, meat-packing, processing, or rendering
- Operating power-driven paper products machines
- Manufacturing brick, tile, and kindred products
- Operating power-driven circular saws, band saws, and guillotine shears
- Working in wrecking, demolition, and shipbreaking operations
- Working in roofing operations
- Working in excavation operations

APPENDIX B

Preventing Deaths and Injuries of Adolescent Workers

The following types of work are especially hazardous to adolescents:

- Working in or around motor vehicles
- Operating tractors and other heavy equipment
- Working near electrical hazards such as overhead power lines while using poles, ladders, pipes, or boomed vehicles
- Working in retail and service businesses where there is a risk of robbery-related homicide
- Working on ladders, scaffolds, roofs, or construction sites
- Working around cooking appliances
- Continuous manual lifting and lifting of heavy objects

Employers

- Comply with child labor laws and occupational safety and health regulations that apply to your business.
- Assess and eliminate hazards for adolescent workers.
- Train adolescent workers to recognize hazards and use safe work practices. Routinely verify that they are using these skills.
- Evaluate equipment used by adolescents to be sure that it is legal and safe for their use.
- Make sure that adolescent workers are appropriately supervised to prevent injuries and hazardous exposures.
- Ask supervisors and experienced workers to help develop an injury and illness prevention program and to help identify and solve safety and health problems.

Parents

- Take an active role in the employment decisions of your children.
- Discuss the types of work involved and the training and supervision provided by the employer.

Educators

- Know the Federal and State child labor laws if you are responsible for signing work permits.
- Talk to students about safety and health hazards in the workplace and their responsibilities as workers.
- Make sure that school-based work experience programs provide jobs in safe and healthful environments and supply information about workers' legal rights and responsibilities.

Adolescents

- Be aware that you have the right to work in a safe and healthful environment.
- Learn to recognize hazards at work.
- Participate in training programs at work or request training if none is offered.
- Seek information about safe work practices from your employer and the State department of labor.
- Use safe work practices.
- Know that you have the right to file a complaint with the U.S. Department of Labor when you feel your rights are being violated or your safety is in jeopardy.

Preventing Homicides in the Workplace

Original Citation: National Institute for Occupational Safety and Health. Publications dissemination. Request for assistance in preventing homicide in the workplace. DHHS (NIOSH) publication no. 93–109.

REQUEST FOR ASSISTANCE IN PREVENTING HOMICIDE IN THE WORKPLACE

The National Institute for Occupational Safety and Health (NIOSH) requests assistance in preventing homicide in the workplace. From 1980 to 1989, homicide was the third leading cause of death from injury in the workplace, according to data from the National Traumatic Occupational Fatalities (NTOF) Surveillance System [NIOSH 1993]. Occupational homicides accounted for approximately 7,600 deaths during this period—or 12% of all deaths from injury in the workplace. Only motor vehicles and machines accounted for more occupational deaths from injury.

NUMBER AND CHARACTERISTICS OF VICTIMS

Number of Victims

During the period 1980–89, nearly 7,600 U.S. workers were victims of homicide in the workplace. Homicide was the leading cause of occupational death from injury for women, and the third leading cause for all workers. The actual number of occupational homicides is higher than reported in this Alert because methods for collecting and reporting death certificate data tend to underestimate the total number of deaths [NIOSH 1993]. NTOF data indicate that for the period 1980–89, the average annual rate of occupational homicide was 0.7/100,000 workers [Castillo and Jenkins 1993]. (See Jenkins et al. [1992] for an overview of work-related homicides based on NTOF data for the years 1980–88.)

Although data are not available to quantify nonfatal assaults in the United States, such intentional injuries to workers occur much more frequently than occupational homicides. Efforts to prevent occupational homicide may also reduce the number of nonfatal assaults.

Sex of Victims

Of the 7,600 homicide victims during the period 1980–89, 80% were male. The homicide rate for male workers was three times that for female workers (1.0/100,000 compared with 0.3/100,000). Nonetheless, homicide was the leading cause of death from occupational injury among women, causing 41% of all such deaths among women compared with 10% among men. (See Bell [1991] for an analysis of NTOF data on occupational homicides among women.)

Age of Victims

Nearly half of the occupational homicides occurred among workers aged 25 to 44, but workers aged 65 and older had the highest rate of occupational homicide (2.0/100,000).

Race of Victims

During the period 1980–89, 75% of occupational homicide victims were white, 19% were black, and 6% were other races. However, the rate of occupational homicide among black workers (1.4/100,000) and other races (1.6/100,000) was more than twice the rate for white workers (0.6/100,000).

Weapons Used

Guns were used in 75% of all occupational homicides from 1980 to 1989. Knives and other types of cutting and piercing instruments accounted for only 14% of these deaths during this period.

HIGH-RISK WORKPLACES AND OCCUPATIONS

Among workplaces, retail trades had the highest number of occupational homicides (2,787) during the period 1980–89, and services had the second highest number (1,275). These two workplaces accounted for 54% of all occupational homicides during this period. Three workplaces had homicide rates that were at least double the average annual rate (0.7/100,000) for the United States: retail trades, public administration, and transportation/communication/public utilities.

Workplaces with the highest rates of occupational homicide were taxicab establishments, liquor stores, gas stations, detective/protective services, justice/public order establishments (including courts, police protection establishments, legal counsel and prosecution establishments, correctional institutions, and fire protection establishments), grocery stores, jewelry stores, hotels/motels, and eating/drinking places (see Table 1). Taxicab establishments had the highest rate of occupational homicide—nearly 40 times the national average and more than three times the rate of liquor stores, which had the next highest rate.

Table 1. Workplaces with the highest rates of occupational homicide, 1980–89

Workplaces and SIC*codes	Number of homicides	Rate[†]
Taxicab establishments (412)	287	26.9
Liquor stores (592)	115	8.0
Gas stations (554)	304	5.6
Detective/protective services (7381, 7382)	152	5.0
Justice/public order establishments (92)	640	3.4
Grocery stores (541)	806	3.2
Jewelry stores (5944)	56	3.2
Hotels/motels (701)	153	1.5
Eating/drinking places (58)	734	1.5

*Standard Industrial Classification. Workplaces were classified according to the Standard Industrial Classification Manual, 1987 [OMB 1987].

[†]Number per 100,000 workers per year.

The occupation with the highest rate of occupational homicide was taxicab driver/chauffeur, with a rate 21 times the national average. Other high-risk occupations were law enforcement officers (police officers/sheriffs), hotel clerks, gas station workers, security guards, stock handlers/baggers, store owners/managers, and bartenders (see Table 2).

Table 2. Occupations with the highest rates of occupational homicide, 1980–89

Occupations and BOC* codes	Number of homicides	Rate[†]
Taxicab drivers/chauffeurs (809)	289	15.1
Law enforcement officers (police officers/sheriffs) (418, 423)	520	9.3
Hotel clerks (317)	40	5.1
Gas station workers (885)	164	4.5
Security guards (426)	253	3.6
Stock handlers/baggers (877)	260	3.1
Store owners/managers (243)	1,065	2.8
Bartenders (434)	84	2.1

*Bureau of Census. Occupations were classified according to the 1980 Census of the Population: Alphabetic Index of Industries and Occupations [U.S. Department of Commerce 1982]

[†]Number per 100,000 workers per year.

CIRCUMSTANCES OF HOMICIDE IN THE WORKPLACE

Information on death certificates does not allow identification of the circumstances of homicide in the workplace. However, the types of high-risk workplaces and occupations identified suggest that robbery is a predominant motive. In addition, some homicides are caused by disgruntled workers and clients or by domestic violence that spills into the workplace.

CURRENT OSHA REGULATIONS

The Occupational Safety and Health Administration (OSHA) has no specific regulations for preventing occupational homicide. However, the OSHA General Duty Clause [29 USC* 654(a)(1)] requires employers to provide a safe and healthful working environment for all workers covered by the Occupational Safety and Health Act of 1970.

POSSIBLE RISK FACTORS AND PREVENTIVE MEASURES

Risk Factors

Researchers have suggested a number of factors that may increase the risk of homicide in the workplace [Kraus 1987; Davis 1987; Davis et al. 1987; Castillo and Jenkins 1993]. The following are examples of these factors:

Exchange of money with the public,
Working alone or in small numbers,
Working late night or early morning hours,
Working in high-crime areas,
Guarding valuable property or possessions, and
Working in community settings (e.g., taxicab drivers and police).

Preventive Measures

Immediate preventive measures are needed to reduce the large number of occupational homicides each year. Although the preventive measures presented in this Alert have not been widely tested, they may provide some protection to workers until research studies can be conducted to evaluate their effectiveness.

A number of environmental and behavioral measures have been proposed for reducing occupational homicides in high-risk establishments and occupations [Chapman 1986; Crow and Erickson 1989; NYCPD 1990; State of Florida 1991]. These measures include the following:

Make high-risk areas visible to more people.
Install good external lighting.
Use drop safes to minimize cash on hand.
Carry small amounts of cash.
Post signs stating that limited cash is on hand.
Install silent alarms.
Install surveillance cameras.
Increase the number of staff on duty.
Provide training in conflict resolution and nonviolent response.
Avoid resistance during a robbery.
Provide bullet-proof barriers or enclosures.
Have police check on workers routinely.
Close establishments during high-risk hours (late at night and early in the morning).

---

* United States Code.

CONCLUSIONS

Occupational homicide is a serious public health problem, but many employers and workers may be unaware of the risk. No current OSHA regulations apply specifically to occupational homicide, but a great need exists for worker protection from intentional injury in the workplace.

High-risk workplaces include taxicab establishments, liquor stores, gas stations, detective/protective services, justice/public order establishments, grocery stores, jewelry stores, hotels/motels, and eating/drinking places. High-risk occupations are taxicab drivers/chauffeurs, law enforcement officers (police officers/sheriffs), hotel clerks, gas station workers, security guards, stock handlers/baggers, store owners/managers, and bartenders. Employers in these high-risk establishments and occupations need to be aware of the risk for homicide and take steps to ensure a safe workplace.

RECOMMENDATIONS

NIOSH recommends that the following steps be taken to prevent occupational homicides:

1. Employers and workers should immediately develop and implement prevention strategies on the basis of available information. They should
   - Evaluate the factors or situations in the workplace that might place workers at risk, and
   - Carefully consider intervention efforts that might minimize or remove the risk.

   Employers and workers may be able to apply some of the preventive measures described in this Alert; they may also identify other preventive measures specific to their workplaces.
2. Researchers should thoroughly evaluate existing or proposed prevention strategies. Few in-depth studies have been conducted to evaluate preventive measures, but such evaluation is critical to homicide prevention efforts [NIOSH 1992].
3. Researchers should further investigate occupational homicide. Research should be conducted on the specific factors associated with occupational homicides. Such research is essential for the development of prevention strategies.
4. Researchers should address the role of guns in occupational homicides. Because of the frequent use of guns in occupational homicides, research should be conducted to
   - Investigate the circumstances surrounding the use of guns in homicides,
   - Evaluate the effectiveness of methods for protecting workers from assaults involving guns, and
   - Evaluate the impact that existing and proposed gun-control regulations might have on protecting workers from occupational homicide.

REFERENCES

Bell CA. Female homicides in United States workplaces, 1980–1985. Am J Public Health 1991;81(6):729–732.
Castillo DN, Jenkins EL. Industries and occupations at high risk for work-related homicides. J Occup Med 1993;36(2):125–132.

Chapman SG. Cops, killers and staying alive: the murder of police officers in America. Springfield, IL: Charles C Thomas, 1986.

Crow WJ, Erickson R. The store safety issue: facts for the future. Alexandria, VA: National Association of Convenience Stores, 1989.

Davis H. Workplace homicides of Texas males. Am J Public Health 1987;77(10):1290–1293.

Davis H, Honchar PA, Suarez L. Fatal occupational injuries of women, Texas 1975–84. Am J Public Health 1987;77(12):1524–1527.

Jenkins EL, Layne LA, Kisner SM. Homicide in the workplace: the U.S. experience, 1980–1988. Am Assoc Occup Health Nurses J 1992;40(5):215–218.

Kraus JF. Homicide while at work: persons, industries, and occupations at high risk. Am J Public Health 1987;77(10):1285–1289.

NIOSH. Homicide in U.S. workplaces: a strategy for prevention and research. Morgantown, WV: U.S. Department of Health and Human Services, Public Health Service, Centers for Disease Control, National Institute for Occupational Safety and Health, 1992:DHHS (NIOSH) Publication No. 92–103.

NIOSH. Fatal injuries to workers in the United States, 1980–1989: a decade of surveillance; national profile. Cincinnati: U.S. Department of Health and Human Services, Public Health Service, Centers for Disease Control and Prevention, National Institute for Occupational Safety and Health, 1993:DHHS (NIOSH) Publication No. 93–108.

NYCPD. Safety tips for the taxi driver and the for-hire vehicle driver. New York: New York City Police Department, 1990.

OMB. Standard industrial classification manual, 1987. Washington, DC: Executive Office of the President, Office of Management and Budget, 1987:NTIS No. PB 87–100012.

State of Florida. Study of safety and security requirements for at-risk businesses. Tallahassee, FL: Office of the Attorney General, 1991.

U.S. Department of Commerce. 1980 Census of population: alphabetical index of industries and occupations. Final ed. Washington, DC: U.S. Department of Commerce, Bureau of the Census, 1982:PHC80-R3.

NIOSH ALERT

Preventing Homicide in the Workplace

Homicide is the third leading cause of death from occupational injury for all workers. Guns are the most commonly used weapon. Employers and workers should take the following steps to protect themselves from homicide in the workplace:

1. Be aware of which workplaces and occupations have the highest risk of work-related homicides:

   Workplaces
   - Taxicab establishments
   - Liquor stores
   - Gas stations
   - Detective/protective services
   - Justice/public order establishments
   - Grocery stores
   - Jewelry stores
   - Hotels/motels
   - Eating/drinking places

   Occupations
   - Taxicab drivers/chauffeurs
   - Law enforcement officers (police officers/sheriffs)
   - Hotel clerks
   - Gas station workers
   - Security guards
   - Stock handlers/baggers
   - Store owners/managers
   - Bartenders

2. Learn the factors that may increase the risk of homicide:
   Exchange of money with the public
   Working alone or in small numbers
   Working late night or early morning hours
   Working in high-crime areas
   Guarding valuable property or possessions
   Working in community settings
3. Evaluate your workplace and take steps that may prevent homicides.
   Preventive measures may include the following:
   Make high-risk areas visible to more people.
   Install good external lighting.
   Use drop safes to minimize cash on hand.
   Carry small amounts of cash.
   Post signs stating that limited cash is on hand.
   Install silent alarms.
   Install surveillance cameras.
   Increase the number of staff on duty.
   Provide training in conflict resolution and nonviolent response.
   Avoid resistance during robbery.
   Provide bullet-proof barriers or enclosures.
   Have police check on workers routinely.
   Close establishments during high-risk hours (late at night and early in the
      morning).

TOPIC 55 / **TAKE-HOME TOXINS**

Workers' Home Contamination Study

Original Citation: Centers for Disease Control and Prevention. Report to Congress on
workers' home contamination study. DHHS (NIOSH) Publication No. 95–123, September,
1995.

EXECUTIVE SUMMARY

The Workers' Family Protection Act of 1992 (Public Law 102–522, 29 U.S.C.
§671a) directed the National Institute for Occupational Safety and Health
(NIOSH) to conduct a study of contamination of workers' homes with hazardous chemicals and substances (including infectious agents) transported
from the workplace. NIOSH found that contamination of workers' homes is a
worldwide problem; incidents have been reported from 28 countries and from
36 States in the United States. Such incidents have resulted in a wide range of
health effects and death among workers' families exposed to toxic substances
and infectious agents. About half of the reports of health effects have appeared
in the last 10 years, revealing new sources of contamination.

Health Effects of Workers' Home Contamination

Workers can inadvertently carry hazardous materials home from work on their
clothes, skin, hair, tools, and in their vehicles. As a result, families of these work-

ers have been exposed to hazardous substances and have developed various health effects. Health effects have also occurred when the home and the workplace are not distinct—such as on farms or in homes that involve cottage industries. For some contaminants, there are other potential sources of home contamination such as air and water pollution and deteriorating lead paint in the home. Only a few of the studies found in the literature used epidemiologic methods to estimate the relative risks of health effects from the contaminant transported home by the worker independent of health risks due to other sources of the contaminant in the home.

Little is known of the full range of health effects or the extent to which they occur as a result of workers' home contamination. There are information systems to enable tracking of illnesses and health conditions resulting from these circumstances. Many of the health effects among workers' family members described below were recognized because of their uniqueness their clear relationship to workplace contaminants, or their serious nature.

Chronic Beryllium Disease

This potentially fatal lung disease has occurred in families of workers exposed to beryllium in the nuclear and aviation industries and workplaces involved in the production of beryllium and fluorescent lights and gyroscopes.

Asbestosis and Mesothelioma

Fatal lung diseases have occurred among family members of workers engaged in manufacture of many products containing asbestos, including thermal insulation materials, asbestos cement, automobile mufflers, shingles, textiles, gas masks, floor tiles, boilers, ovens, and brakeshoes and other friction products for automobiles. Families have also been exposed to asbestos when workers were engaged in mining, shipbuilding, insulating (e.g., pipe laggers and railway workers), maintenance and repair of boilers and vehicles, and asbestos removal operations.

Lead Poisoning, Neurological Effects, Aid Mental Retardation

These health effects have occurred in children of workers engaged in mining, smelting, construction, manufacturing (pottery, ceramics, stained glass, ceramic tiles, electrical components, bullets, and lead batteries), repair and reclamation of lead batteries, repair of radiators, recovery of gold and silver, work on firing ranges, and welding, painting, and splicing of cables.

Deaths and Neurological Effects from Pesticides

Farm families and families of other workers exposed to pesticides have suffered these serious effects.

Chemical Burns from Caustic Substances

Chemical burns of the mouth and esophagus and fatalities from ingesting caustic substances have occurred in farm families when hazardous substances were improperly used and stored on farms.

Chloracne and Other Effects from Chlorinated Hydrocarbons

Family members have been exposed when these substances were transported home on clothing of workers manufacturing or using these compounds in the production of insulated wire, plastic products, ion exchange resins, and textiles. Family members have been similarly exposed when workers' clothes became contaminated during marine electrical work, transformer maintenance, municipal sewage treatment, rail transportation, wood treatment, and application of herbicides.

Neurological Effects from Mercury

Family members have developed various neurological effects as a result of being exposed to mercury carried home on clothing of workers engaged in mining, thermometer manufacture, and cottage-industry gold extraction.

Abnormal Development from Estrogenic Substances

Enlarged breasts have occurred in boys and girls and premature menstruation has occurred in girls from estrogenic substances brought home on contaminated clothing of pharmaceutical and farm workers.

Asthmatic and Allergic Reactions from Dusts

Farm families and others have suffered asthmatic and other allergic effects from animal allergens, mushrooms, grain dust, and platinum salts.

Liver Angiosarcoma from Arsenic

Families of workers engaged in mining, smelting, and wood treatment have been exposed to arsenic from contaminated skin and clothing; one child developed liver angiosarcoma.

Dermatitis from Fibrous Glass

Family members have developed dermatitis when their clothing was contaminated with fibrous glass during laundering of insulation workers' clothing.

Status Epilepticus from Chemical Exposure

A child experienced epileptic seizures following ingestion of an explosive compound brought home on the clothing of a worker engaged in the manufacture of explosives.

Diseases from Infectious Agents

Family members have contracted infectious diseases such as scabies and Q fever from agents brought home on contaminated clothing and skin of workers engaged in agriculture, hospital, and laboratory work. As intended by Congress, infectious agents are included as hazardous substances to the extent that pathogens can be transported on a worker's person or clothing.

Measures for Preventing Home Contamination

Preventive measures that were found to be effective when used in the workplace include:

- Reducing exposures in the workplace;
- Changing clothes before going home and leaving the soiled clothing at work to be laundered by the employer;
- Storing street clothes in separate areas of the workplace to prevent their contamination;
- Showering before leaving work; and
- Prohibiting removal of toxic substances or contaminated items from the workplace.

Preventive measures that have been used successfully at home include:

- Separating work areas of cottage industries from living areas;
- Properly storing and disposing of toxic substances on farms and in cottage industries;
- Preventing family members from visiting the workplace;
- Laundering contaminated clothing separately from family laundry when it is necessary to launder contaminated clothing at home; and
- Informing workers of the risk to family members and of preventive measures.

Other preventive measures that need to be used include:

- Educating physicians and other health professionals to inquire about potential work related causes of disease;
- Developing surveillance programs to track health effects that could be related to home contamination; and
- Educating children, parents, and teachers about the effects of toxic substances.

Procedures for Decontaminating Homes and Clothing

Decontamination procedures include air showers, laundering, airing, vacuuming and other methods of surface, cleaning, and destruction and disposal of contaminated items. These procedures appear to have widely varying effectiveness, depending on the specific methods employed, the contaminants, and the surfaces. In general, hard surfaces can be far more easily decontaminated than clothes, carpets, and soft furniture. In most cases effective decontamination requires relatively intensive methods. Normal house cleaning and laundry practices appear to be inadequate for decontaminating workers' clothes and homes. Lead, asbestos, pesticides, and beryllium contamination can be especially persistent. In some instances even intensive decontamination procedures may be ineffective.

Another serious concern is that decontamination methods can increase the hazard to the person performing the operation and to offers in the household. Home laundering of contaminated clothing exposes the launderer. Vacuuming of floors contaminated with mercury can substantially increase air concentrations, and vacuuming of carpets contaminated with lead can increase lead concentrations on the carpet surface.

The difficulty of decontaminating work clothing, the prominence of clothing as a source of home contamination, and the potential exposure of the launderer are problems that can be avoided through the use of disposable work clothing. The use, availability and cost of this alternative need to be assessed.

Federal and State Laws

Seven statutes provided Federal agencies with some mechanisms for responding to or preventing workers' home contamination. Twenty rules or standards in the Code of Federal Regulations (CFR) address workers' home contamination or have elements that serve to protect workers' families.

Under the Occupational Safety and Health Act of 1970 (Public Law 91–596), NIOSH research assessing the health of workers has also addressed the exposure of their families to workplace contaminants, resulting in recommendations to prevent home contamination. The Occupational Safety and Health Administration (OSHA) regulations and actions intended to protect workers also help assure that families are protected. In addition, OSHA can promulgate standards to protect workers' family members when workers are required to live in housing provided by the employer as a condition of employment. Under the Federal Mine Safety and Health Act of 1977 (Public Law 95–164), the Mine Safety and Health Administration (MSHA) has limited regulatory authority to address issues of workers' home contamination.

The U.S. Environmental Protection Agency (EPA) has broad authority under the Toxic Substances Control Act (Public Law 94–469) to regulate chemicals and to obtain information about the adverse effects of chemicals. In addition, EPA has specific authority and responsibility regarding the use of asbestos and lead. Under the Federal Insecticide, Fungicide and Rodenticide Act (Public Law 92–516), EPA also regulates the use and disposal of pesticides (which also help to protect workers' families). EPA and the Agency for Toxic Substances and Disease Registry (ATSDR) are authorized under the Superfund Amendments and Reauthorization Act of 1986 (Public Law 99–499) to address hazardous waste and releases of hazardous substances that may relate to identifying contamination of workers' homes and assuring decontamination.

Thirty States and Puerto Rico responded to the requests from NIOSH for information about State laws. Most indicated that there were no laws specific to workers' home contamination or protection of workers' family members. Some states identified laws requiring the reporting of cases of elevated blood lead levels and pesticide poisonings to a State agency; other States identified laws related to work at hazardous waste sites and emergency responses to releases of hazardous substances. An examination of occupational safety and health regulations of States with OSHA-approved occupational safety and health programs revealed none more stringent than Federal OSHA regulations—with respect to the protection of workers' families. However, extension of occupational safety and health regulations to State and local government employees in these States also helps protect the families of public employees' in these States.

Limitation of the Report

- The only report found on indoor air quality applicable to workers' family protection involved tetrachloroethylene exposures in living quarters located in the same building as dry-cleaning establishments. Indoor air quality studies would be useful to protect family members in cottage industries.
- Incidents of contamination of fire fighters' homes were not identified. However, NIOSH has conducted several studies of contamination and decontamination of protective clothing used by firefighters. These studies are reviewed in this report and NIOSH will continue to pursue the issues related to potential contamination of firefighters' homes.

Other limitations of the report include:

- Little research has documented the frequency and distribution of health effects among the families of workers in various industries and occupations. NIOSH is undertaking one study addressing lead exposure among families of bridge repair workers.
- Lead and pesticides are the only contaminants for which monitoring or reporting programs help to identify and prevent cases of poisoning from workers home contamination.
- Despite various case reports, the prevalence of health effects from workers' home contamination is not known because there are no surveillance systems in place for tracking or monitoring such health conditions.
- Many diseases have long latency periods between exposure and manifestation of the disease, making identification and intervention difficult.
- The workplace origin of many common diseases that occur in workers' families (such as asthma, dermatitis, and infectious diseases) is probably unrecognized because physicians and other health professionals fail to inquire about the occupation of family members and to consider whether these diseases are work-related.
- The literature reviewed in this report contained only nominal information about contamination levels in workers' homes. Most measurements were of surface dust, for which there are no guidelines for acceptable levels of contamination.

Conclusions

- Worker's home contamination may pose a serious public health problem. Health effects and deaths from contaminants brought home from the workplace have been reported in 28 countries and 36 States.
- The extent to which these health effects occur is not known because there are no information systems to track them, and physicians do not always recognize the occupational contribution to various common diseases.
- About half of the reports of health effects from home contamination are less than 10 years old. The literature on the health effects involved approximately 30 different substances or agents. The potential exists for many of the thousands of other chemicals used in commerce to be transported to workers' homes or home-centered businesses.
- Health effects and deaths from contaminants brought home from the workplace are preventable using known effective measures. Educational programs are needed to promote their use.

- Normal house cleaning and laundry practices are often inadequate for decontaminating workers' homes and clothing and can increase the hazard to the person performing the tasks and others in the household.
- Only two Federal laws have elements that directly address workers' home contamination. However, other laws provide agencies with certain mechanisms for responding to, or preventing workers' home contamination. Operating under existing laws OSHA, MSHA, DOE, ATSDR, EPA, and CDC, including NIOSH and the National Center for Environmental Health have responded to incidents of workers' home contamination, made recommendations to prevent such incidents, and conducted relevant research.

section eight

MISCELLANEOUS

Health Information for International Travel

Original Citation: Centers for Disease Control and Prevention. Health information for international travel, 1995.

Editor's Note: The full book (200 pages) is a must-have for those who care for frequent international travelers; the travelers themselves are encouraged to purchase their own copy ($7; see Appendix B for ordering information). We have excerpted only those parts that change relatively little from year-to-year. The best way to obtain current information on epidemics is online (see Preface), or through CDC's Fax Information service at (404) 332-4559 . Most of the information on immunizations has been excluded as it can be found in its original sources in the Infectious Diseases section of this book.

HEALTH HINTS FOR THE INTERNATIONAL TRAVELER

Introduction

This section includes practical information on how to avoid potential health problems. Some of these recommendations are common-sense precautions; others have been scientifically documented.

Travelers who take prescription medications should carry an adequate supply accompanied by a signed and dated statement from a physician; the statement should indicate the major health problems and dosage of such medications, to provide information for medical authorities in case of emergency. The traveler should take an extra pair of glasses or lens prescription, and a card, tag, or bracelet that identifies any physical condition that may require emergency care.

If Medical Care Is Needed Abroad

If medical care is needed abroad, travel agents or the American Embassy or Consulate can usually provide names of hospitals, physicians, or emergency medical service agencies. Prior to departure, travelers should contact their own insurance companies concerning their coverage.

WHO Blood Transfusion Guidelines for International Travelers

Basic principles:

1. Unexpected, emergency blood transfusion is rarely required. It is needed only in situations of massive hemorrhage like severe trauma, gynecologic and obstetric emergency, or gastrointestinal bleeding.
2. In many cases, resuscitation can be achieved by use of colloid or crystalloid plasma expanders instead of blood.
3. Blood transfusion is not free of risk, even in the best of conditions. In most developing countries, the risk is increased by limited technical resources

for screening blood donors for HIV infection and other diseases transmissible by blood.

4. The international shipment of blood for transfusion is practical only when handled by agreement between two responsible organizations, such as national blood transfusion services. This mechanism is not useful for emergency needs of individual patients and should not be attempted by private individuals or organizations not operating recognized blood programs.

Therefore:

1. There are no medical indications for travelers to take blood with them from their home country.
2. The limited storage period of blood and the need for special equipment negate the feasibility of independent blood banking for individual travelers or small groups.
3. Blood should be transfused only when absolutely indicated. This applies even more forcefully in those countries where screening of blood for transmissible diseases is not yet widely performed.

Proposed Options:

1. When urgent resuscitation is necessary, the use of plasma expanders rather than blood should always be considered.
2. In case of emergency need of blood, use of plasma expanders and urgent evacuation home may be the actions of choice.
3. When blood transfusion cannot be avoided, the attending physician should make every effort to ensure that the blood has been screened for transmissible diseases, including HIV.
4. International travelers should:
   a. take active steps to minimize the risk of injury;
   b. establish a plan for dealing with medical emergencies;
   c. support the development within countries of safe and adequate blood supplies.

Motion Sickness

Travelers with a history of motion sickness or sea sickness can attempt to avoid symptoms by taking anti-motion-sickness pills or antihistaminics before departure.

Protection Against Mosquitoes and Other Arthropod Vectors

Although vaccines or chemoprophylactic drugs are available against important vector-borne diseases such as yellow fever and malaria, there are none for most other mosquito-borne diseases such as dengue, and travelers still should avail themselves of repellents and other general protective measures against arthropods. The effectiveness of malaria chemoprophylaxis is variable, depending on patterns of resistance and compliance with medication, and for many vector-borne diseases, no specific preventatives are available.

General Preventative Measures

The principal approach to prevention of vector-borne diseases is avoidance. Tick- and mite-borne infections characteristically are diseases of "place"; whenever possible, known foci of disease transmission should be avoided. Although many vector-borne infections can be prevented by avoiding rural locations, certain mosquito- and midge-borne arboviral and parasitic infections are transmitted around human residences and in urban locations. Most vector-borne infections are transmitted seasonally and simple changes in itinerary may greatly reduce risk for acquiring certain infections.

Exposure to arthropod bites can be minimized by modifying patterns of activity or behavior. Some vector mosquitoes are most active in twilight periods at dawn and dusk or in the evening. Avoidance of outdoor activity during these periods may reduce risk of exposure. Wearing long-sleeved shirts, long pants and hats will minimize areas of exposed skin. Shirts should be tucked in. Repellents applied to clothing, shoes, tents, mosquito nets and other gear will enhance protection.

When exposure to ticks or mites are a possibility, pants should be tucked into socks and boots should be worn; sandals should be avoided. Permethrin-based repellents applied as directed (see below) will enhance protection. During outdoor activity and at the end of the day, travelers should inspect themselves and their clothing for ticks. Ticks are detected more easily on light colored or white clothing. Prompt removal of attached ticks may prevent infection.

When accommodations are not adequately screened or air-conditioned, bednets are essential to provide protection and comfort. Bednets should be tucked under mattresses and can be sprayed with repellent. Aerosol insecticides and mosquito coils may help to clear rooms of mosquitoes; however, some coils contain DDT and should be used with caution.

Repellents

Permethrin-containing repellents (Permanone) are recommended for use on clothing, shoes, bednets and camping gear. Permethrin is highly effective as an insecticide/acaricide and as a repellent. Permethrin-treated clothing repels and kills ticks, mosquitoes and other arthropods and retains this effect after repeated laundering. There appears to be little potential for toxicity from permethrin-treated clothing.

Permethrin-containing shampoo (Nix) and cream (Elimite), marketed for use against head lice and scabies infestations, potentially could be extremely effective as repellents when applied on the hair and skin. However, they are approved only to treat existing conditions. Most authorities recommend repellents containing deet (N,N-diethylmetatoluamide) as an active ingredient. Deet repels mosquitoes, ticks, and other arthropods when applied to skin or clothing. Formulations containing <30% deet are recommended because the additional gain in repellent effect with higher concentrations is not significant when weighed against the potential for toxicity. A microencapsulated formulation (Skeedadle) may have a longer period of activity than liquid formulations.

Deet is toxic when ingested. High concentrations applied to skin may cause blistering. Rare cases of encephalopathy in children, some fatal, have been reported after cutaneous exposure. Other neurologic side effects also have been reported. Toxicity did not appear to be dose-related in many cases and these may have been idiosyncratic reactions in predisposed individuals. However, a dose-related effect leading to irritability and impaired concentration and memory has been reported.

PREGNANT WOMEN TRAVELING ABROAD

The problems that a pregnant woman might encounter during international travel are basically the same problems that other international travelers have. These have to do with exposure to infectious diseases and availability of good medical care. There is the additional potential problem that air travel late in pregnancy might precipitate labor.

Potential health problems vary from country to country; therefore, if the traveler has specific questions, she should be advised to check with the embassy or local consulate general's office of the country in question before traveling.

DISABLED TRAVELERS

The United States (U.S.) Architectural and Transportation Barriers Compliance Board (Access Board) produces or distributes a variety of publications, at no cost. U.S. air carriers must comply with the U.S. laws or regulations regarding access. Up-to-date information regarding access abroad is more difficult to ascertain. A booklet, Access Travel: Airports, is available free from the Consumer Information Center in Pueblo, Colorado 81009. It lists accessibility features at 553 airports worldwide. U.S. companies or entities conducting programs or tours on cruise ships also have some obligations for access, even if the ship itself is foreign flagged. Write or call, Access Board, Suite 1000, 1331 F Street, NW, Washington, DC 20004-1111, 1–800-USA-ABLE (voice/TDD) for a list of its publications.

Risks from Food and Drink

Water

Water that has been adequately chlorinated, using minimum recommended water-works standards as practiced in the United States, will afford significant protection against viral and bacterial waterborne diseases. However, chlorine treatment alone, as used in the routine disinfection of water, may not kill some enteric viruses and the parasitic organisms that cause giardiasis, amebiasis and cryptosporidiosis. In areas where chlorinated tap water is not available, or where hygiene and sanitation are poor, travelers should be advised that only the following may be safe to drink:

1. Beverages, such as tea and coffee, made with boiled water
2. Canned or bottled carbonated beverages, including carbonated bottled water and soft drinks
3. Beer and wine

Where water may be contaminated, ice (or containers for drinking) also should be considered contaminated. Thus, in these areas ice should not be used in beverages. If ice has been in contact with containers used for drinking, the containers should be thoroughly cleaned, preferably with soap and hot water, after the ice has been discarded.

It is safer to drink directly from a can or bottle of a beverage than from a questionable container. However, water on the outside of cans or bottles of beverages might be contaminated. Therefore, wet cans or bottles should be dried before being opened, and surfaces which are contacted directly by the mouth in drinking should first be wiped clean. Where water may be contaminated, travelers should avoid brushing their teeth with tap water.

Treatment of Water

Boiling is by far the most reliable method to make water of uncertain purity safe for drinking. Water should be brought to a vigorous rolling boil for one minute and allowed to cool to room temperature—do not add ice. At very high altitudes above 6,562 feet (2 km), for an extra margin of safety, boil for three minutes or use chemical disinfection. Adding a pinch of salt to each quart, or pouring the water several times from one container to another will improve the taste.

Chemical disinfection with iodine is an alternative method of water treatment when it is not feasible to boil water. Two well-tested methods for disinfection with iodine are the use of tincture of iodine (Table 24), and the use of tetraglycine hydroperiodide tablets (Globaline, Potable-Agua, Coghlan's, etc.). The tablets are available from pharmacies and sporting goods stores. The manufacturer's instructions should be followed. If water is cloudy, the number of tablets should be doubled; if water is extremely cold, an attempt should be made to warm the water, and the recommended contact time should be increased to achieve reliable disinfection. Cloudy water should be strained through a clean cloth into a container to remove any sediment or floating matter, and then the water should be treated with heat or iodine. Chlorine, in various forms, has also been used for chemical disinfection. However, its germicidal activity varies greatly with pH, temperature, and organic content of the water to be purified, and is less reliable than iodine.

Table 24. Treatment of Water with Tincture of Iodine

Tincture of iodine (from medicine chest or first aid kit)	Drops* to be added per quart or liter	
	Clear water	Cold or clody water+
2%	5	10

*1 drop = 0.05 ml. Let stand for 30 minutes. Water is safe to use.

+Very turbid or very cold water may require prolonged contact time; let stand prior to use, if possible.

There are a variety of portable filters currently on the market which according to the manufacturers' data will provide safe drinking water. Although the iodide-impregnated resins and the microstrainer type filters will kill and/or remove many micoorganisms, very few published reports in the scientific literature deal both with the methods used and the results of the tests employed to evaluate the efficacy of these filters against water-borne pathogens. Until there is sufficient independent verification of the efficacy of these filters, CDC makes no recommendation regarding their use.

As a last resort, if no source of safe drinking water is available or can be obtained, tap water that is uncomfortably hot to touch may be safer than cold tap water, however proper disinfection or boiling is still advised.

Food

To avoid illness, food should be selected with care. All raw food is subject to contamination. Particularly in areas where hygiene and sanitation are inadequate, the traveler should be advised to avoid salads, uncooked vegetables, unpasteurized milk and milk products such as cheese, and to eat only food that has been cooked and is still hot, or fruit that has been peeled by the traveler. Undercooked and raw meat, fish, and shellfish may carry various intestinal pathogens. Cooked food that has been allowed to stand for several hours at ambient temperature may provide a fertile medium for bacterial growth and should be thoroughly reheated before serving. Consumption of food and beverages obtained from street food vendors has been associated with increased risk of illness. The easiest way to guarantee a safe food source for an infant less than 6 months of age is to have the child breast-feed. If the infant has already been weaned from the breast, formula prepared from commercial powder and boiled water is the safest and most practical food.

Some species of fish and shellfish can contain poisonous biotoxins, even when well cooked. The most common type of fish poisoning in travelers is ciguatera fish poisoning. Barracuda is the most toxic fish and should always be avoided. Red snapper, grouper, amberjack, sea bass, and a wide range of tropical reef fish contain the toxin at unpredictable times. The potential for ciguatera poisoning exists in all subtropical and tropical insular areas of the West Indies, Pacific and Indian Oceans where the implicated fish species are consumed.

Recently, cholera cases have occurred among persons who ate crab brought back from Latin America by travelers. Travelers should not bring perishable seafoods with them when they return.

Travelers' Diarrhea

Epidemiology

Travelers' diarrhea (TD) is a syndrome characterized by a twofold or greater increase in the frequency of unformed bowel movements. Commonly associated symptoms include abdominal cramps, nausea, bloating, urgency, fever, and malaise. Episodes of TD usually begin abruptly, occur during travel or soon after returning home, and are generally self-limited. The most important determinant of risk is the destination of the traveler. Attack rates in the range of 20 to 50 percent are commonly reported. High-risk destinations include most of the developing countries of Latin America, Africa, the Middle East, and Asia. Intermediate risk destinations include most of the Southern European countries and a few Caribbean islands. Low risk destinations include Canada, Northern Europe, Australia, New Zealand, the United States and a number of the Caribbean islands.

TD is slightly more common in young adults than in older people. The reasons for this difference are unclear, but may include a lack of acquired immunity, more adventurous travel styles, and different eating habits. Attack rates are similar in men and women. The onset of TD is usually within the first week, but may occur at any time during the visit, and even after returning home.

TD is acquired through ingestion of fecally contaminated food and/or water. Both cooked and uncooked foods may be implicated if improperly handled. Especially risky foods include raw or undercooked meat and seafood, and raw fruits and vegetables. Tap water, ice, and unpasteurized milk and dairy products may be associated with increased risk of TD; safe beverages include bottled carbonated beverages (especially flavored beverages), beer, wine, hot coffee or tea, or water boiled or appropriately treated with iodine or chlorine. The place food is prepared appears to be an important variable; with private homes, restaurants, and street vendors listed in order of increasing risk.

TD typically results in four to five loose or watery stools per day. The median duration of diarrhea is 3 to 4 days. Ten percent of the cases persist longer than 1 week, approximately 2 percent longer than 1 month, and less than 1 percent longer than 3 months. Persistent diarrhea is thus quite uncommon and may differ considerably from acute TD with respect to etiology and risk factors. Approximately 15 percent vomiting, and 2 to 10 percent may have diarrhea accompanied by fever or bloody stools, or both. Travelers may experience more than one attack of TD during a single trip. Rarely is TD life-threatening.

Etiology

Infectious agents are the primary cause of TD. Travelers from industrialized countries to developing countries frequently develop a rapid, dramatic change in the type of organisms in their gastrointestinal tract. These new organisms often include potential enteric pathogens. Those who develop diarrhea have ingested an inoculum of virulent organisms sufficiently large to overcome individual defense mechanisms, resulting in symptoms.

Prevention

There are four possible approaches to prevention of TD. They include instruction regarding food and beverage consumption, immunization, use of nonantimicrobial medications, and prophylactic antimicrobial drugs.

Data indicate that meticulous attention to food and beverage consumption, as mentioned above, can decrease the likelihood of developing TD. Most travelers, however, encounter difficulty in observing the requisite dietary restrictions.

No available vaccines and none that are expected to be available in the next 5 years are effective against TD. Several nonantimicrobial agents have been advocated for prevention of TD. Available controlled studies indicate that prophylactic use of difenoxine, the active metabolite of diphenoxylate (Lomotil), actually increases the incidence of TD in addition to producing other undesirable side effects. Antiperistaltic agents, e.g., Lomotil and Imodium are not effective in preventing TD. No data support the prophylactic use of activated charcoal.

Bismuth subsalicylate, taken as the active ingredient of Pepto-Bismol (2 oz. 4 times daily, or 2 tablets 4 times daily), has decreased the incidence of diarrhea by about 60 percent in several placebo-controlled studies. Side effects include temporary blackening of tongue and stools, occasional nausea and constipation, and rarely, tinnitus. Available data are not extensive enough to exclude a risk to the traveler from the use of such large doses of bismuth subsalicylate for a period of more than three weeks. Bismuth subsalicylate should be avoided by persons with aspirin-allergy, renal insufficiency, gout, and by those who are taking anticoagulants, probenecid, or methotrexate. In patients already taking salicylates for arthritis, large concurrent doses of bismuth subsalicylate can produce toxic serum concentrations of salicylate. Caution should be used in giving bismuth subsalicylate to adolescents and children with chicken pox or flu because of a potential risk of Reye's syndrome. Bismuth subsalicylate has not been approved for children under three years old. Bismuth subsalicylate appears to be an effective prophylactic agent for TD, but is not recommended for prophylaxis of TD for periods of more than three weeks. Further studies of the efficacy and side effects of lower dose regimens are needed.

Controlled data are available on the prophylactic value of several other nonantimicrobial drugs. Enterovioform and related halogenated hydroxyquinoline derivatives, e.g., clioquinol, iodoquinol, Mexaform, Intestopan, and others, are not helpful in preventing TD, may have serious neurological side effects, and should never be used for prophylaxis of TD.

Controlled studies have indicated that a variety of antibiotics, including doxycycline, trimethoprim/sulfamethoxazole (TMP/SMX), trimethoprim alone, and the fluoroquinolone agents ciprofloxacin and norfloxacin, when taken prophylactically have been 52–95% effective in preventing traveler's diarrhea in several areas of the developing world. The effectiveness of these agents, however, depends upon the antibiotic resistance patterns of the pathogenic bacteria in each area of travel, and such information is seldom available. Resistance to the fluoroquinolones is the least common, but this may change as the use of these agents increases worldwide.

While effective in preventing some bacterial causes of diarrhea, antibiotics have no effect on the acquisition of various viral and parasitic diseases. Prophylactic antibiotics may give travelers a false sense of security about the risk associated with consuming certain local foods and beverages.

The benefits of widespread prophylactic use of doxycycline, quinolones, TMP/SMX or TMP alone in several million travelers must be weighed against the potential drawbacks. The known risks include allergic and other side effects (such as common skin rashes, photosensitivity of the skin, blood disorders, Stevens-Johnson syndrome and staining of the teeth in children) as well as other infections that may be induced by antimicrobial therapy (such as antibiotic-associated colitis, Candida vaginitis, and Salmonella enteritis). Because of the uncertain risk of widespread administration of these antimicrobial agents, their prophylactic use is not recommended. While it seems reasonable to use prophylactic antibiotics in certain high risk groups, such as travelers with immunosuppression or immunodeficiency, there are no data which directly support this practice. There is little evidence that other disease entities are worsened sufficiently by an episode of TD to risk the rare undesirable side effects of prophylactic antimicrobial drugs. Therefore, prophylactic antimicrobial agents are not recommended for travelers. Instead, available data support the recommendation that travelers be instructed in sensible dietary practices as a prophylactic measure. This recommendation is justified by the excellent results of early treatment of TD as outlined below. Some travelers may wish to consult with their physician and may elect to use prophylactic antimicrobial agents for travel under special circumstances, once the risks and benefits are clearly understood.

Treatment

Individuals with TD have two major complaints for which they desire relief—abdominal cramps and diarrhea. Many agents have been proposed to control these symptoms, but few have been demonstrated to be effective by rigorous clinical trials.

Nonspecific Agents

A variety of "adsorbents" have been used in treating diarrhea. For example, activated charcoal has been found to be ineffective in the treatment of diarrhea. Kaolin and pectin have been widely used for diarrhea. The combination appears to give the stools more consistency but has not been shown to decrease cramps and frequency of stools nor to shorten the course of infectious diarrhea.

Lactobacillus preparations and yogurt have also been advocated, but no evidence supports use of these treatments for TD.

Bismuth subsalicylate preparation (1 oz of liquid or 2 262.5 mg tablets every 30 minutes for eight doses) decreased the rate of stooling and shortened the duration of illness in several placebo-controlled studies. Treatment was limited to 48 hours at most with no more than 8 doses in a 24-hour period. There is concern about taking, without supervision, large amounts of bismuth and salicylate, especially in individuals who may be intolerant to salicylates, who have renal insufficiency, or who take salicylates for other reasons.

Antimotility Agents

Antimotility agents are widely used in treating diarrhea of all types. Natural opiates (paregoric, deodorized tincture of opium, and codeine) have long been used to control diarrhea and cramps. Synthetic agents, diphenoxylate and loperamide, come in convenient dosage forms and provide prompt symptomatic but temporary relief of uncomplicated TD. However, they should not be used in patients with high fever or with blood in the stool. These drugs should be discontinued if symptoms persist beyond 48 hours. Diphenoxylate and loperamide should not be used in children under the age of 2.

Antimicrobial Treatment

Travelers who develop diarrhea with three or more loose stools in an 8-hour period, especially if associated with nausea, vomiting, abdominal cramps, fever, or blood in the stools, may benefit from antimicrobial treatment. A typical 3- to 5-day illness can often be shortened to 1 day by effective antimicrobial agents. The effectiveness of antibiotic therapy will depend on the etiologic agent and its antibiotic sensitivity. Antibiotic regimens most likely to be effective are TMP/SMX (160 mg TMP and 800 mg SMX) or ciprofloxacin (500 mg) taken twice daily. Other fluoroquinolones such as fleroxacin, norfloxacin and ofloxacin may be equally effective as ciprofloxacin. Fewer side effects and less widespread resistance has been reported with the fluoroquinolones than with TMP/SMX. Three days of treatment is recommended, although 2 days or fewer may be sufficient. Nausea and vomiting without diarrhea should not be treated with antimicrobial drugs.

Travelers should consult a physician, rather than attempt self-medication, if the diarrhea is severe or does not resolve within several days; if there is blood and/or mucus in the stool; if fever occurs with shaking chills; or if there is dehydration with persistent diarrhea.

Oral Fluids

Most cases of diarrhea are self-limited and require only simple replacement of fluids and salts lost in diarrheal stools. This is best achieved by use of an oral rehydration solution such as World Health Organization Oral Rehydration Salts (ORS) solution (Table 25). This solution is appropriate for treating as well as preventing dehydration. ORS packets are available at stores or pharmacies in almost all developing countries. ORS is prepared by adding one packet to boiled or treated water. Packet instructions should be checked carefully to ensure that the salts are added to the correct volume of water. ORS solution should be consumed or discarded within 12 hours if held at room temperature, or 24 hours if held refrigerated.

Table 25. Composition of World Health Organization Oral Rehydration Solution (ORS) for Diarrheal Illness

Ingredient	Amount
Sodium chloride	3.5 grams/liter
Potassium chloride	1.5 grams/liter
Glucose	20.0 grams/liter
Trisodium citrate*	2.9 grams/liter

*An earlier formulation using sodium bicarbonate 2.5 grams/liter had a shorter shelf physiologically equivalent, and may still be produced in some countries.

Iced drinks and noncarbonated bottled fluids made from water of uncertain quality should be avoided. Dairy products aggravate diarrhea in some people and should be avoided.

Infants with Diarrhea

Children aged 0–2 years are at high risk of acquiring traveler's diarrhea. The greatest risk to the infant with diarrhea is dehydration. Dehydration is best prevented by use of WHO ORS solution in addition to the infant's usual food. ORS packets are available at stores or pharmacies in almost all developing countries. ORS is prepared by adding one packet to boiled or treated water. Packet instructions should be checked carefully to ensure that the salts are added to the correct volume of water. ORS solution should be consumed or discarded within 12 hours if held at room temperature, or 24 hours if held refrigerated. The dehydrated child will drink ORS avidly; ORS is given ad lib to the child as long as the dehydration persists. The infant who vomits the ORS will usually keep it down if the ORS is offered by spoon in frequent small sips. Breast-fed infants should continue nursing on demand. For bottle-fed infants, full-strength lactose-free, or lactose-reduced formulas should be administered. Older children receiving semi-solid or solid foods should continue to receive their usual diet during diarrhea. Recommended foods include starches, cereals, yogurt, fruits, and vegetables.

Immediate medical attention is required for the infant with diarrhea who develops signs of moderate to severe dehydration, bloody diarrhea, fever of greater than 102 degrees F, or persistent vomiting. While medical attention is being obtained, the infant should be offered ORS.

More information is available from CDC in a publication entitled, "The management of acute diarrhea in children: oral rehydration, maintenance, and nutritional therapy." (MMWR No. RR-16, October 16, 1992). ORS packets are available in the United States from Jianas Brothers Packaging Company, Kansas City, Missouri (telephone: (816) 421-2880).

Precautions in Children and Pregnant Women

Although children do not make up a large proportion of travelers to high-risk areas, some children do accompany their families. Teenagers should follow the advice given to adults, with possible adjustment of doses of medication. Physicians should be aware of the risks of tetracyclines to children under 12 years of age. There are few data available about usage of antidiarrheal drugs in children. Drugs should be prescribed with caution for pregnant women and nursing mothers.

CRUISE SHIP SANITATION

In 1975, because of several major disease outbreaks on cruise vessels, the Centers for Disease Control and Prevention (CDC) established the Vessel Sanitation Program (VSP) as a cooperative activity with the cruise ship industry. This joint program strives to achieve and maintain a level of sanitation on passenger vessels that will lower the risk of gastrointestinal disease outbreaks and provide a healthful environment for ships' passengers and crew. The program goals are addressed through encouraging industry to establish and maintain a comprehensive sanitation program and oversight of its success through an inspections process. Every vessel with a foreign itinerary that carries 13 or more passengers is subject to twice yearly inspections and when necessary reinspection. Inspections are only conducted at those ports under U.S. control and cover such environmental aspects as:

1. Water supply, storage, distribution, backflow protection and disinfection.
2. Food preparation during storage, preparation, and service and product temperature control.
3. Potential contamination of food, water, and ice.
4. Employee practices and personal hygiene.
5. General cleanliness, facility repair, and vector control.
6. The ship's training programs in general environmental and public health practices.

A score of 86 or higher at the time of the inspection indicates that the ship is providing an accepted standard of sanitation. In general, the lower the score the lower the level of sanitation; however, a low score does not necessarily imply an imminent risk of an outbreak of gastrointestinal disease or other illness related to environmental sanitation. Each ship is required to document a plan for corrective action following each inspection. Inspectors will recommend a ship not sail if they detect an imminent health hazard aboard ship (e.g., inadequate facilities for maintaining safe food temperatures or a contaminated drinking-water system.) Full information on inspection criteria can be obtained by writing to the VSP office at the address listed at the end of this section. At any time, the Director of CDC may determine that failure to implement corrective actions presents a threat of communicable disease being introduced into the United States and may take additional action including detention of the ship in port.

The scores for each ship are published every 2 weeks in the Summary of Sanitation Inspections of International Cruise Ships, commonly referred to as the green sheet. This sheet is distributed to more than 4,500 travel-related services around the world and is a way to communicate a ship's compliance with VSP recommendations to both the cruise ship industry and the consumer. The green sheet is available to the public via Internet, FTP.CDC.GOV//PUB/SHIP_INSPECTIONS/SHIPSCORE.TXT; or by the CDC fax-back service by dialing (404) 332-4565 and requesting Document Number 510051. Interested parties can also obtain the green sheet or a copy of the complete inspection for a specific ship by writing to the Vessel Sanitation Program, National Center for Environmental Health, Centers for Disease Control and Prevention, 1015 North America Way, Room 107, Miami, Florida 33132.

DISINSECTION OF AIRCRAFT

International travelers should be aware that some countries require disinsection of certain passenger aircraft in order to prevent the importation of insects such as mosquitos. Disinsection procedures may include the spraying of the aircraft passenger compartment with insecticide while passengers are present. While the recommended disinsection procedures have been determined to be safe by the World Health Organization, they may aggravate certain health conditions (i.e., allergies). Travelers with such conditions or who are otherwise interested in determining what disinsection procedures may be performed on a particular flight should contact their travel agent or airline.

TUBERCULOSIS RISK IN AIRCRAFT

The Centers for Disease Control and Prevention (CDC) and state and local health departments have conducted six investigations of possible tuberculosis (TB) transmission on commercial aircraft. In all six instances, a passenger or a member of the flight crew traveled on commercial airplanes while infectious with TB. In none of the six instances were the airlines aware of the TB in their passengers. In two of the instances, CDC concluded that TB was probably transmitted to others on the airplane.

TB is spread from person to person through the air. When a person with infectious TB coughs or sneezes, tiny droplets containing TB bacteria may be released into the air. Other people may inhale these droplets and become infected.

The CDC found that the risk of TB transmission from an infectious person to others on an airplane was greater on long flights (i.e., 8 hours or longer). The risk of exposure to TB was higher for passengers and flight crew sitting or working near an infectious person. These persons may inhale droplets containing TB bacteria.

The risk of TB transmission on a airplane does not appear to be greater than in any other enclosed space. To prevent the possibility of exposure to TB on airplanes, CDC recommends that persons known to have infectious TB travel by private transportation (i.e., not by commercial airplanes or other commercial carriers), if travel is required. CDC has issued guidelines for notifying passengers who may have been exposed to TB aboard airplanes. Passengers concerned about a possible exposure to TB should see their primary health care provider for a TB skin test. TB is a treatable and preventable disease.

ENVIRONMENTAL EFFECTS

International travelers may be subject to certain stresses that may lower resistance to disease, such as crowding, disruption of usual eating and drinking habits, and time changes with "jet lag" contributing to a disturbed pattern of the sleep and wakefulness cycle. These conditions of stress can lead to nausea, indigestion, fatigue, or insomnia. Complete adaptation depends on the number of time zones crossed but may take a week or more.

Heat and cold can be directly or indirectly responsible for some diseases and can give rise to serious skin conditions. Dermatophytoses such as athlete's foot are often made worse by warm, humid conditions.

Excessive heat and humidity alone, or immoderate activity under those conditions, may lead to heat exhaustion due to salt and water deficiency and to the more serious heat stroke or hyperthermia. The ultraviolet rays of the sun can cause severe and very debilitating sunburn in lighter-skinned persons.

Excessive cold affects persons who may be inadequately dressed and particularly the elderly; it can lead to hypothermia and to frost-bite of exposed parts of the body.

Breathing and swallowing dust when traveling on unpaved roads or in arid areas may be followed by nausea and malaise, and may cause increased susceptibility to infections of the upper respiratory tract.

Traveling in high altitudes may lead to insomnia, headache, nausea, and altitude sickness, even in young and healthy persons, and can cause distress to those with cardiac or pulmonary conditions. Individual susceptibility to acute mountain sickness is highly variable. Travelers who are at greatest risk are those who ascend rapidly to tourist sites in the Andes and the Himalayas. Acetazolamide has been shown, under both simulated and actual climbing conditions, to hasten the process of acclimatization to high altitudes. The recommended dosage to prevent acute mountain sickness is 250 mg every 8–12 hours, with medication initiated 24–48 hours before, and continued during ascent. Acetazolamide should not be taken by individuals who are allergic to sulfonamides.

Injuries

Trauma caused by injuries, principally that suffered in motor vehicle crashes, is the leading cause of death and disability in both developed and developing countries worldwide. Motor vehicle crashes result from a variety of factors, including inadequate roadway design, hazardous conditions, lack of appropriate vehicles and vehicle maintenance, unskilled or inexperienced drivers, inattention to pedestrians and pedalcyclists, or impairment due to alcohol or drug use; all these factors are preventable or can be abated. Defensive driving is an important preventive measure. When driving or riding, insist on a vehicle equipped with safety belts, and where available, use them. Where available, also insist on a vehicle equipped with airbags and anti-lock brakes. As a high proportion of crashes occur at night when returning from "social events," avoid non-essential night driving, alcohol, and riding with persons who are under the influence of alcohol or drugs. Pedestrian, bicycle, and motorcycle travel are often dangerous, and helmet use is imperative for bicycle and motorcycle travel.

Fire injuries are also a significant cause of injuries and death—inquire about whether hotels have smoke detectors and sprinkler systems, and do not smoke in bed. Travelers may wish to bring their own smoke detectors with them. Upon arrival, always look for a primary and alternate escape route in rooms in which you are meeting or staying. Look for improperly vented heating devices which may cause carbon monoxide poisoning. Remember to escape a fire by crawling low under smoke.

Other major causes of injury trauma include drowning (see Swimming Precautions) and drug reactions. Protection against potentially hazardous drugs is nonexistent in some countries. Do not buy medications "over the counter" unless you are familiar with the product.

Travelers should also be aware of the potential for violence-related injuries. Risk for assault or terrorist attack varies from country to country; heed advice from residents and tour guides about areas to be avoided, going out at night, and going out alone. Do not fight attackers. If confronted, give up your valuables. For more information, contact the U.S. Department of State, Overseas Citizens Emergency Center, at (202) 647-5225.

Animal-Associated Hazards

Animals in general tend to avoid human beings, but they can attack, particularly if they are with young. In areas of endemic rabies, domestic dogs, cats, or other animals should not be petted. Wild animals should be avoided.

The bites, stings, and contact of some insects cause unpleasant reactions. Medical attention should be sought if an insect bite or sting causes redness, swelling, bruising, or persistent pain. Many insects also transmit communicable diseases. Some insects can bite and transmit disease without the person being aware of the bite, particularly when camping or staying in rustic or primitive accommodations. Insect repellents, protective clothing, and mosquito netting are advisable in many parts of the world (see Protection Against Mosquitoes and Other Arthropod Vectors).

Poisonous snakes are hazards in many parts of the world, although deaths from snake bites are relatively rare. The Australian brown snake, Russell's viper and cobras in southern Asia, carpet vipers in the Middle East, and coral and rattlesnakes in the Americas are particularly dangerous. Most snakebites are the direct result of handling or harassing snakes, which bite as a defensive reaction. Attempts to kill snakes are dangerous, often leading to bites on the fingers. The venom of small or immature snakes may be even more concentrated than that of a larger individual, therefore all snakes should be left strictly alone.

Less than half of all snake bite wounds actually contain venom, but medical attention should be sought anytime a bite wound breaks the skin. A pressure bandage, ice (if available), and immobilization of the affected limb are recommended first aid measures while the victim is moved as quickly as possible to a medical facility. Specific therapy for snakebite is controversial, and should be left to the judgement of local emergency medical personnel. Snakes tend to be active at night and in warm weather. As a precaution, boots and long pants may be worn when walking outdoors at night in snake-infested regions. Bites from scorpions may be painful but seldom are dangerous except possibly in infants. In general, exposure to bites can be avoided by sleeping under mosquito nets and by shaking clothing and shoes before putting them on, particularly in the morning. Snakes and scorpions tend to rest in shoes and clothing.

Anthrax-Contaminated Goatskin Handicrafts

Anthrax is a disease caused by a bacterial organism that produces spores that are highly resistant to disinfection. These infectious spores may persist on a contaminated item for many years. Anthrax spores have been found on goatskin handicrafts from Haiti.

Travelers to Caribbean countries are advised not to purchase Haitian goatskin handicrafts. Because of the risk, importation of goatskin handicrafts from Haiti will not be permitted at U.S. ports of entry; they will be confiscated and destroyed.

Swimming Precautions

Swimming in contaminated water may result in skin, eye, ear, and certain intestinal infections, particularly if the swimmer's head is submerged. Generally for infectious disease prevention, only pools that contain chlorinated water can be considered safe places to swim. In certain areas, fatal primary amebic meningoencephalitis has occurred following swimming in warm dirty water. Swimmers should avoid beaches that might be contaminated with human sewage, or with dog feces. Wading or swimming should be avoided in freshwater streams, canals, and lakes liable to be infested with the snail hosts of schistosomiasis (bilharziasis) or contaminated with urine from animals infected with Leptospira. Biting and stinging fish and corals and jelly fish may provide a hazard to the swimmer. Never swim alone or when under the influence of alcohol or drugs, and never dive head first into an unfamiliar body of water.

The Post-Travel Period

Some diseases may not manifest themselves immediately. If travelers become ill after they return home, they should tell their physician where they have traveled. Most persons who acquire viral, bacterial, or parasitic infections abroad become ill within 6 weeks after returning from international travel. However, some diseases may not manifest themselves immediately, e.g., malaria may not cause symptoms for as long as 6 months to a year after the traveler returns to the United States. It is recommended that a traveler always advise a physician of the countries visited within the 12 months preceding onset of illness. Knowledge of such travel and the possibility the patient may be ill with a disease the physician rarely encounters will help the physician arrive at a correct diagnosis.

UNITED STATES PUBLIC HEALTH SERVICE RECOMMENDATIONS

Introduction

Recommendations for individuals engaging in international travel apply primarily to vaccinations and prophylactic measures for U.S. travelers planning to spend time in areas of the world where diseases such as measles, poliomyelitis, typhoid fever, viral hepatitis, and malaria occur, posing a threat to their health. In addition, some countries require an International Certificate of Vaccination against yellow fever as a condition for entry. The majority of U.S. international travelers probably do not need any additional immunizations or prophylaxis, provided their routine immunization status is up-to-date according to the standards of the Public Health Service Advisory Committee on Immunization Practices (ACIP).

The extent to which advisory statements can be made specific for each country and each disease is limited by the lack of reliable data. Although data on the occurrence of many of these diseases are published regularly by WHO, these figures represent only a small percentage of the total number of cases that actually occur. Communicable diseases are not well reported by practicing physicians, and in some countries many cases never come to medical attention. For these reasons, any recommendations must be interpreted with care.

In general, the risk of acquiring illness when engaging in international travel depends on the areas of the world to be visited—travelers in developing countries are at greater risk than those traveling in developed areas. In most developed countries (i.e., Canada, Australia, New Zealand, Japan, and western Europe), the risk to the general health of the traveler will be no greater than that incurred throughout the United States. However, a higher risk of measles, mumps, and rubella may exist. Likewise, in many developed countries such as Germany, Ireland, Italy, Spain, Sweden, and the United Kingdom, pertussis immunization is not as widely practiced as in the United States, and the risk of acquiring pertussis is greater. Living conditions and standards of sanitation and hygiene vary considerably throughout the world, and immunization coverage levels may be low. Thus the risk of acquiring disease also can vary greatly in these locations. Travelers visiting primarily tourist areas on itineraries that do not include travel or visits in rural areas have less risk of exposure to food or water that is of questionable quality. Travelers who visit smaller cities off the usual tourist routes, who spend time in small villages or rural areas for extended periods, or who expect to have extended contact with children are at greater risk of acquiring infectious diseases, because of exposure to water and food of uncertain quality and closer contact with local residents who may harbor the organisms that cause such diseases. Consequently, the added protection of booster or additional doses of certain vaccines and other prophylaxis is recommended for these persons.

General Recommendations on Human Immunodeficiency Virus (HIV) Infection and Acquired Immunodeficiency Syndrome (AIDS)

HIV infection is preventable. HIV is transmitted through sexual intercourse, needle sharing, by medical use of blood or blood components, and perinatally from an infected woman. HIV is not transmitted through casual contact; air, food, or water routes; contact with inanimate objects; or through mosquitoes or other arthropod vectors. The use of any public conveyance (e.g., airplane, automobile, boat, bus, train) by persons with AIDS or HIV infection does not pose a risk of infection for the crew or other passengers.

Travelers are at risk if they:

- have sexual intercourse (heterosexual or homosexual) with an infected person;
- Use or allow the use of contaminated, unsterilized syringes or needles for any injections or other skin-piercing procedures including acupuncture, use of illicit drugs, steroid injections, medical/dental procedures, ear piercing, or tattooing;
- Use infected blood, blood components, or clotting factor concentrates. HIV infection by this route is a rare occurrence in those countries or cities where donated blood/plasma is screened for HIV antibody.

Travelers should avoid sexual encounters with a person who is infected with HIV or whose HIV-infection status is unknown. This includes avoiding sexual activity with intravenous drug users and persons with multiple sexual partners, such as male or female prostitutes. Condoms decrease, but do not entirely eliminate, the risk of transmission of HIV. Persons who engage in vaginal, anal, or oral-genital intercourse with anyone who is infected with HIV or whose infection status is unknown should use a condom.

In many countries, needle sharing by IV drug users is a major source of HIV transmission and other infections such as hepatitis B and C. Do not use drugs intravenously or share needles for any purpose.

In the United States, Australia, New Zealand, Canada, Japan, and western European countries, the risk of infection of transfusion-associated HIV infection has been virtually eliminated through required testing of all donated blood for antibodies to HIV.

If produced in the United States according to procedures approved by the Food and Drug Administration, immune globulin preparations (such as those used for the prevention of hepatitis A and B) and hepatitis B virus vaccine undergo processes that are known to inactivate HIV and therefore these products should be used as indicated.

In less-developed nations, there may not be a formal program for testing blood or biological products for antibody to HIV. In these countries, use of unscreened blood clotting factor concentrates or those of uncertain purity should be avoided (when medically prudent). If transfusion is necessary, the blood should be tested, if at all possible, for HIV antibodies by appropriately-trained laboratory technicians using a reliable test, see earlier section WHO Blood Transfusion Guidelines for International Travelers.

Needles used to draw blood or administer injections should be sterile, preferably of the single-use disposable type, and prepackaged in a sealed container. Insulin-dependent diabetics, hemophiliacs, and other persons who require routine or frequent injections should carry a supply of syringes, needles and disinfectant swabs (e.g., alcohol wipes) sufficient to last their entire stay abroad.

International travelers should be aware that some countries serologically screen incoming travelers (primarily those with extended visits, such as for work or study) and deny entry to persons with AIDS and those whose test results indicate infection with HIV. Persons who are intending to visit a country for a substantial period or to work or study abroad should be informed of the policies and requirements of the particular country. This information is usually available from consular officials of individual nations.

Spacing of Immunobiologics

The General Recommendations on Immunization (MMWR 1994;43(RR-1)) should be consulted for specific guidance on MMR vaccination following use of these products (see chapter 65 of original publication).

Because of imminent exposure to disease, immune globulin administration may become necessary after MMR or its individual component vaccines have been given, and interference can occur. Vaccine virus replication and stimulation of immunity usually will occur within 1–2 weeks after vaccination. If the interval between administration of these vaccines and the subsequent administration of an immune globulin preparation is 14 days or longer, vaccine need not be readministered. If the interval is less than 14 days, the vaccine should be readministered (a) at least 3 months after hepatitis A, hepatitis B, or tetanus prophylaxis, (b) at least 4 months after rabies prophylaxis, and (c) at least 5 months after measles or varicella prophylaxis, unless serologic testing indicates that antibodies have been produced. If administration of immune globulin becomes necessary because of imminent exposure to disease, MMR or its component vaccines can be administered simultaneously with immune globulin, with the recognition that vaccine-induced immunity may be compromised. The vaccine should be administered in a site remote from that chosen for the immune globulin inoculation. Vaccination should be repeated after the interval noted above unless serologic testing indicates antibodies have been produced.

When immune globulin is given with the first dose of hepatitis A vaccine, the proportion of persons who develop protective levels of antibody is not affected, but antibody concentrations are lower. Because the final concentrations of anti-HAV are many-fold higher than that considered protective, this reduced immunogenicity is not expected to be clinically important. Immune globulin preparations interact minimally with other inactivated vaccines and toxoids. Therefore, other inactivated vaccines can be given simultaneously or at any time interval after or before an immune globulin product is used. However, vaccines should be administered at sites different than the immune globulin.

Immunization Schedule Modifications for International Travel for Infants and Inadequately Immunized Young Children <2 Years of Age

Routine Childhood Vaccine Preventable Diseases (Measles, Mumps, Rubella, Polio, Diphtheria, Tetanus, Pertussis, Haemophilus influenzae Type b, and Hepatitis B)

Diphtheria and Tetanus Toxoid and Pertussis Vaccine

Diphtheria is an endemic disease in many developing countries and is currently found throughout the New Independent States of the former Soviet Union. Tetanus is ubiquitous worldwide. Pertussis is common in developing countries and in other countries where routine immunization against pertussis is not practiced widely. Because the risk of contracting pertussis in other countries and of diphtheria in developing countries is higher than in the United States, children who will be leaving the United States should be as well immunized as is possible before departing. Optimum protection against diphtheria, tetanus, and pertussis in the first year of life is achieved with 3 doses of DTP, the first administered at 6–8 weeks of age and the next two at 4–8 week intervals, as is generally the practice in the United States. A fourth dose of DTP 6–12 months after the third dose or diphtheria and tetanus toxoids and acellular pertussis vaccine (DTaP), at 15 months, maintains protection. Infants traveling to areas where diphtheria and/or pertussis are endemic or epidemic preferably should have received 3 doses; the first dose may be given to infants as young as 4 weeks of age and the next 2 doses at intervals of no less than 4 weeks. Two doses of DTP received at intervals of at least 4 weeks may provide some protection particularly against diphtheria and tetanus, while a single dose is of little protective benefit. Parents who are traveling with young infants should be informed that infants who have not received 3 doses of DTP are at greater risk of contracting pertussis than children who have been adequately vaccinated. Infants and other children less than 7 years of age who at the time of travel have received less than 3 doses of DTP and who will remain for extended periods in areas of increased risk of exposure to pertussis and/or diphtheria should complete their remaining doses at 4-week intervals.

For infants and children traveling internationally or remaining in areas of increased risk of exposure, reducing the interval between the third and fourth doses of the primary series to 6 months may be considered.

Measles Vaccine

Measles is an endemic disease in many developing countries and in other countries where measles immunization is not routinely practiced. Because the risk of contracting measles in many countries is far greater than in the United States, children should be as well protected as possible before departing from the United States. Measles vaccine, preferably in combination with rubella and mumps vaccines, i.e., MMR vaccine, should be administered to all children 12–15 months of age and older. A second dose is currently recommended for all children, and is usually given at school entry.

The age at vaccination should be lowered for infants traveling to areas where measles is endemic or epidemic. Infants 6–11 months of age who will be traveling to areas where measles is endemic or epidemic should receive a dose of single measles antigen vaccine before departure, although MMR may be used if single antigen measles vaccine is not available. Children vaccinated prior to their first birthday must be revaccinated with two doses of MMR vaccine on or after their first birthday and at least 1 month apart. The optimal age for the first revaccination is 12–15 months. The second revaccination dose should normally be given at school entry. Since virtually all infants less than 6 months of age will be protected by maternally derived antibodies, no additional means to provide protection against measles is generally necessary in this age group.

Mumps and Rubella Vaccine(s)

Because the risk of serious disease from infection with either mumps or rubella in infants is so small, mumps or rubella vaccine generally should not be administered to children below the age of 12 months, unless measles vaccine is indicated and single antigen measles vaccine is not available. However, parents of children less than 12 months of age should be immune to mumps and rubella so they will not become infected if their infants develop illness.

Polio Vaccine

Trivalent oral polio vaccine (OPV) is the vaccine of choice for all infants and children if there are no contraindications to vaccination. Inactivated polio vaccine (IPV) also is available. When time permits, children traveling to polio-endemic areas should receive at least 3 doses of OPV at intervals of at least 6 weeks. Children who have received 3 prior doses of OPV should receive a fourth dose if at least 6–8 weeks have elapsed since the third dose. In the United States, the Advisory Committee on Immunization Practices (ACIP) recommends that a primary series of 3 doses of oral poliovirus vaccine (OPV) be given at 2, 4, and 6 months of age. The OPV series may start as early as 6 weeks of age and at intervals of at least 6 weeks. However, in polio endemic areas, the "Expanded Programme on Immunization" of the World Health Organization recommends that a dose of OPV be given in the newborn period, e.g., at birth or before 6 weeks of age, with 3 additional doses (the primary series) given subsequently at 6, 10, and 14 weeks of age. While ideally the ACIP recommendations on age and intervals between doses of OPV should be followed, if travel to an endemic country will occur before a child is 6 weeks of age, a dose of OPV should be given prior to travel. A dose of vaccine administered before 6 weeks of age should not be counted as part of the standard 3-dose primary series. If the child remains in an endemic country, the child should receive the first dose of the standard 3-dose primary series no sooner than 4 weeks after the newborn period dose and the remaining 2 doses of the primary series at 4-week intervals. If the child has left the endemic area, the first dose of the primary series should be given 6–8 weeks after the newborn period dose, the second dose 6–8 weeks after the first dose and the third dose of the primary series 6–8 weeks after the second as is now recommended by the ACIP.

Children traveling to an endemic country who have received a first or second dose of the primary series of OPV but lack sufficient time to complete the primary series schedule as generally practiced in the United States should receive their second and/or third doses of OPV 4 weeks after their prior dose(s). Children with less than a primary series at the time of departure to an endemic area and who remain in an endemic area should complete the 3-dose primary series within the endemic area with doses at 4-week intervals.

No data or recommendations are available for the use of IPV prior to 6 weeks of age. Otherwise, if IPV is indicated, a primary series of IPV consists of 3 doses which can be given at 2, 4, and 15–18 months of age. The interval between doses 1 and 2 should be 6–8 weeks and between doses 2 and 3 at least 6 months.

Haemophilus influenzae Type b Conjugate Vaccine

Haemophilus influenzae type b is an endemic disease worldwide. Risk of acquiring disease may be higher in developing countries than in the United States. In the United States, three types of Haemophilus influenzae type b conjugate vaccines (HbCV) are recommended for use in infants beginning at 6 weeks of age, and a fourth is recommended for use as a primary vaccination only in children age 15 months and older. Two of the Hib conjugates vaccines for infants are also available as combined DTP-Hib vaccines. Routine vaccination is recommended beginning at 2 months of age for all U.S. children. The number and timing of remaining doses depend on the type of conjugate vaccine used (see Haemophilus influenzae Type b section for additional details). If vaccination is started at >7 months of age, fewer doses may be required. The same conjugate vaccine should preferably be used for all doses in the primary series. If, however, different vaccines are administered, a total of three doses of Hib conjugate vaccine is adequate. After completion of the primary infant vaccination series, any of the licensed Hib conjugate vaccines may be used for the booster dose at 12–15 months.

Infants and children should have optimal protection prior to travel. If previously unvaccinated, children less than 15 months of age should ideally receive at least 2 vaccine doses prior to travel. An interval as short as 1 month is acceptable.

Children between 15 months and 2 years of age require a single dose of vaccine.

Hepatitis B Vaccine

Since November, 1991, hepatitis B vaccine has been recommended for all infants beginning either at birth or by 2 months of age. Infants and young children who have not previously been vaccinated and who are traveling to areas with highly endemic hepatitis B virus (HBV) infection may be at risk if they are directly exposed to blood from the local population. Circumstances in which HBV transmission could occur include receipt of blood transfusions not screened for HBsAg, exposure to unsterilized needles (or other medical/dental equipment) in local health facilities, or continuous close contact with local children who have open skin lesions (impetigo, scabies, scratched insect bites). Such exposures are most likely to occur if the child is living for long periods in smaller cities or rural areas and in close contact with the local population. Children who will live in an HBV endemic area for six or more months and who are expected to have the above exposures should receive the 3 doses of hepatitis B vaccine. The interval between doses 1 and 2 should be 1–2 months. Between doses 2 and 3 the interval should be a minimum of 2 months however, 4–12 months is preferred.

Other Vaccines and Immune Globulin

Cholera Vaccine

The risk of cholera to U.S. travelers of any age is so low that it is questionable whether vaccination is of benefit. No data are available concerning the efficacy or side effects of cholera vaccine in children less than 6 months of age. Cholera vaccine is not recommended for children less than 6 months of age. Breast-feeding is protective against cholera; careful preparation of formula and food from safe water and foodstuffs should protect nonbreast-fed infants. If a child less than 6 months of age is to travel to areas requiring cholera immunization, a medical waiver should be obtained before travel. For older infants and children traveling to countries that require vaccination, a single dose of vaccine is sufficient to satisfy country requirements.

Typhoid Vaccine

Typhoid vaccination is not required for international travel. No data are available concerning the efficacy of typhoid vaccine in infants. Breast-feeding is likely to be protective against typhoid; careful preparation of formula and food from safe water and foodstuffs should protect nonbreast-fed infants. Typhoid vaccine is recommended for older children traveling to areas where there is a recognized risk of exposure to Salmonella typhi (see Typhoid Fever for information on dosage and route of administration of the vaccines).

Yellow Fever Vaccine

Because infants are at high risk of developing encephalitis from yellow fever vaccine, the recommendations for vaccinating infants should be considered on an individual basis. Although the incidence of these adverse events has not been clearly defined, 14 of 18 reported cases of post-vaccination encephalitis were in infants under 4 months of age. One fatal case confirmed by viral isolation was in a 4-year-old child. The ACIP and the World Health Organization recommend that yellow fever vaccine should never be given to infants <4 months. Yellow fever vaccine can be given to children >9 months of age if they are traveling to or living in areas of South America and Africa where yellow fever infection is officially reported or to countries that require yellow fever immunization. Children 9 months of age or older also should be immunized if they travel outside urban areas within the yellow fever endemic zone. Infants 6–9 months of age should be vaccinated only if they travel to areas of ongoing epidemic yellow fever, and a high level of protection against mosquito bites is not possible. Immunization of children 4–6 months of age should be considered only under unusual circumstances (consult CDC), and in no instance should infants under 4 months of age receive yellow fever vaccine. Information on yellow fever risk is also available from the CDC travel hotline, telephone (404) 332-4559.

Hepatitis A Vaccine or Immune Globulin for Hepatitis A

Infants and children traveling to developing countries are at increased risk of acquiring hepatitis A virus infection, especially if their travel is outside usual tourist routes, if they will be eating food or drinking water in settings of questionable sanitation, or if they will be in contact with local young children in settings of poor sanitation. Although hepatitis A is rarely severe in children under age 5 years, infected children efficiently transmit infection to older children and adults. Immune globulin (IG) should be given to children younger than 2 years old in the same schedule as recommended for adults. Children 2 years of age and older should receive the pediatric formulation of hepatitis A vaccine or IG.

TOPIC 57 / **SYNDROMES OF UNKNOWN ETIOLOGY**

Chronic Fatigue Syndrome

Original Citation: Centers for Disease Control and Prevention. Chronic fatigue syndrome. Centers for Disease Control and Prevention, National Center for Infectious Diseases, Division of Viral and Rickettsial Diseases, 1991.

GENERAL DESCRIPTION

Chronic Fatigue Syndrome, or CFS, comprises a complex of symptoms characterized by chronic, debilitating fatigue and other nonspecific symptoms. It has no known cause and may actually include several similar illnesses with different causes. In some persons, the symptoms of CFS develop following an otherwise self-limited illness, such as influenza, infectious mononucleosis, acute cytomegalovirus (cy-to-meg-lo-virus) infections, or a nonspecific acute viral syndrome. However, in many people CFS symptoms develop gradually over weeks to months, with no recognized precipitating event.

DIAGNOSTIC CRITERIA

CFS was defined by a panel of experts in 1988 as an illness lasting at least 6 months, characterized by chronic or recurrent, debilitating fatigue combined with at least 6 of the following chronic symptoms: headache, fever or feverishness, sore throat, muscle aches, joint pains, generalized muscle weakness, lymph node pain, prolonged fatigue following exercise, sleep alterations, and various nervous system complaints, for which no likely explanation has been identified after thorough medical and laboratory evaluation. Many people have been diagnosed with CFS without fulfilling these criteria or receiving a full evaluation for other chronic diseases.

There is no absolute means of confirming the diagnosis of CFS. No known laboratory tests are of proven positive diagnostic value. As a result, CFS should be considered by the physician only after a thorough evaluation for other potential causes of illness. Some possible causes of CFS-like symptoms include autoimmune diseases such as systemic lupus erythematosus (e-ryth-e-ma-to-sus), malignancies such as breast or ovarian cancer, lymphoma, thyroid disease, brain tumor, infectious diseases such as endocarditis, encephalitis, hepatitis, syphilis, or AIDS, and a variety of chronic diseases of the heart, lungs, liver, kidneys, gastrointestinal tract, endocrine system, or musculoskeletal (mus-cu-lo-skel-e-tal) systems.

DIAGNOSTIC EVALUATION

It is very important for the patient with CFS symptoms to be fully evaluated for other chronic diseases. Chronic fatigue, as an isolated symptom, is common in the general population, and CFS appears to be present in only a small fraction of persons who have complaints of chronic fatigue. Many well-recognized medical diseases, such as lupus, various cancers and lymphomas, chronic heart, lung, and other diseases, and primary psychiatric disorders, such as major depression or anxiety states, can produce chronic fatigue and must be considered in the differential diagnosis of CFS. Most of these diseases can be treated or managed appropriately following diagnosis and some may be progressive or even fatal if untreated, justifying the cost in time and money of a full medical evaluation. It is also advisable to periodically repeat such evaluations—there have been several cases in which patients diagnosed with CFS have later been found to have a specific disease, such as a connective tissue disorder or other chronic illness, that was likely to have caused their CFS symptoms from the beginning.

CDC cannot recommend specific physicians for referral. Our general recommendation is to consult an infectious disease specialist or the infectious disease department at a university affiliated medical center in your area if you feel you need further evaluation, or to ask your county medical society for a referral.

TREATMENT

Although there have been numerous claims of therapeutic breakthroughs, no proven effective cure for CFS now exists. Treatment should be initiated only after a thorough evaluation for other chronic diseases by a reputable physician. Most experts begin by recommending a regimen of balanced diet, adequate rest, and physical conditioning. Moderate exercise, not to the point of exhaustion, is generally helpful. However, CFS patients often report relapses of severe fatigue and other symptoms after over-exerting themselves.

Symptomatic treatment is often helpful in reducing symptoms to tolerable levels. This includes anti-inflammatory agents for headaches, and muscle and joint pains. Low doses of anti-anxiety drugs have been anecdotally reported to be of value.

Many CFS patients suffer from depressive symptoms, such as sleep disturbance, loss of enjoyment of life, and decreased appetite. Low doses of antidepressant drugs, taken at bedtime, have been reported to improve many of these and other CFS symptoms. In persons who have depressive symptoms, formal psychological testing should be performed to confirm their severity. For such patients, full doses of antidepressants may be expected to produce significant improvement. Antidepressant drugs are very potent and have a number of possible side effects. They must be used under the careful guidance of a physician. A variety of antidepressant agents are available, each with its own range of side-effects. If one agent fails to be tolerated, another may be tried.

All treatments have potential side effects, and in many instances the risk of side effects outweighs the potential beneficial effect of treatment. A number of currently used treatments are of no proven value, are often costly, and may actually be harmful. Only one agent, acyclovir, has undergone rigorous clinical testing, and it was recently reported to be no more effective than a placebo in treating CFS patients. Some successes have been reported in small numbers of patients, using a wide range of treatments, including antiviral and immunomodulating (im-mu-no-mod-u-la-ting) drugs, vitamins, holistic remedies, diet mod-ifications, and activity reduction. However, such anecdotal reports are often based upon faulty study design and the results cannot be distinguished from a placebo effect or the natural course of the illness. Several formal treatment tri-als are in planning stages around the country and may shed new light on the treatment of CFS.

FOR FURTHER INFORMATION

There are several national and local non-profit support groups for persons who are thought to have the chronic fatigue syndrome. These groups publish peri-odic newsletters and provide lists of interested physicians and telephone num-bers of other affected persons who can provide assistance in dealing with the illness. The Centers for Disease Control and Prevention does not necessarily endorse these organizations or their published information. They are included as further sources of information. Contact:

1. The National CFS Association, 919 Scott Avenue, Kansas City, KS 66105. Tel. (913) 321-2278.
2. The CFIDS Association, Community Health Services, P.O. Box 220398, Charlotte, NC 28222-0398. Tel. (704) 362-2343
3. The CFIDS Society, Box 230108, Portland, OR 97223.
4. Minann, Inc., Box 582, Glenview, IL 60025.
5. Consult your local newspaper for local support groups.

APPENDIX A / **BOARD MEMBERS**

Listing of Immunizations Practices Advisory Committee (ACIP), Advisory Committee for the Elimination of Tuberculosis (ACET), and Hospital Infection Control Practices Advisory Committee (HIPAC) official and ex-officio members. In addition to the Advisory Committee members, many internal and external reviewers made important contributions to the recommendations; we regret not being able to name them all.

ADVISORY COMMITTEE ON IMMUNIZATIONS PRACTICES (ACIP)

The following served or are serving on the ACIP during the time in which the articles included in this book were compiled.

Members

Ellen S. Alkon, M.D.
Harbor Health Center

Stanley E. Broadnax, M.D.
Cincinnati Health Department

Betty F. Bumpers
Consumer Advocate

James D. Cherry, M.D.
University of California School of Medicine

James Chin, M.D.
University of California, Berkeley

Mary Lou Clements, M.D.
Johns Hopkins University

Jeffery P. Davis, Ph.D.
Wisconsin Department of Health and Social Services, Epidemiologist

Barbara Ann DeBuono, M.D.
Rhode Island Department of Health

John B. DeHoff, M.D.
Baltimore City Health Department

Kathryn M. Edwards, M.D.
Vanderbilt University School of Medicine

David Fedson, Ph. D.
Division of General Medicine, University of Virginia School of Medicine

David W. Fraser, M.D.
Aga Khan Development Network (Europe), Ali Khan Foundation (Europe), Swarthmore College

Anne A. Gershon, M.D.
Department of Pediatrics, New York University Medical Center

William P. Glezen, Ph.D.
Department of Microbiology and Immunology, Baylor College of Medicine

Marie R. Griffin, M.D., M.P.H.
Vanderbilt University Medical Center

Fernando A. Guerra, M.D.
San Antonio Metro Health District

Caroline B. Hall, M.D.
University of Rochester, School of Medicine and Dentistry

Neal A. Halsey, M.D.
Johns Hopkins University School of Hygiene and Public Health

Donald A. Henderson, M.D.
Johns Hopkins University School of Hygiene and Public Health

Carlos E. Hernandez, M.D.
Kentucky Department for Health Services

Gregory R. Istre, M.D.
University of Texas, Health Science Center Department of Pediatrics,
Oklahoma State Department of Health

Rudolph E. Jackson, M.D.
Morehouse School of Medicine

Samuel L. Katz, M.D.
Department of Pediatrics, Duke University Medical Center

Francois M. LaForce, M.D.
Genesee Hospital, Department of Medicine

Joan K. Leavitt, M.D.
Oklahoma State Department of Health

William M. Marine, M.D.
Department of Preventive Medicine, University of Colorado Medical Center

Carlos H. Ramirez-Ronda, M.D.
University of Puerto Rico School of Medicine

Frederick L. Ruben, M.D.
Montefiore Hospital

William Schaffner II, M.D.
Vanderbilt University School of Medicine

Stephen C. Schoenbaum, M.D.
Harvard Community Health Plan of New England

Herbert D. Scott, Ph.D.
Rhode Island Department of Health

Fred E. Thompson, Jr., M.D.
Mississippi State Department of Health

Joel Ira Ward, M.D.
Harbor-UCLA Medical Center

Mary E. Wilson, M.D.
Mount Auburn Hospital

Ex Officio Members

Geoffrey Evans, M.D.
Division of Vaccine Injury Compensation

Carolyn Hardegree, M.D.
Food and Drug Administration

William S. Jordan, Jr., M.D.
Microbiology and Infectious Disease Program

Harry Meyer, Jr., M.D.
National Center for Drugs and Biologics

John La Montagne, Ph.D.
National Institutes of Health

Paul D. Parkman, Ph.D.
Center for Biologics Evaluation and Research, FDA

Jerry Zelinger, M.D.
Health Care Financing Administration

Liaison Representatives

Marvin S. Amstey, M.D.
American College of Obstetricians and Gynecologists

Kenneth J. Bart, M.D.
National Vaccine Program

Philip A. Brunell, M.D.
Division of Infectious Disease, University of Texas Health Science Center

William M. Butler, MC, USN
American Academy of Pediatrics

Keith Clark, D.V.M., Ph.D.
National Association of State Public Health Veterinarians

Jarrett Clinton, M.D.
Office of the Assistant Secretary of Defense

Richard D. Clover, M.D.
Pharmaceutical Research and Association of Teachers of Preventive Medicine

Thomas L. Copmann, Ph.D.
Pharmaceutical Research and Manufacturers of America

J. Michael S. Dixon, M.D.
Provincial Laboratory of Public Health, University of Alberta

Theodore C. Eickhoff, M.D.
St. Luke's Presbyterian Medical Center

David S. Fedson, M.D.
American College of Physicians

David W. Fleming, M.D.
Hospital Infections Control Practices Advisory Committee

Captain Peter A. Flynn, MC, USN
Special Assistant for Professional Activities, QASD

Stanley A. Gall, M.D.
American College of Obstetricians and Gynecologists

Pierce Gardner, M.D.
American Hospital Association, American College of Physicians

William P. Glezen, M.D.
Infectious Diseases Society of America

Caroline B. Hall, M.D.
American College of Physicians

Richard J. Jones, M.D.
Division of Scientific Activities, American Medical Association

Edward A. Mortimer, Jr., M.D.
American Medical Association

Kristin Lee Nichol, M.D., M.P.H.
Hospital Infections Control Practices Advisory Committee, Department of Veterans Affairs

Georges Peter, M.D.
American Academy of Pediatrics

Michael Peterson, D.V.M., M.P.H., Dr.P.H.
Department of Defense

Stanley A. Plotkin, M.D.
Divisions of Infectious Diseases, Children's Hospital of Philadelphia

Albert Pruitt, M.D.
Department of Pediatrics, Medical College of Georgia

Anthony Robbins, M.D.
National Vaccine Program

Chester Robinson
National Vaccine Program

William Schaffner, M.D.
American Hospital Association

David Scheifele, M.D.
Canadian National Advisory Committee on Immunization

Susan E. Tamblyn, M.D., Dr.P.H.
Canadian National Advisory Committee on Immunization

Ronald C. Van Buren, M.D.
American Academy of Family Physicians

Richard Zimmerman, M.D.
American Academy of Family Physicians, Department of Defense

ADVISORY COMMITTEE FOR THE ELIMINATION OF TUBERCULOSIS (ACET)

The following served or are serving on the ACET during the time in which the articles included in this book were compiled.

Members

William C. Banton
Missouri Department of Health

John B. Bass, Jr., M.D.
American Thoracic Society, University of South Alabama

Zenda J. Bowie
American Lung Association of Atlanta

George Comstock
John Hopkins University School of Hygiene and Public Health

Paul T. Davidson, M.D.
Los Angeles County Department of Health Services

Jerrold J. Elner
Case Western Reserve University, Cleveland

Miguel A. Escobedo, M.D.
El Paso City, County Health District

Sue C. Etkind, R.N., M.S.
Massachusetts Department of Public Health

Charles P. Felton, M.D.
Harlem Hospital Center

Kathleen F. Gensheimer, M.D.
Maine Department of Human Services

Jeffrey Glassroth, M.D.
Northwestern University Medical School, Medical College of Pennsylvania
and Hahnemann University

James L. Hadler
Connecticut Department of Health Services

Michael Iseman
National Jewish Center for Immunology and Respiratory Medicine, Denver

Stephen C. Joseph
New York City Department of Health

Reynard McDonald
University of Medicine and Dentistry of New Jersey

James M. Melius, M.D., Dr.P.H.
The Center to Protect Workers' Rights

Kathleen S. Moser, M.D.
San Diego County Department of Health Services

Anthony P. Najera
American Lung Association of California

Charles M. Nolan
Seattle-King County Department of Public Health

Carol J. Pozsik
South Carolina Department of Health and Environmental Control

Robert J. Reza
Suffolk Pulmonary Associates, New York

Alice M. Sarro, R.N., B.S.N.
San Antonio, Texas

John A. Sbarbaro
St. Anthony's Hospital System, Denver

Gisela F. Schecter, M.D., M.P.H.
San Francisco Tuberculosis Control Program

Margaret H. D. Smith
Tulane University School of Medicine

Jeffrey R. Starke, M.D.
Baylor College of Medicine

William W. Stead
Arkansas Department of Health

Fred E. Thompson
Mississippi State Department of Health

Lillian J. Tom-Orme, Ph.D.
Utah Department of Health

Betti Jo Warren, M.D.
King-Drew Medical Center

Patricia N. Whitley
Morehouse School of Medicine

Ex Officio Members

G. Stephen Bowen, M.D.
Health Resources and Services Administration

Michael J. Brennan, Ph.D.
Food and Drug Administration

Georgia S. Buggs
Office of Minority Health, Public Health Service

Carole A. Heilman, Ph.D.
National Institutes of Health

Warren Hewitt, Jr.
Substance Abuse and Mental Health Services Administration

J. Terrell Hoffeld, D.D.S.
Agency for Health Care Policy and Research

Gary A. Roselle, M.D.
Department of Veterans Affairs, VA Medical Center

Zeda Rosenberg, Sc.D.
National Institutes of Health

Bruce D. Tempest, M.D., F.A.C.P.
Indian Health Service

Basil P. Vareldzis, M.D.
Agency for International Development

Liaison Representatives
John B. Bass, Jr., M.D.
American Thoracic Society, University of South Alabama

Nancy E. Dunlap, M.D.
American College of Chest Physicians, University of Alabama at Birmingham

Wafaa M. El-Sadr, M.D., M.P.H.
Infectious Disease Society of America, Harlem Hospital Center

Alice Y. McIntosh
American Lung Association

Norbert P. Rapoza, Ph.D.
American Medical Association

Michael L. Tapper, M.D.
Society for Hospital Epidemiology of America, Lenox Hill Hospital

HOSPITAL INFECTION CONTROL PRACTICES ADVISORY COMMITTEE (HIPAC)

The following served or are serving on the HIPAC during the time in which the articles included in this book were compiled.

Audrey B. Adams, R.N., M.P.H.
Montefiore Medical Center

Larry J. Anderson, M.D.
Centers for Disease Control and Prevention

Roger L. Anderson, Ph.D.
Center for Infectious Diseases
Centers for Disease Control and Prevention

Nancy H. Arden, M.N.
Centers for Disease Control and Prevention

Lee A. Bland, M.A., M.P.H.
Center for Infectious Diseases
Centers for Disease Control and Prevention

Walter W. Bond, M.S.
Center for Infectious Diseases
Centers for Disease Control and Prevention

Robert F. Breiman, M.D.
Centers for Disease Control and Prevention

Dennis Brimhall
University of Utah Hospital

Jay C. Butler, M.D.
University of Wisconsin

Herbert W. Clegg II, M.D.
Children's Hospital Medical Center

Sheila Cram, R.N., M.P.H.
Newton-Wellesley Hospital

Donald E. Craven, M.D.
Boston City Hospital
Boston University School of Medicine

Barry J. Davis, M.S.
Center for Infectious Diseases
Centers for Disease Control and Prevention

T. Grace Emori, R.N., M.S.
Center for Infectious Diseases
Centers for Disease Control and Prevention

Jane DeGroot-Kosolcharoen, R.N., M.S.
William S. Middleton Memorial Veterans Hospital
University of Wisconsin School of Nursing

E. Patchen Dellinger, M.D.
Harborview Medical Center

Martin S. Favero, Ph.D.
Center for Infectious Diseases
Centers for Disease Control and Prevention

David W. Fleming, M.D.
Oregon State Health Department

Susan W. Forlenza, M.D.
New York City Department of Health

Richard Garibaldi, M.D.
University of Utah Medical Center
Salt Lake Veterans Administration Medical Center

Julia S. Garner, R.N., M.N.
Centers for Disease Control and Prevention

Mary J. Gilchrist, Ph.D.
University of Iowa

Donald A. Goldmann, M.D.
The Children's Hospital Medical Center

Robert W. Haley, M.D.
University of Texas Southwestern Medical Center

Teresa C. Horan, M.P.H.
Center for Infectious Diseases
Centers for Disease Control and Prevention

Walter J. Hierholzer, Jr., M.D.
Yale-New Haven Hospital

Douglas C. Hubner, M.D.
Hillcrest Medical Center

James M. Hughes, M.D.
Center for Infectious Diseases
Centers for Disease Control and Prevention

Marguerite M. Jackson, R.N., M.S.
University of California Medical Center

Edward H. Kass, M.D.
Brigham and Women's Hospital

Calvin M. Kunin, M.D.
Ohio State University College of Medicine

Elaine L. Larson, R.N., Ph.D.
Georgetown University School of Nursing and Public Health

Rosemary Lindan, M.D.
Case Western Reserve School of Medicine
Cuyahoga County Hospital

Donald C. Mackel, M.S., M.P.H.
Center for Infectious Diseases
Centers for Disease Control and Prevention

William J. Martone, M.D.
Center for Infectious Diseases
Centers for Disease Control and Prevention

C. Glen Mayhall, M.D.
University of Texas Medical Center Branch at Galveston

Rita D. McCormick, R.N.
University of Wisconsin Hospital and Clinics

Michael M. McNeil, M.D.
Centers for Disease Control and Prevention

Ronald L. Nichols, M.D.
Tulane University School of Medicine

Joyce L. Safian, R.N., F.N.P., M.A.
North Bay Corporate Health Services, Inc.

Christine C. Sanders, Ph.D.
Creighton University School of Medicine

Emily Rhinehart Smith, R.N.
Cleveland Clinic Foundation

Walter E. Stamm, M.D.
University of Washington School of Medicine
Harborview Medical Center

Ofelia C. Tablan, M.D.
Centers for Disease Control and Prevention

William M. Valenti, M.D.
University of Rochester Medical Center
Strong Memorial Hospital

Catherine M. Wilfert, M.D.
Duke University Medical Center

Edward S. Wong, M.D.
McGuire Veterans Administration Hospital

Listing of all articles included on the *CDC Prevention Guidelines* CD-ROM.

1993 Revised Classification System for HIV Infection and Expanded Surveillance Case Definition for AIDS among Adolescents and Adults

1993 Sexually Transmitted Diseases Treatment Guidelines

1994 Revised Classification System for Human Immunodeficiency Virus Infection in Children Less Than 13 Years of Age

1994 Revised Guidelines for the Performance of CD4+ T-Cell Determinations in Persons with Human Immunodeficiency Virus (HIV) Infections

1995 Revised Guidelines for Prophylaxis Against Pneumocystis carinii Pneumonia for Children Infected with or Perinatally Exposed to Human Immunodeficiency Virus

A Framework for Assessing the Effectiveness of Disease and Injury Prevention

A Program for Prevention and Control of Epidemic Dengue and Dengue Hemorrhagic Fever in Puerto Rico and the U.S. Virgin Islands

A Strategic Plan for the Elimination of Tuberculosis in the United States

Acquired Immunodeficiency Syndrome—United States, 1992

Acquired Immunodeficiency Syndrome (AIDS): Precautions for Health-Care Workers and Allied Professionals

Action Plan to Improve Access to Immunization Services, Report of the Interagency Committee on Immunization

Addressing Emerging Infectious Disease Threats: A Prevention Strategy for the United States Executive Summary

Agent Summary Statement for Human Immunodeficiency Viruses (HIVs) Including HTLV-III, LAV, HIV-1, and HIV-2*

Agricultural Auger Related Injuries and Fatalities—Minnesota, 1992-1994

Air-Bag Associated Fatal Injuries to Infants and Children Riding in Front Passenger Seats—United States

Application for Permit to Import or Transport Agents or Vectors of Human Disease

Assessing the Public Health Threat Associated with Waterborne Cryptosporidiosis: Report of a Workshop

Assessment Protocol for Excellence in Public Health (APEXPH)

BB and Pellet Gun-Related Injuries—United States, June 1992-May 1994

Behavioral Risk Factor Survey of Vietnamese—California, 1991

Biosafety in Microbiological and Biomedical Laboratories

Carbon Monoxide Poisoning from Use of Gasoline-Fueled Power Washers in an Underground Parking Garage—District of Columbia, 1994

Carbon Monoxide Poisonings Associated with Snow-Obstructed Vehicle Exhaust Systems—Philadelphia and New York City, January 1996

Case Definitions for Public Health Surveillance

Case Studies in Environmental Medicine: Lead Toxicity

Case-Control Study of HIV Seroconversion in Health-Care Workers after

Deaths Associated with Hurricanes Marilyn and Opal—United States, September–October 1995

Deaths Resulting from Firearm- and Motor-Vehicle-Related Injuries—United States, 1968–1991

Defeating Cholera: Clinical Presentation and Management

Defining the Public Health Impact of Drug-Resistant Streptococcus pneumoniae—Report of a Working Group. Appendix—Laboratory-Based Surveillance System

Dengue Activity in Puerto Rico, 1990

Dengue and Dengue Hemorrhagic Fever

Diagnosis and Management of Mycobacterial Infection and Disease in Persons with Human T-Lymphotropic Virus Type III/ Lymphadenopathy-Associated Virus Infection

Diphtheria, Tetanus, and Pertussis: Recommendations for Vaccine Use and Other Preventive Measures Recommendations of the Immunization Practices Advisory Committee (ACIP)

Effectiveness in Disease and Injury Prevention Control of Excessive Lead Exposure in Radiator Repair Workers

Effectiveness in Disease and Injury Prevention Successful Strategies in Adult Immunization

Effectiveness in Disease and Injury Prevention Use of Folic Acid for Prevention of Spina Bifida and Other Neural Tube Defects—1983–1991

Emerging Infectious Diseases Update: Hantavirus Disease—United States, 1993

Engineering and Administrative Recommendations for Water Fluoridation, 1995

Enhanced Detection of Sporadic Escherichia coli O157:H7 Infections—New Jersey, July 1994

Epidemic Dengue 1 in Brazil, 1986: Evaluation of a Clinically Based Dengue Surveillance System

Epidemiologic Notes and Reports: An Evaluation of the Acquired Immunodeficiency Syndrome (AIDS) Reported in Health-Care Personnel—United States

Epidemiologic Notes and Reports: Encephalitis Associated with Cat Scratch Disease—Broward and Palm Beach Counties, Florida, 1994

Epidemiologic Notes and Reports: HIV-1 Infection and Artificial Insemination with Processed Semen

Epidemiologic Notes and Reports: Human Immunodeficiency Virus Infection Transmitted from an Organ Donor Screened for HIV Antibody—North Carolina

Epidemiologic Notes and Reports: Injuries Associated with Soccer Goalposts—United States, 1979–1993

Epidemiologic Notes and Reports: Nosocomial Transmission of Multidrug-Resistant Tuberculosis to Health-Care Workers and HIV-Infected Patients in an Urban Hospital—Florida

Epidemiologic Notes and Reports: Outbreak of Hepatitis C Associated with Intravenous Immunoglobulin Administration—United States, October 1993–June 1994

Epidemiologic Notes and Reports: Risk for Cervical Disease in HIV-Infected Women—New York City

Epidemiologic Notes and Reports: Testing Donors of Organs, Tissues, and Semen for Antibody to Human T-Lymphotropic Virus Type III/Lymph-adenopathy-Associated Virus

Epidemiologic Notes and Reports: Transmission of HIV Through Bone Transplantation: Case Report and Public Health Recommendations

Epidemiologic Notes and Reports Update: Ebola Related Filovirus Infection in Nonhuman Primates and Interim Guidelines for Handling Nonhuman Primates during Transit and Quarantine

Epidemiologic Notes and Reports Update: Evaluation of Human T-Lymph-otropic Virus Type III/ Lymphadenopathy-Associated Virus Infection in Health-Care Personnel—United States

Epidemiologic Notes and Reports Update: Human Immunodeficiency Virus Infections in Health-Care Workers Exposed to Blood of Infected Patients

Epidemiologic Notes and Reports Update: Transmission of HIV Infection during an Invasive Dental Procedure—Florida

Epidemiologic Notes and Reports Update: Transmission of HIV Infection during Invasive Dental Procedures—Florida

Escherichia coli O157:H7 Outbreak at a Summer Camp—Virginia, 1994

Essential Components of a Tuberculosis Prevention and Control Program Recommendations of the Advisory Council for the Elimination of Tuberculosis

Famine-Affected, Refugee, and Displaced Populations: Recommendations for Public Health Issues

Fatalities Associated with Improper Hitching to Farm Tractors—New York, 1991-1995

Final Recommendations for Protecting the Health and Safety against Potential Adverse Effects of Long-Term Exposure to Low Doses of Agents: GA, BV, VX, Mustard Agent (H, HD, Y), and Lewisite (L)

Flood: A Prevention Guide to Promote Your Personal Health and Safety

Foodborne Hepatitis A—Missouri, Wisconsin, and Alaska, 1990–1992

Forum on Youth Violence in Minority Communities Setting the Agenda for Prevention. Summary of the Proceedings. Public Health Reports

General Recommendations on Immunization Recommendations of the Advisory Committee on Immunization Practices (ACIP)

Guide to Clinical Preventive Services; An Assessment of the Effectiveness of 169 Interventions

Guidelines for AIDS Prevention Program Operations

Guidelines for Effective School Health Education to Prevent the Spread of AIDS

Guidelines for Evaluating Surveillance Systems

Guidelines for Health Education and Risk Reduction Activities

Guidelines for Investigating Clusters of Health Events

Guidelines for Investigating Clusters of Health Events—Appendix. Summary of Methods for Statistically Assessing Clusters of Health Events

Laboratory Management of Agents Associated with Hantavirus Pulmonary Syndrome: Interim Biosafety Guidelines

Lead Poisoning Associated with Use of Traditional Ethnic Remedies—California, 1991–1992

Limited Supplies of Inactivated Poliovirus Vaccine—United States

Lyme Disease—United States, 1994

Malaria among U.S. Military Personnel Returning from Somalia, 1993

Malaria Surveillance—United States, 1992

Malaria: Health Information for International Travel

Management of Patients with Suspected Viral Hemorrhagic Fever

Management of Persons Exposed to Multidrug-Resistant Tuberculosis

Managing Hazardous Materials Incidents Volume I, Emergency Medical Services

Managing Hazardous Materials Incidents Volume II, Hospital Emergency Departments

Mass Treatment of Humans Exposed to Rabies—New Hampshire, 1994

Measles Prevention: Recommendations of the Immunization Practices Advisory Committee (ACIP)

Medical Management Guidelines for Acute Chemical Exposures

Modern Vaccines; Immunization Practice in Developed Countries

National Action Plan to Combat Multidrug-Resistant Tuberculosis

National Adult Immunization Awareness Week

National Laboratory Training Network; Building Alliances to Enhance Training

NIOSH Alert: Request for Assistance in Preventing Organic Dust Toxic Syndrome

NIOSH Recommendations for Occupational Safety and Health Standards 1988

NIOSH Recommendations for Occupational Safety and Health: Compendium of Policy Documents and Statements

Notice to Readers: Availability of NIOSH Criteria Document Hand-Arm Vibration Syndrome

Notice to Readers: Licensure of Inactivated Hepatitis A Vaccine and Recommendations for Use among International Travelers

Notice to Readers: NIOSH Alert: Request for Assistance in Controlling Exposures to Nitrous Oxide during Anesthetic Administration

Notice to Readers: Recommendations for Test Performance and Interpretation from the Second National Conference on Serologic Diagnosis of Lyme Disease

Notice to Readers: Recommended Childhood Immunization Schedule—United States, January–June 1996

Notice to Readers: Reinstatement of Regular Diphtheria-Tetanus-Pertussis Vaccine Schedule

Notice to Readers: Revision of HIV Classification Codes

Notice to Readers Update: Management of Patients with Suspected Viral Hemorrhagic Fever—United States

Notice to Readers Update: Provisional Public Health Service Recommendations for Chemoprophylaxis after Occupational Exposure to HIV

Recommendation of the Immunization Practices Advisory Committee (ACIP): Influenza Vaccines, 1983–1984

Recommendation of the Immunization Practices Advisory Committee (ACIP): Measles Prevention

Recommendation of the Immunization Practices Advisory Committee (ACIP): Postexposure Prophylaxis of Hepatitis B

Recommendation of the Immunization Practices Advisory Committee (ACIP): Prevention and Control of Influenza

Recommendation of the Immunization Practices Advisory Committee (ACIP): Rabies Prevention—United States, 1984

Recommendation of the Immunization Practices Advisory Committee (ACIP): Rubella Prevention

Recommendation of the Immunization Practices Advisory Committee (ACIP): Immunization of Children Infected with Human T-Lymphotropic Virus Type III/ Lymphadenopathy-Associated Virus

Recommendation of the Immunization Practices Advisory Committee (ACIP): Meningococcal Vaccines

Recommendation of the Immunization Practices Advisory Committee (ACIP): Mumps Vaccine

Recommendation of the Immunization Practices Advisory Committee (ACIP): New Recommended Schedule for Active Immunization of Normal Infants and Children

Recommendation of the Immunization Practices Advisory Committee (ACIP): Smallpox Vaccine

Recommendation of the Immunization Practices Advisory Committee (ACIP): Supplementary Statement on Pre-Exposure Rabies Prophylaxis by the Intradermal Route

Recommendations for Collection of Laboratory Specimens Associated with Outbreaks of Gastroenteritis

Recommendations for Counseling Persons Infected with Human T-Lymphotrophic Virus, Types I and II*

Recommendations for HIV Testing Services for Inpatients and Outpatients in Acute-Care Hospital Settings

Recommendations for Preventing the Spread of Vancomycin Resistance Recommendations of the Hospital Infection Control Practices Advisory Committee (HICPAC)

Recommendations for Preventing Transmission of Human Immunodeficiency Virus and Hepatitis B Virus to Patients during Exposure-Prone Invasive Procedures

Recommendations for Preventing Transmission of Infection with Human T-Lymphotropic Virus Type III/ Lymphadenopathy-Associated Virus in the Workplace

Recommendations for Prevention of HIV Transmission in Health-Care Settings

Recommendations for Prophylaxis Against Pneumocystis carinii Pneumonia for Adults and Adolescents Infected with Human Immunodeficiency Virus

Reducing the Health Consequences of Smoking: A Report of the Surgeon General: 25 Years of Progress

Regulations for Implementing the Clinical Laboratory Improvement Amendments of 1988: A Summary

Report from the 1988 Trauma Registry Workshop, Including Recommendations for Hospital-Based Trauma Registries.

Safety of Therapeutic Immune Globulin Preparations with Respect to Transmission of Human T-Lymphotropic Virus Type III/ Lymphadenopathy-Associated Virus Infection

Salmonella enteritis Infection

Screening for Colorectal Cancer—United States, 1992–1993, and New Guidelines

Screening for Tuberculosis and Tuberculosis Infection in High-Risk Populations Recommendations of the Advisory Council for the Elimination of Tuberculosis

Serious Eye Injuries Associated with Fireworks—United States, 1990–1994

Severe Isoniazid-Associated Hepatitis—New York, 1991–1993

Shipping Regulations—Biomedical Materials

Smoking and Health in the Americas: A 1992 report of the Surgeon General in Collaboration with the Pan American Health Organization

Smoking Cessation during Previous Year among Adults—United States, 1990 and 1991

Spina Bifida Incidence at Birth—United States, 1983–1990

Standards for Pediatric Immunization Practices

State Tobacco Prevention and Control Activities: Results of the 1989-1990 Association of State and Territorial Health Officials (ASTHO) Survey Final Report

Suicide Contagion and the Reporting of Suicide: Recommendations from a National Workshop

Surveillance for Dengue and Dengue Hemorrhagic Fever

Surveillance for Diabetes Mellitus—United States, 1980–1989

Surveillance for Ectopic Pregnancy—United States, 1970–1989

Surveillance for Epidemics—United States

Surveillance for Geographic and Secular Trends in Congenital Syphilis—United States, 1983–1991

Surveillance for Pregnancy and Birth Rates among Teenagers, by State—United States, 1980 and 1990

Symposium—Dengue and Dengue Hemorrhagic Fever

SYNOPSIS: Current Guidelines for M. tuberculosis Testing

TB Facts for Health Care Workers

Technical Guidance on HIV Counseling

Testing for Antibodies to Human Immunodeficiency Virus Type 2 in the United States

Tetrodotoxin Poisoning Associated with Eating Puffer Fish Transported from Japan—California, 1996

Update: Barrier Protection Against HIV Infection and Other Sexually Transmitted Diseases

Update: Hantavirus Infection—United States, 1993

Update: Hantavirus Pulmonary Syndrome—United States, 1993

Update: Influenza Activity—United States and Worldwide, and Composition of the 1992-93 Influenza Vaccine

Update: Influenza Activity—Worldwide and Recommendations for Influenza Vaccine Composition for the 1990-91 Influenza Season

Update: Influenza Activity and Vaccine Availability—United States, 1991-92

Update: Influenza Activity—Worldwide and Recommendations for Influenza Vaccine Composition for the 1990-91 Influenza Seasons

Update: Outbreak of Hantavirus Infection—Southwestern United States, 1993

Update: Revised Public Health Service Definition of Persons Who Should Refrain from Donating Blood and Plasma—United States

Use of Race and Ethnicity in Public Health Surveillance Summary of the CDC/ATSDR Workshop

USPHS/IDSA Guidelines for the Prevention of Opportunistic Infections in Persons Infected with Human Immunodeficiency Virus: A Summary

Vaccine Management: Recommendations for Handling and Storage of Selected Biologicals

Varicella

Vector-Borne Diseases (Lyme disease, Japanese Encephalitis, Yellow Fever)

Viral Agents of Gastroenteritis Public Health Importance and Outbreak Management

Why Does My Baby Need Hepatitis B Vaccine?

Workshop on the Public Health Response to Nasopharyngeal Radium Irradiation—September 1995

World Health Organization Consultation on Public Health Issues Related to Bovine Spongiform Encephalopathy and the Emergence of a New Variant of Creutzfeldt-Jakob Disease

World No-Tobacco Day, 1992

Yellow Fever Vaccine; Recommendations of the Immunization Practices Advisory Committee (ACIP)

Youth Suicide Prevention Programs: A Resource Guide

Zidovudine for the Prevention of HIV Transmission from Mother to Infant

APPENDIX C / **ORDERING BOOK-LENGTH DOCUMENTS**

This is a listing of frequently requested book-length documents that are partially excerpted in this book; all but the Surgeon General's Report and the Mantoux Tuberculin Skin Test Wall Chart are on the CD-ROM.

1993—Sexually Transmitted Disease Treatment Guidelines. MMWR 1993;42(RR-14); Contact: MMWR Office, 1600 Clifton Road, MS C-08, Atlanta, Georgia 30333.

A Framework for Assessing the Effectiveness of Disease and Injury Prevention. MMWR 1992;41(RR-3); Contact: MMWR Office, 1600 Clifton Road, MS C-08, Atlanta, Georgia 30333.

Health Information and International Travel ("Yellow Book"). Publication date: 8/1/95; Division of Quarantine, National Center for Chronic Disease Prevention and Health Promotion, 1600 Clifton Road, MS E-03, Atlanta, Georgia 30333.

Management Hazardous Materials Incidents, Volume 1: Emergency Medical Services. Publication Date: 1/1/92; Contact: Scott Wright, Agency for Toxic Substances and Disease Registry, MS E-57, 1600 Clifton Road, Atlanta, Georgia 30333.

Management Hazardous Materials Incidents, Volume 2: Hospital Emergency Departments. Publication Date: 1/1/92; Contact: Scott Wright, Agency for Toxic Substances and Disease Registry, 1600 Clifton Road, MS E-57, Atlanta, Georgia 30333.

The Mantoux Tuberculin Skin Test (Wall Chart in Color). Publication date: 01/01/92; Contact: NCPS Publication Requests (NCPSPUBL) Division of Tuberculosis Elimination, Centers for Disease Control and Prevention, MS E-10, Atlanta, Georgia 30333.

Medical Management Guidelines for Acute Chemical Exposures. Publication Date 8/1/92; Contact: Donna Orti, 1600 Clifton Road, MS E-33, Atlanta, Georgia 30333.

Preventing Lead Poisoning in Young Children. Publication Date 10/1/91; Contact: NCEH Publications, Centers for Disease Control and Prevention, 4770 Buford Highway NE, MS F-29, Atlanta, Georgia 30341-3724.

Prevention and Treatment of Complications of Diabetes Mellitus: A Guide to Primary Care Practitioners. Publication date: 1/1/91; Contact: Patricia Metger, Division of Diabetes Translation, National Center for Chronic Disease Prevention and Health Promotion, 1600 Clifton Road, MS K-10, Atlanta, Georgia 30333.

The Prevention of Youth Violence: A Framework for Community Action. Publication Date: 1/1/92; Contact: Mary-Ann Fenley, National Center for Injury Prevention and Control, 1600 Clifton Road, MS F-36, Atlanta, Georgia 30333.

Publication of Surgeon General's Report on Smoking and Health. Publication date: 02/25/94; Contact: National Center for Chronic Disease Prevention and Health Promotion, Centers for Disease Control and Prevention, MS C-08, Atlanta, Georgia 30333.

Youth Suicide Prevention Programs: A Resource Guide. Publication Date: 9/1/92; Contact: Mary-Ann Fenley, National Center for Injury Prevention and Control, 1600 Clifton Road, MS F-36, Atlanta, Georgia 30333

INDEX

Page numbers in italics refer to figures; those followed by *t* refer to tables.